EUROPEAN PHARMACOPOEIA

5th Edition

published 15 June 2004

replaces the 4th Edition on 1 January 2005

Volumes 1 and 2 of this publication 5.0 constitute the 5th Edition of the European Pharmacopoeia. They will be complemented by **non-cumulative supplements** that are to be kept for the duration of the 5th Edition. 2 supplements will be published in 2004 and 3 supplements in each of the years 2005 and 2006. A cumulative list of reagents will be published in supplements 5.4 and 5.7.

If you are using the 5th Edition at any time later than 1 April 2005, make sure that you have all the published supplements and consult the index of the most recent supplement to ensure that you use the latest versions of the monographs and general chapters.

EUROPEAN PHARMACOPOEIA
ELECTRONIC VERSION

The 5th Edition is also available in an electronic format (CD-ROM and internet version) with all the monographs and general chapters contained in the book. With the publication of each supplement the electronic version is replaced by a new fully updated cumulative version.

PHARMEUROPA
Quarterly Forum Publication

Pharmeuropa contains preliminary drafts of all new and revised monographs proposed for inclusion in the European Pharmacopoeia and gives an opportunity for all interested parties to comment on the specifications before they are finalised. Pharmeuropa also contains information on the work programme and on certificates of suitability to monographs of the European Pharmacopoeia issued by the EDQM, scientific articles on pharmacopoeial matters and other articles of general interest. Pharmeuropa is available on subscription from the EDQM.

INTERNATIONAL HARMONISATION

Refer to information given in chapter *5.8. Pharmacopoeial Harmonisation.*

WEBSITE

http://www.pheur.org
http://book.pheur.org (for prices and orders)

KEY TO MONOGRAPHS

Version date of the text — **01/2005:0884**

Text reference number

Modification to be taken into account from the publication date of volume 5.0 — corrected

CARBIMAZOLE

Carbimazolum

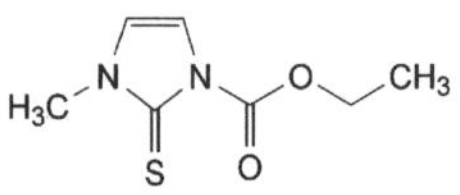

$C_7H_{10}N_2O_2S$ M_r 186.2

Chemical name in accordance with IUPAC nomenclature rules

DEFINITION

Ethyl 3-methyl-2-thioxo-2,3-dihydro-1*H*-imidazole-1-carboxylate.

Content: 98.0 per cent to 102.0 per cent (dried substance).

CHARACTERS

Appearance: white or yellowish-white, crystalline powder.

Solubility: slightly soluble in water, soluble in acetone and in alcohol.

Application of the first and second identification is defined in the General Notices (chapter 1)

IDENTIFICATION

First identification: B.

Second identification: A, C, D.

A. Melting point (*2.2.14*): 122 °C to 125 °C.

B. Infrared absorption spectrophotometry (*2.2.24*).

Preparation: discs.

Comparison: *carbimazole CRS.*

Chemical reference substance available from the Secretariat (see www.pheur.org)

C. Thin-layer chromatography (*2.2.27*).

Test solution. Dissolve 10 mg of the substance to be examined in *methylene chloride R* and dilute to 10 ml with the same solvent.

Reference solution. Dissolve 10 mg of *carbimazole CRS* in *methylene chloride R* and dilute to 10 ml with the same solvent.

Plate: *TLC silica gel GF_{254} plate R.*

Mobile phase: *acetone R*, *methylene chloride R* (20:80 *V/V*).

Reagents described in chapter 4

Application: 10 µl.

Development: over a path of 15 cm.

Drying: in air for 30 min.

Detection: examine in ultraviolet light at 254 nm.

Results: the principal spot in the chromatogram obtained with the test solution is similar in position and size to the principal spot in the chromatogram obtained with the reference solution.

D. Dissolve about 10 mg in a mixture of 50 ml of *water R* and 0.05 ml of *dilute hydrochloric acid R*. Add 1 ml of *potassium iodobismuthate solution R*. A red precipitate is formed.

TESTS

Impurity A and other related substances. Liquid chromatography (*2.2.29*).

Reference to a general chapter

Test solution. Dissolve 5.0 mg of the substance to be examined in 10.0 ml of a mixture of 20 volumes of *acetonitrile R* and 80 volumes of *water R*. Use this solution within 5 min of preparation.

Reference solution (a). Dissolve 5 mg of *thiamazole R* and 0.10 g of *carbimazole CRS* in a mixture of 20 volumes of *acetonitrile R* and 80 volumes of *water R* and dilute to 100.0 ml with the same mixture of solvents. Dilute 1.0 ml of this solution to 10.0 ml with a mixture of 20 volumes of *acetonitrile R* and 80 volumes of *water R*.

Reference solution (b). Dissolve 5.0 mg of *thiamazole R* in a mixture of 20 volumes of *acetonitrile R* and 80 volumes of *water R* and dilute to 10.0 ml with the same mixture of solvents. Dilute 1.0 ml of this solution to 100.0 ml with a mixture of 20 volumes of *acetonitrile R* and 80 volumes of *water R*.

Column:

- *size*: *l* = 0.15 m, Ø = 3.9 mm,
- *stationary phase*: *octadecylsilyl silica gel for chromatography R* (5 µm).

Mobile phase: *acetonitrile R*, *water R* (10:90 *V/V*).

Flow rate: 1 ml/min.

Detection: spectrophotometer at 254 nm.

Injection: 10 µl.

Run time: 1.5 times the retention time of carbimazole.

Retention time: carbimazole = about 6 min.

System suitability: reference solution (a):

- *resolution*: minimum 5.0 between the peaks due to impurity A and carbimazole.

Limits:

- *impurity A*: not more than half the area of the principal peak in the chromatogram obtained with reference solution (b) (0.5 per cent),
- *any other impurity*: not more than 0.1 times the area of the principal peak in the chromatogram obtained with reference solution (b) (0.1 per cent).

Loss on drying (*2.2.32*): maximum 0.5 per cent, determined on 1.000 g by drying in a desiccator over *diphosphorus pentoxide R* at a pressure not exceeding 0.7 kPa for 24 h.

Sulphated ash (*2.4.14*): maximum 0.1 per cent, determined on 1.0 g.

ASSAY

Dissolve 50.0 mg in *water R* and dilute to 500.0 ml with the same solvent. To 10.0 ml add 10 ml of *dilute hydrochloric acid R* and dilute to 100.0 ml with *water R*. Measure the absorbance (*2.2.25*) at the maximum at 291 nm. Calculate the content of $C_7H_{10}N_2O_2S$ taking the specific absorbance to be 557.

IMPURITIES

Specified impurities: A.

Other detectable impurities: B.

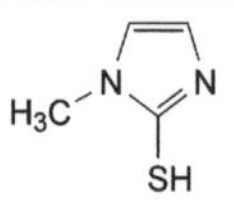

A. 1-methyl-1*H*-imidazole-2-thiol (thiamazole).

List of impurities detected by the tests (see the general monograph Substances for pharmaceutical use (2034) and chapter 5.10. Control of impurities in substances for pharmaceutical use)

General Notices (1) apply to all monographs and other texts

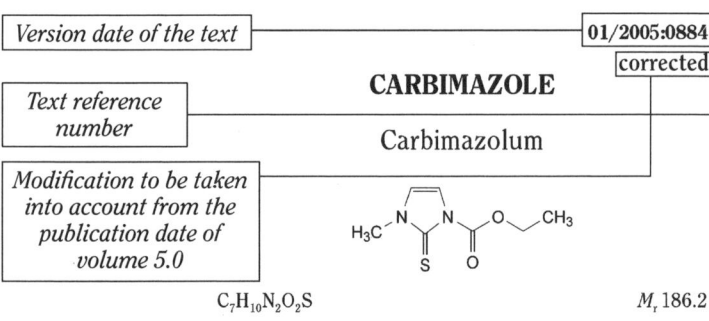

IMPORTANT NOTICE

GENERAL MONOGRAPHS

The European Pharmacopoeia contains a number of general monographs covering classes of products. These general monographs give requirements that are applicable to all products in the given class or, in some cases, to any product in the given class for which there is a specific monograph in the Pharmacopoeia (see *1. General Notices*, General monographs). Where no restriction on scope of a general monograph is given in a preamble, it is applicable to all products in the class defined, irrespective of whether there is an individual monograph for the product in the Pharmacopoeia.

Whenever a monograph is used, it is essential to ascertain whether there is a general monograph applicable to the product in question. The general monographs listed below are published in the section General Monographs (unless otherwise stated). This list is updated where necessary and republished in each Supplement.

Allergen products (1063)

Dosage Forms monographs
(published in the Dosage Forms section)

Extracts (0765)

Herbal drug preparations (1434)

Herbal drugs (1433)

Herbal drugs for homoeopathic preparations (2045)
(published in the Homoeopathy section)

Herbal teas (1435)

Homoeopathic preparations (1038)
(published in the Homoeopathy section)

Immunosera for human use, animal (0084)

Immunosera for veterinary use (0030)

Mother tinctures for homoeopathic preparations (2029)
(published in the Homoeopathy section)

Products of fermentation (1468)

Products with risk of transmitting agents of
animal spongiform encephalopathies (1483)

Radiopharmaceutical preparations (0125)

Recombinant DNA technology, products of (0784)

Substances for pharmaceutical use (2034)

Vaccines for human use (0153)

Vaccines for veterinary use (0062)

Vegetable fatty oils (1579)

Members of the European Pharmacopoeia Commission: Austria, Belgium, Bosnia and Herzegovina, Croatia, Cyprus, Czech Republic, Denmark, Estonia, Finland, France, Germany, Greece, Hungary, Iceland, Ireland, Italy, Latvia, Luxembourg, Netherlands, Norway, Portugal, Romania, Serbia and Montenegro, Slovak Republic, Slovenia, Spain, Sweden, Switzerland, "The former Yugoslav Republic of Macedonia", Turkey, United Kingdom and the European Union.

Observers to the European Pharmacopoeia Commission: Albania, Algeria, Australia, Bulgaria, Canada, China, Georgia, Lithuania, Malaysia, Malta, Morocco, Poland, Senegal, Syria, Tunisia, Ukraine and WHO (World Health Organisation).

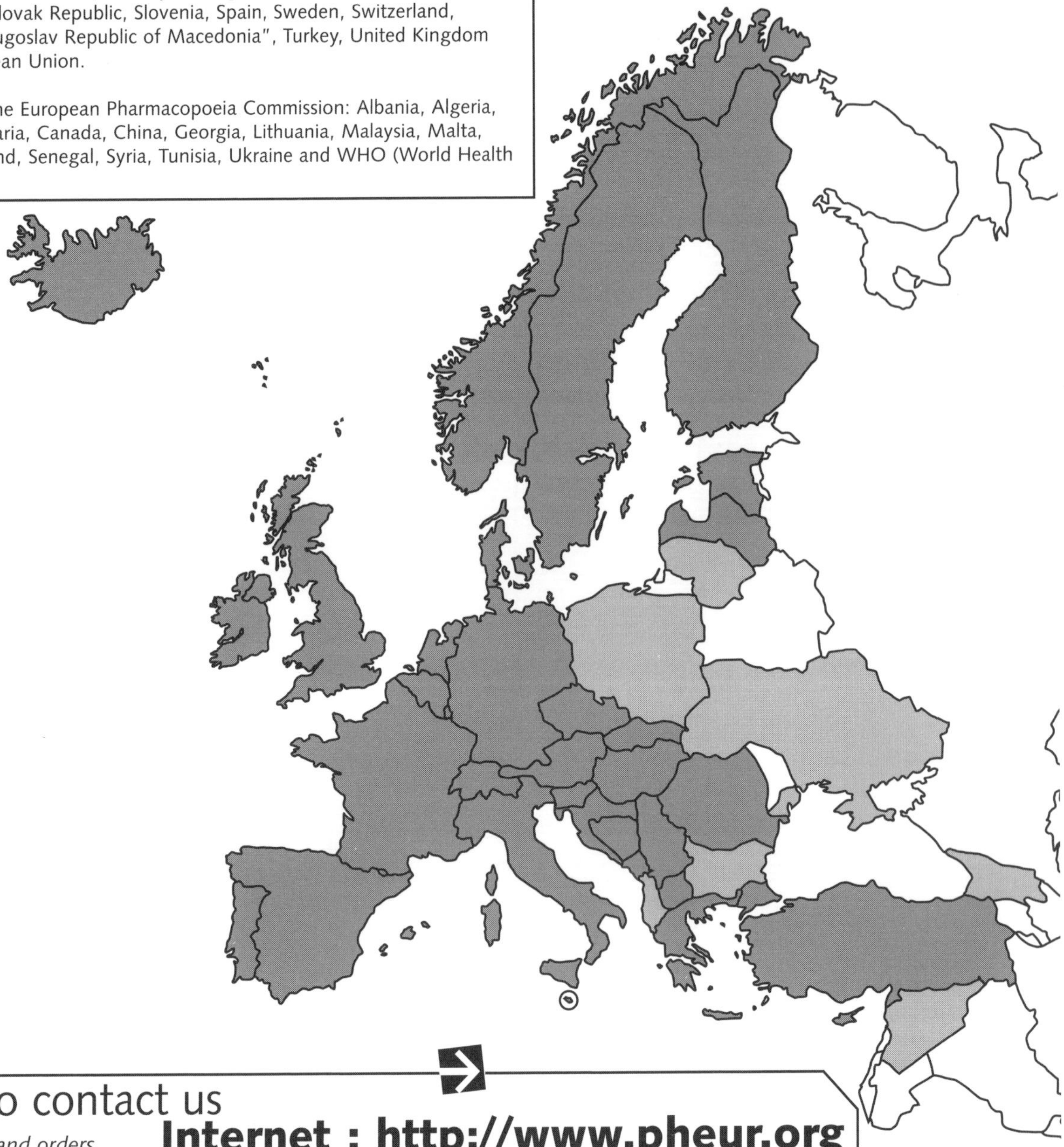

How to contact us

Information and orders **Internet : http://www.pheur.org**

European Directorate for the Quality of Medicines
Council of Europe - 226 avenue de Colmar BP 907
F-67029 STRASBOURG Cedex 1, FRANCE
Tel: +33 (0)3 88 41 30 30*
Fax: +33 (0)3 88 41 27 71*

	E-mail
CD-ROM	cdromtech@pheur.org
Certification	certification@pheur.org
Monographs	monographs@pheur.org
Publications	publications@pheur.org
Reference substances	crs@pheur.org
Conferences	publicrelations@pheur.org
All other correspondence	info@pheur.org

*: Do not dial 0 if calling from outside France.

All reference substances required for application of the monographs are available from the EDQM. A catalogue of reference substances is available on request; the catalogue is included in the Pharmeuropa subscription; it can also be consulted on the EDQM internet site.

EUROPEAN PHARMACOPOEIA

FIFTH EDITION

Volume 1

EUROPEAN PHARMACOPOEIA

FIFTH EDITION

Volume 1

Published in accordance with the
Convention on the Elaboration of a European Pharmacopoeia
(European Treaty Series No. 50)

Council of Europe
Strasbourg

The European Pharmacopoeia is published by the Directorate for the Quality of Medicines of the Council of Europe (EDQM).

ISBN: 92-871-5281-0

Printed in France by Aubin, Ligugé

CONTENTS

VOLUME 1

VOLUME 2

Note : on the first page of each chapter/section there is a list of contents.

I. PREFACE

The European Pharmacopoeia was inaugurated in 1964 through the Convention on the Elaboration of a European Pharmacopoeia. The present Fifth Edition of the European Pharmacopoeia is therefore published at the time where the 40th Anniversary of the Pharmacopoeia can be celebrated. The work on the Pharmacopoeia has gone through a remarkable development since the first difficult years. Elaboration and approval of monographs and other texts proceed by an effective and smoothly running process producing public quality standards that keep pace with scientific progresses. The work is remarkable because of its volume - the Fifth Edition presents close to 2000 monographs and other texts - and because all technical requirements have to be adopted by the European Pharmacopoeia Commission by unanimous decision. The monographs of the Pharmacopoeia are legally enforced in the countries being signatories to the Convention on the Elaboration of a European Pharmacopoeia. In addition to the 31 European countries and the European Union now being parties to the Convention, the work on the Pharmacopoeia is followed by 16 European and non-European countries and the WHO as observers. The quality standards of the European Pharmacopoeia have, therefore, an impact on the quality of medicines, which goes far beyond the European region.

The Fifth Edition of the European Pharmacopoeia will become effective on 1st January 2005. Like the Fourth Edition, the present main volumes will be added to by three annual supplements implementing the decisions of each of the three annual Sessions of the European Pharmacopoeia Commission. The presentation of the Pharmacopoeia in a main volume and three annual supplements was initiated by the publication of the Fourth Edition. The intention was to increase the flexibility of the publication scheme and, in particular, to shorten the time span between adoption and enforcement. The shortening of the time span, which has indeed been successful, is possible only thanks to a very flexible attitude by those countries that make national translations of the European Pharmacopoeia monographs. A very low number of rapid revisions implemented in the past three years is another result of the new publication scheme. The Fourth Edition is completed with the publication of Supplement 4.8 since it is impracticable to work with more than the eight supplements. The Commission decided therefore to proceed to the Fifth Edition by consolidation of the Fourth Edition after three years, only. The change from First to Second Edition was caused by major changes in the general methods, while the change from Second to Third Edition was due to the wish to consolidate the work achieved and to change the form of presentation from a loose-leaf format into a main volume followed by annual supplements. The change from Fourth Edition to Fifth Edition continues the work of making the publication of the Pharmacopoeia as user-friendly as possible. It is assumed that the publication of this Fifth Edition will proceed by publication of supplements over the next three years.

The eight founder countries of the Convention realised in 1964 that manufacturing and quality control standards for medicinal products on the European market had to be harmonised for reasons of public health and to facilitate the free movement of medicines. Since 1964 the world has changed and the market for medicinal products has become global. Accordingly, international harmonisation among the three major pharmacopoeias of the world, the European Pharmacopoeia, the Japanese Pharmacopoeia and the United States Pharmacopeia, has been in progress since 1990 when the Pharmacopoeial Discussion Group was set up to co-ordinate the harmonisation work. In the first years, the work was focused on the harmonisation of monographs on widely used excipients. In the absence of harmonised general methods this was a difficult work, which has now been speeded up by 'harmonisation by attribute' meaning that there may be tests that cannot be fully harmonised before the concerned general method is harmonised. At the stage where the monographs are harmonised, detailed information will be provided in the monograph and in a chapter of the Pharmacopoeia devoted to information on international harmonisation. In recent years, harmonisation of a wide range of general methods has been in progress, partly because of an impact from the International Conference on Harmonisation (ICH). Implementation in the Pharmacopoeia of harmonised general methods, for example for a dosage form specification, needs careful consideration because the specification must be met by products already on the market as well as new products submitted to the regulatory process.

The European Pharmacopoeia Commission supports strongly the international harmonisation. It is not the harmonisation work itself that gives rise to the greatest problems, rather the implementation, which has to be decided in mutual agreement with the registration authorities. The links between the European Pharmacopoeia Commission and European regulators have been steadily strengthened during the years, as have the links with the pharmaceutical manufacturers and their associations.

The new European Directives 2001/82/EC and 2001/83/EC on medicines for human use and veterinary use maintain the mandatory character of the European Pharmacopoeia monographs in the preparation of dossiers for marketing authorisation of medicines, which was instituted in the first directive 75/318/EEC in 1975. It means that the monographs of the European Pharmacopoeia must therefore be updated to keep pace with products on the market, with scientific progress, and with regulatory developments. In the field of active pharmaceutical substances, the European Pharmacopoeia Commission decided at its March 2002 Session that the principles and terminology of the revised ICH Q3A impurity testing guideline *Impurities in new drug substances* should as far as possible be implemented in the monographs on active substances, both new and already published. A change in terminology has been introduced in the Impurities section of monographs published in Supplement 4.6 and later where the term 'specified impurities' is used for impurities that have a defined individual acceptance criterion. A revision of the general monograph *Substances for pharmaceutical use (2034)* was also presented in Supplement 4.6 to implement the threshold values for reporting, identification and qualification of organic impurities in active substances of the revised ICH guideline. For the Fifth Edition a new chapter, *5.10. Control of impurities in substances for pharmaceutical use* has been developed with great assistance by the chairs of the chemical Groups of Experts and other experts from the Commission, and by consultations of the Groups of Experts. The next step will be revision of monographs to ensure that they contain related substances tests and lists on specified and other detectable impurities. Monographs containing a related substances test based on TLC will be considered for revision. Major revision work will thus proceed during the coming years. Hopefully, these revisions can be completed with the publication of the Sixth Edition. In the meantime, users of the Pharmacopoeia must consult the new Chapter *5.10* on impurity control for the interpretation of monographs published in the past and therefore adapted to a style that has now been changed as described above. Users can in addition find information on representative chromatograms, reagents and columns used in drafting the monographs on the EDQM web site.

The aim of the revision is to ensure that the related substances test and impurity lists reflect the purity of pharmaceutical substances being authorised for the European market. The goal cannot be met without close collaboration with the registration authorities and consultations regarding the specifications for impurities. A procedure for co-operation with the CPMP/CVMP Quality Working Party has been established. It will certainly contribute to ensure the validity of the European Pharmacopoeia monographs. The Certification of Suitability of Monographs of the European Pharmacopoeia might be a valuable source of information on the purity of pharmaceutical substances. The procedure is, however, confidential and will be kept so. In cases where a new impurity is present and calls for revision of the monograph, this can be done only when the manufacturer provides the concerned Group of Experts with the information required for updating.

The growing number of monographs on pharmaceutical substances and the need to keep them updated means a great workload on the Groups of Experts. In 2001, the number of chemical groups was increased and some reallocations of experts between the groups took place. There is, however, still a need for more experts with access to experimental facilities as permanent members of the Groups of Experts or as members on an *ad hoc* basis. In addition to the reorganisation of the system of Groups of Experts and Working Parties the working procedures for the elaboration of monographs have been expanded. In addition to Procedure 1, the traditional elaboration by a Group of Experts, and Procedure 2, adaptation of national monographs, which is now considered almost complete, Procedures 3 and 4 have been established in recent years. Procedure 3 applies to substances produced by only one manufacturer and which are close to patent expiry. The manufacturer and the national pharmacopoeia authority of the country where the substance is produced carry out the preliminary drafting stages and check the requirements experimentally. The draft is reviewed by the working party also responsible for the adaptation procedure and then processed in the usual way by public inquiry. Procedure 3 has proved successful. The Commission decided in 2002 to establish a modified version, Procedure 4. This procedure implies collaboration between the manufacturer of the substance and the EDQM on the draft monograph and experimental checking by the EDQM laboratory and laboratories of national pharmacopoeia authorities before publication for public inquiry. At present, Procedure 4 is run as a pilot project supervised by members of the European Pharmacopoeia Commission. It is the aim of the Commission to have a full coverage of monographs on substances no longer subject to a patent and being present on more than one European market. It requires the collaboration with the innovators and manufacturers of active substances, which has been established during recent years.

The Fifth Edition of the European Pharmacopoeia has a number of excipient monographs containing a non-mandatory section on functionality-related characteristics. The aim is to provide users with a list of physical and physicochemical characteristics that are critical to the typical uses of the concerned excipient, and to provide the general methods required to assess these characteristics. The section does not necessarily give acceptance criteria for the concerned properties; this is usually left as an option for labelling by the manufacturers and where specified, the values are indicative only. This is a new development which is in agreement with the policy of the European Pharmacopoeia Commission to make monographs and other texts appropriate to the needs of regulatory authorities and manufacturers of starting materials and medicinal products. The intention is to provide manufacturers of excipient materials and manufacturers of medicinal products a 'common language', to facilitate the establishment of product-specific specifications, and to provide regulators with data generated by methods that have been independently assessed.

It is the intention of the European Pharmacopoeia Commission to continue the work by drafting sections on functionality-related characteristics in monographs on excipients available in more than one physical grade. Introduction of the concept of functionality-related characteristics presupposes that the relevant general methods are available in the Pharmacopoeia. The European Pharmacopoeia Commission has therefore established a Working Party on synthetic polymers to investigate the need for general methods for polymers and a Working Party on powder characterisation methods. The provision of the needed general methods, for example in the field of powder characterisation, is also included in international harmonisation among the pharmacopoeias.

The achievements of the European Pharmacopoeia Commission during the past three years would not have been possible without the participation of the great number of experts from industry, academia and national authorities, who have given their time and expertise to the work of Groups of Experts and Working Parties. The Commission is indebted to all these experts whose work is given on a voluntary basis. The Commission is equally indebted to the Chairs of the Groups and Working Parties who have the responsibility of guiding the work through and bringing it to term according to tight time limits. The Chairs are thanked for their contributions within the Groups and also for their advice and counsel to the Commission itself.

The work of the European Pharmacopoeia Commission is strongly dependent on an effective Secretariat. The role of the Secretariat is to obtain and process all the information and reports needed for the Groups of Experts, Working Parties and for the Commission, to undertake laboratory work to support the experts and to ensure the availability of all the reference standards needed to allow the requirements in the monographs to be tested. The prompt publication of the Pharmacopoeia main volumes and Supplements and the on-line electronic version is possible, only, because of dedicated and hard work by the staff at the Secretariat.

Along with the growing volume of the European Pharmacopoeia and its adjustment to the regulatory process, the use of the Pharmacopoeia and its interpretation has become rather complex. The journal of the European Pharmacopoeia, *Pharmeuropa*, is a valuable source of information. General chapters for information will appear in the Pharmacopoeia during the publication of the Fifth Edition as a result of the international harmonisation, and because the European Pharmacopoeia Commission has agreed on the elaboration of other chapters for information. During the past two years, the staff at the EDQM have offered training courses to users of the Pharmacopoeia. The Commission is grateful to the EDQM for having taken this initiative, which also strengthens the role of the Pharmacopoeia and the links to its users. The links to users of the Pharmacopoeia are also strengthened by the frequent workshops and conferences organised by the EDQM. This activity is highly valued by the Commission as it gives the opportunity to Commission members to exchange viewpoints and to discuss new developments with experts from authorities, industry and academia. The EDQM web site is another valuable source for information on the work programme and other activities of the Commission, its Groups and the EDQM.

During the past three years I have had the honour to serve the European Pharmacopoeia Commission as its elected chair. The task has been challenging but, certainly, rewarding because of the insight it has given me into the many quality aspects of the development, manufacture and marketing of medicinal products. I wish to thank members of the European Pharmacopoeia Commission for their support and collaborative spirit within and in between the Sessions of the Commission. The two vice-chairs of the Commission are thanked for good collaboration and support during the years we have joined the Presidium. I will also thank the staff at the EDQM, in particular the secretaries to the Groups, for their kindness, enthusiasm and hard work for the benefit of the Pharmacopoeia. Finally, I wish to express warm thanks to the Director of EDQM, Dr. Agnes Artiges, and her deputy as secretary to the European Pharmacopoeia Commission, Mr. Peter Castle. I have appreciated our collaboration during the three years and wish to express heartfelt thanks to both for their support to the chair and for the tremendous work they are doing to develop the European Pharmacopoeia and its role in the European regulatory system.

Professor, Dr. Henning G. Kristensen

Chair of the European Pharmacopoeia Commission

II. INTRODUCTION

The European Pharmacopoeia is prepared under the auspices of the Council of Europe in accordance with the terms of the *Convention on the elaboration of a European Pharmacopoeia* (European Treaty Series No. 50) as amended by the Protocol to the Convention (European Treaty Series No. 134), signed by the Governments of Austria, Belgium, Bosnia and Herzegovina, Croatia, Cyprus, the Czech Republic, Denmark, Estonia, Finland, France, Germany, Greece, Hungary, Iceland, Ireland, Italy, Latvia, Luxembourg, the Netherlands, Norway, Portugal, Romania, Serbia and Montenegro, Slovak Republic, Slovenia, Spain, Sweden, Switzerland, "the Former Yugoslav Republic of Macedonia", Turkey, the United Kingdom, and by the European Community.

The preparation of the Pharmacopoeia is the responsibility of the *European Pharmacopoeia Commission* ("the Commission"), appointed in accordance with Article 5 of the above-mentioned Convention. It is composed of delegations appointed by the Contracting Parties. Each delegation consists of not more than 3 members chosen for their competence in matters within the functions of the Commission.

Observers from non-Member States and international organisations are admitted to Sessions of the Commission in accordance with the Rules of Procedures. Observers are at present admitted from: Albania, Algeria, Australia, Bulgaria, Canada, China, Georgia, Lithuania, Malaysia, Malta, Morocco, Poland, Senegal, Syria, Tunisia, Ukraine, and the World Health Organisation.

The functions of the Commission established by Article 6 of the Convention as amended by the Protocol are:

Article 6

"Subject to the provision of Article 4 of the present Convention, the functions of the Commission shall be:

(a) to determine the general principles applicable to the elaboration of the European Pharmacopoeia;

(b) to decide upon methods of analysis for that purpose;

(c) to arrange for the preparation of and to adopt monographs to be included in the European Pharmacopoeia and;

(d) to recommend the fixing of the time limits within which its decisions of a technical character relating to the European Pharmacopoeia shall be implemented within the territories of the Contracting Parties."

In accordance with the terms of the Convention, the Contracting Parties undertake to take the necessary measures to ensure that the monographs of the European Pharmacopoeia shall become the official standards applicable within their respective territories.

PURPOSE OF THE EUROPEAN PHARMACOPOEIA

The purpose of the European Pharmacopoeia is to promote public health by the provision of recognised common standards for use by health-care professionals and others concerned with the quality of medicines. Such standards are to be of appropriate quality as a basis for the safe use of medicines by patients and consumers. Their existence:

- facilitates the free movement of medicinal products in Europe;
- ensures the quality of medicinal products exported from Europe.

European Pharmacopoeia monographs and other texts are designed to be appropriate to the needs of:

- regulatory authorities;
- those engaged in the control of quality;
- manufacturers of starting materials and medicinal products.

The European Pharmacopoeia is widely used internationally. It is the intention of the Commission to work closely with users of the Pharmacopoeia in order to satisfy better their needs and facilitate their co-operation. To this end improved procedures are being developed for obtaining advice on priorities for elaborating new monographs and enhancing the quality of the Pharmacopoeia.

TECHNICAL SECRETARIAT AND LABORATORY

The European Pharmacopoeia Commission has a Technical Secretariat with scientific and administrative staff, situated in Strasbourg. The European Pharmacopoeia Laboratory is situated within the Secretariat and, amongst other duties, is in charge of the establishment and monitoring of all reference substances, preparations and spectra needed for the monographs of the Pharmacopoeia. The Technical Secretariat is an administrative division of the European Directorate for the Quality of Medicines (EDQM) of the Council of Europe.

GENERAL PRINCIPLES

General rules for interpretation of the texts of the Pharmacopoeia are given in the General Notices. The following information should also be noted.

The general principles applied in the elaboration of monographs of the European Pharmacopoeia are laid down in technical guides. The *Technical Guide for the Elaboration of Monographs,* which deals mainly with monographs on chemical substances, is available as a special issue of *Pharmeuropa* (see below under Publications). Other technical guides are being prepared to deal with aspects specific to monographs on other groups of products. The principles applied are revised from time to time without complete retrospective application so that monographs published already may not always follow the latest recommendations, but wherever an issue with impact on public health is identified, monographs are revised.

The procedures for the tests and assays published in the individual monographs have been validated, according to current practice at the time of their elaboration, for the purpose for which they are intended.

It is recognised that general chapters are used elsewhere than in the monographs of the Pharmacopoeia; in these circumstances users are recommended to consult the Technical Guide which gives extensive information on the application of many of the methods.

General monographs. The standards of the European Pharmacopoeia are represented by general and specific monographs. The use of general monographs has developed in recent years to provide standards that best fulfil the aims stated above and meet the needs of users. It is now usually necessary to apply one or more general monographs along with any specific monograph. Since it is not practically possible to include in each specific monograph a cross-reference to applicable or potientially applicable general monographs, cross-referencing has been discontinued except where it is necessary to avoid ambiguity.

A list of general monographs is included in each new edition and supplement to aid users in identifying those that are needed for use with a specific monograph.

Use of animals. In accordance with the *European Convention on the protection of animals used for experimental and other scientific purposes (1986)*, the Commission is committed to the reduction of animal usage, wherever possible, in pharmacopoeia testing and encourages those associated with its work to seek alternative procedures. An alternative or modified method is adopted by the Commission once it has been clearly demonstrated that it offers satisfactory control for pharmacopoeial purposes. Considerable progress was made in this area while the 4th Edition was in force and while the 5th Edition was being prepared.

Hydrates. With the publication of the 4th Edition, the policy on monograph titles for hydrated forms was changed. For all monographs published for the first time in the 4th Edition or subsequent editions, the degree of hydration, where applicable, is indicated in the monograph title. In previous editions, the policy was to indicate the degree of hydration only where several forms exist. If a monograph on both an anhydrous and a hydrated form of a given substance are published, then "anhydrous" will be included in the title of the relevant form. In order to avoid placing an unnecessary burden on manufacturers for relabelling, this policy will not be applied retrospectively to monographs published already, unless there is reason to believe that this is justified as a public health measure, notably for safety reasons where the substance contains a large proportion of water.

Chiral substances. Monographs on chiral substances that describe a particular enantiomer have a test to confirm enantiomeric purity, usually by measurement of optical rotation. Monographs that describe racemates are, in this respect, heterogeneous because of changes of policy during the 3rd Edition. Older monographs do not always have a test to show racemic character. During the course of the 3rd Edition, a test for racemic character was included in all new and revised monographs on racemates, using measurement of optical rotation. When it was shown that in many cases a test for optical rotation, even with narrow limits around zero rotation, was not necessarily sufficiently discriminating because of the low specific optical rotation of the enantiomers, the Commission modified the policy applied. A test for racemic character using optical rotation is now included only if there is information on the specific optical rotation of the enantiomers that indicates that such a test would be discriminating in terms of enantiomeric purity. If other techniques, such as circular dichroism, can serve the intended purpose, they will be prescribed instead of optical rotation.

Polymorphism. Where a substance shows polymorphism, this is usually stated under Characters. In general, no particular crystalline form is required in monographs; exceptionally, in a few monographs, the crystalline form required is specified, for example, via an infrared absorption spectrophotometric identification test where the spectrum is required to be recorded using the substance in the solid state without recrystallisation, the chemical reference substance provided being of the required crystalline form. However, for substances other than these exceptional cases, depending on the use of a given substance in a dosage form, it may be necessary for a manufacturer to ensure that a particular crystalline form is used. The information given under Characters is intended to alert users to the need to evaluate this aspect during the development of a dosage form. The monograph on *Substances for pharmaceutical use (2034)* and *5.9. Polymorphism* should also be consulted.

Specificity of assays. For the elaboration of monographs on chemical substances, the approach generally preferred by the Commission is to provide control of impurities via a well designed Tests section rather than by the inclusion of an assay that is specific for the active moiety. It is therefore the full set of requirements of a monograph that is designed to ensure that the product is of suitable quality.

Impurities. Following a review of policy on control of impurities, a new general chapter *5.10. Control of impurities in substances for pharmaceutical use* has been included in the 5th Edition. Together with the general monograph *Substances for pharmaceutical use (2034)*, it describes the policy of controlling impurities in specific monographs and provides explanations on how the limits in the related substances test should be understood. Currently the test is a limit test (comparison of peaks areas). In the future (next Edition) and in order to be in line with licensing practice and international collaboration, this test will progressively be changed to utilise a quantitative acceptance criterion. At present, some of the current monographs already satisfy this approach.

Except where required for the application of the monograph, in which case the name is followed by "CRS", impurities are not provided as reference substances nor can they be provided for experimental purposes.

Chromatographic columns. As an aid to users, information is made available via the web site www.pheur.org on chromatographic columns that have been found satisfactory during development of monographs and general methods. Information is also given on other equipment and reagents where this is considered useful. This information is given without warranty and does not imply that other columns, equipment or reagents than those specified are not suitable.

Residual solvents. The requirements for residual solvents are given in the monograph *Substances for pharmaceutical use (2034)* together with the general chapters *2.4.24. Identification and control of residual solvents* and *5.4. Residual solvents*. Thus all active substances and excipients are subject to relevant control of residual solvents, even where no test is specified in the individual monograph. The requirements have been aligned with the ICH guideline on this topic.

Reference substances, reference preparations and reference spectra. Where necessary for application of a monograph, reference substances, reference preparations and reference spectra are established and provided to users. They are chosen for their suitability for the purposes stated in the monograph and are not necessarily suitable for other uses. Any necessary information for proper use is given, for example a declared content, but no complete certificate of analysis is provided since this is not relevant for the intended use. No expiry date is attributed to reference substances and preparations, which are subjected to regular periodic monitoring to ensure their continued suitability. Where an assigned value for a given attribute, for example chemical content, is provided, no uncertainty for the assigned value is indicated. The reference substances, preparations and spectra are provided to enable the analyst to determine compliance or otherwise with a monograph. The uncertainty of an assigned value is not to be taken into account when judging compliance, since the uncertainty is already allowed for in the prescribed limits.

Medical devices. All editions of the Pharmacopoeia have contained monographs on articles that are regarded as medical devices. For Member States of the European Union, a unified framework for standardisation of medical devices is now provided by a Directive (93/42/EEC). Following an agreement between the various parties involved, the Commission has decided that the monographs on medical devices will be deleted once standards have been developed as foreseen by the Directive. Specifications included in the section on containers will be adapted to take account of future standards developed within the framework of the Directive. The monographs on surgical sutures remain in the Pharmacopoeia but they have been modified to conform to the requirements of the Directive and are now to be seen as standards of the type foreseen there. This adaptation of the monographs has involved deletion of some monographs on specific types of sutures in favour of a more general approach.

Homoeopathic preparations. A general monograph on homoeopathic preparations was added to the Pharmacopoeia during the 2nd Edition. A number of monographs on substances used in homoeopathic preparations are now also included and further monographs are in preparation. All of these texts have been grouped in a separate section. It is understood that when the same substance is used in both homoeopathic and other preparations then the monograph in the main body of the Pharmacopoeia applies.

Patents. The description in the Pharmacopoeia of articles subject to protection by patent does not confer or imply any right to the use of such patents by any person or persons other than the proprietors of the patents concerned.

Protected species. Monographs, notably those on herbal drugs, may cover material obtained from protected species. Inclusion of these monographs is without prejudice to the provisions for protection of these species by national and international law.

CERTIFICATION PROCEDURE

A procedure for the certification of suitability of monographs of the Pharmacopoeia with respect to control of the purity of a product from a given source has been established [see Public Health Committee (Partial Agreement) Resolution AP-CSP (99) 4 or any subsequent revision available from EDQM and on the web site (www.pheur.org)] as an aid to the use of monographs in applications for marketing authorisation. The certification procedure also applies to herbal drugs, herbal drug preparations and transmissible spongiform encephalopathy (TSE) risk. Certificates may be granted with respect to published monographs. Details of the operation of this scheme are available from the Secretariat and on the EDQM web site. A daily updated list of certificates granted is available on-line on the EDQM web site. A list of voided or suspended certificates is also published in *Pharmeuropa*.

PUBLICATIONS

The European Pharmacopoeia is available in English and French versions in the form of a book with 3 supplements per year, and in electronic form (internet and CD-ROM).

Pharmeuropa, the European Pharmacopoeia Forum, is published 4 times per year as an aid in the elaboration of monographs and as a vehicle for information on pharmacopoeial and related matters. It is available on subscription from EDQM.

Web site. Information on activities and many other aspects of the European Pharmacopoeia is to be found on the EDQM web site (www.pheur.org).

Implementation. The date on which monographs are to be implemented is fixed by a resolution of the Public Health Committee (Partial Agreement) of the Council of Europe, following a recommendation by the Commission. This date is usually about 6 months after publication. Where a monograph is to be implemented at a date earlier than the next publication date of the Pharmacopoeia or a supplement, a Resolution of the Public Health Committee gives the full text to be implemented. The text is also published in *Pharmeuropa* for information and posted on the web site as part of the Resolution.

Revision programme. Monographs and other texts of the Pharmacopoeia are revised as necessary following a decision of the Commission. Revision proposals are published in *Pharmeuropa*.

INTERNATIONAL HARMONISATION

The European Pharmacopoeia is engaged in a process of harmonisation with the Japanese Pharmacopoeia and the United States Pharmacopeia, within an informal structure referred to as the Pharmacopoeial Discussion Group (PDG). The activities are developed in co-ordination with those of the International Conference on Harmonisation (ICH). Information on the status of harmonised texts is given in chapter *5.8. Pharmacopoeial harmonisation*. Harmonised general chapters have a preliminary statement indicating interchangeability with the other two pharmacopoeias.

III. EUROPEAN PHARMACOPOEIA COMMISSION

COMPOSITION OF THE COMMISSION, LIST OF EXPERTS AND OF THE SECRETARIAT AS OF 30 NOVEMBER 2003

CHAIR AND VICE-CHAIRS OF THE COMMISSION

Chair	Henning G.	KRISTENSEN
Vice-chairs	Dries	DE KASTE
	Liisa	TURAKKA

MEMBERS OF THE COMMISSION

Austria	Kristof	LISZKA
	Andreas	MAYRHOFER
	Christian	NOE
Belgium	Luc	ANGENOT
	Jos	HOOGMARTENS
	Paule	JACQMAIN
Bosnia and Herzegovina	Aida	MEHMEDAGIC
Croatia	Dragica	BEGIC
	Ivana	STARESINIC-SERNHORST
	Laila	STEFANINI ORESIC
Cyprus	Louis	PANAYI
Czech Republic	Jiri	PORTYCH
	M.	TRAVNICKOVA
Denmark	Kirsten	BRØNNUM-HANSEN
	Steen Honoré	HANSEN
	Eva	SANDBERG
Estonia	Signe	LEITO
Finland	Jussi	HOLMALAHTI
	Kaarina	SINIVUO
	Liisa	TURAKKA
France	Jean-Paul	FOURNIER
	An	LÊ
	Alain	NICOLAS
Germany	Ulrike	HOLZGRABE
	Dietrich	KRÜGER
	D.	SCHNÄDELBACH
Greece	Michael A.	KOUPPARIS
	Alexandra	TSOKA
Hungary	Hilda	KÖSZEGI-SZALAI
	Jozsef J.	LIPTAK
Iceland	Gudrun	BALDURSDOTTIR
	Ingolf J.	PETERSEN
Ireland	T.A.	McGUINN
	Michael	MORRIS
	Joan	O'RIORDAN
Italy	Maurizio	CIGNITTI
	Anna	FARINA
	Graziella	OREFICI
Latvia	Janis	OZOLINS
Luxembourg	Jacqueline	GENOUX-HAMES
	Jean-Louis	ROBERT
Netherlands	Dries	DE KASTE
	Jan Willem	DORPEMA
	Pieter H.	VREE
Norway	Gunhild	BRUGAARD
	Valborg	HOLTEN
	Randi	WINSNES
Portugal	José Manuel	CORREIA NEVES SOUSA LOBO
	Rui	MORGADO
Romania	Daniele	ENACHE
Serbia and Montenegro	Marija	MASKOVIC
	Stana	MICIC
Slovak Republic	N.	CHALABALA
	Ruzena	MARTINCOVA
	J.	SLANY
Slovenia	Martina	CVELBAR
	Evgen	TOMAZIN
	Uros	URLEB
Spain	Franco	FERNANDEZ GONZALEZ
	Jordi	RUIZ COMBALIA
	Alexandra	VARDULAKI
Sweden	Lennart	AKERBLOM
	Marianne	EK
	Christina	GRAFFNER

Switzerland	Werner	ERNI
	Silvia	WEBER BRUNNER
	Helena	WINDEMANN
"The Former Yugoslav Republic of Macedonia"	Aneta	DIMITROVSKA
	Tatjana	PERUSEVSKA
Turkey	Orhan	CANBOLAT
	Yilmaz	CAPAN
	Hayriye	MIHCAK
United Kingdom	Derek H.	CALAM
	Gerard	LEE
	A.David	WOOLFSON
European Commission	Nicolas	ROSSIGNOL
EMEA	Emer	COOKE

ALTERNATE MEMBERS

Austria	J.	KURZ
	Josef	TRENKER
Belgium	Jacques	DE BEER
	Luc	DELATTRE
	Arnold J.	VLIETINCK
Denmark	Sven	FRØKJAER
	Lars J	HUSAGER
	Lene	THOMSEN
Estonia	Juhan	RUUT
Finland	Hannele	SALOMIES
France	Thierry	BOURQUIN
	Hendrick Jan	DE JONG
	Caroline	VILAIN
Germany	Gerhard	FRANZ
	Rainer	MOHR
	Rainer	SEITZ
Greece	Evangelos	PETRODASKALAKIS
	A.	TSANTILI-KAKOULIDOU
Hungary	Tamas L.	PAÀL
Ireland	Edward	BOURKE
Italy	Massimo	DI MUZIO
	Agostino	MACRI
	Loredana	NICOLETTI
Luxembourg	Mariette	BACKES-LIES
Netherlands	Ellen	DE ROOIJ-LAMME
	Peter M.J.M.	JONGEN
	Jan-Anton	NORDER
Slovak Republic	Daniel	GRANCAI
	Ladislav	SOVIK
Slovenia	Maja	LUSIN
	Barbara	RAZINGER-MIHOVEC
	Ales	ROTAR
Sweden	Torbjörn	ARVIDSSON
Switzerland	Andreas	BRUTSCHE
	Uwe	VÖLKER
	Eugen	WACHBERGER
United Kingdom	Aileen M.T.	LEE
	John M.	MIDGLEY

EXPERTS

Susan	AGERHOLM
Maqbool	AHMED
Jean-Marc	AIACHE
Lennart	AKERBLOM
Ferhan	AKTAN
Concepcion	ALONSO VERDURAS
Hansruedy	ALTORFER
Julio	ALVAREZ-BUILLA
Hanspeter	AMSTUTZ
Cyrille	ANDRES
Luc	ANGENOT
Gunnar	ANTONI
Astrid	ARBIN
Jean-Claude	ARGOUD
Torbjörn	ARVIDSSON
Wilfried	ARZ
Nataliya Nikolaevna	ASMOLOVA
Jérôme	AUCOUTURIER
Sylvie	AUDOLY
Paolo	AURELI
Teresa	AZCONA LLANEZA
Kenneth	BÄCKSTRÖM
Elizabeth Ann	BAKER
K. Hüsnü Can	BASER
Michel	BAUER
Alain	BAYOL
Françoise	BEAUJEAN
Denis	BELLENOT
Leandro	BELLENTANI
David N.	BENTLEY
Brita	BERGH
Kathrin	BERNARD-SUMMERMATTER
Serge	BESSET
Pietro	BIANCHINI
Jean-Pierre	BINDER
Hanno	BINDER
Mikael	BISRAT
Johannes	BLÜMEL
Giovanni	BOCCARDI
Colin	BOOTH
Nicole	BORNSTEIN
Thierry	BOURQUIN
Bernard	BOUYSSIERE

Brigitte	BRAKE
Harald	BREIVIK
Per O.	BREMER
Einar M.	BREVIK
Adrian F.	BRISTOW
Kirsten	BRØNNUM-HANSEN
Lukas	BRUCKNER
Peter	BRUEGGER
Volker	BUEHLER
Marian	BUKOVSKY
Rosario	BULLIDO
Jörg	BUND
Roger	BURGENER
Peter R.	BYRON
Derek H.	CALAM
Kandemir	CANEFE
Salvador	CANIGUERAL
François	CANO
Gunnar	CARLIN
Sergio	CAROLI
A.J.	CAWS
Richard	CAWTHORNE
Pierre	CHAMINADE
Xavier	CHENIVESSE
Vivienne	CHRIST
Maurizio	CIANFRIGLIA
Klaus	CICHUTEK
Juan	CLARAMUNT CAMPANA
Giovanni	COLLI
Laurence	COLLIERE
Pierre-Albert	COMPAGNON
Stéphane	CORNEN
Giordano Bruno	CORSI
Klaus	CUSSLER
Gérard	DAMIEN
Jacques-Christian	DARBORD
Alastair	DAVIDSON
Jacqueline	DAYAN-KENIGSBERG
Jacques	DE BEER
Josep M.	DE CIURANA i GAY
Hendrick Jan	DE JONG
Dries	DE KASTE
Carmen	DE LA MORENA CRIADO
Anna	DE PASQUALE
Ellen	DE ROOIJ-LAMME
Paul	DECLERCK
Clemens	DECRISTOFORO
Louis H.T.	DEDEREN
Luc	DELATTRE
Reto	DELLA CASA
Joseph	DEMEESTER
Jan	DEN HARTIGH
S.	DENYER
Jan J.	DIJKSTERHUIS
Roland	DOBBELAER
Johannes	DODT
Eric	DOELKER
Erik	DOEVENDANS
Milada	DOLEZALOVA
Thomas	DOLL
Jan Willem	DORPEMA

Maria Helena	DOS ANJOS RODRIGUES AMARAL
Robert	DRILLIEN
Anil	DUDANI
Siegfried	EBEL
Erling	EHRIN
Marianne	EK
Torben	ELHAUGE
Ulrich	ENGEL
Magnus	ERICKSON
Bengt	ERLANDSSON
Jean-Pierre	ETCHEGARAY
Øystein	EVENSEN
Bernard M.	EVERETT
Charles J.	FALLAIS
Gemma L.M.	FEENSTRA-BIELDERS
Peter	FEIGENWINTER
Rainer	FENDT
V'Iain	FENTON-MAY
Øystein	FODSTAD
Ton	FÖRCH
Ulf	FORSMAN
Lucien	FOSSE
Isabelle	FOURASTÉ
Jean-Paul	FOURNIER
Bruno	FRANK
Gerhard	FRANZ
Florence	FUCHS
Nicola	FUZZATI
Rose E.	GAINES DAS
Maria Cristina	GALLI
Andreas	GARDI
Jesus	GARICANO AISA
Didier	GARONNAT
Andrea	GAZZANIGA
Olga	GELDOF
Nicole	GIBELIN
Michel	GIRARD
Chris T.	GODDARD
Marcel	GOVERDE
Christina	GRAFFNER
Tatjana	GRAFNETTEROVA
Daniel	GRANCAI
Marta	GRANSTRÖM
Norbert	GREIDZIAK
Gerhard	GROHMANN
Peter	GRONSKI
Kjell-Olov	GRÖNVIK
Jean Louis	GROSSIORD
Emanuel	GUADAGNINO
Giuseppe	GUALANDI
Michèle	GUITTET
Robert	GURNY
Sylvie	GUYOMARD-DEVANLAY
Klaus	HABERER
Lilian	HAMILTON
Franz-Josef	HAMMERSCHMIDT
Steen Honoré	HANSEN
Paul	HARGREAVES
Goetz	HARNISCHFEGER
Vassiliki	HARTOFYLAX
Kaare	HASLOV

Heribert	HÄUSLER
Mary Alice	HEFFORD
Ingrid	HEGGER
Irmtraud	HELD
Keith	HELLIWELL
Peter	HENRYS
Jaakko-Juhani	HIMBERG
B.	HINSCH
François	HIRSCH
Rikke	HOFF-JØRGENSEN
Valborg	HOLTEN
Ulrike	HOLZGRABE
Ronald	HOOGERBRUGGE
Ernö	HORVATH
Rolf	HOVIK
Anthony R.	HUBBARD
Ronny	HÜBINETTE
Lars J	HUSAGER
Herwig	IGEL
Marianne	INZELT-KOVACS
Miia	JAKAVA-VILJANEN
M.B.	JAMES
Jana	JERABKOVA
Christa	JERSCH
Mats E.	JOHANSSON
Edgar	JOHN
Robert	JOHNSON
Peter M.J.M.	JONGEN
Karl-Henrik	JÖNSSON
Juan Ignacio	JORQUERA NIETO
Mats	JOSEFSON
Jan	KARLSEN
Hans	KEEGSTRA
Ernst	KELLER
Lawrence	KELLY
Isabelle	KEMPF
Damien	KERLOC'H
Marylène	KOBISCH
Claus	KOCH
Brigitte	KOPP
Frans	KORSE
Hilda	KÖSZEGI-SZALAI
Katjusa	KREFT
Henning G.	KRISTENSEN
Nikolaus G.	KRIZ
Burt H.	KROES
M.	KROON
Michael	KRÜGER
Ursula	KUKRAL
Harry V.	KUPPERS
Francesco	LA TORRE
Fritz	LACKNER
Reinhard	LANGE
Mervi	LANKINEN
Christophe	LAROCHE
Daniel	LARZUL
Annie	LASSERRE
Maria Grazia	LAVAGGI
John	LAVDIOTIS
Joyce	LAWRENCE
An	LÊ

Marie-Frédérique	LE POTIER
Aileen M.T.	LEE
Eva	LEMBERKOVICS
Ulla	LENNMARKER
Franck	LEVEILLER
Silvano	LONARDI
Céline	LORTEAU-SOURGEN
Patrick	LOUIS
Heiner	LUDWIG
Bruce	MADSEN
Antonio	MANES ARMENGOL
Warren C.	MANN
Georges	MANSVELD
Carla	MARCHIORO
Ana Maria	MARQUES GONCALVES
Andreas	MARTI
Alessandro	MARTINI
D.L.	MASSART
Jos H.A.	MATHÔT
Andreas	MAYRHOFER
Bernard	MAZIERE
Geerd J.	MEYER
Jacques	MICHAUD
John M.	MIDGLEY
Giovanni	MIGLIACCIO
Marianne	MIKAELSSON
Michael	MILCHARD
Miquel	MIR
Tony	MOFFAT
Birgitte	MØLLGAARD
Thomas	MONTAG-LESSING
Patrick	MONTENOISE
Manfred	MOOS
Jacques	MOREL
Laurence	MOUILLOT
Carl	MROZ
Zdenka	MRVOVA
B.W.	MÜLLER
Hartwig	MÜLLER
Michael	MUTZ
Vera	MYSLIVCOVA
Philip S.	NEWLANDS
Ria	NIBBELING
Robin A.J.	NICHOLAS
Steven C.	NICHOLS
Alain	NICOLAS
Loredana	NICOLETTI
Vittorio	NISTRIO
Jochen	NORWIG
Dagmar	NOVA
Ningur	NOYANALPAN
Werner	OBEXER
Hok Liang	OEI
Edgar	OHST
Rose-Marie	ÖLANDER
Bo	OLSSON
Graziella	OREFICI
Carsten	OVERBALLE-PETERSEN
Inge	OVERBY JENSEN
R.A.	PACKER
A.	PADILLA

Béatrice	PANTERNE	Theres	SCHNEIDER
Roya	PARKER	Henrik	SCHULTZ
Berit Smestad	PAULSEN	Dieter	SCHULZ
Maurice	PENSAERT	Harald	SCHULZ
Teresa Caroline	PEPPER	Volker	SCHULZE
J.M.	PERSON	Michael	SCHWANIG
Skevos	PHILIANOS	Roland	SEGONDS
Geoffrey F.	PHILLIPS	Gerhard	SEIPKE
Jean-Paul	PICAULT	Rainer	SEITZ
Roger D.	PICKETT	Carlo	SERAFINI
Aude	PLANTEFEVE	Dorothea	SESARDIC
Wolfgang	POHLER	Carlo	SESSA
Bertrand	POIRIER	Hanfried	SEYFARTH
Gilles	PONCHEL	Ekrem	SEZIK
Stephen	POOLE	François	SIMONDET
Poly	POPOVA	Kaarina	SINIVUO
Agustín	PORTELA MOREIRA	Carl Einar	SJØGREN
Juhani	POSTI	Wenche	SKARE
Roberto	POZZI	Mikael	SKOOG
Brian	PRIESTLY	Jan W.H.	SMEETS
Bernard	PRILLEUX	William Henry	SMITH
Miluse	PSEIDLOVA	Glenn	SMITH
Ivan	PSIKAL	Robert	SOUSSAIN
Martin	PUNZENGRUBER	Axel	STAHLBOM
Ain	RAAL	Juerg	STALDER
Jean	RABIANT	Roland	STERN
Alain	RAGON	Otto	STICHER
H.H.T.	RAYMAKERS	Borut	STRUKELJ
Alessandro	REGOLA	Rainer	SUCHI
Eike	REICH	Adriana	SUPPA
Franz	REIGEL	Maryse	SURGOT
Ascensao Maria	RIBEIRO FARINHA	Karl Gustav	SVENSSON
Markus	RICHTER	Lennart	SVENSSON
Valérie	RIDOUX	Pierre-Cyril	TCHORELOFF
Therese	RINGBOM	Robin C.	THORPE
Hans Peter	RINIKER	Maria	TOLLIS
Jean-Louis	ROBERT	Keith G.	TRUMAN
Yves	ROCHÉ	Liisa	TURAKKA
Eugène	ROETS	Michael	TÜRCK
Joachim	RÖHMEL	Peter	TURECEK
Véronique	ROSILIO	Michel	ULMSCHNEIDER
Michael	RÖSSLER	Uros	URLEB
Ales	ROTAR	Miguel Angel	USERA
D.	RUDD	Lars	VAELDS FREDERIKSEN
Maria-Sol	RUIZ	Luisa	VALVO
Jordi	RUIZ COMBALIA	Anja	VAN ARKENS
Christoph	SAAL	F.J.	VAN DE VAART
Alain	SABOURAUD	Willem G.	VAN DER SLUIS
Michael	SAENGER	Heim	VAN DER VELDE
Corinne	SAINT-REQUIER	Cees	VAN DER VLIES
Piero A.	SALVADORI	Hans	VAN DOORNE
Eva	SANDBERG	Hans P.	VAN EGMOND
Magali	SAUTEL	Bernard M.M.	VAN GENUGTEN
Gabriele	SCHÄFFNER	Daniel	VAN GYSEGEM
Marjolijn	SCHALK	Jos	VAN ROMPAY
J.J.C.	SCHEFFER	Philippe	VANNIER
Jeannot	SCHELCHER	Alexandra	VARDULAKI
Martin	SCHIESTL	Paul	VARLEY
Ernst	SCHLÄFLI	Michel	VEILLARD
Heinz	SCHMITTER	Alfons	VERBRUGGEN
D.	SCHNÄDELBACH	Geert	VERDONK

Christopher H.	VERMAAT
Michel	VERT
Peep	VESKI
Philippe	VILLATTE
Eva	VITKOVA
Arnold J.	VLIETINCK
Pieter H.	VREE
Claude	WASTIEL
Stephen	WATERS
Silvia	WEBER BRUNNER
Marjolein	WEDA
Volker	WESSELY
A.J.	WEST
Elisabeth M.	WILLIAMSON
Randi	WINSNES
Maria	WIRZ
Bengt	WITTGREN
Bernhard	WOLF
David	WOOD
A.David	WOOLFSON
Kaskashan	ZAIDI
Giorgio	ZANNI
Max	ZELLER
Tatjana	ZEUGIN MISEV
Stéphan	ZIENTARA
Ange	ZOLA

SECRETARIAT OF THE EUROPEAN PHARMACOPOEIA COMMISSION

Director (European Directorate for the Quality of Medicines)

Agnès	ARTIGES

Scientific Officers (Technical Secretariat, Laboratory and Biological Standardisation):

Peter	CASTLE (Secretary to the Commission)
John	MILLER
Jean-Marc	SPIESER
Stefan	ALMELING
Anne-Sophie	BOUIN
Karl-Heinz	BUCHHEIT
Catherine	CHAMBERLIN
Emmanuelle	CHARTON
Arnold	DAAS
Marie-Emmanuelle	BEHR-GROSS
Brigitte	JACQUEL
Andrea	LODI
Isabelle	MERCIER
Catherine	MILNE
Ellen	PEL
Pascale	POUKENS-RENWART
Guy	RAUTMANN
Ulrich	ROSE
Monica	SORINAS-JIMENO
Laure	TACONET
Michael	WIERER

Publication

Claude	COUNE
Hans-Joachim	BIGALKE
Stephan	BREHIN
Lynne	HENDERSON
Valérie	MÉAU-BOUDES
Catherine	NICOLAS
Alice	ROBERTS
Rachel	TURNER

Quality Assurance

Vincent	EGLOFF
Pierre	LEVEAU

Translation

Michelle	BACQUE
Benoît	BERNARD
Rex	HUISH

Public relations

Caroline	LARSEN-LE TARNEC

Expert consultants

Syed Laik	ALI
Raymond	BOUDET-DALBIN

The European Pharmacopoeia Commission and the European Directorate for the Quality of Medicines also wishes to thank the Secretariat for their contribution towards the publication:

Isabelle	BYLINSKI
Anne	ESPIN
Sandra	FROMWEILER
Carole	KNAUP

IV. CONTENTS OF THE 5th EDITION

The 5th Edition consists of all texts published in the 4th Edition, which may subsequently have been revised or corrected, and new texts.

For the information of the reader, lists are given below of monographs and general chapters that are new, or that have been revised, corrected or deleted, and texts whose title has been changed for the 5th Edition.

The version date (01/2005 for volume 5.0) and the reference number (four digits for monographs and five digits for general chapters) are specified above the title of each text (monographs and general chapters). The version date makes it possible to identify the successive versions of revised texts in different volumes of the 5th Edition. Corrections that are indicated by the word "corrected" under the version date are to be taken into account from the publication date of the volume.

For the 5th Edition, the following systematic modifications have been made to the texts of the Pharmacopoeia.

- The term "specified impurities" has replaced "qualified impurities" in the Impurities section of monographs in accordance with the texts on *Substances for pharmaceutical use (2034)* and *5.10. Control of impurities in substances for pharmaceutical use*. This term, which is compliant with the ICH guidelines, applies to impurities for which a specific acceptance criterion has been defined.
- In cases covered by the general monograph on *Substances for pharmaceutical use (2034)*, the test for sterility and the corresponding information in the Labelling section are no longer included in specific monographs.
- Chromatograms published for information no longer appear in the Pharmacopoeia; they are now available on the Internet site: www.pheur.org.
- A reference to available biological reference preparations has been added to the monographs concerned.
- The solubility in ether has been deleted from the Characters section and from the reagent descriptions.
- The reference to storage in a cool place has been deleted from the monographs and reagent descriptions.

A vertical line in the margin indicates where part of a text has been revised or corrected. A horizontal line in the margin indicates where part of a text has been deleted. It is to be emphasized that these indications, which are not necessarily exhaustive, are given for information and do not form an official part of the texts. Editorial changes are not indicated.

Individual copies of texts will not be supplied.

NEW TEXTS INCLUDED IN THE 5th EDITION

GENERAL CHAPTERS

2.4.30. Ethylene glycol and diethylene glycol in ethoxylated substances

2.6.24. Avian viral vaccines: tests for extraneous agents in seed lots *(previously texts 2.6.3, 2.6.4, 2.6.5 and 2.6.6)*

2.6.25. Avian live virus vaccines: tests for extraneous agents in batches of finished product *(previously texts 2.6.3, 2.6.4, 2.6.5 and 2.6.6)*

5.9. Polymorphism

5.10. Control of impurities in substances for pharmaceutical use

5.11. Characters section in monographs

MONOGRAPHS

*The monographs below appear for the first time in the European Pharmacopoeia. They will be implemented on **1 January 2005** at the latest.*

Monographs

Botulinum toxin type A for injection (2113)

Ciprofibrate (2013)

Clioquinol (2111)

Clofazimine (2054)

Closantel sodium dihydrate for veterinary use (1716)

Colestyramine (1775)

Coriander oil (1820)

Dipivefrine hydrochloride (1719)

Dodecyl gallate (2078)

Edrophonium chloride (2106)

Formoterol fumarate dihydrate (1724)

Human coagulation factor VIII (rDNA) (1643)

Hydromorphone hydrochloride (2099)

Insulin aspart (2084)

Insulin lispro (2085)

Isradipine (2110)

Lactobionic acid (1647)

Lysine acetate (2114)

Mitomycin (1655)

Octyl gallate (2057)

Oleyl alcohol (2073)

Oxeladin hydrogen citrate (1761)

Propylene glycol dicaprylocaprate (2122)

Pyrantel embonate (1680)
Ribavirin (2109)
Salmon oil, farmed (1910)
Tiamulin for veterinary use (1660)
Tiamulin hydrogen fumarate for veterinary use (1659)
Vinorelbine tartrate (2107)

Vaccines for human use

Meningococcal group C conjugate vaccine (2112)

Vaccines for veterinary use

Avian viral tenosynovitis vaccine (live) (1956)
Bovine leptospirosis vaccine (inactivated) (1939)
Infectious chicken anaemia vaccine (live) (2038)

Radiopharmaceutical preparations

Sodium fluoride (^{18}F) injection (2100)
Sodium iodide (^{131}I) solution for radiolabelling (2121)

REVISED TEXTS IN THE 5th EDITION

GENERAL CHAPTERS

1. General notices
2.2.1. Clarity and degree of opalescence of liquids
2.2.3. Potentiometric determination of pH
2.2.5. Relative density
2.2.24. Absorption spectrophotometry, infrared
2.2.34. Thermal analysis
2.2.40. Near-infrared spectrophotometry
2.2.46. Chromatographic separation techniques
2.4.8. Heavy metals
2.6.9. Abnormal toxicity
2.6.14. Bacterial endotoxins
2.7.16. Assay of pertussis vaccine (acellular)
2.9.11. Test for methanol and 2-propanol
3.2.1. Glass containers for pharmaceutical use
4. Reagents
5.2.8. Minimising the risk of transmitting animal spongiform encephalopathy agents via human and veterinary medicinal products

MONOGRAPHS

*The monographs below have been technically revised since their last publication. They will be implemented on **1 January 2005**.*

General monographs

Substances for pharmaceutical use (2034)

Monographs

Adrenaline tartrate (0254)
Ammonium glycyrrhizate (1772)
Bitter-fennel fruit oil (1826)
Buserelin (1077)
Cefapirin sodium (1650)
Codergocrine mesilate (2060)
Dexpanthenol (0761)
Doxycycline hyclate (0272)
Epirubicin hydrochloride (1590)
Estradiol benzoate (0139)
Etilefrine hydrochloride (1205)
Eucalyptus oil (0390)
Famotidine (1012)
Goserelin (1636)
Human anti-D immunoglobulin (0557)
Hyoscine butylbromide (0737)
Hyoscine hydrobromide (0106)
Hyoscyamine sulphate (0501)
Insulin, human (0838)
Iohexol (1114)
Iopamidol (1115)
Josamycin propionate (1982)
Ketoprofen (0922)
Lactose, anhydrous (1061)
Lactose monohydrate (0187)
Lavender oil (1338)
Paraffin, light liquid (0240)
Paraffin, liquid (0239)
Penbutolol sulphate (1461)
Povidone, iodinated (1142)
Primidone (0584)
Propyl gallate (1039)
Propylene glycol (0430)
Protirelin (1144)
Risperidone (1559)
Sulfamethoxazole (0108)
Thiamazole (1706)

Vaccines for human use

BCG for immunotherapy (1929)
BCG vaccine, freeze-dried (0163)
Diphtheria and tetanus vaccine (adsorbed) (0444)
Diphtheria and tetanus vaccine (adsorbed) for adults and adolescents (0647)
Diphtheria, tetanus and hepatitis B (rDNA) vaccine (adsorbed) (2062)
Diphtheria, tetanus and pertussis vaccine (adsorbed) (0445)

CORRECTED TEXTS IN THE 5th EDITION

The texts below from the 4th Edition have been modified and specify "01/2005:XXXX-corrected" above the title. These modifications are to be taken into account from the publication date of the 5th Edition.

Eleutherococcus (1419)
Erythropoietin concentrated solution (1316)
Fibrin sealant kit (0903)
Fish oil, rich in omega-3-acids (1912)
Foscarnet sodium hexahydrate (1520)
Framycetin sulphate (0180)
Gentamicin sulphate (0331)
Glycerol (0496)
Glycerol (85 per cent) (0497)
Glycine (0614)
Goldenrod (1892)
Goldenrod, European (1893)
Gonadorelin acetate (0827)
Guaifenesin (0615)
Halofantrine hydrochloride (1979)
Heparins, low-molecular-mass (0828)
Heptaminol hydrochloride (1980)
Human anti-D immunoglobulin for intravenous administration (1527)
Human plasma for fractionation (0853)
Human plasma (pooled and treated for virus inactivation) (1646)
Hyaluronidase (0912)
Hydroxycarbamide (1616)
Ifosfamide (1529)
Imipramine hydrochloride (0029)
Insulin, bovine (1637)
Insulin, porcine (1638)
Interferon alfa-2 concentrated solution (1110)
Interferon gamma-1b concentrated solution (1440)
Ioxaglic acid (2009)
Isoflurane (1673)
Ivermectin (1336)
Lemon oil (0620)
Lisinopril dihydrate (1120)
Lobeline hydrochloride (1988)
Lomustine (0928)
Magaldrate (1539)
Maltitol, liquid (1236)
Methylprednisolone hydrogen succinate (1131)
Methylthioninium chloride (1132)
Minoxidil (0937)
Mometasone furoate (1449)
Netilmicin sulphate (1351)
Nifedipine (0627)
Nifuroxazide (1999)
Omega-3-acid ethyl esters 60 (2063)
Papaverine hydrochloride (0102)
Pefloxacin mesilate dihydrate (1460)
Pepsin powder (0682)
Phenoxymethylpenicillin (0148)
Phenoxymethylpenicillin potassium (0149)
Piroxicam (0944)
Polymyxin B sulphate (0203)
Polysorbate 20 (0426)
Potassium acetate (1139)
Potassium clavulanate, diluted (1653)
Povidone (0685)
Pravastatin sodium (2059)
Primaquine diphosphate (0635)
Propanol (2036)
Propranolol hydrochloride (0568)
Propylene glycol dilaurate (2087)
Propylene glycol monolaurate (1915)
Pseudoephedrine hydrochloride (1367)
Rifabutin (1657)
Sodium alendronate (1564)
Sodium hyaluronate (1472)
Sodium polystyrene sulphonate (1909)
Somatropin (0951)
Somatropin bulk solution (0950)
Somatropin for injection (0952)
Sorbitol, liquid (crystallising) (0436)
Sorbitol, liquid (non-crystallising) (0437)
Spiramycin (0293)
Star anise oil (2108)
Sucrose (0204)
Tamoxifen citrate (1046)
Thiamine hydrochloride (0303)
Ticlopidine hydrochloride (1050)
DL-α-Tocopheryl hydrogen succinate (1258)
RRR-α-Tocopheryl hydrogen succinate (1259)
Tramazoline hydrochloride monohydrate (1597)
Triacetin (1106)
Vancomycin hydrochloride (1058)
Vinblastine sulphate (0748)
Vincristine sulphate (0749)
Water for injections (0169)
Water, highly purified (1927)
Water, purified (0008)
Willow bark (1583)
Xylose (1278)
Zopiclone (1060)

Vaccines for human use

Measles, mumps and rubella vaccine (live) (1057)

Measles vaccine (live) (0213)

Mumps vaccine (live) (0538)

Pertussis vaccine (acellular, co-purified, adsorbed) (1595)

Rubella vaccine (live) (0162)

Vaccines for veterinary use

Clostridium novyi (type B) vaccine for veterinary use (0362)

Clostridium perfringens vaccine for veterinary use (0363)

Clostridium septicum vaccine for veterinary use (0364)

Equine influenza vaccine (inactivated) (0249)

Foot-and-mouth disease (ruminants) vaccine (inactivated) (0063)

Swine erysipelas vaccine (inactivated) (0064)

Tetanus vaccine for veterinary use (0697)

Radiopharmaceutical preparations

Iobenguane (^{123}I) injection (1113)

L-Methionine ([^{11}C]methyl) injection (1617)

Homoeopathic preparations

Iron for homoeopathic preparations (2026)

TEXTS WHOSE TITLE HAS CHANGED FOR THE 5th EDITION

The titles of the following texts have been changed in the 5th Edition.

GENERAL CHAPTERS

2.2.34. Thermal analysis *(previously Thermogravimetry)*

2.7.4. Assay of human coagulation factor VIII *(previously Assay of blood coagulation factor VIII)*

3.1.4. Polyethylene without additives for containers for parenteral preparations and for ophthalmic preparations *(previously Polyethylene without additives for containers for preparations for parenteral use and for ophthalmic preparations)*

3.1.5. Polyethylene with additives for containers for parenteral preparations and for ophthalmic preparations *(previously Polyethylene with additives for containers for preparations for parenteral use and for ophthalmic preparations)*

3.1.6. Polypropylene for containers and closures for parenteral preparations and ophthalmic preparations *(previously Polypropylene for containers and closures for preparations for parenteral and ophthalmic use)*

5.2.8. Minimising the risk of transmitting animal spongiform encephalopathy agents via human and veterinary medicinal products *(previously Minimising the risk of transmitting animal spongiform encephalopathy agents via medicinal products)*

MONOGRAPHS

Monographs

Amfetamine sulphate (0368) *(previously Amphetamine sulphate)*

Riboflavin (0292) (*previously Riboflavine*)

Riboflavin sodium phosphate (0786) (*previously Riboflavine sodium phosphate)*

Tosylchloramide sodium (0381) (*previously Chloramine*)

Triacetin (1106) (*previously Glycerol triacetate*)

Vaccines for veterinary use

Avian infectious bronchitis vaccine (live) (0442) *(previously Avian infectious bronchitis vaccine (live), freeze-dried)*

Avian infectious bursal disease vaccine (live) (0587) *(previously Avian infectious bursal disease (Gumboro disease) vaccine (live), freeze-dried)*

Avian infectious laryngotracheitis vaccine (live) (1068) *(previously Avian infectious laryngotracheitis vaccine (live) for chickens)*

Canine leptospirosis vaccine (inactivated) (0447) *(previously Leptospira vaccine for veterinary use)*

Duck viral hepatitis type I vaccine (live) (1315) *(previously Duck viral hepatitis vaccine (live))*

Fowl-pox vaccine (live) (0649) *(previously Fowl-pox vaccine (live), freeze-dried)*

Newcastle disease vaccine (live) (0450) *(previously Newcastle disease vaccine (live), freeze-dried)*

TEXTS DELETED FOR THE 5th EDITION

*The following texts were deleted on **1 January 2005**.*

GENERAL CHAPTERS

2.6.3. Tests for extraneous viruses using fertilised eggs
2.6.4. Test for leucosis viruses
2.6.5. Test for extraneous viruses using cell cultures
2.6.6. Test for extraneous agents using chicks

MONOGRAPHS

Carbenicillin sodium (0812)

1. GENERAL NOTICES

1. GENERAL NOTICES

01/2005:10100

1.1. GENERAL STATEMENTS

The General Notices apply to all monographs and other texts of the European Pharmacopoeia.

The official texts of the European Pharmacopoeia are published in English and French. Translations in other languages may be prepared by the signatory States of the European Pharmacopoeia Convention. In case of doubt or dispute, the English and French versions are alone authoritative.

In the texts of the European Pharmacopoeia, the word "Pharmacopoeia" without qualification means the European Pharmacopoeia. The official abbreviation Ph. Eur. may be used to indicate the European Pharmacopoeia.

The use of the title or the subtitle of a monograph implies that the article complies with the requirements of the relevant monograph. Such references to monographs in the texts of the Pharmacopoeia are shown using the monograph title and reference number in *italics*.

A preparation must comply throughout its period of validity; a distinct period of validity and/or specifications for opened or broached containers may be decided by the competent authority. The subject of any other monograph must comply throughout its period of use. The period of validity that is assigned to any given article and the time from which that period is to be calculated are decided by the competent authority in the light of experimental results of stability studies.

Unless otherwise indicated in the General Notices or in the monographs, statements in monographs constitute mandatory requirements. General chapters become mandatory when referred to in a monograph, unless such reference is made in a way that indicates that it is not the intention to make the text referred to mandatory but rather to cite it for information.

The active ingredients (medicinal substances), excipients (auxiliary substances), pharmaceutical preparations and other articles described in the monographs are intended for human and veterinary use (unless explicitly restricted to one of these uses). An article is not of Pharmacopoeia quality unless it complies with all the requirements stated in the monograph. This does not imply that performance of all the tests in a monograph is necessarily a prerequisite for a manufacturer in assessing compliance with the Pharmacopoeia before release of a product. The manufacturer may obtain assurance that a product is of Pharmacopoeia quality from data derived, for example, from validation studies of the manufacturing process and from in-process controls. Parametric release in circumstances deemed appropriate by the competent authority is thus not precluded by the need to comply with the Pharmacopoeia.

The tests and assays described are the official methods upon which the standards of the Pharmacopoeia are based. With the agreement of the competent authority, alternative methods of analysis may be used for control purposes, provided that the methods used enable an unequivocal decision to be made as to whether compliance with the standards of the monographs would be achieved if the official methods were used. In the event of doubt or dispute, the methods of analysis of the Pharmacopoeia are alone authoritative.

Certain materials that are the subject of a pharmacopoeial monograph may exist in different grades suitable for different purposes. Unless otherwise indicated in the monograph, the requirements apply to all grades of the material. In some monographs, particularly those on excipients, a list of functionality-related characteristics that are important for the use of the substance may be appended to the monograph for information. Test methods for determination of one or more of these characteristics may be given, also for information.

General monographs. Substances and preparations that are the subject of an individual monograph are also required to comply with relevant, applicable general monographs. Cross-references to applicable general monographs are not normally given in individual monographs.

General monographs apply to all substances and preparations within the scope of the Definition section of the general monograph, except where a preamble limits the application, for example to substances and preparations that are the subject of a monograph of the Pharmacopoeia.

General monographs on dosage forms apply to all preparations of the type defined. The requirements are not necessarily comprehensive for a given specific preparation and requirements additional to those prescribed in the general monograph may be imposed by the competent authority.

Conventional terms. The term "competent authority" means the national, supranational or international body or organisation vested with the authority for making decisions concerning the issue in question. It may, for example, be a national pharmacopoeia authority, a licensing authority or an official control laboratory.

The expression "unless otherwise justified and authorised" means that the requirements have to be met, unless the competent authority authorises a modification or an exemption where justified in a particular case.

Statements containing the word "should" are informative or advisory.

In certain monographs or other texts, the terms "suitable" and "appropriate" are used to describe a reagent, micro-organism, test method etc.; if criteria for suitability are not described in the monograph, suitability is demonstrated to the satisfaction of the competent authority.

Interchangeable methods. Certain general chapters contain a statement that the text in question is harmonised with the corresponding text of the Japanese Pharmacopoeia and/or the United States Pharmacopeia and that these texts are interchangeable. This implies that if a substance or preparation is found to comply with a requirement using an interchangeable method from one of these pharmacopoeias it complies with the requirements of the European Pharmacopoeia. In the event of doubt or dispute, the text of the European Pharmacopoeia is alone authoritative.

01/2005:10200

1.2. OTHER PROVISIONS APPLYING TO GENERAL CHAPTERS AND MONOGRAPHS

Quantities. In tests with numerical limits and assays, the quantity stated to be taken for examination is approximate. The amount actually used, which may deviate by not more than 10 per cent from that stated, is accurately weighed or measured and the result is calculated from this exact quantity. In tests where the limit is not numerical, but usually depends upon comparison with the behaviour of a reference in the same conditions, the stated quantity is taken for examination. Reagents are used in the prescribed amounts.

Quantities are weighed or measured with an accuracy commensurate with the indicated degree of precision. For weighings, the precision corresponds to plus or minus 5 units after the last figure stated (for example, 0.25 g is to be interpreted as 0.245 g to 0.255 g). For the measurement of volumes, if the figure after the decimal point is a zero or ends in a zero (for example, 10.0 ml or 0.50 ml), the volume is measured using a pipette, a volumetric flask or a burette, as appropriate; otherwise, a graduated measuring cylinder or a graduated pipette may be used. Volumes stated in microlitres are measured using a micropipette or microsyringe.

It is recognised, however, that in certain cases the precision with which quantities are stated does not correspond to the number of significant figures stated in a specified numerical limit. The weighings and measurements are then carried out with a sufficiently improved accuracy.

Apparatus and procedures. Volumetric glassware complies with Class A requirements of the appropriate International Standard issued by the International Organisation for Standardisation.

Unless otherwise prescribed, analytical procedures are carried out at a temperature between 15 °C and 25 °C.

Unless otherwise prescribed, comparative tests are carried out using identical tubes of colourless, transparent, neutral glass with a flat base; the volumes of liquid prescribed are for use with tubes having an internal diameter of 16 mm but tubes with a larger internal diameter may be used provided the volume of liquid used is adjusted (*2.1.5*). Equal volumes of the liquids to be compared are examined down the vertical axis of the tubes against a white background, or if necessary against a black background. The examination is carried out in diffuse light.

Any solvent required in a test or assay in which an indicator is to be used is previously neutralised to the indicator, unless a blank test is prescribed.

Water-bath. The term "water-bath" means a bath of boiling water unless water at another temperature is indicated. Other methods of heating may be substituted provided the temperature is near to but not higher than 100 °C or the indicated temperature.

Drying and ignition to constant mass. The terms "dried to constant mass" and "ignited to constant mass" mean that 2 consecutive weighings do not differ by more than 0.5 mg, the second weighing following an additional period of drying or of ignition respectively appropriate to the nature and quantity of the residue.

Where drying is prescribed using one of the expressions "in a desiccator" or "*in vacuo*", it is carried out using the conditions described under *2.2.32. Loss on drying.*

REAGENTS

The proper conduct of the analytical procedures described in the Pharmacopoeia and the reliability of the results depend, in part, upon the quality of the reagents used. The reagents are described in general chapter *4.* It is assumed that reagents of analytical grade are used; for some reagents, tests to determine suitability are included in the specifications.

SOLVENTS

Where the name of the solvent is not stated, the term "solution" implies a solution in water.

Where the use of water is specified or implied in the analytical procedures described in the Pharmacopoeia or for the preparation of reagents, water complying with the requirements of the monograph on *Purified water (0008)* is used, except that for many purposes the requirements for bacterial endotoxins (*Purified water in bulk*) and microbial contamination (*Purified water in containers)* are not relevant. The term "distilled water" indicates purified water prepared by distillation.

The term "ethanol" without qualification means anhydrous ethanol. The term "alcohol" without qualification means ethanol (96 per cent). Other dilutions of ethanol are indicated by the term "ethanol" or "alcohol" followed by a statement of the percentage by volume of ethanol (C_2H_6O) required.

EXPRESSION OF CONTENT

In defining content, the expression "per cent" is used according to circumstances with one of two meanings:

- per cent *m/m* (percentage, mass in mass) expresses the number of grams of substance in 100 grams of final product,
- per cent *V/V* (percentage, volume in volume) expresses the number of millilitres of substance in 100 millilitres of final product.

The expression "parts per million (ppm)" refers to mass in mass, unless otherwise specified.

TEMPERATURE

Where an analytical procedure describes temperature without a figure, the general terms used have the following meaning:

- in a deep-freeze: below − 15 °C,
- in a refrigerator: 2 °C to 8 °C,
- cold or cool: 8 °C to 15 °C,
- room temperature: 15 °C to 25 °C.

01/2005:10300

1.3. GENERAL CHAPTERS

CONTAINERS

Materials used for containers are described in general chapter *3.1.* General names used for materials, particularly plastic materials, each cover a range of products varying not only in the properties of the principal constituent but also in the additives used. The test methods and limits for materials depend on the formulation and are therefore applicable only for materials whose formulation is covered by the preamble to the specification. The use of materials with different formulations, and the test methods and limits applied to them, are subject to agreement by the competent authority.

The specifications for containers in general chapter *3.2* have been developed for general application to containers of the stated category but in view of the wide variety of containers available and possible new developments, the publication of a specification does not exclude the use, in justified circumstances, of containers that comply with other specifications, subject to agreement by the competent authority.

Reference may be made within the monographs of the Pharmacopoeia to the definitions and specifications for containers provided in chapter *3.2. Containers.* The general monographs for pharmaceutical dosage forms may, under the heading Definition/Production, require the use of certain types of container; certain other monographs may, under the heading Storage, indicate the type of container that is recommended for use.

01/2005:10400

1.4. MONOGRAPHS

TITLES

Monograph titles are in English and French in the respective versions and there is a Latin subtitle.

RELATIVE ATOMIC AND MOLECULAR MASSES

The relative atomic mass (A_r) or the relative molecular mass (M_r) is shown, as and where appropriate, at the beginning of each monograph. The relative atomic and molecular masses and the molecular and graphic formulae do not constitute analytical standards for the substances described.

DEFINITION

Statements under the heading Definition constitute an official definition of the substance, preparation or other article that is the subject of the monograph.

Limits of content. Where limits of content are prescribed, they are those determined by the method described under Assay.

Vegetable drugs. In monographs on vegetable drugs, the definition indicates whether the subject of the monograph is, for example, the whole drug or the drug in powdered form. Where a monograph applies to the drug in several states, for example both to the whole drug and the drug in powdered form, the definition states this.

PRODUCTION

Statements under the heading Production draw attention to particular aspects of the manufacturing process but are not necessarily comprehensive. They constitute instructions to manufacturers. They may relate, for example, to source materials, to the manufacturing process itself and its validation and control, to in-process testing or to testing that is to be carried out by the manufacturer on the final article either on selected batches or on each batch prior to release. These statements cannot necessarily be verified on a sample of the final article by an independent analyst. The competent authority may establish that the instructions have been followed, for example, by examination of data received from the manufacturer, by inspection of manufacture or by testing appropriate samples.

The absence of a section on Production does not imply that attention to features such as those referred to above is not required. A product described in a monograph of the Pharmacopoeia is manufactured in accordance with a suitable quality system in accordance with relevant international agreements and supranational and national regulations governing medicinal products for human or veterinary use.

Where in the section under the heading Production a monograph on a vaccine defines the characteristics of the vaccine strain to be used, any test methods given for confirming these characteristics are provided for information as examples of suitable methods. Similarly, test methods for choice of vaccine composition are provided for information as examples of suitable methods.

CHARACTERS

The statements under the heading Characters are not to be interpreted in a strict sense and are not requirements.

Solubility. In statements of solubility in the section headed Characters, the terms used have the following significance referred to a temperature between 15 °C and 25 °C.

Descriptive term	Approximate volume of solvent in millilitres per gram of solute			
Very soluble	less than	1		
Freely soluble	from	1	to	10
Soluble	from	10	to	30
Sparingly soluble	from	30	to	100
Slightly soluble	from	100	to	1000
Very slightly soluble	from	1000	to	10 000
Practically insoluble	more than			10 000

The term "partly soluble" is used to describe a mixture where only some of the components dissolve. The term "miscible" is used to describe a liquid that is miscible in all proportions with the stated solvent.

IDENTIFICATION

The tests given in the identification section are not designed to give a full confirmation of the chemical structure or composition of the product; they are intended to give confirmation, with an acceptable degree of assurance, that the article conforms to the description on the label.

Certain monographs have subdivisions entitled "First identification" and "Second identification". The test or tests that constitute the "First identification" may be used for identification in all circumstances. The test or tests that constitute the "Second identification" may be used for identification provided it can be demonstrated that the substance or preparation is fully traceable to a batch certified to comply with all the other requirements of the monograph.

TESTS AND ASSAYS

Scope. The requirements are not framed to take account of all possible impurities. It is not to be presumed, for example, that an impurity that is not detectable by means of the prescribed tests is tolerated if common sense and good pharmaceutical practice require that it be absent. See also below under Impurities.

Calculation. Where the result of a test or assay is required to be calculated with reference to the dried or anhydrous substance or on some other specified basis, the determination of loss on drying, water content or other property is carried out by the method prescribed in the relevant test in the monograph. The words "dried substance" or "anhydrous substance" etc. appear in parenthesis after the result.

Limits. The limits prescribed are based on data obtained in normal analytical practice; they take account of normal analytical errors, of acceptable variations in manufacture and compounding and of deterioration to an extent considered acceptable. No further tolerances are to be applied to the limits prescribed to determine whether the article being examined complies with the requirements of the monograph.

In determining compliance with a numerical limit, the calculated result of a test or assay is first rounded to the number of significant figures stated, unless otherwise prescribed. The last figure is increased by one when the part rejected is equal to or exceeds one half-unit, whereas it is not modified when the part rejected is less than a half-unit.

Indication of permitted limit of impurities. For comparative tests, the approximate content of impurity tolerated, or the sum of impurities, may be indicated for information only. Acceptance or rejection is determined on the basis of compliance or non-compliance with the stated test. If the use of a reference substance for the named impurity is not prescribed, this content may be expressed as a nominal concentration of the substance used to prepare the reference solution specified in the monograph, unless otherwise described.

Vegetable drugs. For vegetable drugs, the sulphated ash, total ash, water-soluble matter, alcohol-soluble matter, water content, content of essential oil and content of active principle are calculated with reference to the drug that has not been specially dried, unless otherwise prescribed in the monograph.

Equivalents. Where an equivalent is given, for the purposes of the Pharmacopoeia only the figures shown are to be used in applying the requirements of the monograph.

STORAGE

The information and recommendations given under the heading Storage do not constitute a pharmacopoeial requirement but the competent authority may specify particular storage conditions that must be met.

The articles described in the Pharmacopoeia are stored in such a way as to prevent contamination and, as far as possible, deterioration. Where special conditions of storage are recommended, including the type of container (see *1.3. General chapters*) and limits of temperature, they are stated in the monograph.

The following expressions are used in monographs under Storage with the meaning shown.

In an airtight container means that the product is stored in an airtight container (*3.2*). Care is to be taken when the container is opened in a damp atmosphere. A low moisture content may be maintained, if necessary, by the use of a desiccant in the container provided that direct contact with the product is avoided.

Protected from light means that the product is stored either in a container made of a material that absorbs actinic light sufficiently to protect the contents from change induced by such light or in a container enclosed in an outer cover that provides such protection or stored in a place from which all such light is excluded.

LABELLING

In general, labelling of medicines is subject to supranational and national regulation and to international agreements. The statements under the heading Labelling therefore are not comprehensive and, moreover, for the purposes of the Pharmacopoeia only those statements that are necessary to demonstrate compliance or non-compliance with the monograph are mandatory. Any other labelling statements are included as recommendations. When the term "label" is used in the Pharmacopoeia, the labelling statements may appear on the container, the package, a leaflet accompanying the package or a certificate of analysis accompanying the article, as decided by the competent authority.

WARNINGS

Materials described in monographs and reagents specified for use in the Pharmacopoeia may be injurious to health unless adequate precautions are taken. The principles of good quality control laboratory practice and the provisions of any appropriate regulations are to be observed at all times. Attention is drawn to particular hazards in certain monographs by means of a warning statement; absence of such a statement is not to be taken to mean that no hazard exists.

IMPURITIES

A list of all known and potential impurities that have been shown to be detected by the tests in a monograph may be given for information. See also *5.10. Control of impurities in substances for pharmaceutical use*.

FUNCTIONALITY-RELATED CHARACTERISTICS

A list of functionality-related characteristics that are not the subject of official requirements but which are nevertheless important for the use of a substance may be appended to a monograph, for information (see also above *1.1. General statements*).

REFERENCE SUBSTANCES, REFERENCE PREPARATIONS AND REFERENCE SPECTRA

Certain monographs require the use of a reference substance, a reference preparation or a reference spectrum. These are chosen with regard to their intended use as prescribed in the monographs of the Pharmacopoeia and are not necessarily suitable in other circumstances. The European Pharmacopoeia Commission does not accept responsibility for any errors arising from use other than as prescribed.

The reference substances, the reference preparations and the reference spectra are established by the European Pharmacopoeia Commission and may be obtained from the Technical Secretariat. They are the official standards to be used in cases of arbitration. A list of reference substances, reference preparations and reference spectra may be obtained from the Technical Secretariat.

Local standards may be used for routine analysis, provided they are calibrated against the standards established by the European Pharmacopoeia Commission.

Any information necessary for proper use of the reference substance or reference preparation is given on the label or in the accompanying leaflet or brochure. Where no drying conditions are stated in the leaflet or on the label, the substance is to be used as received. No certificate of analysis or other data not relevant to the prescribed use of the product are provided. No expiry date is indicated: the products are guaranteed to be suitable for use when dispatched. The stability of the contents of opened containers cannot be guaranteed.

Chemical Reference Substances. The abbreviation CRS indicates a Chemical Reference Substance established by the European Pharmacopoeia Commission. Some Chemical Reference Substances are used for the microbiological assay of antibiotics and their activity is stated, in International Units, on the label or on the accompanying leaflet and defined in the same manner as for Biological Reference Preparations.

Biological Reference Preparations. The majority of the primary biological reference preparations referred to in the European Pharmacopoeia are the appropriate International Standards and Reference Preparations established by the World Health Organisation. Because these reference materials are usually available only in limited quantities, the Commission has established Biological Reference Preparations (indicated by the abbreviation BRP) where appropriate. Where applicable, the potency of the Biological Reference Preparations is expressed in International Units. For some Biological Reference Preparations, where an international standard or reference preparation does not exist, the potency is expressed in European Pharmacopoeia Units.

Reference spectra. The reference spectrum is accompanied by information concerning the conditions used for sample preparation and recording the spectrum.

01/2005:10500

1.5. ABBREVIATIONS AND SYMBOLS

A	Absorbance
$A_{1\,\text{cm}}^{1\,\text{per cent}}$	Specific absorbance
A_r	Relative atomic mass
$[\alpha]_D^{20}$	Specific optical rotation
bp	Boiling point
BRP	Biological Reference Preparation
CRS	Chemical Reference Substance
d_{20}^{20}	Relative density
IU	International Unit
λ	Wavelength
M	Molarity
M_r	Relative molecular mass
mp	Melting point
n_D^{20}	Refractive index
Ph. Eur. U.	European Pharmacopoeia Unit
ppm	Parts per million
R	Substance or solution defined under *4. Reagents*
R_f	Used in chromatography to indicate the ratio of the distance travelled by a substance to the distance travelled by the solvent front
R_{st}	Used in chromatography to indicate the ratio of the distance travelled by a substance to the distance travelled by a reference substance
RV	Substance used as a primary standard in volumetric analysis (chapter *4.2.1*)

Abbreviations used in the monographs on immunoglobulins, immunosera and vaccines

LD_{50}	The statistically determined quantity of a substance that, when administered by the specified route, may be expected to cause the death of 50 per cent of the test animals within a given period
MLD	Minimum lethal dose
L+/10 dose	The smallest quantity of a toxin that, in the conditions of the test, when mixed with 0.1 IU of antitoxin and administered by the specified route, causes the death of the test animals within a given period
L+ dose	The smallest quantity of a toxin that, in the conditions of the test, when mixed with 1 IU of antitoxin and administered by the specified route, causes the death of the test animals within a given period
lr/100 dose	The smallest quantity of a toxin that, in the conditions of the test, when mixed with 0.01 IU of antitoxin and injected intracutaneously causes a characteristic reaction at the site of injection within a given period
Lp/10 dose	The smallest quantity of toxin that, in the conditions of the test, when mixed with 0.1 IU of antitoxin and administered by the specified route, causes paralysis in the test animals within a given period
Lo/10 dose	The largest quantity of a toxin that, in the conditions of the test, when mixed with 0.1 IU of antitoxin and administered by the specified route, does not cause symptoms of toxicity in the test animals within a given period
Lf dose	The quantity of toxin or toxoid that flocculates in the shortest time with 1 IU of antitoxin
$CCID_{50}$	The statistically determined quantity of virus that may be expected to infect 50 per cent of the cell cultures to which it is added
EID_{50}	The statistically determined quantity of virus that may be expected to infect 50 per cent of fertilised eggs into which it is inoculated
ID_{50}	The statistically determined quantity of a virus that may be expected to infect 50 per cent of the animals into which it is inoculated
PD_{50}	The statistically determined dose of a vaccine that, in the conditions of the tests, may be expected to protect 50 per cent of the animals against a challenge dose of the micro-organisms or toxins against which it is active
ED_{50}	The statistically determined dose of a vaccine that, in the conditions of the tests, may be expected to induce specific antibodies in 50 per cent of the animals for the relevant vaccine antigens
PFU	Pock-forming units or plaque-forming units
SPF	Specified-pathogen-free.

Collections of micro-organisms

ATCC	American Type Culture Collection 10801 University Boulevard Manassas, Virginia 20110-2209, USA
C.I.P.	Collection de Bactéries de l'Institut Pasteur B.P. 52, 25 rue du Docteur Roux 75724 Paris Cedex 15, France
IMI	International Mycological Institute Bakeham Lane Surrey TW20 9TY, Great Britain
I.P.	Collection Nationale de Culture de Microorganismes (C.N.C.M.) Institut Pasteur 25, rue du Docteur Roux 75724 Paris Cedex 15, France
NCIMB	National Collection of Industrial and Marine Bacteria Ltd 23 St Machar Drive Aberdeen AB2 1RY, Great Britain

NCPF National Collection of Pathogenic Fungi
London School of Hygiene and Tropical Medicine
Keppel Street
London WC1E 7HT, Great Britain

NCTC National Collection of Type Cultures
Central Public Health Laboratory
Colindale Avenue
London NW9 5HT, Great Britain

NCYC National Collection of Yeast Cultures
AFRC Food Research Institute
Colney Lane
Norwich NR4 7UA, Great Britain

S.S.I. Statens Serum Institut
80 Amager Boulevard, Copenhagen, Denmark

01/2005:10600

1.6. UNITS OF THE INTERNATIONAL SYSTEM (SI) USED IN THE PHARMACOPOEIA AND EQUIVALENCE WITH OTHER UNITS

INTERNATIONAL SYSTEM OF UNITS (SI)

The International System of Units comprises 3 classes of units, namely base units, derived units and supplementary units(1). The base units and their definitions are set out in Table 1.6-1.

The derived units may be formed by combining the base units according to the algebraic relationships linking the corresponding quantities. Some of these derived units have special names and symbols. The SI units used in the European Pharmacopoeia are shown in Table 1.6-2.

Some important and widely used units outside the International System are shown in Table 1.6-3.

The prefixes shown in Table 1.6-4 are used to form the names and symbols of the decimal multiples and submultiples of SI units.

NOTES

1. In the Pharmacopoeia, the Celsius temperature is used (symbol *t*). This is defined by the equation:

$$t = T - T_0$$

where T_0 = 273.15 K by definition. The Celsius or centigrade temperature is expressed in degree Celsius (symbol °C). The unit "degree Celsius" is equal to the unit "kelvin".

2. The practical expressions of concentrations used in the Pharmacopoeia are defined in the General Notices.

3. The radian is the plane angle between two radii of a circle which cut off on the circumference an arc equal in length to the radius.

4. In the Pharmacopoeia, conditions of centrifugation are defined by reference to the acceleration due to gravity (*g*):

$$g = 9.806\,65\ m \cdot s^{-2}$$

5. Certain quantities without dimensions are used in the Pharmacopoeia: relative density (*2.2.5*), absorbance (*2.2.25*), specific absorbance (*2.2.25*) and refractive index (*2.2.6*).

6. The microkatal is defined as the enzymic activity which, under defined conditions, produces the transformation (e.g. hydrolysis) of 1 micromole of the substrate per second.

Table 1.6.-1. – *SI base units*

Quantity		Unit		Definition
Name	**Symbol**	**Name**	**Symbol**	
Length	*l*	metre	m	The metre is the length of the path travelled by light in a vacuum during a time interval of 1/299 792 458 of a second.
Mass	*m*	kilogram	kg	The kilogram is equal to the mass of the international prototype of the kilogram.
Time	*t*	second	s	The second is the duration of 9 192 631 770 periods of the radiation corresponding to the transition between the two hyperfine levels of the ground state of the caesium-133 atom.
Electric current	*I*	ampere	A	The ampere is that constant current which, maintained in two straight parallel conductors of infinite length, of negligible circular cross-section and placed 1 metre apart in vacuum would produce between these conductors a force equal to 2×10^{-7} newton per metre of length.
Thermodynamic temperature	*T*	kelvin	K	The kelvin is the fraction 1/273.16 of the thermodynamic temperature of the triple point of water.
Amount of substance	*n*	mole	mol	The mole is the amount of substance of a system containing as many elementary entities as there are atoms in 0.012 kilogram of carbon-12*.
Luminous intensity	I_v	candela	cd	The candela is the luminous intensity in a given direction of a source emitting monochromatic radiation with a frequency of 540×10^{12} hertz and whose energy intensity in that direction is 1/683 watt per steradian.

* When the mole is used, the elementary entities must be specified and may be atoms, molecules, ions, electrons, other particles or specified groups of such particles.

(1) The definitions of the units used in the International System are given in the booklet " Le Système International d'Unités (SI) " published by the Bureau International des Poids et Mesures, Pavillon de Breteuil, F-92310 Sèvres.

Table 1.6.-2. – *SI units used in the European Pharmacopoeia and equivalence with other units*

Quantity		Unit				
Name	**Symbol**	**Name**	**Symbol**	**Expression in SI base units**	**Expression in other SI units**	**Conversion of other units into SI units**
Wave number	ν	one per metre	1/m	m^{-1}		
Wavelength	λ	micrometre nanometre	µm nm	10^{-6}m 10^{-9}m		
Area	A, S	square metre	m^2	m^2		
Volume	V	cubic metre	m^3	m^3		1 ml = 1 cm^3 = 10^{-6} m^3
Frequency	ν	hertz	Hz	s^{-1}		
Density	ρ	kilogram per cubic metre	kg/m^3	$kg{\cdot}m^{-3}$		1 g/ml = 1 g/cm^3 = 10^3 $kg{\cdot}m^{-3}$
Velocity	v	metre per second	m/s	$m{\cdot}s^{-1}$		
Force	F	newton	N	$m{\cdot}kg{\cdot}s^{-2}$		1 dyne = 1 $g{\cdot}cm{\cdot}s^{-2}$ = 10^{-5} N 1 kp = 9.806 65 N
Pressure	p	pascal	Pa	$m^{-1}{\cdot}kg{\cdot}s^{-2}$	$N{\cdot}m^{-2}$	1 dyne/cm^2 = 10^{-1} Pa = 10^{-1} $N{\cdot}m^{-2}$ 1 atm = 101 325 Pa = 101.325 kPa 1 bar = 10^5 Pa = 0.1 MPa 1 mm Hg = 133.322 387 Pa 1 Torr = 133.322 368 Pa 1 psi = 6.894 757 kPa
Dynamic viscosity	η	pascal second	Pa·s	$m^{-1}{\cdot}kg{\cdot}s^{-1}$	$N{\cdot}s{\cdot}m^{-2}$	1 P = 10^{-1} Pa·s = 10^{-1} $N{\cdot}s{\cdot}m^{-2}$ 1 cP = 1 mPa·s
Kinematic viscosity	ν	square metre per second	m^2/s	$m^2{\cdot}s^{-1}$	$Pa{\cdot}s{\cdot}m^3{\cdot}kg^{-1}$ $N{\cdot}m{\cdot}s{\cdot}kg^{-1}$	1 St = 1 $cm^2{\cdot}s^{-1}$ = 10^{-4} $m^2{\cdot}s^{-1}$
Energy	W	joule	J	$m^2{\cdot}kg{\cdot}s^{-2}$	N·m	1 erg = 1 $cm^2{\cdot}g{\cdot}s^{-2}$ = 1 dyne·cm = 10^{-7} J 1 cal = 4.1868 J
Power Radiant flux	P	watt	W	$m^2{\cdot}kg{\cdot}s^{-3}$	$N{\cdot}m{\cdot}s^{-1}$ $J{\cdot}s^{-1}$	1 erg/s = 1 dyne·cm·s^{-1} = 10^{-7} W = 10^{-7} $N{\cdot}m{\cdot}s^{-1}$ = 10^{-7} $J{\cdot}s^{-1}$
Absorbed dose (of radiant energy)	D	gray	Gy	$m^2{\cdot}s^{-2}$	$J{\cdot}kg^{-1}$	1 rad = 10^{-2} Gy
Electric potential, electromotive force	U	volt	V	$m^2{\cdot}kg{\cdot}s^{-3}{\cdot}A^{-1}$	$W{\cdot}A^{-1}$	
Electric resistance	R	ohm	Ω	$m^2{\cdot}kg{\cdot}s^{-3}{\cdot}A^{-2}$	$V{\cdot}A^{-1}$	
Quantity of electricity	Q	coulomb	C	A·s		
Activity of a radionuclide	A	becquerel	Bq	s^{-1}		1 Ci = 37·10^9 Bq = 37·10^9 s^{-1}
Concentration (of amount of substance), molar concentration	c	mole per cubic metre	mol/m^3	$mol{\cdot}m^{-3}$		1 mol/l = 1M = 1 mol/dm^3 = 10^3 $mol{\cdot}m^{-3}$
Mass concentration	ρ	kilogram per cubic metre	kg/m^3	$kg{\cdot}m^{-3}$		1 g/l = 1 g/dm^3 = 1 $kg{\cdot}m^{-3}$

Table 1.6.-3. – *Units used with the International System*

Quantity	**Unit**		**Value in SI units**
	Time	**Symbol**	
Time	minute	min	1 min = 60 s
	hour	h	1 h = 60 min = 3600 s
	day	d	1 d = 24 h = 86 400 s
Plan angle	degree	°	1° = (π/180) rad
Volume	litre	l	1 l = 1 dm^3 = 10^{-3} m^3
Mass	tonne	t	1 t = 10^3 kg
Rotational frequency	revolution per minute	r/min	1 r/min = (1/60) s^{-1}

Table 1.6.-4. – *Decimal multiples and sub-multiples of units*

Factor	**Prefix**	**Symbol**	**Factor**	**Prefix**	**Symbol**
10^{18}	exa	E	10^{-1}	deci	d
10^{15}	peta	P	10^{-2}	centi	c
10^{12}	tera	T	10^{-3}	milli	m
10^9	giga	G	10^{-6}	micro	µ
10^6	mega	M	10^{-9}	nano	n
10^3	kilo	k	10^{-12}	pico	p
10^2	hecto	h	10^{-15}	femto	f
10^1	deca	da	10^{-18}	atto	a

2. METHODS OF ANALYSIS

2.1. APPARATUS

2.1. APPARATUS

01/2005:20101

2.1.1. DROPPERS

The term "drops" means standard drops delivered from a standard dropper as described below.

Standard droppers (Figure 2.1.1-1) are constructed of practically colourless glass. The lower extremity has a circular orifice in a flat surface at right angles to the axis.

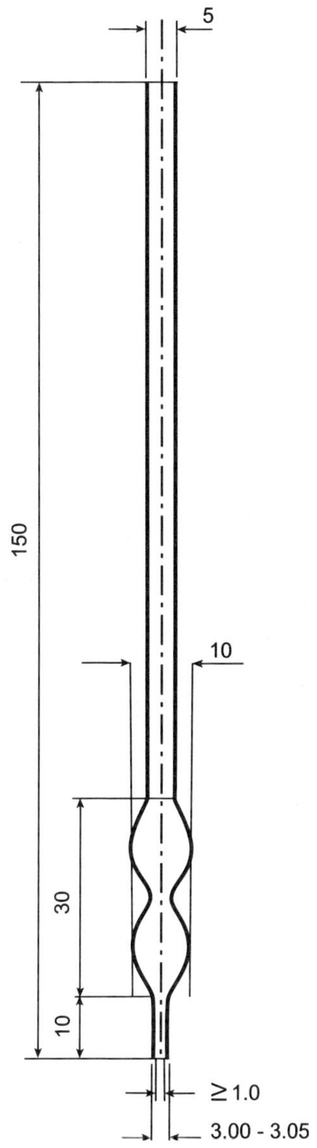

Figure 2.1.1.-1. – *Standard dropper*
Dimensions in millimetres

Other droppers may be used provided they comply with the following test.

Twenty drops of *water R* at 20 ± 1 °C flowing freely from the dropper held in the vertical position at a constant rate of one drop per second weighs 1000 ± 50 mg.

The dropper must be carefully cleaned before use. Carry out three determinations on any given dropper. No result may deviate by more than 5 per cent from the mean of the three determinations.

01/2005:20102

2.1.2. COMPARATIVE TABLE OF POROSITY OF SINTERED-GLASS FILTERS(1)

Table 2.1.2.-1

Porosity number (Ph. Eur.) (2)	Maximum diameter of pores in micrometres	Germany	France	United Kingdom
1.6	less than 1.6	5f	–	–
–	1 - 2.5	5	–	5
4	1.6 - 4	–	–	–
–	4 - 6	–	5	–
10	4 - 10	4f	–	4
16	10 - 16	4	4	–
40	16 - 40	3	3	3
–	40 - 50	–	–	2
100	40 - 100	2	2	–
–	100 - 120	–	–	1
160	100 - 160	1	1	–
–	150 - 200	0	0	–
250	160 - 250	–	–	–
–	200 - 500	–	00	–

Special Uses

Diameters in micrometres

< 2.5	Bacteriological filtration
4 - 10	Ultra-fine filtration, separation of micro-organisms of large diameter
10 - 40	Analytical filtration, very fine filtration of mercury, very fine dispersion of gases
40 - 100	Fine filtration, filtration of mercury, fine dispersion of gases
100 - 160	Filtration of coarse materials, dispersion and washing of gases, support for other filter materials
160 - 500	Filtration of very coarse materials, dispersion and washing of gases.

01/2005:20103

2.1.3. ULTRAVIOLET RAY LAMPS FOR ANALYTICAL PURPOSES

Mercury vapour in quartz lamps is used as the source of ultraviolet light. A suitable filter may be fitted to eliminate the visible part of the spectrum emitted by the lamp. When the Pharmacopoeia prescribes in a test the use of ultraviolet light of wavelength 254 nm or 365 nm, an instrument consisting of a mercury vapour lamp and a filter which gives an emission band with maximum intensity at about 254 nm or 365 nm is used. The lamp used should be capable of revealing without doubt a standard spot of sodium salicylate with a diameter of about 5 mm on a support of *silica gel G R*, the spot being examined while in a position normal to the radiation.

(1) The given limits are only approximate.
(2) The European Pharmacopoeia has adopted the system proposed by the International Organisation for Standardisation (ISO).

For this purpose apply 5 µl of a 0.4 g/l solution of *sodium salicylate R* in *alcohol R*[3] for lamps of maximum output at 254 nm and 5 µl of a 2 g/l solution in *alcohol R*[1] for lamps of maximum output at 365 nm. The distance between the lamp and the chromatographic plate under examination used in a pharmacopoeial test should never exceed the distance used to carry out the above test.

01/2005:20104

2.1.4. SIEVES

Sieves are constructed of suitable materials with square meshes. For purposes other than analytical procedures, sieves with circular meshes may be used, the internal diameters of which are 1.25 times the aperture of the square mesh of the corresponding sieve size. There must be no reaction between the material of the sieve and the substance being sifted. Degree of comminution is prescribed in the monograph using the sieve number, which is the size of the mesh in micrometres, given in parenthesis after the name of the substance (Table 2.1.4.-1).

Maximum tolerance[4] for an aperture (+ X): no aperture size shall exceed the nominal size by more than X, where:

$$X = \frac{2\left(w^{0.75}\right)}{3} + 4\left(w^{0.25}\right)$$

w = width of aperture.

Tolerance for mean aperture (± Y): the average aperture size shall not depart from the nominal size by more than ± Y, where:

$$Y = \frac{w^{0.98}}{27} + 1.6$$

Intermediary tolerance (+ Z): not more than 6 per cent of the total number of apertures shall have sizes between "nominal + X" and "nominal + Z", where:

$$Z = \frac{X + Y}{2}$$

Wire diameter d: the wire diameters given in Table 2.1.4.-1 apply to woven metal wire cloth mounted in a frame. The nominal sizes of the wire diameters may depart from these values within the limits d_{max} and d_{min}. The limits define a permissible range of choice ± 15 per cent of the recommended nominal dimensions. The wires in a test sieve shall be of a similar diameter in warp and weft directions.

Table 2.1.4.-1 (*values in micrometers*)

Sieve numbers (Nominal dimensions of apertures)	**Tolerances for apertures**			**Wire diameters**		
	Maximum tolerance for an aperture	**Tolerance for mean aperture**	**Intermediary tolerance**	**Recommended nominal dimensions**	**Admissible limits**	
	+ X	**± Y**	**+ Z**	**d**	**d_{max}**	**d_{min}**
11 200	770	350	560	2500	2900	2100
8000	600	250	430	2000	2300	1700
5 600	470	180	320	1600	1900	1300
4000	370	130	250	1400	1700	1200
2 800	290	90	190	1120	1300	950
2000	230	70	150	900	1040	770
1 400	180	50	110	710	820	600
1000	140	30	90	560	640	480
710	112	25	69	450	520	380
500	89	18	54	315	360	270
355	72	13	43	224	260	190
250	58	9.9	34	160	190	130
180	47	7.6	27	125	150	106
125	38	5.8	22	90	104	77
90	32	4.6	18	63	72	54
63	26	3.7	15	45	52	38
45	22	3.1	13	32	37	27
38	–	–	–	30	35	24

(3) The *alcohol R* used must be free from fluorescence.
(4) See the International Standard ISO 3310/1 (1975).

01/2005:20105

2.1.5. TUBES FOR COMPARATIVE TESTS

Tubes used for comparative tests are matched tubes of colourless glass with a uniform internal diameter. The base is transparent and flat.

A column of the liquid is examined down the vertical axis of the tube against a white background, or if necessary, against a black background. The examination is carried out in diffused light.

It is assumed that tubes with an internal diameter of 16 mm will be used. Tubes with a larger internal diameter may be used instead but the volume of liquid examined must then be increased so that the depth of liquid in the tubes is not less than where the prescribed volume of liquid and tubes 16 mm in internal diameter are used.

01/2005:20106

2.1.6. GAS DETECTOR TUBES

Gas detector tubes are cylindrical, sealed tubes consisting of an inert transparent material and are constructed to allow the passage of gas. They contain reagents adsorbed onto inert substrates that are suitable for the visualisation of the substance to be detected and, if necessary, they also contain preliminary layers and/or adsorbent filters to eliminate substances that interfere with the substance to be detected. The layer of indicator contains either a single reagent for the detection of a given impurity or several reagents for the detection of several substances (monolayer tube or multilayer tube).

The test is carried out by passing the required volume of the gas to be examined through the indicator tube. The length of the coloured layer or the intensity of a colour change on a graduated scale gives an indication of the impurities present.

The calibration of the detector tubes is verified according to the manufacturer's instructions.

Operating conditions. Examine according to the manufacturer's instructions or proceed as follows:

The gas supply is connected to a suitable pressure regulator and needle valve. Connect the flexible tubing fitted with a Y-piece to the valve and adjust the flow of gas to be examined to purge the tubing in order to obtain an appropriate flow (Figure 2.1.6.-1). Prepare the indicator tube and fit to the metering pump, following the manufacturer's instructions. Connect the open end of the indicator tube to the short leg of the tubing and operate the pump by the appropriate number of strokes to pass a suitable volume of gas to be examined through the tube. Read the value corresponding to the length of the coloured layer or the intensity of the colour on the graduated scale. If a negative result is achieved, indicator tubes can be verified with a calibration gas containing the appropriate impurity.

In view of the wide variety of available compressor oils, it is necessary to verify the reactivity of the oil detector tubes for the oil used. Information on the reactivity for various oils is given in the leaflet supplied with the tube. If the oil used is not cited in the leaflet, the tube manufacturer must verify the reactivity and if necessary provide a tube specific for this oil.

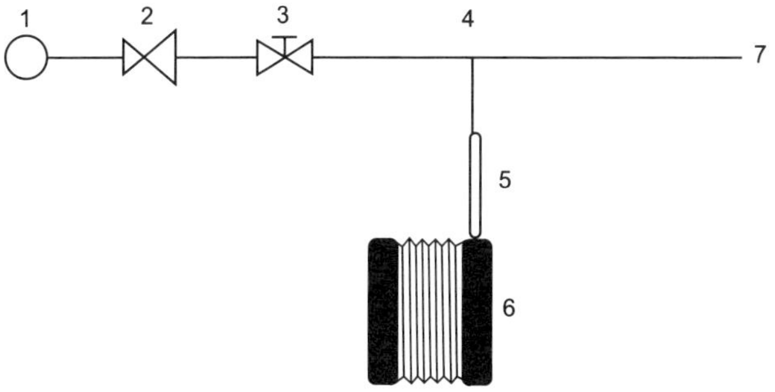

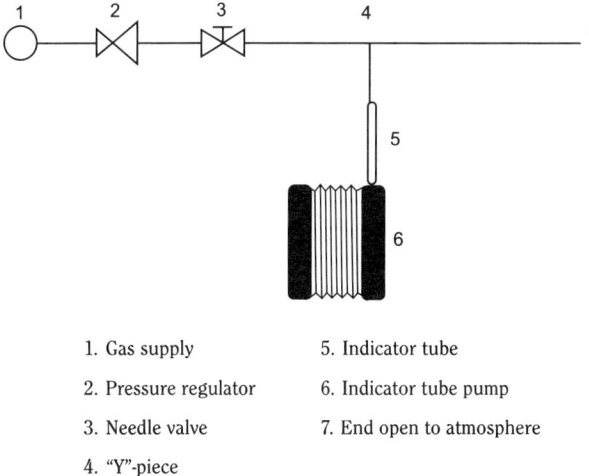

1. Gas supply
2. Pressure regulator
3. Needle valve
4. "Y"-piece
5. Indicator tube
6. Indicator tube pump
7. End open to atmosphere

Figure 2.1.6.-1. – *Apparatus for gas detector tubes*

Carbon dioxide detector tube. Sealed glass tube containing adsorbent filters and suitable supports for hydrazine and crystal violet indicators. The minimum value indicated is 100 ppm with a relative standard deviation of at most ± 15 per cent.

Sulphur dioxide detector tube. Sealed glass tube containing adsorbent filters and suitable supports for the iodine and starch indicator. The minimum value indicated is 0.5 ppm with a relative standard deviation of at most ± 15 per cent.

Oil detector tube. Sealed glass tube containing adsorbent filters and suitable supports for the sulphuric acid indicator. The minimum value indicated is 0.1 mg/m^3 with a relative standard deviation of at most ± 30 per cent.

Nitrogen monoxide and nitrogen dioxide detector tube. Sealed glass tube containing adsorbent filters and suitable supports for an oxidising layer (Cr(VI) salt) and the diphenylbenzidine indicator. The minimum value indicated is 0.5 ppm with a relative standard deviation of at most ± 15 per cent.

Carbon monoxide detector tube. Sealed glass tube containing adsorbent filters and suitable supports for di-iodine pentoxide, selenium dioxide and fuming sulphuric acid indicators. The minimum value indicated is 5 ppm or less, with a relative standard deviation of at most ± 15 per cent.

Hydrogen sulphide detector tube. Sealed glass tube containing adsorbent filters and suitable supports for an appropriate lead salt indicator. The minimum value indicated is 1 ppm or less, with a relative standard deviation of at most ± 10 per cent.

Water vapour detector tube. Sealed glass tube containing adsorbent filters and suitable supports for the magnesium perchlorate indicator. The minimum value indicated is 67 ppm or less, with a relative standard deviation of at most ± 20 per cent.

2.2. PHYSICAL AND PHYSICOCHEMICAL METHODS

2.2. PHYSICAL AND PHYSICOCHEMICAL METHODS

01/2005:20201

2.2.1. CLARITY AND DEGREE OF OPALESCENCE OF LIQUIDS

VISUAL METHOD

Using identical test tubes of colourless, transparent, neutral glass with a flat base and an internal diameter of 15-25 mm, compare the liquid to be examined with a reference suspension freshly prepared as described below, the depth of the layer being 40 mm. Compare the solutions in diffused daylight 5 min after preparation of the reference suspension, viewing vertically against a black background. The diffusion of light must be such that reference suspension I can readily be distinguished from *water R*, and that reference suspension II can readily be distinguished from reference suspension I.

A liquid is considered *clear* if its clarity is the same as that of *water R* or of the solvent used when examined under the conditions described above, or if its opalescence is not more pronounced than that of reference suspension I.

Hydrazine sulphate solution. Dissolve 1.0 g of *hydrazine sulphate R* in *water R* and dilute to 100.0 ml with the same solvent. Allow to stand for 4-6 h.

Hexamethylenetetramine solution. In a 100 ml glass-stoppered flask, dissolve 2.5 g of *hexamethylenetetramine R* in 25.0 ml of *water R*.

Primary opalescent suspension (formazin suspension). To the solution of hexamethylenetetramine in the flask add 25.0 ml of hydrazine sulphate solution. Mix and allow to stand for 24 h. This suspension is stable for 2 months, provided it is stored in a glass container free from surface defects. The suspension must not adhere to the glass and must be well mixed before use.

Standard of opalescence. Dilute 15.0 ml of the primary opalescent suspension to 1000.0 ml with *water R*. This suspension is freshly prepared and may be stored for at most 24 h.

Reference suspensions. Prepare the reference suspensions according to Table 2.2.1.-1. Mix and shake before use.

Table 2.2.1.-1

	I	II	III	IV
Standard of opalescence	5.0 ml	10.0 ml	30.0 ml	50.0 ml
Water R	95.0 ml	90.0 ml	70.0 ml	50.0 ml

Turbidity standard. The formazin suspension prepared by mixing equal volumes of the hydrazine sulphate solution and the hexamethylenetetramine solution is defined as a 4000 NTU (nephelometric turbidity units) primary reference standard. Reference suspensions I, II, III and IV have values of 3 NTU, 6 NTU, 18 NTU and 30 NTU respectively. Stabilised formazin suspensions that can be used to prepare stable, diluted turbidity standards are available commercially and may be used after comparison with the standards prepared as described.

Formazin has several desirable characteristics that make it an excellent turbidity standard. It can be reproducibly prepared from assayed raw materials. The physical characteristics make it a desirable light-scatter calibration standard. The formazin polymer consists of chains of different lengths, which fold into random configurations. This results in a wide assay of particle shapes and sizes, which analytically fits the possibility of different particle sizes and shapes that are found in the real samples. Due to formazin's reproducibility, scattering characteristics and traceability, instrument calibration algorithms and performance criteria are mostly based on this standard.

INSTRUMENTAL METHODS

INTRODUCTION

The degree of opalescence may also be determined by instrumental measurement of the light absorbed or scattered on account of submicroscopic optical density inhomogeneities of opalescent solutions and suspensions. 2 such techniques are nephelometry and turbidimetry. For turbidity measurement of coloured samples, ratio turbidimetry and nephelometry with ratio selection are used.

The light scattering effect of suspended particles can be measured by observation of either the transmitted light (turbidimetry) or the scattered light (nephelometry). Ratio turbidimetry combines the principles of both nephelometry and turbidimetry. Turbidimetry and nephelometry are useful for the measurement of slightly opalescent suspensions. Reference suspensions produced under well-defined conditions must be used. For quantitative measurements the construction of calibration curves is essential, since the relationship between the optical properties of the suspension and the concentration of the dispersed phase is at best semi-empirical.

The determination of opalescence of coloured liquids is done with ratio turbidimeters or nephelometers with ratio selection since colour provides a negative interference, attenuating both incident and scattered light and lowering the turbidity value. The effect is so great for even moderately coloured samples that conventional nephelometers cannot be used.

The instrumental assessment of clarity and opalescence provides a more discriminatory test that does not depend on the visual acuity of the analyst. Numerical results are more useful for quality monitoring and process control, especially in stability studies. For example, previous numerical data on stability can be projected to determine whether a given batch of dosage formulation or active pharmaceutical ingredient will exceed shelf-life limits prior to the expiry date.

NEPHELOMETRY

When a suspension is viewed at right angles to the direction of the incident light, the system appears opalescent due to the reflection of light from the particles of the suspension (Tyndall effect). A certain portion of the light beam entering a turbid liquid is transmitted, another portion is absorbed and the remaining portion is scattered by the suspended particles. If measurement is made at 90° to the light beam, the light scattered by the suspended particles can be used for the determination of their concentration, provided the number and size of particles influencing the scattering remain constant. The reference suspension must maintain a constant degree of turbidity and the sample and reference suspensions must be prepared under identical conditions. The Tyndall effect depends both upon the number of particles and their size. Nephelometric measurements are more reliable in low turbidity ranges, where there is a linear relationship between nephelometric turbidity unit (NTU) values and relative detector signals. As the degree of turbidity increases, not all the particles are exposed to the incident light and the scattered radiation of other particles is hindered on its way to the detector. The maximum nephelometric values at which reliable measurements can be made lie between 1750-2000 NTU. Linearity must be demonstrated by constructing a calibration curve using at least 4 concentrations.

TURBIDIMETRY

The optical property expressed as turbidity is the interaction between light and suspended particles in liquid. This is an expression of the optical property that causes light to be scattered and absorbed rather than transmitted in a straight line through the sample. The quantity of a solid material in suspension can be determined by the measurement of the transmitted light. A linear relationship between turbidity and concentration is obtained when the particle sizes are uniform and homogeneous in the suspension. This is true only in very dilute suspensions containing small particles. Linearity between turbidity and concentration must be established by constructing a calibration curve using at least 4 concentrations.

RATIO TURBIDIMETRY

In ratio turbidimetry the relationship of the transmission measurement to the 90° scattered light measurement is determined. This procedure compensates for the light that is diminished by the colour of the sample. The influence of colour of the sample may also be eliminated by using an infrared light-emitting diode (IR LED) at 860 nm as light source of the instrument. The instrument's photodiode detectors receive and measure scattered light at a 90° angle from the sample as well as measuring the forward scatter (light reflected) in front of the sample along with the measurement of light transmitted directly through the sample. The measuring results are given in NTU(ratio) and are obtained by calculating the ratio of the 90° angle scattered light measured to the sum of the components of forward scattered and transmitted light values. In ratio turbidimetry the influence of stray light becomes negligible. Nephelometers are used for measurements of the degree of opalescence of colourless liquids.

Measurements of reference suspensions I-IV with a ratio turbidimeter show a linear relationship between the concentrations and measured NTU values. Reference suspensions I-IV (Ph. Eur.) may be used as calibrators for the instrument.

Table 2.2.1.-2

Formazin suspensions	Opalescent values (NTU)
Reference suspension I	3
Reference suspensions II	6
Reference suspension III	18
Reference suspension IV	30
Standard of opalescence	60
Primary opalescent suspension	4000

INSTRUMENTAL DETERMINATION OF OPALESCENCE

Requirements in monographs are expressed in terms of the visual examination method with the defined reference suspensions. Instrumental methods may also be used for determining compliance with monograph requirements once the suitability of the instrument as described below has been established and calibration with reference suspensions I-IV and with *water R* or the solvent used has been performed.

Apparatus. Ratio turbidimeters or nephelometers with selectable ratio application use as light source a tungsten lamp with spectral sensitivity at about 550 nm operating at a filament colour temperature of 2700 K or IR LED having an emission maximum at 860 nm with a 60 nm spectral bandwidth. Other suitable light sources may also be used. Silicon photodiodes and photomultipliers are commonly used as detectors and record changes in light scattered or transmitted by the sample. The light scattered at 90 ± 2.5° is detected by the primary detector. Other detectors are those to detect back and forward scatter as well as transmitted light. The instruments used are calibrated against standards of known turbidity and are capable of automatic determination of turbidity. The test results expressed in NTU units are obtained directly from the instrument and compared to the specifications in the individual monographs.

Instruments complying with the following specifications are suitable.

- *Measuring units*: NTU. NTU is based on the turbidity of a primary reference standard of formazin. FTU (Formazin Turbidity Units) or FNU (Formazin Nephelometry Units) are also used which are equivalent to NTU in low regions (up to 40 NTU). These units are used in all 3 instrumental methods, nephelometry, turbidimetry and ratio turbidimetry.
- *Measuring range*: 0.01-1100 NTU.
- *Resolution*: 0.01 NTU within the range of 0-10 NTU, 0.1 NTU within the range of 10-100 NTU and 1 NTU for the range > 100 NTU. The instrument is calibrated and controlled with reference standards of formazin.
- *Accuracy*: 0-10 NTU: ± 0.01 NTU. 10-1000 NTU: ± 5 per cent.
- *Repeatability*: 0-10 NTU: ± 0.01 NTU. 10-1000 NTU: ± 2 per cent of the measured value.
- *Calibration*: with 4 reference suspensions of formazin in the range of interest. Reference suspensions described in this chapter or suitable reference standards calibrated against the primary reference suspensions may be used.
- *Stray light*: this is a significant source of error in low level turbidimetric measurement; stray light reaches the detector of an optical system, but does not come from the sample < 0.15 NTU for the range 0-10 NTU, < 0.5 NTU for the range 10-1000 NTU.

Instruments complying with the above characteristics and verified using the reference suspensions described under Visual method may be used instead of visual examination for determination of compliance with monograph requirements.

Instruments with range or resolution, accuracy and repeatability capabilities other than those mentioned above may be used provided they are sufficiently validated and are capable for the intended use. The test methodology for the specific substance/product to be analysed must also be validated to demonstrate its analytical capability. The instrument and methodology should be consistent with the attributes of the product to be tested.

01/2005:20202

2.2.2. DEGREE OF COLORATION OF LIQUIDS

The examination of the degree of coloration of liquids in the range brown-yellow-red is carried out by one of the 2 methods below, as prescribed in the monograph.

A solution is *colourless* if it has the appearance of *water R* or the solvent or is not more intensely coloured than reference solution B_9.

METHOD I

Using identical tubes of colourless, transparent, neutral glass of 12 mm external diameter, compare 2.0 ml of the liquid to be examined with 2.0 ml of *water R* or of the solvent or of the reference solution (see Tables of reference solutions) prescribed in the monograph. Compare the colours in diffused daylight, viewing horizontally against a white background.

METHOD II

Using identical tubes of colourless, transparent, neutral glass with a flat base and an internal diameter of 15 mm to 25 mm, compare the liquid to be examined with *water R* or the solvent or the reference solution (see Tables of reference solutions) prescribed in the monograph, the depth of the layer being 40 mm. Compare the colours in diffused daylight, viewing vertically against a white background.

REAGENTS

Primary solutions

Yellow solution. Dissolve 46 g of *ferric chloride R* in about 900 ml of a mixture of 25 ml of *hydrochloric acid R* and 975 ml of *water R* and dilute to 1000.0 ml with the same mixture. Titrate and adjust the solution to contain 45.0 mg of $FeCl_3,6H_2O$ per millilitre by adding the same acidic mixture. Protect the solution from light.

Titration. Place in a 250 ml conical flask fitted with a ground-glass stopper, 10.0 ml of the solution, 15 ml of *water R,* 5 ml of *hydrochloric acid R* and 4 g of *potassium iodide R,* close the flask, allow to stand in the dark for 15 min and add 100 ml of *water R.* Titrate the liberated iodine with *0.1 M sodium thiosulphate,* using 0.5 ml of *starch solution R,* added towards the end of the titration, as indicator.

1 ml of *0.1 M sodium thiosulphate* is equivalent to 27.03 mg of $FeCl_3,6H_2O$.

Red solution. Dissolve 60 g of *cobalt chloride R* in about 900 ml of a mixture of 25 ml of *hydrochloric acid R* and 975 ml of *water R* and dilute to 1000.0 ml with the same mixture. Titrate and adjust the solution to contain 59.5 mg of $CoCl_2,6H_2O$ per millilitre by adding the same acidic mixture.

Titration. Place in a 250 ml conical flask fitted with a ground-glass stopper, 5.0 ml of the solution, 5 ml of *dilute hydrogen peroxide solution R* and 10 ml of a 300 g/l solution of *sodium hydroxide R.* Boil gently for 10 min, allow to cool and add 60 ml of *dilute sulphuric acid R* and 2 g of *potassium iodide R.* Close the flask and dissolve the precipitate by shaking gently. Titrate the liberated iodine with *0.1 M sodium thiosulphate,* using 0.5 ml of *starch solution R,* added towards the end of the titration, as indicator. The end-point is reached when the solution turns pink.

1 ml of *0.1 M sodium thiosulphate* is equivalent to 23.79 mg of $CoCl_2,6H_2O$.

Blue primary solution. Dissolve 63 g of *copper sulphate R* in about 900 ml of a mixture of 25 ml of *hydrochloric acid R* and 975 ml of *water R* and dilute to 1000.0 ml with the same mixture. Titrate and adjust the solution to contain 62.4 mg of $CuSO_4,5H_2O$ per millilitre by adding the same acidic mixture.

Titration. Place in a 250 ml conical flask fitted with a ground-glass stopper, 10.0 ml of the solution, 50 ml of *water R,* 12 ml of *dilute acetic acid R* and 3 g of *potassium iodide R.* Titrate the liberated iodine with *0.1 M sodium thiosulphate,* using 0.5 ml of *starch solution R,* added towards the end of the titration, as indicator. The end-point is reached when the solution shows a slight pale brown colour.

1 ml of *0.1 M sodium thiosulphate* is equivalent to 24.97 mg of $CuSO_4,5H_2O$.

Standard solutions

Using the 3 primary solutions, prepare the 5 standard solutions as follows:

Table 2.2.2.-1

Standard solution	Volume in millilitres			
	Yellow solution	Red solution	Blue solution	Hydrochloric acid (10 g/l HCl)
B (brown)	3.0	3.0	2.4	1.6
BY (brownish-yellow)	2.4	1.0	0.4	6.2
Y (yellow)	2.4	0.6	0.0	7.0
GY (greenish-yellow)	9.6	0.2	0.2	0.0
R (red)	1.0	2.0	0.0	7.0

Reference solutions for Methods I and II

Using the 5 standard solutions, prepare the following reference solutions.

Table 2.2.2.-2. - *Reference solutions B*

Reference solution	Volumes in millilitres	
	Standard solution B	Hydrochloric acid (10 g/l HCl)
B_1	75.0	25.0
B_2	50.0	50.0
B_3	37.5	62.5
B_4	25.0	75.0
B_5	12.5	87.5
B_6	5.0	95.0
B_7	2.5	97.5
B_8	1.5	98.5
B_9	1.0	99.0

Table 2.2.2.-3. - *Reference solutions BY*

Reference solution	Volumes in millilitres	
	Standard solution BY	Hydrochloric acid (10 g/l HCl)
BY_1	100.0	0.0
BY_2	75.0	25.0
BY_3	50.0	50.0
BY_4	25.0	75.0
BY_5	12.5	87.5
BY_6	5.0	95.0
BY_7	2.5	97.5

Table 2.2.2.-4. - *Reference solutions Y*

Reference solution	Volumes in millilitres	
	Standard solution Y	Hydrochloric acid (10 g/l HCl)
Y_1	100.0	0.0
Y_2	75.0	25.0
Y_3	50.0	50.0
Y_4	25.0	75.0
Y_5	12.5	87.5
Y_6	5.0	95.0
Y_7	2.5	97.5

Table 2.2.2.-5. - *Reference solutions GY*

Reference solution	Volumes in millilitres	
	Standard solution GY	Hydrochloric acid (10 g/l HCl)
GY_1	25.0	75.0
GY_2	15.0	85.0
GY_3	8.5	91.5
GY_4	5.0	95.0
GY_5	3.0	97.0
GY_6	1.5	98.5
GY_7	0.75	99.25

Table 2.2.2.-6. - *Reference solutions R*

Reference solution	Volumes in millilitres	
	Standard solution R	Hydrochloric acid (10 g/l HCl)
R_1	100.0	0.0
R_2	75.0	25.0
R_3	50.0	50.0
R_4	37.5	62.5
R_5	25.0	75.0
R_6	12.5	87.5
R_7	5.0	95.0

Storage

For Method I, the reference solutions may be stored in sealed tubes of colourless, transparent, neutral glass of 12 mm external diameter, protected from light.

For Method II, prepare the reference solutions immediately before use from the standard solutions.

01/2005:20203

2.2.3. POTENTIOMETRIC DETERMINATION OF pH

The pH is a number which represents conventionally the hydrogen ion concentration of an aqueous solution. For practical purposes, its definition is an experimental one. The pH of a solution to be examined is related to that of a reference solution (pH_s) by the following equation:

$$pH = pH_s - \frac{E - E_s}{k}$$

in which E is the potential, expressed in volts, of the cell containing the solution to be examined and E_s is the potential, expressed in volts, of the cell containing the solution of known pH (pH_s), k is the change in potential per unit change in pH expressed in volts, and calculated from the Nernst equation.

Table 2.2.3.-1. – *Values of k at different temperatures*

Temperature (°C)	*k* (V)
15	0.0572
20	0.0582
25	0.0592
30	0.0601
35	0.0611

The potentiometric determination of pH is made by measuring the potential difference between 2 appropriate electrodes immersed in the solution to be examined: 1 of these electrodes is sensitive to hydrogen ions (usually a glass electrode) and the other is the reference electrode (for example, a saturated calomel electrode).

Apparatus. The measuring apparatus is a voltmeter with an input resistance at least 100 times that of the electrodes used. It is normally graduated in pH units and has a sensitivity such that discrimination of at least 0.05 pH unit or at least 0.003 V may be achieved.

Method. Unless otherwise prescribed in the monograph, all measurements are made at the same temperature (20-25 °C). Table 2.2.3.-2 shows the variation of pH with respect to temperature of a number of reference buffer solutions used for calibration. For the temperature correction, when necessary, follow the manufacturer's instructions. The apparatus is calibrated with the buffer solution of potassium hydrogen phthalate (primary standard) and 1 other buffer solution of different pH (preferably one shown in Table 2.2.3.-2). The pH of a third buffer solution of intermediate pH read off on the scale must not differ by more than 0.05 pH unit from the value corresponding to this solution. Immerse the electrodes in the solution to be examined and take the reading in the same conditions as for the buffer solutions.

When the apparatus is in frequent use, checks must be carried out regularly. If not, such checks should be carried out before each measurement.

All solutions to be examined and the reference buffer solutions must be prepared using *carbon dioxide-free water R*.

PREPARATION OF REFERENCE BUFFER SOLUTIONS

Potassium tetraoxalate 0.05 M. Dissolve 12.61 g of $C_4H_3KO_8,2H_2O$ in *carbon dioxide-free water R* and dilute to 1000.0 ml with the same solvent.

Potassium hydrogen tartrate, saturated at 25 °C. Shake an excess of $C_4H_5KO_6$ vigorously with *carbon dioxide-free water R* at 25 °C. Filter or decant. Prepare immediately before use.

Potassium dihydrogen citrate 0.05 M. Dissolve 11.41 g of $C_6H_7KO_7$ in *carbon dioxide-free water R* and dilute to 1000.0 ml with the same solvent. Prepare immediately before use.

Potassium hydrogen phthalate 0.05 M. Dissolve 10.13 g of $C_8H_5KO_4$, previously dried for 1 h at 110 ± 2 °C, in *carbon dioxide-free water R* and dilute to 1000.0 ml with the same solvent.

Table 2.2.3.-2. – *pH of reference buffer solutions at various temperatures*

Temperature (°C)	Potassium tetraoxalate 0.05 M	Potassium hydrogen tartrate saturated at 25 °C	Potassium dihydrogen citrate 0.05 M	Potassium hydrogen phthalate 0.05 M	Potassium dihydrogen phosphate 0.025 M + disodium hydrogen phosphate 0.025 M	Potassium dihydrogen phosphate 0.0087 M + disodium hydrogen phosphate 0.0303 M	Disodium tetraborate 0.01 M	Sodium carbonate 0.025 M + sodium bicarbonate 0.025 M	Calcium hydroxide, saturated at 25°C
	$C_4H_3KO_8,2H_2O$	$C_4H_5KO_6$	$C_6H_7KO_7$	$C_8H_5KO_4$	KH_2PO_4+ Na_2HPO_4	KH_2PO_4+ Na_2HPO_4	$Na_2B_4O_7$, $10H_2O$	Na_2CO_3+ $NaHCO_3$	$Ca(OH)_2$
15	1.67		3.80	4.00	6.90	7.45	9.28	10.12	12.81
20	1.68		3.79	4.00	6.88	7.43	9.23	10.06	12.63
25	1.68	3.56	3.78	4.01	6.87	7.41	9.18	10.01	12.45
30	1.68	3.55	3.77	4.02	6.85	7.40	9.14	9.97	12.29
35	1.69	3.55	3.76	4.02	6.84	7.39	9.10	9.93	12.13
$\frac{\Delta pH^{(1)}}{\Delta t}$	+ 0.001	−0.0014	−0.0022	+ 0.0012	−0.0028	−0.0028	−0.0082	−0.0096	−0.034

(1) pH variation per degree Celsius.

Potassium dihydrogen phosphate 0.025 M + disodium hydrogen phosphate 0.025 M. Dissolve 3.39 g of KH_2PO_4 and 3.53 g of Na_2HPO_4, both previously dried for 2 h at 120 ± 2 °C, in *carbon dioxide-free water R* and dilute to 1000.0 ml with the same solvent.

Potassium dihydrogen phosphate 0.0087 M + disodium hydrogen phosphate 0.0303 M. Dissolve 1.18 g of KH_2PO_4 and 4.30 g of Na_2HPO_4, both previously dried for 2 h at 120 ± 2 °C, in *carbon dioxide-free water R* and dilute to 1000.0 ml with the same solvent.

Disodium tetraborate 0.01 M. Dissolve 3.80 g of $Na_2B_4O_7,10H_2O$ in *carbon dioxide-free water R* and dilute to 1000.0 ml with the same solvent. Store protected from atmospheric carbon dioxide.

Sodium carbonate 0.025 M + sodium hydrogen carbonate 0.025 M. Dissolve 2.64 g of Na_2CO_3 and 2.09 g of $NaHCO_3$ in *carbon dioxide-free water R* and dilute to 1000.0 ml with the same solvent. Store protected from atmospheric carbon dioxide.

Calcium hydroxide, saturated at 25 °C. Shake an excess of *calcium hydroxide R* with *carbon dioxide-free water R* and decant at 25 °C. Store protected from atmospheric carbon dioxide.

STORAGE

Store buffer solutions in suitable chemically resistant, tight containers, such as type I glass bottles or plastic containers suitable for aqueous solutions.

01/2005:20204

2.2.4. RELATIONSHIP BETWEEN REACTION OF SOLUTION, APPROXIMATE pH AND COLOUR OF CERTAIN INDICATORS

To 10 ml of the solution to be examined, add 0.1 ml of the indicator solution, unless otherwise prescribed in Table 2.2.4.-1.

Table 2.2.4.-1

Reaction	pH	Indicator	Colour
Alkaline	> 8	*Litmus paper red R*	Blue
		Thymol blue solution R (0.05 ml)	Grey or violet-blue
Slightly alkaline	8.0 – 10.0	*Phenolphthalein solution R* (0.05 ml)	Colourless or pink
		Thymol blue solution R (0.05 ml)	Grey
Strongly alkaline	> 10	*Phenolphthalein paper R*	Red
		Thymol blue solution R (0.05 ml)	Violet-blue
Neutral	6.0 – 8.0	*Methyl red solution R*	Yellow
		Phenol red solution R (0.05 ml)	
Neutral to methyl red	4.5 – 6.0	*Methyl red solution R*	Orange-red
Neutral to phenolphtalein	< 8.0	*Phenolphthalein solution R* (0.05 ml)	Colourless; pink or red after adding 0.05 ml of 0.1 M base
Acid	< 6	*Methyl red solution R*	Orange or red
		Bromothymol blue solution R1	Yellow
Faintly acid	4.0 – 6.0	*Methyl red solution R*	Orange
		Bromocresol green solution R	Green or blue
Strongly acid	< 4	*Congo red paper R*	Green or blue

01/2005:20205

2.2.5. RELATIVE DENSITY

The relative density $d_{t_2}^{t_1}$ of a substance is the ratio of the mass of a certain volume of a substance at temperature t_1 to the mass of an equal volume of water at temperature t_2.

Unless otherwise indicated, the relative density d_{20}^{20} is used. Relative density is also commonly expressed as d_4^{20}. Density ρ_{20}, defined as the mass of a unit volume of the substance at 20 °C may also be used, expressed in kilograms per cubic metre or grams per cubic centimetre

(1 kg·m^{-3} = 10^{-3} g·cm^{-3}). These quantities are related by the following equations where density is expressed in grams per cubic centimetre:

$$\rho_{20} = 0.998203 \times d_{20}^{20} \text{ or } d_{20}^{20} = 1.00180 \times \rho_{20}$$

$$\rho_{20} = 0.999972 \times d_{4}^{20} \text{ or } d_{4}^{20} = 1.00003 \times \rho_{20}$$

$$d_{4}^{20} = 0.998230 \times d_{20}^{20}$$

Relative density or density are measured with the precision to the number of decimals prescribed in the monograph using a density bottle (solids or liquids), a hydrostatic balance (solids), a hydrometer (liquids) or a digital density meter with an oscillating transducer (liquids and gases). When the determination is made by weighing, the buoyancy of air is disregarded, which may introduce an error of 1 unit in the 3rd decimal place. When using a density meter, the buoyancy of air has no influence.

Oscillating transducer density meter. The apparatus consists of:

– a U-shaped tube, usually of borosilicate glass, which contains the liquid to be examined;
– a magneto-electrical or piezo-electrical excitation system that causes the tube to oscillate as a cantilever oscillator at a characteristic frequency depending on the density of the liquid to be examined;
– a means of measuring the oscillation period (*T*), which may be converted by the apparatus to give a direct reading of density, or used to calculate density using the constants *A* and *B* described below.

The resonant frequency (*f*) is a function of the spring constant (*c*) and the mass (*m*) of the system:

$$f^2 = \frac{1}{T^2} = \frac{c}{m} \times \frac{1}{4\pi^2}$$

Hence:

$$T^2 = \left(\frac{M}{c} + \frac{\rho \times V}{c}\right) \times 4\pi^2$$

M = mass of the tube,

V = inner volume of the tube.

Introduction of 2 constants $A = c/\left(4\pi^2 \times V\right)$ and $B = M/V$, leads to the classical equation for the oscillating transducer:

$$\rho = A \times T^2 - B$$

The constants *A* and *B* are determined by operating the instrument with the U-tube filled with 2 different samples of known density, for example, degassed *water R* and air. Control measurements are made daily using degassed *water R*. The results displayed for the control measurement using degassed *water R* shall not deviate from the reference value (ρ_{20} = 0.998203 g·cm^{-3}, d_{20}^{20} = 1.000000) by more than its specified error. For example, an instrument specified to ± 0.0001 g·cm^{-3} shall display 0.9982 ± 0.0001 g·cm^{-3} in order to be suitable for further measurement. Otherwise a re-adjustment is necessary. Calibration with certified reference materials is carried out regularly. Measurements are made using the same procedure as for calibration. The liquid to be examined is equilibrated in a thermostat at 20 °C before introduction into the tube, if necessary, to avoid the formation of bubbles and to reduce the time required for measurement.

Factors affecting accuracy include:

– temperature uniformity throughout the tube,
– non-linearity over a range of density,
– parasitic resonant effects,
– viscosity, whereby solutions with a higher viscosity than the calibrant have a density that is apparently higher than the true value.

The effects of non-linearity and viscosity may be avoided by using calibrants that have density and viscosity close to those of the liquid to be examined (± 5 per cent for density, ± 50 per cent for viscosity). The density meter may have functions for automatic viscosity correction and for correction of errors arising from temperature changes and non-linearity.

Precision is a function of the repeatability and stability of the oscillator frequency, which is dependent on the stability of the volume, mass and spring constant of the cell.

Density meters are able to achieve measurements with an error of the order of 1 × 10^{-3} g·cm^{-3} to 1 × 10^{-5} g·cm^{-3} and a repeatability of 1 × 10^{-4} g·cm^{-3} to 1 × 10^{-6} g·cm^{-3}.

01/2005:20206

2.2.6. REFRACTIVE INDEX

The refractive index of a medium with reference to air is equal to the ratio of the sine of the angle of incidence of a beam of light in air to the sine of the angle of refraction of the refracted beam in the given medium.

Unless otherwise prescribed, the refractive index is measured at 20 ± 0.5 °C, with reference to the wavelength of the D-line of sodium (λ = 589.3 nm); the symbol is then n_{D}^{20}.

Refractometers normally determine the critical angle. In such apparatus the essential part is a prism of known refractive index in contact with the liquid to be examined. Calibrate the apparatus using certified reference materials. When white light is used, the refractometer is provided with a compensating system. The apparatus gives readings accurate to at least the third decimal place and is provided with a means of operation at the temperature prescribed. The thermometer is graduated at intervals of 0.5 °C or less.

01/2005:20207

2.2.7. OPTICAL ROTATION

Optical rotation is the property displayed by chiral substances of rotating the plane of polarisation of polarised light.

Optical rotation is considered to be positive (+) for dextrorotatory substances (i.e. those that rotate the plane of polarisation in a clockwise direction) and negative (−) for laevorotatory substances.

The specific optical rotation $[\alpha_m]_{\lambda}^{t}$ is the rotation, expressed in radians (rad), measured at the temperature *t* and at the wavelength λ given by a 1 m thickness of liquid or a solution containing 1 kg/m^3 of optically active substance. For practical reasons the specific optical rotation $[\alpha_m]_{\lambda}^{t}$ is normally expressed in milliradians metre squared per kilogram (mrad·m^2·kg^{-1}).

The Pharmacopoeia adopts the following conventional definitions.

The *angle of optical rotation* of a neat liquid is the angle of rotation α, expressed in degrees (°), of the plane of polarisation at the wavelength of the D-line of sodium (λ = 589.3 nm) measured at 20 °C using a layer of 1 dm; for a solution, the method of preparation is prescribed in the monograph.

The *specific optical rotation* $[\alpha]_D^{20}$ of a liquid is the angle of rotation α, expressed in degrees (°), of the plane of polarisation at the wavelength of the D-line of sodium (λ = 589.3 nm) measured at 20 °C in the liquid substance to be examined, calculated with reference to a layer of 1 dm and divided by the density expressed in grams per cubic centimetre.

The *specific optical rotation* $[\alpha]_D^{20}$ of a substance in solution is the angle of rotation α, expressed in degrees (°), of the plane of polarisation at the wavelength of the D-line of sodium (λ = 589.3 nm) measured at 20 °C in a solution of the substance to be examined and calculated with reference to a layer of 1 dm containing 1 g/ml of the substance. The specific optical rotation of a substance in solution is always expressed with reference to a given solvent and concentration.

In the conventional system adopted by the Pharmacopoeia the specific optical rotation is expressed by its value without units; the actual units, degree millilitres per decimetre gram [(°)·ml·dm^{-1}·g^{-1}] are understood.

The conversion factor from the International System to the Pharmacopoeia system is the following:

$$[\alpha_m]_\lambda^t = [\alpha]_\lambda^t \times 0.1745$$

In certain cases specified in the monograph the angle of rotation may be measured at temperatures other than 20 °C and at other wavelengths.

The polarimeter must be capable of giving readings to the nearest 0.01°. The scale is usually checked by means of certified quartz plates. The linearity of the scale may be checked by means of sucrose solutions.

Method. Determine the zero of the polarimeter and the angle of rotation of polarised light at the wavelength of the D-line of sodium (λ = 589.3 nm) at 20 ± 0.5 °C. Measurements may be carried out at other temperatures only where the monograph indicates the temperature correction to be made to the measured optical rotation. Determine the zero of the apparatus with the tube closed; for liquids the zero is determined with the tube empty and for solids filled with the prescribed solvent.

Calculate the specific optical rotation using the following formulae.

For neat liquids:

$$[\alpha]_D^{20} = \frac{\alpha}{l \cdot \rho_{20}}$$

For substances in solution:

$$[\alpha]_D^{20} = \frac{1000\alpha}{l \cdot c}$$

where *c* is the concentration of the solution in g/l.

Calculate the content *c* in g/l or the content *c′* in per cent *m/m* of a dissolved substance using the following formulae:

$$c = \frac{1000\alpha}{l \cdot [\alpha]_D^{20}} \qquad c' = \frac{1000\alpha}{l \cdot [\alpha]_D^{20} \cdot \rho_{20}}$$

α = angle of rotation in degrees read at 20 ± 0.5°C,

l = length in decimetres of the polarimeter tube,

ρ_{20} = density at 20 °C in grams per cubic centimetre. For the purposes of the Pharmacopoeia, density is replaced by relative density (*2.2.5*),

c = concentration of the substance in g/l,

c′ = content of the substance in per cent *m/m*.

01/2005:20208

2.2.8. VISCOSITY

The *dynamic* viscosity or *viscosity coefficient* η is the tangential force per unit surface, known as *shearing stress* τ and expressed in pascals, necessary to move, parallel to the sliding plane, a layer of liquid of 1 square metre at a rate (v) of 1 metre per second relative to a parallel layer at a distance (x) of 1 metre.

The ratio dv/dx is a speed gradient giving the *rate of shear D* expressed in reciprocal seconds (s^{-1}), so that $\eta = \tau/D$.

The unit of dynamic viscosity is the pascal second (Pa·s). The most commonly used submultiple is the millipascal second (mPa·s).

The *kinematic viscosity* v, expressed in square metres per second, is obtained by dividing the dynamic viscosity η by the density ρ expressed in kilograms per cubic metre, of the liquid measured at the same temperature, i.e. $v = \eta/\rho$. The kinematic viscosity is usually expressed in square millimetres per second.

A capillary viscometer may be used for determining the viscosity of Newtonian liquids and a rotating viscometer for determining the viscosity of Newtonian and non-Newtonian liquids. Other viscometers may be used provided that the accuracy and precision is not less than that obtained with the viscometers described below.

01/2005:20209

2.2.9. CAPILLARY VISCOMETER METHOD

The determination of viscosity using a suitable capillary viscometer is carried out at a temperature of 20 ± 0.1 °C, unless otherwise prescribed. The time required for the level of the liquid to drop from one mark to the other is measured with a stop-watch to the nearest one-fifth of a second. The result is valid only if two consecutive readings do not differ by more than 1 per cent. The average of not fewer than three readings gives the flow time of the liquid to be examined.

Calculate the dynamic viscosity η (*2.2.8*) in millipascal seconds using the formula:

$$\eta = k\rho t$$

k = constant of the viscometer, expressed in square millimetres per second squared,

ρ = density of the liquid to be examined expressed in milligrams per cubic millimetre, obtained by multiplying its relative density (d_{20}^{20}) by 0.9982,

t = flow time, in seconds, of the liquid to be examined.

The constant *k* is determined using a suitable viscometer calibration liquid.

To calculate the kinematic viscosity (mm^2·s^{-1}), use the following formula: $v = kt$.

2. Methods of analysis

The determination may be carried out with an apparatus (Figure 2.2.9.-1) having the specifications described in Table 2.2.9.-1(1):

Table 2.2.9.-1

Size number	Nominal constant of viscometer	Kinematic viscosity range	Internal diameter of tube *R*	Volume of bulb *C*	Internal diameter of tube *N*
	$mm^2 \cdot s^{-2}$	$mm^2 \cdot s^{-1}$	mm (± 2 %)	ml (± 5 %)	mm
1	0.01	3.5 to 10	0.64	5.6	2.8 to 3.2
1A	0.03	6 to 30	0.84	5.6	2.8 to 3.2
2	0.1	20 to 100	1.15	5.6	2.8 to 3.2
2A	0.3	60 to 300	1.51	5.6	2.8 to 3.2
3	1.0	200 to 1000	2.06	5.6	3.7 to 4.3
3A	3.0	600 to 3000	2.74	5.6	4.6 to 5.4
4	10	2000 to 10 000	3.70	5.6	4.6 to 5.4
4A	30	6000 to 30 000	4.07	5.6	5.6 to 6.4
5	100	20 000 to 100 000	6.76	5.6	6.8 to 7.5

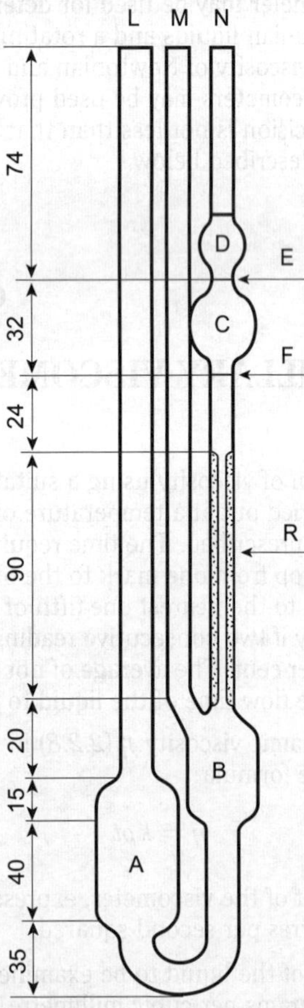

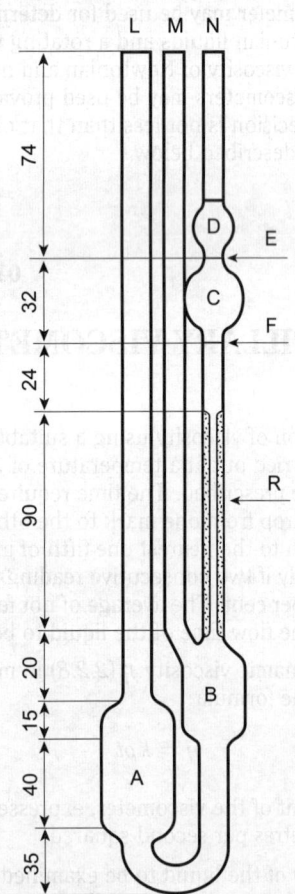

Figure 2.2.9.- 1. – *Suspended level viscometer*

Dimensions in millimetres

The minimum flow time should be 350 s for size no. 1 and 200 s for all other sizes.

Method. Fill the viscometer through tube (*L*) with a sufficient quantity of the liquid to be examined, previously brought to 20 °C unless otherwise prescribed, to fill bulb (*A*) but ensuring that the level of liquid in bulb (*B*) is below the exit to ventilation tube (*M*). Immerse the viscometer in the bath of water at 20 ± 0.1 °C, unless otherwise prescribed, maintain it in the upright position and allow to stand for not less than 30 min to allow the temperature to reach equilibrium. Close tube (*M*) and raise the level of the liquid in tube (*N*) up to a level about 8 mm above mark (*E*). Keep the liquid at this level by closing tube (*N*) and opening tube (*M*). Open tube (*N*) and measure, with a stop-watch to the nearest one-fifth of a second, the time required for the level of the liquid to drop from mark (*E*) to (*F*).

01/2005:20210

2.2.10. ROTATING VISCOMETER METHOD

Commonly used types of rotating viscometers are based on the measurement of shearing forces in a liquid medium placed between two coaxial cylinders, one of which is driven by a motor and the other is made to revolve by the rotation of the first. Under these conditions, the viscosity (or apparent viscosity) becomes a measurement (*M*) of the angle of deflection of the cylinder made to revolve, which corresponds to a moment of force expressed in Newton metres.

For laminar flow, the dynamic viscosity η expressed in pascal seconds is given by the formula:

$$\eta = \frac{1}{\omega}\left(\frac{M}{4\pi \cdot h}\right) \cdot \left(\frac{1}{R_A^2} - \frac{1}{R_B^2}\right)$$

where h is the height of immersion in metres of the cylinder made to revolve in the liquid medium, R_A and R_B are the radii in metres of the cylinders, R_A being smaller than R_B, and ω is the angular velocity in radians per second. The constant k of the apparatus(2) may be determined at various speeds of rotation using a suitable viscometer calibration liquid. The viscosity then corresponds to the formula:

$$\eta = k\frac{M}{\omega}$$

Method. Measure the viscosity according to the instructions for the operation of the rotating viscometer. The temperature for measuring the viscosity is indicated in the monograph. For pseudoplastic and other non-Newtonian systems, the monograph indicates the type of viscometer to be used and the angular velocity or the shear rate at which the measurement is made. If it is impossible to obtain the indicated shear rate exactly, use a shear rate slightly higher and a shear rate slightly lower and interpolate.

01/2005:20211

2.2.11. DISTILLATION RANGE

The distillation range is the temperature interval, corrected for a pressure of 101.3 kPa (760 Torr), within which a liquid, or a specified fraction of a liquid, distils in the following conditions.

Apparatus. The apparatus (see Figure 2.2.11.-1) consists of a distillation flask (*A*), a straight tube condenser (*B*) which fits on to the side arm of the flask and a plain-bend adaptor (*C*) attached to the end of the condenser. The lower end of the condenser may, alternatively, be bent to replace the

(1) The European Pharmacopoeia describes the system proposed by the International Organisation for Standardisation (ISO).

(2) Commercially available apparatus is supplied with tables giving the constants of the apparatus in relation to the surface area of the cylinders used and their speed of rotation.

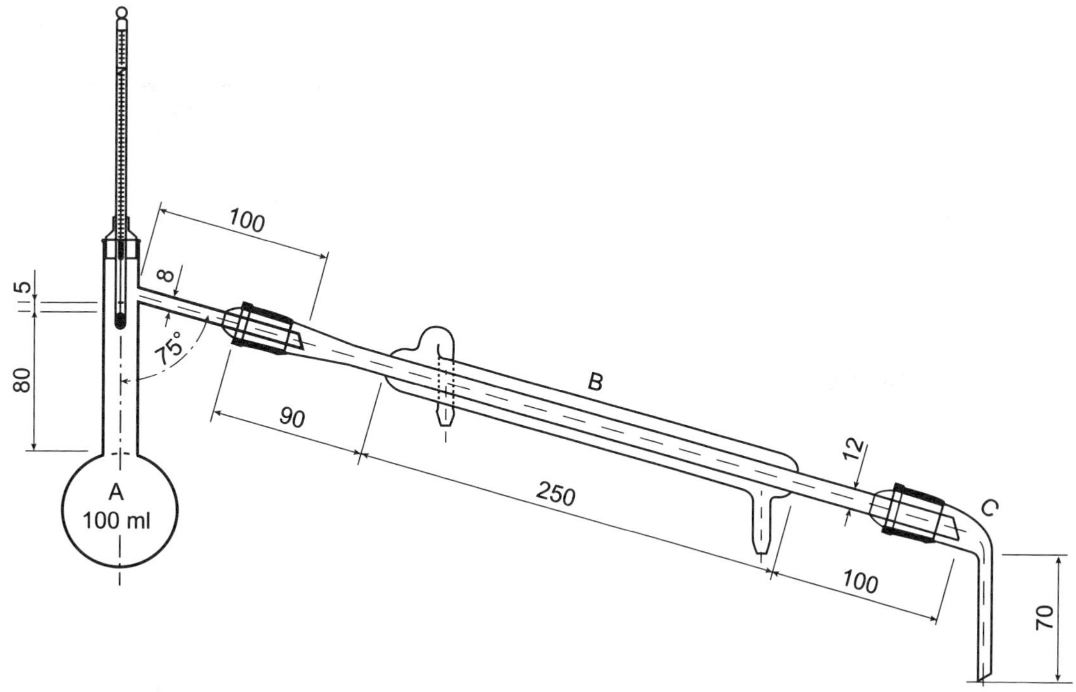

Figure 2.2.11.-1. – *Apparatus for the determination of distillation range*

Dimensions in millimetres

adaptor. A thermometer is inserted in the neck of the flask so that the upper end of the mercury reservoir is 5 mm lower than the junction of the lower wall of the lateral tube. The thermometer is graduated at 0.2 °C intervals and the scale covers a range of about 50 °C. During the determination, the flask, including its neck, is protected from draughts by a suitable screen.

Method. Place in the flask (*A*) 50.0 ml of the liquid to be examined and a few pieces of porous material. Collect the distillate in a 50 ml cylinder graduated in 1 ml. Cooling by circulating water is essential for liquids distilling below 150 °C. Heat the flask so that boiling is rapidly achieved and note the temperature at which the first drop of distillate falls into the cylinder. Adjust the heating to give a regular rate of distillation of 2-3 ml/min and note the temperature when the whole or the prescribed fraction of the liquid, measured at 20 °C, has distilled.

Table 2.2.11.-1. – *Temperature correction in relation to the pressure*

Distillation temperature	Correction factor *k*
up to 100 °C	0.30
above 100 °C up to 140 °C	0.34
above 140 °C up to 190 °C	0.38
above 190 °C up to 240 °C	0.41
above 240 °C	0.45

Correct the observed temperatures for barometric pressure by means of the formula:

$$t_1 = t_2 + k\,(101.3 - b)$$

t_1 = the corrected temperature,

t_2 = the observed temperature, at the barometric pressure b,

k = the correction factor taken from Table 2.2.11.-1 unless the factor is given,

b = the barometric pressure, expressed in kilopascals, during the distillation.

01/2005:20212

2.2.12. BOILING POINT

The boiling point is the corrected temperature at which the vapour pressure of a liquid is equal to 101.3 kPa.

Apparatus. The apparatus is that used for Distillation Range (*2.2.11*) with the exception that the thermometer is inserted in the neck of the flask so that the lower end of the mercury reservoir is level with the lower end of the neck of the distillation flask and that the flask is placed on a plate of isolating material pierced by a hole 35 mm in diameter.

Method. Place in the flask (*A*) 20 ml of the liquid to be examined and a few pieces of porous material. Heat the flask so that boiling is rapidly achieved and record the temperature at which liquid runs from the side-arm into the condenser.

Correct the observed temperature for barometric pressure by means of the formula:

$$t_1 = t_2 + k\,(101.3 - b)$$

t_1 = the corrected temperature,

t_2 = the observed temperature at barometric pressure b,

k = the correction factor as shown in Table 2.2.11.-1 under Distillation Range,

b = the barometric pressure, in kilopascals, at the time of the determination.

01/2005:20213

2.2.13. DETERMINATION OF WATER BY DISTILLATION

The apparatus (see Figure 2.2.13.-1) consists of a glass flask (*A*) connected by a tube (*D*) to a cylindrical tube (*B*) fitted with a graduated receiving tube (*E*) and reflux condenser (*C*). The receiving tube (*E*) is graduated in 0.1 ml. The source of heat is preferably an electric heater with rheostat control or an oil bath. The upper portion of the flask and the connecting tube may be insulated.

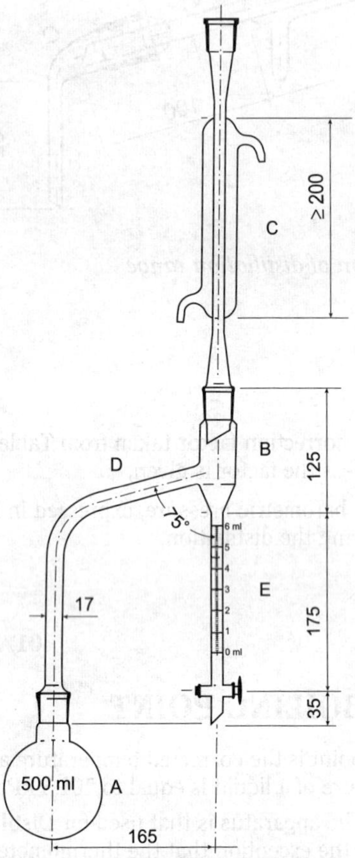

Figure 2.2.13.-1. – *Apparatus for the determination of water by distillation*

Dimensions in millimetres

Method. Clean the receiving tube and the condenser of the apparatus, thoroughly rinse with water, and dry.

Introduce 200 ml of *toluene R* and about 2 ml of *water R* into the dry flask. Distil for 2 h, then allow to cool for about 30 min and read the water volume to the nearest 0.05 ml. Place in the flask a quantity of the substance, weighed with an accuracy of 1 per cent, expected to give about 2 ml to 3 ml of water. If the substance has a pasty consistency, weigh it in a boat of metal foil. Add a few pieces of porous material and heat the flask gently for 15 min. When the toluene begins to boil, distil at the rate of about two drops per second until most of the water has distilled over, then increase the rate of distillation to about four drops per second. When the water has all distilled over, rinse the inside of the condenser tube with *toluene R*. Continue the distillation for 5 min, remove the heat, allow the receiving tube to cool to room temperature and dislodge any droplets of water which adhere to the walls of the receiving tube. When the water and toluene have completely separated, read the volume of water and calculate the content present in the substance as millilitre per kilogram, using the formula:

$$\frac{1000\,(n_2 - n_1)}{m}$$

m = the mass in grams of the substance to be examined,

n_1 = the number of millilitres of water obtained in the first distillation,

n_2 = the total number of millilitres of water obtained in the 2 distillations.

01/2005:20214

2.2.14. MELTING POINT - CAPILLARY METHOD

The melting point determined by the capillary method is the temperature at which the last solid particle of a compact column of a substance in a tube passes into the liquid phase.

When prescribed in the monograph, the same apparatus and method are used for the determination of other factors, such as meniscus formation or melting range, that characterise the melting behaviour of a substance.

Apparatus. The apparatus consists of:

– a suitable glass vessel containing a liquid bath (for example, water, liquid paraffin or silicone oil) and fitted with a suitable means of heating,

– a suitable means of stirring, ensuring uniformity of temperature within the bath,

– a suitable thermometer with graduation at not more than 0.5 °C intervals and provided with an immersion mark. The range of the thermometer is not more than 100 °C,

– alkali-free hard-glass capillary tubes of internal diameter 0.9 mm to 1.1 mm with a wall 0.10 mm to 0.15 mm thick and sealed at one end.

Method. Unless otherwise prescribed, dry the finely powdered substance *in vacuo* and over *anhydrous silica gel R* for 24 h. Introduce a sufficient quantity into a capillary tube to give a compact column 4 mm to 6 mm in height. Raise the temperature of the bath to about 10 °C below the presumed melting point and then adjust the rate of heating to about 1 °C/min. When the temperature is 5 °C below the presumed melting point, correctly introduce the capillary tube into the instrument. For the apparatus described above, immerse the capillary tube so that the closed end is near the centre of the bulb of the thermometer, the immersion mark of which is at the level of the surface of the liquid. Record the temperature at which the last particle passes into the liquid phase.

Calibration of the apparatus. The apparatus may be calibrated using melting point reference substances such as those of the World Health Organisation or other appropriate substances.

01/2005:20215

2.2.15. MELTING POINT - OPEN CAPILLARY METHOD

For certain substances, the following method is used to determine the melting point (also referred to as slip point and rising melting point when determined by this method).

Use glass capillary tubes open at both ends, about 80 mm long, having an external diameter of 1.4 mm to 1.5 mm and an internal diameter of 1.0 mm to 1.2 mm.

Introduce into each of 5 capillary tubes a sufficient amount of the substance, previously treated as described, to form in each tube a column about 10 mm high and allow the tubes to stand for the appropriate time and at the prescribed temperature.

Unless otherwise prescribed, substances with a waxy consistency are carefully and completely melted on a water-bath before introduction into the capillary tubes. Allow the tubes to stand at 2-8 °C for 2 h.

Attach one of the tubes to a thermometer graduated in 0.5 °C so that the substance is close to the bulb of the thermometer. Introduce the thermometer with the attached tube into a beaker so that the distance between the bottom of the beaker and the lower part of the bulb of the thermometer is 1 cm. Fill the beaker with water to a depth of 5 cm. Increase the temperature of the water gradually at a rate of 1 °C/min.

The temperature at which the substance begins to rise in the capillary tube is regarded as the melting point.

Repeat the operation with the other 4 capillary tubes and calculate the result as the mean of the 5 readings.

01/2005:20216

2.2.16. MELTING POINT - INSTANTANEOUS METHOD

The instantaneous melting point is calculated using the expression:

$$\frac{t_1 + t_2}{2}$$

in which t_1 is the first temperature and t_2 the second temperature read under the conditions stated below.

Apparatus. The apparatus consists of a metal block resistant to the substance to be examined, of good heat-conducting capacity, such as brass, with a carefully polished plane upper surface. The block is uniformly heated throughout its mass by means of a micro-adjustable gas heater or an electric heating device with fine adjustment. The block has a cylindrical cavity, wide enough to accomodate a thermometer, which should be maintained with the mercury column in the same position during the calibration of the apparatus and the determination of the melting point of the substance to be examined. The cylindrical cavity is parallel to the upper polished surface of the block and about 3 mm from it. The apparatus is calibrated using appropriate substances of known melting point.

Method. Heat the block at a suitably rapid rate to a temperature about 10 °C below the presumed melting temperature, then adjust the heating rate to about 1 °C/min. At regular intervals drop a few particles of powdered and, where appropriate, dried substance, prepared as for the capillary tube method, onto the block in the vicinity of the thermometer bulb, cleaning the surface after each test. Record the temperature t_1 at which the substance melts instantaneously for the first time in contact with the metal. Stop the heating. During cooling drop a few particles of the substance at regular intervals on the block, cleaning the surface after each test. Record the temperature t_2 at which the substance ceases to melt instantaneously when it comes in contact with the metal

Calibration of the apparatus. The apparatus may be calibrated using melting point reference substances such as those of the World Health Organisation or other appropriate substances.

01/2005:20217

2.2.17. DROP POINT

The drop point is the temperature at which the first drop of the melting substance to be examined falls from a cup under defined conditions.

Apparatus. The apparatus (see Figure 2.2.17.-1)

consists of 2 metal sheaths (*A*) and (*B*) screwed together. Sheath (*A*) is fixed to a mercury thermometer. A metal cup (*F*) is loosely fixed to the lower part of sheath (*B*) by means of 2 tightening bands (*E*). Fixed supports (*D*) 2 mm long determine the exact position of the cup in addition to which they are used to centre the thermometer. A hole (*C*) pierced in the wall of sheath (*B*) is used to balance the pressure. The draining surface of the cup must be flat and the edges of the outflow orifice must be at right angles to it. The lower part of the mercury thermometer has the form and size shown in the Figure; it covers a range from 0 °C to 110 °C and on its scale a distance of 1 mm represents a difference of 1 °C. The mercury reservoir of the thermometer has a diameter of 3.5 ± 0.2 mm and a height of 6.0 ± 0.3 mm. The apparatus is placed in the axis of a tube about 200 mm long and with an external diameter of about 40 mm. It is fixed to the test-tube by means of a stopper through which the thermometer passes, and is provided with a side groove. The opening of the cup is placed about 15 mm from the bottom of the test-tube. The whole device is immersed in a beaker with a capacity of about 1 litre, filled with water. The bottom of the test-tube is placed about 25 mm from the bottom of the beaker. The water level reaches the upper part of sheath (*A*). A stirrer is used to ensure that the temperature of the water remains uniform.

Method. Fill the cup to the brim with the substance to be examined, without melting it, unless otherwise prescribed. Remove the excess substance at the 2 ends of the cup with a spatula. When sheaths (*A*) and (*B*) have been assembled press the cup into its housing in sheath (*B*) until it touches the supports. Remove with a spatula the substance pushed out by the thermometer. Place the apparatus in the water-bath as described above. Heat the water-bath and when the temperature is at about 10 °C below the presumed drop point, adjust the heating rate to about 1 °C/min. Note the temperature at the fall of the first drop. Carry out at least 3 determinations, each time with a fresh sample of the substance. The difference between the readings must not exceed 3 °C. The mean of three readings is the drop point of the substance.

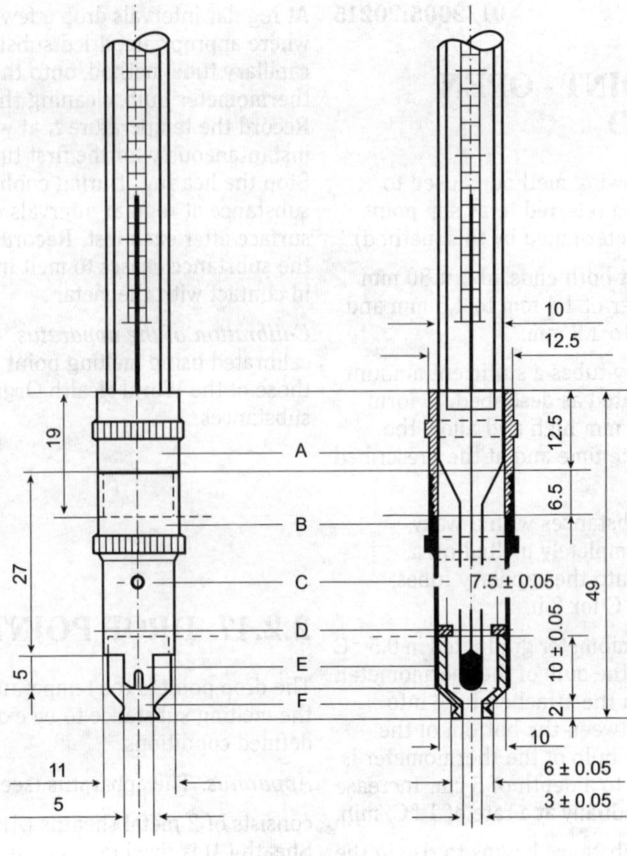

Figure 2.2.17.-1. – *Apparatus for the determination of drop point*
Dimensions in millimetres

01/2005:20218

2.2.18. FREEZING POINT

The freezing point is the maximum temperature occurring during the solidification of a supercooled liquid.

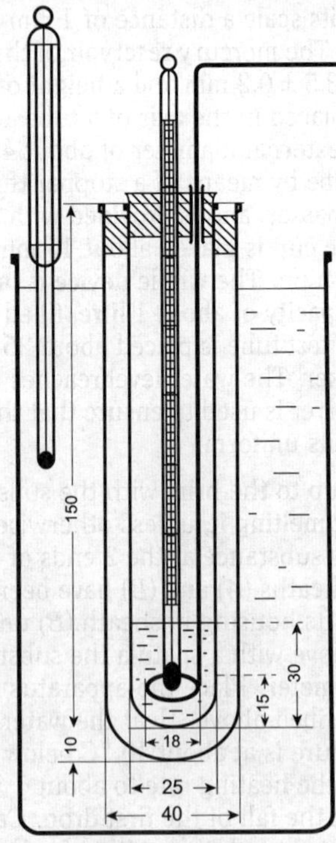

Figure 2.2.18.-1. – *Apparatus for the determination of freezing point*
Dimensions in millimetres

Apparatus. The apparatus (see Figure 2.2.18.-1) consists of a test-tube about 25 mm in diameter and 150 mm long placed inside a test-tube about 40 mm in diameter and 160 mm long. The inner tube is closed by a stopper which carries a thermometer about 175 mm long and graduated in 0.2 °C fixed so that the bulb is about 15 mm above the bottom of the tube. The stopper has a hole allowing the passage of the stem of a stirrer made from a glass rod or other suitable material formed at one end into a loop of about 18 mm overall diameter at right angles to the rod. The inner tube with its jacket is supported centrally in a 1 litre beaker containing a suitable cooling liquid to within 20 mm of the top. A thermometer is supported in the cooling bath.

Method. Place in the inner tube sufficient quantity of the liquid or previously melted substance to be examined, to cover the thermometer bulb and determine the approximate freezing point by cooling rapidly. Place the inner tube in a bath about 5 °C above the approximate freezing point until all but the last traces of crystals are melted. Fill the beaker with water or a saturated solution of sodium chloride, at a temperature about 5 °C lower than the expected freezing point, insert the inner tube into the outer tube, ensuring that some seed crystals are present, and stir thoroughly until solidification takes place. Note the highest temperature observed during solidification.

01/2005:20219

2.2.19. AMPEROMETRIC TITRATION

In amperometric titration the end-point is determined by following the variation of the current measured between 2 electrodes (either one indicator electrode and one reference electrode or 2 indicator electrodes) immersed in the solution to be examined and maintained at a constant potential difference as a function of the quantity of titrant added.

The potential of the measuring electrode is sufficient to ensure a diffusion current for the electroactive substance.

Apparatus. The apparatus comprises an adjustable voltage source and a sensitive microammeter; the detection system generally consists of an indicator electrode (for example, a platinum electrode, a dropping-mercury electrode, a rotating-disc electrode or a carbon electrode) and a reference electrode (for example, a calomel electrode or a silver-silver chloride electrode).

A three-electrode apparatus is sometimes used, consisting of an indicator electrode, a reference electrode and a polarised auxiliary electrode.

Method. Set the potential of the indicator electrode as prescribed and plot a graph of the initial current and the values obtained during the titration as functions of the quantity of titrant added. Add the titrant in not fewer than 3 successive quantities equal to a total of about 80 per cent of the theoretical volume corresponding to the presumed equivalence point. The 3 values must fall on a straight line. Continue adding the titrant beyond the presumed equivalence point in not fewer than 3 successive quantities. The values obtained must fall on a straight line. The point of intersection of the 2 lines represents the end-point of the titration.

For amperometric titration with 2 indicator electrodes, the whole titration curve is recorded and used to determine the end-point.

01/2005:20220

2.2.20. POTENTIOMETRIC TITRATION

In a potentiometric titration the end-point of the titration is determined by following the variation of the potential difference between 2 electrodes (either one indicator electrode and one reference electrode or 2 indicator electrodes) immersed in the solution to be examined as a function of the quantity of titrant added.

The potential is usually measured at zero or practically zero current.

Apparatus. The apparatus used (a simple potentiometer or electronic device) comprises a voltmeter allowing readings to the nearest millivolt.

The indicator electrode to be used depends on the substance to be determined and may be a glass or metal electrode (for example, platinum, gold, silver or mercury). The reference electrode is generally a calomel or a silver-silver chloride electrode.

For acid-base titrations and unless otherwise prescribed, a glass-calomel or glass-silver-silver chloride electrode combination is used.

Method. Plot a graph of the variation of potential difference as a function of the quantity of the titrant added, continuing the addition of the titrant beyond the presumed equivalence point. The end-point corresponds to a sharp variation of potential difference.

01/2005:20221

2.2.21. FLUORIMETRY

Fluorimetry is a procedure which uses the measurement of the intensity of the fluorescent light emitted by the substance to be examined in relation to that emitted by a given standard.

Method. Dissolve the substance to be examined in the solvent or mixture of solvents prescribed in the monograph, transfer the solution to the cell or the tube of the fluorimeter and illuminate it with an excitant light beam of the wavelength prescribed in the monograph and as near as possible monochromatic.

Measure the intensity of the emitted light at an angle of 90° to the excitant beam, after passing it through a filter which transmits predominantly light of the wavelength of the fluorescence. Other types of apparatus may be used provided that the results obtained are identical.

For quantitative determinations, first introduce into the apparatus the solvent or mixture of solvents used to dissolve the substance to be examined and set the instrument to zero. Introduce the standard solution and adjust the sensitivity of the instrument so that the reading is greater than 50. If the second adjustment is made by altering the width of the slits, a new zero setting must be made and the intensity of the standard must be measured again. Finally introduce the solution of unknown concentration and read the result on the instrument. Calculate the concentration c_x of the substance in the solution to be examined, using the formula:

$$c_x = \frac{I_x c_s}{I_s}$$

c_x = concentration of the solution to be examined,

c_s = concentration of the standard solution,

I_x = intensity of the light emitted by the solution to be examined,

I_s = intensity of the light emitted by the standard solution.

If the intensity of the fluorescence is not strictly proportional to the concentration, the measurement may be effected using a calibration curve.

In some cases, measurement can be made with reference to a fixed standard (for example a fluorescent glass or a solution of another fluorescent substance). In such cases, the concentration of the substance to be examined must be determined using a previously drawn calibration curve under the same conditions.

01/2005:20222

2.2.22. ATOMIC EMISSION SPECTROMETRY

Atomic emission spectrometry is a method for determining the concentration of an element in a substance by measuring the intensity of one of the emission lines of the atomic vapour of the element generated from the substance. The determination is carried out at the wavelength corresponding to this emission line.

Apparatus. This consists essentially of an atomic generator of the element to be determined (flame, plasma, arc, etc.), a monochromator and a detector. If the generator is a flame, *water R* is the solvent of choice for preparing test and reference solutions, although organic solvents may also be used if precautions are taken to ensure that the solvent does not interfere with the stability of the flame.

Method. Operate an atomic emission spectrometer in accordance with the manufacturer's instructions at the prescribed wavelength setting. Introduce a blank solution into the atomic generator and adjust the instrument reading to zero. Introduce the most concentrated reference solution and adjust the sensitivity to obtain a suitable reading.

Determinations are made by comparison with reference solutions with known concentrations of the element to be determined either by the Method of Direct Calibration (Method I) or the Method of Standard Additions (Method II).

METHOD I - DIRECT CALIBRATION

Prepare the solution of the substance to be examined (test solution) as prescribed. Prepare not fewer than 3 reference solutions of the element to be determined the concentrations of which span the expected value in the test solution. Any reagents used in the preparation of the test solution are added to the reference solutions at the same concentration. Introduce the test solution and each reference solution into the instrument at least 3 times and record the steady reading. Rinse the apparatus with blank solution each time and ascertain that the reading returns to its initial blank value.

Prepare a calibration curve from the mean of the readings obtained with the reference solutions and determine the concentration of the element in the test solution from the curve so obtained.

METHOD II - STANDARD ADDITIONS

Add to at least 3 similar volumetric flasks equal volumes of the solution of the substance to be examined (test solution) prepared as prescribed. Add to all but one of the flasks progressively larger volumes of a reference solution containing a known concentration of the element to be determined to produce a series of solutions containing steadily increasing concentrations of that element known to give responses in the linear part of the curve. Dilute the contents of each flask to volume with solvent.

Introduce each of the solutions into the instrument at least 3 times and record the steady reading. Rinse the apparatus with solvent each time and ascertain that the reading returns to its initial blank value.

Calculate the linear equation of the graph using a least-squares fit, and derive from it the concentration of the element to be determined in the test solution.

Alternatively, plot on a graph the mean of readings against the added quantity of the element to be determined. Extrapolate the line joining the points on the graph until it meets the concentration axis. The distance between this point and the intersection of the axes represents the concentration of the element to be determined in the test solution.

If a solid sampling technique is required, full details of the procedure to be followed are provided in the monograph.

01/2005:20223

2.2.23. ATOMIC ABSORPTION SPECTROMETRY

Atomic absorption spectrometry is a method for determining the concentration of an element in a substance by measuring the absorption of radiation by the atomic vapour of the element generated from the substance. The determination is carried out at the wavelength of one of the absorption lines of the element concerned.

Apparatus. This consists essentially of a source of radiation, an atomic generator of the element to be determined (flame, furnace, etc.), a monochromator and a detector.

The method of introducing the substance to be analysed depends on the type of atomic generator used. If it is a flame, substances are nebulised and *water R* is the solvent of choice for preparing test and reference solutions although organic solvents may also be used if precautions are taken to ensure that the solvent does not interfere with the stability of the flame. When a furnace is used, substances may be introduced dissolved in *water R* or an organic solvent, but with this technique, solid sampling is also possible.

The atomic vapour may also be generated outside the spectrometer, for example, the cold vapour method for mercury or certain hydrides. For mercury, atoms are generated by chemical reduction and the atomic vapour is swept by a stream of an inert gas into an absorption cell mounted in the optical path of the instrument. Hydrides are either mixed with the gas feeding the burner or swept by an inert gas into a heated cell in which they are dissociated into atoms.

Method. Operate an atomic absorption spectrometer in accordance with the manufacturer's instructions at the prescribed wavelength setting. Introduce a blank solution into the atomic generator and adjust the instrument reading so that it indicates maximum transmission. Introduce the most concentrated reference solution and adjust the sensitivity to obtain a suitable absorbance reading.

Determinations are made by comparison with reference solutions with known concentrations of the element to be determined either by the Method of Direct Calibration (Method I) or the Method of Standard Additions (Method II).

METHOD I - DIRECT CALIBRATION

Prepare the solution of the substance to be examined (test solution) as prescribed. Prepare not fewer than 3 reference solutions of the element to be determined the concentrations of which span the expected value in the test solution. Any reagents used in the preparation of the test solution are added to the reference and blank solutions at the same concentration.

Introduce the test solution and each reference solution into the instrument at least 3 times and record the steady reading. Rinse the apparatus with the blank solution each time and ascertain that the reading returns to its initial blank value. If a furnace is being used, it is fired between readings.

Prepare a calibration curve from the mean of the readings obtained with the reference solutions and determine the concentration of the element to be determined in the test solution from the curve so obtained.

If a solid sampling technique is required, full details of the procedure to be followed are provided in the monograph.

METHOD II - STANDARD ADDITIONS

Add to at least 3 similar volumetric flasks equal volumes of the solution of the substance to be examined (test solution) prepared as prescribed. Add to all but one of the flasks progressively larger volumes of a reference solution containing a known concentration of the element to be determined to produce a series of solutions containing increasing concentrations of that element known to give responses in the linear part of the curve. Dilute the contents of each flask to volume with solvent.

Introduce each of the solutions into the instrument at least 3 times and record the steady reading. Rinse the apparatus with solvent each time and ascertain that the reading returns to its initial blank value.

If a furnace is being used, it is fired between readings.

Calculate the linear equation of the graph using a least-squares fit, and derive from it the concentration of the element to be determined in the test solution.

Alternatively, plot on a graph the mean of readings against the added quantity of the element to be determined. Extrapolate the line joining the points on the graph until it meets the concentration axis. The distance between this point and the intersection of the axes represents the concentration of the element to be determined in the test solution.

If a solid sampling technique is required, full details of the procedure to be followed are provided in the monograph.

01/2005:20224

2.2.24. ABSORPTION SPECTROPHOTOMETRY, INFRARED

Infrared spectrophotometers are used for recording spectra in the region of 4000-650 cm^{-1} (2.5-15.4 µm) or in some cases down to 200 cm^{-1} (50 µm).

APPARATUS

Spectrophotometers for recording spectra consist of a suitable light source, monochromator or interferometer and detector.

Fourier transform spectrophotometers use polychromatic radiation and calculate the spectrum in the frequency domain from the original data by Fourier transformation. Spectrophotometers fitted with an optical system capable of producing monochromatic radiation in the measurement region may also be used. Normally the spectrum is given as a function of transmittance, the quotient of the intensity of the transmitted radiation and the incident radiation. It may also be given in absorbance.

The absorbance (A) is defined as the logarithm to base 10 of the reciprocal of the transmittance (T):

$$A = \log_{10}\left(\frac{1}{T}\right) = \log_{10}\left(\frac{I_0}{I}\right)$$

T = $\frac{I}{I_0}$,

I_0 = intensity of incident radiation,

I = intensity of transmitted radiation.

PREPARATION OF THE SAMPLE

FOR RECORDING BY TRANSMISSION OR ABSORPTION

Prepare the substance by one of the following methods.

Liquids. Examine a liquid either in the form of a film between 2 plates transparent to infrared radiation, or in a cell of suitable path length, also transparent to infrared radiation.

Liquids or solids in solution. Prepare a solution in a suitable solvent. Choose a concentration and a path length of the cell which give a satisfactory spectrum. Generally, good results are obtained with concentrations of 10-100 g/l for a path length of 0.5-0.1 mm. Absorption due to the solvent is compensated by placing in the reference beam a similar cell containing the solvent used. If an FT-IR instrument is used, the absorption is compensated by recording the spectra for the solvent and the sample successively. The solvent absorbance, corrected by a compensation factor, is subtracted using calculation software.

Solids. Examine solids dispersed in a suitable liquid (mull) or in a solid (halide disc), as appropriate. If prescribed in the monograph, make a film of a molten mass between 2 plates transparent to infrared radiation.

A. Mull

Triturate a small quantity of the substance to be examined with the minimum quantity of *liquid paraffin R* or other suitable liquid; 5-10 mg of the substance to be examined is usually sufficient to make an adequate mull using one drop of *liquid paraffin R*. Compress the mull between 2 plates transparent to infrared radiation.

B. Disc

Triturate 1-2 mg of the substance to be examined with 300-400 mg, unless otherwise specified, of finely powdered and dried *potassium bromide R* or *potassium chloride R*. These quantities are usually sufficient to give a disc of 10-15 mm diameter and a spectrum of suitable intensity. If the substance is a hydrochloride, it is recommended to use *potassium chloride R*. Carefully grind the mixture, spread it uniformly in a suitable die, and submit it to a pressure of about 800 MPa (8 $t{\cdot}cm^{-2}$). For substances that are unstable under normal atmospheric conditions or are hygroscopic, the disc is pressed *in vacuo*. Several factors may cause the formation of faulty discs, such as insufficient or excessive grinding, humidity or other impurities in the dispersion medium or an insufficient reduction of particle size. A disc is rejected if visual examination shows lack of uniform transparency or when transmittance at about 2000 cm^{-1} (5 µm) in the absence of a specific absorption band is less than 60 per cent without compensation, unless otherwise prescribed.

Gases. Examine gases in a cell transparent to infrared radiation and having an optical path length of about 100 mm. Evacuate the cell and fill to the desired pressure through a stopcock or needle valve using a suitable gas transfer line between the cell and the container of the gas to be examined.

If necessary adjust the pressure in the cell to atmospheric pressure using a gas transparent to infrared radiation (for example *nitrogen R* and *argon R*). To avoid absorption interferences due to water, carbon dioxide or other atmospheric gases, place in the reference beam, if possible, an identical cell that is either evacuated or filled with the gas transparent to infrared radiation.

FOR RECORDING BY DIFFUSE REFLECTANCE

Solids. Triturate a mixture of the substance to be examined with finely powdered and dried *potassium bromide R* or *potassium chloride R*. Use a mixture containing approximately 5 per cent of the substance, unless otherwise specified. Grind the mixture, place it in a sample cup and examine the reflectance spectrum.

The spectrum of the sample in absorbance mode may be obtained after mathematical treatment of the spectra by the Kubelka-Munk function.

FOR RECORDING BY ATTENUATED TOTAL REFLECTION

Attenuated total reflection (including multiple reflection) involves light being reflected internally by a transmitting medium, typically for a number of reflections. However, several accessories exist where only one reflection occurs. Prepare the substance as follows. Place the substance to be examined in close contact with an internal reflection element (IRE) such as diamond, germanium, zinc selenide, thallium bromide-thallium iodide (KRS-5) or another suitable material of high refractive index. Ensure close and uniform contact between the substance and the whole crystal surface of the internal reflection element, either by applying pressure or by dissolving the substance in an appropriate solvent, then covering the IRE with the obtained solution and evaporating to dryness. Examine the attenuated total reflectance (ATR) spectrum.

IDENTIFICATION USING REFERENCE SUBSTANCES

Prepare the substance to be examined and the reference substance by the same procedure and record the spectra between 4000-650 cm^{-1} (2.5-15.4 µm) under the same operational conditions. The transmission minima (absorption maxima) in the spectrum obtained with the substance to be examined correspond in position and relative size to those in the spectrum obtained with the reference substance (*CRS*).

When the spectra recorded in the solid state show differences in the positions of the transmission minima (absorption maxima), treat the substance to be examined and the reference substance in the same manner so that they crystallise or are produced in the same form, or proceed as prescribed in the monograph, then record the spectra.

IDENTIFICATION USING REFERENCE SPECTRA

Control of resolution performance. For instruments having a monochromator, record the spectrum of a polystyrene film approximately 35 μm in thickness. The difference *x* (see Figure 2.2.24.-1) between the percentage transmittance at the transmission maximum *A* at 2870 cm^{-1} (3.48 μm) and that at the transmission minimum *B* at 2849.5 cm^{-1} (3.51 μm) must be greater than 18. The difference *y* between the percentage transmittance at the transmission maximum *C* at 1589 cm^{-1} (6.29 μm) and that at the transmission minimum *D* at 1583 cm^{-1} (6.32 μm) must be greater than 10.

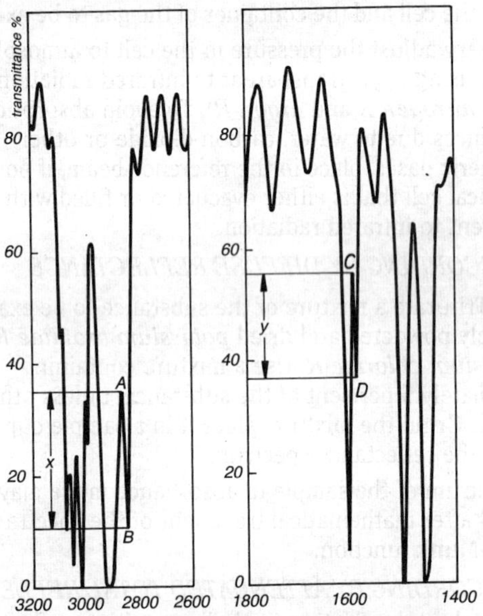

Figure 2.2.24.-1. – *Typical spectrum of polystyrene used to verify the resolution performance*

For Fourier-transform instruments, use suitable instrument resolution with the appropriate apodisation prescribed by the manufacturer. The resolution is checked by suitable means, for example by recording the spectrum of a polystyrene film approximately 35 μm in thickness. The difference between the absorbances at the absorption minimum at 2870 cm^{-1} and the absorption maximum at 2849.5 cm^{-1} is greater than 0.33. The difference between the absorbances at the absorption minimum at 1589 cm^{-1} and the absorption maximum at 1583 cm^{-1} is greater than 0.08.

Verification of the wave-number scale. The wave-number scale may be verified using a polystyrene film, which has transmission minima (absorption maxima) at the wave numbers (in cm^{-1}) shown in Table 2.2.24.-1.

Table 2.2.24.-1. – *Transmission minima and acceptable tolerances of a polystyrene film*

Transmission minima (cm^{-1})	Acceptable tolerance (cm^{-1})	
	Monochromator instruments	Fourier-transform instruments
3060.0	± 1.5	± 1.0
2849.5	± 2.0	± 1.0
1942.9	± 1.5	± 1.0
1601.2	± 1.0	± 1.0
1583.0	± 1.0	± 1.0
1154.5	± 1.0	± 1.0
1028.3	± 1.0	± 1.0

Method. Prepare the substance to be examined according to the instructions accompanying the reference spectrum/reference substance. Using the operating conditions that were used to obtain the reference spectrum, which will usually be the same as those for verifying the resolution performance, record the spectrum of the substance to be examined.

The positions and the relative sizes of the bands in the spectrum of the substance to be examined and the reference spectrum are concordant in the 2 spectra.

Compensation for water vapour and atmospheric carbon dioxide. For Fourier-transform instruments, spectral interference from water vapour and carbon dioxide is compensated using suitable algorithms according to the manufacturer's instructions. Alternatively, spectra can be acquired using suitable purged instruments or ensuring that sample and background single beam spectra are acquired under exactly the same conditions.

IMPURITIES IN GASES

For the analysis of impurities, use a cell transparent to infrared radiation and of suitable optical path length (for example, 1-20 m). Fill the cell as prescribed under Gases. For detection and quantification of the impurities, proceed as prescribed in the monograph.

01/2005:20225

2.2.25. ABSORPTION SPECTROPHOTOMETRY, ULTRAVIOLET AND VISIBLE

Determination of absorbance. The absorbance (*A*) of a solution is defined as the logarithm to base 10 of the reciprocal of the transmittance (*T*) for monochromatic radiation:

$$A = \log_{10}\left(\frac{1}{T}\right) = \log_{10}\left(\frac{I_0}{I}\right)$$

T = I/I_0,

I_0 = intensity of incident monochromatic radiation,

I = intensity of transmitted monochromatic radiation.

In the absence of other physico-chemical factors, the measured absorbance (A) is proportional to the path length (b) through which the radiation passes and to the concentration (c) of the substance in solution in accordance with the equation:

$$A = \varepsilon \cdot c \cdot b$$

ε = molar absorptivity, if b is expressed in centimetres and c in moles per litre.

The expression $A_{1\,\mathrm{cm}}^{1\ \mathrm{per\ cent}}$ representing the specific absorbance of a dissolved substance refers to the absorbance of a 10 g/l solution in a 1 cm cell and measured at a defined wavelength so that:

$$A_{1\,\mathrm{cm}}^{1\ \mathrm{per\ cent}} = \frac{10\varepsilon}{M_r}$$

Unless otherwise prescribed, measure the absorbance at the prescribed wavelength using a path length of 1 cm and at 20 ± 1 °C. Unless otherwise prescribed, the measurements are carried out with reference to the same solvent or the same mixture of solvents. The absorbance of the solvent measured against air and at the prescribed wavelength shall not exceed 0.4 and is preferably less than 0.2. Plot the absorption spectrum with absorbance or function of absorbance as ordinate against wavelength or function of wavelength as abscissa.

Where a monograph gives a single value for the position of an absorption maximum, it is understood that the value obtained may differ by not more than ± 2 nm.

Apparatus. Spectrophotometers suitable for measuring in the ultraviolet and visible range of the spectrum consist of an optical system capable of producing monochromatic radiation in the range of 200 nm to 800 nm and a device suitable for measuring the absorbance.

Control of wavelengths. Verify the wavelength scale using the absorption maxima of *holmium perchlorate solution R*, the line of a hydrogen or deuterium discharge lamp or the lines of a mercury vapour shown in Table 2.2.25.-1. The permitted tolerance is ± 1 nm for the ultraviolet range and ± 3 nm for the visible range.

Table 2.2.25.-1. – *Absorption maxima for control of wavelength scale*

241.15 nm (Ho)	404.66 nm (Hg)
253.7 nm (Hg)	435.83 nm (Hg)
287.15 nm (Ho)	486.0 nm (Dβ)
302.25 nm (Hg)	486.1 nm (Hβ)
313.16 nm (Hg)	536.3 nm (Ho)
334.15 nm (Hg)	546.07 nm (Hg)
361.5 nm (Ho)	576.96 nm (Hg)
365.48 nm (Hg)	579.07 nm (Hg)

Control of absorbance. Check the absorbance using suitable filters or a solution of *potassium dichromate R* at the wavelengths indicated in Table 2.2.25.-2 which gives for each wavelength the exact values and the permitted limits of the specific absorbance. The tolerance for the absorbance is ± 0.01.

For the control of absorbance, use a solution of potassium dichromate prepared as follows. Dissolve 57.0 mg to 63.0 mg of *potassium dichromate R*, previously dried to constant mass at 130 °C, in *0.005 M sulphuric acid* and dilute to 1000.0 ml with the same acid.

Table 2.2.25.-2

Wavelength (nm)	Specific absorbance $A_{1\,\mathrm{cm}}^{1\ \mathrm{per\ cent}}$	Maximum tolerance
235	124.5	122.9 to 126.2
257	144.5	142.8 to 146.2
313	48.6	47.0 to 50.3
350	107.3	105.6 to 109.0

Limit of stray light. Stray light may be detected at a given wavelength with suitable filters or solutions: for example the absorbance of a 12 g/l solution of *potassium chloride R* in a 1 cm cell increases steeply between 220 nm and 200 nm and is greater than 2 at a wavelength between 198 nm and 202 nm when compared with water as compensation liquid.

Resolution (for qualitative analysis). When prescribed in a monograph, measure the resolution of the apparatus as follows: record the spectrum of a 0.02 per cent *V/V* solution of *toluene R* in *hexane R*. The minimum ratio of the absorbance at the maximum at 269 nm to that at the minimum at 266 nm is stated in the monograph.

Spectral slit-width (for quantitative analysis). To avoid errors due to spectral slit-width, when using an instrument on which the slit-width is variable at the selected wavelength, the slit-width must be small compared with the half-width of the absorption band but it must be as large as possible to obtain a high value of I_0. Therefore, a slit-width is chosen such that further reduction does not result in a change in absorbance reading.

Cells. The tolerance on the path length of the cells used is ± 0.005 cm. When filled with the same solvent, the cells intended to contain the solution to be examined and the compensation liquid must have the same transmittance. If this is not the case, an appropriate correction must be applied.

The cells must be cleaned and handled with care.

DERIVATIVE SPECTROPHOTOMETRY

Derivative spectrophotometry involves the transformation of absorption spectra (zero-order) into first-, second- or higher-order-derivative spectra.

A *first-derivative spectrum* is a plot of the gradient of the absorption curve (rate of change of the absorbance with wavelength, $dA/d\lambda$) against wavelength.

A *second-derivative spectrum* is a plot of the curvature of the absorption spectrum against wavelength ($d^2A/d\lambda^2$). The second derivative at any wavelength λ is related to concentration by the following equations:

$$\frac{d^2A}{d\lambda^2} = \frac{d^2A_{1\,\mathrm{cm}}^{1\ \mathrm{per\ cent}}}{d\lambda^2} \times \frac{c'b}{10} = \frac{d^2A\varepsilon}{d\lambda^2} \times \frac{cb}{10}$$

c' = concentration of the absorbing solute, in grams per litre.

Apparatus. Use a spectrophotometer complying with the requirements prescribed above and equipped with an analogue resistance-capacitance differentiation module or a digital differentiator or other means of producing derivative spectra. Some methods of producing second-derivative spectra produce a wavelength shift relative to the zero-order spectrum and this is to be taken into account where applicable.

Resolution power. When prescribed in a monograph, record the second-derivative spectrum of a 0.2 g/l solution of *toluene R* in *methanol R*, using *methanol R* as the compensation liquid. The spectrum shows a small negative extremum located between 2 large negative extrema at 261 nm and 268 nm, respectively, as shown in Figure 2.2.25.-1. Unless otherwise prescribed in the monograph, the ratio *A/B* (see Figure 2.2.25.-1) is not less than 0.2.

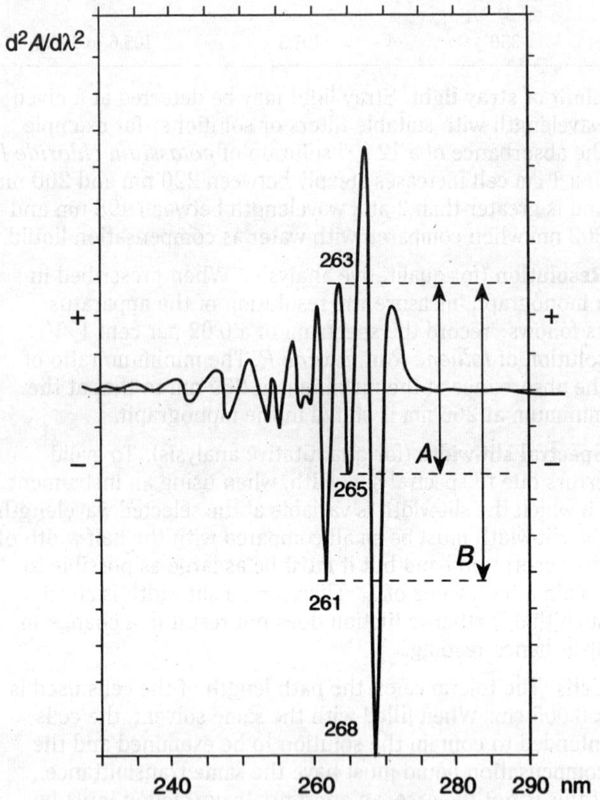

Figure 2.2.25.-1

Procedure. Prepare the solution of the substance to be examined, adjust the various instrument settings according to the manufacturer's instructions and calculate the amount of the substance to be determined as prescribed in the monograph.

01/2005:20226

2.2.26. PAPER CHROMATOGRAPHY

ASCENDING PAPER CHROMATOGRAPHY

Apparatus. The apparatus consists of a glass tank of suitable size for the chromatographic paper used, ground at the top to take a closely fitting lid. In the top of the tank is a device which suspends the chromatographic paper and is capable of being lowered without opening the chamber. In the bottom of the tank is a dish to contain the mobile phase into which the paper may be lowered. The chromatographic paper consists of suitable filter paper, cut into strips of sufficient length and not less than 2.5 cm wide; the paper is cut so that the mobile phase runs in the direction of the grain of the paper.

Method. Place in the dish a layer 2.5 cm deep of the mobile phase prescribed in the monograph. If prescribed in the monograph, pour the stationary phase between the walls of the tank and the dish. Close the tank and allow to stand for 24 h at 20 °C to 25 °C. Maintain the tank at this temperature throughout the subsequent procedure. Draw a fine pencil line horizontally across the paper 3 cm from one end. Using a micro pipette, apply to a spot on the pencil line the volume of the solution prescribed in the monograph. If the total volume to be applied would produce a spot more than 10 mm in diameter, apply the solution in portions allowing each to dry before the next application. When more than one chromatogram is to be run on the same strip of paper, space the solutions along the pencil line at points not less than 3 cm apart. Insert the paper into the tank, close the lid and allow to stand for 1 h 30 min. Lower the paper into the mobile phase and allow elution to proceed for the prescribed distance or time. Remove the paper from the tank and allow to dry in air. Protect the paper from bright light during the elution process.

DESCENDING PAPER CHROMATOGRAPHY

Apparatus. The apparatus consists of a glass tank of suitable size for the chromatographic paper used, ground at the top to take a closely fitting glass lid. The lid has a central hole about 1.5 cm in diameter closed by a heavy glass plate or a stopper. In the upper part of the tank is suspended a solvent trough with a device for holding the chromatographic paper. On each side of the trough, parallel to and slightly above its upper edges, are two glass guide rods to support the paper in such a manner that no part of it is in contact with the walls of the tank. The chromatographic paper consists of suitable filter paper, cut into strips of sufficient length, and of any convenient width between 2.5 cm and the length of the trough; the paper is cut so that the mobile phase runs in the direction of the grain of the paper.

Method. Place in the bottom of the tank a layer 2.5 cm deep of the solvent prescribed in the monograph, close the tank and allow to stand for 24 h at 20 °C to 25 °C. Maintain the tank at this temperature throughout the subsequent procedure. Draw a fine pencil line horizontally across the paper at such a distance from one end that when this end is secured in the solvent trough and the remainder of the paper is hanging freely over the guide rod, the line is a few centimetres below the guide rod and parallel with it. Using a micro-pipette, apply on the pencil line the volume of the solution prescribed in the monograph. If the total volume to be applied would produce a spot more than 10 mm in diameter, apply the solution in portions, allowing each to dry before the next application. When more than one chromatogram is to be run on the same strip of paper, space the solutions along the pencil line at points not less than 3 cm apart. Insert the paper in the tank, close the lid, and allow to stand for 1 h 30 min. Introduce into the solvent trough, through the hole in the lid, a sufficient quantity of the mobile phase, close the tank and allow elution to proceed for the prescribed distance or time. Remove the paper from the tank and allow to dry in air. The paper should be protected from bright light during the elution process.

01/2005:20227

2.2.27. THIN-LAYER CHROMATOGRAPHY

Thin-layer chromatography is a separation technique in which a stationary phase consisting of an appropriate material is spread in a uniform thin layer on a support (plate) of glass, metal or plastic. Solutions of analytes are deposited on the plate prior to development. The separation is based on adsorption, partition, ion-exchange or on combinations of these mechanisms and is carried out by migration (development) of solutes (solutions of analytes) in a solvent or a suitable mixture of solvents (mobile phase) through the thin-layer (stationary phase).

APPARATUS

Plates. The chromatography is carried out using pre-coated plates as described under *Reagents (4.1.1)*.

Preconditioning of the plates. It may be necessary to wash the plates prior to separation. This can be done by migration of an appropriate solvent. The plates may also be impregnated by procedures such as development, immersion or spraying. At the time of use, the plates may be activated, if necessary, by heating in an oven at 100-105 °C for 1 h.

A chromatographic tank with a flat bottom or twin trough, of inert, transparent material, of a size suitable for the plates used and provided with a tightly fitting lid. For horizontal development the tank is provided with a trough for the mobile phase and it additionally contains a device for directing the mobile phase to the stationary phase.

Micropipettes, microsyringes, calibrated disposable capillaries or other application devices suitable for the proper application of the solutions.

Fluorescence detection device to measure direct fluorescence or the inhibition of fluorescence.

Visualisation reagents to detect the separated spots by spraying, exposure to vapour or immersion.

METHOD

Vertical development. Line the walls of the chromatographic tank with filter paper. Pour into the chromatographic tank a sufficient quantity of the mobile phase for the size of the tank to give after impregnation of the filter paper a layer of appropriate depth related to the dimension of the plate to be used. For saturation of the chromatographic tank, replace the lid and allow to stand at 20-25 °C for 1 h. Unless otherwise indicated, the chromatographic separation is performed in a saturated tank.

Apply the prescribed volume of the solutions in sufficiently small portions to obtain bands or circular spots at an appropriate distance from the lower edge and from the sides of the plate. Apply the solutions on a line parallel to the lower edge of the plate with an interval of at least 10 mm between the spots.

When the solvent has evaporated from the applied solutions, place the plate in the chromatographic tank, ensuring that the plate is as vertical as possible and that the spots or bands are above the surface of the mobile phase. Close the chromatographic tank, maintain it at 20-25 °C and protect from sunlight. Remove the plate when the mobile phase has moved over the prescribed distance. Dry the plate and visualise the chromatograms as prescribed.

For two-dimensional chromatography, dry the plates after the first development and carry out a second development in a direction perpendicular to that of the first development.

Horizontal development. Apply the prescribed volume of the solutions in sufficiently small portions to obtain circular spots 1 mm to 2 mm in diameter, or bands 5 mm to 10 mm by 1 mm to 2 mm, at an appropriate distance from the lower edge and from the sides of the plate. Apply the solutions on a line parallel to the lower edge of the plate with an interval of at least 5 mm between the spots. When the solvent has evaporated from the applied solutions, introduce a sufficient quantity of the mobile phase into the trough of the chamber using a syringe or pipette, place the plate horizontally in the chamber and connect the mobile phase direction device according to the manufacturer's instructions. If prescribed, develop the plate starting simultaneously at both ends. Close the chamber and maintain it at 20-25 °C. Remove the plate when the mobile phase has moved over the distance prescribed in the monograph. Dry the plate and visualise the chromatograms as prescribed.

For two-dimensional chromatography, dry the plates after the first development and carry out a second development in a direction perpendicular to that of the first development.

VISUAL ESTIMATION

Identification. The principal spot in the chromatogram obtained with the test solution is visually compared to the corresponding spot in the chromatogram obtained with the reference solution by comparing the colour, the size and the retention factor (R_f) of both spots.

The retention factor (R_f) is defined as the ratio of the distance from the point of application to the centre of the spot and the distance travelled by the solvent front from the point of application.

Verification of the separating power for identification. Normally the performance given by the suitability test described in *Reagents (4.1.1)* is sufficient. Only in special cases an additional performance criterion is prescribed in the monograph.

Related substances test. The secondary spot(s) in the chromatogram obtained with the test solution is (are) visually compared to either the corresponding spot(s) in the chromatogram obtained with the reference solution containing the impurity(ies) or the spot in the chromatogram obtained with the reference solution prepared from a dilution of the test solution.

Verification of the separating power. The requirements for the verification of the separating power are prescribed in the monographs concerned.

Verification of the detecting power. The detecting power is satisfactory if a spot or band is clearly visible in the chromatogram obtained with the most dilute reference solution.

QUANTITATIVE MEASUREMENT

The requirements for resolution and separation are prescribed in the monographs concerned.

Substances separated by thin-layer chromatography and responding to UV-Vis irradiation can be determined directly on the plate, using appropriate instrumentation. While moving the plate or the measuring device, examine the plate by measuring the reflectance or transmittance of the incident light. Similarly, fluorescence may be measured using an appropriate optical system. Substances containing radionuclides can be quantified in three ways: either directly by moving the plate alongside a suitable counter or vice versa (see *Radiopharmaceutical preparations (0125)*), by cutting the plates into strips and measuring the radioactivity on each individual strip using a suitable counter or by scraping off the stationary phase, dissolving it in a suitable scintillation cocktail and measuring the radioactivity using a liquid scintillation counter.

Apparatus. The apparatus for direct measurement on the plate consists of:

- a device for exact positioning and reproducible dispensing of the amount of substances onto the plate,
- a mechanical device to move the plate or the measuring device along the *x*-axis or the *y*-axis,
- a recorder and a suitable integrator or a computer,
- *for substances responding to UV-Vis irradiation*: a photometer with a source of light, an optical device able to generate monochromatic light and a photo cell of adequate sensitivity are used for the measurement of reflectance or transmittance. In the case where

fluorescence is measured, a monochromatic filter is required in addition, to select a particular spectral region of the emitted light,

- *for substances containing radionuclides*: a suitable counter for radioactivity. The linearity range of the counting device is to be verified.

Method. Prepare the solution of the substance to be examined (test solution) as prescribed in the monograph and, if necessary, prepare the reference solutions of the substance to be determined using the same solvent as in the test solution. Apply the same volume of each solution to the plate and develop.

Substances responding to UV-Vis irradiation: Prepare and apply not fewer than three reference solutions of the substance to be examined, the concentrations of which span the expected value in the test solution (about 80, 100 and 120 per cent). Spray with the prescribed reagent, if necessary, and record the reflectance, the transmittance or fluorescence in the chromatograms obtained with the test and reference solutions. Use the measured results for the calculation of the amount of substance in the test solution.

Substances containing radionuclides: Prepare and apply a test solution containing about 100 per cent of the expected value. Determine the radioactivity as a function of the path length and report the radioactivity in each resulting peak as a percentage of the total amount of radioactivity.

Criteria for assessing the suitability of the system are described in the chapter on *Chromatographic separation techniques* (*2.2.46*). The extent to which adjustments of parameters of the chromatographic system can be made to satisfy the criteria of system suitability are also given in this chapter.

01/2005:20228

2.2.28. GAS CHROMATOGRAPHY

Gas chromatography (GC) is a chromatographic separation technique based on the difference in the distribution of species between two non-miscible phases in which the mobile phase is a carrier gas moving through or passing the stationary phase contained in a column. It is applicable to substances or their derivatives which are volatilised under the temperatures employed.

GC is based on mechanisms of adsorption, mass distribution or size exclusion.

APPARATUS

The apparatus consists of an injector, a chromatographic column contained in an oven, a detector and a data acquisition system (or an integrator or a chart recorder). The carrier gas flows through the column at a controlled rate or pressure and then through the detector.

The chromatography is carried out either at a constant temperature or according to a given temperature programme.

INJECTORS

Direct injections of solutions are the usual mode of injection, unless otherwise prescribed in the monograph. Injection may be carried out either directly at the head of the column using a syringe or an injection valve, or into a vaporisation chamber which may be equipped with a stream splitter.

Injections of vapour phase may be effected by static or dynamic head-space injection systems.

Dynamic head-space (purge and trap) injection systems include a sparging device by which volatile substances in solution are swept into an absorbent column maintained at a low temperature. Retained substances are then desorbed into the mobile phase by rapid heating of the absorbent column.

Static head-space injection systems include a thermostatically controlled sample heating chamber in which closed vials containing solid or liquid samples are placed for a fixed period of time to allow the volatile components of the sample to reach equilibrium between the non-gaseous phase and the vapour phase. After equilibrium has been established, a predetermined amount of the head-space of the vial is flushed into the gas chromatograph.

STATIONARY PHASES

Stationary phases are contained in columns which may be:

- a capillary column of fused-silica whose wall is coated with the stationary phase,
- a column packed with inert particles impregnated with the stationary phase,
- a column packed with solid stationary phase.

Capillary columns are 0.1 mm to 0.53 mm in internal diameter (Ø) and 5 m to 60 m in length. The liquid or stationary phase, which may be chemically bonded to the inner surface, is a film 0.1 µm to 5.0 µm thick.

Packed columns, made of glass or metal, are usually 1 m to 3 m in length with an internal diameter (Ø) of 2 mm to 4 mm. Stationary phases usually consist of porous polymers or solid supports impregnated with liquid phase.

Supports for analysis of polar compounds on columns packed with low-capacity, low-polarity stationary phase must be inert to avoid peak tailing. The reactivity of support materials can be reduced by silanising prior to coating with liquid phase. Acid-washed, flux-calcinated diatomaceous earth is often used. Materials are available in various particle sizes, the most commonly used particles are in the ranges of 150 µm to 180 µm and 125 µm to 150 µm.

MOBILE PHASES

Retention time and peak efficiency depend on the carrier gas flow rate; retention time is directly proportional to column length and resolution is proportional to the square root of the column length. For packed columns, the carrier gas flow rate is usually expressed in millilitres per minute at atmospheric pressure and room temperature. Flow rate is measured at the detector outlet, either with a calibrated mechanical device or with a bubble tube, while the column is at operating temperature. The linear velocity of the carrier gas through a packed column is inversely proportional to the square root of the internal diameter of the column for a given flow volume. Flow rates of 60 ml/min in a 4 mm internal diameter column and 15 ml/min in a 2 mm internal diameter column, give identical linear velocities and thus similar retention times.

Helium or nitrogen are usually employed as the carrier gas for packed columns, whereas commonly used carrier gases for capillary columns are nitrogen, helium and hydrogen.

DETECTORS

Flame-ionisation detectors are usually employed but additional detectors which may be used include: electron-capture, nitrogen-phosphorus, mass spectrometric, thermal conductivity, Fourier transform infrared spectrophotometric, and others, depending on the purpose of the analysis.

METHOD

Equilibrate the column, the injector and the detector at the temperatures and the gas flow rates specified in the monograph until a stable baseline is achieved. Prepare the test solution(s) and the reference solution(s) as prescribed. The solutions must be free from solid particles.

Criteria for assessing the suitability of the system are described in the chapter on *Chromatographic separation techniques* (*2.2.46*). The extent to which adjustments of parameters of the chromatographic system can be made to satisfy the criteria of system suitability are also given in this chapter.

Static head-space gas chromatography

Static head-space gas chromatography is a technique particularly suitable for separating and determining volatile compounds present in solid or liquid samples. The method is based on the analysis of the vapour phase in equilibrium with the solid or liquid phase.

APPARATUS

The apparatus consists of a gas chromatograph provided with a device for introducing the sample that may be connected to a module that automatically controls the pressure and the temperature. If necessary, a device for eliminating solvents can be added.

The sample to be analysed is introduced into a container fitted with a suitable stopper and a valve-system which permits the passage of the carrier gas. The container is placed in a thermostatically controlled chamber at a temperature set according to the substance to be examined.

The sample is held at this temperature long enough to allow equilibrium to be established between the solid or liquid phase and the vapour phase.

The carrier gas is introduced into the container and, after the prescribed time, a suitable valve is opened so that the gas expands towards the chromatographic column taking the volatilised compounds with it.

Instead of using a chromatograph specifically equipped for the introduction of samples, it is also possible to use airtight syringes and a conventional chromatograph. Equilibration is then carried out in a separate chamber and the vapour phase is carried onto the column, taking the precautions necessary to avoid any changes in the equilibrium.

METHOD

Using the reference preparations, determine suitable instrument settings to produce an adequate response.

DIRECT CALIBRATION

Separately introduce into identical containers the preparation to be examined and each of the reference preparations, as prescribed in the monograph, avoiding contact between the sampling device and the samples.

Close the containers hermetically and place in the thermostatically controlled chamber set to the temperature and pressure prescribed in the monograph; after equilibration, carry out the chromatography under the prescribed conditions.

STANDARD ADDITIONS

Add to a set of identical suitable containers equal volumes of the preparation to be examined. Add to all but one of the containers, suitable quantities of a reference preparation containing a known concentration of the substance to be determined so as to produce a series of preparations containing steadily increasing concentrations of the substance.

Close the containers hermetically and place in the thermostatically controlled chamber set to the temperature and pressure prescribed in the monograph; after equilibration, carry out the chromatography under the prescribed conditions.

Calculate the linear equation of the graph using a least-squares fit, and derive from it the concentration of the substance to be determined in the preparation to be examined.

Alternatively, plot on a graph the mean of readings against the added quantity of the substance to be determined. Extrapolate the line joining the points on the graph until it meets the concentration axis. The distance between this point and the intersection of the axes represents the concentration of the substance to be determined in the preparation to be examined.

SUCCESSIVE WITHDRAWALS (MULTIPLE HEAD-SPACE EXTRACTION)

If prescribed, the successive withdrawal method is fully described in the monograph.

01/2005:20229

2.2.29. LIQUID CHROMATOGRAPHY

Liquid chromatography (LC) is a method of chromatographic separation based on the difference in the distribution of species between two non-miscible phases, in which the mobile phase is a liquid which percolates through a stationary phase contained in a column.

LC is mainly based on mechanisms of adsorption, mass distribution, ion exchange, size exclusion or stereochemical interaction.

APPARATUS

The apparatus consists of a pumping system, an injector, a chromatographic column (a column temperature controller may be used), a detector and a data acquisition system (or an integrator or a chart recorder). The mobile phase is supplied from one or several reservoirs and flows through the column, usually at a constant rate, and then through the detector.

PUMPING SYSTEMS

LC pumping systems are required to deliver the mobile phase at a constant flow rate. Pressure fluctuations are to be minimised, e.g. by passing the pressurised solvent through a pulse-dampening device. Tubing and connections are capable of withstanding the pressures developed by the pumping system. LC pumps may be fitted with a facility for "bleeding" the system of entrapped air bubbles.

Microprocessor controlled systems are capable of accurately delivering a mobile phase of either constant (isocratic elution) or varying composition (gradient elution), according to a defined programme. In the case of gradient elution, pumping systems which deliver solvent(s) from several reservoirs are available and solvent mixing can be achieved on either the low or high-pressure side of the pump(s).

INJECTORS

The sample solution is introduced into the flowing mobile phase at or near the head of the column using an injection system which can operate at high pressure. Fixed-loop and variable volume devices operated manually or by an auto-sampler are used. Manual partial filling of loops may lead to poorer injection volume precision.

STATIONARY PHASES

There are many types of stationary phases employed in LC, including:

– silica, alumina or porous graphite, used in normal-phase chromatography, where the separation is based on differences in adsorption and/or mass distribution,

– resins or polymers with acid or basic groups, used in ion-exchange chromatography, where separation is based on competition between the ions to be separated and those in the mobile phase,

– porous silica or polymers, used in size-exclusion chromatography, where separation is based on differences between the volumes of the molecules, corresponding to steric exclusion,

– a variety of chemically modified supports prepared from polymers, silica or porous graphite, used in reversed-phase LC, where the separation is based principally on partition of the molecules between the mobile phase and the stationary phase,

– special chemically modified stationary phases, e.g. cellulose or amylose derivatives, proteins or peptides, cyclodextrins etc., for the separation of enantiomers (chiral chromatography).

Most separations are based upon partition mechanisms utilising chemically modified silica as the stationary phase and polar solvents as the mobile phase. The surface of the support, e.g. the silanol groups of silica, is reacted with various silane reagents to produce covalently bound silyl derivatives covering a varying number of active sites on the surface of the support. The nature of the bonded phase is an important parameter for determining the separation properties of the chromatographic system.

Commonly used bonded phases are shown below:

octyl	= $Si\text{-}[CH_2]_7\text{-}CH_3$	C_8
octadecyl	= $Si\text{-}[CH_2]_{17}\text{-}CH_3$	C_{18}
phenyl	= $Si\text{-}[CH_2]_n\text{-}C_6H_5$	C_6H_5
cyanopropyl	= $Si\text{-}[CH_2]_3\text{-}CN$	CN
aminopropyl	= $Si\text{-}[CH_2]_3\text{-}NH_2$	NH_2
diol	= $Si\text{-}[CH_2]_3\text{-}O\text{-}CH(OH)\text{-}CH_2\text{-}OH$	

Unless otherwise stated by the manufacturer, silica based reversed-phase columns are considered to be stable in mobile phases having an apparent pH in the range 2.0 to 8.0. Columns containing porous graphite or particles of polymeric materials such as styrene-divinylbenzene copolymer are stable over a wider pH range.

Analysis using normal-phase chromatography with unmodified silica, porous graphite or polar chemically modified silica, e.g. cyanopropyl or diol, as the stationary phase with a non-polar mobile phase is applicable in certain cases.

For analytical separations, the particle size of the most commonly used stationary phases varies between 3 μm and 10 μm. The particles may be spherical or irregular, of varying porosity and specific surface area. These parameters contribute to the chromatographic behaviour of a particular stationary phase. In the case of reversed phases, the nature of the stationary phase, the extent of bonding, e.g. expressed as the carbon loading, and whether the stationary phase is end-capped (i.e. residual silanol groups are silylated) are additional determining factors. Tailing of peaks, particularly of basic substances, can occur when residual silanol groups are present.

Columns, made of stainless steel unless otherwise prescribed in the monograph, of varying length and internal diameter (Ø) are used for analytical chromatography. Columns with internal diameters of less than 2 mm are often referred to as microbore columns. The temperature of the mobile phase and the column must be kept constant during an analysis. Most separations are performed at room temperature, but columns may be heated to give higher efficiency. It is recommended that columns not be heated above 60 °C because of the potential for stationary phase degradation or changes occurring to the composition of the mobile phase.

MOBILE PHASES

For normal-phase chromatography, less polar solvents are employed. The presence of water in the mobile phase is to be strictly controlled to obtain reproducible results. In reversed-phase LC, aqueous mobile phases, with or without organic modifiers, are employed.

Components of the mobile phase are usually filtered to remove particles greater than 0.45 μm. Multicomponent mobile phases are prepared by measuring the required volumes (unless masses are specified) of the individual components, followed by mixing. Alternatively, the solvents may be delivered by individual pumps controlled by proportioning valves by which mixing is performed according to the desired proportion. Solvents are normally degassed before pumping by sparging with helium, sonication or using on-line membrane/vacuum modules to avoid the creation of gas bubbles in the detector cell.

Solvents for the preparation of the mobile phase are normally free of stabilisers and are transparent at the wavelength of detection, if an ultraviolet detector is employed. Solvents and other components employed are to be of appropriate quality. Adjustment of the pH, if necessary, is effected using only the aqueous component of the mobile phase and not the mixture. If buffer solutions are used, adequate rinsing of the system is carried out with a mixture of water and the organic modifier of the mobile phase (5 per cent *V/V*) to prevent crystallisation of salts after completion of the chromatography.

Mobile phases may contain other components, e.g. a counter-ion for ion-pair chromatography or a chiral selector for chromatography using an achiral stationary phase.

DETECTORS

Ultraviolet/visible (UV/Vis) spectrophotometers, including diode array detectors, are the most commonly employed detectors. Fluorescence spectrophotometers, differential refractometers, electrochemical detectors, mass spectrometers, light scattering detectors, radioactivity detectors or other special detectors may also be used.

METHOD

Equilibrate the column with the prescribed mobile phase and flow rate, at room temperature or at the temperature specified in the monograph, until a stable baseline is achieved. Prepare the solution(s) of the substance to be examined and the reference solution(s) required. The solutions must be free from solid particles.

Criteria for assessing the suitability of the system are described in the chapter on *Chromatographic separation techniques (2.2.46)*. The extent to which adjustments of parameters of the chromatographic system can be made to satisfy the criteria of system suitability are also given in this chapter.

01/2005:20230

2.2.30. SIZE-EXCLUSION CHROMATOGRAPHY

Size-exclusion chromatography is a chromatographic technique which separates molecules in solution according to their size. With organic mobile phases, the technique is known as *gel-permeation chromatography* and with aqueous mobile phases, the term *gel-filtration chromatography* has been used. The sample is introduced into a column, which is filled with a gel or a porous particle packing material, and is carried by the mobile phase through the column. The size separation takes place by repeated exchange of the solute molecules between the solvent of the mobile phase and the same solvent in the stagnant liquid phase (stationary phase) within the pores of the packing material. The pore-size range of the packing material determines the molecular-size range within which separation can occur.

Molecules small enough to penetrate all the pore spaces elute at the *total permeation volume* (V_t). On the other hand, molecules apparently larger than the maximum pore size of the packing material migrate along the column only through the spaces between the particles of the packing material without being retained and elute at the *exclusion volume* (V_0 void volume). Separation according to molecular size occurs between the exclusion volume and the total permeation volume, with useful separation usually occurring in the first two thirds of this range.

Apparatus. The apparatus consists essentially of a chromatographic column of varying length and internal diameter (Ø), if necessary temperature-controlled, packed with a separation material that is capable of fractionation in the appropriate range of molecular sizes and through which the eluent is passed at a constant rate. One end of the column is usually fitted with a suitable device for applying the sample such as a flow adapter, a syringe through a septum or an injection valve and may also be connected to a suitable pump for controlling the flow of the eluent. Alternatively the sample may be applied directly to the drained bed surface or, where the sample is denser than the eluent, it may be layered beneath the eluent. The outlet of the column is usually connected to a suitable detector fitted with an automatic recorder which enables the monitoring of the relative concentrations of separated components of the sample. Detectors are usually based on photometric, refractometric or luminescent properties. An automatic fraction collector may be attached, if necessary.

The packing material may be a soft support such as a swollen gel or a rigid support composed of a material such as glass, silica or a solvent-compatible, cross-linked organic polymer. Rigid supports usually require pressurised systems giving faster separations. The mobile phase is chosen according to sample type, separation medium and method of detection. Before carrying out the separation, the packing material is treated, and the column is packed, as described in the monograph, or according to the manufacturer's instructions.

Criteria for assessing the suitability of the system are described in the chapter on *Chromatographic separation techniques* (*2.2.46*). The extent to which adjustments of parameters of the chromatographic system can be made to satisfy the criteria of system suitability are also given in this chapter.

DETERMINATION OF RELATIVE COMPONENT COMPOSITION OF MIXTURES

Carry out the separation as stated in the monograph. If possible, monitor the elution of the components continuously and measure the corresponding peak areas. If the sample is monitored by a physico-chemical property to which all the components of interest exhibit equivalent responses (for example if they have the same specific absorbance), calculate the relative amount of each component by dividing the respective peak area by the sum of the peak areas of all the components of interest. If the responses to the property used for detection of the components of interest are not equivalent, calculate the content by means of calibration curves obtained with the calibration standards prescribed in the monograph.

DETERMINATION OF MOLECULAR MASSES

Size-exclusion chromatography may be used to determine molecular masses by comparison with appropriate calibration standards specified in the monograph. The retention volumes of the calibration standards may be plotted against the logarithm of their molecular masses. The plot usually approximates a straight line within the exclusion and total permeation limits for the separation medium used. From the calibration curve, molecular masses may be estimated. The molecular-mass calibration is valid only for the particular macromolecular solute/solvent system used under the specified experimental conditions.

DETERMINATION OF MOLECULAR SIZE DISTRIBUTION OF POLYMERS

Size-exclusion chromatography may be used to determine the distribution of the molecular size of polymers. However, sample comparison may be valid only for results obtained under the same experimental conditions. The reference substances used for the calibration and the methods for determination of the distribution of molecular sizes of polymers are specified in the monograph.

01/2005:20231

2.2.31. ELECTROPHORESIS

GENERAL PRINCIPLE

Under the influence of an electrical field, charged particles dissolved or dispersed in an electrolyte solution migrate in the direction of the electrode bearing the opposite polarity. In gel electrophoresis, the movements of the particles are retarded by interactions with the surrounding gel matrix, which acts as a molecular sieve. The opposing interactions of the electrical force and molecular sieving result in differential migration rates according to sizes, shapes and charges of particles. Because of their different physico-chemical properties, different macromolecules of a mixture will migrate at different speeds during electrophoresis and will thus be separated into discrete fractions. Electrophoretic separations can be conducted in systems without support phases (e.g. free solution separation in capillary electrophoresis) and in stabilising media such as thin-layer plates, films or gels.

FREE OR MOVING BOUNDARY ELECTROPHORESIS

This method is mainly used for the determination of mobility, the experimental characteristics being directly measurable and reproducible. It is chiefly employed with substances of high relative molecular mass and low diffusibility. The boundaries are initially located by a physical process such as refractometry or conductimetry. After applying a given electric field for an accurately measured time, the new boundaries and their respective positions are observed. The operating conditions must be such as to make it possible to determine as many boundaries as there are components.

ZONE ELECTROPHORESIS USING A SUPPORTING MEDIUM

This method requires the use of small samples only.

The nature of the support, such as paper, agar gel, cellulose acetate, starch, agarose, methacrylamide, mixed gel, introduces a number of additional factors modifying the mobility:

a) owing to channelling in the supporting medium, the apparent distance covered is less than the real distance,

b) some supporting media are not electrically neutral. As the medium is a stationary phase it may sometimes give rise to a considerable electro-endosmotic flow,

c) any heating due to the joule effect may cause some evaporation of the liquid from the supporting medium which, by capillarity, causes the solution to move from the ends towards the centre. The ionic strength therefore tends to increase gradually.

The rate of migration then depends on four main factors: the mobility of the charged particle, the electro-endosmotic flow, the evaporation flow, and the field strength. Hence it is necessary to operate under clearly defined experimental conditions and to use, wherever possible, reference substances.

An *apparatus* for electrophoresis consists of:

– a *generator supplying direct current* whose voltage can be controlled and, preferably, stabilised,

– an *electrophoresis chamber*. This is usually rectangular and made of glass or rigid plastic, with two separate compartments, the anodic and the cathodic, containing the electrolyte solution. In each compartment is immersed an electrode, for example of platinum or graphite. These are connected by means of an appropriately isolated circuit to the corresponding terminal of the power supply to form the anode and the cathode. The level of the liquid in the two compartments is kept equal to prevent siphoning.

  The electrophoresis chamber is fitted with an airtight lid which maintains a moisture-saturated atmosphere during operation and reduces evaporation of the solvent. A safety device may be used to cut off the power when the lid is removed. If the electrical power measured across the strip exceeds 10 W, it is preferable to cool the support.

– a *support-carrying device*:

  Strip electrophoresis. The supporting strip, previously wetted with the same conducting solution and dipped at each end into an electrode compartment is appropriately tightened and fixed on to a suitable carrier designed to prevent diffusion of the conducting electrolyte, such as a horizontal frame, inverted-V stand or a uniform surface with contact points at suitable intervals.

  Gel electrophoresis. The device consists essentially of a glass plate (for example, a microscope slide) over the whole surface of which is deposited a firmly adhering layer of gel of uniform thickness. The connection between the gel and the conducting solution is effected in various ways according to the type of apparatus used. Precautions must be taken to avoid condensation of moisture or drying of the solid layer.

– measuring *device or means of detection*.

Method. Introduce the electrolyte solution into the electrode compartments. Place the support suitably impregnated with electrolyte solution in the chamber under the conditions prescribed for the type of apparatus used. Locate the starting line and apply the sample. Apply the electric current for the prescribed time. After the current has been switched off, remove the support from the chamber, dry and visualise.

POLYACRYLAMIDE ROD GEL ELECTROPHORESIS

In polyacrylamide rod gel electrophoresis, the stationary phase is a gel which is prepared from a mixture of acrylamide and *N,N′*-methylenebisacrylamide. Rod gels are prepared in tubes 7.5 cm long and 0.5 cm in internal diameter, one solution being applied to each rod.

Apparatus. This consists of two buffer solution reservoirs made of suitable material such as poly(methyl methacrylate) and mounted vertically one above the other. Each reservoir is fitted with a platinum electrode. The electrodes are connected to a power supply allowing operation either at constant current or at constant voltage. The apparatus has in the base of the upper reservoir a number of holders equidistant from the electrode.

Method. The solutions should usually be degassed before polymerisation and the gels used immediately after preparation. Prepare the gel mixture as prescribed and pour into suitable glass tubes, stoppered at the bottom, to an equal height in each tube and to about 1 cm from the top, taking care to ensure that no air bubbles are trapped in the tubes. Cover the gel mixture with a layer of *water R* to exclude air and allow to set. Gel formation usually takes about 30 min and is complete when a sharp interface appears between the gel and the water layer. Remove the water layer. Fill the lower reservoir with the prescribed buffer solution and remove the stoppers from the tubes. Fit the tubes into the holders of the upper reservoir and adjust so that the bottom of the tubes are immersed in the buffer solution in the lower reservoir. Carefully fill the tubes with the prescribed buffer solution. Prepare the test and reference solutions containing the prescribed marker dye and make them dense by dissolving in them *sucrose R*, for example. Apply the solutions to the surface of a gel using a different tube for each solution. Add the same buffer to the upper reservoir. Connect the electrodes to the power supply and allow electrophoresis to proceed at the prescribed temperature and using the prescribed constant voltage or current. Switch off the power supply when the marker dye has migrated almost into the lower reservoir. Immediately remove each tube from the apparatus and extrude the gel. Locate the position of the bands in the electropherogram as prescribed.

SODIUM DODECYL SULPHATE POLYACRYLAMIDE GEL ELECTROPHORESIS (SDS-PAGE)

Scope. Polyacrylamide gel electrophoresis is used for the qualitative characterisation of proteins in biological preparations, for control of purity and quantitative determinations.

Purpose. Analytical gel electrophoresis is an appropriate method with which to identify and to assess the homogeneity of proteins in pharmaceutical preparations. The method is routinely used for the estimation of protein subunit molecular masses and for determining the subunit compositions of purified proteins.

Ready-to-use gels and reagents are widely available on the market and can be used instead of those described in this text, provided that they give equivalent results and that they meet the validity requirements given below under Validation of the test.

CHARACTERISTICS OF POLYACRYLAMIDE GELS

The sieving properties of polyacrylamide gels are established by the three-dimensional network of fibres and pores which is formed as the bifunctional bisacrylamide cross-links adjacent polyacrylamide chains. Polymerisation is catalysed by a free radical-generating system composed of ammonium persulphate and tetramethylethylenediamine.

As the acrylamide concentration of a gel increases, its effective pore size decreases. The effective pore size of a gel is operationally defined by its sieving properties; that is, by the resistance it imparts to the migration of macromolecules. There are limits on the acrylamide concentrations that can be used. At high acrylamide concentrations, gels break much more easily and are difficult to handle. As the pore size of a gel decreases, the migration rate of a protein through the gel decreases. By adjusting the pore size of a gel, through manipulating the acrylamide concentration, the resolution of the method can be optimised for a given protein product. Thus, a given gel is physically characterised by its respective composition in acrylamide and bisacrylamide.

In addition to the composition of the gel, the state of the protein is an important component to the electrophoretic mobility. In the case of proteins, the electrophoretic mobility is dependent on the pK value of the charged groups and the size of the molecule. It is influenced by the type, concentration and pH of the buffer, by the temperature and the field strength as well as by the nature of the support material.

DENATURING POLYACRYLAMIDE GEL ELECTROPHORESIS

The method cited as an example is limited to the analysis of monomeric polypeptides with a mass range of 14 000 to 100 000 daltons. It is possible to extend this mass range by various techniques (e.g. gradient gels, particular buffer system) but those techniques are not discussed in this chapter.

Denaturing polyacrylamide gel electrophoresis using sodium dodecyl sulphate (SDS-PAGE) is the most common mode of electrophoresis used in assessing the pharmaceutical quality of protein products and will be the focus of the example method. Typically, analytical electrophoresis of proteins is carried out in polyacrylamide gels under conditions that ensure dissociation of the proteins into their individual polypeptide subunits and that minimise aggregation. Most commonly, the strongly anionic detergent sodium dodecyl sulphate (SDS) is used in combination with heat to dissociate the proteins before they are loaded on the gel. The denatured polypeptides bind to SDS, become negatively charged and exhibit a consistent charge-to-mass ratio regardless of protein type. Because the amount of SDS bound is almost always proportional to the molecular mass of the polypeptide and is independent of its sequence, SDS-polypeptide complexes migrate through polyacrylamide gels with mobilities dependent on the size of the polypeptide.

The electrophoretic mobilities of the resultant detergent-polypeptide complexes all assume the same functional relationship to their molecular masses. Migration of SDS complexes is toward the anode in a predictable manner, with low-molecular-mass complexes migrating faster than larger ones. The molecular mass of a protein can therefore be estimated from its relative mobility in calibrated SDS-PAGE and the occurrence of a single band in such a gel is a criterion of purity.

Modifications to the polypeptide backbone, such as *N*- or *O*-linked glycosylation, however, have a significant impact on the apparent molecular mass of a protein since SDS does not bind to a carbohydrate moiety in a manner similar to a polypeptide. Thus, a consistent charge-to-mass ratio is not maintained. The apparent molecular mass of proteins having undergone post-translational modifications is not a true reflection of the mass of the polypeptide chain.

Reducing conditions. Polypeptide subunits and three-dimensional structure is often maintained in proteins by the presence of disulphide bonds. A goal of SDS-PAGE analysis under reducing conditions is to disrupt this structure by reducing disulphide bonds. Complete denaturation and dissociation of proteins by treatment with 2-mercaptoethanol or dithiothreitol (DTT) will result in unfolding of the polypeptide backbone and subsequent complexation with SDS. In these conditions, the molecular mass of the polypeptide subunits can be calculated by linear regression in the presence of suitable molecular-mass standards.

Non-reducing conditions. For some analyses, complete dissociation of the protein into subunit peptides is not desirable. In the absence of treatment with reducing agents such as 2-mercaptoethanol or DTT, disulphide covalent bonds remain intact, preserving the oligomeric form of the protein. Oligomeric SDS-protein complexes migrate more slowly than their SDS-polypeptide subunits. In addition, non-reduced proteins may not be completely saturated with SDS and, hence, may not bind the detergent in a constant mass ratio. This makes molecular-mass determinations of these molecules by SDS-PAGE less straightforward than analyses of fully denatured polypeptides, since it is necessary that both standards and unknown proteins be in similar configurations for valid comparisons. However, the staining of a single band in such a gel is a criterion of purity.

CHARACTERISTICS OF DISCONTINUOUS BUFFER SYSTEM GEL ELECTROPHORESIS

The most popular electrophoretic method for the characterisation of complex mixtures of proteins involves the use of a discontinuous buffer system consisting of two contiguous, but distinct gels: a resolving or separating (lower) gel and a stacking (upper) gel. The two gels are cast with different porosities, pH, and ionic strengths. In addition, different mobile ions are used in the gel and electrode buffers. The buffer discontinuity acts to concentrate large volume samples in the stacking gel, resulting in improved resolution. When power is applied, a voltage drop develops across the sample solution which drives the proteins into the stacking gel. Glycinate ions from the electrode buffer follow the proteins into the stacking gel. A moving boundary region is rapidly formed with the highly mobile chloride ions in the front and the relatively slow glycinate ions in the rear. A localised high-voltage gradient forms between the leading and trailing ion fronts, causing the SDS-protein complexes to form into a thin zone (stack) and migrate between the chloride and glycinate phases. Within broad limits, regardless of the height of the applied sample, all SDS-proteins condense into a very narrow region and enter the resolving gel as a well-defined, thin zone of high protein density. The large-pore stacking gel does not retard the migration of most proteins and serves mainly as an anticonvective medium. At the interface of the stacking and resolving gels, the proteins experience a sharp increase in retardation due to the restrictive pore size of the resolving gel. Once in the resolving gel, proteins continue to be slowed by the sieving of the matrix. The glycinate ions overtake the proteins, which then move in a space of uniform pH formed by the tris(hydroxymethyl)aminomethane and glycine. Molecular sieving causes the SDS-polypeptide complexes to separate on the basis of their molecular masses.

PREPARING VERTICAL DISCONTINUOUS BUFFER SDS POLYACRYLAMIDE GELS

Assembling of the gel moulding cassette. Clean the two glass plates (size: e.g. 10 cm × 8 cm), the polytetrafluoroethylene comb, the two spacers and the silicone rubber tubing (diameter e.g. 0.6 mm × 35 cm) with mild detergent and rinse extensively with water. Dry all the items with a paper towel or tissue. Lubricate the spacers and the tubing with non-silicone grease. Apply the spacers along each of the two short sides of the glass plate 2 mm away from the edges and 2 mm away from the long side corresponding to the bottom of the gel. Begin to lay the tubing on the glass plate by using one spacer as a guide. Carefully twist the tubing at the bottom of the spacer and follow the long side of the glass plate. While holding the tubing with one finger along the long side twist again the tubing and lay it on the second short side of the glass plate, using the spacer as a guide. Place the second glass plate in perfect alignment and hold the mould together by hand pressure. Apply two clamps on each of the two short sides of the mould. Carefully apply four clamps on the longer side of the gel mould thus forming the bottom of the gel mould. Verify that the tubing is running along the edge of the glass plates and has not been extruded while placing the clamps. The gel mould is now ready for pouring the gel.

Preparation of the gel. In a discontinuous buffer SDS polyacrylamide gel, it is recommended to pour the resolving gel, let the gel set, and then pour the stacking gel since the composition of the two gels in acrylamide-bisacrylamide, buffer and pH are different.

Preparation of the resolving gel. In a conical flask, prepare the appropriate volume of solution containing the desired concentration of acrylamide for the resolving gel, using the values given in Table 2.2.31.-1. Mix the components in the order shown. Where appropriate, before adding the ammonium persulphate solution and the tetramethylethylenediamine (TEMED), filter the solution if necessary under vacuum through a cellulose acetate membrane (pore diameter 0.45 μm); keep the solution under vacuum by swirling the filtration unit until no more bubbles are formed in the solution. Add appropriate amounts of ammonium persulphate solution and TEMED as indicated in Table 2.2.31.-1, swirl and pour immediately into the gap between the two glass plates of the mould. Leave sufficient space for the stacking gel (the length of the teeth of the comb plus 1 cm). Using a tapered glass pipette, carefully overlay the solution with water-saturated isobutanol. Leave the gel in a vertical position at room temperature to allow polymerisation.

Preparation of the stacking gel. After polymerisation is complete (about 30 min), pour off the isobutanol and wash the top of the gel several times with water to remove the isobutanol overlay and any unpolymerised acrylamide. Drain as much fluid as possible from the top of the gel, and then remove any remaining water with the edge of a paper towel.

In a conical flask, prepare the appropriate volume of solution containing the desired concentration of acrylamide, using the values given in Table 2.2.31.-2. Mix the components in the order shown. Where appropriate, before adding the ammonium persulphate solution and the TEMED, filter the solution if necessary under vacuum through a cellulose acetate membrane (pore diameter: 0.45 μm); keep the solution under vacuum by swirling the filtration unit until no more bubbles are formed in the solution. Add appropriate amounts of ammonium persulphate solution and TEMED as indicated in Table 2.2.31.-2, swirl and pour immediately into the gap between the two glass plates of the mould directly onto the surface of the polymerised resolving gel. Immediately insert a clean polytetrafluoroethylene comb into the stacking gel solution, being careful to avoid trapping air bubbles. Add more stacking gel solution to fill the spaces of the comb completely. Leave the gel in a vertical position and allow to polymerise at room temperature.

Table 2.2.31.-1. – *Preparation of resolving gel*

Solution components	Component volumes (ml) per gel mould volume of							
	5 ml	10 ml	15 ml	20 ml	25 ml	30 ml	40 ml	50 ml
6 per cent acrylamide								
Water R	2.6	5.3	7.9	10.6	13.2	15.9	21.2	26.5
Acrylamide solution(1)	1.0	2.0	3.0	4.0	5.0	6.0	8.0	10.0
1.5 M Tris (pH 8.8)(2)	1.3	2.5	3.8	5.0	6.3	7.5	10.0	12.5
100 g/l SDS(3)	0.05	0.1	0.15	0.2	0.25	0.3	0.4	0.5
100 g/l APS(4)	0.05	0.1	0.15	0.2	0.25	0.3	0.4	0.5
TEMED(5)	0.004	0.008	0.012	0.016	0.02	0.024	0.032	0.04
8 per cent acrylamide								
Water R	2.3	4.6	6.9	9.3	11.5	13.9	18.5	23.2
Acrylamide solution(1)	1.3	2.7	4.0	5.3	6.7	8.0	10.7	13.3
1.5 M Tris (pH 8.8)(2)	1.3	2.5	3.8	5.0	6.3	7.5	10.0	12.5
100 g/l SDS(3)	0.05	0.1	0.15	0.2	0.25	0.3	0.4	0.5
100 g/l APS(4)	0.05	0.1	0.15	0.2	0.25	0.3	0.4	0.5
TEMED(5)	0.003	0.006	0.009	0.012	0.015	0.018	0.024	0.03
10 per cent acrylamide								
Water R	1.9	4.0	5.9	7.9	9.9	11.9	15.9	19.8
Acrylamide solution(1)	1.7	3.3	5.0	6.7	8.3	10.0	13.3	16.7
1.5 M Tris (pH 8.8)(2)	1.3	2.5	3.8	5.0	6.3	7.5	10.0	12.5
100 g/l SDS(3)	0.05	0.1	0.15	0.2	0.25	0.3	0.4	0.5
100 g/l APS(4)	0.05	0.1	0.15	0.2	0.25	0.3	0.4	0.5
TEMED(5)	0.002	0.004	0.006	0.008	0.01	0.012	0.016	0.02

Solution components	Component volumes (ml) per gel mould volume of							
	5 ml	**10 ml**	**15 ml**	**20 ml**	**25 ml**	**30 ml**	**40 ml**	**50 ml**
12 per cent acrylamide								
Water R	1.6	3.3	4.9	6.6	8.2	9.9	13.2	16.5
Acrylamide solution(1)	2.0	4.0	6.0	8.0	10.0	12.0	16.0	20.0
1.5 M Tris (pH 8.8)(2)	1.3	2.5	3.8	5.0	6.3	7.5	10.0	12.5
100 g/l SDS(3)	0.05	0.1	0.15	0.2	0.25	0.3	0.4	0.5
100 g/l APS(4)	0.05	0.1	0.15	0.2	0.25	0.3	0.4	0.5
TEMED(5)	0.002	0.004	0.006	0.008	0.01	0.012	0.016	0.02
14 per cent acrylamide								
Water R	1.4	2.7	3.9	5.3	6.6	8.0	10.6	13.8
Acrylamide solution(1)	2.3	4.6	7.0	9.3	11.6	13.9	18.6	23.2
1.5 M Tris (pH 8.8)(2)	1.2	2.5	3.6	5.0	6.3	7.5	10.0	12.5
100 g/l SDS(3)	0.05	0.1	0.15	0.2	0.25	0.3	0.4	0.5
100 g/l APS(4)	0.05	0.1	0.15	0.2	0.25	0.3	0.4	0.5
TEMED(5)	0.002	0.004	0.006	0.008	0.01	0.012	0.016	0.02
15 per cent acrylamide								
Water R	1.1	2.3	3.4	4.6	5.7	6.9	9.2	11.5
Acrylamide solution(1)	2.5	5.0	7.5	10.0	12.5	15.0	20.0	25.0
1.5 M Tris (pH 8.8)(2)	1.3	2.5	3.8	5.0	6.3	7.5	10.0	12.5
100 g/l SDS(3)	0.05	0.1	0.15	0.2	0.25	0.3	0.4	0.5
100 g/l APS(4)	0.05	0.1	0.15	0.2	0.25	0.3	0.4	0.5
TEMED(5)	0.002	0.004	0.006	0.008	0.01	0.012	0.016	0.02

(1) *Acrylamide solution: 30 per cent acrylamide/bisacrylamide(29:1) solution R.*
(2) 1.5 M Tris (pH 8.8): *1.5 M tris-hydrochloride buffer solution pH 8.8 R.*
(3) 100 g/l SDS: a 100 g/l solution of *sodium dodecyl sulphate R.*
(4) 100 g/l APS: a 100 g/l solution of *ammonium persulphate R.* Ammonium persulphate provides the free radicals that drive polymerisation of acrylamide and bisacrylamide. Since ammonium persulphate solution decomposes slowly, fresh solutions must be prepared weekly.
(5) TEMED: *tetramethylethylenediamine R.*

Mounting the gel in the electrophoresis apparatus and electrophoretic separation. After polymerisation is complete (about 30 min), remove the polytetrafluoroethylene comb carefully. Rinse the wells immediately with water or with the *SDS-PAGE running buffer R* to remove any unpolymerised acrylamide. If necessary, straighten the teeth of the stacking gel with a blunt hypodermic needle attached to a syringe. Remove the clamps on one short side, carefully pull out the tubing and replace the clamps. Proceed similarly on the other short side. Remove the tubing from the bottom part of the gel. Mount the gel in the electrophoresis apparatus. Add the electrophoresis buffers to the top and bottom reservoirs. Remove any bubbles that become trapped at the bottom of the gel between the glass plates. This is best done with a bent hypodermic needle attached to a syringe. Never pre-run the gel before loading the samples, since this will destroy the discontinuity of the buffer systems. Before loading the sample carefully rinse the slot with *SDS-PAGE running buffer R.* Prepare the test and reference solutions in the recommended sample buffer and treat as specified in the

Table 2.2.31.-2. – *Preparation of stacking gel*

Solution components	Component volumes (ml) per gel mould volume of							
	1 ml	**2 ml**	**3 ml**	**4 ml**	**5 ml**	**6 ml**	**8 ml**	**10 ml**
Water R	0.68	1.4	2.1	2.7	3.4	4.1	5.5	6.8
Acrylamide solution(1)	0.17	0.33	0.5	0.67	0.83	1.0	1.3	1.7
1.0 M Tris (pH 6.8)(2)	0.13	0.25	0.38	0.5	0.63	0.75	1.0	1.25
100 g/l SDS(3)	0.01	0.02	0.03	0.04	0.05	0.06	0.08	0.1
100 g/l APS(4)	0.01	0.02	0.03	0.04	0.05	0.06	0.08	0.1
TEMED(5)	0.001	0.002	0.003	0.004	0.005	0.006	0.008	0.01

(1) Acrylamide solution: *30 per cent acrylamide/bisacrylamide (29:1) solution R.*
(2) 1.0 M Tris (pH 6.8): *1 M tris-hydrochloride buffer solution pH 6.8 R.*
(3) 100 g/l SDS: a 100 g/l solution of *sodium dodecyl sulphate R.*
(4) 100 g/l APS: a 100 g/l solution of *ammonium persulphate R.* Ammonium persulphate provides the free radicals that drive polymerisation of acrylamide and bisacrylamide. Since ammonium persulphate solution decomposes slowly, fresh solutions must be prepared weekly.
(5) TEMED: *tetramethylethylenediamine R.*

individual monograph. Apply the appropriate volume of each solution to the stacking gel wells. Start the electrophoresis using the conditions recommended by the manufacturer of the equipment. Manufacturers of SDS-PAGE equipment may provide gels of different surface area and thickness. Electrophoresis running time and current/voltage may need to vary as described by the manufacturer of the apparatus in order to achieve optimum separation. Check that the dye front is moving into the resolving gel. When the dye is reaching the bottom of the gel, stop the electrophoresis. Remove the gel assembly from the apparatus and separate the glass plates. Remove the spacers, cut off and discard the stacking gel and immediately proceed with staining.

DETECTION OF PROTEINS IN GELS

Coomassie staining is the most common protein staining method with a detection level of the order of 1 µg to 10 µg of protein per band. Silver staining is the most sensitive method for staining proteins in gels and a band containing 10 ng to 100 ng can be detected.

All of the steps in gel staining are done at room temperature with gentle shaking (e.g. on an orbital shaker platform) in any convenient container. Gloves must be worn when staining gels, since fingerprints will stain.

Coomassie staining. Immerse the gel in a large excess of *Coomassie staining solution R* and allow to stand for at least 1 h. Remove the staining solution.

Destain the gel with a large excess of *destaining solution R*. Change the destaining solution several times, until the stained protein bands are clearly distinguishable on a clear background. The more thoroughly the gel is destained, the smaller is the amount of protein that can be detected by the method. Destaining can be speeded up by including a few grams of anion-exchange resin or a small sponge in the *destaining solution R*.

NOTE: the acid-alcohol solutions used in this procedure do not completely fix proteins in the gel. This can lead to losses of some low-molecular-mass proteins during the staining and destaining of thin gels. Permanent fixation is obtainable by allowing the gel to stand in a mixture of 1 volume of trichloroacetic acid R, 4 volumes of methanol R and 5 volumes of water R for 1 h before it is immersed in the Coomassie staining solution R.

Silver staining. Immerse the gel in a large excess of *fixing solution R* and allow to stand for 1 h. Remove the fixing solution, add fresh fixing solution and incubate either for at least 1 h or overnight, if convenient. Discard the fixing solution and wash the gel in a large excess of *water R* for 1 h. Soak the gel for 15 min in a 1 per cent *V/V* solution of *glutaraldehyde R*. Wash the gel twice for 15 min in a large excess of *water R*. Soak the gel in fresh *silver nitrate reagent R* for 15 min, in darkness. Wash the gel three times for 5 min in a large excess of *water R*. Immerse the gel for about 1 min in *developer solution R* until satisfactory staining has been obtained. Stop the development by incubation in the *blocking solution R* for 15 min. Rinse the gel with *water R*.

DRYING OF STAINED SDS POLYACRYLAMIDE GELS

Depending on the staining method used, gels are treated in a slightly different way. For Coomassie staining, after the destaining step, allow the gel to stand in a 100 g/l solution of *glycerol R* for at least 2 h (overnight incubation is possible). For silver staining, add to the final rinsing a step of 5 min in a 20 g/l solution of *glycerol R*.

Immerse two sheets of porous cellulose film in *water R* and incubate for 5 min to 10 min. Place one of the sheets on a drying frame. Carefully lift the gel and place it on the cellulose film. Remove any trapped air bubbles and pour a few millilitres of *water R* around the edges of the gel. Place the second sheet on top and remove any trapped air bubbles. Complete the assembly of the drying frame. Place in an oven or leave at room temperature until dry.

MOLECULAR-MASS DETERMINATION

Molecular masses of proteins are determined by comparison of their mobilities with those of several marker proteins of known molecular weight. Mixtures of proteins with precisely known molecular masses blended for uniform staining are available for calibrating gels. They are obtainable in various molecular mass ranges. Concentrated stock solutions of proteins of known molecular mass are diluted in the appropriate sample buffer and loaded on the same gel as the protein sample to be studied.

Immediately after the gel has been run, the position of the bromophenol blue tracking dye is marked to identify the leading edge of the electrophoretic ion front. This can be done by cutting notches in the edges of the gel or by inserting a needle soaked in India ink into the gel at the dye front. After staining, measure the migration distances of each protein band (markers and unknowns) from the top of the resolving gel. Divide the migration distance of each protein by the distance travelled by the tracking dye. The normalised migration distances so obtained are called the relative mobilities of the proteins (relative to the dye front) and conventionally denoted as R_f. Construct a plot of the logarithm of the relative molecular masses (M_r) of the protein standards as a function of the R_f values. Note that the graphs are slightly sigmoid. Unknown molecular masses can be estimated by linear regression analysis or interpolation from the curves of log M_r against R_f as long as the values obtained for the unknown samples are positioned along the linear part of the graph.

VALIDATION OF THE TEST

The test is not valid unless the proteins of the molecular mass marker are distributed along 80 per cent of the length of the gel and over the required separation range (e.g. the range covering the product and its dimer or the product and its related impurities) the separation obtained for the relevant protein bands shows a linear relationship between the logarithm of the molecular mass and the R_f. Additional validation requirements with respect to the solution under test may be specified in individual monographs.

QUANTIFICATION OF IMPURITIES

Where the impurity limit is specified in the individual monograph, a reference solution corresponding to that level of impurity should be prepared by diluting the test solution. For example, where the limit is 5 per cent, a reference solution would be a 1:20 dilution of the test solution. No impurity (any band other than the main band) in the electropherogram obtained with the test solution may be more intense than the main band obtained with the reference solution.

Under validated conditions impurities may be quantified by normalisation to the main band using an integrating densitometer. In this case, the responses must be validated for linearity.

01/2005:20232

2.2.32. LOSS ON DRYING

Loss on drying is the loss of mass expressed as per cent *m/m*.

Method. Place the prescribed quantity of the substance to be examined in a weighing bottle previously dried under the conditions prescribed for the substance to be examined. Dry the substance to constant mass or for the prescribed time by one of the following procedures. Where the drying temperature is indicated by a single value rather than a range, drying is carried out at the prescribed temperature ± 2 °C.

a) "in a desiccator": the drying is carried out over *diphosphorus pentoxide R* at atmospheric pressure and at room temperature;

b) "*in vacuo*": the drying is carried out over *diphosphorus pentoxide R*, at a pressure of 1.5 kPa to 2.5 kPa at room temperature;

c) "*in vacuo* within a specified temperature range": the drying is carried out over *diphosphorus pentoxide R*, at a pressure of 1.5 kPa to 2.5 kPa within the temperature range prescribed in the monograph;

d) "in an oven within a specified temperature range": the drying is carried out in an oven within the temperature range prescribed in the monograph;

e) "under high vacuum": the drying is carried out over *diphosphorus pentoxide R* at a pressure not exceeding 0.1 kPa, at the temperature prescribed in the monograph.

If other conditions are prescribed, the procedure to be used is described in full in the monograph.

01/2005:20233

2.2.33. NUCLEAR MAGNETIC RESONANCE SPECTROMETRY

Nuclear magnetic resonance (NMR) spectrometry is based on the fact that nuclei such as ^{1}H, ^{13}C, ^{19}F, ^{31}P possess a permanent nuclear magnetic moment. When placed in an external magnetic field (main field), they take certain well-defined orientations with respect to the direction of this field which correspond to distinct energy levels. For a given field value, transitions between neighbouring energy levels take place due to absorption of electromagnetic radiation of characteristic wavelengths at radio frequencies.

The determination of these frequencies may be made either by sequential search of the resonance conditions (continuous-wave spectrometry) or by simultaneous excitation of all transitions with a multifrequency pulse followed by computer analysis of the free-induction decay of the irradiation emitted as the system returns to the initial state (pulsed spectrometry).

A *proton* magnetic resonance spectrum appears as a set of signals which correspond to protons and are characteristic of their nuclear and electronic environment within the molecule. The separation between a given signal and that of a reference compound is called a chemical shift (δ) and is expressed in parts per million (ppm); it characterises the kind of proton in terms of electronic environment. Signals are frequently split into groups of related peaks, called doublets, triplets, multiplets; this splitting is due to the presence of permanent magnetic fields emanating from adjacent nuclei, particularly from other protons within two to five valence bonds. The intensity of each signal, determined from the area under the signal, is proportional to the number of equivalent protons.

Apparatus. A nuclear magnetic resonance spectrometer for continuous-wave spectrometry consists of a magnet, a low-frequency sweep generator, a sample holder, a radio-frequency transmitter and receiver, a recorder and an electronic integrator. A pulsed spectrometer is additionally equipped with a pulse transmitter and a computer for the acquisition, storage and mathematical transformation of the data into a conventional spectrum.

Use a nuclear magnetic resonance spectrometer operating at not less than 60 MHz for ^{1}H. Unless otherwise prescribed, follow the instructions of the manufacturer.

Before recording the spectrum, verify that:

1) The resolution is equal to 0.5 Hz or less by measuring the peak width at half-height using an adequate scale expansion of:

– either the band at δ 7.33 ppm or at δ 7.51 ppm of the symmetrical multiplet of a 20 per cent *V/V* solution of *dichlorobenzene R* in *deuterated acetone R*,

– or the band at δ 0.00 ppm of a 5 per cent *V/V* solution of *tetramethylsilane R* in *deuterated chloroform R*.

2) The signal-to-noise ratio (*S/N*), measured over the range from δ 2 ppm to δ 5 ppm on the spectrum obtained with a 1 per cent *V/V* solution of *ethylbenzene R* in *deuterated chloroform R*, is at least 25:1. This ratio is calculated as the mean of five successive determinations from the expression:

$$\frac{S}{N} = 2.5\frac{A}{H}$$

A = amplitude, measured in millimetres, of the largest peak of the methylene quartet of ethylbenzene centred at δ 2.65 ppm. The amplitude is measured from a base line constructed from the centre of the noise on either side of this quartet and at a distance of at least 1 ppm from its centre.

H = peak to peak amplitude of the base line noise measured in millimetres obtained between δ 4 ppm and δ 5 ppm.

3) The amplitude of spinning side bands is not greater than 2 per cent of the sample peak height in a tube rotating at a speed appropriate for the spectrometer used.

4) For quantitative measurements verify the repeatability of the integrator responses, using a 5 per cent *V/V* solution of *ethylbenzene R* in *deuterated chloroform R*. Carry out five successive scans of the protons of ethyl groups and determine the mean of the values obtained. None of the individual values differs by more than 2.5 per cent from the mean.

Method. Dissolve the substance to be examined as prescribed and filter; the solution must be clear. Use a chemical shift internal reference compound, which, unless otherwise prescribed, is a solution containing 0.5 per cent *V/V* to 1.0 per cent *V/V* of *tetramethylsilane R* (TMS) in deuterated organic solvents or 5 g/l to 10 g/l of *sodium tetradeuteriodimethylsilapentanoate acid R* (TSP) in *deuterium oxide R*. Take the necessary quantity and record the spectrum.

CONTINUOUS-WAVE SPECTROMETRY

Adjust the spectrometer so that it is operating as closely as possible in the pure absorption mode and use a radio-frequency setting which avoids saturation of the signals. Adjust the controls of the spectrometer so that the strongest peak in the spectrum of the substance to be examined occupies almost the whole of the scale on the recorder chart and that the signal of the internal reference compound corresponds to a chemical shift of δ 0.00 ppm. Record the spectrum over the prescribed spectral width and, unless otherwise specified, at a sweep rate of not more than 2 Hz per second. Record the integral spectrum over the same spectral width and at a suitable sweep rate according to the instrument used. When quantitative measurements are required, these should be obtained as prescribed.

PULSED SPECTROMETRY

Set the spectrometer controls, e.g. pulse flip angle, pulse amplitude, pulse interval, spectral width, number of data points (resolution) and data acquisition rate, as indicated in the manufacturer's instructions and collect the necessary number of free induction decays. After mathematical transformation of the data by the computer, adjust the phase control in order to obtain as far as possible a pure absorption spectrum and calibrate the spectrum relative to the resonance frequency of the chemical shift internal reference compound. Display the spectrum stored in the computer on a suitable output device and, for quantitative measurements, process the integral according to the facility of the instrument.

01/2005:20234

2.2.34. THERMAL ANALYSIS

Thermal analysis is a group of techniques in which the variation of a physical property of a substance is measured as a function of temperature. The most commonly used techniques are those which measure changes of mass or changes in energy of a sample of a substance.

THERMOGRAVIMETRY

Thermogravimetry is a technique in which the mass of a sample of a substance is recorded as a function of temperature according to a controlled temperature programme.

Apparatus. The essential components of a thermobalance are a device for heating or cooling the substance according to a given temperature program, a sample holder in a controlled atmosphere, an electrobalance and a recorder. In some cases the instrument may be coupled to a device permitting the analysis of volatile products.

Temperature verification. Check the temperature scale using a suitable material according to the manufacturer's instructions.

Calibration of the electrobalance. Place a suitable quantity of a suitable certified reference material in the sample holder and record the mass. Set the heating rate according to the manufacturer's instructions and start the temperature increase. Record the thermogravimetric curve as a graph with temperature, or time, on the abscissa, increasing from left to right, and mass on the ordinate, increasing upwards. Stop the temperature increase at about 230 °C. Measure the difference on the graph between the initial and final mass-temperature plateaux, or mass-time plateaux, which corresponds to the loss of mass. The declared loss of mass for the certified reference material is stated on the label.

Method. Apply the same procedure to the substance to be examined, using the conditions prescribed in the monograph. Calculate the loss of mass of the substance to be examined from the difference measured in the graph obtained. Express the loss of mass as per cent $\Delta\ m/m$.

If the apparatus is in frequent use, carry out temperature verification and calibration regularly. Otherwise, carry out such checks before each measurement.

Since the test atmosphere is critical, the following parameters are noted for each measurement: pressure or flow rate, composition of the gas.

DIFFERENTIAL SCANNING CALORIMETRY

Differential Scanning Calorimetry (DSC) is a technique that can be used to demonstrate the energy phenomena produced during heating (or cooling) of a substance (or a mixture of substances) and to determine the changes in enthalpy and specific heat and the temperatures at which these occur.

The technique is used to determine the difference in the flow of heat (with reference to the temperature) evolved or absorbed by the test sample compared with the reference cell, as a function of the temperature. Two types of DSC apparatuses are available, those using power compensation to maintain a null temperature difference between sample and reference and those that apply a constant rate of heating and detect temperature differential as a difference in heat flow between sample and reference.

Apparatus. The apparatus for the power compensation DSC consists of a furnace containing a sample holder with a reference cell and a test cell. The apparatus for the heat flow DSC consists of a furnace containing a single cell with a sample holder for the reference crucible and the test crucible.

A temperature-programming device, thermal detector(s) and a recording system which can be connected to a computer are attached. The measurements are carried out under a controlled atmosphere.

Calibration of the apparatus. Calibrate the apparatus for temperature and enthalpy change, using indium of high purity or any other suitable certified material, according to the manufacturer's instructions. A combination of 2 metals, e.g. indium and zinc may be used to control linearity.

Operating procedure. Weigh in a suitable crucible an appropriate quantity of the substance to be examined; place it in the sample holder. Set the initial and final temperatures, and the heating rate according to the operating conditions prescribed in the monograph.

Begin the analysis and record the differential thermal analysis curve, with the temperature or time on the abscissa (values increasing from left to right) and the energy change on the ordinate (specify whether the change is endothermic or exothermic).

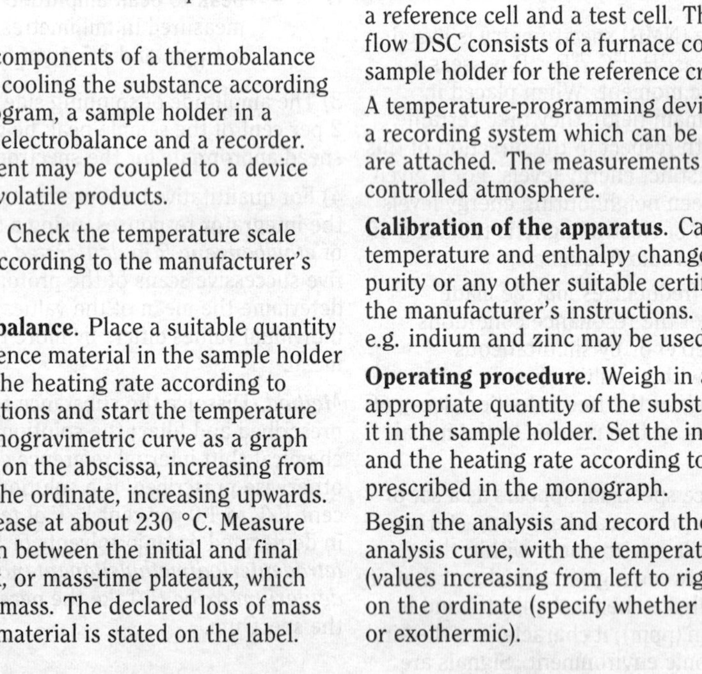

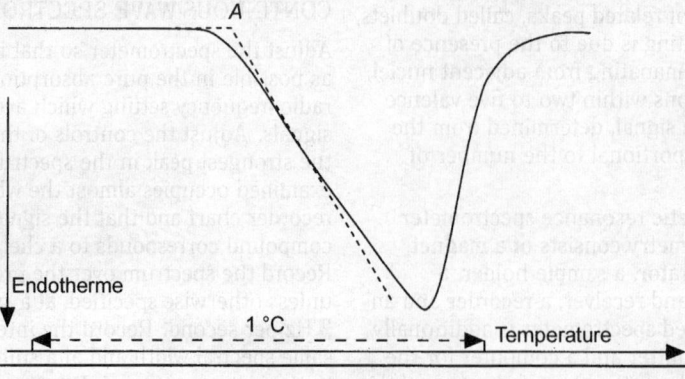

Figure 2.2.34.-1. – *Thermogram*

The temperature at which the phenomenon occurs (the onset temperature) corresponds to the intersection (A) of the extension of the baseline with the tangent at the point of greatest slope (inflexion point) of the curve (see Figure 2.2.34.-1). The end of the thermal phenomenon is indicated by the peak of the curve.

The enthalpy of the phenomenon is proportional to the area under the curve limited by the baseline; the proportionality factor is determined from the measurement of the heat of fusion of a known substance (e.g., indium) under the same operating conditions.

Each thermogram may be accompanied by the following data: conditions employed, record of last calibration, sample size and identification (including thermal history), container, atmosphere (identity, flow rate, pressure), direction and rate of temperature change, instrument and recorder sensitivity.

Applications

Phase changes. Determination of the temperature, heat capacity change and enthalpy of phase changes undergone by a substance as a function of temperature.

solid - solid transition:	allotropy - polymorphism glass transition desolvation amorphous-crystalline
solid - liquid transition:	melting
solid - gas transition:	sublimation
liquid - solid transition:	freezing recrystallisation
liquid - gas transition:	evaporation

Changes in chemical composition. Measurement of heat and temperatures of reaction under given experimental conditions, so that, for example, the kinetics of decomposition or of desolvation can be determined.

Application to phase diagrams. Establishment of phase diagrams for solid mixtures. The establishment of a phase diagram may be an important step in the preformulation and optimisation of the freeze-drying process.

Determination of purity. The measurement of the heat of fusion and the melting point by DSC enables the impurity content of a substance to be determined from a single thermal diagram, requiring the use of only a few milligrams of sample with no need for repeated accurate measurements of the true temperature.

In theory, the melting of an entirely crystalline, pure substance at constant pressure is characterised by a heat of fusion ΔH_f in an infinitely narrow range, corresponding to the melting point T_0. A broadening of this range is a sensitive indicator of impurities. Hence, samples of the same substance, whose impurity contents vary by a few tenths of a per cent, give thermal diagrams that are visually distinct (see Figure 2.2.34.-2).

The determination of the molar purity by DSC is based on the use of a mathematical approximation of the integrated form of the Van't Hoff equation applied to the concentrations (not the activities) in a binary system [$\ln(1 - x_2) = -x_2$ and $T \times T_0 = T_0^2$]:

$$T = T_0 - \frac{RT_0^2}{\Delta H_f} \times x_2 \qquad (1)$$

x_2 = mole fraction of the impurity i.e. the number of molecules of the impurity divided by the total number of molecules in the liquid phase (or molten phase) at temperature T (expressed in kelvins),

T_0 = melting point of the chemically pure substance, in kelvins,

ΔH_f = molar heat of fusion of the substance, in joules,

R = gas constant for ideal gases, in joules·kelvin^{-1}·mole^{-1}.

Hence, the determination of purity by DSC is limited to the detection of impurities forming a eutectic mixture with the principal compound and present at a mole fraction of less than 2 per cent in the substance to be examined.

This method cannot be applied to:

- amorphous substances,
- solvates or polymorphic compounds that are unstable within the experimental temperature range,
- impurities forming solid solutions with the principal substance,
- impurities that are insoluble in the liquid phase or in the melt of the principal substance.

During the heating of the substance to be examined, the impurity melts completely at the temperature of the eutectic mixture. Above this temperature, the solid phase contains

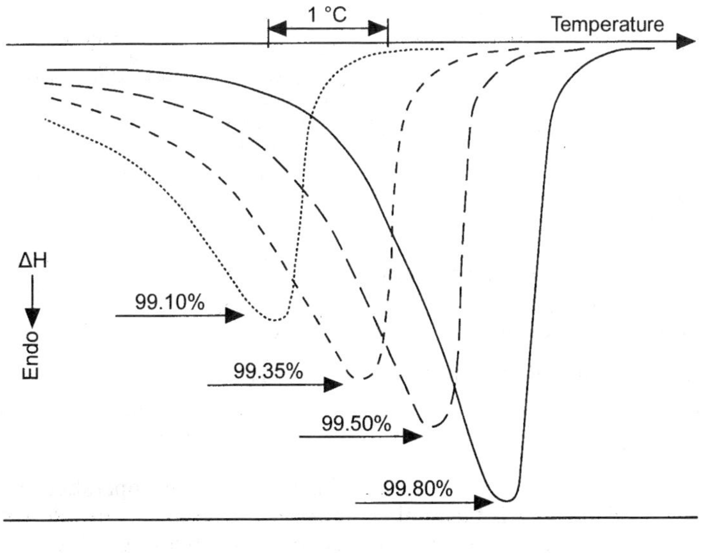

Figure 2.2.34.-2. – *Thermal diagrams according to purity*

only the pure substance. As the temperature increases progressively from the temperature of the eutectic mixture to the melting point of the pure substance, the mole fraction of impurity in the liquid decreases constantly, since the quantity of liquified pure substance increases constantly. For all temperatures above the eutectic point:

$$x_2 = \frac{1}{F} \times x_2^* \quad (2)$$

F = molten fraction of the analysed sample,

x_2^* = mole fraction of the impurity in the analysed sample.

When the entire sample has melted, $F = 1$ and $x_2 = x_2^*$.

If equation (2) is combined with equation (1), the following equation is obtained:

$$T = T_0 - \frac{x_2^* R T_0^2}{\Delta H_f} \times \frac{1}{F}$$

The value of the heat of fusion is obtained by integrating the melting peak.

The melting point T_0 of the pure substance is extrapolated from the plot of $1/F$ versus the temperature expressed in kelvins. The slope α of the curve, obtained after linearisation, if necessary, corresponding to $RT_0^2 \frac{x_2^*}{\Delta H_f}$ allows x_2^* to be evaluated.

The fraction x_2^*, multiplied by 100 gives the mole fraction in per cent for the total eutectic impurities.

THERMOMICROSCOPY

Phase changes may be visualised by thermomicroscopy, a method which enables a sample subjected to a programmed temperature change to be examined, in polarised light, under a microscope.

The observations made in thermomicroscopy allow the nature of the phenomena detected using thermogravimetry and differential thermal analysis to be clearly identified.

Apparatus. The apparatus consists of a microscope fitted with a light polariser, a hot plate, a temperature and heating rate and/or cooling rate programmer and a recording system for the transition temperatures. A video camera and video recorder may be added.

01/2005:20235

2.2.35. OSMOLALITY

Osmolality is a practical means of giving an overall measure of the contribution of the various solutes present in a solution to the osmotic pressure of the solution.

An acceptable approximation for the osmolality ξ_m of a given aqueous solution is given by:

$$\xi_m = \upsilon m \Phi$$

If the solute is not ionised, $\upsilon = 1$; otherwise υ is the total number of ions already present or formed by solvolysis from one molecule of solute.

m = molality of the solution, that is the number of moles of solute per kilogram of solvent,

Φ = molal osmotic coefficient which takes account of the interactions between ions of opposite charge in the solution. It is dependent on the value of m. As the complexity of solutions increases, Φ becomes difficult to measure.

The unit of osmolality is osmole per kilogram (osmol/kg), but the submultiple milliosmole per kilogram (mosmol/kg) is usually used.

Unless otherwise prescribed, osmolality is determined by measurement of the depression of freezing point. The following relationship exists between the osmolality and the depression of freezing point ΔT:

$$\xi_m = \frac{\Delta T}{1.86} \times 1000 \text{ mosmol/kg}$$

Apparatus. The apparatus (osmometer) consists of:

- a means of cooling the container used for the measurement,
- a system for measuring temperature consisting of a resistor sensitive to temperature (thermistor), with an appropriate current or potential-difference measurement device that may be graduated in temperature depression or directly in osmolality,
- a means of mixing the sample is usually included.

Method. Prepare reference solutions as described in Table 2.2.35.-1, as required. Determine the zero of the apparatus using *water R*. Calibrate the apparatus using the reference solutions: introduce 50 µl to 250 µl of sample into the measurement cell and start the cooling system. Usually, the mixing device is programmed to operate at a temperature below that expected through cryoscopic depression to prevent supercooling. A suitable device indicates attainment of equilibrium. Before each measurement, rinse the measurement cell with the solution to be examined.

Table 2.2.35.-1. – *Reference solutions for osmometer calibration*

Mass in grams of *sodium chloride R* per kilogram of *water R*	Real osmolality (mosmol/kg)	Ideal osmolality (mosmol/kg)	Molal osmotic coefficient	Cryoscopic depression (°C)
3.087	100	105.67	0.9463	0.186
6.260	200	214.20	0.9337	0.372
9.463	300	323.83	0.9264	0.558
12.684	400	434.07	0.9215	0.744
15.916	500	544.66	0.9180	0.930
19.147	600	655.24	0.9157	1.116
22.380	700	765.86	0.9140	1.302

Carry out the same operations with the test sample. Read directly the osmolality or calculate it from the measured depression of freezing point. The test is not valid unless the value found is within two values of the calibration scale.

01/2005:20236

2.2.36. POTENTIOMETRIC DETERMINATION OF IONIC CONCENTRATION USING ION-SELECTIVE ELECTRODES

Ideally, the potential E of an ion-selective electrode varies linearly with the logarithm of the activity a_i of a given ion, as expressed by the Nernst equation:

$$E = E_0 + 2.303\frac{RT}{z_i F}\log a_i$$

E_0 = part of the constant potential due to the apparatus used,

R = gas constant,

T = absolute temperature,

F = Faraday's number,

z_i = charge number of the ion including its sign.

At a constant ionic strength, the following holds:

$$E = E_0 + \frac{k}{z_i}\log f C_i$$

C_i = molar concentration of the ion,

f = the activity coefficient ($a_i = fC_i$),

k = $\frac{RT}{F}$

If: $E_0 + \frac{k}{z_i}\log f = E'_0$ and $S = \frac{k}{z_i}$

S = slope of the calibration curve of the electrode,

the following holds: $E = E'_0 + S\log C_i$

and for $-\log C_i = pC_i$: $E = E'_0 - SpC_i$.

The potentiometric determination of the ion concentration is carried out by measuring the potential difference between two suitable electrodes immersed in the solution to be examined; the indicator electrode is selective for the ion to be determined and the other is a reference electrode.

Apparatus. Use a voltmeter allowing measurements to the nearest 0.1 millivolt and whose input impedance is at least one hundred times greater than that of the electrodes used.

Ion-selective electrodes may be primary electrodes with a crystal or non-crystal membrane or with a rigid matrix (for example, glass electrodes), or electrodes with charged (positive or negative) or uncharged mobile carriers, or sensitised electrodes (enzymatic-substrate electrodes, gas-indicator electrodes). The reference electrode is generally a silver–silver chloride electrode or a calomel electrode, with suitable junction liquids producing no interference.

Procedure. Carry out each measurement at a temperature constant to ± 0.5 °C, taking into account the variation of the slope of the electrode with temperature (see Table 2.2.36.-1). Adjust the ionic strength and possibly the pH of the solution to be analysed using the buffer reagent described in the monograph and equilibrate the electrode by immersing it in the solution to be analysed, under slow and uniform stirring, until a constant reading is obtained.

Table 2.2.36.-1. - *Values of k at different temperatures*

Temperature (°C)	k
20	0.0582
25	0.0592
30	0.0602

If the electrode system is used frequently, check regularly the repeatability and the stability of responses, and the linearity of the calibration curve or the calculation algorithm in the range of concentrations of the test solution; if not, carry out the test before each set of measurements. The response of the electrode may be regarded as linear if the slope S of the calibration curve is approximately equal to k/z_i, per unit of pC_i.

METHOD I (DIRECT CALIBRATION)

Measure at least three times in succession the potential of at least three reference solutions spanning the expected concentration of the test solution. Calculate the calibration curve, or plot on a chart the mean potential E obtained against the concentration of the ion to be determined expressed as $-\log C_i$ or pC_i.

Prepare the test solution as prescribed in the monograph; measure the potential three times and, from the mean potential, calculate the concentration of the ion to be determined using the calibration curve.

METHOD II (MULTIPLE STANDARD ADDITIONS)

Prepare the test solution as prescribed in the monograph. Measure the potential at equilibrium E_T of a volume V_T of this solution of unknown concentration C_T of the ion to be determined. Make at least three consecutive additions of a volume V_S negligible compared to V_T ($V_S \leq 0.01V_T$) of a reference solution of a concentration C_S known to be within the linear part of the calibration curve. After each addition, measure the potential and calculate the difference of potential ΔE between the measured potential and E_T. ΔE is related to the concentration of the ion to be determined by the equation:

$$\Delta E = S\log\left(1 + \frac{C_S V_S}{C_T V_T}\right)$$

or

$$10^{\frac{\Delta E}{S}} = 1 + \frac{C_S V_S}{C_T V_T}$$

V_T = volume of the test solution,

C_T = concentration of the ion to be determined in the test solution,

V_S = added volume of the reference solution,

C_S = concentration of the ion to be determined in the reference solution,

S = slope of the electrode determined experimentally, at constant temperature, by measuring the difference between the potentials obtained with two reference solutions whose concentrations differ by a factor of ten and are situated within the range where the calibration curve is linear.

Plot on a graph $10^{\frac{\Delta E}{S}}$ (y-axis) against V_S (x-axis) and extrapolate the line obtained until it intersects the x-axis. At the intersection, the concentration C_T of the test solution in the ion to be determined is given by the equation:

$$C_T = \frac{C_S V_S}{V_T}$$

METHOD III (SINGLE STANDARD ADDITION)

To a volume V_T of the test solution prepared as prescribed in the monograph, add a volume V_S of a reference solution containing an amount of the ion to be determined known to give a response situated in the linear part of the calibration curve. Prepare a blank solution in the same conditions. Measure at least three times the potentials of the test solution and the blank solution, before and after adding the reference solution. Calculate the concentration C_T of the ion to be analysed using the following equation and making the necessary corrections for the blank:

$$C_T = \frac{C_S V_S}{10^{\frac{\Delta E}{S}}(V_T + V_S) - V_T}$$

V_T = volume of the test solution or the blank,

C_T = concentration of the ion to be determined in the test solution,

V_S = added volume of the reference solution,

C_S = concentration of the ion to be determined in the reference solution,

ΔE = difference between the average potentials measured before and after adding V_S,

S = slope of the electrode determined experimentally, at constant temperature, by measuring the difference between the potentials obtained from two reference solutions whose concentrations differ by a factor of ten and are situated within the range where the calibration curve is linear.

01/2005:20237

2.2.37. X-RAY FLUORESCENCE SPECTROMETRY(3)

Wavelength dispersive X-ray fluorescence spectrometry is a procedure that uses the measurement of the intensity of the fluorescent radiation emitted by an element having an atomic number between 11 and 92 excited by a continuous primary X-ray radiation. The intensity of the fluorescence produced by a given element depends on the concentration of this element in the sample but also on the absorption by the matrix of the incident and fluorescent radiation.

At trace levels, where the calibration curve is linear, the intensity of the fluorescent radiation emitted by an element in a given matrix, at a given wavelength, is proportional to the concentration of this element and inversely proportional to the mass absorption coefficient of the matrix at this wavelength.

Method. Set and use the instrument in accordance with the instructions given by the manufacturer. Liquid samples are placed directly in the instrument; solid samples are first compressed into pellets, sometimes after mixing with a suitable binder.

To determine the concentration of an element in a sample, it is necessary to measure the net impulse rate produced by one or several standard preparations containing known amounts of this element in given matrices and to calculate or measure the mass absorption coefficient of the matrix of the sample to be analysed.

Calibration. From a calibration solution or a series of dilutions of the element to be analysed in various matrices, determine the slope of the calibration curve b_0 from the following equation:

$$b_0 \frac{1}{\mu_M} = \frac{I_C^N}{C}$$

μ_M = absorption coefficient of the matrix M, calculated or measured,

I_C^N = net impulse rate,

C = concentration of the element to be assayed in the standard preparation.

Mass absorption coefficent of the matrix of the sample. If the empirical formula of the sample to be analysed is known, calculate its mass absorption coefficient from the known elemental composition and the tabulated elemental mass absorption coefficients. If the elemental composition is unknown, determine the mass absorption coefficient of the sample matrix by measuring the intensity of the scattered X-radiation I_U (Compton scattering) from the following equation:

$$\frac{1}{\mu_{MP}} = a + bI_U$$

μ_{MP} = mass absorption coefficient of the sample,

I_U = scattered X-radiation.

Determination of the net pulse rate of the element to be determined in the sample. Calculate the net impulse rate I_{EP}^N of the element to be determined from the measured intensity of the fluorescence line and the intensity of the background line(s), allowing for any tube contaminants present.

Calculation of the trace content. If the concentration of the element is in the linear part of the calibration curve, it can be calculated using the following equation:

$$C = \frac{I_{EP}^N}{b_0 \frac{1}{\mu_{MP}}} \times f$$

f = dilution factor.

01/2005:20238

2.2.38. CONDUCTIVITY

The conductivity of a solution (κ) is, by definition, the reciprocal of resistivity (ρ). Resistivity is defined as the quotient of the electric field and the density of the current. The resistance R (Ω) of a conductor of cross-section S (cm^2) and length L (cm) is given by the expression:

$$R = \rho \frac{L}{S}$$

(3) G. Andermann &M.W. Kemp, Analytical Chemistry 30 1306 (1958). Z.H. Kalman & L. Heller, Analytical Chemistry 34 946 (1962). R.C. Reynolds, Jr., The American Mineralogist 46 1133 (1963). R.O. Müller, Spectrochimica Acta 20 143 (1964). R.O. Müller, Spectrochemische Analyse mit Röntgenfluoreszenz, R. Oldenburg München-Wien (1967).

thus: $R = \frac{1}{\kappa} \cdot \frac{L}{S}$ or $\kappa = \frac{1}{R} \cdot \frac{L}{S}$

The unit of conductivity in the International System is the siemens per metre ($S \cdot m^{-1}$). In practice, the electrical conductivity of a solution is expressed in siemens per centimetre ($S \cdot cm^{-1}$) or in microsiemens per centimetre ($\mu S \cdot cm^{-1}$). The unit of resistivity in the International System is the ohm-metre (Ωm). The resistivity of a solution is generally expressed in ohm-centimetres (Ωcm). Unless otherwise prescribed, the reference temperature for the expression of conductivity or resistivity is 20 °C.

APPARATUS

The apparatus used (conductivity meter or resistivity meter) measures the resistance of the column of liquid between the electrodes of the immersed measuring device (conductivity cell). The apparatus is supplied with alternating current to avoid the effects of electrode polarisation. It is equipped with a temperature compensation device or a precision thermometer.

The conductivity cell contains two parallel platinum electrodes coated with platinum black, each with a surface area *S*, and separated from the other by a distance *L*. Both are generally protected by a glass tube that allows good exchange between the solution and the electrodes.

The cell constant *C* of the conductivity cell is given in cm^{-1} according to the equation:

$$C = \alpha \frac{L}{S}$$

α = a dimensionless numerical coefficient, which is characteristic of the cell design.

REAGENTS

Prepare three standard solutions of *potassium chloride R* containing 0.7455 g, 0.0746 g and 0.0149 g, respectively, of *potassium chloride R* per 1000.0 g of solution, using *carbon dioxide-free water R*, prepared from *distilled water R* whose conductivity does not exceed 2 $\mu S \cdot cm^{-1}$.

The conductivity and resistivity of these three solutions at 20 °C are given below:

Table 2.2.38.-1. - *Conductivity and resistivity of potassium chloride solutions*

Concentration in g per 1000.0 g of solution	Conductivity $\mu S \cdot cm^{-1}$	Resistivity Ωcm
0.7455	1330	752
0.0746	133.0	7519
0.0149	26.6	37594

If the determination cannot be made at the temperature of 20 °C, use the following equation to correct the conductivity of the potassium chloride solutions indicated in the table. This equation is valid only for temperatures in the range 20 ± 5 °C.

$$C_T = C_{20}\left[1 + 0.021\,(T - 20)\right]$$

T = measurement temperature prescribed in the monograph,

C_T = Conductivity of the solution at T °C,

C_{20} = Conductivity of the solution at 20 °C.

OPERATING PROCEDURE

Determination of the cell constant

Choose a conductivity cell that is appropriate for the conductivity of the solution to be examined. The higher the expected conductivity, the higher the cell constant that must be chosen (low ρ) so that the value *R* measured is as large as possible for the apparatus used. Commonly used conductivity cells have cell constants of the order of 0.1 cm^{-1}, 1 cm^{-1} and 10 cm^{-1}. Use a standard solution of *potassium chloride R* that is appropriate for the measurement. Rinse the cell several times with *carbon dioxide-free water R* prepared from *distilled water R* and at least twice with the potassium chloride solution used for the determination of the cell constant of the conductivity cell. Measure the resistance of the conductivity cell using the potassium chloride solution at 20 ± 0.1 °C or at the temperature prescribed in the monograph. The constant *C* (in cm^{-1}) of the conductivity cell is given by the expression:

$$C = R_{KCl} \cdot \kappa_{KCl}$$

R_{KCl} = measured resistance, expressed in mega-ohms,

κ_{KCl} = conductivity of the standard solution of *potassium chloride R* used, expressed in $\mu S \cdot cm^{-1}$.

The measured constant *C* of the conductivity cell must be within 5 per cent of the given value.

Determination of the conductivity of the solution to be examined

After calibrating the apparatus with one of the standard solutions, rinse the conductivity cell several times with *carbon dioxide-free water R* prepared from *distilled water R* and at least twice with the aqueous solution to be examined at 20 ± 0.1 °C or at the temperature prescribed in the monograph. Carry out successive measurements as described in the monograph.

01/2005:20239

2.2.39. MOLECULAR MASS DISTRIBUTION IN DEXTRANS

Examine by size-exclusion chromatography (*2.2.30*).

Test solution. Dissolve 0.200 g of the substance to be examined in the mobile phase and dilute to 10 ml with the mobile phase.

Marker solution. Dissolve 5 mg of *glucose R* and 2 mg of *dextran V_0 CRS* in 1 ml of the mobile phase.

Calibration solutions. Dissolve separately in 1 ml of the mobile phase 15 mg of *dextran 4 for calibration CRS*, 15 mg of *dextran 10 for calibration CRS*, 20 mg of *dextran 40 for calibration CRS*, 20 mg of *dextran 70 for calibration CRS* and 20 mg of *dextran 250 for calibration CRS*.

System suitability solution. Dissolve either 20 mg of *dextran 40 for performance test CRS* (for dextran 40) or 20 mg of *dextran 60/70 for performance test CRS* (for dextran 60 and dextran 70) in 1 ml of the mobile phase.

The chromatographic procedure may be carried out using:

- a column 0.3 m long and 10 mm in internal diameter, packed with *cross-linked agarose for chromatography R* or a series of columns, 0.3 m long and 10 mm in internal diameter, packed with *polyether hydroxylated gel for chromatography R*,
- as the mobile phase, at a flow rate of 0.5-1 ml/min, kept constant to ± 1 per cent per hour, a solution containing 7 g of *anhydrous sodium sulphate R* and 1 g of *chlorobutanol R* in 1 litre of *water R*,

2. Methods of analysis

– as detector a differential refractometer,

– a 100 µl to 200 µl loop injector,

maintaining the system at a constant temperature (± 0.1 °C).

CALIBRATION OF THE CHROMATOGRAPHIC SYSTEM

Carry out replicate injections of the chosen volume of the marker solution. The chromatogram shows 2 peaks, the first of which corresponds to *dextran V_0 CRS* and the second of which corresponds to *dextrose R*. From the elution volume of the peak corresponding to dextran V_0, calculate the void volume V_0 and from the peak corresponding to dextrose, calculate the total volume V_t.

Inject the chosen volume of each of the calibration solutions. Draw carefully the baseline of each of the chromatograms. Divide each chromatogram into *p* (at least 60) equal vertical sections (corresponding to equal elution volumes). In each section *i*, corresponding to an elution volume V_i measure the height (y_i) of the chromatogram line above the baseline and calculate the coefficient of distribution K_i using the expression:

$$\frac{(V_i - V_0)}{(V_t - V_0)} \qquad (1)$$

V_0 = void volume of the column, determined using the peak corresponding to *dextran V_0 CRS* in the chromatogram obtained with the marker solution,

V_t = total volume of the column, determined using the peak corresponding to glucose in the chromatogram obtained with the marker solution,

V_i = elution volume of section *i* in the chromatogram obtained with each of the calibration solutions.

Carry out the calibration using either of the following methods.

Calibration by plotting of the curve. For each of the dextrans for calibration calculate the coefficient of distribution K_{max} corresponding to the maximum height of the chromatographic line, using expression (1). Plot on semilogarithmic paper the values of K_{max} (on the *x*-axis) against the declared molecular mass at the maximum height of the chromatographic line (M_{max}) of each of the dextrans for calibration and glucose. Draw a first calibration curve through the points obtained, extrapolating it from the point K_{max} obtained with *dextran 250 for calibration CRS* to the lowest *K* value obtained for this CRS (Figure 2.2.39.-1). Using this first calibration curve, transform, for each chromatogram, all K_i values into the corresponding molecular mass M_i, thus obtaining the molecular mass distribution. Calculate for each dextran for calibration the average molecular mass M_w using equation (3) below. If the calculated values for M_w do not differ by more than 5 per cent from those declared for each of the dextrans for calibration and the mean difference is within ± 3 per cent, the calibration curve is approved. If not, move the calibration curve along the y-axis and repeat the procedure above until the calculated and the declared values for M_w do not differ by more than 5 per cent.

Calibration by calculation of the curve. Calculate from equations (2) and (3) below, using a suitable method[(4)], values for b_1, b_2, b_3, b_4 and b_5 that give values of M_w within 5 per cent of the declared values of each of the dextrans for calibration and 180 ± 2 for glucose:

$$M_i = b_5 + e^{\left(b_4 + b_1 K_i + b_2 K_i^2 + b_3 K_i^3\right)} \qquad (2)$$

$$\overline{M}_w = \frac{\sum_{i=1}^{p} (y_i M_i)}{\sum_{i=1}^{p} y_i} \qquad (3)$$

p = number of sections dividing the chromatograms,

y_i = height of the chromatographic line above the baseline in section *i*,

M_i = molecular mass in section *i*.

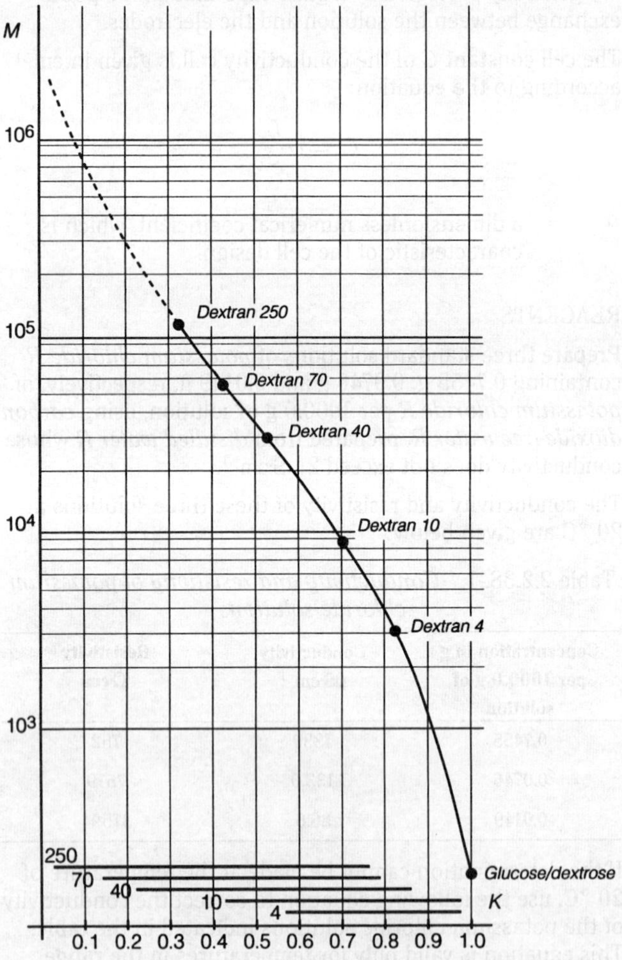

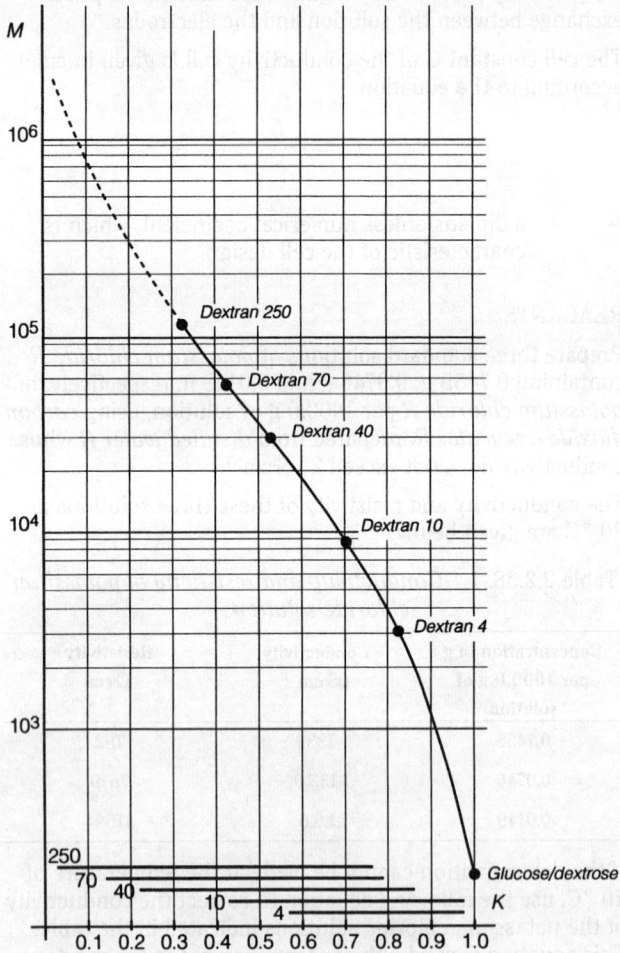

Figure 2.2.39.-1. - *Example of a calibration curve.*

The dotted line corresponds to the part of the curve that is extrapolated. Horizontal lines at the bottom of the figure represent the width and the position of the chromatographic line obtained with each of the dextrans for calibration.

(4) An iterative method such as the Gauss-Newton method modified by Hartley is suitable (see O. Hartley, Tecnometrics, 3 (1961) and G. Nilsson and K. Nilsson, J. Chromat. 101, 137 (1974)). A curve-fitting programme for microcomputers, capable of non-linear regression, may be used.

SYSTEM SUITABILITY

Inject the chosen volume of the appropriate system suitability solution.

Average molecular mass of dextran for performance test CRS. Calculate the average molecular mass M_w as indicated under Calibration of the chromatographic system, using either the plotted calibration curve or the values obtained above for b_1, b_2, b_3, b_4 and b_5. The test is not valid unless M_w is:

- 41 000 to 47 000 (*dextran 40 for performance test CRS*),
- 67 000 to 75 000 (*dextran 60/70 for performance test CRS*).

Average molecular mass of the 10 per cent high-fraction dextran. Calculate M_w for the 10 per cent high-fraction dextran eluted through section n using the equation:

$$M_w = \frac{\sum_{i=1}^{n} (y_i M_i)}{\sum_{i=1}^{n} y_i} \quad (4)$$

in which n is defined by the expressions:

$$\sum_{i=1}^{n} y_i \leq 0.1 \left(\sum_{i=1}^{p} y_i \right) \quad (5)$$

$$\sum_{i=1}^{n+1} y_i > 0.1 \left(\sum_{i=1}^{p} y_i \right) \quad (6)$$

p = number of sections dividing the chromatograms,

y_i = height of the chromatographic line above the baseline in section i,

M_i = molecular mass in section i.

The test is not valid unless M_w of the 10 per cent high fraction dextran is:

- 110 000 to 130 000 (*dextran 40 for performance test CRS*),
- 190 000 to 230 000 (*dextran 60/70 for performance test CRS*).

Average molecular mass of the 10 per cent low-fraction dextran. Calculate M_w for the 10 per cent low-fraction dextran eluted in and after section m using the expression:

$$M_w = \frac{\sum_{i=m}^{p} (y_i M_i)}{\sum_{i=m}^{p} y_i} \quad (7)$$

in which m is defined by the expressions:

$$\sum_{i=m}^{p} y_i \leq 0.1 \left(\sum_{i=1}^{p} y_i \right) \quad (8)$$

$$\sum_{i=m-1}^{p} y_i > 0.1 \left(\sum_{i=1}^{p} y_i \right) \quad (9)$$

p = number of sections dividing the chromatograms,

y_i = height of the chromatographic line above the baseline in section i,

M_i = molecular mass in section i.

The test is not valid unless M_w of the 10 per cent low-fraction dextran is:

- 6000 to 8500 (*dextran 40 for performance test CRS*),
- 7000 to 11 000 (*dextran 60/70 for performance test CRS*).

MOLECULAR MASS DISTRIBUTION OF THE DEXTRAN TO BE ANALYSED

Inject the chosen volume of the test solution and calculate M_w of the total molecular mass distribution, M_w of the 10 per cent high-fraction dextran and M_w of the 10 per cent low-fraction dextran as indicated under System suitability.

01/2005:20240

2.2.40. NEAR-INFRARED SPECTROPHOTOMETRY

Near-infrared (NIR) spectrophotometry is a technique with wide and varied applications in pharmaceutical analysis. The NIR spectral range extends from about 780 nm to about 2500 nm (from about 12 800 cm^{-1} to about 4000 cm^{-1}). In some cases the most useful information is found in the spectral range from about 1700 nm to about 2500 nm (from about 6000 cm^{-1} to 4000 cm^{-1}). NIR spectra are dominated by C-H, N-H, O-H and S-H overtone resonances and combinations of fundamental vibrational modes; they have a high informative character if the information is extracted by suitable chemometric algorithms. NIR bands are much weaker than the fundamental mid-IR vibrations from which they originate. Because molar absorptivities in the NIR range are low, radiation typically penetrates several millimeters into materials, including solids. Furthermore, many materials such as glass are relatively transparent in this region.

Measurements can be made directly on *in situ* samples, in addition to standard sampling and testing procedures. Physical as well as chemical information, both qualitative and quantitative, is available from NIR spectra. However, direct comparison of the spectrum obtained with the substance being examined with a reference spectrum of a chemical reference substance, as used in infrared absorption spectrophotometry, is not appropriate. Suitable validated mathematical treatment of the data is required.

NIR spectrophotometry has a wide variety of applications for both chemical and physical analysis, for example:

chemical analysis

- identification of active substances, excipients, dosage forms, manufacturing intermediates, chemical raw materials and packaging materials,
- quantification of active substances and excipients, determination of chemical values such as hydroxyl value, iodine value, acid value, determination of water content, determination of degree of hydroxylation, control of solvent content,
- process control.

physical analysis

- crystalline form and crystallinity, polymorphism, pseudopolymorphism, particle size,
- dissolution behaviour, disintegration pattern, hardness,
- examination of film properties,
- process control, for example monitoring of blending and granulation.

Measurements in the NIR region are influenced by many chemical and physical factors as described below; reproducibility and relevance of results depend on control of these factors and measurements are usually valid only for a defined calibration model.

APPARATUS

NIR spectrophotometers are used for recording spectra in the region of about 780 nm to about 2500 nm (about 12 800 cm^{-1} to about 4000 cm^{-1}). All NIR measurements are based on passing light through or into a sample and measuring the attenuation of the emerging (transmitted, scattered or reflected) beam. Spectrophotometers for measurement in the NIR region consist of a suitable light source, a monochromator or interferometer. Common monochromators are acousto-optical tuneable filters (AOTF), gratings or prisms. High intensity light sources such as quartz or tungsten lamps or similar are used. The tungsten lamp light source can be highly stabilised. Therefore many NIR instruments have the single-beam design. Silicon, lead sulphide, indium arsenide, indium gallium arsenide, mercury cadmium telluride (MCT) and deuterated triglycine sulphate are commonly used detector materials. Conventional cuvette sample holders, fibre-optic probes, transmission dip cells and spinning or traversing sample holders are a few common sampling devices. The selection is based on the intended application, paying particular attention to the suitability of the sampling system for the type of sample to be analysed. Suitable data processing and evaluation units are usually part of the system.

MEASUREMENT METHODS

Transmission mode. Transmittance (*T*) is a measure of the decrease in radiation intensity at given wavelengths when radiation is passed through the sample. The sample is placed in the optical beam between the source and detector. The arrangement is analogous to that in many conventional spectrophotometers and the result can be presented directly in terms of transmittance (*T*) or/and absorbance (*A*).

$T = \frac{I}{I_0}$,

I_0 = intensity of incident radiation,

I = intensity of transmitted radiation,

$$A = -\log_{10} T = \log_{10}\left(\frac{1}{T}\right) = \log_{10}\left(\frac{I_0}{I}\right).$$

Diffuse reflection mode. The diffuse reflection mode gives a measure of reflectance (*R*), the ratio of the intensity of light reflected from the sample (*I*) to that reflected from a background or reference reflective surface (I_r). NIR radiation can penetrate a substantial distance into the sample, where it can be absorbed by vibrational combinations and overtone resonances of the analyte species present in the sample. Non-absorbed radiation is reflected back from the sample to the detector. NIR reflectance spectra are typically obtained by calculating and plotting log (1/*R*) versus the wavelength or wavenumbers.

$R = \frac{I}{I_r}$,

I = intensity of light diffusively reflected from the sample,

I_r = intensity of light reflected from the background or reference reflective surface,

$$A_R = \log_{10}\left(\frac{1}{R}\right) = \log_{10}\left(\frac{I_r}{I}\right).$$

Transflection mode. This mode is a combination of transmittance and reflectance. In the measurement of transflectance (T^*) a mirror or a diffuse reflectance surface is used to reflect the radiation transmitted through the sample a second time and thus doubling the pathlength. Non-absorbed radiation is reflected back from the sample to the detector.

$T^* = \frac{I}{I_T}$,

I_T = intensity of transflected radiation, without sample

I = intensity of transmitted and reflected radiation measured with the sample,

$$A^* = \log_{10}\left(\frac{1}{T^*}\right).$$

SAMPLE PREPARATION/PRESENTATION

Transmission mode. The measurement of transmittance (*T*) is dependent on a background transmittance spectrum for its calculation. A background reference can be air, an empty cell, and a solvent blank or in special cases a reference sample. The method generally applies to liquids, diluted or undiluted, dispersions, solutions and solids. For transmittance measurements of solids, a suitable sample accessory is to be used. The samples are examined in a cell of suitable pathlength (generally 0.5-4 mm), transparent to NIR radiation, or by immersion of a fibre optic probe of a suitable configuration, which yields a spectrum situated in a zone of transmission compatible with the specifications of the apparatus and appropriate for the intended purpose.

Diffuse reflection mode. This method generally applies to solids. The sample is examined in a suitable device. Care must be taken to make the measuring conditions as reproducible as possible from one sample to another. When immersing a fibre optic probe in the sample, care must be taken in the positioning of the probe to ensure that it remains stationary during the acquisition of the spectra and that the measuring conditions are as reproducible as possible from one sample to another. The reflected radiation of a background reference is scanned to obtain the baseline, and then the reflectance of one or more analytical samples is measured. Common reflectance references are ceramic tiles, perfluorinated polymers and gold. Other suitable materials may be used. Only spectra measured against a background possessing the same optical properties can be directly compared with one another. The particle size, water of hydration and state of solvation must be taken into consideration.

Transflection mode. A reflector is placed behind the sample so as to double the pathlength. This configuration can be adopted to share the same instrument geometry with reflectance and fibre optic probe systems where the source and the detector are on the same side of the sample. The sample is examined in a cell with a mirror or a suitable diffusive reflector, made either of metal or of an inert substance (for example titanium dioxide) not absorbing in the NIR region.

FACTORS AFFECTING SPECTRAL RESPONSE

Sample temperature. This parameter is important for aqueous solutions and many liquids, where a difference of a few degrees can result in substantial spectral changes. Temperature is also an important parameter for solids and powders containing water.

Moisture and solvent residues. Moisture and solvent residues present in the samples will contribute significant absorption bands in the NIR region.

Sample thickness. Sample thickness is a known source of spectral variability and must be understood and/or controlled. For example, in a reflection measurement the sample may be "infinitely" thick, or thinner samples of constant thickness must have a stable, diffusively reflecting backing material of constant, and preferably high reflectivity.

Sample optical properties. In solids, both surface and bulk scattering properties of samples must be taken into account. Spectra of physically, chemically or optically heterogeneous samples may require sample averaging by increasing the beam size or examining multiple samples or spinning the probe. Certain factors such as differing degree of compaction or particle size in powdered materials and surface finish can cause significant spectral differences.

Polymorphism. The variations in crystalline structure (polymorphism) influence the spectra. Hence different crystalline forms as well as the amorphous form of a solid may be distinguished from one another on the basis of their NIR spectra. Where multiple crystalline forms are present, care must be taken to ensure that the calibration standards have a distribution of forms relevant to the intended application.

Age of samples. Samples may exhibit changes in their chemical, physical or optical properties over time. Care must be taken to ensure that samples for NIR analysis are representative of those used for calibration. If samples of different age are to be analysed, potential differences in the properties must be accounted for.

CONTROL OF INSTRUMENT PERFORMANCE

Use the apparatus according to the manufacturer's instructions and carry out the prescribed verification at regular intervals, according to the use of the apparatus and the substances to be tested.

Verification of the wavelength scale (except for filter apparatus). Verify the wavelength scale employed, generally in the region between about 780 nm and about 2500 nm (about 12 800 cm^{-1} to about 4000 cm^{-1}) or in the intended spectral range using one or more suitable wavelength standards which have characteristic maxima or minima within the range of wavelengths to be used. For example, methylene chloride or a mixture of rare-earth oxides are suitable reference materials. Take one spectrum with the same spectral resolution used to obtain the certified value, and measure the position of at least 3 peaks distributed over the range used. Acceptable tolerances are ± 1 nm at 1200 nm, ± 1 nm at 1600 nm and ± 1.5 nm at 2000 nm (± 8 cm^{-1} at 8300 cm^{-1}, ± 4 cm^{-1} at 6250 cm^{-1} and ± 4 cm^{-1} at 5000 cm^{-1}). For the reference material used, apply the tolerance for the nearest wavelength (wavenumber) from the above for each peak used. For FT instruments, the calibration of the wavenumber scale may be performed using a narrow water-vapour line at 7299.86 cm^{-1} or a narrow line from a certified material. For rare-earth oxides, NIST 1920 (a) is the most appropriate reference.

Measurement in transmission mode. Methylene chloride R may be used at an optical pathlength of 1.0 mm. Methylene chloride has characteristic sharp bands at 1155 nm, 1366 nm, 1417 nm, 1690 nm, 1838 nm, 1894 nm, 2068 nm and 2245 nm. The bands at 1155 nm, 1417 nm, 1690 nm and 2245 nm are used for calibration. Other suitable standards may also be used.

Measurement in diffuse reflection (reflectance) mode. A mixture of dysprosium, holmium and erbium oxides (1+1+1 by mass) or other certified material may be used. This reference material exhibits characteristic peaks at 1261 nm, 1681 nm and 1935 nm. If it is not possible to use external solid standards and if measurements of diffuse reflection are carried out in cells or if fibre optic probes are used, a suspension of 1.2 g of *titanium dioxide R* in about 4 ml of *methylene chloride R*, vigorously shaken, is used directly in the cell or probe. The spectrum is recorded after 2 min. Titanium dioxide has no absorption in the NIR range. Spectra are recorded with a maximum nominal instrument bandwidth of 10 nm at 2500 nm (16 cm^{-1} at 4000 cm^{-1}). Measurement is made of the position of at least 3 peaks distributed over the range used. The acceptance tolerances are given under Verification of the wavelength scale. For the reference material used, apply the tolerance for the nearest wavelength (wavenumber) for each peak used.

Verification of the wavelength repeatability (except for filter apparatus). Verify the wavelength repeatability using suitable standards. The standard deviation of the wavelength is consistent with the specifications of the instrument manufacturer.

Verification of photometric linearity and response stability. Verification of photometric linearity is demonstrated with a set of transmission or reflection standards with known values of transmittance or reflectance in percentage. For reflectance measurements, carbon-doped polymer standards are available. At least 4 reference standards in the range of 10-90 per cent such as 10 per cent, 20 per cent, 40 per cent and 80 per cent with respective absorbance values of 1.0, 0.7, 0.4 and 0.1 are used. If the system is used for analytes with absorbances higher than 1.0, a 2 per cent and/or 5 per cent standard is added to the set. Plot the observed absorbance values against the reference absorbance values and perform a linear regression. Acceptable tolerances are 1.00 ± 0.05 for the slope and 0.00 ± 0.05 for the intercept.

Spectra obtained from reflectance standards are subject to variability due to the difference between the experimental conditions under which they were factory-calibrated and those under which they are subsequently put to use. Hence, the percentage reflectance values supplied with a set of calibration standards may not be useful in the attempt to establish an "absolute" calibration for a given instrument. But as long as the standards do not change chemically or physically and the same reference background is used as was used to obtain the certified values, subsequent measurements of the same standards under identical conditions including precise sample positioning give information on long-term stability of the photometric response. A tolerance of ± 2 per cent is acceptable for long-term stability; this is only necessary if spectra are used without pre-treatment.

Verification of photometric noise. Determine the photometric noise using a suitable reflectance standard, for example white reflective ceramic tiles or reflective thermoplastic resins (for example, PTFE). Scan the reflection standard over a suitable wavelength/wavenumber range in accordance with the manufacturer's recommendation and calculate the photometric noise as peak-to-peak noise. The value is approximately twice the standard deviation. The photometric noise is consistent with the specification of the spectrophotometer.

IDENTIFICATION AND CHARACTERISATION (QUALITATIVE ANALYSIS)

Establishment of a spectral reference library. Record the spectra of a suitable number of batches of the substance which have been fully tested according to established specifications and which exhibit the variation typical for the substance to be analysed (for example, manufacturer, physical form, particle size). The set of spectra represents the information for identification and characterisation that defines the similarity border for that substance and is the entry for that substance in the spectral library used to identify the substance. The number of substances in the library depends on the specific application, but libraries that are too big can cause some difficulties in discriminating between different materials and in validation. All spectra in the library used have the same:

– spectral range and number of data points,
– technique of measurement,
– data pre-treatment.

If sub-groups (libraries) are created, the above criteria are applied independently for each group. The collection of spectra in the library may be represented in different ways defined by the mathematical technique used for identification. These may be:

– all individual spectra representing the substance,
– a mean spectrum of each batch of substance,
– if necessary, a description of the variability within the substance spectra.

Electronic raw data for the preparation of the spectral library must be archived.

Pre-treatment of data. In many cases, and particularly for reflection mode spectra, some form of mathematical pretreatment of the spectrum may be useful before the development of a classification or calibration model. The aim can be, for example, to reduce baseline variations, to reduce the impact of known variations that are interfering in the subsequent mathematical models, or to compress data before use. Typical methods are multiplicative scatter correction (MSC), the Kubelka-Munk transforms, spectral compression techniques that may include windowing and noise reduction and the numerical calculation of the first- or second-order derivative of the spectrum. Higher-order derivatives are not recommended. In some cases spectra may also be normalised, for example against the maximum absorbance, the mean absorbance or the integrated absorbance area under the spectrum.

Caution must be excercised when performing any mathematical transformation, as artefacts can be introduced or essential information (important with qualification methods) can be lost. An understanding of the algorithm is required and in all cases the rationale for the use of transform must be documented.

Data evaluation. Direct comparison of the spectrum of the substance under investigation is made with the individual or mean reference spectra of all substances in the database on the basis of their mathematical correlation or other suitable algorithms. A set of known reference mean spectra and the variability around this mean can be used with an algorithm for classification. There are different algorithms based on principal component analysis (PCA) combined with cluster analysis, SIMCA (soft independent modelling by class analogy), COMPARE functions using filters or UNEQ (unequal dispersed class) and others used in the software of NIR instruments or supplied as third-party software. The reliability of the algorithm chosen for a particular application has to be validated. For example, correlation coefficient, the sum of squared residuals or the distance using cluster analysis must comply with the acceptance limits defined in the validation procedure.

Validation of the database

Specificity. The selectivity of the classification using database spectra for positive identification of a given material and adequate discrimination against other materials in the database is to be established during the validation procedure. Acceptance thresholds are established. High thresholds achieve a higher discriminatory power, but may cause some errors due to the own variability of materials. Lower thresholds solve these problems, but could produce ambiguous results. Potential challenges must be addressed to the spectral database. These can be materials received on site that are similar to database members in visual appearance, chemical structure or by name. This challenge must fail identification. Independent samples of materials represented in the database, but not used to create it (i.e. different batches, blends) must give positive identification when analysed.

Robustness. The robustness of the qualitative procedure must also be challenged to test the effect of minor changes to normal operating conditions on the analysis. There must be no changes to pre-processing and calibration algorithm parameters. Typical challenges are:

– effect of differences across operators on variations in environmental conditions (for example, temperature and humidity in the laboratory),
– effect of sample temperature, sample positioning on the optical window and probe depth and compression/packing of material,
– replacement of instrument parts or sampling presentation devices.

QUANTITATIVE ANALYSIS

Establishment of a spectral reference library for a calibration model. Calibration is the process of constructing a mathematical model to relate the response from an analytical instrument to the properties of the samples. Any calibration algorithm that can be clearly defined in an exact mathematical expression and gives suitable results can be used. Record spectra of a suitable number of samples with known values of the content throughout the range to be measured (for example, content of water). Wavelengths used in the calibration model can be compared to the known bands of the analyte and those of the matrix to verify that the bands of the analyte of interest are being used by the calibration. Establish the calibration model with about two-thirds of the measured samples. Compare the remaining one-third of the measured samples with the database. All samples must give quantitative results within a precision interval as defined by the intended purpose of the method. Correct quantification must be demonstrated in the presence of variations in the matrix within the specified range. Multiple linear regression (MLR), partial least squares (PLS) and principal component regression (PCR) are commonly used. For PLS or PCR calibrations, the coefficients or the loadings can be plotted and the regions of large coefficients compared with the spectrum of the analyte. Raw data for the preparation of the calibration model must be archived, without data pretreatment.

Pre-treatment of data. Data pre-treatment can be defined as the mathematical transformation of the NIR spectral data to enhance spectral features and/or remove or reduce unwanted sources of variation prior to the development of the calibration model. Many suitable algorithms for data pre-treatment and calibration exist. The selection is based on the suitability for the intended use. Wavelength selection may enhance the efficiency of calibration models such as MLR (for example, in particle-size determination). It is useful to delete certain ranges of the wavelength scale in some cases, for example in the determination of water of hydration. Wavelength compression may be applied to the data.

Validation parameters. Analytical performance characteristics to be considered for demonstrating the validation of NIR methods are similar to those required for any analytical procedure. Specific acceptance criteria for each validation parameter must be consistent with the intended use of the method.

Specificity. The relative discriminatory power and selectivity for quantitative determination must be similar to those mentioned under Qualitative analysis. The extent of specificity testing is dependent on the application and the risks being controlled. Variations in matrix concentrations within the operating range of the method must not affect the quantitative measurement significantly.

Linearity. The validation of linearity involves the correlation of NIR results calculated from NIR responses within the used algorithms to reference method results distributed throughout the defined range of the calibration model. Actual NIR responses that are non-linear may still be valid.

Range. The range of analyte reference values defines the range of the NIR method and quantitation limits of the method. Controls must be in place to ensure that results outside the validated range are not accepted.

Accuracy. This can be determined by comparison with the validation method or with known samples (samples of blank and added amounts of tested substance). Accuracy can be indicated by the standard error of prediction (SEP) of the NIR method that should be in close agreement with the data of the validated method. The SEP is the standard deviation of the residuals obtained from comparing the NIR results with analytical reference data for the specified samples. It is demonstrated by correlation of NIR results with analytical reference data, by comparison of the SEP to the reference method used for validation. Alternatively statistical comparison methods may be used to compare NIR results with reference values (paired *t*-test, bias evaluation).

Precision. This expresses the closeness of agreement between a series of measurements under the prescribed conditions. It is assessed by a minimum of 6 measurements performed according to the developed analytical method. Precision may be considered at 2 levels, repeatability (replicate measurements of the same sample with or without variation in sample positioning) and intermediate precision (replicate measurements by different analysts, different days of measurements).

Robustness. This includes the effects of variations of temperature, humidity, sample handling and the influence of instrument changes.

Outliers. Outlier results from NIR measurements of a sample containing an analyte outside the calibration range indicates that further testing is required. If further testing of the sample by an appropriate analytical method gives the analyte content within the specifications, this may be accepted and considered to have met the specifications. Thus an outlier result generated by NIR measurements of the sample may still meet specifications for the analyte of interest.

ONGOING MODEL EVALUATION

NIR models validated for use are subjected to ongoing performance evaluation and monitoring of validation parameters. If discrepancies are found, corrective action will be necessary. The degree of revalidation required depends on the nature of the changes. Revalidation of a qualitative model will be necessary when a new material is added to the reference library and may be necessary when changes in the physical properties of the material occur and when changes in the source of supply take place. Revalidation of a quantitative model is required on account of changes in the composition of the finished product, in the manufacturing process and in sources/grades of raw materials.

TRANSFER OF DATABASES

When databases are transferred to another instrument, spectral range, number of data points, spectral resolution and other parameters have to be taken into consideration. Further procedures and criteria must be applied to demonstrate that the model remains valid with the new database or new instrument.

DATA STORAGE

Store the electronic NIR spectra, libraries and data according to the current regulations.

Store the NIR spectra with the necessary data pre-treatment for the special use (for example identification, particle size analysis, content of water etc.) according to the current specifications.

01/2005:20241

2.2.41. CIRCULAR DICHROISM

The difference in absorbance of optically active substances within an absorption band for left and right circularly polarised light is referred to as circular dichroism.

Direct measurement gives a mean algebraic value:

$$\Delta A = A_{\mathrm{L}} - A_{\mathrm{R}}$$

ΔA = circular dichroic absorbance,

A_{L} = absorbance of left circularly polarised light,

A_{R} = absorbance of right circularly polarised light.

Circular dichroism is calculated using the equation:

$$\Delta\varepsilon = \varepsilon_{\mathrm{L}} - \varepsilon_{\mathrm{R}} = \frac{\Delta A}{c \times l}$$

$\Delta\varepsilon$ = molar circular dichroism or molar differential dichroic absorptivity expressed in litre·mole^{-1}·cm^{-1},

ε_{L} = molar absorptivity (*2.2.25*) of left circularly polarised light,

ε_{R} = molar absorptivity of right circularly polarised light,

c = concentration of the test solution in mole·litre^{-1},

l = optical path of the cell in centimetres.

The following units may also be used to characterise circular dichroism:

Dissymmetry factor:

$$g = \frac{\Delta\varepsilon}{\varepsilon}$$

ε = molar absorptivity (*2.2.25*).

Molar ellipticity:

Certain types of instruments display directly the value of ellipticity Θ, expressed in degrees. When such instruments are used, the molar ellipticity $[\Theta]$ may be calculated using the following equation:

$$[\Theta] = \frac{\Theta \times M}{c \times l \times 10}$$

$[\Theta]$ = molar ellipticity, expressed in degrees·cm^2·decimole^{-1},

Θ = value of ellipticity given by the instrument,

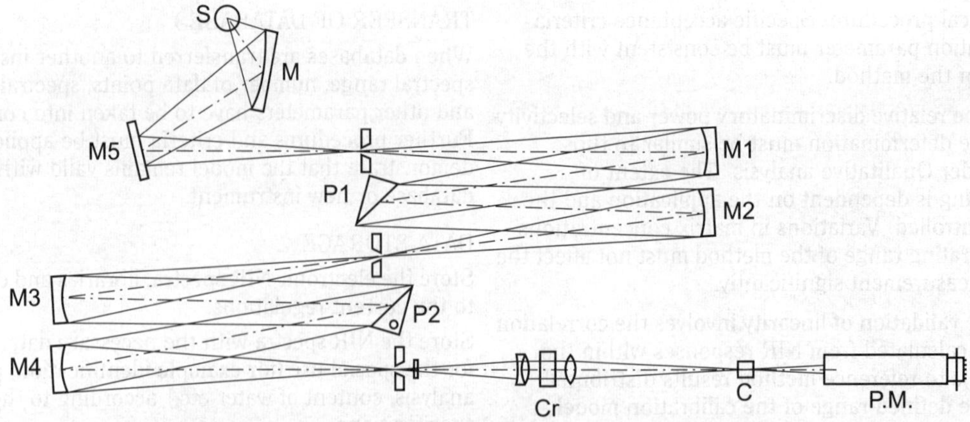

Figure 2.2.41.-1. – *Optical scheme of a dichrograph*

M = relative molecular mass of the substance to be examined,

c = concentration of the solution to be examined in g/ml,

l = optical path of the cell in centimetres.

Molar ellipticity is also related to molar circular dichroism by the following equation:

$$[\Theta] = 2.303\Delta\varepsilon\frac{4500}{\pi} \approx 3300\Delta\varepsilon$$

Molar ellipticity is often used in the analysis of proteins and nucleic acids. In this case, molar concentration is expressed in terms of monomeric residue, calculated using the expression:

$$\frac{\text{molecular mass}}{\text{number of amino acids}}$$

The mean relative molecular mass of the monomeric residue is 100 to 120 (generally 115) for proteins and about 330 for nucleic acids (as the sodium salt).

Apparatus. The light source (S) is a xenon lamp (Figure 2.2.41.-1); the light passes through a double monochromator (M) equipped with quartz prisms (P1, P2).

The linear beam from the first monochromator is split into 2 components polarised at right angles in the second monochromator. The exit slit of the monochromator eliminates the extraordinary beam.

The polarised and monochromatic light passes through a birefringent modulator (Cr): the result is alternating circularly polarised light.

The beam then passes through the sample to be examined (C) and reaches a photomultiplier (PM) followed by an amplifier circuit which produces 2 electrical signals: one is a direct current V_c and the other is an alternating current at the modulation frequency V_{ac} characteristic of the sample to be examined. The phase gives the sign of the circular dichroism. The ratio V_{ac}/V_c is proportional to the differential absorption ΔA which created the signal. The region of wavelengths normally covered by a dichrograph is 170 nm to 800 nm.

Calibration of the apparatus

Accuracy of absorbance scale. Dissolve 10.0 mg of *isoandrosterone R* in *dioxan R* and dilute to 10.0 ml with the same solvent. Record the circular dichroism spectrum of the solution between 280 nm and 360 nm. Measured at the maximum at 304 nm, $\Delta\varepsilon$ is + 3.3.

The solution of *(1S)-(+)-10-camphorsulphonic acid R* may also be used.

Linearity of modulation. Dissolve 10.0 mg of *(1S)-(+)-10-camphorsulphonic acid R* in *water R* and dilute to 10.0 ml with the same solvent. Determine the exact concentration of camphorsulphonic acid in the solution by ultraviolet spectrophotometry (*2.2.25*), taking the specific absorbance to be 1.49 at 285 nm.

Record the circular dichroism spectrum between 185 nm and 340 nm. Measured at the maximum at 290.5 nm, $\Delta\varepsilon$ is + 2.2 to + 2.5. Measured at the maximum at 192.5 nm, $\Delta\varepsilon$ is − 4.3 to − 5.

(1S)-(+)- or antipodal *(1R)-(−)-ammonium 10-camphorsulphonate R* can also be used.

01/2005:20242

2.2.42. DENSITY OF SOLIDS

The density of solids corresponds to their average mass per unit volume and typically is expressed in grams per cubic centimetre (g/cm^3) although the International Unit is the kilogram per cubic meter ($1\ g/cm^3 = 1000\ kg/m^3$).

Unlike gases and liquids whose density depends only on temperature and pressure, the density of a solid particle also depends on its molecular assembly and therefore varies with the crystal structure and degree of crystallinity.

When a solid particle is amorphous or partially amorphous, its density may further depend upon the history of preparation and treatment.

Therefore, unlike fluids, the densities of two chemically equivalent solids may be different, and this difference reflects a difference in solid-state structure. The density of constituent particles is an important physical characteristic of pharmaceutical powders.

The density of a solid particle can assume different values depending on the method used to measure the volume of the particle. It is useful to distinguish three levels of expression of density:

- the *crystal density* which only includes the solid fraction of the material; the crystal density is also called *true density*;
- the *particle density* which also includes the volume due to intraparticulate pores,
- the *bulk density* which further includes the interparticulate void volume formed in the powder bed; the bulk density is also called *apparent density.*

CRYSTAL DENSITY

The crystal density of a substance is the average mass per unit volume, exclusive of all voids that are not a fundamental part of the molecular packing arrangement. It is an intrinsic property of the substance, and hence should be independent of the method of determination. The crystal density can be determined either by calculation or by simple measurement.

A. The *calculated crystal density* is obtained using crystallographic data (size and composition of the unit cell) of a perfect crystal, from for example X-ray diffraction data, and the molecular mass of the substance.

B. The *measured crystal density* is the mass to volume ratio after measuring the monocrystal mass and volume.

PARTICLE DENSITY

The particle density takes into account both the crystal density and the intraparticulate porosity (sealed and/or open pores). Thus, particle density depends on the value of the volume determined which in turn depends on the method of measurement. The particle density can be determined using one of the two following methods.

A. The *pycnometric density* is determined by measuring the volume occupied by a known mass of powder which is equivalent to the volume of gas displaced by the powder using a gas displacement pycnometer (*2.9.23*). In pycnometric density measurements, the volume determined includes the volume occupied by open pores; however, it excludes the volume occupied by sealed pores or pores inaccessible to the gas. Due to the high diffusivity of helium, which is the preferred choice of gas, most open pores are accessible to the gas. Therefore, the pycnometric density of a finely milled powder is generally not very different from the crystal density.

B. The *mercury porosimeter density* is also called *granular density*. With this method the volume determined also excludes contributions from sealed pores; however, it includes the volume only from open pores larger than some size limit. This pore size limit or minimal access diameter depends on the maximal mercury intrusion pressure applied during the measurement and under normal operating pressures the mercury does not penetrate the finest pores accessible to helium. Various granular densities can be obtained from one sample since, for each applied mercury intrusion pressure, a density can be determined that corresponds to the pore size limit at that pressure.

BULK AND TAPPED DENSITY

The bulk density of a powder includes the contribution of interparticulate void volume. Hence, the bulk density depends on both the density of powder particles and the space arrangement of particles in the powder bed.

The bulk density of a powder is often very difficult to measure since the slightest disturbance of the bed may result in a new density. Thus, it is essential in reporting bulk density to specify how the determination was made.

A. The *bulk density* is determined by measuring the volume of a known mass of powder, that has been passed through a screen, into a graduated cylinder (*2.9.15*).

B. The *tapped density* is achieved by mechanically tapping a measuring cylinder containing a powder sample. After observing the initial volume, the cylinder is mechanically tapped, and volume readings are taken until little further volume change is observed (*2.9.15*).

01/2005:20243

2.2.43. MASS SPECTROMETRY

Mass spectrometry is based on the direct measurement of the ratio of the mass to the number of positive or negative elementary charges of ions (m/z) in the gas phase obtained from the substance to be analysed. This ratio is expressed in atomic mass units (1 a.m.u. = one twelfth the mass of ^{12}C) or in daltons (1 Da = the mass of the hydrogen atom).

The ions, produced in the ion *source* of the apparatus, are accelerated and then separated by the *analyser* before reaching the *detector*. All of these operations take place in a chamber where a pumping system maintains a vacuum of 10^{-3} to 10^{-6} Pa.

The resulting spectrum shows the relative abundance of the various ionic species present as a function of m/z. The signal corresponding to an ion will be represented by several peaks corresponding to the statistical distribution of the various isotopes of that ion. This pattern is called the *isotopic profile* and (at least for small molecules) the peak representing the most abundant isotopes for each atom is called the *monoisotopic peak*.

Information obtained in mass spectrometry is essentially qualitative (determination of the molecular mass, information on the structure from the fragments observed) or quantitative (using internal or external standards) with limits of detection ranging from the picomole to the femtomole.

INTRODUCTION OF THE SAMPLE

The very first step of an analysis is the introduction of the sample into the apparatus without overly disturbing the vacuum. In a common method, called *direct liquid introduction*, the sample is placed on the end of a cylindrical rod (in a quartz crucible, on a filament or on a metal surface). This rod is introduced into the spectrometer after passing through a vacuum lock where a primary intermediate vacuum is maintained between atmospheric pressure and the secondary vacuum of the apparatus.

Other introduction systems allow the components of a mixture to be analysed as they are separated by an appropriate apparatus connected to the mass spectrometer.

Gas chromatography/mass spectrometry. The use of suitable columns (capillary or semi-capillary) allows the end of the column to be introduced directly into the source of the apparatus without using a separator.

Liquid chromatography/mass spectrometry. This combination is particularly useful for the analysis of polar compounds, which are insufficiently volatile or too heat-labile to be analysed by gas chromatography coupled with mass spectrometry. This method is complicated by the difficulty of obtaining ions in the gas phase from a liquid phase, which requires very special interfaces such as:

- *direct liquid introduction*: the mobile phase is nebulised, and the solvent is evaporated in front of the ion source of the apparatus,
- *particle-beam interface*: the mobile phase, which may flow at a rate of up to 0.6 ml/min, is nebulised in a desolvation chamber such that only the analytes, in neutral form, reach the ion source of the apparatus; this technique is used for compounds of relatively low polarity with molecular masses of less than 1000 Da,
- *moving-belt interface*: the mobile phase, which may flow at a rate of up to 1 ml/min, is applied to the surface of a moving belt; after the solvent evaporates, the components to be analysed are successively carried to the ion source of the apparatus where they are ionised; this technique is rather poorly suited to very polar or heat-labile compounds.

Other types of coupling (electrospray, thermospray, atmospheric-pressure chemical ionisation) are considered to be ionisation techniques in their own right and are described in the section on modes of ionisation.

Supercritical fluid chromatography/mass spectrometry. The mobile phase, usually consisting of supercritical carbon dioxide enters the gas state after passing a heated restrictor between the column and the ion source.

Capillary electrophoresis/mass spectrometry. The eluent is introduced into the ion source, in some cases after adding another solvent so that flow rates of the order of a few microlitres per minute can be attained. This technique is limited by the small quantities of sample introduced and the need to use volatile buffers.

MODES OF IONISATION

Electron impact. The sample, in the gas state, is ionised by a beam of electrons whose energy (usually 70 eV) is greater than the ionisation energy of the sample. In addition to the molecular ion M^+, fragments characteristic of the molecular structure are observed. This technique is limited mainly by the need to vaporise the sample. This makes it unsuited to polar, heat-labile or high molecular mass compounds. Electron impact is compatible with the coupling of gas chromatography to mass spectrometry and sometimes with the use of liquid chromatography.

Chemical ionisation. This type of ionisation involves a reagent gas such as methane, ammonia, nitrogen oxide, nitrogen dioxide or oxygen. The spectrum is characterised by ions of the $(M + H)^+$ or $(M - H)^-$ types, or adduct ions formed from the analyte and the gas used. Fewer fragments are produced than with electron impact. A variant of this technique is used when the substance is heat-labile: the sample, applied to a filament, is very rapidly vaporised by the Joule-Thomson effect (desorption chemical ionisation).

Fast-atom bombardment (FAB) or fast-ion bombardment ionisation (liquid secondary-ion mass spectrometry LSIMS). The sample, dissolved in a viscous matrix such as glycerol, is applied to a metal surface and ionised by a beam of neutral atoms such as argon or xenon or high-kinetic-energy caesium ions. Ions of the $(M + H)^+$ or $(M - H)^-$ types or adduct ions formed from the matrix or the sample are produced. This type of ionisation, well suited to polar and heat-labile compounds, allows molecular masses of up to 10 000 Da to be obtained. The technique can be combined with liquid chromatography by adding 1 per cent to 2 per cent of glycerol to the mobile phase; however, the flow rates must be very low (a few microlitres per minute). These ionisation techniques also allow thin-layer chromatography plates to be analysed by applying a thin layer of matrix to the surface of these plates.

Field desorption and field ionisation. The sample is vaporised near a tungsten filament covered with microneedles (*field ionisation*) or applied to this filament (*field desorption*). A voltage of about 10 kV, applied between this filament and a counter-electrode, ionises the sample. These two techniques mainly produce molecular ions M^+, and $(M + H)^+$ ions and are used for low polarity and/or heat-labile compounds.

Matrix-assisted laser desorption ionisation (MALDI). The sample, in a suitable matrix and deposited on a metal support, is ionised by a pulsed laser beam whose wavelength may range from UV to IR (impulses lasting from a picosecond to a few nanoseconds). This mode of ionisation plays an essential role in the analysis of very high molecular mass compounds (more than 100 000 Da) but is limited to time-of flight analysers (see below).

Electrospray. This mode of ionisation is carried out at atmospheric pressure. The samples, in solution, are introduced into the source through a capillary tube, the end of which has a potential of the order of 5 kV. A gas can be used to facilitate nebulisation. Desolvation of the resulting microdroplets produces singly or multiply charged ions in the gas phase. The flow rates vary from a few microlitres per minute to 1 ml/min. This technique is suited to polar compounds and to the investigation of biomolecules with molecular masses of up to 100 000 Da. It can be coupled to liquid chromatography or capillary electrophoresis.

Atmospheric-pressure chemical ionisation (APCI). Ionisation is carried out at atmospheric pressure by the action of an electrode maintained at a potential of several kilovolts and placed in the path of the mobile phase, which is nebulised both by thermal effects and by the use of a stream of nitrogen. The resulting ions carry a single charge and are of the $(M + H)^+$ type in the positive mode and of the $(M - H)^-$ type in the negative mode. The high flow rates that can be used with this mode of ionisation (up to 2 ml/min) make this an ideal technique for coupling to liquid chromatography.

Thermospray. The sample, in the mobile phase consisting of water and organic modifiers and containing a volatile electrolyte (generally ammonium acetate) is introduced in nebulised form after having passed through a metal capillary tube at controlled temperature. Acceptable flow rates are of the order of 1 ml/min to 2 ml/min. The ions of the electrolyte ionise the compounds to be analysed. This ionisation process may be replaced or enhanced by an electrical discharge of about 800 volts, notably when the solvents are entirely organic. This technique is compatible with the use of liquid chromatography coupled with mass spectrometry.

ANALYSERS

Differences in the performance of analysers depend mainly on two parameters:

- the range over which m/z ratios can be measured, ie, the *mass range*,
- their *resolving power* characterised by the ability to separate two ions of equal intensity with m/z ratios differing by ΔM, and whose overlap is expressed as a given percentage of valley definition; for example, a resolving power ($M/\Delta M$) of 1000 with 10 per cent valley definition allows the separation of m/z ratios of 1000 and 1001 with the intensity returning to 10 per cent above baseline. However, the resolving power may in some cases (time-of-flight analysers, quadrupoles, ion-trap analysers) be defined as the ratio between the molecular mass and peak width at half height (50 per cent valley definition).

Magnetic and electrostatic analysers. The ions produced in the ion source are accelerated by a voltage *V*, and focused towards a magnetic analyser (magnetic field *B*) or an electrostatic analyser (electrostatic field *E*), depending on the configuration of the instrument. They follow a trajectory of radius *r* according to Laplace's law:

$$\frac{m}{z} = \frac{B^2 r^2}{2V}$$

Two types of scans can be used to collect and measure the various ions produced by the ion source: a scan of *B* holding *V* fixed or a scan of *V* with constant *B*. The magnetic analyser is usually followed by an electric sector that acts as a kinetic energy filter and allows the resolving power of the instrument to be increased appreciably. The maximum resolving power of such an instrument (double sector) ranges from 10 000 to 150 000 and in most cases allows the value of m/z ratios to be calculated accurately enough to determine the elemental composition of the corresponding ions. For monocharged ions, the mass range is from 2000 Da to 15 000 Da. Some ions may decompose spontaneously (metastable transitions) or by colliding with a gas (collision-activated dissociation

(CAD)) in field-free regions between the ion source and the detector. Examination of these decompositions is very useful for the determination of the structure as well as the characterisation of a specific compound in a mixture and involves tandem mass spectrometry. There are many such techniques depending on the region where these decompositions occur:

- *daughter-ion mode* (determination of the decomposition ions of a given parent ion): B/E = constant, *MIKES (Mass-analysed Ion Kinetic Energy Spectroscopy)*,
- *parent-ion mode* (determination of all ions which by decomposition give an ion with a specific m/z ratio): B^2/E = constant,
- *neutral-loss mode* (detection of all the ions that lose the same fragment):

  $B/E(1 - E/E_0)^{1/2}$ = constant, where E_0 is the basic voltage of the electric sector.

Quadrupoles. The analyser consists of four parallel metal rods, which are cylindrical or hyperbolic in cross-section. They are arranged symmetrically with respect to the trajectory of the ions; the pairs diagonally opposed about the axis of symmetry of rods are connected electrically. The potentials to the two pairs of rods are opposed. They are the resultant of a constant component and an alternating component. The ions produced at the ion source are transmitted and separated by varying the voltages applied to the rods so that the ratio of continuous voltage to alternating voltage remains constant. The quadrupoles usually have a mass range of 1 a.m.u. to 2000 a.m.u., but some may range up to 4000 a.m.u. Although they have a lower resolving power than magnetic sector analysers, they nevertheless allow the monoisotopic profile of single charged ions to be obtained for the entire mass range. It is possible to obtain spectra using three quadrupoles arranged in series, Q_1, Q_2, Q_3 (Q_2 serves as a collision cell and is not really an analyser; the most commonly used collision gas is argon).

The most common types of scans are the following:

- *daughter-ion mode*: Q_1 selects an m/z ion whose fragments obtained by collision in Q_2 are analysed by Q_3,
- *parent-ion mode*: Q_3 filters only a specific m/z ratio, while Q_1 scans a given mass range. Only the ions decomposing to give the ion selected by Q_3 are detected,
- *neutral loss mode*: Q_1 and Q_3 scan a certain mass range but at an offset corresponding to the loss of a fragment characteristic of a product or family of compounds.

It is also possible to obtain spectra by combining quadrupole analysers with magnetic or electrostatic sector instruments; such instruments are called *hybrid mass spectrometers*.

Ion-trap analyser. The principle is the same as for a quadrupole, this time with the electric fields in three dimensions. This type of analyser allows product-ion spectra over several generations (MS^n) to be obtained.

Ion-cyclotron resonance analysers. Ions produced in a cell and subjected to a uniform, intense magnetic field move in circular orbits at frequencies which can be directly correlated to their m/z ratio by applying a Fourier transform algorithm. This phenomenon is called ion-cyclotron resonance. Analysers of this type consist of superconducting magnets and are capable of very high resolving power (up to 1000 000 and more) as well as MS^n spectra. However, very low pressures are required (of the order of 10^{-7} Pa).

Time-of-flight analysers. The ions produced at the ion source are accelerated at a voltage V of 10 kV to 20 kV. They pass through the analyser, consisting of a field-free tube, 25 cm to 1.5 m long, generally called a *flight tube*. The time (t) for an ion to travel to the detector is proportional to the square root of the m/z ratio. Theoretically the mass range of such an analyser is infinite. In practice, it is limited by the ionisation or desorption method. Time-of-flight analysers are mainly used for high molecular mass compounds (up to several hundred thousand daltons). This technique is very sensitive (a few picomoles of product are sufficient). The accuracy of the measurements and the resolving power of such instruments may be improved considerably by using an electrostatic mirror (reflectron).

SIGNAL ACQUISITION

There are essentially three possible modes.

Complete spectrum mode. The entire signal obtained over a chosen mass range is recorded. The spectrum represents the relative intensity of the different ionic species present as a function of m/z. The results are essentially qualitative. The use of spectral reference libraries for more rapid identification is possible.

Fragmentometric mode (Selected-ion monitoring). The acquired signal is limited to one (single-ion monitoring (SIM)) or several (multiple-ion monitoring (MIM)) ions characteristic of the substance to be analysed. The limit of detection can be considerably reduced in this mode. Quantitative or semiquantitative tests can be carried out using external or internal standards (for example, deuterated standards). Such tests cannot be carried out with time-of-flight analysers.

Fragmentometric double mass spectrometry mode (multiple reaction monitoring (MRM)). The unimolecular or bimolecular decomposition of a chosen precursor ion characteristic of the substance to be analysed is followed specifically. The selectivity and the highly specific nature of this mode of acquisition provide excellent sensitivity levels and make it the most appropriate for quantitative studies using suitable internal standards (for example, deuterated standards). This type of analysis can be performed only on apparatus fitted with three quadrupoles in series, ion-trap analysers or cyclotron-resonance analysers.

CALIBRATION

Calibration allows the corresponding m/z value to be attributed to the detected signal. As a general rule, this is done using a reference substance. This calibration may be external (acquisition file separate from the analysis) or internal (the reference substance(s) are mixed with the substance to be examined and appear on the same acquisition file). The number of ions or points required for reliable calibration depends on the type of analyser and on the desired accuracy of the measurement, for example, in the case of a magnetic analyser where the m/z ratio varies exponentially with the value of the magnetic field, there should be as many points as possible.

SIGNAL DETECTION AND DATA PROCESSING

Ions separated by an analyser are converted into electric signals by a detection system such as a photomultiplier or an electron multiplier. These signals are amplified before being re-converted into digital signals for data processing, allowing various functions such as calibration, reconstruction of spectra, automatic quantification, archiving, creation or use of libraries of mass spectra. The various physical parameters required for the functioning of the apparatus as a whole are controlled by computer.

01/2005:20244

2.2.44. TOTAL ORGANIC CARBON IN WATER FOR PHARMACEUTICAL USE

Total organic carbon (TOC) determination is an indirect measure of organic substances present in water for pharmaceutical use. TOC determination can also be used to monitor the performance of various operations in the preparation of medicines.

A variety of acceptable methods is available for determining TOC. Rather than prescribing a given method to be used, this general chapter describes the procedures used to qualify the chosen method and the interpretation of results in limit tests. A standard solution is analysed at suitable intervals, depending on the frequency of measurements; the solution is prepared with a substance that is expected to be easily oxidisable (for example, sucrose) at a concentration adjusted to give an instrument response corresponding to the TOC limit to be measured. The suitability of the system is determined by analysis of a solution prepared with a substance expected to be oxidisable with difficulty (for example, 1,4-benzoquinone).

The various types of apparatus used to measure TOC in water for pharmaceutical use have in common the objective of completely oxidising the organic molecules in the sample water to produce carbon dioxide followed by measurement of the amount of carbon dioxide produced, the result being used to calculate the carbon concentration in the water.

The apparatus used must discriminate between organic and inorganic carbon, the latter being present as carbonate. The discrimination may be effected either by measuring the inorganic carbon and subtracting it from the total carbon, or by purging inorganic carbon from the sample before oxidisation. Purging may also entrain organic molecules, but such purgeable organic carbon is present in negligible quantities in water for pharmaceutical use.

Apparatus. Use a calibrated instrument installed either on-line or off-line. Verify the system suitability at suitable intervals as described below. The apparatus must have a limit of detection specified by the manufacturer of 0.05 mg or less of carbon per litre.

TOC water. Use highly purified water complying with the following specifications:

– conductivity: not greater than 1.0 μS·cm^{-1} at 25 °C,
– total organic carbon: not greater than 0.1 mg/l.

Depending on the type of apparatus used, the content of heavy metals and copper may be critical. The manufacturer's instructions should be followed.

Glassware preparation. Use glassware that has been scrupulously cleaned by a method that will remove organic matter. Use *TOC water* for the final rinse of glassware.

Standard solution. Dissolve *sucrose R*, dried at 105 °C for 3 h in *TOC water* to obtain a solution containing 1.19 mg of sucrose per litre (0.50 mg of carbon per litre).

Test solution. Using all due care to avoid contamination, collect water to be tested in an airtight container leaving minimal head-space. Examine the water with minimum delay to reduce contamination from the container and its closure.

System suitability solution. Dissolve *1,4-benzoquinone R* in *TOC water* to obtain a solution having a concentration of 0.75 mg of 1,4-benzoquinone per litre (0.50 mg of carbon per litre).

TOC water control. Use *TOC water* obtained at the same time as that used to prepare the standard solution and the system suitability solution.

Control solutions. In addition to the *TOC water control*, prepare suitable blank solutions or other solutions needed for establishing the baseline or for calibration adjustments following the manufacturer's instructions; run the appropriate blanks to zero the instrument.

System suitability. Run the following solutions and record the responses: *TOC water* (r_w); *standard solution* (r_s); *system suitability solution* (r_{ss}). Calculate the percentage response efficiency using the expression:

$$\frac{r_{ss} - r_w}{r_s - r_w} \times 100$$

The system is suitable if the response efficiency is not less than 85 per cent and not more than 115 per cent of the theoretical response.

Procedure. Run the test solution and record the response (r_u). The test solution complies with the test if r_u is not greater than $r_s - r_w$.

The method can also be applied using on-line instrumentation that has been adequately calibrated and shown to have acceptable system suitability. The location of instrumentation must be chosen to ensure that the responses are representative of the water used.

01/2005:20245

2.2.45. SUPERCRITICAL FLUID CHROMATOGRAPHY

Supercritical fluid chromatography (SFC) is a method of chromatographic separation in which the mobile phase is a fluid in a supercritical or a subcritical state. The stationary phase, contained in a column, consists of either finely divided solid particles, such as a silica or porous graphite, a chemically modified stationary phase, as used in liquid chromatography, or, for capillary columns, a cross-linked liquid film evenly coated on the walls of the column.

SFC is based on mechanisms of adsorption or mass distribution.

APPARATUS

The apparatus usually consists of a cooled pumping system, an injector, a chromatographic column, contained in an oven, a detector, a pressure regulator and a data acquisition device (or an integrator or a chart recorder).

Pumping system

Pumping systems are required to deliver the mobile phase at a constant flow rate. Pressure fluctuations are to be minimised, e.g. by passing the pressurised solvent through a pulse-damping device. Tubing and connections are capable of withstanding the pressures developed by the pumping system.

Microprocessor controlled systems are capable of accurately delivering a mobile phase in either constant or varying conditions, according to a defined programme. In the case of gradient elution, pumping systems which deliver solvent(s) from several reservoirs are available and solvent mixing can be achieved on either the low or high-pressure side of the pump(s).

Injectors

Injection may be carried out directly at the head of the column using a valve.

Stationary phases

Stationary phases are contained in columns which have been described in the chapters on *Liquid chromatography (2.2.29)* (packed columns) and *Gas chromatography (2.2.28)* (capillary columns). A capillary column has a maximum internal diameter (Ø) of 100 µm.

Mobile phases

Usually the mobile phase is carbon-dioxide which may contain a polar modifier such as methanol, 2-propanol or acetonitrile. The composition, pressure (density), temperature and flow rate of the prescribed mobile phase may either be constant throughout the whole chromatographic procedure (isocratic, isodense, isothermic elution) or may vary according to a defined programme (gradient elution of the modifier, pressure (density), temperature or flow rate).

Detectors

Ultraviolet/visible (UV/Vis) spectrophotometers and flame ionisation detectors are the most commonly employed detectors. Light scattering detectors, infrared absorption spectrophotometers, thermal conductivity detectors or other special detectors may be used.

METHOD

Prepare the test solution(s) and the reference solution(s) as prescribed. The solutions must be free from solid particles.

Criteria for assessing the suitability of the system are described in the chapter on *Chromatographic separation techniques* (*2.2.46*). The extent to which adjustments of parameters of the chromatographic system can be made to satisfy the criteria of system suitability are also given in this chapter.

01/2005:20246

2.2.46. CHROMATOGRAPHIC SEPARATION TECHNIQUES

Chromatographic separation techniques are multi-stage separation methods in which the components of a sample are distributed between 2 phases, one of which is stationary, while the other is mobile. The stationary phase may be a solid or a liquid supported on a solid or a gel. The stationary phase may be packed in a column, spread as a layer, or distributed as a film, etc. The mobile phase may be gaseous or liquid or supercritical fluid. The separation may be based on adsorption, mass distribution (partition), ion exchange, etc., or may be based on differences in the physico-chemical properties of the molecules such as size, mass, volume, etc.

This chapter contains definitions and calculations of common parameters and generally applicable requirements for system suitability. Principles of separation, apparatus and methods are given in the following general methods:

- paper chromatography (*2.2.26*),
- thin-layer chromatography (*2.2.27*),
- gas chromatography (*2.2.28*),
- liquid chromatography (*2.2.29*),
- size-exclusion chromatography (*2.2.30*),
- supercritical fluid chromatography (*2.2.45*).

DEFINITIONS

The following definitions have been used to calculate the limits in monographs.

With some equipment, certain parameters, such as the signal-to-noise ratio, can be calculated using software provided by the manufacturer. It is the responsibility of the user to ensure that the calculation methods used in the software are compatible with the requirements of the European Pharmacopoeia. If not, the necessary corrections must be made.

Chromatogram

A chromatogram is a graphical or other representation of detector response, effluent concentration or other quantity used as a measure of effluent concentration, versus time, volume or distance. Idealised chromatograms are represented as a sequence of gaussian peaks on a baseline.

RETENTION DATA

Retention time and retention volume

Retention measurements in elution chromatography may be given as the retention time (t_R) directly defined by the position of the maximum of the peak in the chromatogram. From the retention time, the retention volume (V_R) may be calculated.

$$V_R = v \times t_R$$

t_R = retention time or distance along the baseline from the point of injection to the perpendicular dropped from the maximum of the peak corresponding to the component,

v = flow rate of the mobile phase.

Mass distribution ratio

The mass distribution ratio (D_m) (also known as the capacity factor *k'* or retention factor k) is defined as:

$$D_m = \frac{\text{amount of solute in stationary phase}}{\text{amount of solute in mobile phase}} = K_C \frac{V_S}{V_M}$$

K_C = equilibrium distribution coefficient (also known as distribution constant),

V_S = volume of the stationary phase,

V_M = volume of the mobile phase.

The mass distribution ratio of a component may be determined from the chromatogram using the expression:

$$D_m = \frac{t_R - t_M}{t_M}$$

t_R = retention time (or volume) or distance along the baseline from the point of injection to the perpendicular dropped from the maximum of the peak corresponding to the component,

t_M = hold-up time (or volume): time (or volume) or distance along the baseline from the point of injection to the perpendicular dropped from the maximum of the peak corresponding to an unretained component.

Distribution coefficient

The elution characteristics of a component in a particular column, in size-exclusion chromatography, may be given by the distribution coefficient (K_o) which is calculated from the expression:

$$K_o = \frac{t_R - t_o}{t_t - t_o}$$

t_R = retention time (or volume) or distance along the baseline from the point of injection to the perpendicular dropped from the maximum of the peak corresponding to the component,

t_o = hold-up time (or volume): time (or volume) or distance along the baseline from the point of injection to the perpendicular dropped from the maximum of the peak corresponding to an unretained component,

t_t = retention time (or volume) or distance along the baseline from the point of injection to the perpendicular dropped from the maximum of the peak corresponding to a component which has full access to the pores of the stationary phase.

Retardation factor

The retardation factor (R_F) (also known as retention factor R_f), used in planar chromatography, is the ratio of the distance from the point of application to the centre of the spot and the distance travelled by the solvent front from the point of application.

$$R_F = \frac{b}{a}$$

b = migration distance of the analyte,

a = migration distance of the solvent front.

CHROMATOGRAPHIC DATA

The peak may be defined by the *peak area (A)* or the *peak height (h)* and the *peak width at half- height (w_h)* or the *peak height (h)* and the *peak width between the points of inflection (w_i)*. In gaussian peaks (Figure 2.2.46.-1) there is the relationship:

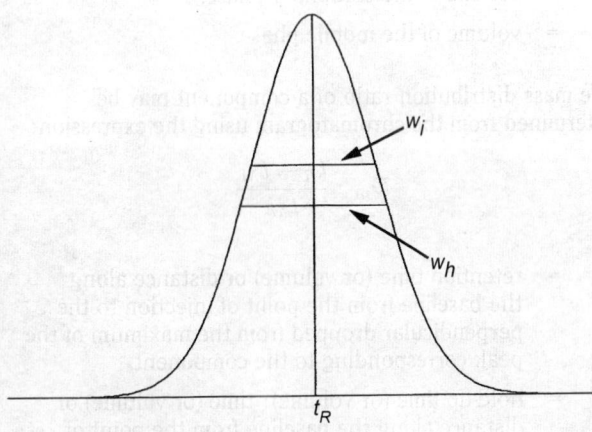

$$w_h = 1.18 w_i$$

Figure 2.2.46.-1.

Symmetry factor

The symmetry factor (A_s) (or tailing factor) of a peak (Figure 2.2.46.-2) is calculated from the expression:

$$A_s = \frac{w_{0.05}}{2d}$$

$w_{0.05}$ = width of the peak at one-twentieth of the peak height,

d = distance between the perpendicular dropped from the peak maximum and the leading edge of the peak at one-twentieth of the peak height.

A value of 1.0 signifies complete (ideal) symmetry.

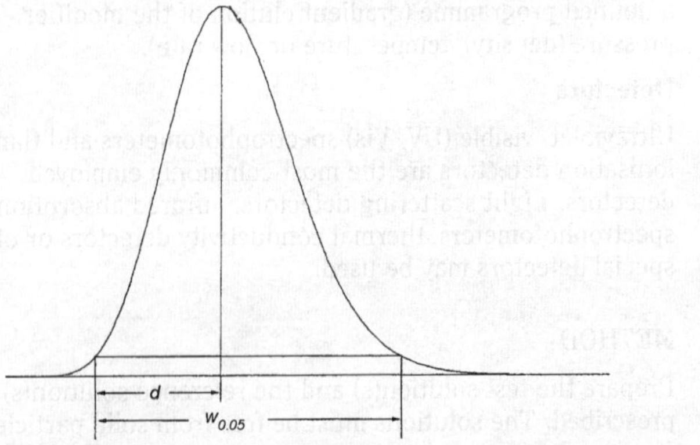

Figure 2.2.46.-2.

Column performance and apparent number of theoretical plates

The column performance (apparent efficiency) may be calculated from data obtained under either isothermal, isocratic or isodense conditions, depending on the technique, as the apparent number of theoretical plates (N) from the following expression, where the values of t_R and w_h have to be expressed in the same units (time, volume or distance).

$$N = 5.54 \left(\frac{t_R}{w_h}\right)^2$$

t_R = retention time (or volume) or distance along the baseline from the point of injection to the perpendicular dropped from the maximum of the peak corresponding to the component,

w_h = width of the peak at half-height.

The apparent number of theoretical plates varies with the component as well as with the column and the retention time.

SEPARATION DATA

Resolution

The resolution (R_s) between peaks of 2 components may be calculated from the expression:

$$R_s = \frac{1.18\,(t_{R2} - t_{R1})}{w_{h1} + w_{h2}}$$

$$t_{R2} > t_{R1}$$

t_{R1} and t_{R2} = retention times or distances along the baseline from the point of injection to the perpendiculars dropped from the maxima of 2 adjacent peaks,

w_{h1} and w_{h2} = peak widths at half-height.

A resolution of greater than 1.5 corresponds to baseline separation.

The expression given above may not be applicable if the peaks are not baseline separated.

In quantitative planar chromatography, the migration distances are used instead of retention times and the resolution may be calculated using the expression:

$$R_s = \frac{1.18\,a\,(R_{F2} - R_{F1})}{w_{h1} + w_{h2}}$$

R_{F1} and R_{F2} = ratios of the distances from the point of application to the centres of the spots and the distance travelled by the solvent front from the point of application (retardation factor),

w_{h1} and w_{h2} = peak widths at half-height,

a = migration distance of the solvent front.

Peak-to-valley ratio

The peak-to-valley ratio (p/v) may be employed as a system suitability requirement in a test for related substances when baseline separation between 2 peaks is not reached (Figure 2.2.46.-3).

$$p/v = \frac{H_p}{H_v}$$

H_p = height above the extrapolated baseline of the minor peak,

H_v = height above the extrapolated baseline at the lowest point of the curve separating the minor and major peaks.

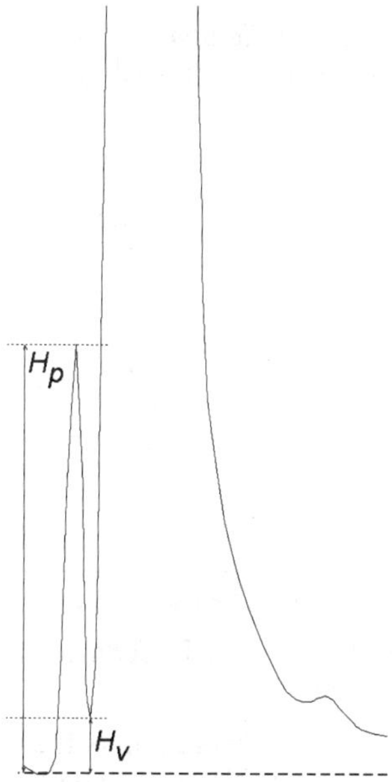

Figure 2.2.46.-3.

Relative retention

The relative retention (r) is calculated as an estimate from the expression:

$$r = \frac{t_{R2} - t_M}{t_{R1} - t_M}$$

t_{R2} = retention time of the peak of interest,

t_{R1} = retention time of the reference peak (usually the peak corresponding to the substance to be examined),

t_M = hold-up time: time or distance along the baseline from the point of injection to the perpendicular dropped from the maximum of the peak corresponding to an unretained component.

The unadjusted relative retention (r_G) is calculated from the expression:

$$r_G = \frac{t_{R2}}{t_{R1}}$$

Unless otherwise indicated, values for relative retention stated in monographs correspond to unadjusted relative retention.

In planar chromatography, the retardation factors R_{F2} and R_{F1} are used instead of t_{R2} and t_{R1}.

PRECISION OF QUANTIFICATION

Signal-to-noise ratio

The signal-to-noise ratio (S/N) influences the precision of quantification and is calculated from the equation:

$$S/N = \frac{2H}{h}$$

H = height of the peak (Figure 2.2.46.-4) corresponding to the component concerned, in the chromatogram obtained with the prescribed reference solution, measured from the maximum of the peak to the extrapolated baseline of the signal observed over a distance equal to 20 times the width at half-height,

h = range of the background noise in a chromatogram obtained after injection or application of a blank, observed over a distance equal to 20 times the width at half-height of the peak in the chromatogram obtained with the prescribed reference solution and, if possible, situated equally around the place where this peak would be found.

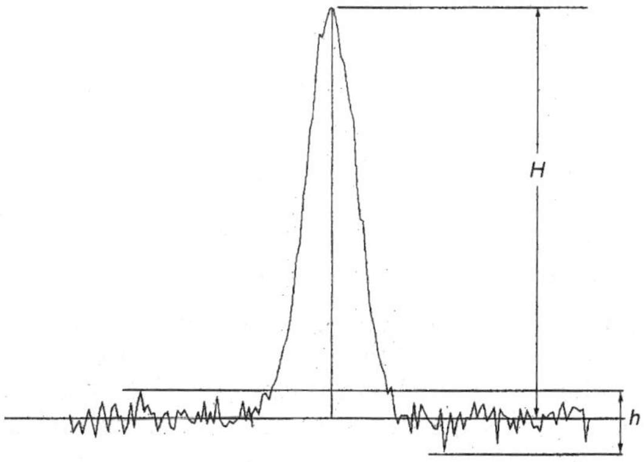

Figure 2.2.46.-4.

Repeatability

The repeatability of response is expressed as an estimated percentage relative standard deviation ($RSD_{\%}$) of a consecutive series of measurement of injections or applications of a reference solution and is calculated from the expression:

$$RSD_{\%} = \frac{100}{\bar{y}}\sqrt{\frac{\sum (y_i - \bar{y})^2}{n-1}}$$

y_i = individual values expressed as peak area, peak height, or ratio of areas by the internal standardisation method,

$\bar{y}$ = mean of individual values,

n = number of individual values.

The maximal permitted relative standard deviation (RSD_{max}) is calculated for a series of injections of the reference solution for defined limits using the following expression:

$$RSD_{\max} = \frac{KB\sqrt{n}}{t_{90\%,n-1}}$$

K = constant (0.349), obtained from the expression $K = \frac{0.6}{\sqrt{2}} \times \frac{t_{90\%,5}}{\sqrt{6}}$ in which $\frac{0.6}{\sqrt{2}}$ represents the required RSD after 6 injections for B = 1.0,

B = upper limit given in the definition of the individual monograph minus 100 per cent,

n = number of replicate injections of the reference solution ($3 \leq n \leq 6$),

$t_{90\%,n-1}$ = Student's t at the 90 per cent probability level (double sided) with $n - 1$ degrees of freedom.

SYSTEM SUITABILITY

The system suitability tests represent an integral part of the method and are used to ensure adequate performance of the chromatographic system. Apparent efficiency, mass distribution ratio, resolution, relative retention and the symmetry factor are the parameters which are usually employed in assessing the performance of the column. Factors which may affect the chromatographic behaviour include the composition, ionic strength, temperature and apparent pH of the mobile phase, flow rate, column length, temperature and pressure, and stationary phase characteristics including porosity, particle size, type of particles, specific surface area and, in the case of reverse-phase supports, the extent of chemical modification (as expressed by end-capping, carbon loading etc.).

The various components of the equipment employed must be qualified and be capable of achieving the precision required to conduct the test or assay.

The following requirements are to be fulfilled unless otherwise stated in the monograph.

- The symmetry factor of the principal peak is to be between 0.8 and 1.5 unless otherwise stated in the monograph. This requirement has general applicability to tests or assays described in the monographs.
- Maximal permitted relative standard deviation for replicate injections of the prescribed reference solution do not exceed the values given in Table 2.2.46.-1. This requirement is applicable to assays for content only and does not apply to the test for related substances.
- The limit of detection of the peak (corresponding to a signal-to-noise ratio of 3) is below the disregard limit of the test for related substances.
- The limit of quantitation of the peak (corresponding to a signal-to-noise ratio of 10) is equal to or less than the disregard limit of the test for related substances.

Table 2.2.46.-1. – *Repeatability requirements*

	Number of individual injections			
	3	4	5	6
B (per cent)	**Maximal permitted relative standard deviation**			
2.0	0.41	0.59	0.73	0.85
2.5	0.52	0.74	0.92	1.06
3.0	0.62	0.89	1.10	1.27

ADJUSTMENT OF CHROMATOGRAPHIC CONDITIONS

The extent to which the various parameters of a chromatographic test may be adjusted to satisfy the system suitability criteria without fundamentally modifying the methods are listed below for information. The chromatographic conditions described have been validated during the elaboration of the monograph. The system suitability tests are included to ensure the separation required for satisfactory performance of the test or assay. Nonetheless, since the stationary phases are described in a general way and there is such a variety available commercially, with differences in chromatographic behaviour, some adjustments of the chromatographic conditions may be necessary to achieve the prescribed system suitability requirements. With reverse-phase liquid chromatographic methods, in particular, adjustment of the various parameters will not always result in satisfactory chromatography. In that case, it may be necessary to replace the column with another of the same type (e.g. octadecylsilyl silica gel) which exhibits the desired chromatographic behaviour.

For critical parameters the adjustments are defined clearly in the monograph to ensure the system suitability.

Multiple adjustments which may have a cumulative effect in the performance of the system are to be avoided.

Thin-layer chromatography and paper chromatography

Composition of the mobile phase: the amount of the minor solvent component may be adjusted by ± 30 per cent relative or ± 2 per cent absolute, whichever is the larger; for a minor component at 10 per cent of the mobile phase, a 30 per cent relative adjustment allows a range of 7-13 per cent whereas a 2 per cent absolute adjustment allows a range of 8-12 per cent, the relative value being therefore the larger; for a minor component at 5 per cent of the mobile phase, a 30 per cent relative adjustment allows a range of 3.5-6.5 per cent whereas a 2 per cent absolute adjustment allows a range of 3-7 per cent, the absolute value being in this case the larger. No other component is altered by more than 10 per cent absolute.

pH of the aqueous component of the mobile phase: ± 0.2 pH, unless otherwise stated in the monograph, or ± 1.0 pH when neutral substances are to be examined.

Concentration of salts in the buffer component of a mobile phase: ± 10 per cent.

Application volume: 10-20 per cent of the prescribed volume if using fine particle size plates (2-10 μm).

Migration distance of the solvent front is to be not less than 50 mm or 30 mm on high-performance plates.

Liquid chromatography

Composition of the mobile phase: the amount of the minor solvent component may be adjusted by ± 30 per cent relative or ± 2 per cent absolute, whichever is the larger (see example above). No other component is altered by more than 10 per cent absolute.

pH of the aqueous component of the mobile phase: ± 0.2 pH, unless otherwise stated in the monograph, or ± 1.0 pH when neutral substances are to be examined.

Concentration of salts in the buffer component of a mobile phase: ± 10 per cent.

Detector wavelength: no adjustment permitted.

Stationary phase:

- *column length*: ± 70 per cent,
- *column internal diameter*: ± 25 per cent,
- *particle size*: maximal reduction of 50 per cent, no increase permitted.

Flow rate: ± 50 per cent. When in a monograph the retention time of the principle peak is indicated, the flow rate has to be adjusted if the column internal diameter has been changed. No decrease of flow rate is permitted if the monograph uses apparent number of theoretical plates in the qualification section.

Temperature: ± 10 per cent, to a maximum of 60 °C.

Injection volume: may be decreased, provided detection and repeatability of the peak(s) to be determined are satisfactory.

Gradient elution: the configuration of the equipment employed may significantly alter the resolution, retention time and relative retentions described in the method. Should this occur, it may be due to excessive dwell volume which is the volume between the point at which the 2 eluants meet and the top of the column.

Gas chromatography

Stationary phase:

- *column length*: ± 70 per cent,
- *column internal diameter*: ± 50 per cent,
- *particle size*: maximal reduction of 50 per cent, no increase permitted,
- *film thickness*: −50 per cent to + 100 per cent.

Flow rate: ± 50 per cent.

Temperature: ± 10 per cent.

Injection volume: may be decreased, provided detection and repeatability are satisfactory.

Supercritical fluid chromatography

Composition of the mobile phase: for packed columns, the amount of the minor solvent component may be adjusted by ± 30 per cent relative or ± 2 per cent absolute, whichever is the larger. No adjustment is permitted for a capillary column system.

Detector wavelength: no adjustment permitted.

Stationary phase:

- *column length*: ± 70 per cent,
- *column internal diameter*:

  ± 25 per cent (packed columns),

  ± 50 per cent (capillary columns),
- *particle size*: maximal reduction of 50 per cent, no increase permitted (packed columns).

Flow rate: ± 50 per cent.

Temperature: ± 10 per cent.

Injection volume: may be decreased, provided detection and repeatability are satisfactory.

QUANTIFICATION

- *Detector response.* The detector sensitivity is the signal output per unit concentration or unit mass of a substance in the mobile phase entering the detector. The relative detector response factor, commonly referred to as *response factor*, expresses the sensitivity of a detector relative to a standard substance. The *correction factor* is the reciprocal of the response factor.
- *External standard method.* The concentration of the component(s) to be analysed is determined by comparing the response(s) (peak(s)) obtained with the test solution to the response(s) (peak(s)) obtained with a reference solution.
- *Internal standard method.* Equal amounts of a component that is resolved from the substance to be examined (the internal standard) is introduced into the test solution and a reference solution. The internal standard should not react with the substance to be examined; it must be stable and must not contain impurities with a retention time similar to that of the substance to be examined. The concentration of the substance to be examined is determined by comparing the ratio of the peak areas or peak heights due to the substance to be examined and the internal standard in the test solution with the ratio of the peak areas or peak heights due to the substance to be examined and the internal standard in the reference solution.
- *Normalisation procedure.* The percentage content of one or more components of the substance to be examined is calculated by determining the area of the peak or peaks as a percentage of the total area of all the peaks, excluding those due to solvents or any added reagents and those below the disregard limit.
- *Calibration procedure.* The relationship between the measured or evaluated signal *(y)* and the amount (concentration, mass, etc.) of substance *(x)* is determined and the calibration function is calculated. The analytical results are calculated from the measured signal or evaluated signal of the analyte by means of the inverse function.

For assays and for quantitative determination of components the external standard method, the internal standard method or the calibration procedure may be described in the monograph, and the normalisation procedure is not normally applied. In tests for related substances, either the external standard method with a single reference solution or the normalisation procedure is generally applied. However, with both the normalisation procedure or the external standard method, when a dilution of the test solution is used for comparison, the responses of the related substances are similar to the substance itself (response factor of 0.8 to 1.2), otherwise correction factors are included in the text.

When the related substances test prescribes the summation of impurities or there is quantitative determination of an impurity, it is important to choose an appropriate threshold setting and appropriate conditions for the integration of the peak areas. In such tests the *disregard limit*, e.g. the areas of peaks whose areas are below the limit are not taken into account, is generally 0.05 per cent. Thus, the threshold setting of the data collection system corresponds to, at least, half of the disregard limit. Integration of the peak areas of the impurities, which are not completely separated from the main peak, are preferably performed by valley-to-valley extrapolation (tangential skim). Peaks due to the solvent(s) used to dissolve the sample are also to be disregarded.

01/2005:20247

2.2.47. CAPILLARY ELECTROPHORESIS

GENERAL PRINCIPLES

Capillary electrophoresis is a physical method of analysis based on the migration, inside a capillary, of charged analytes dissolved in an electrolyte solution, under the influence of a direct-current electric field.

The migration velocity of an analyte under an electric field of intensity E, is determined by the electrophoretic mobility of the analyte and the electro-osmotic mobility of the buffer inside the capillary. The electrophoretic mobility of a solute (μ_{ep}) depends on the characteristics of the solute (electric charge, molecular size and shape) and those of the buffer in which the migration takes place (type and ionic strength of the electrolyte, pH, viscosity and additives). The electrophoretic velocity (ν_{ep}) of a solute, assuming a spherical shape, is given by the equation:

$$\nu_{ep} = \mu_{ep} \times E = \left(\frac{q}{6\pi\eta r}\right) \times \left(\frac{V}{L}\right)$$

- q = effective charge of the solute,
- η = viscosity of the electrolyte solution,
- r = Stoke's radius of the solute,
- V = applied voltage,
- L = total length of the capillary.

When an electric field is applied through the capillary filled with buffer, a flow of solvent is generated inside the capillary, called electro-osmotic flow. The velocity of the electro-osmotic flow depends on the electro-osmotic mobility (μ_{eo}) which in turn depends on the charge density on the capillary internal wall and the buffer characteristics. The electro-osmotic velocity (ν_{eo}) is given by the equation:

$$\nu_{eo} = \mu_{eo} \times E = \left(\frac{\varepsilon\zeta}{\eta}\right) \times \left(\frac{V}{L}\right)$$

- ε = dielectric constant of the buffer,
- ζ = zeta potential of the capillary surface.

The velocity of the solute (ν) is given by:

$$\nu = \nu_{ep} + \nu_{eo}$$

The electrophoretic mobility of the analyte and the electro-osmotic mobility may act in the same direction or in opposite directions, depending on the charge of the solute. In normal capillary electrophoresis, anions will migrate in the opposite direction to the electro-osmotic flow and their velocities will be smaller than the electro-osmotic velocity. Cations will migrate in the same direction as the electro-osmotic flow and their velocities will be greater than the electro-osmotic velocity. Under conditions in which there is a fast electro-osmotic velocity with respect to the electrophoretic velocity of the solutes, both cations and anions can be separated in the same run.

The time (t) taken by the solute to migrate the distance (l) from the injection end of the capillary to the detection point (capillary effective length) is given by the expression:

$$t = \frac{l}{\nu_{ep} + \nu_{eo}} = \frac{l \times L}{(\mu_{ep} + \mu_{eo}) \times V}$$

In general, uncoated fused-silica capillaries above pH 3 have negative charge due to ionised silanol groups in the inner wall. Consequently, the electro-osmotic flow is from anode to cathode. The electro-osmotic flow must remain constant from run to run if good reproducibility is to be obtained in the migration velocity of the solutes. For some applications, it may be necessary to reduce or suppress the electro-osmotic flow by modifying the inner wall of the capillary or by changing the concentration, composition and/or pH of the buffer solution.

After the introduction of the sample into the capillary, each analyte ion of the sample migrates within the background electrolyte as an independent zone, according to its electrophoretic mobility. Zone dispersion, that is the spreading of each solute band, results from different phenomena. Under ideal conditions the sole contribution to the solute-zone broadening is molecular diffusion of the solute along the capillary (longitudinal diffusion). In this ideal case the efficiency of the zone, expressed as the number of theoretical plates (N), is given by:

$$N = \frac{(\mu_{ep} + \mu_{eo}) \times V \times l}{2 \times D \times L}$$

- D = molecular diffusion coefficient of the solute in the buffer.

In practice, other phenomena such as heat dissipation, sample adsorption onto the capillary wall, mismatched conductivity between sample and buffer, length of the injection plug, detector cell size and unlevelled buffer reservoirs can also significantly contribute to band dispersion.

Separation between 2 bands (expressed as the resolution, R_s) can be obtained by modifying the electrophoretic mobility of the analytes, the electro-osmotic mobility induced in the capillary and by increasing the efficiency for the band of each analyte, according to the equation:

$$R_s = \frac{\sqrt{N}\,(\mu_{epb} - \mu_{epa})}{4\,(\overline{\mu}_{ep} + \mu_{eo})}$$

- μ_{epa} and μ_{epb} = electrophoretic mobilities of the 2 analytes separated,
- $\overline{\mu}_{ep}$ = mean electrophoretic mobility of the 2 analytes $\overline{\mu}_{ep} = \frac{1}{2}(\mu_{epb} + \mu_{epa})$.

APPARATUS

An apparatus for capillary electrophoresis is composed of:

- a high-voltage, controllable direct-current power supply;
- 2 buffer reservoirs, held at the same level, containing the prescribed anodic and cathodic solutions;
- 2 electrode assemblies (the cathode and the anode), immersed in the buffer reservoirs and connected to the power supply;
- a separation capillary (usually made of fused-silica) which, when used with some specific types of detectors, has an optical viewing window aligned with the detector. The ends of the capillary are placed in the buffer reservoirs. The capillary is filled with the solution prescribed in the monograph;
- a suitable injection system;
- a detector able to monitor the amount of substances of interest passing through a segment of the separation capillary at a given time; it is usually based on absorption spectrophotometry (UV and visible) or fluorimetry, but conductimetric, amperometric or mass spectrometric

detection can be useful for specific applications; indirect detection is an alternative method used to detect non-UV-absorbing and non-fluorescent compounds;

- a thermostatic system able to maintain a constant temperature inside the capillary is recommended to obtain a good separation reproducibility;
- a recorder and a suitable integrator or a computer.

The definition of the injection process and its automation are critical for precise quantitative analysis. Modes of injection include gravity, pressure or vacuum injection and electrokinetic injection. The amount of each sample component introduced electrokinetically depends on its electrophoretic mobility, leading to possible discrimination using this injection mode.

Use the capillary, the buffer solutions, the preconditioning method, the sample solution and the migration conditions prescribed in the monograph of the considered substance. The employed electrolytic solution is filtered to remove particles and degassed to avoid bubble formation that could interfere with the detection system or interrupt the electrical contact in the capillary during the separation run. A rigorous rinsing procedure should be developed for each analytical method to achieve reproducible migration times of the solutes.

CAPILLARY ZONE ELECTROPHORESIS

PRINCIPLE

In capillary zone electrophoresis, analytes are separated in a capillary containing only buffer without any anticonvective medium. With this technique, separation takes place because the different components of the sample migrate as discrete bands with different velocities. The velocity of each band depends on the electrophoretic mobility of the solute and the electro-osmotic flow in the capillary (see General Principles). Coated capillaries can be used to increase the separation capacity of those substances adsorbing on fused-silica surfaces.

Using this mode of capillary electrophoresis, the analysis of both small (M_r < 2000) and large molecules (2000 < M_r < 100 000) can be accomplished. Due to the high efficiency achieved in capillary zone electrophoresis, separation of molecules having only minute differences in their charge-to-mass ratio can be effected. This separation mode also allows the separation of chiral compounds by addition of chiral selectors to the separation buffer.

OPTIMISATION

Optimisation of the separation is a complex process where several separation parameters can play a major role. The main factors to be considered in the development of separations are instrumental and electrolytic solution parameters.

Instrumental parameters

Voltage. A Joule heating plot is useful in optimising the applied voltage and capillary temperature. Separation time is inversely proportional to applied voltage. However, an increase in the voltage used can cause excessive heat production, giving rise to temperature and, as a result thereof, viscosity gradients in the buffer inside the capillary. This effect causes band broadening and decreases resolution.

Polarity. Electrode polarity can be normal (anode at the inlet and cathode at the outlet) and the electro-osmotic flow will move toward the cathode. If the electrode polarity is reversed, the electro-osmotic flow is away from the outlet and only charged analytes with electrophoretic mobilities greater than the electro-osmotic flow will pass to the outlet.

Temperature. The main effect of temperature is observed on buffer viscosity and electrical conductivity, and therefore on migration velocity. In some cases, an increase in capillary temperature can cause a conformational change in proteins, modifying their migration time and the efficiency of the separation.

Capillary. The dimensions of the capillary (length and internal diameter) contribute to analysis time, efficiency of separations and load capacity. Increasing both effective length and total length can decrease the electric fields (working at constant voltage) which increases migration time. For a given buffer and electric field, heat dissipation, and hence sample band-broadening, depend on the internal diameter of the capillary. The latter also affects the detection limit, depending on the sample volume injected and the detection system employed.

Since the adsorption of the sample components on the capillary wall limits efficiency, methods to avoid these interactions should be considered in the development of a separation method. In the specific case of proteins, several strategies have been devised to avoid adsorption on the capillary wall. Some of these strategies (use of extreme pH and adsorption of positively charged buffer additives) only require modification of the buffer composition to prevent protein adsorption. In other strategies, the internal wall of the capillary is coated with a polymer, covalently bonded to the silica, that prevents interaction between the proteins and the negatively charged silica surface. For this purpose, ready-to-use capillaries with coatings consisting of neutral-hydrophilic, cationic and anionic polymers are available.

Electrolytic solution parameters

Buffer type and concentration. Suitable buffers for capillary electrophoresis have an appropriate buffer capacity in the pH range of choice and low mobility to minimise current generation.

Matching buffer-ion mobility to solute mobility, whenever possible, is important for minimising band distortion. The type of sample solvent used is also important to achieve on-column sample focusing, which increases separation efficiency and improves detection.

An increase in buffer concentration (for a given pH) decreases electro-osmotic flow and solute velocity.

Buffer pH. The pH of the buffer can affect separation by modifying the charge of the analyte or additives, and by changing the electro-osmotic flow. In protein and peptide separation, changing the pH of the buffer from above to below the isoelectric point (pI) changes the net charge of the solute from negative to positive. An increase in the buffer pH generally increases the electro-osmotic flow.

Organic solvents. Organic modifiers (methanol, acetonitrile, etc.) may be added to the aqueous buffer to increase the solubility of the solute or other additives and/or to affect the degree of ionisation of the sample components. The addition of these organic modifiers to the buffer generally causes a decrease in the electro-osmotic flow.

Additives for chiral separations. For the separation of optical isomers, a chiral selector is added to the separation buffer. The most commonly used chiral selectors are cyclodextrins, but crown ethers, polysaccharides and proteins may also be used. Since chiral recognition is governed by the different interactions between the chiral selector and each of the enantiomers, the resolution achieved for the chiral compounds depends largely on the type of chiral selector used. In this regard, for the development of a given separation it may be useful to test cyclodextrins having a different cavity size (α-, β-, or γ-cyclodextrin) or modified cyclodextrins with neutral (methyl, ethyl, hydroxyalkyl, etc.) or ionisable (aminomethyl, carboxymethyl, sulphobutyl ether, etc.) groups. When using modified cyclodextrins, batch-to-batch variations in the degree of substitution of the cyclodextrins must be taken into account since it will influence the selectivity. Other factors controlling the resolution in chiral separations are concentration of chiral selector, composition and pH of the buffer and temperature. The use of organic additives, such as methanol or urea can also modify the resolution achieved.

CAPILLARY GEL ELECTROPHORESIS

PRINCIPLE

In capillary gel electrophoresis, separation takes place inside a capillary filled with a gel that acts as a molecular sieve. Molecules with similar charge-to-mass ratios are separated according to molecular size since smaller molecules move more freely through the network of the gel and therefore migrate faster than larger molecules. Different biological macromolecules (for example, proteins and DNA fragments), which often have similar charge-to-mass ratios, can thus be separated according to their molecular mass by capillary gel electrophoresis.

CHARACTERISTICS OF GELS

2 types of gels are used in capillary electrophoresis: permanently coated gels and dynamically coated gels. Permanently coated gels, such as cross-linked polyacrylamide, are prepared inside the capillary by polymerisation of the monomers. They are usually bonded to the fused-silica wall and cannot be removed without destroying the capillary. If the gels are used for protein analysis under reducing conditions, the separation buffer usually contains sodium dodecyl sulphate and the samples are denatured by heating in a mixture of sodium dodecyl sulphate and 2-mercaptoethanol or dithiothreitol before injection. When non-reducing conditions are used (for example, analysis of an intact antibody), 2-mercaptoethanol and dithiothreitol are not used. Separation in cross-linked gels can be optimised by modifying the separation buffer (as indicated in the capillary zone electrophoresis section) and controlling the gel porosity during the gel preparation. For cross-linked polyacrylamide gels, the porosity can be modified by changing the concentration of acrylamide and/or the proportion of cross-linker. As a rule, a decrease in the porosity of the gel leads to a decrease in the mobility of the solutes. Due to the rigidity of these gels, only electrokinetic injection can be used.

Dynamically coated gels are hydrophilic polymers, such as linear polyacrylamide, cellulose derivatives, dextran, etc., which can be dissolved in aqueous separation buffers giving rise to a separation medium that also acts as a molecular sieve. These separation media are easier to prepare than cross-linked polymers. They can be prepared in a vial and filled by pressure in a wall-coated capillary (with no electro-osmotic flow). Replacing the gel before every injection generally improves the separation reproducibility. The porosity of the gels can be increased by using polymers of higher molecular mass (at a given polymer concentration) or by decreasing the polymer concentration (for a given polymer molecular mass). A reduction in the gel porosity leads to a decrease in the mobility of the solute for the same buffer. Since the dissolution of these polymers in the buffer gives low viscosity solutions, both hydrodynamic and electrokinetic injection techniques can be used.

CAPILLARY ISOELECTRIC FOCUSING

PRINCIPLE

In isoelectric focusing, the molecules migrate under the influence of the electric field, so long as they are charged, in a pH gradient generated by ampholytes having pI values in a wide range (poly-aminocarboxylic acids), dissolved in the separation buffer.

The three basic steps of isoelectric focusing are loading, focusing and mobilisation.

Loading step. Two methods may be employed:

- loading in one step: the sample is mixed with ampholytes and introduced into the capillary either by pressure or vacuum;
- sequential loading: a leading buffer, then the ampholytes, then the sample mixed with ampholytes, again ampholytes alone and finally the terminating buffer are introduced into the capillary. The volume of the sample must be small enough not to modify the pH gradient.

Focusing step. When the voltage is applied, ampholytes migrate toward the cathode or the anode, according to their net charge, thus creating a pH gradient from anode (lower pH) to cathode (higher pH). During this step the components to be separated migrate until they reach a pH corresponding to their isoelectric point (pI) and the current drops to very low values.

Mobilisation step. If mobilisation is required for detection, use one of the following methods.

- in the first method, mobilisation is accomplished during the focusing step under the effect of the electro-osmotic flow; the electro-osmotic flow must be small enough to allow the focusing of the components;
- in the second method, mobilisation is accomplished by applying positive pressure after the focusing step;
- in the third method, mobilisation is achieved after the focusing step by adding salts to the cathode reservoir or the anode reservoir (depending on the direction chosen for mobilisation) in order to alter the pH in the capillary when the voltage is applied. As the pH is changed, the proteins and ampholytes are mobilised in the direction of the reservoir which contains the added salts and pass the detector.

The separation achieved, expressed as ΔpI, depends on the pH gradient (dpH/dx), the number of ampholytes having different pI values, the molecular diffusion coefficient (*D*), the intensity of the electric field (*E*) and the variation of the electrophoretic mobility of the analyte with the pH ($-d\mu/dpH$):

$$\Delta pI = 3 \times \sqrt{\frac{D\,(dpH/dx)}{E\,(-d\mu/dpH)}}$$

OPTIMISATION

The main parameters to be considered in the development of separations are:

Voltage. Capillary isoelectric focusing utilises very high electric fields, 300 V/cm to 1000 V/cm in the focusing step.

Capillary. The electro-osmotic flow must be reduced or suppressed depending on the mobilisation strategy (see above). Coated capillaries tend to reduce the electro-osmotic flow.

Solutions. The anode buffer reservoir is filled with a solution with a pH lower than the pI of the most acidic ampholyte and the cathode reservoir is filled with a solution with a pH higher than the pI of the most basic ampholyte. Phosphoric acid for the anode and sodium hydroxide for the cathode are frequently used.

Addition of a polymer, such as methylcellulose, in the ampholyte solution tends to suppress convective forces (if any) and electro-osmotic flow by increasing the viscosity. Commercial ampholytes are available covering many pH ranges and may be mixed if necessary to obtain an expanded pH range. Broad pH ranges are used to estimate the isoelectric point whereas narrower ranges are employed to improve accuracy. Calibration can be done by correlating migration time with isoelectric point for a series of protein markers.

During the focusing step precipitation of proteins at their isoelectric point can be prevented, if necessary, using buffer additives such as glycerol, surfactants, urea or zwitterionic buffers. However, depending on the concentration, urea denatures proteins.

MICELLAR ELECTROKINETIC CHROMATOGRAPHY (MEKC)

PRINCIPLE

In micellar electrokinetic chromatography, separation takes place in an electrolyte solution which contains a surfactant at a concentration above the critical micellar concentration (*cmc*). The solute molecules are distributed between the aqueous buffer and the pseudo-stationary phase composed of micelles, according to the partition coefficient of the solute. The technique can therefore be considered as a hybrid of electrophoresis and chromatography. It is a technique that can be used for the separation of both neutral and charged solutes, maintaining the efficiency, speed and instrumental suitability of capillary electrophoresis. One of the most widely used surfactants in MEKC is the anionic surfactant sodium dodecyl sulphate, although other surfactants, for example cationic surfactants such as cetyltrimethylammonium salts, are also used.

The separation mechanism is as follows. At neutral and alkaline pH, a strong electro-osmotic flow is generated and moves the separation buffer ions in the direction of the cathode. If sodium dodecyl sulphate is employed as the surfactant, the electrophoretic migration of the anionic micelle is in the opposite direction, towards the anode. As a result, the overall micelle migration velocity is slowed down compared to the bulk flow of the electrolytic solution. In the case of neutral solutes, since the analyte can partition between the micelle and the aqueous buffer, and has no electrophoretic mobility, the analyte migration velocity will depend only on the partition coefficient between the micelle and the aqueous buffer. In the electropherogram, the peaks corresponding to each uncharged solute are always between that of the electro-osmotic flow marker and that of the micelle (the time elapsed between these two peaks is called the separation window). For electrically charged solutes, the migration velocity depends on both the partition coefficient of the solute between the micelle and the aqueous buffer, and on the electrophoretic mobility of the solute in the absence of micelle.

Since the mechanism in MEKC of neutral and weakly ionised solutes is essentially chromatographic, migration of the solute and resolution can be rationalised in terms of the retention factor of the solute (k), also referred to as mass distribution ratio (D_m), which is the ratio of the number of moles of solute in the micelle to those in the mobile phase. For a neutral compound, k is given by:

$$k = \frac{t_R - t_0}{t_0 \times \left(1 - \frac{t_R}{t_{mc}}\right)} = K \times \frac{V_S}{V_M}$$

t_R = migration time of the solute,

t_0 = analysis time of an unretained solute (determined by injecting an electro-osmotic flow marker which does not enter the micelle, for instance methanol),

t_{mc} = micelle migration time (measured by injecting a micelle marker, such as Sudan III, which migrates while continuously associated in the micelle),

K = partition coefficient of the solute,

V_S = volume of the micellar phase,

V_M = volume of the mobile phase.

Likewise, the resolution between 2 closely-migrating solutes (R_s) is given by:

$$R_s = \frac{\sqrt{N}}{4} \times \frac{\alpha - 1}{\alpha} \times \frac{k_b}{k_b + 1} \times \frac{1 - \left(\frac{t_0}{t_{mc}}\right)}{1 + k_a \times \left(\frac{t_0}{t_{mc}}\right)}$$

N = number of theoretical plates for one of the solutes,

α = selectivity,

k_a and k_b = retention factors for both solutes, respectively ($k_b > k_a$).

Similar, but not identical, equations give k and R_s values for electrically charged solutes.

OPTIMISATION

The main parameters to be considered in the development of separations by MEKC are instrumental and electrolytic solution parameters.

Instrumental parameters

Voltage. Separation time is inversely proportional to applied voltage. However, an increase in voltage can cause excessive heat production that gives rise to temperature gradients and viscosity gradients of the buffer in the cross-section of the capillary. This effect can be significant with high conductivity buffers such as those containing micelles. Poor heat dissipation causes band broadening and decreases resolution.

Temperature. Variations in capillary temperature affect the partition coefficient of the solute between the buffer and the micelles, the critical micellar concentration and the viscosity of the buffer. These parameters contribute to the migration time of the solutes. The use of a good cooling system improves the reproducibility of the migration time for the solutes.

Capillary. As in capillary zone electrophoresis, the dimensions of the capillary (length and internal diameter) contribute to analysis time and efficiency of separations. Increasing both effective length and total length can decrease the electric fields (working at constant voltage), increase migration time and improve the separation efficiency. The internal diameter controls heat dissipation (for a given buffer and electric field) and consequently the sample band broadening.

Electrolytic solution parameters

Surfactant type and concentration. The type of surfactant, in the same way as the stationary phase in chromatography, affects the resolution since it modifies separation selectivity.

Also, the log k of a neutral compound increases linearly with the concentration of surfactant in the mobile phase. Since resolution in MEKC reaches a maximum when k approaches the value of $\sqrt{t_{mc}/t_0}$, modifying the concentration of surfactant in the mobile phase changes the resolution obtained.

Buffer pH. Although pH does not modify the partition coefficient of non-ionised solutes, it can modify the electro-osmotic flow in uncoated capillaries. A decrease in the buffer pH decreases the electro-osmotic flow and therefore increases the resolution of the neutral solutes in MEKC, resulting in a longer analysis time.

Organic solvents. To improve MEKC separation of hydrophobic compounds, organic modifiers (methanol, propanol, acetonitrile, etc.) can be added to the electrolytic solution. The addition of these modifiers usually decreases migration time and the selectivity of the separation. Since the addition of organic modifiers affects the critical micellar concentration, a given surfactant concentration can be used only within a certain percentage of organic modifier before the micellisation is inhibited or adversely affected, resulting in the absence of micelles and, therefore, in the absence of partition. The dissociation of micelles in the presence of a high content of organic solvent does not always mean that the separation will no longer be possible; in some cases the hydrophobic interaction between the ionic surfactant monomer and the neutral solutes forms solvophobic complexes that can be separated electrophoretically.

Additives for chiral separations. For the separation of enantiomers using MEKC, a chiral selector is included in the micellar system, either covalently bound to the surfactant or added to the micellar separation electrolyte. Micelles that have a moiety with chiral discrimination properties include salts of *N*-dodecanoyl-L-amino acids, bile salts, etc. Chiral resolution can also be achieved using chiral discriminators, such as cyclodextrins, added to the electrolytic solutions which contain micellised achiral surfactants.

Other additives. Several strategies can be carried out to modify selectivity, by adding chemicals to the buffer. The addition of several types of cyclodextrins to the buffer can also be used to reduce the interaction of hydrophobic solutes with the micelle, thus increasing the selectivity for this type of compound.

The addition of substances able to modify solute-micelle interactions by adsorption on the latter, is used to improve the selectivity of the separations in MEKC. These additives may be a second surfactant (ionic or non-ionic) which gives rise to mixed micelles or metallic cations which dissolve in the micelle and form co-ordination complexes with the solutes.

QUANTIFICATION

Peak areas must be divided by the corresponding migration time to give the corrected area in order to:

- compensate for the shift in migration time from run to run, thus reducing the variation of the response,
- compensate for the different responses of sample constituents with different migration times.

Where an internal standard is used, verify that no peak of the substance to be examined is masked by that of the internal standard.

CALCULATIONS

From the values obtained, calculate the content of the component or components being examined. When prescribed, the percentage content of one or more components of the sample to be examined is calculated by determining the corrected area(s) of the peak(s) as a percentage of the total of the corrected areas of all peaks, excluding those due to solvents or any added reagents (normalisation procedure). The use of an automatic integration system (integrator or data acquisition and processing system) is recommended.

SYSTEM SUITABILITY

In order to check the behaviour of the capillary electrophoresis system, system suitability parameters are used. The choice of these parameters depends on the mode of capillary electrophoresis used. They are: retention factor (k) (only for micellar electrokinetic chromatography), apparent number of theoretical plates (N), symmetry factor (A_s) and resolution (R_s). In previous sections, the theoretical expressions for N and R_s have been described, but more practical equations that allow these parameters to be calculated from the electropherograms are given below.

APPARENT NUMBER OF THEORETICAL PLATES

The apparent number of theoretical plates (N) may be calculated using the expression:

$$N = 5.54 \times \left(\frac{t_R}{w_h}\right)^2$$

t_R = migration time or distance along the baseline from the point of injection to the perpendicular dropped from the maximum of the peak corresponding to the component,

w_h = width of the peak at half-height.

RESOLUTION

The resolution (R_s) between peaks of similar height of 2 components may be calculated using the expression:

$$R_s = \frac{1.18 \times (t_{R2} - t_{R1})}{w_{h1} + w_{h2}}$$

$$t_{R2} > t_{R1}$$

t_{R1} and t_{R2} = migration times or distances along the baseline from the point of injection to the perpendiculars dropped from the maxima of two adjacent peaks,

w_{h1} and w_{h2} = peak widths at half-height.

When appropriate, the resolution may be calculated by measuring the height of the valley (H_v) between 2 partly resolved peaks in a standard preparation and the height of the smaller peak (H_p) and calculating the peak-to-valley ratio:

$$\frac{p}{v} = \frac{H_p}{H_v}$$

SYMMETRY FACTOR

The symmetry factor (A_s) of a peak may be calculated using the expression:

$$A_s = \frac{w_{0.05}}{2d}$$

$w_{0.05}$ = width of the peak at one-twentieth of the peak height,

d = distance between the perpendicular dropped from the peak maximum and the leading edge of the peak at one-twentieth of the peak height.

Tests for area repeatability (standard deviation of areas or of the area/migration-time ratio) and for migration time repeatability (standard deviation of migration time) are introduced as suitability parameters. Migration time repeatability provides a test for the suitability of the capillary washing procedures. An alternative practice to avoid the lack of repeatability of the migration time is to use migration time relative to an internal standard.

A test for the verification of the signal-to-noise ratio for a standard preparation (or the determination of the limit of quantification) may also be useful for the determination of related substances.

SIGNAL-TO-NOISE RATIO

The detection limit and quantification limit correspond to signal-to-noise ratios of 3 and 10 respectively. The signal-to-noise ratio (S/N) is calculated using the expression:

$$\frac{S}{N} = \frac{2H}{h}$$

H = height of the peak corresponding to the component concerned, in the electropherogram obtained with the prescribed reference solution, measured from the maximum of the peak to the extrapolated baseline of the signal observed over a distance equal to twenty times the width at half-height,

h = range of the background in an electropherogram obtained after injection of a blank, observed over a distance equal to twenty times the width at the half-height of the peak in the electropherogram obtained with the prescribed reference solution and, if possible, situated equally around the place where this peak would be found.

01/2005:20248

2.2.48. RAMAN SPECTROMETRY

Raman spectrometry (inelastic light scattering) is a light-scattering process in which the specimen under examination is irradiated with intense monochromatic light (usually laser light) and the light scattered from the specimen is analysed for frequency shifts.

Raman spectrometry is complementary to infrared spectrometry in the sense that the two techniques both probe the molecular vibrations in a material. However, Raman and infrared spectrometry have different relative sensitivities for different functional groups. Raman spectrometry is particularly sensitive to non-polar bonds (e.g. C-C single or multiple bonds) and less sensitive to polar bonds. Hence, water, which has a strong infrared absorption spectrum, is a weak Raman scatterer and is thus well suited as a solvent for Raman spectrometry.

Apparatus: Spectrometers for recording Raman spectra typically consist of the following components:

- a monochromatic light source, typically a laser, with a wavelength in the ultraviolet, visible or near-infrared region,
- suitable optics (lens, mirrors or optical-fibre assembly) which directs the irradiating light to and collects the scattered light from the sample,
- an optical device (monochromator or filter) that transmits the frequency-shifted Raman scattering and prevents the intense incident frequency (Rayleigh scattering) from reaching the detector,
- a dispersing device (grating or prism monochromator) combined with wavelength-selecting slits and a detector (usually a photomultiplier tube),

  or:
- a dispersing device (grating or prism) combined with a multichannel detector (usually a charge-coupled device (CCD)),

  or:
- an interferometer with a detector that records the intensity of the scattered light over time, and a data-handling device that converts the data to the frequency or wavenumber domain by a Fourier-transform calculation.

PREPARATION OF THE SAMPLE

Raman spectra can be obtained from solids, liquids and gases either directly, or in glass containers or tubes, generally without prior sample preparation or dilution.

A major limitation of Raman spectrometry is that impurities may cause fluorescence that interferes with the detection of the much weaker Raman signal. Fluorescence may be avoided by choosing a laser source with a longer wavelength, for example in the near infrared, as the exciting line. The intensity of certain Raman lines may be enhanced in a number of ways, for instance in Resonance Raman (RR) and by Surface Enhanced Raman Spectrometry (SERS).

Due to the narrow focus of the irradiating laser beam, the spectrum is typically obtained from only a few microlitres of sample. Hence, sample inhomogeneities must be considered, unless the sample volume is increased, for example by rotation of the sample.

IDENTIFICATION AND QUANTITATION USING REFERENCE SUBSTANCES

Prepare the substance to be examined and the reference substance by the same procedure and record the spectra under the same operational conditions. The maxima in the spectrum obtained with the substance to be examined correspond in position and relative intensity to those in the spectrum obtained with the reference substance (CRS).

When the spectra recorded in the solid state show differences in the positions of the maxima, treat the substance to be examined and the reference substance in the same manner so that they crystallise or are produced in the same form, or proceed as described in the monograph, then record the spectra.

While Beer-Lambert's law is not valid for Raman spectrometry, Raman intensity is directly proportional to the concentration of the scattering species. As for other spectroscopic techniques, quantitation can be performed using known amounts or concentrations of reference substances. Owing to the small spatial resolution of the technique, care must be taken to ensure representative samples of standards and unknowns, for example by making sure that they are in the same physical state or by using an internal standard for liquid samples.

IDENTIFICATION AND QUANTITATION USING SPECTRAL LIBRARIES AND STATISTICAL METHODS FOR CLASSIFICATION AND CALIBRATION

Control of instrument performance. Use the apparatus according to the manufacturer's instructions and carry out the prescribed calibrations and system performance tests at regular intervals, depending on the use of the apparatus and the substances to be examined. When using Raman spectrometry for quantitative determinations, or when setting up spectral reference libraries for (chemometric) classification or calibration, particular care should be taken to ensure that corrections are made or measures are taken to control the variability in wavenumber and response-intensity of the instrumentation.

Verification of the wavenumber scale. Verify the wavenumber scale of the Raman shift (normally expressed in reciprocal centimetres) using a suitable standard which has characteristic maxima at the wavenumbers under investigation, for example, an organic substance, an Ne lamp or Ar^+ plasma lines from an argon-ion laser.

The calibration measurement should be matched to the sample type, i.e. a solid calibration sample should be used for solid samples and a liquid calibration sample for liquid samples. Choose a suitable substance (e.g. indene, cyclohexane or naphthalene) for which accurate wavenumber shifts have been established. The indene sample can favourably be placed in an NMR tube, evacuated and sealed under inert gas, and stored cool in the dark to avoid degradation of the sample.

Table 2.2.48.-1. – *Wavenumber shifts (and acceptable tolerances) of cyclohexane, indene and naphthalene.*

cyclohexane [A]	indene [B]	naphthalene [A]
		3056.4 (± 1.5)
2938.3 (± 1.5)		
2923.8 (± 1.5)		
2852.9 (± 1.5)		
	1609.7 (± 1.0)	1576.6 (± 1.0)
1444.4 (± 1.0)	1552.6 (± 1.0)	1464.5 (± 1.0)
1266.4 (± 1.0)	1205.2 (± 1.0)	1382.2 (± 1.0)
1157.6 (± 1.0)		1147.2 (± 1.0)
1028.3 (± 1.0)	1018.6 (± 1.0)	1021.6 (± 1.0)
801.3 (± 1.0)	730.5 (± 1.0)	763.8 (± 1.0)
	533.9 (± 1.0)	513.8 (± 1.0)

[A] *Standard guide for Raman shift standards for spectrometer calibration* (American Society for Testing and Materials ASTM E 1840).

[B] D. A. Carter, W. R. Thompson, C. E. Taylor and J. E. Pemberton, *Applied Spectroscopy*, 1995, 49 (11), 1561-1576.

Verification of the response-intensity scale. The absolute and relative intensities of the Raman bands are affected by several factors including:

- the state of polarisation of the irradiating light,
- the state of polarisation of the collection optics,
- the intensity of the irradiating light,
- differences in instrument response,
- differences in focus and geometry at sample,
- differences in packing density for solid samples.

Appropriate acceptance criteria will vary with the application but a day-to-day variation of ± 10 per cent in relative band intensities is achievable in most cases.

Establishment of a spectral reference library. Record the spectra of a suitable number of materials which have been fully tested (e.g. as prescribed in a monograph) and which exhibit the variation (manufacturer, batch, crystal modification, particle size, etc.) typical of the material to be analysed. The set of spectra represents the information that defines the similarity border or quantitative limits, which may be used, e.g. to identify the substance or control the amount formed in a manufacturing process. The number of substances in the database depends on the specific application. The collection of spectra in the database may be represented in different ways defined by the mathematical technique used for classification or quantitation.

The selectivity of the database which makes it possible to identify positively a given material and distinguish it adequately from other materials in the database is to be established during the validation procedure. This selectivity must be challenged on a regular basis to ensure ongoing validity of the database; this is especially necessary after any major change in a substance (e.g. change in supplier or in the manufacturing process of the material) or in the set-up of the Raman instrument (e.g. verification of the wavenumber and response repeatability of the spectrometer).

This database is then valid for use only with the originating instrument, or with a similar instrument, provided the transferred database has been demonstrated to remain valid.

Method. Prepare and examine the sample in the same manner as for the establishment of the database. A suitable mathematical transformation of the Raman spectrum may be calculated to facilitate spectrum comparison or quantitative prediction.

Comparison of the spectra or transforms of the spectra or quantitative prediction of properties or amounts in the material in question may involve the use of a suitable chemometric or statistical classification or calibration technique.

01/2005:20249

2.2.49. FALLING BALL VISCOMETER METHOD

The determination of dynamic viscosity of Newtonian liquids using a suitable falling ball viscometer is performed at 20 ± 0.1 °C, unless otherwise prescribed in the monograph. The time required for a test ball to fall in the liquid to be examined from one ring mark to the other is determined. If no stricter limit is defined for the equipment used the result is valid only if 2 consecutive measures do not differ by more than 1.5 per cent.

Apparatus. The falling ball viscometer consists of: a glass tube enclosed in a mantle, which allow precise control of temperature; six balls made of glass, nickel-iron or steel with different densities and diameters. The tube is fixed in such a way that the axis is inclined by 10 ± 1° with regard to the vertical. The tube has 2 ring marks which define the distance the ball has to roll. Commercially available apparatus is supplied with tables giving the constants, the density of the balls and the suitability of the different balls for the expected range of viscosity.

Method. Fill the clean, dry tube of the viscometer, previously brought to 20 ± 0.1 °C, with the liquid to be examined, avoiding bubbles. Add the ball suitable for the range of viscosity of the liquid so as to obtain a falling time not less than 30 s. Close the tube and maintain the solution at 20 ± 0.1 °C for at least 15 min. Let the ball run through the liquid between the 2 ring marks once without measurement. Let it run again and measure with a stop-watch, to the nearest one-fifth of a second, the time required for the ball to roll from the upper to the lower ring mark. Repeat the test run at least 3 times.

Calculate the dynamic viscosity η in millipascal seconds using the formula:

$$\eta = k(\rho_1 - \rho_2) \times t$$

k = constant, expressed in millimeter squared per second squared,

ρ_1 = density of the ball used, expressed in grams per cubic centimetre,

ρ_2 = density of the liquid to be examined, expressed in grams per cubic centimetre, obtained by multiplying its relative density d_{20}^{20} by 0.9982,

t = falling time of the ball, in seconds.

01/2005:20254

2.2.54. ISOELECTRIC FOCUSING

GENERAL PRINCIPLES

Isoelectric focusing (IEF) is a method of electrophoresis that separates proteins according to their isoelectric point. Separation is carried out in a slab of polyacrylamide or agarose gel that contains a mixture of amphoteric electrolytes (ampholytes). When subjected to an electric field, the ampholytes migrate in the gel to create a pH gradient. In some cases gels containing an immobilised pH gradient, prepared by incorporating weak acids and bases to specific regions of the gel network during the preparation of the gel, are used. When the applied proteins reach the gel fraction that has a pH that is the same as their isoelectric point (pI), their charge is neutralised and migration ceases. Gradients can be made over various ranges of pH, according to the mixture of ampholytes chosen.

THEORETICAL ASPECTS

When a protein is at the position of its isoelectric point, it has no net charge and cannot be moved in a gel matrix by the electric field. It may, however, move from that position by diffusion. The pH gradient forces a protein to remain in its isoelectric point position, thus concentrating it; this concentrating effect is called "focusing". Increasing the applied voltage or reducing the sample load result in improved separation of bands. The applied voltage is limited by the heat generated, which must be dissipated. The use of thin gels and an efficient cooling plate controlled by a thermostatic circulator prevents the burning of the gel whilst allowing sharp focusing. The separation is estimated by determining the minimum pI difference (ΔpI), which is necessary to separate 2 neighbouring bands:

$$\Delta\mathrm{pI} = 3 \times \sqrt{\frac{D\,(\mathrm{dpH}/\mathrm{d}x)}{E\,(-\mathrm{d}\mu/\mathrm{dpH})}}$$

D = diffusion coefficient of the protein,

$\frac{\mathrm{dpH}}{\mathrm{d}x}$ = pH gradient,

E = intensity of the electric field, in volts per centimetre,

$-\frac{\mathrm{d}\mu}{\mathrm{dpH}}$ = variation of the solute mobility with the pH in the region close to the pI.

Since D and $-\frac{\mathrm{d}\mu}{\mathrm{dpH}}$ for a given protein cannot be altered, the separation can be improved by using a narrower pH range and by increasing the intensity of the electric field.

Resolution between protein bands on an IEF gel prepared with carrier ampholytes can be quite good. Improvements in resolution may be achieved by using immobilised pH gradients where the buffering species, which are analogous to carrier ampholytes, are copolymerised within the gel matrix. Proteins exhibiting pIs differing by as little as 0.02 pH units may be resolved using a gel prepared with carrier ampholytes while immobilised pH gradients can resolve proteins differing by approximately 0.001 pH units.

PRACTICAL ASPECTS

Special attention must be paid to sample characteristics and/or preparation. Having salt in the sample can be problematic and it is best to prepare the sample, if possible, in deionised water or 2 per cent ampholytes, using dialysis or gel filtration if necessary.

The time required for completion of focusing in thin-layer polyacrylamide gels is determined by placing a coloured protein (e.g. haemoglobin) at different positions on the gel surface and by applying the electric field: the steady state is reached when all applications give an identical band pattern. In some protocols the completion of the focusing is indicated by the time elapsed after the sample application.

The IEF gel can be used as an identity test when the migration pattern on the gel is compared to a suitable standard preparation and IEF calibration proteins, the IEF gel can be used as a limit test when the density of a band on IEF is compared subjectively with the density of bands appearing in a standard preparation, or it can be used as a quantitative test when the density is measured using a densitometer or similar instrumentation to determine the relative concentration of protein in the bands subject to validation.

APPARATUS

An apparatus for IEF consists of:

- a controllable generator for constant potential, current and power; potentials of 2500 V have been used and are considered optimal under a given set of operating conditions; a supply of up to 30 W of constant power is recommended;
- a rigid plastic IEF chamber that contains a cooled plate, of suitable material, to support the gel;
- a plastic cover with platinum electrodes that are connected to the gel by means of paper wicks of suitable width, length and thickness, impregnated with solutions of anodic and cathodic electrolytes.

ISOELECTRIC FOCUSING IN POLYACRYLAMIDE GELS: DETAILED PROCEDURE

The following method is a detailed description of an IEF procedure in thick polyacrylamide slab gels, which is used unless otherwise stated in the monograph.

PREPARATION OF THE GELS

Mould. The mould (see Figure 2.2.54.-1) is composed of a glass plate (A) on which a polyester film (B) is placed to facilitate handling of the gel, one or more spacers (C), a second glass plate (D) and clamps to hold the structure together.

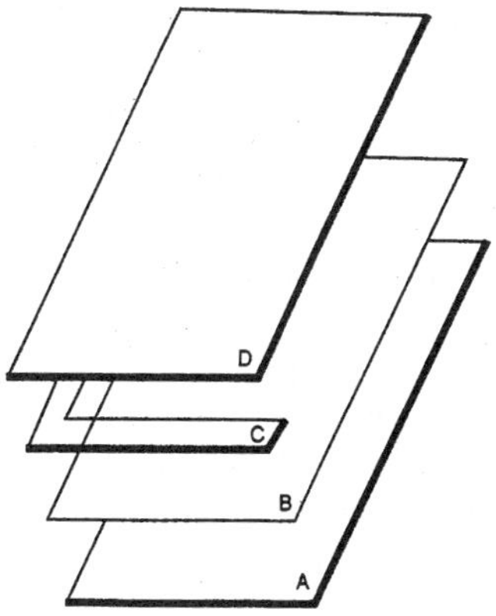

Figure 2.2.54.-1 – *Mould*

7.5 per cent polyacrylamide gel. Dissolve 29.1 g of *acrylamide R* and 0.9 g of *methylenebisacrylamide R* in 100 ml of *water R*. To 2.5 volumes of this solution, add the mixture of ampholytes specified in the monograph and dilute to 10 volumes with *water R*. Mix carefully and degas the solution.

Preparation of the mould. Place the polyester film on the lower glass plate, apply the spacer, place the second glass plate and fit the clamps. Before use, place the solution on a magnetic stirrer and add 0.25 volumes of a 100 g/l solution of *ammonium persulphate R* and 0.25 volumes of *tetramethylethylenediamine R*. Immediately fill the space between the glass plates of the mould with the solution.

METHOD

Dismantle the mould and, making use of the polyester film, transfer the gel onto the cooled support, wetted with a few millilitres of a suitable liquid, taking care to avoid forming air bubbles. Prepare the test solutions and reference solutions as specified in the monograph. Place strips of paper for sample application, about 10 mm × 5 mm in size, on the gel and impregnate each with the prescribed amount of the test and reference solutions. Also apply the prescribed quantity of a solution of proteins with known isoelectric points as pH markers to calibrate the gel. In some protocols the gel has pre-cast slots where a solution of the sample is applied instead of using impregnated paper strips. Cut 2 strips of paper to the length of the gel and impregnate them with the electrolyte solutions: acid for the anode and alkaline for the cathode. The compositions of the anode and cathode solutions are given in the monograph. Apply these paper wicks to each side of the gel several millimetres from the edge. Fit the cover so that the electrodes are in contact with the wicks (respecting the anodic and cathodic poles). Proceed with the isoelectric focusing by applying the electrical parameters described in the monograph. Switch off the current when the migration of the mixture of standard proteins has stabilised. Using forceps, remove the sample application strips and the 2 electrode wicks. Immerse the gel in *fixing solution for isoelectric focusing in polyacrylamide gel R*. Incubate with gentle shaking at room temperature for 30 min. Drain off the solution and add 200 ml of *destaining solution R*. Incubate with shaking for 1 h. Drain the gel, add *coomassie staining solution R*. Incubate for 30 min. Destain the gel by passive diffusion with *destaining solution R* until the bands are well visualised against a clear background. Locate the position and intensity of the bands in the electropherogram as prescribed in the monograph.

VARIATIONS TO THE DETAILED PROCEDURE (SUBJECT TO VALIDATION)

Where reference to the general method on isoelectric focusing is made, variations in methodology or procedure may be made subject to validation. These include:

- the use of commercially available pre-cast gels and of commercial staining and destaining kits,
- the use of immobilised pH gradients,
- the use of rod gels,
- the use of gel cassettes of different dimensions, including ultra-thin (0.2 mm) gels,
- variations in the sample application procedure, including different sample volumes or the use of sample application masks or wicks other than paper,
- the use of alternate running conditions, including variations in the electric field depending on gel dimensions and equipment, and the use of fixed migration times rather than subjective interpretation of band stability,
- the inclusion of a pre-focusing step,
- the use of automated instrumentation,
- the use of agarose gels.

VALIDATION OF ISO-ELECTRIC FOCUSING PROCEDURES

Where alternative methods to the detailed procedure are employed they must be validated. The following criteria may be used to validate the separation:

- formation of a stable pH gradient of desired characteristics, assessed for example using coloured pH markers of known isoelectric points,
- comparison with the electropherogram provided with the chemical reference substance for the preparation to be examined,
- any other validation criteria as prescribed in the monograph.

SPECIFIED VARIATIONS TO THE GENERAL METHOD

Variations to the general method required for the analysis of specific substances may be specified in detail in monographs. These include:

- the addition of urea in the gel (3 M concentration is often satisfactory to keep protein in solution but up to 8 M can be used): some proteins precipitate at their isoelectric point; in this case, urea is included in the gel formulation to keep the protein in solution; if urea is used, only fresh solutions should be used to prevent carbamylation of the protein;
- the use of alternative staining methods;
- the use of gel additives such as non-ionic detergents (e.g. octylglucoside) or zwitterionic detergents (e.g., CHAPS or CHAPSO), and the addition of ampholyte to the sample, to prevent proteins from aggregating or precipitating.

POINTS TO CONSIDER

Samples can be applied to any area on the gel, but to protect the proteins from extreme pH environments samples should not be applied close to either electrode. During method development the analyst can try applying the protein in 3 positions on the gel (i.e. middle and both ends); the pattern of a protein applied at opposite ends of the gel may not be identical.

A phenomenon known as cathodic drift, where the pH gradient decays over time, may occur if a gel is focused too long. Although not well understood, electroendoosmosis and absorption of carbon dioxide may be factors that lead to cathodic drift. Cathodic drift is observed as focused protein migrating off the cathode end of the gel. Immobilised pH gradients may be used to address this problem.

Efficient cooling (approximately 4 °C) of the bed that the gel lies on during focusing is important. High field strengths used during isoelectric focusing can lead to overheating and affect the quality of the focused gel.

01/2005:20255

2.2.55. PEPTIDE MAPPING

Peptide mapping is an identity test for proteins, especially those obtained by rDNA technology. It involves the chemical or enzymatic treatment of a protein resulting in the formation of peptide fragments followed by separation and identification of these fragments in a reproducible manner. It is a powerful test that is capable of identifying almost any single amino acid changes resulting from events such as errors in the reading of complementary DNA (cDNA) sequences or point mutations. Peptide mapping is a comparative procedure because the information obtained, compared to a reference substance similarly treated, confirms the primary structure of the protein, is capable of detecting whether alterations in structure have occurred, and demonstrates process consistency and genetic stability. Each protein presents unique characteristics which must be well understood so that the scientific and analytical approaches permit validated development of a peptide map that provides sufficient specificity.

This chapter provides detailed assistance in the application of peptide mapping and its validation to characterise the desired protein, to evaluate the stability of the expression construct of cells used for recombinant DNA products and to evaluate the consistency of the overall process, to assess product stability as well as to ensure the identity of the protein, or to detect the presence of protein variant.

Peptide mapping is not a general method, but involves developing specific maps for each unique protein. Although the technology is evolving rapidly, there are certain methods that are generally accepted. Variations of these methods will be indicated, when appropriate, in specific monographs.

A peptide map may be viewed as a fingerprint of a protein and is the end product of several chemical processes that provide a comprehensive understanding of the protein being analysed. 4 principal steps are necessary for the development of the procedure: isolation and purification of the protein, if the protein is part of a formulation; selective cleavage of the peptide bonds; chromatographic separation of the peptides; and analysis and identification of the peptides. A test sample is digested and assayed in parallel with a reference substance. Complete cleavage of peptide bonds is more likely to occur when enzymes such as endoproteases (e.g., trypsin) are used, instead of chemical cleavage reagents. A map must contain enough peptides to be meaningful. On the other hand, if there are too many fragments, the map might lose its specificity because many proteins will then have the same profiles.

ISOLATION AND PURIFICATION

Isolation and purification are necessary for analysis of bulk drugs or dosage forms containing interfering excipients and carrier proteins and, when required, will be specified in the monograph. Quantitative recovery of protein from the dosage form must be validated.

SELECTIVE CLEAVAGE OF PEPTIDE BONDS

The selection of the approach used for the cleavage of peptide bonds will depend on the protein under test. This selection process involves determination of the type of cleavage to be employed, enzymatic or chemical, and the type of cleavage agent within the chosen category. Several cleavage agents and their specificity are shown in Table 2.2.55.-1. This list is not all-inclusive and will be expanded as other cleavage agents are identified.

Pretreatment of sample. Depending on the size or the configuration of the protein, different approaches in the pretreatment of samples can be used. If trypsin is used as a cleavage agent for proteins with a molecular mass greater than 100 000 Da, lysine residues must be protected by citraconylation or maleylation; otherwise, too many peptides will be generated.

Pretreatment of the cleavage agent. Pretreatment of cleavage agents, especially enzymatic agents, might be necessary for purification purposes to ensure reproducibility of the map. For example, trypsin used as a cleavage agent will have to be treated with tosyl-L-phenylalanine chloromethyl ketone to inactivate chymotrypsin. Other methods, such as purification of trypsin by high performance liquid chromatography (HPLC) or immobilisation of enzyme on a gel support, have been successfully used when only a small amount of protein is available.

Pretreatment of the protein. Under certain conditions, it might be necessary to concentrate the sample or to separate the protein from added substances and stabilisers used in formulation of the product, if these interfere with the mapping procedure. Physical procedures used for pretreatment can include ultrafiltration, column chromatography and lyophilization. Other pretreatments, such as the addition of chaotropic agents (e.g. urea) can be used to unfold the protein prior to mapping. To allow the enzyme to have full access to cleavage sites and permit some unfolding of the protein, it is often necessary to reduce and alkylate the disulphide bonds prior to digestion.

Digestion with trypsin can introduce ambiguities in the peptide map due to side reactions occurring during the digestion reaction, such as non-specific cleavage, deamidation, disulphide isomerisation, oxidation of methionine residues, or formation of pyroglutamic groups created from the deamidation of glutamine at the *N*-terminal side of a peptide. Furthermore, peaks may be produced by

Table 2.2.55.-1. – *Examples of cleavage agents*

Type	Agent	Specificity
Enzymatic	Trypsin (EC 3.4.21.4)	*C*-terminal side of Arg and Lys
	Chymotrypsin (EC 3.4.21.1)	*C*-terminal side of hydrophobic residues (e.g. Leu, Met, Ala, aromatics)
	Pepsin (EC 3.4.23.1 and 2)	Non-specific digest
	Lysyl endopeptidase (Lys-C endopeptidase) (EC 3.4.21.50)	*C*-terminal side of Lys
	Glutamyl endopeptidase (from *S. aureus* strain V8) (EC 3.4.21.19)	*C*-terminal side of Glu and Asp
	Peptidyl-Asp metallo-endopeptidase (endoproteinase Asp-N)	*N*-terminal side of Asp
	Clostripain (EC 3.4.22.8)	*C*-terminal side of Arg
Chemical	Cyanogen bromide	*C*-terminal side of Met
	2-Nitro-5-thio-cyanobenzoic acid	*N*-terminal side of Cys
	O-Iodosobenzoic acid	*C*-terminal side of Trp and Tyr
	Dilute acid	Asp and Pro
	BNPS-skatole	Trp

autohydrolysis of trypsin. Their intensities depend on the ratio of trypsin to protein. To avoid autohydrolysis, solutions of proteases may be prepared at a pH that is not optimal (e.g. at pH 5 for trypsin), which would mean that the enzyme would not become active until diluted with the digest buffer.

Establishment of optimal digestion conditions. Factors that affect the completeness and effectiveness of digestion of proteins are those that could affect any chemical or enzymatic reactions.

pH of the reaction milieu. The pH of the digestion mixture is empirically determined to ensure the optimisation of the performance of the given cleavage agent. For example, when using cyanogen bromide as a cleavage agent, a highly acidic environment (e.g. pH 2, formic acid) is necessary; however, when using trypsin as a cleavage agent, a slightly alkaline environment (pH 8) is optimal. As a general rule, the pH of the reaction milieu must not alter the chemical integrity of the protein during the digestion and must not change during the course of the fragmentation reaction.

Temperature. A temperature between 25 °C and 37 °C is adequate for most digestions. The temperature used is intended to minimise chemical side reactions. The type of protein under test will dictate the temperature of the reaction milieu, because some proteins are more susceptible to denaturation as the temperature of the reaction increases. For example, digestion of recombinant bovine somatropin is conducted at 4 °C, because at higher temperatures it will precipitate during digestion.

Time. If sufficient sample is available, a time course study is considered in order to determine the optimum time to obtain a reproducible map and avoid incomplete digestion. Time of digestion varies from 2 h to 30 h. The reaction is stopped by the addition of an acid which does not interfere in the map or by freezing.

Amount of cleavage agent used. Although excessive amounts of cleavage agent are used to accomplish a reasonably rapid digestion time (i.e. 6-20 hours), the amount of cleavage agent is minimised to avoid its contribution to the chromatographic map pattern. A protein to protease ratio between 20:1 and 200:1 is generally used. It is recommended that the cleavage agent is added in 2 or more stages to optimise cleavage. Nonetheless, the final reaction volume remains small enough to facilitate the next step in peptide mapping, the separation step. To sort out digestion artifacts that might interfere with the subsequent analysis, a blank determination is performed, using a digestion control with all the reagents, except the test protein.

CHROMATOGRAPHIC SEPARATION

Many techniques are used to separate peptides for mapping. The selection of a technique depends on the protein being mapped. Techniques that have been successfully used for separation of peptides are shown in Table 2.2.55-2. In this section, a most widely used reversed-phase HPLC method is described as one of the procedures of chromatographic separation.

The purity of solvents and mobile phases is a critical factor in HPLC separation. HPLC-grade solvents and water that are commercially available, are recommended for reversed-phase HPLC. Dissolved gases present a problem in gradient systems where the solubility of the gas in a solvent may be less in a mixture than in a single solvent. Vacuum degassing and agitation by sonication are often used as useful degassing procedures. When solid particles in the solvents are drawn into the HPLC system, they can damage the sealing of pump valves or clog the top of the chromatographic column. Both pre- and post-pump filtration is also recommended.

Table 2.2.55-2. – *Techniques used for the separation of peptides*

Reversed-phase high performance liquid chromatography (HPLC)
Ion-exchange chromatography (IEC)
Hydrophobic interaction chromatography (HIC)
Polyacrylamide gel electrophoresis (PAGE), non-denaturating
Sodium dodecyl sulphate polyacrylamide gel electrophoresis (SDS-PAGE)
Capillary electrophoresis (CE)
Paper chromatography-high voltage (PCHV)
High voltage-paper electrophoresis (HVPE)

Chromatographic column. The selection of a chromatographic column is empirically determined for each protein. Columns with 10 nm or 30 nm pore size with silica support can give optimal separation. For smaller peptides, *octylsilyl silica gel for chromatography R* (3-10 µm) and *octadecylsilyl silica gel for chromatography R* (3-10 µm) column packings are more efficient than *butylsilyl silica gel for chromatography R* (5-10 µm).

Solvent. The most commonly used solvent is water with acetonitrile as the organic modifier to which not more than 0.1 per cent trifluoroacetic acid is added. If necessary, add propyl alcohol or isopropyl alcohol to solubilise the digest components, provided that the addition does not unduly increase the viscosity of the components.

Mobile phase. Buffered mobile phases containing phosphate are used to provide some flexibility in the selection of pH conditions, since shifts of pH in the 3.0-5.0 range enhance the separation of peptides containing acidic residues (e.g. glutamic and aspartic acids). Sodium or potassium phosphates, ammonium acetate, phosphoric acid at a pH between 2 and 7 (or higher for polymer-based supports) have also been used with acetonitrile gradients. Acetonitrile containing trifluoroacetic acid is used quite often.

Gradient. Gradients can be linear, nonlinear, or include step functions. A shallow gradient is recommended in order to separate complex mixtures. Gradients are optimised to provide clear resolution of 1 or 2 peaks that will become "marker" peaks for the test.

Isocratic elution. Isocratic HPLC systems using a single mobile phase are used on the basis of their convenience of use and improved detector responses. Optimal composition of a mobile phase to obtain clear resolution of each peak is sometimes difficult to establish. Mobile phases for which slight changes in component ratios or in pH significantly affect retention times of peaks in peptide maps must not be used in isocratic HPLC systems.

Other parameters. Temperature control of the column is usually necessary to achieve good reproducibility. The flow rates for the mobile phases range from 0.1-2.0 ml/min, and the detection of peptides is performed with a UV detector at 200-230 nm. Other methods of detection have been used (e.g. post-column derivatisation), but they are not as robust or versatile as UV detection.

Validation. This section provides an experimental means for measuring the overall performance of the test method. The acceptance criteria for system suitability depend on the identification of critical test parameters that affect data interpretation and acceptance. These critical parameters are also criteria that monitor peptide digestion and peptide analysis. An indicator that the desired digestion endpoint has been achieved is shown by comparison with a reference standard, which is treated in the same manner as the test protein. The use of a reference substance in parallel with the test protein is critical in the development and establishment of system suitability limits. In addition, a specimen chromatogram is included with the reference substance for additional comparison purposes. Other indicators may include visual inspection of protein or peptide solubility, the absence of intact protein, or measurement of responses of a digestion-dependent peptide. The critical system suitability parameters for peptide analysis will depend on the particular mode of peptide separation and detection and on the data analysis requirements.

When peptide mapping is used as an identification test, the system suitability requirements for the identified peptides cover selectivity and precision. In this case, as well as when identification of variant protein is done, the identification of the primary structure of the peptide fragments in the peptide map provides both a verification of the known primary structure and the identification of protein variants by comparison with the peptide map of the reference substance for the specified protein. The use of a digested reference substance for a given protein in the determination of peptide resolution is the method of choice. For an analysis of a variant protein, a characterised mixture of a variant and a reference substance can be used, especially if the variant peptide is located in a less-resolved region of the map. The index of pattern consistency can be simply the number of major peptides detected. Peptide pattern consistency can be best defined by the resolution of peptide peaks. Chromatographic parameters, such as peak-to-peak resolution, maximum peak width, peak area, peak tailing factors, and column efficiency, may be used to define peptide resolution. Depending on the protein under test and the method of separation used, single peptide or multiple peptide resolution requirements may be necessary.

The replicate analysis of the digest of the reference substance for the protein under test yields measures of precision and quantitative recovery. Recovery of the identified peptides is generally ascertained by the use of internal or external peptide standards. The precision is expressed as the relative standard deviation (RSD). Differences in the recovery and precision of the identified peptides are to be expected; therefore, the system suitability limits will have to be established for both the recovery and the precision of the identified peptides. These limits are unique for a given protein and will be specified in the individual monograph.

Visual comparison of the relative retentions, the peak responses (the peak area or the peak height), the number of peaks, and the overall elution pattern is completed initially. It is then complemented and supported by mathematical analysis of the peak response ratios and by the chromatographic profile of a 1:1 (*V/V*) mixture of sample and reference substance digest. If all peaks in the sample digest and in the reference substance digest have the same relative retentions and peak response ratios, then the identity of the sample under test is confirmed.

If peaks that initially eluted with significantly different relative retentions are then observed as single peaks in the 1:1 mixture, the initial difference would be an indication of system variability. However, if separate peaks are observed in the 1:1 mixture, this would be evidence of the nonequivalence of the peptides in each peak. If a peak in the 1:1 mixture is significantly broader than the corresponding peak in the sample and reference substance digest, it may indicate the presence of different peptides. The use of computer-aided pattern recognition software for the analysis of peptide mapping data has been proposed and applied, but issues related to the validation of the computer software preclude its use in a compendial test in the near future. Other automated approaches have been used that employ mathematical formulas, models, and pattern recognition. Such approaches are, for example, the automated identification of compounds by IR spectroscopy and the application of diode-array UV spectral analysis for identification of peptides. These methods have limitations due to inadequate resolutions, co-elution of fragments, or absolute peak response differences between reference substance and sample digest fragments.

The numerical comparison of the peak retention times and peak areas or peak heights can be done for a selected group of relevant peaks that have been correctly identified in the peptide maps. Peak areas can be calculated using 1 peak showing relatively small variation as an internal reference, keeping in mind that peak area integration is sensitive to baseline variation and likely to introduce error in the analysis. Alternatively, the percentage of each peptide peak height relative to the sum of all peak heights can be calculated for the sample under test. The percentage is then compared to that of the corresponding peak of the reference substance. The possibility of auto-hydrolysis of trypsin is monitored by producing a blank peptide map, that is, the peptide map obtained when a blank solution is treated with trypsin.

The minimum requirement for the qualification of peptide mapping is an approved test procedure that includes system suitability as a test control. In general, early in the regulatory process, qualification of peptide mapping for a protein is sufficient. As the regulatory approval process for the protein progresses, additional qualifications of the test can include a partial validation of the analytical procedure to provide assurance that the method will perform as intended in the development of a peptide map for the specified protein.

ANALYSIS AND IDENTIFICATION OF PEPTIDES

This section gives guidance on the use of peptide mapping during development in support of regulatory applications.

The use of a peptide map as a qualitative tool does not require the complete characterisation of the individual peptide peaks. However, validation of peptide mapping in support of regulatory applications requires rigorous characterisation of each of the individual peaks in the peptide map. Methods to characterise peaks range from *N*-terminal sequencing of each peak followed by amino acid analysis to the use of mass spectroscopy (MS).

For characterisation purposes, when *N*-terminal sequencing and amino acids analysis are used, the analytical separation is scaled up. Since scale-up might affect the resolution of peptide peaks, it is necessary, using empirical data, to assure that there is no loss of resolution due to scale-up. Eluates corresponding to specific peptide peaks are collected, vacuum-concentrated, and chromatographed again, if necessary. Amino acid analysis of fragments may be limited by the peptide size. If the *N*-terminus is blocked, it may need to be cleared before sequencing. *C*-terminal sequencing of proteins in combination with carboxypeptidase and matrix-assisted laser desorption ionisation coupled to time-of-flight analyser (MALDI-TOF) can also be used for characterisation purposes.

The use of MS for characterisation of peptide fragments is by direct infusion of isolated peptides or by the use of on-line LC-MS for structure analysis. In general, it includes electrospray and MALDI-TOF-MS, as well as fast-atom bombardment (FAB). Tandem MS has also been used to sequence a modified protein and to determine the type of amino acid modification that has occurred. The comparison of mass spectra of the digests before and after reduction provides a method to assign the disulphide bonds to the various sulphydryl-containing peptides.

If regions of the primary structure are not clearly demonstrated by the peptide map, it might be necessary to develop a secondary peptide map. The goal of a validated method of characterisation of a protein through peptide mapping is to reconcile and account for at least 95 per cent of the theoretical composition of the protein structure.

01/2005:20256

2.2.56. AMINO ACID ANALYSIS

Amino acid analysis refers to the methodology used to determine the amino acid composition or content of proteins, peptides, and other pharmaceutical preparations. Proteins and peptides are macromolecules consisting of covalently bonded amino acid residues organised as a linear polymer. The sequence of the amino acids in a protein or peptide determines the properties of the molecule. Proteins are considered large molecules that commonly exist as folded structures with a specific conformation, while peptides are smaller and may consist of only a few amino acids. Amino acid analysis can be used to quantify proteins and peptides, to determine the identity of proteins or peptides based on their amino acid composition, to support protein and peptide structure analysis, to evaluate fragmentation strategies for peptide mapping, and to detect atypical amino acids that might be present in a protein or peptide. It is necessary to hydrolyse a protein/peptide to its individual amino acid constituents before amino acid analysis. Following protein/peptide hydrolysis, the amino acid analysis procedure can be the same as that practiced for free amino acids in other pharmaceutical preparations. The amino acid constituents of the test sample are typically derivatised for analysis.

APPARATUS

Methods used for amino acid analysis are usually based on a chromatographic separation of the amino acids present in the test sample. Current techniques take advantage of the automated chromatographic instrumentation designed for analytical methodologies. An amino acid analysis instrument will typically be a low-pressure or high-pressure liquid chromatograph capable of generating mobile phase gradients that separate the amino acid analytes on a chromatographic column. The instrument must have post-column derivatisation capability, unless the sample is analysed using precolumn derivatisation. The detector is usually an ultraviolet/visible or fluorescence detector depending on the derivatisation method used. A recording device (e.g., integrator) is used for transforming the analogue signal from the detector and for quantitation. It is preferred that instrumentation be dedicated particularly for amino acid analysis.

GENERAL PRECAUTIONS

Background contamination is always a concern for the analyst in performing amino acid analysis. High purity reagents are necessary (e.g., low purity hydrochloric acid can contribute to glycine contamination). Analytical reagents are changed routinely every few weeks using only high-pressure liquid chromatography (HPLC) grade solvents. Potential microbial contamination and foreign material that might be present in the solvents are reduced by filtering solvents before use, keeping solvent reservoirs covered, and not placing amino acid analysis instrumentation in direct sunlight.

Laboratory practices can determine the quality of the amino acid analysis. Place the instrumentation in a low traffic area of the laboratory. Keep the laboratory clean. Clean and calibrate pipets according to a maintenance schedule. Keep pipet tips in a covered box; the analysts may not handle pipet tips with their hands. The analysts may wear powder-free latex or equivalent gloves. Limit the number of times a test sample vial is opened and closed because dust can contribute to elevated levels of glycine, serine, and alanine.

A well-maintained instrument is necessary for acceptable amino acid analysis results. If the instrument is used on a routine basis, it is to be checked daily for leaks, detector and lamp stability, and the ability of the column to maintain resolution of the individual amino acids. Clean or replace all instrument filters and other maintenance items on a routine schedule.

REFERENCE MATERIAL

Acceptable amino acid standards are commercially available for amino acid analysis and typically consist of an aqueous mixture of amino acids. When determining amino acid composition, protein or peptide standards are analysed with the test material as a control to demonstrate the integrity of the entire procedure. Highly purified bovine serum albumin has been used as a protein standard for this purpose.

CALIBRATION OF INSTRUMENTATION

Calibration of amino acid analysis instrumentation typically involves analysing the amino acid standard, which consists of a mixture of amino acids at a number of concentrations, to determine the response factor and range of analysis for each amino acid. The concentration of each amino acid in the standard is known. In the calibration procedure, the analyst dilutes the amino acid standard to several different analyte levels within the expected linear range of the amino acid analysis technique. Then, replicates at each of the different analyte levels can be analysed. Peak areas obtained for each amino acid are plotted versus the known concentration for each of the amino acids in the standard dilution. These results will allow the analyst to determine the range of amino acid concentrations where the peak area of a given amino acid is an approximately linear function of the amino acid concentration. It is important that the analyst prepare the samples for amino acid analysis so that they are within the analytical limits (e.g., linear working range) of the technique employed in order to obtain accurate and repeatable results.

4 to 6 amino acid standard levels are analysed to determine a response factor for each amino acid. The response factor is calculated as the average peak area or peak height per nanomole of amino acid present in the standard. A calibration file consisting of the response factor for each amino acid is prepared and used to calculate the concentration of each amino acid present in the test sample. This calculation involves dividing the peak area corresponding to a given amino acid by the response factor for that amino acid to give the nanomoles of the amino acid. For routine analysis, a single-point calibration may be sufficient; however, the calibration file is updated frequently and tested by the analysis of analytical controls to ensure its integrity.

REPEATABILITY

Consistent high quality amino acid analysis results from an analytical laboratory require attention to the repeatability of the assay. During analysis of the chromatographic separation of the amino acids or their derivatives, numerous peaks can be observed on the chromatogram that correspond to the amino acids. The large number of peaks makes it necessary to have an amino acid analysis system that can repeatedly identify the peaks based on retention time and integrate the peak areas for quantitation. A typical repeatability evaluation involves preparing a standard amino acid solution and analysing many replicates (e.g., 6 analyses or more) of the same standard solution. The relative standard deviation (RSD) is determined for the retention time and integrated peak area of each amino acid. An evaluation of the repeatability is expanded to include multiple assays conducted over several days by different analysts. Multiple assays include the preparation of standard dilutions from starting materials to determine the variation due to sample handling. The amino acid composition of a standard protein (e.g., bovine serum albumin) is often analysed as part of the repeatability evaluation. By evaluating the replicate variation (i.e., RSD), the laboratory can establish analytical limits to ensure that the analyses from the laboratory are under control. It is desirable to establish the lowest practical variation limits to ensure the best results. Areas to focus on to lower the variability of the amino acid analysis include sample preparation, high background spectral interference due to quality of reagents and/or laboratory practices, instrument performance and maintenance, data analysis and interpretation, and analyst performance and habits. All parameters involved are fully investigated in the scope of the validation work.

SAMPLE PREPARATION

Accurate results from amino acid analysis require purified protein and peptide samples. Buffer components (e.g., salts, urea, detergents) can interfere with the amino acid analysis and are removed from the sample before analysis. Methods that utilise post-column derivatisation of the amino acids are generally not affected by buffer components to the extent seen with pre-column derivatisation methods. It is desirable to limit the number of sample manipulations to reduce potential background contamination, to improve analyte recovery, and to reduce labour. Common techniques used to remove buffer components from protein samples include the following methods: (1) injecting the protein sample onto a reversed-phase HPLC system, removing the protein with a volatile solvent containing a sufficient organic component, and drying the sample in a vacuum centrifuge; (2) dialysis against a volatile buffer or water; (3) centrifugal ultrafiltration for buffer replacement with a volatile buffer or water; (4) precipitating the protein from the buffer using an organic solvent (e.g., acetone); (5) gel filtration.

INTERNAL STANDARDS

It is recommended that an internal standard be used to monitor physical and chemical losses and variations during amino acid analysis. An accurately known amount of internal standard can be added to a protein solution prior to hydrolysis. The recovery of the internal standard gives the general recovery of the amino acids of the protein solution. Free amino acids, however, do not behave in the same way as protein-bound amino acids during hydrolysis, whose rates of release or destruction are variable. Therefore, the use of an internal standard to correct for losses during hydrolysis may give unreliable results. It will be necessary to take this point into consideration when interpreting the results. Internal standards can also be added to the mixture of amino acids after hydrolysis to correct for differences in sample application and changes in reagent stability and flow rates. Ideally, an internal standard is an unnaturally occurring primary amino acid that is commercially available and inexpensive. It should also be stable during hydrolysis, its response factor should be linear with concentration, and it needs to elute with a unique retention time without overlapping other amino acids. Commonly used amino acid standards include norleucine, nitrotyrosine, and α-aminobutyric acid.

PROTEIN HYDROLYSIS

Hydrolysis of protein and peptide samples is necessary for amino acid analysis of these molecules. The glassware used for hydrolysis must be very clean to avoid erroneous results. Glove powders and fingerprints on hydrolysis tubes may cause contamination. To clean glass hydrolysis tubes, boil tubes for 1 h in 1 M hydrochloric acid or soak tubes in concentrated nitric acid or in a mixture of equal volumes of concentrated hydrochloric acid and nitric acid. Clean hydrolysis tubes are rinsed with high-purity water followed by a rinse with HPLC grade methanol, dried overnight in an oven, and stored covered until use. Alternatively, pyrolysis of clean glassware at 500 °C for 4 h may also be used to eliminate contamination from hydrolysis tubes. Adequate disposable laboratory material can also be used.

Acid hydrolysis is the most common method for hydrolysing a protein sample before amino acid analysis. The acid hydrolysis technique can contribute to the variation of the analysis due to complete or partial destruction of several amino acids: tryptophan is destroyed; serine and threonine are partially destroyed; methionine might undergo oxidation; and cysteine is typically recovered as cystine (but cystine recovery is usually poor because of partial destruction or reduction to cysteine). Application of adequate vacuum (less than 200 μm of mercury or 26.7 Pa) or introduction of an inert gas (argon) in the headspace of the reaction vessel can reduce the level of oxidative destruction. In peptide bonds involving isoleucine and valine the amido bonds of Ile-Ile, Val-Val, Ile-Val, and Val-Ile are partially cleaved; and asparagine and glutamine are deamidated, resulting in aspartic acid and glutamic acid, respectively. The loss of tryptophan, asparagine, and glutamine during an acid hydrolysis limits quantitation to 17 amino acids. Some of the hydrolysis techniques described are used to address these concerns. Some of the hydrolysis techniques described (i.e., Methods 4-11) may cause modifications to other amino acids. Therefore, the benefits of using a given hydrolysis technique are weighed against the concerns with the technique and are tested adequately before employing a method other than acid hydrolysis.

A time-course study (i.e., amino acid analysis at acid hydrolysis times of 24 h, 48 h and 72 h) is often employed to analyse the starting concentration of amino acids that are partially destroyed or slow to cleave. By plotting the observed concentration of labile amino acids (e.g., serine and threonine) versus hydrolysis time, the line can be extrapolated to the origin to determine the starting concentration of these amino acids. Time-course hydrolysis studies are also used with amino acids that are slow to cleave (e.g., isoleucine and valine). During the hydrolysis time course, the analyst will observe a plateau in these residues. The level of this plateau is taken as the residue concentration. If the hydrolysis time is too long, the residue concentration of the sample will begin to decrease, indicating destruction by the hydrolysis conditions.

An acceptable alternative to the time-course study is to subject an amino acid calibration standard to the same hydrolysis conditions as the test sample. The amino acid in free form may not completely represent the rate of destruction of labile amino acids within a peptide or protein during the hydrolysis. This is especially true for peptide bonds that are slow to cleave (e.g., Ile-Val bonds). However, this technique will allow the analyst to account for some residue destruction. Microwave acid hydrolysis has been used and is rapid but requires special equipment as well as special precautions. The optimal conditions for microwave hydrolysis must be investigated for each individual protein/peptide sample. The microwave hydrolysis technique typically requires only a few minutes, but even a deviation of one minute may give inadequate results (e.g., incomplete hydrolysis or destruction of labile amino acids). Complete proteolysis, using a mixture of proteases, has been used but can be complicated, requires the proper controls, and is typically more applicable to peptides than proteins.

During initial analyses of an unknown protein, experiments with various hydrolysis time and temperature conditions are conducted to determine the optimal conditions.

METHOD 1

Acid hydrolysis using hydrochloric acid containing phenol is the most common procedure used for protein/peptide hydrolysis preceding amino acid analysis. The addition of phenol to the reaction prevents the halogenation of tyrosine.

Hydrolysis solution. 6 M hydrochloric acid containing 0.1 per cent to 1.0 per cent of phenol.

Procedure

Liquid phase hydrolysis. Place the protein or peptide sample in a hydrolysis tube, and dry (the sample is dried so that water in the sample will not dilute the acid used for the hydrolysis). Add 200 µl of hydrolysis solution per 500 µg of lyophilised protein. Freeze the sample tube in a dry ice-acetone bath, and flame seal *in vacuo*. Samples are typically hydrolysed at 110 °C for 24 h *in vacuo* or in an inert atmosphere to prevent oxidation. Longer hydrolysis times (e.g., 48 h and 72 h) are investigated if there is a concern that the protein is not completely hydrolysed.

Vapour phase hydrolysis. This is one of the most common acid hydrolysis procedures, and it is preferred for microanalysis when only small amounts of the sample are available. Contamination of the sample from the acid reagent is also minimised by using vapour phase hydrolysis. Place vials containing the dried samples in a vessel that contains an appropriate amount of hydrolysis solution. The hydrolysis solution does not come in contact with the test sample. Apply an inert atmosphere or vacuum (less than 200 µm of mercury or 26.7 Pa) to the headspace of the vessel, and heat to about 110 °C for a 24 h hydrolysis time. Acid vapour hydrolyses the dried sample. Any condensation of the acid in the sample vials is to be minimised. After hydrolysis, dry the test sample *in vacuo* to remove any residual acid.

METHOD 2

Tryptophan oxidation during hydrolysis is decreased by using mercaptoethanesulfonic acid as the reducing acid.

Hydrolysis solution. 2.5 M mercaptoethanesulfonic acid solution.

Vapour phase hydrolysis. Dry about 1 µg to 100 µg of the protein/peptide under test in a hydrolysis tube. Place the hydrolysis tube in a larger tube with about 200 µl of the hydrolysis solution. Seal the larger tube *in vacuo* (about 50 µm of mercury or 6.7 Pa) to vaporise the hydrolysis solution. Heat the hydrolysis tube to 170-185 °C for about 12.5 min. After hydrolysis, dry the hydrolysis tube *in vacuo* for 15 min to remove the residual acid.

METHOD 3

Tryptophan oxidation during hydrolysis is prevented by using thioglycollic acid (TGA) as the reducing acid.

Hydrolysis solution. 7 M hydrochloric acid containing 1 per cent of phenol, 10 per cent of trifluoroacetic acid and 20 per cent of thioglycollic acid.

Vapour phase hydrolysis. Dry about 10 µg to 50 µg of the protein/peptide under test in a sample tube. Place the sample tube in a larger tube with about 200 µl of the hydrolysis solution. Seal the larger tube *in vacuo* (about 50 µm of mercury or 6.7 Pa) to vaporise the TGA. Heat the sample tube to 166 °C for about 15-30 min. After hydrolysis, dry the sample tube *in vacuo* for 5 min to remove the residual acid. Recovery of tryptophan by this method may be dependent on the amount of sample present.

METHOD 4

Cysteine/cystine and methionine oxidation is performed with performic acid before the protein hydrolysis.

Oxidation solution. Use performic acid freshly prepared by mixing 1 volume of hydrogen peroxide solution (30 per cent) and 9 volumes of anhydrous formic acid and incubating at room temperature for 1 h.

Procedure. Dissolve the protein/peptide sample in 20 µl of anhydrous formic acid and heat at 50 °C for 5 min; then add 100 µl of the oxidation solution. Allow the oxidation to proceed for 10-30 min. In this reaction, cysteine is converted to cysteic acid and methionine is converted to methionine-sulphone. Remove the excess reagent from the sample in a vacuum centrifuge. The oxidised protein can then be acid hydrolysed using Method 1 or Method 2. This technique may cause modifications to tyrosine residues in the presence of halides.

METHOD 5

Cysteine/cystine oxidation is accomplished during the liquid phase hydrolysis with sodium azide.

Hydrolysis solution. To 6 M hydrochloric acid containing 0.2 per cent of phenol, add sodium azide to obtain a final concentration of 2 g/l. The added phenol prevents halogenation of tyrosine.

Liquid phase hydrolysis. Conduct the protein/peptide hydrolysis at about 110 °C for 24 h. During the hydrolysis, the cysteine/cystine present in the sample is converted to cysteic acid by the sodium azide present in the hydrolysis solution. This technique allows better tyrosine recovery than Method 4, but it is not quantitative for methionine. Methionine is converted to a mixture of the parent methionine and its 2 oxidative products, methionine-sulphoxide and methionine-sulphone.

METHOD 6

Cysteine/cystine oxidation is accomplished with dimethyl sulphoxide (DMSO).

Hydrolysis solution. To 6 M hydrochloric acid containing 0.1 per cent to 1.0 per cent of phenol, add dimethyl sulphoxide to obtain a final concentration of 2 per cent *V/V*.

Vapour phase hydrolysis. Conduct the protein/peptide hydrolysis at about 110 °C for 24 h. During the hydrolysis, the cysteine/cystine present in the sample is converted to cysteic acid by the DMSO present in the hydrolysis solution. As an approach to limit variability and compensate for partial destruction, it is recommended to evaluate the cysteic acid recovery from oxidative hydrolysis of standard proteins containing 1-8 mol of cysteine. The response factors from protein/peptide hydrolysates are typically about 30 per cent lower than those for non-hydrolysed cysteic acid standards. Because histidine, methionine, tyrosine, and tryptophan are also modified, a complete compositional analysis is not obtained with this technique.

METHOD 7

Cysteine/cystine reduction and alkylation is accomplished by a vapour phase pyridylethylation reaction.

Reducing solution. Transfer 83.3 µl of pyridine, 16.7 µl of 4-vinylpyridine, 16.7 µl of tributylphosphine, and 83.3 µl of water to a suitable container and mix.

Procedure. Add the protein/peptide (between 1 and 100 µg) to a hydrolysis tube, and place in a larger tube. Transfer the reducing solution to the large tube, seal *in vacuo* (about

50 µm of mercury or 6.7 Pa), and heat at about 100 °C for 5 min. Then remove the inner hydrolysis tube, and dry it in a vacuum desiccator for 15 min to remove residual reagents. The pyridylethylated sample can then be acid hydrolysed using previously described procedures. The pyridylethylation reaction is performed simultaneously with a protein standard sample containing 1-8 mol of cysteine to evaluate the pyridylethyl-cysteine recovery. Longer incubation times for the pyridylethylation reaction can cause modifications to the α-amino terminal group and the ε-amino group of lysine in the protein.

METHOD 8

Cysteine/cystine reduction and alkylation is accomplished by a liquid phase pyridylethylation reaction.

Stock solutions. Prepare and filter 3 solutions: 1 M Tris-hydrochloride pH 8.5 containing 4 mM disodium edetate (stock solution A), 8 M guanidine hydrochloride (stock solution B), and 10 per cent of 2-mercaptoethanol (stock solution C).

Reducing solution. Prepare a mixture of 1 volume of stock solution A and 3 volumes of stock solution B to obtain a buffered solution of 6 M guanidine hydrochloride in 0.25 M tris-hydrochloride.

Procedure. Dissolve about 10 µg of the test sample in 50 µl of the reducing solution, and add about 2.5 µl of stock solution C. Store under nitrogen or argon for 2 h at room temperature in the dark. To achieve the pyridylethylation reaction, add about 2 µl of 4-vinylpyridine to the protein solution, and incubate for an additional 2 h at room temperature in the dark. Desalt the protein/peptide by collecting the protein/peptide fraction from a reversed-phase HPLC separation. The collected sample can be dried in a vacuum centrifuge before acid hydrolysis.

METHOD 9

Cysteine/cystine reduction and alkylation is accomplished by a liquid phase carboxymethylation reaction.

Stock solutions. Prepare as directed for Method 8.

Carboxymethylation solution. Prepare a 100 g/l solution of iodoacetamide in alcohol.

Buffer solution. Use the reducing solution, prepared as described for Method 8.

Procedure. Dissolve the test sample in 50 µl of the buffer solution, and add about 2.5 µl of stock solution C. Store under nitrogen or argon for 2 h at room temperature in the dark. Add the carboxymethylation solution in a ratio 1.5 fold per total theoretical content of thiols, and incubate for an additional 30 min at room temperature in the dark. If the thiol content of the protein is unknown, then add 5 µl of 100 mM iodoacetamide for every 20 nmol of protein present. The reaction is stopped by adding excess of 2-mercaptoethanol. Desalt the protein/peptide by collecting the protein/peptide fraction from a reversed-phase HPLC separation. The collected sample can be dried in a vacuum centrifuge before acid hydrolysis. The *S*-carboxyamidomethyl-cysteine formed will be converted to *S*-carboxymethyl-cysteine during acid hydrolysis.

METHOD 10

Cysteine/cystine is reacted with dithiodiglycolic acid or dithiodipropionic acid to produce a mixed disulphide. The choice of dithiodiglycolic acid or dithiodipropionic acid depends on the required resolution of the amino acid analysis method.

Reducing solution. A 10 g/l solution of dithiodiglycolic acid (or dithiodipropionic acid) in 0.2 M sodium hydroxide.

Procedure. Transfer about 20 µg of the test sample to a hydrolysis tube, and add 5 µl of the reducing solution. Add 10 µl of isopropyl alcohol, and then remove all of the sample liquid by vacuum centrifugation. The sample is then hydrolysed using Method 1. This method has the advantage that other amino acid residues are not derivatised by side reactions, and that the sample does not need to be desalted prior to hydrolysis.

METHOD 11

Asparagine and glutamine are converted to aspartic acid and glutamic acid, respectively, during acid hydrolysis. Asparagine and aspartic acid residues are added and represented by *Asx*, while glutamine and glutamic acid residues are added and represented by *Glx*. Proteins/peptides can be reacted with bis(1,1-trifluoroacetoxy)iodobenzene (BTI) to convert the asparagine and glutamine residues to diaminopropionic acid and diaminobutyric acid residues, respectively, upon acid hydrolysis. These conversions allow the analyst to determine the asparagine and glutamine content of a protein/peptide in the presence of aspartic acid and glutamic acid residues.

Reducing solutions. Prepare and filter 3 solutions: a solution of 10 mM trifluoroacetic acid (Solution A), a solution of 5 M guanidine hydrochloride and 10 mM trifluoroacetic acid (Solution B), and a freshly prepared solution of dimethylformamide containing 36 mg of BTI per millilitre (Solution C).

Procedure. In a clean hydrolysis tube, transfer about 200 µg of the test sample, and add 2 ml of Solution A or Solution B and 2 ml of Solution C. Seal the hydrolysis tube *in vacuo*. Heat the sample at 60 °C for 4 h in the dark. The sample is then dialysed with water to remove the excess reagents. Extract the dialysed sample 3 times with equal volumes of butyl acetate, and then lyophilise. The protein can then be acid hydrolysed using previously described procedures. The α,β-diaminopropionic and α,γ-diaminobutyric acid residues do not typically resolve from the lysine residues upon ion-exchange chromatography based on amino acid analysis. Therefore, when using ion-exchange as the mode of amino acid separation, the asparagine and glutamine contents are the quantitative difference in the aspartic acid and glutamic acid content assayed with underivatised and BTI-derivatised acid hydrolysis. The threonine, methionine, cysteine, tyrosine, and histidine assayed content can be altered by BTI derivatisation; a hydrolysis without BTI will have to be performed if the analyst is interested in the composition of these other amino acid residues of the protein/peptide.

METHODOLOGIES OF AMINO ACID ANALYSIS: GENERAL PRINCIPLES

Many amino acid analysis techniques exist, and the choice of any one technique often depends on the sensitivity required from the assay. In general, about one-half of the amino acid analysis techniques employed rely on the separation of the free amino acids by ion-exchange chromatography followed by post-column derivatisation (e.g., with ninhydrin or *o*-phthalaldehyde). Post-column derivatisation techniques can be used with samples that contain small amounts of buffer components, (such as salts and urea) and generally require between 5 µg and 10 µg of protein sample per analysis. The remaining amino acid techniques typically involve pre-column derivatisation of the free amino acids (e.g., phenyl isothiocyanate; 6-aminoquinolyl-*N*-hydroxysuccinimidyl carbamate or *o*-phthalaldehyde; (dimethylamino)azobenzenesulphonyl chloride; 9-fluorenylmethyl chloroformate; and 7-fluoro-4-nitrobenzo-2-oxa-1,3-diazole) followed by reversed-phase HPLC. Pre-column derivatisation techniques are very sensitive and usually require between 0.5 µg and 1.0 µg of protein sample per analysis but may be influenced by buffer salts in the samples. Pre-column derivatisation techniques may also result in multiple derivatives of a given amino acid, which complicates the result interpretation. Post-column derivatisation techniques are generally influenced less by performance variation of the assay than pre-column derivatisation techniques.

The following methods may be used for quantitative amino acid analysis. Instruments and reagents for these procedures are available commercially. Furthermore, many modifications of these methodologies exist with different reagent preparations, reaction procedures, chromatographic systems, etc. Specific parameters may vary according to the exact equipment and procedure used. Many laboratories will use more than one amino acid analysis technique to exploit the advantages offered by each. In each of these methods, the analogue signal is visualised by means of a data acquisition system, and the peak areas are integrated for quantification purposes.

METHOD 1 - POST-COLUMN NINHYDRIN DERIVATISATION

Ion-exchange chromatography with post-column ninhydrin derivatisation is one of the most common methods employed for quantitative amino acid analysis. As a rule, a lithium-based cation-exchange system is employed for the analysis of the more complex physiological samples, and the faster sodium-based cation-exchange system is used for the more simplistic amino acid mixtures obtained with protein hydrolysates (typically containing 17 amino acid components). Separation of the amino acids on an ion-exchange column is accomplished through a combination of changes in pH and cation strength. A temperature gradient is often employed to enhance separation.

When the amino acid reacts with ninhydrin, the reactant has a characteristic purple or yellow colour. Amino acids, except imino acid, give a purple colour, and show an absorption maximum at 570 nm. The imino acids such as proline give a yellow colour, and show an absorption maximum at 440 nm. The post-column reaction between ninhydrin and amino acids eluted from the column is monitored at 440 nm and 570 nm, and the chromatogram obtained is used for the determination of amino acid composition.

The detection limit is considered to be 10 pmol for most of the amino acid derivatives, but 50 pmol for the proline derivative. Response linearity is obtained in the range of 20-500 pmol with correlation coefficients exceeding 0.999. To obtain good composition data, samples larger than 1 µg before hydrolysis are best suited for this amino acid analysis of protein/peptide.

METHOD 2 - POST-COLUMN OPA DERIVATISATION

o-Phthalaldehyde (OPA) reacts with primary amines in the presence of thiol compound, to form highly fluorescent isoindole products. This reaction is used for the post-column derivatisation in analysis of amino acids by ion-exchange chromatography. The rule of the separation is the same as Method 1.

Although OPA does not react with secondary amines (imino acids such as proline) to form fluorescent substances, the oxidation with sodium hypochlorite or chloramine T allows secondary amines to react with OPA. The procedure employs a strongly acidic cation-exchange column for separation of free amino acids followed by post-column oxidation with sodium hypochlorite or chloramine T and post-column derivatisation using OPA and a thiol compound such as *N*-acetyl-L-cysteine or 2-mercaptoethanol. The derivatisation of primary amino acids is not noticeably affected by the continuous supply of sodium hypochlorite or chloramine T.

Separation of the amino acids on an ion-exchange column is accomplished through a combination of changes in pH and cation strength. After post-column derivatisation of eluted amino acids with OPA, the reactant passes through the fluorometric detector. Fluorescence intensity of OPA-derivatised amino acids are monitored with an excitation wavelength of 348 nm and an emission wavelength of 450 nm.

The detection limit is considered to be a few tens of picomole level for most of the OPA-derivatised amino acids. Response linearity is obtained in the range of a few picomole level to a few tens of nanomole level. To obtain good compositional data, samples larger than 500 ng of protein/peptide before hydrolysis are recommended.

METHOD 3 - PRE-COLUMN PITC DERIVATISATION

Phenylisothiocyanate (PITC) reacts with amino acids to form phenylthiocarbamyl (PTC) derivatives which can be detected with high sensitivity at 254 nm. Therefore, pre-column derivatisation of amino acids with PITC followed by a reversed-phase HPLC separation with UV detection is used to analyse the amino acid composition.

After the reagent is removed under vacuum, the derivatised amino acids can be stored dry and frozen for several weeks with no significant degradation. If the solution for injection is kept cold, no noticeable loss in chromatographic response occurs after 3 days.

Separation of the PTC-amino acids on a reversed-phase HPLC with an octadecylsilyl (ODS) column is accomplished through a combination of changes in concentrations of acetonitrile and buffer ionic strength. PTC-amino acids eluted from the column are monitored at 254 nm.

The detection limit is considered to be 1 pmol for most of the PTC-amino acids. Response linearity is obtained in the range of 20-500 pmol with correlation coefficients exceeding 0.999. To obtain good compositional data, samples larger than 500 ng of protein/peptide before hydrolysis are recommended.

METHOD 4 - PRE-COLUMN AQC DERIVITISATION

Pre-column derivatisation of amino acids with 6-aminoquinolyl-*N*-hydroxysuccinimidyl carbamate (AQC) followed by reversed-phase HPLC separation with fluorometric detection is used.

AQC reacts with amino acids to form stable, fluorescent unsymmetric urea derivatives (AQC-amino acids) which are readily amenable to analysis by reversed-phase HPLC. Therefore, pre-column derivatisation of amino acids with AQC followed by reversed-phase HPLC separation with fluorimetric detection is used to analyse the amino acid composition.

Separation of the AQC-amino acids on a reversed-phase HPLC with an ODS column is accomplished through a combination of changes in concentrations of acetonitrile and buffer ionic strengh. Selective fluorescence detection of the derivatives with an excitation wavelength at 250 nm and an emission wavelength at 395 nm allows for the direct injection of the reaction mixture with no significant interference from the only major fluorescent reagent by-product, 6-aminoquinoline. Excess reagent is rapidly hydrolysed ($t_{1/2}$<15 s) to yield 6-aminoquinoline, *N*-hydroxysuccinimide and carbon dioxide, and after 1 min no further derivatisation can take place.

Peak areas for AQC-amino acids are essentially unchanged for at least 1 week at room temperature. Therefore AQC-amino acids have more than sufficient stability to allow for overnight automated chromatographic analysis.

The detection limit is considered to range from about 40 fmol to 320 fmol for each amino acid, except for cystein. The detection limit for cystein is approximately 800 fmol. Response linearity is obtained in the range of 2.5-200 µM with correlation coefficients exceeding 0.999. Good compositional data can be obtained from the analysis of derivatised protein hydrolysates derived from as little as 30 ng of protein/peptide.

METHOD 5 - PRE-COLUMN OPA DERIVATISATION

Pre-column derivatisation of amino acids with *o*-phthalaldehyde (OPA) followed by reversed-phase HPLC separation with fluorometric detection is used. This technique does not detect amino acids that exist as secondary amines (e.g., proline).

OPA in conjunction with a thiol reagent reacts with primary amine groups to form highly fluorescent isoindole products. 2-Mercaptoethanol or 3-mercaptopropionic acid can be used as the thiol. OPA itself does not fluoresce and consequently produces no interfering peaks. In addition, its solubility and stability in aqueous solution, along with the rapid kinetics for the reaction, make it amenable to automated derivatisation and analysis using an autosampler to mix the sample with the reagent. However, lack of reactivity with secondary amino acids has been a predominant drawback. This method does not detect amino acids that exist as secondary amines (e.g., proline). To compensate for this drawback, this technique may be combined with another technique described in Method 7 or Method 8.

Pre-column derivatisation of amino acids with OPA is followed by a reversed-phase HPLC separation. Because of the instability of the OPA-amino acid derivative, HPLC separation and analysis are performed immediately following derivatisation. The liquid chromatograph is equipped with a fluorometric detector for the detection of derivatised amino acids. Fluorescence intensity of OPA-derivatised amino acids is monitored with an excitation wavelength of 348 nm and an emission wavelength of 450 nm.

Detection limits as low as 50 fmol via fluorescence have been reported, although the practical limit of analysis remains at 1 pmol.

METHOD 6 - PRE-COLUMN DABS-Cl DERIVATISATION

Pre-column derivatisation of amino acids with (dimethylamino)azobenzenesulphonyl chloride (DABS-Cl) followed by reversed-phase HPLC separation with visible light detection is used.

DABS-Cl is a chromophoric reagent employed for the labelling of amino acids. Amino acids labelled with DABS-Cl (DABS-amino acids) are highly stable and show an absorption maximum at 436 nm.

DABS-amino acids, all naturally occurring amino acid derivatives, can be separated on an ODS column of a reversed-phase HPLC by employing gradient systems consisting of acetonitrile and aqueous buffer mixture. Separated DABS-amino acids eluted from the column are detected at 436 nm in the visible region.

This method can analyse the imino acids such as proline together with the amino acids at the same degree of sensitivity, DABS-Cl derivatisation method permits the simultaneous quantification of tryptophan residues by previous hydrolysis of the protein/peptide with sulphonic acids such as mercaptoethanesulphonic acid, *p*-toluenesulphonic acid or methanesulphonic acid described in Method 2 under Protein hydrolysis. The other acid-labile residues, asparagine and glutamine, can also be analysed by previous conversion into diaminopropionic acid and diaminobutyric acid, respectively, by treatment of protein/peptide with BTI described in Method 11 under Protein hydrolysis.

The non-proteinogenic amino acid norleucine cannot be used as an internal standard in this method as this compound is eluted in a chromatographic region crowded with peaks of primary amino acids. Nitrotyrosine can be used as an internal standard because it is eluted in a clean region.

The detection limit of DABS-amino acid is about 1 pmol. As little as 2-5 pmol of an individual DABS-amino acid can be quantitatively analysed with reliability, and only 10-30 ng of the dabsylated protein hydrolysate is required for each analysis.

METHOD 7 - PRE-COLUMN FMOC-Cl DERIVATISATION

Pre-column derivatisation of amino acids with 9-fluorenylmethyl chloroformate (FMOC-Cl) followed by reversed-phase HPLC separation with fluorometric detection is used.

FMOC-Cl reacts with both primary and secondary amino acids to form highly fluorescent products. The reaction proceeds under mild conditions in aqueous solution and is completed in 30 s. The derivatives are stable, only the histidine derivative showing any breakdown. Although FMOC-Cl is fluorescent itself, the reagent excess and fluorescent side-products can be eliminated without loss of FMOC-amino acids.

FMOC-amino acids are separated by a reversed-phase HPLC using an ODS column. The separation is carried out by gradient elution varied linearly from a mixture of 10 volumes of acetonitrile, 40 volumes of methanol and 50 volumes of acetic acid buffer to a mixture of 50 volumes of acetonitrile and 50 volumes of acetic acid buffer and 20 amino acid derivatives are separated in 20 min. Each derivative eluted from the column is monitored by a fluorometric detector set at an excitation wavelength of 260 nm and an emission wavelength of 313 nm.

The detection limit is in the low femtomole range. A linearity range of 0.1-50 µM is obtained for most of the amino acids.

METHOD 8 - PRE-COLUMN NBD-F DERIVATISATION

Pre-column derivatisation of amino acids with 7-fluoro-4-nitrobenzo-2-oxa-1,3-diazole (NBD-F) followed by reversed-phase HPLC separation with fluorometric detection is used.

NBD-F reacts with both primary and secondary amino acids to form highly fluorescent products. Amino acids are derivatised with NBD-F by heating to 60 °C for 5 min.

NBD-amino acid derivatives are separated on an ODS column of a reversed-phase HPLC by employing a gradient elution system consisting of acetonitrile and aqueous buffer mixture, and 17 amino acid derivatives are separated in 35 min. ε-Aminocaproic acid can be used as an internal standard, because it is eluted in a clean chromatographic region. Each derivative eluted from the column is monitored by a fluorometric detector set at an excitation wavelength of 480 nm and an emission wavelength of 530 nm.

The sensitivity of this method is almost the same as for the pre-column OPA derivatisation method (Method 5), excluding proline to which OPA is not reactive, and might be advantageous for NBD-F against OPA. The detection limit for each amino acid is about 10 fmol. Profile analysis can be achieved with about 1.5 mg of protein hydrolysates in the pre-column reaction mixture.

DATA CALCULATION AND ANALYSIS

When determining the amino acid content of a protein/peptide hydrolysate, it should be noted that the acid hydrolysis step destroys tryptophan and cysteine. Serine and threonine are partially destroyed by acid hydrolysis, while isoleucine and valine residues may be only partially cleaved. Methionine can undergo oxidation during acid hydrolysis, and some amino acids (e.g., glycine and serine) are common contaminants. Application of adequate vacuum (less than 200 µm of mercury or 26.7 Pa) or introduction of inert gas (argon) in the headspace of the reaction vessel during vapour phase hydrolysis can reduce the level of oxidative destruction. Therefore, the quantitative results obtained for cysteine, tryptophan, threonine, isoleucine, valine, methionine, glycine, and serine from a protein/peptide hydrolysate may be variable and may warrant further investigation and consideration.

Amino Acid Mole Percent. This is the number of specific amino acid residues per 100 residues in a protein. This result may be useful for evaluating amino acid analysis data when the molecular mass of the protein under investigation is unknown. This information can be used to corroborate the identity of a protein/peptide and has other applications. Carefully identify and integrate the peaks obtained as directed for each procedure. Calculate the mole percent for each amino acid present in the test sample using the formula:

$$\frac{100 r_U}{r}$$

in which r_U is the peak response, in nanomoles, of the amino acid under test; and r is the sum of peak responses, in nanomoles, for all amino acids present in the test sample. Comparison of the mole percent of the amino acids under test to data from known proteins can help establish or corroborate the identity of the sample protein.

Unknown Protein Samples. This data analysis technique can be used to estimate the protein concentration of an unknown protein sample using the amino acid analysis data. Calculate the mass, in micrograms, of each recovered amino acid using the formula:

$$\frac{m M_r}{1000}$$

in which m is the recovered quantity, in nanomoles, of the amino acid under test; and M_r is the average molecular mass for that amino acid, corrected for the mass of the water molecule that was eliminated during peptide bond formation. The sum of the masses of the recovered amino acids will give an estimate of the total mass of the protein analysed after appropriate correction for partially and completely destroyed amino acids. If the molecular mass of the unknown protein is available (i.e., by SDS-PAGE analysis or mass spectroscopy), the amino acid composition of the unknown protein can be predicted. Calculate the number of residues of each amino acid using the formula:

$$\frac{m}{\left(\frac{1000M}{M_{rt}}\right)}$$

in which m is the recovered quantity, in nanomoles, of the amino acid under test; M is the total mass, in micrograms, of the protein; and M_{rt} is the molecular mass of the unknown protein.

Known protein samples. This data analysis technique can be used to investigate the amino acid composition and protein concentration of a protein sample of known molecular mass and amino acid composition using the amino acid analysis data. When the composition of the protein being analysed is known, one can exploit the fact that some amino acids are recovered well, while other amino acid recoveries may be compromised because of complete or partial destruction (e.g., tryptophan, cysteine, threonine, serine, methionine), incomplete bond cleavage (i.e., for isoleucine and valine) and free amino acid contamination (i.e., by glycine and serine). Because those amino acids that are recovered best represent the protein, these amino acids are chosen to quantify the amount of protein. Well-recovered amino acids are, typically, aspartate-asparagine, glutamate-glutamine, alanine, leucine, phenylalanine, lysine, and arginine. This list can be modified based on experience with one's own analysis system. Divide the quantity, in nanomoles, of each of the well-recovered amino acids by the expected number of residues for that amino acid to obtain the protein content based on each well-recovered amino acid. Average the protein content results calculated. The protein content determined for each of the well-recovered amino acids should be evenly distributed about the mean. Discard protein content values for those amino acids that have an unacceptable deviation from the mean. Typically greater than 5 per cent variation from the mean is considered unacceptable. Recalculate the mean protein content from the remaining values to obtain the protein content of the sample. Divide the content of each amino acid by the calculated mean protein content to determine the amino acid composition of the sample by analysis.

Calculate the relative compositional error, in percentage, using the formula:

$$\frac{100m}{m_S}$$

in which m is the experimentally determined quantity, in nanomoles per amino acid residue, of the amino acid under test; and m_S is the known residue value for that amino acid. The average relative compositional error is the average of the absolute values of the relative compositional errors of the individual amino acids, typically excluding tryptophan and cysteine from this calculation. The average relative compositional error can provide important information on the stability of analysis run over time. The agreement in the amino acid composition between the protein sample and the known composition can be used to corroborate the identity and purity of the protein in the sample.

2.3. IDENTIFICATION

2.3. IDENTIFICATION

01/2005:20301

2.3.1. IDENTIFICATION REACTIONS OF IONS AND FUNCTIONAL GROUPS

ACETATES

a) Heat the substance to be examined with an equal quantity of *oxalic acid R*. Acid vapours with the characteristic odour of acetic acid are liberated, showing an acid reaction (*2.2.4*).

b) Dissolve about 30 mg of the substance to be examined in 3 ml of *water R* or use 3 ml of the prescribed solution. Add successively 0.25 ml of *lanthanum nitrate solution R*, 0.1 ml of *0.05 M iodine* and 0.05 ml of *dilute ammonia R2*. Heat carefully to boiling. Within a few minutes a blue precipitate is formed or a dark blue colour develops.

ACETYL

In a test-tube about 180 mm long and 18 mm in external diameter, place about 15 mg of the substance to be examined, or the prescribed quantity, and 0.15 ml of *phosphoric acid R*. Close the tube with a stopper through which passes a small test-tube about 100 mm long and 10 mm in external diameter containing *water R* to act as a condenser. On the outside of the smaller tube, hang a drop of *lanthanum nitrate solution R*. Except for substances hydrolysable only with difficulty, place the apparatus in a water-bath for 5 min, then take out the smaller tube. Remove the drop and mix it with 0.05 ml of *0.01 M iodine* on a tile. Add at the edge 0.05 ml of *dilute ammonia R2*. After 1 min to 2 min, a blue colour develops at the junction of the two drops; the colour intensifies and persists for a short time.

For *substances hydrolysable only with difficulty* heat the mixture slowly to boiling over an open flame and then proceed as prescribed above.

ALKALOIDS

Dissolve a few milligrams of the substance to be examined, or the prescribed quantity, in 5 ml of *water R*, add *dilute hydrochloric acid R* until an acid reaction occurs (*2.2.4*), then 1 ml of *potassium iodobismuthate solution R*. An orange or orange-red precipitate is formed immediately.

ALUMINIUM

Dissolve about 15 mg of the substance to be examined in 2 ml of *water R* or use 2 ml of the prescribed solution. Add about 0.5 ml of *dilute hydrochloric acid R* and about 0.5 ml of *thioacetamide reagent R*. No precipitate is formed. Add dropwise *dilute sodium hydroxide solution R*. A gelatinous white precipitate is formed which dissolves on further addition of *dilute sodium hydroxide solution R*. Gradually add *ammonium chloride solution R*. The gelatinous white precipitate is re-formed.

AMINES, PRIMARY AROMATIC

Acidify the prescribed solution with *dilute hydrochloric acid R* and add 0.2 ml of *sodium nitrite solution R*. After 1 min to 2 min, add 1 ml of *β-naphthol solution R*. An intense orange or red colour and usually a precipitate of the same colour are produced.

AMMONIUM SALTS

To the prescribed solution add 0.2 g of *magnesium oxide R*. Pass a current of air through the mixture and direct the gas that escapes just beneath the surface of a mixture of 1 ml of *0.1 M hydrochloric acid* and 0.05 ml of *methyl red solution R*. The colour of the indicator changes to yellow. On addition of 1 ml of a freshly prepared 100 g/l solution of *sodium cobaltinitrite R* a yellow precipitate is formed.

AMMONIUM SALTS AND SALTS OF VOLATILE BASES

Dissolve about 20 mg of the substance to be examined in 2 ml of *water R* or use 2 ml of the prescribed solution. Add 2 ml of *dilute sodium hydroxide solution R*. On heating, the solution gives off vapour that can be identified by its odour and by its alkaline reaction (*2.2.4*).

ANTIMONY

Dissolve with gentle heating about 10 mg of the substance to be examined in a solution of 0.5 g of *sodium potassium tartrate R* in 10 ml of *water R* and allow to cool: to 2 ml of this solution, or to 2 ml of the prescribed solution, add *sodium sulphide solution R* dropwise; an orange-red precipitate is formed which dissolves on addition of *dilute sodium hydroxide solution R*.

ARSENIC

Heat 5 ml of the prescribed solution on a water-bath with an equal volume of *hypophosphorous reagent R*. A brown precipitate is formed.

BARBITURATES, NON-NITROGEN SUBSTITUTED

Dissolve about 5 mg of the substance to be examined in 3 ml of *methanol R*, add 0.1 ml of a solution containing 100 g/l of *cobalt nitrate R* and 100 g/l of *calcium chloride R*. Mix and add, with shaking, 0.1 ml of *dilute sodium hydroxide solution R*. A violet-blue colour and precipitate are formed.

BENZOATES

a) To 1 ml of the prescribed solution add 0.5 ml of *ferric chloride solution R1*. A dull-yellow precipitate, soluble in *ether R*, is formed.

b) Place 0.2 g of the substance to be examined, treated if necessary as prescribed, in a test-tube. Moisten with 0.2 ml to 0.3 ml of *sulphuric acid R*. Gently warm the bottom of the tube. A white sublimate is deposited on the inner wall of the tube.

c) Dissolve 0.5 g of the substance to be examined in 10 ml of *water R* or use 10 ml of the prescribed solution. Add 0.5 ml of *hydrochloric acid R*. The precipitate obtained, after crystallisation from warm *water R* and drying *in vacuo*, has a melting point (*2.2.14*) of 120 °C to 124 °C.

BISMUTH

a) To 0.5 g of the substance to be examined add 10 ml of *dilute hydrochloric acid R* or use 10 ml of the prescribed solution. Heat to boiling for 1 min. Cool and filter if necessary. To 1 ml of the solution obtained add 20 ml of *water R*. A white or slightly yellow precipitate is formed which on addition of 0.05 ml to 0.1 ml of *sodium sulphide solution R* turns brown.

b) To about 45 mg of the substance to be examined add 10 ml of *dilute nitric acid R* or use 10 ml of the prescribed solution. Boil for 1 min. Allow to cool and filter if necessary. To 5 ml of the solution obtained add 2 ml of a 100 g/l solution of *thiourea R*. A yellowish-orange colour or an orange precipitate is formed. Add 4 ml of a 25 g/l solution of *sodium fluoride R*. The solution is not decolorised within 30 min.

BROMIDES

a) Dissolve in 2 ml of *water R* a quantity of the substance to be examined equivalent to about 3 mg of bromide (Br^-) or use 2 ml of the prescribed solution. Acidify with *dilute nitric acid R* and add 0.4 ml of *silver nitrate solution R1*.

Shake and allow to stand. A curdled, pale yellow precipitate is formed. Centrifuge and wash the precipitate with three quantities, each of 1 ml, of *water R*. Carry out this operation rapidly in subdued light disregarding the fact that the supernatant solution may not become perfectly clear. Suspend the precipitate obtained in 2 ml of *water R* and add 1.5 ml of *ammonia R*. The precipitate dissolves with difficulty.

b) Introduce into a small test-tube a quantity of the substance to be examined equivalent to about 5 mg of bromide (Br^-) or the prescribed quantity. Add 0.25 ml of *water R*, about 75 mg of *lead dioxide R*, 0.25 ml of *acetic acid R* and shake gently. Dry the inside of the upper part of the test-tube with a piece of filter paper and allow to stand for 5 min. Prepare a strip of suitable filter paper of appropriate size. Impregnate it by capillarity, by dipping the tip in a drop of *decolorised fuchsin solution R* and introduce the impregnated part immediately into the tube. Starting from the tip, a violet colour appears within 10 s that is clearly distinguishable from the red colour of fuchsin, which may be visible on a small area at the top of the impregnated part of the paper strip.

CALCIUM

a) To 0.2 ml of a neutral solution containing a quantity of the substance to be examined equivalent to about 0.2 mg of calcium (Ca^{2+}) per millilitre or to 0.2 ml of the prescribed solution add 0.5 ml of a 2 g/l solution of *glyoxal-hydroxyanil R* in *alcohol R*, 0.2 ml of *dilute sodium hydroxide solution R* and 0.2 ml of *sodium carbonate solution R*. Shake with 1 ml to 2 ml of *chloroform R* and add 1 ml to 2 ml of *water R*. The chloroform layer is coloured red.

b) Dissolve about 20 mg of the substance to be examined or the prescribed quantity in 5 ml of *acetic acid R*. Add 0.5 ml of *potassium ferrocyanide solution R*. The solution remains clear. Add about 50 mg of *ammonium chloride R*. A white, crystalline precipitate is formed.

CARBONATES AND BICARBONATES

Introduce into a test-tube 0.1 g of the substance to be examined and suspend in 2 ml of *water R* or use 2 ml of the prescribed solution. Add 3 ml of *dilute acetic acid R*. Close the tube immediately using a stopper fitted with a glass tube bent twice at right angles. The solution or the suspension becomes effervescent and gives off a colourless and odourless gas. Heat gently and collect the gas in 5 ml of *barium hydroxide solution R*. A white precipitate is formed that dissolves on addition of an excess of *hydrochloric acid R1*.

CHLORIDES

a) Dissolve in 2 ml of *water R* a quantity of the substance to be examined equivalent to about 2 mg of chloride (Cl^-) or use 2 ml of the prescribed solution. Acidify with *dilute nitric acid R* and add 0.4 ml of *silver nitrate solution R1*. Shake and allow to stand. A curdled, white precipitate is formed. Centrifuge and wash the precipitate with three quantities, each of 1 ml, of *water R*. Carry out this operation rapidly in subdued light, disregarding the fact that the supernatant solution may not become perfectly clear. Suspend the precipitate in 2 ml of *water R* and add 1.5 ml of *ammonia R*. The precipitate dissolves easily with the possible exception of a few large particles which dissolve slowly.

b) Introduce into a test-tube a quantity of the substance to be examined equivalent to about 15 mg of chloride (Cl^-) or the prescribed quantity. Add 0.2 g of *potassium dichromate R* and 1 ml of *sulphuric acid R*. Place a filter-paper strip impregnated with 0.1 ml of *diphenylcarbazide solution R* over the opening of the test-tube. The paper turns violet-red. The impregnated paper must not come into contact with the potassium dichromate.

CITRATES

Dissolve in 5 ml of *water R* a quantity of the substance to be examined equivalent to about 50 mg of citric acid or use 5 ml of the prescribed solution. Add 0.5 ml of *sulphuric acid R* and 1 ml of *potassium permanganate solution R*. Warm until the colour of the permanganate is discharged. Add 0.5 ml of a 100 g/l solution of *sodium nitroprusside R* in *dilute sulphuric acid R* and 4 g of *sulphamic acid R*. Make alkaline with *concentrated ammonia R*, added dropwise until all the sulphamic acid has dissolved. Addition of an excess of *concentrated ammonia R* produces a violet colour, turning to violet-blue.

ESTERS

To about 30 mg of the substance to be examined or the prescribed quantity add 0.5 ml of a 70 g/l solution of *hydroxylamine hydrochloride R* in *methanol R* and 0.5 ml of a 100 g/l solution of *potassium hydroxide R* in *alcohol R*. Heat to boiling, cool, acidify with *dilute hydrochloric acid R* and add 0.2 ml of *ferric chloride solution R1* diluted ten times. A bluish-red or red colour is produced.

IODIDES

a) Dissolve a quantity of the substance to be examined equivalent to about 4 mg of iodide (I^-) in 2 ml of *water R* or use 2 ml of the prescribed solution. Acidify with *dilute nitric acid R* and add 0.4 ml of *silver nitrate solution R1*. Shake and allow to stand. A curdled, pale-yellow precipitate is formed. Centrifuge and wash with three quantities, each of 1 ml, of *water R*. Carry out this operation rapidly in subdued light disregarding the fact that the supernatant solution may not become perfectly clear. Suspend the precipitate in 2 ml of *water R* and add 1.5 ml of *ammonia R*. The precipitate does not dissolve.

b) To 0.2 ml of a solution of the substance to be examined containing about 5 mg of iodide (I^-) per millilitre, or to 0.2 ml of the prescribed solution, add 0.5 ml of *dilute sulphuric acid R*, 0.1 ml of *potassium dichromate solution R*, 2 ml of *water R* and 2 ml of *chloroform R*. Shake for a few seconds and allow to stand. The chloroform layer is coloured violet or violet-red.

IRON

a) Dissolve a quantity of the substance to be examined equivalent to about 10 mg of iron (Fe^{2+}) in 1 ml of *water R* or use 1 ml of the prescribed solution. Add 1 ml of *potassium ferricyanide solution R*. A blue precipitate is formed that does not dissolve on addition of 5 ml of *dilute hydrochloric acid R*.

b) Dissolve a quantity of the substance to be examined equivalent to about 1 mg of iron (Fe^{3+}) in 30 ml of *water R*. To 3 ml of this solution or to 3 ml of the prescribed solution, add 1 ml of *dilute hydrochloric acid R* and 1 ml of *potassium thiocyanate solution R*. The solution is coloured red. Take two portions, each of 1 ml, of the mixture. To one portion add 5 ml of *isoamyl alcohol R* or 5 ml of *ether R*. Shake and allow to stand. The organic layer is coloured pink. To the other portion add 2 ml of *mercuric chloride solution R*. The red colour disappears.

c) Dissolve a quantity of the substance to be examined equivalent to not less than 1 mg of iron (Fe^{3+}) in 1 ml of *water R* or use 1 ml of the prescribed solution. Add 1 ml of *potassium ferrocyanide solution R*. A blue precipitate is formed that does not dissolve on addition of 5 ml of *dilute hydrochloric acid R*.

LACTATES

Dissolve a quantity of the substance to be examined equivalent to about 5 mg of lactic acid in 5 ml of *water R* or use 5 ml of the prescribed solution. Add 1 ml of *bromine water R* and 0.5 ml of *dilute sulphuric acid R*. Heat on a water-bath until the colour is discharged, stirring occasionally with a glass rod. Add 4 g of *ammonium sulphate R* and mix. Add dropwise and without mixing 0.2 ml of a 100 g/l solution of *sodium nitroprusside R* in *dilute sulphuric acid R*. Still without mixing add 1 ml of *concentrated ammonia R*. Allow to stand for 30 min. A dark green ring appears at the junction of the two liquids.

LEAD

a) Dissolve 0.1 g of the substance to be examined in 1 ml of *acetic acid R* or use 1 ml of the prescribed solution. Add 2 ml of *potassium chromate solution R*. A yellow precipitate is formed that dissolves on addition of 2 ml of *strong sodium hydroxide solution R*.

b) Dissolve 50 mg of the substance to be examined in 1 ml of *acetic acid R* or use 1 ml of the prescribed solution. Add 10 ml of *water R* and 0.2 ml of *potassium iodide solution R*. A yellow precipitate is formed. Heat to boiling for 1 min to 2 min. The precipitate dissolves. Allow to cool. The precipitate is re-formed as glistening, yellow plates.

MAGNESIUM

Dissolve about 15 mg of the substance to be examined in 2 ml of *water R* or use 2 ml of the prescribed solution. Add 1 ml of *dilute ammonia R1*. A white precipitate is formed that dissolves on addition of 1 ml of *ammonium chloride solution R*. Add 1 ml of *disodium hydrogen phosphate solution R*. A white crystalline precipitate is formed.

MERCURY

a) Place about 0.1 ml of a solution of the substance to be examined on well-scraped copper foil. A dark-grey stain that becomes shiny on rubbing is formed. Dry the foil and heat in a test-tube. The spot disappears.

b) To the prescribed solution add *dilute sodium hydroxide solution R* until strongly alkaline (*2.2.4*). A dense yellow precipitate is formed (mercuric salts).

NITRATES

To a mixture of 0.1 ml of *nitrobenzene R* and 0.2 ml of *sulphuric acid R*, add a quantity of the powdered substance equivalent to about 1 mg of nitrate (NO_3^-) or the prescribed quantity. Allow to stand for 5 min. Cool in iced water and add slowly and with mixing 5 ml of *water R*, then 5 ml of *strong sodium hydroxide solution R*. Add 5 ml of *acetone R*. Shake and allow to stand. The upper layer is coloured deep violet.

PHOSPHATES (ORTHOPHOSPHATES)

a) To 5 ml of the prescribed solution, neutralised if necessary, add 5 ml of *silver nitrate solution R1*. A yellow precipitate is formed whose colour is not changed by boiling and which dissolves on addition of *ammonia R*.

b) Mix 1 ml of the prescribed solution with 2 ml of *molybdovanadic reagent R*. A yellow colour develops.

POTASSIUM

a) Dissolve 0.1 g of the substance to be examined in 2 ml of *water R* or use 2 ml of the prescribed solution. Add 1 ml of *sodium carbonate solution R* and heat. No precipitate is formed. Add to the hot solution 0.05 ml of *sodium sulphide solution R*. No precipitate is formed. Cool in iced water and add 2 ml of a 150 g/l solution of *tartaric acid R*. Allow to stand. A white crystalline precipitate is formed.

b) Dissolve about 40 mg of the substance to be examined in 1 ml of *water R* or use 1 ml of the prescribed solution. Add 1 ml of *dilute acetic acid R* and 1 ml of a freshly prepared 100 g/l solution of *sodium cobaltinitrite R*. A yellow or orange-yellow precipitate is formed immediately.

SALICYLATES

a) To 1 ml of the prescribed solution add 0.5 ml of *ferric chloride solution R1*. A violet colour is produced that persists after the addition of 0.1 ml of *acetic acid R*.

b) Dissolve 0.5 g of the substance to be examined in 10 ml of *water R* or use 10 ml of the prescribed solution. Add 0.5 ml of *hydrochloric acid R*. The precipitate obtained, after recrystallisation from hot *water R* and drying *in vacuo*, has a melting point (*2.2.14*) of 156 °C to 161 °C.

SILICATES

Mix the prescribed quantity of the substance to be examined in a lead or platinum crucible by means of a copper wire with about 10 mg of *sodium fluoride R* and a few drops of *sulphuric acid R* to give a thin slurry. Cover the crucible with a thin, transparent plate of plastic under which a drop of *water R* is suspended and warm gently. Within a short time a white ring is rapidly formed around the drop of water.

SILVER

Dissolve about 10 mg of the substance to be examined in 10 ml of *water R* or use 10 ml of the prescribed solution. Add 0.3 ml of *hydrochloric acid R1*. A curdled, white precipitate is formed that dissolves on addition of 3 ml of *dilute ammonia R1*.

SODIUM

a) Dissolve 0.1 g of the substance to be examined in 2 ml of *water R* or use 2 ml of the prescribed solution. Add 2 ml of a 150 g/l solution of *potassium carbonate R* and heat to boiling. No precipitate is formed. Add 4 ml of *potassium pyroantimonate solution R* and heat to boiling. Allow to cool in iced water and if necessary rub the inside of the test-tube with a glass rod. A dense white precipitate is formed.

b) Dissolve a quantity of the substance to be examined equivalent to about 2 mg of sodium (Na^+) in 0.5 ml of *water R* or use 0.5 ml of the prescribed solution. Add 1.5 ml of *methoxyphenylacetic reagent R* and cool in ice-water for 30 min. A voluminous, white, crystalline precipitate is formed. Place in water at 20 °C and stir for 5 min. The precipitate does not disappear. Add 1 ml of *dilute ammonia R1*. The precipitate dissolves completely. Add 1 ml of *ammonium carbonate solution R*. No precipitate is formed.

SULPHATES

a) Dissolve about 45 mg of the substance to be examined in 5 ml of *water R* or use 5 ml of the prescribed solution. Add 1 ml of *dilute hydrochloric acid R* and 1 ml of *barium chloride solution R1*. A white precipitate is formed.

b) To the suspension obtained during reaction (a), add 0.1 ml of *0.05 M iodine*. The suspension remains yellow (distinction from sulphites and dithionites), but is decolorised by adding dropwise *stannous chloride solution R* (distinction from iodates). Boil the mixture. No coloured precipitate is formed (distinction from selenates and tungstates).

TARTRATES

a) Dissolve about 15 mg of the substance to be examined in 5 ml of *water R* or use 5 ml of the prescribed solution. Add 0.05 ml of a 10 g/l solution of *ferrous sulphate R* and 0.05 ml of *dilute hydrogen peroxide solution R*. A transient yellow colour is produced. After the colour has disappeared add *dilute sodium hydroxide solution R* dropwise. An intense blue colour is produced.

b) To 0.1 ml of a solution of the substance to be examined containing the equivalent of about 15 mg of tartaric acid per millilitre or to 0.1 ml of the prescribed solution add 0.1 ml of a 100 g/l solution of *potassium bromide R*, 0.1 ml of a 20 g/l solution of *resorcinol R* and 3 ml of *sulphuric acid R*. Heat on a water-bath for 5 min to 10 min. A dark-blue colour develops. Allow to cool and pour the solution into *water R*. The colour changes to red.

XANTHINES

To a few milligrams of the substance to be examined or the prescribed quantity add 0.1 ml of *strong hydrogen peroxide solution R* and 0.3 ml of *dilute hydrochloric acid R*. Heat to dryness on a water-bath until a yellowish-red residue is obtained. Add 0.1 ml of *dilute ammonia R2*. The colour of the residue changes to violet-red.

ZINC

Dissolve 0.1 g of the substance to be examined in 5 ml of *water R* or use 5 ml of the prescribed solution. Add 0.2 ml of *strong sodium hydroxide solution R*. A white precipitate is formed. Add a further 2 ml of *strong sodium hydroxide solution R*. The precipitate dissolves. Add 10 ml of *ammonium chloride solution R*. The solution remains clear. Add 0.1 ml of *sodium sulphide solution R*. A flocculent white precipitate is formed.

01/2005:20302

2.3.2. IDENTIFICATION OF FATTY OILS BY THIN-LAYER CHROMATOGRAPHY

Examine by thin-layer chromatography (*2.2.27*), using as the coating substance a suitable octadecylsilyl silica gel for high performance thin-layer chromatography.

Test solution. Unless otherwise prescribed, dissolve about 20 mg (1 drop) of the fatty oil in 3 ml of *methylene chloride R*.

Reference solution. Dissolve about 20 mg (1 drop) of *maize oil R* in 3 ml of *methylene chloride R*.

Apply separately to the plate 1 µl of each solution. Develop twice over a path of 0.5 cm using *ether R*. Develop twice over a path of 8 cm using a mixture of 20 volumes of *methylene chloride R*, 40 volumes of *glacial acetic acid R* and 50 volumes of *acetone R*. Allow the plate to dry in air and spray with a 100 g/l solution of *phosphomolybdic acid R* in *alcohol R*. Heat the plate at 120 °C for about 3 min and examine in daylight.

The chromatogram obtained typically shows spots comparable to those in Figure 2.3.2.-1.

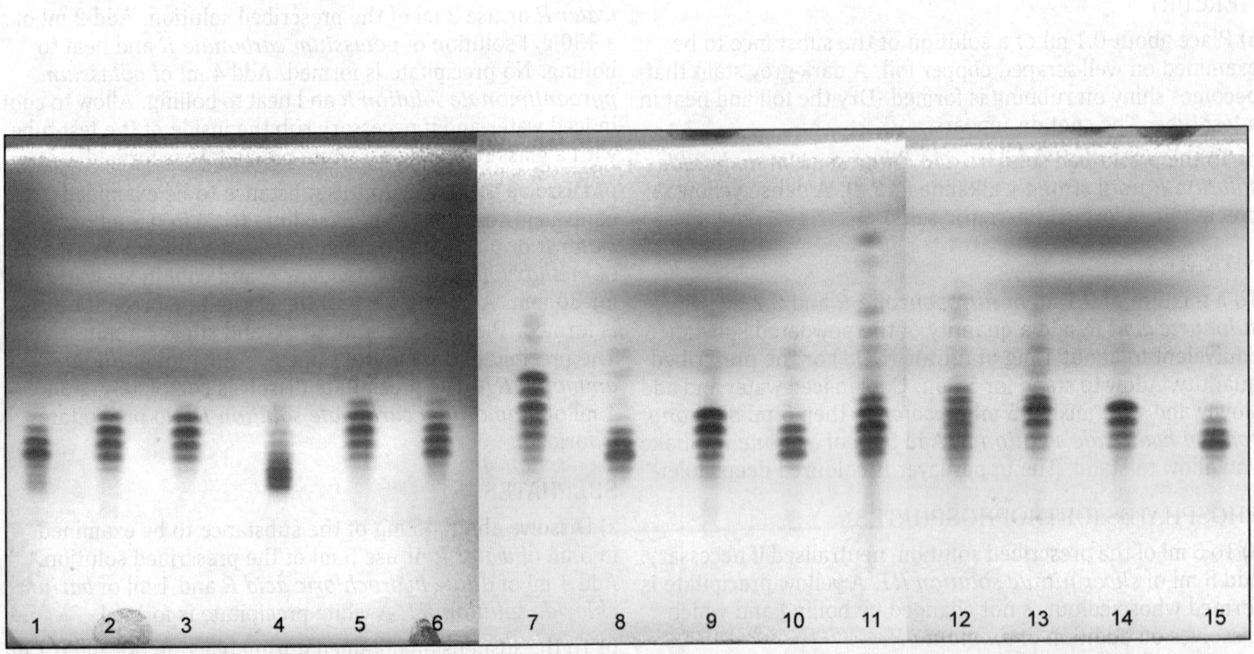

1. arachis oil
2. sesame oil
3. maize oil
4. rapeseed oil
5. soya-bean oil
6. rapeseed oil (erucic acid-free)
7. linseed oil
8. olive oil
9. sunflower oil
10. almond oil
11. wheat-germ oil
12. borage oil
13. evening primrose oil
14. safflower oil (type I)
15. safflower oil (type II)

Figure 2.3.2.-1. – *Chromatograms for the identification of fatty oils*

01/2005:20303

2.3.3. IDENTIFICATION OF PHENOTHIAZINES BY THIN-LAYER CHROMATOGRAPHY

Examine by thin-layer chromatography (*2.2.27*) using *kieselguhr G R* as the coating substance. Impregnate the plate by placing it in a closed tank containing the necessary quantity of the impregnation mixture composed of a solution containing 10 per cent *V/V* of *phenoxyethanol R* and 50 g/l of *macrogol 300 R* in *acetone R* so that the plate dips about 5 mm beneath the surface of the liquid. When the impregnation mixture has risen at least 17 cm from the lower edge of the plate, remove the plate and use immediately for chromatography. Carry out the chromatography in the same direction as the impregnation.

Test solution. Dissolve 20 mg of the substance to be examined in *chloroform R* and dilute to 10 ml with the same solvent.

Reference solution. Dissolve 20 mg of the corresponding chemical reference substance (CRS) in *chloroform R* and dilute to 10 ml with the same solvent.

Apply separately to the plate 2 μl of each solution and develop in the dark over a path of 15 cm using a mixture of 50 ml of *light petroleum R* and 1 ml of *diethylamine R* saturated with *phenoxyethanol R* (i.e. add about 3 ml to 4 ml of *phenoxyethanol R* to the above mixture of solvents to give a persistent cloudiness on shaking, decant, and use the supernatant liquid, even if it is cloudy). After development place the plate under ultraviolet light at 365 nm and examine after a few minutes. The spot in the chromatogram obtained with the test solution is similar in position, fluorescence and size to the spot in the chromatogram obtained with the reference solution. Spray with a 10 per cent *V/V* solution of *sulphuric acid R* in *alcohol R*. The spot in the chromatogram obtained with the test solution is of the same colour as that in the chromatogram obtained with the reference solution and has similar stability over a period of at least 20 min.

01/2005:20304

2.3.4. ODOUR

On a watch-glass 6 cm to 8 cm in diameter, spread in a thin layer 0.5 g to 2.0 g of the substance to be examined. After 15 min, determine the odour or verify the absence of odour.

2.4. LIMIT TESTS

2.4. LIMIT TESTS

01/2005:20401

2.4.1. AMMONIUM

Unless otherwise prescribed, use method A.

METHOD A

Dissolve the prescribed quantity of the substance to be examined in 14 ml of *water R* in a test-tube, make alkaline if necessary by the addition of *dilute sodium hydroxide solution R* and dilute to 15 ml with *water R*. To the solution add 0.3 ml of *alkaline potassium tetraiodomercurate solution R*. Prepare a standard by mixing 10 ml of *ammonium standard solution (1 ppm NH_4) R* with 5 ml of *water R* and 0.3 ml of *alkaline potassium tetraiodomercurate solution R*. Stopper the test-tubes.

After 5 min, any yellow colour in the test solution is not more intense than that in the standard.

METHOD B

In a 25 ml jar fitted with a cap, place the prescribed quantity of the finely powdered substance to be examined and dissolve or suspend in 1 ml of *water R*. Add 0.30 g of *heavy magnesium oxide R*. Close immediately after placing a piece of *silver manganese paper R* 5 mm square, wetted with a few drops of *water R*, under the polyethylene cap. Swirl, avoiding projections of liquid, and allow to stand at 40 °C for 30 min. If the silver manganese paper shows a grey colour, it is not more intense than that of a standard prepared at the same time and in the same manner using the prescribed volume of *ammonium standard solution (1 ppm NH_4) R*, 1 ml of *water R* and 0.30 g of *heavy magnesium oxide R*.

01/2005:20402

2.4.2. ARSENIC

METHOD A

The apparatus (see Figure 2.4.2.-1) consists of a 100 ml conical flask closed with a ground-glass stopper through which passes a glass tube about 200 mm long and of internal diameter 5 mm. The lower part of the tube is drawn to an internal diameter of 1.0 mm, and 15 mm from its tip is a lateral orifice 2 mm to 3 mm in diameter. When the tube is in position in the stopper, the lateral orifice should be at least 3 mm below the lower surface of the stopper. The upper end of the tube has a perfectly flat, ground surface at right angles to the axis of the tube. A second glass tube of the same internal diameter and 30 mm long, with a similar flat ground surface, is placed in contact with the first, and is held in position by two spiral springs. Into the lower tube insert 50 mg to 60 mg of *lead acetate cotton R*, loosely packed, or a small plug of cotton and a rolled piece of *lead acetate paper R* weighing 50 mg to 60 mg. Between the flat surfaces of the tubes place a disc or a small square of *mercuric bromide paper R* large enough to cover the orifice of the tube (15 mm × 15 mm).

In the conical flask dissolve the prescribed quantity of the substance to be examined in 25 ml of *water R*, or in the case of a solution adjust the prescribed volume to 25 ml with *water R*. Add 15 ml of *hydrochloric acid R*, 0.1 ml of *stannous chloride solution R* and 5 ml of *potassium iodide solution R*, allow to stand for 15 min and introduce 5 g of *activated zinc R*. Assemble the two parts of the apparatus immediately and immerse the flask in a bath of water at a temperature such that a uniform evolution of gas is maintained. Prepare a standard in the same manner, using 1 ml of *arsenic standard solution (1 ppm As) R*, diluted to 25 ml with *water R*.

After not less than 2 h the stain produced on the mercuric bromide paper in the test is not more intense than that in the standard.

METHOD B

Introduce the prescribed quantity of the substance to be examined into a test-tube containing 4 ml of *hydrochloric acid R* and about 5 mg of *potassium iodide R* and add 3 ml of *hypophosphorous reagent R*. Heat the mixture on a water-bath for 15 min, shaking occasionally. Prepare a standard in the same manner, using 0.5 ml of *arsenic standard solution (10 ppm As) R*.

After heating on the water-bath, any colour in the test solution is not more intense than that in the standard.

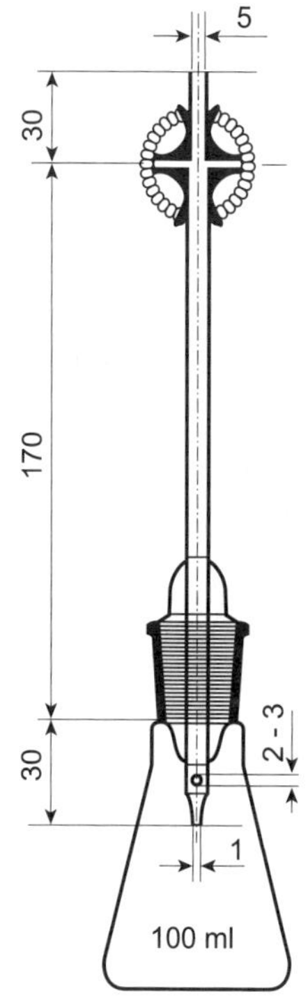

Figure 2.4.2.-1. - *Apparatus for limit test A for arsenic*
Dimensions in millimetres

01/2005:20403

2.4.3. CALCIUM

All solutions used for this test should be prepared with distilled water R.

To 0.2 ml of *alcoholic calcium standard solution (100 ppm Ca) R*, add 1 ml of *ammonium oxalate solution R*. After 1 min, add a mixture of 1 ml of *dilute acetic acid R* and 15 ml of a solution containing the prescribed quantity of the substance to be examined and shake. Prepare a standard in the same manner using a mixture of 10 ml of *aqueous calcium standard solution (10 ppm Ca) R*, 1 ml of *dilute acetic acid R* and 5 ml of *distilled water R*.

After 15 min, any opalescence in the test solution is not more intense than that in the standard.

01/2005:20404

2.4.4. CHLORIDES

To 15 ml of the prescribed solution add 1 ml of *dilute nitric acid R* and pour the mixture as a single addition into a test-tube containing 1 ml of *silver nitrate solution R2*. Prepare a standard in the same manner using 10 ml of *chloride standard solution (5 ppm Cl) R* and 5 ml of *water R*. Examine the tubes laterally against a black background.

After standing for 5 min protected from light, any opalescence in the test solution is not more intense than that in the standard.

01/2005:20405

2.4.5. FLUORIDES

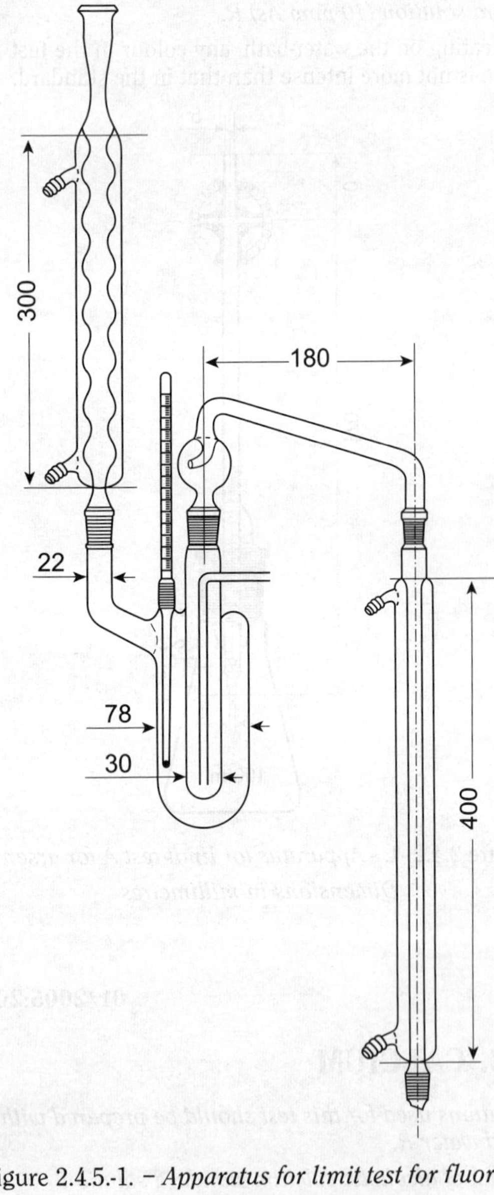

Figure 2.4.5.-1. – *Apparatus for limit test for fluorides*
Dimensions in millimetres

Introduce into the inner tube of the apparatus (see Figure 2.4.5.-1) the prescribed quantity of the substance to be examined, 0.1 g of acid-washed *sand R* and 20 ml of a mixture of equal volumes of *sulphuric acid R* and *water R*. Heat the jacket containing *tetrachloroethane R* maintained at its boiling point (146 °C). Heat the steam generator and distil, collecting the distillate in a 100 ml volumetric flask containing 0.3 ml of *0.1 M sodium hydroxide* and 0.1 ml of *phenolphthalein solution R*. Maintain a constant volume (20 ml) in the tube during distillation and ensure that the distillate remains alkaline, adding *0.1 M sodium hydroxide* if necessary. Dilute the distillate to 100 ml with *water R* (test solution). Prepare a standard in the same manner by distillation, using 5 ml of *fluoride standard solution (10 ppm F) R* instead of the substance to be examined. Into two glass-stoppered cylinders introduce 20 ml of the test solution and 20 ml of the standard and 5 ml of *aminomethylalizarindiacetic acid reagent R*.

After 20 min, any blue colour in the test solution (originally red) is not more intense than that in the standard.

01/2005:20406

2.4.6. MAGNESIUM

To 10 ml of the prescribed solution add 0.1 g of *disodium tetraborate R*. Adjust the solution, if necessary, to pH 8.8 to pH 9.2 using *dilute hydrochloric acid R* or *dilute sodium hydroxide solution R*. Shake with 2 quantities, each of 5 ml, of a 1 g/l solution of *hydroxyquinoline R* in *chloroform R*, for 1 min each time. Allow to stand. Separate and discard the organic layer. To the aqueous solution add 0.4 ml of *butylamine R* and 0.1 ml of *triethanolamine R*. Adjust the solution, if necessary, to pH 10.5 to pH 11.5. Add 4 ml of the solution of hydroxyquinoline in chloroform, shake for 1 min, allow to stand and separate. Use the lower layer for comparison. Prepare a standard in the same manner using a mixture of 1 ml of *magnesium standard solution (10 ppm Mg) R* and 9 ml of *water R*.

Any colour in the solution obtained from the substance to be examined is not more intense than that in the standard.

01/2005:20407

2.4.7. MAGNESIUM AND ALKALINE-EARTH METALS

To 200 ml of *water R* add 0.1 g of *hydroxylamine hydrochloride R*, 10 ml of *ammonium chloride buffer solution pH 10.0 R*, 1 ml of *0.1 M zinc sulphate* and about 15 mg of *mordant black 11 triturate R*. Heat to about 40 °C. Titrate with *0.01 M sodium edetate* until the violet colour changes to full blue. To the solution add the prescribed quantity of the substance to be examined dissolved in 100 ml of *water R* or use the prescribed solution. If the colour of the solution changes to violet, titrate with *0.01 M sodium edetate* until the full blue colour is again obtained.

The volume of *0.01 M sodium edetate* used in the second titration does not exceed the prescribed quantity.

01/2005:20408

2.4.8. HEAVY METALS

The methods described below require the use of *thioacetamide reagent R*. As an alternative, *sodium sulphide solution R1* (0.1 ml) is usually suitable. Since tests prescribed in monographs have been developed using *thioacetamide reagent R*, if *sodium sulphide solution R1* is used instead, it is necessary to include also for methods A and B a monitor solution, prepared from the quantity of the substance to be examined prescribed for the test, to which has been added the volume of lead standard solution prescribed for preparation of the reference solution. The test is invalid if the monitor solution is not comparable with the reference solution.

METHOD A

Test solution. 12 ml of the prescribed aqueous solution of the substance to be examined.

Reference solution (standard). A mixture of 10 ml of *lead standard solution (1 ppm Pb) R* or *lead standard solution (2 ppm Pb) R,* as prescribed, and 2 ml of the prescribed aqueous solution of the substance to be examined.

Blank solution. A mixture of 10 ml of *water R* and 2 ml of the prescribed aqueous solution of the substance to be examined.

To each solution, add 2 ml of *buffer solution pH 3.5 R.* Mix. Add 1.2 ml of *thioacetamide reagent R.* Mix immediately. Examine the solutions after 2 min. The test is invalid if the reference solution does not show a slight brown colour compared to the blank solution. The substance to be examined complies with the test if any brown colour in the test solution is not more intense than that in the reference solution.

If the result is difficult to judge, filter the solutions through a membrane filter (pore size 3 µm; see Figure 2.4.8.-1, without the prefilter). Carry out the filtration slowly and uniformly, applying moderate and constant pressure to the piston. Compare the spots on the filters obtained with the different solutions.

METHOD B

Test solution. 12 ml of the prescribed solution of the substance to be examined prepared using an organic solvent containing a minimum percentage of water (for example, dioxan containing 15 per cent of water or acetone containing 15 per cent of water).

Reference solution (standard). A mixture of 10 ml of lead standard solution (1 or 2 ppm Pb), as prescribed, and 2 ml of the prescribed solution of the substance to be examined in an organic solvent. Prepare the lead standard solution (1 or 2 ppm Pb) by dilution of *lead standard solution (100 ppm Pb) R* with the solvent used for the substance to be examined.

Blank solution. A mixture of 10 ml of the solvent used for the substance to be examined and 2 ml of the prescribed solution of the substance to be examined in an organic solvent.

To each solution, add 2 ml of *buffer solution pH 3.5 R.* Mix. Add 1.2 ml of *thioacetamide reagent R.* Mix immediately. Examine the solutions after 2 min. The test is invalid if the reference solution does not show a slight brown colour compared to the blank solution. The substance to be examined complies with the test if any brown colour in the test solution is not more intense than that in the reference solution.

If the result is difficult to judge, filter the solutions through a membrane filter (pore size 3 µm; see Figure 2.4.8.-1, without the prefilter). Carry out the filtration slowly and uniformly, applying moderate and constant pressure to the piston. Compare the spots on the filters obtained with the different solutions.

METHOD C

Test solution. Place the prescribed quantity (not more than 2 g) of the substance to be examined in a silica crucible with 4 ml of a 250 g/l solution of *magnesium sulphate R* in *dilute sulphuric acid R.* Mix using a fine glass rod. Heat cautiously. If the mixture is liquid, evaporate gently to dryness on a water-bath. Progressively heat to ignition and continue heating until an almost white or at most greyish residue is obtained. Carry out the ignition at a temperature not exceeding 800 °C. Allow to cool. Moisten the residue with a few drops of *dilute sulphuric acid R.* Evaporate, ignite again and allow to cool. The total period of ignition must not exceed 2 h. Take up the residue in 2 quantities, each of 5 ml, of *dilute hydrochloric acid R.* Add 0.1 ml of *phenolphthalein solution R,* then *concentrated ammonia R* until a pink colour is obtained. Cool, add *glacial acetic acid R* until the solution is decolorised and add 0.5 ml in excess. Filter if necessary and wash the filter. Dilute to 20 ml with *water R.*

Reference solution (standard). Prepare as described for the test solution, using the prescribed volume of *lead standard solution (10 ppm Pb) R* instead of the substance to be examined. To 10 ml of the solution obtained add 2 ml of the test solution.

Monitor solution. Prepare as described for the test solution, adding to the substance to be examined the volume of *lead standard solution (10 ppm Pb) R* prescribed for preparation of the reference solution. To 10 ml of the solution obtained add 2 ml of the test solution.

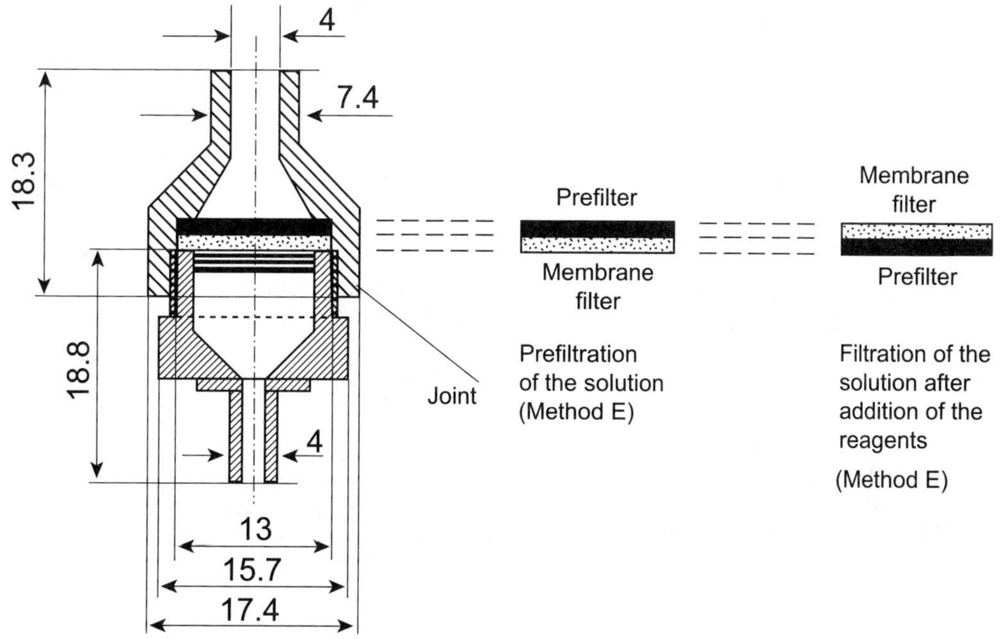

Figure 2.4.8.-1. – *Apparatus for the test for heavy metals*
Dimensions in millimetres

Blank solution. A mixture of 10 ml of *water R* and 2 ml of the test solution.

To 12 ml of each solution, add 2 ml of *buffer solution pH 3.5 R*. Mix. Add 1.2 ml of *thioacetamide reagent R*. Mix immediately. Examine the solutions after 2 min. The test is invalid if the reference solution does not show a slight brown colour compared to the blank solution or if the monitor solution is not comparable with the reference solution. The substance to be examined complies with the test if any brown colour in the test solution is not more intense than that in the reference solution.

If the result is difficult to judge, filter the solutions through a membrane filter (pore size 3 μm; see Figure 2.4.8.-1, without the prefilter). Carry out the filtration slowly and uniformly, applying moderate and constant pressure to the piston. Compare the spots on the filters obtained with the different solutions.

METHOD D

Test solution. In a silica crucible, mix thoroughly the prescribed quantity of the substance to be examined with 0.5 g of *magnesium oxide R1*. Ignite to dull redness until a homogeneous white or greyish-white mass is obtained. If after 30 min of ignition the mixture remains coloured, allow to cool, mix using a fine glass rod and repeat the ignition. If necessary repeat the operation. Heat at 800 °C for about 1 h. Take up the residue in 2 quantities, each of 5 ml, of a mixture of equal volumes of *hydrochloric acid R1* and *water R*. Add 0.1 ml of *phenolphthalein solution R* and then *concentrated ammonia R* until a pink colour is obtained. Cool, add *glacial acetic acid R* until the solution is decolorised and add 0.5 ml in excess. Filter if necessary and wash the filter. Dilute to 20 ml with *water R*.

Reference solution (standard). Prepare as described for the test solution using the prescribed volume of *lead standard solution (10 ppm Pb) R* instead of the substance to be examined and drying in an oven at 100-105 °C. To 10 ml of the solution obtained add 2 ml of the test solution.

Monitor solution. Prepare as described for the test solution, adding to the substance to be examined the volume of *lead standard solution (10 ppm Pb) R* prescribed for preparation of the reference solution and drying in an oven at 100-105 °C. To 10 ml of the solution obtained add 2 ml of the test solution.

Blank solution. A mixture of 10 ml of *water R* and 2 ml of the test solution.

To 12 ml of each solution, add 2 ml of *buffer solution pH 3.5 R*. Mix. Add 1.2 ml of *thioacetamide reagent R*. Mix immediately. Examine the solutions after 2 min. The test is invalid if the reference solution does not show a slight brown colour compared to the blank solution or if the monitor solution is not comparable with the reference solution. The substance to be examined complies with the test if any brown colour in the test solution is not more intense than that in the reference solution.

If the result is difficult to judge, filter the solutions through a membrane filter (pore size 3 μm; see Figure 2.4.8.-1, without the prefilter). Carry out the filtration slowly and uniformly, applying moderate and constant pressure to the piston. Compare the spots on the filters obtained with the different solutions.

METHOD E

Test solution. Dissolve the prescribed quantity of the substance to be examined in 30 ml of *water R* or the prescribed volume.

Reference solution (standard). Unless otherwise prescribed, dilute the prescribed volume of *lead standard solution (1 ppm Pb) R* to the same volume as the test solution.

Prepare the filtration apparatus by adapting the barrel of a 50 ml syringe without its piston to a support containing, on the plate, a membrane filter (pore size 3 μm) and above it a prefilter (Figure 2.4.8.-1).

Transfer the test solution into the syringe barrel, put the piston in place and then apply an even pressure on it until the whole of the liquid has been filtered. In opening the support and removing the prefilter, check that the membrane filter remains uncontaminated with impurities. If this is not the case replace it with another membrane filter and repeat the operation under the same conditions.

To the prefiltrate or to the prescribed volume of the prefiltrate add 2 ml of *buffer solution pH 3.5 R*. Add to 1.2 ml of *thioacetamide reagent R*. Mix and allow to stand for 10 min and again filter as described above, but inverting the order of the filters, the liquid passing first through the membrane filter before passing through the prefilter (Figure 2.4.8.-1). The filtration must be carried out slowly and uniformly by applying moderate and constant pressure to the piston of the syringe. After complete filtration, open the support, remove the membrane filter, and dry using filter paper.

In parallel, treat the reference solution in the same manner as the test solution.

The colour of the spot obtained with the test solution is not more intense than that obtained with the reference solution.

METHOD F

Test solution. Place the prescribed quantity or volume of the substance to be examined in a clean, dry, 100 ml long-necked combustion flask (a 300 ml flask may be used if the reaction foams excessively). Clamp the flask at an angle of 45°. If the substance to be examined is a solid, add a sufficient volume of a mixture of 8 ml of *sulphuric acid R* and 10 ml of *nitric acid R* to moisten the substance thoroughly; if the substance to be examined is a liquid, add a few millilitres of a mixture of 8 ml of *sulphuric acid R* and 10 ml of *nitric acid R*. Warm gently until the reaction commences, allow the reaction to subside and add additional portions of the same acid mixture, heating after each addition, until a total of 18 ml of the acid mixture has been added. Increase the amount of heat and boil gently until the solution darkens. Cool, add 2 ml of *nitric acid R* and heat again until the solution darkens. Continue the heating, followed by the addition of *nitric acid R* until no further darkening occurs, then heat strongly until dense, white fumes are produced. Cool, cautiously add 5 ml of *water R*, boil gently until dense, white fumes are produced and continue heating to reduce to 2-3 ml. Cool, cautiously add 5 ml of *water R* and examine the colour of the solution. If the colour is yellow, cautiously add 1 ml of *strong hydrogen peroxide solution R* and again evaporate until dense, white fumes are produced and reduce to a volume of 2-3 ml. If the solution is still yellow in colour, repeat the addition of 5 ml of *water R* and 1 ml of *strong hydrogen peroxide solution R* until the solution is colourless. Cool, dilute cautiously with *water R* and rinse into a 50 ml colour comparison tube, ensuring that the total volume does not exceed 25 ml. Adjust the solution to pH 3.0-4.0, using short range pH indicator paper as external indicator, with *concentrated ammonia R1* (*dilute ammonia R1* may be used, if desired, as the specified range is approached), dilute with *water R* to 40 ml and mix. Add 2 ml of *buffer solution pH 3.5 R* and 1.2 ml of *thioacetamide reagent R*. Mix immediately. Dilute to 50 ml with *water R* and mix.

Reference solution (standard). Prepare at the same time and in the same manner as the test solution, using the prescribed volume of *lead standard solution (10 ppm Pb) R*.

Monitor solution. Prepare as described for the test solution, adding to the substance to be examined the volume of *lead standard solution (10 ppm Pb) R* prescribed for the preparation of the reference solution.

Blank solution. Prepare as described for the test solution, omitting the substance to be examined.

Examine the solutions vertically against a white background. After 2 min, any brown colour in the test solution is not more intense than that in the reference solution.

The test is invalid if the reference solution does not show a brown colour compared to the blank solution or if the monitor solution is not comparable with the reference solution.

If the result is difficult to judge, filter the solutions through a membrane filter (pore size 3 µm; see Figure 2.4.8-1, without the prefilter). Carry out the filtration slowly and uniformly, applying moderate and constant pressure to the piston. Compare the spots on the filters obtained with the different solutions.

METHOD G

CAUTION: when using high-pressure digestion vessels the safety precautions and operating instructions given by the manufacturer must be followed. The digestion cycles have to be elaborated depending on the type of microwave oven to be used (for example, energy-controlled microwave ovens, temperature-controlled microwave ovens or high-pressure ovens). The cycle must be conform to the manufacturer's instructions. The digestion cycle is suitable if a clear solution is obtained.

Test solution. Place the prescribed amount of the substance to be examined (not more than 0.5 g) in a suitable, clean beaker. Add successively 2.7 ml of *sulphuric acid R*, 3.3 ml of *nitric acid R* and 2.0 ml of *strong hydrogen peroxide solution R* using a magnetic stirrer. Allow the substance to react with a reagent before adding the next one. Transfer the mixture to a dry high-pressure-resistant digestion vessel (fluoropolymer or quartz glass).

Reference solution (standard). Prepare as described for the test solution, using the prescribed volume of *lead standard solution (10 ppm Pb) R* instead of the substance to be examined.

Monitor solution. Prepare as prescribed for the test solution, adding to the substance to be examined the volume of *lead standard solution (10 ppm Pb) R* prescribed for the preparation of the reference solution.

Blank solution. Prepare as described for the test solution, omitting the substance to be examined.

Close the vessels and place in a laboratory microwave oven. Digest using a sequence of 2 separate suitable programmes. Design the programmes in several steps in order to control the reaction, monitoring pressure, temperature or energy depending on the type of microwave oven available. After the first programme allow the digestion vessels to cool before opening. Add to each vessel 2.0 ml of *strong hydrogen peroxide solution R* and digest using the second programme. After the second programme allow the digestion vessels to cool before opening. If necessary to obtain a clear solution, repeat the addition of *strong hydrogen peroxide solution R* and the second digestion programme.

Cool, dilute cautiously with *water R* and rinse into a flask, ensuring that the total volume does not exceed 25 ml.

Using short-range pH indicator paper as external indicator, adjust the solutions to pH 3.0-4.0 with *concentrated ammonia R1* (*dilute ammonia R1* may be used as the specified range is approached). To avoid heating of the solutions use an ice-bath and a magnetic stirrer. Dilute to 40 ml with *water R* and mix. Add 2 ml of *buffer solution pH 3.5 R* and 1.2 ml of *thioacetamide reagent R*. Mix immediately. Dilute to 50 ml with *water R*, mix and allow to stand for 2 min.

Filter the solutions through a membrane filter (pore size 3 µm; see Figure 2.4.8.-1, without the prefilter). Carry out the filtration slowly and uniformly, applying moderate and constant pressure to the piston. Compare the spots on the filters obtained with the different solutions.

Examine the spots on the filters. The brown colour from the spot of the test solution is not more intense than that from the reference solution.

The test is invalid if the reference solution spot does not show a brown colour compared to the blank spot, or if the spot from the monitor solution is not comparable with the spot from the reference solution.

01/2005:20409

2.4.9. IRON

Dissolve the prescribed quantity of the substance to be examined in *water R* and dilute to 10 ml with the same solvent or use 10 ml of the prescribed solution. Add 2 ml of a 200 g/l solution of *citric acid R* and 0.1 ml of *thioglycollic acid R*. Mix, make alkaline with *ammonia R* and dilute to 20 ml with *water R*. Prepare a standard in the same manner, using 10 ml of *iron standard solution (1 ppm Fe) R*.

After 5 min, any pink colour in the test solution is not more intense than that in the standard.

01/2005:20410

2.4.10. LEAD IN SUGARS

Determine the lead by atomic absorption spectrometry (*2.2.23, Method II*).

Test solution. Dissolve 20.0 g of the substance to be examined in a mixture of equal volumes of *dilute acetic acid R* and *water R* and dilute to 100.0 ml with the same mixture of solvents. Add 2.0 ml of a clear 10 g/l solution of *ammonium pyrrolidinedithiocarbamate R* and 10.0 ml of *methyl isobutyl ketone R* and then shake for 30 s protected from bright light. Allow the layers to separate and use the methyl isobutyl ketone layer.

Reference solutions. Prepare 3 reference solutions in the same manner as the test solution but adding 0.5 ml, 1.0 ml and 1.5 ml respectively of *lead standard solution (10 ppm Pb) R* in addition to the 20.0 g of the substance to be examined.

Set the zero of the instrument using *methyl isobutyl ketone R* treated as described for the test solution without the substance to be examined. Measure the absorbance at 283.3 nm using a lead hollow-cathode lamp as source of radiation and an air-acetylene flame.

The substance to be examined contains not more than 0.5 ppm of lead, unless otherwise prescribed.

2. Methods of analysis

01/2005:20411

2.4.11. PHOSPHATES

To 100 ml of the solution prepared and, if necessary, neutralised as prescribed add 4 ml of *sulphomolybdic reagent R3*. Shake and add 0.1 ml of *stannous chloride solution R1*. Prepare a standard in the same manner using 2 ml of *phosphate standard solution (5 ppm PO_4) R* and 98 ml of *water R*. After 10 min, compare the colours using 20 ml of each solution.

Any colour in the test solution is not more intense than that in the standard.

01/2005:20412

2.4.12. POTASSIUM

To 10 ml of the prescribed solution add 2 ml of a freshly prepared 10 g/l solution of *sodium tetraphenylborate R*. Prepare a standard in the same manner using a mixture of 5 ml of *potassium standard solution (20 ppm K) R* and 5 ml of *water R*.

After 5 min, any opalescence in the test solution is not more intense than that in the standard.

01/2005:20413

2.4.13. SULPHATES

All solutions used for this test must be prepared with distilled water R.

Add 3 ml of a 250 g/l solution of *barium chloride R* to 4.5 ml of *sulphate standard solution (10 ppm SO_4) R1*. Shake and allow to stand for 1 min. To 2.5 ml of this solution, add 15 ml of the solution to be examined and 0.5 ml of *acetic acid R*. Prepare a standard in the same manner using 15 ml of *sulphate standard solution (10 ppm SO_4) R* instead of the solution to be examined.

After 5 min, any opalescence in the test solution is not more intense than that in the standard.

01/2005:20414

2.4.14. SULPHATED ASH

Ignite a suitable crucible (silica, platinum, porcelain or quartz) at 600 ± 50 °C for 30 min, allow to cool in a desiccator over silica gel and weigh. Place the prescribed amount of the substance to be examined in the crucible and weigh. Moisten the substance to be examined with a small amount of *sulphuric acid R* (usually 1 ml) and heat gently at as low a temperature as practicable until the sample is thoroughly charred. After cooling, moisten the residue with a small amount of *sulphuric acid R*, heat gently until white fumes are no longer evolved and ignite at 600 ± 50 °C until the residue is completely incinerated. Ensure that flames are not produced at any time during the procedure. Allow the crucible to cool in a desiccator over silica gel, weigh it again and calculate the mass of the residue.

If the mass of the residue so obtained exceeds the prescribed limit, repeat the moistening with *sulphuric acid R* and ignition, as previously, to constant mass, unless otherwise prescribed.

01/2005:20415

2.4.15. NICKEL IN POLYOLS

Determine the nickel by atomic absorption spectrometry (*2.2.23, Method II*).

Test solution. Dissolve 20.0 g of the substance to be examined in a mixture of equal volumes of *dilute acetic acid R* and *water R* and dilute to 100.0 ml with the same mixture of solvents. Add 2.0 ml of a saturated solution of *ammonium pyrrolidinedithiocarbamate R* (about 10 g/l) and 10.0 ml of *methyl isobutyl ketone R* and then shake for 30 s protected from bright light. Allow the layers to separate and use the methyl isobutyl ketone layer.

Reference solutions. Prepare 3 reference solutions in the same manner as the test solution but adding 0.5 ml, 1.0 ml and 1.5 ml respectively of *nickel standard solution (10 ppm Ni) R* in addition to the 20.0 g of the substance to be examined.

Set the zero of the instrument using *methyl isobutyl ketone R* treated as described for preparation of the test solution omitting the substance to be examined. Measure the absorbance at 232.0 nm using a nickel hollow-cathode lamp as source of radiation and an air-acetylene flame.

The substance to be examined contains not more than 1 ppm of nickel, unless otherwise prescribed.

01/2005:20416

2.4.16. TOTAL ASH

Heat a silica or platinum crucible to redness for 30 min, allow to cool in a desiccator and weigh. Unless otherwise prescribed, evenly distribute 1.00 g of the substance or the powdered vegetable drug to be examined in the crucible. Dry at 100 °C to 105 °C for 1 h and ignite to constant mass in a muffle furnace at 600 °C ± 25 °C, allowing the crucible to cool in a desiccator after each ignition. Flames should not be produced at any time during the procedure. If after prolonged ignition the ash still contains black particles, take up with hot water, filter through an ashless filter paper and ignite the residue and the filter paper. Combine the filtrate with the ash, carefully evaporate to dryness and ignite to constant mass.

01/2005:20417

2.4.17. ALUMINIUM

Place the prescribed solution in a separating funnel and shake with 2 quantities, each of 20 ml, and then with one 10 ml quantity of a 5 g/l solution of *hydroxyquinoline R* in *chloroform R*. Dilute the combined chloroform solutions to 50.0 ml with *chloroform R* (test solution).

Prepare a standard in the same manner using the prescribed reference solution.

Prepare a blank in the same manner using the prescribed blank solution.

Measure the intensity of the fluorescence (*2.2.21*) of the test solution (I_1), of the standard (I_2) and of the blank (I_3) using an excitant beam at 392 nm and a secondary filter with a transmission band centred on 518 nm or a monochromator set to transmit at this wavelength.

The fluorescence ($I_1 - I_3$) of the test solution is not greater than that of the standard ($I_2 - I_3$).

01/2005:20418
corrected

2.4.18. FREE FORMALDEHYDE

Use method A, unless otherwise prescribed. Method B is suitable for vaccines where sodium metabisulphite has been used to neutralise excess formaldehyde.

METHOD A

For vaccines for human use, prepare a 1 in 10 dilution of the vaccine to be examined. For bacterial toxoids for veterinary use, prepare a 1 in 25 dilution of the vaccine to be examined.

To 1 ml of the dilution, add 4 ml of *water R* and 5 ml of *acetylacetone reagent R1*. Place the tube in a water-bath at 40 °C for 40 min. Examine the tubes down their vertical axes. The solution is not more intensely coloured than a standard, prepared at the same time and in the same manner, using 1 ml of a dilution of *formaldehyde solution R* containing 20 µg of formaldehyde (CH_2O) per millilitre, instead of the dilution of the vaccine to be examined.

METHOD B

Test solution. Prepare a 1 in 200 dilution of the vaccine to be examined with *water R*. If the vaccine is an emulsion, prepare an equivalent dilution using the aqueous phase separated by a suitable procedure (see below). If one of the methods described below is used for separation of the aqueous phase, a 1 in 20 dilution of the latter is used.

Reference solutions. Prepare solutions containing 0.25 g/l, 0.50 g/l, 1.00 g/l and 2.00 g/l of CH_2O by dilution of *formaldehyde solution R* with *water R*. Prepare a 1 in 200 dilution of each solution with *water R*.

To 0.5 ml of the test solution and of each of the reference solutions in test-tubes, add 5.0 ml of a freshly prepared 0.5 g/l solution of *methylbenzothiazolone hydrazone hydrochloride R*. Close the tubes, shake and allow to stand for 60 min. Add 1 ml of *ferric chloride-sulphamic acid reagent R* and allow to stand for 15 min. Measure the absorbance (*2.2.25*) of the solutions at 628 nm. Calculate the content of formaldehyde in the vaccine to be examined from the calibration curve established using the reference solutions. The test is invalid if the correlation coefficient (r) of the calibration curve is less than 0.97.

Emulsions. If the vaccine to be examined is an emulsion, the aqueous phase is separated using a suitable procedure and used for preparation of the test solution. The following procedures have been found suitable.

(a) Add 1.0 ml of the vaccine to be examined to 1.0 ml of *isopropyl myristate R* and mix. Add 1.3 ml of *1 M hydrochloric acid*, 2.0 ml of *chloroform R* and 2.7 ml of a 9 g/l solution of *sodium chloride R*. Mix thoroughly. Centrifuge at 15 000 *g* for 60 min. Transfer the aqueous phase to a 10 ml volumetric flask and dilute to volume with *water R*. If this procedure fails to separate the aqueous phase, add 100 g/l of *polysorbate 20 R* to the sodium chloride solution and repeat the procedure but centrifuge at 22 500 *g*.

(b) Add 1.0 ml of the vaccine to be examined to 1.0 ml of a 100 g/l solution of *sodium chloride R* and mix. Centrifuge at 1000 *g* for 15 min. Transfer the aqueous phase to a 10 ml volumetric flask and dilute to volume with *water R*.

(c) Add 1.0 ml of the vaccine to be examined to 2.0 ml of a 100 g/l solution of *sodium chloride R* and 3.0 ml of *chloroform R* and mix. Centrifuge at 1000 *g* for 5 min. Transfer the aqueous phase to a 10 ml volumetric flask and dilute to volume with *water R*.

01/2005:20419

2.4.19. ALKALINE IMPURITIES IN FATTY OILS

In a test-tube mix 10 ml of recently distilled *acetone R* and 0.3 ml of *water R* and add 0.05 ml of a 0.4 g/l solution of *bromophenol blue R* in *alcohol R*. Neutralise the solution if necessary with *0.01 M hydrochloric acid* or *0.01 M sodium hydroxide*. Add 10 ml of the oil to be examined, shake and allow to stand. Not more than 0.1 ml of *0.01 M hydrochloric acid* is required to change the colour of the upper layer to yellow.

01/2005:20421

2.4.21. FOREIGN OILS IN FATTY OILS BY THIN-LAYER CHROMATOGRAPHY

Examine by thin-layer chromatography (*2.2.27*) using *kieselguhr G R* as the coating substance. Impregnate a plate by placing it in a chromatographic tank containing the necessary quantity of a mixture of 10 volumes of *liquid paraffin R* and 90 volumes of *light petroleum R* so that the plate dips about 5 mm beneath the surface of the liquid. When the impregnation mixture has risen by at least 12 cm from the lower edge of the plate, remove the plate and allow the solvent to evaporate for 5 min. Carry out the chromatography in the same direction as the impregnation.

Preparation of the mixture of fatty acids. Heat 2 g of the oil with 30 ml of *0.5 M alcoholic potassium hydroxide* under a reflux condenser for 45 min. Add 50 ml of *water R*, allow to cool, transfer to a separating funnel and extract with three quantities, each of 50 ml, of *ether R*. Discard the ether extracts, acidify the aqueous layer with *hydrochloric acid R* and extract with three quantities, each of 50 ml, of *ether R*. Combine the ether extracts and wash with three quantities, each of 10 ml, of *water R*; discard the washings, dry the ether over *anhydrous sodium sulphate R* and filter. Evaporate the ether on a water-bath. Use the residue to prepare the test solution. The fatty acids may also be obtained from the soap solution prepared during the determination of the unsaponifiable matter.

Test solution. Dissolve 40 mg of the mixture of fatty acids obtained from the substance to be examined in 4 ml of *chloroform R*.

Reference solution. Dissolve 40 mg of the mixture of fatty acids obtained from a mixture of 19 volumes of *maize oil R* and 1 volume of *rapeseed oil R* in 4 ml of *chloroform R*.

Apply to the plate 3 µl of each solution. Develop over a path of 8 cm using a mixture of 10 volumes of *water R* and 90 volumes of *glacial acetic acid R*. Dry the plate at 110 °C for 10 min. Allow to cool and, unless otherwise prescribed, place the plate in a chromatographic chamber, with a tightly fitting lid, that has previously been saturated with iodine vapour by placing *iodine R* in an evaporating dish at the bottom of the chamber. After some time brown or yellowish-brown spots become visible. Remove the plate and allow to stand for a few minutes. When the brown background colour has disappeared, spray with *starch solution R*. Blue spots appear which may become brown on drying and again become blue after spraying with *water R*. The chromatogram obtained with the test solution always shows a spot with an R_f of about 0.5 (oleic acid) and a spot with an R_f of about 0.65 (linoleic acid) corresponding to the spots in the chromatogram obtained with the reference solution. With some oils a spot with an R_f of about 0.75 may be present (linolenic acid). By comparison with the spot in the chromatogram obtained with the reference solution, verify the absence in the chromatogram obtained with the test solution of a spot with an R_f of about 0.25 (erucic acid).

01/2005:20422

2.4.22. COMPOSITION OF FATTY ACIDS BY GAS CHROMATOGRAPHY

The test for foreign oils is carried out on the methyl esters of the fatty acids contained in the oil to be examined by gas chromatography (*2.2.28*).

METHOD A

This method is not applicable to oils that contain glycerides of fatty acids with an epoxy-, hydroepoxy-, cyclopropyl or cyclopropenyl group, or those that contain a large proportion of fatty acids of chain length less than 8 carbon atoms or to oils with an acid value greater than 2.0.

Test solution. When prescribed in the monograph, dry the oil to be examined before the methylation step. Weigh 1.0 g of the oil into a 25 ml round-bottomed flask with a ground-glass neck fitted with a reflux condenser and a gas port into the flask. Add 10 ml of *anhydrous methanol R* and 0.2 ml of a 60 g/l solution of *potassium hydroxide R* in *methanol R*. Attach the reflux condenser, pass *nitrogen R* through the mixture at a rate of about 50 ml/min, shake and heat to boiling. When the solution is clear (usually after about 10 min), continue heating for a further 5 min. Cool the flask under running water and transfer the contents to a separating funnel. Rinse the flask with 5 ml of *heptane R* and transfer the rinsings to the separating funnel and shake. Add 10 ml of a 200 g/l solution of *sodium chloride R* and shake vigorously. Allow to separate and transfer the organic layer to a vial containing *anhydrous sodium sulphate R*. Allow to stand, then filter.

Reference solution (a). Prepare 0.50 g of the mixture of calibrating substances with the composition described in one of the tables 2.4.22, as prescribed in the individual monograph (if the monograph does not mention a specific solution, use the composition described in Table 2.4.22.-1). Dissolve in *heptane R* and dilute to 50.0 ml with the same solvent.

Reference solution (b). Dilute 1.0 ml of reference solution (a) to 10.0 ml with *heptane R*.

Reference solution (c). Prepare 0.50 g of a mixture of fatty acid methyl esters(1), which corresponds in composition to the mixture of fatty acids indicated in the monograph of the substance to be examined. Dissolve in *heptane R* and dilute to 50.0 ml with the same solvent. Commercially available mixtures of fatty acid methyl esters may also be used.

Column:

- *material*: fused silica, glass or quartz,
- *size*: l = 10-30 m, Ø = 0.2-0.8 mm,
- *stationary phase*: *poly[(cyanopropyl)(methyl)][(phenyl)(methyl)]siloxane R* or *macrogol 20 000 R* (film thickness 0.1-0.5 µm) or some other suitable stationary phase.

Carrier gas: *helium for chromatography R* or *hydrogen for chromatography R.*

Flow rate: 1.3 ml/min (for a column Ø = 0.32 mm).

Split ratio: 1:100 or less, according to the internal diameter of the column used (1:50 when Ø = 0.32 mm).

Temperature:

- *column*: 160-200 °C, according to the length and type of column used (200 °C for a column 30 m long and coated with a layer of *macrogol 20 000 R*); if necessary, or where prescribed, raise the temperature of the column at a rate of 3 °C/min from 170 °C to 230 °C (for the *macrogol 20 000 R* column),
- *injection port*: 250 °C,
- *detector*: 250 °C.

Detection: flame ionisation.

Injection: 1 µl.

Sensitivity: the height of the principal peak in the chromatogram obtained with reference solution (a) is 50 per cent to 70 per cent of the full scale of the recorder.

System suitability when using the mixture of calibrating substances in Table 2.4.22.-1 or 2.4.22.-3:

- *resolution*: minimum 1.8 between the peaks due to methyl oleate and methyl stearate in the chromatogram obtained with reference solution (a),
- *signal-to-noise ratio*: minimum 5 for the peak due to methyl myristate in the chromatogram obtained with reference solution (b),
- *number of theoretical plates*: minimum 30 000 calculated for the peak due to methyl stearate in the chromatogram obtained with reference solution (a).

System suitability when using the mixture of calibrating substances in Table 2.4.22.-2:

- *resolution*: minimum 4.0 between the peaks due to methyl caprylate and methyl caprate in the chromatogram obtained with reference solution (a),
- *signal-to-noise ratio*: minimum 5 for the peak due to methyl caproate in the chromatogram obtained with reference solution (b),
- *number of theoretical plates*: minimum 15 000 calculated for the peak due to methyl caprate in the chromatogram obtained with reference solution (a).

ASSESSMENT OF CHROMATOGRAMS

Avoid working conditions tending to give masked peaks (presence of constituents with small differences between retention times, for example linolenic acid and arachidic acid).

Qualitative analysis. Identify the peaks in the chromatogram obtained with reference solution (c); the peaks may also be identified by drawing calibration curves using the chromatogram obtained with reference solution (a) and the information given in Tables 2.4.22.-1, 2.4.22.-2 and 2.4.22.-3:

a) using isothermal operating conditions giving the logarithms of reduced retention times as a function of the number of carbon atoms of the fatty acid; identify the peaks by means of the straight line thus obtained and the "equivalent chain lengths" of the different peaks. The calibration curve of the saturated acids is a straight line. The logarithms of reduced retention times of unsaturated acids are situated on this line at points corresponding to non-integer values of carbon atoms known as "equivalent chain lengths";

b) using linear temperature programming giving the retention time according to the number of carbon atoms of the fatty acid; identify by reference to the calibration curve.

Quantitative analysis. In general, the normalisation procedure is used in which the sum of the areas of the peaks in the chromatogram, except that of the solvent, is set at 100 per cent. The content of a constituent is calculated

(1) The fatty acid methyl esters used show a quality at least as good as that guaranteed by the BCR (Community Bureau of Reference) of the European Union.

by determining the area of the corresponding peak as a percentage of the sum of the areas of all the peaks. Disregard any peak with an area less than 0.05 per cent of the total area.

In certain cases, for example in the presence of fatty acids with 12 or less carbon atoms, correction factors can be prescribed in the individual monograph to convert peak areas in per cent *m/m*.

METHOD B

This method is not applicable to oils that contain glycerides of fatty acids with an epoxy-, hydroepoxy-, cyclopropyl or cyclopropenyl group or to oils with an acid value greater than 2.0.

Test solution. Introduce 0.100 g of the substance to be examined in a 10 ml centrifuge tube with a screw cap. Dissolve with 1 ml of *heptane R* and 1 ml of *dimethyl carbonate R* and mix vigorously under gentle heating (50-60 °C). Add, while still warm, 1 ml of a 12 g/l solution of *sodium R* in *anhydrous methanol R*, prepared with the necessary precautions and mix vigorously for about 5 min. Add 3 ml of *distilled water R* and mix vigorously for about 30 s. Centrifuge for 15 min at 1500 *g*. Inject 1 µl of the organic phase.

Reference solutions and assessment of chromatograms. Without specific prescription in the individual monograph, proceed as described under Method A.

Column:

- *material*: fused silica,
- *size*: l = 30 m, Ø = 0.25 mm,
- *stationary phase*: *macrogol 20 000 R* (film thickness 0.25 µm),

Carrier gas: *helium for chromatography R.*

Flow rate: 0.9 ml/min.

Split ratio: 1:100.

Temperature:

	Time (min)	Temperature (°C)
Column	0 - 15	100
	15 - 36	100 → 225
	36 - 61	225
Injection port		250
Detector		250

Detection: flame ionisation.

Injection: 1 µl.

METHOD C

This method is not applicable to oils that contain glycerides of fatty acids with epoxy-, hydroperoxy-, aldehyde, ketone, cyclopropyl and cyclopropenyl groups, and conjugated polyunsaturated and acetylenic compounds because of partial or complete destruction of these groups.

Test solution. Dissolve 0.10 g of the substance to be examined in 2 ml of a 20 g/l solution of *sodium hydroxide R* in *methanol R* in a 25 ml conical flask and boil under a reflux condenser for 30 min. Add 2.0 ml of *boron trifluoride-methanol solution R* through the condenser and boil for 30 min. Add 4 ml of *heptane R* through the condenser and boil for 5 min. Cool and add 10.0 ml of *saturated sodium chloride solution R*, shake for about 15 s and add a quantity of *saturated sodium chloride solution R* such that the upper phase is brought into the neck of the flask. Collect 2 ml of the upper phase, wash with 3 quantities, each of 2 ml, of *water R* and dry over *anhydrous sodium sulphate R.*

Reference solutions, chromatographic procedure and assessment of chromatograms. Without specific prescription in the individual monograph, proceed as described under Method A.

Table 2.4.22.-1. – *Mixture of calibrating substances*(2)

Mixture of the following substances	Equivalent chain length(3)	Composition (per cent m/m) Isothermal	Linear temperature programme
Methyl laurate R	12.0	5	10
Methyl myristate R	14.0	5	15
Methyl palmitate R	16.0	10	15
Methyl stearate R	18.0	20	20
Methyl arachidate R	20.0	40	20
Methyl oleate R	18.3	20	20

Table 2.4.22.-2. – *Mixture of calibrating substances*(2)

Mixture of the following substances	Equivalent chain length(3)	Composition (per cent m/m) Isothermal	Linear temperature programme
Methyl caproate R	6.0	5	10
Methyl caprylate R	8.0	5	35
Methyl caprate R	10.0	10	35
Methyl laurate R	12.0	20	10
Methyl myristate R	14.0	40	10

Table 2.4.22.-3. – *Mixture of calibrating substances*(2)

Mixture of the following substances	Equivalent chain length(3)	Composition (per cent m/m) Isothermal	Linear temperature programme
Methyl myristate R	14.0	5	15
Methyl palmitate R	16.0	10	15
Methyl stearate R	18.0	15	20
Methyl arachidate R	20.0	20	15
Methyl oleate R	18.3	20	15
Methyl eicosenoate R	20.2	10	10
Methyl behenate R	22.0	10	5
Methyl lignocerate R	24.0	10	5

01/2005:20423

2.4.23. STEROLS IN FATTY OILS

SEPARATION OF THE STEROL FRACTION

Prepare the unsaponifiable matter and then isolate the sterol fraction of the fatty oil by thin-layer chromatography (*2.2.27*), using *silica gel G R* in a 0.3 mm to 0.5 mm layer as the coating substance.

(2) For GC with capillary column and split inlet system, it is recommended that the component with the longest chain length of the mixture to be examined be added to the calibration mixture, when the qualitative analysis is done using calibration curves.

(3) This value, which is to be calculated using calibration curves, is given as an example for a column of *macrogol 20 000 R.*

Test solution (a). In a 150 ml flask fitted with a reflux condenser, place a volume of a 2 g/l solution of *betulin R* in *methylene chloride R* containing betulin corresponding to about 10 per cent of the sterol content of the sample used for the determination (e.g. in the case of olive oil add 500 µl, in the case of other vegetable oils add 1500 µl of the betulin solution). If the monograph requires the content of the individual sterols as a percentage of the sterol fraction, the addition of betulin may be omitted. Evaporate to dryness under a current of *nitrogen R*. Add 5.00 g (*m* g) of the substance to be examined. Add 50 ml of *2 M alcoholic potassium hydroxide R* and heat on a water-bath for 1 h, swirling frequently. Cool to a temperature below 25 °C and transfer the contents of the flask to a separating funnel with 100 ml of *water R*. Shake the liquid carefully with 3 quantities, each of 100 ml, of *peroxide-free ether R*. Combine the ether layers in another separating funnel containing 40 ml of *water R*, shake gently for a few minutes, allow to separate and reject the aqueous phase. Wash the ether phase with several quantities, each of 40 ml, of *water R*, until the aqueous phase is no longer alkaline to phenolphthalein. Transfer the ether phase to a tared flask, washing the separating funnel with *peroxide-free ether R*. Distil off the ether with suitable precautions and add 6 ml of *acetone R*. Carefully remove the solvent in a current of *nitrogen R*. Dry to constant mass at 100 °C to 105 °C. Allow to cool in a desiccator and weigh. Dissolve the residue in a minimal volume of *methylene chloride R*.

Test solution (b). Treat 5.00 g of *rapeseed oil R* as prescribed for the substance to be examined, beginning at the words "Add 50 ml of *2 M alcoholic potassium hydroxide R*".

Test solution (c). Treat 5.00 g of *sunflower oil R* as prescribed for the substance to be examined, beginning at the words "Add 50 ml of *2 M alcoholic potassium hydroxide R*".

Reference solution. Dissolve 25 mg of *cholesterol R* and 10 mg of *betulin R* in 1 ml of *methylene chloride R*.

Use a separate plate for each test solution. Apply separately as a band 20 mm by 3 mm 20 µl of the reference solution and as a band 40 mm by 3 mm 0.4 ml of test solution (a), test solution (b) or test solution (c). Develop over a path of 18 cm using a mixture of 35 volumes of *ether R* and 65 volumes of *hexane R*. Dry the plates in a current of *nitrogen R*. Spray the plates with a 2 g/l solution of *dichlorofluorescein R* in *ethanol R* and examine in ultraviolet light at 254 nm. The chromatogram obtained with the reference solution shows bands corresponding to cholesterol and betulin. The chromatograms obtained with the test solutions show bands with similar R_f values due to sterols. From each of the chromatograms, remove an area of coating corresponding to the area occupied by the sterol bands and additionally the area of the zones 2 mm to 3 mm above and below the visible zones corresponding to the reference solution. Place separately in three 50 ml flasks. To each flask add 15 ml of hot *methylene chloride R* and shake. Filter each solution through a sintered-glass filter (40) or suitable filter paper and wash each filter with three quantities, each of 15 ml, of *methylene chloride R*. Place the combined filtrate and washings from each filter separately in three tared flasks, evaporate to dryness under a stream of *nitrogen R* and weigh.

DETERMINATION OF THE STEROLS

Examine by gas chromatography *(2.2.28)*. *Carry out the operations protected from humidity and prepare the solutions immediately before use.*

Test solution. To the sterols separated from the substance to be examined by thin-layer chromatography add, per milligram of residue, 0.02 ml of a freshly prepared mixture of 1 volume of *chlorotrimethylsilane R*, 3 volumes of *hexamethyldisilazane R* and 9 volumes of *anhydrous pyridine R*. Shake carefully until the sterols are completely dissolved. Allow to stand in a desiccator over *diphosphorus pentoxide R* for 30 min. Centrifuge if necessary and use the supernatant liquid.

Reference solution (a). To 9 parts of the sterols separated from *rapeseed oil R* by thin-layer chromatography add 1 part of *cholesterol R*. To the mixture add, per milligram of residue, 0.02 ml of a freshly prepared mixture of 1 volume of *chlorotrimethylsilane R*, 3 volumes of *hexamethyldisilazane R* and 9 volumes of *anhydrous pyridine R*. Shake carefully until the sterols are completely dissolved. Allow to stand in a desiccator over *diphosphorus pentoxide R* for 30 min. Centrifuge if necessary and use the supernatant liquid.

Reference solution (b). To the sterols separated from *sunflower oil R* by thin-layer chromatography add, per milligram of residue, 0.02 ml of a freshly prepared mixture of 1 volume of *chlorotrimethylsilane R*, 3 volumes of *hexamethyldisilazane R* and 9 volumes of *anhydrous pyridine R*. Shake carefully until the sterols are completely dissolved. Allow to stand in a desiccator over *diphosphorus pentoxide R* for 30 min. Centrifuge if necessary and use the supernatant liquid.

The chromatographic procedure may be carried out using:

- a fused-silica column 20 m to 30 m long and 0.25 mm to 0.32 mm in internal diameter, coated with *poly[methyl(95)phenyl(5)]siloxane R* or of *poly[methyl(94)phenyl(5) vinyl(1)]siloxane R* (film thickness 0.25 µm),

- *hydrogen for chromatography R* at a velocity of 30 cm to 50 cm per second or *helium for chromatography R* at a velocity of 20 cm to 35 cm per second as the carrier gas. Measure the velocity as follows: maintaining the indicated operating conditions for the determination of the sterols, inject 1 µl to 3 µl of methane or propane. Measure the time in seconds required by the gas to pass through the column from the moment of the injection to the appearance of the peak (t_M). The velocity is given by L/t_M, where L is the length of the column in centimetres,

- a flame-ionisation detector,

- a split injector (1:50 or 1:100),

maintaining the temperature of the column at 260 °C, that of the injection port at 280 °C and that of the detector at 290 °C.

Inject 1 µl of each solution.

The chromatogram obtained with reference solution (a) shows 4 principal peaks corresponding to cholesterol, brassicasterol, campesterol and β-sitosterol and the chromatogram obtained with reference solution (b) shows 4 principal peaks corresponding to campesterol, stigmasterol, β-sitosterol and Δ7-stigmastenol. The retention times of the sterols relative to β-sitosterol are given in Table 2.4.23.-1.

The peak of the internal standard (betulin) must be clearly separated from the peaks of the sterols to be determined.

Table 2.4.23.-1. – *Retention times of sterols relative to β-sitosterol for 2 different columns*

	Poly[methyl(95)-phenyl(5)]siloxane	Poly[methyl(94)-phenyl(5)vinyl(1)]siloxane
Cholesterol	0.63	0.67
Brassicasterol	0.71	0.73
24-Methylenecholesterol	0.80	0.82
Campesterol	0.81	0.83
Campestanol	0.82	0.85
Stigmasterol	0.87	0.88
Δ7-Campesterol	0.92	0.93
Δ5,23-Stigmastadienol	0.95	0.95
Clerosterol	0.96	0.96
β-Sitosterol	1	1
Sitostanol	1.02	1.02
Δ5-Avenasterol	1.03	1.03
Δ5,24-Stigmastadienol	1.08	1.08
Δ7-Stigmastenol[(1)]	1.12	1.12
Δ7-Avenasterol	1.16	1.16
Betulin	1.4	1.6

(1) This sterol may also be referred to as Δ7-stigmasterol in literature.

For the chromatogram obtained with the test solution, identify the peaks and calculate the percentage content of each sterol in the sterol fraction of the substance to be examined using the following expression:

$$\frac{A}{S} \times 100$$

A = area of the peak corresponding to the component to be determined,

S = sum of the areas of the peaks corresponding to the components indicated in Table 2.4.23.-1.

If required in the monograph, calculate the content of each sterol in milligrams per 100 grams of the substance to be examined using the following expression:

$$\frac{A \times m_S \times 100}{A_S \times m}$$

A = area of the peak corresponding to the component to be determined,

A_S = area of the peak corresponding to betulin,

m = mass of the sample of the substance to be examined in grams,

m_S = mass of *betulin R* added in milligrams.

01/2005:20424 corrected

2.4.24. IDENTIFICATION AND CONTROL OF RESIDUAL SOLVENTS

The test procedures described in this general method may be used:

i. for the identification of the majority of Class 1 and Class 2 residual solvents in an active substance, excipient or medicinal product when the residual solvents are unknown;

ii. as a limit test for Class 1 and Class 2 solvents when present in an active substance, excipient or medicinal product;

iii. for the quantification of Class 2 solvents when the limits are greater than 1000 ppm (0.1 per cent) or for the quantification of Class 3 solvents when required.

Class 1, Class 2 and Class 3 residual solvents are listed in general chapter *5.4. Residual solvents.*

Three diluents are described for sample preparation and the conditions to be applied for head-space injection of the gaseous sample onto the chromatographic system. Two chromatographic systems are prescribed but System A is preferred whilst System B is employed normally for confirmation of identity. The choice of sample preparation procedure depends on the solubility of the substance to be examined and in certain cases the residual solvents to be controlled.

The following residual solvents are not readily detected by the head-space injection conditions described: formamide, 2-ethoxyethanol, 2-methoxyethanol, ethylene glycol, *N*-methylpyrrolidone and sulfolane. Other appropriate procedures should be employed for the control of these residual solvents.

When the test procedure is applied quantitatively to control residual solvents in a substance, then it must be validated.

PROCEDURE

Examine by gas chromatography with static head-space injection (*2.2.28*).

Sample preparation 1. This is intended for the control of residual solvents in water-soluble substances.

Sample solution (1). Dissolve 0.200 g of the substance to be examined in *water R* and dilute to 20.0 ml with the same solvent.

Sample preparation 2. This is intended for the control of residual solvents in water-insoluble substances.

Sample solution (2). Dissolve 0.200 g of the substance to be examined in *N,N-dimethylformamide R* (DMF) and dilute to 20.0 ml with the same solvent.

Sample preparation 3. This is intended for the control of *N,N*-dimethylacetamide and/or *N,N*-dimethylformamide, when it is known or suspected that one or both of these substances are present in the substance to be examined.

Sample solution (3). Dissolve 0.200 g of the substance to be examined in *1,3-dimethyl-2-imidazolidinone R* (DMI) and dilute to 20.0 ml with the same solvent.

In some cases none of the above sample preparation procedures are appropriate, in which case the diluent to be used for the preparation of the sample solution and the static head-space conditions to be employed must be demonstrated to be suitable.

Solvent solution (a). To 1.0 ml of *Class 1 residual solvent solution CRS*, add 9 ml of *dimethyl sulphoxide R* and dilute to 100.0 ml with *water R*. Dilute 1.0 ml of this solution to 100 ml with *water R*. Dilute 1.0 ml of this solution to 10.0 ml with *water R*.

The reference solutions correspond to the following limits:

- benzene: 2 ppm,
- carbon tetrachloride: 4 ppm,
- 1,2-dichloroethane: 5 ppm,
- 1,1-dichloroethene: 8 ppm,
- 1,1,1-trichloroethane: 10 ppm.

2. Methods of analysis

Solvent solution (b). Dissolve appropriate quantities of the Class 2 residual solvents in *dimethyl sulphoxide R* and dilute to 100.0 ml with *water R*. Dilute to give a concentration of 1/20 of the limits stated in Table 2 (see *5.4. Residual solvents*).

Solvent solution (c). Dissolve 1.00 g of the solvent or solvents present in the substance to be examined in *dimethyl sulphoxide R* or *water R*, if appropriate, and dilute to 100.0 ml with *water R*. Dilute to give a concentration of 1/20 of the limit(s) stated in Table 1 or 2 (see *5.4. Residual solvents*).

Blank solution. Prepare as described for solvent solution (c) but without the addition of solvent(s) (used to verify the absence of interfering peaks).

Test solution. Introduce 5.0 ml of the sample solution and 1.0 ml of the blank solution into an injection vial.

Reference solution (a) (Class 1). Introduce 1.0 ml of solvent solution (a) and 5.0 ml of the appropriate diluent into an injection vial.

Reference solution (a_1) (Class 1). Introduce 5.0 ml of the sample solution and 1.0 ml of solvent solution (a) into an injection vial.

Reference solution (b) (Class 2). Introduce 1.0 ml of solvent solution (b) and 5.0 ml of the appropriate diluent into an injection vial.

Reference solution (c). Introduce 5.0 ml of the sample solution and 1.0 ml of solvent solution (c) into an injection vial.

Reference solution (d). Introduce 1.0 ml of the blank solution and 5.0 ml of the appropriate diluent into an injection vial.

Close the vials with a tight rubber membrane stopper coated with polytetrafluoroethylene and secure with an aluminium crimped cap. Shake to obtain a homogeneous solution.

The following static head-space injection conditions may be used:

Operating parameters	Sample preparation procedure 1	2	3
Equilibration temperature (°C)	80	105	80
Equilibration time (min)	60	45	45
Transfer-line temperature (°C)	85	110	105
Carrier gas: *Nitrogen for chromatography R* or *Helium for chromatography R* at an appropriate pressure			
Pressurisation time (s)	30	30	30
Injection volume (ml)	1	1	1

The chromatographic procedure may be carried out using:

SYSTEM A

- a fused-silica capillary or wide-bore column 30 m long and 0.32 mm or 0.53 mm in internal diameter coated with cross-linked 6 per cent polycyanopropylphenylsiloxane and 94 per cent polydimethylsiloxane (film thickness: 1.8 μm or 3 μm),
- *nitrogen for chromatography R* or *helium for chromatography R* as the carrier gas, split ratio 1:5 with a linear velocity of about 35 cm/s,
- a flame-ionisation detector (a mass spectrometer may also be used or an electron-capture detector for the chlorinated residual solvents of Class 1),

maintaining the temperature of the column at 40 °C for 20 min, then raising the temperature at a rate of 10 °C per min to 240 °C and maintaining it at 240 °C for 20 min and maintaining the temperature of the injection port at 140 °C and that of the detector at 250 °C, or, where there is interference from the matrix, use:

SYSTEM B

- a fused-silica capillary or wide-bore column 30 m long and 0.32 mm or 0.53 mm in internal diameter coated with *macrogol 20 000 R* (film thickness: 0.25 μm),
- *nitrogen for chromatography R* or *helium for chromatography R* as the carrier gas, split ratio 1:5 with a linear velocity of about 35 cm/s.
- a flame-ionisation detector (a mass spectrophotometer may also be used or an electron-capture detector for the chlorinated residual solvents of Class 1),

maintaining the temperature of the column at 50 °C for 20 min, then raising the temperature at a rate of 6 °C per min to 165 °C and maintaining it at 165 °C for 20 min and maintaining the temperature of the injection port at 140 °C and that of the detector at 250 °C.

Inject 1 ml of the gaseous phase of reference solution (a) onto the column described in System A and record the chromatogram under such conditions that the signal-to-noise ratio for 1,1,1-trichloroethane can be measured. The signal-to-noise ratio must be at least five. A typical chromatogram is shown in Figure 2.4.24.-1.

Inject 1 ml of the gaseous phase of reference solution (a_1) onto the column described in System A. The peaks due to the Class 1 residual solvents are still detectable.

Inject 1 ml of the gaseous phase of reference solution (b) onto the column described in System A and record the chromatogram under such conditions that the resolution between acetonitrile and methylene chloride can be determined. The system is suitable if the chromatogram obtained resembles the chromatogram shown in Figure 2.4.24.-2 and the resolution between acetonitrile and methylene chloride is at least 1.0.

Inject 1 ml of the gaseous phase of the test solution onto the column described in System A. If in the chromatogram obtained, there is no peak which corresponds to one of the residual solvent peaks in the chromatograms obtained with reference solution (a) or (b), then the substance to be examined meets the requirements of the test. If any peak in the chromatogram obtained with the test solution corresponds to any of the residual solvent peaks obtained with reference solution (a) or (b) then System B is to be employed.

Inject 1 ml of the gaseous phase of reference solution (a) onto the column described in System B and record the chromatogram under such conditions that the signal-to-noise ratio for benzene can be measured. The signal-to-noise ratio must be at least five. A typical chromatogram is shown in Figure 2.4.24.-3.

Inject 1 ml of the gaseous phase of reference solution (a_1) onto the column described in System B. The peaks due to the Class I residual solvents are still detectable.

Inject 1 ml of the gaseous phase of reference solution (b) onto the column described in System B and record the chromatogram under such conditions that the resolution between acetonitrile and trichloroethene can be determined. The system is suitable if the chromatogram obtained resembles the chromatogram shown in Figure 2.4.24-4 and the resolution between acetonitrile and trichloroethene is at least 1.0.

Inject 1 ml of the gaseous phase of the test solution onto the column described in System B. If in the chromatogram obtained, there is no peak which corresponds to any of the residual solvent peaks in the chromatogram obtained with the reference solution (a) or (b), then the substance

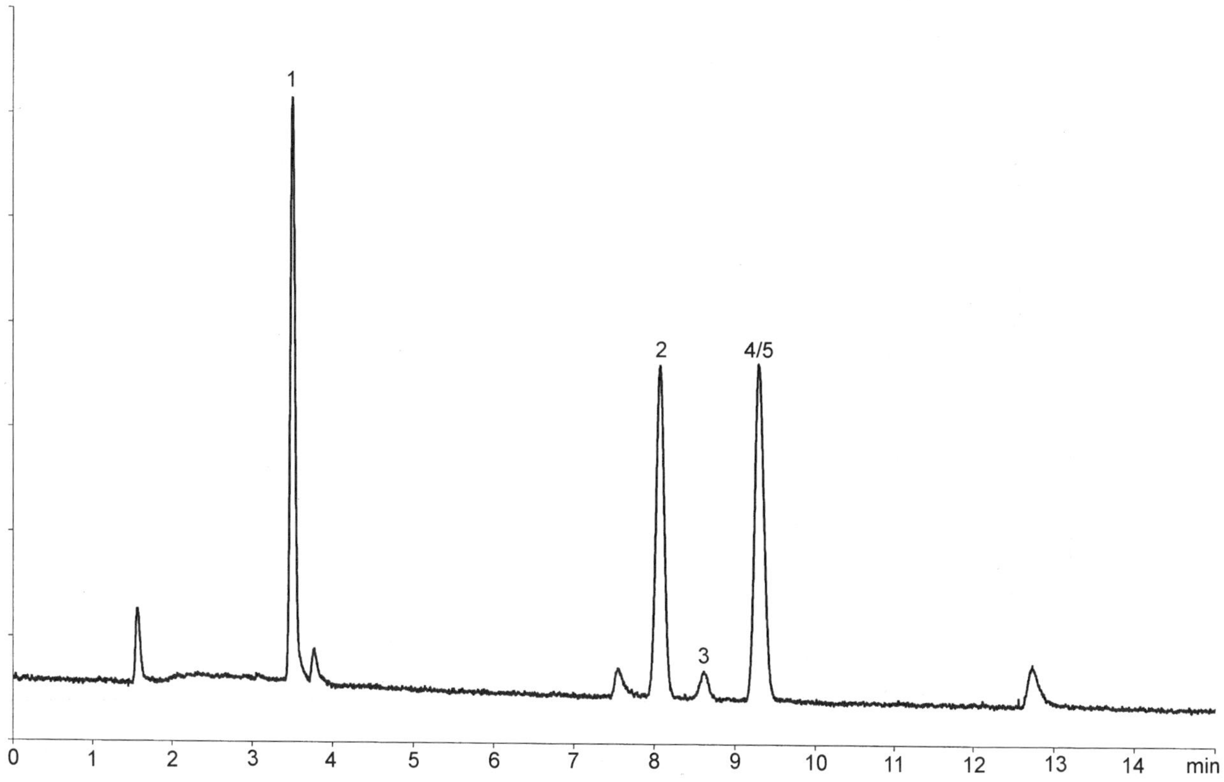

1. 1,1-dichloroethene 2. 1,1,1-trichloroethane 3. carbon tetrachloride 4. benzene 5. 1,2-dichloroethane

Figure 2.4.24.-1. – *Typical chromatogram of class 1 solvents using the conditions described for System A and Procedure 1. Flame-ionisation detector.*

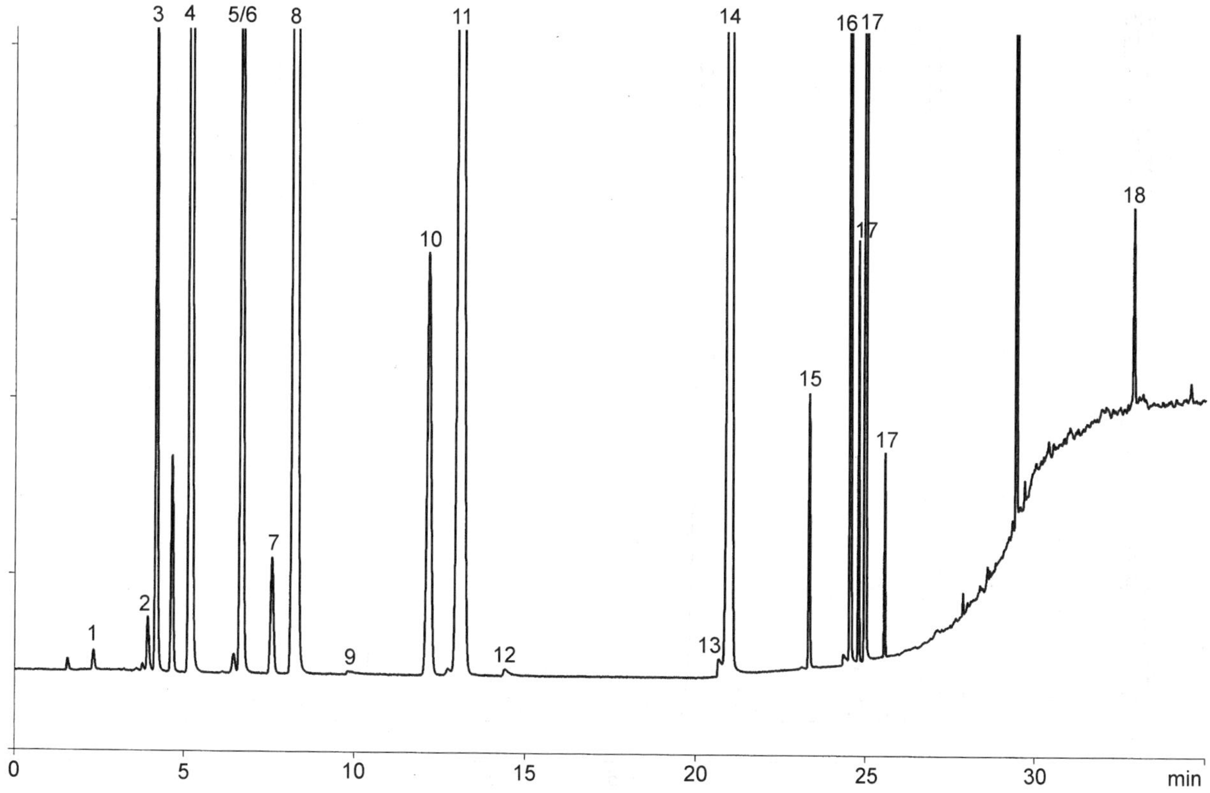

1. methanol
2. acetonitrile
3. dichloromethane
4. hexane
5. *cis*-1,2-dichloroethene
6. nitromethane
7. chloroform
8. cyclohexane
9. 1,2-dimethoxymethane
10. 1,1,2-trichloroethene
11. methylcyclohexane
12. 1,4-dioxan
13. pyridine
14. toluene
15. 2-hexanone
16. chlorobenzene
17. xylene *ortho, meta, para*
18. tetralin

Figure 2.4.24.-2. – *Chromatogram of Class 2 solvents using the conditions described for System A and Procedure 1. Flame-ionisation detector.*

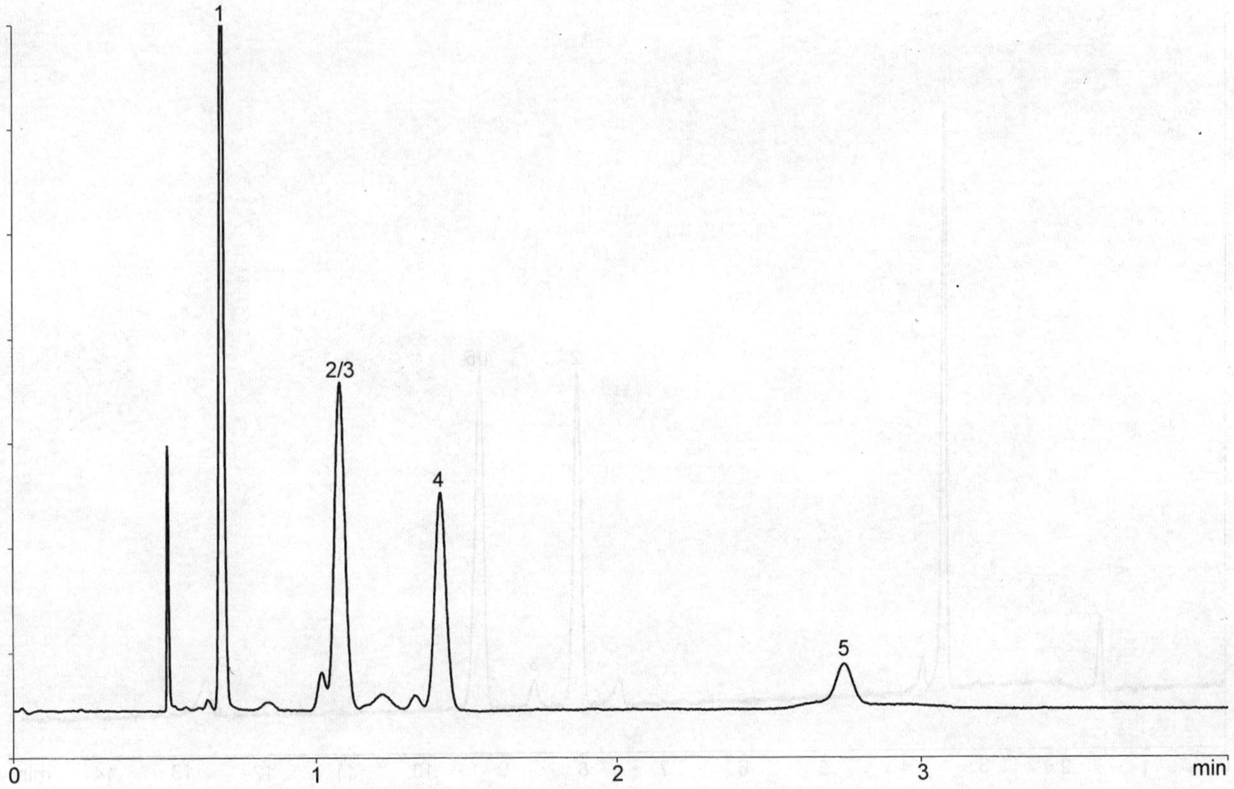

1. 1,1-dichloroethene 2. 1,1,1-trichloroethane 3. carbon tetrachloride 4. benzene 5. 1,2-dichloroethane

Figure 2.4.24.-3. – *Chromatogram of Class 1 residual solvents using the conditions described for System B and Procedure 1. Flame-ionisation detector.*

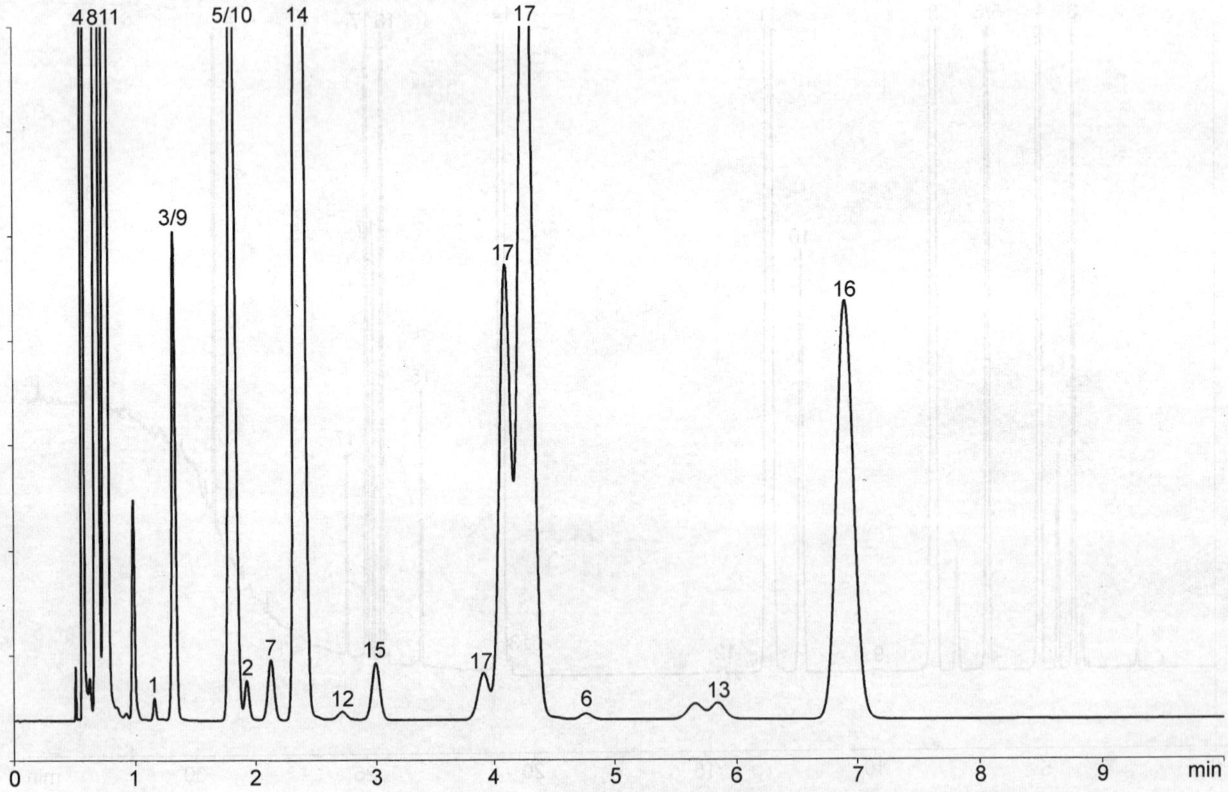

1. methanol
2. acetonitrile
3. dichloromethane
4. hexane
5. *cis*-1,2-dichloroethene
6. nitromethane
7. chloroform
8. cyclohexane
9. 1,2-dimethoxyethane
10. 1,1,2-trichloroethene
11. methylcyclohexane
12. 1,4-dioxan
13. pyridine
14. toluene
15. 2-hexanone
16. chlorobenzene
17. xylene *ortho, meta, para*
18. tetralin (t_R = 28 min)

Figure 2.4.24.-4. – *Typical chromatogram of class 2 residual solvents using the conditions described for System B and Procedure 1. Flame-ionisation detector.*

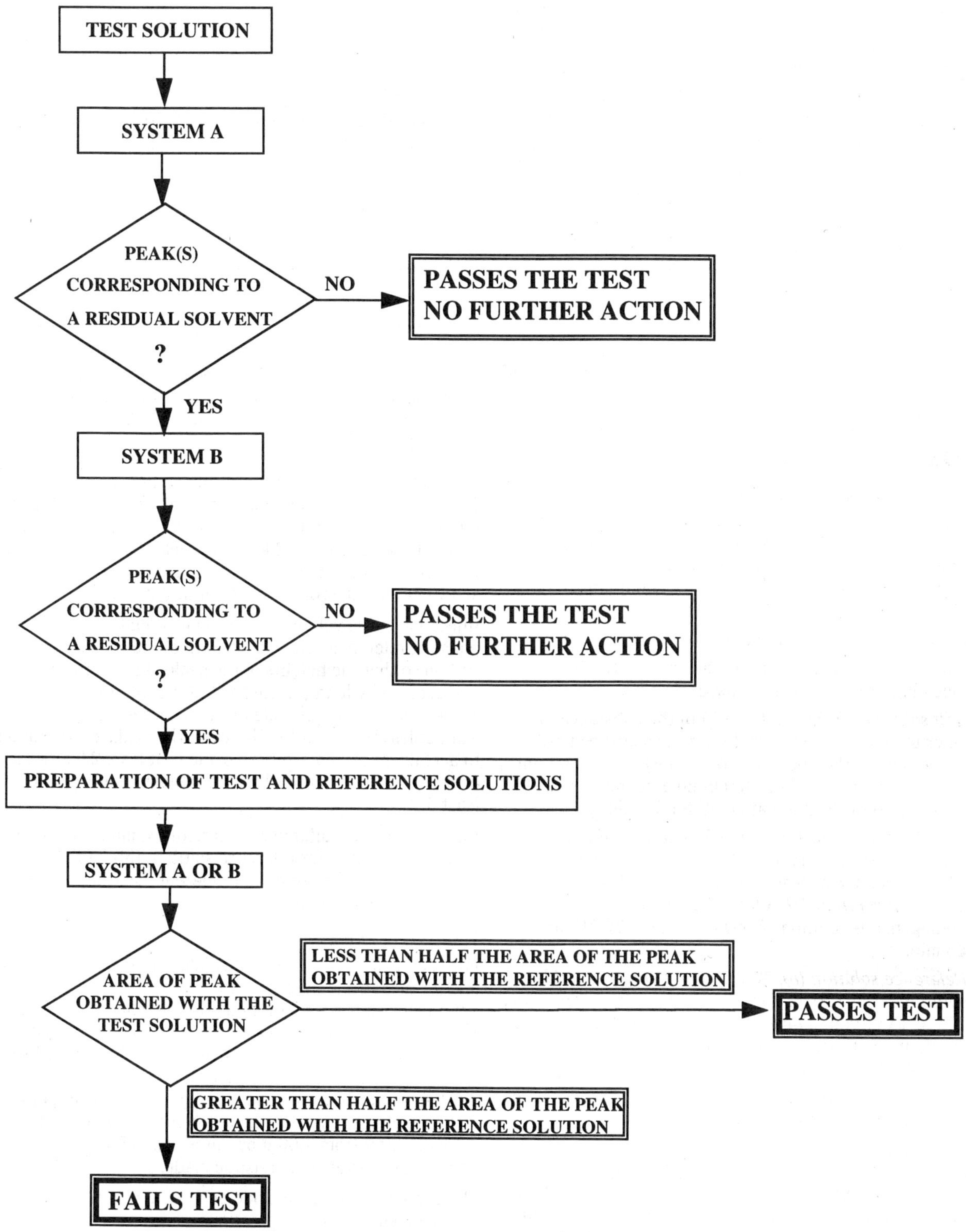

Figure 2.4.24.-5. – *Diagram relating to the identification of residual solvents and the application of limit tests*

to be examined meets the requirements of the test. If any peak in the chromatogram obtained with the test solution corresponds to any of the residual solvent peaks obtained with reference solution (a) or (b) and confirms the correspondence obtained when using System A, then proceed as follows.

Inject 1 ml of the gaseous phase of reference solution (c) onto the column described for System A or System B. If necessary, adjust the sensitivity of the system so that the height of the peak corresponding to the identified residual solvent(s) is at least 50 per cent of the full scale of the recorder.

Inject 1 ml of the gaseous phase of reference solution (d) onto the column. No interfering peaks should be observed.

Inject 1 ml of the gaseous phase of the test solution and 1 ml of the gaseous phase of reference solution (c) on to the column. Repeat these injections twice more.

The mean area of the peak of the residual solvent(s) in the chromatograms obtained with the test solution is not greater than half the mean area of the peak of the corresponding residual solvent(s) in the chromatograms obtained with reference solution (c). The test is not valid unless the relative standard deviation of the differences in areas between the analyte peaks obtained from three replicate paired injections of reference solution (c) and the test solution, is at most 15 per cent.

A flow diagram of the procedure is shown in Figure 2.4.24.-5.

When a residual solvent (Class 2 or Class 3) is present at a level of 0.1 per cent or greater then the content may be quantitatively determined by the method of standard additions.

01/2005:20425

2.4.25. ETHYLENE OXIDE AND DIOXAN

The test is intended for the determination of residual ethylene oxide and dioxan in samples soluble in water or dimethylacetamide. For substances that are insoluble or insufficiently soluble in these solvents, the preparation of the sample solution and the head-space conditions to be employed are given in the individual monograph.

Examine by head-space gas chromatography (*2.2.28*).

A. For samples soluble in or miscible with water, the following procedure may be used.

Test solution. Weigh 1.00 g (M_T) of the substance to be examined in a 10 ml vial (other sizes may be used depending on the operating conditions) and add 1.0 ml of *water R*. Close and mix to obtain a homogeneous solution. Allow to stand at 70 °C for 45 min.

Reference solution (a). Weigh 1.00 g (M_R) of the substance to be examined into an identical 10 ml vial, add 0.50 ml of *ethylene oxide solution R3* and 0.50 ml of *dioxan solution R1*. Close and mix to obtain a homogeneous solution. Allow to stand at 70 °C for 45 min.

Reference solution (b). To 0.50 ml of *ethylene oxide solution R3* in a 10 ml vial add 0.1 ml of a freshly prepared 10 mg/l solution of *acetaldehyde R* and 0.1 ml of *dioxan solution R1*. Close and mix to obtain a homogeneous solution. Allow to stand at 70 °C for 45 min.

B. For samples soluble in or miscible with dimethylacetamide, the following procedure may be used.

Test solution. Weigh 1.00 g (M_T) of the substance to be examined in a 10 ml vial (other sizes may be used depending on the operating conditions) and add 1.0 ml of *dimethylacetamide R* and 0.20 ml of *water R*. Close and mix to obtain a homogeneous solution. Allow to stand at 90 °C for 45 min.

Reference solution (a). Weigh 1.00 g (M_R) of the substance to be examined into a 10 ml vial, add 1.0 ml of *dimethylacetamide R*, 0.10 ml of *dioxan solution R* and 0.10 ml of *ethylene oxide solution R2*. Close and mix to obtain a homogeneous solution. Allow to stand at 90 °C for 45 min.

Reference solution (b). To 0.10 ml of *ethylene oxide solution R2* in a 10 ml vial, add 0.1 ml of a freshly prepared 10 mg/l solution of *acetaldehyde R* and 0.10 ml of *dioxan solution R*. Close and mix to obtain a homogeneous solution. Allow to stand at 70 °C for 45 min.

The following static head-space injection conditions may be used:

- equilibration temperature: 70 °C (90 °C for solutions in dimethylacetamide),
- equilibration time: 45 min,
- transfer-line temperature: 75 °C (150 °C for solutions in dimethylacetamide),
- carrier gas: *helium for chromatography R*,
- pressurisation time: 1 min,
- injection time: 12 s.

The chromatographic procedure may be carried out using:

- a capillary glass or quartz column 30 m long and 0.32 mm in internal diameter the inner surface of which is coated with a 1.0 μm thick layer of *poly(dimethyl)siloxane R*,
- *helium for chromatography R* or *nitrogen for chromatography R* as the carrier gas with a linear velocity of about 20 cm/s and a split ratio of 1:20,
- a flame-ionisation detector,

maintaining the temperature of the column at 50 °C for 5 min, then raising the temperature at a rate of 5 °C per minute to 180 °C and then raising the temperature at a rate of 30 °C per minute to 230 °C and maintaining at 230 °C for 5 min; maintaining the temperature of the injection port at 150 °C and that of the detector at 250 °C.

Inject a suitable volume, for example 1.0 ml, of the gaseous phase of reference solution (b). Adjust the sensitivity of the system so that the heights of the peaks due to ethylene oxide and acetaldehyde in the chromatogram obtained are at least 15 per cent of the full scale of the recorder. The test is not valid unless the resolution between the peaks corresponding to acetaldehyde and ethylene oxide is at least 2.0 and the peak of dioxan is detected with a signal-to-noise ratio of at least 5.

Inject separately suitable volumes, for example 1.0 ml (or the same volume used for reference solution (b)), of the gaseous phases of the test solution and reference solution (a). Repeat the procedure twice more.

Verification of precision

For each pair of injections, calculate for ethylene oxide and for dioxan the difference in area between the peaks obtained with the test solution and reference solution (a). The test is not valid unless the relative standard deviation of the 3 values obtained for ethylene oxide is not greater than 15 per cent and the relative standard deviation of the 3 values obtained for dioxan is not greater than 10 per cent. If the weighings used for the test solution and reference solution differ from 1.00 g by more than 0.5 per cent, the appropriate corrections must be made.

The content of ethylene oxide or dioxan in parts per million is calculated from the expressions:

$$\frac{A_T \times C}{(A_R \times M_T) - (A_T \times M_R)}$$

A_T = area of the peak corresponding to ethylene oxide in the chromatogram obtained with the test solution,

A_R = area of the peak corresponding to ethylene oxide in the chromatogram obtained with reference solution (a),

M_T = mass of the substance to be examined in the test solution, in grams,

M_R = mass of the substance to be examined in the reference solution, in grams,

C = the amount of ethylene oxide added to reference solution (a), in micrograms.

$$\frac{D_T \times C}{(D_R \times M_T) - (D_T \times M_R)}$$

D_T = area of the peak corresponding to dioxan in the chromatogram obtained with the test solution,

D_R = area of the peak corresponding to dioxan in the chromatogram obtained with reference solution (a),

C = the amount of dioxan added to reference solution (a) in micrograms.

01/2005:20426

2.4.26. *N,N*-DIMETHYLANILINE

METHOD A

Examine by gas chromatography (*2.2.28*), using *N,N-diethylaniline R* as the internal standard.

Internal standard solution. Dissolve 50 mg of *N,N-diethylaniline R* in 4 ml of *0.1 M hydrochloric acid* and dilute to 50 ml with *water R*. Dilute 1 ml of this solution to 100 ml with *water R*.

Test solution. Dissolve in a ground-glass-stoppered tube 0.50 g of the substance to be examined in 30.0 ml of *water R*. Add 1.0 ml of the internal standard solution. Adjust the solution to a temperature of 26 °C to 28 °C. Add 1.0 ml of *strong sodium hydroxide solution R* and mix until completely dissolved. Add 2.0 ml of *trimethylpentane R*. Shake for 2 min and allow the phases to separate. Use the upper layer.

Reference solution. Dissolve 50.0 mg of *N,N-dimethylaniline R* in 4.0 ml of *0.1 M hydrochloric acid* and dilute to 50.0 ml with *water R*. Dilute 1.0 ml of this solution to 100.0 ml with *water R*. Dilute 1.0 ml of this solution to 30.0 ml with *water R*. Add 1.0 ml of the internal standard solution and 1.0 ml of *strong sodium hydroxide solution R*. Add 2.0 ml of *trimethylpentane R*. Shake for 2 min and allow the phases to separate. Use the upper layer.

The chromatographic procedure may be carried out using:

- a fused-silica capillary column 25 m long and 0.32 mm in internal diameter coated with cross-linked *polymethylphenylsiloxane R* (film thickness 0.52 µm),
- *helium for chromatography R* as the carrier gas with a split ratio 1:20, a column head pressure of 50 kPa and a split vent of 20 ml/min,
- a flame-ionisation detector,
- a split-liner consisting of a column about 1 cm long packed with *diatomaceous earth for gas chromatography R* impregnated with 10 per cent *m/m* of *poly(dimethyl)siloxane R*,

maintaining the temperature of the column at 150 °C for 5 min, then raising the temperature at a rate of 20 °C per min to 275 °C and maintaining it at 275 °C for 3 min and maintaining the temperature of the detector at 300 °C and that of the injection port at 220 °C.

The retention times are: *N,N*-dimethylaniline about 3.6 min, *N,N*-diethylaniline about 5.0 min.

Inject 1 µl of the test solution and 1 µl of the reference solution.

METHOD B

Examined by gas chromatography (*2.2.28*), using *naphthalene R* as the internal standard.

Internal standard solution. Dissolve 50 mg of *naphthalene R* in *cyclohexane R* and dilute to 50 ml with the same solvent. Dilute 5 ml of this solution to 100 ml with *cyclohexane R*.

Test solution. To 1.00 g of the substance to be examined in a ground-glass-stoppered tube add 5 ml of *1 M sodium hydroxide* and 1.0 ml of the internal standard solution. Stopper the tube and shake vigorously for 1 min. Centrifuge if necessary and use the upper layer.

Reference solution. To 50.0 mg of *N,N-dimethylaniline R* add 2 ml of *hydrochloric acid R* and 20 ml of *water R*, shake to dissolve and dilute to 50.0 ml with *water R*. Dilute 5.0 ml of this solution to 250.0 ml with *water R*. To 1.0 ml of the latter solution in a ground-glass-stoppered tube add 5 ml of *1 M sodium hydroxide* and 1.0 ml of the internal standard solution. Stopper the tube and shake vigorously for 1 min. Centrifuge if necessary and use the upper layer.

The chromatographic procedure may be carried out using:

- a glass column 2 m long and 2 mm in internal diameter packed with *silanised diatomaceous earth for gas chromatography R* impregnated with 3 per cent *m/m* of *polymethylphenylsiloxane R*,
- *nitrogen for chromatography R* as the carrier gas at a flow rate of 30 ml/min,
- a flame-ionisation detector,

maintaining the temperature of the column at 120 °C and that of the injection port and of the detector at 150 °C.

Inject 1 µl of the test solution and 1 µl of the reference solution.

01/2005:20427

2.4.27. HEAVY METALS IN HERBAL DRUGS AND FATTY OILS

Examine by atomic absorption spectrometry (*2.2.23*).

CAUTION: when using closed high-pressure digestion vessels and microwave laboratory equipment, be familiar with the safety and operating instructions given by the manufacturer.

APPARATUS

The apparatus typically consists of the following:

- as digestion flasks, polytetrafluoroethylene flasks with a volume of about 120 ml, fitted with an airtight closure, a valve to adjust the pressure inside the container and a polytetrafluoroethylene tube to allow release of gas,
- a system to make flasks airtight, using the same torsional force for each of them,
- a microwave oven, with a magnetron frequency of 2450 MHz, with a selectable output from 0 to 630 ± 70 W in 1 per cent increments, a programmable digital computer, a polytetrafluoroethylene-coated microwave cavity with a variable speed exhaust fan, a rotating turntable drive system and exhaust tubing to vent fumes,
- an atomic absorption spectrometer, equipped with hollow-cathode lamps as source of radiation and a deuterium lamp as background corrector; the system is fitted with:

  (a) a graphite furnace as atomisation device for cadmium, copper, iron, lead, nickel and zinc.

  (b) an automated continuous-flow hydride vapour generation system for arsenic and mercury.

METHOD

In case alternative apparatus is used, an adjustment of the instrument parameters may be necessary.

Clean all the glassware and laboratory equipment with a 10 g/l solution of *nitric acid R* before use.

Test solution. In a digestion flask place the prescribed quantity of the substance to be examined (about 0.50 g of powdered drug (1400) or 0.50 g of fatty oil). Add 6 ml of *heavy metal-free nitric acid R* and 4 ml of *heavy metal-free hydrochloric acid R*. Make the flask airtight.

Place the digestion flasks in the microwave oven. Carry out the digestion in 3 steps according to the following programme, used for 7 flasks each containing the test solution: 80 per cent power for 15 min, 100 per cent power for 5 min, 80 per cent power for 20 min.

At the end of the cycle allow the flasks to cool in air and to each add 4 ml of *heavy metal-free sulphuric acid R*. Repeat the digestion programme. After cooling in air, open each digestion flask and introduce the clear, colourless solution obtained into a 50 ml volumetric flask. Rinse each digestion flask with 2 quantities, each of 15 ml, of *water R* and collect the rinsings in the volumetric flask. Add 1.0 ml of a 10 g/l solution of *magnesium nitrate R* and 1.0 ml of a 100 g/l solution of *ammonium dihydrogen phosphate R* and dilute to 50.0 ml with *water R*.

Blank solution. Mix 6 ml of *heavy metal-free nitric acid R* and 4 ml of *heavy metal-free hydrochloric acid R* in a digestion flask. Carry out the digestion in the same manner as for the test solution.

CADMIUM, COPPER, IRON, LEAD, NICKEL AND ZINC

Measure the content of cadmium, copper, iron, lead, nickel and zinc by the standard additions method (*2.2.23, Method II*), using reference solutions of each heavy metal and the instrumental parameters described in Table 2.4.27.-1.

The absorbance value of the blank solution is automatically subtracted from the value obtained with the test solution.

Table 2.4.27.-1

		Cd	Cu	Fe	Ni	Pb	Zn
Wavelength	nm	228.8	324.8	248.3	232	283.5	213.9
Slit width	nm	0.5	0.5	0.2	0.2	0.5	0.5
Lamp current	mA	6	7	5	10	5	7
Ignition temperature	°C	800	800	800	800	800	800
Atomisation temperature	°C	1800	2300	2300	2500	2200	2000
Background corrector		on	off	off	off	off	off
Nitrogen flow	l/min	3	3	3	3	3	3

ARSENIC AND MERCURY

Measure the content of arsenic and mercury in comparison with the reference solutions of arsenic or mercury at a known concentration by direct calibration (*2.2.23, Method I*) using an automated continuous-flow hydride vapour generation system.

The absorbance value of the blank solution is automatically subtracted from the value obtained with the test solution.

Arsenic

Sample solution. To 19.0 ml of the test solution or of the blank solution as prescribed above, add 1 ml of a 200 g/l solution of *potassium iodide R*. Allow the test solution to stand at room temperature for about 50 min or at 70 °C for about 4 min.

Acid reagent. Heavy metal-free hydrochloric acid R.

Reducing reagent. A 6 g/l solution of *sodium tetrahydroborate R* in a 5 g/l solution of *sodium hydroxide R*.

The instrumental parameters in Table 2.4.27.-2 may be used.

Mercury

Sample solution. Test solution or blank solution, as prescribed above.

Acid reagent. A 515 g/l solution of *heavy metal-free hydrochloric acid R*.

Reducing reagent. A 10 g/l solution of *stannous chloride R* in *dilute heavy metal-free hydrochloric acid R*.

The instrumental parameters in Table 2.4.27.-2 may be used.

Table 2.4.27.-2

		As	Hg
Wavelength	nm	193.7	253.7
Slit width	nm	0.2	0.5
Lamp current	mA	10	4
Acid reagent flow rate	ml/min	1.0	1.0
Reducing reagent flow rate	ml/min	1.0	1.0
Sample solution flow rate	ml/min	7.0	7.0
Absorption cell		Quartz (heated)	Quartz (unheated)
Background corrector		off	off
Nitrogen flow rate	l/min	0.1	0.1

01/2005:20428

2.4.28. 2-ETHYLHEXANOIC ACID

Examine by gas chromatography (*2.2.28*), using *3-cyclohexylpropionic acid R* as the internal standard.

Internal standard solution. Dissolve 100 mg of *3-cyclohexylpropionic acid R* in *cyclohexane R* and dilute to 100 ml with the same solvent.

Test solution. To 0.300 g of the substance to be examined, add 4.0 ml of a 33 per cent *V/V* solution of *hydrochloric acid R*. Shake vigorously for 1 min with 1.0 ml of the internal standard solution. Allow the phases to separate (if necessary, centrifuge for a better separation). Use the upper layer.

Reference solution. Dissolve 75.0 mg of *2-ethylhexanoic acid R* in the internal standard solution and dilute to 50.0 ml with the same solution. To 1.0 ml of the solution add 4.0 ml of a 33 per cent *V/V* solution of *hydrochloric acid R*. Shake vigorously for 1 min. Allow the phases to separate (if necessary, centrifuge for a better separation). Use the upper layer.

The chromatographic procedure may be carried out using:

– a wide-bore fused-silica column 10 m long and 0.53 mm in internal diameter coated with *macrogol 20 000 2-nitroterephthalate R* (film thickness 1.0 µm),
– *helium for chromatography R* as the carrier gas at a flow rate of 10 ml/min,
– a flame-ionisation detector,

with the following temperature programme:

	Time (min)	Temperature (°C)	Rate (°C/min)	Comment
Column	0 - 2	40	-	isothermal
	2 - 7.3	40 → 200	30	linear gradient
	7.3 - 10.3	200	-	isothermal
Injection port		200		
Detector		300		

Inject 1 µl of the test solution and 1 µl of the reference solution.

The test is not valid unless the resolution between the peaks corresponding to 2-ethylhexanoic acid (first peak) and the internal standard is at least 2.0.

Calculate the percentage content of 2-ethylhexanoic acid from the expression:

$$\frac{A_T \times I_R \times m_R \times 2}{A_R \times I_T \times m_T}$$

A_T = area of the peak corresponding to 2-ethylhexanoic acid in the chromatogram obtained with the test solution,

A_R = area of the peak corresponding to 2-ethylhexanoic acid in the chromatogram obtained with the reference solution,

I_T = area of the peak corresponding to the internal standard in the chromatogram obtained with the test solution,

I_R = area of the peak corresponding to the internal standard in the chromatogram obtained with the reference solution,

m_T = mass of the substance to be examined in the test solution, in grams,

m_R = mass of 2-ethylhexanoic acid in the reference solution, in grams.

01/2005:20429

2.4.29. COMPOSITION OF FATTY ACIDS IN OILS RICH IN OMEGA-3-ACIDS

The assay may be used for quantitative determination of the EPA and DHA content in omega-3-containing products of fish oil in different concentrations. The method is applicable to triglycerides or ethyl esters and the results are expressed as triglycerides or ethyl esters, respectively.

EPA AND DHA

Gas chromatography (*2.2.28*). *Carry out the operations as rapidly as possible, avoiding exposure to actinic light, oxidising agents, oxidation catalysts (for example, copper and iron) and air.*

The assay is carried out on the methyl or ethyl esters of (all-*Z*)-eicosa-5,8,11,14,17-pentaenoic acid (EPA; 20:5 n-3) and (all-*Z*)-docosa-4,7,10,13,16,19-hexaenoic acid (DHA; 22:6 n-3) in the substance to be examined.

Internal standard. Methyl tricosanoate R.

Test solution (a)

A. Dissolve the mass of sample to be examined according to Table 2.4.29.-1 and about 70.0 mg of the internal standard in a 50 mg/l solution of *butylhydroxytoluene R* in *trimethylpentane R* and dilute to 10.0 ml with the same solution.

Table 2.4.29.-1.

Approximative sum EPA + DHA (per cent)	Amount sample to be weighed (grams)
30 - 50	0.4 - 0.5
50 - 70	0.3
70 - 90	0.25

Ethyl esters are now ready for analysis. For triglycerides continue as described in step B.

B. Introduce 2.0 ml of the solution obtained into a quartz tube and evaporate the solvent with a gentle current of *nitrogen R*. Add 1.5 ml of a 20 g/l solution of *sodium hydroxide R* in *methanol R*, cover with *nitrogen R*, cap tightly with a polytetrafluoroethylene-lined cap, mix and heat on a water-bath for 7 min. Allow to cool. Add 2 ml of *boron trichloride-methanol solution R*, cover with *nitrogen R*, cap tightly, mix and heat on a water-bath for 30 min. Cool to 40-50 °C, add 1 ml of *trimethylpentane R*, cap and shake vigorously for at least 30 s. Immediately add 5 ml of a *saturated sodium chloride solution R*, cover with *nitrogen R*, cap and shake thoroughly for at least 15 s. Transfer the upper layer to a separate tube. Shake the methanol layer once more with 1 ml of *trimethylpentane R*. Wash the combined trimethylpentane extracts with 2 quantities, each of 1 ml, of *water R* and dry over *anhydrous sodium sulphate R*. Prepare 3 solutions for each sample.

Test solution (b). Dissolve 0.300 g of the sample to be examined in a 50 mg/l solution of *butylhydroxytoluene R* in *trimethylpentane R* and dilute to 10.0 ml with the same solution. Proceed as described for test solution (a).

Reference solution (a). Dissolve 60.0 mg of *docosahexaenoic acid ethyl ester CRS*, about 70.0 mg of the internal standard and 90.0 mg of *eicosapentaenoic acid ethyl ester CRS* in a 50 mg/l solution of *butylhydroxytoluene R* in *trimethylpentane R* and dilute to 10.0 ml with the same solution. Proceed as described for test solution (a) step A when analysing ethyl esters. For analysis of triglycerides, continue with step B in the same manner as for test solution (a). Prepare 3 solutions for each sample.

Reference solution (b). Into a 10 ml volumetric flask dissolve 0.3 g of *methyl palmitate R*, 0.3 g of *methyl stearate R*, 0.3 g of *methyl arachidate R* and 0.3 g of *methyl behenate R*, in a 50 mg/l solution of *butylhydroxytoluene R* in *trimethylpentane R* and dilute to 10.0 ml with the same solution.

Reference solution (c). Into a 10 ml volumetric flask dissolve a sample containing about 55.0 mg of *docosahexaenoic acid methyl ester R* and about 5.0 mg of *tetracos-15-enoic acid methyl ester R* in a 50 mg/l solution of *butylhydroxytoluene R* in *trimethylpentane R* and dilute to 10.0 ml with the same solution.

Column:

- *material*: fused silica,
- *dimensions*: *l* = at least 25 m, Ø = 0.25 mm,
- *stationary phase*: bonded *macrogol 20 000 R* (film thickness 0.2 µm).

Carrier gas: *hydrogen for chromatography R* or *helium for chromatography R.*

2. Methods of analysis

Split ratio: 1:200, alternatively splitless with temperature control (sample solutions need to be diluted 1/200 with a 50 mg/l solution of *butylhydroxytoluene R* in *trimethylpentane R* before injection).

Temperature:

	Time (min)	Temperature (°C)
Column	0 - 2	170
	2 - 25.7	170 → 240
	25.7 - 28	240
Injection port		250
Detector		270

Detection: flame ionisation.

Injection: 1 µl, twice.

System suitability:

- in the chromatogram obtained with reference solution (b), the area per cent composition increases in the following order: methyl palmitate, methyl stearate, methyl arachidate, methyl behenate; the difference between the percentage area of methyl palmitate and that of methyl behenate is less than 2 area per cent units,
- *resolution*: minimum of 1.2 between the peaks due to docosahexaenoic acid methyl ester and to tetracos-15-enoic acid methyl ester in the chromatogram obtained with reference solution (c),
- in the chromatogram obtained with test solution (a), the peaks due to methyl tricosanoate and any heneicosapentaenoic acid methyl ester or ethyl ester (C21:5) present when compared with the chromatogram obtained with test solution (b) are clearly separated (if not, a correction factor has to be used),
- in the chromatogram obtained with test solution (a) the recovery for the added *eicosapentaenoic acid ethyl ester CRS* and *docosahexaenoic acid ethyl ester CRS* is greater than 95 per cent when due consideration has been given to the correction by the internal standard, and the standard addition method is used.

Calculate the percentage content of EPA and DHA using the following expression and taking into account the assigned value of the reference substances:

$$A_x \times \frac{A_3}{m_3} \times \frac{m_1}{A_1} \times \frac{m_{x,r}}{A_{x,r}} \times \frac{1}{m_2} \times C \times 100$$

m_1 = mass of the internal standard in test solution (a), in milligrams,

m_2 = mass of the sample to be examined in test solution (a), in milligrams,

m_3 = mass of the internal standard in reference solution (a), in milligrams,

$m_{x,r}$ = mass of *eicosapentaenoic acid ethyl ester CRS* or *docosahexaenoic acid ethyl ester CRS* in reference solution (a), in milligrams,

A_x = area of the peak due to eicosapentaenoic acid ester or docosahexaenoic acid ester in the chromatogram obtained with test solution (a),

$A_{x,r}$ = area of the peak due to eicosapentaenoic acid ester or docosahexaenoic acid ester in the chromatogram obtained with reference solution (a),

A_1 = area of the peak due to the internal standard in the chromatogram obtained with test solution (a),

A_3 = area of the peak due to the internal standard in the chromatogram obtained with reference solution (a),

C = conversion factor between ethyl ester and triglycerides,
C = 1.00 for ethyl esters,
C = 0.954 for EPA,
C = 0.957 for DHA.

TOTAL OMEGA-3-ACIDS

From the assay for EPA and DHA, calculate the percentage content of the total omega-3-acids using the following expression and identifying the peaks from the chromatograms:

$$EPA + DHA + \frac{A_{n-3}\,(EPA + DHA)}{A_{\mathrm{EPA}} + A_{\mathrm{DHA}}}$$

EPA = percentage content of EPA,

DHA = percentage content of DHA,

$A_{n\text{-}3}$ = sum of the areas of the peaks due to C18:3 n-3, C18:4 n-3, C20:4 n-3, C21:5 n-3 and C22:5 n-3 methyl esters in the chromatogram obtained with test solution (b),

A_{EPA} = area of the peak due to EPA ester in the chromatogram obtained with test solution (b),

A_{DHA} = area of the peak due to DHA ester in the chromatogram obtained with test solution (b).

01/2005:20430

2.4.30. ETHYLENE GLYCOL AND DIETHYLENE GLYCOL IN ETHOXYLATED SUBSTANCES

Ethoxylated substances may contain varied amounts of ethylene glycol and diethylene glycol, as a result of the manufacturing process. The following method may be used for the quantitative determination of these substances, in particular in the case of the following surfactants: macrogolglycerol ricinoleate, macrogolglycerol hydroxystearate, macrogol 15 hydroxystearate, nonoxinol 9 and macrogol cetostearyl ether.

Gas chromatography (*2.2.28*).

Internal standard solution. Dissolve 30.0 mg of *1,2-pentanediol R* in *acetone R* and dilute to 30.0 ml with the same solvent. Dilute 1.0 ml of this solution to 20.0 ml with *acetone R*.

Test solution. Dissolve 0.500 g of the substance to be examined in the internal standard solution and dilute to 10.0 ml with the same solution.

Reference solution (a). Mix 30.0 mg of *ethylene glycol R* with *acetone R* and dilute to 100.0 ml with the same solvent. Dilute 1.0 ml to 10.0 ml with the internal standard solution.

Reference solution (b). Prepare a solution of *diethylene glycol R* with a concentration corresponding to the prescribed limit and using the same solvents as for the preparation of reference solution (a).

Column:

- *material*: fused silica,
- *size*: l = 30 m, Ø = 0.53 mm,

– *stationary phase*: *macrogol 20 000 R* (film thickness 1 μm).

Carrier gas: *helium for chromatography R.*

Flow rate: 30 ml/min.

Split ratio: 1:3.

Temperature:

	Time (min)	Temperature (°C)
Column	0 - 40	80 → 200
	40 - 45	200 → 230
	45 - 65	230
Injection port		250
Detector		250

Detection: flame ionisation.

Injection: 2 μl.

Relative retentions with reference to 1,2-pentanediol (retention time = about 19 min): ethylene glycol = about 0.7; diethylene glycol = about 1.3.

2.5. ASSAYS

2.5. ASSAYS

01/2005:20501

2.5.1. ACID VALUE

The acid value I_A is the number that expresses in milligrams the quantity of potassium hydroxide required to neutralise the free acids present in 1 g of the substance.

Dissolve 10.00 g of the substance to be examined, or the quantity prescribed (*m* g) in 50 ml of a mixture of equal volumes of *alcohol R* and *ether R*, previously neutralised with *0.1 M potassium hydroxide*, unless otherwise specified, using 0.5 ml of *phenolphthalein solution R1* as indicator. When the substance to be examined has dissolved, titrate with *0.1 M potassium hydroxide* until the pink colour persists for at least 15 s (*n* ml of *0.1 M potassium hydroxide*).

$$I_A = \frac{5.610n}{m}$$

01/2005:20502

2.5.2. ESTER VALUE

The ester value I_E is the number that expresses in milligrams the quantity of potassium hydroxide required to saponify the esters present in 1 g of the substance. It is calculated from the saponification value I_S and the acid value I_A:

$$I_E = I_S - I_A$$

01/2005:20503

2.5.3. HYDROXYL VALUE

The hydroxyl value I_{OH} is the number that expresses in milligrams the quantity of potassium hydroxide required to neutralise the acid combined by acylation in 1 g of the substance.

METHOD A

Introduce the quantity of the substance to be examined shown in Table 2.5.3.-1 (*m* g) into a 150 ml acetylation flask fitted with an air condenser, unless another quantity is prescribed in the monograph. Add the quantity of *acetic anhydride solution R1* stated in Table 2.5.3.-1 and attach the air condenser.

Table 2.5.3.-1

Presumed value I_{OH}	Quantity of sample (g)	Volume of acetylating reagent (ml)
10 - 100	2.0	5.0
100 - 150	1.5	5.0
150 - 200	1.0	5.0
200 - 250	0.75	5.0
250 - 300	0.60 or 1.20	5.0 or 10.0
300 - 350	1.0	10.0
350 - 700	0.75	15.0
700 - 950	0.5	15.0

Heat the flask in a water-bath for 1 h keeping the level of the water about 2.5 cm above the level of the liquid in the flask. Withdraw the flask and allow to cool. Add 5 ml of *water R* through the upper end of the condenser. If a cloudiness appears add sufficient *pyridine R* to clear it, noting the volume added. Shake the flask and replace in the water-bath for 10 min. Withdraw the flask and allow to cool. Rinse the condenser and the walls of the flask with 5 ml of *alcohol R*, previously neutralised to *phenolphthalein solution R1*. Titrate with *0.5 M alcoholic potassium hydroxide* using 0.2 ml of *phenolphthalein solution R1* as indicator (n_1 ml of *0.5 M alcoholic potassium hydroxide*). Carry out a blank test under the same conditions (n_2 ml of *0.5 M alcoholic potassium hydroxide*).

$$I_{OH} = \frac{28.05\,(n_2 - n_1)}{m} + I_A$$

METHOD B

Introduce the prescribed quantity of the substance to be examined (*m* g) into a perfectly dry 5 ml conical flask fitted with a ground-glass or suitable plastic stopper and add 2.0 ml of *propionic anhydride reagent R*. Close the flask and shake gently to dissolve the substance. Allow to stand for 2 h unless otherwise prescribed. Remove the stopper and transfer the flask and its contents into a wide-mouthed 500 ml conical flask containing 25.0 ml of a 9 g/l solution of *aniline R* in *cyclohexane R* and 30 ml of *glacial acetic acid R*. Swirl the contents of the flask, allow to stand for 5 min, add 0.05 ml of *crystal violet solution R* and titrate with *0.1 M perchloric acid* until an emerald-green colour is obtained (n_1 ml of *0.1 M perchloric acid*). Carry out a blank test under the same conditions (n_2 ml of *0.1 M perchloric acid*).

$$I_{OH} = \frac{5.610\,(n_1 - n_2)}{m}$$

To take account of any water present, determine this (*y* per cent) by the semi-micro determination of water (*2.5.12*). The hydroxyl value is then given by the equation:

$$I_{OH} = (\text{hydroxyl value as determined}) - 31.1y$$

01/2005:20504

2.5.4. IODINE VALUE

The iodine value I_I is the number that expresses in grams the quantity of halogen, calculated as iodine, that can be fixed in the prescribed conditions by 100 g of the substance.

When the monograph does not specify the method to be used, method A is applied. Any change from method A to method B is validated.

METHOD A

Unless otherwise prescribed, use the following quantities (Table 2.5.4.-1) for the determination.

Table 2.5.4.-1

Presumed value I_I	Quantity of sample (g)
less than 20	1.0
20 - 60	0.5 - 0.25
60 - 100	0.25 - 0.15
more than 100	0.15 - 0.10

Introduce the prescribed quantity of the substance to be examined (*m* g) into a 250 ml flask fitted with a ground-glass stopper and previously dried or rinsed with *glacial acetic acid R*, and dissolve it in 15 ml of *chloroform R* unless otherwise prescribed. Add very slowly 25.0 ml of *iodine bromide solution R*. Close the flask and keep it in the dark for 30 min unless otherwise prescribed, shaking frequently. Add 10 ml of a 100 g/l solution of *potassium iodide R* and 100 ml of *water R*. Titrate with *0.1 M sodium*

2. Methods of analysis

thiosulphate, shaking vigorously until the yellow colour is almost discharged. Add 5 ml of *starch solution R* and continue the titration adding the *0.1 M sodium thiosulphate* dropwise until the colour is discharged (n_1 ml of *0.1 M sodium thiosulphate*). Carry out a blank test under the same conditions (n_2 ml of *0.1 M sodium thiosulphate*).

$$I_I = \frac{1.269\,(n_2 - n_1)}{m}$$

METHOD B

Unless otherwise prescribed, use the following quantities (Table 2.5.4.-2) for the determination.

Table 2.5.4.-2

Presumed value I_I	Mass (g) (corresponding to an excess of 150 per cent ICl)	Mass (g) (corresponding to an excess of 100 per cent ICl)	Iodine chloride solution (ml)
<3	10	10	25
3	8.4613	10.5760	25
5	5.0770	6.3460	25
10	2.5384	3.1730	20
20	0.8461	1.5865	20
40	0.6346	0.7935	20
60	0.4321	0.5288	20
80	0.3173	0.3966	20
100	0.2538	0.3173	20
120	0.2115	0.2644	20
140	0.1813	0.2266	20
160	0.1587	0.1983	20
180	0.1410	0.1762	20
200	0.1269	0.1586	20

The mass of the sample is such that there will be an excess of *iodine chloride solution R* of 50 per cent to 60 per cent of the amount added, i.e. 100 per cent to 150 per cent of the amount absorbed.

Introduce the prescribed quantity of the substance to be examined (*m* g) into a 250 ml flask fitted with a ground-glass stopper and previously rinsed with *glacial acetic acid R* or dried, and dissolve it in 15 ml of a mixture of equal volumes of *cyclohexane R* and *glacial acetic acid R*, unless otherwise prescribed. If necessary, melt the substance before dissolution (melting point greater than 50 °C). Add very slowly the volume of *iodine chloride solution R* stated in Table 2.5.4.-2. Close the flask and keep it in the dark for 30 min, unless otherwise prescribed, shaking frequently. Add 10 ml of a 100 g/l solution of *potassium iodide R* and 100 ml of *water R*. Titrate with *0.1 M sodium thiosulphate*, shaking vigorously until the yellow colour is almost discharged. Add 5 ml of *starch solution R* and continue the titration adding the *0.1 M sodium thiosulphate* dropwise until the colour is discharged (n_1 ml of *0.1 M sodium thiosulphate*). Carry out a blank test under the same conditions (n_2 ml of *0.1 M sodium thiosulphate*).

$$I_I = \frac{1.269\,(n_2 - n_1)}{m}$$

01/2005:20505

2.5.5. PEROXIDE VALUE

The peroxide value I_P is the number that expresses in milliequivalents of active oxygen the quantity of peroxide contained in 1000 g of the substance, as determined by the methods described below.

When the monograph does not specify the method to be used, method A is applied. Any change from method A to method B is validated.

METHOD A

Place 5.00 g of the substance to be examined (*m* g) in a 250 ml conical flask fitted with a ground-glass stopper. Add 30 ml of a mixture of 2 volumes of *chloroform R* and 3 volumes of *glacial acetic acid R*. Shake to dissolve the substance and add 0.5 ml of *saturated potassium iodide solution R*. Shake for exactly 1 min then add 30 ml of *water R*. Titrate with *0.01 M sodium thiosulphate*, adding the titrant slowly with continuous vigorous shaking, until the yellow colour is almost discharged. Add 5 ml of *starch solution R* and continue the titration, shaking vigorously, until the colour is discharged (n_1 ml of *0.01 M sodium thiosulphate*). Carry out a blank test under the same conditions (n_2 ml of *0.01 M sodium thiosulphate*). The volume of *0.01 M sodium thiosulphate* used in the blank titration must not exceed 0.1 ml.

$$I_P = \frac{10\,(n_1 - n_2)}{m}$$

METHOD B

Carry out the operations avoiding exposure to actinic light. Place 50 ml of a mixture of 2 volumes of *trimethylpentane R* and 3 volumes of *glacial acetic acid R* in a conical flask and replace the stopper. Swirl the flask until the substance to be examined (*m* g; see Table 2.5.5.-1) has dissolved. Using a suitable volumetric pipette, add 0.5 ml of *saturated potassium iodide solution R* and replace the stopper. Allow the solution to stand for 60 ± 1 s, thoroughly shaking the solution continuously, then add 30 ml of *water R*.

Table 2.5.5.-1

Expected peroxide value I_p	Mass of substance to be examined (g)
0 to 12	2.00 to 5.00
12 to 20	1.20 to 2.00
20 to 30	0.80 to 1.20
30 to 50	0.500 to 0.800
50 to 90	0.300 to 0.500

Titrate the solution with *0.01 M sodium thiosulphate* (V_1 ml), adding it gradually and with constant, vigorous shaking, until the yellow iodine colour has almost disappeared. Add about 0.5 ml of *starch solution R1* and continue the titration, with constant shaking especially near the end-point, to liberate all of the iodine from the solvent layer. Add the sodium thiosulphate solution dropwise until the blue colour just disappears.

Depending on the volume of *0.01 M sodium thiosulphate* used, it may be necessary to titrate with *0.1 M sodium thiosulphate*.

NOTE: there is a 15 s to 30 s delay in neutralising the starch indicator for peroxide values of 70 and greater, due to the tendency of trimethylpentane to float on the surface of the aqueous medium and the time necessary to adequately mix the solvent and the aqueous titrant, thus liberating the last traces of iodine. It is recommended to use *0.1 M sodium thiosulphate* for peroxide values greater than 150. A small amount (0.5 per cent to 1.0 per cent (*m/m*)) of high HLB emulsifier (for example polysorbate 60) may be added to the mixture to retard the phase separation and decrease the time lag in the liberation of iodine.

Carry out a blank determination (V_0 ml). If the result of the blank determination exceeds 0.1 ml of titration reagent, replace the impure reagents and repeat the determination.

$$I_p = \frac{1000\,(V_1 - V_0)\,c}{m}$$

c = concentration of the sodium thiosulphate solution in moles, per litre.

01/2005:20506

2.5.6. SAPONIFICATION VALUE

The saponification value I_S is the number that expresses in milligrams the quantity of potassium hydroxide required to neutralise the free acids and to saponify the esters present in 1 g of the substance.

Unless otherwise prescribed, use the quantities indicated in Table 2.5.6.-1 for the determination.

Table 2.5.6.-1

Presumed value I_S	Quantity of sample (g)
<3	20
3 to 10	12 to 15
10 to 40	8 to 12
40 to 60	5 to 8
60 to 100	3 to 5
100 to 200	2.5 to 3
200 to 300	1 to 2
300 to 400	0.5 to 1

Introduce the prescribed quantity of the substance to be examined (*m* g) into a 250 ml borosilicate glass flask fitted with a reflux condenser. Add 25.0 ml of *0.5 M alcoholic potassium hydroxide* and a few glass beads. Attach the condenser and heat under reflux for 30 min, unless otherwise prescribed. Add 1 ml of *phenolphthalein solution R1* and titrate immediately (while still hot) with *0.5 M hydrochloric acid* (n_1 ml of *0.5 M hydrochloric acid*). Carry out a blank test under the same conditions (n_2 ml of *0.5 M hydrochloric acid*).

$$I_S = \frac{28.05\,(n_2 - n_1)}{m}$$

01/2005:20507

2.5.7. UNSAPONIFIABLE MATTER

The term "unsaponifiable matter" is applied to the substances non-volatile at 100-105 °C obtained by extraction with an organic solvent from the substance to be examined after it has been saponified. The result is calculated as per cent *m/m*.

Use ungreased ground-glass glassware.

Introduce the prescribed quantity of the substance to be examined (*m* g) into a 250 ml flask fitted with a reflux condenser. Add 50 ml of *2 M alcoholic potassium hydroxide R* and heat on a water-bath for 1 h, swirling frequently. Cool to a temperature below 25 °C and transfer the contents of the flask to a separating funnel with the aid of 100 ml of *water R*. Shake the liquid carefully with 3 quantities, each of 100 ml, of *peroxide-free ether R*. Combine the ether layers in another separating funnel containing 40 ml of *water R*, shake gently for a few minutes, allow to separate and reject the aqueous phase. Wash the ether phase with 2 quantities, each of 40 ml, of *water R* then wash successively with 40 ml of a 30 g/l solution of *potassium hydroxide R* and 40 ml of *water R*; repeat this procedure 3 times. Wash the ether phase several times, each with 40 ml of *water R*, until the aqueous phase is no longer alkaline to phenolphthalein. Transfer the ether phase to a tared flask, washing the separating funnel with *peroxide-free ether R*.

Distil off the ether with suitable precautions and add 6 ml of *acetone R* to the residue. Carefully remove the solvent in a current of air. Dry to constant mass at 100-105 °C. Allow to cool in a desiccator and weigh (*a* g).

$$\text{Unsaponifiable matter} = \frac{100a}{m} \text{ per cent}$$

Dissolve the residue in 20 ml of *alcohol R*, previously neutralised to *phenolphthalein solution R* and titrate with *0.1 M ethanolic sodium hydroxide*. If the volume of *0.1 M ethanolic sodium hydroxide* used is greater than 0.2 ml, the separation of the layers has been incomplete; the residue weighed cannot be considered as "unsaponifiable matter". In case of doubt, the test must be repeated.

01/2005:20508

2.5.8. DETERMINATION OF PRIMARY AROMATIC AMINO-NITROGEN

Dissolve the prescribed quantity of the substance to be examined in 50 ml of *dilute hydrochloric acid R* or in another prescribed solvent and add 3 g of *potassium bromide R*. Cool in ice-water and titrate by slowly adding *0.1 M sodium nitrite* with constant stirring.

Determine the end-point electrometrically or by the use of the prescribed indicator.

01/2005:20509

2.5.9. DETERMINATION OF NITROGEN BY SULPHURIC ACID DIGESTION

SEMI-MICRO METHOD

Place a quantity of the substance to be examined (*m* g) containing about 2 mg of nitrogen in a combustion flask, add 4 g of a powdered mixture of 100 g of *dipotassium sulphate R*, 5 g of *copper sulphate R* and 2.5 g of *selenium R*, and three glass beads. Wash any adhering particles from the neck into the flask with 5 ml of *sulphuric acid R*, allowing it to run down the sides of the flask, and mix the contents by rotation. Close the mouth of the flask loosely, for example by means of a glass bulb with a short stem, to avoid excessive loss of sulphuric acid. Heat gradually at first, then increase the temperature until there is vigorous boiling with condensation of sulphuric acid in the neck of the flask; precautions should be taken to prevent the upper part of the flask from becoming overheated. Continue the heating for 30 min, unless otherwise prescribed. Cool, dissolve the solid material by cautiously adding to the mixture 25 ml of *water R*, cool again and place in a steam-distillation apparatus. Add 30 ml of *strong sodium hydroxide solution R* and distil immediately by passing steam through the mixture. Collect about 40 ml of distillate in 20.0 ml of *0.01 M hydrochloric acid* and enough *water R* to cover the tip of the condenser. Towards the end of the distillation, lower the receiver so that the tip of the condenser is above the surface of the acid. Take precautions to prevent any water on the outer surface of the condenser from reaching the contents of the receiver. Titrate the distillate with *0.01 M sodium hydroxide*, using *methyl red mixed solution R* as indicator (n_1 ml of *0.01 M sodium hydroxide*).

Repeat the test using about 50 mg of *glucose R* in place of the substance to be examined (n_2 ml of *0.01 M sodium hydroxide*).

$$\text{Content of nitrogen} = \frac{0.01401\,(n_2 - n_1)}{m}\ \text{per cent}$$

01/2005:20510

2.5.10. OXYGEN-FLASK METHOD

Unless otherwise prescribed the combustion flask is a conical flask of at least 500 ml capacity of borosilicate glass with a ground-glass stopper fitted with a suitable carrier for the sample, for example in platinum or platinum-iridium. Finely grind the substance to be examined, place the prescribed quantity in the centre of a piece of filter paper measuring about 30 mm by 40 mm provided with a small strip about 10 mm wide and 30 mm long. If paper impregnated with lithium carbonate is prescribed, moisten the centre of the paper with a saturated solution of *lithium carbonate R* and dry in an oven before use. Envelop the substance to be examined in the paper and place it in the sample carrier. Introduce into the flask *water R* or the prescribed solution designed to absorb the combustion products, displace the air with oxygen by means of a tube having its end just above the liquid, moisten the neck of the flask with *water R* and close with its stopper. Ignite the paper strip by suitable means with the usual precautions. Keep the flask firmly closed during the combustion. Shake the flask vigorously to completely dissolve the combustion products. Cool and after about 5 min, unless otherwise prescribed, carefully unstopper the flask. Wash the ground parts and the walls of the flask, as well as the sample carrier, with *water R*. Combine the combustion products and the washings and proceed as prescribed in the monograph.

01/2005:20511

2.5.11. COMPLEXOMETRIC TITRATIONS

ALUMINIUM

Introduce 20.0 ml of the prescribed solution into a 500 ml conical flask, add 25.0 ml of *0.1 M sodium edetate* and 10 ml of a mixture of equal volumes of a 155 g/l solution of *ammonium acetate R* and *dilute acetic acid R*. Boil for 2 min, then cool. Add 50 ml of *ethanol R* and 3 ml of a freshly prepared 0.25 g/l solution of *dithizone R* in *ethanol R*. Titrate the excess of sodium edetate with *0.1 M zinc sulphate* until the colour changes from greenish-blue to reddish-violet.

1 ml of *0.1 M sodium edetate* is equivalent to 2.698 mg of Al.

BISMUTH

Introduce the prescribed solution into a 500 ml conical flask. Dilute to 250 ml with *water R* and then, unless otherwise prescribed, add dropwise, with shaking, *concentrated ammonia R* until the mixture becomes cloudy. Add 0.5 ml of *nitric acid R*. Heat to about 70 °C until the cloudiness disappears completely. Add about 50 mg of *xylenol orange triturate R* and titrate with *0.1 M sodium edetate* until the colour changes from pinkish-violet to yellow.

1 ml of *0.1 M sodium edetate* is equivalent to 20.90 mg of Bi.

CALCIUM

Introduce the prescribed solution into a 500 ml conical flask, and dilute to 300 ml with *water R*. Add 6.0 ml of *strong sodium hydroxide solution R* and about 15 mg of *calconecarboxylic acid triturate R*. Titrate with *0.1 M sodium edetate* until the colour changes from violet to full blue.

1 ml of *0.1 M sodium edetate* is equivalent to 4.008 mg of Ca.

MAGNESIUM

Introduce the prescribed solution into a 500 ml conical flask and dilute to 300 ml with *water R*. Add 10 ml of *ammonium chloride buffer solution pH 10.0 R* and about 50 mg of *mordant black 11 triturate R*. Heat to about 40 °C then titrate at this temperature with *0.1 M sodium edetate* until the colour changes from violet to full blue.

1 ml of *0.1 M sodium edetate* is equivalent to 2.431 mg of Mg.

LEAD

Introduce the prescribed solution into a 500 ml conical flask and dilute to 200 ml with *water R*. Add about 50 mg of *xylenol orange triturate R* and *hexamethylenetetramine R* until the solution becomes violet-pink. Titrate with *0.1 M sodium edetate* until the violet-pink colour changes to yellow.

1 ml of *0.1 M sodium edetate* is equivalent to 20.72 mg of Pb.

ZINC

Introduce the prescribed solution into a 500 ml conical flask and dilute to 200 ml with *water R*. Add about 50 mg of *xylenol orange triturate R* and *hexamethylenetetramine R* until the solution becomes violet-pink. Add 2 g of *hexamethylenetetramine R* in excess. Titrate with *0.1 M sodium edetate* until the violet-pink colour changes to yellow.

1 ml of *0.1 M sodium edetate* is equivalent to 6.54 mg of Zn.

01/2005:20512

2.5.12. WATER: SEMI-MICRO DETERMINATION

The titration vessel, of about 60 ml capacity, is fitted with 2 platinum electrodes, a nitrogen inlet tube, a stopper which accommodates the burette tip, and a vent-tube protected by a desiccant. The substance to be examined is introduced through a side-arm which can be closed by a ground stopper. Stirring is effected magnetically or by means of a stream of dried nitrogen passed through the solution during the titration.

The end-point is determined by amperometry. A suitable circuit consists of a potentiometer of about 2000 Ω connected across a 1.5 V battery to supply a variable potential. This potential is adjusted so that an initial low current passes through the platinum electrodes connected in series with a microammeter. On adding the reagent, the needle of the microammeter shows a deflection but returns immediately to its starting position. At the end of the reaction, a deflection is obtained which persists for not less than 30 s.

Use the *iodosulphurous reagent R* after determination of the water equivalent (*4.1.1*). The reagents and solutions used must be kept anhydrous and precautions must be taken throughout to prevent exposure to atmospheric moisture.

The *iodosulphurous reagent R* is protected from light, preferably stored in a bottle to which is fitted an automatic burette.

The composition of commercially available iodosulphurous reagents often differs from that of iodosulphurous reagent R by the replacement of pyridine with various other basic compounds. The use of these reagents must previously be validated, in order to verify, in each individual case, the stoichiometry and the absence of incompatibility between the substance under test and the reagent (1.1. General Notices).

Unless otherwise prescribed, use Method A.

Method A. Add about 20 ml of *anhydrous methanol R* or the solvent prescribed in the monograph to the titration vessel and titrate to the amperometric end-point with the *iodosulphurous reagent R*. Quickly transfer the prescribed amount of the substance to be examined to the titration vessel. Stir for 1 min and titrate again to the amperometric end-point using *iodosulphurous reagent R*.

Method B. Add about 10 ml of *anhydrous methanol R* or the solvent prescribed in the monograph to the titration vessel and titrate to the amperometric end-point with *iodosulphurous reagent R*. Quickly transfer the prescribed amount of the substance to be examined in a suitable state of division followed by an accurately measured volume of *iodosulphurous reagent R*, sufficient to give an excess of about 1 ml or the volume prescribed in the monograph. Allow the stoppered flask to stand protected from light for 1 min or the time prescribed in the monograph, stirring from time to time. Titrate the excess of *iodosulphurous reagent R* until the initial low current is again obtained, using *anhydrous methanol R* or the solvent prescribed in the monograph, to which has been added an accurately known amount of *water R* equivalent to about 2.5 g/l.

01/2005:20513

2.5.13. ALUMINIUM IN ADSORBED VACCINES

Homogenise the preparation to be examined and transfer a suitable quantity, presumed to contain 5 mg to 6 mg of aluminium, to a 50 ml combustion flask. Add 1 ml of *sulphuric acid R*, 0.1 ml of *nitric acid R* and some glass beads. Heat the solution until thick, white fumes are evolved. If there is charring at this stage add a few more drops of *nitric acid R* and continue boiling until the colour disappears. Allow to cool for a few minutes, carefully add 10 ml of *water R* and boil until a clear solution is obtained. Allow to cool, add 0.05 ml of *methyl orange solution R* and neutralise with *strong sodium hydroxide solution R* (6.5 ml to 7 ml). If a precipitate forms dissolve it by adding, dropwise, sufficient *dilute sulphuric acid R*. Transfer the solution to a 250 ml conical flask, rinsing the combustion flask with 25 ml of *water R*. Add 25.0 ml of *0.02 M sodium edetate*, 10 ml of *acetate buffer solution pH 4.4 R* and a few glass beads and boil gently for 3 min. Add 0.1 ml of *pyridylazonaphthol solution R* and titrate the hot solution with *0.02 M copper sulphate* until the colour changes to purplish-brown. Carry out a blank titration omitting the vaccine.

1 ml of *0.02 M sodium edetate* is equivalent to 0.5396 mg of Al.

01/2005:20514

2.5.14. CALCIUM IN ADSORBED VACCINES

All solutions used for this test must be prepared using water R.

Determine the calcium by atomic emission spectrometry (*2.2.22, Method I*). Homogenise the preparation to be examined. To 1.0 ml add 0.2 ml of *dilute hydrochloric acid R* and dilute to 3.0 ml with *water R*. Measure the absorbance at 620 nm.

01/2005:20515

2.5.15. PHENOL IN IMMUNOSERA AND VACCINES

Homogenise the preparation to be examined. Dilute an appropriate volume with *water R* so as to obtain a solution presumed to contain 15 µg of phenol per millilitre. Prepare a series of reference solutions with *phenol R* containing 5 µg, 10 µg, 15 µg, 20 µg and 30 µg of phenol per millilitre respectively. To 5 ml of the solution to be examined and to 5 ml of each of the reference solutions respectively, add 5 ml of *buffer solution pH 9.0 R*, 5 ml of *aminopyrazolone solution R* and 5 ml of *potassium ferricyanide solution R*. Allow to stand for 10 min and measure the intensity of colour at 546 nm.

Plot the calibration curve and calculate the phenol content of the preparation to be examined.

01/2005:20516

2.5.16. PROTEIN IN POLYSACCHARIDE VACCINES

Test solution. Use a volumetric flask with a suitable volume for preparation of a solution containing about 5 mg per millilitre of dry polysaccharide. Transfer the contents of a container quantitatively to the flask and dilute to volume with *water R*. Place 1 ml of the solution in a glass tube and add 0.15 ml of a 400 g/l solution of *trichloroacetic acid R*. Shake, allow to stand for 15 min, centrifuge for 10 min at 5000 r/min and discard the supernatant. Add 0.4 ml of *0.1 M sodium hydroxide* to the centrifugation residue.

Reference solutions. Dissolve 0.100 g of *bovine albumin R* in 100 ml of *0.1 M sodium hydroxide* (stock solution containing 1 g of protein per litre). Dilute 1 ml of the stock solution to 20 ml with *0.1 M sodium hydroxide* (working dilution 1: 50 mg of protein per litre). Dilute 1 ml of the stock solution to 4 ml with *0.1 M sodium hydroxide* (working dilution 2: 250 mg of protein per litre). Place in 6 glass tubes 0.10 ml, 0.20 ml and 0.40 ml of working dilution 1 and 0.15 ml, 0.20 ml and 0.25 ml of working dilution 2. Make up the volume in each tube to 0.40 ml using *0.1 M sodium hydroxide*.

Prepare a blank using 0.40 ml of *0.1 M sodium hydroxide*.

Add 2 ml of *cupri-tartaric solution R3* to each tube, shake and allow to stand for 10 min. Add to each tube 0.2 ml of a mixture of equal volumes of *phosphomolybdotungstic reagent R* and *water R*, prepared immediately before use. Stopper the tubes, mix by inverting and allow to stand in the dark for 30 min. The blue colour is stable for 60 min. If necessary, centrifuge to obtain clear solutions.

Measure the absorbance (*2.2.25*) of each solution at 760 nm using the blank as the compensation liquid. Draw a calibration curve from the absorbances of the 6 reference solutions and the corresponding protein contents and read from the curve the content of protein in the test solution.

01/2005:20517

2.5.17. NUCLEIC ACIDS IN POLYSACCHARIDE VACCINES

Test solution. Use a volumetric flask with a suitable volume for preparation of a solution containing about 5 mg per millilitre of dry polysaccharide. Transfer the contents of a container quantitatively to the flask and dilute to volume with *water R*.

Dilute the test solution if necessary to obtain an absorbance value suitable for the instrument used. Measure the absorbance (*2.2.25*) at 260 nm using *water R* as the compensation liquid.

The absorbance of a 1 g/l solution of nucleic acid at 260 nm is 20.

01/2005:20518

2.5.18. PHOSPHORUS IN POLYSACCHARIDE VACCINES

Test solution. Use a volumetric flask with a suitable volume for preparation of a solution containing about 5 mg per millilitre of dry polysaccharide. Transfer the contents of a container quantitatively to the flask and dilute to volume with *water R*. Dilute the solution so that the volume used in the test (1 ml) contains about 6 µg of phosphorus. Transfer 1.0 ml of the solution to a 10 ml ignition tube.

Reference solutions. Dissolve 0.2194 g of *potassium dihydrogen phosphate R* in 500 ml of *water R* to give a solution containing the equivalent of 0.1 mg of phosphorus per millilitre. Dilute 5.0 ml of the solution to 100.0 ml with *water R*. Introduce 0.5 ml, 1.0 ml and 2.0 ml of the dilute solution into 3 ignition tubes.

Prepare a blank solution using 2.0 ml of *water R* in an ignition tube.

To all the tubes add 0.2 ml of *sulphuric acid R* and heat in an oil bath at 120 °C for 1 h and then at 160 °C until white fumes appear (about 1 h). Add 0.1 ml of *perchloric acid R* and heat at 160 °C until the solution is decolorised (about 90 min). Cool and add to each tube 4 ml of *water R* and 4 ml of *ammonium molybdate reagent R*. Heat in a water-bath at 37 °C for 90 min and cool. Adjust the volume to 10.0 ml with *water R*. The blue colour is stable for several hours.

Measure the absorbance (*2.2.25*) of each solution at 820 nm using the blank solution as the compensation liquid. Draw a calibration curve with the absorbances of the 3 reference solutions as a function of the quantity of phosphorus in the solutions and read from the curve the quantity of phosphorus in the test solution.

01/2005:20519

2.5.19. *O*-ACETYL IN POLYSACCHARIDE VACCINES

Test solution. Use a volumetric flask with a suitable volume for preparation of a solution containing about 5 mg per millilitre of dry polysaccharide. Transfer the contents of a container quantitatively to the flask and dilute to volume with *water R*. Dilute the solution so that the volumes used in the test contain 30 µg to 600 µg of acetylcholine chloride (*O*-acetyl). Introduce 0.3 ml, 0.5 ml and 1.0 ml in duplicate into 6 tubes (3 reaction solutions and 3 correction solutions).

Reference solutions. Dissolve 0.150 g of *acetylcholine chloride R* in 10 ml of *water R* (stock solution containing 15 g of acetylcholine chloride per litre). Immediately before use, dilute 1 ml of the stock solution to 50 ml with *water R* (working dilution 1: 300 µg of acetylcholine chloride per millilitre). Immediately before use, dilute 1 ml of the stock solution to 25 ml with *water R* (working dilution 2: 600 µg of acetylcholine chloride per millilitre). Introduce 0.1 ml and 0.4 ml of working dilution 1 in duplicate (reaction and correction solutions) in 4 tubes and 0.6 ml and 1.0 ml of working dilution 2 in duplicate (reaction and correction solutions) in another 4 tubes.

Prepare a blank using 1 ml of *water R*.

Make up the volume in each tube to 1 ml with *water R*. Add 1.0 ml of *4 M hydrochloric acid* to each of the correction tubes and to the blank. Add 2.0 ml of *alkaline hydroxylamine solution R* to each tube. Allow the reaction to proceed for exactly 2 min and add 1.0 ml of *4 M hydrochloric acid* to each of the reaction tubes. Add 1.0 ml of a 100 g/l solution of *ferric chloride R* in *0.1 M hydrochloric acid* to each tube, stopper the tubes and shake vigorously to remove bubbles.

Measure the absorbance (*2.2.25*) of each solution at 540 nm using the blank as the compensation liquid. For each reaction solution, subtract the absorbance of the corresponding correction solution. Draw a calibration curve from the corrected absorbances for the 4 reference solutions and the corresponding content of acetylcholine chloride and read from the curve the content of acetylcholine chloride in the test solution for each volume tested. Calculate the mean of the 3 values.

1 mole of acetylcholine chloride (181.7 g) is equivalent to 1 mole of *O*-acetyl (43.05 g).

01/2005:20520

2.5.20. HEXOSAMINES IN POLYSACCHARIDE VACCINES

Test solution. Use a volumetric flask with a suitable volume for preparation of a solution containing about 5 mg per millilitre of dry polysaccharide. Transfer the contents of a container quantitatively to the flask and dilute to volume with *water R*. Dilute the solution so that the volumes used in the test contain 125 µg to 500 µg of glucosamine (hexosamine). Introduce 1.0 ml of the diluted solution into a graduated tube.

Reference solutions. Dissolve 60 mg of *glucosamine hydrochloride R* in 100 ml of *water R* (stock solution containing 0.500 g of glucosamine per litre). Introduce 0.25 ml, 0.50 ml, 0.75 ml, and 1.0 ml of the working dilution into 4 graduated tubes.

Prepare a blank using 1 ml of *water R*.

Make up the volume in each tube to 1 ml with *water R*. Add 1 ml of a solution of *hydrochloric acid R* (292 g/l) to each tube. Stopper the tubes and place in a water-bath for 1 h. Cool to room temperature. Add to each tube 0.05 ml of a 5 g/l solution of *thymolphthalein R* in *alcohol R*; add a solution of *sodium hydroxide R* (200 g/l) until a blue colour is obtained and then *1 M hydrochloric acid* until the solution is colourless. Dilute the volume in each tube to 10 ml with *water R* (neutralised hydrolysates).

In a second series of 10 ml graduated tubes, place 1 ml of each neutralised hydrolysate. Add 1 ml of acetylacetone reagent (a mixture, prepared immediately before use, of 1 volume of *acetylacetone R* and 50 volumes of a 53 g/l solution of *anhydrous sodium carbonate R*) to each tube. Stopper the tubes and place in a water-bath at 90 °C for 45 min. Cool to room temperature. Add to each tube 2.5 ml of *alcohol R* and 1.0 ml of dimethylaminobenzaldehyde solution (immediately before use dissolve 0.8 g of *dimethylaminobenzaldehyde R* in 15 ml of *alcohol R* and add 15 ml of *hydrochloric acid R*) and dilute the volume in each tube to 10 ml with *alcohol R*. Stopper the tubes, mix by inverting and allow to stand in the dark for 90 min. Measure the absorbance (*2.2.25*) of each solution at 530 nm using the blank as the compensation liquid.

Draw a calibration curve from the absorbances for the 4 reference solutions and the corresponding content of hexosamine and read from the curve the quantity of hexosamine in the test solution.

01/2005:20521

2.5.21. METHYLPENTOSES IN POLYSACCHARIDE VACCINES

Test solution. Use a volumetric flask with a suitable volume for preparation of a solution containing about 5 mg per millilitre of dry polysaccharide. Transfer the contents of a container quantitatively to the flask and dilute to volume with *water R*. Dilute the solution so that the volumes used in the test contain 2 μg to 20 μg of rhamnose (methylpentoses). Introduce 0.25 ml, 0.50 ml and 1.0 ml of the diluted solution into 3 tubes.

Reference solutions. Dissolve 0.100 g of *rhamnose R* in 100 ml of *water R* (stock solution containing 1 g of methylpentose per litre). Immediately before use, dilute 1 ml of the stock solution to 50 ml with *water R* (working dilution: 20 mg of methylpentose per litre). Introduce 0.10 ml, 0.25 ml, 0.50 ml, 0.75 ml and 1.0 ml of the working dilution into 5 tubes.

Prepare a blank using 1 ml of *water R*.

Make up the volume in each tube to 1 ml with *water R*. Place the tubes in iced water and add dropwise and with continuous stirring to each tube 4.5 ml of a cooled mixture of 1 volume of *water R* and 6 volumes of *sulphuric acid R*. Warm the tubes to room temperature and place in a water-bath for a few minutes. Cool to room temperature. Add to each tube 0.10 ml of a 30 g/l solution of *cysteine hydrochloride R*, prepared immediately before use. Shake and allow to stand for 2 h.

Measure the absorbance (*2.2.25*) of each solution at 396 nm and at 430 nm using the blank as compensation liquid. For each solution, calculate the difference between the absorbance measured at 396 nm and that measured at 430 nm. Draw a calibration curve from the absorbance differences for the 5 reference solutions and the corresponding content of methylpentose and read from the curve the quantity of methylpentose in the test solution for each volume tested. Calculate the mean of the 3 values.

01/2005:20522

2.5.22. URONIC ACIDS IN POLYSACCHARIDE VACCINES

Test solution. Use a volumetric flask with a suitable volume for preparation of a solution containing about 5 mg per millilitre of dry polysaccharide. Transfer the contents of a container quantitatively to the flask and dilute to volume with *water R*. Dilute the solution so that the volumes used in the test contain 4 μg to 40 μg of glucuronic acid (uronic acids). Introduce 0.25 ml, 0.50 ml and 1.0 ml of the diluted solution into 3 tubes.

Reference solutions. Dissolve 50 mg of *sodium glucuronate R* in 100 ml of *water R* (stock solution containing 0.4 g of glucuronic acid per litre). Immediately before use, dilute 5 ml of the stock solution to 50 ml with *water R* (working dilution: 40 mg of glucuronic acid per litre). Introduce 0.10 ml, 0.25 ml, 0.50 ml, 0.75 ml, and 1.0 ml of the working dilution into 5 tubes.

Prepare a blank using 1 ml of *water R*.

Make up the volume in each tube to 1 ml with *water R*. Place the tubes in iced water and add dropwise and with continuous stirring to each tube 5.0 ml of *borate solution R*. Stopper the tubes and place in a water-bath for 15 min. Cool to room temperature. Add 0.20 ml of a 1.25 g/l solution of *carbazole R* in *ethanol R* to each tube. Stopper the tubes and place in a water-bath for 15 min. Cool to room temperature. Measure the absorbance (*2.2.25*) of each solution at 530 nm using the blank as the compensation liquid.

Draw a calibration curve from the absorbances for the 5 reference solutions and the corresponding content of glucuronic acid and read from the curve the quantity of glucuronic acid in the test solution for each volume tested. Calculate the mean of the 3 values.

01/2005:20523

2.5.23. SIALIC ACID IN POLYSACCHARIDE VACCINES

Test solution. Transfer quantitatively the contents of one or several containers to a volumetric flask of a suitable volume that will give a solution with a known concentration of about 250 μg per millilitre of polysaccharide and dilute to volume with *water R*. Using a syringe, transfer 4.0 ml of this solution to a 10 ml ultrafiltration cell suitable for the passage of molecules of relative molecular mass less than 50 000. Rinse the syringe twice with *water R* and transfer the rinsings to the ultrafiltration cell. Carry out the ultrafiltration, with constant stirring, under *nitrogen R* at a pressure of about 150 kPa. Refill the cell with *water R* each time the volume of liquid in it has decreased to 1 ml and continue until 200 ml has been filtered and the remaining volume in the cell is about 2 ml. Using a syringe, transfer this residual liquid to a 10 ml volumetric flask. Wash the cell with 3 quantities, each of 2 ml, of *water R*, transfer the washings to the flask and dilute to 10.0 ml with *water R* (test solution). In each of 2 test-tubes place 2.0 ml of the test solution.

Reference solutions. Use the reference solutions prescribed in the monograph.

Prepare 2 series of 3 test-tubes, place in the tubes of each series 0.5 ml, 1.0 ml and 1.5 ml respectively, of the reference solution corresponding to the type of vaccine to be examined and adjust the volume in each tube to 2.0 ml with *water R*.

Prepare blank solutions using 2.0 ml of *water R* in each of 2 test-tubes.

To all the tubes add 5.0 ml of *resorcinol reagent R*. Heat at 105 °C for 15 min, cool in cold water and transfer the tubes to a bath of iced water. To each tube add 5 ml of *isoamyl alcohol R* and mix thoroughly. Place in the bath of iced water for 15 min. Centrifuge the tubes and keep them in the bath of iced water until the examination by absorption spectrophotometry. Measure the absorbance (*2.2.25*) of each supernatant solution at 580 nm and 450 nm using *isoamyl*

2. Methods of analysis

2. Methods of analysis

alcohol R as the compensation liquid. For each wavelength, calculate the absorbance as the mean of the values obtained with 2 identical solutions. Subtract the mean value for the blank solution from the mean values obtained for the other solutions.

Draw a graph showing the difference between the absorbances at 580 nm and 450 nm of the reference solutions as a function of the content of *N*-acetylneuraminic acid and read from the graph the quantity of *N*-acetylneuraminic acid (sialic acid) in the test solution.

01/2005:20524

2.5.24. CARBON DIOXIDE IN GASES

Carbon dioxide in gases is determined using an infrared analyser (see Figure 2.5.24.-1).

The infrared analyser comprises 2 generators of identical infrared beams. The generators are equipped with reflectors and coils electrically heated to low red heat. One beam crosses a sample cell and the other beam crosses a reference cell. The sample cell receives a stream of the gas to be analysed and the reference cell contains *nitrogen R1*. The 2 chambers of the detector are filled with *carbon dioxide R1* and the radiation is automatically received selectively. The absorption of this radiation produces heat and differential expansion of the gas in the 2 chambers, owing to absorption of some of the emitted radiation by the carbon dioxide in the gas to be examined. The pressure difference between the 2 chambers of the detector causes distension of the metal diaphragm that separates them. This diaphragm is part of a capacitor, whose capacitance varies with the pressure difference, which itself depends on the carbon dioxide content in the gas to be examined. Since the infrared beams are periodically blocked by a rotating chopper, the electric signal is frequency modulated.

01/2005:20525

2.5.25. CARBON MONOXIDE IN GASES

METHOD I

Apparatus. The apparatus (see Figure 2.5.25.-1) consists of the following parts connected in series:

- a U-tube (U_1) containing *anhydrous silica gel R* impregnated with *chromium trioxide R*,
- a wash bottle (F_1) containing 100 ml of a 400 g/l solution of *potassium hydroxide R*,
- a U-tube (U_2) containing pellets of *potassium hydroxide R*,
- a U-tube (U_3) containing *diphosphorus pentoxide R* dispersed on previously granulated, fused pumice,
- a U-tube (U_4) containing 30 g of *recrystallised iodine pentoxide R* in granules, previously dried at 200 °C and kept at a temperature of 120 °C (*T*) during the test. The iodine pentoxide is packed in the tube in 1 cm columns separated by 1 cm columns of glass wool to give an effective length of 5 cm,
- a reaction tube (F_2) containing 2.0 ml of *potassium iodide solution R* and 0.15 ml of *starch solution R*.

Method. Flush the apparatus with 5.0 litres of *argon R* and, if necessary, discharge the blue colour in the iodide solution by adding the smallest necessary quantity of freshly prepared *0.002 M sodium thiosulphate*. Continue flushing until not more than 0.045 ml of *0.002 M sodium thiosulphate* is required after passage of 5.0 litres of *argon R*. Pass the gas to be examined from the cylinder through the apparatus, using the prescribed volume and the flow rate. Flush the last traces of liberated iodine into the reaction tube by passing through the apparatus 1.0 litre of *argon R*. Titrate the liberated iodine with *0.002 M sodium thiosulphate*. Carry out a blank test, using the prescribed volume of *argon R*. The difference between the volumes of *0.002 M sodium thiosulphate* used in the titrations is not greater than the prescribed limit.

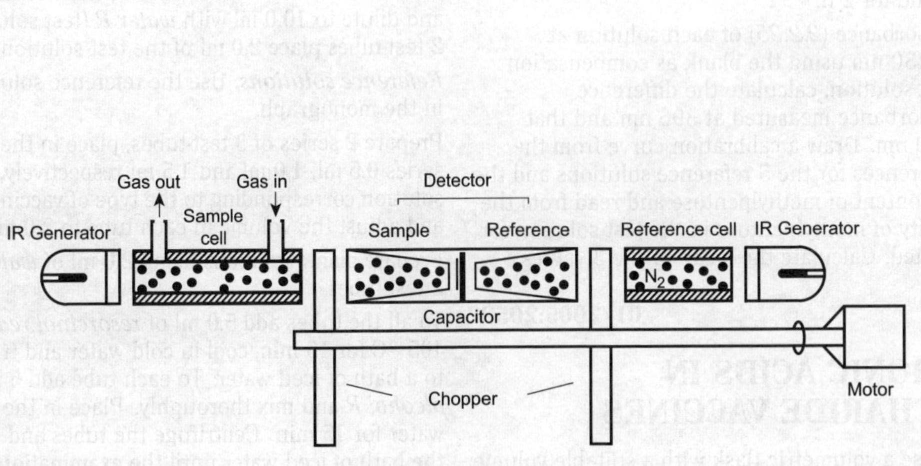

Figure 2.5.24.-1. – *Infrared analyser*

METHOD II

Carbon monoxide in gases may also be determined using an infrared analyser (see Figure 2.5.25.-2).

The infrared analyser comprises 2 generators of identical infrared beams. The generators are equipped with reflectors and coils electrically heated to low red heat. One beam crosses a sample cell and the other beam crosses a reference cell. The sample cell receives a current of the gas to be analysed and the reference cell contains *nitrogen R1*. The 2 chambers of the detector are filled with *carbon monoxide R* and the radiation is automatically received selectively. The absorption of this radiation produces heat and differential expansion of the gas in the two chambers, owing to absorption of some of the emitted radiation by the carbon monoxide in the gas to be examined. The pressure difference between the two chambers of the detector causes distension of the metal diaphragm that separates them. This diaphragm is part of a capacitor, whose capacitance varies with the pressure difference, which itself depends on the carbon monoxide content in the gas to be examined. Since the infrared beams are periodically blocked by a rotating chopper, the electric signal is frequency modulated.

01/2005:20526

2.5.26. NITROGEN MONOXIDE AND NITROGEN DIOXIDE IN GASES

Nitrogen monoxide and nitrogen dioxide in gases are determined using a chemiluminescence analyser (Figure 2.5.26.-1).

The apparatus consists of the following:

- a device for filtering, checking and controlling the flow of the gas to be examined,
- a converter that reduces nitrogen dioxide to nitrogen monoxide, to determine the combined content of nitrogen monoxide and nitrogen dioxide. The efficiency of the converter has to be verified prior to use,
- a controlled-flow-rate ozone generator; the ozone is produced by high-voltage electric discharges across two electrodes; the ozone generator is supplied with pure oxygen or with dehydrated ambient air and the concentration of ozone obtained must greatly exceed the maximum content of any detectable nitrogen oxides,
- a chamber in which nitrogen monoxide and ozone can react,
- a system for detecting light radiation emitted at a wavelength of 1.2 µm, consisting of a selective optical filter and a photomultiplier tube.

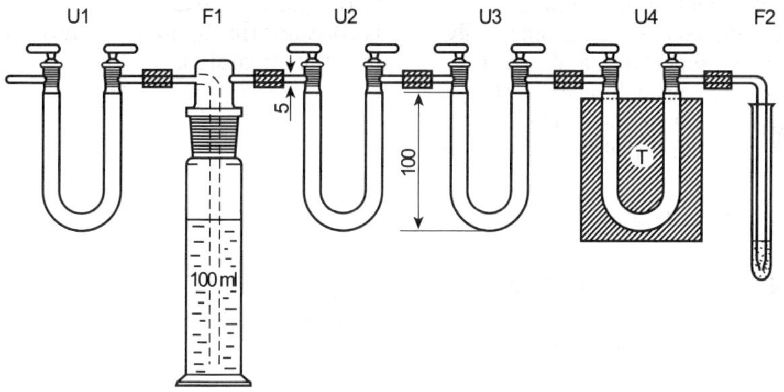

Figure 2.5.25.-1. – *Apparatus for the determination of carbon monoxide*

Dimensions in millimetres

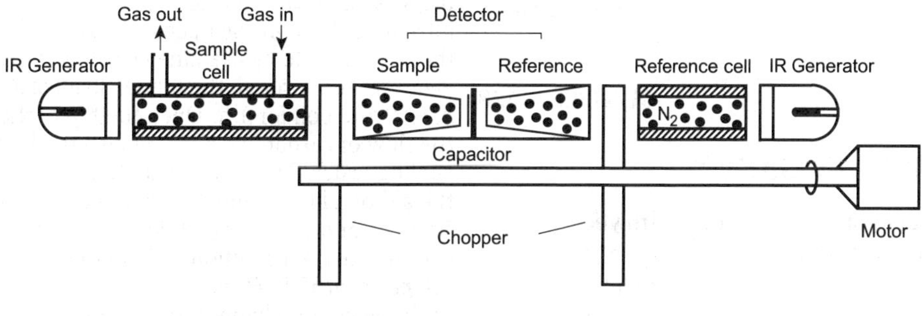

Figure 2.5.25.- 2. – *Infrared analyser*

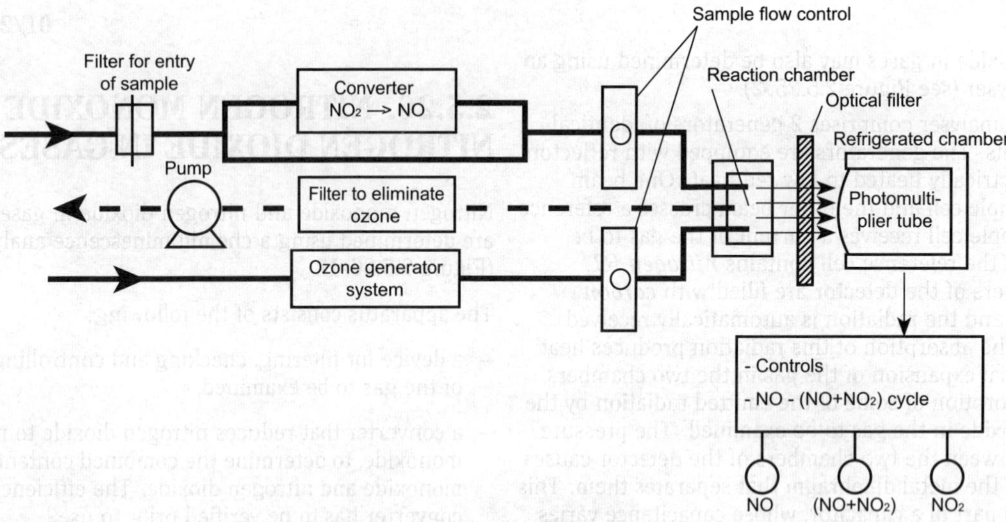

Figure 2.5.26.-1. – *Chemiluminescence analyser*

01/2005:20527

2.5.27. OXYGEN IN GASES

Oxygen in gases is determined using a paramagnetic analyser.

The principle of the method is based on the high paramagnetic sensitivity of the oxygen molecule. Oxygen exerts a strong interaction on magnetic fields, which is measured electronically, amplified and converted to a reading of oxygen concentration. The measurement of oxygen concentration is dependent upon the pressure and temperature and, if the analyser is not automatically compensated for variations in temperature and pressure, it must be calibrated immediately prior to use. As the paramagnetic effect of oxygen is linear the instrument must have a suitable range with a readability of 0.1 per cent or better.

Calibration of the instrument. Make the setting in the following manner:

– set the zero by passing *nitrogen R1* through the instrument at a suitable flow rate until a constant reading is obtained. It should be set to zero according to the manufacturer's instructions;

– set the appropriate limit by passing air (20.9 per cent *V/V* O_2) through the instrument at a suitable flow rate until a constant reading is obtained. The limit should be set to 20.9 per cent *V/V* in accordance with the manufacturer's instructions.

Assay. Pass the gas to be examined through the instrument at a constant flow rate until a suitable reading is obtained.

01/2005:20528

2.5.28. WATER IN GASES

Water in gases is determined using an electrolytic hygrometer, described below.

The measuring cell consists of a thin film of diphosphorus pentoxide, between 2 coiled platinum wires which act as electrodes. The water vapour in the gas to be examined is absorbed by the diphosphorus pentoxide, which is transformed to phosphoric acid, an electrical conductor. A continuous voltage applied across the electrodes produces electrolysis of the water and the regeneration of the diphosphorus pentoxide. The resulting electric current, which is proportional to the water content in the gas to be examined, is measured. This system is self-calibrating since it obeys Faraday's law.

Take a sample of the gas to be examined. Allow the gas to stabilise at room temperature. Purge the cell continuously until a stable reading is obtained. Measure the water content in the gas to be examined, making sure that the temperature is constant throughout the device used to introduce the gas into the apparatus.

01/2005:20529

2.5.29. SULPHUR DIOXIDE

Introduce 150 ml of *water R* into the flask (*A*) (see Figure 2.5.29.-1) and pass *carbon dioxide R* through the whole system for 15 min at a rate of 100 ml/min. To 10 ml of *dilute hydrogen peroxide solution R* add 0.15 ml of a 1 g/l solution of *bromophenol blue R* in *alcohol (20 per cent V/V) R*. Add *0.1 M sodium hydroxide* until a violet-blue colour is obtained, without exceeding the end-point. Place the solution in the test-tube (*D*). Without interrupting the stream of carbon dioxide, remove the funnel (*B*) and introduce through the opening into the flask (*A*) 25.0 g of the substance to be examined (*m* g) with the aid of 100 ml of *water R*. Add through the funnel 80 ml of *dilute hydrochloric acid R* and boil for 1 h. Open the tap of the funnel and stop the flow of carbon dioxide and also the heating and the cooling water. Transfer the contents of the test-tube with the aid of a little *water R* to a 200 ml wide-necked, conical flask. Heat on a water-bath for 15 min and allow to cool. Add 0.1 ml of a 1 g/l solution of *bromophenol blue R* in *alcohol (20 per cent V/V) R* and titrate with *0.1 M sodium hydroxide* until the colour changes from yellow to violet-blue (V_1 ml). Carry out a blank titration (V_2 ml).

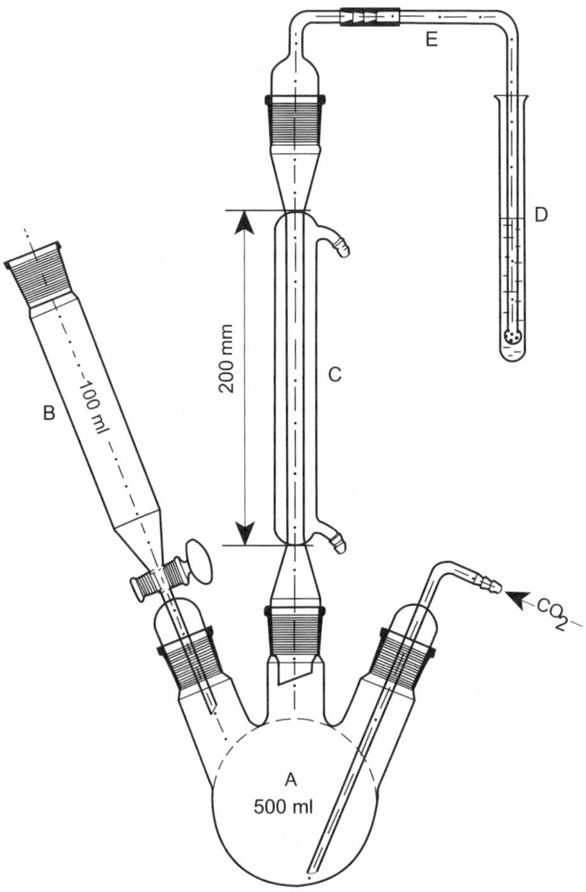

Figure 2.5.29.-1.– *Apparatus for the determination of sulphur dioxide*

Calculate the content of sulphur dioxide in parts per million from the expression:

$$32\,030 \times (V_1 - V_2) \times \frac{n}{m}$$

n = molarity of the sodium hydroxide solution used as titrant.

01/2005:20530

2.5.30. OXIDISING SUBSTANCES

Transfer 4.0 g to a glass-stoppered, 125 ml conical flask and add 50.0 ml of *water R*. Insert the stopper and swirl for 5 min. Transfer to a glass-stoppered 50 ml centrifuge tube and centrifuge. Transfer 30.0 ml of the clear supernatant liquid to a glass-stoppered 125 ml conical flask. Add 1 ml of *glacial acetic acid R* and 0.5 g to 1.0 g of *potassium iodide R*. Insert the stopper, swirl, and allow to stand for 25 min to 30 min in the dark. Add 1 ml of *starch solution R* and titrate with *0.002 M sodium thiosulphate* until the starch-iodine colour disappears. Carry out a blank determination. Not more than 1.4 ml of *0.002 M sodium thiosulphate* is required (0.002 per cent, calculated as H_2O_2).

1 ml of *0.002 M sodium thiosulphate* is equivalent to 34 µg of oxidising substances, calculated as hydrogen peroxide.

01/2005:20531

2.5.31. RIBOSE IN POLYSACCHARIDE VACCINES

Test solution. Use a volumetric flask with a suitable volume for preparation of a solution containing about 5 mg per millilitre of dry polysaccharide. Transfer the contents of a container quantitatively to the flask and dilute to volume with *water R*. Dilute the solution so that the volumes used in the test contain 2.5 µg to 25 µg of ribose. Introduce 0.20 ml and 0.40 ml of the diluted solution into tubes in triplicate.

Reference solutions. Dissolve 25 mg of *ribose R* in *water R* and dilute to 100.0 ml with the same solvent (stock solution containing 0.25 g/l of ribose). Immediately before use, dilute 1 ml of the stock solution to 10.0 ml with *water R* (working dilution: 25 mg/l of ribose). Introduce 0.10 ml, 0.20 ml, 0.40 ml, 0.60 ml, 0.80 ml and 1.0 ml of the working dilution into 6 tubes.

Prepare a blank using 2 ml of *water R*.

Make up the volume in each tube to 2 ml with *water R*. Shake. Add 2 ml of a 0.5 g/l solution of *ferric chloride R* in *hydrochloric acid R* to each tube. Shake. Add 0.2 ml of a 100 g/l solution of *orcinol R* in *ethanol R*. Place the tubes in a water-bath for 20 min. Cool in iced water. Measure the absorbance (*2.2.25*) of each solution at 670 nm using the blank as the compensation liquid. Draw a calibration curve from the absorbance readings for the 6 reference solutions and the corresponding content of ribose and read from the curve the quantity of ribose in the test solution for each volume tested. Calculate the mean of the 3 values.

01/2005:20532

2.5.32. WATER: MICRO DETERMINATION

PRINCIPLE

The coulometric titration of water is based upon the quantitative reaction of water with sulphur dioxide and iodine in an anhydrous medium in the presence of a base with sufficient buffering capacity. In contrast to the volumetric method described under (*2.5.12*), iodine is produced electrochemically in the reaction cell by oxidation of iodide. The iodine produced at the anode reacts immediately with the water and the sulphur dioxide contained in the reaction cell. The amount of water in the substance is directly proportional to the quantity of electricity up until the titration end-point. When all of the water in the cell has been consumed, the end-point is reached and thus an excess of iodine appears. 1 mole of iodine corresponds to 1 mole of water, a quantity of electricity of 10.71 C corresponds to 1 mg of water.

Moisture is eliminated from the system by pre-electrolysis. Individual determinations can be carried out successively in the same reagent solution, under the following conditions:

– each component of the test mixture is compatible with the other components,

– no other reactions take place,

– the volume and the water capacity of the electrolyte reagent are sufficient.

Coulometric titration is restricted to the quantitative determination of small amounts of water, a range of 10 µg up to 10 mg of water is recommended.

Accuracy and precision of the method are predominantly governed by the extent to which atmospheric moisture is excluded from the system. Control of the system must be monitored by measuring the amount of baseline drift.

APPARATUS

The apparatus consists of a reaction cell, electrodes and magnetic stirrer. The reaction cell consists of a large anode compartment and a smaller cathode compartment. Depending on the design of the electrode, both compartments can be separated by a diaphragm. Each compartment contains a platinum electrode. Liquid or solubilised samples are introduced through a septum, using a syringe. Alternatively, an evaporation technique may be used in which the sample is heated in a tube (oven) and the water is evaporated and carried into the cell by means of a stream of dry inert gas. The introduction of solid samples into the cell should in general be avoided. However, if it has to be done it is effected through a sealable port; appropriate precautions must be taken to avoid the introduction of moisture from air, such as working in a glove box in an atmosphere of dry inert gas. The analytical procedure is controlled by a suitable electronic device, which also displays the results.

METHOD

Fill the compartments of the reaction cell with *electrolyte reagent for the micro determination of water R* according to the manufacturer's instructions and perform the coulometric titration to a stable end-point. Introduce the prescribed amount of the substance to be examined into the reaction cell, stir for 30 s, if not otherwise indicated in the monograph, and titrate again to a stable end-point. In case an oven is used, the prescribed sample amount is introduced into the tube and heated. After evaporation of the water from the sample into the titration cell, the titration is started. Read the value from the instrument's output and calculate if necessary the percentage or amount of water that is present in the substance. When appropriate to the type of sample and the sample preparation, perform a blank titration.

VERIFICATION OF THE ACCURACY

Between two successive sample titrations, introduce an accurately weighed amount of water in the same order of magnitude as the amount of water in the sample, either as *water R* or in the form of *standard solution for the micro determination of water R*, and perform the coulometric titration. The recovery rate is within the range from 97.5 per cent to 102.5 per cent for an addition of 1000 µg of H_2O and in the range from 90.0 per cent to 110.0 per cent for the addition of 100 µg of H_2O.

01/2005:20533

2.5.33. TOTAL PROTEIN

Many of the assay methods described in this chapter can be performed using kits from commercial sources.

METHOD 1

Protein in solution absorbs ultraviolet light at a wavelength of 280 nm, due to the presence of aromatic amino acids, mainly tyrosine and tryptophan, in the protein structure. This property can be used for assay purposes. If the buffer used to dissolve the protein has a high absorbance relative to that of water, an interfering substance is present. This interference may be obviated by using the buffer as compensation liquid but if the interfering substance produces a high absorbance, the results may nevertheless be compromised. At low concentrations, protein adsorbed onto the cell may significantly reduce the content in solution. This can be prevented by preparing samples at higher concentration or by using a non-ionic detergent in the preparation.

Test solution. Dissolve a suitable quantity of the substance to be examined in the prescribed buffer to obtain a solution having a protein concentration between 0.2 mg/ml and 2 mg/ml.

Reference solution. Prepare a solution of a suitable reference substance for the protein to be determined, in the same buffer and at the same protein concentration as the test solution.

Procedure. Keep the test solution, the reference solution and the compensation liquid at the same temperature during the performance of this test. Determine the absorbances (*2.2.25*) of the test solution and the reference solution in quartz cells at 280 nm, using the prescribed buffer as the compensation liquid. The response must be linear in the range of protein concentrations to be assayed to obtain accurate results.

Light scattering. The accuracy of the determination of protein can be diminished by the scattering of light by the test sample. If the proteins in solution exist as particles comparable in size to the wavelength of the measuring light (250 nm to 300 nm), scattering of the light beam results in an apparent increase in absorbance of the test sample. To calculate the absorbance at 280 nm due to light scattering, determine the absorbances of the test solution at wavelengths of 320 nm, 325 nm, 330 nm, 335 nm, 340 nm, 345 nm and 350 nm. Plot the logarithm of the observed absorbance against the logarithm of the wavelength and determine the standard curve best fitting the plotted points by linear regression. Extrapolate the curve to determine the logarithm of the absorbance at 280 nm. The antilogarithm of this value is the absorbance attributed to light scattering. Correct the observed values by subtracting the absorbance attributed to light scattering from the total absorbance at 280 nm to obtain the absorbance value of the protein in solution. Filtration with a 0.2 µm filter that does not adsorb protein or clarification by centrifugation may be performed to reduce the effect of light scattering, especially if the solution is noticeably turbid.

Calculations. Use corrected values for the calculations. Calculate the concentration of protein in the test solution (C_U) from the following equation:

$$C_U = C_S \, (A_U / A_S)$$

where C_S is the concentration of protein in the reference solution and A_U and A_S are the corrected absorbances of the test solution and the reference solution, respectively.

METHOD 2

This method (commonly referred to as the Lowry assay) is based on the reduction by protein of the phosphomolybdotungstic mixed acid chromogen in the phosphomolybdotungstic reagent, which results in an absorbance maximum at 750 nm. The phosphomolybdotungstic reagent reacts primarily with tyrosine residues in the protein. Colour development reaches a maximum in 20 min to 30 min at room temperature, after which there is a gradual loss of colour. Because the method is sensitive to interfering substances, a procedure for precipitation of the protein from the test sample may be used. Most interfering substances cause a lower colour yield; however, some detergents cause a slight increase in colour. A high salt concentration may cause a precipitate to form. Because different protein species may give different colour response intensities, the reference substance and test protein must be the same. Where separation of interfering substances from the protein in the test sample is necessary, proceed as directed below for interfering substances prior to preparation of the test solution. The effect of interfering substances may be minimised by dilution, provided the concentration of the test protein remains sufficient for accurate measurement.

Use *distilled water R* to prepare all buffers and reagents used for this method.

Test solution. Dissolve a suitable quantity of the substance to be examined in the prescribed buffer to obtain a solution having a concentration within the range of the standard curve. A suitable buffer will produce a solution of pH 10.0 to 10.5.

Reference solutions. Dissolve the reference substance for the protein to be determined in the prescribed buffer. Dilute portions of this solution with the same buffer to obtain not fewer than five reference solutions having protein concentrations evenly spaced over a suitable range situated between 5 μg/ml and 100 μg/ml.

Blank. Use the buffer used to prepare the test solution and the reference solutions.

Copper sulphate reagent. Dissolve 100 mg of *copper sulphate R* and 0.2 g of *sodium tartrate R* in *distilled water R* and dilute to 50 ml with the same solvent. Dissolve 10 g of *anhydrous sodium carbonate R* in *distilled water R* and dilute to 50 ml with the same solvent. Slowly pour the sodium carbonate solution into the copper sulphate solution with mixing. Use within 24 h.

Alkaline copper reagent. Mix 1 volume of copper sulphate reagent, 2 volumes of a 50 g/l solution of *sodium dodecyl sulphate R* and 1 volume of a 32 g/l solution of *sodium hydroxide R*. Store at room temperature and use within 2 weeks.

Diluted phosphomolybdotungstic reagent. Mix 5 ml of *phosphomolybdotungstic reagent R* with 55 ml of *distilled water R*. Store in an amber bottle, at room temperature.

Procedure. To 1.0 ml of each reference solution, of the test solution and of the blank, add 1.0 ml of alkaline copper reagent and mix. Allow to stand for 10 min. Add 0.5 ml of the diluted phosphomolybdotungstic reagent, mix and allow to stand at room temperature for 30 min. Determine the absorbances (*2.2.25*) of the solutions at 750 nm, using the solution from the blank as compensation liquid.

Calculations. The relationship of absorbance to protein concentration is non-linear; however, if the range of concentrations used to prepare the standard curve is sufficiently small, the latter will approach linearity. Plot the absorbances of the reference solutions against the protein concentrations and use linear regression to establish the standard curve. From the standard curve and the absorbance of the test solution, determine the concentration of protein in the test solution.

Interfering substances. In the following procedure, deoxycholate-trichloroacetic acid is added to a test sample to remove interfering substances by precipitation of proteins before determination; this technique can also be used to concentrate proteins from a dilute solution.

Add 0.1 ml of a 1.5 g/l solution of *sodium deoxycholate R* to 1 ml of a solution of the substance to be examined. Mix using a vortex mixer and allow to stand at room temperature for 10 min. Add 0.1 ml of a 720 g/l solution of *trichloroacetic acid R* and mix using a vortex mixer. Centrifuge at 3000 *g* for 30 min, decant the liquid and remove any residual liquid with a pipette. Redissolve the protein pellet in 1 ml of alkaline copper reagent.

METHOD 3

This method (commonly referred to as the Bradford assay) is based on the absorption shift from 470 nm to 595 nm observed when the acid blue 90 dye binds to protein. The acid blue 90 dye binds most readily to arginine and lysine residues in the protein which can lead to variation in the response of the assay to different proteins. The protein used as reference substance must therefore be the same as the protein to be determined. There are relatively few interfering substances, but it is preferable to avoid detergents and ampholytes in the test sample. Highly alkaline samples may interfere with the acidic reagent.

Use *distilled water R* to prepare all buffers and reagents used for this method.

Test solution. Dissolve a suitable quantity of the substance to be examined in the prescribed buffer to obtain a solution having a concentration within the range of the standard curve.

Reference solutions. Dissolve the reference substance for the protein to be determined in the prescribed buffer. Dilute portions of this solution with the same buffer to obtain not fewer than five reference solutions having protein concentrations evenly spaced over a suitable range situated between 0.1 mg/ml and 1 mg/ml.

Blank. Use the buffer used to prepare the test solution and the reference solutions.

Acid blue 90 reagent. Dissolve 0.10 g of *acid blue 90 R* in 50 ml of *alcohol R*. Add 100 ml of *phosphoric acid R*, dilute to 1000 ml with *distilled water R* and mix. Filter the solution and store in an amber bottle at room temperature. Slow precipitation of the dye occurs during storage. Filter the reagent before using.

Procedure. Add 5 ml of acid blue 90 reagent to 0.100 ml of each reference solution, of the test solution and of the blank. Mix by inversion. Avoid foaming, which will lead to poor reproducibility. Determine the absorbances (*2.2.25*) of the standard solutions and of the test solution at 595 nm, using the blank as compensation liquid. Do not use quartz (silica) spectrophotometer cells because the dye binds to this material.

Calculations. The relationship of absorbance to protein concentration is non-linear; however, if the range of concentrations used to prepare the standard curve is sufficiently small, the latter will approach linearity. Plot the absorbances of the reference solutions against protein concentrations and use linear regression to establish the standard curve. From the standard curve and the absorbance of the test solution, determine the concentration of protein in the test solution.

METHOD 4

This method (commonly referred to as the bicinchoninic acid or BCA assay) is based on reduction of the cupric (Cu^{2+}) ion to cuprous (Cu^{1+}) ion by protein. The bicinchoninic acid reagent is used to detect the cuprous ion. Few substances interfere with the reaction. When interfering substances are present their effect may be minimised by dilution, provided that the concentration of the protein to be determined remains sufficient for accurate measurement. Alternatively, the protein precipitation procedure given in Method 2 may be used to remove interfering substances. Because different protein species may give different colour response intensities, the reference protein and protein to be determined must be the same.

Use *distilled water R* to prepare all buffers and reagents used for this method.

Test solution. Dissolve a suitable quantity of the substance to be examined in the prescribed buffer to obtain a solution having a concentration within the range of the concentrations of the reference solutions.

Reference solutions. Dissolve the reference substance for the protein to be determined in the prescribed buffer. Dilute portions of this solution with the same buffer to obtain not fewer than five reference solutions having protein concentrations evenly spaced over a suitable range situated between 10 µg/ml and 1200 µg/ml.

Blank. Use the buffer used to prepare the test solution and the reference solutions.

BCA reagent. Dissolve 10 g of *disodium bicinchoninate R*, 20 g of *sodium carbonate monohydrate R*, 1.6 g of *sodium tartrate R*, 4 g of *sodium hydroxide R*, and 9.5 g of *sodium hydrogen carbonate R* in *distilled water R*. Adjust, if necessary, to pH 11.25 with a solution of *sodium hydroxide R* or a solution of *sodium hydrogen carbonate R*. Dilute to 1000 ml with *distilled water R* and mix.

Copper-BCA reagent. Mix 1 ml of a 40 g/l solution of *copper sulphate R* and 50 ml of BCA reagent.

Procedure. Mix 0.1 ml of each reference solution, of the test solution and of the blank with 2 ml of the copper-BCA reagent. Incubate the solutions at 37 °C for 30 min, note the time and allow the mixtures to cool to room temperature. Within 60 min of the end of incubation, determine the absorbances (*2.2.29*) of the reference solutions and of the test solution in quartz cells at 562 nm, using the blank as compensation liquid. After the solutions have cooled to room temperature, the colour intensity continues to increase gradually.

Calculations. The relationship of absorbance to protein concentration is non-linear; however, if the range of concentrations used to prepare the standard curve is sufficiently small, the latter will approach linearity. Plot the absorbances of the reference solutions against protein concentrations and use linear regression to establish the standard curve. From the standard curve and the absorbance of the test solution, determine the concentration of protein in the test solution.

METHOD 5

This method (commonly referred to as the biuret assay) is based on the interaction of cupric (Cu^{2+}) ion with protein in alkaline solution and resultant development of absorbance at 545 nm. This test shows minimal difference between equivalent IgG and albumin samples. Addition of the sodium hydroxide and the biuret reagent as a combined reagent, insufficient mixing after the addition of the sodium hydroxide, or an extended time between the addition of the sodium hydroxide solution and the addition of the biuret reagent will give IgG samples a higher response than albumin samples. The trichloroacetic acid method used to minimise the effects of interfering substances also can be used to determine the protein content in test samples at concentrations below 500 µg/ml.

Use *distilled water R* to prepare all buffers and reagents used for this method.

Test solution. Dissolve a suitable quantity of the substance to be examined in a 9 g/l solution of *sodium chloride R* to obtain a solution having a concentration within the range of the concentrations of the reference solutions.

Reference solutions. Dissolve the reference substance for the protein to be determined in a 9 g/l solution of *sodium chloride R*. Dilute portions of this solution with a 9 g/l solution of *sodium chloride R* to obtain not fewer than three reference solutions having protein concentrations evenly spaced over a suitable range situated between 0.5 mg/ml and 10 mg/ml.

Blank. Use a 9 g/l solution of *sodium chloride R*.

Biuret reagent. Dissolve 3.46 g of *copper sulphate R* in 10 ml of hot *distilled water R*, and allow to cool (Solution A). Dissolve 34.6 g of *sodium citrate R* and 20.0 g of *anhydrous sodium carbonate R* in 80 ml of hot *distilled water R*, and allow to cool (Solution B). Mix solutions A and B and dilute to 200 ml with *distilled water R*. Use within 6 months. Do not use the reagent if it develops turbidity or contains any precipitate.

Procedure. To one volume of the test solution add an equal volume of a 60 g/l solution of *sodium hydroxide R* and mix. Immediately add biuret reagent equivalent to 0.4 volumes of the test solution and mix rapidly. Allow to stand at a temperature between 15 °C and 25 °C for not less than 15 min. Within 90 min of addition of the biuret reagent, determine the absorbances (*2.2.29*) of the reference solutions and of the test solution at the maximum at 545 nm, using the blank as compensation liquid. Any solution that develops turbidity or a precipitate is not acceptable for calculation of protein concentration.

Calculations. The relationship of absorbance to protein concentration is approximately linear within the indicated range of protein concentrations for the reference solutions. Plot the absorbances of the reference solutions against protein concentrations and use linear regression to establish the standard curve. Calculate the correlation coefficient for the standard curve. A suitable system is one that yields a line having a correlation coefficient not less than 0.99. From the standard curve and the absorbance of the test solution, determine the concentration of protein in the test solution.

Interfering substances. To minimise the effect of interfering substances, the protein can be precipitated from the test sample as follows: add 0.1 volumes of a 500 g/l solution of *trichloroacetic acid R* to 1 volume of a solution of the test sample, withdraw the supernatant layer and dissolve the precipitate in a small volume of *0.5 M sodium hydroxide*. Use the solution obtained to prepare the test solution.

METHOD 6

This fluorimetric method is based on the derivatisation of the protein with *o*-phthalaldehyde, which reacts with the primary amines of the protein (*N*-terminal amino acid and the ε-amino group of lysine residues). The sensitivity of the assay can be increased by hydrolysing the protein before adding *o*-phthalaldehyde. Hydrolysis makes the α-amino group of the constituent amino acids available for reaction with the phthalaldehyde reagent. The method requires very small quantities of the protein. Primary amines, such as tris(hydroxymethyl)aminomethane and amino acid buffers, react with phthalaldehyde and must be avoided or removed. Ammonia at high concentrations reacts with phthalaldehyde. The fluorescence obtained when amine reacts with phthalaldehyde can be unstable. The use of automated procedures to standardise this procedure may improve the accuracy and precision of the test.

Use *distilled water R* to prepare all buffers and reagents used for this method.

Test solution. Dissolve a suitable quantity of the substance to be examined in a 9 g/l solution of *sodium chloride R* to obtain a solution having a concentration within the range of the concentrations of the reference solutions. Adjust the solution to pH 8 to 10.5 before addition of the phthalaldehyde reagent.

Reference solutions. Dissolve the reference substance for the protein to be determined in a 9 g/l solution of *sodium chloride R*. Dilute portions of this solution with a 9 g/l solution of *sodium chloride R* to obtain not fewer than five reference solutions having protein concentrations evenly spaced over a suitable range situated between 10 µg/ml and 200 µg/ml. Adjust the solutions to pH 8 to 10.5 before addition of the phthalaldehyde reagent.

Blank solution. Use a 9 g/l solution of *sodium chloride R*.

Borate buffer solution. Dissolve 61.83 g of *boric acid R* in *distilled water R* and adjust to pH 10.4 with a solution of *potassium hydroxide R*. Dilute to 1000 ml with *distilled water R* and mix.

Phthalaldehyde stock solution. Dissolve 1.20 g of *phthalaldehyde R* in 1.5 ml of *methanol R*, add 100 ml of borate buffer solution and mix. Add 0.6 ml of a 300 g/l solution of *macrogol 23 lauryl ether R* and mix. Store at room temperature and use within 3 weeks.

Phthalaldehyde reagent. To 5 ml of phthalaldehyde stock solution add 15 µl of *2-mercaptoethanol R*. Prepare at least 30 min before use. Use within 24 h.

Procedure. Mix 10 µl of the test solution and of each of the reference solutions with 0.1 ml of phthalaldehyde reagent and allow to stand at room temperature for 15 min. Add 3 ml of *0.5 M sodium hydroxide* and mix. Determine the fluorescent intensities (*2.2.21*) of solutions from the reference solutions and from the test solution at an excitation wavelength of 340 nm and an emission wavelength between 440 and 455 nm. Measure the fluorescent intensity of a given sample only once, since irradiation decreases the fluorescence intensity.

Calculations. The relationship of fluorescence to protein concentration is linear. Plot the fluorescent intensities of the reference solutions against protein concentrations and use linear regression to establish the standard curve. From the standard curve and the fluorescent intensity of the test solution, determine the concentration of protein in the test solution.

METHOD 7

This method is based on nitrogen analysis as a means of protein determination. Interference caused by the presence of other nitrogen-containing substances in the test sample can affect the determination of protein by this method. Nitrogen analysis techniques destroy the test sample during the analysis but are not limited to protein presentation in an aqueous environment.

Procedure A. Proceed as prescribed for the determination of nitrogen by sulphuric acid digestion (*2.5.9*) or use commercial instrumentation for Kjeldahl nitrogen assay.

Procedure B. Commercial instrumentation is available for nitrogen analysis. Most nitrogen analysis instruments use pyrolysis (i.e. combustion of the sample in oxygen at temperatures approaching 1000 °C), which produces nitric oxide (NO) and other oxides of nitrogen (NO_x) from the nitrogen present in the substance to be examined. Some instruments convert the nitric oxides to nitrogen gas, which is quantified using a thermal-conductivity detector. Other instruments mix nitric oxide (NO) with ozone (O_3) to produce excited nitrogen dioxide (NO_2^*), which emits light when it decays and can be quantified with a chemiluminescence detector. A protein reference material that is relatively pure and is similar in composition to the test proteins is used to optimise the injection and pyrolysis parameters and to evaluate consistency in the analysis.

Calculations. The protein concentration is calculated by dividing the nitrogen content of the sample by the known nitrogen content of the protein. The known nitrogen content of the protein can be determined from the chemical composition of the protein or by comparison with a suitable reference substance.

01/2005:20534
corrected

2.5.34. ACETIC ACID IN SYNTHETIC PEPTIDES

Examine by liquid chromatography (*2.2.29*).

Test solution. Prepare as described in the monograph. The concentration of peptide in the solution may be adapted, depending on the expected amount of acetic acid in the sample.

Reference solution. Prepare a 0.10 g/l solution of *glacial acetic acid R* in a mixture of 5 volumes of mobile phase B and 95 volumes of mobile phase A.

The chromatographic procedure may be carried out using:

– a stainless steel column 0.25 m long and 4.6 mm in internal diameter packed with *octadecylsilyl silica gel for chromatography R* (5 µm),

– as mobile phase at a flow rate of 1.2 ml/min:

Mobile phase A. Dilute 0.7 ml of *phosphoric acid R* to 1000 ml with *water R*; adjust the pH to 3.0 with *strong sodium hydroxide solution R*,

Mobile phase B. *Methanol R2*,

Time (min)	Mobile phase A (per cent *V/V*)	Mobile phase B (per cent *V/V*)
0 - 5	95	5
5 - 10	95 → 50	5 → 50
10 - 20	50	50
20 - 22	50 → 95	50 → 5
22 - 30	95	5

– as detector a spectrophotometer set at 210 nm.

Inject 10 µl of the reference solution and 10 µl of the test solution. In the chromatograms obtained, the peak corresponding to acetic acid has a retention time of 3-4 min. The baseline presents a steep rise after the start of the linear gradient, which corresponds to the elution of the peptide from the column. Determine the content of acetic acid in the peptide.

01/2005:20535

2.5.35. NITROUS OXIDE IN GASES

Nitrous oxide in gases is determined using an infrared analyser (see Figure 2.5.35.-1).

The infrared analyser comprises 2 generators of identical infrared beams. The generators are equipped with reflectors and coils electrically heated to low red heat. One beam crosses a sample cell and the other beam crosses a reference cell. The sample cell receives a stream of the gas to be examined and the reference cell contains *nitrogen R1*. The 2 chambers of the detector are filled with *nitrous oxide R* and the radiation is automatically received selectively. The absorption of this radiation produces heat and differential expansion of the gas in the 2 chambers, owing to absorption of some of the emitted radiation by the nitrous oxide in the gas to be examined. The pressure difference between the

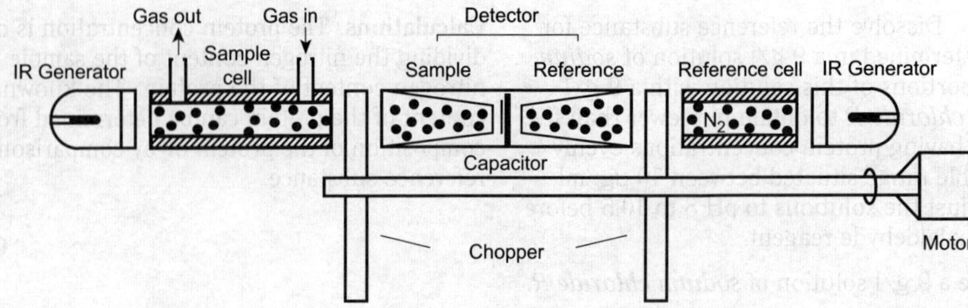

Figure 2.5.35.-1. – *Infrared analyser*

2 chambers of the detector causes distension of the metal diaphragm that separates them. This diaphragm is part of a capacitor, whose capacitance varies with the pressure difference, which itself depends on the nitrous oxide content in the gas to be examined. Since the infrared beams are periodically blocked by a rotating chopper, the electric signal is frequency modulated.

01/2005:20536

2.5.36. ANISIDINE VALUE

The anisidine value is defined as 100 times the optical density measured in a 1 cm cell of a solution containing 1 g of the substance to be examined in 100 ml of a mixture of solvents and reagents according to the following method.

Carry out the operations as rapidly as possible, avoiding exposure to actinic light.

Test solution (a). Dissolve 0.500 g of the substance to be examined in *trimethylpentane R* and dilute to 25.0 ml with the same solvent.

Test solution (b). To 5.0 ml of test solution (a) add 1.0 ml of a 2.5 g/l solution of *p-anisidine R* in *glacial acetic acid R*, shake and store protected from light.

Reference solution. To 5.0 ml of *trimethylpentane R* add 1.0 ml of a 2.5 g/l solution of *p-anisidine R* in *glacial acetic acid R*, shake and store protected from light.

Measure the absorbance (*2.2.25*) of test solution (a) at the maximum at 350 nm using *trimethylpentane R* as the compensation liquid. Measure the absorbance of test solution (b) at 350 nm exactly 10 min after its preparation, using the reference solution as the compensation liquid.

Calculate the anisidine value from the expression:

$$\frac{25 \times (1.2A_1 - A_2)}{m}$$

A_1 = absorbance of test solution (b) at 350 nm,

A_2 = absorbance of test solution (a) at 350 nm,

m = mass of the substance to be examined in test solution (a), in grams.

2.6. BIOLOGICAL TESTS

2.6. BIOLOGICAL TESTS

01/2005:20601

2.6.1. STERILITY

The test is applied to substances, preparations or articles which, according to the Pharmacopoeia, are required to be sterile. However, a satisfactory result only indicates that no contaminating micro-organism has been found in the sample examined in the conditions of the test. Guidance for using the test for sterility is given at the end of this text.

PRECAUTIONS AGAINST MICROBIAL CONTAMINATION

The test for sterility is carried out under aseptic conditions. In order to achieve such conditions, the test environment has to be adapted to the way in which the sterility test is performed. The precautions taken to avoid contamination are such that they do not affect any micro-organisms which are to be revealed in the test. The working conditions in which the tests are performed are monitored regularly by appropriate sampling of the working area and by carrying out appropriate controls (such as those indicated in the appropriate European Community Directives and associated guidance documents on GMP).

CULTURE MEDIA AND INCUBATION TEMPERATURES

Media for the test may be prepared as described below, or equivalent commercial media may be used provided that they comply with the growth promotion test.

The following culture media have been found to be suitable for the test for sterility. Fluid thioglycollate medium is primarily intended for the culture of anaerobic bacteria; however, it will also detect aerobic bacteria. Soya-bean casein digest medium is suitable for the culture of both fungi and aerobic bacteria.

Other media may be used provided that they pass the growth promotion and the validation tests.

Fluid thioglycollate medium

L-Cystine	0.5 g
Agar, granulated (moisture content not in excess of 15 per cent)	0.75 g
Sodium chloride	2.5 g
Glucose monohydrate/anhydrous	5.5 g/5.0 g
Yeast extract (water-soluble)	5.0 g
Pancreatic digest of casein	15.0 g
Sodium thioglycollate or	0.5 g
Thioglycollic acid	0.3 ml
Resazurin sodium solution (1 g/l of resazurin sodium), freshly prepared	1.0 ml
Water R	1000 ml

pH of the medium after sterilisation 7.1 ± 0.2

Mix the L-cystine, agar, sodium chloride, glucose, water-soluble yeast extract and pancreatic digest of casein with the *water R* and heat until solution is effected. Dissolve the sodium thioglycollate or thioglycollic acid in the solution and, if necessary, add *1 M sodium hydroxide* so that, after sterilisation, the solution will have a pH of 7.1 ± 0.2. If filtration is necessary, heat the solution again without boiling and filter while hot through moistened filter paper. Add the resazurin sodium solution, mix and place the medium in suitable vessels which provide a ratio of surface to depth of medium such that not more than the upper half of the medium has undergone a colour change indicative of oxygen uptake at the end of the incubation period. Sterilise using a validated process. If the medium is stored, store at 2-25 °C in a sterile, airtight container. If more than the upper third of the medium has acquired a pink colour, the medium may be restored once by heating the containers in a water-bath or in free-flowing steam until the pink colour disappears and cooling quickly, taking care to prevent the introduction of non-sterile air into the container. Do not use the medium for a longer storage period than has been validated.

Fluid thioglycollate medium is to be incubated at 30-35 °C.

Soya-bean casein digest medium

Pancreatic digest of casein	17.0 g
Papaic digest of soya-bean meal	3.0 g
Sodium chloride	5.0 g
Dipotassium hydrogen phosphate	2.5 g
Glucose monohydrate/anhydrous	2.5 g/2.3 g
Water R	1000 ml

pH of the medium after sterilisation 7.3 ± 0.2

Dissolve the solids in *water R*, warming slightly to effect solution. Cool the solution to room temperature. Add *1 M sodium hydroxide*, if necessary, so that after sterilisation the medium will have a pH of 7.3 ± 0.2. Filter, if necessary, to clarify, distribute into suitable vessels and sterilise using a validated process. Store at 2-25 °C in a sterile well-closed container, unless it is intended for immediate use. Do not use the medium for a longer storage period than has been validated.

Soya-bean casein digest medium is to be incubated at 20-25 °C.

The media used comply with the following tests, carried out before or in parallel with the test on the product to be examined.

Sterility. Incubate portions of the media for 14 days. No growth of micro-organisms occurs.

Growth promotion test of aerobes, anaerobes and fungi. Test each batch of ready-prepared medium and each batch of medium prepared either from dehydrated medium or from the ingredients. Suitable strains of micro-organisms are indicated in Table 2.6.1.-1.

Inoculate portions of fluid thioglycollate medium with a small number (not more than 100 CFU) of the following micro-organisms, using a separate portion of medium for each of the following species of micro-organism: *Clostridium sporogenes, Pseudomonas aeruginosa, Staphylococcus aureus*. Inoculate portions of soya-bean casein digest medium with a small number (not more than 100 CFU) of the following micro-organisms, using a separate portion of medium for each of the following species of micro-organism: *Aspergillus niger, Bacillus subtilis, Candida albicans*. Incubate for not more than 3 days in the case of bacteria and not more than 5 days in the case of fungi.

Seed lot culture maintenance techniques (seed-lot systems) are used so that the viable micro-organisms used for inoculation are not more than 5 passages removed from the original master seed-lot.

The media are suitable if a clearly visible growth of the micro-organisms occurs.

VALIDATION TEST

Carry out a test as described below under Test for sterility of the product to be examined using exactly the same methods except for the following modifications.

Table 2.6.1.-1 – *Strains of the test micro-organisms suitable for use in the Growth Promotion Test and the Validation Test*

Aerobic bacteria	
Staphylococcus aureus	ATCC 6538, CIP 4.83, NCTC 10788, NCIMB 9518
Bacillus subtilis	ATCC 6633, CIP 52.62, NCIMB 8054
Pseudomonas aeruginosa	ATCC 9027, NCIMB 8626, CIP 82.118
Anaerobic bacterium	
Clostridium sporogenes	ATCC 19404, CIP 79.3, NCTC 532 *or* ATCC 11437
Fungi	
Candida albicans	ATCC 10231, IP 48.72, NCPF 3179
Aspergillus niger	ATCC 16404, IP 1431.83, IMI 149007

Membrane filtration. After transferring the contents of the container or containers to be tested to the membrane add an inoculum of a small number of viable micro-organisms (not more than 100 CFU) to the final portion of sterile diluent used to rinse the filter.

Direct inoculation. After transferring the contents of the container or containers to be tested (for catgut and other surgical sutures for veterinary use: strands) to the culture medium add an inoculum of a small number of viable micro-organisms (not more than 100 CFU) to the medium.

In both cases use the same micro-organisms as those described above under Growth promotion test of aerobes, anaerobes and fungi. Perform a growth promotion test as a positive control. Incubate all the containers containing medium for not more than 5 days.

If clearly visible growth of micro-organisms is obtained after the incubation, visually comparable to that in the control vessel without product, either the product possesses no antimicrobial activity under the conditions of the test or such activity has been satisfactorily eliminated. The test for sterility may then be carried out without further modification.

If clearly visible growth is not obtained in the presence of the product to be tested, visually comparable to that in the control vessels without product, the product possesses antimicrobial activity that has not been satisfactorily eliminated under the conditions of the test. Modify the conditions in order to eliminate the antimicrobial activity and repeat the validation test.

This validation is performed:

a) when the test for sterility has to be carried out on a new product,

b) whenever there is a change in the experimental conditions of the test.

The validation may be performed simultaneously with the test for sterility of the product to be examined.

TEST FOR STERILITY OF THE PRODUCT TO BE EXAMINED

The test may be carried out using the technique of membrane filtration or by direct inoculation of the culture media with the product to be examined. Appropriate negative controls are included. The technique of membrane filtration is used whenever the nature of the product permits, that is, for filterable aqueous preparations, for alcoholic or oily preparations and for preparations miscible with or soluble in aqueous or oily solvents provided these solvents do not have an antimicrobial effect in the conditions of the test.

Membrane filtration. Use membrane filters having a nominal pore size not greater than 0.45 µm whose effectiveness to retain micro-organisms has been established. Cellulose nitrate filters, for example, are used for aqueous, oily and weakly alcoholic solutions and cellulose acetate filters, for example, for strongly alcoholic solutions. Specially adapted filters may be needed for certain products, e.g. for antibiotics.

The technique described below assumes that membranes about 50 mm in diameter will be used. If filters of a different diameter are used the volumes of the dilutions and the washings should be adjusted accordingly. The filtration apparatus and membrane are sterilised by appropriate means. The apparatus is designed so that the solution to be examined can be introduced and filtered under aseptic conditions; it permits the aseptic removal of the membrane for transfer to the medium or it is suitable for carrying out the incubation after adding the medium to the apparatus itself.

Aqueous solutions. If appropriate, transfer a small quantity of a suitable, sterile diluent such as a 1 g/l neutral solution of meat or casein peptone pH 7.1 ± 0.2 onto the membrane in the apparatus and filter. The diluent may contain suitable neutralising substances and/or appropriate inactivating substances for example in the case of antibiotics.

Transfer the contents of the container or containers to be tested to the membrane or membranes, if necessary after diluting to the volume used in the validation test with the chosen sterile diluent but in any case using not less than the quantities of the product to be examined prescribed in Table 2.6.1.-2. Filter immediately. If the product has antimicrobial properties, wash the membrane not less than 3 times by filtering through it each time the volume of the chosen sterile diluent used in the validation test. Do not exceed a washing cycle of 5 times 200 ml, even if during validation it has been demonstrated that such a cycle does not fully eliminate the antimicrobial activity. Transfer the whole membrane to the culture medium or cut it aseptically into 2 equal parts and transfer one half to each of 2 suitable media. Use the same volume of each medium as in the validation test. Alternatively, transfer the medium onto the membrane in the apparatus. Incubate the media for not less than 14 days.

Soluble solids. Use for each medium not less than the quantity prescribed in Table 2.6.1.-2 of the product dissolved in a suitable solvent such as a 1 g/l neutral solution of meat or casein peptone and proceed with the test as described above for aqueous solutions using a membrane appropriate to the chosen solvent.

Oils and oily solutions. Use for each medium not less than the quantity of the product prescribed in Table 2.6.1.-2. Oils and oily solutions of sufficiently low viscosity may be filtered without dilution through a dry membrane. Viscous oils may be diluted as necessary with a suitable sterile diluent such as isopropyl myristate shown not to have antimicrobial activity in the conditions of the test. Allow the oil to penetrate the membrane by its own weight then filter, applying the pressure or suction gradually. Wash the membrane at least

Table 2.6.1.-2 – *Minimum quantity to be used for each medium*

Quantity per container	Minimum quantity to be used for each medium unless otherwise justified and authorised
Liquids	
– less than 1 ml	The whole contents of each container
– 1-40 ml	Half the contents of each container but not less than 1 ml
– greater than 40 ml and not greater than 100 ml	20 ml
– greater than 100 ml	10 per cent of the contents of the container but not less than 20 ml
Antibiotic liquids	1 ml
Other preparations soluble in water or in isopropyl myristate	The whole contents of each container to provide not less than 200 mg
Insoluble preparations, creams and ointments to be suspended or emulsified	The whole contents of each container to provide not less than 200 mg
Solids	
– less than 50 mg	The whole contents of each container
– 50 mg or more but less than 300 mg	Half the contents of each container but not less than 50 mg
– 300 mg to 5 g	150 mg
– greater than 5 g	500 mg
Catgut and other surgical sutures for veterinary use	3 sections of a strand (each 30 cm long)

3 times by filtering through it each time about 100 ml of a suitable sterile solution such as 1 g/l neutral meat or casein peptone containing a suitable emulsifying agent at a concentration shown to be appropriate in the validation of the test, for example polysorbate 80 at a concentration of 10 g/l. Transfer the membrane or membranes to the culture medium or media or vice versa as described above for aqueous solutions, and incubate at the same temperatures and for the same times.

Ointments and creams. Use for each medium not less than the quantities of the product prescribed in Table 2.6.1.-2. Ointments in a fatty base and emulsions of the water-in-oil type may be diluted to 1 per cent in isopropyl myristate as described above, by heating, if necessary, to not more than 40 °C. In exceptional cases it may be necessary to heat to not more than 44 °C. Filter as rapidly as possible and proceed as described above for oils and oily solutions.

Direct inoculation of the culture medium. Transfer the quantity of the preparation to be examined prescribed in Table 2.6.1.-2 directly into the culture medium so that the volume of the product is not more than 10 per cent of the volume of the medium, unless otherwise prescribed.

If the product to be examined has antimicrobial activity, carry out the test after neutralising this with a suitable neutralising substance or by dilution in a sufficient quantity of culture medium. When it is necessary to use a large volume of the product it may be preferable to use a concentrated culture medium prepared in such a way that it takes account of the subsequent dilution. Where appropriate, the concentrated medium may be added directly to the product in its container.

Oily liquids. Use media to which have been added a suitable emulsifying agent at a concentration shown to be appropriate in the validation of the test, for example polysorbate 80 at a concentration of 10 g/l.

Ointments and creams. Prepare by diluting to about 1 in 10 by emulsifying with the chosen emulsifying agent in a suitable sterile diluent such as a 1 g/l neutral solution of meat or casein peptone. Transfer the diluted product to a medium not containing an emulsifying agent.

Incubate the inoculated media for not less than 14 days. Observe the cultures several times during the incubation period. Shake cultures containing oily products gently each day. However when thioglycollate medium or other similar medium is used for the detection of anaerobic micro-organisms keep shaking or mixing to a minimum in order to maintain anaerobic conditions.

Catgut and other surgical sutures for veterinary use. Use for each medium not less than the quantities of the product prescribed in Table 2.6.1.-2. Open the sealed package using aseptic precautions and remove 3 sections of the strand for each culture medium. Carry out the test on 3 sections, each 30 cm long, cut off from the beginning, the centre and the end of the strand. Use whole strands from freshly opened cassette packs. Transfer each section of the strand to the selected medium. Use sufficient medium to cover adequately the material to be tested (20 ml to 150 ml).

OBSERVATION AND INTERPRETATION OF RESULTS

At intervals during the incubation period and at its conclusion, examine the media for macroscopic evidence of microbial growth. If the material being tested renders the medium turbid so that the presence or absence of microbial growth cannot be readily determined by visual examination, 14 days after the beginning of incubation transfer portions (each not less than 1 ml) of the medium to fresh vessels of the same medium and then incubate the original and transfer vessels for not less than 4 days.

If no evidence of microbial growth is found, the product to be examined complies with the test for sterility. If evidence of microbial growth is found the product to be examined does not comply with the test for sterility, unless it can be clearly demonstrated that the test was invalid for causes unrelated to the product to be examined. The test may be considered invalid only if one or more of the following conditions are fulfilled:

a) the data of the microbiological monitoring of the sterility testing facility show a fault,

b) a review of the testing procedure used during the test in question reveals a fault,

c) microbial growth is found in the negative controls,

d) after determination of the identity of the micro-organisms isolated from the test, the growth of this species or these species may be ascribed unequivocally to faults with respect to the material and/or the technique used in conducting the sterility test procedure.

If the test is declared to be invalid it is repeated with the same number of units as in the original test.

If no evidence of microbial growth is found in the repeat test the product examined complies with the test for sterility.

If microbial growth is found in the repeat test the product examined does not comply with the test for sterility.

APPLICATION OF THE TEST TO PARENTERAL PREPARATIONS, OPHTHALMIC AND OTHER NON-INJECTABLE PREPARATIONS REQUIRED TO COMPLY WITH THE TEST FOR STERILITY

When using the technique of membrane filtration, use, whenever possible, the whole contents of the container, but not less than the quantities indicated in Table 2.6.1.-2, diluting where necessary to about 100 ml with a suitable sterile solution, such as 1 g/l neutral meat or casein peptone.

When using the technique of direct inoculation of media, use the quantities shown in Table 2.6.1.-2, unless otherwise justified and authorised. The tests for bacterial and fungal sterility are carried out on the same sample of the product to be examined. When the volume or the quantity in a single container is insufficient to carry out the tests, the contents of 2 or more containers are used to inoculate the different media.

GUIDELINES FOR USING THE TEST FOR STERILITY

The purpose of the test for sterility, as that of all pharmacopoeial tests, is to provide an independent control analyst with the means of verifying that a particular material meets the requirements of the European Pharmacopoeia. A manufacturer is neither obliged to carry out such tests nor precluded from using modifications of, or alternatives to, the stated method, provided he is satisfied that, if tested by the official method, the material in question would comply with the requirements of the European Pharmacopoeia.

Precautions against microbial contamination. Aseptic conditions for performance of the test can be achieved using, for example, a class A laminar-air-flow cabinet located within a class B clean-room, or an isolator.

Guidance to manufacturers. The level of assurance provided by a satisfactory result of a test for sterility (the absence of contaminated units in the sample) as applied to the quality of the batch is a function of the homogeneity of the batch, the conditions of manufacture and the efficiency of the adopted sampling plan. Hence for the purpose of this text a batch is defined as a homogeneous collection of sealed containers prepared in such a manner that the risk of contamination is the same for each of the units contained therein.

In the case of terminally sterilised products, physical proofs, biologically based and automatically documented, showing correct treatment throughout the batch during sterilisation are of greater assurance than the sterility test. The circumstances in which parametric release may be considered appropriate are described under Methods of preparation of sterile products (*5.1.1*). The method of media-fill runs may be used to evaluate the process of aseptic production. Apart from that the sterility test is the only analytical method available for products prepared under aseptic conditions and furthermore it is, in all cases, the only analytical method available to the authorities who have to examine a specimen of a product for sterility.

The probability of detecting micro-organisms by the test for sterility increases with their number present in the sample tested and varies according to the readiness of growth of micro-organism present. The probability of detecting very low levels of contamination even when it is homogenous throughout the batch is very low. The interpretation of the results of the test for sterility rests on the assumption that the contents of every container in the batch, had they been tested, would have given the same result. Since it is manifest that every container cannot be tested, an appropriate sampling plan should be adopted. In the case of aseptic production, it is recommended to include samples filled at the beginning and at the end of the batch and after significant intervention.

Guidance on the minimum number of items recommended to be tested in relation to the size of the batch is given in Table 2.6.1-3. The application of the recommendations must have regard to the volume of preparation per container, to the validation of the sterilisation method and to any other special considerations concerning the intended sterility of the product.

Table 2.6.1.-3. – *Minimum number of items to be tested*

Number of items in the batch	Minimum number of items to be tested for each medium, unless otherwise justified and authorised*
Parenteral preparations	
– Not more than 100 containers	10 per cent or 4 containers, whichever is the greater
– More than 100 but not more than 500 containers	10 containers
– More than 500 containers	2 per cent or 20 containers, whichever is less
Ophthalmic and other non-injectable preparations	
– Not more than 200 containers	5 per cent or 2 containers, whichever is the greater
– More than 200 containers	10 containers
– If the product is presented in the form of single-dose containers, apply the scheme shown above for preparations for parenteral use	
Catgut and other surgical sutures for veterinary use	2 per cent or 5 packages whichever is the greater, up to a maximum total of 20 packages
Bulk solid products	
– Up to 4 containers	Each container
– More than 4 containers but not more than 50 containers	20 per cent or 4 containers, whichever is the greater
– More than 50 containers	2 per cent or 10 containers, whichever is the greater
Pharmacy bulk packages of antibiotics (greater than 5 g)	6 containers

*If the contents of one container are enough to inoculate the two media, this column gives the number of containers needed for both the media together.

Observation and interpretation of results. Conventional microbiological/biochemical techniques are generally satisfactory for identification of micro-organisms recovered from a sterility test. However, if a manufacturer wishes to use condition (d) as the sole criterion for invalidating a sterility test, it may be necessary to employ sensitive typing techniques to demonstrate that a micro-organism isolated from the product test is identical to a micro-organism isolated from the test materials and/or the testing environment. While routine microbiological/biochemical identification techniques can demonstrate that 2 isolates are not identical, these methods may not be sufficiently sensitive or reliable enough to provide unequivocal evidence that two isolates are from the same source. More sensitive tests, for example, molecular typing with RNA/DNA homology, may be necessary to determine that micro-organisms are clonally related and have a common origin.

01/2005:20602

2.6.2. MYCOBACTERIA

If the sample to be examined may be contaminated by micro-organisms other than mycobacteria, treat it with a suitable decontamination solution, such as acetylcysteine-sodium hydroxide solution or sodium laurilsulfate solution.

Inoculate 0.2 ml of the sample in triplicate onto each of 2 suitable solid media (Löwenstein-Jensen medium and Middlebrook 7H10 medium are considered suitable). Inoculate 0.5 ml in triplicate into a suitable liquid medium. Incubate all media at 37 °C for 56 days.

Establish the fertility of the media in the presence of the preparation to be examined by inoculation of a suitable strain of a *Mycobacterium* sp. such as BCG and if necessary use a suitable neutralising substance.

If contaminating micro-organisms develop during the first 8 days of incubation, repeat the test and carry out at the same time a bacteriological sterility test.

If at the end of the incubation time no growth of mycobacteria occurs in any of the test media, the preparation complies with the test.

01/2005:20607

2.6.7. MYCOPLASMAS

Where the test for mycoplasmas is prescribed for a master cell bank, for a working cell bank, for a virus seed lot or for control cells, both the culture method and the indicator cell culture method are used. Where the test for mycoplasmas is prescribed for a virus harvest, for a bulk vaccine or for the final lot (batch), the culture method is used. The indicator cell culture method may also be used, where necessary, for screening of media.

CULTURE METHOD

CHOICE OF CULTURE MEDIA

The test is carried out using a sufficient number of both solid and liquid media to ensure growth in the chosen incubation conditions of small numbers of mycoplasmas that may be present in the product to be examined. Liquid media must contain phenol red. The range of media chosen is shown to have satisfactory nutritive properties for at least the organisms shown below. The nutritive properties of each new batch of medium are verified for the appropriate organisms in the list.

Acholeplasma laidlawii (vaccines for human and veterinary use where an antibiotic has been used during production)

Mycoplasma gallisepticum (where avian material has been used during production or where the vaccine is intended for use in poultry)

Mycoplasma hyorhinis (non-avian veterinary vaccines)

Mycoplasma orale (vaccines for human and veterinary use)

Mycoplasma pneumoniae (vaccines for human use) or other suitable species of D-glucose fermenter

Mycoplasma synoviae (where avian material has been used during production or where the vaccine is intended for use in poultry).

The test strains are field isolates having undergone not more than fifteen subcultures and are stored frozen or freeze-dried. After cloning the strains are identified as being of the required species by a suitable method, by comparison with type cultures, for example:

A. laidlawii	NCTC 10116	CIP 75.27	ATCC 23206
M. gallisepticum	NCTC 10115	CIP 104967	ATCC 19610
M. hyorhinis	NCTC 10130	CIP 104968	ATCC 17981
M. orale	NCTC 10112	CIP 104969	ATCC 23714
M. pneumoniae	NCTC 10119	CIP 103766	ATCC 15531
M. synoviae	NCTC 10124	CIP 104970	ATCC 25204

INCUBATION CONDITIONS

Divide inoculated media into two equal parts and incubate one in aerobic conditions and the other in microaerophilic conditions; for solid media maintain an atmosphere of adequate humidity to prevent desiccation of the surface. For aerobic conditions, incubate in an atmosphere of air containing, for solid media, 5 to 10 per cent of carbon dioxide. For microaerophilic conditions, incubate in an atmosphere of nitrogen containing, for solid media, 5 to 10 per cent of carbon dioxide.

NUTRITIVE PROPERTIES

Carry out the test for nutritive properties for each new batch of medium. Inoculate the chosen media with the appropriate test organisms; use not more than 100 CFU (colony-forming units) per 60 mm plate containing 9 ml of solid medium and not more than 40 CFU per 100 ml container of the corresponding liquid medium; use a separate plate and container for each species of organism. Incubate the media in the conditions that will be used for the test of the product to be examined (aerobically, microaerophilically or both, depending on the requirements of the test organism). The media comply with the test for nutritive properties if there is adequate growth of the test organisms accompanied by an appropriate colour change in liquid media.

INHIBITORY SUBSTANCES

Carry out the test for nutritive properties in the presence of the product to be examined. If growth of the test organisms is notably less than that found in the absence of the product to be examined, the latter contains inhibitory substances that must be neutralised (or their effect otherwise countered, for example, by dilution) before the test for mycoplasmas is carried out. The effectiveness of the neutralisation or other process is checked by repeating the test for inhibitory substances after neutralisation.

TEST FOR MYCOPLASMAS IN THE PRODUCT TO BE EXAMINED

For solid media, use plates 60 mm in diameter and containing 9 ml of medium. Inoculate each of not fewer than two plates of each solid medium with 0.2 ml of the product to be examined and inoculate 10 ml per 100 ml of each liquid medium. Incubate at 35 °C to 38 °C, aerobically and microaerophilically, for 21 days and at the same time incubate an uninoculated 100 ml portion of each liquid medium for use as a control. If any significant pH change occurs on addition of the product to be examined, restore the liquid medium to its original pH value by the addition of a solution of either sodium hydroxide or hydrochloric acid. On the first, second or third day after inoculation subculture each liquid culture by inoculating each of two plates of each solid medium with 0.2 ml and incubating at 35 °C to 38 °C aerobically and microaerophilically for not less than 21 days. Repeat the procedure on the sixth, seventh or eighth day and again on the thirteenth or fourteenth day of the test. Observe the liquid media every 2 or 3 days and if any colour change occurs subculture immediately. Observe solid media once per week.

If the liquid media show bacterial or fungal contamination, repeat the test. If, not earlier than 7 days after inoculation, not more than one plate at each stage of the test is accidentally contaminated with bacteria or fungi, or broken, that plate may be ignored provided that on immediate examination it shows no evidence of mycoplasmal growth. If, at any stage of the test, more than one plate is accidentally contaminated with bacteria or fungi, or broken, the test is invalid and must be repeated.

Include in the test positive controls prepared by inoculating not more than 100 CFU of suitable species such as *M. orale* and *M. pneumoniae*.

At the end of the incubation periods, examine all the inoculated solid media microscopically for the presence of mycoplasmas. The product passes the test if growth of mycoplasmas has not occurred in any of the inoculated media. If growth of mycoplasmas has occurred, the test may be repeated once using twice the amount of inoculum, media and plates; if growth of mycoplasmas does not occur, the product complies with the test. The test is invalid if the positive controls do not show growth of the relevant test organism.

INDICATOR CELL CULTURE METHOD

Cell cultures are stained with a fluorescent dye that binds to DNA. Mycoplasmas are detected by their characteristic particulate or filamentous pattern of fluorescence on the cell surface and, if contamination is heavy, in surrounding areas.

VERIFICATION OF THE SUBSTRATE

Using a Vero cell culture substrate, pretest the procedure using an inoculum of not more than 100 CFU (colony-forming units) of a strain growing readily in liquid or solid medium and demonstrate its ability to detect potential mycoplasma contaminants such as suitable strains of *Mycoplasma hyorhinis* and *Mycoplasma orale*. A different cell substrate may be used, for example the production cell line, if it has been demonstrated that it will provide at least equal sensitivity for the detection of potential mycoplasma contaminants.

Test method

Take not less than 1 ml of the product to be examined and use it to inoculate in duplicate, as described under Procedure, indicator cell cultures representing not less than 25 cm² of cell culture area at confluence.

Include in the test a negative (non-infected) control and two positive mycoplasma controls, such as *M. hyorhinis* and *M. orale*. Use an inoculum of not more than 100 CFU for the positive controls.

If for viral suspensions the interpretation of results is affected by marked cytopathic effects, the virus may be neutralised using a specific antiserum that has no inhibitory effects on mycoplasmas or a cell culture substrate that does not allow growth of the virus may be used. To demonstrate the absence of inhibitory effects of serum, carry out the positive control tests in the presence and absence of the antiserum.

Procedure

1. Seed culture at a regular density (2×10^4 to 2×10^5 cells/ml, 4×10^3 to 2.5×10^4 cells/cm²) and incubate at 36 ± 1 °C for at least 2 days. Inoculate the product to be examined and incubate for at least 2 days; make not fewer than one subculture. Grow the last subculture on coverslips in suitable containers or on some other surface suitable for the test procedure. Do not allow the last subculture to reach confluence since this would inhibit staining and impair visualisation of mycoplasmas.
2. Remove and discard the medium.
3. Rinse the monolayer with *phosphate buffered saline pH 7.4 R*, then with a mixture of equal volumes of *phosphate buffered saline pH 7.4 R* and a suitable fixing solution and finally with the fixing solution; when *bisbenzimide R* is used for staining, a freshly prepared mixture of 1 volume of *glacial acetic acid R* and 3 volumes of *methanol R* is a suitable fixing solution.
4. Add the fixing solution and allow to stand for 10 min.
5. Remove the fixing solution and discard.
6. If the monolayer is to be stained later, dry it completely. (Particular care is needed for staining of the slides after drying because of artefacts that may be produced.)
7. If the monolayer is to be stained directly, wash off the fixing solution twice with sterile water and discard the wash.
8. Add *bisbenzimide working solution R* or some other suitable DNA staining agent and allow to stand for 10 min.
9. Remove the stain and rinse the monolayer with water.
10. Mount each coverslip, where applicable, with a drop of a mixture of equal volumes of *glycerol R* and *phosphate-citrate buffer solution pH 5.5 R*; blot off surplus mountant from the edge of the coverslip.
11. Examine by epifluorescence (330 nm/380 nm excitation filter, LP 440 nm barrier filter) at 100-400 × magnification or greater.
12. Compare the microscopic appearance of the test cultures with that of the negative and positive controls, examining for extranuclear fluorescence. Mycoplasmas give pinpoints or filaments over the cytoplasm and sometimes in intercellular spaces.

The product to be examined complies with the test if there is no evidence of the presence of mycoplasmas in the test cultures inoculated with it. The test is invalid if the positive controls do not show the presence of the appropriate test organisms.

The following section is published for information.

RECOMMENDED MEDIA FOR THE CULTURE METHOD

The following media are recommended. Other media may be used providing their ability to sustain the growth of mycoplasmas has been demonstrated on each batch in the presence and absence of the product to be examined.

RECOMMENDED MEDIA FOR THE DETECTION OF MYCOPLASMA GALLISEPTICUM

Liquid medium

Beef heart infusion broth (1)	90.0 ml
Horse serum (unheated)	20.0 ml

Yeast extract (250 g/l)	10.0 ml
Thallium acetate (10 g/l solution)	1.0 ml
Phenol red (0.6 g/l solution)	5.0 ml
Penicillin (20 000 IU/ml)	0.25 ml
Deoxyribonucleic acid (2 g/l solution)	1.2 ml

Adjust to pH 7.8.

Solid medium

Prepare as described above replacing beef heart infusion broth by beef heart infusion agar containing 15 g/l of agar.

RECOMMENDED MEDIA FOR THE DETECTION OF MYCOPLASMA SYNOVIAE

Liquid medium

Beef heart infusion broth (1)	90.0 ml
Essential vitamins (2)	0.025 ml
Glucose monohydrate (500 g/l solution)	2.0 ml
Swine serum (inactivated at 56 °C for 30 min)	12.0 ml
β-Nicotinamide adenine dinucleotide (10 g/l solution)	1.0 ml
Cysteine hydrochloride (10 g/l solution)	1.0 ml
Phenol red (0.6 g/l solution)	5.0 ml
Penicillin (20 000 IU/ml)	0.25 ml

Mix the solutions of β-nicotinamide adenine dinucleotide and cysteine hydrochloride and after 10 min add to the other ingredients. Adjust to pH 7.8.

Solid medium

Beef heart infusion broth (1)	90.0 ml
Ionagar (3)	1.4 g

Adjust to pH 7.8, sterilise by autoclaving then add:

Essential vitamins (2)	0.025 ml
Glucose monohydrate (500 g/l solution)	2.0 ml
Swine serum (unheated)	12.0 ml
β-Nicotinamide adenine dinucleotide (10 g/l solution)	1.0 ml
Cysteine hydrochloride (10 g/l solution)	1.0 ml
Phenol red (0.6 g/l solution)	5.0 ml
Penicillin (20 000 IU/ml)	0.25 ml

RECOMMENDED MEDIA FOR THE DETECTION OF NON-AVIAN MYCOPLASMAS

Liquid medium

Hanks' balanced salt solution (modified) (4)	800 ml
Distilled water	67 ml
Brain heart infusion (5)	135 ml
PPLO Broth (6)	248 ml
Yeast extract (170 g/l)	60 ml
Bacitracin	250 mg
Meticillin	250 mg
Phenol red (5 g/l)	4.5 ml
Thallium acetate (56 g/l)	3 ml
Horse serum	165 ml
Swine serum	165 ml

Adjust to pH 7.4 - 7.45.

Solid medium

Hanks' balanced salt solution (modified) (4)	200 ml
DEAE-dextran	200 mg
Ionagar (3)	15.65 mg

Mix well and sterilise by autoclaving. Cool to 100 °C. Add to 1740 ml of liquid medium as described above.

(1) *Beef heart infusion broth*

Beef heart (for preparation of the infusion)	500 g
Peptone	10 g
Sodium chloride	5 g
Distilled water to	1000 ml

Sterilise by autoclaving.

(2) *Essential vitamins*

Biotin	100 mg
Calcium pantothenate	100 mg
Choline chloride	100 mg
Folic acid	100 mg
i-Inositol	200 mg
Nicotinamide	100 mg
Pyridoxal hydrochloride	100 mg
Riboflavine	10 mg
Thiamine hydrochloride	100 mg
Distilled water to	1000 ml

(3) *Ionagar*

A highly refined agar for use in microbiology and immunology prepared by an ion-exchange procedure which results in a product having superior purity, clarity and gel strength.

It contains about:

Water	12.2 per cent
Ash	1.5 per cent
Acid-insoluble ash	0.2 per cent
Chlorine	0
Phosphate (calculated as P_2O_5)	0.3 per cent
Total nitrogen	0.3 per cent
Copper	8 ppm
Iron	170 ppm
Calcium	0.28 per cent
Magnesium	0.32 per cent

(4) *Hanks' balanced salt solution (modified)*

Sodium chloride	6.4 g
Potassium chloride	0.32 g
Magnesium sulphate heptahydrate	0.08 g
Magnesium chloride hexahydrate	0.08 g
Calcium chloride, anhydrous	0.112 g
Disodium hydrogen phosphate dihydrate	0.0596 g
Potassium dihydrogen phosphate, anhydrous	0.048 g
Distilled water to	800 ml

(5) *Brain heart infusion*

Calf-brain infusion	200 g
Beef-heart infusion	250 g
Proteose peptone	10 g
Glucose monohydrate	2 g
Sodium chloride	5 g
Disodium hydrogen phosphate, anhydrous	2.5 g
Distilled water to	1000 ml

(6) *PPLO broth*

Beef-heart infusion	50 g
Peptone	10 g
Sodium chloride	5 g
Distilled water to	1000 ml

01/2005:20608

2.6.8. PYROGENS

The test consists of measuring the rise in body temperature evoked in rabbits by the intravenous injection of a sterile solution of the substance to be examined.

Selection of animals. Use healthy, adult rabbits of either sex weighing not less than 1.5 kg, fed a complete and balanced diet not containing antibiotics, and not showing loss of body mass during the week preceding the test. A rabbit is not be used in a pyrogen test:

a) if it has been used in a negative pyrogen test in the preceding 3 days, or

b) if it has been used in the preceding 3 weeks in a pyrogen test in which the substance under examination failed to pass the test.

Animals' quarters. Keep the rabbits individually in a quiet area with a uniform appropriate temperature. Withhold food from the rabbits overnight and until the test is completed; withhold water during the test. Carry out the test in a quiet room where there is no risk of disturbance exciting the animals and in which the room temperature is within 3 °C of that of the rabbits' living quarters, or in which the rabbits have been kept for at least 18 h before the test.

Materials. Glassware, syringes and needles. Thoroughly wash all glassware, syringes and needles with water for injections and heat in a hot-air oven at 250 °C for 30 min or at 200 °C for 1 h.

Retaining boxes. The retaining boxes for rabbits whose temperature is being measured by an electrical device are made in such a way that the animals are retained only by loosely fitting neck-stocks; the rest of the body remains relatively free so that the rabbits may sit in a normal position. They are not restrained by straps or other similar methods which may harm the animal. The animals are put into the boxes not less than 1 h before the first record of the temperature and remain in them throughout the test.

Thermometers. Use a thermometer or electrical device which indicates the temperature with a precision of 0.1 °C and insert into the rectum of the rabbit to a depth of about 5 cm. The depth of insertion is constant for any one rabbit in any one test. When an electrical device is used it may be left in position throughout the test.

Preliminary test. After selection of the animals, one to three days before testing the product to be examined, treat those animals that have not been used during the previous 2 weeks by intravenous injection of 10 ml per kilogram of body mass of a pyrogen-free 9 g/l solution of *sodium chloride R* warmed to about 38.5 °C. Record the temperatures of the animals, beginning at least 90 min before injection and continuing for 3 h after the injection of the solution. Any animal showing a temperature variation greater than 0.6 °C is not used in the main test.

Main test. Carry out the test using a group of three rabbits. Preparation and injection of the product. Warm the liquid to be examined to approximately 38.5 °C before the injection. The product to be examined may be dissolved in, or diluted with, a pyrogen-free 9 g/l solution of *sodium chloride R* or another prescribed liquid. Inject the solution slowly into the marginal vein of the ear of each rabbit over a period not exceeding 4 min, unless otherwise prescribed in the monograph. The amount of the product to be injected varies according to the product to be examined and is prescribed in the monograph. The volume injected is not less than 0.5 ml per kilogram and not more than 10 ml per kilogram of body mass.

Determination of the initial and maximum temperatures. The "initial temperature" of each rabbit is the mean of two temperature readings recorded for that rabbit at an interval of 30 min in the 40 min immediately preceding the injection of the product to be examined. The "maximum temperature" of each rabbit is the highest temperature recorded for that rabbit in the 3 h after the injection. Record the temperature of each rabbit at intervals of not more than 30 min, beginning at least 90 min before the injection of the product to be examined and continuing 3 h after the injection. The difference between the maximum temperature and the initial temperature of each rabbit is taken to be its response. When this difference is negative, the result is counted as a zero response.

Rabbits showing a temperature variation greater than 0.2 °C between two successive readings in the determination of the initial temperature are withdrawn from the test. In any one test, only rabbits having initial temperatures which do not differ from one another by more than 1 °C are used. All rabbits having an initial temperature higher than 39.8 °C or less than 38.0 °C are withdrawn from the test.

Interpretation of results. Having carried out the test first on a group of three rabbits, repeat if necessary on further groups of three rabbits to a total of four groups, depending on the results obtained. If the summed response of the first group does not exceed the figure given in the second column of the Table 2.6.8.-1, the substance passes the test. If the summed response exceeds the figure given in the second column of the table but does not exceed the figure given in the third column of the table, repeat the test as indicated above. If the summed response exceeds the figure given in the third column of the table, the product fails the test.

Table 2.6.8.-1

Number of rabbits	Product passes if summed response does not exceed	Product fails if summed response exceeds
3	1.15 °C	2.65 °C
6	2.80 °C	4.30 °C
9	4.45 °C	5.95 °C
12	6.60 °C	6.60 °C

Rabbits used in a test for pyrogens where the mean rise in the rabbits' temperature has exceeded 1.2 °C are permanently excluded.

01/2005:20609

2.6.9. ABNORMAL TOXICITY

GENERAL TEST

Inject intravenously into each of 5 healthy mice, weighing 17 g to 22 g, the quantity of the substance to be examined prescribed in the monograph, dissolved in 0.5 ml of *water for injections R* or of a 9 g/l sterile solution of *sodium chloride R*. Inject the solution over a period of 15 s to 30 s, unless otherwise prescribed.

The substance passes the test if none of the mice die within 24 h or within such time as is specified in the individual monograph. If more than one animal dies the preparation fails the test. If one of the animals dies, repeat the test. The substance passes the test if none of the animals in the second group die within the time interval specified.

IMMUNOSERA AND VACCINES FOR HUMAN USE

Unless otherwise prescribed, inject intraperitoneally 1 human dose but not more than 1.0 ml into each of 5 healthy mice, weighing 17 g to 22 g. The human dose is that stated on the label of the preparation to be examined or on the accompanying leaflet. Observe the animals for 7 days.

The preparation passes the test if none of the animals shows signs of ill health. If more than one animal dies, the preparation fails the test. If one of the animals dies or shows signs of ill health, repeat the test. The preparation passes the test if none of the animals in the second group die or shows signs of ill health in the time interval specified.

The test must also be carried out on 2 healthy guinea-pigs weighing 250 g to 350 g. Inject intraperitoneally into each animal 1 human dose but not more than 5.0 ml. The human dose is that stated on the label of the preparation to be examined or on the accompanying leaflet. Observe the animals for 7 days.

The preparation passes the test if none of the animals shows signs of ill health. If more than one animal dies the preparation fails the test. If one of the animals dies or shows signs of ill health, repeat the test. The preparation passes the test if none of the animals in the second group die or shows signs of ill health in the time interval specified.

01/2005:20610

2.6.10. HISTAMINE

Kill a guinea-pig weighing 250 g to 350 g that has been deprived of food for the preceding 24 h. Remove a portion of the distal small intestine 2 cm in length and empty the isolated part by rinsing carefully with solution B described below using a syringe. Attach a fine thread to each end and make a small transverse incision in the middle of the piece of intestine. Place it in an organ bath with a capacity of 10 ml to 20 ml, containing solution B maintained at a constant temperature (34 °C to 36 °C) and pass through the solution a current of a mixture of 95 parts of oxygen and 5 parts of carbon dioxide. Attach one of the threads near to the bottom of the organ bath. Attach the other thread to an isotonic myograph and record the contractions of the organ on a kymograph or other suitable means of giving a permanent record. If a lever is used, its length is such that the movements of the organ are amplified about 20 times. The tension on the intestine should be about 9.8 mN (1 g) and it should be adjusted to the sensitivity of the organ. Flush out the organ bath with solution B. Allow it to stand for 10 min. Flush 2 or 3 times more with solution B. Stimulate a series of contractions by the addition of measured volumes between 0.2 ml and 0.5 ml of a solution of *histamine dihydrochloride R* having a strength which produces reproducible submaximal responses. This dose is termed the "high dose". Flush the organ bath (preferably by overflow without emptying the bath) 3 times with solution B before each addition of histamine. The successive additions should be made at regular intervals allowing a complete relaxation between additions (about 2 min). Add equal volumes of a weaker dilution of *histamine dihydrochloride R* which produces reproducible responses approximately half as great as the "high dose". This dose is termed the "low dose". Continue the regular additions of "high" and "low" doses of histamine solution as indicated above, and alternate each addition with an equal volume of a dilution of the solution to be examined, adjusting the dilution so that the contraction of the intestine, if any, is smaller than that due to the "high dose" of histamine. Determine whether the contraction, if any, is reproducible and that the responses to the "high" and "low" doses of histamine are unchanged. Calculate the activity of the substance to be examined in terms of its equivalent in micrograms of histamine base from the dilution determined as above.

The quantity so determined does not exceed the quantity prescribed in the monograph.

If the solution to be examined does not produce a contraction, prepare a fresh solution adding a quantity of histamine corresponding to the maximum tolerated in the monograph and note whether the contractions produced by the preparation with the added histamine correspond to the amount of histamine added. If this is not the case, or if the contractions caused by the substance to be examined are not reproducible or if subsequent responses to "high" and "low" doses of histamine are diminished, the results of the tests are invalid and the test for depressor substances (*2.6.11*) must be carried out.

Solution A

Sodium chloride	160.0 g
Potassium chloride	4.0 g
Calcium chloride, anhydrous	2.0 g
Magnesium chloride, anhydrous	1.0 g
Disodium hydrogen phosphate dodecahydrate	0.10 g
Water for injections R sufficient to produce	1000 ml

Solution B

Solution A	50.0 ml
Atropine sulphate	0.5 mg
Sodium hydrogen carbonate	1.0 g
Glucose monohydrate	0.5 g
Water for injections R sufficient to produce	1000 ml

Solution B should be freshly prepared and used within 24 h.

01/2005:20611

2.6.11. DEPRESSOR SUBSTANCES

Carry out the test on a cat weighing not less than 2 kg and anaesthetised with chloralose or with a barbiturate that allows the maintenance of uniform blood pressure. Protect the animal from loss of body heat and maintain it so that the rectal temperature remains within physiological limits. Introduce a cannula into the trachea. Insert a cannula filled with a heparinised 9 g/l solution of sodium chloride into the common carotid artery and connect it to a device capable of giving a continuous record of the blood pressure. Insert into the femoral vein another cannula, filled with a heparinised 9 g/l solution of sodium chloride, through which can be injected the solutions of histamine and of the substance to be examined. Determine the sensitivity of the animal to histamine by injecting intravenously at regular intervals, doses of *histamine solution R* corresponding to 0.1 µg and 0.15 µg of histamine base per kilogram of body mass. Repeat the lower dose at least 3 times. Administer the second and subsequent injections not less than 1 min after the blood pressure has returned to the level it was at immediately before the previous injection. The animal is used for the test only if a readily discernible decrease in blood pressure that is constant for the lower dose is obtained and if the higher dose causes greater responses. Dissolve the substance to be examined in sufficient of a 9 g/l solution of sodium chloride or other prescribed solvent, to give the prescribed concentration. Inject intravenously per kilogram of body mass 1.0 ml of *histamine solution R*, followed by 2 successive injections of the prescribed amount of the solution to be examined and, finally, 1.0 ml of *histamine solution R*. The second, third and fourth injections are given not less than 1 min after the blood pressure has returned to the level it was at immediately before the preceding injection. Repeat this series of injections twice and conclude the test by giving 1.5 ml of *histamine solution R* per kilogram of body mass.

If the response to 1.5 ml of *histamine solution R* per kilogram of body mass is not greater than that to 1.0 ml the test is invalid. The substance to be examined fails the test if the mean of the series of responses to the substance is greater than the mean of the responses to 1.0 ml of *histamine solution R* per kilogram of body mass or if any one dose of the substance causes a greater depressor response than the concluding dose of the histamine solution. The test animal must not be used in another test for depressor substances if the second criterion applies or if the response to the high dose of histamine given after the administration of the substance to be examined is less than the mean response to the low doses of histamine previously injected.

01/2005:20612

2.6.12. MICROBIOLOGICAL EXAMINATION OF NON-STERILE PRODUCTS (TOTAL VIABLE AEROBIC COUNT)

The tests described hereafter will allow quantitative enumeration of mesophilic bacteria and fungi which may grow under aerobic conditions.

The tests are designed primarily to determine whether or not a substance that is the subject of a monograph in the Pharmacopoeia complies with the microbiological requirements specified in the monograph in question. When used for such purposes follow the instructions given below, including the number of samples to be taken and interpret the results as stated below. The tests may also be used for the test for *Efficacy of antimicrobial preservation* (*5.1.3*) as described in the Pharmacopoeia. They may furthermore be used for monitoring raw material quality and may be used in association with guidelines on *Microbiological quality of pharmaceutical preparations* (*5.1.4*). When used for such purposes, for example by a manufacturer for raw materials and/or finished product monitoring or for process validation, the conduct of the tests including the number of samples to be taken and the interpretation of the results are matters for agreement between the manufacturer and the competent authority.

Carry out the determination under conditions designed to avoid accidental contamination of the product to be examined. The precautions taken to avoid contamination must be such that they do not affect any micro-organisms which are revealed in the test. If the product to be examined has antimicrobial activity this must be adequately neutralised. If inactivators are used for this purpose their efficacy and non-toxicity versus micro-organisms are demonstrated.

Determine the total viable aerobic count by the membrane filtration method, or the plate-count method as prescribed in the monograph.

The Most Probable Number (MPN) method is reserved for bacterial counts when no other method is available. The choice of a method may be based on factors such as the nature of the product and the expected number of micro-organisms. Any method which is chosen must be properly validated.

When used in conjunction with chapter *5.1.3* or *5.1.4*, the pour-plate method, the surface-spread method and the membrane filtration method may be used.

PREPARATION OF THE SAMPLE

Sampling plan. Sampling of the product must follow a well-defined sampling plan. The sampling plan will be dependent on factors such as batch size, health hazard associated with unacceptably highly contaminated products, the characteristics of the product and the expected level of contamination. Unless otherwise prescribed, use sample(s) of 10 g or 10 ml of the substance or preparation to be examined taken with the precautions referred to above. Select the sample(s) at random from the bulk material or from the available containers of the preparation. If necessary, to obtain the required quantity, mix the contents of a sufficient number of containers to provide each sample, depending on the nature of the substance or preparation to be examined.

An example of a sampling plan applicable to products where homogeneity with respect to the distribution of micro-organisms may be a problem, is the three-class sampling plan. In this case five samples from each batch are drawn and investigated separately. The three recognised classes are:

(i) acceptable samples, i.e. samples containing less than *m* CFU (colony-forming units) per gram or millilitre, where *m* is the limit specified in the relevant monograph;

(ii) marginal samples, i.e. with more than *m* CFU, but less than 10*m* CFU per gram or millilitre;

(iii) defective samples, i.e. containing more than 10*m* CFU per gram or millilitre.

Water-soluble products. Dissolve or dilute 10 g or 10 ml of the product to be examined in buffered sodium chloride-peptone solution pH 7.0 or in another suitable liquid. In general a one in ten dilution is prepared. However, the characteristics of the product, or the required sensitivity may necessitate the use of other ratios. If the product is known to have antimicrobial activity, an inactivating agent may be added to the diluent. If necessary adjust the pH to about pH 7 and prepare further serial tenfold dilutions using the same diluent.

Non-fatty products insoluble in water. Suspend 10 g or 10 ml of the product to be examined in buffered sodium chloride-peptone solution pH 7.0 or in another suitable liquid. In general a one in ten suspension is prepared, but the characteristics of some products may necessitate the use of larger volumes. A suitable surface-active agent such as 1 g/l of polysorbate 80 may be added to assist the suspension of poorly wettable substances. If the product is known to have antimicrobial activity, an inactivating agent may be added to the diluent. If necessary adjust the pH to about pH 7 and prepare further serial tenfold dilutions using the same diluent.

Fatty products. Homogenise 10 g or 10 ml of the product to be examined with not more than half its weight of sterile polysorbate 80 or another suitable sterile surface-active agent, heated if necessary to not more than 40 °C, in exceptional cases to not more than 45 °C. Mix carefully and if necessary maintain the temperature in a water-bath or in an incubator. Add sufficient pre-warmed buffered sodium chloride-peptone solution pH 7.0 to make a one in ten dilution of the original product. Mix carefully whilst maintaining the temperature for the shortest time necessary for the formation of an emulsion and in any case for not more than 30 min. Further serial tenfold dilutions may be prepared using buffered sodium chloride-peptone solution pH 7.0 containing a suitable concentration of sterile polysorbate 80 or another sterile surface-active agent.

Transdermal patches. Remove the protective cover sheets ("release liner") of ten patches of the transdermal preparation by using sterile forceps and place them, the adhesive side upwards, on sterile glass or plastic trays. Cover the adhesive surface with sterile gauze (or woven-filter type monofilament polymer grid), if necessary, and transfer the ten patches to a minimum volume of 500 ml of buffered sodium chloride-peptone solution pH 7.0 containing suitable inactivators such as polysorbate 80 and/or lecithin. Shake vigorously the preparation for at least 30 min (preparation A). Prepare another ten patches in the same way, place them in a minimum volume of 500 ml of broth medium D and shake vigorously for at least 30 min (preparation B).

EXAMINATION OF THE SAMPLE

Membrane filtration. Use membrane filters having a nominal pore size not greater than 0.45 µm and whose effectiveness to retain bacteria has been established. The type of filter material is chosen in such a way that the bacteria retaining efficiency is not affected by the components of the sample to be investigated. Cellulose nitrate filters, for example, may be used for aqueous, oily and weakly alcoholic solutions and cellulose acetate filters, for example, for strongly alcoholic solutions. The filtration apparatus is designed to allow the transfer of the filter to the culture medium.

Transfer a suitable amount of the sample prepared as described in the section Preparation of the sample (preferably representing 1 g of the product, or less if large numbers of colony-forming units are expected) to each of two membrane filters and filter immediately. Wash each filter with three quantities, each of about 100 ml of a suitable liquid such as buffered sodium chloride-peptone solution pH 7.0. To this solution, surface-active agents such as polysorbate 80, or inactivators of antimicrobial agents may be added. If validated, less than three washes may be applied. Transfer one of the membrane filters, intended primarily for the enumeration of bacteria, to the surface of a suitable agar medium, such as medium B and the other, intended primarily for the enumeration of fungi, to the surface of a suitable agar medium, such as medium C. Incubate the plate of agar medium B at 30 °C to 35 °C, and the plate of agar medium C at 20 °C to 25 °C for five days, unless a reliable count is obtained in a shorter time. Select plates with the highest number less than 100 colonies and calculate the number of colony-forming units per gram or millilitre of product.

When examining transdermal patches, filter 50 ml of preparation A separately through each of two sterile filter membranes. Place one membrane to agar medium B for total aerobic microbial count, the other membrane to agar medium C for the count of fungi.

PLATE-COUNT METHODS

a. Pour-plate method. Using Petri dishes 9 cm in diameter, add to each dish 1 ml of the sample prepared as described in the section Preparation of the sample and 15 ml to 20 ml of a liquefied agar medium suitable for the cultivation of bacteria (such as medium B), or 15 ml to 20 ml of a liquefied agar medium suitable for the cultivation of fungi (such as medium C) at not more than 45 °C. If larger Petri dishes are used the amount of agar is increased accordingly. Prepare for each medium at least two Petri dishes for each level of dilution. Incubate the plates at 30 °C to 35 °C (20 °C to 25 °C for fungi) for five days, unless a reliable count is obtained in a shorter time. Select the plates corresponding to one dilution and showing the highest number of colonies less than 300 (100 colonies for fungi). Take the arithmetic average of the counts and calculate the number of colony-forming units per gram or millilitre.

b. Surface-spread method. Using Petri dishes 9 cm in diameter, add 15 ml to 20 ml of a liquefied agar medium suitable for the cultivation of bacteria (such as medium B) or a liquefied agar medium suitable for the cultivation of fungi (such as medium C) at about 45 °C to each Petri dish and allow to solidify. If larger Petri dishes are used, the volume of the agar is increased accordingly. Dry the plates, for example in a LAF bench or in an incubator. Spread a measured volume of not less than 0.1 ml of the sample prepared as described in the section Preparation of the sample over the surface of the medium. Use at least two Petri dishes for each medium and each level of dilution. For incubation and calculation of the number of colony-forming units proceed as described for the pour-plate method.

MOST-PROBABLE-NUMBER METHOD

The precision and accuracy of the most-probable-number method (MPN) is less than that of the membrane filtration method or the plate-count methods. Unreliable results are obtained particularly for the enumeration of moulds. For these reasons the MPN method is reserved for the enumeration of bacteria in situations where no other method is available. If the use of the method is justified, proceed as follows.

Prepare a series of at least three subsequent tenfold dilutions of the product as described in the section Preparation of the sample. From each level of dilution three aliquots of 1 g or 1 ml are used to inoculate three tubes with 9 ml to 10 ml of a suitable liquid medium (such as broth medium A). If necessary a surface-active agent such as polysorbate 80, or an inactivator of antimicrobial agents may be added to the medium. Thus, if three levels of dilution are prepared nine tubes are inoculated. Incubate all tubes for five days at 30 °C to 35 °C. Record for each level of dilution the number of tubes showing microbial growth. If the reading of the results is difficult or uncertain owing to the nature of the product to be examined, subculture in the same broth, or on a suitable agar medium (such as agar medium B), for 18 h to 24 h at the same temperature and use these results. Determine the most probable number of bacteria per gram or millilitre of the product to be examined from Table 2.6.12.-1.

Table 2.6.12.-1. – *Most-probable-number values of bacteria*

Three tubes at each level of dilution							
Number of positive tubes			MPN per gram	Category*		95 per cent confidence limits	
0.1 g	0.01 g	0.001 g		1	2		
0	0	0	< 3			–	–
0	1	0	3		x	< 1	17
1	0	0	3	x		1	21
1	0	1	7		x	2	27
1	1	0	7	x		2	28
1	2	0	11		x	4	35
2	0	0	9	x		2	38
2	0	1	14		x	5	48
2	1	0	15	x		5	50
2	1	1	20		x	8	61
2	2	0	21	x		8	63
3	0	0	23	x		7	129
3	0	1	38	x		10	180
3	1	0	43	x		20	210
3	1	1	75	x		20	280
3	2	0	93	x		30	390
3	2	1	150	x		50	510
3	2	2	210		x	80	640
3	3	0	240	x		100	1400
3	3	1	460	x		200	2400
3	3	2	1100	x		300	4800
3	3	3	> 1100			–	–

Category 1: Normal results, obtained in 95 per cent of the cases.

Category 2: Less likely results, obtained in only 4 per cent of cases. These are not to be used for important decisions. Results that are even less likely than those of category 2 are not mentioned and are always unacceptable.

EFFECTIVENESS OF CULTURE MEDIA AND VALIDITY OF THE COUNTING METHOD

Grow the bacterial test strains separately in containers containing a suitable liquid medium (such as broth medium A) at 30 °C to 35 °C for 18 h to 24 h. Grow the fungal test strains separately on a suitable agar medium (such as medium C without antibiotics) at 20 °C to 25 °C for 48 h for *Candida albicans* and at 20 °C to 25 °C for 7 days for *Aspergillus niger*.

Staphylococcus aureus	such as ATCC 6538 (NCIMB 9518, CIP 4.83)
Escherichia coli	such as ATCC 8739 (NCIMB 8545, CIP 53.126)
Bacillus subtilis	such as ATCC 6633 (NCIMB 8054, CIP 52.62)
Candida albicans	such as ATCC 10231 (NCPF 3179, IP 48.72)
Aspergillus niger	such as ATCC 16404 (IMI 149007, IP 1431.83)

Use buffered sodium chloride-peptone solution pH 7.0 to make reference suspensions containing about 100 colony-forming units per millilitre. Use the suspension of each of the micro-organisms separately as a control of the counting methods, in the presence and absence of the product to be examined. When testing the membrane filtration method or the plate-count method, a count of any of the test organisms differing by not more than a factor of five from the calculated value from the inoculum is to be obtained. When testing the most-probable-number method the calculated value from the inoculum is to be within the 95 per cent confidence limits of the results obtained. To test the sterility of the medium and of the diluent and the aseptic performance of the test, carry out the method using sterile sodium chloride-peptone solution pH 7.0 as the test preparation. There must be no growth of micro-organisms.

INTERPRETATION OF THE RESULTS

The bacterial count will be considered to be equal to the average number of colony-forming units found on agar medium B. The fungal count will be considered to be equal to the average number of colony-forming units on agar medium C. The total viable aerobic count is the sum of the bacterial count and the fungal count as described above. If there is evidence that the same types of micro-organisms grow on both media this may be corrected. If the count is carried out by the most-probable-number method the calculated value is the bacterial count.

When a limit is prescribed in a monograph it is interpreted as follows:

10^2 micro-organisms: maximum acceptable limit: 5×10^2,

10^3 micro-organisms: maximum acceptable limit: 5×10^3,

and so forth.

If a sampling plan such as the three-class sampling plan for example, is used, proceed as follows:

Calculate the total viable aerobic count separately for each of the five samples. The substance or preparation passes the test if the following conditions are fulfilled:

(i) none of the individual total viable aerobic counts exceeds the prescribed limit by a factor of ten or more (i.e. no "unacceptable samples"),

(ii) and not more than two of the individual total viable aerobic counts are between the prescribed limit and ten times this limit (i.e. no more than two "marginal samples").

The solutions and culture mediums recommended are described in the general chapter *2.6.13.*

01/2005:20613

2.6.13. MICROBIOLOGICAL EXAMINATION OF NON-STERILE PRODUCTS (TEST FOR SPECIFIED MICRO-ORGANISMS)

In this general method the use of certain selective media is proposed. A feature common to all selective media is that sub-lethally injured organisms are not detected. As sub-lethally injured organisms are relevant for the quality of the product a resuscitation must be included in examination procedures that rely on selective media.

If the product to be examined has antimicrobial activity this must be adequately neutralised.

Enterobacteria and certain other gram-negative bacteria

Although the test has been designed to detect bacteria belonging to the family of Enterobacteriaceae, it is recognised that other types of organisms (e.g. *Aeromonas, Pseudomonas*) may be recovered.

Detection of bacteria. Prepare the product to be examined as described in the general method *2.6.12*, but using broth medium D in place of buffered sodium chloride-peptone solution pH 7.0, homogenise and incubate at 35-37 °C for a time sufficient to revive the bacteria but not sufficient to encourage multiplication of the organisms (usually 2 h but not more than 5 h). Shake the container, transfer the quantity of the contents (homogenate A) corresponding to 1 g or 1 ml of the product to 100 ml of enrichment medium E and incubate at 35-37 °C for 18-48 h. Subculture on plates of agar medium F. Incubate at 35-37 °C for 18-24 h. The product passes the test if there is no growth of colonies of gram-negative bacteria on any plate.

Quantitative evaluation. Inoculate suitable quantities of enrichment broth medium E with homogenate A and/or dilutions of it containing respectively 0.1 g, 0.01 g and 0.001 g (or 0.1 ml, 0.01 ml and 0.001 ml) of the product to be examined. Incubate at 35-37 °C for 24-48 h. Subculture each of the cultures on a plate of agar medium F to obtain selective isolation. Incubate at 35-37 °C for 18-24 h. Growth of well-developed colonies, generally red or reddish, of gram-negative bacteria constitutes a positive result. Note the smallest quantity of the product which gives a positive result and the largest quantity that gives a negative result. Determine from Table 2.6.13.-1 the probable number of bacteria.

Table 2.6.13.-1

Results for each quantity of product			**Probable number of bacteria per gram of product**
0.1 g or 0.1 ml	**0.01 g or 0.01 ml**	**0.001 g or 0.001 ml**	
+	+	+	More than 10^3
+	+	–	Less than 10^3 and more than 10^2
+	–	–	Less than 10^2 and more than 10
–	–	–	Less than 10

When testing transdermal patches, filter 50 ml of preparation B as described in the general method *2.6.12* through a sterile filter membrane, place the membrane in 100 ml of enrichment broth medium E and incubate at 35-37 °C for 18-24 h. After incubation, spread on agar medium F for the detection of Enterobacteria and other gram-negative micro-organisms.

Escherichia coli

Prepare the product to be examined as described in the general method *2.6.12* and use 10 ml or the quantity corresponding to 1 g or 1 ml to inoculate 100 ml of broth medium A, homogenise and incubate at 35-37 °C for 18-48 h. Shake the container, transfer 1 ml to 100 ml of broth medium G and incubate at 43-45 °C for 18-24 h. Subculture on plates of agar medium H at 35-37 °C for 18-72 h. Growth of red, non-mucoid colonies of gram-negative rods indicates the possible presence of *E. coli*. This is confirmed by suitable biochemical tests, such as indole production. The product passes the test if such colonies are not seen or if the confirmatory biochemical tests are negative.

Salmonella

Prepare the product to be examined as described in the general method *2.6.12*, but using broth medium A in place of buffered sodium chloride-peptone solution pH 7.0, homogenise and incubate at 35-37 °C for 18-24 h. Transfer 1 ml of the enrichment culture to 10 ml of broth medium I and incubate at 41-43 °C for 18-24 h. Subculture on at least 2 different agar media chosen from agar medium J, agar medium K and agar medium L. Incubate at 35-37 °C for 18-72 h. The probable presence of salmonellae is indicated by the growth of cultures having the following appearance:

- agar medium J: well-developed, colourless colonies,
- agar medium K: well-developed, red colonies, with or without black centres,
- agar medium L: small, transparent, colourless or pink or opaque-white colonies, often surrounded by a pink or red zone.

Transfer separately a few of the suspect colonies to agar medium M in tubes, using surface and deep inoculation. The presence of salmonellae is provisionally confirmed if in the deep inoculation but not in the surface culture there is a change of colour from red to yellow and usually a formation of gas, with or without production of hydrogen sulphide in the agar. Precise confirmation may be carried out by appropriate biochemical and serological tests. The product passes the test if colonies of the type described do not appear or if the confirmatory biochemical and serological tests are negative.

Pseudomonas aeruginosa

Prepare the product to be examined as described in the general method *2.6.12* and use 10 ml or the quantity corresponding to 1 g or 1 ml to inoculate 100 ml of broth medium A, homogenise and incubate at 35-37 °C for 18-48 h. Subculture on a plate of agar medium N and incubate at 35-37 °C for 18-72 h. If no growth of micro-organisms is detected, the product passes the test. If growth of gram-negative rods occurs, transfer some material of morphologically different, isolated colonies to broth medium A and incubate at 41-43 °C for 18-24 h. The product passes the test if no growth occurs at 41-43 °C.

When testing transdermal patches, filter 50 ml of preparation A as described in the general method *2.6.12* through a sterile filter membrane and place in 100 ml of broth medium A and incubate at 35-37 °C for 18-48 h. After incubation spread on agar medium N.

Staphylococcus aureus

Prepare the product to be examined as described in the general method *2.6.12* and use 10 ml or the quantity corresponding to 1 g or 1 ml to inoculate 100 ml of broth medium A, homogenise and incubate at 35-37 °C for 18-48 h. Subculture on a plate of agar medium O and incubate at 35-37 °C for 18-72 h. Black colonies of gram-positive cocci, surrounded by a clear zone indicate the presence of *S. aureus*. Confirmation may be effected by suitable biochemical tests such as the coagulase test and the deoxyribonuclease test. The product passes the test if colonies of the type described do not appear on agar medium O or if the confirmatory biochemical tests are negative.

When testing transdermal patches, filter 50 ml of preparation A as described in the general method *2.6.12* through a sterile filter membrane and place in 100 ml of broth medium A and incubate at 35-37 °C for 18-48 h. After incubation spread on agar medium O.

Nutritive and selective properties of the media and validity of the test

The tests described hereafter must be performed at least on each lot of dehydrated media.

Proceed as follows. Grow the following test strains separately, in tubes containing suitable media such as those indicated, at 30-35 °C for 18-24 h:

Staphylococcus aureus such as ATCC 6538 (NCIMB 9518, CIP 4.83): broth medium A,

Pseudomonas aeruginosa such as ATCC 9027 (NCIMB 8626, CIP 82.118): broth medium A,

Escherichia coli — such as ATCC 8739 (NCIMB 8545, CIP 53.126): broth medium A,

Salmonella typhimurium — no strain number is recommended (a salmonella not pathogenic for man, such as *Salmonella abony* (NCTC 6017, CIP 80.39), may also be used): broth medium A.

Dilute portions of each of the cultures using buffered sodium chloride-peptone solution pH 7.0 to make test suspensions containing about 1000 viable micro-organisms per millilitre. Mix equal volumes of each suspension and use 0.4 ml (approximately 100 micro-organisms of each strain) as an inoculum in tests for *S. aureus, P. aeruginosa, E. coli* and *Salmonellae* in the presence and in the absence of the product to be examined. A positive result for the respective micro-organisms must be obtained.

Clostridia

The tests described below are intended for distinct purposes. The first method is intended for products where exclusion of pathogenic clostridia is essential and it is necessary to test for their absence. The products generally have a low total count. The second method is a semi-quantitative test for *Clostridium perfringens* and is intended for products where the level of this species is a criterion of quality.

1. *Test for Clostridia*

Prepare the product to be examined as described in the general method *2.6.12*. Take 2 equal portions corresponding to 1 g or 1 ml of the product to be examined. Heat 1 portion to 80 °C for 10 min and cool rapidly. Do not heat the other portion. Transfer 10 ml of each of the homogenised portions to 2 containers (38 mm × 200 mm) or other suitable containers containing 100 ml of medium P. Incubate under anaerobic conditions at 35-37 °C for 48 h. After incubation, make subcultures from each tube on medium Q to which gentamicin has been added and incubate under anaerobic conditions at 35-37 °C for 48 h. If no growth of micro-organisms is detected, the product passes the test.

Where growth occurs, subculture each distinct colony form on culture medium Q, without gentamicin, and incubate in both aerobic and anaerobic conditions. The occurrence of only anaerobic growth of gram-positive bacilli (with or without endospores) giving a negative catalase reaction indicates the presence of *Clostridium spp.* Compare, if necessary, colony morphology on the 2 plates and apply the catalase test to eliminate aerobic and facultatively anaerobic *Bacillus spp.* which give a positive catalase reaction. This test may be applied to discrete colonies on agar, or indirectly following transfer to a glass slide, by application of a drop of *dilute hydrogen peroxide solution R*. The formation of gas bubbles indicates a positive catalase reaction.

2. *Count of Clostridium perfringens*

Prepare the product to be examined as described in the general method *2.6.12*, and prepare 1:100 and 1:1000 dilutions in buffered sodium chloride-peptone solution pH 7.0. Determine the most probable number of bacteria as described under total viable aerobic count *2.6.12*, using culture medium R in tubes or other suitable containers with a small Durham tube. Mix with minimum shaking and incubate at 45.5-46.5 °C for 24-48 h. The containers showing a blackening due to iron sulphide and abundant formation of gas in the Durham tube (at least 1/10 of the volume) indicate the presence of *Cl. perfringens*. Estimate the most probable number of *Cl. perfringens* by means of Table 2.6.13.-2.

Table 2.6.13.-2. – *Most-probable-number (MPN) values of bacteria*

3 tubes at each level of dilution							
Number of positive tubes			MPN per gram	Category*		95 per cent confidence limits	
0.1 g	0.01 g	0.001 g		1	2		
0	0	0	< 3				–
0	1	0	3		x	< 1	17
1	0	0	3	x		1	21
1	0	1	7		x	2	27
1	1	0	7	x		2	28
1	2	0	11		x	4	35
2	0	0	9	x		2	38
2	0	1	14		x	5	48
2	1	0	15	x		5	50
2	1	1	20		x	8	61
2	2	0	21	x		8	63
3	0	0	23	x		7	129
3	0	1	38	x		10	180
3	1	0	43	x		20	210
3	1	1	75	x		20	280
3	2	0	93	x		30	390
3	2	1	150	x		50	510
3	2	2	210		x	80	640
3	3	0	240	x		100	1400
3	3	1	460	x		200	2400
3	3	2	1100	x		300	4800
3	3	3	> 1100			–	–

* Category 1: normal results, obtained in 95 per cent of cases.
Category 2: less likely results, obtained in only 4 per cent of cases. These are not to be used for important decisions. Results that are even less likely than those of category 2 are not mentioned and are always unacceptable.

Controls

Use the following test strains:

For method 1: *Clostridium sporogenes*, e.g. ATCC 19404 (NCTC 532) or CIP 79.3,

For method 2: *Clostridium perfringens*, e.g. ATCC 13124 (NCIMB 6125, NCTC 8237, CIP 103 409).

If necessary combine with *Cl. sporogenes* to check selectivity and anaerobic conditions.

The following section is published for information.

RECOMMENDED SOLUTION AND CULTURE MEDIA

The following solution and culture media have been found satisfactory for the purposes for which they are prescribed in the test for microbial contamination in the Pharmacopoeia. Other media may be used if they have similar nutritive and selective properties for the micro-organisms to be tested for.

Buffered sodium chloride-peptone solution pH 7.0

Potassium dihydrogen phosphate	3.6 g
Disodium hydrogen phosphate dihydrate	7.2 g, equivalent to 0.067 M phosphate
Sodium chloride	4.3 g
Peptone (meat or casein)	1.0 g
Purified water	1000 ml

To this solution surface-active agents or inactivators of antimicrobial agents may be added, such as:

Polysorbate 80	1 g/l to 10 g/l

Sterilise by heating in an autoclave at 121 °C for 15 min.

Broth medium A (Casein soya bean digest broth)

Pancreatic digest of casein	17.0 g
Papaic digest of soya bean	3.0 g
Sodium chloride	5.0 g
Dipotassium hydrogen phosphate	2.5 g
Glucose monohydrate	2.5 g
Purified water	1000 ml

Adjust the pH so that after sterilisation it is 7.3 ± 0.2. Sterilise by heating in an autoclave at 121 °C for 15 min.

Agar medium B (Casein soya bean digest agar)

Pancreatic digest of casein	15.0 g
Papaic digest of soya bean	5.0 g
Sodium chloride	5.0 g
Agar	15.0 g
Purified water	1000 ml

Adjust the pH so that after sterilisation it is 7.3 ± 0.2. Sterilise by heating in an autoclave at 121 °C for 15 min.

Agar medium C (Sabouraud-glucose agar with antibiotics)

Peptones (meat and casein)	10.0 g
Glucose monohydrate	40.0 g
Agar	15.0 g
Purified water	1000 ml

Adjust the pH so that after sterilisation it is 5.6 ± 0.2. Sterilise by heating in an autoclave at 121 °C for 15 min. Immediately before use, add 0.10 g of benzylpenicillin sodium and 0.10 g of tetracycline per litre of medium as sterile solutions or, alternatively, add 50 mg of chloramphenicol per litre of medium before sterilisation.

Broth medium D (Lactose monohydrate broth)

Beef extract	3.0 g
Pancreatic digest of gelatin	5.0 g
Lactose monohydrate	5.0 g
Purified water	1000 ml

Adjust the pH so that after sterilisation it is 6.9 ± 0.2. Sterilise by heating in an autoclave at 121 °C for 15 min and cool immediately.

Enrichment broth medium E (Enterobacteria enrichment broth-Mossel)

Pancreatic digest of gelatin	10.0 g
Glucose monohydrate	5.0 g
Dehydrated ox bile	20.0 g
Potassium dihydrogen phosphate	2.0 g
Disodium hydrogen phosphate dihydrate	8.0 g
Brilliant green	15 mg
Purified water	1000 ml

Adjust the pH so that after heating it is 7.2 ± 0.2. Heat at 100 °C for 30 min and cool immediately.

Agar medium F (Crystal violet, neutral red, bile agar with glucose)

Yeast extract	3.0 g
Pancreatic digest of gelatin	7.0 g
Bile salts	1.5 g
Lactose monohydrate	10.0 g
Sodium chloride	5.0 g
Glucose monohydrate	10.0 g
Agar	15.0 g
Neutral red	30 mg
Crystal violet	2 mg
Purified water	1000 ml

Adjust the pH so that after heating it is 7.4 ± 0.2. Heat to boiling; do not heat in an autoclave.

Broth medium G (MacConkey broth)

Pancreatic digest of gelatin	20.0 g
Lactose monohydrate	10.0 g
Dehydrated ox bile	5.0 g
Bromocresol purple	10 mg
Purified water	1000 ml

Adjust the pH so that after sterilisation it is 7.3 ± 0.2. Sterilise by heating in an autoclave at 121 °C for 15 min.

Agar medium H (MacConkey agar)

Pancreatic digest of gelatin	17.0 g
Peptones (meat and casein)	3.0 g
Lactose monohydrate	10.0 g
Sodium chloride	5.0 g
Bile salts	1.5 g
Agar	13.5 g
Neutral red	30.0 mg
Crystal violet	1 mg
Purified water	1000 ml

Adjust the pH so that after sterilisation it is 7.1 ± 0.2. Boil for 1 min with constant shaking then sterilise by heating in an autoclave at 121 °C for 15 min.

Broth medium I (Tetrathionate bile brilliant green broth)

Peptone	8.6 g
Ox bile, dried	8.0 g
Sodium chloride	6.4 g
Calcium carbonate	20.0 g
Potassium tetrathionate	20.0 g
Brilliant green	70 mg
Purified water	1000 ml

Adjust the pH so that after heating it is 7.0 ± 0.2. Heat just to boiling. Do not re-heat.

Agar medium J (Deoxycholate citrate agar)

Beef extract	10.0 g
Meat peptone	10.0 g
Lactose monohydrate	10.0 g
Sodium citrate	20.0 g

Ferric citrate	1.0 g
Sodium deoxycholate	5.0 g
Agar	13.5 g
Neutral red	20 mg
Purified water	1000 ml

Adjust the pH so that after heating it is 7.3 ± 0.2. Heat gently to boiling and boil for 1 min, cool to 50 °C and pour into Petri dishes. Do not heat in an autoclave.

Agar medium K (Xylose, lysine, deoxycholate agar)

Xylose	3.5 g
L-Lysine	5.0 g
Lactose monohydrate	7.5 g
Sucrose	7.5 g
Sodium chloride	5.0 g
Yeast extract	3.0 g
Phenol red	80 mg
Agar	13.5 g
Sodium deoxycholate	2.5 g
Sodium thiosulphate	6.8 g
Ferric ammonium citrate	0.8 g
Purified water	1000 ml

Adjust the pH so that after heating it is 7.4 ± 0.2. Heat just to boiling, cool to 50 °C and pour into Petri dishes. Do not heat in an autoclave.

Agar medium L (Brilliant green, phenol red, lactose monohydrate, sucrose agar)

Peptones (meat and casein)	10.0 g
Yeast extract	3.0 g
Sodium chloride	5.0 g
Lactose monohydrate	10.0 g
Sucrose	10.0 g
Agar	20.0 g
Phenol red	80 mg
Brilliant green	12.5 mg
Purified water	1000 ml

Heat to boiling for 1 min. Adjust the pH so that after sterilisation it is 6.9 ± 0.2. Immediately before use, sterilise by heating in an autoclave at 121 °C for 15 min, cool to 50 °C and pour into Petri dishes.

Agar medium M (Triple sugar, iron agar)

Beef extract	3.0 g
Yeast extract	3.0 g
Peptones (casein and beef)	20.0 g
Sodium chloride	5.0 g
Lactose monohydrate	10.0 g
Sucrose	10.0 g
Glucose monohydrate	1.0 g
Ferric ammonium citrate	0.3 g
Sodium thiosulphate	0.3 g
Phenol red	25 mg
Agar	12.0 g
Purified water	1000 ml

Heat to boiling for 1 min with shaking. Adjust the pH so that after sterilisation it is 7.4 ± 0.2. Fill into tubes to one-third of their height, sterilise by heating in an autoclave at 121 °C for 15 min and allow to cool in a position that gives a deep portion and a sloping surface.

Agar medium N (Cetrimide agar)

Pancreatic digest of gelatin	20.0 g
Magnesium chloride	1.4 g
Dipotassium sulphate	10.0 g
Cetrimide	0.3 g
Agar	13.6 g
Purified water	1000 ml
Glycerol	10.0 ml

Heat to boiling for 1 min with shaking. Adjust the pH so that after sterilisation it is 7.2 ± 0.2. Sterilise by heating in an autoclave at 121 °C for 15 min.

Agar medium O (Baird-Parker agar)

Pancreatic digest of casein	10.0 g
Beef extract	5.0 g
Yeast extract	1.0 g
Lithium chloride	5.0 g
Agar	20.0 g
Glycine	12.0 g
Sodium pyruvate	10.0 g
Purified water	950 ml

Heat to boiling for 1 min with shaking. Adjust the pH so that after sterilisation it is 6.8 ± 0.2. Sterilise by heating in an autoclave at 121 °C for 15 min, cool to 45-50 °C and add 10 ml of a sterile 10 g/l solution of potassium tellurite and 50 ml of egg-yolk emulsion.

Medium P (Reinforced medium for clostridia)

Beef extract	10.0 g
Peptone	10.0 g
Yeast extract	3.0 g
Soluble starch	1.0 g
Glucose monohydrate	5.0 g
Cysteine hydrochloride	0.5 g
Sodium chloride	5.0 g
Sodium acetate	3.0 g
Agar	0.5 g
Purified water	1000 ml

Hydrate the agar, dissolve by heating to boiling with continuous stirring. If necessary, adjust the pH so that after sterilisation it is about 6.8. Sterilise by heating in an autoclave at 121 °C for 15 min.

Medium Q (Columbia agar)

Pancreatic digest of casein	10.0 g
Meat peptic digest	5.0 g
Heart pancreatic digest	3.0 g
Yeast extract	5.0 g

Maize starch	1.0 g
Sodium chloride	5.0 g
Agar, according to gelling power	10.0 g to 15.0 g
Purified water	1000 ml

Hydrate the agar, dissolve by heating to boiling with continuous stirring. If necessary, adjust the pH so that after sterilisation it is 7.3 ± 0.2. Sterilise by heating in an autoclave at 121 °C for 15 min. Allow to cool to 45-50 °C; add, where necessary, gentamicin sulphate corresponding to 20 mg of gentamicin base and pour into Petri dishes.

Medium R (Lactose monohydrate sulphite medium)

Pancreatic digest of casein	5.0 g
Yeast extract	2.5 g
Sodium chloride	2.5 g
Lactose monohydrate	10.0 g
Cysteine hydrochloride	0.3 g
Purified water	1000 ml

Dissolve, adjust to pH 7.1 ± 0.1 and fill to 8 ml in 16 mm × 160 mm tubes containing a small Durham tube. Sterilise by heating in an autoclave at 121 °C for 15 min and store at 4 °C.

Before use, heat the medium for 5 min in a water-bath and cool. Add to each tube 0.5 ml of a 12 g/l solution of *sodium metabisulphite R* and 0.5 ml of a 10 g/l solution of ferric ammonium citrate, both solutions being freshly prepared and filtered through membranes (pore size: 0.45 μm).

Agar medium S (R2A)

Yeast extract	0.5 g
Proteose peptone	0.5 g
Casein hydrolysate	0.5 g
Glucose	0.5 g
Starch	0.5 g
Dipotassium hydrogen phosphate	0.3 g
Magnesium sulphate, anhydrous	0.024 g
Sodium pyruvate	0.3 g
Agar	15.0 g
Purified water	1000 ml

Adjust the pH so that after sterilisation it is 7.2 ± 0.2. Sterilise by heating in an autoclave at 121 °C for 15 min.

NEUTRALISING AGENTS

Neutralising agents may be used to neutralise the activity of antimicrobial agents. They may be added to buffered sodium chloride-peptone solution pH 7.0, preferably before sterilisation. If utilised their efficacy and non-toxicity towards micro-organisms are demonstrated.

A typical neutralising fluid has the following composition:

Polysorbate 80	30 g
Lecithin (egg)	3 g
Histidine hydrochloride	1 g
Peptone (meat or casein)	1 g
Sodium chloride	4.3 g
Potassium dihydrogen phosphate	3.6 g
Disodium hydrogen phosphate dihydrate	7.2 g
Purified water	1000 ml

Sterilise by heating in an autoclave at 121 °C for 15 min.

If the solution has insufficient neutralising capacity the concentration of polysorbate 80 or lecithin may be increased. Alternatively, the neutralisers mentioned in Table 2.6.13.-3 may be added.

Table 2.6.13.-3. – *Inactivators for antimicrobial agents to be added to buffered sodium chloride-peptone solution pH 7.0*

Type of antimicrobial agent	Inactivator	Concentration	Comment
Phenolics	Sodium laurilsulfate	4 g/l	Add after sterilisation of buffered sodium chloride-peptone solution pH 7.0
	Polysorbate 80 and lecithin	30 g/l and 3 g/l	
	Egg yolk	5 ml/l - 50 ml/l	
Organo-mercurals	Sodium thioglycolate	0.5 g/l - 5 g/l	
Halogens	Sodium thiosulphate	5 g/l	
Quaternary ammonium compounds	Egg yolk	5 ml/l - 50 ml/l	Add after sterilisation of buffered sodium chloride-peptone solution pH 7.0

01/2005:20614

2.6.14. BACTERIAL ENDOTOXINS

The test for bacterial endotoxins is used to detect or quantify endotoxins of gram-negative bacterial origin using amoebocyte lysate from horseshoe crab (*Limulus polyphemus* or *Tachypleus tridentatus*). There are 3 techniques for this test: the gel-clot technique, which is based on gel formation; the turbidimetric technique, based on the development of turbidity after cleavage of an endogenous substrate; and the chromogenic technique, based on the development of colour after cleavage of a synthetic peptide-chromogen complex.

The following 6 methods are described in the present chapter:

Method A. Gel-clot method: limit test

Method B. Gel-clot method: semi-quantitative test

Method C. Turbidimetric kinetic method

Method D. Chromogenic kinetic method

Method E. Chromogenic end-point method

Method F. Turbidimetric end-point method

Proceed by any of the 6 methods for the test. In the event of doubt or dispute, the final decision is made based upon method A unless otherwise indicated in the monograph.

The test is carried out in a manner that avoids endotoxin contamination.

Apparatus

Depyrogenate all glassware and other heat-stable apparatus in a hot-air oven using a validated process. A commonly used minimum time and temperature is 30 minutes at 250 °C. If employing plastic apparatus, such as microtitre plates and pipette tips for automatic pipetters, use apparatus shown to be free of detectable endotoxin and of interfering effects for the test.

NOTE: In this chapter, the term 'tube' includes all types of receptacles, for example microtitre plate wells.

Preparation of the standard endotoxin stock solution

The standard endotoxin stock solution is prepared from an endotoxin reference standard that has been calibrated against the International Standard, for example *endotoxin standard BRP*.

Endotoxin is expressed in International Units (IU). The equivalence in IU of the International Standard is stated by the World Health Organisation.

NOTE: One International Unit (IU) of endotoxin is equal to one Endotoxin Unit (E.U.).

Follow the specifications in the package leaflet and on the label for preparation and storage of the standard endotoxin stock solution.

Preparation of the standard endotoxin solutions

After vigorously mixing the standard endotoxin stock solution, prepare appropriate serial dilutions of this solution using water for bacterial endotoxins test (water for BET).

Use the solutions as soon as possible to avoid loss of activity by adsorption.

Preparation of the test solutions

Prepare the test solutions by dissolving or diluting active substances or medicinal products using water for BET. Some substances or preparations may be more appropriately dissolved or diluted in other aqueous solutions. If necessary, adjust the pH of the test solution (or dilution thereof) so that the pH of the mixture of the lysate and test solution falls within the pH range specified by the lysate manufacturer. This usually applies to a product with a pH in the range of 6.0 to 8.0. The pH may be adjusted by the use of acid, base or a suitable buffer, as recommended by the lysate manufacturer. Acids and bases may be prepared from concentrates or solids with water for BET in containers free of detectable endotoxin. Buffers must be validated to be free of detectable endotoxin and interfering factors.

Determination of the Maximum Valid Dilution

The Maximum Valid Dilution (MVD) is the maximum allowable dilution of a sample at which the endotoxin limit can be determined. Determine the MVD using the following formulae:

$$\text{MVD} = \frac{\text{endotoxin limit} \times \text{concentration of test solution}}{\lambda}$$

Endotoxin limit: the endotoxin limit for active substances administered parenterally, defined on the basis of dose, is equal to:

$$\frac{K}{M}$$

K = threshold pyrogenic dose of endotoxin per kilogram of body mass in a single hour period,

M = maximum recommended dose of product per kilogram of body mass in a single hour period.

The endotoxin limit for active substances administered parenterally is specified in units such as IU/ml, IU/mg, IU/Unit of biological activity, etc., in monographs.

Concentration of test solution:

- in mg/ml if the endotoxin limit is specified by mass (IU/mg),
- in Units/ml if the endotoxin limit is specified by unit of biological activity (IU/Unit),
- in ml/ml if the endotoxin limit is specified by volume (IU/ml).

λ = the labelled lysate sensitivity in the gel-clot technique (IU/ml) or the lowest point used in the standard curve of the turbidimetric or chromogenic techniques.

GEL-CLOT TECHNIQUE (METHODS A AND B)

The gel-clot technique allows detection or quantification of endotoxins and is based on clotting of the lysate in the presence of endotoxins. The concentration of endotoxins required to cause the lysate to clot under standard conditions is the labelled lysate sensitivity. To ensure both the precision and validity of the test, confirm the labelled lysate sensitivity and perform the test for interfering factors as described under *1. Preparatory testing.*

1. PREPARATORY TESTING

(i) Confirmation of the labelled lysate sensitivity

Confirm in 4 replicates the labelled sensitivity λ, expressed in IU/ml, of the lysate solution prior to use in the test. Confirmation of the lysate sensitivity is carried out when a new batch of lysate is used or when there is any change in the experimental conditions which may affect the outcome of the test.

Prepare standard solutions of at least 4 concentrations equivalent to 2λ, λ, 0.5λ and 0.25λ by diluting the standard endotoxin stock solution with water for BET.

Mix a volume of the lysate solution with an equal volume of 1 of the standard solutions (such as 0.1 ml aliquots) in each tube. When single test vials or ampoules containing lyophilised lysate are employed, add solutions directly to the vial or ampoule. Incubate the reaction mixture for a constant period according to the recommendations of the lysate manufacturer (usually at 37 ± 1 °C for 60 ± 2 min), avoiding vibration. Test the integrity of the gel: for tubes, take each tube in turn directly from the incubator and invert it through approximately 180° in one smooth motion. If a firm gel has formed that remains in place upon inversion, record the result as positive. A result is negative if an intact gel is not formed.

The test is not valid unless the lowest concentration of the standard solutions shows a negative result in all replicate tests.

The end-point is the last positive result in the series of decreasing concentrations of endotoxin. Calculate the mean value of the logarithms of the end-point concentrations and then the antilogarithm of the mean value using the following expression:

$$\text{Geometric mean end-point concentration} = \text{antilog} \frac{\sum e}{f}$$

$\sum e$ = sum of the log end-point concentrations of the dilution series used,

f = number of replicates.

The geometric mean end-point concentration is the measured sensitivity of the lysate solution (IU/ml). If this is not less than 0.5λ and not more than 2λ, the labelled sensitivity is confirmed and is used in the tests performed with this lysate.

(ii) Test for interfering factors

Prepare solutions A, B, C and D as shown in Table 2.6.14.-1, and use the test solutions at a dilution less than the MVD, not containing any detectable endotoxins, operating as described under 1. Preparatory testing, (i) Confirmation of the labelled lysate sensitivity.

Table 2.6.14.-1

Solution	Endotoxin concentration/ Solution to which endotoxin is added	Diluent	Dilution factor	Initial endotoxin concentration	Number of replicates
A	None/Test solution	-	-	-	4
B	2λ/Test solution	Test solution	1	2λ	4
			2	1λ	4
			4	0.5λ	4
			8	0.25λ	4
C	2λ/Water for BET	Water for BET	1	2λ	2
			2	1λ	2
			4	0.5λ	2
			8	0.25λ	2
D	None/Water for BET	-	-	-	2

Solution A = solution of the preparation being examined that is free of detectable endotoxins.
Solution B = test for interference.
Solution C = control of the labelled lysate sensitivity.
Solution D = negative control (water for BET).

The geometric mean end-point concentrations of solutions B and C are determined using the expression described in 1. Preparatory testing, (i) Confirmation of the labelled lysate sensitivity.

The test for interfering factors is repeated when any changes are made to the experimental conditions that are likely to influence the result of the test.

The test is not valid unless all replicates of solutions A and D show no reaction and the result of solution C confirms the labelled lysate sensitivity.

If the sensitivity of the lysate determined with solution B is not less than 0.5λ and not greater than 2λ, the test solution does not contain interfering factors under the experimental conditions used. Otherwise, the solution interferes with the test.

If the preparation being examined interferes with the test at a dilution less than the MVD, repeat the test for interfering factors using a greater dilution, not exceeding the MVD. The use of a more sensitive lysate permits a greater dilution of the preparation being examined and this may contribute to the elimination of interference.

Interference may be overcome by suitable treatment, such as filtration, neutralisation, dialysis or heat treatment. To establish that the treatment chosen effectively eliminates interference without loss of endotoxins, repeat the test for interfering factors using the preparation being examined to which the standard endotoxin has been added and which has then been submitted to the chosen treatment.

2. LIMIT TEST (METHOD A)

(i) Procedure

Prepare solutions A, B, C and D as shown in Table 2.6.14.-2, and perform the test on these solutions following the procedure described under 1. Preparatory testing, (i) Confirmation of the labelled lysate sensitivity.

Table 2.6.14.-2

Solution	Endotoxin concentration/ Solution to which endotoxin is added	Number of replicates
A	None/Diluted test solution	2
B	2λ/Diluted test solution	2
C	2λ/Water for BET	2
D	None/Water for BET	2

Prepare solution A and solution B (positive product control) using a dilution not greater than the MVD and treatments as described in 1. Preparatory testing, (ii) Test for interfering factors. Solutions B and C (positive controls) contain the standard endotoxin at a concentration corresponding to twice the labelled lysate sensitivity. Solution D (negative control) consists of water for BET.

(ii) Interpretation

The test is not valid unless both replicates of the 2 positive control solutions B and C are positive and those of the negative control solution D are negative.

The preparation being examined complies with the test when a negative result is found for both replicates of solution A.

When a positive result is found for both replicates of solution A:

– if the preparation being examined is diluted to the MVD, it does not comply with the test,
– if the preparation being examined is diluted to a dilution less than the MVD, the test is repeated at a dilution not greater than the MVD.

Repeat the test if a positive result is found for one replicate of solution A and a negative result is found for the other. The preparation being examined complies with the test if a negative result is found for both replicates of solution A in the repeat test.

3. SEMI-QUANTITATIVE TEST (METHOD B)

(i) Procedure

The test quantifies bacterial endotoxins in the test solution by titration to an end-point. Prepare solutions A, B, C and D as shown in Table 2.6.14.-3, and test these solutions according to the procedure described under 1. Preparatory testing, (i) Confirmation of the labelled lysate sensitivity.

(ii) Calculation and interpretation

The test is not valid unless the following 3 conditions are met:

(a) both replicates of solution D (negative control) are negative,

(b) both replicates of solution B (positive product control) are positive,

(c) the geometric mean end-point concentration of solution C is in the range of 0.5λ to 2λ.

To determine the endotoxin concentration of solution A, calculate the end-point concentration for each replicate series of dilutions by multiplying each end-point dilution factor by λ.

The endotoxin concentration in the test solution is the geometric mean end-point concentration of the replicates (see the expression given under 1. Preparatory testing, (i) Confirmation of the labelled lysate sensitivity). If the test is conducted with a diluted test solution, calculate the concentration of endotoxin in the original solution by multiplying the result by the dilution factor.

If none of the dilutions of the test solution is positive in a valid test, record the endotoxin concentration as less than λ (or, if a diluted sample was tested, as less than λ × the lowest dilution factor of the sample). If all dilutions are positive, the endotoxin concentration is recorded as equal to or greater than the greatest dilution factor multiplied by λ (e.g. in Table 2.6.14.-3, the initial dilution factor × 8 × λ).

The preparation meets the requirements of the test if the endotoxin concentration is less than that specified in the individual monograph.

PHOTOMETRIC TECHNIQUES (METHODS C, D, E AND F)

1. TURBIDIMETRIC TECHNIQUE (METHODS C AND F)

This technique is a photometric test to measure the increase in turbidity. Based on the test principle employed, this technique is classified as being the end-point-turbidimetric test or the kinetic-turbidimetric test.

The end-point-turbidimetric test (Method F) is based on the quantitative relationship between the endotoxin concentration and the turbidity (absorbance or transmission) of the reaction mixture at the end of an incubation period.

The kinetic-turbidimetric test (Method C) is a method to measure either the time (onset time) needed for the reaction mixture to reach a predetermined absorbance, or the rate of turbidity development.

The test is carried out at the incubation temperature recommended by the lysate manufacturer (usually 37 ± 1 °C).

2. CHROMOGENIC TECHNIQUE (METHODS D AND E)

This technique is used to measure the chromophore released from a suitable chromogenic peptide by the reaction of endotoxins with the lysate. Depending on the test principle employed, this technique is classified as being the end-point-chromogenic test or the kinetic-chromogenic test.

The end-point-chromogenic test (Method E) is based on the quantitative relationship between the endotoxin concentration and the quantity of chromophore released at the end of an incubation period.

The kinetic-chromogenic test (Method D) measures either the time (onset time) needed for the reaction mixture to reach a predetermined absorbance, or the rate of colour development.

The test is carried out at the incubation temperature recommended by the lysate manufacturer (usually 37 ± 1 °C).

3. PREPARATORY TESTING

To assure the precision or validity of the turbidimetric and chromogenic tests, preparatory tests are conducted to assure that the criteria for the standard curve are satisfied and that the test solution does not interfere with the test.

Validation of the test method is required when any changes are made to the experimental conditions that are likely to influence the result of the test.

(i) Assurance of criteria for the standard curve

Using the standard endotoxin solution, prepare at least 3 endotoxin concentrations to generate the standard curve. Perform the test using at least 3 replicates of each standard endotoxin solution as recommended by the lysate manufacturer (volume ratios, incubation time, temperature, pH, etc.).

If the desired range is greater than 2 log in the kinetic methods, additional standards must be included to bracket each log increase in the range of the standard curve.

The absolute value of the correlation coefficient, | r |, must be greater than or equal to 0.980, for the range of endotoxin concentrations indicated by the lysate manufacturer.

(ii) Test for interfering factors

Select an endotoxin concentration at or near the middle of the endotoxin standard curve.

Prepare solutions A, B, C and D as shown in Table 2.6.14.-4. Perform the test on at least 2 replicates of these solutions as recommended by the lysate manufacturer (volume of test solution and lysate solution, volume ratio of test solution to lysate solution, incubation time, etc.).

Table 2.6.14.-3

Solution	Endotoxin concentration/ Solution to which endotoxin is added	Diluent	Dilution factor	Initial endotoxin concentration	Number of replicates
A	None/Test solution	Water for BET	1	-	2
			2	-	2
			4	-	2
			8	-	2
B	2λ/Test solution		1	2λ	2
C	2λ/Water for BET	Water for BET	1	2λ	2
			2	1λ	2
			4	0.5λ	2
			8	0.25λ	2
D	None/Water for BET	-	-	-	2

Solution A = test solution at the dilution, not exceeding the MVD, with which the test for interfering factors was carried out. Subsequent dilution of the test solution must not exceed the MVD. Use water for BET to make two dilution series of 1, 1/2, 1/4 and 1/8, relative to the dilution with which the test for interfering factors was carried out. Other dilutions may be used as appropriate.

Solution B = solution A containing standard endotoxin at a concentration of 2λ (positive product control).

Solution C = 2 series of water for BET containing the standard endotoxin at concentrations of 2λ, λ, 0.5λ and 0.25λ.

Solution D = water for BET (negative control).

Table 2.6.14.-4.

Solution	Endotoxin concentration	Solution to which endotoxin is added	Number of replicates
A	None	Test solution	Not less than 2
B	Middle concentration of the standard curve	Test solution	Not less than 2
C	At least 3 concentrations (lowest concentration is designated λ)	Water for BET	Each concentration not less than 2
D	None	Water for BET	Not less than 2

Solution A = test solution, that may be diluted not to exceed the MVD.

Solution B = preparation to be examined at the same dilution as solution A, containing added endotoxin at a concentration equal to or near the middle of the standard curve.

Solution C = standard endotoxin solution at the concentrations used in the validation of the method as described under 3. Preparatory testing, (i) Assurance of criteria for the standard curve (positive controls.

Solution D = water for BET (negative control).

Calculate the mean recovery of the added endotoxin by subtracting the mean endotoxin concentration in the solution (if any) from that in the solution containing the added endotoxin.

The test solution is considered free of interfering factors if under the conditions of the test, the measured concentration of the endotoxin added to the test solution is within 50-200 per cent of the known added endotoxin concentration, after subtraction of any endotoxin detected in the solution without added endotoxin.

When the endotoxin recovery is out of the specified ranges, the interfering factors must be removed as described in the section Gel-clot technique, under 1. Preparatory testing, (ii) Test for interfering factors. The efficiency of the treatment is verified by repeating the test for interfering factors.

4. TEST

(i) Procedure

Follow the procedure described in 3. Preparatory testing, (ii) Test for interfering factors.

(ii) Calculation

Calculate the endotoxin concentration of each replicate of solution A using the standard curve generated by the series of positive controls, solution C.

The test is not valid unless the following 3 requirements are met:

(a) the result obtained with solution D (negative control) does not exceed the limit of the blank value required in the description of the lysate employed,

(b) the results obtained with the series of positive controls, solution C, comply with the requirements for validation defined under 3. Preparatory testing, (i) Assurance of criteria for the standard curve,

(c) the endotoxin recovery, calculated from the endotoxin concentration found in solution B after subtracting the endotoxin concentration found in solution A, is within the range of 50-200 per cent.

(iii) Interpretation

The preparation being examined complies with the test if the mean endotoxin concentration of the replicates of solution A, after correction for dilution and concentration, is less than the endotoxin limit for the product.

5. REAGENTS

(i) Lysate solution

Dissolve amoebocyte lysate in water for BET or in a buffer, as recommended by the lysate manufacturer, by gentle stirring. Store the reconstituted lysate, refrigerated or frozen, as indicated by the manufacturer.

(ii) Amoebocyte lysate

Amoebocyte lysate is a lyophilised product obtained from amoebocyte lysate from Horseshoe Crab (*Limulus polyphemus* or *Tachypleus tridentatus*). This reagent refers only to a product manufactured in accordance with the regulations of the competent authority.

Amoebocyte lysate reacts with some β-glucans in addition to endotoxins. Amoebocyte lysate preparations which do not react with glucans are available; they are prepared by removing from amoebocyte lysate the G factor, which reacts with glucans, or by inhibiting the G factor reacting system of amoebocyte lysate. These preparations may be used for endotoxin testing in the presence of glucans.

(iii) Water for BET (water for bacterial endotoxins test)

Water for BET is *water for injections R* or water produced by other procedures that shows no reaction with the lysate employed at the detection limit of the reagent.

The following section is published for information.

Test for bacterial endotoxins: guidelines

1. INTRODUCTION

Endotoxins from gram-negative bacteria are the most common cause of toxic reactions resulting from contamination of pharmaceutical products with pyrogens; their pyrogenic activity is much higher than that of most other pyrogenic substances. These endotoxins are lipo-polysaccharides. Although there are a small number of pyrogens which possess a different structure, the conclusion is generally justified that the absence of bacterial endotoxins in a product implies the absence of pyrogenic components, provided the presence of non-endotoxin pyrogenic substances can be ruled out.

The presence of endotoxins in a product may be masked by factors interfering with the reaction between the endotoxins and the amoebocyte lysate. Hence, the analyst who wishes to replace the rabbit pyrogen test required in a pharmacopoeial monograph by a test for bacterial endotoxins has to demonstrate that a valid test can be carried out on the product concerned; this may entail a procedure for removing interfering factors.

As indicated in the test for bacterial endotoxins, information must be available on the 2 following aspects before a test on a sample can be regarded as valid.

1.1. The suitability of the material to be used for the test has to be established. The absence of endotoxins in the water for BET and in the other reagents must be assured and the sensitivity of the amoebocyte lysate must be checked to confirm the sensitivity declared by the manufacturer.

1.2. As the product to be examined may interfere with the test, the sensitivity of the amoebocyte lysate is determined in the presence and in the absence of the product under examination. There must be no significant difference between the 2 sensitivity values.

The test for bacterial endotoxins (*2.6.14*) indicates methods for removing interfering factors; in the case of interference, another test must be carried out after such a method has been applied to check whether the interference has indeed been neutralised or removed.

This annex explains the reasons for the requirements in the test for bacterial endotoxins, then deals with the reading and interpretation of the results.

Substitution of the rabbit pyrogen test required in a pharmacopoeial monograph by an amoebocyte lysate test constitutes the use of an alternative method of analysis and hence requires validation; some guidance on how to proceed is given in section 11.

The reference method for bacterial endotoxins is stated in the monograph on a given product; where no method is stated, method A is the reference method. If a method other than the reference method is to be used, the analyst must demonstrate that the method is appropriate for this product and gives a result consistent with that obtained with the reference method (see also Section 13).

2. METHOD

The addition of endotoxins to amoebocyte lysate may result in turbidity, precipitation or gelation (gel-clot); only the gel-clot method was used in the Pharmacopoeia as an evaluation criterion in the first type of test for bacterial endotoxins. The advantage was the simplicity of basing the decision to pass or fail the product under examination on the absence or presence of a gel-clot, visible with the naked eye. The quantitative methods described as methods C, D, E and F were developed later: they require more instrumentation, but they are easier to automate for the regular testing of large numbers of samples of the same product.

Endotoxins may be adsorbed onto the surface of tubes or pipettes made from certain plastics or types of glass. Interference may appear due to the release of substances from plastic materials. Hence, the materials used should be checked; subsequent batches of tubes or pipettes may have a slightly different composition, and therefore the analyst is advised to repeat such tests on starting with new batches of materials.

The decision to use the test for bacterial endotoxins as a limit test implies first, that a threshold endotoxin concentration must be defined for the product to be tested and second, that the objective of the test is to know whether the endotoxin concentration in the product under examination is below or above this threshold. The quantitative methods C, D, E and F make it possible to determine the endotoxin concentration in the sample under examination, but for compliance with the Pharmacopoeia and in routine quality control the final question is whether or not this concentration exceeds a defined limit.

In setting a threshold concentration of endotoxin for the product to be tested, due attention should be paid to the dose of the product: the threshold should be set so as to ensure that as long as the endotoxin concentration in the product remains below this threshold even the maximal dose administered by the intended route per hour does not contain sufficient endotoxin to cause a toxic reaction.

When the endotoxin concentration in the product exactly equals the threshold value, gelation will occur, as is the case when the endotoxin concentration is much higher, and the product will fail the test, because the all-or-none character of the test makes it impossible to differentiate between a concentration exactly equal to the threshold concentration and one that is higher. It is only when no gelation occurs that the analyst may conclude that the endotoxin concentration is below the threshold concentration.

For products in the solid state, this threshold concentration of endotoxin per mass unit or per International Unit (IU) of product has to be translated into a concentration of endotoxin per millilitre of solution to be tested, as the test can only be carried out on a solution. The case of products that already exist in the liquid state (such as infusion fluids) is discussed below.

Endotoxin limit: the endotoxin limit for active substances administered parenterally, defined on the basis of dose, is equal to, where:

$$\frac{K}{M}$$

K = threshold pyrogenic dose of endotoxin per kilogram of body mass in a single hour period,

M = maximum recommended dose of product per kilogram of body mass in a single hour period.

The endotoxin limit depends on the product and its route of administration and is stated in monographs. Values for K are suggested in Table 2.6.14.-5.

For other routes, the acceptance criterion for bacterial endotoxins is generally determined on the basis of results obtained during the development of the preparation.

Table 2.6.14.-5

Route of administration	K (IU of endotoxin per kilogram of body mass per hour)
Intravenous	5.0
Intravanous, for radiopharmaceuticals	2.5
Intrathecal	0.2

Which dilution of the product is to be used in the test to obtain maximal assurance that a negative result means that the endotoxin concentration of the product is less than the endotoxin limit and that a positive result means that the lysate detected an endotoxin concentration equal to or greater than the endotoxin limit? This dilution depends on the endotoxin limit and on the sensitivity of the lysate: it is called the Maximum Valid Dilution (MVD) and its value may be calculated as follows:

$$\text{MVD} = \frac{\text{endotoxin limit} \times \text{concentration of test solution}}{\lambda}$$

Concentration of test solution:

- in mg/ml if the endotoxin limit is specified by mass (IU/mg),
- in Units/ml if the endotoxin limit is specified by unit of biological activity (IU/Unit),
- in ml/ml if the endotoxin limit is specified by volume (IU/ml).

λ = the labelled lysate sensitivity in the gel-clot technique (IU/ml) or the lowest point used in the standard curve of the turbidimetric or chromogenic techniques.

When the value of the maximum valid dilution is not a whole number, a convenient whole number smaller than the MVD may be used for routine purposes (which means preparing a solution of the product which is less diluted than the MVD indicates). In this case, a negative result indicates that the endotoxin concentration of the product lies below the limit value. However, when the endotoxin concentration of the product in such a test is less than the endotoxin limit but high enough to make the reaction with the lysate result in a clot, the test may be positive under these conditions. Hence, when a test with this 'convenient' dilution factor is positive, the product should be diluted to the MVD and the test should be repeated. In any case of doubt or dispute the MVD must be used.

This stresses the importance of the confirmation of the sensitivity of the lysate.

Example

A 50 mg/ml solution of phenytoin sodium (intended for intravenous injection) has to be tested. Determine the MVD, given the following variables:

M = maximum human dose = 15 mg per kilogram of body mass per hour,

c = 50 mg/ml,

K = 5 IU of endotoxin per kilogram of body mass per hour,

λ = 0.4 IU of endotoxin per millilitre.

$$\text{MVD} = \frac{5 \times 50}{15} \times \frac{1}{0.4} = 41.67$$

For routine tests on this product, it may be expedient to dilute 1 ml of the solution to be tested to 20 ml (MVD/2 rounded to the next lower whole number). However, if this test result is positive the analyst will have to dilute 1 ml to 41.67 ml and repeat the test. A dilution to 41.67 ml is also necessary when the test is performed to settle a dispute.

3. REFERENCE MATERIAL

Endotoxin standard BRP is intended for use as the reference preparation. It has been assayed against the WHO International Standard for Endotoxin and its potency is expressed in International Units of endotoxin per ampoule. The International Unit of endotoxin is defined as the specific activity of a defined mass of the International Standard.

For routine purposes, another preparation of endotoxin may be used, provided it has been assayed against the International Standard for Endotoxin or the BRP and its potency is expressed in International Units of endotoxin.

NOTE: 1 International Unit (IU) of endotoxin is equal to 1 Endotoxin Unit (E.U.).

4. WATER FOR BET

Testing the absence of endotoxin in this reagent by a technique derived from the rabbit pyrogen test was rejected for practical and theoretical reasons:

4.1. The rabbit test is not sensitive enough to detect endotoxin in water for BET intended for tests on products with a very low endotoxin limit.

4.2. The relatively low precision of the rising temperature response in rabbits would call for many replications in rabbits.

4.3. The terms 'pyrogens' and 'endotoxins' denote groups of entities that do not coincide completely.

The text of the test for bacterial endotoxins indicates that methods other than triple distillation may be used to prepare water for BET. Reverse osmosis has been used with good results; some analysts may prefer to distil the water more than three times. Whatever method is used, the resultant product must be free of detectable endotoxins.

5. pH OF THE MIXTURE

In the test for bacterial endotoxins, optimum gel-clot occurs for a mixture at pH 6.0 to 8.0. However, the addition of the lysate to the sample may result in a lowering of the pH.

6. VALIDATION OF THE LYSATE

It is important to follow the manufacturer's instructions for the preparation of the solutions of the lysate.

The positive end-point dilution factors in the gel-clot methods A and B are converted to logarithms. The reason is that if the frequency distribution of these logarithmic values is plotted, it usually approaches a normal distribution curve much more closely than the frequency distribution of the dilution factors themselves; in fact it is so similar that it is acceptable to use the normal frequency distribution as a mathematical model and to calculate confidence limits with Student's *t*-test.

7. PRELIMINARY TEST FOR INTERFERING FACTORS

Some products cannot be tested directly for the presence of endotoxins because they are not miscible with the reagents, they cannot be adjusted to pH 6.0 to 8.0 or they inhibit or activate gel formation. Therefore a preliminary test is required to check for the presence of interfering factors; when these are found the analyst must demonstrate that the procedure to remove them has been effective.

The object of the preliminary test is to test the null hypothesis that the sensitivity of the lysate in the presence of the product under examination does not differ significantly from the sensitivity of the lysate in the absence of the product. A simple criterion is used in methods A and B: the null hypothesis is accepted when the sensitivity of the lysate in the presence of the product is at least 0.5 times and not more than twice the sensitivity of the lysate by itself.

A classical approach would have been to calculate the means of the log dilution factor for the lysate sensitivity with and without the product and to test the difference between the two means with Student's *t*-test.

The test for interfering factors in gel-clot methods A and B requires the use of a sample of the product in which no endotoxins are detectable. This presents a theoretical problem when an entirely new product has to be tested. Hence, a different approach was designed for quantitative methods C, D, E and F.

8. REMOVAL OF INTERFERING FACTORS

The procedures to remove interfering factors must not increase or decrease (for example, by adsorption) the amount of endotoxin in the product under examination. The correct way of checking this is to apply the procedures to a spiked sample of the product, that is, a sample to which a known amount of endotoxin has been added, and then to measure the recovery of the endotoxin.

Methods C and D. If the nature of the product to be analysed shows interference which cannot be removed by classical methods, it may be possible to carry out the standard curve in the same type of product freed from endotoxins by appropriate treatment or by dilution of the product. The endotoxins test is then carried out by comparison with this standard curve.

Ultrafiltration with cellulose triacetate asymmetric membrane filters has been found to be suitable in most cases. The filters should be properly validated, because under some circumstances cellulose derivatives (β-D-glucans) can cause false positive results.

Polysulphone filters have been found to be unsuitable because false positive results had been obtained by some users.

9. THE PURPOSE OF THE CONTROLS

The purpose of the control made up with water for BET and the reference preparation of endotoxin at twice the concentration of the labelled lysate sensitivity is to verify the activity of the lysate at the time and under the conditions of the test. The purpose of the negative control is to verify the absence of a detectable concentration of endotoxin in water for BET.

The positive control, which contains the product to be examined at the concentration used in the test, is intended to show the absence of inhibiting factors at the time and under the conditions of the test.

10. READING AND INTERPRETATION OF THE RESULTS

Minute amounts of endotoxin in the water for BET, or in any other reagent or material to which the lysate is exposed during the test, may escape detection as long as they do not reach the sensitivity limit of the lysate. However, they may raise the amount of endotoxin in the solution containing the product under examination to just above the sensitivity limit and cause a positive reaction.

The risk of this happening may be reduced by testing the water for BET and the other reagents and materials with the most sensitive lysate available, or at least one that is more sensitive than the one used in the test on the product. Even then, the risk of such a 'false positive result' cannot be ruled out completely. It should be realised, however, that in this respect the test design is 'fail-safe' in contrast to a test design permitting a false negative result, which could lead to the release of an unsatisfactory product, thus endangering the patient's health.

11. REPLACEMENT OF THE RABBIT PYROGEN TEST BY A TEST FOR BACTERIAL ENDOTOXINS

Monographs on pharmaceutical products intended for parenteral use that may contain toxic amounts of bacterial endotoxins require either a test for bacterial endotoxins or a rabbit pyrogen test. As a general policy:

11.1. In any individual monograph, when a test is required, only one test is included, either that for pyrogens or that for bacterial endotoxins.

11.2. In the absence of evidence to the contrary, the test for bacterial endotoxins is preferred over the test for pyrogens, since it is usually considered to provide equal or better protection to the patient.

11.3. Before including a test for bacterial endotoxins in a monograph, evidence is required that one of the tests described in chapter *2.6.14* can be applied satisfactorily to the product in question.

11.4. The necessary information is sought from manufacturers. Companies are invited to provide any validation data that they have concerning the applicability of the test for bacterial endotoxins to the substances and formulations of interest. Such data include details of sample preparation and of any procedures necessary to eliminate interfering factors. In addition, any available parallel data for rabbit pyrogen testing that would contribute to an assurance that the replacement of a rabbit pyrogen test by the test for bacterial endotoxin is appropriate, must be provided.

Additional requirements are defined in the following sections.

12. USE OF A DIFFERENT BACTERIAL ENDOTOXIN TEST FROM THAT PRESCRIBED IN THE MONOGRAPH

When a test for bacterial endotoxins is prescribed in a monograph and none of the six methods (A to F) described in chapter *2.6.14* is specified, then method A, the gel-clot method limit test, has been validated for this product. If one of the other methods (B to F) is specified, this is the one which has been validated for this product.

13. VALIDATION OF ALTERNATIVE METHODS

Replacement of a rabbit pyrogen test by a bacterial endotoxin test, or replacement of a stated or implied method for bacterial endotoxins by another method, is to be regarded as the use of an alternative method in the replacement of a pharmacopoeial test, as described in the General Notices:

> "The test and assays described are the official methods upon which the standards of the Pharmacopoeia are based. With the agreement of the competent authority, alternative methods of analysis may be used for control purposes, provided that the methods used enable an unequivocal decision to be made as to whether compliance with the standards of the monographs would be achieved if the official methods were used. In the event of doubt or dispute, the methods of analysis of the Pharmacopoeia are alone authoritative."

The following procedures are suggested for validating a method for bacterial endotoxins other than the one implied or indicated in the monograph.

13.1. The procedure and the materials and reagents used in the method should be validated as described for the test concerned.

13.2. The presence of interfering factors (and, if needed, the procedure for removing them) should be tested on samples of at least three production batches. It should be borne in mind that methods D and E, using a chromogenic peptide, require reagents that are absent in methods A, B, C and F, and hence compliance of methods A, B, C or F with the requirements for interfering factors cannot be extrapolated to method D or method E without further testing.

14. VALIDATION OF THE TEST FOR NEW PRODUCTS

The procedures described under 13.1 and 13.2 should be applied to all new products intended for parenteral use that have to be tested for the presence of bacterial endotoxins according to the requirements of the Pharmacopoeia.

01/2005:20615
corrected

2.6.15. PREKALLIKREIN ACTIVATOR

Prekallikrein activator (PKA) activates prekallikrein to kallikrein and may be assayed by its ability to cleave a chromophore from a synthetic peptide substrate so that the rate of cleavage can be measured spectrophotometrically and the concentration of PKA calculated by comparison with a reference preparation calibrated in International Units.

The International Unit is the activity of a stated amount of the International Standard which consists of freeze-dried prekallikrein activator. The equivalence in International Units of the International Standard is stated by the World Health Organisation.

Prekallikrein activator in albumin BRP is calibrated in International Units by comparison with the International Standard.

PREPARATION OF PREKALLIKREIN SUBSTRATE

To avoid coagulation activation, blood or plasma used for the preparation of prekallikrein must come into contact only with plastics or silicone-treated glass surfaces.

Draw 9 volumes of human blood into 1 volume of anticoagulant solution (ACD, CPD or 38 g/l *sodium citrate R*) to which 1 mg/ml of *hexadimethrine bromide R* has been added. Centrifuge the mixture at 3600 *g* for 5 min. Separate the plasma and centrifuge again at 6000 *g* for 20 min to sediment platelets. Separate the platelet-poor plasma and dialyse against 10 volumes of buffer A for 20 h. Apply the dialysed plasma to a chromatography column containing *agarose-DEAE for ion exchange chromatography R* which has been equilibrated in buffer A and is equal to twice the volume of the plasma. Elute from the column with buffer A at 20 ml/cm^2/h. Collect the eluate in fractions and record the absorbance at 280 nm (*2.2.25*). Pool the fractions containing the first protein peak so that the volume of the pool is about 1.2 times the volume of the platelet-poor plasma.

Test the substrate pool for absence of kallikrein activity by mixing 1 part with 20 parts of the pre-warmed chromogenic substrate solution to be used in the assay and incubate at 37 °C for 2 min. The substrate is suitable if the increase in absorbance is less than 0.001 per minute. Add to the pooled solution 7 g/l of *sodium chloride R* and filter using a membrane filter (porosity 0.45 µm). Freeze the filtrate in portions and store at − 25 °C; the substrate may be freeze-dried before storage.

Carry out all procedures from the beginning of the chromatography to freezing in portions during a single working day.

ASSAY

The assay is preferably carried out using an automated enzyme analyser at 37 °C, with volumes, concentration of substrates and incubation times adjusted so that the reaction rate is linear at least up to 35 IU/ml. Standards, samples and prekallikrein substrate may be diluted as necessary using buffer B.

Incubate diluted standards or samples with prekallikrein substrate for 10 min such that the volume of the undiluted sample does not exceed 1/10 of the total volume of the incubation mixture to avoid errors caused by variation in ionic strength and pH in the incubation mixture. Incubate the mixture or a part thereof with at least an equal volume of a solution of a suitable synthetic chromogenic substrate, known to be specific for kallikrein (for example, *N-benzoyl-L-prolyl-L-phenylalanyl-L-arginine 4-nitroanilide acetate R* or *D-prolyl-L-phenylalanyl-L-arginine-4-nitroanilide-dihydrochloride R*), dissolved in buffer B. Record the rate of change in absorbance per minute for 2 min to 10 min at the wavelength specific for the substrate used. Prepare a blank for each mixture of sample or standard using buffer B instead of prekallikrein substrate.

Correct ΔA/min by subtracting the value obtained for the corresponding blank. Plot a calibration curve using the values thus obtained for the reference preparation and the respective concentrations; use the curve to determine the PKA activity of the preparation to be examined.

Buffer A

Tris(hydroxymethyl)aminomethane R	6.055 g
Sodium chloride R	1.17 g
Hexadimethrine bromide R	50 mg
Sodium azide R	0.100 g

Dissolve the ingredients in *water R,* adjust to pH 8.0 with *2 M hydrochloric acid* and dilute to 1000 ml with *water R.*

Buffer B

Tris(hydroxymethyl)aminomethane R	6.055 g
Sodium chloride R	8.77 g

Dissolve the ingredients in *water R,* adjust to pH 8.0 with *2 M hydrochloric acid* and dilute to 1000 ml with *water R.*

01/2005:20616

2.6.16. TESTS FOR EXTRANEOUS AGENTS IN VIRAL VACCINES FOR HUMAN USE

In those tests that require prior neutralisation of the virus, use specific antibodies of non-human, non-simian origin; if the virus has been propagated in avian tissues, the antibodies must also be of non-avian origin. To prepare antiserum, use an immunising antigen produced in cell culture from a species different from that used for the production of the vaccine and free from extraneous agents. Where the use of SPF eggs is prescribed, the eggs are obtained from a flock free from specified pathogens (*5.2.2*).

VIRUS SEED LOT

Take samples of the virus seed lot at the time of harvesting and, if they are not tested immediately, keep them at a temperature below − 40 °C.

Adult mice. Inoculate each of at least ten adult mice, each weighing 15 g to 20 g, intracerebrally with 0.03 ml and intraperitoneally with 0.5 ml of the virus seed lot. Observe the mice for at least 21 days. Carry out an autopsy of all mice that die after the first 24 h of the test or that show signs of illness and examine for evidence of viral infection, both by direct macroscopical observation and by subinoculation of appropriate tissue suspensions by the intracerebral and intraperitoneal routes into at least five additional mice which are observed for 21 days. The virus seed lot complies with the test if no mouse shows evidence of infection attributable to the seed lot. The test is not valid unless at least 80 per cent of the original inoculated mice survive the observation period.

Suckling mice. Inoculate each of at least twenty mice, less than 24 h old, intracerebrally with 0.01 ml and intraperitoneally with at least 0.1 ml of the virus seed lot. Observe the mice daily for at least 14 days. Carry out an autopsy of all mice that die after the first 24 h of the test or that show signs of illness and examine for evidence of viral infection, both by direct macroscopical observation and by subinoculation of appropriate tissue suspensions by the intracerebral and intraperitoneal routes into at least five additional suckling mice which are observed daily for 14 days. The virus seed lot passes the test if no mouse shows evidence of infection attributable to the seed lot. The test is not valid unless at least 80 per cent of the original inoculated mice survive the observation period.

Guinea-pigs. Inoculate intraperitoneally into each of at least five guinea pigs, each weighing 350 g to 450 g, 5.0 ml of the virus seed lot. Observe the animals for at least 42 days for signs of disease. Carry out an autopsy of all guinea-pigs that die after the first 24 h of the test, or that show signs of illness and examine macroscopically; examine the tissues both microscopically and culturally for evidence of infection. Kill animals that survive the observation period and examine in a similar manner. The virus seed lot passes the test if no guinea-pig shows evidence of infection attributable to the seed lot. The test is not valid unless at least 80 per cent of the guinea-pigs survive the observation period.

VIRUS SEED LOT AND VIRUS HARVESTS

Take samples at the time of harvesting and, if not tested immediately, keep them at a temperature below − 40 °C.

Bacterial and fungal sterility. A 10 ml sample complies with the test for sterility (*2.6.1*).

Mycoplasmas. A 10 ml sample complies with the test for mycoplasmas (*2.6.7*).

Mycobacteria (*2.6.2*). A 5 ml sample is tested for the presence of *Mycobacterium spp.* by culture methods known to be sensitive for the detection of these organisms.

Test in cell culture for other extraneous agents. Neutralised samples equivalent, unless otherwise prescribed, to 500 human doses of vaccine or 50 ml, whichever is the greater, are tested for the presence of extraneous agents by inoculation into continuous simian kidney and human cell cultures. If the virus is grown in human diploid cells, the neutralised virus harvest is also tested on a separate culture of the diploid cells. If the vaccine virus is grown in a cell system other than simian or human, cells of that species, from a separate batch, are also inoculated. The cells are incubated at 36 ± 1 °C and observed for a period of 14 days. The virus seed lot or harvest passes the tests if none of the cell cultures shows evidence of the presence of any extraneous agents not attributable to accidental contamination. The test is not valid unless at least 80 per cent of the cell cultures remain viable.

Avian viruses (only required for virus propagated in avian tissues). Neutralise a sample equivalent to 100 human doses or 10 ml, whichever is the greater. Using 0.5 ml per egg, inoculate a group of fertilised SPF eggs, 9 to 11 days old, by the allantoic route and a second group, 5 to 7 days old, into the yolk sac. Incubate for 7 days. The virus seed lot or harvest complies with the test if the allantoic and yolk sac fluids show no sign of the presence of any haemagglutinating agent and if all embryos and chorio-allantoic membranes, examined for gross pathology, are normal. The test is not valid unless at least 80 per cent of the inoculated eggs survive for 7 days.

PRODUCTION CELL CULTURE: CONTROL CELLS

Examine the control cells microscopically for freedom from any virus causing cytopathic degeneration throughout the time of incubation of the inoculated production cell cultures or for not less than 14 days beyond the time of inoculation of the production vessels, whichever is the longer. The test is not valid unless at least 80 per cent of the control cell cultures survive to the end of the observation period.

At 14 days or at the time of the last virus harvest, whichever is the longer, carry out the tests described below.

Test for haemadsorbing viruses. Examine not fewer than 25 per cent of the control cultures for the presence of haemadsorbing viruses by the addition of guinea-pig red blood cells. If the guinea-pig red blood cells have been stored, they shall have been stored at 5 ± 3 °C for not more than 7 days. Read half of the cultures after incubation at 5 ± 3 °C for 30 min and the other half after incubation at 20 °C to 25 °C for 30 min. No evidence of haemadsorbing agents is found.

Tests in cell cultures for other extraneous agents. Pool the supernatant fluids from the control cells and examine for the presence of extraneous agents by inoculation of simian kidney and human cell cultures. If the vaccine virus is grown in a cell system other than simian or human, cells of that species, but from a separate batch, are also inoculated. In each cell system, at least 5 ml is tested. Incubate the inoculated cultures at a temperature of 36 ± 1 °C and observe for a period of 14 days. No evidence of extraneous agents is found.

If the production cell culture is maintained at a temperature different from 36 ± 1 °C, a supplementary test for extraneous agents is carried out at the production temperature using the same type of cells as used for growth of the virus.

Avian leucosis viruses (required only if the virus is propagated in avian tissues). Carry out a test for avian leucosis viruses using 5 ml of the supernatant fluid from the control cells.

CONTROL EGGS

Haemagglutinating agents. Examine 0.25 ml of the allantoic fluid from each egg for haemagglutinating agents by mixing directly with chicken red blood cells and after a passage in SPF eggs carried out as follows: inoculate a 5 ml sample of the pooled amniotic fluids from the control eggs in 0.5 ml volumes into the allantoic cavity and into the amniotic cavity of SPF eggs. The control eggs comply with the test if no evidence of the presence of haemagglutinating agents is found in either test.

Avian leucosis viruses. Use a 10 ml sample of the pooled amniotic fluids from the control eggs. Carry out amplification by five passages in leucosis-free chick-embryo cell cultures; carry out a test for avian leucosis using cells from the fifth passage. The control eggs comply with the test if no evidence of the presence of avian leucosis viruses is found.

Other extraneous agents. Inoculate 5 ml samples of the pooled amniotic fluids from the control eggs into human and simian cell cultures. Observe the cell cultures for 14 days. The control eggs comply with the test if no evidence of the presence of extraneous agents is found. The test is not valid unless 80 per cent of the inoculated cultures survive to the end of the observation period.

01/2005:20617

2.6.17. TEST FOR ANTICOMPLEMENTARY ACTIVITY OF IMMUNOGLOBULIN

For the measurement of anticomplementary activity (ACA) of immunoglobulin, a defined amount of test material (10 mg of immunoglobulin) is incubated with a defined amount of guinea-pig complement (20 CH_{50}) and the remaining complement is titrated; the anticomplementary activity is expressed as the percentage consumption of complement relative to the complement control considered as 100 per cent.

The haemolytic unit of complement activity (CH_{50}) is the amount of complement that, in the given reaction conditions, will produce the lysis of 2.5×10^8 out of a total of 5×10^8 optimally sensitised red blood cells.

Magnesium and calcium stock solution. Dissolve 1.103 g of *calcium chloride R* and 5.083 g of *magnesium chloride R* in *water R* and dilute to 25 ml with the same solvent.

Barbital buffer stock solution. Dissolve 207.5 g of *sodium chloride R* and 25.48 g of *barbital sodium R* in 4000 ml of *water R* and adjust to pH 7.3 using *1 M hydrochloric acid.* Add 12.5 ml of magnesium and calcium stock solution and dilute to 5000 ml with *water R*. Filter through a membrane filter (pore size 0.22 µm). Store at 4 °C in glass containers.

Gelatin solution. Dissolve 12.5 g of *gelatin R* in about 800 ml of *water R* and heat to boiling in a water-bath. Cool to 20 °C and dilute to 10 litres with *water R*. Filter through a membrane filter (pore size: 0.22 µm). Store at 4 °C. Use clear solutions only.

Citrate solution. Dissolve 8.0 g of *sodium citrate R*, 4.2 g of *sodium chloride R* and 20.5 g of *glucose R* in 750 ml of *water R*. Adjust to pH 6.1 using a 100 g/l solution of *citric acid R* and dilute to 1000 ml with *water R*.

Gelatin barbital buffer solution. Add 4 volumes of gelatin solution to 1 volume of barbital buffer stock solution and mix. Adjust to pH 7.3, if necessary, using *1 M sodium hydroxide* or *1 M hydrochloric acid.* Maintain at 4 °C. Prepare fresh solutions daily.

Stabilised sheep blood. Collect one volume of sheep blood into one volume of citrate solution and mix. Store at 4 °C for not less than 7 days and not more than 28 days. (Stabilised sheep blood and sheep red blood cells are available from a number of commercial sources.)

Haemolysin. Antiserum against sheep red blood cells prepared in rabbits. (Such antisera are available from a number of commercial sources.)

Guinea-pig complement. Prepare a pool of serum from the blood of not fewer than ten guinea-pigs. Separate the serum from the clotted blood by centrifugation at about 4 °C. Store the serum in small amounts below − 70 °C.

METHOD

Preparation of standardised 5 per cent sheep red blood cell suspension. Separate sheep red blood cells by centrifuging an appropriate volume of stabilised sheep blood and wash the cells at least three times with gelatin barbital buffer solution and prepare as a 5 per cent *V/V* suspension in the same solution. Measure the cell density of the suspension as follows: add 0.2 ml to 2.8 ml of *water R* and centrifuge the lysed solution for 5 min at 1000 *g*; the cell density is suitable if the absorbance (*2.2.25*) of the supernatant liquid at 541 nm is 0.62 ± 0.01. Correct the cell density by adding gelatin barbital buffer solution according to the formula:

$$V_f = \frac{V_i \times A}{0.62}$$

V_f = final adjusted volume,

V_i = the initial volume,

A = absorbance of the original suspension at 541 nm.

The adjusted suspension contains about 1×10^9 cells/ml.

Haemolysin titration

Prepare haemolysin dilutions as shown in Table 2.6.17.-1.

Table 2.6.17.-1

Required dilution of haemolysin	Prepared using		
	Gelatin barbital buffer solution		Haemolysin
	Volume (millilitres)	Dilution (1: ...)	Volume (millilitres)
7.5	0.65	undiluted	0.1
10	0.90	undiluted	0.1
75	1.80	7.5	0.2
100	1.80	10	0.2
150	1.00	75	1.0
200	1.00	100	1.0
300	1.00	150	1.0
400	1.00	200	1.0
600	1.00	300	1.0
800	1.00	400	1.0
1200	1.00	600	1.0
1600	1.00	800	1.0
2400	1.00	1200	1.0
3200*	1.00	1600	1.0
4800*	1.00	2400	1.0

* discard 1.0 ml of the mixture.

Add 1.0 ml of 5 per cent sheep red blood cell suspension to each tube of the haemolysin dilution series, starting at the 1:75 dilution, and mix. Incubate at 37 °C for 30 min.

Transfer 0.2 ml of each of these incubated mixtures to new tubes and add 1.10 ml of gelatin barbital buffer solution and 0.2 ml of diluted guinea-pig complement (for example, 1:150). Perform this in duplicate.

As the unhaemolysed cell control, prepare three tubes with 1.4 ml of gelatin barbital buffer solution and 0.1 ml of 5 per cent sheep red blood cell suspension.

As the fully haemolysed control, prepare three tubes with 1.4 ml of *water R* and 0.1 ml of 5 per cent sheep red cell suspension.

Incubate all tubes at 37 °C for 60 min and centrifuge at 1000 *g* for 5 min. Measure the absorbance (*2.2.25*) of the supernatants at 541 nm and calculate the percentage degree of haemolysis in each tube using the expression:

$$\frac{A_a - A_1}{A_b - A_1} \times 100$$

A_a = absorbance of tubes with haemolysin dilution,

A_b = mean absorbance of the three tubes with full haemolysis,

A_1 = mean absorbance of the three tubes with no haemolysis.

Plot the percentage degree of haemolysis as the ordinate against the corresponding reciprocal value of the haemolysin dilution as the abscissa on linear graph paper. Determine the optimal dilution of the haemolysin from the graph by inspection. Select a dilution such that further increase in the amount of haemolysin does not cause appreciable change in the degree of haemolysis. This dilution is defined as one minimal haemolytic unit (1 MHU) in 1.0 ml. The optimal haemolytic haemolysin dilution for preparation of sensitised sheep red blood cells contains 2 MHU/ml.

The haemolysin titration is not valid unless the maximum degree of haemolysis is 50 per cent to 70 per cent. If the maximum degree of haemolysis is not in this range, repeat the titration with more or less diluted complement solution.

Preparation of optimised sensitised sheep red blood cells (haemolytic system)

Prepare an appropriate volume of diluted haemolysin containing 2 MHU/ml and an equal volume of standardised 5 per cent sheep red blood cell suspension. Add the haemolysin dilution to the standardised cell suspension and mix. Incubate at 37 °C for 15 min, store at 2 °C to 8 °C and use within 6 h.

Titration of complement

Prepare an appropriate dilution of complement (for example, 1:250) with gelatin barbital buffer solution and perform the titration in duplicate as shown in Table 2.6.17.-2.

Add 0.2 ml of sensitised sheep red blood cells to each tube, mix well and incubate at 37 °C for 60 min. Cool the tubes in an ice-bath and centrifuge at 1000 *g* for 5 min. Measure the absorbance of the supernatant liquid at 541 nm and calculate the degree of haemolysis (Y) using the expression:

$$\frac{A_c - A_1}{A_b - A_1}$$

A_c = absorbance of tubes 1 to 12,

A_b = mean absorbance of tubes with 100 per cent haemolysis,

A_1 = mean absorbance of cell controls with 0 per cent haemolysis.

Plot $Y/(1-Y)$ as the abscissa against the amount of diluted complement in millilitres as the ordinate on log–log graph paper. Fit the best line to the points and determine the

2. Methods of analysis

ordinate for the 50 per cent haemolytic complement dose where $Y/(1-Y) = 1.0$. Calculate the activity in haemolytic units (CH_{50}/ml) from the expression:

$$\frac{C_d}{C_a \times 5}$$

C_d = reciprocal value of the complement dilution,

C_a = volume of diluted complement in millilitres resulting in 50 per cent haemolysis,

5 = scaling factor to take account of the number of red blood cells.

The test is not valid unless the plot is a straight line between 15 per cent and 85 per cent haemolysis and the slope is 0.15 to 0.40, and preferably 0.18 to 0.30.

Table 2.6.17.-2

Tube Number	Volume of diluted complement in millilitres (for example 1:250)	Volume of gelatin barbital buffer solution in millilitres
1	0.1	1.2
2	0.2	1.1
3	0.3	1.0
4	0.4	0.9
5	0.5	0.8
6	0.6	0.7
7	0.7	0.6
8	0.8	0.5
9	0.9	0.4
10	1.0	0.3
11	1.1	0.2
12	1.2	0.1
Three tubes as cell control at 0 per cent haemolysis	–	1.3
Three tubes at 100 per cent haemolysis	–	1.3 ml of water

Test for anticomplementary activity

Prepare a complement dilution having 100 CH_{50}/ml by diluting titrated guinea-pig complement with gelatin barbital buffer solution. If necessary, adjust the immunoglobulin to be examined to pH 7. Prepare incubation mixtures as follows for an immunoglobulin containing 50 mg/ml:

Table 2.6.17.-3

	Immunoglobulin to be examined	Complement control (in duplicate)
Immunoglobulin (50 mg/ml)	0.2 ml	–
Gelatin barbital buffer	0.6 ml	0.8 ml
Complement	0.2 ml	0.2 ml

Carry out the test on the immunoglobulin to be examined and prepare ACA negative and positive controls using *human immunoglobulin BRP*, as indicated in the leaflet accompanying the reference preparation. Higher or lower volumes of sample and of gelatin barbital buffer solution are added if the immunoglobulin concentration varies from 50 mg/ml; for example, 0.47 ml of gelatin barbital buffer solution is added to 0.33 ml of immunoglobulin containing 30 mg/ml to give 0.8 ml. Close the tubes and incubate at 37 °C for 60 min. Add 0.2 ml of each incubation mixture to 9.8 ml of gelatin barbital buffer solution to dilute the complement. Perform complement titrations as described above on each tube to determine the remaining complement activity (Table 2.6.17.-2). Calculate the anticomplementary activity of the preparation to be examined relative to the complement control considered as 100 per cent, from the expression:

$$\frac{a-b}{a} \times 100$$

a = mean complement activity (CH_{50}/ml) of complement control,

b = complement activity (CH_{50}/ml) of tested sample.

The test is not valid unless:

– the anticomplementary activities found for ACA negative control and ACA positive control are within the limits stated in the leaflet accompanying the reference preparation,

– the complement activity of the complement control (a) is in the range 80 to 120 CH_{50}/ml.

01/2005:20618

2.6.18. TEST FOR NEUROVIRULENCE OF LIVE VIRUS VACCINES

For each test, use not fewer than ten monkeys that are seronegative for the virus to be tested. For each monkey, inject not more than 0.5 ml of the material to be examined into the thalamic region of each hemisphere, unless otherwise prescribed. The total amount of virus inoculated in each monkey must be not less than the amount contained in the recommended single human dose of the vaccine. As a check against the introduction of wild neurovirulent virus, keep a group of not fewer than four control monkeys as cage-mates or in the immediate vicinity of the inoculated monkeys. Observe the inoculated monkeys for 17 to 21 days for symptoms of paralysis and other evidence of neurological involvement; observe the control monkeys for the same period plus 10 days. Animals that die within 48 h of injection are considered to have died from non-specific causes and may be replaced. The test is not valid if: more than 20 per cent of the inoculated monkeys die from nonspecific causes; serum samples taken from the control monkeys at the time of inoculation of the test animals and 10 days after the latter are killed show evidence of infection by wild virus of the type to be tested or by measles virus. At the end of the observation period, carry out autopsy and histopathological examinations of appropriate areas of the brain for evidence of central nervous system involvement. The material complies with the test if there is no unexpected clinical or histopathological evidence of involvement of the central nervous system attributable to the inoculated virus.

01/2005:20619

2.6.19. TEST FOR NEUROVIRULENCE OF POLIOMYELITIS VACCINE (ORAL)

Monkeys used in the neurovirulence test comply with the requirements given in the monograph on *Poliomyelitis vaccine oral (0215)* and weigh not less than 1.5 kg. The pathogenicity for *Macaca* or *Cercopithecus monkeys* is tested in comparison with that of a reference virus preparation for neurovirulence testing by inoculation into the lumbar region of the central nervous system after sedation with a suitable substance, for example, ketamine hydrochloride. A sample of serum taken before the injection shall be shown not to contain neutralising antibody at a dilution of 1:4 when tested against not more than 1000 $CCID_{50}$ of each of the three types of poliovirus.

Number of monkeys. The vaccine and the appropriate homotypic reference virus are tested concurrently in the same group of monkeys. Equal numbers of animals are inoculated with the vaccine to be examined and the reference preparation. The animals are allocated randomly to treatment groups and cages and their identity is coded so that the treatment received by each animal is concealed from the observers and the evaluators of the sections. The number of monkeys inoculated is such that in the evaluation of both the vaccine and the reference preparation not fewer than eleven positive monkeys are included for type 1 and type 2 virus and not fewer than eighteen positive monkeys for type 3 virus (positive monkeys are those that show specific neuronal lesions of poliovirus in the central nervous system). More than one batch of vaccine may be tested with the same homotypic reference. Monkeys from the same quarantine group are used wherever possible, otherwise monkeys from two groups are used and equal numbers from each group are treated with the vaccine and the reference preparation. If the test is carried out on two working days, an equal number of monkeys from each group are inoculated on each day with the vaccine and the homotypic reference preparation.

Virus content. The virus contents of the vaccine and the homotypic reference preparation are adjusted so as to be as near as possible equal and between $10^{5.5}$ and $10^{6.5}$ $CCID_{50}$/0.1 ml.

Observation. All monkeys are observed for 17 to 22 days for signs of poliomyelitis or other virus infection. Monkeys that survive the first 24 h but die before the 11th day after inoculation are autopsied to determine whether poliomyelitis was the cause of death. Animals that die from causes other than poliomyelitis are excluded from the evaluation. Animals that become moribund or are severely paralysed are killed and autopsied. All animals that survive until the end of the observation period are autopsied. The test is not valid if more than 20 per cent of the animals show intercurrent infection during the observation period.

Number of sections examined. The lumbar cord, the cervical cord, the lower and upper medulla oblongata, the midbrain, the thalamus and the motor cortex of each monkey, as a minimum, are subjected to histological examination. Sections are cut with a thickness of 15 μm and stained with gallocyanin. The minimum number of sections examined is as follows:

(a) 12 sections representative of the whole of the lumbar enlargement,

(b) 10 sections representative of the whole of the cervical enlargement,

(c) 2 sections from the medulla oblongata,

(d) 1 section from the pons and cerebellum,

(e) 1 section from the midbrain,

(f) 1 section from the left and the right of the thalamus,

(g) 1 section from the left and the right motor cerebral cortex.

Scoring of virus activity. For the evaluation of virus activity in the hemisections of the spinal cord and brain-stem, a score system for the severity of lesions is used, differentiating cellular infiltration and destruction of neurons as follows:

1. Cellular infiltration only (the monkey is not counted as positive),
2. Cellular infiltration with minimal neuronal damage,
3. Cellular infiltration with extensive neuronal damage,
4. Massive neuronal damage with or without cellular infiltration.

The scores are recorded on a standard form(1). A monkey with neuronal lesions in the sections but that shows no needle tract is counted as positive. A monkey showing a needle tract in the sections, but no neuronal lesions is not regarded as positive. A section that shows damage from trauma but no specific virus lesions is not included in the score.

Severity scores are based on hemisection readings of the lumbar (L), cervical (C) and brain (B) histological sections. The lesion score (LS) for each positive monkey is calculated as follows:

$$LS = \frac{\left[\frac{\text{Sum of L score}}{\text{Number of hemisections}}\right] + \left[\frac{\text{Sum of C score}}{\text{Number of hemisections}}\right] + \left[\frac{\text{Sum of B score}}{\text{Number of hemisections}}\right]}{3}$$

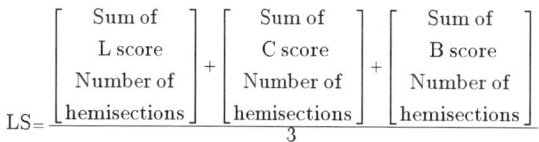

A mean lesion score is calculated for each group of positive monkeys.

Evaluation. The comparison of the virus activity in the vaccine and the reference preparation is based on the activity in the lumbar enlargement of the cord and the degree of spread of activity from this region to the cervical enlargement and the brain. Acceptance or rejection is based on the total score of all the test animals. Individual animals showing evidence of unusually high activity, either in the lumbar region or as the result of spread from this region, are also taken into consideration in the final evaluation. The monovalent bulk passes the test if the required number of animals is positive and if none of the clinical and histopathological examinations shows a significant difference in pathogenicity between the vaccine virus and the reference material. Criteria for acceptance are given below.

Criteria. A suitable number of neurovirulence qualifying tests (for example, four tests) is carried out on each reference vaccine (types 1, 2 and 3) to provide data on the activity of such vaccines that will serve as the basis of the criteria for vaccines to be tested. The overall mean lesion score (M) for the replicate tests on each reference virus is calculated together with the pooled estimate of the within-test variance (s^2) and the within-test deviation (s).

Validity criteria for the results of a test on a reference preparation are established on the basis of the cumulative data from the qualifying tests. No generally applicable criteria can be given; for laboratories with limited experience, the following empirical method for setting acceptable limits for the mean lesion score for the reference preparation (X_{ref}) may be helpful (see Table 2.6.19.-1):

Table 2.6.19.-1

	Lower limit	Upper limit
Types 1 and 2	$M - s$	$M + s$
Type 3	$M - s/2$	$M + s$

If the mean lesion score for the vaccine to be tested is X_{test} and C_1, C_2 and C_3 are constants determined as described below, then:

the vaccine is not acceptable if:

$$X_{test} - X_{ref} > C_1$$

the vaccine may be retested once if:

$$C_1 < X_{test} - X_{ref} < C_2$$

(1) A suitable form is shown in the Requirements for Poliomyelitis Vaccine (Oral) (Requirements for Biological Substances No. 7, World Health Organization).

If the vaccine is retested, the means of the lesion scores for the vaccine to be tested and the reference vaccine are recalculated. The vaccine is not acceptable if:

$$\frac{X_{(\text{test }1+\text{test }2)} - X_{(\text{ref }1+\text{ref }2)}}{2} > C_3$$

The constants C_1, C_2 and C_3 are calculated from the expressions:

$$C_1 = 2.3\sqrt{\frac{2s^2}{N_1}}$$

$$C_2 = 2.6\sqrt{\frac{2s^2}{N_1}}$$

$$C_3 = 1.6\sqrt{\frac{2s^2}{N_1}}$$

N_1 = number of positive monkeys per vaccine test,
N_2 = number of positive monkeys in the two tests,
2.3 = normal deviate at the 1 per cent level,
2.6 = normal deviate at the 0.5 per cent level,
1.6 = normal deviate at the 5 per cent level.

A neurovirulence test in which the mean lesion score for the reference (X_{ref}) is not compatible with previous experience is not used for assessing a test vaccine. If the test is valid, the mean lesion score for the vaccine to be tested (X_{test}) is calculated and compared with that of the homotypic reference vaccine.

01/2005:20620

2.6.20. ANTI-A AND ANTI-B HAEMAGGLUTININS (INDIRECT METHOD)

Prepare in duplicate serial dilutions of the preparation to be examined in a 9 g/l solution of *sodium chloride R*. To each dilution of one series add an equal volume of a 5 per cent *V/V* suspension of group A_1 red blood cells previously washed three times with the sodium chloride solution. To each dilution of the other series add an equal volume of a 5 per cent *V/V* suspension of group B red blood cells previously washed three times with the sodium chloride solution. Incubate the suspensions at 37 °C for 30 min then wash the cells three times with the sodium chloride solution. Leave the cells in contact with a polyvalent anti-human globulin reagent for 30 min. Without centrifuging, examine each suspension for agglutination under a microscope.

01/2005:20621
corrected

2.6.21. NUCLEIC ACID AMPLIFICATION TECHNIQUES

1. INTRODUCTION

Nucleic acid amplification techniques are based on two different approaches:

1. amplification of a target nucleic acid sequence using, for example, polymerase chain reaction (PCR), ligase chain reaction (LCR), or isothermal ribonucleic acid (RNA) amplification,
2. amplification of a hybridisation signal using, for example, for deoxyribonucleic acid (DNA), the branched DNA (bDNA) method. In this case signal amplification is achieved without subjecting the nucleic acid to repetitive cycles of amplification.

In this general chapter, the PCR method is described as the reference technique. Alternative methods may be used, if they comply with the quality requirements described below.

2. SCOPE

This section establishes the requirements for sample preparation, *in vitro* amplification of DNA sequences and detection of the specific PCR product. With the aid of PCR, defined DNA sequences can be detected. RNA sequences can also be detected following reverse transcription of the RNA to complementary DNA (cDNA) and subsequent amplification.

3. PRINCIPLE OF THE METHOD

PCR is a procedure that allows specific *in vitro* amplification of segments of DNA or of RNA after reverse transcription into cDNA.

Following denaturation of double-stranded DNA into single-stranded DNA, two synthetic oligonucleotide primers of opposite polarity, anneal to their respective complementary sequences in the DNA to be amplified. The short double-stranded regions which form as a result of specific base pairing between the primers and the complementary DNA sequence, border the DNA segment to be amplified and serve as starting positions for *in vitro* DNA synthesis by means of a heat-stable DNA polymerase.

Amplification of the DNA occurs in cycles consisting of:

- heat denaturation of the nucleic acid (target sequence) into two single strands;
- specific annealing of the primers to the target sequence under suitable reaction conditions;
- extension of the primers, which are bound to both single strands, by DNA polymerase at a suitable temperature (DNA synthesis).

Repeated cycles of heat denaturation, primer annealing and DNA synthesis results in an exponential amplification of the DNA segment limited by the primers.

The specific PCR product known as an amplicon can be detected by a variety of methods of appropriate specificity and sensitivity.

4. TEST MATERIAL

Because of the high sensitivity of PCR, the samples must be optimally protected against external contamination with target sequences. Sampling, storage and transport of the test material are performed under conditions that minimise degradation of the target sequence. In the case of RNA target sequences, special precautions are necessary since RNA is highly sensitive to degradation by ribonucleases. Care must be taken since some added reagents, such as anticoagulants or preservatives, may interfere with the test procedure.

5. TEST METHOD

5.1. Prevention of contamination

The risk of contamination requires a strict segregation of the areas depending on the material handled and the technology used. Points to consider include movement of personnel, gowning, material flow and air supply and decontamination procedures.

The system should be sub-divided into compartments such as:

- master-mix area (area where exclusively template-free material is handled, e.g. primers, buffers, etc.),

- pre-PCR (area where reagents, samples and controls are handled),
- PCR amplification (amplified material is handled in a closed system),
- post-PCR detection (the only area where the amplified material is handled in an open system).

5.2. Sample preparation

When preparing samples, the target sequence to be amplified needs to be efficiently extracted or liberated from the test material in a reproducible manner and in such a way that amplification under the selected reaction conditions is possible. A variety of physico-chemical extraction procedures and/or enrichment procedures may be employed.

Additives present in test material may interfere with PCR. The procedures described under 7.3.2. must be used as a control for the presence of inhibitors originating from the test material.

In the case of RNA-templates, care must be taken to avoid ribonuclease activity.

5.3. Amplification

PCR amplification of the target sequence is conducted under optimised cycling conditions (temperature profile for denaturation of double-stranded DNA, annealing and extension of primers; incubation times at selected temperatures; ramp rates). These depend on various parameters such as:

- the length and base composition of primer and target sequences;
- the type of DNA polymerase, buffer composition and reaction volume used for the amplification;
- the type of thermocycler used and the thermal conductivity rate between the apparatus, reaction tube and reaction fluid.

5.4. Detection

The amplicon generated by PCR may be identified by size, sequence, chemical modification or a combination of these parameters. Characterisation by size may be achieved by gel electrophoresis (using agarose or polyacrylamide slab gels or capillary electrophoresis) or column chromatography (for example, HPLC). Characterisation by sequence composition may be achieved by the specific hybridisation of probes having a sequence complementary to the target sequence or by cleavage of the amplified material reflecting target-specific restriction-enzyme sites. Characterisation by chemical modification may be achieved, for example, by incorporation of a fluorophore into the amplicons and subsequent detection of fluorescence following excitation.

Detection of amplicons may also be achieved by using probes labelled to permit a subsequent radioisotopic or immuno-enzyme-coupled detection.

6. EVALUATION AND INTERPRETATION OF RESULTS

A valid result is obtained within a test only if the positive control(s) is unambiguously positive and the negative control(s) is unambiguously negative. Due to the very high sensitivity of the PCR method and the inherent risk of contamination, it is necessary to confirm positive results by repeating the complete test procedure in duplicate, where possible on a new aliquot of the sample. The sample is considered positive if at least one of the repeat tests gives a positive result.

7. QUALITY ASSURANCE

7.1. Validation of the PCR assay system

The validation programme must include validation of instrumentation and the PCR method employed. Reference should be made to the *ICH guidelines* (topic Q2B) Validation of Analytical Method: Methodology.

Appropriate official working reference preparations or in-house reference preparations calibrated against International Standards for the target sequences for which the test system will be used are indispensable for validation of a PCR test.

During validation the positive cut-off point must be determined. The positive cut-off point is defined as the minimum number of target sequences per volume sample which can be detected in 95 per cent of test runs. The positive cut-off point depends on interrelated factors such as the volume of the sample extracted and the efficacy of the extraction methodology, the transcription of the target RNA into cDNA, the amplification process and the detection.

To define the detection limit of the assay system, reference must be made to the positive cut-off point for each target sequence and the test performance above and below the positive cut-off point.

7.2. Quality control of reagents

All reagents crucial for the methodology used have to be controlled prior to use in routine applications. Their acceptance/withdrawal is based on pre-defined quality criteria.

Primers are a crucial component of the PCR assay and as such their design, purity and the validation of their use in a PCR assay require careful attention. Each new batch of primers is tested for specificity, amplification efficiency and absence of inhibitory impurities before acceptance. Primers may be modified (for example, by conjugation with a fluorophore or antigen) in order to permit a specific method of detection of the amplicon, provided such modifications do not inhibit accurate and efficient amplification of the target sequence.

7.3. Run controls

7.3.1. External controls

In order to minimise the risk of contamination and to ensure adequate sensitivity, the following external controls are included in each PCR test:

- positive control: this contains a defined number of target-sequence copies, the number being determined individually for each assay system and indicated as a multiple of the positive cut-off value of the test system;
- negative control: a sample of the same matrix already proven to be free of the target sequences;

7.3.2. Internal control

Internal controls are defined nucleic acid sequences containing the primer binding sites. Internal controls must be amplified with similar efficacy as the target sequence to be tested, but the amplicons must be clearly discernible. Internal controls must be of the same type of nucleic acid (DNA/RNA) as the material to be tested. The internal control is preferably added to the test material before isolating the nucleic acid and therefore acts as an overall control (extraction, reverse transcription, amplification, detection).

7.4. External quality assessment

Participation in external quality assessment programmes is an important PCR quality assurance procedure for each laboratory and each operator.

The following section is published for information.

Validation of nucleic acid amplification techniques (NAT) for the detection of hepatitis C virus (HCV) RNA in plasma pools: guidelines

1. SCOPE

The majority of nucleic acid amplification analytical procedures are qualitative (quantal) tests for the presence of nucleic acid with some quantitative tests (either in-house or commercial) being available. For the detection of HCV RNA contamination of plasma pools, qualitative tests are adequate and may be considered to be a limit test for the control of impurities as described in the *Pharmeuropa* Technical Guide for the elaboration of monographs, December 1999, Chapter III "Validation of analytical procedures". These guidelines describe methods to validate only qualitative nucleic acid amplification analytical procedures for assessing HCV RNA contamination of plasma pools. Therefore, the two characteristics regarded as the most important for validation of the analytical procedure are the specificity and the detection limit. In addition, the robustness of the analytical procedure should be evaluated.

However, this document may also be used as a basis for the validation of nucleic acid amplification in general.

For the purpose of this document, an analytical procedure is defined as the complete procedure from extraction of nucleic acid to detection of the amplified products.

Where commercial kits are used for part of or the complete analytical procedure, documented validation points already covered by the kit manufacturer can substitute for the validation by the user. Nevertheless, the performance of the kit with respect to its intended use has to be demonstrated by the user (e.g. detection limit, robustness, cross contamination).

2. SPECIFICITY

Specificity is the ability to unequivocally assess nucleic acid in the presence of components which may be expected to be present.

The specificity of nucleic acid amplification analytical procedures is dependent on the choice of primers, the choice of probe (for analysis of the final product) and the stringency of the test conditions (for both the amplification and detection steps).

When designing primers and probes, the specificity of the primers and probes to detect only HCV RNA should be investigated by comparing the chosen sequences with sequences in published data banks. For HCV, primers (and probes) will normally be chosen from areas of the 5' non-coding region of the HCV genome which are highly conserved for all genotypes.

The amplified product should be unequivocally identified by using one of a number of methods such as amplification with nested primers, restriction enzyme analysis, sequencing or hybridisation with a specific probe.

In order to validate the specificity of the analytical procedure, at least 100 HCV RNA-negative plasma pools should be tested and shown to be non-reactive. Suitable samples of non-reactive pools are available from the European Directorate for the Quality of Medicines.

The ability of the analytical procedure to detect all HCV genotypes will again depend on the choice of primers, probes and method parameters. This ability should be demonstrated using characterised reference panels. However, in view of the difficulty in obtaining samples of some genotypes (e.g. genotype 6), the most prevalent genotypes (e.g. genotype 1 and 3 in Europe) should be detected at a suitable level.

3. DETECTION LIMIT

The detection limit of an individual analytical procedure is the lowest amount of nucleic acid in a sample which can be detected but not necessarily quantitated as an exact value.

The nucleic acid amplification analytical procedure used for the detection of HCV RNA in plasma pools usually yields qualitative results. The number of possible results is limited to two, either positive or negative. Although the determination of the detection limit is recommended, for practical purposes, a positive cut-off point should be determined for the nucleic acid amplification analytical procedure. The positive cut-off point (as defined in the General Chapter (*2.6.21*)) is the minimum number of target sequences per volume sample which can be detected in 95 per cent of test runs. This positive cut-off point is influenced by the distribution of viral genomes in the individual samples being tested and by factors such as enzyme efficiency and can result in different 95 per cent cut-off values for individual analytical test runs.

In order to determine the positive cut-off point, a dilution series of a working reagent or of the *hepatitis C virus RNA for NAT testing BRP*, which has been calibrated against the WHO HCV International Standard 96/790, should be tested on different days to examine variation between test runs. At least 3 independent dilution series should be tested with a sufficient number of replicates at each dilution to give a total number of 24 test results for each dilution to enable a statistical analysis of the results.

For example, a laboratory could test 3 dilution series on different days with 8 replicates for each dilution, 4 dilution series on different days with 6 replicates for each dilution, or 6 dilution series on different days with 4 replicates for each dilution. In order to keep the number of dilutions at a manageable level, a preliminary test (using, for example, log dilutions of the plasma pool sample) should be done in order to obtain a preliminary value for the positive cut-off point (i.e. the highest dilution giving a positive signal). The range of dilutions can then be chosen around the predetermined preliminary cut-off point (using, for example, a dilution factor of 0.5 log or less and a negative plasma pool for the dilution matrix). The concentration of HCV RNA which can be detected in 95 per cent of test runs can then be calculated using an appropriate statistical evaluation.

These results may also serve to demonstrate the intra-assay variation and the day-to-day variation of the analytical procedure.

4. ROBUSTNESS

The robustness of an analytical procedure is a measure of its capacity to remain unaffected by small but deliberate variations in method parameters and provides an indication of its reliability during normal usage.

The evaluation of robustness should be considered during the development phase. It should show the reliability of the analytical procedure with respect to deliberate variations in method parameters. For NAT, small variations in the method parameters can be crucial. However, the robustness of the method can be demonstrated during its development when small variations in the concentrations of reagents (e.g. $MgCl_2$, primers or dNTP) are tested. To demonstrate robustness, at least 20 HCV RNA negative plasma pools (selected at random) spiked with HCV RNA to a final concentration of 3 times the previously determined 95 per cent cut-off value should be tested and found positive.

Problems with robustness may also arise with methods which use an initial ultracentrifugation step prior to extraction of the viral RNA. Therefore, to test the robustness of such methods, at least 20 plasma pools containing varying levels of HCV RNA, but lacking HCV specific antibodies, should be tested and found positive.

Cross contamination prevention should be demonstrated by the accurate detection of a panel of at least 20 samples consisting of alternate samples of negative plasma pools and negative plasma pools spiked with high concentrations of HCV (at least 10^2 times the 95 per cent cut-off value or at least 10^4 IU/ml).

Human plasma pools for NAT validation BRP are suitable for use as a negative control.

5. QUALITY ASSURANCE

For biological tests such as NAT, specific problems may arise which may influence both the validation and interpretation of results. The test procedures must be described precisely in the form of standard operating procedures (SOPs). These should cover:

- the mode of sampling (type of container, etc.),
- the preparation of mini-pools (where appropriate),
- the conditions of storage before analysis,
- the exact description of the test conditions, including precautions taken to prevent cross contamination or destruction of the viral RNA, reagents and reference preparations used,
- the exact description of the apparatus used,
- the detailed formulae for calculation of results, including statistical evaluation.

The use of a suitable run control (for example, an appropriate dilution of *hepatitis C virus RNA for NAT testing BRP* or plasma spiked with an HCV sample calibrated against the WHO HCV International Standard 96/790) can be considered a satisfactory system suitability check and ensures that the reliability of the analytical procedure is maintained whenever used.

Technical qualification: an appropriate installation and operation qualification programme should be implemented for each critical piece of the equipment used. Confirmation of analytical procedure performance after change of critical equipment (e.g. thermocyclers) should be documented by conducting a parallel test on 8 replicate samples of a plasma pool spiked with HCV RNA to a final concentration of 3 times the previously determined 95 per cent cut-off value. All results should be positive.

Operator qualification: an appropriate qualification programme should be implemented for each operator involved in the testing. To confirm successful training each operator should test at least 8 replicate samples of a plasma pool spiked with HCV RNA to a final concentration of 3 times the previously determined 95 per cent cut-off value. This test (8 replicate samples) should be repeated twice on two separate days, i.e. a total of 24 tests performed on three different days. All results should be positive.

01/2005:20622

2.6.22. ACTIVATED COAGULATION FACTORS

Where applicable, determine the amount of heparin present (*2.7.12*) and neutralise the heparin by addition of *protamine sulphate R* (10 μg of protamine sulphate neutralises 1 IU of heparin). Prepare 1 to 10 and 1 to 100 dilutions of the preparation to be examined using *tris(hydroxymethyl)aminomethane buffer solution pH 7.5 R*. Place a series of polystyrene tubes in a water-bath at 37 °C and add to each tube 0.1 ml of *platelet-poor plasma R* and 0.1 ml of a suitable dilution of *cephalin R* or *platelet substitute R*. Allow to stand for 60 s. Add to each tube either 0.1 ml of one of the dilutions or 0.1 ml of the buffer solution (control tube). To each tube add immediately 0.1 ml of a 3.7 g/l solution of *calcium chloride R* (previously warmed to 37 °C) and measure, within 30 min of the original dilution, the time that elapses between addition of the calcium chloride solution and the formation of a clot. The test is not valid unless the coagulation time measured for the control tube is 200 s to 350 s.

01/2005:20624

2.6.24. AVIAN VIRAL VACCINES: TESTS FOR EXTRANEOUS AGENTS IN SEED LOTS

GENERAL PROVISIONS

a) In the following tests, chickens and/or chicken material such as eggs and cell cultures shall be derived from chicken flocks free from specified pathogens (SPF) (*5.2.2*).

b) Cell cultures for the testing of extraneous agents comply with the requirements for the master cell seed of chapter *5.2.4. Cell cultures for the production of veterinary vaccines*, with the exception of the karyotype test and the tumorigenicity test, which do not have to be carried out.

c) In tests using cell cultures, precise specifications are given for the number of replicates, monolayer surface areas and minimum survival rate of the cultures. Alternative numbers of replicates and cell surface areas are possible as well, provided that a minimum of 2 replicates are used, the total surface area and the total volume of test substance applied are not less than that prescribed here and the survival rate requirements are adapted accordingly.

d) For a freeze-dried preparation, reconstitute using a suitable liquid. Unless otherwise stated or justified, the test substance must contain a quantity of virus equivalent to at least 10 doses of vaccine in 0.1 ml of inoculum.

e) If the virus of the seed lot would interfere with the conduct and sensitivity of the test, neutralise the virus in the preparation with a monospecific antiserum.

f) Monospecific antiserum and serum of avian origin used for cell culture or any other purpose, in any of these tests, shall be free of antibodies against and free from inhibitory effects on the organisms listed hereafter under 7. Antibody specifications for sera used in extraneous agents testing.

g) Where specified in a monograph or otherwise justified, if neutralisation of the virus of the seed lot is required but difficult to achieve, the *in vitro* tests described below are adapted, as required, to provide the necessary guarantees of freedom from contamination with an extraneous agent.

h) Other types of tests than those indicated may be used provided they are at least as sensitive as those indicated and of appropriate specificity. Nucleic acid amplification techniques (*2.6.21*) give specific detection for many agents and can be used after validation for sensitivity and specificity.

1. TEST FOR EXTRANEOUS AGENTS USING EMBRYONATED HENS' EGGS

Use a test substance, diluted if necessary, containing a quantity of neutralised virus equivalent to at least 10 doses of vaccine in 0.2 ml of inoculum. Suitable antibiotics may be added. Inoculate the test substance into 3 groups of 10 embryonated hens' eggs as follows:

– group 1: 0.2 ml into the allantoic cavity of each 9- to 11-day-old embryonated egg,
– group 2: 0.2 ml onto the chorio-allantoic membrane of each 9- to 11-day-old embryonated egg,
– group 3: 0.2 ml into the yolk sac of each 5- to 6-day-old embryonated egg.

Candle the eggs in groups 1 and 2 daily for 7 days and the eggs in group 3 for 12 days. Discard embryos that die during the first 24 h as non-specific deaths; the test is not valid unless at least 6 embryos in each group survive beyond the first 24 h after inoculation. Examine macroscopically for abnormalities all embryos which die more than 24 h after inoculation, or which survive the incubation period. Examine also the chorio-allantoic membranes of these eggs for any abnormality and test the allantoic fluids for the presence of haemagglutinating agents.

Carry out a further embryo passage. Pool separately material from live and from the dead and abnormal embryos. Inoculate each pool into 10 eggs for each route as described above, chorio-allantoic membrane material being inoculated onto chorio-allantoic membranes, allantoic fluids into the allantoic cavity and embryo material into the yolk sac. For eggs inoculated by the allantoic and chorio-allantoic routes, candle the eggs daily for 7 days, proceeding and examining the material as described above. For eggs inoculated by the yolk sac route, candle the eggs daily for 12 days, proceeding and examining the material as described above.

The seed lot complies with the test if no test embryo shows macroscopic abnormalities or dies from causes attributable to the seed lot and if examination of the chorio-allantoic membranes and testing of the allantoic fluids show no evidence of the presence of any extraneous agent.

2. TEST IN CHICKEN KIDNEY CELLS

Prepare 7 monolayers of chicken kidney cells, each monolayer having an area of about 25 cm². Maintain 2 monolayers as negative controls and treat these in the same way as the 5 monolayers inoculated with the test substance, as described below. Remove the culture medium when the cells reach confluence. Inoculate 0.1 ml of test substance onto each of the 5 monolayers. Allow adsorption for 1 h, add culture medium and incubate the cultures for a total of at least 21 days, subculturing at 4- to 7-day intervals. Each passage is made with pooled cells and fluids from all 5 monolayers after carrying out a freeze-thaw cycle. Inoculate 0.1 ml of pooled material onto each of 5 recently prepared monolayers of about 25 cm² each, at each passage. For the last subculture, grow the cells also on a suitable substrate so as to obtain an area of about 10 cm² of cells from each of the monolayers for test A. The test is not valid if less than 80 per cent of the monolayers survive after any passage.

Examine microscopically all the cell cultures frequently throughout the entire incubation period for any signs of cytopathic effect or other evidence of the presence of contaminating agents in the test substance. At the end of the total incubation period, carry out the following procedures.

A. Fix and stain (with Giemsa or haematoxylin and eosin) about 10 cm² of confluent cells from each of the 5 monolayers. Examine the cells microscopically for any cytopathic effect, inclusion bodies, syncytial formation, or any other evidence of the presence of contaminating agents from the test substance.

B. Drain and wash about 25 cm² of cells from each of the 5 monolayers. Cover these cells with a 0.5 per cent suspension of washed chicken erythrocytes (using at least 1 ml of suspension for each 5 cm² of cells). Incubate the cells at 4 °C for 20 min and then wash gently in phosphate buffered saline pH 7.4. Examine the cells microscopically for haemadsorption attributable to the presence of a haemadsorbing agent in the test substance.

C. Test pooled cell culture fluids using chicken erythrocytes for haemagglutination attributable to the presence of a haemagglutinating agent in the test substance.

The test is not valid if there are any signs of extraneous agents in the negative control cultures. The seed lot complies with the test if there is no evidence of the presence of any extraneous agent.

3. TEST FOR AVIAN LEUCOSIS VIRUSES

Prepare at least 13 replicate monolayers of primary or secondary chick embryo fibroblasts from the tissues of 9- to 11-day-old embryos that are known to be genetically susceptible to subgroups A, B and J of avian leucosis viruses and that support the growth of exogenous but not endogenous avian leucosis viruses (cells from C/E strain chickens are suitable). Each replicate shall have an area of about 50 cm².

Remove the culture medium when the cells reach confluence. Inoculate 0.1 ml of the test substance onto each of 5 of the replicate monolayers. Allow adsorption for 1 h, and add culture medium. Inoculate 2 of the replicate monolayers with subgroup A avian leucosis virus (not more than 10 $CCID_{50}$ in 0.1 ml), 2 with subgroup B avian leucosis virus (not more than 10 $CCID_{50}$ in 0.1 ml) and 2 with subgroup J avian leucosis virus (not more than 10 $CCID_{50}$ in 0.1 ml) as positive controls. Maintain not fewer than 2 non-inoculated replicate monolayers as negative controls.

Incubate the cells for a total of at least 9 days, subculturing at 3- to 4-day intervals. Retain cells from each passage level and harvest the cells at the end of the total incubation period. Wash cells from each passage level from each replicate and resuspend the cells at 10^7 cells per millilitre in barbital-buffered saline for subsequent testing by a Complement Fixation for Avian Leucosis (COFAL) test or in phosphate buffered saline for testing by Enzyme-Linked Immunosorbent Assay (ELISA). Then, carry out 3 cycles of freezing and thawing to release any group-specific antigen and perform a COFAL test or an ELISA test on each extract to detect group-specific avian leucosis antigen if present.

The test is not valid if group-specific antigen is detected in fewer than 5 of the 6 positive control replicate monolayers or if a positive result is obtained in any of the negative control monolayers, or if the results for both of the 2 negative control monolayers are inconclusive. If the results for more than 1 of the test replicate monolayers are inconclusive, then further subcultures of reserved portions of the fibroblast monolayers shall be made and tested until an unequivocal result is obtained. If a positive result is obtained for any of the test monolayers, then the presence of avian leucosis virus in the test substance has been detected.

The seed lot complies with the test if there is no evidence of the presence of any avian leucosis virus.

4. TEST FOR AVIAN RETICULOENDOTHELIOSIS VIRUS

Prepare 11 monolayers of primary or secondary chick embryo fibroblasts from the tissues of 9- to 11-day old chick embryos or duck embryo fibroblasts from the tissues of 13- to 14-day-old embryos, each monolayer having an area of about 25 cm².

Remove the culture medium when the cells reach confluence. Inoculate 0.1 ml of the test substance onto each of 5 of the monolayers. Allow adsorption for 1 h, and add culture medium. Inoculate 4 of the monolayers with avian reticuloendotheliosis virus as positive controls (not more than 10 $CCID_{50}$ in 0.1 ml). Maintain 2 non-inoculated monolayers as negative controls.

Incubate the cells for a total of at least 10 days, subculturing twice at 3- to 4-day intervals. The test is not valid if fewer than 3 of the 4 positive controls or fewer than 4 of the 5 test monolayers or neither of the 2 negative controls survive after any passage.

For the last subculture, grow the fibroblasts on a suitable substrate so as to obtain an area of about 10 cm^2 of confluent fibroblasts from each of the original 11 monolayers for the subsequent test: test about 10 cm^2 of confluent fibroblasts derived from each of the original 11 monolayers by immunostaining for the presence of avian reticuloendotheliosis virus. The test is not valid if avian reticuloendotheliosis virus is detected in fewer than 3 of the 4 positive control monolayers or in any of the negative control monolayers, or if the results for both of the 2 negative control monolayers are inconclusive. If the results for more than 1 of the test monolayers are inconclusive then further subcultures of reserved portions of the fibroblast monolayers shall be made and tested until an unequivocal result is obtained.

The seed lot complies with the test if there is no evidence of the presence of avian reticuloendotheliosis virus.

5. TEST FOR CHICKEN ANAEMIA VIRUS

Prepare eleven 20 ml suspensions of the MDCC-MSBI cell line or another cell line of equivalent sensitivity in 25 ml flasks containing about 5×10^5 cells/ml. Inoculate 0.1 ml of test substance into each of 5 flasks. Inoculate 4 of the suspensions with 10 $CCID_{50}$ chicken anaemia virus as positive controls. Maintain not fewer than 2 non-inoculated suspensions. Maintain all the cell cultures for a total of at least 24 days, subculturing 8 times at 3- to 4-day intervals. During the subculturing the presence of chicken anaemia virus may be indicated by a metabolic colour change in the infected cultures, the culture fluids become red in comparison with the control cultures. Examine the cells microscopically for cytopathic effect. At this time or at the end of the incubation period, centrifuge the cells from each flask at low speed and resuspend at about 10^6 cells/ml and place 25 μl in each of 10 wells of a multi-well slide. Examine the cells by immunostaining.

The test is not valid if chicken anaemia virus is detected in fewer than 3 of the 4 positive controls or in any of the non-inoculated controls. If the results for more than 1 of the test suspensions are inconclusive, then further subcultures of reserved portions of the test suspensions shall be made and tested until an unequivocal result is obtained.

The seed lot complies with the test if there is no evidence of the presence of chicken anaemia virus.

6. TEST FOR EXTRANEOUS AGENTS USING CHICKS

Inoculate each of at least 10 chicks, with the equivalent of 100 doses of vaccine by the intramuscular route and with the equivalent of 10 doses by eye-drop. Chicks that are 2 weeks of age are used in the test except that if the seed virus is pathogenic for birds of this age, older birds may be used, if required and justified. In exceptional cases, for inactivated vaccines, the virus may be neutralised by specific antiserum if the seed virus is pathogenic for birds at the age of administration. Repeat these inoculations 2 weeks later. Observe the chicks for a period of 5 weeks from the day of the first inoculation. No antimicrobial agents shall be administered to the chicks during the test period. The test is not valid if fewer than 80 per cent of the chicks survive to the end of the test period.

Collect serum from each chick at the end of the test period. Test each serum sample for antibodies against each of the agents listed below (with the exception of the virus type of the seed lot) using one of the methods indicated for testing for the agent.

A. Standard tests

AGENT	TYPE OF TEST
Avian adenoviruses, group 1	SN, EIA, AGP
Avian encephalomyelitis virus	AGP, EIA
Avian infectious bronchitis virus	EIA, HI
Avian infectious laryngotracheitis virus	SN, EIA, IS
Avian leucosis viruses	SN, EIA
Avian nephritis virus	IS
Avian reoviruses	IS, EIA
Avian reticuloendotheliosis virus	AGP, IS, EIA
Chicken anaemia virus	IS, EIA, SN
Egg drop syndrome virus	HI, EIA
Avian infectious bursal disease virus	AGP, EIA
Influenza A virus	AGP, EIA
Marek's disease virus	AGP
Newcastle disease virus	HI, EIA
Turkey rhinotracheitis virus	EIA
Salmonella pullorum	Agg

Agg: agglutination

AGP: agar gel precipitation

EIA: enzyme immunoassay (e.g. ELISA)

IS: immunostaining (e.g. fluorescent antibody)

HI: haemagglutination inhibition

SN: serum neutralisation

B. Additional tests for turkey extraneous agents

If the seed virus is of turkey origin or was propagated in turkey substrates, tests for antibodies against the following agents are also carried out.

AGENT	TYPE OF TEST
Chlamydia spp.	EIA
Avian infectious haemorrhagic enteritis virus	AGP
Avian paramyxovirus 3	HI
Avian infectious bursal disease virus type 2	SN

A test for freedom from turkey lympho-proliferative disease virus is carried out by intraperitoneal inoculation of twenty 4-week-old turkey poults. Observe the poults for 40 days. The test is not valid if more than 20 per cent of the poults die from non-specific causes. The seed lot complies with the test if sections of spleen and thymus taken from 10 poults 2 weeks after inoculation show no macroscopic or microscopic lesions (other than those attributable to the seed lot virus) and no poult dies from causes attributable to the seed lot.

C. Additional tests for duck extraneous agents

If the seed virus is of duck origin or was propagated in duck substrates, tests for antibodies against the following agents are also carried out.

AGENT	TYPE OF TEST
Chlamydia spp.	EIA
Duck and goose parvoviruses	SN
Duck enteritis virus	SN
Duck hepatitis virus type I	SN

The seed lot complies with the test if there is no evidence of the presence of any extraneous agent.

The test is not valid if antibodies are detected in the chicks to any of the test agents before inoculation.

Clinical signs of disease in the chicks during the test period (other than signs attributable to the virus of the seed lot) and the detection of antibodies in the chicks after inoculation, (with the exception of antibodies to the virus of the seed lot) are classed as evidence of the presence of an extraneous agent in the seed lot.

It is recommended that sera from these birds is retained so that additional testing may be carried out if requirements change.

7. ANTIBODY SPECIFICATIONS FOR SERA USED IN EXTRANEOUS AGENTS TESTING

All batches of serum to be used in extraneous agents testing either to neutralise the vaccine virus (seed lot or batch of finished product) and all batches of avian serum used as a supplement for culture media used for tissue culture propagation, shall be shown to be free of antibodies against and free from inhibitory effects on the following micro-organisms by suitably sensitive tests:

Avian adenoviruses

Avian encephalomyelitis virus

Avian infectious bronchitis viruses

Avian infectious bursal disease virus types 1 and 2

Avian infectious haemorrhagic enteritis virus

Avian infectious laryngotracheitis virus

Avian leucosis viruses

Avian nephritis virus

Avian paramyxoviruses 1 to 9

Avian reoviruses

Avian reticuloendotheliosis virus

Chicken anaemia virus

Duck enteritis virus

Duck hepatitis virus type I

Egg drop syndrome virus

Fowl pox virus

Influenza viruses

Marek's disease virus

Turkey herpesvirus

Turkey rhinotracheitis virus

Non-immune serum for addition to culture media can be assumed to be free of antibodies against any of these viruses if the agent is known not to infect the species of origin of the serum and it is not necessary to test the serum for such antibodies. Monospecific antisera for virus neutralisation can be assumed to be free of the antibodies against any of these viruses if it can be shown that the immunising antigen could not have been contaminated with antigens derived from that virus and if the virus is known not to infect the species of origin of the serum; it is not necessary to test the serum for such antibodies. It is not necessary to retest sera obtained from birds from SPF chicken flocks (*5.2.2*).

Batches of sera prepared for neutralising the vaccine virus must not be prepared from any passage level derived from the virus isolate used to prepare the master seed lot or from an isolate cultured in the same cell line.

01/2005:20625

2.6.25. AVIAN LIVE VIRUS VACCINES: TESTS FOR EXTRANEOUS AGENTS IN BATCHES OF FINISHED PRODUCT

GENERAL PROVISIONS

a) In the following tests, chickens and/or chicken material such as eggs and cell cultures shall be derived from chicken flocks free from specified pathogens (SPF) (*5.2.2*).

b) Cell cultures for the testing of extraneous agents comply with the requirements for the master cell seed of chapter *5.2.4. Cell cultures for the production of veterinary vaccines*, with the exception of the karyotype test and the tumorigenicity test, which do not have to be carried out.

c) In tests using cell cultures, precise specifications are given for the number of replicates, monolayer surface areas and minimum survival rate of the cultures. Alternative numbers of replicates and cell surface areas are possible as well, provided that a minimum of 2 replicates are used, the total surface area and the total volume of vaccine test applied are not less than that prescribed here and the survival rate requirements are adapted accordingly.

d) In these tests, use the liquid vaccine or reconstitute a quantity of the freeze-dried preparation to be tested with the liquid stated on the label or another suitable diluent such as water for injections. Unless otherwise stated or justified, the test substance contains the equivalent of 10 doses in 0.1 ml of inoculum.

e) If the vaccine virus would interfere with the conduct and sensitivity of the test, neutralise the virus in the preparation with a monospecific antiserum.

f) Where specified in a monograph or otherwise justified, if neutralisation of the vaccine virus is required but difficult to achieve, the *in vitro* tests described below are adapted, as required, to provide the necessary guarantees of freedom from contamination with an extraneous agent. Alternatively, or in addition to *in vitro* tests conducted on the batch, a test for extraneous agents may be conducted on chick sera obtained from testing the batch of vaccine, as decribed under 6. Test for extraneous agents using chicks of chapter *2.6.24. Test for extraneous agents in seed lots.*

g) Monospecific antiserum and serum of avian origin used for cell culture and any other purpose, in any of these tests, shall be free of antibodies against and free from inhibitory effects on the organisms listed under 7. Antibody specifications for sera used in extraneous agents testing (*2.6.24*).

h) Other types of tests than those indicated may be used provided they are at least as sensitive as those indicated and of appropriate specificity. Nucleic acid amplification techniques (*2.6.21*) give specific detection for many agents and can be used after validation for sensitivity and specificity.

1. TEST FOR EXTRANEOUS AGENTS USING EMBRYONATED HENS' EGGS

Prepare the test vaccine, diluted if necessary, to contain neutralised virus equivalent to 10 doses of vaccine in 0.2 ml of inoculum. Suitable antibiotics may be added. Inoculate the test vaccine into 3 groups of 10 embryonated hens' eggs as follows:

– group 1: 0.2 ml into the allantoic cavity of each 9- to 11-day-old embryonated egg,

– group 2: 0.2 ml onto the chorio-allantoic membrane of each 9- to 11-day-old embryonated egg,
– group 3: 0.2 ml into the yolk sac of each 5- to 6-day-old embryonated egg.

Candle the eggs in groups 1 and 2 daily for 7 days and the eggs in group 3 for 12 days. Discard embryos that die during the first 24 h as non-specific deaths; the test is not valid unless at least 6 embryos in each group survive beyond the first 24 h after inoculation. Examine macroscopically for abnormalities all embryos which die more than 24 h after inoculation, or which survive the incubation period. Examine also the chorio-allantoic membranes of these eggs for any abnormality and test the allantoic fluids for the presence of haemagglutinating agents.

Carry out a further embryo passage. Pool separately material from live and from the dead and abnormal embryos. Inoculate each pool into 10 eggs for each route as described above, chorio-allantoic membrane material being inoculated onto chorio-allantoic membranes, allantoic fluids into the allantoic cavity and embryo material into the yolk sac. For eggs inoculated by the allantoic and chorio-allantoic routes, candle the eggs daily for 7 days, proceeding and examining the material as described above. For eggs inoculated by the yolk sac route, candle the eggs daily for 12 days, proceeding and examining the material as described above.

The batch of vaccine complies with the test if no test embryo shows macroscopic abnormalities or dies from causes attributable to the vaccine and if examination of the chorio-allantoic membranes and testing of the allantoic fluids show no evidence of the presence of extraneous agents.

2. TEST IN CHICKEN EMBRYO FIBROBLAST CELLS

Prepare 7 monolayers of primary or secondary chicken embryo fibroblasts, from the tissues of 9- to 11-day-old embryos, each monolayer having an area of about 25 cm^2. Maintain 2 monolayers as negative controls and treat these in the same way as the 5 monolayers inoculated with the test vaccine, as described below. Remove the culture medium when the cells reach confluence. Inoculate 0.1 ml of test vaccine onto each of 5 of the monolayers. Allow adsorption for 1 h and add culture medium. Incubate the cultures for a total of at least 21 days, subculturing at 4- to 5-day intervals. Each passage is made with pooled cells and fluids from all 5 monolayers after carrying out a freeze-thaw cycle. Inoculate 0.1 ml of pooled material onto each of 5 recently prepared monolayers of chicken embryo fibroblast cells, each monolayer having an area of about 25 cm^2 each as before. For the last subculture, grow the cells also on a suitable substrate so as to obtain an area of about 10 cm^2 of cells from each of the monolayers, for test A. The test is not valid if less than 80 per cent of the test monolayers, or neither of the 2 negative control monolayers survive after any passage.

Examine microscopically all the cell cultures frequently throughout the entire incubation period for any signs of cytopathic effect or other evidence of the presence of contaminating agents in the test vaccine. At the end of the total incubation period, carry out the following procedures.

A. Fix and stain (with Giemsa or haematoxylin and eosin) about 10 cm^2 of confluent cells from each of the 5 original monolayers. Examine the cells microscopically for any cytopathic effect, inclusion bodies, syncytial formation, or any other evidence of the presence of a contaminating agent from the test vaccine.

B. Drain and wash about 25 cm^2 of cells from each of the 5 monolayers. Cover these cells with a 0.5 per cent suspension of washed chicken red blood cells (using at least 1 ml of suspension for each 5 cm^2 of cells). Incubate the cells at 4 °C for 20 min and then wash gently in phosphate buffered saline pH 7.4. Examine the cells microscopically for haemadsorption attributable to the presence of a haemadsorbing agent in the test vaccine.

C. Test pooled cell culture fluids using chicken red blood cells for haemagglutination attributable to the presence of a haemagglutinating agent in the test vaccine.

The test is not valid if there are any signs of extraneous agents in the negative control cultures. The batch of vaccine complies with the test if there is no evidence of the presence of any extraneous agent.

3. TEST FOR EGG DROP SYNDROME VIRUS

Prepare 11 monolayers of chicken embryo liver cells, from the tissues of 14- to 16-day-old embryos, each monolayer having an area of about 25 cm^2. Remove the culture medium when the cells reach confluence. Inoculate 0.1 ml of test vaccine onto each of 5 of the monolayers (test monolayers). Allow adsorption for 1 h, add culture medium. Inoculate 4 of the monolayers with a suitable strain of egg drop syndrome virus (not more than 10 $CCID_{50}$ in 0.1 ml) to serve as positive control monolayers. Maintain 2 non-inoculated monolayers as negative control monolayers.

Incubate the cells for a total of at least 21 days, subculturing every 4-5 days. Each passage is made as follows: carry out a freeze-thaw cycle; prepare separate pools of the cells plus fluid from the test monolayers, from the positive control monolayers and from the negative control monolayers; inoculate 0.1 ml of the pooled material onto each of 5, 4 and 2 recently prepared monolayers of chicken embryo liver cells, each monolayer having an area of about 25 cm^2 as before. The test is not valid if fewer than 4 of the 5 test monolayers or fewer than 3 of the 4 positive controls or neither of the 2 negative control monolayers survive after any passage.

Examine microscopically all the cell cultures at frequent intervals throughout the entire incubation period for any signs of cytopathic effect or other evidence of the presence of a contaminating agent in the test vaccine. At the end of the total incubation period, carry out the following procedure: test separately, cell culture fluid from the test monolayers, positive control monolayers and negative control monolayers, using chicken red blood cells, for haemagglutination attributable to the presence of haemagglutinating agents.

The test is not valid if egg drop syndrome virus is detected in fewer than 3 of the 4 positive control monolayers or in any of the negative control monolayers, or if the results for both of the 2 negative control monolayers are inconclusive. If the results for more than 1 of the test monolayers are inconclusive then further subcultures of reserved portions of the monolayers shall be made and tested until an unequivocal result is obtained.

The batch of vaccine complies with the test if there is no evidence of the presence of egg drop syndrome virus or any other extraneous agent.

4. TEST FOR MAREK'S DISEASE VIRUS

Prepare 11 monolayers of primary or secondary chick embryo fibroblasts from the tissues of 9- to 11-day-old embryos, each monolayer having an area of about 25 cm^2. Remove the culture medium when the cells reach confluence. Inoculate 0.1 ml of test vaccine onto each of 5 of the monolayers (test monolayers). Allow adsorption for 1 h, and add culture medium. Inoculate 4 of the monolayers with a suitable strain of Marek's disease virus (not more than 10 $CCID_{50}$ in 0.1 ml) to serve as positive controls. Maintain 2 non-inoculated monolayers as negative controls.

Incubate the cultures for a total of at least 21 days, subculturing at 4- to 5-day intervals. Each passage is made as follows: trypsinise the cells, prepare separate pools of the cells from the test monolayers, from the positive control monolayers and from the negative control monolayers. Mix an appropriate quantity of each with a suspension of freshly prepared primary or secondary chick embryo fibroblasts and prepare 5, 4 and 2 monolayers, as before. The test is not valid if fewer than 4 of the 5 test monolayers or fewer than 3 of the 4 positive controls or neither of the 2 negative control monolayers survive after any passage.

Examine microscopically all the cell cultures frequently throughout the entire incubation period for any signs of cytopathic effect or other evidence of the presence of a contaminating agent in the test vaccine.

For the last subculture, grow the cells on a suitable substrate so as to obtain an area of about 10 cm² of confluent cells from each of the original 11 monolayers for the subsequent test: test about 10 cm² of confluent cells derived from each of the original 11 monolayers by immunostaining for the presence of Marek's disease virus. The test is not valid if Marek's disease virus is detected in fewer than 3 of the 4 positive control monolayers or in any of the negative control monolayers, or if the results for both of the 2 negative control monolayers are inconclusive.

The batch of vaccine complies with the test if there is no evidence of the presence of Marek's disease virus or any other extraneous agent.

5. TESTS FOR TURKEY RHINOTRACHEITIS VIRUS

A. In chicken embryo fibroblasts

NOTE: this test can be combined with Test 2 by using the same test monolayers and negative controls, for all stages up to the final specific test for turkey rhinotracheitis virus on cells prepared from the last subculture.

Prepare 11 monolayers of primary or secondary chick embryo fibroblasts from the tissues of 9- to 11-day-old embryos, each monolayer having an area of about 25 cm². Remove the culture medium when the cells reach confluence. Inoculate 0.1 ml of test vaccine onto each of 5 of the monolayers (test monolayers). Allow adsorption for 1 h, and add culture medium. Inoculate 4 of the monolayers with a suitable strain of turkey rhinotracheitis virus as positive controls (not more than 10 $CCID_{50}$ in 0.1 ml). Maintain 2 non-inoculated monolayers as negative controls.

Incubate the cultures for a total of at least 21 days, subculturing at 4- to 5-day intervals. Each passage is made as follows: carry out a freeze-thaw cycle; prepare separate pools of the cells plus fluid from the test monolayers, from the positive control monolayers and from the negative control monolayers; inoculate 0.1 ml of the pooled material onto each of 5, 4 and 2 recently prepared monolayers of chicken embryo fibroblasts cells, each monolayer having an area of about 25 cm² as before. The test is not valid if fewer than 4 of the 5 test monolayers or fewer than 3 of the 4 positive controls or neither of the 2 negative control monolayers survive after any passage.

For the last subculture, grow the cells on a suitable substrate so as to obtain an area of about 10 cm² of confluent cells from each of the original 11 monolayers for the subsequent test: test about 10 cm² of confluent cells derived from each of the original 11 monolayers by immunostaining for the presence of turkey rhinotracheitis virus. The test is not valid if turkey rhinotracheitis virus is detected in fewer than 3 of the 4 positive control monolayers or in any of the negative control monolayers, or if the results for both of the 2 negative control monolayers are inconclusive. If the results for both of the 2 test monolayers are inconclusive then further subcultures of reserved portions of the fibroblasts shall be made and tested until an unequivocal result is obtained.

The batch of vaccine complies with the test if there is no evidence of the presence of turkey rhinotracheitis virus or any other extraneous agent.

B. In Vero cells

Prepare 11 monolayers of Vero cells, each monolayer having an area of about 25 cm². Remove the culture medium when the cells reach confluence. Inoculate 0.1 ml of test vaccine onto each of 5 of the monolayers (test monolayers). Allow adsorption for 1 h, and add culture medium. Inoculate 4 of the monolayers with a suitable strain of turkey rhinotracheitis virus (not more than 10 $CCID_{50}$ in 0.1 ml) to serve as positive controls. Maintain 2 non-inoculated monolayers as negative controls.

Incubate the cultures for a total of at least 21 days, subculturing at 4- to 5-day intervals. Each passage is made as follows: carry out a freeze-thaw cycle. Prepare separate pools of the cells plus fluid from the test monolayers, from the positive control monolayers and from the negative control monolayers. Inoculate 0.1 ml of the pooled material onto each of 5, 4 and 2 recently prepared monolayers of Vero cells, each monolayer having an area of about 25 cm² as before. The test is not valid if fewer than 4 of the 5 test monolayers or fewer than 3 of the 4 positive controls or neither of the 2 negative controls survive after any passage.

For the last subculture, grow the cells on a suitable substrate so as to obtain an area of about 10 cm² of confluent cells from each of the original 11 monolayers for the subsequent test: test about 10 cm² of confluent cells derived from each of the original 11 monolayers by immunostaining for the presence of turkey rhinotracheitis virus. The test is not valid if turkey rhinotracheitis virus is detected in fewer than 3 of the 4 positive control monolayers or in any of the negative control monolayers, or if the results for both of the 2 negative control monolayers are inconclusive. If the results for more than 1 of the test monolayers are inconclusive then further subcultures of reserved portions of the monolayers shall be made and tested until an unequivocal result is obtained.

The batch of vaccine complies with the test if there is no evidence of the presence of turkey rhinotracheitis virus or any other extraneous agent.

6. TEST FOR CHICKEN ANAEMIA VIRUS

Prepare eleven 20 ml suspensions of the MDCC-MSBI cell line or another cell line of equivalent sensitivity in 25 ml flasks containing about 5×10^5 cells/ml. Inoculate 0.1 ml of test vaccine into each of 5 of these flasks. Inoculate 4 other suspensions with 10 $CCID_{50}$ chicken anaemia virus as positive controls. Maintain not fewer than 2 non-inoculated suspensions. Maintain all the cell cultures for a total of at least 24 days, subculturing 8 times at 3- to 4-day intervals. During the subculturing the presence of chicken anaemia virus may be indicated by a metabolic colour change in the infected cultures, the culture fluids becoming red in comparison with the control cultures. Examine the cells microscopically for cytopathic effect. At this time or at the end of the incubation period, centrifuge the cells from each flask at low speed, resuspend at about 10^6 cells per millilitre and place 25 µl in each of 10 wells of a multi-well slide. Examine the cells by immunostaining.

The test is not valid if chicken anaemia virus is detected in fewer than 3 of the 4 positive controls or in any of the non-inoculated controls. If the results for more than 1 of the test suspensions are inconclusive then further subcultures of reserved portions of the test suspensions shall be made and tested until an unequivocal result is obtained.

The batch of vaccine complies with the test if there is no evidence of the presence of chicken anaemia virus.

7. TEST FOR DUCK ENTERITIS VIRUS

This test is carried out for vaccines prepared on duck or goose substrates.

Prepare 11 monolayers of primary or secondary Muscovy duck embryo liver cells, from the tissues of 21- or 22-day-old embryos, each monolayer having an area of about 25 cm^2. Remove the culture medium when the cells reach confluence. Inoculate 0.1 ml of test vaccine onto each of 5 of the monolayers (test monolayers). Allow adsorption for 1 h and add culture medium. Inoculate 4 of the monolayers with a suitable strain of duck enteritis virus (not more than 10 $CCID_{50}$ in 0.1 ml) to serve as positive controls. Maintain 2 non-inoculated monolayers as negative controls.

Incubate the cultures for a total of at least 21 days, subculturing at 4- to 5-day intervals. Each passage is made as follows: trypsinise the cells and prepare separate pools of the cells from the test monolayers, from the positive control monolayers and from the negative control monolayers. Mix a portion of each with a suspension of freshly prepared primary or secondary Muscovy duck embryo liver cells to prepare 5, 4 and 2 monolayers, as before. The test is not valid if fewer than 4 of the 5 test monolayers or fewer than 3 of the 4 positive controls or neither of the 2 negative controls survive after any passage.

For the last subculture, grow the cells on a suitable substrate so as to obtain an area of about 10 cm^2 of confluent cells from each of the original 11 monolayers for the subsequent test: test about 10 cm^2 of confluent cells derived from each of the original 11 monolayers by immunostaining for the presence of duck enteritis virus. The test is not valid if duck enteritis virus is detected in fewer than 3 of the 4 positive control monolayers or in any of the negative control monolayers, or if the results for both of the 2 negative control monolayers are inconclusive. If the results for more than 1 of the test monolayers are inconclusive then further subcultures of reserved portions of the monolayers shall be made and tested until an unequivocal result is obtained.

The batch of vaccine complies with the test if there is no evidence of the presence of duck enteritis virus or any other extraneous agent.

8. TEST FOR DUCK AND GOOSE PARVOVIRUSES

This test is carried out for vaccines prepared on duck or goose substrates.

Prepare a suspension of sufficient primary or secondary Muscovy duck embryo fibroblasts from the tissues of 16- to 18-day-old embryos, to obtain not fewer than 11 monolayers, each having an area of about 25 cm^2. Inoculate 0.5 ml of test vaccine into an aliquot of cells for 5 monolayers and seed into 5 replicate containers to form 5 test monolayers. Inoculate 0.4 ml of a suitable strain of duck parvovirus (not more than 10 $CCID_{50}$ in 0.1 ml) into an aliquot of cells for 4 monolayers and seed into 4 replicate containers to form 4 positive control monolayers. Prepare 2 non-inoculated monolayers as negative controls.

Incubate the cultures for a total of at least 21 days, subculturing at 4- to 5-day intervals. Each passage is made as follows: carry out a freeze-thaw cycle. Prepare separate pools of the cells plus fluid from the test monolayers, from the positive control monolayers and from the negative control monolayers. Inoculate 0.5 ml, 0.4 ml and 0.2 ml of the pooled materials into aliquots of a fresh suspension of sufficient primary or secondary Muscovy duck embryo fibroblast cells to prepare 5, 4 and 2 monolayers, as before. The test is not valid if fewer than 4 of the 5 test monolayers or fewer than 3 of the 4 positive controls or neither of the 2 negative controls survive after any passage.

For the last subculture, grow the cells on a suitable substrate so as to obtain an area of about 10 cm^2 of confluent cells from each of the original 11 monolayers for the subsequent test: test about 10 cm^2 of confluent cells derived from each of the original 11 monolayers by immunostaining for the presence of duck or goose parvovirus. The test is not valid if duck parvovirus is detected in fewer than 3 of the 4 positive control monolayers or in any of the negative control monolayers, or if the results for both of the 2 negative control monolayers are inconclusive.

The batch of vaccine complies with the test if there is no evidence of the presence of duck (or goose) parvovirus or any other extraneous agent.

2.7. BIOLOGICAL ASSAYS

2.7. BIOLOGICAL ASSAYS

01/2005:20701

2.7.1. IMMUNOCHEMICAL METHODS

Immunochemical methods are based on the selective, reversible and non-covalent binding of antigens by antibodies. These methods are employed to detect or quantify either antigens or antibodies. The formation of an antigen-antibody complex may be detected, and the amount of complex formed may be measured by a variety of techniques. The provisions of this general method apply to immunochemical methods using labelled or unlabelled reagents, as appropriate.

The results of immunochemical methods depend on the experimental conditions and the nature and quality of the reagents used. It is essential to standardise the components of an immunoassay and to use, wherever available, international reference preparations for immunoassays.

The reagents necessary for many immunochemical methods are available as commercial assay kits, that is, a set including reagents (particularly the antigen or the antibody) and materials intended for the *in vitro* estimation of a specified substance as well as instructions for their proper use. The kits are used in accordance with the manufacturers' instructions; it is important to ascertain that the kits are suitable for the analysis of the substance to be examined, with particular reference to selectivity and sensitivity. Guidance concerning immunoassay kits is provided by the World Health Organisation, Technical Report Series 658 (1981).

METHODS IN WHICH A LABELLED ANTIGEN OR A LABELLED ANTIBODY IS USED

Methods using labelled substances may employ suitable labels such as enzymes, fluorophores, luminophores and radioisotopes. Where the label is a radioisotope, the method is described as a "radio-immunoassay". The recommendations for the measurement of radioactivity given in the monograph on *Radiopharmaceutical Preparations (0125)* are applicable to immunoassays involving radioisotopes. All work with radioactive materials must be carried out in conformity with national legislation and internationally accepted codes of practice for protection against radiation hazards.

METHODS IN WHICH AN UNLABELLED ANTIGEN OR ANTIBODY IS USED

Immunoprecipitation methods

Immunoprecipitation methods include flocculation and precipitation reactions. When a solution of an antigen is mixed with its corresponding antibody under suitable conditions, the reactants form flocculating or precipitating aggregates. The ratio of the reactants which gives the shortest flocculation time or the most marked precipitation is called the optimal ratio, and is usually produced by equivalent amounts of antigen and antibody. Immunoprecipitation can be assessed visually or by light-scattering techniques (nephelometric or turbidimetric assay). An increase in sensitivity can be obtained by using antigen- or antibody-coated particles (e.g. latex) as reactants.

In flocculation methods, stepwise dilutions of one of the reactants is usually used whereas, in immunodiffusion (ID) methods, the dilution is obtained by diffusion in a gel medium: concentration gradients of one or both of the reactants are obtained, thus creating zones in the gel medium where the ratio of the reactants favours precipitation. While flocculation methods are performed in tubes, immunodiffusion methods may be performed using different supports such as tubes, plates, slides, cells or chambers.

Where the immunoprecipitating system consists of one antigen combining with its corresponding antibody, the system is referred to as *simple*; when it involves related but not serologically identical reactants, the system is *complex* and where several serologically unrelated reactants are involved, the system is *multiple*.

In *simple diffusion methods,* a concentration gradient is established for only one of the reactants diffusing from an external source into the gel medium containing the corresponding reactant at a comparatively low concentration.

Single radial immunodiffusion (SRID) is a simple quantitative immunodiffusion technique. When the equilibrium between the external and the internal reactant has been established, the circular precipitation area, originating from the site of the external reactant, is directly proportional to the amount of the antigen applied and inversely proportional to the concentration of the antibody in the gel.

In *double diffusion methods,* concentration gradients are established for both reactants. Both antigen and antibody diffuse from separate sites into an initially immunologically neutral gel.

Comparative double diffusion methods are used for qualitatively comparing various antigens versus a suitable antibody or vice versa. The comparison is based on the presence or absence of interaction between the precipitation patterns. Reactions of identity, non-identity or partial identity of antigens/antibodies can be distinguished.

Immunoelectrophoretic methods

Immunoelectrophoresis (IE) is a qualitative technique combining 2 methods: gel electrophoresis followed by immunodiffusion.

Crossed immunoelectrophoresis is a modification of the IE method. It is suitable both for qualitative and quantitative analysis. The first part of the procedure is an ordinary gel electrophoresis, after which a longitudinal gel strip, containing the separated fractions to be determined, is cut out and transferred to another plate. The electrophoresis in the second direction is carried out perpendicular to the previous electrophoretic run in a gel containing a comparatively low concentration of antibodies corresponding to the antigens. For a given antibody concentration and gel thickness, the relationship between the area of the respective precipitation peaks and the amount of the corresponding antigen is linear.

Electroimmunoassay, often referred to as *rocket immuno-electrophoresis* is a rapid quantitative method for determining antigens with a charge differing from that of the antibodies or vice versa. The electrophoresis of the antigen to be determined is carried out in a gel containing a comparatively lower concentration of the corresponding antibody. The test material and dilutions of a standard antigen used for calibration are introduced into different wells in the gel. During electrophoresis, migrating peak-shaped precipitation zones originating from the wells are developed. The front of the precipitate becomes stationary when the antigen is no longer in excess. For a given antibody concentration, the relationship between the distance travelled by the precipitate and the amount of antigen applied is linear.

Counter-immunoelectrophoresis is a rapid quantitative method allowing concentration gradients of external antigen and external antibody to be established in an electric field depending on the different charges. Dilutions of a standard for calibration and dilutions of the test material are introduced into a row of wells in a gel and a fixed amount of the corresponding reactant is introduced into an opposite row of wells. The titre of the test material may be determined as the highest dilution showing a precipitation line.

A number of modifications of crossed immunoelectrophoresis and electroimmunoassay methods exist.

Other techniques combine separation of antigens by molecular size and serological properties.

Visualisation and characterisation of immunoprecipitation lines

These may be performed by selective or non-selective stains, by fluorescence, by enzyme or isotope labelling or other relevant techniques. Selective staining methods are usually performed for characterisation of non-protein substances in the precipitates.

In translucent gels such as agar or agarose, the precipitation line becomes clearly visible in the gel, provided that the concentration of each of the reactants is appropriate.

VALIDATION OF THE METHOD

Validation criteria

A quantitative immunochemical method is not valid unless:

1) The antibody or antigen does not significantly discriminate between the test and standard. For a labelled reactant, the corresponding reactant does not significantly discriminate between the labelled and unlabelled compound,

2) The method is not affected by the assay matrix, that is, any component of the test sample or its excipients, which can vary between samples. These may include high concentrations of other proteins, salts, preservatives or contaminating proteolytic activity,

3) The limit of quantitation is below the acceptance criteria stated in the individual monograph,

4) The precision of the assay is such that the variance of the results meets the requirements stated in the individual monographs,

5) The order in which the assay is performed does not give rise to systematic errors.

Validation methods

In order to verify these criteria, the validation design includes the following elements:

1) The assay is performed at least in triplicate,

2) The assay includes at least 3 different dilutions of the standard preparation and 3 dilutions of sample preparations of presumed activity similar to the standard preparation,

3) The assay layout is randomised,

4) If the test sample is presented in serum or formulated with other components, the standard is likewise prepared,

5) The test includes the measurement of non-specific binding of the labelled reactant,

6) For displacement immunoassay:

(a) maximum binding (zero displacement) is determined,

(b) dilutions cover the complete response range from values close to non-specific binding to maximum binding, preferably for both standard and test preparations.

STATISTICAL CALCULATION

To analyse the results, response curves for test and standard may be analysed by the methods described in *5.3. Statistical Analysis of Results of Biological Assays and Tests*.

Significant non-parallelism indicates that the antibody or antigen discriminates between test and standard, and the results are not valid.

In displacement immunoassays, the values for non-specific binding and maximum displacement at high test or standard concentration must not be significantly different. Differences may indicate effects due to the matrix, either inhibition of binding or degradation of tracer.

01/2005:20702

2.7.2. MICROBIOLOGICAL ASSAY OF ANTIBIOTICS

The potency of an antibiotic is estimated by comparing the inhibition of growth of sensitive micro-organisms produced by known concentrations of the antibiotic to be examined and a reference substance.

The reference substances used in the assays are substances whose activity has been precisely determined with reference to the corresponding international standard or international reference preparation.

The assay must be designed in a way that will permit examination of the validity of the mathematical model on which the potency equation is based. If a parallel-line model is chosen, the 2 log dose-response (or transformed response) lines of the preparation to be examined and the reference preparation must be parallel; they must be linear over the range of doses used in the calculation. These conditions must be verified by validity tests for a given probability, usually $P = 0.05$. Other mathematical models, such as the slope ratio model, may be used provided that proof of validity is demonstrated.

Unless otherwise stated in the monograph, the confidence limits ($P = 0.95$) of the assay for potency are not less than 95 per cent and not more than 105 per cent of the estimated potency.

Carry out the assay by method A or method B.

A. DIFFUSION METHOD

Liquefy a medium suitable for the conditions of the assay and inoculate it at a suitable temperature, for example 48 °C to 50 °C for vegetative forms, with a known quantity of a suspension of micro-organisms sensitive to the antibiotic to be examined, such that clearly defined zones of inhibition of suitable diameter are produced with the concentrations of the antibiotic used for the assay. Immediately pour into Petri dishes or large rectangular dishes a quantity of the inoculated medium to form a uniform layer 2 mm to 5 mm thick. Alternatively, the medium may consist of 2 layers, only the upper layer being inoculated.

Store the dishes so that no appreciable growth or death of the micro-organisms occurs before the dishes are used and so that the surface of the medium is dry at the time of use.

Using the solvent and the buffer solution indicated in Table 2.7.2.-1, prepare solutions of the reference substance and of the antibiotic to be examined having known concentrations and presumed to be of equal activity. Apply the solutions to the surface of the medium, for example, in sterile cylinders of porcelain, stainless steel or other suitable material, or in cavities prepared in the agar. The same volume of solution must be added to each cylinder or cavity. Alternatively, use sterile absorbent paper discs of suitable quality; impregnate the discs with the solutions of the reference substance or the solutions of the antibiotic to be examined and place on the surface of the agar.

In order to assess the validity of the assay, use not fewer than 3 doses of the reference substance and 3 doses of the antibiotic to be examined having the same presumed activity as the doses of the reference substance. It is preferable to use a series of doses in geometric progression.

In routine assays when the linearity of the system has been demonstrated over an adequate number of experiments using a three-point assay, a two-point assay may be sufficient, subject to agreement by the competent authority. However, in all cases of dispute, a three-point assay as described above must be applied.

Table 2.7.2.-1. – *Diffusion assay*

Antibiotic	**Reference substance**	**Solvent to be used in preparing the stock solution**	**Buffer solution (pH)**	**Micro-organism**	**Medium and final pH (± 0.1 pH unit)**	**Incubation temperature**
Amphotericin B	*Amphotericin B CRS*	*Dimethyl sulphoxide R*	pH 10.5 (0.2 M)	*Saccharomyces cerevisiae* ATCC 9763 IP 1432-83	F - pH 6.1	35-37 °C
Bacitracin zinc	*Bacitracin zinc CRS*	*0.01 M hydrochloric acid*	pH 7.0 (0.05 M)	*Micrococcus luteus* NCTC 7743 CIP 53.160 ATCC 10240	A - pH 7.0	35-39 °C
Bleomycin sulphate	*Bleomycin sulphate CRS*	*Water R*	pH 6.8 (0.1 M)	*Mycobacterium smegmatis* ATCC 607	G - pH 7.0	35-37 °C
Colistimethate sodium	*Colistimethate sodium CRS*	*Water R*	pH 6.0 (0.05 M)	*Bordetella bronchiseptica* NCTC 8344 CIP 53.157 ATCC 4617 *Escherichia coli* NCIB 8879 CIP 54.127 ATCC 10536	B - pH 7.3	35-39 °C
Dihydrostreptomycin sulphate	*Dihydrostreptomycin sulphate CRS*	*Water R*	pH 8.0 (0.05 M)	*Bacillus subtilis* NCTC 8236 CIP 1.83 *Bacillus subtilis* NCTC 10400 CIP 52.62 ATCC 6633	A - pH 7.9 A - pH 7.9	30-37 °C 30-37 °C
Erythromycin estolate	*Erythromycin CRS*	*Methanol R* (see the monographs)	pH 8.0 (0.05 M)	*Bacillus pumilus* NCTC 8241 CIP 76.18 *Bacillus subtilis* NCTC 10400 CIP 52.62 ATCC 6633	A - pH 7.9	30-37 °C
Framycetin sulphate	*Framycetin sulphate CRS*	*Water R*	pH 8.0 (0.05 M)	*Bacillus subtilis* NCTC 10400 CIP 52.62 ATCC 6633 *Bacillus pumilus* NCTC 8241 CIP 76.18	E - pH 7.9 E - pH 7.9	30-37 °C 30-37 °C
Gentamicin sulphate	*Gentamicin sulphate CRS*	*Water R*	pH 8.0 (0.05 M)	*Bacillus pumilus* NCTC 8241 CIP 76.18 *Staphylococcus epidermidis* NCIB 8853 CIP 68.21 ATCC 12228	A - pH 7.9 A - pH 7.9	35-39 °C 35-39 °C
Josamycin	*Josamycin CRS*	*Methanol R* (see the monograph)	pH 5.6	*Bacillus subtilis* CIP 52.62 ATCC 6633 NCTC 10400	A - pH 6.6	35-37 °C
Josamycin propionate	*Josamycin propionate CRS*	*Methanol R* (see the monograph)	pH 5.6	*Bacillus subtilis* CIP 52.62 ATCC 6633 NCTC 10400	A - pH 6.6	35-37 °C

Antibiotic	Reference substance	Solvent to be used in preparing the stock solution	Buffer solution (pH)	Micro-organism	Medium and final pH (± 0.1 pH unit)	Incubation temperature
Kanamycin monosulphate Kanamycin acid sulphate	*Kanamycin monosulphate CRS*	*Water R*	pH 8.0 (0.05 M)	*Bacillus subtilis* NCTC 10400 CIP 52.62 ATCC 6633	A - pH 7.9	30-37 °C
				Staphylococcus aureus NCTC 7447 CIP 53.156 ATCC 6538 P	A - pH 7.9	35-39 °C
Neomycin sulphate	*Neomycin sulphate for microbiological assay CRS*	*Water R*	pH 8.0 (0.05 M)	*Bacillus pumilus* NCTC 8241 CIP 76.18	E - pH 7.9	30-37 °C
				Bacillus subtilis NCTC 10400 CIP 52.62 ATCC 6633	E - pH 7.9	30-37 °C
Netilmicin sulphate	*Netilmicin sulphate CRS*	*Water R*	pH 8.0 ± 0.1	*Staphylococcus aureus* ATCC 6538P CIP 53.156	A - pH 7.9	32-35 °C
Nystatin	*Nystatin CRS*	*Dimethylformamide R*	pH 6.0 (0.05 M) containing 5 per cent *V/V* of *dimethylformamide R*	*Candida tropicalis* CIP 1433-83 NCYC 1393	F - pH 6.0	30-37 °C
				Saccharomyces cerevisiae NCYC 87 CIP 1432-83 ATCC 9763	F - pH 6.0	30-32 °C
Rifamycin sodium	*Rifamycin sodium CRS*	*Methanol R*	pH 7.0 (0.05 M)	*Micrococcus luteus* NCTC 8340 CIP 53.45 ATCC 9341	A - pH 6.6	35-39 °C
Spiramycin	*Spiramycin CRS*	*Methanol R*	pH 8.0 (0.05 M)	*Bacillus subtilis* NCTC 10400 CIP 52.62 ATCC 6633	A - pH 7.9	30-32 °C
Streptomycin sulphate	*Streptomycin sulphate CRS*	*Water R*	pH 8.0 (0.05 M)	*Bacillus subtilis* NCTC 8236 CIP 1.83	A - pH 7.9	30-37 °C
				Bacillus subtilis NCTC 10400 CIP 52.62 ATCC 6633	A - pH 7.9	30-37 °C
Tylosin for veterinary use Tylosin tartrate for veterinary use	*Tylosin CRS*	2.5 per cent *V/V* solution of *methanol R* in *0.1 M phosphate buffer solution pH 7.0 R*	A mixture of 40 volumes of *methanol R* and 60 volumes of *0.1 M phosphate buffer solution pH 8.0 R*	*Micrococcus luteus* NCTC 8340 CIP 53.45 ATCC 9341	A - pH 8.0	32-35 °C
Vancomycin hydrochloride	*Vancomycin hydrochloride CRS*	*Water R*	pH 8.0	*Bacillus subtilis* NCTC 8236 CIP 52.62 ATCC 6633	A - pH 8.0	37-39 °C

Arrange the solutions on each Petri dish or on each rectangular dish according to a statistically suitable design, except for small Petri dishes that cannot accommodate more than 6 solutions, arrange the solutions of the antibiotic to be examined and the solutions of the reference substance in an alternate manner to avoid interaction of the more concentrated solutions.

Incubate at a suitable temperature for about 18 h. A period of diffusion prior to incubation, usually 1 h to 4 h, at room temperature or at about 4 °C, as appropriate, may be used to minimise the effects of the variation in time between the application of the solutions and to improve the regression slope.

Measure the diameters with a precision of at least 0.1 mm or the areas of the circular inhibition zones with a corresponding precision and calculate the potency using appropriate statistical methods.

Use in each assay the number of replications per dose sufficient to ensure the required precision. The assay may be repeated and the results combined statistically to obtain the required precision and to ascertain whether the potency of the antibiotic to be examined is not less than the minimum required.

B. TURBIDIMETRIC METHOD

Inoculate a suitable medium with a suspension of the chosen micro-organism having a sensitivity to the antibiotic to be examined such that a sufficiently large inhibition of microbial growth occurs in the conditions of the test. Use a known quantity of the suspension chosen so as to obtain a readily measurable opacity after an incubation period of about 4 h.

Use the inoculated medium immediately after its preparation.

Using the solvent and the buffer solution indicated in Table 2.7.2.-2 prepare solutions of the reference substance and of the antibiotic to be examined having known concentrations presumed to be of equal activity.

In order that the validity of the assay may be assessed, use not fewer than 3 doses of the reference substance and 3 doses of the antibiotic to be examined having the same presumed activity as the doses of the reference substance. It is preferable to use a series of doses in geometric progression. In order to obtain the required linearity, it may be necessary to select from a large number 3 consecutive doses, using corresponding doses for the reference substance and the antibiotic to be examined.

Distribute an equal volume of each of the solutions into identical test-tubes and add to each tube an equal volume of inoculated medium (for example, 1 ml of the solution and 9 ml of the medium). For the assay of tyrothricin add 0.1 ml of the solution to 9.9 ml of inoculated medium.

Prepare at the same time 2 control tubes without antibiotic, both containing the inoculated medium and to one of which is added immediately 0.5 ml of *formaldehyde R*. These tubes are used to set the optical apparatus used to measure the growth.

Place all the tubes, randomly distributed or in a Latin square or randomised block arrangement, in a water-bath or other suitable apparatus fitted with a means of bringing all the tubes rapidly to the appropriate incubation temperature and maintain them at that temperature for 3 h to 4 h, taking precautions to ensure uniformity of temperature and identical incubation time.

After incubation, stop the growth of the micro-organisms by adding 0.5 ml of *formaldehyde R* to each tube or by heat treatment and measure the opacity to 3 significant figures using suitable optical apparatus. Alternatively use a method which allows the opacity of each tube to be measured after exactly the same period of incubation.

Calculate the potency using appropriate statistical methods.

Linearity of the dose-response relationship, transformed or untransformed, is often obtained only over a very limited range. It is this range which must be used in calculating the activity and it must include at least 3 consecutive doses in order to permit linearity to be verified. In routine assays when the linearity of the system has been demonstrated over an adequate number of experiments using a three-point assay, a two-point assay may be sufficient, subject to agreement by the competent authority. However, in all cases of dispute, a three-point assay must be applied.

Use in each assay the number of replications per dose sufficient to ensure the required precision. The assay may be repeated and the results combined statistically to obtain the required precision and to ascertain whether the potency of the antibiotic to be examined is not less than the minimum required.

Table 2.7.2.-2. – *Turbidimetric assay*

Antibiotic	**Reference substance**	**Solvent to be used in preparing the stock solution**	**Buffer solution (pH)**	**Micro-organism**	**Medium and final pH (± 0.1 pH unit)**	**Incubation temperature**
Colistimethate sodium	*Colistimethate sodium CRS*	*Water R*	pH 7.0	*Escherichia coli* NCIB 8666 CIP 2.83 ATCC 9637	C - pH 7.0	35-37 °C
Dihydrostreptomycin sulphate	*Dihydrostreptomycin sulphate CRS*	*Water R*	pH 8.0	*Klebsiella pneumoniae* NCTC 7427 CIP 53.153 ATCC 10031	C - pH 7.0	35-37 °C
Erythromycin estolate Erythromycin ethylsuccinate	*Erythromycin CRS*	*Methanol R* (see the monographs)	pH 8.0	*Klebsiella pneumoniae* NCTC 7427 CIP 53.153 ATCC 10031	D - pH 7.0	35-37 °C
				Staphylococcus aureus NCTC 7447 CIP 53.156 ATCC 6538 P	C - pH 7.0	35-37 °C
Framycetin sulphate	*Framycetin sulphate CRS*	*Water R*	pH 8.0	*Staphylococcus aureus* NCTC 7447 CIP 53.156 ATCC 6538 P	C - pH 7.0	35-37 °C

Antibiotic	Reference substance	Solvent to be used in preparing the stock solution	Buffer solution (pH)	Micro-organism	Medium and final pH (± 0.1 pH unit)	Incubation temperature
Gentamicin sulphate	*Gentamicin sulphate CRS*	*Water R*	pH 7.0	*Staphylococcus aureus* NCTC 7447 CIP 53.156 ATCC 6538 P	C - pH 7.0	35-37 °C
Gramicidin	*Gramicidin CRS*	*Methanol R*	pH 7.0*	*Enterococcus hirae* CIP 58.55 ATCC 10541 *Staphylococcus aureus* ATCC 6538 P	C - pH 7.0	35-37 °C
Josamycin	*Josamycin CRS*	*Methanol R* (see the monograph)	pH 5.6	*Staphylococcus aureus* CIP 53.156 ATCC 6538 P NCTC 7447	C - pH 8.0	35-37 °C
Josamycin propionate	*Josamycin propionate CRS*	*Methanol R* (see the monograph)	pH 5.6	*Staphylococcus aureus* CIP 53.156 ATCC 6538 P NCTC 7447	C - pH 8.0	35-37 °C
Kanamycin monosulphate Kanamycin acid sulphate	*Kanamycin monosulphate CRS*	*Water R*	pH 8.0	*Staphylococcus aureus* NCTC 7447 CIP 53.156 ATCC 6538 P	C - pH 7.0	35-37 °C
Neomycin sulphate	*Neomycin sulphate for microbiological assay CRS*	*Water R*	pH 8.0	*Staphylococcus aureus* NCTC 7447 CIP 53.156 ATCC 6538 P	C - pH 7.0	35-37 °C
Rifamycin sodium	*Rifamycin sodium CRS*	*Methanol R*	pH 7.0	*Escherichia coli* NCIB 8879 CIP 54.127 ATCC 10536	C - pH 7.0	35-37 °C
Spiramycin	*Spiramycin CRS*	*Methanol R*	pH 7.0	*Staphylococcus aureus* NCTC 7447 CIP 53.156 ATCC 6538 P	C - pH 7.0	35-37 °C
Streptomycin sulphate	*Streptomycin sulphate CRS*	*Water R*	pH 8.0	*Klebsiella pneumoniae* NCTC 7427 CIP 53.153 ATCC 10031	C - pH 7.0	35-37 °C
Tylosin for veterinary use Tylosin tartrate for veterinary use	*Tylosin CRS*	2.5 per cent *V/V* solution of *methanol R* in *0.1 M phosphate buffer solution pH 7.0 R*	pH 7.0	*Staphylococcus aureus* NCTC 6571 ATCC 9144 CIP 53.154	C - pH 7.0	37 °C
Tyrothricin	*Gramicidin CRS*	*Alcohol R*	*Alcohol R*	*Enterococcus hirae* ATCC 10541	C - pH 7.0	37 °C
Vancomycin hydrochloride	*Vancomycin hydrochloride CRS*	*Water R*	pH 8.0	*Staphylococcus aureus* CIP 53.156 ATCC 6538 P	C - pH 7.0	37-39 °C

*Addition of a detergent may be necessary to avoid adsorption on the material during the dilutions, for example 0.1 mg/ml of *polysorbate 80 R*

The following section is published for information.

RECOMMENDED MICRO-ORGANISMS

The following text details the recommended micro-organisms and the conditions of use. Other micro-organisms may be used provided that they are shown to be sensitive to the antibiotic to be examined and are used in appropriate media and appropriate conditions of temperature and pH. The concentrations of the solutions used should be chosen so as to ensure that a linear relationship exists between the logarithm of the dose and the response in the conditions of the test.

Preparation of inocula. *Bacillus cereus* var. *mycoides*; *Bacillus subtilis*; *Bacillus pumilus*. Spore suspensions of the organisms to be used as inocula are prepared as follows.

Grow the organism at 35-37 °C for 7 days on the surface of a suitable medium to which has been added 0.001 g/l of *manganese sulphate R*. Using sterile *water R*, wash off the growth, which consists mainly of spores. Heat the suspension at 70 °C for 30 min and dilute to give an appropriate concentration of spores, usually 10×10^6 to 100×10^6 per millilitre. The spore suspensions may be stored for long periods at a temperature not exceeding 4 °C.

Alternatively, spore suspensions may be prepared by cultivating the organisms in medium C at 26 °C for 4-6 days, then adding, aseptically, sufficient *manganese sulphate R* to give a concentration of 0.001 g/l and incubating for a further 48 h. Examine the suspension microscopically to ensure that adequate spore formation has taken place (about 80 per cent) and centrifuge. Re-suspend the sediment in sterile *water R* to give a concentration of 10×10^6 to 100×10^6 spores per millilitre, and then heat to 70 °C for 30 min. Store the suspension at a temperature not exceeding 4 °C.

Bordetella bronchiseptica. Grow the test organism on medium B at 35-37 °C for 16-18 h. Wash off the bacterial growth with sterile *water R* and dilute to a suitable opacity.

Staphylococcus aureus; *Klebsiella pneumoniae*; *Escherichia coli*; *Micrococcus luteus*; *Staphylococcus epidermidis*. Prepare as described above for *B. bronchiseptica* but using medium A and adjusting the opacity to one which has been shown to produce a satisfactory dose-response relationship in the turbidimetric assay, or to produce clearly defined zones of inhibition of convenient diameter in the diffusion assay, as appropriate.

Saccharomyces cerevisiae; *Candida tropicalis*. Grow the test organism on medium F at 30-37 °C for 24 h. Wash off the growth with a sterile 9 g/l solution of *sodium chloride R*. Dilute to a suitable opacity with the same solution.

Buffer solutions. Buffer solutions having a pH between 5.8 and 8.0 are prepared by mixing 50.0 ml of *0.2 M potassium dihydrogen phosphate R* with the quantity of *0.2 M sodium hydroxide* indicated in Table 2.7.2.-3. Dilute with freshly prepared *distilled water R* to produce 200.0 ml.

Table 2.7.2.-3.

pH	*0.2 M Sodium hydroxide* (ml)
5.8	3.72
6.0	5.70
6.2	8.60
6.4	12.60
6.6	17.80
6.8	23.65
7.0	29.63
7.2	35.00
7.4	39.50
7.6	42.80
7.8	45.20
8.0	46.80

These buffer solutions are used for all microbiological assays shown in Table 2.7.2.-1 with the exception of bleomycin sulphate and amphotericin B.

For bleomycin sulphate, prepare the buffer solution pH 6.8 as follows: dissolve 6.4 g of *potassium dihydrogen phosphate R* and 18.9 g of *disodium hydrogen phosphate R* in *water R* and dilute to 1000 ml with *water R*.

For amphotericin B, prepare the 0.2 M phosphate buffer solution pH 10.5 as follows: dissolve 35 g of *dipotassium hydrogen phosphate R* in 900 ml of *water R*, add 20 ml of *1 M sodium hydroxide* and dilute to 1000.0 ml with *water R*.

Culture media. The following media or equivalent media may be used.

Medium A

Peptone	6 g
Pancreatic digest of casein	4 g
Beef extract	1.5 g
Yeast extract	3 g
Glucose monohydrate	1 g
Agar	15 g
Water to produce	1000 ml

Medium B

Pancreatic digest of casein	17 g
Papaic digest of soya bean	3 g
Sodium chloride	5 g
Dipotassium hydrogen phosphate	2.5 g
Glucose monohydrate	2.5 g
Agar	15 g
Polysorbate 80	10 g
Water to produce	1000 ml

The polysorbate 80 is added to the hot solution of the other ingredients after boiling, and immediately before adjusting to volume.

Medium C

Peptone	6 g
Beef extract	1.5 g
Yeast extract	3 g
Sodium chloride	3.5 g
Glucose monohydrate	1 g
Dipotassium hydrogen phosphate	3.68 g
Potassium dihydrogen phosphate	1.32 g
Water to produce	1000 ml

Medium D

Heart extract	1.5 g
Yeast extract	1.5 g
Peptone-casein	5 g
Glucose monohydrate	1 g
Sodium chloride	3.5 g
Dipotassium hydrogen phosphate	3.68 g
Potassium dihydrogen phosphate	1.32 g
Potassium nitrate	2 g
Water to produce	1000 ml

Medium E

Peptone	5 g
Meat extract	3 g
Disodium hydrogen phosphate,12H_2O	26.9 g
Agar	10 g
Water to produce	1000 ml

The disodium hydrogen phosphate is added as a sterile solution after sterilisation of the medium.

Medium F

Peptone	9.4 g
Yeast extract	4.7 g
Beef extract	2.4 g
Sodium chloride	10.0 g
Glucose monohydrate	10.0 g
Agar	23.5 g
Water to produce	1000 ml

Medium G

Glycerol	10 g
Peptone	10 g
Meat extract	10 g
Sodium chloride	3 g
Agar	15 g
Water to produce	1000 ml

pH 7.0 ± 0.1 after sterilisation.

01/2005:20704

2.7.4. ASSAY OF HUMAN COAGULATION FACTOR VIII

Human coagulation factor VIII is assayed by its biological activity as a cofactor in the activation of factor X by activated factor IX (factor IXa) in the presence of calcium ions and phospholipids. The potency of a factor VIII preparation is estimated by comparing the quantity necessary to achieve a certain rate of factor Xa formation in a test mixture containing the substances that take part in the activation of factor X, and the quantity of the International Standard, or of a reference preparation calibrated in International Units, required to produce the same rate of factor Xa formation.

The International Unit is the factor VIII activity of a stated amount of the International Standard which consists of a freeze-dried human coagulation factor VIII concentrate. The equivalence in International Units of the International Standard is stated by the World Health Organisation.

Human coagulation factor VIII BRP is calibrated in International Units by comparison with the International Standard.

The chromogenic assay method consists of two consecutive steps: the factor VIII-dependent activation of factor X in a coagulation-factor reagent composed of purified components, and the enzymatic cleavage of a chromogenic factor Xa substrate to yield a chromophore that can be quantified spectrophotometrically. Under appropriate assay conditions, there is a linear relation between the rate of factor Xa formation and the factor VIII concentration. The assay is summarised by the following scheme:

$$\text{Step 1 Factor X} \xrightarrow[\text{factor IXa, phospholipid Ca}^{++}]{\text{(activated) factor VIII}} \text{factor Xa}$$

$$\text{Step 2 chromogenic substrate} \xrightarrow{\text{factor Xa}} \text{peptide + chromophore}$$

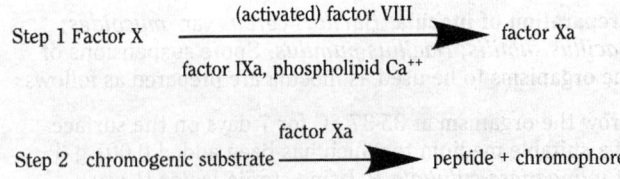

Both steps employ reagents that may be obtained commercially from a variety of sources. Although the composition of individual reagents may be subject to some variation, their essential features are described in the following specification. Deviations from this description may be permissible provided that it has been shown, using the International Standard for Human Blood Coagulation Factor VIII concentrate as the standard, that the results obtained do not differ significantly.

Commercial assay kits are to be used in accordance with the manufacturers' instructions; it is important to ascertain the suitability for the assay of the kit used.

REAGENTS

The coagulation factor reagent comprises purified proteins derived from human or bovine sources. These include factor X, factor IXa, and a factor VIII activator, usually thrombin. These proteins are partly purified, preferably to at least 50 per cent, and do not contain impurities that interfere with the activation of factor VIII or factor X. Factor X is present in amounts giving a final concentration during the first step of the assay of 10-350 nmol/l, preferably 15-30 nmol/l. Factor IXa is prepared by activating purified factor IX to factor IXaβ using factor XIa, and by subsequent purification of factor IXaβ from the reaction mixture. Its final concentration during factor Xa generation is less than 30 per cent of the factor X concentration, usually 1-100 nmol/l, preferably 1-10 nmol/l. Thrombin may be present in its precursor form prothrombin, provided that its activation in the reagent is sufficiently rapid to give almost instantaneous, complete activation of factor VIII in the assay. Phospholipids may be obtained from natural sources such as bovine brain or spinal cord or soya-bean extract, or synthetically prepared, and must consist to a substantial extent, usually 15 per cent to 35 per cent, of the species phosphatidylserine. The final phospholipid concentration during factor Xa generation is 1-50 µmol/l, preferably 10-35 µmol/l. The reagent contains calcium ions to give a final concentration of 5-15 mmol/l. The final factor Xa generation is performed in a solution containing at least 1 mg/ml of human or bovine albumin which is appropriately buffered, at a pH of 7.3–8.0. The components of the complete reagent are usually divided into at least two separate reagents each lacking the ability to generate factor Xa on its own. After reconstitution, these may be combined provided that no substantial amounts of factor Xa are generated in the absence of factor VIII. In the final incubation mixture, factor VIII must be the only rate-limiting component.

The second step comprises the quantification of the formed factor Xa employing a chromogenic substrate that is specific for factor Xa. Generally this consists of a derivatised short peptide of between three and five amino acids, joined to a chromophore group. On cleavage of this group from the peptide substrate, its chromophoric properties shift to a wavelength allowing its spectrophotometric quantification. The substrate is usually dissolved in water and used at a final concentration of 0.2-2 mmol/l. The substrate may further contain appropriate inhibitors to stop further factor Xa generation and to suppress thrombin activity, thereby improving selectivity for factor Xa.

ASSAY PROCEDURE

Reconstitute the entire contents of one ampoule of the reference preparation and the preparation to be examined by adding the appropriate quantity of *water R*; use immediately. Add sufficient prediluent to the reconstituted preparations to produce solutions containing between 0.5 IU/ml and 2.0 IU/ml.

The prediluent consists of plasma from a patient with severe haemophilia A, or of an artificially prepared reagent that gives results that do not differ significantly from those obtained employing haemophilic plasma and the same reference and test preparations. The prediluted materials must be stable beyond the time required for the assay, for at least 30 min at 20 °C and must be used within 15 min.

Prepare further dilutions of reference and test preparations using an isotonic non-chelating buffer containing 1 per cent of human or bovine albumin and for example, tris(hydroxy-methyl)aminomethane or imidazole, buffered preferably between pH 7.3 and 8.0. Prepare at least three separate, independent dilutions for each material, preferably with each one prepared in duplicate. Prepare the dilutions such that the final factor VIII concentration is below 0.03 IU/ml, and preferably below 0.01 IU/ml, during the step of factor Xa generation.

Prepare a control solution that includes all components except factor VIII.

Prepare all dilutions in plastic tubes and use without delay.

Step 1. Mix prewarmed dilutions of the factor VIII reference preparation and the preparation to be examined with an appropriate volume of the prewarmed coagulation factor reagent or a combination of its separate constituents, and incubate the mixture in plastic tubes or microplate wells at 37 °C. The concentrations of the various components during the factor Xa generation must be as specified above under the description of the reagents. Allow the activation of factor X to proceed for a suitable time, preferably terminating the reaction before the factor Xa concentration has reached its maximal level in order to obtain a satisfactory linear dose-response relationship. The activation time is also chosen to achieve linear production of factor Xa in time. Appropriate activation times are usually between 2 min and 5 min, but deviations are permissible if better linearity of the dose-response relationship is thus obtained.

Step 2. Terminate the activation by addition of a prewarmed reagent containing a chromogenic substrate. Quantify the rate of substrate cleavage, which must be linear with the concentration of factor Xa formed, by measuring the absorbance change at an appropriate wavelength using a spectrophotometer, either monitoring the absorbance continuously, thus allowing the initial rate of substrate cleavage to be calculated, or terminating the hydrolysis reaction after a suitable interval by lowering the pH by addition of a suitable reagent, such as acetic acid (50 per cent *V/V* $C_2H_4O_2$) or a citrate solution (1 mol/l) at pH 3. Adjust the hydrolysis time to achieve a linear development of chromophore in time. Appropriate hydrolysis times usually are between 3 min and 15 min, but deviations are permissible if better linearity of the dose-response relationship is thus obtained.

Check the validity of the assay and calculate the potency of the test preparation by the usual statistical methods (for example, *5.3. Statistical analysis of results of biological assays and tests*).

01/2005:20705

2.7.5. ASSAY OF HEPARIN

The anticoagulant activity of heparin is determined *in vitro* by comparing its ability in given conditions to delay the clotting of recalcified citrated sheep plasma with the same ability of a reference preparation of heparin calibrated in International Units.

The International Unit is the activity contained in a stated amount of the International Standard, which consists of a quantity of freeze-dried heparin sodium from pork intestinal mucosa. The equivalence in International Units of the International Standard is stated by the World Health Organisation.

Heparin sodium BRP is calibrated in International Units by comparison with the International Standard by means of the assay given below.

Carry out the assay using one of the following methods for determining the onset of clotting and using tubes and other equipment appropriate to the chosen method:

a) direct visual inspection, preferably using indirect illumination and viewing against a matt black background;

b) spectrophotometric recording of the change in optical density at a wavelength of approximately 600 nm;

c) visual detection of the change in fluidity on manual tilting of the tubes;

d) mechanical recording of the change in fluidity on stirring, care being taken to cause the minimum disturbance of the solution during the earliest phase of clotting.

ASSAY PROCEDURE

The volumes in the text are given as examples and may be adapted to the apparatus used provided that the ratios between the different volumes are respected.

Dilute *heparin sodium BRP* with a 9 g/l solution of *sodium chloride R* to contain a precisely known number of International Units per millilitre and prepare a similar solution of the preparation to be examined which is expected to have the same activity. Using a 9 g/l solution of *sodium chloride R*, prepare from each solution a series of dilutions in geometric progression such that the clotting time obtained with the lowest concentration is not less than 1.5 times the blank recalcification time, and that obtained with the highest concentration is such as to give a satisfactory log dose-response curve, as determined in a preliminary test.

Place 12 tubes in a bath of iced water, labelling them in duplicate: T_1, T_2 and T_3 for the dilutions of the preparation to be examined and S_1, S_2 and S_3 for the dilutions of the reference preparation. To each tube add 1.0 ml of thawed *plasma substrate R1* and 1.0 ml of the appropriate dilution of the preparation to be examined or the reference preparation. After each addition, mix but do not allow bubbles to form. Treating the tubes in the order S_1, S_2, S_3, T_1, T_2, T_3, transfer each tube to a water-bath at 37 °C, allow to equilibrate at 37 °C for about 15 min and add to each tube 1 ml of a dilution of *cephalin R* to which has been added an appropriate activator such as kaolin so that a suitable blank recalcification time not exceeding 60 s is obtained. When kaolin is used, prepare just before use, a mixture of equal volumes of *cephalin R* and a 4 g/l suspension of *light kaolin R* in a 9 g/l solution of *sodium chloride R*. After exactly 2 min add 1 ml of a 3.7 g/l solution of *calcium chloride R* and record as the clotting time the interval in seconds between this last addition and the onset of clotting determined by the chosen technique. Determine the blank recalcification time at the beginning and at the end of the procedure in a similar manner, using 1 ml of a 9 g/l solution of *sodium chloride R* in place of one of the heparin dilutions; the 2 blank values obtained should not differ significantly. Transform the clotting times to logarithms, using the mean value for the duplicate tubes. Repeat the procedure using fresh dilutions and carrying out the incubation in the order T_1, T_2, T_3, S_1, S_2, S_3. Calculate the results by the usual statistical methods.

Carry out not fewer than 3 independent assays. For each such assay prepare fresh solutions of the reference preparation and the preparation to be examined and use another, freshly thawed portion of plasma substrate. Calculate the potency of the preparation to be examined by combining the results of these assays by the usual statistical methods. When the variance due to differences between assays is significant at $P = 0.01$ a combined estimate of potency may be obtained by calculating the non-weighted mean of potency estimates.

01/2005:20706
corrected

2.7.6. ASSAY OF DIPHTHERIA VACCINE (ADSORBED)

The potency of diphtheria vaccine (adsorbed) is determined by comparing the dose of the vaccine required to protect guinea-pigs from the effects of either an erythrogenic dose of diphtheria toxin administered intradermally or a lethal dose of diphtheria toxin administered subcutaneously with the dose of a reference preparation, calibrated in International Units, needed to give the same protection.

The International Unit is the activity contained in a stated amount of the International Standard which consists of a quantity of diphtheria toxoid adsorbed on aluminium hydroxide. The equivalence in International Units of the International Standard is stated by the World Health Organisation.

Diphtheria vaccine (adsorbed) BRP is suitable for use as a reference preparation.

The design of the assay described below follows a parallel-line model with 3 dilutions for the test and reference preparations. Once the analyst has sufficient experience with this method for a given vaccine, it is possible to apply a simplified model using a single dilution for both test and reference preparations. Such a model enables the analyst to determine whether the potency of the test preparation is significantly higher than the minimum required but does not give information on linearity, parallelism and the dose-response curve. The simplified model leads to a considerable reduction in the number of experimental animals required and must be considered by each analyst in accordance with the provisions of the European Convention for the Protection of Vertebrate Animals used for Experimental and other Scientific Purposes.

METHOD OF INTRADERMAL CHALLENGE

Selection and distribution of the test animals. Use in the test, healthy, white guinea-pigs from the same stock and of a size suitable for the prescribed number of challenge sites, the difference in body mass between the heaviest and the lightest animal being not greater than 100 g. Distribute the guinea-pigs in not fewer than 6 equal groups; use groups containing a number of animals sufficient to obtain results that fulfil the requirements for a valid assay prescribed below. If the challenge toxin to be used has not been shown to be stable or has not been adequately standardised, include 5 guinea-pigs as unvaccinated controls. Use guinea-pigs of the same sex or with males and females equally distributed between the groups.

Selection of the challenge toxin. Select a preparation of diphtheria toxin containing 67 to 133 lr/100 in 1 Lf and 25 000 to 50 000 minimal reacting doses for guinea-pig skin in 1 Lf. If the challenge toxin preparation has been shown to be stable, it is not necessary to verify the activity for every assay.

Preparation of the challenge toxin solution. Immediately before use, dilute the challenge toxin with a suitable diluent to obtain a challenge toxin solution containing about 0.0512 Lf in 0.2 ml. Prepare from this a further series of 5 four-fold dilutions containing about 0.0128, 0.0032, 0.0008, 0.0002 and 0.00005 Lf in 0.2 ml.

Determination of potency of the vaccine. Using a 9 g/l solution of *sodium chloride R*, prepare dilutions of the vaccine to be examined and of the reference preparation, such that for each, the dilutions form a series differing by not more than 2.5-fold steps and in which the intermediate dilutions, when injected subcutaneously at a dose of 1.0 ml per guinea-pig, will result in an intradermal score of approximately 3 when the animals are challenged. Allocate the dilutions 1 to each of the groups of guinea-pigs and inject subcutaneously 1.0 ml of each dilution into each guinea-pig in the group to which that dilution is allocated. After 28 days, shave both flanks of each guinea-pig and inject 0.2 ml of each of the 6 toxin dilutions intradermally into 6 separate sites on each of the vaccinated guinea-pigs in such a way as to minimise interference between adjacent sites.

Determination of the activity of the challenge toxin. If necessary, inject the unvaccinated control animals with dilutions containing 80, 40, 20, 10 and 5 millionths of an Lf of the challenge toxin.

Reading and interpretation of results. Examine all injection sites 48 h after injection of the challenge toxin and record the incidence of specific diphtheria erythema. Record also the number of sites free from such reactions as the intra-dermal challenge score. Tabulate together the intradermal challenge scores for all the animals receiving the same dilution of vaccine and use those data with a suitable transformation, such as $(\text{score})^2$ or $\arcsin((\text{score}/6)^2)$, to obtain an estimate of the relative potency for each of the test preparations by parallel-line quantitative analysis.

Requirements for a valid assay. The test is not valid unless:

- for both the vaccine to be examined and the reference preparation, the mean score obtained at the lowest dose level is less than 3 and the mean score at the highest dose level is more than 3,
- if applicable, the toxin dilution that contains 40 millionths of an Lf gives a positive erythema in at least 80 per cent of the control guinea-pigs and the dilution containing 20 millionths of an Lf gives a positive erythema in less than 80 per cent of the guinea-pigs (if these criteria are not met a different toxin has to be selected),
- the confidence limits ($P = 0.95$) are not less than 50 per cent and not more than 200 per cent of the estimated potency,
- the statistical analysis shows no deviation from linearity and parallelism.

The test may be repeated but when more than 1 test is performed the results of all valid tests must be combined in the estimate of potency.

METHOD OF LETHAL CHALLENGE

Selection and distribution of the test animals. Use in the test healthy guinea-pigs from the same stock, each weighing 250 g to 350 g. Distribute the guinea-pigs in not fewer than 6 equal groups; use groups containing a number of animals sufficient to obtain results that fulfil the requirements for a valid assay prescribed below. If the challenge toxin to be used has not been shown to be stable or has not been adequately standardised, include 4 further groups of 5 guinea-pigs as unvaccinated controls. Use guinea-pigs of the same sex or with males and females equally distributed between the groups.

Selection of the challenge toxin. Select a preparation of diphtheria toxin containing not less than 100 LD_{50} per millilitre. If the challenge toxin preparation has been shown to be stable, it is not necessary to verify the lethal dose for every assay.

Preparation of the challenge toxin solution. Immediately before use, dilute the challenge toxin with a suitable diluent to obtain a challenge toxin solution containing approximately 100 LD_{50} per millilitre. If necessary, dilute portions of the challenge toxin solution 1 in 32, 1 in 100 and 1 in 320 with the same diluent.

Determination of potency of the vaccine. Using a 9 g/l solution of *sodium chloride R*, prepare dilutions of the vaccine to be examined and of the reference preparation, such that for each, the dilutions form a series differing by not more than 2.5-fold steps and in which the intermediate dilutions, when injected subcutaneously at a dose of 1.0 ml per guinea-pig, protect approximately 50 per cent of the animals from the lethal effects of the subcutaneous injection of the quantity of diphtheria toxin prescribed for this test. Allocate the dilutions 1 to each of the groups of guinea-pigs and inject subcutaneously 1.0 ml of each dilution into each guinea-pig in the group to which that dilution is allocated. After 28 days, inject subcutaneously into each animal 1.0 ml of the challenge toxin solution (100 LD_{50}).

Determination of the activity of the challenge toxin. If necessary, allocate the challenge toxin solution and the 3 dilutions made from it, 1 to each of the 4 groups of 5 guinea-pigs and inject subcutaneously 1.0 ml of each solution into each guinea-pig in the group to which that solution is allocated.

Reading and interpretation of results. Count the number of surviving guinea-pigs 4 days after injection of the challenge toxin. Calculate the potency of the vaccine to be examined relative to the potency of the reference preparation on the basis of the proportion of animals surviving in each of the groups of vaccinated guinea-pigs, using the usual statistical methods.

Requirements for a valid assay. The test is not valid unless:

- for the vaccine to be examined and the reference preparation the 50 per cent protective dose lies between the largest and smallest doses of the preparations given to the guinea-pigs,
- if applicable, the number of animals that die in the 4 groups of 5 injected with the challenge toxin solution and its dilutions indicates that the challenge dose was approximately 100 LD_{50},
- the confidence limits ($P = 0.95$) are not less than 50 per cent and not more than 200 per cent of the estimated potency,
- the statistical analysis shows no deviation from linearity and parallelism.

The test may be repeated but when more than 1 test is performed the results of all valid tests must be combined in the estimate of potency.

01/2005:20707

2.7.7. ASSAY OF PERTUSSIS VACCINE

The potency of pertussis vaccine is determined by comparing the dose necessary to protect mice against the effects of a lethal dose of *Bordetella pertussis*, administered intracerebrally, with the quantity of a reference preparation, calibrated in International Units, needed to give the same protection.

The International Unit is the activity contained in a stated amount of the International Standard which consists of a quantity of dried pertussis vaccine. The equivalence in International Units of the International Standard is stated by the World Health Organisation.

Selection and distribution of the test animals. Use in the test, healthy mice less than 5 weeks old of a suitable strain from the same stock, the difference in mass between the heaviest and the lightest being not greater than 5 g. Distribute the mice in 6 groups of not fewer than 16 and 4 groups of 10. The mice must all be of the same sex or the males and females should be distributed equally between the groups.

Selection of the challenge strain and preparation of the challenge suspension. Select a suitable strain of *B. pertussis* capable of causing the death of mice within 14 days of intracerebral injection. If more than 20 per cent of the mice die within 48 h of the injection the strain is not suitable. Make one subculture from the strain and suspend the harvested *B. pertussis* in a solution containing 10 g/l of *casein hydrolysate R* and 6 g/l of *sodium chloride R* and having a pH of 7.0 to 7.2 or in another suitable solution. Determine the opacity of the suspension. Prepare a series of dilutions in the same solution and allocate each dilution to a group of ten mice. Inject intracerebrally into each mouse a dose (0.02 ml or 0.03 ml) of the dilution allocated to its group. After 14 days, count the number of mice surviving in each group. From the results, calculate the expected opacity of a suspension containing 100 LD_{50} in each challenge dose. For the test of the vaccine to be examined make a fresh subculture from the same strain of *B. pertussis* and prepare a suspension of the harvested organisms with an opacity corresponding to about 100 LD_{50} in each challenge dose. Prepare 3 dilutions of the challenge suspension.

Determination of potency. Prepare 3 serial dilutions of the vaccine to be examined and 3 similar dilutions of the reference preparation such that in each the intermediate dilution may be expected to protect about 50 per cent of the mice from the lethal effects of the challenge dose of *B. pertussis*. Suggested doses are 1/8, 1/40 and 1/200 of the human dose of the vaccine to be examined and 0.5 IU, 0.1 IU and 0.02 IU of the reference preparation, each dose being contained in a volume not exceeding 0.5 ml. Allocate 6 dilutions one to each of the groups of not fewer than 16 mice and inject intraperitoneally into each mouse one dose of the dilution allocated to its group. After 14 to 17 days inject intracerebrally into each animal in the groups of not fewer than 16, one dose of the challenge suspension. Allocate the challenge suspension and the 3 dilutions made from it one to each of the groups of 10 mice and inject intracerebrally one dose of each suspension into each mouse in the group to which that suspension is allocated.

Exclude from consideration any mice that die within 48 h of challenge. Count the number of mice surviving in each of the groups after 14 days. Calculate the potency of the vaccine to be examined relative to the potency of the reference preparation on the basis of the numbers of animals surviving in each of the groups of not fewer than 16.

The test is not valid unless:

- for both the vaccine to be examined and the reference preparation, the 50 per cent protective dose lies between the largest and the smallest doses given to the mice;
- the number of animals which die in the four groups of ten injected with the challenge suspension and its dilutions indicates that the challenge dose is approximately 100 LD_{50};
- and the statistical analysis shows no deviation from linearity or parallelism.

The test may be repeated but when more than one test is performed the results of all valid tests must be combined.

01/2005:20708

2.7.8. ASSAY OF TETANUS VACCINE (ADSORBED)

The potency of tetanus vaccine is determined by administration of the vaccine to animals (guinea-pigs or mice) followed either by challenge with tetanus toxin (method A or B) or by determination of the titre of antibodies against tetanus toxoid in the serum of the guinea-pigs (method C). In both cases the potency of the vaccine is calculated by comparison with a reference vaccine, calibrated in International Units. For methods A and B, in countries where the paralysis method is not obligatory the LD_{50} method may be used. For the LD_{50} method, the number of animals and the procedure are identical with those described for the paralysis method but the end-point is the death of the animal rather than paralysis.

The International Unit is the activity contained in a stated amount of the International Standard for tetanus toxoid (adsorbed). The equivalence in International Units of the International Standard is stated by the World Health Organisation.

Tetanus vaccine (adsorbed) BRP is calibrated in International Units with reference to the International Standard.

The method chosen for assay of tetanus vaccine (adsorbed) depends on the intended purpose. Method A or B is used:

1. during development of a vaccine, to assay batches produced to validate the production;
2. wherever revalidation is needed following a significant change in the manufacturing process.

Method A or B may also be used for routine assay of batches of vaccine but in the interests of animal welfare, method C is used wherever possible.

Method C may be used, except as specified under 1 and 2 above, after verification of the suitability of the method for the product. For this purpose, a suitable number of batches (usually 3) are assayed by method C and method A or B. Where different vaccines (monovalent or combinations) are prepared from tetanus toxoid of the same origin, suitability demonstrated for the combination with the highest number of components can be assumed to be valid for combinations with fewer components and for monovalent vaccine. For combinations with a whole-cell pertussis component, a separate demonstration of equivalence must be made for the highest combination.

The design of the assays described below uses multiple dilutions for the test and reference preparations. Based on the potency data obtained in multidilution assays, it may be possible to decrease the number of animals needed to obtain a statistically significant result by applying a simplified model using a single dilution for both test and reference preparations. Such a model enables the analyst to determine whether the potency of the test preparation is significantly higher than the minimum required but does not give information on the dose-response curves and their linearity, parallelism and significant slope. The simplified model may lead to a considerable reduction in the number of animals required and its use must be considered in accordance with the provisions of the European Convention for the protection of vertebrate animals used for experimental and other scientific purposes.

Where a single-dilution assay is used, production and test consistency over time are monitored via suitable indicators and by carrying out a full multiple-dilution assay periodically, for example every 2 years. For serological assays, suitable indicators to monitor test consistency are:

- mean and standard deviation of relative antitoxin titres or scores of the serum samples obtained after administration of a fixed dose of the vaccine reference preparation,
- antitoxin titres or scores of run controls (positive and negative serum samples),
- ratio of antitoxin titres or scores for the positive serum control and the serum samples corresponding to the reference vaccine.

METHOD A. CHALLENGE TEST IN GUINEA-PIGS

SELECTION AND DISTRIBUTION OF THE TEST ANIMALS

Use in the test healthy guinea-pigs from the same stock, each weighing 250-350 g. Distribute the guinea-pigs in not fewer than 6 equal groups; use groups containing a number of animals sufficient to obtain results that fulfil the requirements for a valid assay prescribed below. If the activity of the challenge toxin has to be determined, include 3 further groups of 5 guinea-pigs as unvaccinated controls. Use guinea-pigs of the same sex or with the males and females equally distributed between the groups.

SELECTION OF THE CHALLENGE TOXIN

Select a preparation of tetanus toxin containing not less than 50 times the 50 per cent paralytic dose per millilitre. If the challenge toxin preparation has been shown to be stable, it is not necessary to verify the paralytic dose for every assay.

PREPARATION OF THE CHALLENGE TOXIN SOLUTION

Immediately before use, dilute the challenge toxin with a suitable diluent (for example, peptone buffered saline solution pH 7.4) to obtain a stable challenge toxin solution containing approximately 50 times the 50 per cent paralytic dose per millilitre. If necessary, use portions of the challenge toxin solution diluted 1 to 16, 1 to 50 and 1 to 160 with the same diluent to determine the activity of the toxin.

DILUTION OF THE TEST AND REFERENCE PREPARATIONS

Using a 9 g/l solution of *sodium chloride R*, prepare dilutions of the vaccine to be examined and of the reference preparation, such that for each, the dilutions form a series differing by not more than 2.5-fold steps and in which the intermediate dilutions, when injected subcutaneously at a dose of 1.0 ml per guinea-pig, protect approximately 50 per cent of the animals from the paralytic effects of the subcutaneous injection of the quantity of tetanus toxin prescribed for this test.

IMMUNISATION AND CHALLENGE

Allocate the dilutions, 1 to each of the groups of guinea-pigs and inject subcutaneously, 1.0 ml of each dilution into each guinea-pig in the group to which that dilution is allocated. After 28 days, inject subcutaneously into each animal 1.0 ml of the challenge toxin solution (containing 50 times the 50 per cent paralytic dose).

DETERMINATION OF THE ACTIVITY OF THE CHALLENGE TOXIN

If necessary, allocate the 3 dilutions made from the challenge toxin solution, 1 to each of the 3 groups of 5 guinea-pigs, and inject subcutaneously 1.0 ml of each solution into each guinea-pig in the group to which that solution is allocated. The activity and stability of the challenge toxin are determined by carrying out a suitable number of determinations of the 50 per cent paralytic dose. It is then not necessary to repeat the determination for each assay.

READING AND INTERPRETATION OF RESULTS

Examine the guinea-pigs twice daily. Remove and humanely kill all animals showing definite signs of tetanus paralysis. Count the number of guinea-pigs without paralysis 5 days after injection of the challenge toxin. Calculate the potency of the vaccine to be examined relative to the potency of the reference preparation on the basis of the proportion of challenged animals without paralysis in each of the groups of vaccinated guinea-pigs, using the usual statistical methods.

REQUIREMENTS FOR A VALID ASSAY

The test is not valid unless:

- for both the vaccine to be examined and the reference preparation the 50 per cent protective dose lies between the largest and smallest doses of the preparations given to the guinea-pigs,
- if applicable, the number of paralysed animals in the 3 groups of 5 injected with the dilutions of the challenge toxin solution indicates that the challenge was approximately 50 times the 50 per cent paralytic dose,
- the confidence limits ($P = 0.95$) are not less than 50 per cent and not more than 200 per cent of the estimated potency,
- the statistical analysis shows significant slope and no deviation from linearity and parallelism of the dose-response lines (chapter *5.3* describes possible alternatives if significant deviations are observed).

The test may be repeated but when more than 1 test is performed the results of all valid tests must be combined in the estimate of potency.

METHOD B. CHALLENGE TEST IN MICE

SELECTION AND DISTRIBUTION OF THE TEST ANIMALS

Use in the test healthy mice from the same stock, about 5 weeks old and from a strain shown to be suitable. Distribute the mice in not fewer than 6 equal groups; use groups containing a number of animals sufficient to obtain results that fulfil the requirements for a valid assay prescribed below. If the challenge toxin to be used has not been shown to be stable or has not been adequately standardised, include 3 groups of not fewer than 5 mice to serve as unvaccinated controls. Use mice of the same sex or with males and females equally distributed between the groups.

SELECTION OF THE CHALLENGE TOXIN

Select a preparation of tetanus toxin containing not less than 100 times the 50 per cent paralytic dose per millilitre. If the challenge toxin preparation has been shown to be stable, it is not necessary to verify the paralytic dose for every assay.

PREPARATION OF THE CHALLENGE TOXIN SOLUTION

Immediately before use, dilute the challenge toxin with a suitable diluent (for example, peptone buffered saline solution pH 7.4) to obtain a stable challenge toxin solution containing approximately 50 times the 50 per cent paralytic dose in 0.5 ml. If necessary, use portions of the challenge toxin solution diluted 1 to 16, 1 to 50 and 1 to 160 with the same diluent to determine the activity of the toxin.

DILUTION OF THE TEST AND REFERENCE PREPARATIONS

Using a 9 g/l solution of *sodium chloride R*, prepare dilutions of the vaccine to be examined and of the reference preparation, such that for each, the dilutions form a series differing by not more than 2.5-fold steps and in which the intermediate dilutions, when injected subcutaneously at a dose of 0.5 ml per mouse, protect approximately 50 per cent of the animals from the paralytic effects of the subcutaneous injection of the quantity of tetanus toxin prescribed for this test.

IMMUNISATION AND CHALLENGE

Allocate the dilutions, 1 to each of the groups of mice and inject subcutaneously 0.5 ml of each dilution into each mouse in the group to which that dilution is allocated. After 28 days, inject subcutaneously into each animal 0.5 ml of the challenge toxin solution (containing 50 times the 50 per cent paralytic dose).

DETERMINATION OF THE ACTIVITY OF THE CHALLENGE TOXIN

If necessary, allocate the 3 dilutions made from the challenge toxin solution, 1 to each of the 3 groups of not fewer than 5 mice and inject subcutaneously 0.5 ml of each solution into each mouse in the group to which that solution is allocated.

READING AND INTERPRETATION OF RESULTS

Examine the mice twice daily. Remove and humanely kill all animals showing definite signs of tetanus paralysis. Count the number of mice without paralysis 4 days after injection of the challenge toxin. Calculate the potency of the vaccine to be examined relative to the potency of the reference preparation on the basis of the proportion of challenged animals without paralysis in each group of vaccinated mice, using the usual statistical methods.

REQUIREMENTS FOR A VALID ASSAY

The test is not valid unless:

- for both the vaccine to be examined and the reference preparation the 50 per cent protective dose lies between the largest and smallest doses of the preparations given to the mice,
- if applicable, the number of paralysed animals in the 3 groups of not fewer than 5 injected with the dilutions of the challenge toxin solution, indicates that the challenge dose was approximately 50 times the 50 per cent paralytic dose,
- the confidence limits ($P = 0.95$) are not less than 50 per cent and not more than 200 per cent of the estimated potency,
- the statistical analysis shows a significant slope and no deviation from linearity and parallelism of the dose-response lines (chapter *5.3* describes possible alternatives if significant deviations are observed).

The test may be repeated but when more than 1 test is performed the results of all valid tests must be combined in the estimate of potency.

METHOD C. DETERMINATION OF ANTIBODIES IN GUINEA-PIGS

SELECTION AND DISTRIBUTION OF THE TEST ANIMALS

Use in the test healthy guinea-pigs from the same stock, each weighing 250-350 g. Use guinea-pigs of the same sex or with males and females equally distributed between groups. Distribute the guinea-pigs in not fewer than 6 equal groups; use groups containing a number of animals sufficient to obtain results that fulfil the requirements for a valid assay. Use a further group of non-vaccinated guinea-pigs of the same origin to provide a negative serum control. If test consistency has been demonstrated, a reference negative serum control may be used.

REFERENCE PREPARATION

Use a suitable reference preparation such as *tetanus vaccine (adsorbed) BRP* or a batch of vaccine shown to be effective in clinical studies, or a batch representative thereof, and which has been calibrated in International Units with reference to *tetanus vaccine (adsorbed) BRP* or the International Standard for tetanus toxoid (adsorbed).

DILUTION OF THE TEST AND REFERENCE PREPARATIONS

Using a 9 g/l solution of *sodium chloride R* as diluent, prepare serial dilutions of the vaccine to be examined and the reference preparation; series differing by 2.5- to 5-fold steps have been found suitable. Use not fewer than 3 dilutions within the range for example 0.5-16 IU/ml for each series. Use dilutions for immunisation preferably within 1 h of preparation. Allocate 1 dilution to each group of guinea-pigs.

IMMUNISATION

Inject subcutaneously in the nape of each guinea-pig 1.0 ml of the dilution allocated to its group.

BLOOD SAMPLING

35-42 days after immunisation, take a blood sample from each vaccinated and control guinea-pig using a suitable method.

PREPARATION OF SERUM SAMPLES

Avoid frequent freezing and thawing of serum samples. To avoid microbial contamination, it is preferable to carry out manipulations in a laminar-flow cabinet.

DETERMINATION OF ANTIBODY TITRE

Determine the relative antibody titre or score of each serum sample by a suitable immunochemical method (*2.7.1*). The methods shown below (enzyme-linked immunosorbent assay (ELISA) and toxin-binding inhibition (ToBI)) have been found suitable.

CALCULATION OF POTENCY

Calculate the potency of the vaccine to be examined in International Units relative to the reference preparation, using the usual statistical methods (for example *5.3*).

NOTE: International Units of potency refer to the reference vaccine and not to the International Units of antitoxin of the reference guinea-pig serum.

Requirements for a valid assay. The test is not valid unless:

- the confidence limits ($P = 0.95$) are not less than 50 per cent and not more than 200 per cent of the estimated potency,
- the statistical analysis shows significant slope and no deviation from linearity and parallelism of the dose-response lines (chapter *5.3* describes possible alternatives if significant deviations are observed).

The test may be repeated but when more than 1 test is performed the results of all valid tests must be combined in the estimate of potency.

Assay of tetanus vaccine (adsorbed): guidelines

METHOD A. CHALLENGE TEST IN GUINEA-PIGS

READING AND INTERPRETATION OF RESULTS

In order to minimise suffering in the test animals, it is recommended to note the degree of paralysis on a scale such as that shown below. The scale gives typical signs when injection of the challenge toxin is made mid-ventrally directly behind the sternum with the needle pointing towards the neck of the guinea-pig. Grade T3 is taken as the end-point, but with experience grade T2 can be used instead. Tetanus toxin produces in at least 1 of the forelimbs paralysis that can be recognised at an early stage. The tetanus grades in guinea-pigs are characterised by the following signs:

- T1: slight stiffness of 1 forelimb, but difficult to observe;
- T2: paresis of 1 forelimb which still can function;
- T3: paralysis of 1 forelimb. The animal moves reluctantly, the body is often slightly banana-shaped owing to scoliosis;
- T4: the forelimb is completely stiff and the toes are immovable. The muscular contraction of the forelimb is very pronounced and usually scoliosis is observed;
- T5: tetanus seizures, continuous tonic spasm of muscles;
- D: death.

METHOD B. CHALLENGE TEST IN MICE

READING AND INTERPRETATION OF RESULTS

In order to minimise suffering in the test animals, it is recommended to note the degree of paralysis on a scale such as that shown below. The scale gives typical signs when injection of the challenge toxin is made in the dorsal region, close to one of the hind legs. Grade T3 is taken as the end-point, but with experience grade T2 can be used instead. Tetanus toxin produces in the toxin-injected hind leg paresis followed by paralysis that can be recognised at an early stage. The tetanus grades in mice are characterised by the following signs:

- T1: slight stiffness of toxin-injected hind leg, only observed when the mouse is lifted by the tail;
- T2: paresis of the toxin-injected hind leg, which still can function for walking;
- T3: paralysis of the toxin-injected hind leg, which does not function for walking;
- T4: the toxin-injected hind leg is completely stiff with immovable toes;
- T5: tetanus seizures, continuous tonic spasm of muscles;
- D: death.

METHOD C. DETERMINATION OF ANTIBODIES IN GUINEA-PIGS

PREPARATION OF SERUM SAMPLES

For preparation of serum samples, the following technique has been found suitable. Invert the tubes containing blood samples 6 times and allow to stand at 37 °C for 2 h, then at 4 °C for 2 h. Centrifuge at room temperature at 800 *g* for 20 min. Transfer the serum to sterile tubes and store at a temperature below − 20 °C. At least 40 per cent yield of serum is obtained by this procedure.

DETERMINATION OF ANTIBODY TITRE

The ELISA and ToBI tests shown below are given as examples of immunochemical methods that have been found suitable for the determination of antibody titre.

Determination of antibody titre in guinea-pig serum by enzyme-linked immunosorbent assay (ELISA). Dilutions of test and reference sera are made on ELISA plates coated with tetanus toxoid. A positive guinea-pig serum control and a negative guinea-pig serum control are included on each plate to monitor the assay performance. Peroxidase-conjugated rabbit or goat antibody directed against guinea-pig-IgG is added followed by a peroxidase substrate. Optical density is measured and the relative antibody titre is calculated using the usual statistical methods (for example *5.3*).

Reagents and equipment

- ELISA plates: 96 wells, columns 1-12, rows A-H.
- *Clostridium tetani guinea-pig antiserum (for vaccines-human use) BRP* (positive control serum).
- Peroxidase conjugate. Peroxidase-conjugated rabbit or goat antibody directed against guinea-pig IgG.
- Tetanus toxoid.
- Carbonate coating buffer pH 9.6. Dissolve 1.59 g of *anhydrous sodium carbonate R* and 2.93 g of *sodium hydrogen carbonate R* in 1000 ml of *water R*. Distribute into 150 ml bottles and sterilise by autoclaving at 121 °C for 15 min.
- Phosphate buffered saline pH 7.4 (PBS). Dissolve with stirring 80.0 g of *sodium chloride R*, 2.0 g of *potassium dihydrogen phosphate R*, 14.3 g of *disodium hydrogen phosphate dihydrate R* and 2.0 g of *potassium chloride R* in 1000 ml of *water R*. Store at room temperature to prevent crystallisation. Dilute to 10 times its volume with *water R* before use.
- Citric acid solution. Dissolve 10.51 g of *citric acid R* in 1000 ml of *water R* and adjust the solution to pH 4.0 with a 400 g/l solution of *sodium hydroxide R*.
- Washing buffer. PBS containing 0.5 g/l of *polysorbate 20 R*.
- Diluent block buffer. PBS containing 0.5 g/l of *polysorbate 20 R* and 25 g/l of dried skimmed milk.
- Peroxidase substrate. Shortly before use, dissolve 10 mg of *diammonium 2,2′-azinobis(3-ethylbenzothiazoline-6-sulphonate) R* (ABTS) in 20 ml of citric acid solution. Immediately before use add 5 μl of *strong hydrogen peroxide solution R*.

Method

The description below is given as an example of a suitable plate lay-out but others may be used. Wells 1A-H are for negative control serum and wells 2A-H and 3A-H are for positive control serum for assay monitoring. Wells 4-12A-H are for test samples.

Coat each well of the ELISA plates with 100 μl of tetanus toxoid solution (0.5 Lf/ml in carbonate coating buffer). Allow to stand overnight at 4 °C in a humid atmosphere. To avoid interference from temperature gradient, do not stack more than 4 plates high. On the following day, wash the plates thoroughly with washing buffer. Block the plates by addition of 100 μl of diluent block buffer to each well. Incubate in a humid atmosphere at 37 °C for 1 h. Wash the plates thoroughly with washing buffer. Place 100 μl of diluent block buffer in each well of the plates, except those of row A. Prepare suitable dilutions of negative control serum, positive control serum (from about 0.01 IU/ml) and test sera. Allocate the negative control serum to column 1, positive control serum to columns 2 and 3 and test sera to columns 4-12 and add 100 μl of each serum to the first 2 wells of the column to which it is allocated. Using a multichannel micropipette, make twofold serial dilutions from row B down the plate to row H by transferring 100 μl to the following well. Discard 100 μl from the last row so that all wells contain 100 μl. Incubate at 37 °C for 2 h. Wash thoroughly with washing buffer. Prepare a suitable dilution (a 1 in 2000 dilution has been found suitable) of peroxidase conjugate in diluent block buffer and add 100 μl to each well. Incubate at 37 °C in a humid atmosphere for 1 h. Wash the plates thoroughly with washing buffer. Add 100 μl of peroxidase substrate to each well. Allow to stand at room temperature, protected from light, for 30 min. Read the plates at 405 nm in the same order as addition of substrate was made.

Determination of antibody titre in guinea-pig serum by toxin- or toxoid-binding inhibition (ToBI). Tetanus toxin or toxoid is added to serial dilutions of test and reference sera; the serum/antigen mixtures are incubated overnight. To determine unbound toxin or toxoid, the mixtures are transferred to an ELISA plate coated with tetanus antitoxin. Peroxidase-conjugated equine anti-tetanus IgG is added followed by a peroxidase substrate. Optical density is measured and the antibody titre is calculated using the usual statistical methods (for example *5.3*). A positive control serum and a negative control serum are included on each plate to monitor assay performance.

Reagents and equipment

- Round-bottomed, rigid polystyrene microtitre plates.
- Flat-bottomed ELISA plates.
- Tetanus toxin or tetanus toxoid.
- *Clostridium tetani guinea-pig antiserum (for vaccines-human use) BRP.*
- Equine anti-tetanus IgG.
- Peroxidase-conjugated equine anti-tetanus IgG.
- Carbonate buffer pH 9.6. Dissolve 1.5 g of *anhydrous sodium carbonate R*, 2.39 g of *sodium hydrogen carbonate R* and 0.2 g of *sodium azide R* in 1000 ml of *water R*, adjust to pH 9.6 and autoclave at 121 °C for 20 min.
- Sodium acetate buffer pH 5.5. Dissolve 90.2 g of *anhydrous sodium acetate R* in 900 ml of *water R*, adjust to pH 5.5 using a saturated solution of *citric acid monohydrate R* and dilute to 1000 ml with *water R*.
- Phosphate buffered saline pH 7.2 (PBS). Dissolve 135.0 g of *sodium chloride R*, 20.55 g of *disodium hydrogen phosphate dihydrate R* and 4.80 g of *sodium dihydrogen phosphate monohydrate R* in *water R* and dilute to 15 litres with the same solvent. Autoclave at 100 °C for 60 min.
- Diluent buffer. PBS containing 5 g/l of *bovine albumin R* and 0.5 g/l of *polysorbate 80 R*.
- Block buffer. PBS containing 5 g/l of *bovine albumin R*.
- Tetramethylbenzidine solution. 6 g/l solution of *tetramethylbenzidine R* in *alcohol R*. The substance dissolves within 30-40 min at room temperature.
- Peroxidase substrate. Mix 90 ml of *water R*, 10 ml of sodium acetate buffer pH 5.5, 1.67 ml of tetramethylbenzidine solution and 20 μl of *strong hydrogen peroxide solution R*.
- Washing solution. Tap water containing 0.5 g/l of *polysorbate 80 R*.

Method

Block the round-bottomed polystyrene microtitre plates by placing in each well 150 μl of block buffer. Cover the plates with a lid or sealer. Incubate in a humid atmosphere at 37 °C for 1 h. Wash the plates thoroughly with washing solution. Place 100 μl of PBS in each well. Place 100 μl of reference guinea-pig tetanus antitoxin in the first well of a row. Place 100 μl of undiluted test sera in the first well of the required number of rows. Using a multichannel micropipette, make twofold serial dilutions across the plate (up to column 10), by transfer of 100 µl to the following well. Discard 100 µl from the last column so that all wells contain 100 µl. Prepare a 0.1 Lf/ml solution of tetanus toxin or toxoid using PBS as diluent. Add 40 µl of this solution to all wells except those of column 12. The wells of row 11 are a positive control. Add 40 µl of PBS to the wells of column 12 (negative control). Shake the plates gently and cover them with lids. Coat the ELISA plates: immediately before use make a suitable dilution of equine anti-tetanus IgG in carbonate buffer pH 9.6 and add 100 µl to all wells. Incubate the 2 series of plates overnight in a humid atmosphere at 37 °C. To avoid temperature gradient effects, do not stack more than 4 plates high. Cover the plates with lids. On the following day, wash the ELISA plates thoroughly with washing solution. Block the plates by placing in each well 125 µl of block buffer. Incubate at 37 °C in a humid atmosphere for 1 h. Wash the plates thoroughly with washing solution. Transfer 100 µl of the pre-incubation mixture from the polystyrene plates to the corresponding wells of the ELISA plates, starting with column 12 and then from 1 to 11. Cover the plates with a lid. Incubate at 37 °C in a humid atmosphere for 2 h. Wash the ELISA plates thoroughly with washing solution. Make a suitable dilution (a 1 in 4000 dilution has been found suitable) of the peroxidase-conjugated equine anti-tetanus IgG in diluent buffer. Add 100 µl of the dilution to each well and cover the plates with a lid. Incubate at 37 °C in a humid atmosphere for 1.5 h. Wash the ELISA plates thoroughly with washing solution. Add 100 µl of peroxidase substrate to each well. A blue colour develops. Incubate the plates at room temperature. Stop the reaction at a given time (within 10 min) by the addition of 100 µl of *2 M sulphuric acid* to each well in the same order as the addition of substrate. The colour changes from blue to yellow. Measure the absorbance at 450 nm immediately after addition of the sulphuric acid or maintain the plates in the dark until reading.

01/2005:20709

2.7.9. TEST FOR Fc FUNCTION OF IMMUNOGLOBULIN

Stabilised human blood. Collect group O human red blood into ACD anticoagulant solution. Store the stabilised blood at 4 °C for not more than 3 weeks.

Phosphate buffered saline pH 7.2. Dissolve 1.022 g of *anhydrous disodium hydrogen phosphate R*, 0.336 g of *anhydrous sodium dihydrogen phosphate R* and 8.766 g of *sodium chloride R* in 800 ml of *water R* and dilute to 1000 ml with the same solvent.

Magnesium and calcium stock solution. Dissolve 1.103 g of *calcium chloride R* and 5.083 g of *magnesium chloride R* in *water R* and dilute to 25 ml with the same solvent.

Barbital buffer stock solution. Dissolve 207.5 g of *sodium chloride R* and 25.48 g of *barbital sodium R* in 4000 ml of *water R* and adjust to pH 7.3 using *1 M hydrochloric acid.* Add 12.5 ml of magnesium and calcium stock solution and dilute to 5000 ml with *water R*. Filter through a membrane filter (pore size 0.22 µm). Store at 4 °C in glass containers.

Albumin barbital buffer solution. Dissolve 0.150 g of *bovine albumin R* in 20 ml of barbital buffer stock solution and dilute to 100 ml with *water R*.

Tannic acid solution. Dissolve 10 mg of *tannic acid R* in 100 ml of phosphate-buffered saline pH 7.2. Prepare immediately before use.

Guinea-pig complement. Prepare a pool of serum from the blood of not fewer than 10 guinea-pigs. Separate the serum from the clotted blood by centrifugation at about 4 °C. Store the serum in small amounts below − 70 °C. Immediately before starting complement-initiated haemolysis, dilute to 125-200 CH_{50} per millilitre with albumin barbital buffer solution and store in an ice-bath during the test.

Rubella antigen. Suitable rubella antigen for haemagglutination-inhibition titre (HIT). Titre > 256 HA units.

Preparation of tanned human red blood cells. Separate human red blood cells by centrifuging an appropriate volume of stabilised human blood and wash the cells at least 3 times with phosphate-buffered saline pH 7.2 and suspend at 2 per cent *V/V* in phosphate-buffered saline pH 7.2. Dilute 0.1 ml of tannic acid solution to 7.5 ml with phosphate-buffered saline pH 7.2 (final concentration 1.3 mg/l). Mix 1 volume of the freshly prepared dilution with 1 volume of human red blood cell suspension and incubate at 37 °C for 10 min. Collect the cells by centrifugation (400-800 *g* for 10 min), discard the supernatant and wash the cells once with phosphate-buffered saline pH 7.2. Resuspend the tanned cells at 1 per cent *V/V* in phosphate-buffered saline pH 7.2.

Antigen coating of tanned human red blood cells. Take a suitable volume (V_s) of tanned cells, add 0.2 ml of rubella antigen per 1.0 ml of tanned cells and incubate at 37 °C for 30 min. Collect the cells by centrifugation (400-800 *g* for 10 min) and discard the supernatant, leaving a volume of 200 µl. Add a volume of albumin barbital buffer solution equivalent to the discarded supernatant, resuspend and collect the cells as described and repeat the washing procedure. Make up the remaining 200 µl to three-quarters of V_s, thereby obtaining the initial volume (V_i). Mix 900 µl of albumin barbital buffer solution with 100 µl of V_i, which is thereby reduced to the residual volume (V_r), and determine the initial absorbance at 541 nm (*A*). Dilute V_r by a factor equal to *A* using albumin barbital buffer solution, thereby obtaining the final adjusted volume $V_f = V_r \times A$ of sensitised human red blood cells and adjusting *A* to 1.0 ± 0.1 for a tenfold dilution.

Antibody binding of antigen-coated tanned human red blood cells. Prepare the following solutions in succession and in duplicate, using for each solution a separate half-micro cuvette (for example, disposable type) or test-tube:

(1) *Test solutions.* If necessary, adjust the immunoglobulin to be examined to pH 7, for example by addition of *1 M sodium hydroxide.* Dilute volumes of the preparation to be examined containing 30 mg and 40 mg of immunoglobulin with albumin barbital buffer solution and adjust the volume to 900 µl.

(2) *Reference solutions.* Prepare as for the test solutions using *human immunoglobulin BRP*.

(3) *Complement control.* 900 µl of albumin barbital buffer solution.

Add to each cuvette/test-tube 100 µl of sensitised human red blood cells and mix well.

Incubate at room temperature for 15 min, add 1000 µl of albumin barbital buffer solution, collect the cells by centrifugation (1000 *g* for 10 min) of the cuvette/test-tube and remove 1900 µl of the supernatant. Replace the 1900 µl with albumin barbital buffer solution and repeat the whole of the washing procedure, finally leaving a volume of 200 µl. Test samples may be stored in sealed cuvette/test-tubes at 4 °C for 24 h.

Complement-initiated haemolysis. To measure haemolysis, add 600 µl of albumin barbital buffer solution warmed to 37 °C to the test sample, resuspend the cells carefully by repeated pipetting (not fewer than 5 times) and place the cuvette in the thermostatted cuvette holder of a spectrophotometer. After 2 min, add 200 µl of diluted guinea-pig complement (125-200 CH_{50}/ml), mix thoroughly by pipetting twice and start immediately after the second pipetting the time-dependent recording of absorbance at 541 nm, using albumin barbital buffer solution as the compensation liquid. Stop the measurement if absorbance as a function of time has clearly passed the inflexion point.

Evaluation. Determine the slope (S) of the haemolysis curve at the approximate inflexion point by segmenting the steepest section in suitable time intervals Δt (for example, Δt = 1 min) and calculate S between adjacent intersection points, expressed as ΔA per minute. The largest value for S serves as (S_{exp}). In addition, determine the absorbance at the start of measurement (A_s) by extrapolating the curve, which is almost linear and parallel to the time axis within the first few minutes. Correct (S_{exp}) using the expression:

$$S' = \frac{S_{\mathrm{exp}}}{A_s}$$

Calculate the arithmetic mean of the values of S' for each preparation. Calculate the index of Fc function (I_{Fc}) from the expression:

$$I_{Fc} = \frac{100 \times \left(\overline{S'} - \overline{S'_c}\right)}{\overline{S'_s} - \overline{S'_c}}$$

$\overline{S'}$ = arithmetic mean of the corrected slope for the preparation to be examined,

$\overline{S'_s}$ = arithmetic mean of the corrected slope for the reference preparation,

$\overline{S'_c}$ = arithmetic mean of the corrected slope for the complement control.

Calculate the index of Fc function for the preparation to be examined: the value is not less than that stated in the leaflet accompanying the reference preparation.

01/2005:20710

2.7.10. ASSAY OF HUMAN COAGULATION FACTOR VII

Human coagulation factor VII is assayed by its biological activity as a factor VIIa-tissue factor complex in the activation of factor X in the presence of calcium ions and phospholipids. The potency of a factor VII preparation is estimated by comparing the quantity necessary to achieve a certain rate of factor Xa formation in a test mixture containing the substances that take part in the activation of factor X, and the quantity of the International Standard, or of a reference preparation calibrated in International Units, required to produce the same rate of factor Xa formation.

The International Unit is the factor VII activity of a stated amount of the International Standard which consists of freeze-dried plasma. The equivalence in International Units of the International Standard is stated by the World Health Organisation.

The chromogenic assay method consists of two consecutive steps: the factor VII-dependent activation of factor X reagent mixture containing tissue factor, phospholipids and calcium ion, followed by enzymatic cleavage of a chromogenic factor Xa substrate into a chromophore that can be quantified spectrophotometrically. Under appropriate assay conditions, there is a linear relation between the rate of factor Xa formation and the factor VII concentration. The assay is summarised in Figure 2.7.10.-1.

Step 1

a) Factor VII $\xrightarrow{\text{Tissue Factor} + Ca^{++}}$ Factor VIIa

b) Factor X $\xrightarrow{\text{Factor VIIa} + Ca^{++} + \text{Tissue factor/Phospholipid}}$ Factor Xa

Step 2

Chromogenic substrate $\xrightarrow{\text{Factor Xa}}$ Peptide + chromophore

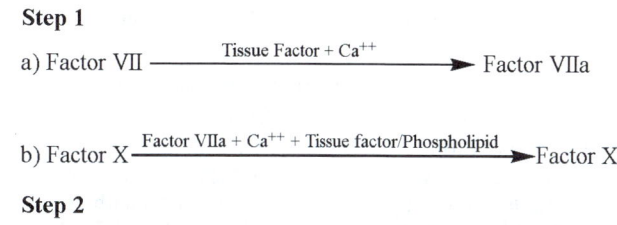

Figure 2.7.10.-1. – *Schematic representation of the assay of human coagulation factor VII*

Both steps employ reagents that may be obtained commercially from a variety of sources. Although the composition of individual reagents may be subject to some variation, their essential features are described in the following specification.

REAGENTS

The coagulation factor reagent comprises purified proteins derived from human or bovine sources. These include factor X and thromboplastin tissue factor/phospholipid as factor VII activator. These proteins are partly purified and do not contain impurities that interfere with the activation of factor VII or factor X. Factor X is present in amounts giving a final concentration during the first step of the assay of 10 nmol/litre to 350 nmol/litre, preferably 14 nmol/litre to 70 nmol/litre. Thromboplastin from natural sources (bovine or rabbit brain) or synthetic preparations may be used as the tissue factor/phospholipid component. Thromboplastin suitable for use in prothrombin time determination is diluted 1:5 to 1:50 in buffer such that the final concentration of Ca^{2+} is 15 mmol/litre to 25 mmol/litre. The final factor Xa generation is performed in a solution containing human or bovine albumin at a concentration such that adsorption losses do not occur and which is appropriately buffered at pH 7.3 to 8.0. In the final incubation mixture, factor VII must be the only rate-limiting component and each reagent component must lack the ability to generate factor Xa on its own.

The second step comprises the quantification of the formed factor Xa employing a chromogenic substrate that is specific for factor Xa. Generally this consists of a short peptide of between three and five amino acids, bound to a chromophore group. On cleavage of this group from the peptide substrate, its absorption maximum shifts to a wavelength allowing its spectrophotometric quantification. The substrate is usually dissolved in *water R* and used at a final concentration of 0.2 mmol/litre to 2 mmol/litre. The substrate may also contain appropriate inhibitors to stop further factor Xa generation (addition of edetate).

ASSAY PROCEDURE

Reconstitute the entire contents of one ampoule of the reference preparation and the preparation to be examined by adding the appropriate quantity of *water R*; use within 1 h. Add sufficient prediluent to the reconstituted preparations to produce solutions containing between 0.5 IU and 2.0 IU of factor VII per millilitre.

Prepare further dilutions of reference and test preparations using an isotonic non-chelating buffer containing 1 per cent of bovine or human albumin, buffered preferably between pH 7.3 and 8.0. Prepare at least three separate, independent dilutions for each material, preferably in duplicate. Prepare the dilutions such that the final factor VII concentration is below 0.005 IU/ml.

Prepare a control solution that includes all components except factor VII.

Prepare all dilutions in plastic tubes and use within 1 h.

Step 1. Mix dilutions of the factor VII reference preparation and the preparation to be examined with an appropriate volume of the prewarmed coagulation factor reagent or a combination of its separate constituents, and incubate the mixture in plastic tubes or microplate wells at 37 °C. The concentrations of the various components during the factor Xa generation must be as specified above under the description of the reagents.

Allow the activation of factor X to proceed for a suitable time, usually terminating the reaction before the factor Xa concentration has reached its maximal level in order to obtain a satisfactory linear dose-response relationship. The activation time is also chosen to achieve linear production of factor Xa in time. Appropriate activation times are usually between 2 min and 5 min, but deviations are permissible if acceptable linearity of the dose-response relationship is thus obtained.

Step 2. Terminate the activation by the addition of a prewarmed reagent containing a chromogenic substrate. Quantify the rate of substrate cleavage, which must be linear with the concentration of factor Xa formed, by measuring the absorbance change at an appropriate wavelength using a spectrophotometer, either monitoring the absorbance continuously, thus allowing the initial rate of substrate cleavage to be calculated, or terminating the hydrolysis reaction after a suitable interval by lowering the pH by the addition of a suitable reagent, such as acetic acid (500 g/l $C_2H_4O_2$) or a citrate solution (1 mol/l) at pH 3. Adjust the hydrolysis time to achieve a linear development of chromophore with time. Appropriate hydrolysis times are usually between 3 min and 15 min, but deviations are permissible if better linearity of the dose-response relationship is thus obtained.

Check the validity of the assay and calculate the potency of the test preparation by the usual statistical methods (for example, *5.3. Statistical analysis of results of biological assays and tests*).

01/2005:20711
corrected

2.7.11. ASSAY OF HUMAN COAGULATION FACTOR IX

The potency is determined by comparing the quantity of the preparation to be examined necessary to reduce the coagulation time of a test mixture containing the substances, other than factor IX, that take part in the coagulation of blood and the quantity of a reference preparation, calibrated in International Units, required to produce the same effect.

The International Unit is the activity of a stated amount of the International Standard, which consists of a freeze-dried concentrate of human coagulation factor IX. The equivalence in International Units of the International Standard is stated by the World Health Organisation.

Human coagulation factor IX concentrate BRP is calibrated in International Units by comparison with the International Standard.

Reconstitute separately the preparation to be examined and the reference preparation as stated on the label and use immediately. Where applicable, determine the amount of heparin present (*2.7.12*) and neutralise the heparin by addition of *protamine sulphate R* (10 µg of protamine sulphate neutralises 1 IU of heparin). Dilute the preparation to be examined and the reference preparation with a sufficient quantity of *imidazole buffer solution pH 7.3 R* to produce solutions containing 0.5 IU to 2.0 IU per millilitre. Prepare twofold dilutions in the range 1 to 10 to 1 to 80 using a mixture of 1 volume of a 38 g/l solution of *sodium citrate R* and 5 volumes of *imidazole buffer solution pH 7.3 R*. Make these dilutions accurately and use immediately.

Use, for example, incubation tubes maintained in a water-bath at 37 °C. Place in each tube 0.1 ml of *plasma substrate R2* and 0.1 ml of one of the dilutions of the reference preparation or of the preparation to be examined. Add to each tube 0.1 ml of a suitable dilution of *cephalin R* or *platelet substitute R* and 0.1 ml of a suspension of 0.5 g of *light kaolin R* in 100 ml of a 9 g/l solution of *sodium chloride R* and allow to stand for about 10 min, tilting the tubes regularly. To each tube, add 0.1 ml of a 7.4 g/l solution of *calcium chloride R*. Using a timer, measure the coagulation time, i.e. the interval between the moment of the addition of the calcium chloride and the first indication of the formation of fibrin, which may be observed visually or by the use of a suitable apparatus. Calculate the potency using the usual statistical methods (for example, *5.3. Statistical analysis of results of biological assays and tests*).

To ensure that there is no appreciable contamination of *plasma substrate R2* by factor IX, carry out a blank test using, instead of the preparation to be examined, a corresponding volume of a mixture of 1 volume of a 38 g/l solution of *sodium citrate R* and 5 volumes of *imidazole buffer solution pH 7.3 R*. The test is not valid unless the coagulation time measured in the blank test is 100 s to 200 s.

01/2005:20712

2.7.12. ASSAY OF HEPARIN IN COAGULATION FACTORS

Heparin is assayed as a complex with antithrombin III (AT) via its inhibition of coagulation factor Xa (anti-Xa activity). An excess of AT is maintained in the reaction mixture to ensure a constant concentration of the heparin-AT complex. Factor Xa is neutralised by the heparin-AT complex and the residual factor Xa hydrolyses a specific chromogenic peptide substrate to release a chromophore. The quantity of chromophore is inversely proportional to the activity of the heparin.

Factor Xa chromogenic substrate. Specific chromogenic substrate for factor Xa such as: *N*-benzoyl-L-isoleucyl-L-glutamyl-glycyl-L-arginine-4-nitroanilide hydrochloride. Reconstitute according to the manufacturer's instructions.

Dilution buffer. 6.05 g/l solution of *tris(hydroxy-methyl)aminomethane R*. Adjust to pH 8.4 if necessary using *hydrochloric acid R*.

Test solution. Dilute the preparation to be examined with dilution buffer to obtain a solution expected to contain 0.1 IU of heparin per millilitre.

Reference solution. Dilute the heparin reference preparation with dilution buffer to obtain a solution containing 0.1 IU of heparin per millilitre.

The following working conditions apply to microtitre plates. If the assay is carried out in tubes, the volumes are adjusted while maintaining the proportions in the mixture.

Warm all solutions to 37 °C in a water-bath shortly before the test.

Distribute in a series of wells, 20 µl of normal human plasma and 20 µl of *antithrombin III solution R1*. Add to the wells a series of volumes (20 µl, 60 µl, 100 µl and 140 µl) of the test solution or the reference solution and make up the volume in each well to 200 µl using dilution buffer (0.02-0.08 IU of heparin per millilitre in the final reaction mixture).

End-point method. Transfer 40 µl from each well to a second series of wells, add 20 µl of *bovine factor Xa solution R* and incubate at 37 °C for 30 s. Add 40 µl of a 1 mmol/l solution of factor Xa chromogenic substrate and incubate at 37 °C for 3 min. Terminate the reaction by lowering the pH by the addition of a suitable reagent, such as a 20 per cent *V/V* solution of *glacial acetic acid R* and measure the absorbance at 405 nm (*2.2.25*). Appropriate reaction times are usually between 3 min and 15 min, but deviations are permissible if better linearity of the dose-response relationship is thus obtained.

Kinetic method. Transfer 40 µl from each well to a second series of wells, add 20 µl of *bovine factor Xa solution R* and incubate at 37 °C for 30 s. Add 40 µl of a 2 mmol/l solution of factor Xa chromogenic substrate, incubate at 37 °C and measure the rate of substrate cleavage by continuous measurement of the absorbance change at 405 nm (*2.2.25*), thus allowing the initial rate of substrate cleavage to be calculated. This rate must be linear with the concentration of residual factor Xa.

Check the validity of the assay and calculate the heparin activity of the test preparation by the usual statistical methods for a slope-ratio assay (for example, *5.3. Statistical analysis of results of biological assays and tests*).

01/2005:20713

2.7.13. ASSAY OF HUMAN ANTI-D IMMUNOGLOBULIN

METHOD A

The potency of human anti-D immunoglobulin is determined by comparing the quantity necessary to produce agglutination of D-positive red blood cells with the quantity of a reference preparation, calibrated in International Units, required to produce the same effect.

The International Unit is the activity contained in a stated amount of the International Reference Preparation. The equivalence in International Units of the International Reference Preparation is stated by the World Health Organisation.

Human anti-D immunoglobulin BRP is calibrated in International Units by comparison with the International Standard and intended for use in the assay of human anti-D immunoglobulin.

Use pooled D-positive red blood cells, collected not more than 7 days earlier and suitably stored, obtained from not fewer than 4 group O R_1R_1 donors. To a suitable volume of the cells, previously washed 3 times with a 9 g/l solution of *sodium chloride R*, add an equal volume of *bromelains solution R*, allow to stand at 37 °C for 10 min, centrifuge, remove the supernatant liquid and wash 3 times with a 9 g/l solution of *sodium chloride R*. Suspend 20 volumes of the red blood cells in a mixture of 15 volumes of inert serum, 20 volumes of a 300 g/l solution of *bovine albumin R* and 45 volumes of a 9 g/l solution of *sodium chloride R*. Stand the resulting suspension in iced water, stirring continuously.

Using a calibrated automated dilutor, prepare suitable dilutions of the preparation to be examined and of the reference preparation using as diluent a solution containing 5 g/l of *bovine albumin R* and 9 g/l of *sodium chloride R*.

Use a suitable apparatus for automatic continuous analysis. The following protocol is usually suitable: maintain the temperature in the manifold, except for the incubation coils, at 15.0 °C. Pump into the manifold of the apparatus the red blood cell suspension at a rate of 0.1 ml/min and a 3 g/l solution of *methylcellulose 450 R* at a rate of 0.05 ml/min. Introduce the dilutions of the preparation to be examined and the reference preparation at a rate of 0.1 ml/min for 2 min, followed by the diluent solution at a rate of 0.1 ml/min for 4 min before the next dilution is introduced.

Introduce air at a rate of 0.6 ml/min. Incubate at 37 °C for 18 min and then disperse the rouleaux by introducing at a rate of 1.6 ml/min a 9 g/l solution of *sodium chloride R* containing a suitable wetting agent (for example, *polysorbate 20 R* at a final concentration of 0.2 g/l) to prevent disruption of the bubble pattern. Allow the agglutinates to settle and decant twice, first at 0.4 ml/min and then at 0.6 ml/min. Lyse the unagglutinated red blood cells with a solution containing 5 g/l of *octoxinol 10 R*, 0.2 g/l of *potassium ferricyanide R*, 1 g/l of *sodium hydrogen carbonate R* and 0.05 g/l of *potassium cyanide R* at a rate of 2.5 ml/min. A ten-minute delay coil is introduced to allow for conversion of the haemoglobin. Continuously record the absorbance (*2.2.25*) of the haemolysate at a wavelength between 540 nm and 550 nm. Determine the range of antibody concentrations over which there is a linear relationship between concentration and the resultant change in absorbance (ΔA). From the results, prepare a standard curve and use the linear portion of the curve to determine the activity of the preparation to be examined.

Calculate the potency of the preparation to be examined using the usual statistical methods (*5.3*).

METHOD B

The potency of human anti-D immunoglobulin is determined by competitive enzyme-linked immunoassay on erythrocyte-coated microtitre plates. The method is based on the competitive binding between a polyclonal anti-D immunoglobulin preparation and a biotinylated monoclonal anti-D antibody directed against a D-antigen specific epitope. The activity of the preparation to be examined is compared with a reference preparation calibrated in International Units.

The International Unit is the activity of a stated amount of International Reference Preparation. The equivalence in International Units of the International Reference Preparation is stated by the World Health Organisation.

Human anti-D immunoglobulin BRP is calibrated in International Units by comparison with the International Standard and intended for use in the assay of human anti-D immunoglobulin.

MATERIALS

Reagents not specified are of analytical grade.

PBS (Phosphate-buffered saline). Dissolve 8.0 g of *sodium chloride R*, 0.76 g of *anhydrous disodium hydrogen phosphate R*, 0.2 g of *potassium chloride R*, 0.2 g of *potassium dihydrogen phosphate R* and 0.2 g of *sodium azide R* in *water R* and dilute to 1000 ml with the same solvent.

TBS (Tris-buffered saline). Dissolve 8.0 g of *sodium chloride R* and 0.6 g of *tris(hydroxymethyl) aminomethane R* in *water R*. Adjust to pH 7.2 (*2.2.3*) with *1 M hydrochloric acid* and dilute to 1000 ml with the same solvent.

Papain solution. Prepare a solution by stirring 1 g of *papain R* at 37 °C for 30 min in 10 ml of *0.067 M phosphate buffer solution pH 5.4 R*, centrifuge at 10 000 *g* for 5 min and filter through a membrane with a pore size of 0.22 µm. To activate, combine 1 ml of the filtrate with 1 ml of a 48.44 g/l solution of *L-cysteine R* and 1 ml of a 3.72 g/l solution of *sodium edetate R* and dilute to 10 ml with *0.067 M phosphate buffer solution pH 5.4 R*. Freeze in aliquots at − 20 °C or below.

Red blood cells. Use pooled D-positive red blood cells obtained from not fewer than 3 group O R_2R_2 donors. Wash the cells 4 times with PBS. Centrifuge the cells at 1800 *g* for 5 min, mix a suitable volume of prewarmed packed cells with a suitable volume of prewarmed papain solution (2 volumes to 1 volume has been found suitable) and incubate at 37 °C for 10 min. Wash the cells 4 times with PBS. Store at 4 °C in an appropriate stabiliser for up to 1 week.

Biotinylated Brad-5. Use according to instructions.

Alkaline phosphatase-conjugated avidin/streptavidin reagent. Preferably modified to combine high specific activity with low non-specific binding. Use according to instructions.

Substrate solution. Use *para*-nitrophenyl phosphate according to instructions.

Cell fixation buffer. Dissolve 18.02 g of *glucose R*, 4.09 g of *sodium chloride R*, 1.24 g of *boric acid R*, 10.29 g of *sodium citrate R* and 0.74 g of *sodium edetate R* in *water R*. Adjust to pH 7.2-7.3 (*2.2.3*) using *1 M sodium hydroxide* or *1 M hydrochloric acid*, and dilute to 1000 ml with *water R*. Use directly from storage at 4 °C.

Glutaraldehyde solution. Immediately before use, add 90 µl of a 250 g/l solution of *glutaraldehyde R* to 24 ml of cold PBS.

Microtitre plates. Plates to be coated with red blood cells are flat-bottomed polystyrene plates with surface properties optimised for enzyme immunoassay and high protein-binding capacity. Plates used to prepare immunoglobulin dilutions are U or V-bottomed polystyrene or poly(vinyl chloride) plates.

METHOD

Prepare a 0.1 per cent (*V/V*) suspension of papain-treated red blood cells in cold cell fixation buffer. Pipette 50 µl into each well of the flat-bottomed microtitre plate.

Centrifuge the plate at 350 *g* for 3 min, preferably at 4 °C. Without removing the supernatant, gently add 100 µl of glutaraldehyde solution to each well and leave for 10 min.

Drain the wells by quickly inverting the plate and wash 3 times with 250-300 µl of PBS. This may be done manually or using a suitable automated plate washer. Either carry out the assay as described below, or store the plate at 4 °C after draining off the PBS and adding 100 µl of cell fixation buffer per well and sealing with plastic film. Plates can be stored at 4 °C for up to 1 month.

Test solutions. For freeze-dried preparations, reconstitute as stated on the label. Prepare 4 independent replicates of 5 serial two-fold dilutions starting with 30 IU/ml in PBS containing 10 g/l of *bovine albumin R*. If necessary, adjust the starting dilution to obtain responses falling in the linear portion of the dose-response curve.

Reference solutions. Reconstitute the reference preparation according to instructions. Prepare 4 independent replicates of 5 serial two-fold dilutions starting with 30 IU/ml in PBS containing 10 g/l of *bovine albumin R*.

Using U or V-bottomed microtitre plates, add 35 µl of each of the dilutions of the test solution or reference solution to each of a series of wells. To each well add 35 µl of biotinylated Brad-5 at 250 ng/ml.

Empty the wells of the red cell-coated plate by inverting and draining on a paper towel. Add 250 µl of PBS containing 20 g/l of *bovine albumin R* and leave at room temperature for 30 min.

Empty the wells of the red cell-coated plate by inverting and draining on a paper towel and transfer 50 µl from each of the dilutions of the test solution or reference solution containing biotinylated Brad-5 into the wells. Use 50 µl of PBS containing 10 g/l of *bovine albumin R* as negative control. Seal the plate with plastic film and incubate at room temperature for 1 h.

Remove liquid from the wells of the red cell-coated plate and wash 3 times with 250-300 µl of TBS.

Dilute the alkaline phosphatase-conjugated avidin/streptavidin reagent in TBS containing 10 g/l of *bovine albumin R* and add 50 µl to each well. Incubate for 30 min at room temperature.

Remove liquid from the wells of the red cell-coated plate and wash 3 times with 250-300 µl of TBS.

Add 100 µl of substrate solution to each of the wells and incubate at room temperature for 10 min in the dark. To stop the reaction, add 50 µl of *3 M sodium hydroxide* to each of the wells.

Measure the absorbances at 405 nm. and substract the negative control reading. Use the absorbance values in the linear range of the titration curve to estimate the potency of the preparation to be examined by the usual statistical methods (*5.3*).

METHOD C

The potency of human anti-D immunoglobulin is determined by flow cytometry in a microtitre plate format. The method is based on the specific binding between anti-D immunoglobulin and D-positive red blood cells. The activity of the preparation to be examined is compared with a reference preparation calibrated in International Units.

The International Unit is the activity of a stated amount of International Reference Preparation. The equivalence in International Units of the International Reference preparation is stated by the World Health Organisation.

Human anti-D immunoglobulin BRP is calibrated in International Units by comparison with the International Standard and intended for use in the assay of human anti-D immunoglobulin.

MATERIALS

Reagents not specified are of analytical grade.

PBS. Dissolve 8.0 g of *sodium chloride R*, 0.76 g of *disodium hydrogen phosphate R*, 0.2 g of *potassium chloride R* and 0.2 g of *potassium dihydrogen phosphate R* in *water R* and dilute to 1000 ml with the same solvent.

PBS-BSA solution. PBS containing 10.0 g/l of *bovine albumin R*.

Red blood cells. Use D-positive red blood cells obtained from a group O R_1R_1 donor within 2 weeks of collection. Store if necessary in an appropriate stabiliser at 4 °C. Wash the cells at least twice with PBS-BSA solution and prepare a suspension containing 1×10^4 cells per microlitre but not more than 5×10^4 cells per microlitre in PBS-BSA solution.

Use D-negative red blood cells obtained from a group O rr donor and prepared similarly.

Secondary antibody. Use a suitable fluorescent dye conjugated anti-IgG antibody-fragment specific for human IgG or parts of it. Store and use according to the manufacturer's instructions.

Microtitres plates. Use flat-bottomed plates without surface treatment for enzyme immunoassays.

METHOD

Test solutions. For freeze-dried preparations, reconstitute as stated on the label. Prepare at least 3 independent replicates of at least 3 serial 1.5 or two-fold dilutions starting with a concentration in the range of 1.2-0.15 IU/ml using PBS/BSA solution as diluent. If necessary, adjust the starting dilution to obtain responses falling in the linear portion of the dose-response curve.

Reference solutions. Reconstitute the reference preparation according to instructions. Prepare at least 3 independent replicates of at least 3 serial 1.5 or two-fold dilutions starting with a concentration in the range of 1.2-0.15 IU/ml using PBS-BSA solution as diluent. If necessary, adjust the starting dilution to obtain responses falling in the linear portion of the dose-response curve.

Distribute 50 µl of the D-positive red blood cells into each well of a microtitre plate. Add 50 µl of each of the dilutions of the test solution or reference solution to each of a series of wells. Use 50 µl of PBS-BSA solution as negative control. Distribute 50 µl of the D-negative red blood cells into 4 wells of the same microtitre plate and add 50 µl of the lowest dilution of the test preparation. To monitor spurious reactions distribute 50 µl of the D-positive red blood cells into 4 wells of the same microtitre plate and add 50 µl of PBS-BSA solution. Seal with plastic film and incubate at 37 °C for 40 min.

Centrifuge the plates at 50 *g* for 3 min, discard the supernatant and wash the cells with 200-250 µl of PBS-BSA solution. Repeat this at least once.

Centrifuge the plates at 50 *g* for 3 min, discard the supernatant and add 50 µl of the secondary antibody diluted with PBS-BSA solution to a suitable protein concentration. Seal with plastic film and incubate, protected from light, at room temperature for 20 min.

Centrifuge the plates at 50 *g* for 3 min, discard the supernatant and wash the cells with 200-250 µl of PBS-BSA solution. Repeat this at least once.

Centrifuge the plates at 50 *g* for 3 min, resuspend the cells into 200-250 µl of PBS. Transfer the cell suspension into a tube suitable for the flow cytometry equipment available and further dilute by adding PBS to allow a suitable flow rate.

Proceed immediately with measurement of the median fluorescence intensity in a flow cytometer. Record at least 10 000 events without gating but excluding debris.

Use the median fluorescence intensity in the linear range of the dose response curve to estimate the potency of the preparation to be examined by the usual statistical methods, (*5.3*).

01/2005:20714
corrected

2.7.14. ASSAY OF HEPATITIS A VACCINE

The assay of hepatitis A vaccine is carried out either *in vivo*, by comparing in given conditions its capacity to induce specific antibodies in mice with the same capacity of a reference preparation, or *in vitro*, by an immunochemical determination of antigen content.

IN VIVO ASSAY

The test in mice shown below is given as an example of a method that has been found suitable for a given vaccine; other validated methods may also be used.

Selection and distribution of the test animals. Use in the test healthy mice from the same stock, about 5 weeks old and from a strain shown to be suitable. Use animals of the same sex. Distribute the animals in at least 7 equal groups of a number suitable for the requirements of the assay.

Determination of potency of the vaccine to be examined. Using a 9 g/l solution of *sodium chloride R* containing the aluminium adjuvant used for the vaccine, prepare at least three dilutions of the vaccine to be examined and matching dilutions of the reference preparation. Allocate the dilutions one to each of the groups of animals and inject subcutaneously not more than 1.0 ml of each dilution into each animal in the group to which that dilution is allocated. Maintain a group of unvaccinated controls, injected subcutaneously with the same volume of diluent. After 28 to 32 days, anaesthetise and bleed all animals, keeping the individual sera separate. Assay the individual sera for specific antibodies against hepatitis A virus by a suitable immunochemical method (*2.7.1*).

Calculations. Carry out the calculations by the usual statistical methods for an assay with a quantal response (*5.3*).

From the distribution of reaction levels measured on all the sera in the unvaccinated group, determine the maximum reaction level that can be expected to occur in an unvaccinated animal for that particular assay. Any response in vaccinated animals that exceeds this level is by definition a seroconversion.

Make a suitable transformation of the percentage of animals showing seroconversion in each group (for example, a probit transformation) and analyse the data according to a parallel-line log dose-response model. Determine the potency of the test preparation relative to the reference preparation.

Validity conditions. The test is not valid unless:

- for both the test and the reference vaccine, the ED_{50} lies between the smallest and the largest doses given to the animals,
- the statistical analysis shows no significant deviation from linearity or parallelism,
- the confidence limits (P = 0.95) are not less than 33 per cent and not more than 300 per cent of the estimated potency.

Potency requirement. The upper confidence limit (P = 0.95) of the estimated relative potency is not less than 1.0.

IN VITRO ASSAY

Carry out an immunochemical determination (*2.7.1*) of antigen content with acceptance criteria validated against the *in vivo* test. The acceptance criteria are approved for a given reference preparation by the competent authority in the light of the validation data.

Hepatitis A vaccine (inactivated, adsorbed) type A BRP, *hepatitis A vaccine (inactivated, adsorbed) type B BRP* and *hepatitis A vaccine (inactivated, adsorbed) type C BRP* are suitable for the *in vitro* assay of certain vaccines as described in the accompanying leaflet.

01/2005:20715
corrected

2.7.15. ASSAY OF HEPATITIS B VACCINE (rDNA)

The assay of hepatitis B vaccine (rDNA) is carried out either *in vivo*, by comparing in given conditions its capacity to induce specific antibodies against hepatitis B surface antigen (HBsAg) in mice or guinea-pigs with the same capacity of a reference preparation, or *in vitro*, by an immunochemical determination of the antigen content.

IN VIVO ASSAY

Selection and distribution of the test animals. Use in the test healthy mice from the same stock, about 5 weeks old. The strain of mice used for this test must give a significant slope for the dose-response curve to the antigen; mice with haplotype H-2^q or H-2^d are suitable. Healthy guinea-pigs weighing 300 g to 350 g (about 7 weeks old) from the same stock are also suitable. Use animals of the same sex. Distribute the animals in at least 7 equal groups of a number appropriate to the requirements of the assay.

Determination of potency of the vaccine to be examined. Using a 9 g/l solution of *sodium chloride R* containing the aluminium adjuvant used for the vaccine or another appropriate diluent, prepare at least three dilutions of the vaccine to be examined and matching dilutions of the reference preparation. Allocate the dilutions one to each of the groups of animals and inject intraperitoneally not more than 1.0 ml of each dilution into each animal in the group to which that dilution is allocated. One group of animals remains unvaccinated and is injected intraperitoneally with the same volume of diluent. After an appropriate time interval (for example, 4 to 6 weeks), anaesthetise and bleed the animals, keeping the individual sera separate. Assay the individual sera for specific antibodies against HBsAg by a suitable immunochemical method (*2.7.1*).

Calculations. Calculations are carried out by the usual statistical methods for an assay with a quantal response (*5.3*).

From the distribution of reaction levels measured on all the sera in the unvaccinated group, the maximum reaction level that can be expected to occur in an unvaccinated animal for that particular assay is determined. Any response in vaccinated animals that exceeds this level is by definition a seroconversion.

Make a suitable transformation of the percentage of animals showing seroconversion in each group (for example, a probit transformation) and analyse the data according to a parallel-line log dose-response model. Determine the potency of the test preparation relative to the reference preparation.

Validity conditions. The test is not valid unless:

- for both the test and the reference vaccine, the ED_{50} lies between the smallest and the largest doses given to the animals,
- the statistical analysis shows no significant deviation from linearity or parallelism,
- the confidence limits (P = 0.95) are not less than 33 per cent and not more than 300 per cent of the estimated potency.

Potency requirement. The upper confidence limit (P = 0.95) of the estimated relative potency is not less than 1.0.

IN VITRO ASSAY

Carry out an immunochemical determination (*2.7.1*) of antigen content with acceptance criteria validated against the *in vivo* test.

Enzyme-linked immunosorbent assay (ELISA) and radio-immunoassay (RIA) using monoclonal antibodies specific for protection-inducing epitopes of HBsAg have been shown to be suitable. Suitable numbers of dilutions of the vaccine to be examined and the reference preparation are used and a parallel-line model is used to analyse the data which may be suitably transformed. Kits for measuring HBsAg *in vitro* are commercially available and it is possible to adapt their test procedures for use as an *in vitro* potency assay.

The acceptance criteria are approved for a given reference preparation by the competent authority in the light of the validation data.

Hepatitis B vaccine (rDNA) method A BRP and *hepatitis B vaccine (rDNA) method B BRP* are suitable for the *in vitro* assay of certain vaccines as described in the accompanying leaflet.

01/2005:20716

2.7.16. ASSAY OF PERTUSSIS VACCINE (ACELLULAR)

The capacity of the vaccine to induce the formation of specific antibodies is compared with the same capacity of a reference preparation examined in parallel; antibodies are determined using suitable immunochemical methods (*2.7.1*) such as enzyme-linked immunosorbent assay (ELISA). The test in mice shown below uses a three-point model but, after validation, for routine testing a single-dilution method may be used.

Reference vaccine. A batch of vaccine shown to be effective in clinical trials or a batch representative thereof is used as a reference vaccine. For the preparation of a representative batch, strict adherence to the production process used for the batch tested in clinical trials is necessary. The stability of the reference vaccine shall be documented.

Reference antiserum. Bordetella pertussis mouse antiserum BRP is suitable for use as a reference antiserum.

Requirement. The capacity of the vaccine to induce antibodies is not significantly (P = 0.95) less than that of the reference vaccine.

The following test model is given as an example of a method that has been found to be satisfactory.

Selection and distribution of test animals. Use in the test healthy mice (for example, CD1 strain) of the same stock, about 5 weeks old. Distribute the animals in 6 groups of a number appropriate to the requirements of the assay. Use 3 dilutions of the vaccine to be examined and 3 dilutions of a reference preparation and attribute each dilution to a group of mice. Inject intraperitoneally or subcutaneously into each mouse 0.5 ml of the dilution attributed to its group.

Collection of serum samples. 4 to 5 weeks after vaccination, bleed the mice individually under anaesthesia. Store the sera at − 20 °C until tested for antibody content.

Antibody determination. Assay the individual sera for content of specific antibodies to each component using a validated method such as the ELISA test shown below.

ELISA test. Microtitre plates (poly(vinyl chloride) or polystyrene as appropriate for the specific antigen) are coated with the purified antigen at a concentration of 100 ng per well. After washing, unreacted sites are blocked by incubating with a solution of bovine serum albumin and then washed. Two-fold dilutions of sera from mice immunised with test or reference vaccines are made on the plates. After incubation at 22-25 °C for 1 h, the plates are washed. A suitable solution of anti-mouse IgG enzyme conjugate is added to each well and incubated at 22-25 °C for 1 h. After washing, a chromogenic substrate is added from which the bound enzyme conjugate liberates a chromophore which can be quantified by measurement of absorbance (*2.2.25*). The test conditions are designed to obtain a linear response for absorbance with respect to antibody content over the range of measurement used and absorbance values within the range 0.1 to 2.0.

A reference antiserum of assigned potency is used in the test and serves as the basis for calculation of the antibody levels in test sera. A standardised control serum is also included in the test.

The test is not valid if:

- the value found for the control serum differs by more than 2 standard deviations from the assigned value,
- the confidence limits (P = 0.95) are less than 50 per cent or more than 200 per cent of the estimated potency.

Calculations. The antibody titres in the sera of mice immunised with reference and test vaccines are calculated and from the values obtained the potency of the test vaccine in relation to the reference vaccine is calculated by the usual statistical methods (*5.3*).

01/2005:20717

2.7.17. ASSAY OF HUMAN ANTITHROMBIN III

The antithrombin III content of the preparation to be examined is determined by comparing its ability to inactivate thrombin in the presence of an excess of heparin with the same ability of a reference preparation of human antithrombin III concentrate calibrated in International Units. Varying quantities of the preparation to be examined are mixed with a given quantity of thrombin and the remaining thrombin activity is determined using a suitable chromogenic substrate.

The International Unit is the activity of a stated amount of the International Standard for human antithrombin III concentrate. The equivalence in International Units of the International Standard is stated by the World Health Organisation.

Method. Prepare 2 independent series of 3 or 4 dilutions in the range 1/75 to 1/200 from 1 IU/ml, for both the preparation to be examined and the reference preparation, using *tris-EDTA BSA buffer solution pH 8.4 R* containing 15 IU of heparin per millilitre.

Warm 200 µl of each dilution at 37 °C for 1-2 min. Add to each dilution 200 µl of a solution of *bovine thrombin R* containing 2 IU/ml in *tris-EDTA BSA buffer solution pH 8.4 R*. Mix and maintain at 37 °C for exactly 1 min. Add 500 µl of a suitable chromogenic substrate (for example, D-phenylalanyl-L-pipecolyl-L-arginine-4-nitroanilide, reconstituted in *water R* to give a solution containing 4 mmol/l and further diluted to a concentration suitable for the assay using *tris-EDTA BSA buffer solution pH 8.4 R* without albumin). Immediately start measurement of the change in absorbance at 405 nm (*2.2.25*), continuing the measurement for at least 30 s. Calculate the rate of change of absorbance (ΔA/min). (Alternatively, an end-point assay may be used by stopping the reaction with acetic acid and measuring the absorbance at 405 nm.)

The rate of change of absorbance (ΔA/min) is inversely proportional to antithrombin III activity.

Check the validity of the assay and calculate the potency of the test preparation by the usual statistical methods (*5.3.*).

01/2005:20718

2.7.18. ASSAY OF HUMAN COAGULATION FACTOR II

Human coagulation factor II is assayed following specific activation to form factor IIa. Factor IIa is estimated by comparing its activity in cleaving a specific chromogenic peptide substrate with the same activity of the International Standard or of a reference preparation calibrated in International Units.

The International Unit is the factor II activity of a stated amount of the International Standard which consists of a freeze-dried concentrate of human blood coagulation factor II. The equivalence in International Units of the International Standard is stated by the World Health Organisation.

The chromogenic assay method consists of 2 steps: snake venom-dependent activation of factor II, followed by enzymatic cleavage of a chromogenic factor IIa substrate to form a chromophore that can be quantified spectrophotometrically. Under appropriate assay conditions, there is a linear relation between factor IIa activity and the cleavage of the chromogenic substrate.

REAGENTS

Viper venom specific factor II activator (Ecarin). A protein derived from the venom of the saw-scaled viper (*Echis carinatus*) which specifically activates factor II. Reconstitute according to the manufacturer's instructions. Store the reconstituted preparation at 4 °C and use within 1 month.

Factor IIa chromogenic substrate. Specific chromogenic substrate for factor IIa such as: *H*-D-phenylalanyl-L-pipecolyl-L-arginine-4-nitroanilide dihydrochloride, 4-toluenesulphonyl-glycyl-prolyl-L-arginine-4-nitroanilide, *H*-D-cyclohexylglycyl-α-aminobutyryl-L-arginine-4-nitroanilide, D-cyclohexylglycyl-L-alanyl-L-arginine-4-nitroanilide diacetate. Reconstitute according to the manufacturer's instructions.

Dilution buffer. Solution containing 6.06 g/l of *tris(hydroxymethyl)aminomethane R*, 17.53 g/l of *sodium chloride R*, 2.79 g/l of *(ethylenedinitrilo)tetra-acetic acid R* and 1 g/l of *bovine albumin R* or *human albumin R*. Adjust to pH 8.4 if necessary, using *hydrochloric acid R*.

METHOD

Test solution. Dilute the preparation to be examined with dilution buffer to obtain a solution containing 0.015 IU of factor II per millilitre. Prepare at least 3 further dilutions in dilution buffer.

Reference solution. Dilute the reference preparation to be examined with dilution buffer to obtain a solution containing 0.015 IU of factor II per millilitre. Prepare at least 3 further dilutions in dilution buffer.

Warm all solutions to 37 °C in a water-bath shortly before the test.

The following working conditions apply to microtitre plates. If the assay is carried out in tubes, the volumes are adjusted while maintaining the proportions in the mixture.

Using a microtitre plate maintained at 37 °C, add 25 µl of each dilution of the test solution or the reference solution to each of a series of wells. To each well add 125 µl of dilution buffer, then 25 µl of ecarin and incubate for exactly 2 min. To each well add 25 µl of factor IIa chromogenic substrate.

Read the rate of change of absorbance (*2.2.25*) at 405 nm continuously over a period of 3 min and obtain the mean rate of change of absorbance (ΔA/min). If continuous monitoring is not possible, read the absorbance at 405 nm at suitable consecutive intervals, for instance 40 s, plot the absorbances against time on a linear graph and calculate ΔA/min as the slope of the line. From the ΔA/min values of each individual dilution of standard and test preparations, calculate the potency of the preparation to be examined and check the validity of the assay by the usual statistical methods (*5.3*).

2. Methods of analysis

01/2005:20719

2.7.19. ASSAY OF HUMAN COAGULATION FACTOR X

Human coagulation factor X is assayed following specific activation to form factor Xa. Factor Xa is estimated by comparing its activity in cleaving a specific chromogenic peptide substrate with the same activity of the International Standard or of a reference preparation calibrated in International Units.

The International Unit is the factor X activity of a stated amount of the International Standard which consists of a freeze-dried concentrate of human coagulation factor X. The equivalence in International Units of the International Standard is stated by the World Health Organisation.

The chromogenic assay method consists of 2 steps: snake venom-dependent activation of factor X, followed by enzymatic cleavage of a chromogenic factor Xa substrate to form a chromophore that can be quantified spectrophotometrically. Under appropriate assay conditions, there is a linear relation between factor Xa activity and the cleavage of the chromogenic substrate.

REAGENTS

Russell's viper venom specific factor X activator (RVV). A protein derived from the venom of Russell's viper (*Vipera russelli*) which specifically activates factor X. Reconstitute according to the manufacturer's instructions. Store the reconstituted preparation at 4 °C and use within 1 month.

Factor Xa chromogenic substrate. Specific chromogenic substrate for factor Xa such as: *N*-α-benzyloxycarbonyl-D-arginyl-L-glycyl-L-arginine-4-nitroanilide dihydrochloride, *N*-benzoyl-L-isoleucyl-L-glutamyl-glycyl-L-arginine-4-nitroanilide hydrochloride, methanesulphonyl-D-leucyl-glycyl-L-arginine-4-nitroanilide, methoxycarbonyl-D-cyclohexylalanyl-glycyl-L-arginine-4-nitroanilide acetate. Reconstitute according to the manufacturer's instructions.

Dilution buffer. Solution containing 3.7 g/l of *tris(hydroxymethyl)aminomethane R*, 18.0 g/l of *sodium chloride R*, 2.1 g/l of *imidazole R*, 0.02 g/l of *hexadimethrine bromide R* and 1 g/l of *bovine albumin R* or *human albumin R*. Adjust to pH 8.4 if necessary using *hydrochloric acid R*.

METHOD

Test solution. Dilute the preparation to be examined with dilution buffer to obtain a solution containing 0.18 IU of factor X per millilitre. Prepare at least 3 further dilutions in dilution buffer.

Reference solution. Dilute the reference preparation to be examined with dilution buffer to obtain a solution containing 0.18 IU of factor X per millilitre. Prepare at least 3 further dilutions in dilution buffer.

Warm all solutions to 37 °C in a water-bath shortly before the test.

The following working conditions apply to microtitre plates. If the assay is carried out in tubes, the volumes are adjusted while maintaining the proportions in the mixture.

Using a microtitre plate maintained at 37 °C, add 12.5 µl of each dilution of the test solution or the reference solution to each of a series of wells. To each well add 25 µl of RVV and incubate for exactly 90 s. To each well add 150 µl of factor Xa chromogenic substrate, diluted 1 in 6 in dilution buffer.

Read the rate of change of absorbance (*2.2.25*) (at 405 nm continuously over a period of 3 min and obtain the mean rate of change of absorbance (ΔA/min). If continuous monitoring is not possible, read the absorbance at 405 nm at suitable consecutive intervals, for instance 40 s, plot the absorbances against time on a linear graph and calculate ΔA/min as the slope of the line. From the ΔA/min values of each individual dilution of standard and test preparations, calculate the potency of the preparation to be examined and check the validity of the assay by the usual statistical methods (*5.3*).

01/2005:20720

2.7.20. *IN VIVO* ASSAY OF POLIOMYELITIS VACCINE (INACTIVATED)

The capacity of the vaccine to induce the formation of neutralising antibodies is determined, *in vivo* by one of the following methods.

TEST IN CHICKS OR GUINEA-PIGS

Prepare a suitable series of not fewer than 3 dilutions of the vaccine to be examined using a suitable buffered saline solution. Distribute either guinea-pigs weighing 250-350 g or 3-week-old chicks into groups of 10, and allocate a group to each dilution of the vaccine. Inject intramuscularly into each animal 0.5 ml of the dilution intended for its group. Bleed the animals after 5-6 days and separate the sera. Examine the sera for the presence of neutralising antibodies, at a dilution of 1 in 4, to each of the human polioviruses 1, 2 and 3. Mix 100 $CCID_{50}$ of virus with the dilution of serum and incubate at 37 °C for 4.5-6 h. Keep at 5 ± 3 °C for 12-18 h where necessary for consistency of results. Inoculate the mixtures into cell cultures for the detection of unneutralised virus and read the results up to 7 days after inoculation. For each group of animals, note the number of sera which have neutralising antibodies and calculate the dilution of the vaccine giving an antibody response in 50 per cent of the animals. Carry out in parallel a control test using a suitable reference preparation. The vaccine complies with the test if a dilution of 1 in 100 or more produces an antibody response for each of the 3 types of virus in 50 per cent of the animals.

TEST IN RATS

A suitable *in vivo* assay method consists of intramuscular injection into the hind limb(s) of not fewer than 3 dilutions of the vaccine to be examined and a reference vaccine, using for each dilution a group of 10 specific pathogen-free rats of a suitable strain. Use of 4 dilutions is often necessary to obtain valid results for all 3 serotypes. The number of animals per group must be sufficient to obtain results that meet the validity criteria; groups of 10 rats are usually sufficient although valid results may be obtained with fewer animals per group. If animals of different sex are used, males and females are evenly distributed between all groups. A weight range of 175-250 g has been found suitable. An inoculum of 0.5 ml per rat is used. The dose range is chosen such that a dose response to all 3 poliovirus types is obtained. Bleed the animals after 20-22 days. Neutralising titres against all 3 poliovirus types are measured separately using 100 $CCID_{50}$ of the Sabin strains as challenge viruses, Vero or Hep2 as indicator cells, and neutralisation conditions of 3 h at 35-37 °C followed by 18 h at 2-8 °C where necessary for consistency of results. Results are read following fixation and staining after 7 days of incubation at 35 °C. For a valid antibody assay, the titre of each challenge virus must be shown to be within the range 10 $CCID_{50}$ to 1000 $CCID_{50}$

and the neutralising antibody titre of a control serum must be within 2 twofold dilutions of the geometric mean titre of the serum. The potency is calculated by comparison of the proportion of responders for the vaccine to be examined and the reference vaccine by the probit method or, after validation, using a parallel-line model. For the probit method it is necessary to establish a cut-off neutralising antibody titre for each poliovirus type to define a responder. Due to interlaboratory variation, it is not possible to define cut-off values that could be applied by all laboratories. Rather, the cut-off values are determined for each laboratory based on a minimum series of 3 tests with the reference vaccine. The mid-point on a $\log_2$ scale of the minimum and maximum geometric mean titres of the series of 3 or more tests is used as the cut-off value. For each of the 3 poliovirus types, the potency of the vaccine is not significantly less than that of the reference preparation. The test is not valid unless:

- for both the test and reference vaccines the ED_{50} lies between the smallest and the largest doses given to the animals,
- the statistical analysis shows no significant deviation from linearity or parallelism,
- the confidence limits (P = 0.95) are not less than 25 per cent and not more than 400 per cent of the estimated potency.

01/2005:20721

2.7.21. ASSAY OF HUMAN VON WILLEBRAND FACTOR

The potency of human von Willebrand factor is determined by comparing, in given conditions its activity in collagen binding or as ristocetin cofactor with the same activity of a reference preparation calibrated against the International Standard, in International Units where applicable.

The International Unit is the activity of a stated amount of the International Standard for von Willebrand factor in human blood coagulation factor VIII concentrate. The equivalence in International Units of the International Standard is stated by the World Health Organisation.

COLLAGEN-BINDING ASSAY

Collagen-binding is determined by an enzyme-linked immunosorbent assay on collagen-coated microtitre plates. The method is based on the specific binding of von Willebrand factor to collagen fibrils and the subsequent binding of polyclonal anti-von Willebrand factor antibody conjugated to an enzyme, which on addition of a chromogenic substrate yields a product that can be quantitated spectrophotometrically. Under appropriate conditions, there is a linear relationship between von Willebrand factor collagen-binding and absorbance.

MATERIALS

Collagen. Use native equine or human fibrils of collagen type I or III. For the ease of handling, collagen solutions may be used.

Collagen diluent. Dissolve 50 g of *glucose R* in *water R*, adjust to pH 2.7-2.9 with *1 M hydrochloric acid* and dilute to 1000 ml with *water R*.

Phosphate-buffered saline solution (PBS). Dissolve 8.0 g of *sodium chloride R*, 1.05 g of *disodium hydrogen phosphate dihydrate R*, 0.2 g of *sodium dihydrogen phosphate R* and 0.2 g of *potassium chloride R* in *water R*. Adjust to pH 7.2 using *1 M sodium hydroxide* or *1 M hydrochloric acid* and dilute to 1000 ml with *water R*.

Washing buffer. PBS containing 1 g/l of *polysorbate 20 R*.

Blocking reagent. PBS containing 1 g/l of *polysorbate 20 R* and 10 g/l of *bovine serum albumin R*.

Dilution buffer. PBS containing 1 g/l of *polysorbate 20 R* and 50 g/l of *bovine serum albumin R*.

Conjugate. Rabbit anti-human von Willebrand factor serum horse-radish peroxidase conjugate. Use according to the manufacturer's instructions.

Substrate solution. Immediately before use, dissolve a tablet of *o*-phenylenediamine dihydrochloride and a tablet of urea hydrogen peroxide in 20 ml of *water R* or use a suitable volume of hydrogen peroxide. Protect from light.

Microtitre plates. Flat-bottomed polystyrene plates with surface properties optimised for enzyme immunoassay and high protein-binding capacity.

METHOD

Test solutions. Reconstitute the preparation to be examined as stated on the label. Dilute with dilution buffer to produce a solution containing approximately 1 IU of von Willebrand factor. Prepare 2 independent series of not fewer than 3 dilutions using dilution buffer.

Reference solutions. Reconstitute the reference preparation as directed. Dilute with dilution buffer to produce a solution containing approximately 1 IU of von Willebrand factor. Prepare 2 independent series of not fewer than 3 dilutions using dilution buffer.

Allow the solution of collagen to warm to room temperature. Dilute with collagen diluent to obtain a solution containing 30-75 µg/ml of collagen, mix gently to produce a uniform suspension of collagen fibrils. Pipette 100 µl into each well of the microtitre plate. Cover the plate with plastic film and incubate at 37 °C overnight. Empty the wells of the collagen-coated plate by inverting and draining on a paper towel. Add 250 µl of washing buffer. Empty the wells of the plate by inverting and draining on a paper towel. Repeat this operation 3 times. Add 250 µl of blocking reagent to each well, cover the plate with plastic film and incubate at 37 °C for 1 h. Empty the wells of the plate by inverting and draining on a paper towel. Add 250 µl of washing buffer. Empty the wells of the plate by inverting and draining on a paper towel. Repeat this operation 3 times.

Add 100 µl each of the test solutions or reference solutions to the wells. Add 100 µl of dilution buffer to a series of wells to serve as negative control. Cover the plate with plastic film and incubate at 37 °C for 2 h. Empty the wells of the plate by inverting and draining on a paper towel. Add 250 µl of washing buffer. Empty the wells of the plate by inverting and draining on a paper towel. Repeat this operation 3 times.

Prepare a suitable dilution of the conjugate with PBS containing 5 g/l of *bovine serum albumin R* and add 100 µl to each well. Cover the plate with plastic film and incubate at 37 °C for 2 h. Empty the wells of the plate by inverting and draining on a paper towel. Add 250 µl of washing buffer. Empty the wells of the plate by inverting and draining on a paper towel. Repeat this operation 3 times.

Add 100 µl of substrate solution to each of the wells and incubate at room temperature for 20 min in the dark. Add 100 µl of *1 M hydrochloric acid* to each of the wells.

Measure the absorbance at 492 nm. Use the absorbance values to estimate the potency of the preparation to be examined by the usual statistical methods (*5.3*).

The assay is invalid if the absorbances measured for the negative controls are greater than 0.05.

RISTOCETIN COFACTOR ASSAY

Carry out appropriate dilutions of the preparation to be examined and of the reference preparation using as diluent a solution containing 9 g/l of *sodium chloride R* and 10-50 g/l of *human albumin R*. Add to each dilution suitable amounts of a von Willebrand reagent containing stabilised human platelets and ristocetin A. Mix on a glass slide by moving it gently in circles for 1 min. Allow to stand for a further 1 min and read the result against a dark background with side lighting. The last dilution which clearly shows visible agglutination indicates the ristocetin cofactor titre of the sample. Use diluent as a negative control.

01/2005:20722

2.7.22. ASSAY OF HUMAN COAGULATION FACTOR XI

The potency of human coagulation factor XI is determined by comparing the quantity of the preparation to be examined necessary to reduce the coagulation time of a test mixture containing the substances other than factor XI that take part in the coagulation of blood, and the quantity of human normal plasma required to produce the same effect. 1 unit of factor XI is equal to the activity of 1 ml of human normal plasma.

Reconstitute separately the preparation to be examined and the reference preparation as stated on the label and use without delay. Where applicable, determine the amount of heparin present (*2.7.12*) and neutralise the heparin by addition of *protamine sulphate R* (10 µg of protamine sulphate neutralises 1 IU of heparin). Dilute the preparation to be examined and the reference preparation with a sufficient quantity of *imidazole buffer solution pH 7.3 R* containing 1 per cent of albumin to produce solutions containing 0.5 units/ml to 2.0 units/ml. Prepare twofold dilutions in the range 1 to 10 to 1 to 80 using *imidazole buffer solution pH 7.3 R*. Make these dilutions accurately and use without delay.

Use, for example, incubation tubes maintained in a water-bath at 37 °C. Place in each tube 0.1 ml of *plasma substrate R3* and 0.1 ml of one of the dilutions of the reference preparation or of the preparation to be examined. Add to each tube 0.1 ml of a suitable dilution of *cephalin R* or *platelet substitute R* and 0.1 ml of a suspension of 0.5 g of *light kaolin R* in 100 ml of a 3.7 g/l solution of *sodium chloride R* and allow to stand for about 10 min, tilting the tubes regularly. To each tube, add 0.1 ml of a 7.4 g/l solution of *calcium chloride R*. Using a timer, measure the coagulation time, i.e. the interval between the moment of the addition of the calcium chloride and the first indication of the formation of fibrin, which may be observed visually or by the use of a suitable apparatus. Calculate the potency using the usual statistical methods (*5.3.*).

To ensure that there is no appreciable contamination of *plasma substrate R3* by factor XI, carry out a blank test using, instead of the preparation to be examined, a corresponding volume of *imidazole buffer solution pH 7.3 R*. The test is not valid unless the coagulation time measured in the blank test is 100 s to 200 s.

2.8. METHODS IN PHARMACOGNOSY

2.8. METHODS IN PHARMACOGNOSY

01/2005:20801

2.8.1. ASH INSOLUBLE IN HYDROCHLORIC ACID

Ash insoluble in hydrochloric acid is the residue obtained after extracting the sulphated or total ash with hydrochloric acid, calculated with reference to 100 g of drug.

To the crucible containing the residue from the determination of sulphated or total ash, add 15 ml of *water R* and 10 ml of *hydrochloric acid R*, cover with a watch-glass, boil the mixture gently for 10 min and allow to cool. Filter through an ashless filter, wash the residue with hot *water R* until the filtrate is neutral, dry, ignite to dull redness, allow to cool in a desiccator and weigh. Reheat until the difference between 2 consecutive weighings is not more than 1 mg.

01/2005:20802

2.8.2. FOREIGN MATTER

Vegetable drugs should be free from moulds, insects and other animal contamination.

Unless otherwise prescribed, the amount of foreign matter is not more than 2 per cent *m/m*.

Foreign matter is material consisting of any or all of the following:

1) *Foreign organs*: matter coming from the source plant but not defined as the drug,

2) *Foreign elements*: matter not coming from the source plant and either of vegetable or mineral origin.

DETERMINATION OF FOREIGN MATTER

Weigh 100 g to 500 g of the substance to be examined, or the minimum quantity prescribed in the monograph, and spread it out in a thin layer. Examine for foreign matter by inspection with the unaided eye or by use of a lens (6 ×). Separate foreign matter and weigh it and calculate the percentage present.

01/2005:20803

2.8.3. STOMATA AND STOMATAL INDEX

STOMATA

There are several types of stomata (see Figure 2.8.3.-1), distinguished by the form and arrangement of the surrounding cells:

(1) The *anomocytic* (irregular-celled) type: the stoma is surrounded by a varying number of cells in no way differing from those of the epidermis generally,

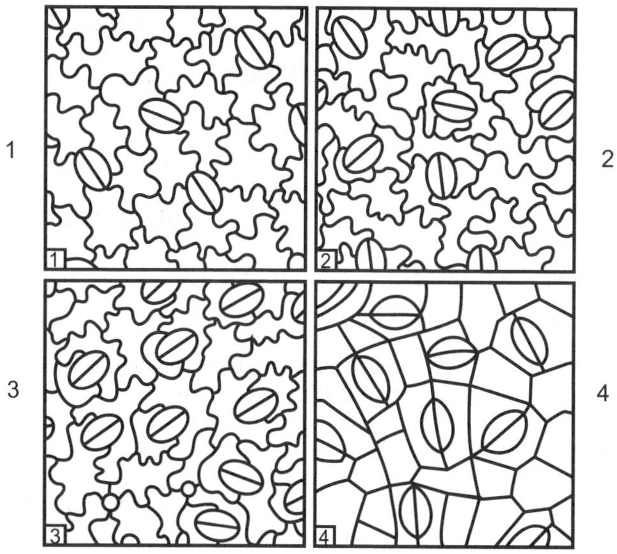

Figure 2.8.3.-1

(2) The *anisocytic* (unequal-celled) type: the stoma is usually surrounded by 3 subsidiary cells, of which one is markedly smaller than the others,

(3) The *diacytic* (cross-celled) type: the stoma is accompanied by 2 subsidiary cells, whose common wall is at right angles to the guard cells,

(4) The *paracytic* (parallel-celled) type: the stoma has on each side one or more subsidiary cells parallel to the long axis of the pore and guard cells.

STOMATAL INDEX

$$\text{Stomatal Index} = \frac{100 \times S}{E + S}$$

S = the number of stomata in a given area of leaf,

E = the number of epidermal cells (including trichomes) in the same area of leaf.

For each sample of leaf, make not fewer than 10 determinations and calculate the mean.

01/2005:20804

2.8.4. SWELLING INDEX

The swelling index is the volume in millilitres occupied by 1 gram of a drug, including any adhering mucilage, after it has swollen in an aqueous liquid for 4 h.

In a 25 ml ground-glass stoppered cylinder graduated over a height of 125 ± 5 mm in 0.5 ml divisions, place 1.0 g of the drug, whole or of the degree of comminution prescribed in the monograph. Unless otherwise prescribed, moisten the drug with 1.0 ml of *alcohol R*, add 25 ml of *water R* and close the cylinder. Shake vigorously every 10 min for 1 h. Allow to stand for 3 h. At 90 min after the beginning of the test, release any large volumes of liquid retained in the layer of the drug and any particles of the drug floating at the surface of the liquid by rotating the cylinder about a vertical axis. Measure the volume occupied by the drug, including any adhering mucilage. Carry out 3 tests at the same time.

The swelling index is given by the mean of the 3 tests.

01/2005:20805

2.8.5. WATER IN ESSENTIAL OILS

Mix 10 drops of the essential oil with 1 ml of *carbon disulphide R*. The solution remains clear on standing.

01/2005:20806

2.8.6. FOREIGN ESTERS IN ESSENTIAL OILS

Heat 1 ml of the essential oil for 2 min on a water-bath with 3.0 ml of a freshly prepared 100 g/l solution of *potassium hydroxide R* in *alcohol R*. No crystals are formed within 30 min, even after cooling.

01/2005:20807

2.8.7. FATTY OILS AND RESINIFIED ESSENTIAL OILS IN ESSENTIAL OILS

Allow 1 drop of the essential oil to fall onto filter paper. The drop evaporates completely within 24 h without leaving any translucent or greasy spot.

01/2005:20808

2.8.8. ODOUR AND TASTE OF ESSENTIAL OILS

Mix 3 drops of the essential oil with 5 ml of *90 per cent V/V alcohol R* and stir in 10 g of powdered *sucrose R*. The odour and taste are similar to that of the plant or parts of the plant from which the essential oil has been obtained.

01/2005:20809

2.8.9. RESIDUE ON EVAPORATION OF ESSENTIAL OILS

The residue on evaporation of an essential oil is the percentage by mass of the oil which remains after evaporation on a water-bath under the conditions specified below.

Apparatus. The apparatus (see Figure 2.8.9.-1) consists of:

- Water-bath with a cover having holes of 70 mm diameter,
- Evaporating dish of heat-resistant glass which is inert to the contents,
- Desiccator.

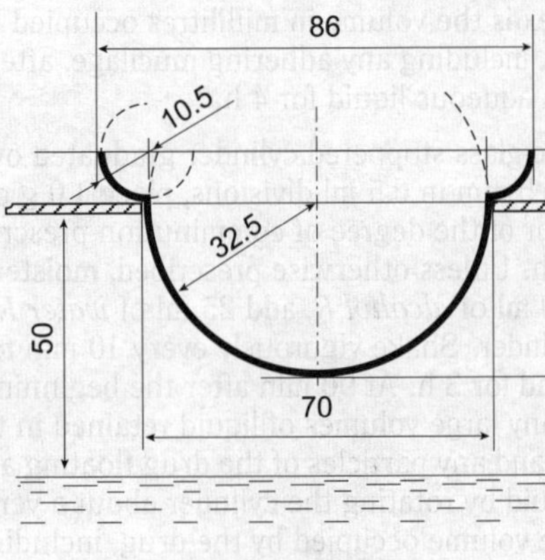

Figure 2.8.9.-1.
Dimensions in millimetres

Method. Weigh the evaporating dish after having heated it on the water-bath for 1 h and cooled it in the desiccator. Weigh into the evaporating dish 5.00 g of the essential oil, unless otherwise prescribed. Heat the oil on the vigorously boiling water-bath in a draught-free atmosphere for the prescribed time. Allow to cool in the desiccator and weigh.

During the test, the level of water in the bath is maintained about 50 mm beneath the level of the cover.

01/2005:20810

2.8.10. SOLUBILITY IN ALCOHOL OF ESSENTIAL OILS

Place 1.0 ml of the essential oil in a 25 ml or 30 ml glass-stoppered cylinder. Place in a constant temperature device, maintained at a temperature of 20 ± 0.2 °C. Using a burette of at least 20 ml capacity, add the alcohol of the strength prescribed in the monograph by increments of 0.1 ml until solution is complete and then continue adding by increments of 0.5 ml to a total of 20 ml, shaking frequently and vigorously. Record the volume of alcohol added when a clear solution has been obtained and, if the solution becomes cloudy or opalescent before 20 ml of alcohol has been added, record the volume added when the cloudiness or opalescence appears and, where applicable, the volume added when the cloudiness or opalescence disappears.

If a clear solution has not been obtained when 20 ml of alcohol of the prescribed strength has been added, repeat the test using the next highest concentration of alcohol.

An essential oil is said to be "soluble in n volumes or more of alcohol of given strength t" when the clear solution in n volumes remains clear when compared with the undiluted oil after further addition of alcohol of the same strength up to a total of 20 volumes of alcohol.

An essential oil is said to be "soluble in n volumes of alcohol of given strength t, becoming cloudy when diluted" when the clear solution in n volumes becomes cloudy in n_1 volumes (n_1 less than 20) and stays so after further gradual addition of alcohol of the same strength up to a total of 20 volumes of alcohol.

An essential oil is said to be "soluble in n volumes of alcohol of given strength t with cloudiness between n_1 and n_2 volumes" when the clear solution in n volumes becomes cloudy in n_1 volumes (n_1 less than 20) and stays so after further gradual addition of alcohol of the same strength up to a total of n_2 volumes of alcohol and then becomes clear (n_2 less than 20).

An essential oil is said to be "soluble with opalescence" when the alcoholic solution shows a bluish tinge, similar to that of a standard of opalescence freshly prepared as follows: mix 0.5 ml of *silver nitrate solution R2* and 0.05 ml of *nitric acid R*; add 50 ml of a 12 mg/l solution of *sodium chloride R*; mix and allow to stand protected from light for 5 min.

01/2005:20811

2.8.11. ASSAY OF 1,8-CINEOLE IN ESSENTIAL OILS

Weigh 3.00 g of the oil, recently dried with *anhydrous sodium sulphate R*, into a dry test-tube and add 2.10 g of melted *cresol R*. Place the tube in the apparatus for the determination of freezing point (*2.2.18*) and allow to cool, stirring continuously. When crystallisation takes place there is a small rise in temperature. Note the highest temperature reached (t_1).

Remelt the mixture on a water-bath at a temperature that does not exceed t_1 by more than 5 °C and place the tube in the apparatus, maintained at a temperature 5 °C below t_1. When crystallisation takes place, or when the temperature of the mixture has fallen 3 °C below t_1, stir continuously. Note the highest temperature at which the mixture crystallises (t_2). Repeat the operation until 2 highest values obtained for t_2 do not differ by more than 0.2 °C. If supercooling occurs, induce crystallisation by adding a small crystal of the complex consisting of 3.00 g of *cineole R* and 2.10 g of melted *cresol R*. If t_2 is below 27.4 °C, repeat the determination after the addition of 5.10 g of the complex.

The content of cineole corresponding to the highest temperature observed (t_2) is given in Table 2.8.11.-1. If 5.10 g of the complex has been added, calculate the cineole content per cent *m/m* from the expression:

$$2(A - 50)$$

where A is the value found in Table 2.8.11.-1.

The content of cineole, corresponding to the highest temperature observed (t_2), is obtained, where necessary, by interpolation.

Table 2.8.11.-1

t_2 °C	cineole per cent *m/m*	t_2 °C	cineole per cent *m/m*	t_2 °C	cineole per cent *m/m*	t_2 °C	cineole per cent *m/m*
24	45.5	32	56.0	40	67.0	48	82.0
25	47.0	33	57.0	41	68.5	49	84.0
26	48.5	34	58.5	42	70.0	50	86.0
27	49.5	35	60.0	43	72.5	51	88.5
28	50.5	36	61.0	44	74.0	52	91.0
29	52.0	37	62.5	45	76.0	53	93.5
30	53.5	38	63.5	46	78.0	54	96.0
31	54.5	39	65.0	47	80.0	55	99.0

01/2005:20812

2.8.12. DETERMINATION OF ESSENTIAL OILS IN VEGETABLE DRUGS

The determination of essential oils in vegetable drugs is carried out by steam distillation in a special apparatus in the conditions described below. The distillate is collected in the graduated tube, using xylene to take up the essential oil; the aqueous phase is automatically returned to the distillation flask.

Apparatus. The apparatus comprises the following parts:

(a) a suitable round-bottomed flask with a short, ground-glass neck having an internal diameter of about 29 mm at the wide end;

(b) a condenser assembly (see Figure 2.8.12.-1) that closely fits the flask, the different parts being fused into one piece; the glass used has a low coefficient of expansion:

- the stopper *K′* is vented and the tube *K* has an orifice of diameter about 1 mm that coincides with the vent; the wide end of the tube *K* is of ground-glass and has an internal diameter of 10 mm;
- a pear-shaped swelling, *J*, of 3 ml capacity;
- the tube *JL* is graduated in 0.01 ml;
- the bulb-shaped swelling *L* has a capacity of about 2 ml;
- *M* is a three-way tap;
- the junction *B* is at a level 20 mm higher than the uppermost graduation;

(c) a suitable heating device, allowing a fine control;

(d) a vertical support with a horizontal ring covered with insulating material.

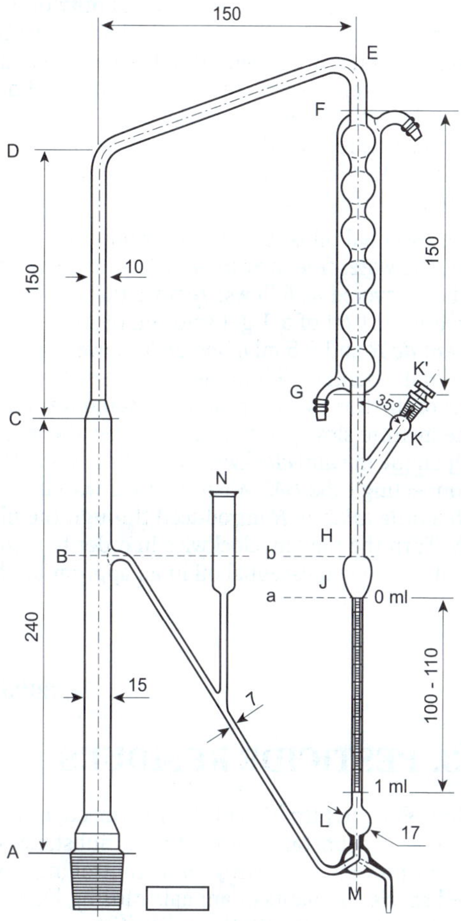

Figure 2.8.12.-1. - *Apparatus for the determination of essential oils in vegetable drugs*

Dimensions in millimetres

Method. Use a thoroughly cleaned apparatus. Carry out the assay according to the nature of the drug to be examined. Place the prescribed volume of distillation liquid in the flask, add a few pieces of porous porcelain and attach the condenser assembly. Introduce *water R* through the filling funnel *N* until it is at the level *B*. Remove the stopper *K′* and introduce the prescribed quantity of *xylene R*, using a pipette with its tip at the bottom of the tube *K*. Replace the stopper *K′* and ensure that the orifice coincides with the vent. Heat the liquid in the flask to boiling and adjust the distillation rate to 2-3 ml/min, unless otherwise prescribed.

To determine the rate of distillation, during distillation lower the level of the water by means of the three-way tap until the meniscus is at the level of the lower mark (a) (see Figure 2.8.12.-2). Close the tap and measure the time taken for the liquid to reach the upper mark (b). Open the tap and continue the distillation, modifying the heat to regulate the distillation rate. Distil for 30 min. Stop the heating and after at least 10 min read off the volume of xylene in the graduated tube.

2. Methods of analysis

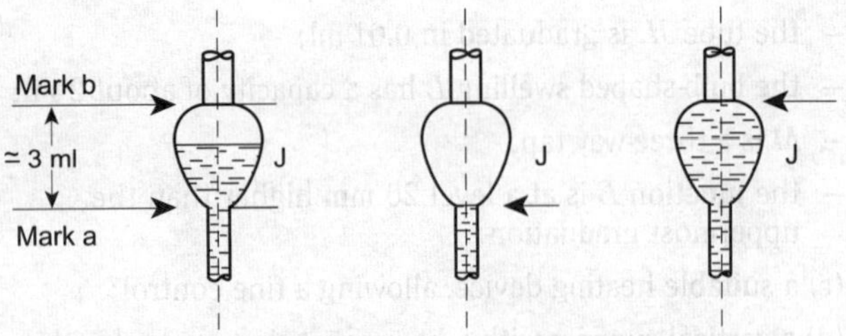

Figure 2.8.12.-2

Introduce into the flask the prescribed quantity of the drug and continue the distillation as described above for the time and at the rate prescribed. Stop the heating and after 10 min read the volume of liquid collected in the graduated tube and subtract the volume of xylene previously noted. The difference represents the quantity of essential oil in the mass of the drug taken. Calculate the result as millilitres per kilogram of drug.

When the essential oil is to be used for other analytical purposes, the water-free mixture of xylene and essential oil may be recovered as follows: remove the stopper *K′* and introduce 0.1 ml of a 1 g/l solution of *sodium fluoresceinate R* and 0.5 ml of *water R*. Lower the mixture of xylene and essential oil into the bulb-shaped swelling *L* by means of the three-way tap, allow to stand for 5 min and lower the mixture slowly until it just reaches the level of the tap *M*. Open the tap anti-clockwise so that the water flows out of the connecting tube *BM*. Wash the tube with *acetone R* and with a little *toluene R* introduced through the filling funnel *N*. Turn the tap anti-clockwise in order to recover the mixture of xylene and essential oil in an appropriate flask.

01/2005:20813

2.8.13. PESTICIDE RESIDUES

Definition. For the purposes of the Pharmacopoeia, a pesticide is any substance or mixture of substances intended for preventing, destroying or controlling any pest, unwanted species of plants or animals causing harm during or otherwise interfering with the production, processing, storage, transport or marketing of vegetable drugs. The item includes substances intended for use as growth-regulators, defoliants or desiccants and any substance applied to crops either before or after harvest to protect the commodity from deterioration during storage and transport.

Limits. Unless otherwise indicated in the monograph, the drug to be examined at least complies with the limits indicated in Table 2.8.13.-1. The limits applying to pesticides that are not listed in the table and whose presence is suspected for any reason comply with the limits set by European Community directives 76/895 and 90/642, including their annexes and successive updates. Limits for pesticides that are not listed in Table 2.8.13.-1 nor in EC directives are calculated using the following expression:

$$\frac{ADI \times M}{MDD \times 100}$$

ADI = acceptable daily intake, as published by FAO-WHO, in milligrams per kilogram of body mass,

M = body mass in kilograms (60 kg),

MDD = daily dose of the drug, in kilograms.

If the drug is intended for the preparation of extracts, tinctures or other pharmaceutical forms whose preparation method modifies the content of pesticides in the finished product, the limits are calculated using the following expression:

$$\frac{ADI \times M \times E}{MDD \times 100}$$

E = extraction factor of the method of preparation, determined experimentally.

Higher limits can also be authorised, in exceptional cases, especially when a plant requires a particular cultivation method or has a metabolism or a structure that gives rise to a higher than normal content of pesticides.

The competent authority may grant total or partial exemption from the test when the complete history (nature and quantity of the pesticides used, date of each treatment during cultivation and after the harvest) of the treatment of the batch is known and can be checked precisely.

Sampling

Method. For containers up to 1 kg, take one sample from the total content, thoroughly mixed, sufficient for the tests. For containers between 1 kg and 5 kg, take three samples, equal in volume, from the upper, middle and lower parts of the container, each being sufficient to carry out the tests. Thoroughly mix the samples and take from the mixture an amount sufficient to carry out the tests. For containers of more than 5 kg, take three samples, each of at least 250 g from the upper, middle and lower parts of the container. Thoroughly mix the samples and take from the mixture an amount sufficient to carry out the tests.

Size of sampling. If the number (n) of containers is three or fewer, take samples from each container as indicated above under Method. If the number of containers is more than three, take $\sqrt{n} + 1$ samples from containers as indicated under Method, rounding up to the nearest unit if necessary.

The samples are to be analysed immediately to avoid possible degradation of the residues. If this is not possible, the samples are stored in airtight containers suitable for food contact, at a temperature below 0 °C, protected from light.

Reagents. All reagents and solvents are free from any contaminants, especially pesticides, that might interfere with the analysis. It is often necessary to use special quality solvents or, if this is not possible, solvents that have recently been re-distilled in an apparatus made entirely of glass. In any case, suitable blank tests must be carried out.

Apparatus. Clean the apparatus and especially glassware to ensure that they are free from pesticides, for example, soak for at least 16 h in a solution of phosphate-free detergent, rinse with large quantities of *distilled water R* and wash with acetone and hexane or heptane.

Qualitative and quantitative analysis of pesticide residues. The analytical procedures used are validated according to the regulations in force. In particular, they satisfy the following criteria:

- the chosen method, especially the purification steps, are suitable for the combination pesticide residue/substance to be analysed, and not susceptible to interference from co-extractives; the limits of detection and quantification are measured for each pesticide-matrix combination to be analysed,
- between 70 per cent to 110 per cent of each pesticide is recovered,
- the repeatability of the method is not less than the values indicated in Table 2.8.13.-2,

– the reproducibility of the method is not less than the values indicated in Table 2.8.13.-2,

– the concentration of test and reference solutions and the setting of the apparatus are such that a linear response is obtained from the analytical detector.

Table 2.8.13.-1

Substance	Limit (mg/kg)
Alachlor	0.02
Aldrin and Dieldrin (sum of)	0.05
Azinphos-methyl	1.0
Bromopropylate	3.0
Chlordane (sum of *cis*-, *trans* - and Oxythlordane)	0.05
Chlorfenvinphos	0.5
Chlorpyrifos	0.2
Chlorpyrifos-methyl	0.1
Cypermethrin (and isomers)	1.0
DDT (sum of *p,p*´-DDT, *o,p*´-DDT, *p,p*´-DDE and *p,p*´-TDE)	1.0
Deltamethrin	0.5
Diazinon	0.5
Dichlorvos	1.0
Dithiocarbamates (as CS_2)	2.0
Endosulfan (sum of isomers and Endosulfan sulphate)	3.0
Endrin	0.05
Ethion	2.0
Fenitrothion	0.5
Fenvalerate	1.5
Fonofos	0.05
Heptachlor (sum of Heptachlor and Heptachlorepoxide)	0.05
Hexachlorobenzene	0.1
Hexachlorocyclohexane isomers (other than γ)	0.3
Lindane (γ-Hexachlorocyclohexane)	0.6
Malathion	1.0
Methidathion	0.2
Parathion	0.5
Parathion-methyl	0.2
Permethrin	1.0
Phosalone	0.1
Piperonyl butoxide	3.0
Pirimiphos-methyl	4.0
Pyrethrins (sum of)	3.0
Quintozene (sum of quintozene, pentachloroaniline and methyl pentachlorophenyl sulphide)	1.0

Table 2.8.13.-2

Concentration of the pesticide (mg/kg)	Repeatability (difference, ± mg/kg)	Reproducibility (difference, ± mg/kg)
0.010	0.005	0.01
0.100	0.025	0.05
1.000	0.125	0.25

The following section is published for information.

Test for pesticides

ORGANOCHLORINE, ORGANOPHOSPHORUS AND PYRETHROID INSECTICIDES

The following methods may be used, in connection with the general method above. Depending on the substance being examined, it may be necessary to modify, sometimes extensively, the procedure described hereafter. In any case, it may be necessary to use, in addition, another column with a different polarity or another detection method (mass spectrometry...) or a different method (immunochemical methods...) to confirm the results obtained.

This procedure is valid only for the analysis of samples of vegetable drugs containing less than 15 per cent of water. Samples with a higher content of water may be dried, provided it has been shown that the drying procedure does not affect significantly the pesticide content.

1. EXTRACTION

To 10 g of the substance being examined, coarsely powdered, add 100 ml of *acetone R* and allow to stand for 20 min. Add 1 ml of a solution containing 1.8 µg/ml of *carbophenothion R* in *toluene R*. Homogenise using a high-speed blender for 3 min. Filter and wash the filter cake with two quantities, each of 25 ml, of *acetone R*. Combine the filtrate and the washings and heat using a rotary evaporator at a temperature not exceeding 40 °C until the solvent has almost completely evaporated. To the residue add a few millilitres of *toluene R* and heat again until the acetone is completely removed. Dissolve the residue in 8 ml of *toluene R*. Filter through a membrane filter (45 µm), rinse the flask and the filter with *toluene R* and dilute to 10.0 ml with the same solvent (solution A).

2. PURIFICATION

2.1. Organochlorine, organophosphorus and pyrethroid insecticides. Examine by size-exclusion chromatography (*2.2.30*).

The chromatographic procedure may be carried out using:

– a stainless steel column 0.30 m long and 7.8 mm in internal diameter packed with *styrene-divinylbenzene copolymer R* (5 µm),

– as mobile phase *toluene R* at a flow rate of 1 ml/min.

Performance of the column. Inject 100 µl of a solution containing 0.5 g/l of *methyl red R* and 0.5 g/l of *oracet blue 2R R* in *toluene R* and proceed with the chromatography. The column is not suitable unless the colour of the eluate changes from orange to blue at an elution volume of about 10.3 ml. If necessary calibrate the column, using a solution containing, in *toluene R*, at a suitable concentration, the insecticide to be analysed with the lowest molecular mass (for example, dichlorvos) and that with the highest molecular mass (for example, deltamethrin). Determine which fraction of the eluate contains both insecticides.

Purification of the test solution. Inject a suitable volume of solution A (100 µl to 500 µl) and proceed with the chromatography. Collect the fraction as determined above (solution B). Organophosphorus insecticides are usually eluted between 8.8 ml and 10.9 ml. Organochlorine and pyrethroid insecticides are usually eluted between 8.5 ml and 10.3 ml.

2.2. Organochlorine and pyrethroid insecticides. In a chromatography column, 0.10 m long and 5 mm in internal diameter, introduce a piece of defatted cotton and 0.5 g of silica gel treated as follows: heat *silica gel for chromatography R* in an oven at 150 °C for at least 4 h.

Allow to cool and add dropwise a quantity of *water R* corresponding to 1.5 per cent of the mass of silica gel used; shake vigorously until agglomerates have disappeared and continue shaking for 2 h using a mechanical shaker. Condition the column using 1.5 ml of *hexane R*. Prepacked columns containing about 0.50 g of a suitable silica gel may also be used provided they are previously validated.

Concentrate solution B in a current of *helium for chromatography R* or *oxygen-free nitrogen R* almost to dryness and dilute to a suitable volume with *toluene R* (200 µl to 1 ml according to the volume injected in the preparation of solution B). Transfer quantitatively onto the column and proceed with the chromatography using 1.8 ml of *toluene R* as the mobile phase. Collect the eluate (solution C).

3. QUANTITATIVE ANALYSIS

3.1. Organophosphorus insecticides. Examine by gas chromatography (*2.2.28*), using *carbophenothion R* as internal standard. It may be necessary to use a second internal stan-dard to identify possible interference with the peak corresponding to carbophenothion.

Test solution. Concentrate solution B in a current of *helium for chromatography R* almost to dryness and dilute to 100 µl with *toluene R*.

Reference solution. Prepare at least three solutions in *toluene R* containing the insecticides to be determined and carbophenothion at concentrations suitable for plotting a calibration curve.

The chromatographic procedure may be carried out using:

– a fused-silica column 30 m long and 0.32 mm in internal diameter the internal wall of which is covered with a layer 0.25 µm thick of *poly(dimethyl)siloxane R*,

– *hydrogen for chromatography R* as the carrier gas. Other gases such as *helium for chromatography R* or *nitrogen for chromatography R* may also be used provided the chromatography is suitably validated.

– a phosphorus-nitrogen flame-ionisation detector or a atomic emission spectrometry detector,

maintaining the temperature of the column at 80 °C for 1 min, then raising it at a rate of 30 °C/min to 150 °C, maintaining at 150 °C for 3 min, then raising the temperature at a rate of 4 °C/min to 280 °C and maintaining at this temperature for 1 min, and maintaining the temperature of the injector port at 250 °C and that of the detector at 275 °C. Inject the chosen volume of each solution. When the chromatograms are recorded in the prescribed conditions, the relative retention times are approximately those listed in Table 2.8.13.-3. Calculate the content of each insecticide from the peak areas and the concentrations of the solutions.

3.2. Organochlorine and pyrethroid insecticides. Examine by gas chromatography (*2.2.28*), using carbophenothion as the internal standard. It may be necessary to use a second internal standard to identify possible interference with the peak corresponding to carbophenothion

Test solution. Concentrate solution C in a current of *helium for chromatography R* or *oxygen-free nitrogen R* almost to dryness and dilute to 500 µl with *toluene R*.

Reference solution. Prepare at least three solutions in *toluene R* containing the insecticides to be determined and carbophenothion at concentrations suitable for plotting a calibration curve.

Table 2.8.13.-3

Substance	Relative retention times
Dichlorvos	0.20
Fonofos	0.50
Diazinon	0.52
Parathion-methyl	0.59
Chlorpyrifos-methyl	0.60
Pirimiphos-methyl	0.66
Malathion	0.67
Parathion	0.69
Chlorpyrifos	0.70
Methidathion	0.78
Ethion	0.96
Carbophenothion	1.00
Azinphos-methyl	1.17
Phosalon	1.18

The chromatographic procedure may be carried out using:

– a fused silica column 30 m long and 0.32 mm in internal diameter the internal wall of which is covered with a layer 0.25 µm thick of *poly(dimethyl)(diphenyl)siloxane R*,

– *hydrogen for chromatography R* as the carrier gas. Other gases such as *helium for chromatography R* or *nitrogen for chromatography R* may also be used, provided the chromatography is suitably validated,

– an electron-capture detector,

– a device allowing direct cold on-column injection,

maintaining the temperature of the column at 80 °C for 1 min, then raising it at a rate of 30 °C/min to 150 °C, maintaining at 150 °C for 3 min, then raising the temperature at a rate of 4 °C/min to 280 °C and maintaining at this temperature for 1 min, and maintaining the temperature of the injector port at 250 °C and that of the detector at 275 °C. Inject the chosen volume of each solution. When the chromatograms are recorded in the prescribed conditions, the relative retention times are approximately those listed in Table 2.8.13.-4. Calculate the content of each insecticide from the peak areas and the concentrations of the solutions.

Table 2.8.13.-4

Substance	Relative rentention times
α-Hexachlorocyclohexane	0.44
Hexachlorobenzene	0.45
β-Hexachlorocyclohexane	0.49
Lindane	0.49
δ-Hexachlorocyclohexane	0.54
ε-Hexachlorocyclohexane	0.56
Heptachlor	0.61
Aldrin	0.68
cis-Heptachlor-epoxide	0.76
o,p'-DDE	0.81
α-Endosulfan	0.82
Dieldrin	0.87
p,p'-DDE	0.87
o,p'-DDD	0.89
Endrin	0.91

Substance	Relative rentention times
β-Endosulfan	0.92
o,p'-DDT	0.95
Carbophenothion	1.00
p,p'-DDT	1.02
cis-Permethrin	1.29
trans-Permethrin	1.31
Cypermethrin*	1.40
Fenvalerate*	1.47 and 1.49
Deltamethrin	1.54

* The substance shows several peaks.

01/2005:20814

2.8.14. DETERMINATION OF TANNINS IN HERBAL DRUGS

Carry out all the extraction and dilution operations protected from light.

In the case of a herbal drug or a dry extract, to the stated amount of the powdered drug (180) or the extract in a 250 ml round-bottomed flask add 150 ml of *water R*. Heat on a water-bath for 30 min. Cool under running water and transfer quantitatively to a 250 ml volumetric flask. Rinse the round-bottomed flask and collect the washings in the volumetric flask, then dilute to 250.0 ml with *water R*. Allow the solids to settle and filter the liquid through a filter paper 125 mm in diameter. Discard the first 50 ml of the filtrate.

In the case of a liquid extract or a tincture, dilute the stated amount of the liquid extract or tincture to 250.0 ml with *water R*. Filter the mixture through a filter paper 125 mm in diameter. Discard the first 50 ml of the filtrate.

Total polyphenols. Dilute 5.0 ml of the filtrate to 25.0 ml with *water R*. Mix 2.0 ml of this solution with 1.0 ml of *phosphomolybdotungstic reagent R* and 10.0 ml of *water R* and dilute to 25.0 ml with a 290 g/l solution of *sodium carbonate R*. After 30 min measure the absorbance (*2.2.25*) at 760 nm (A_1), using *water R* as the compensation liquid.

Polyphenols not adsorbed by hide powder. To 10.0 ml of the filtrate, add 0.10 g of *hide powder CRS* and shake vigorously for 60 min. Filter and dilute 5.0 ml of the filtrate to 25.0 ml with *water R*. Mix 2.0 ml of this solution with 1.0 ml of *phosphomolybdotungstic reagent R* and 10.0 ml of *water R* and dilute to 25.0 ml with a 290 g/l solution of *sodium carbonate R*. After 30 min measure the absorbance (*2.2.25*) at 760 nm (A_2), using *water R* as the compensation liquid.

Standard. Dissolve immediately before use 50.0 mg of *pyrogallol R* in *water R* and dilute to 100.0 ml with the same solvent. Dilute 5.0 ml of the solution to 100.0 ml with *water R*. Mix 2.0 ml of this solution with 1.0 ml of *phosphomolybdotungstic reagent R* and 10.0 ml of *water R* and dilute to 25.0 ml with a 290 g/l solution of *sodium carbonate R*. After 30 min measure the absorbance (*2.2.25*) at 760 nm (A_3), using *water R* as the compensation liquid.

Calculate the percentage content of tannins expressed as pyrogallol from the expression:

$$\frac{62.5\,(A_1 - A_2)\,m_2}{A_3 \times m_1}$$

m_1 = mass of the sample to be examined, in grams,

m_2 = mass of pyrogallol, in grams.

01/2005:20815

2.8.15. BITTERNESS VALUE

The bitterness value is the reciprocal of the dilution of a compound, a liquid or an extract that still has a bitter taste. It is determined by comparison with quinine hydrochloride, the bitterness value of which is set at 200 000.

Determination of the correction factor

A taste panel comprising at least 6 persons is recommended. The mouth must be rinsed with *water R* before tasting.

To correct for individual differences in tasting bitterness amongst the panel members it is necessary to determine a correction factor for each panel member.

Stock solution. Dissolve 0.100 g of *quinine hydrochloride R* in *water R* and dilute to 100.0 ml with the same solvent. Dilute 1.0 ml of this solution to 100.0 ml with *water R*.

Reference solutions. Prepare a series of dilutions by placing in a first tube 3.6 ml of the stock solution and increasing the volume by 0.2 ml in each subsequent tube to a total of 5.8 ml; dilute the contents of each tube to 10.0 ml with *water R*.

Determine as follows the dilution with the lowest concentration that still has a bitter taste. Take 10.0 ml of the weakest solution into the mouth and pass it from side to side over the back of the tongue for 30 s. If the solution is not found to be bitter, spit it out and wait for 1 min. Rinse the mouth with *water R*. After 10 min, use the next dilution in order of increasing concentration.

Calculate the correction factor *k* for each panel member from the expression:

$$k = \frac{n}{5.00}$$

n = number of millilitres of the stock solution in the dilution of lowest concentration that is judged to be bitter.

Persons who are unable to taste any bitterness when using the reference solution prepared from 5.8 ml of stock solution have to be excluded from the panel.

Sample preparation

If necessary, reduce the sample to a powder (710). To 1.0 g of sample add 100 ml of boiling *water R*. Heat on a water-bath for 30 min, stirring continuously. Allow to cool and dilute to 100 ml with *water R*. Shake vigorously and filter, discarding the first 2 ml of the filtrate. The filtrate is labelled C-1 and has a dilution factor (DF) of 100.

If liquids have to be examined, 1 ml of the liquid is diluted with a suitable solvent to 100 ml and designated C-1.

Determination of the bitterness value

Test solutions:

10.0 ml of C-1 is diluted with *water R* to 100 ml: C-2	(DF = 1000)
10.0 ml of C-2 is diluted with *water R* to 100 ml: C-3	(DF = 10 000)
20.0 ml of C-3 is diluted with *water R* to 100 ml: C-3A	(DF = 50 000)
10.0 ml of C-3 is diluted with *water R* to 100 ml: C-4	(DF = 100 000)

Starting with dilution C-4 each panel member determines the dilution which still has a bitter taste. This solution is designated D. Note the DF of solution D is Y.

2. Methods of analysis

Starting with solution D prepare the following sequence of dilutions:

Solution D (ml)	1.2	1.5	2.0	3.0	6.0	8.0
water R (ml)	8.8	8.5	8.0	7.0	4.0	2.0

Determine the number of millilitres of solution D which, when diluted to 10.0 ml with *water R*, still has a bitter taste (X).

Calculate the bitterness value for each panel member from the expression:

$$\left(\frac{\mathrm{Y} \times k}{\mathrm{X} \times 0.1}\right)$$

Calculate the bitterness value of the sample to be examined as the average value for all panel members.

01/2005:20816

2.8.16. DRY RESIDUE OF EXTRACTS

In a flat-bottomed dish about 50 mm in diameter and about 30 mm in height, introduce rapidly 2.00 g or 2.0 ml of the extract to be examined. Evaporate to dryness on a water-bath and dry in an oven at 100-105 °C for 3 h. Allow to cool in a desiccator over *diphosphorus pentoxide R* or *anhydrous silica gel R* and weigh. Calculate the result as a mass percentage or in grams per litre.

01/2005:20817

2.8.17. LOSS ON DRYING OF EXTRACTS

In a flat-bottomed dish about 50 mm in diameter and about 30 mm in height, weigh rapidly 0.50 g of the extract to be examined, finely powdered. Dry in an oven at 100-105 °C for 3 h. Allow to cool in a desiccator over *diphosphorus pentoxide R* or *anhydrous silica gel R* and weigh. Calculate the result as a mass percentage.

2.9. PHARMACEUTICAL TECHNICAL PROCEDURES

2.9. PHARMACEUTICAL TECHNICAL PROCEDURES

01/2005:20901

2.9.1. DISINTEGRATION OF TABLETS AND CAPSULES

The disintegration test determines whether tablets or capsules disintegrate within the prescribed time when placed in a liquid medium in the experimental conditions prescribed below.

Disintegration is considered to be achieved when:

a) no residue remains on the screen, or

b) if there is a residue, it consists of a soft mass having no palpably firm, unmoistened core, or

c) only fragments of coating (tablets) or only fragments of shell (capsules) remain on the screen; if a disc has been used (capsules), fragments of shell may adhere to the lower surface of the disc.

Use apparatus A for tablets and capsules that are not greater than 18 mm long. For larger tablets or capsules use apparatus B.

TEST A - TABLETS AND CAPSULES OF NORMAL SIZE

Apparatus. The main part of the apparatus (Figure 2.9.1.-1) is a rigid basket-rack assembly supporting 6 cylindrical transparent tubes 77.5 ± 2.5 mm long, 21.5 mm in internal diameter, and with a wall thickness of about 2 mm. Each tube is provided with a cylindrical disc 20.7 ± 0.15 mm in diameter and 9.5 ± 0.15 mm thick, made of transparent plastic with a relative density of 1.18 to 1.20 or weighing 3.0 ± 0.2 g. Each disc is pierced by 5 holes 2 mm in diameter, 1 in the centre and the other 4 spaced equally on a circle of radius 6 mm from the centre of the disc. On the lateral surface of the disc, 4 equally spaced grooves are cut in such a way that at the upper surface of the disc they are 9.5 mm wide and 2.55 mm deep and at the lower surface 1.6 mm square. The tubes are held vertically by 2 separate and superimposed rigid plastic plates 90 mm in diameter and 6 mm thick with 6 holes. The holes are equidistant from the centre of the plate and equally spaced. Attached to the under side of the lower plate is a piece of woven gauze made from stainless steel wire 0.635 mm in diameter and having mesh apertures of 2.00 mm. The plates are held rigidly in position and 77.5 mm apart by vertical metal rods at the periphery, a metal rod is also fixed to the centre of the upper plate to enable the assembly to be attached to a mechanical device

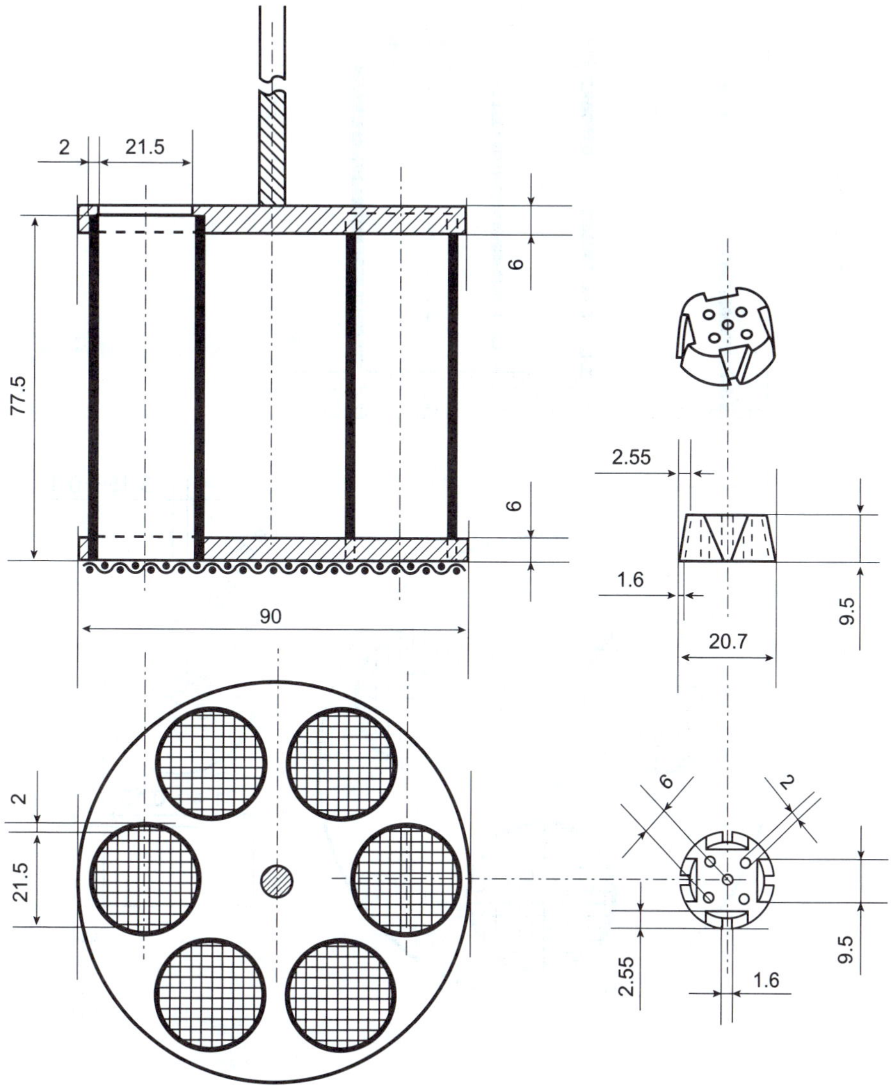

Figure 2.9.1.-1. – *Apparatus A*

Dimensions in millimetres

capable of raising and lowering it smoothly at a constant frequency between 29 and 32 cycles per minute, through a distance of 50 mm to 60 mm.

The assembly is suspended in the specified liquid in a suitable vessel, preferably a 1 litre beaker. The volume of the liquid is such that when the assembly is in the highest position the wire mesh is at least 15 mm below the surface of the liquid, and when the assembly is in the lowest position the wire mesh is at least 25 mm above the bottom of the beaker and the upper open ends of the tubes remain above the surface of the liquid. A suitable device maintains the temperature of the liquid at 35-39 °C.

The design of the basket-rack assembly may be varied provided the specifications for the tubes and wire mesh are maintained.

Method. In each of the 6 tubes, place one tablet or capsule and, if prescribed, add a disc; suspend the assembly in the beaker containing the specified liquid. Operate the apparatus for the prescribed period, withdraw the assembly and examine the state of the tablets or capsules. To pass the test, all the tablets or capsules must have disintegrated.

TEST B – LARGE TABLETS AND LARGE CAPSULES

Apparatus. The main part of the apparatus (Figure 2.9.1.-2) is a rigid basket-rack assembly supporting 3 cylindrical transparent tubes 77.5 ± 2.5 mm long, 33.0 mm ± 0.5 mm in internal diameter, and with a wall thickness of 2.5 ± 0.5 mm. Each tube is provided with a cylindrical disc 31.4 ± 0.13 mm in diameter and 15.3 ± 0.15 mm thick, made of transparent plastic with a relative density of 1.18 to 1.20 or weighing 13.0 ± 0.2 g. Each disc is pierced by 7 holes, each 3.15 ± 0.1 mm in diameter, 1 in the centre and the other 6 spaced equally on a circle of radius 4.2 mm from the centre of the disc. The tubes are held vertically by 2 separate and superimposed rigid plastic plates 97 mm in diameter and 9 mm thick, with 3 holes. The holes are equidistant from the centre of the plate and equally spaced. Attached to the under side of the lower plate is a piece of woven gauze made from stainless steel wire 0.63 ± 0.03 mm in diameter and having mesh apertures of 2.0 ± 0.2 mm. The plates are held rigidly in position and 77.5 mm apart by vertical metal rods at the periphery, a metal rod is also fixed to the centre of the upper plate to enable the assembly to be attached

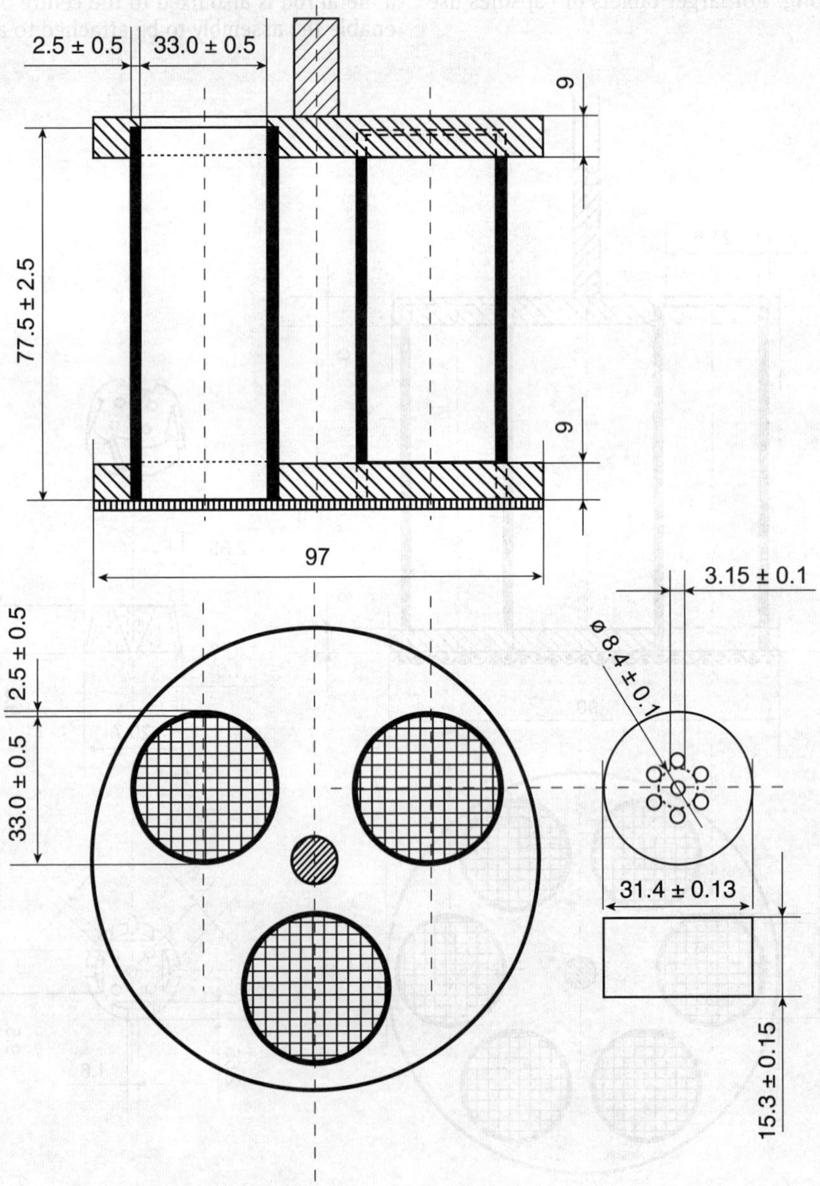

Figure 2.9.1.-2. – *Apparatus B*

Dimensions in millimetres

to a mechanical device capable of raising and lowering it smoothly at constant frequency between 29 and 32 cycles per minute, through a distance of 55 ± 2 mm.

The assembly is suspended in the specified liquid medium in a suitable vessel, preferably a 1 litre beaker. The volume of the liquid is such that when the assembly is in the highest position the wire mesh is at least 15 mm below the surface of the liquid, and when the assembly is in the lowest position the wire mesh is at least 25 mm above the bottom of the beaker and the upper open ends of the tubes remain above the surface of the liquid. A suitable device maintains the temperature of the liquid at 35-39 °C.

The design of the basket-rack assembly may be varied provided the specifications for the tubes and wire mesh are maintained.

Method. Test 6 tablets or capsules either by using 2 basket-rack assemblies in parallel or by repeating the procedure. In each of the 3 tubes, place one tablet or capsule and, if prescribed, add a disc; suspend the assembly in the beaker containing the specified liquid. Operate the apparatus for the prescribed period, withdraw the assembly and examine the state of the tablets or capsules. To pass the test, all 6 of the tablets or capsules must have disintegrated.

01/2005:20902

2.9.2. DISINTEGRATION OF SUPPOSITORIES AND PESSARIES

The disintegration test determines whether the suppositories or pessaries soften or disintegrate within the prescribed time when placed in a liquid medium in the experimental conditions described below.

Disintegration is considered to be achieved when:

a) dissolution is complete,

b) the components of the suppository or pessary have separated: melted fatty substances collect on the surface of the liquid, insoluble powders fall to the bottom and soluble components dissolve, depending on the type of preparation, the components may be distributed in one or more of these ways,

c) there is softening of the sample that may be accompanied by appreciable change of shape without complete separation of the components, the softening is such that the suppository or pessary no longer has a solid core offering resistance to pressure of a glass rod,

d) rupture of the gelatin shell of rectal or vaginal capsules occurs allowing release of the contents,

e) no residue remains on the perforated disc or if a residue remains, it consists only of a soft or frothy mass having no solid core offering resistance to pressure of a glass rod (vaginal tablets).

Apparatus. The apparatus (Figure 2.9.2.-1) consists of a sleeve of glass or suitable transparent plastic, of appropriate thickness, to the interior of which is attached by means of three hooks a metal device consisting of two perforated stainless metal discs each containing 39 holes 4 mm in diameter; the diameter of the discs is similar to that of the interior of the sleeve; the discs are about 30 mm apart. The test is carried out using three such apparatuses each containing a single sample. Each apparatus is placed in a beaker with a capacity of at least 4 litres filled with water maintained at 36-37 °C, unless otherwise prescribed. The apparatuses may also be placed together in a vessel with a capacity of at least 12 litres. The beaker is fitted with a slow stirrer and a device that will hold the cylinders vertically not less than 90 mm below the surface of the water and allow them to be inverted without emerging from the water.

Method. Use three suppositories or pessaries. Place each one on the lower disc of a device, place the latter in the sleeve and secure. Invert the apparatuses every 10 min. Examine the samples after the period prescribed in the monograph. To pass the test all the samples must have disintegrated.

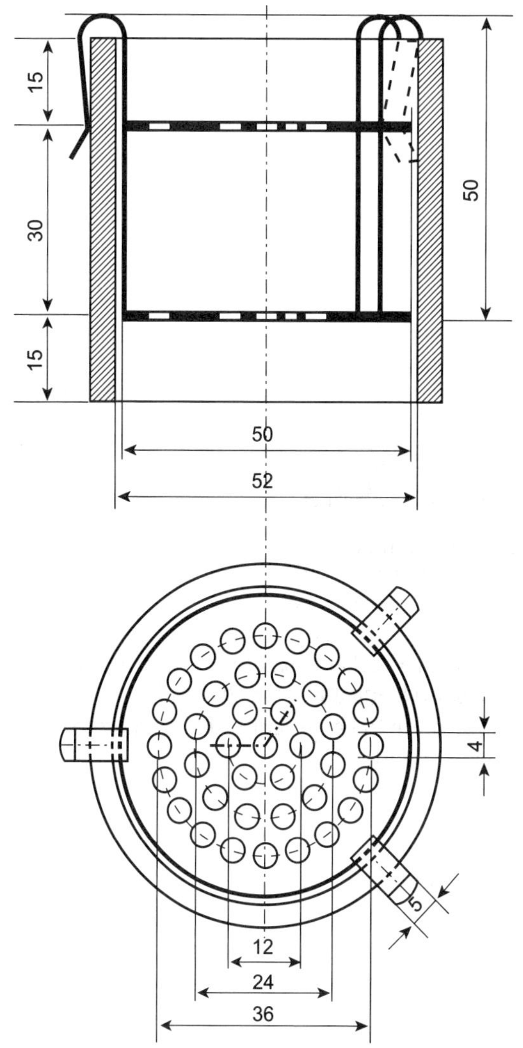

Figure 2.9.2.-1. – *Apparatus for disintegration of suppositories and pessaries*

Dimensions in millimetres

METHOD OF OPERATION FOR VAGINAL TABLETS

Use the apparatus described above, arranged so as to rest on the hooks (see Figure 2.9.2.-2). Place it in a beaker of suitable diameter containing water maintained at 36-37 °C with the level just below the upper perforated disc. Using a pipette, adjust the level with water at 36-37 °C until a uniform film covers the perforations of the disc. Use three vaginal tablets. Place each one on the upper plate of an apparatus and cover the latter with a glass plate to maintain appropriate conditions of humidity. Examine the state of the samples after the period prescribed in the monograph. To pass the test all the samples must have disintegrated.

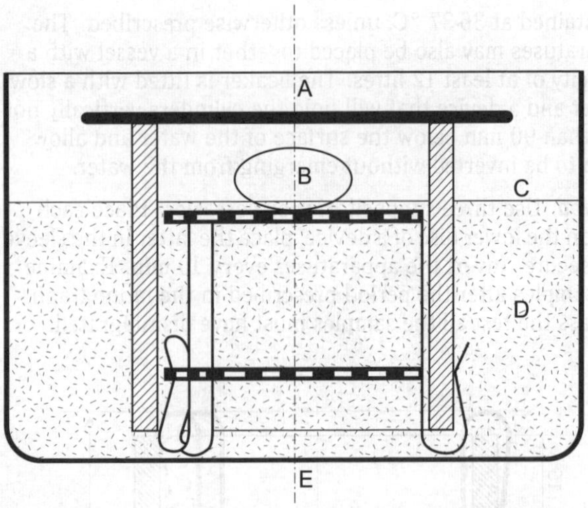

A. glass plate

B. vaginal tablet

C. water surface

D. water

E. dish, beaker

Figure 2.9.2.-2.

01/2005:20903

2.9.3. DISSOLUTION TEST FOR SOLID DOSAGE FORMS

The test is used to determine the dissolution rate of the active ingredients of solid dosage forms (for example, tablets, capsules and suppositories).

Unless otherwise justified and authorised, either the paddle apparatus or the basket apparatus or in special cases, the flow-through cell apparatus may be used.

The following are to be prescribed for each preparation to which the dissolution test is applied:

- the apparatus to be used, including in those cases where the flow-through cell apparatus is prescribed, which flow-through cell (Figures 2.9.3.-4/5/6) is to be used,
- the composition, the volume and the temperature of the dissolution medium,
- the rotation speed or the flow rate of the dissolution medium,
- the time, the method and the amount for sampling of the test solution or the conditions for continuous monitoring,
- the method of analysis,
- the quantity or quantities of active ingredients required to dissolve within a prescribed time.

APPARATUS

The choice of the apparatus to be used depends on the physico-chemical characteristics of the dosage form. All parts of the apparatus that may come into contact with the preparation or the dissolution medium are chemically inert and do not adsorb or react or interfere with the test sample. All metal parts of the apparatus that may come into contact with the preparation or the dissolution medium must be made from a suitable stainless steel or coated with a suitable material to ensure that such parts do not react or interfere with the preparation or the dissolution medium. No part of the assembly or its environment contributes significant motion, agitation or vibration beyond that resulting from the smoothly rotating element or from the flow-through system.

An apparatus that permits observation of the preparation to be examined and the stirrer during the test is preferable.

Paddle apparatus. The apparatus (see Figure 2.9.3.-1) consists of:

- a cylindrical vessel of borosilicate glass or other suitable transparent material with a hemispherical bottom and a nominal capacity of 1000 ml; a cover is fitted to retard evaporation; the cover has a central hole to accommodate the shaft of the stirrer and other holes for the thermometer and the devices used to withdraw liquid;
- a stirrer consisting of a vertical shaft to the lower end of which is attached a blade having the form of that part of a circle subtended by 2 parallel chords; the blade passes through the diameter of the shaft so that the bottom of the blade is flush with the bottom of the shaft; the shaft is placed so that its axis is within 2 mm of the axis of the vessel and the bottom of the blade is 25 ± 2 mm from the inner bottom of the vessel; the upper part of the shaft is connected to a motor provided with a speed regulator; the stirrer rotates smoothly without significant wobble;
- a water-bath that will maintain the dissolution medium at 37 ± 0.5 °C.

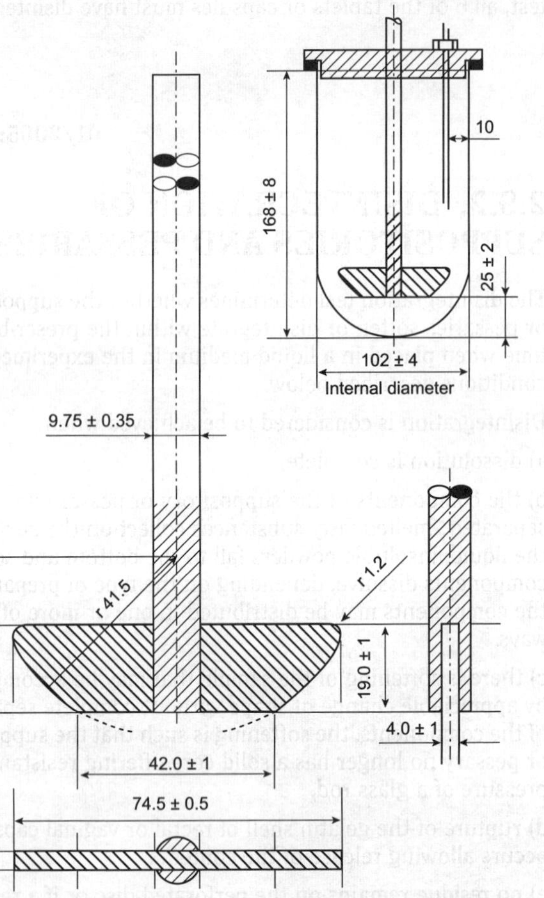

Figure 2.9.3.-1. – *Paddle apparatus*
Dimensions in millimetres

Basket apparatus. The apparatus (see Figure 2.9.3.-2) consists of:

- a vessel identical with that described for the paddle apparatus;
- a stirrer consisting of a vertical shaft to the lower part of which is attached a cylindrical basket; the basket has 2 parts: the upper part, with a 2 mm vent, is welded to the shaft and has 3 spring clips or other suitable device that allows removal of the lower part of the basket for introduction of the preparation to be examined and firmly

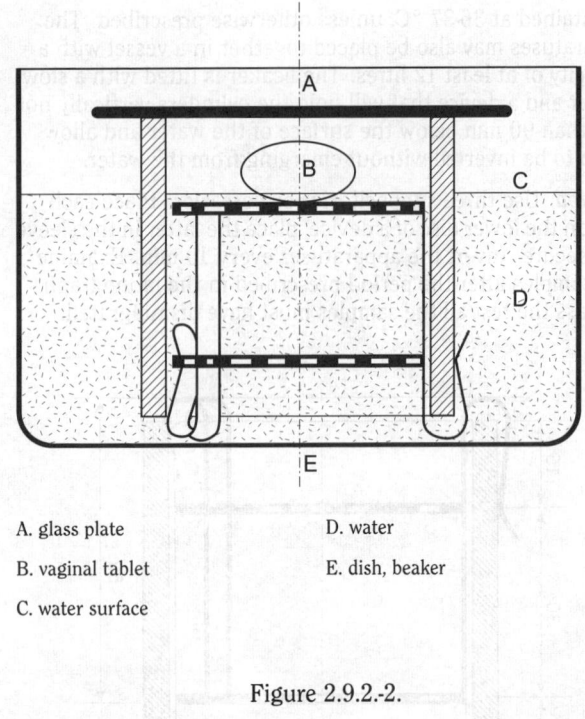

holds the lower part concentric with the axis of the vessel during rotation; the lower part of the basket is made of welded-seam cloth formed into a cylinder with a narrow rim of sheet metal around the top and bottom; unless otherwise prescribed, the cloth has a wire thickness of 0.254 mm in diameter and 0.381 mm square openings; a basket with a gold coating 2.5 µm thick may be used for tests carried out in dilute acid medium; the bottom of the basket is 25 ± 2 mm from the inner bottom of the vessel during the test; the upper part of the shaft is connected to a motor provided with a speed regulator; the stirrer rotates smoothly without significant wobble;

– a water-bath that will maintain the dissolution medium at 37 ± 0.5 °C.

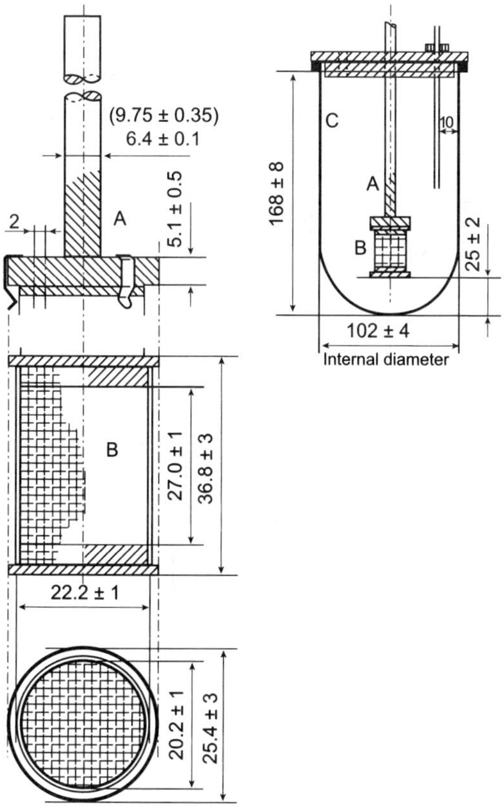

Figure 2.9.3.-2. – *Basket apparatus*
Dimensions in millimetres

Flow-through apparatus. The apparatus (see Figure 2.9.3.-3) consists of:

– a reservoir for the dissolution medium;

– a pump that forces the dissolution medium upwards through the flow-through cell;

– a flow-through cell (see Figures 2.9.3.-4/5/6) of transparent material mounted vertically with a filter system preventing escape of undissolved particles.

The flow-through cell shown in Figure 2.9.3.-6 is specifically intended for lipophilic solid dosage forms such as supposi-tories and soft capsules. It consists of 3 transparent parts which fit into each other. The lower part (1) is made up of 2 adjacent chambers connected to an overflow device.

The dissolution medium passes through chamber A and is subjected to an upwards flow. The flow in chamber B is downwards directed to a small-size bore exit which leads upwards to a filter assembly. The middle part (2) of the cell has a cavity designed to collect lipophilic excipients which float on the dissolution medium. A metal grill serves as a rough filter. The upper part (3) holds a filter unit for paper, glass fibre or cellulose filters.

– a water-bath that will maintain the dissolution medium at 37 ± 0.5 °C.

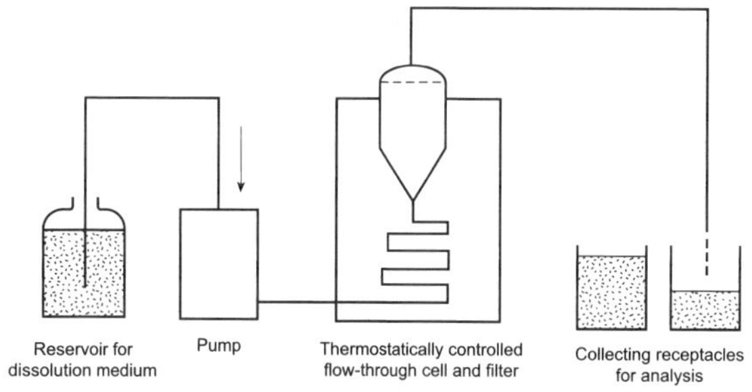

Figure 2.9.3.-3. – *Flow-through apparatus*

Dissolution medium. If the dissolution medium is buffered, adjust its pH to within ± 0.05 units of the prescribed value. Remove any dissolved gases from the dissolution medium before the test since they can cause the formation of bubbles that significantly affect the results.

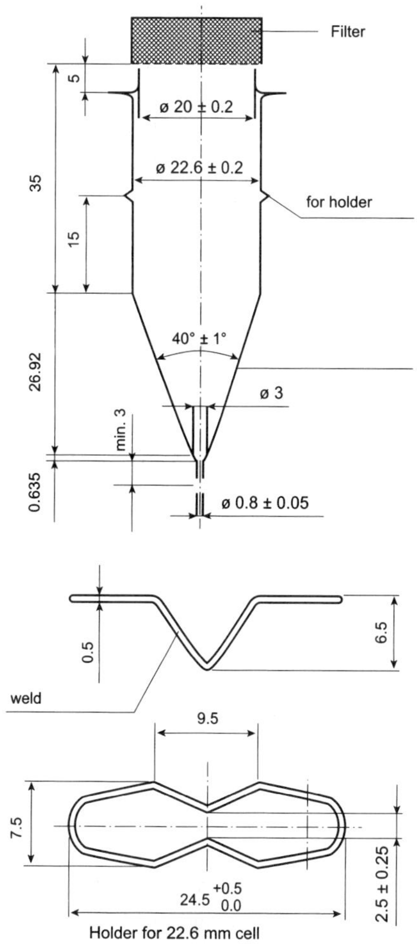

Figure 2.9.3.-4. – *Flow-through cell*
Dimensions in millimetres

METHOD

Paddle and basket apparatus

Place the prescribed volume of dissolution medium in the vessel, assemble the apparatus, warm the dissolution medium to 37 ± 0.5 °C and remove the thermometer.

Place one unit of the preparation to be examined in the apparatus. For the paddle apparatus, place the preparation at the bottom of the vessel before starting rotation of the blade; dosage forms that would otherwise float are kept horizontal at the bottom of the vessel using a suitable device, such as a wire or glass helix.

For the basket apparatus, place the preparation in a dry basket and lower into position before starting rotation.

Take care to avoid the presence of air bubbles on the surface of the preparation. Start the rotation of the apparatus immediately at the prescribed rate (± 4 per cent).

Flow-through apparatus

– Cells (see Figures 2.9.3.-4/5)

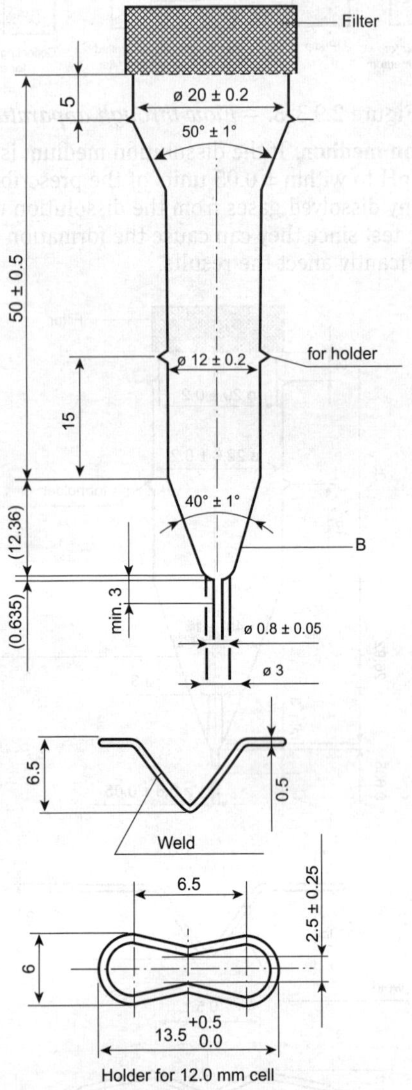

Figure 2.9.3.-5. – *Flow-through cell*

Dimensions in millimetres

Place 1 bead of 5 mm (± 0.5 mm) diameter at the bottom of the cone to protect the fluid entry of the tube and then glass beads of suitable size, preferably 1 mm (± 0.1 mm) diameter. Introduce 1 unit of the preparation in the cell on or within the layer of glass beads, by means of a holder. Assemble the filter head. Heat the dissolution medium to 37 ± 0.5 °C. Using a suitable pump, introduce the dissolution medium through the bottom of the cell to obtain a suitable continuous flow through an open or closed circuit at the prescribed rate (± 5 per cent).

– Cell (Figure 2.9.3.-6)

Place 1 unit of the preparation to be examined in chamber A. Close the cell with the prepared filter assembly. At the beginning of the test, chamber A requires air removal via a small orifice connected to the filter assembly. Heat the dissolution medium to an appropriate temperature taking the melting point of the preparation into consideration. Using a suitable pump, introduce the warmed dissolution medium through the bottom of the cell to obtain a suitable continuous flow through an open or closed circuit at the prescribed rate (± 5 per cent). When the dissolution medium reaches the overflow, air starts to escape through the capillary and chamber B fills with the dissolution medium. The preparation spreads through the dissolution medium according to its physico-chemical properties.

In justified and authorised cases, representative fractions of large volume suppositories may be tested.

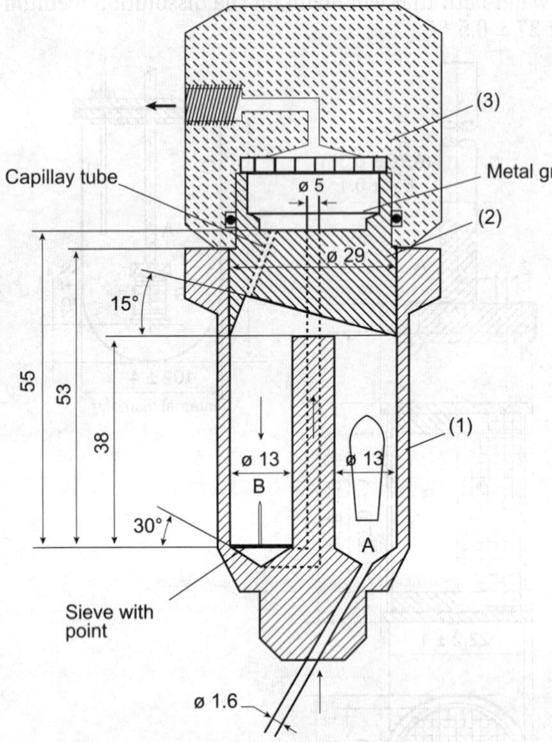

Figure 2.9.3.-6. – *Flow-through cell*

Dimensions in millimetres

SAMPLING AND EVALUATION

In the case of the paddle apparatus and the basket apparatus, withdraw at the prescribed time, or at the prescribed intervals or continuously, the prescribed volume or volumes from a position midway between the surface of the dissolution medium and the top of the basket or blade and not less than 10 mm from the vessel wall.

In the case of the flow-through apparatus, samples are always collected at the outlet of the cell, irrespective of whether the circuit is opened or closed.

Except where continuous measurement is used with the paddle or basket method (the liquid removed being returned to the vessel) or where a single portion of liquid is removed, add a volume of dissolution medium equal to the volume of liquid removed or compensate by calculation.

Filter the liquid removed using an inert filter of appropriate pore size that does not cause significant adsorption of the active ingredient from the solution and does not contain substances extractable by the dissolution medium that would interfere with the prescribed analytical method. Proceed with analysis of the filtrate as prescribed.

The quantity of the active ingredient dissolved in a specified time is expressed as a percentage of the content stated on the label.

01/2005:20904

2.9.4. DISSOLUTION TEST FOR TRANSDERMAL PATCHES

This test is used to determine the dissolution rate of the active ingredients of transdermal patches.

1. DISK ASSEMBLY METHOD

Equipment. Use the paddle and vessel assembly from the paddle apparatus described in the dissolution test for solid oral dosage forms (*2.9.3*) with the addition of a stainless steel disk assembly (SSDA) in the form of a net with an aperture of 125 µm (see Figure 2.9.4.-1).

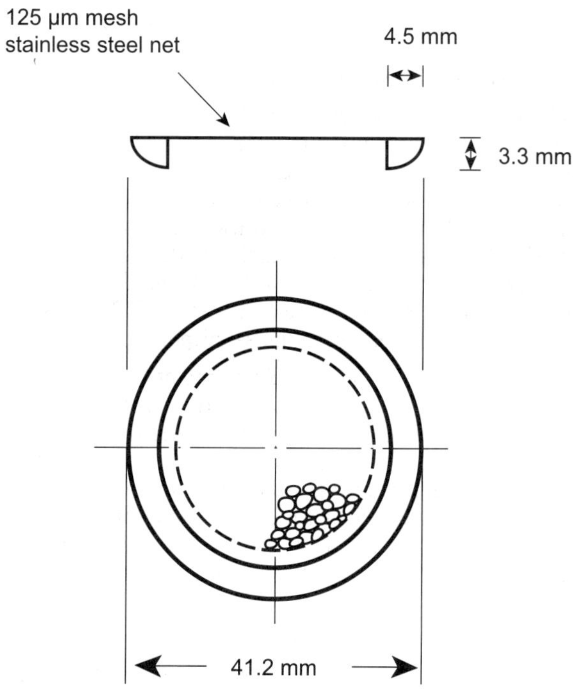

Figure 2.9.4.-1. – *Disk assembly*

The SSDA holds the system at the bottom of the vessel and is designed to minimise any dead volume between the SSDA and the bottom of the vessel. The SSDA holds the patch flat, with the release surface uppermost and parallel to the bottom of the paddle blade. A distance of 25 ± 2 mm between the bottom of the paddle blade and the surface of the SSDA is maintained during the test (see Figure 2.9.4.-2). The temperature is maintained at 32 ± 0.5 °C. The vessel may be covered during the test to minimise evaporation.

Procedure. Place the prescribed volume of the dissolution medium in the vessel and equilibrate the medium to the prescribed temperature. Apply the patch to the SSDA, ensuring that the release surface of the patch is as flat as possible. The patch may be attached to the SSDA by a prescribed adhesive or by a strip of a double-sided adhesive tape. The adhesive or tape are previously tested for the absence of interference with the assay and of adsorption of the active ingredient(s). Press the patch, release surface facing up, onto the side of the SSDA made adhesive. The applied patch must not overlap the borders of the SSDA. For this purpose and provided that the preparation is homogeneous and uniformly spread on the outer covering, an appropriate and exactly measured piece of the patch may be cut and used for testing the dissolution rate. This procedure may also be necessary to achieve appropriate sink conditions. This procedure must not be applied to membrane-type patches. Place the patch mounted on the SSDA flat at the bottom of the vessel with the release surface facing upwards. Immediately rotate the paddle at 100 r/min, for example. At predetermined intervals, withdraw a sample from the zone midway between the surface of the dissolution medium and the top of the blade, not less than 1 cm from the vessel wall.

Perform the assay on each sample, correcting for any volume losses, as necessary. Repeat the test with additional patches.

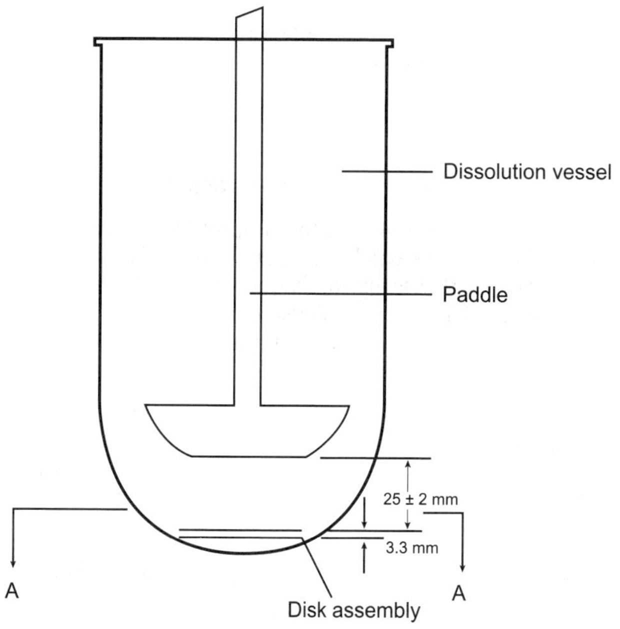

Figure 2.9.4.-2. – *Paddle and disk*

2. CELL METHOD

Equipment. Use the paddle and vessel assembly from the paddle apparatus described in the dissolution test for solid oral dosage forms (*2.9.3*) with the addition of the extraction cell (*cell*).

The *cell* is made of chemically inert materials and consists of a *support*, a *cover* and, if necessary, a *membrane* placed on the patch to isolate it from the medium that may modify or adversely affect the physico-chemical properties of the patch (see Figure 2.9.4.-3).

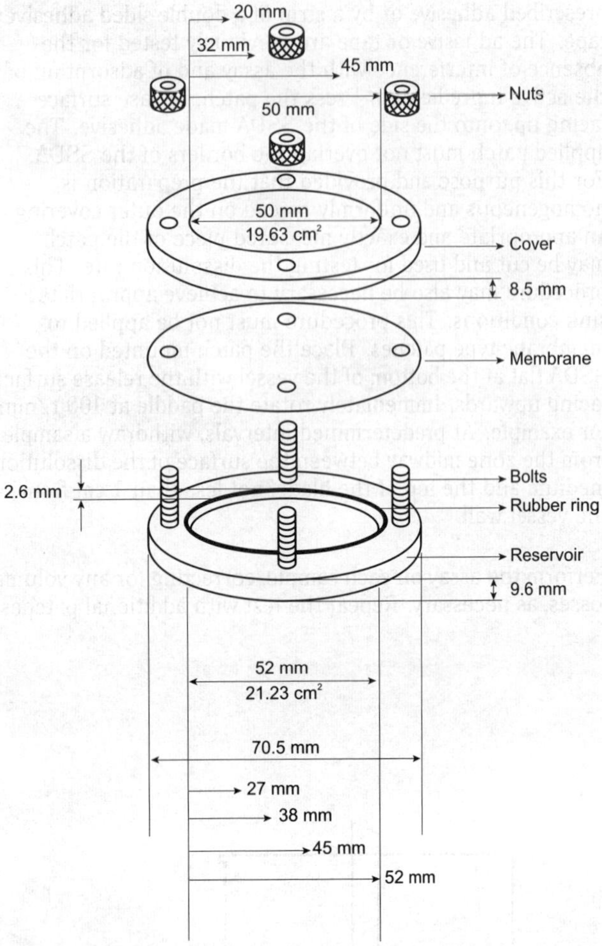

Figure 2.9.4.-3. – *Extraction cell*

Support. The central part of the support forms a cavity intended to hold the patch. The cavity has a depth of 2.6 mm and a diameter that is appropriate to the size of the patch to be examined. The following diameters can be used: 27 mm, 38 mm, 45 mm, 52 mm, corresponding to volumes of 1.48 ml, 2.94 ml, 4.13 ml, 5.52 ml, respectively.

Cover. The cover has a central opening with a diameter selected according to the size of the patch to be examined. The patch can thus be precisely centred, and its releasing surface limited. The following diameters may be used: 20 mm, 32 mm, 40 mm, 50 mm corresponding to areas of 3.14 cm², 8.03 cm², 12.56 cm², 19.63 cm², respectively. The cover is held in place by nuts screwed onto bolts projecting from the support. The cover is sealed to the support by a rubber ring set on the reservoir.

Extraction cell. The *cell* holds the patch flat, with the release surface uppermost and parallel to the bottom of the paddle blade. A distance of 25 ± 2 mm is maintained between the paddle blade and the surface of the patch (see Figure 2.9.4.-4). The temperature is maintained at 32 ± 0.5 °C. The vessel may be covered during the test to minimise evaporation.

Procedure. Place the prescribed volume of the dissolution medium in the vessel and equilibrate the medium to the prescribed temperature. Precisely centre the patch in the *cell* with the releasing surface uppermost. Close the *cell*, if necessary applying a hydrophobic substance (for example, petrolatum) to the flat surfaces to ensure the seal, and ensure that the patch stays in place. Introduce the cell flat into the bottom of the vessel with the cover facing upwards. Immediately rotate the paddle, at 100 r/min for example. At predetermined intervals, withdraw a sample from the zone midway between the surface of the dissolution medium and the top of the paddle blade, not less than 1 cm from the vessel wall.

Perform the assay on each sample, correcting for any volume losses, as necessary. Repeat the test with additional patches.

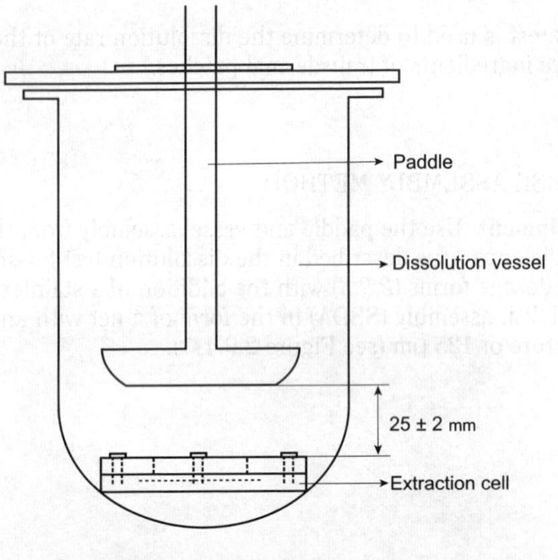

Figure 2.9.4.-4. – *Paddle over extraction cell*

3. ROTATING CYLINDER METHOD

Equipment. Use the assembly of the paddle apparatus described in the dissolution test for solid oral dosage forms (*2.9.3*). Replace the paddle and shaft with a stainless steel cylinder stirring element (*cylinder*) (see Figure 2.9.4.-5). The patch is placed on the *cylinder* at the beginning of each test. The distance between the inside bottom of the vessel and the *cylinder* is maintained at 25 ± 2 mm during the test. The temperature is maintained at 32 ± 0.5 °C. The vessel is covered during the test to minimise evaporation.

Procedure. Place the prescribed volume of the dissolution medium in the vessel and equilibrate the medium to the prescribed temperature. Remove the protective liner from the patch and place the adhesive side on a piece of suitable inert porous membrane that is at least 1 cm larger on all sides than the patch. Place the patch on a clean surface with the membrane in contact with this surface. Two systems for adhesion to the *cylinder* may be used:

- apply a suitable adhesive to the exposed membrane borders and, if necessary, to the back of the patch,
- apply a double-sided adhesive tape to the external wall of the *cylinder*.

Using gentle pressure, carefully apply the non-adhesive side of the patch to the *cylinder*, so that the release surface is in contact with the dissolution medium and the long axis of the patch fits around the circumference of the *cylinder*.
The system for adhesion used is previously tested for absence of interference with the assay and of adsorption of the active ingredient(s).

Place the *cylinder* in the apparatus, and immediately rotate the *cylinder* at 100 r/min, for example. At determined intervals, withdraw a sample of dissolution medium from a zone midway between the surface of the dissolution medium and the top of the rotating *cylinder*, and not less than 1 cm from the vessel wall.

Perform the assay on each sample as directed in the individual monograph, correcting for any volume withdrawn, as necessary. Repeat the test with additional patches.

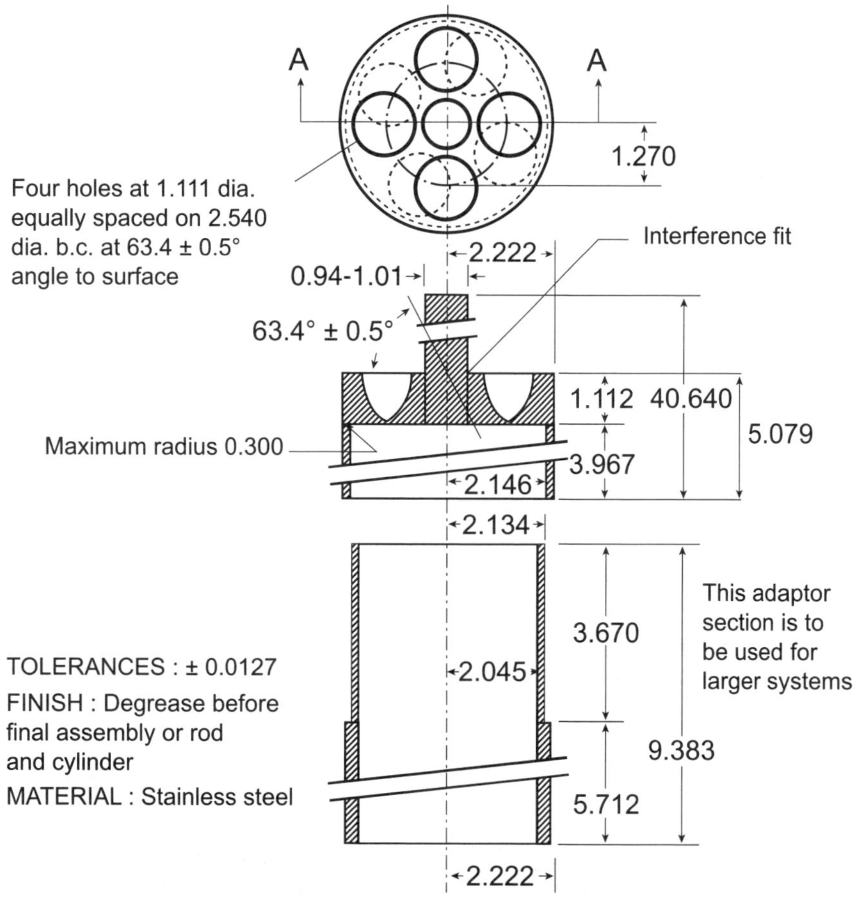

Figure 2.9.4.-5. – *Cylinder stirring element*
Dimensions in centimetres

Interpretation. The requirements are met if the quantity of active ingredient(s) released from the patch, expressed as the amount per surface area per time unit, is within the prescribed limits at the defined sampling times.

01/2005:20905

2.9.5. UNIFORMITY OF MASS OF SINGLE-DOSE PREPARATIONS

Weigh individually 20 units taken at random or, for single-dose preparations presented in individual containers, the contents of 20 units, and determine the average mass. Not more than 2 of the individual masses deviate from the average mass by more than the percentage deviation shown in Table 2.9.5.-1 and none deviates by more than twice that percentage.

For capsules and powders for parenteral use, proceed as described below.

Table 2.9.5.-1

Pharmaceutical Form	Average Mass	Percentage deviation
Tablets (uncoated and film-coated)	80 mg or less	10
	More than 80 mg and less than 250 mg	7.5
	250 mg or more	5
Capsules, granules (uncoated, single-dose) and powders (single-dose)	Less than 300 mg	10
	300 mg or more	7.5
Powders for parenteral use* (single-dose)	More than 40 mg	10
Suppositories and pessaries	All masses	5
Powders for eye-drops and powders for eye lotions (single-dose)	Less than 300 mg	10
	300 mg or more	7.5

* When the average mass is equal to or below 40 mg, the preparation is not submitted to the test for uniformity of mass but to the test for uniformity of content of single-dose preparations (*2.9.6*).

CAPSULES

Weigh an intact capsule. Open the capsule without losing any part of the shell and remove the contents as completely as possible. For soft shell capsules, wash the shell with a suitable solvent and allow to stand until the odour of the solvent is no longer perceptible. Weigh the shell. The mass of the contents is the difference between the weighings. Repeat the procedure with another 19 capsules.

POWDERS FOR PARENTERAL USE

Remove any paper labels from a container and wash and dry the outside. Open the container and without delay weigh the container and its contents. Empty the container as completely as possible by gentle tapping, rinse it if necessary with *water R* and then with *alcohol R* and dry at 100-105 °C for 1 h, or, if the nature of the container precludes heating at this temperature, dry at a lower temperature to constant mass. Allow to cool in a desiccator and weigh. The mass of the contents is the difference between the weighings. Repeat the procedure with another 19 containers.

01/2005:20906

2.9.6. UNIFORMITY OF CONTENT OF SINGLE-DOSE PREPARATIONS

The test for uniformity of content of single-dose preparations is based on the assay of the individual contents of active substance(s) of a number of single-dose units to determine whether the individual contents are within limits set with reference to the average content of the sample.

The test is not required for multivitamin and trace-element preparations and in other justified and authorised circumstances.

Method. Using a suitable analytical method, determine the individual contents of active substance(s) of 10 dosage units taken at random.

Apply the criteria of test A, test B or test C as specified in the monograph for the dosage form in question.

TEST A

Tablets, powders for parenteral use, ophthalmic inserts, suspensions for injection. The preparation complies with the test if each individual content is between 85 per cent and 115 per cent of the average content. The preparation fails to comply with the test if more than one individual content is outside these limits or if one individual content is outside the limits of 75 per cent to 125 per cent of the average content.

If one individual content is outside the limits of 85 per cent to 115 per cent but within the limits of 75 per cent to 125 per cent, determine the individual contents of another 20 dosage units taken at random. The preparation complies with the test if not more than one of the individual contents of the 30 units is outside 85 per cent to 115 per cent of the average content and none is outside the limits of 75 per cent to 125 per cent of the average content.

TEST B

Capsules, powders other than for parenteral use, granules, suppositories, pessaries. The preparation complies with the test if not more than one individual content is outside the limits of 85 per cent to 115 per cent of the average content and none is outside the limits of 75 per cent to 125 per cent of the average content. The preparation fails to comply with the test if more than 3 individual contents are outside the limits of 85 per cent to 115 per cent of the average content or if one or more individual contents are outside the limits of 75 per cent to 125 per cent of the average content.

If 2 or 3 individual contents are outside the limits of 85 per cent to 115 per cent but within the limits of 75 per cent to 125 per cent, determine the individual contents of another 20 dosage units taken at random. The preparation complies with the test if not more than 3 individual contents of the 30 units are outside the limits of 85 per cent to 115 per cent of the average content and none is outside the limits of 75 per cent to 125 per cent of the average content.

TEST C

Transdermal patches. The preparation complies with the test if the average content of the 10 dosage units is between 90 per cent and 110 per cent of the content stated on the label and if the individual content of each dosage unit is between 75 per cent and 125 per cent of the average content.

01/2005:20907

2.9.7. FRIABILITY OF UNCOATED TABLETS

This test is intended to determine, under defined conditions, the friability of uncoated tablets, the phenomenon whereby tablet surfaces are damaged and/or show evidence of lamination or breakage when subjected to mechanical shock or attrition.

APPARATUS

Use a drum with an internal diameter between 283 and 291 mm and a depth between 36 mm and 40 mm, made of a transparent synthetic polymer with polished internal surfaces and not subject to static build-up (see Figure 2.9.7.-1). One side of the drum is removable. The tablets are tumbled at each turn of the drum by a curved projection with an inside radius between 75.5 mm and 85.5 mm that extends from the middle of the drum to the outer wall. The drum is attached to the horizontal axis of a device that rotates at 25 ± 1 r/min. Thus, at each turn the tablets roll or slide and fall onto the drum wall or onto each other.

METHOD

For tablets weighing up to 0.65 g each, take a sample of twenty tablets; for tablets weighing more than 0.65 g each, take ten tablets. Place the tablets on a sieve no. 1000 and remove any loose dust with the aid of air pressure or a soft brush. Accurately weigh the tablet sample and place the tablets in the drum. Rotate the drum 100 times and remove the tablets. Remove any loose dust from the tablets as before. If no tablets are cracked, split or broken, weigh the tablets to the nearest milligram.

Generally the test is run once. If the results are doubtful or if the mass loss is greater than 1 per cent, repeat the test twice and determine the mean of the 3 tests. A maximum loss of 1 per cent of the mass of the tablets tested is considered to be acceptable for most products.
For tablets having a diameter of 13 mm or greater, problems of reproducibility may be encountered due to frequent irregular tumbling. In such cases, adjust the drum so that the tablets may fall freely and do not bind together when lying next to each other, adjusting the drum so that the axis forms a 10° angle with the base is usually satisfactory.

EXPRESSION OF THE RESULTS

The friability is expressed as the loss of mass and it is calculated as a percentage of the initial mass.
Indicate the number of tablets used.

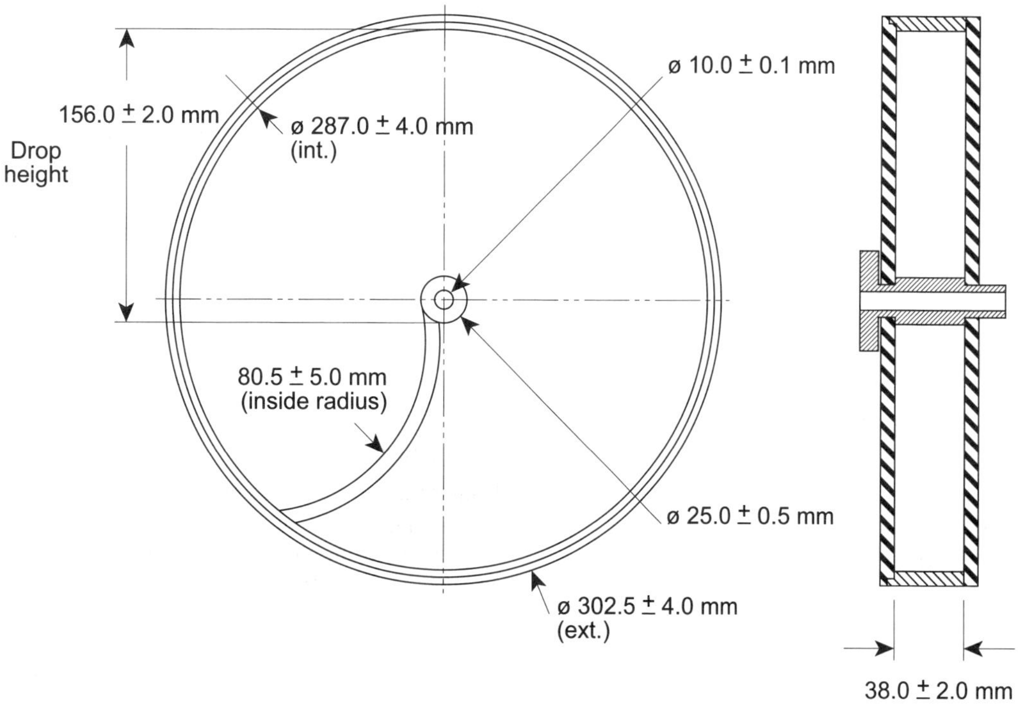

Figure 2.9.7.-1. – *Tablet friability apparatus*

01/2005:20908

2.9.8. RESISTANCE TO CRUSHING OF TABLETS

This test is intended to determine, under defined conditions, the resistance to crushing of tablets, measured by the force needed to disrupt them by crushing.

APPARATUS

The apparatus consists of 2 jaws facing each other, one of which moves towards the other. The flat surfaces of the jaws are perpendicular to the direction of movement. The crushing surfaces of the jaws are flat and larger than the zone of contact with the tablet. The apparatus is calibrated using a system with a precision of 1 newton.

OPERATING PROCEDURE

Place the tablet between the jaws, taking into account, where applicable, the shape, the break-mark and the inscription; for each measurement orient the tablet in the same way with respect to the direction of application of the force. Carry out the measurement on 10 tablets, taking care that all fragments of tablets have been removed before each determination.

This procedure does not apply when fully automated equipment is used.

EXPRESSION OF RESULTS

Express the results as the mean, minimum and maximum values of the forces measured, all expressed in newtons.

Indicate the type of apparatus and, where applicable, the orientation of the tablets.

01/2005:20909

2.9.9. MEASUREMENT OF CONSISTENCY BY PENETROMETRY

This test is intended to measure, under determined and validated conditions, the penetration of an object into the product to be examined in a container with a specified shape and size.

APPARATUS

The apparatus consists of a penetrometer made up of a stand and a penetrating object. A suitable apparatus is shown in Figure 2.9.9.-1.

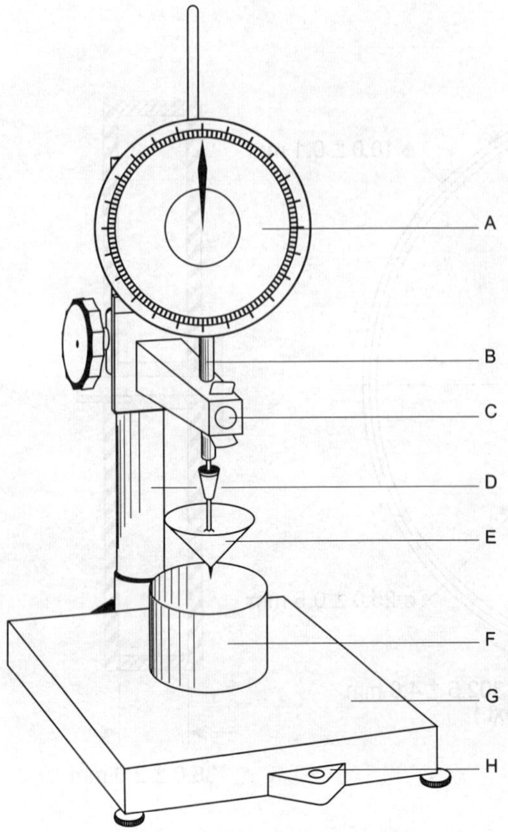

Figure 2.9.9.-1. – *Penetrometer*

A. Scale showing the depth of penetration, graduated in tenths of millimetres.

B. Vertical shaft to maintain and guide the penetrating object.

C. Device to retain and to release the penetrating object automatically and for a constant time.

D. Device to ensure that the penetrating object is vertical and that the base is horizontal.

E. Penetrating object (see Figures 2.9.9.-2 and 3).

F. Container.

G. Horizontal base.

H. Control for the horizontal base.

The stand is made up of:

– a vertical shaft to maintain and guide the penetrating object,

– a horizontal base,

– a device to ensure that the penetrating object is vertical,

– a device to check that the base is horizontal,

– a device to retain and release the penetrating object,

– a scale showing the depth of penetration, graduated in tenths of a millimetre.

The penetrating object, made of a suitable material, has a smooth surface, and is characterised by its shape, size and mass.

Suitable penetrating objects are shown in Figures 2.9.9.-2 and 2.9.9.-3.

PROCEDURE

Prepare the test samples by one of the following procedures:

A. Carefully and completely fill three containers, without forming air bubbles. Level if necessary to obtain a flat surface. Store the samples at 25 ± 0.5 °C for 24 h, unless otherwise prescribed.

B. Store three samples at 25 ± 0.5 °C for 24 h. Apply a suitable shear to the samples for 5 min. Carefully and completely fill three containers, without forming air bubbles, and level if necessary to obtain a flat surface.

C. Melt three samples and carefully and completely fill three containers, without forming air bubbles. Store the samples at 25 ± 0.5 °C for 24 h, unless otherwise prescribed.

Determination of penetration. Place the test sample on the base of the penetrometer. Verify that its surface is perpendicular to the vertical axis of the penetrating object. Bring the temperature of the penetrating object to 25 ± 0.5 °C and then adjust its position such that its tip just touches the surface of the sample. Release the penetrating object and hold it free for 5 s. Clamp the penetrating object and measure the depth of penetration. Repeat the test with the two remaining containers.

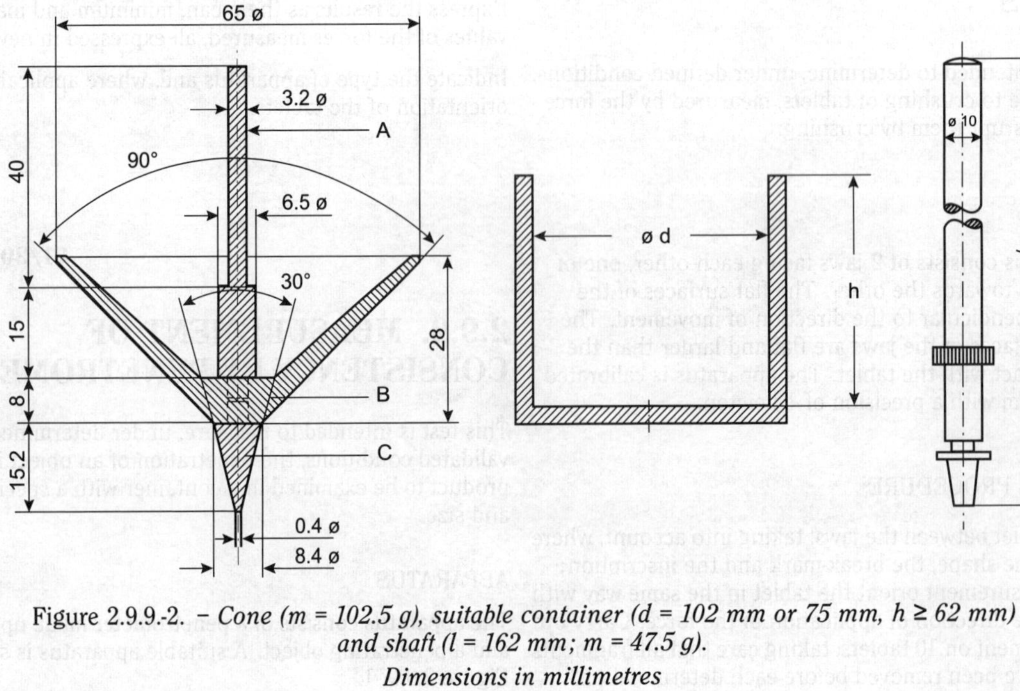

Figure 2.9.9.-2. – *Cone (m = 102.5 g), suitable container (d = 102 mm or 75 mm, h ≥ 62 mm) and shaft (l = 162 mm; m = 47.5 g).*

Dimensions in millimetres

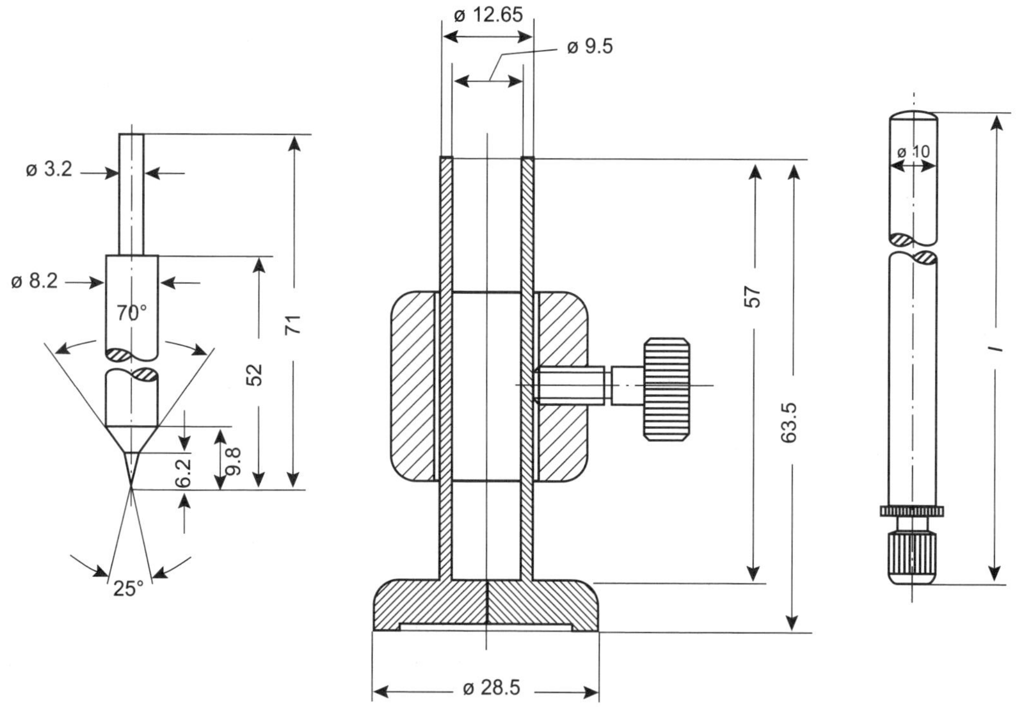

Figure 2.9.9.-3 – *Micro-cone (m = 7.0 g), suitable container and shaft (l = 116 mm; m = 16.8 g)*

Dimensions in millimetres

EXPRESSION OF THE RESULTS

The penetration is expressed in tenths of a millimetre as the arithmetic mean of the three measurements. If any of the individual results differ from the mean by more than 3 per cent, repeat the test and express the results of the six measurements as the mean and the relative standard deviation.

01/2005:20910

2.9.10. ETHANOL CONTENT AND ALCOHOLIMETRIC TABLES

This method is intended only for the examination of liquid pharmaceutical preparations containing ethanol. These preparations also contain dissolved substances which must be separated from the ethanol to be determined by distillation. When distillation would distil volatile substances other than ethanol and water the appropriate precautions are stated in the monograph.

The ethanol content of a liquid is expressed as the number of volumes of ethanol contained in 100 volumes of the liquid, the volumes being measured at 20 ± 0.1 °C. This is known as the "percentage of ethanol by volume" (per cent *V/V*). The content may also be expressed in grams of ethanol per 100 g of the liquid. This is known as the "percentage of ethanol by mass" (per cent *m/m*).

The relation between the density at 20 ± 0.1 °C, the relative density (corrected to vacuum) and the ethanol content of a mixture of water and ethanol is given in the tables of the International Organisation for Legal Metrology (1972), International Recommendation No. 22.

Apparatus. The apparatus (see Figure 2.9.10.-1) consists of a round-bottomed flask (*A*) fitted with a distillation head (*B*) with a steam trap and attached to a vertical condenser (*C*). The latter is fitted at its lower part with a tube (*D*) which carries the distillate into the lower part of a 100 ml or 250 ml volumetric flask. The volumetric flask is immersed in a mixture of ice and water (*E*) during the distillation. A disc having a circular aperture 6 cm in diameter is placed under flask (*A*) to reduce the risk of charring of any dissolved substances.

Method

Pycnometer method. Transfer 25.0 ml of the preparation to be examined, measured at 20 ± 0.1 °C, to the distillation flask. Dilute with 100 ml to 150 ml of *distilled water R* and add a few pieces of pumice. Attach the distillation head and condenser. Distil and collect not less than 90 ml of distillate in a 100 ml volumetric flask. Adjust the temperature to 20 ± 0.1 °C and dilute to 100.0 ml with *distilled water R* at 20 ± 0.1 °C. Determine the relative density at 20 ± 0.1 °C using a pycnometer.

The values indicated in Table 2.9.10.-1, column 3, are multiplied by four to obtain the percentage of ethanol by volume (*V/V*) contained in the preparation. After calculation of the ethanol content using the Table, round off the result to one decimal place.

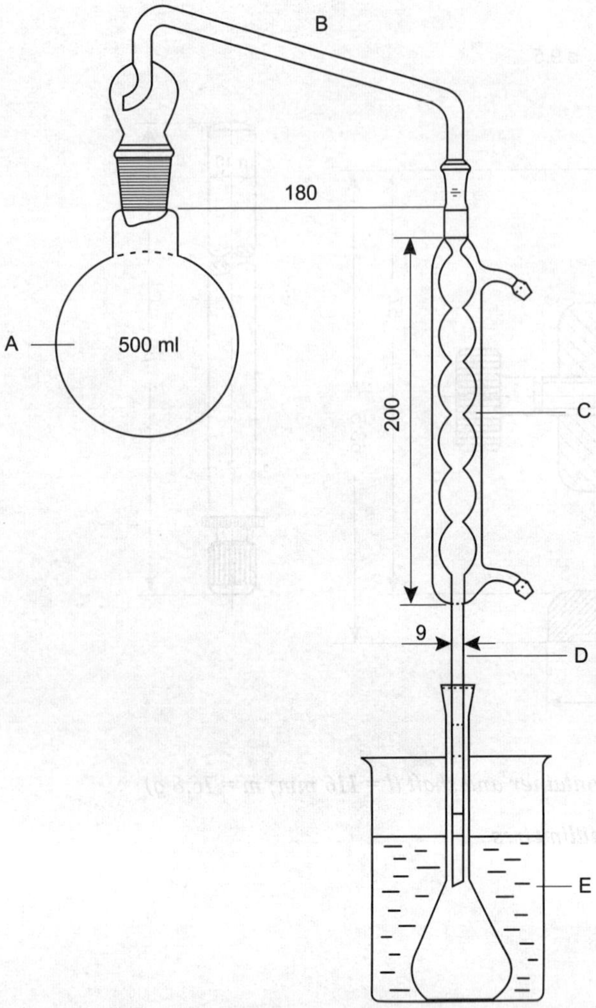

Figure 2.9.10.-1. – *Apparatus for the determination of ethanol content*

Dimensions in millimetres

Table 2.9.10.-1. - *Relationship between density, relative density and ethanol content*

ρ_{20} (kg·m^{-3})	Relative density of the distillate measured in air d_{20}^{20}	Ethanol content in per cent *V/V* at 20 °C
968.0	0.9697	25.09
968.5	0.9702	24.64
969.0	0.9707	24.19
969.5	0.9712	23.74
970.0	0.9717	23.29
970.5	0.9722	22.83
971.0	0.9727	22.37
971.5	0.9733	21.91
972.0	0.9738	21.45
972.5	0.9743	20.98
973.0	0.9748	20.52
973.5	0.9753	20.05
974.0	0.9758	19.59
974.5	0.9763	19.12
975.0	0.9768	18.66
975.5	0.9773	18.19
976.0	0.9778	17.73
976.5	0.9783	17.25
977.0	0.9788	16.80
977.5	0.9793	16.34
978.0	0.9798	15.88
978.5	0.9803	15.43
979.0	0.9808	14.97
979.5	0.9813	14.52
980.0	0.9818	14.07
980.5	0.9823	13.63
981.0	0.9828	13.18
981.5	0.9833	12.74
982.0	0.9838	12.31
982.5	0.9843	11.87
983.0	0.9848	11.44
983.5	0.9853	11.02
984.0	0.9858	10.60
984.5	0.9863	10.18
985.0	0.9868	9.76
985.5	0.9873	9.35
986.0	0.9878	8.94
986.5	0.9883	8.53
987.0	0.9888	8.13
987.5	0.9893	7.73
988.0	0.9898	7.34
988.5	0.9903	6.95
989.0	0.9908	6.56
989.5	0.9913	6.17
990.0	0.9918	5.79
990.5	0.9923	5.42
991.0	0.9928	5.04
991.5	0.9933	4.67
992.0	0.9938	4.30
992.5	0.9943	3.94
993.0	0.9948	3.58
993.5	0.9953	3.22
994.0	0.9958	2.86
994.5	0.9963	2.51
995.0	0.9968	2.16
995.5	0.9973	1.82
996.0	0.9978	1.47
996.5	0.9983	1.13
997.0	0.9988	0.80
997.5	0.9993	0.46
998.0	0.9998	0.13

Hydrometer method. Transfer 50.0 ml of the preparation to be examined, measured at 20 ± 0.1 °C, to the distillation flask, add 200 ml to 300 ml of *distilled water R* and distil, as described above, into a volumetric flask until at least 180 ml has been collected. Adjust the temperature to 20 ± 0.1 °C and dilute to 250.0 ml with *distilled water R* at 20 ± 0.1 °C.

Transfer the distillate to a cylinder whose diameter is at least 6 mm wider than the bulb of the hydrometer. If the volume is insufficient, double the quantity of the sample and dilute the distillate to 500.0 ml with *distilled water R* at 20 ± 0.1 °C.

Multiply the strength by five to allow for the dilution during the determination. After calculation of the ethanol content using the Table 2.9.10.-1 round off the result to one decimal place.

01/2005:20911

2.9.11. TEST FOR METHANOL AND 2-PROPANOL

Examine by gas chromatography (*2.2.28*).

Internal standard solution. Prepare a solution containing 2.5 per cent *V/V* of *propanol R* in *ethanol R1*.

Test solution (a). To a certain amount of the distillate add 2.0 ml of the internal standard solution; adjust the ethanol content (*2.9.10*) to 10.0 per cent *V/V* by dilution to 50 ml with *water R* or addition of *ethanol R1*.

Test solution (b). Adjust the ethanol content (*2.9.10*) of a certain amount of the distillate to 10.0 per cent *V/V* by dilution to 50 ml with *water R* or addition of *ethanol R1*.

Reference solution (a). Prepare 50 ml of a solution containing 2.0 ml of the internal standard solution, 3.0 ml of *ethanol R1*, 0.05 per cent *V/V* of *2-propanol R* and sufficient *anhydrous methanol R* to give a total of 0.05 per cent *V/V* of methanol taking into account the methanol content of *ethanol R1*.

Reference solution (b). Prepare a 10.0 per cent *V/V* solution of *ethanol R1* containing 0.0025 per cent *V/V* of each *methanol R* and *2-propanol R*.

Column:
- *material*: fused silica,
- *size*: l = 30 m, Ø = 0.53 mm,
- *stationary phase*: *poly(cyanopropyl)(7)(phenyl)(7)(methyl)(86)siloxane R* (film thickness 3 μm).

Carrier gas: *helium for chromatography R.*

Flow rate: 2 ml/min.

Split ratio: 1:10.

Temperature:

	Time (min)	Temperature (°C)
Column	0 - 5	35
	5 - 15	35 - 85
Injection port		250
Detector		250

Detection: flame ionisation.

Injection: 1.0 μl.

System suitability:
- *propanol*: there is no peak corresponding to propanol in the chromatogram obtained with test solution (b),
- *peak-to-valley ratio*: minimum 15, where H_p = height above the baseline of the peak due to 2-propanol and H_v = height above the baseline of the lowest point of the curve separating this peak from the peak due to ethanol in the chromatogram obtained with the reference solution (a),
- *signal-to-noise ratio*: minimum 10 for the peaks due to methanol and 2-propanol in the chromatogram obtained with reference solution (b).

The content of methanol and 2-propanol is calculated with reference to the original sample.

01/2005:20912

2.9.12. SIEVE TEST

The degree of fineness of a powder may be expressed by reference to sieves that comply with the specifications for non-analytical sieves (*2.1.4*).

Where the degree of fineness of powders is determined by sieving, it is defined in relation to the sieve number(s) used either by means of the following terms or, where such terms cannot be used, by expressing the fineness of the powder as a percentage *m/m* passing the sieve(s) used.

The following terms are used in the description of powders:

Coarse powder. Not less than 95 per cent by mass passes through a number 1400 sieve and not more than 40 per cent by mass passes through a number 355 sieve.

Moderately fine powder. Not less than 95 per cent by mass passes through a number 355 sieve and not more than 40 per cent by mass passes through a number 180 sieve.

Fine powder. Not less than 95 per cent by mass passes through a number 180 sieve and not more than 40 per cent by mass passes through a number 125 sieve.

Very fine powder. Not less than 95 per cent by mass passes through a number 125 sieve and not more than 40 per cent by mass passes through a number 90 sieve.

If a single sieve number is given, not less than 97 per cent of the powder passes through the sieve of that number, unless otherwise prescribed.

Assemble the sieves and operate in a suitable manner until sifting is practically complete. Weigh the separated fractions of the powder.

01/2005:20913

2.9.13. LIMIT TEST OF PARTICLE SIZE BY MICROSCOPY

Weigh a suitable quantity of the powder to be examined (for example 10 mg to 100 mg) and suspend it in 10.0 ml of a suitable medium in which the powder does not dissolve, adding, if necessary, a wetting agent. Introduce a portion of the homogeneous suspension into a suitable counting cell and scan under a microscope an area corresponding to not less than 10 μg of the powder to be examined. Count all the particles having a maximum dimension greater than the prescribed size limit. The size limit and the permitted number of particles exceeding the limit are stated in the monograph.

01/2005:20914

2.9.14. SPECIFIC SURFACE AREA BY AIR PERMEABILITY

The test is intended for the determination of the specific surface area of dry powders expressed in square metres per gram in the sub-sieve region. The effect of molecular flow ("slip flow") which may be important when testing powders consisting of particles less than a few micrometres is not taken into account in the equation used to calculate the specific surface area.

APPARATUS

The apparatus consists of the following parts:

(a) a *permeability cell* (see Figure 2.9.14.-1), which consists of a cylinder with an inner diameter of 12.6 ± 0.1 mm (*A*), constructed of glass or non-corroding metal. The bottom of the cell forms an airtight connection (for example, via an adapter) with the manometer (Figure 2.9.14.-2). A ledge 0.5 mm to 1 mm in width is located 50 ± 15 mm from the top of the cell. It is an integral part of the cell or firmly fixed so as to be airtight. It supports a perforated metal disk (*B*), constructed of non-corroding metal. The disk has a thickness of 0.9 ± 0.1 mm and is perforated with thirty to forty holes 1 mm in diameter evenly distributed over this area.

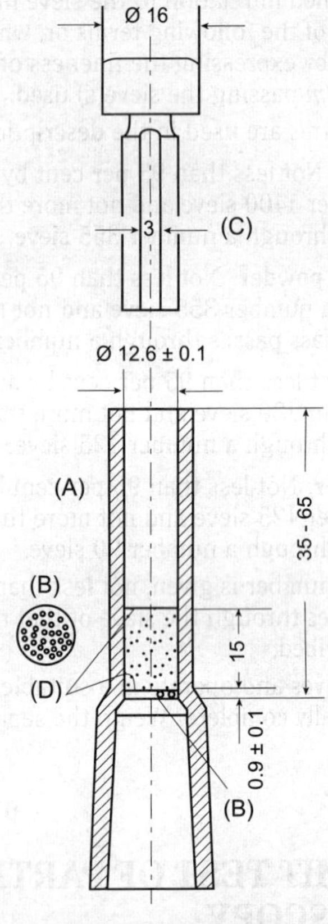

Figure 2.9.14.-1. – *Permeability cell*
Dimensions in millimetres

The plunger (*C*) is made of non-corroding metal and fits into the cell with a clearance of not more than 0.1 mm. The bottom of the plunger has sharp square edges at right angles to the principal axis. There is an air vent 3 mm long and 0.3 mm deep on one side of the plunger. The top of the plunger has a collar such that when the plunger is placed in the cell and the collar is brought into contact with the top of the cell, the distance between the bottom of the plunger and the top of the perforated disk (*B*) is 15 ± 1 mm.

The filter paper disks (*D*) have smooth edges and the same diameter as the inside of the cell.

(b) a *U-tube manometer* (*E*) (Figure 2.9.14.-2) is made of nominal 9 mm outer diameter and 7 mm inner diameter glass tubing with standard walls. The top of one arm of the manometer forms an airtight connection with the permeability cell (*F*). The manometer arm connected to the permeability cell has a line etched around the tube at 125 mm to 145 mm below the top of the side outlet and three other lines at distances of 15 mm, 70 mm and 110 mm above that line (*G*). The side outlet 250 mm to 305 mm above the bottom of the manometer is used to evacuate the manometer arm connected to the permeability cell. A tap is provided on the side outlet not more than 50 mm from the manometer arm.

The manometer is mounted firmly in such a manner that the arms are vertical. It is filled to the lowest mark with *dibutyl phthalate R* containing a lipophilic dye.

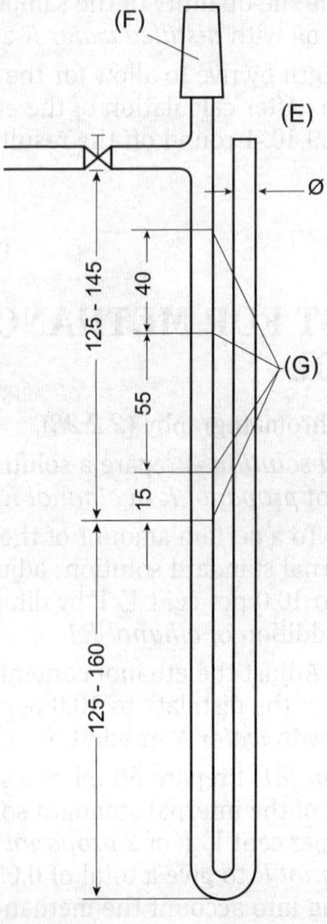

Figure 2.9.14.-2. – *Manometer*
Dimensions in millimetres

METHOD

If prescribed, dry the powder to be examined and sift through a suitable sieve (for example no. 125) to disperse agglomerates. Calculate the mass (*M*) of the powder to be used from the following expression:

$$M = V \times \rho \times (1 - \varepsilon) \qquad (1)$$

V = bulk volume of the compacted bed of powder,

ρ = density of the substance to be examined in grams per millilitre,

ε = porosity of the compacted bed of powder.

Assume first a porosity of 0.5 and introduce this value in Eq. 1 to calculate the mass (*M*) of the powder to be examined.

Place a filter paper disk on top of the perforated metal disk (*B*). Weigh the calculated mass (*M*) of the powder to be examined to the nearest 1 mg. Carefully transfer the powder into the cleaned, tared permeability cell and carefully tap the cell so that the surface of the powder bed is level and cover it with a second filter paper disk. Slowly compact the powder by means of the plunger, avoiding rotary movement. Maintain the pressure until the plunger is completely inserted into the permeability cell. If this is not possible, decrease the quantity of the powder used. If, on the contrary, there is not enough resistance, increase the quantity of the powder. In this case calculate the porosity again. After at least 10 s, remove the plunger.

Attach the permeability cell to the tube of the manometer by means of an airtight connection. Evacuate the air from the manometer by means of a rubber bulb until the level of the coloured liquid is at the highest mark. Close the tap and check that the apparatus is airtight by closing the upper end of the cell, for example with a rubber stopper. Remove the stopper and, using a timer, measure the time taken for the liquid to fall from the second to the third mark.

Using the measured flow time, calculate the specific surface area (S), expressed in square metres per gram, from the following expression:

$$S = \frac{K \times \sqrt{\varepsilon^3} \times \sqrt{t}}{\rho \times (1 - \varepsilon) \times \sqrt{\eta}} \qquad (2)$$

t = flow time in seconds,

η = dynamic viscosity of air in millipascal seconds (see Table 2.9.14.-1),

K = apparatus constant determined according to Equation (4),

ρ = density of the substance to be examined in grams per millilitre,

ε = porosity of the compacted bed of powder.

CALIBRATION OF THE APPARATUS

The bulk volume of the compacted bed of powder is determined by the mercury displacement method as follows:

Place two filter paper disks in the permeability cell, pressing down the edges with a rod slightly smaller than the cell diameter until the filter disks lie flat on the perforated metal disk; fill the cell with mercury, removing any air bubbles adhering to the wall of the cell and wipe away the excess to create a plane surface of mercury at the top of the cell. If the cell is made of material that will amalgamate, grease the cell and the metal disk first with a thin layer of liquid paraffin. Pour out the mercury into a tared beaker and determine the mass (M_A) and the temperature of the mercury.

Make a compacted bed using the reference powder and again fill the cell with mercury with a planar surface at the top of the cell. Pour out the mercury in a tared beaker and again determine the mass of the mercury (M_B). Calculate the bulk volume (V) of the compacted bed of powder from the following expression:

$$V = \frac{M_A - M_B}{\rho_{Hg}} \qquad (3)$$

$M_A - M_B$ = difference between the determined masses of mercury in grams,

ρ_{Hg} = density of mercury at the determined temperature in grams per millilitre.

Repeat the procedure twice, changing the powder each time; the range of values for the calculated volume (V) is not greater than 0.01 ml. Use the mean value of the three determined volumes for the calculations.

The apparatus constant *K* is determined using a reference powder with known specific surface area and density as follows:

Calculate the required quantity of the reference powder to be used (Eq. 1) using the stated density and the determined volume of the compacted powder bed (Eq. 3).

Homogenise and loosen up the powder by shaking it for 2 min in a 100 ml bottle. Prepare a compacted powder bed and measure the flow time of air as previously described. Calculate the apparatus constant (K) from the following expression:

$$K = \frac{S_{sp} \times \rho \times (1 - \varepsilon) \times \sqrt{\eta}}{\sqrt{\varepsilon^3} \times \sqrt{t}} \qquad (4)$$

S_{sp} = stated specific surface area of the reference powder,

ρ = density of the substance to be examined in grams per millilitre,

ε = porosity of the compacted bed of powder,

t = flow time in seconds,

η = dynamic viscosity of air in millipascal seconds (see Table 2.9.14.-1).

The density of mercury and the viscosity of air over a range of temperatures are shown in Table 2.9.14.-1.

Table 2.9.14.-1.

Temperature (°C)	**Density of mercury (g/ml)**	**Viscosity of air (η) (mPa·s)**	$\sqrt{\eta}$
16	13.56	0.01800	0.1342
17	13.56	0.01805	0.1344
18	13.55	0.01810	0.1345
19	13.55	0.01815	0.1347
20	13.55	0.01819	0.1349
21	13.54	0.01824	0.1351
22	13.54	0.01829	0.1353
23	13.54	0.01834	0.1354
24	13.54	0.01839	0.1356

01/2005:20915

2.9.15. APPARENT VOLUME

The test for apparent volume is intended to determine under defined conditions the apparent volumes, before and after settling, the ability to settle and the apparent densities of divided solids (for example, powders, granules).

APPARATUS

The apparatus (see Figure 2.9.15.-1) consists of the following:

- a settling apparatus capable of producing in 1 min 250 ± 15 taps from a height of 3 ± 0.2 mm. The support for the graduated cylinder, with its holder, has a mass of 450 ± 5 g;
- a 250 ml graduated cylinder (2 ml intervals) with a mass of 220 ± 40 g.

METHOD

Into the dry cylinder, introduce without compacting 100.0 g (m g) of the substance to be examined. If this is not possible, select a test sample with an apparent volume between 50 ml and 250 ml and specify the mass in the expression of results. Secure the cylinder in its holder. Read the unsettled apparent volume V_0 to the nearest millilitre. Carry out 10, 500 and 1250 taps and read the corresponding volumes V_{10}, V_{500} and V_{1250}, to the nearest millilitre. If the difference between V_{500} and V_{1250} is greater than 2 ml, carry out another 1250 taps.

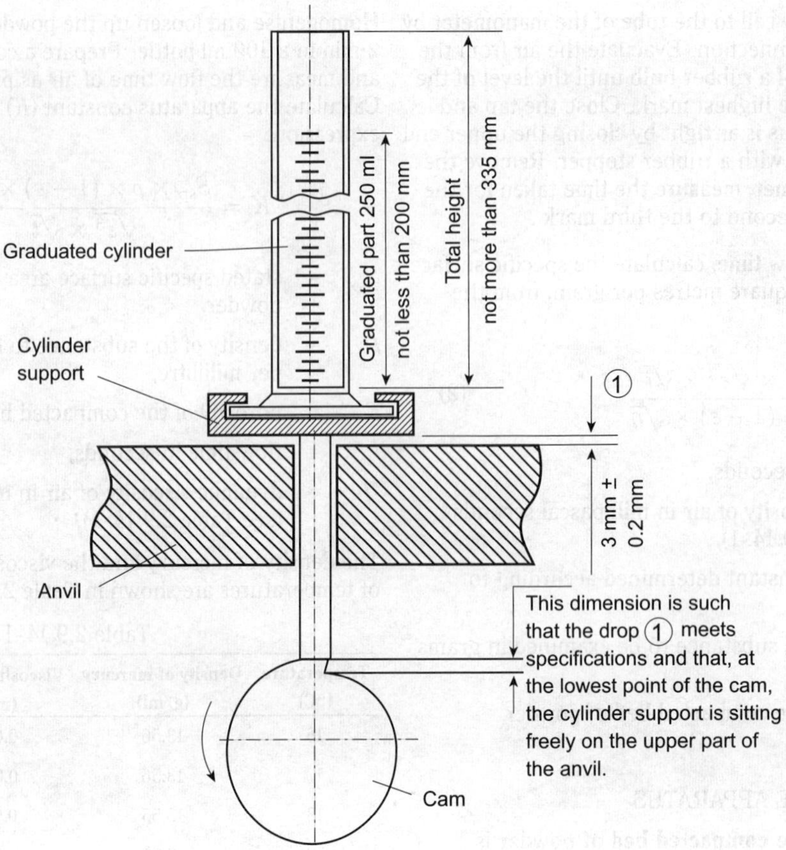

Figure 2.9.15.-1

EXPRESSION OF THE RESULTS

a) Apparent volumes:

– apparent volume before settling or bulk volume: V_0 ml.

– apparent volume after settling or settled volume: V_{1250} ml or V_{2500} ml.

b) Ability to settle: difference V_{10} ml – V_{500} ml.

c) Apparent densities:

The apparent densities are expressed as follows:

– apparent density before settling or density of bulk product: m/V_0 (grams per millilitre) (poured density).

– apparent density after settling or density of settled product: m/V_{1250} or m/V_{2500} (grams per millilitre) (tapped density).

01/2005:20916

2.9.16. FLOWABILITY

The test for flowability is intended to determine the ability of divided solids (for example, powders and granules) to flow vertically under defined conditions.

APPARATUS

According to the flow properties of the material to be tested, funnels with or without stem, with different angles and orifice diameters are used. Typical apparatuses are shown in Figures 2.9.16.-1 and 2.9.16.-2. The funnel is maintained upright by a suitable device. The assembly must be protected from vibrations.

METHOD

Into a dry funnel, whose bottom opening has been blocked by suitable means, introduce without compacting a test sample weighed with 0.5 per cent accuracy. The amount of the sample depends on the apparent volume and the apparatus used. Unblock the bottom opening of the funnel and measure the time needed for the entire sample to flow out of the funnel. Carry out three determinations.

EXPRESSION OF RESULTS

The flowability is expressed in seconds and tenths of seconds, related to 100 g of sample.

The results depend on the storage conditions of the material to be tested.

The results can be expressed as the following:

a) the mean of the determinations, if none of the individual values deviates from the mean value by more than 10 per cent;

b) as a range, if the individual values deviate from the mean value by more than 10 per cent;

c) as a plot of the mass against the flow time;

d) as an infinite time, if the entire sample fails to flow through.

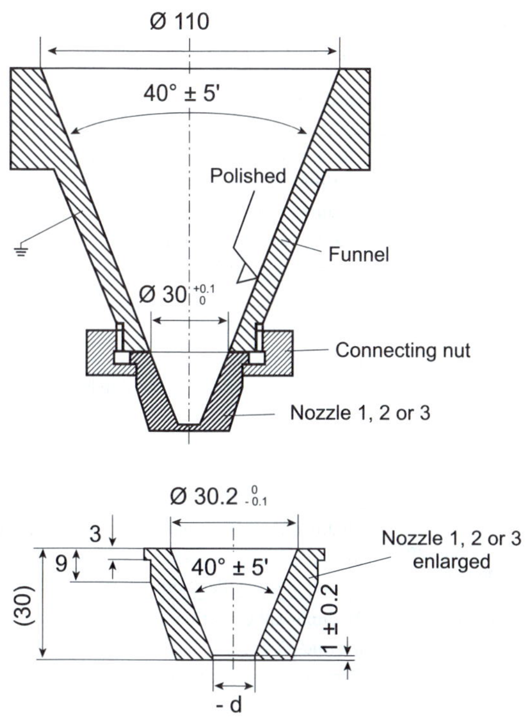

Nozzle	Diameter (*d*) of the outflow opening (millimetres)
1	10 ± 0.01
2	15 ± 0.01
3	25 ± 0.01

Figure 2.9.16.-1. – *Flow funnel and nozzle. Nozzle is made of stainless, acid-resistant steel (V4A,CrNi)*

Dimensions in millimetres

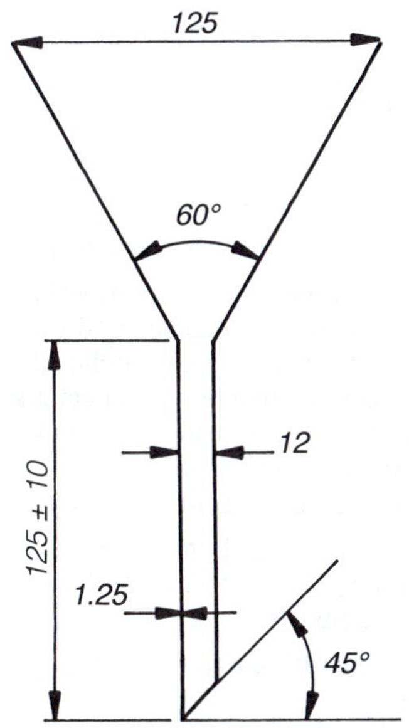

Figure 2.9.16.-2

Dimensions in millimetres

01/2005:20917

2.9.17. TEST FOR EXTRACTABLE VOLUME OF PARENTERAL PREPARATIONS

Injections may be supplied in single-dose containers such as ampoules, cartridges or prefilled syringes filled with a volume of injection which is sufficient to permit administration of the nominal volume declared on the label.

Compliance with the requirements for extractable volume is assured by filling with a volume in slight excess of the nominal volume to be withdrawn. The excess volume is determined by the characteristics of the product. The single-dose container does not hold a quantity relative to the nominal volume that would present a risk should the whole contents be administered.

Suspensions and emulsions are shaken before withdrawal of the contents and before the determination of the density. Oily and viscous preparations may be warmed according to the instructions on the label, if necessary, and thoroughly shaken immediately before removing the contents. The contents are then cooled to 25 °C before measuring the volume.

SINGLE-DOSE CONTAINERS

Select one container if the nominal volume is 10 ml or more, 3 containers if the nominal volume is more than 3 ml and less than 10 ml, or 5 containers if the nominal volume is 3 ml or less. Take up individually the total contents of each container selected into a dry hypodermic syringe of a capacity not exceeding 3 times the volume to be measured, and fitted with a 21-gauge needle not less than 2.5 cm in length. Expel any air bubbles from the syringe and needle, then discharge the contents of the syringe without emptying the needle into a standardised dry cylinder (graduated to contain rather than to deliver the designated volumes) of such size that the volume to be measured occupies at least 40 per cent of its graduated volume. Alternatively, the volume of the contents in millilitres may be calculated as the mass in grams divided by the density.

The contents of 2 or 3 containers with a nominal volume of 2 ml or less may be pooled for the measurement provided that a separate, dry syringe assembly is used for each container. The contents of containers holding 10 ml or more may be determined by opening them and emptying the contents directly into the graduated cylinder or tared beaker.

The volume is not less than the nominal volume in the case of containers examined individually, or, in the case of containers with a nominal volume of 2 ml or less, is not less than the sum of the nominal volumes of the containers taken collectively.

MULTI-DOSE CONTAINERS

For injections in multidose containers labelled to yield a specific number of doses of a stated volume, select one container and proceed as directed for single-dose containers using the same number of separate syringe assemblies as the number of doses specified.

The volume is such that each syringe delivers not less than the stated dose.

CARTRIDGES AND PREFILLED SYRINGES

Select one container if the nominal volume is 10 ml or more, 3 containers if the nominal volume is more than 3 ml and less than 10 ml, or 5 containers if the nominal volume is 3 ml or less. If necessary, fit the containers with the accessories required for their use (needle, piston, syringe) and transfer the entire contents of each container without emptying the needle into a dry tared beaker by slowly and constantly depressing the piston. Determine the volume in millilitres calculated as the mass in grams divided by the density.

The volume measured for each of the containers is not less than the nominal volume.

PARENTERAL INFUSIONS

Select one container. Transfer the contents into a dry measuring cylinder of such a capacity that the volume to be determined occupies at least 40 per cent of the nominal volume of the cylinder. Measure the volume transferred. The volume is not less than the nominal volume.

01/2005:20918

2.9.18. PREPARATIONS FOR INHALATION: AERODYNAMIC ASSESSMENT OF FINE PARTICLES

This test is used to determine the fine particle characteristics of the aerosol clouds generated by preparations for inhalation.

Unless otherwise justified and authorised, one of the following apparatus and test procedures is used.

APPARATUS A - GLASS IMPINGER

The apparatus is shown in Figure 2.9.18.-1 (see also Table 2.9.18.-1).

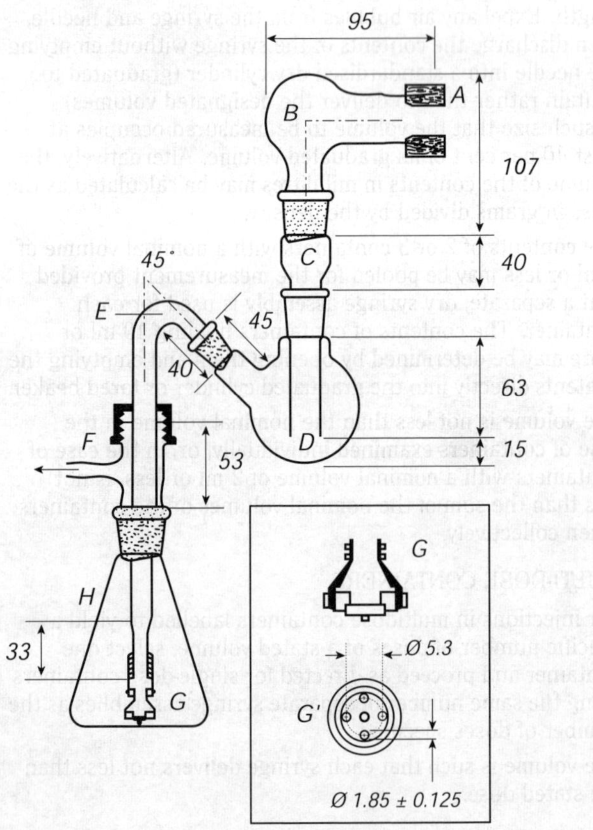

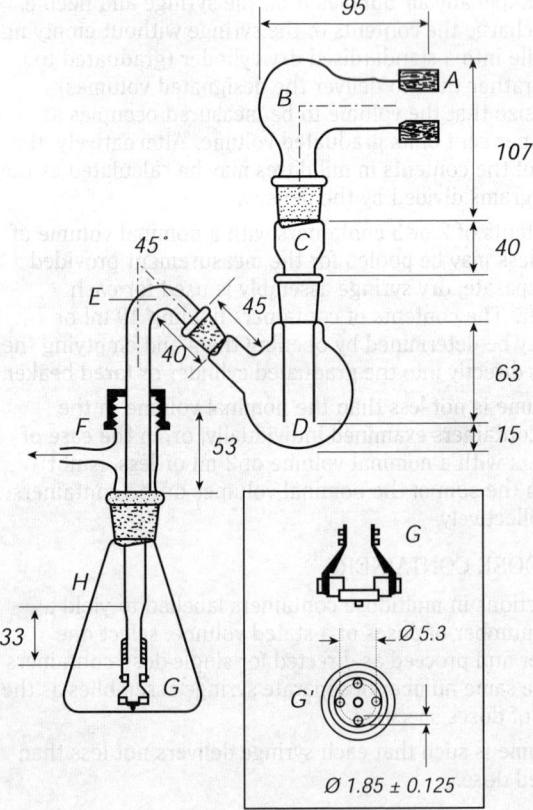

Figure 2.9.18.-1. – *Apparatus A for the aerodynamic assessment of fine particles*
Dimensions in millimetres
(tolerances ± 1 mm unless otherwise prescribed)

Table 2.9.18.-1. – *Component specification for Figure 2.9.18.-1*

Code	Item	Description	Dimensions*
A	Mouthpiece adaptor	Moulded rubber adapter for actuator mouthpiece	
B	Throat	Modified round-bottomed flask	50 ml
		ground-glass inlet socket	29/32
		ground-glass outlet cone	24/29
C	Neck	Modified glass adapter	
		ground-glass inlet socket	24/29
		ground-glass outlet cone	24/29
		Lower outlet section of precision-bore glass tubing	
		bore diameter	14
		Selected bore light-wall glass tubing	
		external diameter	17
D	Upper impingement chamber	Modified round-bottomed flask	100 ml
		ground-glass inlet socket	24/29
		ground-glass outlet cone	24/29
E	Coupling tube	Medium-wall glass tubing	
		ground-glass cone	14/23
		Bent section and upper vertical section	
		external diameter	13
		Lower vertical section	
		external diameter	8
F	Screwthread, side-arm adaptor	Plastic screw cap	28/13
		Silicone rubber ring	28/11
		PTFE washer	28/11
		Glass screwthread, *thread size*	28
		Side-arm outlet to vacuum pump, *minimum bore diameter*	5
G	Lower jet assembly	Modified polypropylene filter holder connected to lower vertical section of coupling tube by PTFE tubing	see Figure 2.9.18.-1
		Acetal circular disc with the centres of four jets arranged on a projected circle of diameter 5.3 mm with an integral jet spacer peg	10
		peg diameter	2
		peg protrusion	2
H	Lower impingement chamber	Conical flask	250 ml
		ground-glass inlet socket	24/29

* Dimensions in millimetres, unless otherwise stated.

Procedure for nebulisers

Introduce 7 ml and 30 ml of a suitable solvent into the upper and lower impingement chambers, respectively.

Connect all the component parts, ensure that the assembly is vertical and adequately supported and that the jet spacer peg of the lower jet assembly just touches the bottom of the lower impingement chamber. Connect a suitable pump fitted with a filter (of suitable pore size) to the outlet of the apparatus and adjust the air flow through the apparatus, as measured at the inlet to the throat, to 60 ± 5 litres/min.

Introduce the liquid preparation for inhalation into the reservoir of the nebuliser. Fit the mouthpiece and connect it by means of an adapter to the device.

Switch on the pump of the apparatus and after 10 s switch on the nebuliser.

After 60 s, unless otherwise justified, switch off the nebuliser, wait for about 5 s and then switch off the pump of the apparatus. Dismantle the apparatus and wash the inner surface of the upper impingement chamber collecting the washings in a volumetric flask. Wash the inner surface of the lower impingement chamber collecting the washings in a second volumetric flask. Finally, wash the filter preceding the pump and its connections to the lower impingement chamber and combine the washings with those obtained from the lower impingement chamber. Determine the amount of active ingredient collected in each of the two flasks. Express the results for each of the two parts of the apparatus as a percentage of the total amount of active ingredient.

Procedure for pressurised inhalers

Place the actuator adapter in position at the end of the throat so that the mouthpiece end of the actuator, when inserted to a depth of about 10 mm, lines up along the horizontal axis of the throat and the open end of the actuator, which accepts the pressurised container, is uppermost and in the same vertical plane as the rest of the apparatus.

Introduce 7 ml and 30 ml of a suitable solvent into the upper and lower impingement chambers, respectively.

Connect all the component parts and ensure that the assembly is vertical and adequately supported and that the lower jet-spacer peg of the lower jet assembly just touches the bottom of the lower impingement chamber. Connect a suitable pump to the outlet of the apparatus and adjust the air flow through the apparatus, as measured at the inlet to the throat, to 60 ± 5 litres/min.

Prime the metering valve by shaking for 5 s and discharging once to waste; after not less than 5 s, shake and discharge again to waste. Repeat a further three times.

Shake for about 5 s, switch on the pump to the apparatus and locate the mouthpiece end of the actuator in the adapter, discharge once immediately. Remove the assembled inhaler from the adapter, shake for not less than 5 s, relocate the mouthpiece end of the actuator in the adapter and discharge again. Repeat the discharge sequence for a further eight times, shaking between actuations. After discharging the tenth delivery, wait for not less than 5 s and then switch off the pump. Dismantle the apparatus.

Wash the inner surface of the inlet tube to the lower impingement chamber and its outer surface that projects into the chamber with a suitable solvent collecting the washings in the lower impingement chamber. Determine the content of active ingredient in this solution. Calculate the amount of active ingredient collected in the lower impingement chamber per actuation of the valve and express the results as a percentage of the dose stated on the label.

Procedure for powder inhalers

Introduce 7 ml and 30 ml of a suitable solvent into the upper and lower impingement chambers, respectively.

Connect all the component parts and ensure that the assembly is vertical and adequately supported and that the jet spacer peg of the lower jet assembly just touches the bottom of the lower impingement chamber. Without the inhaler in place, connect a suitable pump to the outlet of the apparatus and adjust the air flow through the apparatus, as measured at the inlet to the throat, to 60 ± 5 litres/min.

Prepare the inhaler for use and locate the mouthpiece in the apparatus by means of a suitable adapter. Switch on the pump for 5 s. Switch off the pump and remove the inhaler. Repeat for a further nine discharges. Dismantle the apparatus.

Wash the inner surface of the inlet tube to the lower impingement chamber and its outer surface that projects into the chamber with a suitable solvent, collecting the washings in the lower impingement chamber. Determine the content of active ingredient in this solution. Calculate the amount of active ingredient collected in the lower impingement chamber per discharge and express the results as a percentage of the dose stated on the label.

APPARATUS B - METAL IMPINGER

The apparatus is shown in Figures 2.9.18.-2/3.

Procedure for nebulisers

The deposition of emitted droplets is tested using the impingement apparatus, which is connected to the filled nebuliser by means of a suitable adapter. The outlet of the apparatus to the pump is fitted with a suitable filter (for example pores of 0.25 μm).

In this procedure, the impingement chamber is used dry. Connect all the component parts and ensure that the base of the impinger is placed on a flat, horizontal and adequately supported surface. Connect a suitable pump to the outlet of the apparatus and adjust the air flow through the apparatus, as measured at the inlet to the throat, to 60 ± 5 litres/min.

Introduce the liquid preparation for inhalation into the reservoir of a suitable nebuliser. Fit the mouth piece and connect it to the adapter of the device.

Switch on the pump of the apparatus and after 10 s, switch on the nebuliser.

After 60 s, unless otherwise justified, switch off the nebuliser, wait for about 5 s and then switch off the pump of the apparatus. Dismantle the apparatus. Wash the inner surface of the throat, the top and bottom portions of the chamber collecting the washings in a volumetric flask. Wash the filter assembly by passing a suitable solvent through the filter and collecting in a suitable graduated flask. Determine the content of active ingredient in these solutions. Express the results for each of the two parts of the apparatus as a percentage of the total amount of active ingredient.

Procedure for pressurised inhalers

Place the actuator adapter in position at the end of the throat so that the mouthpiece end of the actuator, when inserted, lines up along the horizontal axis of the throat and the open end of the actuator, which accepts the pressurised container, is uppermost and in the same vertical plane as the rest of the apparatus.

In this procedure, the impingement chamber is used dry. Connect all the component parts and ensure that the base of the impinger is placed on a flat, horizontal and adequately supported surface so that the open end of the actuator, which accepts the pressurised container is in a vertical position. Connect a suitable pump to the outlet of the apparatus and adjust the air flow through the apparatus, as measured at the inlet to the throat, to 60 ± 5 litres/min.

Prime the metering valve by shaking for 5 s and discharging once to waste; after not less than 5 s, shake and discharge again to waste. Repeat a further three times.

Shake for about 5 s, switch on the pump to the apparatus and locate the mouthpiece end of the actuator in the adapter and discharge once immediately. Remove the assembled inhaler from the adapter, shake for about 5 s, relocate the mouthpiece end of the actuator in the adapter and discharge again.

Repeat the discharge sequence for a further eight times shaking between actuations. After discharging the tenth delivery, wait for about 5 s and then switch off the pump. Dismantle the apparatus.

Wash the filter assembly by passing a suitable solvent through the filter. Determine the content of active ingredient in this solution. Calculate the amount of active ingredient

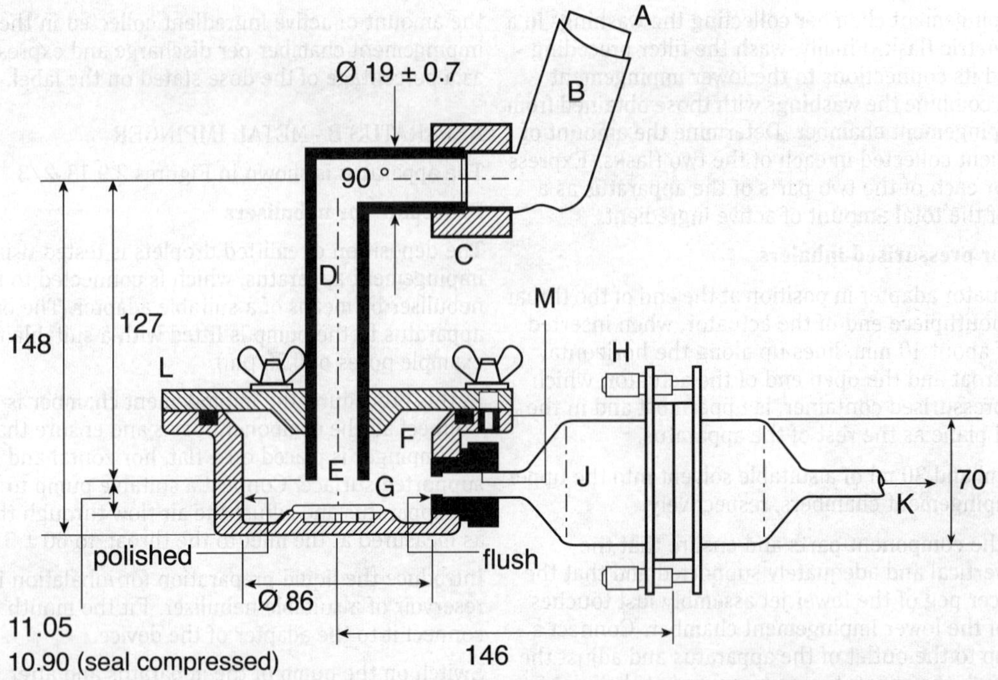

A. Pressurised inhalation container
B. Actuator
C. Adapter
D. Throat
E. Jet
F. Impingement chamber
G. Sintered-glass disc (BS porosity No. 1)
H. Stainless steel filter clamp
J. Glass filter assembly
K. Vacuum pump
L. Aluminium impingement chamber lid
M. Rubber O-rings

Figure 2.9.18.-2. – *Apparatus B for the aerodynamic assessment of fine particles*
Dimensions in millimetres

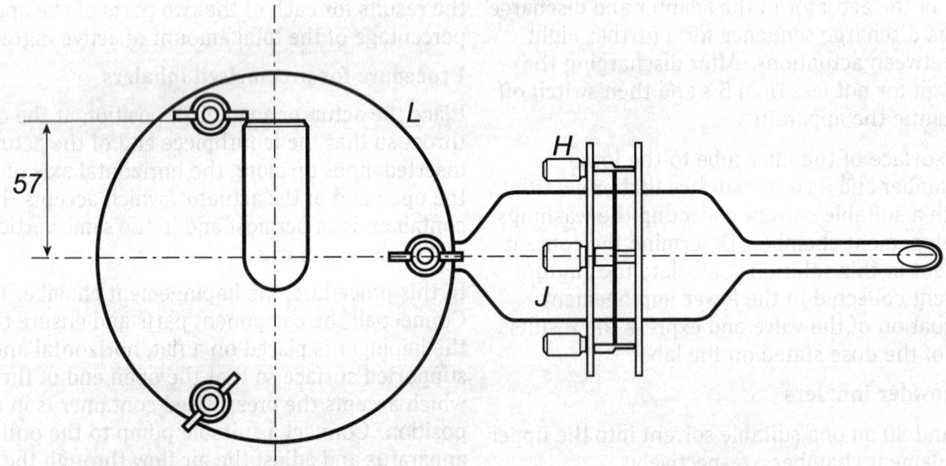

Figure 2.9.18.-3. – *Apparatus B for the aerodynamic assessment of fine particles (top elevation)*
Dimensions in millimetres

collected on the filter assembly per actuation of the valve and express the results as a percentage of the dose stated on the label.

Procedure for powder inhalers

Introduce 25 ml amounts of a suitable solvent into the impingement chamber so as to cover the sintered-glass disk. Connect all the component parts and ensure that the base of the impinger is placed on a flat, horizontal and adequately supported surface. Without the inhaler in place, connect a suitable pump to the outlet of the apparatus and adjust the air flow through the apparatus, as measured at the inlet to the throat, to 60 ± 5 litres/min.

Prepare the inhaler for use and locate the mouthpiece in the apparatus by means of a suitable adapter. Switch on the pump for 5 s. Switch off the pump and remove the inhaler. Repeat the discharge for a further nine discharges. Dismantle the apparatus.

Wash the filter assembly by passing a suitable solvent through the filter. Determine the content of active ingredient in this solution. Calculate the amount of active ingredient collected on the filter assembly per discharge and express the results as a percentage of the dose stated on the label.

Fine particle dose and particle size distribution

APPARATUS C – MULTI-STAGE LIQUID IMPINGER

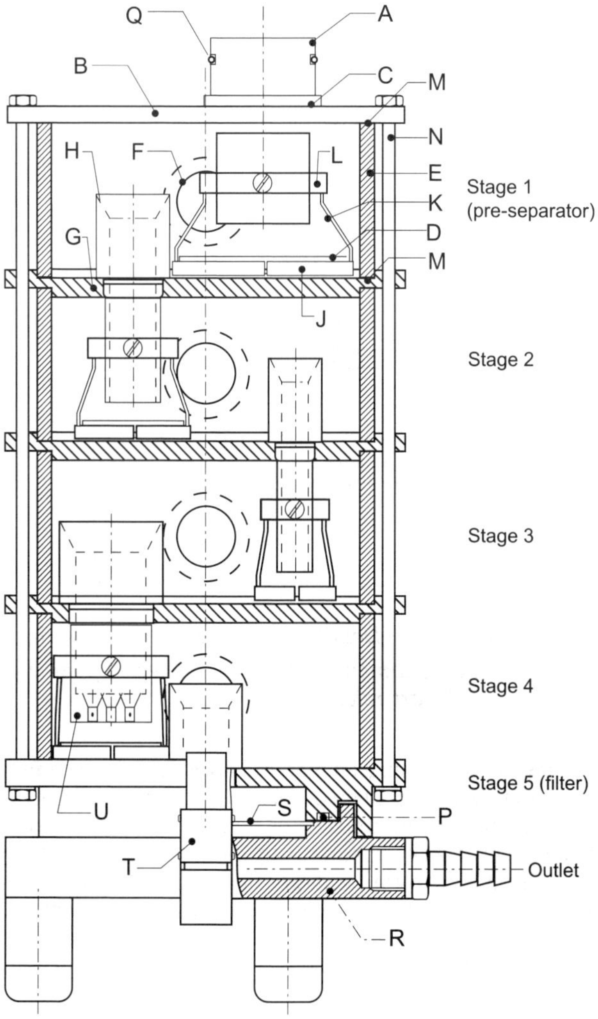

Figure 2.9.18.-4. – *The Multi-stage Liquid Impinger*

Table 2.9.18.-2. – *Component specification for Figures 2.9.18.-4 to -6*

Code*	Item	Description	Dimensions**
A,H	Jet tube	Metal tube screwed onto partition wall sealed by gasket (C), polished inner surface	see Figure 2.9.18.-5
B,G	Partition wall	Circular metal plate - thickness - diameter - thickness	 120 see Figure 2.9.18.-5
C	Gasket	e.g. PTFE	to fit jet tube
D	Impaction plate	Porosity 0 sintered-glass disk, diameter	see Figure 2.9.18.-5
E	Glass cylinder	Plane polished cut glass tube - height, including gaskets - outer diameter - wall thickness - sampling port (F) diameter - stopper in sampling port	 46 100 3.5 18 ISO 24/25
J	Metal frame	L-profiled circular frame with slit - inner diameter - height - thickness of horizontal section - thickness of vertical section	 to fit impaction plate 4 0.5 2
K	Wire	Steel wire interconnecting metal frame and sleeve (two for each frame) - diameter	 1
L	Sleeve	Metal sleeve secured on jet tube by screw - inner diameter - height - thickness	 to fit jet tube 6 5
M	Gasket	e.g. silicone	to fit glass cylinder
N	Bolt	Metal bolt with nut (six pairs) - length - diameter	 205 4
P	O-ring	Rubber O-ring, diameter × thickness	66.34 × 2.62
Q	O-ring	Rubber O-ring, diameter × thickness	29.1 × 1.6
R	Filter holder	Metal housing with stand and outlet	see Figure 2.9.18.-6
S	Filter support	Perforated sheet metal - diameter - hole diameter - distance between holes (centre-points)	 65 3 4
T	Snap-locks		
U	Multi-jet tube	Jet tube (H) ending in multi-jet arrangement	see inserts Figure 2.9.18.-5

* Refers to Figure 2.9.18.–4.

** Measures in mm with tolerances according to ISO 2768-m unless otherwise stated.

The Multi-stage Liquid Impinger consists of impaction stages 1 (pre-separator), 2, 3 and 4 and an integral filter stage (stage 5), see Figures 2.9.18.-4 to -6. An impaction stage comprises an upper horizontal metal partition wall (B) through which a metal inlet jet tube (A) with its impaction plate (D) is protruding, a glass cylinder (E) with sampling port (F) forming the vertical wall of the stage, and a lower horizontal metal partition wall (G) through which the tube (H) connects to the next lower stage. The tube into stage 4 (U) ends in a multi-jet arrangement. The impaction plate (D) is secured in a metal frame (J) which is fastened by two wires (K) to a sleeve (L) secured on the jet tube (C). The horizontal face of the collection plate is perpendicular to the axis of the jet tube and centrally aligned. The upper surface of the impaction plate is slightly raised above the edge of the metal frame. A recess around the perimeter of the horizontal partition wall guides the position of the glass cylinder. The glass cylinders are sealed against the horizontal partition walls with gaskets (M) and clamped together by six bolts (N). The sampling ports are sealed by stoppers. The bottom-side of the lower partition wall of stage 4 has a concentrical protrusion fitted with a rubber O-ring (P) which seals against the edge of a filter placed in the filter holder. The filter holder (R) is constructed as a basin with a concentrical recess in which a perforated filter support (S) is flush-fitted. The filter holder is dimensioned for 76 mm diameter filters.

The assembly of impaction stages is clamped onto the filter holder by two snap-locks (T). Connect a right-angle bend metal tube induction port according to Figure 2.9.18.-7 onto the stage 1 inlet jet tube of the impinger. A rubber O-ring on the jet tube provides an airtight connection to the induction port. A suitable mouthpiece adapter should be used to provide an airtight seal between the inhaler and the induction port. The front face of the inhaler mouthpiece must be flush with the front face of the induction port.

Table 2.9.18.-3. – *Dimensions*[1] *of jet tube with impaction plate*

Type	Code[2]	Stage 1	Stage 2	Stage 3	Stage 4	Filter (stage 5)
Distance	1	9.5 (-.0+.5)	5.5 (-.0+.5)	4.0 (-.0+.5)	6.0 (-.0+.5)	n.a.
Distance	2	26	31	33	30.5	0
Distance	3	8	5	5	5	5
Distance	4	3	3	3	3	n.a.
Distance	5	0	3	3	3	3
Distance	6 [3]	20	25	25	25	25
Distance	7	n.a.	n.a.	n.a.	8.5	n.a.
Diameter	c	25	14	8.0(± .1)	21	14
Diameter	d	50	30	20	30	n.a.
Diameter	e	27.9	16.5	10.5	23.9	n.a.
Diameter	f	31.75 (-.0+.5)	22	14	31	22
Diameter	g	25.4	21	13	30	21
Diameter	h	n.a.	n.a.	n.a.	2.70 (± .5)	n.a.
Diameter	j	n.a.	n.a.	n.a.	6.3	n.a.
Diameter	k	n.a.	n.a.	n.a.	12.6	n.a.
Radius[4]	r	16	22	27	28.5	0
Radius	s	46	46	46	46	n.a.
Radius	t	n.a.	50	50	50	50
Angle	w	10°	53°	53°	53°	53°
Angle	u	n.a.	n.a.	n.a.	45°	n.a.
Angle	v	n.a.	n.a.	n.a.	60°	n.a.

(1) Measures in mm with tolerances according to ISO 2768-m unless otherwise stated

(2) Refer to Figure 2.9.18-5

(3) Including gasket

(4) Relative centreline of stage compartment

n.a. = not applicable

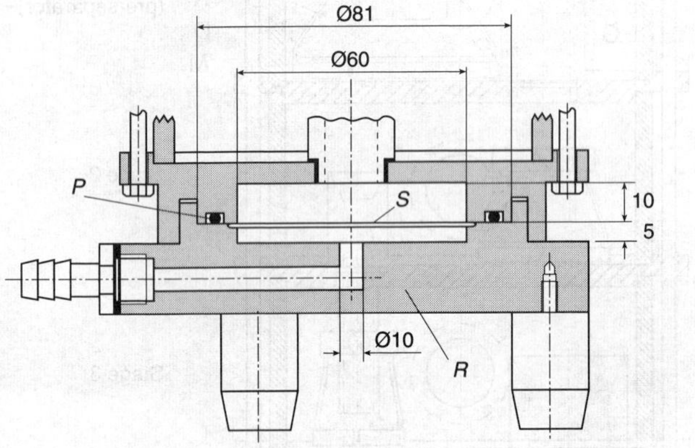

Figure 2.9.18.-6. – *Details of the filter stage (stage 5). Numbers refer to dimensions (Ø = diameter). Uppercase letters refer to Table 2.9.18.-2.*

Procedure for pressurised metered-dose preparations for inhalation. Dispense 20 ml of a solvent, capable of dissolving the active ingredient into each of stages 1 to 4 and replace the stoppers. Tilt the apparatus to wet the stoppers, thereby neutralising electrostatic charge. Place a suitable filter capable of quantitatively collecting the active ingredient in stage 5 and assemble the apparatus. Place a suitable mouthpiece adapter in position at the end of the induction

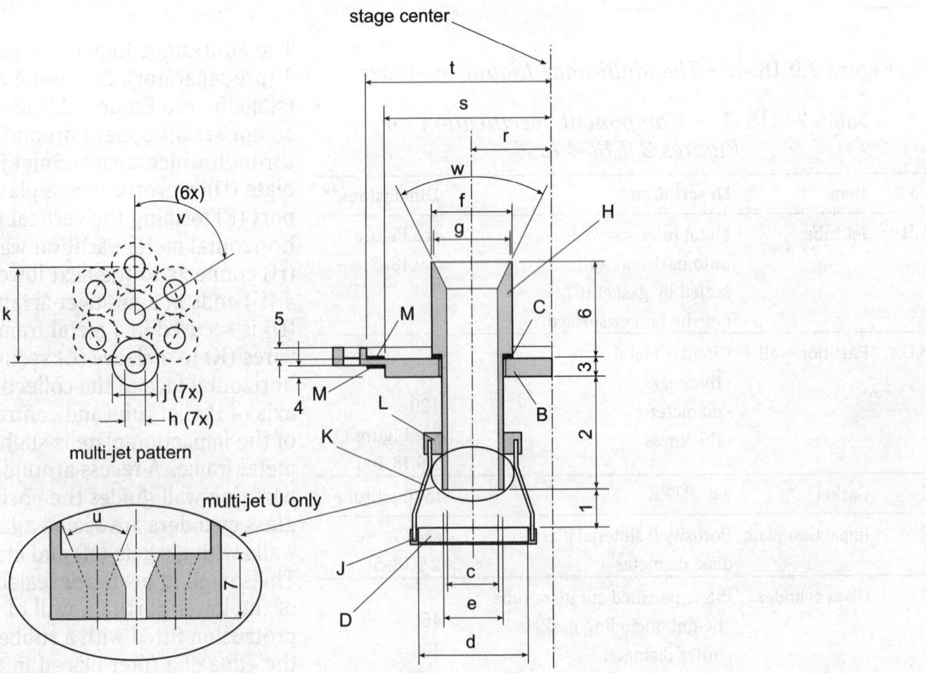

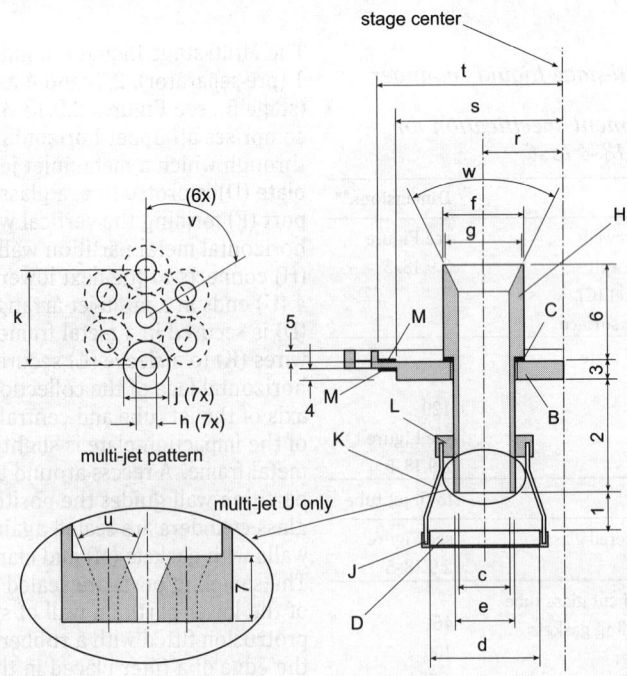

Figure 2.9.18.-5. – *Details of jet tube and impaction plate. Inserts show end of multi-jet tube U leading to stage 4 (numbers and lowercase letters refer to Table 2.9.18.-3 and uppercase letters refer to Figure 2.9.18.-4).*

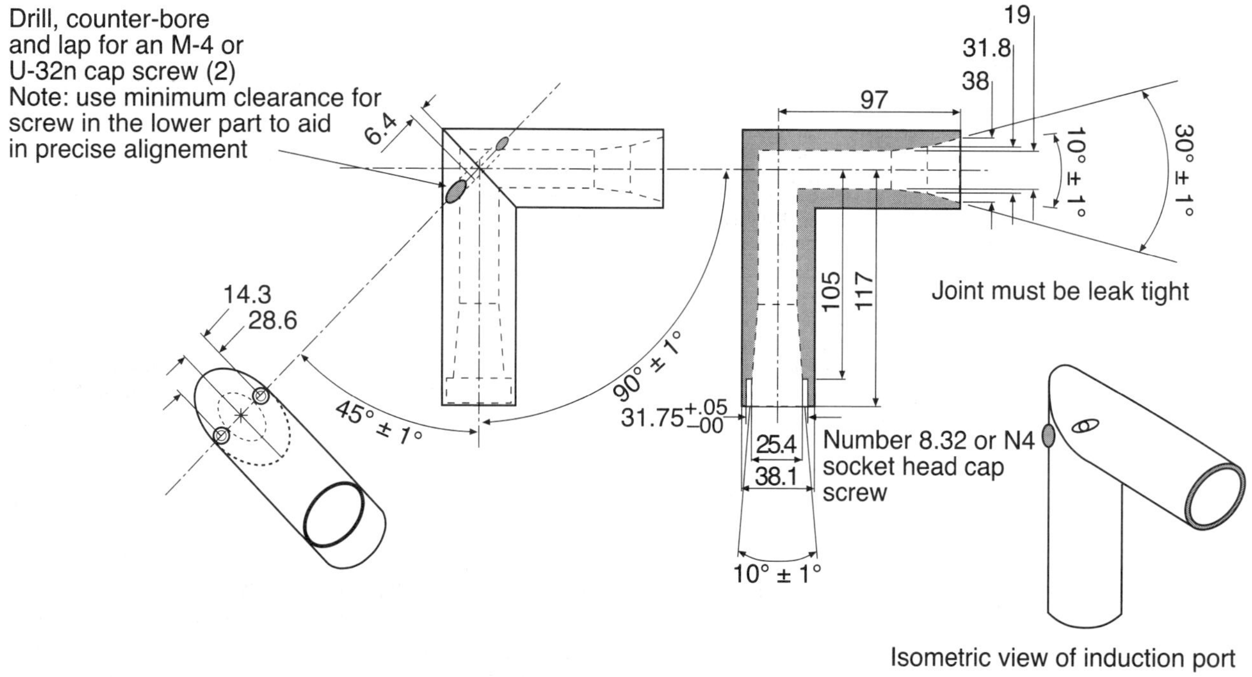

Note

(1)	Material may be aluminium or stainless steel.
(2)	Machine from 38 mm (1.5″) bar stock.
(3)	Bore 19 mm hole through bar.
(4)	Cut tube to exact 45° as shown.
(5)	The inner bores and tapers should be smooth – approximate 0.40 µm (16 µm) finish.
(6)	Mill joining cads of stock to provide a liquid tight leak-free seal.
(7)	Set up a holding fixture for aligning the inner 19 mm bore and for drilling and tapping M4 × 0.7 or 8-32 threads. There must be virtually no mismatch of the inner bores in the miter joint.

Figure 2.9.18.-7. – *Induction port*
Dimensions in millimetres unless otherwise stated

port so that the mouthpiece end of the actuator, when inserted, lines up along the horizontal axis of the induction port and the inhaler is positioned in the same orientation intended for use. Connect a suitable vacuum pump to the outlet of the apparatus and adjust the air flow through the apparatus, as measured at the inlet to the induction port, to 30 ± 1.5 litres/min. Switch off the air flow.

Unless otherwise prescribed in the patient instructions, shake the inhaler for 5 s and discharge one delivery to waste. Switch on the pump to the apparatus, locate the mouthpiece end of the actuator in the adapter and discharge the inhaler into the apparatus, depressing the valve for a sufficient time to ensure complete discharge. Remove the assembled inhaler from the adapter. Repeat the procedure. The number of discharges should be minimised and typically would not be greater than ten. The number of discharges should be sufficient to ensure an accurate and precise determination of the fine particle dose. After the final discharge, wait for 5 s and then switch off the pump.

Dismantle the filter stage of the apparatus. Carefully remove the filter and extract the active ingredient into an aliquot of the solvent. Remove the induction port and mouthpiece adapter from the apparatus and extract the active ingredient into an aliquot of the solvent. If necessary, rinse the inside of the inlet jet tube to stage 1 with solvent, allowing the solvent to flow into the stage. Extract the active ingredient from the inner walls and the collection plate of each of the four upper stages of the apparatus into the solution in the respective stage by carefully tilting and rotating the apparatus, observing that no liquid transfer occurs between the stages.

Using a suitable method of analysis, determine the quantity of active ingredient contained in each of the six volumes of solvent.

Calculate the fine particle dose (see below).

Procedure for powder inhalers. Place a suitable low resistance filter capable of quantitatively collecting the drug in stage 5 and assemble the apparatus. Connect the apparatus to a flow system according to the scheme specified in Figure 2.9.18.-8. Unless otherwise defined, conduct the test at the flow rate, Q, used in the test for uniformity of delivered dose, drawing 4 litres of air through the apparatus.

Table 2.9.18.-4. – *Component specification for Figure 2.9.18.-8*

Code	Item	Description
A	Connector	ID ≥ 8 mm, e.g., short metal coupling, with low-diameter branch to P3.
B	Vacuum tubing	8 ± 0.5 mm ID × 50 ± 10 cm length, e.g., silicon tubing with an OD of 14 mm and an ID of 8 mm.
C	Two-way solenoid valve	Minimum airflow resistance orifice having an internal diameter of ≥ 8 mm and a maximum response time 100 milliseconds (e.g. type 256-A08, Bürkert GmbH, D-74653 Ingelfingen), or equivalent.

Code	Item	Description
D	Vacuum pump	Pump must be capable of drawing the required flow rate through the assembled apparatus with the dry powder inhaler in the mouthpiece adapter (e.g. product type 1023, 1423 or 2565, Gast Manufacturing Inc., Benton Harbor, MI 49022), or equivalent. Connect the pump to the solenoid valve using short and/or wide (≥ 10 mm ID) vacuum tubing and connectors to minimise pump capacity requirements.
E	Timer	Timer capable to drive the solenoid valve for the required duration (e.g. type G814, RS Components International, Corby, NN17 9RS, UK), or equivalent.
P2 P3	Pressure measurements	Determine under steady-state flow condition with an absolute pressure transducer.
F	Flow control valve	Adjustable regulating valve with maximum $C_v \geq 1$, (e.g. type 8FV12LNSS, Parker Hannifin plc., Barnstaple, EX31 1NP, UK), or equivalent.

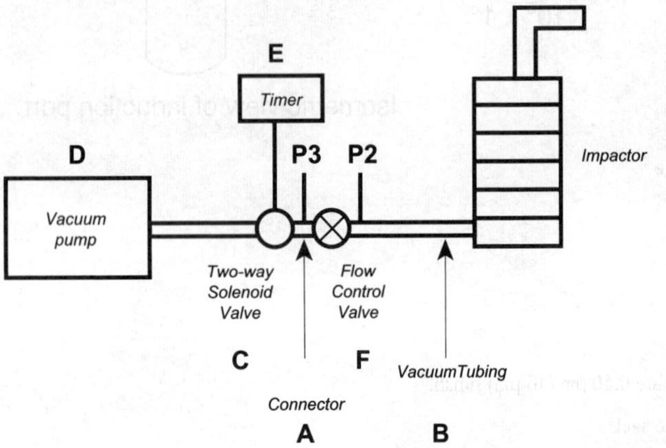

Figure 2.9.18.-8. – *Experimental set-up for testing powders for inhalation*

Connect a flow meter, calibrated for the volumetric flow leaving the meter, to the induction port. Adjust the flow control valve to achieve steady flow through the system at the required rate, Q (± 5 per cent). Switch off the flow. Ensure that critical flow occurs in the flow control valve by the following procedure. With the inhaler in place and the test flow rate established, measure the absolute pressure on both sides of the control valve (pressure reading points P2 and P3 in Figure 2.9.18.-8). A ratio P3/P2 ≤ 0.5 indicates critical flow. Switch to a more powerful pump and re-measure the test flow rate if critical flow is not indicated.

Dispense 20 ml of a solvent, capable of dissolving the active ingredient into each of the four upper stages of the apparatus and replace the stoppers. Tilt the apparatus to wet the stoppers, thereby neutralising electrostatic charge. Place a suitable mouthpiece adapter in position at the end of the induction port.

Prepare the dry-powder inhaler for use according to patient instructions. With the pump running and the two-way valve closed, locate the mouthpiece of the inhaler in the mouthpiece adapter. Discharge the powder into the apparatus by opening the valve for the required time, T (± 5 per cent). Repeat the procedure. The number of discharges should be minimised and typically would not be greater than ten. The number of discharges should be sufficient to ensure an accurate and precise determination of fine particle dose. After the final discharge, wait for 5 s and then switch off the pump.

Dismantle the filter stage of the apparatus. Carefully remove the filter and extract the active ingredient into an aliquot of the solvent. Remove the induction port and mouthpiece adapter from the apparatus and extract the active ingredient into an aliquot of the solvent. If necessary, rinse the inside of the inlet jet tube to stage 1 with solvent, allowing the solvent to flow into the stage. Extract the active ingredient from the inner walls and the collection plate of each of the four upper stages of the apparatus into the solution in the respective stage by carefully tilting and rotating the apparatus, observing that no liquid transfer occurs between the stages.

Using a suitable method of analysis, determine the amount of active ingredient contained in each of the six volumes of solvent.

Calculate the fine particle dose (see below).

APPARATUS D – "ANDERSEN" SIZING SAMPLER

The "Andersen" 1 ACFM non-viable ambient sizing sampler consists of 8 aluminium stages together with a final filter. The stages are clamped together and sealed with O-rings. In the configuration used for pressurised inhalers, Figure 2.9.18.-9, the entry cone of the sampler is connected to a right-angle bend metal induction port defined in Figure 2.9.18.-7. A suitable mouthpiece adapter should be used to provide an airtight seal between the inhaler and the induction port. The front face of the inhaler mouthpiece must be flush with the front face of the induction port.

In the configuration for powder inhalers, a pre-separator is placed above the top stage to collect large masses of non-respirable powder. It is connected to the induction port as shown in Figure 2.9.18.-10. To accommodate high flow rates through the sampler, the outlet nipple, used to connect the sampler to the vacuum system is enlarged to have an internal diameter ≥ 8 mm.

Procedure for pressurised inhalers. Assemble the "Andersen" Sampler with a suitable filter in place and ensure that the system is airtight. Place a suitable mouthpiece adapter in position at the end of the induction port so that the mouthpiece end of the actuator, when inserted, lines up along the horizontal axis of the induction port and the inhaler unit is positioned in the same orientation as the intended use. Connect a suitable pump to the

Table 2.9.18.-5. – *Calculations for Apparatus C. Use* $q_1 = \sqrt{(60/Q)}$, *where Q is the flow rate in litres per minute*

Cut-off diameter (µm)	Mass of active ingredient deposited per discharge	Cumulative mass of active ingredient deposited per discharge	Cumulative fraction of active ingredient (per cent)
$d_4 = 1.7 \cdot q_1$	mass from stage 5, m_5*	$c_4 = m_5$	$f_4 = (c_4/c) \cdot 100$
$d_3 = 3.1 \cdot q_1$	mass from stage 4, m_4	$c_3 = c_4 + m_4$	$f_3 = (c_3/c) \cdot 100$
$d_2 = 6.8 \cdot q_1$	mass from stage 3, m_3	$c_2 = c_3 + m_3$	$f_2 = (c_2/c) \cdot 100$
	mass from stage 2, m_2	$c = c_2 + m_2$	100

* stage 5 is the filter stage

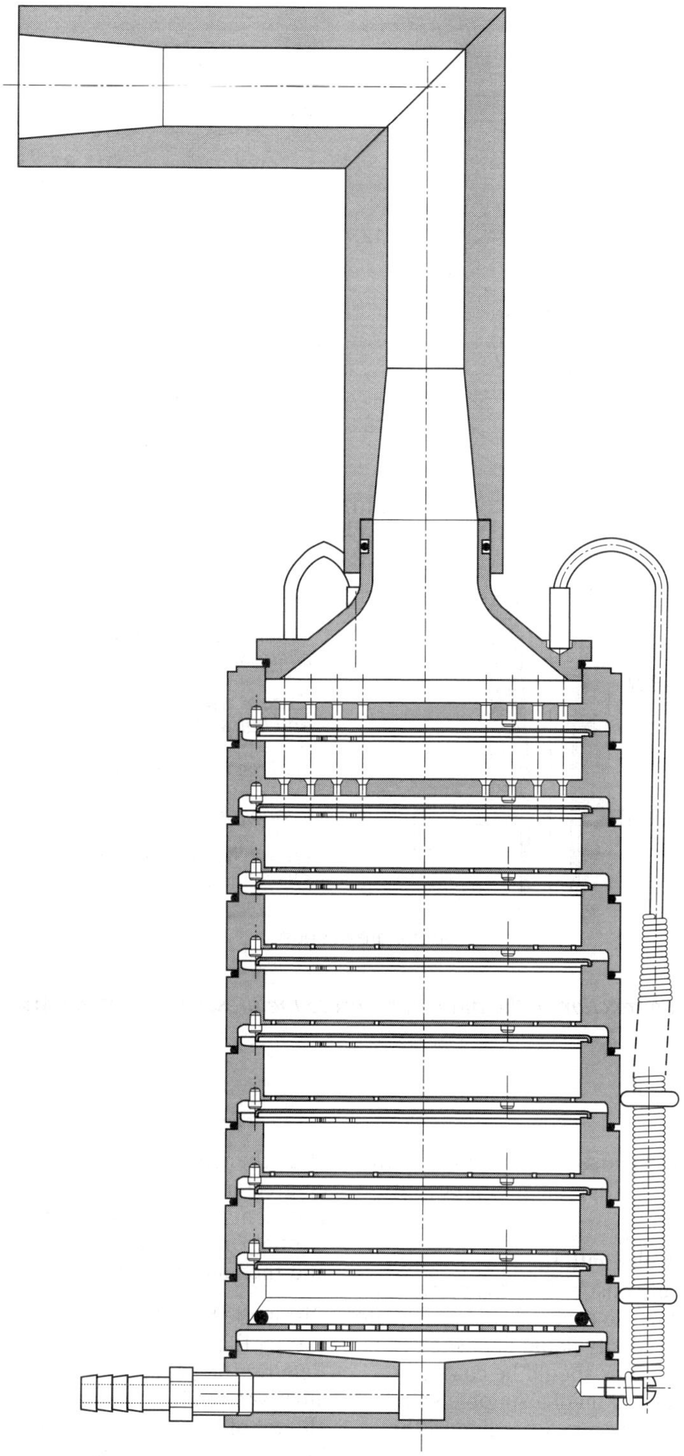

Figure 2.9.18.-9. – *"Andersen" sizing sampler adapted for pressurised inhalers*

outlet of the apparatus and adjust the air flow through the apparatus, as measured at the inlet to the induction port, to 28.3 ± 1.5 litres/min. Switch off the air flow.

Unless otherwise prescribed in the patient instructions, shake the inhaler for 5 s and discharge one delivery to waste. Switch on the pump to the apparatus, locate the mouthpiece end of the actuator in the adapter and discharge the inverted inhaler into the apparatus, depressing the valve for a sufficient time to ensure complete discharge. Remove the assembled inhaler from the adapter. Repeat the procedure. The number of discharges should be minimised and typically would not be greater than ten. The number of discharges should be sufficient to ensure an accurate and precise determination of the fine particle dose. After the final discharge, wait for 5 s and then switch off the pump.

Dismantle the apparatus. Carefully remove the filter and extract the drug into an aliquot of the solvent. Remove the induction port and mouthpiece adapter from the apparatus and extract the drug into an aliquot of the solvent. Extract the drug from the inner walls and the collection plate of each of the stages of the apparatus into aliquots of solvent.

Using a suitable method of analysis, determine the quantity of drug contained in each of the nine volumes of solvent.

Calculate the fine particle dose (see below).

Procedure for powder inhalers. In order to assess powder inhalers, the "Andersen" Sampler may be used at flow rates other than 28.3 litres/min. However, no general calibration data is presently available. In the absence of published data,

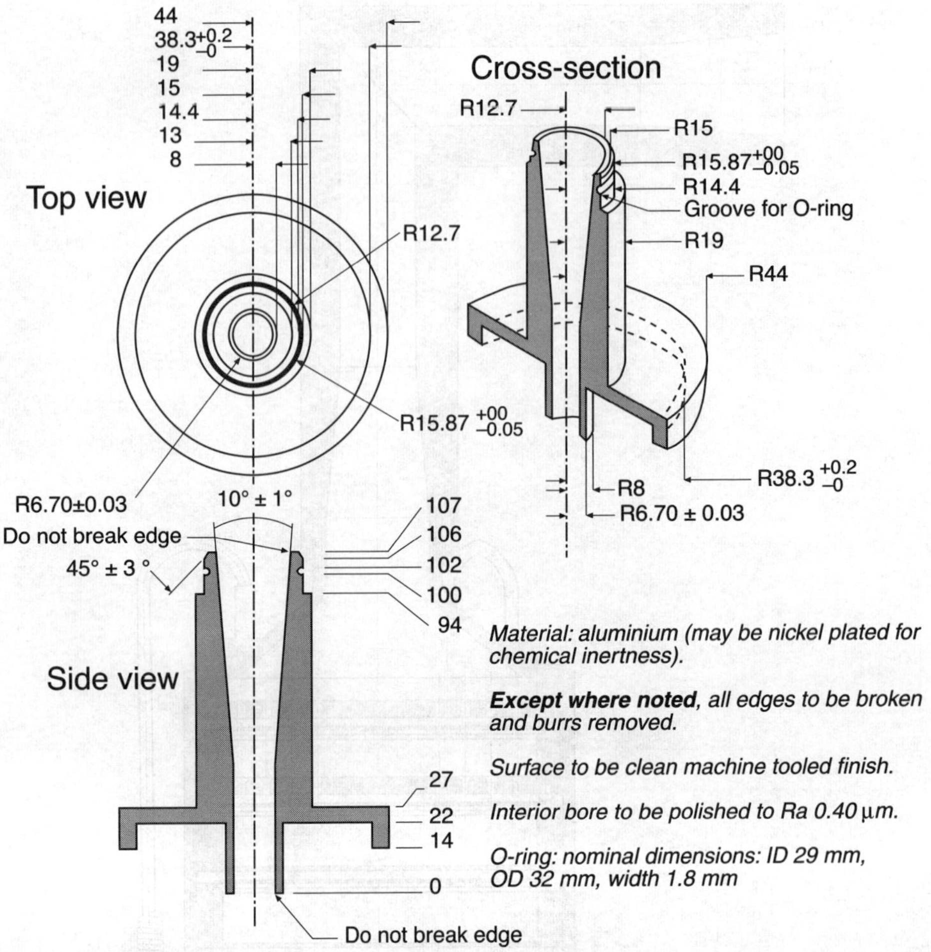

Figure 2.9.18.-10. – *Connection of the induction port to the preseparator of the Andersen sizing sampler*

users must, therefore, validate the use of the sampler in the chosen conditions. The following experimental procedure may then be adopted.

Assemble the "Andersen" Sampler with the pre-separator and a suitable filter in place and ensure that the system is airtight. To ensure efficient particle capture, coat each plate with glycerol or similar high viscosity liquid deposited from a volatile solvent. The pre-separator should be coated in the same way or should contain 10 ml of a suitable solvent. Connect the apparatus to a flow system according to the scheme specified in Figure 2.9.18.-8.

Unless otherwise defined conduct the test at the flow rate used in the test for uniformity of delivered dose drawing 4 litres of air through the apparatus. At high flow rates it may be necessary to remove the lowest stages from the stack. Connect a flow meter, calibrated for the volumetric flow leaving the meter, to the induction port. Adjust the flow control valve to achieve steady flow through the system at the required rate, Q (± 5 per cent). Ensure that critical flow occurs in the flow control valve by the procedure described for Apparatus C. Switch off the airflow.

Prepare the dry-powder inhaler for use according to the patient instructions. With the pump running and the two-way valve closed, locate the mouthpiece of the inhaler in the mouthpiece adapter. Discharge the powder into the apparatus by opening the valve for the required time, T (± 5 per cent). Repeat the discharge sequence. The number of discharges should be minimised and typically would not be greater than ten. The number of discharges should be sufficient to ensure an accurate and precise determination of fine particle dose. After the final discharge, wait for 5 s and then switch off the pump.

Dismantle the apparatus. Carefully remove the filter and extract the active ingredient into an aliquot of the solvent. Remove the pre-separator, induction port and mouthpiece adapter from the apparatus and extract the drug into an aliquot of the solvent. Extract the active ingredient from the inner walls and the collection plate of each of the stages of the apparatus into aliquots of solvent.

Using a suitable method of analysis, determine the quantity of active ingredient contained in each of the nine volumes of solvent.

Calculate the fine particle dose (see below).

Calculations

From the analyses of the solutions, calculate the mass of active ingredient deposited on each stage per discharge and the mass of active ingredient per discharge deposited in the induction port, mouthpiece adapter and where used the pre-separator. The total mass of the active ingredient is not less than 75 per cent and not more than 125 per cent of the average delivered dose determined during testing for uniformity of delivered dose. If the total mass is outside this range the test must be repeated.

Table 2.9.18.-6. – *Calculations for Apparatus D when used at 28.3 litres/min*

Cut-off diameter (µm)	Mass of active ingredient deposited per discharge	Cumulative mass of active ingredient deposited per discharge	Cumulative fraction of active ingredient (per cent)
d_7 = 0.4	mass from stage 8, m_8	$c_7 = m_8$	$f_7 = (c_7/c) \cdot 100$
d_6 = 0.7	mass from stage 7, m_7	$c_6 = c_7 + m_7$	$f_6 = (c_6/c) \cdot 100$
d_5 = 1.1	mass from stage 6, m_6	$c_5 = c_6 + m_6$	$f_5 = (c_5/c) \cdot 100$
d_4 = 2.1	mass from stage 5, m_5	$c_4 = c_5 + m_5$	$f_4 = (c_4/c) \cdot 100$
d_3 = 3.3	mass from stage 4, m_4	$c_3 = c_4 + m_4$	$f_3 = (c_3/c) \cdot 100$
d_2 = 4.7	mass from stage 3, m_3	$c_2 = c_3 + m_3$	$f_2 = (c_2/c) \cdot 100$
d_1 = 5.8	mass from stage 2, m_2	$c_1 = c_2 + m_2$	$f_1 = (c_1/c) \cdot 100$
d_0 = 9.0	mass from stage 1, m_1	$c_0 = c_1 + m_1$	$f_0 = (c_0/c) \cdot 100$
	mass from stage 0, m_0	$c = c_0 + m_0$	100

Starting at the filter, derive a cumulative mass vs. cut-off diameter of the respective stages (see Table 2.9.18.-5 for Apparatus C or Table 2.9.18.-6 for Apparatus D). Calculate by interpolation the mass of active ingredient less than 5 µm. This is the Fine Particle Dose (FPD).

If necessary, and where appropriate, plot the cumulative fraction of active ingredient versus cut-off diameter (see Tables 2.9.18.-5/6) on log probability paper, and use this plot to determine values for the Mass Median Aerodynamic Diameter (MMAD) and the Geometric Standard Deviation (GSD), as appropriate. Appropriate computational methods may also be used.

01/2005:20919

2.9.19. PARTICULATE CONTAMINATION: SUB-VISIBLE PARTICLES

Particulate contamination of injections and infusions consists of extraneous, mobile undissolved particles, other than gas bubbles, unintentionally present in the solutions.

For the determination of particulate contamination 2 procedures, Method 1 (Light Obscuration Particle Count Test) and Method 2 (Microscopic Particle Count Test), are specified hereinafter. When examining injections and infusions for sub-visible particles, Method 1 is preferably applied. However, it may be necessary to test some preparations by the light obscuration particle count test followed by the microscopic particle count test to reach a conclusion on conformance to the requirements.

Not all parenteral preparations can be examined for sub-visible particles by one or both of these methods. When Method 1 is not applicable, e.g. in case of preparations having reduced clarity or increased viscosity, the test is carried out according to Method 2. Emulsions, colloids, and liposomal preparations are examples. Similarly, products that produce air or gas bubbles when drawn into the sensor may also require microscopic particle count testing. If the viscosity of the preparation to be tested is sufficiently high so as to preclude its examination by either test method, a quantitative dilution with an appropriate diluent may be made to decrease viscosity, as necessary, to allow the analysis to be performed.

The results obtained in examining a discrete unit or group of units for particulate contamination cannot be extrapolated with certainty to other units that remain untested. Thus, statistically sound sampling plans must be developed if valid inferences are to be drawn from observed data to characterise the level of particulate contamination in a large group of units.

METHOD 1. LIGHT OBSCURATION PARTICLE COUNT TEST

Use a suitable apparatus based on the principle of light blockage which allows an automatic determination of the size of particles and the number of particles according to size.

The apparatus is calibrated using suitable certified reference materials consisting of dispersions of spherical particles of known sizes between 10 µm and 25 µm. These standard particles are dispersed in *particle-free water R*. Care must be taken to avoid aggregation of particles during dispersion.

General precautions

The test is carried out under conditions limiting particulate contamination, preferably in a laminar-flow cabinet.

Very carefully wash the glassware and filtration equipment used, except for the membrane filters, with a warm detergent solution and rinse with abundant amounts of water to remove all traces of detergent. Immediately before use, rinse the equipment from top to bottom, outside and then inside, with *particle-free water R*.

Take care not to introduce air bubbles into the preparation to be examined, especially when fractions of the preparation are being transferred to the container in which the determination is to be carried out.

In order to check that the environment is suitable for the test, that the glassware is properly cleaned and that the water to be used is particle-free, the following test is carried out: determine the particulate contamination of 5 samples of *particle-free water R*, each of 5 ml, according to the method described below. If the number of particles of 10 µm or greater size exceeds 25 for the combined 25 ml, the precautions taken for the test are not sufficient. The preparatory steps must be repeated until the environment, glassware and water are suitable for the test.

Method

Mix the contents of the sample by slowly inverting the container 20 times successively. If necessary, cautiously remove the sealing closure. Clean the outer surfaces of the container opening using a jet of *particle-free water R* and remove the closure, avoiding any contamination of the contents. Eliminate gas bubbles by appropriate measures such as allowing to stand for 2 min or sonicating.

For large-volume parenterals, single units are tested. For small-volume parenterals less than 25 ml in volume, the contents of 10 or more units are combined in a cleaned container to obtain a volume of not less than 25 ml; where justified and authorised, the test solution may be prepared by mixing the contents of a suitable number of vials and diluting to 25 ml with *particle-free water R* or with an appropriate solvent without contamination of particles when *particle-free water R* is not suitable. Small-volume parenterals having a volume of 25 ml or more may be tested individually.

Powders for parenteral use are reconstituted with *particle-free water R* or with an appropriate solvent without contamination of particles when *particle-free water R* is not suitable.

The number of test specimens must be adequate to provide a statistically sound assessment. For large-volume parenterals or for small-volume parenterals having a volume of 25 ml or more, fewer than 10 units may be tested, based on an appropriate sampling plan.

Remove 4 portions, each of not less than 5 ml, and count the number of particles equal to or greater than 10 μm and 25 μm. Disregard the result obtained for the first portion, and calculate the mean number of particles for the preparation to be examined.

Evaluation

For preparations supplied in containers with a nominal volume of more than 100 ml, apply the criteria of test 1.A.

For preparations supplied in containers with a nominal volume of less than 100 ml, apply the criteria of test 1.B.

For preparations supplied in containers with a nominal volume of 100 ml, apply the criteria of test 1.B

If the average number of particles exceeds the limits, test the preparation by the microscopic particle count test.

Test 1.A – Solutions for infusion or solutions for injection supplied in containers with a nominal content of more than 100 ml

The preparation complies with the test if the average number of particles present in the units tested does not exceed 25 per millilitre equal to or greater than 10 μm and does not exceed 3 per millilitre equal to or greater than 25 μm.

Test 1.B – Solutions for infusion or solutions for injection supplied in containers with a nominal content of less than 100 ml

The preparation complies with the test if the average number of particles present in the units tested does not exceed 6000 per container equal to or greater than 10 μm and does not exceed 600 per container equal to or greater than 25 μm.

METHOD 2. MICROSCOPIC PARTICLE COUNT TEST

Use a suitable binocular microscope, filter assembly for retaining particulate contamination and membrane filter for examination.

The microscope is equipped with an ocular micrometer calibrated with an objective micrometer, a mechanical stage capable of holding and traversing the entire filtration area of the membrane filter, 2 suitable illuminators to provide episcopic illumination in addition to oblique illumination, and is adjusted to 100 ± 10 magnifications.

The ocular micrometer is a circular diameter graticule (see Figure 2.9.19.-1) and consists of a large circle divided by crosshairs into quadrants, transparent and black reference circles 10 μm and 25 μm in diameter at 100 magnifications, and a linear scale graduated in 10 μm increments. It is calibrated using a stage micrometer that is certified by either a domestic or international standard institution. A relative error of the linear scale of the graticule within ± 2 per cent is acceptable. The large circle is designated the graticule field of view (GFOV).

2 illuminators are required. One is an episcopic brightfield illuminator internal to the microscope, the other is an external, focusable auxiliary illuminator adjustable to give reflected oblique illumination at an angle of 10-20°.

The filter assembly for retaining particulate contamination consists of a filter holder made of glass or other suitable material, and is equipped with a vacuum source and a suitable membrane filter.

The membrane filter is of suitable size, black or dark grey in colour, non-gridded or gridded, and 1.0 μm or finer in nominal pore size.

General precautions

The test is carried out under conditions limiting particulate contamination, preferably in a laminar-flow cabinet.

Very carefully wash the glassware and filter assembly used, except for the membrane filter, with a warm detergent solution and rinse with abundant amounts of water to remove

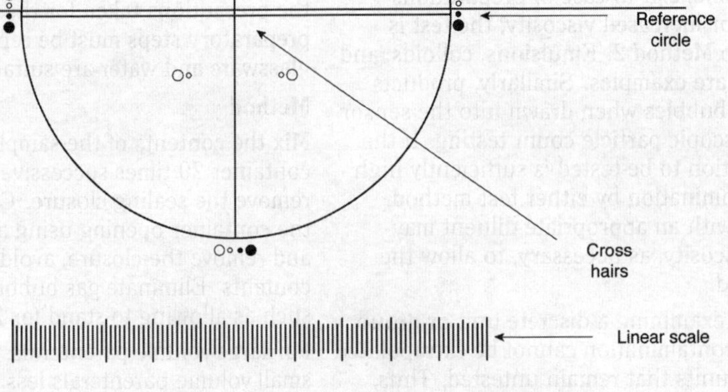

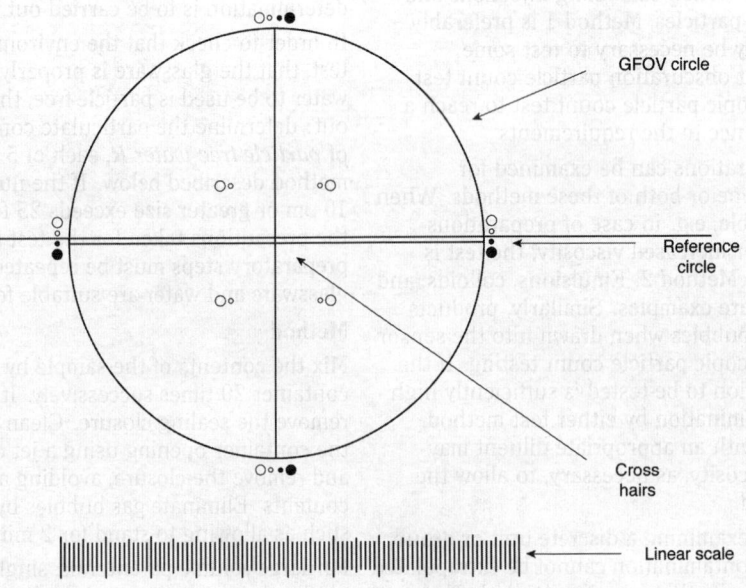

Figure 2.9.19.-1. – *Circular diameter graticule*

all traces of detergent. Immediately before use, rinse both sides of the membrane filter and the equipment from top to bottom, outside and then inside, with *particle-free water R*.

In order to check that the environment is suitable for the test, that the glassware and the membrane filter are properly cleaned and that the water to be used is particle-free, the following test is carried out: determine the particulate contamination of a 50 ml volume of *particle-free water R* according to the method described below. If more than 20 particles 10 μm or larger in size or if more than 5 particles 25 μm or larger in size are present within the filtration area, the precautions taken for the test are not sufficient. The preparatory steps must be repeated until the environment, glassware, membrane filter and water are suitable for the test.

Method

Mix the contents of the samples by slowly inverting the container 20 times successively. If necessary, cautiously remove the sealing closure. Clean the outer surfaces of the container opening using a jet of *particle-free water R* and remove the closure, avoiding any contamination of the contents.

For large-volume parenterals, single units are tested. For small-volume parenterals less than 25 ml in volume, the contents of 10 or more units are combined in a cleaned container; where justified and authorised, the test solution may be prepared by mixing the contents of a suitable number of vials and diluting to 25 ml with *particle-free water R* or with an appropriate solvent without contamination of particles when *particle-free water R* is not suitable. Small-volume parenterals having a volume of 25 ml or more may be tested individually.

Powders for parenteral use are constituted with *particle-free water R* or with an appropriate solvent without contamination of particles when *particle-free water R* is not suitable.

The number of test specimens must be adequate to provide a statistically sound assessment. For large-volume parenterals or for small-volume parenterals having a volume of 25 ml or more, fewer than 10 units may be tested, based on an appropriate sampling plan.

Wet the inside of the filter holder fitted with the membrane filter with several millilitres of *particle-free water R*. Transfer to the filtration funnel the total volume of a solution pool or of a single unit, and apply vacuum. If needed, add stepwise a portion of the solution until the entire volume is filtered. After the last addition of solution, begin rinsing the inner walls of the filter holder by using a jet of *particle-free water R*. Maintain the vacuum until the surface of the membrane filter is free from liquid. Place the filter in a Petri dish and allow the filter to air-dry with the cover slightly ajar. After the filter has been dried, place the Petri dish on the stage of the microscope, scan the entire membrane filter under the reflected light from the illuminating device, and count the number of particles that are equal to or greater than 10 μm and the number of particles that are equal to or greater than 25 μm. Alternatively, partial filter count and determination of the total filter count by calculation is allowed. Calculate the mean number of particles for the preparation to be examined.

The particle sizing process with the use of the circular diameter graticule is carried out by transforming mentally the image of each particle into a circle and then comparing it to the 10 μm and 25 μm graticule reference circles. Thereby the particles are not moved from their initial locations within the graticule field of view and are not superimposed on the reference circles for comparison. The inner diameter of the transparent graticule reference circles is used to size white and transparent particles, while dark particles are sized by using the outer diameter of the black opaque graticule reference circles.

In performing the microscopic particle count test do not attempt to size or enumerate amorphous, semi-liquid, or otherwise morphologically indistinct materials that have the appearance of a stain or discoloration on the membrane filter. These materials show little or no surface relief and present a gelatinous or film-like appearance. In such cases the interpretation of enumeration may be aided by testing a sample of the solution by the light obscuration particle count test.

Evaluation

For preparations supplied in containers with a nominal volume of more than 100 ml, apply the criteria of test 2.A.

For preparations supplied in containers with a nominal volume of less than 100 ml, apply the criteria of test 2.B.

For preparations supplied in containers with a nominal volume of 100 ml, apply the criteria of test 2.B.

Test 2.A — Solutions for infusion or solutions for injection supplied in containers with a nominal content of more than 100 ml

The preparation complies with the test if the average number of particles present in the units tested does not exceed 12 per millilitre equal to or greater than 10 μm and does not exceed 2 per millilitre equal to or greater than 25 μm.

Test 2.B — Solutions for infusion or solutions for injection supplied in containers with a nominal content of less than 100 ml

The preparation complies with the test if the average number of particles present in the units tested does not exceed 3000 per container equal to or greater than 10 μm and does not exceed 300 per container equal to or greater than 25 μm.

01/2005:20920

2.9.20. PARTICULATE CONTAMINATION: VISIBLE PARTICLES

Particulate contamination of injections and infusions consists of extraneous, mobile undissolved particles, other than gas bubbles, unintentionally present in the solutions.

The test is intended to provide a simple procedure for the visual assessment of the quality of parenteral solutions as regards visible particles. Other validated methods may be used.

APPARATUS

The apparatus (see Figure 2.9.20.-1) consists of a viewing station comprising:

- a matt black panel of appropriate size held in a vertical position,
- a non-glare white panel of appropriate size held in a vertical position next to the black panel,
- an adjustable lampholder fitted with a suitable, shaded, white-light source and with a suitable light diffuser (a viewing illuminator containing two 13 W fluorescent tubes, each 525 mm in length, is suitable). The intensity of illumination at the viewing point is maintained between 2000 lux and 3750 lux, although higher values are preferable for coloured glass and plastic containers.

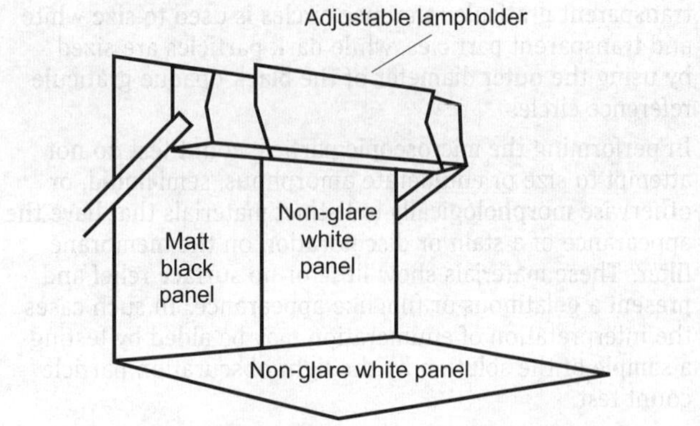

Figure 2.9.20.-1. – *Apparatus for visible particles*

METHOD

Remove any adherent labels from the container and wash and dry the outside. Gently swirl or invert the container, ensuring that air bubbles are not introduced, and observe for about 5 s in front of the white panel. Repeat the procedure in front of the black panel. Record the presence of any particles.

01/2005:20922

2.9.22. SOFTENING TIME DETERMINATION OF LIPOPHILIC SUPPOSITORIES

The test is intended to determine, under defined conditions, the time which elapses until a suppository maintained in water softens to the extent that it no longer offers resistance when a defined weight is applied.

APPARATUS A

The apparatus (see Figure 2.9.22.-1) consists of a glass tube 15.5 mm in internal diameter with a flat bottom and a length of about 140 mm. The tube is closed by a removable plastic cover having an opening 5.2 mm in diameter. The apparatus comprises a rod 5.0 mm in diameter which becomes wider towards the lower end, reaching a diameter of 12 mm. A metal needle 2 mm in length and 1 mm in diameter is fixed on the flat underside.

The rod consists of 2 parts, a lower part made of plastic material and an upper part made of plastic material or metal with a weight disk. The upper and lower parts are either fitted together (manual version) or separate (automated version). The weight of the entire rod is 30 ± 0.4 g. The upper part of the rod carries a sliding mark ring. When the rod is introduced into the glass tube so that it touches the bottom, the mark ring is adjusted to coincide with the upper level of the plastic cover.

Method. Place the glass tube containing 10 ml of water in a water-bath and equilibrate at 36.5 ± 0.5 °C. Fix the glass tube vertically and immerse to a depth of at least 7 cm below the surface but without touching the bottom of the water-bath. Introduce a suppository, tip first, into the tube followed by the rod with the free gliding plastic cover into the glass tube until the metal needle touches the flat end of the suppository. Put the cover on the tube (beginning of time measurement). Note the time which elapses until the rod sinks down to the bottom of the glass tube and the mark ring reaches the upper level of the plastic cover.

APPARATUS B

The apparatus (see Figure 2.9.22.-2) consists of a water-bath (B) into which an inner tube (A) is inserted and fixed with a stopper. The inner tube is closed by a stopper at the bottom. The apparatus is fitted with a thermometer. 2 insets are available:

– a glass rod (C1) in the form of a tube sealed at both ends, carrying a rim at its lower end weighed with lead shot, which has a weight of 30 ± 0.4 g,

– a penetration inset (C2) consisting of a rod (7.5 ± 0.1 g) in a tube which has an enlargement for the suppository, both made of stainless steel.

Method. Pour 5 ml of water at 36.5 ± 0.5 °C into the inner tube (A), introduce a suppository with the tip downwards and onto that, place the inset (C1 or C2). Note the time which elapses between this moment and the moment when the lower, rimmed end of the glass rod (C1) or the steel rod (C2) reaches the narrowed part of the inner glass tube. Melting or dissolution is then considered as complete.

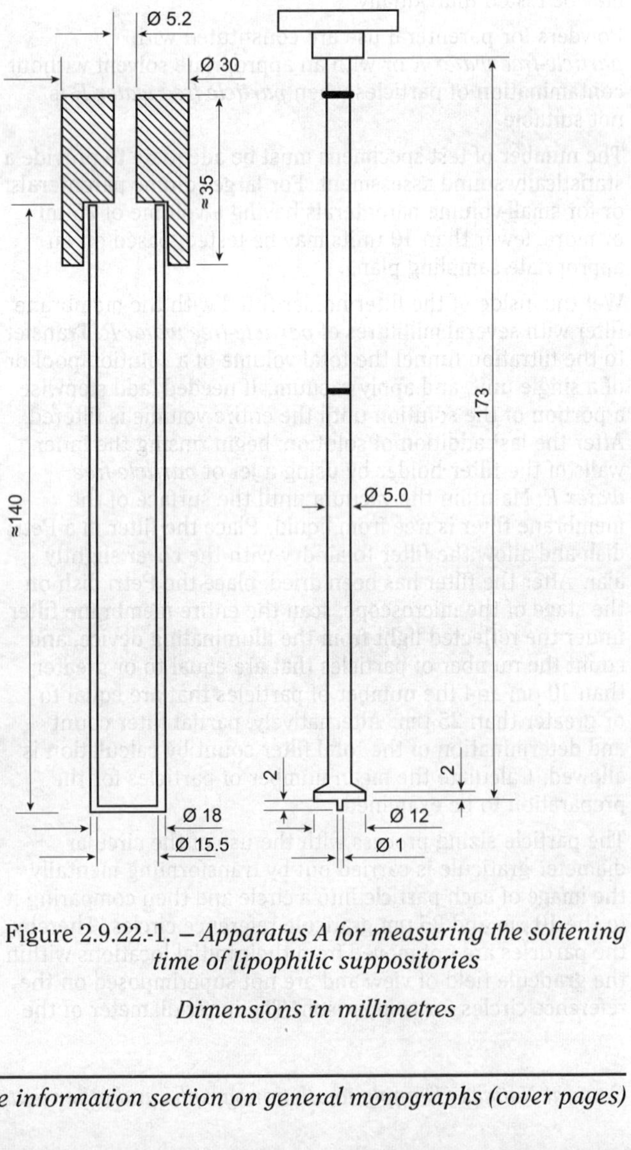

Figure 2.9.22.-1. – *Apparatus A for measuring the softening time of lipophilic suppositories*

Dimensions in millimetres

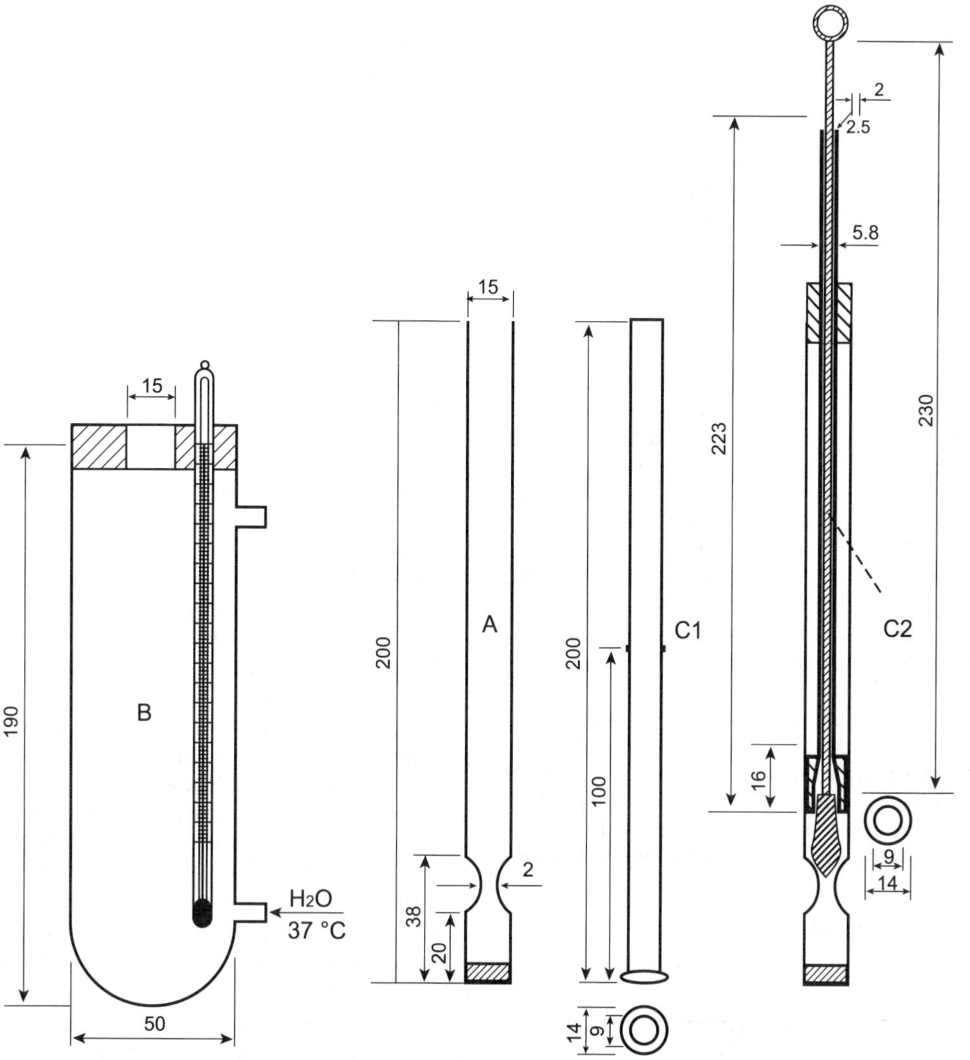

Figure 2.9.22.-2. – *Apparatus B for measuring the softening time of lipophilic suppositories*
Dimensions in millimetres

01/2005:20923

2.9.23. PYCNOMETRIC DENSITY OF SOLIDS

The test for pycnometric density of solids is intended to determine the volume occupied by a known mass of powder by measuring the volume of gas displaced under defined conditions. Hence, its pycnometric density is calculated.

APPARATUS

The apparatus (see Figure 2.9.23.-1) consists of the following:

- a sealed test cell, with an empty cell volume (V_c), connected through a valve to a reference cell, with a reference volume (V_r),
- a system capable of pressurising the test cell with the measurement gas until a defined pressure (*P*) indicated by a manometer,
- the system is connected to a source of measurement gas, which is preferably helium, unless another gas is specified[(1)].

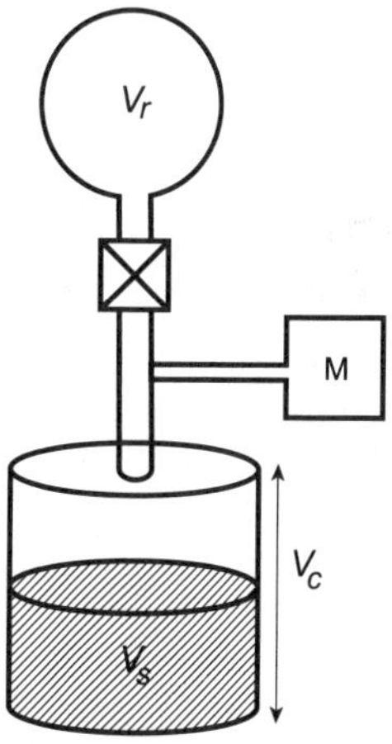

V_r = reference volume
V_c = cell volume
V_s = sample volume
M = manometer

Figure 2.9.23.-1. – *Schematic diagram of a gas pycnometer*

(1) If gases other than helium are used, it would not be surprising to obtain values different from those obtained with helium, since the penetration of the gas is dependent on the size of the pore as well as the cross-sectional area of the penetrating molecule. For example, the pycnometric density of porous materials will be overestimated by a measure using nitrogen by comparison with helium.

The temperature of the gas pycnometer is between 15 °C and 30 °C and must not vary by more than 2 °C during the course of measurement.

The apparatus is calibrated which means that the volumes (V_c) and (V_r) are determined, using calibrated, polished steel balls having a total volume (around 6 cm³) known to the nearest 0.001 cm³. The procedure described below is followed in two runs. Firstly, with an empty test cell and secondly with the steel balls placed in the test cell. The volumes (V_c) and (V_r) are calculated using the equation for the sample volume taking into account that the volume is zero in the first run.

METHOD

Weigh the test cell of the pycnometer and record the mass. Fill the test cell with a given mass of powder of the substance to be examined. Seal the test cell in the pycnometer. Remove volatile contaminants in the powder by degassing the powder under a constant purge of gas; occasionally, powders may initially have to be degassed under vacuum. Record the system reference pressure (P_r) as indicated by the manometer while the valve that connects the reference cell with the test cell is open. Close the valve to separate the reference cell from the test cell. Pressurise the test cell with the gas to an initial pressure (P_i) and record the value obtained. Open the valve to connect the reference cell with the test cell. Record the final pressure (P_f). Repeat the measurement sequence for the same powder sample until consecutive measurements of the sample volume (V_s) agree to within 0.5 per cent. The sample volume is expressed in cubic centimetres. Unload the test cell and measure the final powder mass (m) expressed in grams.

EXPRESSION OF THE RESULTS

The sample volume (V_s) is given by the expression:

$$V_s = V_c - \frac{V_r}{\dfrac{P_i - P_r}{P_f - P_r} - 1}$$

The density (ρ) is given by the equation:

$$\rho = \frac{m}{V_s}$$

01/2005:20924

2.9.24. RESISTANCE TO RUPTURE OF SUPPOSITORIES AND PESSARIES

This test determines, under defined conditions, the resistance to rupture of suppositories and pessaries measured by the mass needed to rupture them by crushing.

This test applies to suppositories and pessaries based on fatty excipients. It is not suited to suppositories and pessaries based on hydrophilic excipients such as a gelatin-glycerol mixture.

Apparatus. The apparatus (see Figures 2.9.24.-1/2) consists of:

- a thermostatted chamber closed in front by a glass window and containing a device that is to hold the suppository or pessary,
- two opposed jaws, the upper jaw descending vertically towards the lower jaw. The crushing surfaces of the jaws are flat, perpendicular to the direction of movement and larger than the zone of contact with the suppository or pessary. A plastic sample holder is fixed in the centre of the jaws (half a holder on each jaw). The upper jaw (top pressure block) is connected to a suspension to which discs can be added, each of which weighs 200 g. The initial mass of the device is 600 g. Crushing of the sample is carried out by successively adding 200 g discs to the initial mass of 600 g.

Method. Check that the apparatus is vertical. Heat the thermostatted chamber to 25 °C.

The dosage form to be tested has been maintained for at least 24 h at the required measuring temperature. Place the suppository or pessary vertically between the jaws in the sample holder with the point upwards. The top pressure block of the suspension loading rod is carefully positioned and the test chamber is closed with its glass window; for each determination, position the suppository or pessary in the same manner with respect to the direction of the force applied.

Wait for 1 min and add the first 200 g disc. Again wait for 1 min and add another disc. Repeat the operation until the suppository or pessary collapses.

The mass required to crush the suppository or pessary is calculated by the sum of the masses weighing on the suppository or pessary when it collapses (including the initial mass of the device) assessed as follows:

- if the suppository or pessary collapses within 20 s of placing the last disc, do not take this mass into account,
- if the suppository or pessary collapses between 20 s and 40 s of placing the last disc, use only half of this mass in the calculation, i.e. 100 g,
- if the suppository or pessary remains uncrushed for more than 40 s after the last disc is placed, use all the mass in the calculation.

Carry out each measurement on ten suppositories or ten pessaries, making sure that no residue remains before each determination.

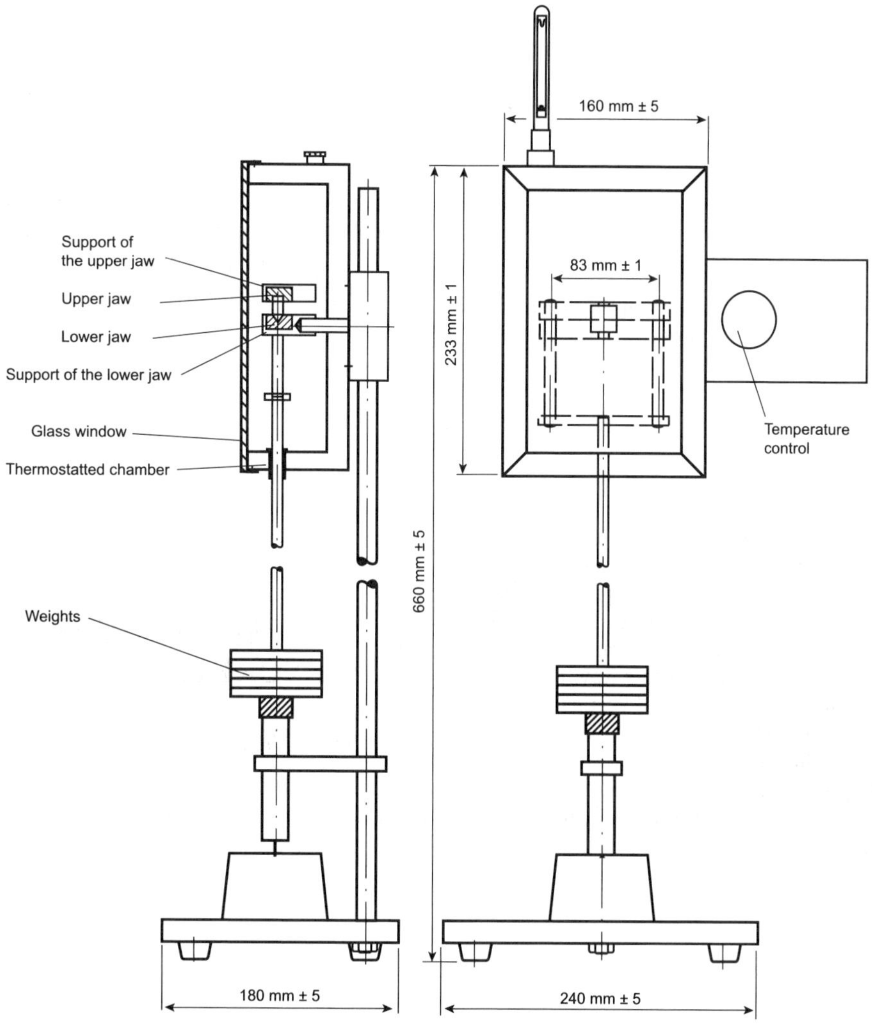

Figure 2.9.24.-1. – *Apparatus for the determination of the resistance to rupture of suppositories and pessaries*

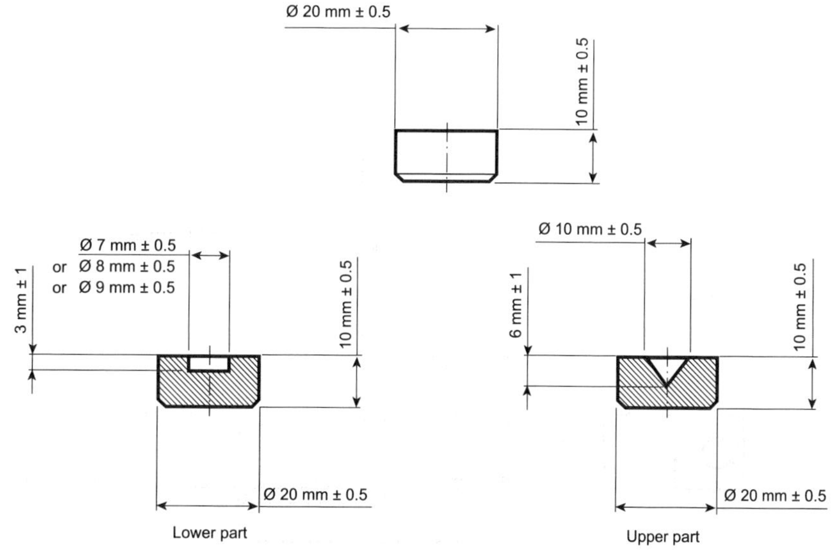

Figure 2.9.24.-2. – *Lower and upper jaws*

01/2005:20925

2.9.25. CHEWING GUM, MEDICATED, DRUG RELEASE FROM

PRINCIPLE

The drug release from medicated chewing gum is determined by applying a mechanical kneading procedure to a piece of gum placed in a small chewing chamber containing a known volume of buffer solution.

APPARATUS

The chewing apparatus (see Figure 2.9.25.-1) comprises a chewing chamber of approximately 40 ml in which the gum is artificially chewed by two horizontal pistons; the pistons operate together at a constant speed. At the end of a chew, the pistons can rotate around their own axes in opposite directions to each other. In this way, the gum is subjected to maximum chewing. A third vertical piston ("tongue") operates alternately with the two horizontal pistons and makes sure that the gum stays in the right place between chews. The pistons are driven by compressed air and their mutual movements are controlled. All materials are composed of stainless steel.

PROCEDURE

Adjust the temperature of the chewing chamber (37 ± 0.5 °C) and the speed of the pistons. Add 20 ml of buffer (generally close to pH 6) into the chewing chamber. Start the machine and let it run for 2 min with buffer, but no chewing gum. Remove all the buffer by pipette and replace it by 20 ml of fresh buffer. The buffer which has been removed is analysed as a control for the cleaning procedure. Weigh precisely a piece of chewing gum, put it into the chewing chamber and start the machine. At specified time intervals, remove samples from the reservoir to determine the drug release. The chewing frequency is usually set at 60 cycles/min. Sometimes the chewing residue is taken out and placed in a bag for later analysis.

01/2005:20926

2.9.26. SPECIFIC SURFACE AREA BY GAS ADSORPTION

I. INTRODUCTION

The specific surface area of a powder is determined by physical adsorption of a gas on the surface of the solid and by measuring the amount of adsorbate gas corresponding to

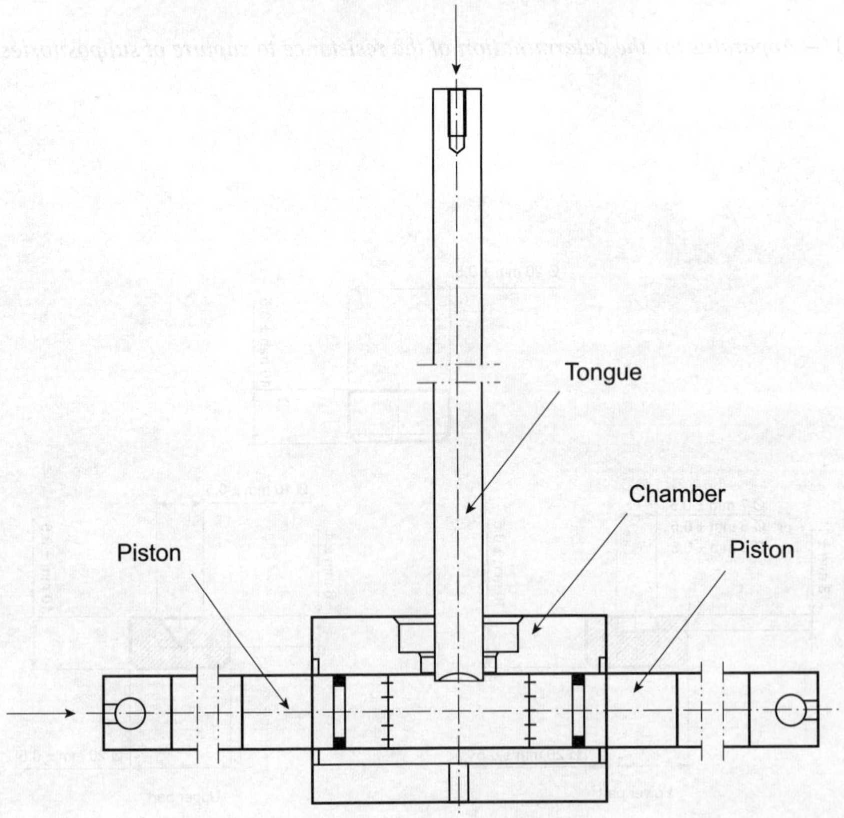

Figure 2.9.25.-1. – *Apparatus for the determination of drug release from medicated chewing gum*

a monomolecular layer on the surface. Physical adsorption results from relatively weak forces (van der Waals forces) between the adsorbate gas molecules and the adsorbent surface of the test powder. The amount of gas adsorbed can be measured by a gravimetric, volumetric or continuous flow procedure.

II. BRUNAUER, EMMETT AND TELLER (BET) THEORY AND SPECIFIC SURFACE AREA DETERMINATION

II.1. MULTI-POINT MEASUREMENT

The data are treated according to the Brunauer, Emmett and Teller (BET) adsorption isotherm equation:

$$\frac{1}{\left[V_a\left(\frac{P_o}{P}-1\right)\right]}=\frac{C-1}{V_m C}\times\frac{P}{P_o}+\frac{1}{V_m C} \qquad (1)$$

P = partial vapour pressure of adsorbate gas in equilibrium with the surface at − 196 °C, in pascals,

P_o = saturated pressure of adsorbate gas, in pascals,

V_a = volume of gas adsorbed at standard temperature and pressure (STP) [273.15 K and atmospheric pressure (1.013 × 10^5 Pa)], in millilitres,

V_m = volume of gas adsorbed at STP to produce an apparent monolayer on the sample surface, in millilitres,

C = dimensionless constant that is related to the enthalpy of adsorption of the adsorbate gas on the powder sample.

A value of V_a is measured at each of not less than three values of P/P_o.

Then the BET value

$$\frac{1}{\left[V_a\left(\frac{P_o}{P}-1\right)\right]}$$

is plotted against P/P_0 according to equation (1). This plot should yield a straight line usually in the approximate relative pressure range 0.05 to 0.3. The data are considered acceptable if the correlation coefficient, *r*, of the linear regression is not less than 0.9975; that is, r^2 is not less than 0.995. From the resulting linear plot, the slope, which is equal to $(C-1)/V_mC$, and the intercept, which is equal to $1/V_mC$, are evaluated by linear regression analysis. From these values, V_m is calculated as 1/(*slope* + *intercept*), while *C* is calculated as (*slope/intercept*) + 1. From the value of V_m so determined, the specific surface area, *S*, in $m^2 \cdot g^{-1}$, is calculated by the equation:

$$S=\frac{V_m\times N\times a}{m\times 22400} \qquad (2)$$

N = Avogadro constant (6.023 × 10^{23} mol^{-1}),

a = effective cross-sectional area of one adsorbate molecule, in square metres (0.162 nm^2 for nitrogen and 0.195 nm^2 for krypton),

m = mass of test powder, in grams,

22400 = volume, in millilitres, occupied by the adsorbate gas at STP allowing for minor departures from the ideal.

II.2. SINGLE-POINT MEASUREMENT

Normally, at least three measurements of V_a each at different values of P/P_o are required for the determination of specific surface area by the dynamic flow gas adsorption technique (*Method I*) or by volumetric gas adsorption (*Method II*). However, under certain circumstances described below, it may be acceptable to determine the specific surface area of a powder from a single value of V_a measured at a single value of P/P_o such as 0.300 (corresponding to 0.300 mole of nitrogen or 0.001038 mole fraction of krypton), using the following equation for calculating V_m:

$$V_m=V_a\left(1-\frac{P}{P_o}\right) \qquad (3)$$

The specific surface area is then calculated from the value of V_m by equation (2) given above.

The single-point method may be employed directly for a series of powder samples of a given material for which the material constant *C* is much greater than unity. These circumstances may be verified by comparing values of specific surface area determined by the single-point method with that determined by the multiple-point method for the series of powder samples. Close similarity between the single-point values and multiple-point values suggests that $1/C$ approaches zero.

The single-point method may be employed indirectly for a series of very similar powder samples of a given material for which the material constant *C* is not infinite but may be assumed to be invariant. Under these circumstances, the error associated with the single-point method can be reduced or eliminated by using the multiple-point method to evaluate *C* for one of the samples of the series from the BET plot, from which *C* is calculated as (1 + *slope/intercept*). Then V_m is calculated from the single value of V_a measured at a single value of P/P_o by the equation:

$$V_m=V_a\left(\frac{P_o}{P}-1\right)\left[\frac{1}{c}+\frac{c-1}{c}\times\left(\frac{P}{P_o}\right)\right] \qquad (4)$$

The specific surface area is calculated from V_m by equation (2) given above.

III. EXPERIMENTAL TECHNIQUES

This section describes the methods to be used for the sample preparation, the dynamic flow gas adsorption technique (*Method I*) and the volumetric gas adsorption technique (*Method II*).

III.1. SAMPLE PREPARATION

III.1.1. Outgassing

Before the specific surface area of the sample can be determined, it is necessary to remove gases and vapours that may have become physically adsorbed onto the surface after manufacture and during treatment, handling and storage. If outgassing is not achieved, the specific surface area may be reduced or may be variable because an intermediate area of the surface is covered with molecules of the previously adsorbed gases or vapours. The outgassing conditions are critical for obtaining the required precision and accuracy of specific surface area measurements on pharmaceuticals because of the sensitivity of the surface of the materials.

Conditions. The outgassing conditions must be demonstrated to yield reproducible BET plots, a constant weight of test powder, and no detectable physical or chemical changes in the test powder.

The outgassing conditions defined by the temperature, pressure and time should be so chosen that the original surface of the solid is reproduced as closely as possible. Outgassing of many substances is often achieved by applying a vacuum or by purging the sample in a flowing stream of a non-reactive, dry gas. In either case, elevated temperatures are sometimes applied to increase the rate at which the contaminants leave the surface. Outgassing by heating the powder sample may change the nature of the surface and should be avoided, unless specifically indicated.

If heating is employed, the recommended temperature and time of outgassing are as low as possible so as to achieve reproducibly high measures of specific surface area within an acceptable time span. For outgassing sensitive samples, other outgassing methods such as the desorption-adsorption cycling method may be employed.

III.1.2. Adsorbate

The standard technique is the adsorption of nitrogen at liquid nitrogen temperature.

For powders of low specific surface area (< 1 $m^2 \cdot g^{-1}$) the proportion adsorbed is low, the use of krypton at liquid nitrogen temperature is preferred in such cases since the low vapour pressure exerted by this gas greatly reduces the error. All gases used must be free from moisture.

III.1.3. Quantity of sample

Accurately weigh a quantity of the test powder such that the total surface of the sample is at least 1 m^2 when adsorbate is nitrogen and 0.5 m^2 when the adsorbate is krypton.

III.2. MEASUREMENTS

Since the amount of gas adsorbed under a given pressure tends to increase on decreasing the temperature, adsorption measurements are usually made at a low temperature. Measurement is performed at − 196 °C, the boiling point of liquid nitrogen.

III.2.1. Method I: the dynamic flow method

III.2.1.1. *Principle of the method*

In the dynamic flow method (see Figure 2.9.26.-1), the recommended adsorbate gas is dry nitrogen or krypton, while helium is employed as a diluent gas, which is not adsorbed under the recommended conditions.

A minimum of three mixtures of the appropriate adsorbate gas with helium are required within the P/P_o range 0.05 to 0.30.

The gas detector-integrator should provide a signal that is approximately proportional to the volume of the gas passing through it under defined conditions of temperature and pressure. For this purpose, a thermal conductivity detector with an electronic integrator is one among various suitable types. A minimum of three data points within the recommended range of 0.05 to 0.30 for P/P_o is to be determined.

III.2.1.2. *Procedure*

A known mixture of the gases, usually nitrogen and helium, is passed through a thermal conductivity cell, through the sample again through the thermal conductivity cell and then to a recording potentiometer.

Immerse the sample cell in liquid nitrogen, then the sample adsorbs nitrogen from the mobile phase. This unbalances the thermal conductivity cell, and a pulse is generated on a recorder chart.

Remove from the coolant; this gives a desorption peak equal in area and in the opposite direction to the adsorption peak. Since this is better defined than the adsorption peak, it is the one used for the determination.

To effect the calibration, inject sufficient air into the system to give a peak of similar magnitude to the desorption peak and obtain the proportion of gas adsorbed per unit peak area (air can be used instead of nitrogen since it has the same thermal conductivity).

Use a nitrogen/helium mixture for a single-point determination and several such mixtures or premixing two streams of gas for a multiple-point determination.

Calculation is essentially the same as for the volumetric method.

III.2.2. Method II: the volumetric method

III.2.2.1. *Principle of the method*

In the volumetric method (see Figure 2.9.26.-2), the recommended adsorbate gas is nitrogen which is admitted into the evacuated space above the previously outgassed powder sample to give a defined equilibrium pressure, *P*, of

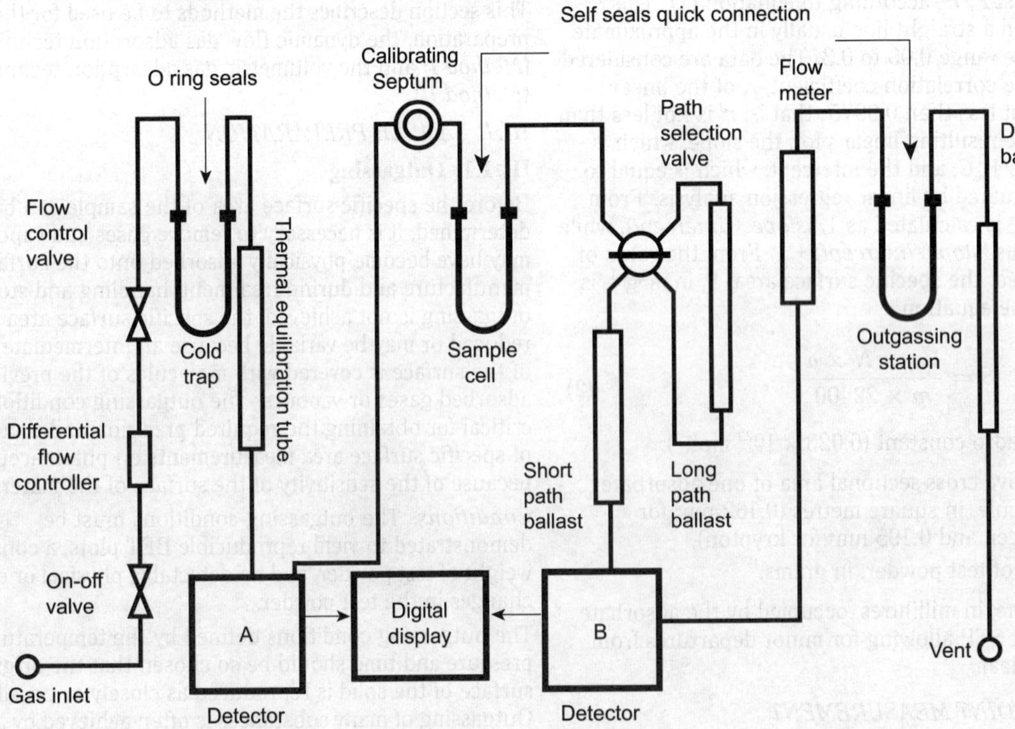

Figure 2.9.26.-1. – *Schematic diagram of the dynamic flow method apparatus*

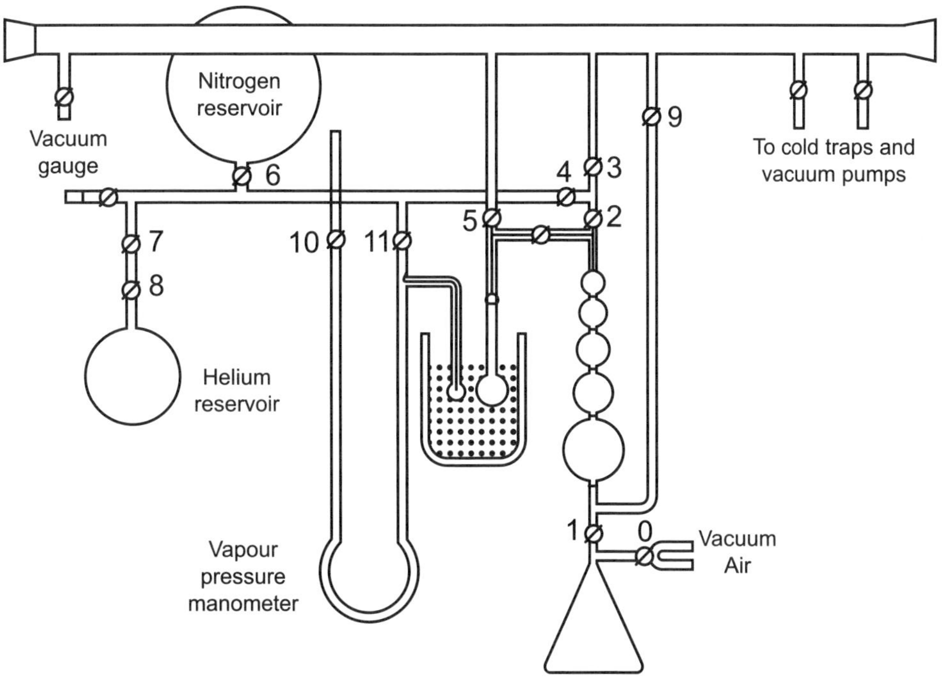

Figure 2.9.26.-2. – *Schematic diagram of the volumetric method apparatus*

the gas. The use of a diluent gas, such as helium, is therefore unnecessary, although helium may be employed for other purposes, such as to measure the void volume.

Since only pure adsorbate gas, instead of a gas mixture, is employed, interfering effects of thermal diffusion are avoided in this method.

III.2.2.2. *Procedure*

Admit a small amount of dry nitrogen into the sample tube to prevent contamination of the clean surface, remove the sample tube, insert the stopper, and weigh it. Calculate the weight of the sample. Attach the sample tube to the volumetric apparatus. Cautiously evacuate the sample down to a pressure of 2.66 Pa or less.

If the principle of operation of the instrument requires the determination of the void volume in the sample tube, for example, by the admission of a non-adsorbed gas, such as helium, this procedure is carried out at this point, followed by evacuation of the sample down to 2.66 Pa or less. The adsorption of nitrogen gas is then measured as described below.

Raise a Dewar vessel containing liquid nitrogen at − 196 °C up to a defined point on the sample cell. Admit a sufficient volume of nitrogen gas to give a relative pressure, P/P_0 equal to 0.10 ± 0.02. Measure the volume adsorbed, V_a. Repeat the measurement of V_a at P/P_0 values of 0.20 ± 0.02 and 0.30 ± 0.02.

A minimum of three data points is required. Additional measurements may be carried out, especially on those rare occasions when non-linearity is obtained at a P/P_0 value close to 0.3. Since non-linearity is often obtained at P/P_0 or below 0.05, values in this region are not recommended. The test for linearity, the treatment of the data, and the calculation of the specific surface area of the sample are described above.

IV. REFERENCE MATERIALS

Periodically verify the functioning of the apparatus using appropriate reference materials of known surface area which should have a specific surface area similar to that of the sample to be examined.

01/2005:20927

2.9.27. UNIFORMITY OF MASS OF DELIVERED DOSES FROM MULTIDOSE CONTAINERS

The following test is intended for oral dosage forms such as granules, powders for oral use and liquids for oral use, which are supplied in multidose containers provided at manufacture with a measuring device.

Weigh individually 20 doses taken at random from one or more containers with the measuring device provided and determine the individual and average masses. Not more than 2 of the individual masses deviate from the average mass by more than 10 per cent and none deviates by more than 20 per cent.

01/2005:20928

2.9.28. TEST FOR DELIVERABLE MASS OR VOLUME OF LIQUID AND SEMI-SOLID PREPARATIONS

The test applies to liquid (solutions, emulsions and suspensions) and semi-solid preparations supplied in single-dose containers where only part of the contents is used.

LIQUID PREPARATIONS

Empty as completely as possible the contents of one container and determine the mass or volume of the contents as appropriate. In the case of emulsions and suspensions, shake the container before the determination. The mass or volume is not less than the amount stated on the label.

SEMI-SOLID PREPARATIONS

Empty as completely as possible the contents of one container. The mass of the contents is not less than that which is stated on the label.

3. MATERIALS FOR CONTAINERS AND CONTAINERS

3.1. MATERIALS USED FOR THE MANUFACTURE OF CONTAINERS

01/2005:30100

3.1. MATERIALS USED FOR THE MANUFACTURE OF CONTAINERS

The materials described in this chapter are used for the manufacture of containers for pharmaceutical use. Their use may also be considered for the manufacture of part or all of objects used for medico-surgical purposes.

Materials and polymers other than those described in the Pharmacopoeia may be used subject to approval in each case by the competent authority responsible for the licensing for sale of the preparation in the container.

01/2005:30101

3.1.1. MATERIALS FOR CONTAINERS FOR HUMAN BLOOD AND BLOOD COMPONENTS

NOTE: for materials based on plasticised poly(vinyl chloride) for containers for aqueous solutions for intravenous infusion, see text 3.1.14.

Plastic containers for the collection, storage, processing and administration of blood and its components may be manufactured from one or more polymers, if necessary with certain additives.

If all or part of the container consists of a material described in a text of the Pharmacopoeia, the quality of the material is controlled by the methods indicated in that text. (See *3.1.1.1. Materials based on plasticised poly(vinyl chloride) for containers for human blood and blood components*).

In normal conditions of use the materials and containers made from such materials do not release monomers, or other substances, in amounts likely to be harmful nor do they lead to any abnormal modifications of the blood or blood components.

01/2005:90001

3.1.1.1. MATERIALS BASED ON PLASTICISED POLY(VINYL CHLORIDE) FOR CONTAINERS FOR HUMAN BLOOD AND BLOOD COMPONENTS

DEFINITION

Materials based on plasticised poly(vinyl chloride) contain not less than 55 per cent of poly(vinyl chloride) and contain various additives, in addition to the high-molecular-mass polymer obtained by polymerisation of vinyl chloride.

Materials based on plasticised poly(vinyl chloride) for containers for human blood and blood components are defined by the nature and the proportions of the substances used in their manufacture.

PRODUCTION

Materials based on plasticised poly(vinyl chloride) are produced by polymerisation methods which guarantee a residual vinyl chloride content of less than 1 ppm. The production method used is validated in order to demonstrate that the product complies with the following test:

Vinyl chloride. Not more than 1 ppm, determined by head-space gas chromatography (*2.2.28*), using *ether R* as the internal standard.

Internal standard solution. Using a microsyringe, inject 10 µl of *ether R* into 20.0 ml of *dimethylacetamide R*, immersing the tip of the needle in the solvent. Immediately before use, dilute the solution to 1000 times its volume with *dimethylacetamide R*.

Test solution. Place 1.000 g of the material to be examined in a 50 ml vial and add 10.0 ml of the internal standard solution. Close the vial and secure the stopper. Shake, avoiding contact between the stopper and the liquid. Place the vial in a water-bath at 60 ± 1 °C for 2 h.

Vinyl chloride primary solution. Prepare under a ventilated hood. Place 50.0 ml of *dimethylacetamide R* in a 50 ml vial, stopper the vial, secure the stopper and weigh to the nearest 0.1 mg. Fill a 50 ml polyethylene or polypropylene syringe with gaseous *vinyl chloride R*, allow the gas to remain in contact with the syringe for about 3 min, empty the syringe and fill again with 50 ml of gaseous *vinyl chloride R*. Fit a hypodermic needle to the syringe and reduce the volume of gas in the syringe from 50 ml to 25 ml. Inject the remaining 25 ml of vinyl chloride slowly into the vial shaking gently and avoiding contact between the liquid and the needle. Weigh the vial again; the increase in mass is about 60 mg (1 µl of the solution thus obtained contains about 1.2 µg of vinyl chloride). Allow to stand for 2 hours. Keep the primary solution in a refrigerator.

Vinyl chloride standard solution. To 1 volume of the vinyl chloride primary solution add 3 volumes of *dimethylacetamide R*.

Reference solutions. Place 10.0 ml of the internal standard solution in each of six 50 ml vials. Close the vials and secure the stoppers. Inject 1 µl, 2 µl, 3 µl, 5 µl and 10 µl, respectively, of the vinyl chloride standard solution into five of the vials. The six solutions thus obtained contain, respectively, 0 µg, about 0.3 µg, 0.6 µg, 0.9 µg, 1.5 µg and 3 µg of vinyl chloride. Shake, avoiding contact between the stopper and the liquid. Place the vials in a water-bath at 60 ± 1 °C for 2 h.

The chromatographic procedure may be carried out using:

- a stainless steel column 3 m long and 3 mm in internal diameter packed with *silanised diatomaceous earth for gas chromatography R* impregnated with 5 per cent *m/m* of *dimethylstearylamide R* and 5 per cent *m/m* of *macrogol 400 R*,
- *nitrogen for chromatography R* as the carrier gas at a flow rate of 30 ml/min,
- a flame-ionisation detector,

maintaining the temperature of the column at 45 °C, that of the injection port at 100 °C and that of the detector at 150 °C.

Inject 1 ml of the head-space of each vial. Calculate the content of vinyl chloride.

Additives

A certain number of additives are added to the polymers to optimise their chemical, physical and mechanical properties in order to adapt them for the intended use. All these additives are chosen from the following list which specifies for each product the maximum allowable content:

- not more than 40 per cent of di(2-ethylhexyl)phthalate (plastic additive 01),
- not more than 1 per cent of zinc octanoate (zinc 2-ethylhexanoate) (plastic additive 02),
- not more than 1 per cent of calcium stearate or zinc stearate or 1 per cent of a mixture of the two,

3. Materials/ Containers

- not more than 1 per cent of *N,N'*-diacylethylenediamines (plastic additive 03),
- not more than 10 per cent of one of the following epoxidised oils or 10 per cent of a mixture of the two:
  - epoxidised soya oil (plastic additive 04), of which the oxiran oxygen content is 6 per cent to 8 per cent and the iodine value is not greater than 6,
  - epoxidised linseed oil (plastic additive 05), of which the oxiran oxygen content is not greater than 10 per cent and the iodine value is not greater than 7.

Very low amounts of antioxidants added to the vinyl chloride monomer may be detected in the polymer.

No antioxidant additive may be added to the polymer.

Ultramarine blue is the only colouring material permitted to be added.

The supplier of the material must be able to demonstrate that the qualitative and quantitative composition of the type sample is satisfactory for each production batch.

CHARACTERS

Colourless or pale yellow powder, beads, granules or, after transformation, translucent sheets of varying thickness or containers, with a slight odour. On combustion it gives off dense, black smoke.

IDENTIFICATION

If necessary, before use, cut the samples of the material to be examined into pieces of maximum dimension on a side of not greater than 1 cm.

To 2.0 g of the material to be examined add 200 ml of *peroxide-free ether R* and heat under a reflux condenser for 8 h. Separate the residue B and the solution A by filtration. Evaporate solution A to dryness under reduced pressure in a water-bath at 30 °C. Dissolve the residue in 10 ml of *toluene R* (solution A1). Dissolve the residue B in 60 ml of *ethylene chloride R*, heating on a water-bath under a reflux condenser. Filter. Add the solution dropwise and with vigorous shaking to 600 ml of *heptane R* heated almost to boiling. Separate the coagulum B1 and the organic solution by hot filtration. Allow the latter to cool; separate the precipitate B2 that forms and filter through a tared sintered-glass filter (40).

A. Dissolve the coagulum B1 in 30 ml of *tetrahydrofuran R* and add, in small volumes with shaking, 40 ml of *ethanol R*. Separate the precipitate B3 by filtration and dry *in vacuo* at a temperature not exceeding 50 °C over *diphosphorus pentoxide R*. Dissolve a few milligrams of precipitate B3 in 1 ml of *tetrahydrofuran R*, place a few drops of the solution obtained on a sodium chloride plate and evaporate to dryness in an oven at 100 °C to 105 °C. Examine by infrared absorption spectrophotometry (*2.2.24*), comparing with the spectrum obtained with *poly(vinyl chloride) CRS*.

B. Examine the residue C obtained in the test for plastic additives 01, 04 and 05 by infrared absorption spectrophotometry (*2.2.24*), comparing with the spectrum obtained with *plastic additive 01 CRS*.

TESTS

If necessary, before use, cut samples of the material to be examined into pieces of maximum dimension on a side of not greater than l cm.

Solution S1. Place 5.0 g of the material to be examined in a combustion flask. Add 30 ml of *sulphuric acid R* and heat until a black, syrupy mass is obtained. Cool and add carefully 10 ml of *strong hydrogen peroxide solution R*. Heat gently. Allow to cool and add 1 ml of *strong hydrogen peroxide solution R*; repeat by alternating evaporation and addition of hydrogen peroxide solution until a colourless liquid is obtained. Reduce the volume to about 10 ml. Cool and dilute to 50.0 ml with *water R*.

Solution S2. Place 25 g of the material to be examined in a borosilicate-glass flask. Add 500 ml of *water for injections R* and cover the neck of the flask with a borosilicate-glass beaker. Heat in an autoclave at 121 ± 2 °C for 20 min. Allow to cool and decant the solution. Make the volume up to 500 ml.

Appearance of solution S2. Solution S2 is clear (*2.2.1*) and colourless (*2.2.2, Method II*).

Acidity or alkalinity. To 100 ml of solution S2, add 0.15 ml of *BRP indicator solution R*. Not more than 1.5 ml of *0.01 M sodium hydroxide* is required to change the colour of the indicator to blue. To 100 ml of solution S2 add 0.2 ml of *methyl orange solution R*. Not more than 1.0 ml of *0.01 M hydrochloric acid* is required to initiate the colour change of the indicator from yellow to orange.

Absorbance (*2.2.25*). Evaporate 100.0 ml of solution S2 to dryness. Dissolve the residue in 5.0 ml of *hexane R*. From 250 nm to 310 nm the absorbance is not greater than 0.25.

Reducing substances. *Carry out the test within 4 h of preparation of solution S2.* To 20.0 ml of solution S2 add 1 ml of *dilute sulphuric acid R* and 20.0 ml of *0.002 M potassium permanganate.* Boil under a reflux condenser for 3 min and cool immediately. Add 1 g of *potassium iodide R* and titrate immediately with *0.01 M sodium thiosulphate,* using 0.25 ml of *starch solution R* as indicator. Carry out a blank titration using 20 ml of *water for injections R*. The difference between the two titration volumes is not more than 2.0 ml.

Primary aromatic amines. To 2.5 ml of solution A1 obtained during the identification, add 6 ml of *water R* and 4 ml of *0.1 M hydrochloric acid*. Shake vigorously and discard the upper layer. To the aqueous layer add 0.4 ml of a freshly prepared 10 g/l solution of *sodium nitrite R*. Mix and allow to stand for 1 min. Add 0.8 ml of a 25 g/l solution of *ammonium sulphamate R*, allow to stand for 1 min and add 2 ml of a 5 g/l solution of *naphthylethylenediamine dihydrochloride R*. After 30 min, any colour in the solution is not more intense than that in a standard prepared at the same time in the same manner replacing the aqueous layer with a mixture of 1 ml of a 0.01 g/l solution of *naphthylamine R* in *0.1 M hydrochloric acid*, 5 ml of *water R* and 4 ml of *0.1 M hydrochloric acid* instead of the aqueous layer (20 ppm).

Plastic additives 01, 04 and 05. Examine by thin-layer chromatography (*2.2.27*), using a *TLC silica gel GF_{254} plate R* (1 mm thick).

Reference solutions. Prepare 0.1 mg/ml solutions of *plastic additive 01 CRS, plastic additive 04 CRS* and *plastic additive 05 CRS*, respectively, in *toluene R*.

Apply to the plate as a band 30 mm by 3 mm, 0.5 ml of solution A1 obtained during the identification. Apply to the plate 5 µl of each reference solution. Develop over a path of 15 cm using *toluene R*. Dry the plate carefully. Examine in ultraviolet light at 254 nm and locate the zone corresponding to plastic additive 01 (R_f about 0.4). Remove the area of silica gel corresponding to this zone and shake with 40 ml of *ether R* for 1 min. Filter, rinse with two quantities, each of 10 ml of *ether R*, add the rinsings to the filtrate and evaporate to dryness. The residue C weighs not more than 40 mg.

Expose the plate to iodine vapour for 5 min. Examine the chromatogram and locate the band corresponding to plastic additives 04 and 05 (R_f = 0). Remove the area of silica gel corresponding to this zone. Similarly remove a corresponding area of silica gel as a blank reference. Separately shake both samples for 15 min with 40 ml of *methanol R*. Filter, rinse with two quantities, each of 10 ml of *methanol R*, add the rinsings to the filtrate and evaporate to dryness. The difference between the masses of both residues is not more than 10 mg.

Plastic additive 03. Wash precipitate B2 obtained during the identification and contained in the tared sintered-glass filter (40) with *ethanol R*. Dry to constant mass over *diphosphorus pentoxide R* and weigh the filter. The precipitate weighs not more than 20 mg.

Examine the residue by infrared absorption spectrophotometry (*2.2.24*), comparing with the spectrum obtained with *plastic additive 03 CRS*.

Barium. Not more than 5 ppm of Ba, examined by atomic emission spectrometry in an argon plasma (*2.2.22, Method I*).

Test solution. Ignite 1.0 g of the substance to be examined in a silica crucible. Take up the residue with 10 ml of *hydrochloric acid R* and evaporate to dryness on a water-bath. Take up the residue with 20 ml of *0.1 M hydrochloric acid*.

Reference solution. A solution containing 0.25 ppm of barium prepared by dilution of *barium standard solution (50 ppm Ba) R* with *0.1 M hydrochloric acid*.

Carry out the determination using the emission of barium at 455.40 nm, the spectral background being taken at 455.30 nm.

Verify the absence of barium in the hydrochloric acid used.

Cadmium. Not more than 0.6 ppm of Cd, determined by atomic absorption spectrometry (*2.2.23, Method I*).

Test solution. Evaporate 10 ml of solution S1 to dryness. Take up the residue using 5 ml of a 1 per cent *V/V* solution of *hydrochloric acid R*, filter and dilute the filtrate to 10.0 ml with the same acid solution.

Reference solutions. Prepare the reference solutions using *cadmium standard solution (0.1 per cent Cd) R*, diluted with a 1 per cent *V/V* solution of *hydrochloric acid R*.

Measure the absorbance at 228.8 nm using a cadmium hollow-cathode lamp as the source of radiation and an air-acetylene flame.

Verify the absence of cadmium in the hydrochloric acid used.

Calcium. Not more than 0.07 per cent of Ca, examined by atomic emission spectrometry in an argon plasma (*2.2.22, Method I*).

Test solution. Use the test solution prepared for the determination of barium.

Reference solution. A solution containing 50.0 ppm of calcium prepared by dilution of *calcium standard solution (400 ppm Ca) R* with *0.1 M hydrochloric acid*.

Carry out the determination using the emission of calcium at 315.89 nm, the spectral background being taken at 315.60 nm.

Verify the absence of calcium in the hydrochloric acid used.

Tin. Not more than 20 ppm of Sn, examined by atomic emission spectrometry in an argon plasma (*2.2.22, Method I*).

Test solution. Dilute solution S1 ten times with *water R* immediately before use.

Reference solution. Introduce 2 ml of *tin standard solution (5 ppm (Sn) R)* into a 50 ml flask containing 5 ml of a 20 per cent *V/V* solution of *sulphuric acid R* and dilute to 50 ml with *water R* immediately before use.

Carry out the determination using the emission of tin at 189.99 nm, the spectral background being taken at 190.10 nm.

Verify the absence of tin in the sulphuric acid used.

Zinc. Not more than 0.2 per cent of Zn, determined by atomic absorption spectrometry (*2.2.23, Method I*).

Test solution. Dilute solution S1 100 times with *0.1 M hydrochloric acid*.

Reference solutions. Prepare the reference solutions using *zinc standard solution (100 ppm Zn) R*, diluted with *0.1 M hydrochloric acid*.

Measure the absorbance at 213.9 nm using a zinc hollow-cathode lamp as the source of radiation and an air-acetylene flame.

Verify the absence of zinc in the hydrochloric acid used.

Heavy metals (*2.4.8*). To 10 ml of solution S1 add 0.5 ml of *phenolphthalein solution R* and then *strong sodium hydroxide solution R* until a pale pink colour is obtained. Dilute to 25 ml with *water R*. 12 ml of the solution complies with limit test A (50 ppm). Prepare the standard using *lead standard solution (2 ppm Pb) R*.

Water extractable substances. Evaporate 50 ml of solution S2 to dryness on a water-bath and dry in an oven at 100-105 °C to constant mass. Carry out a blank test with 50.0 ml of *water for injections R*. The residue weighs not more than 7.5 mg (0.3 per cent) taking into account the blank test.

ASSAY

Carry out the oxygen-flask method (*2.5.10*) using 50.0 mg. Absorb the combustion products in 20 ml of *1 M sodium hydroxide*. To the solution obtained add 2.5 ml of *nitric acid R*, 10.0 ml of *0.1 M silver nitrate*, 5 ml of *ferric ammonium sulphate solution R2* and 1 ml of *dibutyl phthalate R*. Titrate with *0.05 M ammonium thiocyanate* until a reddish-yellow colour is obtained. Carry out a blank test.

1 ml of *0.1 M silver nitrate* is equivalent to 6.25 mg of poly(vinyl chloride).

In addition, the following tests are carried out on the sterile and empty containers.

Solution S3. If the container to be examined contains an anticoagulant solution, empty the container and wash the inside with 250 ml of *water for injections R* at 20 ± 1 °C and discard the washings before the preparation of solution S3. Introduce into the container a volume of *water for injections R* corresponding to the volume of solution. Close the container and heat in an autoclave so that the temperature of the liquid is maintained at 110 °C for 30 min. After cooling, fill the container with *water for injections R* to its nominal volume and homogenise.

Reference solution. Heat *water for injections R* in a borosilicate-glass flask in an autoclave at 110 °C for 30 min.

Reducing substances. Immediately after preparation of solution S3, transfer to a borosilicate-glass flask a volume corresponding to 8 per cent of the nominal volume of the container. At the same time, prepare a blank using an equal volume of the freshly prepared reference solution in another borosilicate-glass flask. To each solution add 20.0 ml of *0.002 M potassium permanganate* and 1 ml of *dilute sulphuric acid R*. Allow to stand protected from light for 15 min. To each solution add 0.1 g of *potassium iodide R*. Allow to stand protected from light for 5 min and titrate immediately with *0.01 M sodium thiosulphate*, using 0.25 ml of *starch solution R* as indicator. The difference between the two titrations is not more than 2.0 ml.

3. Materials/ Containers

Acidity or alkalinity. To a volume of solution S3 corresponding to 4 per cent of the nominal capacity of the container add 0.1 ml of *phenolphthalein solution R*. The solution remains colourless. Add 0.4 ml of *0.01 M sodium hydroxide*. The solution is pink. Add 0.8 ml of *0.01 M hydrochloric acid* and 0.1 ml of *methyl red solution R*. The solution is orange-red or red.

Chlorides (*2.4.4*). 15 ml of solution S3 complies with the limit test for chlorides (0.4 ppm). Prepare the standard using a mixture of 1.2 ml of *chloride standard solution (5 ppm Cl) R* and 13.8 ml of *water R*.

Ammonium (*2.4.1*). Dilute 5 ml of solution S3 to 14 ml with *water R*. The solution complies with limit test A (2 ppm).

Water extractable substances. Evaporate 100 ml of solution S3 to dryness on a water-bath. Dry in an oven to constant mass at 100-105 °C. Carry out a blank test using 100 ml of the reference solution. The residue from solution S3 weighs not more than 3 mg, taking into account the blank test.

Absorbance (*2.2.25*). Measure the absorbance of solution S3 from 230 nm to 360 nm, using the reference solution as compensation liquid. At wavelengths from 230 nm to 250 nm, the absorbance is not greater than 0.30. At wavelengths from 251 nm to 360 nm, the absorbance is not greater than 0.10.

Extractable plastic additive 01. Use as the extraction solvent, *alcohol R* diluted with *water R* to have a relative density (*2.2.5*) of 0.9389 to 0.9395, measured with a densimeter.

Stock solution. Dissolve 0.100 g of *plastic additive 01 CRS* in the extraction solvent and dilute to 100.0 ml with the same solvent.

Standard solutions:

(*a*) Dilute 20.0 ml of the stock solution to 100.0 ml with the extraction solvent,

(*b*) Dilute 10.0 ml of the stock solution to 100.0 ml with the extraction solvent,

(*c*) Dilute 5.0 ml of the stock solution to 100.0 ml with the extraction solvent,

(*d*) Dilute 2.0 ml of the stock solution to 100.0 ml with the extraction solvent,

(*e*) Dilute 1.0 ml of the stock solution to 100.0 ml with the extraction solvent.

Measure the absorbances (*2.2.25*) of the standard solutions at the maximum at 272 nm, using the extraction solvent as compensation liquid and plot a curve of absorbance against the concentration of plastic additive 01.

Extraction procedure. Using the donor tubing and the needle or adapter, fill the empty container with a volume equal to half the nominal volume with the extraction solvent, previously heated to 37 °C in a well-stoppered flask. Expel the air completely from the container and seal the donor tubing. Immerse the filled container in a horizontal position in a water-bath maintained at 37 ± 1 °C for 60 ± 1 min without shaking. Remove the container from the water-bath, invert it gently ten times and transfer the contents to a glass flask. Immediately measure the absorbance at the maximum at 272 nm, using the extraction solvent as compensation liquid.

Determine the concentration of plastic additive 01 in milligrams per 100 ml of extract from the calibration curve. The concentration does not exceed:

– 10 mg per 100 ml for containers of nominal volume greater than 300 ml but not greater than 500 ml;
– 13 mg per 100 ml for containers of nominal volume greater than 150 ml but not greater than 300 ml;
– 14 mg per 100 ml for containers of nominal volume up to 150 ml.

Where containers contain an anticoagulant solution, this solution complies with the monograph on Anticoagulant and preservative solutions for human blood (0209) and the following additional test.

Absorbance (*2.2.25*). Measure the absorbance of the anticoagulant solution from the container between 250 nm and 350 nm, using as the compensation liquid an anticoagulant solution of the same composition that has not been in contact with a plastic material. The absorbance at the maximum at 280 nm is not greater than 0.5.

01/2005:90002

3.1.1.2. MATERIALS BASED ON PLASTICISED POLY(VINYL CHLORIDE) FOR TUBING USED IN SETS FOR THE TRANSFUSION OF BLOOD AND BLOOD COMPONENTS

DEFINITION

Materials based on plasticised poly(vinyl chloride) for transfusion of blood and blood components contain not less than 55 per cent of poly(vinyl chloride) with di(2-ethylhexyl) phthalate (plastic additive 01) as plasticiser.

PRODUCTION

Materials based on plasticised poly(vinyl chloride) are produced by polymerisation methods which guarantee a residual vinyl chloride content of less than 1 ppm. The production method used is validated in order to demonstrate that the product complies with the following test:

Vinyl chloride. Not more than 1 ppm, determined by head-space gas chromatography (*2.2.28*), using *ether R* as the internal standard.

Internal standard solution. Using a microsyringe, inject 10 μl of *ether R* into 20.0 ml of *dimethylacetamide R*, immersing the tip of the needle in the solvent. Immediately before use, dilute the solution to 1000 times its volume with *dimethylacetamide R*.

Test solution. Place 1.000 g of the material to be examined in a 50 ml vial and add 10.0 ml of the internal standard solution. Close the vial and secure the stopper. Shake, avoiding contact between the stopper and the liquid. Place the vial in a water-bath at 60 ± 1 °C for 2 h.

Vinyl chloride primary solution. Prepare under a ventilated hood. Place 50.0 ml of *dimethylacetamide R* in a 50 ml vial, stopper the vial, secure the stopper and weigh to the nearest 0.1 mg. Fill a 50 ml polyethylene or polypropylene syringe with gaseous *vinyl chloride R*, allow the gas to remain in contact with the syringe for about 3 min, empty the syringe and fill again with 50 ml of gaseous *vinyl chloride R*. Fit a hypodermic needle to the syringe and reduce the volume of gas in the syringe from 50 ml to 25 ml. Inject the remaining 25 ml of vinyl chloride slowly into the vial shaking gently and avoiding contact between the liquid and the needle. Weigh the vial again; the increase in mass is about 60 mg (1 μl of the solution thus obtained contains about 1.2 μg of vinyl chloride). Allow to stand for 2 h. Keep the primary solution in a refrigerator.

Vinyl chloride standard solution. To 1 volume of the vinyl chloride primary solution add 3 volumes of *dimethylacetamide R*.

Reference solutions. Place 10.0 ml of the internal standard solution in each of six 50 ml vials. Close the vials and secure the stoppers. Inject 1 µl, 2 µl, 3 µl, 5 µl and 10 µl, respectively, of the vinyl chloride standard solution into five of the vials. The six solutions thus obtained contain respectively, 0 µg, about 0.3 µg, 0.6 µg, 0.9 µg, 1.5 µg and 3 µg of vinyl chloride. Shake, avoiding contact between the stopper and the liquid. Place the vials in a water-bath at 60 ± 1 °C for 2 h.

The chromatographic procedure may be carried out using:

– a stainless steel column 3 m long and 3 mm in internal diameter packed with *silanised diatomaceous earth for gas chromatography R* impregnated with 5 per cent *m/m* of *dimethylstearylamide R* and 5 per cent *m/m* of *macrogol 400 R*,
– *nitrogen for chromatography R* as the carrier gas at a flow rate of 30 ml/min,
– a flame-ionisation detector,

maintaining the temperature of the column at 45 °C, that of the injection port at 100 °C and that of the detector at 150 °C.

Inject 1 ml of the head-space of each vial. Calculate the content of vinyl chloride.

The supplier of the material must be able to demonstrate that the qualitative and quantitative composition of the type sample is satisfactory for each production batch.

CHARACTERS

Almost colourless or pale-yellow material in the form of powder, beads, granules or, after transformation, tubes with a slight odour. On combustion it gives off dense, black smoke.

IDENTIFICATION

If necessary, cut samples of the material to be examined into pieces of maximum dimension on a side of not greater than 1 cm.

A. To 0.5 g add 30 ml of *tetrahydrofuran R*. Heat with stirring on a water-bath under a hood for 10 min. The material dissolves completely. Add *methanol R* dropwise with stirring. A granular precipitate is formed. Filter the precipitate and dry at 60 °C. Examine the precipitate by infrared absorption spectrophotometry (*2.2.24*). Dissolve 50 mg in 2 ml of *tetrahydrofuran R* and pour on a glass slide. Dry in an oven at 80 °C, remove the film and fix on a suitable mount. Examine by infrared absorption spectrophotometry (*2.2.24*), comparing with the spectrum obtained with *poly(vinyl chloride) CRS*.

B. Examine the residue obtained in the test Plastic additive 01 by infrared absorption spectrophotometry (*2.2.24*), comparing with the spectrum obtained with *plastic additive 01 CRS*.

TESTS

If necessary, cut the material to be examined into pieces with a maximum dimension on a side of not greater than 1 cm.

Solution S1. Place 5.0 g of the material to be examined in a combustion flask. Add 30 ml of *sulphuric acid R* and heat until a black, syrupy mass is obtained. Cool and add carefully 10 ml of *strong hydrogen peroxide solution R*. Heat gently. Allow to cool and add 1 ml of *strong hydrogen peroxide solution R*; repeat by alternating evaporation and addition of hydrogen peroxide solution until a colourless liquid is obtained. Reduce the volume to about 10 ml. Cool and dilute to 50.0 ml with *water R*.

Solution S2. Place 25 g of the material to be examined in a borosilicate-glass flask. Add 500 ml of *water R* and cover the neck of the flask with a borosilicate-glass beaker. Heat in an autoclave at 121 ± 2 °C for 20 min. Allow to cool and decant the solution and make up to a volume of 500 ml.

Appearance of solution S2. Solution S2 is clear (*2.2.1*) and colourless (*2.2.2, Method II*).

Plastic additive 01. Examine by thin-layer chromatography (*2.2.27*), using a *TLC silica gel G plate R*.

Test solution. To 2.0 g of the material to be examined add 200 ml of *peroxide-free ether R* and heat under a reflux condenser for 8 h. Separate the residue and the solution by filtration and evaporate the solution to dryness under reduced pressure in a water-bath at 30 °C. Dissolve the residue in 10 ml of *toluene R*.

Reference solution. Dissolve 0.8 g of *plastic additive 01 CRS* in *toluene R* and dilute to 10 ml with the same solvent.

Apply separately to the plate as a band 30 mm by 3 mm 0.5 ml of the test solution and 5 µl of the reference solution. Develop over a path of 15 cm using *toluene R*. Dry the plate carefully. Examine the chromatogram obtained in ultraviolet light at 254 nm and locate the zone corresponding to plastic additive 01. Remove the area of silica gel corresponding to this zone and shake with 40 ml of *ether R*. Filter without loss and evaporate to dryness. The residue weighs not more than 40 mg.

Barium. Not more than 5 ppm of Ba, examined by atomic emission spectrometry in an argon plasma (*2.2.22, Method I*).

Test solution. Ignite 1.0 g of the substance to be examined in a silica crucible. Take up the residue with 10 ml of *hydrochloric acid R* and evaporate to dryness on a water-bath. Take up the residue with 20 ml of *0.1 M hydrochloric acid*.

Reference solution. A solution containing 0.25 ppm of barium prepared by dilution of *barium standard solution (50 ppm Ba) R* with *0.1 M hydrochloric acid*.

Carry out the determination using the emission of barium at 455.40 nm, the spectral background being taken at 455.30 nm.

Verify the absence of barium in the hydrochloric acid used.

Cadmium. Not more than 0.6 ppm of Cd, determined by atomic absorption spectrophotometry (*2.2.23, Method I*).

Test solution. Evaporate 10.0 ml of solution S1 to dryness. Take up the residue using 5 ml of a 1 per cent *V/V* solution of *hydrochloric acid R*, filter and dilute the filtrate to 10.0 ml with the same acid.

Reference solutions. Prepare the reference solutions using *cadmium standard solution (0.1 per cent Cd) R*, diluted with a 1 per cent *V/V* solution of *hydrochloric acid R*.

Measure the absorbance at 228.8 nm using a cadmium hollow-cathode lamp as source of radiation and an air-acetylene flame.

Verify the absence of cadmium in the hydrochloric acid used.

Tin. Not more than 20 ppm of Sn, examined by atomic emission spectrometry in an argon plasma (*2.2.22, Method I*).

Test solution. Dilute solution S1 ten times with *water R* immediately before use.

Reference solution. Introduce 2 ml of *tin standard solution (5 ppm Sn) R* into a 50 ml flask containing 5 ml of a 20 per cent *V/V* solution of *sulphuric acid R* and dilute to 50 ml with *water R* immediately before use.

Carry out the determination using the emission of tin at 189.99 nm, the spectral background being taken at 190.10 nm.

Verify the absence of tin in the sulphuric acid used.

Heavy metals (*2.4.8*). To 10 ml of solution S1 add 0.5 ml of *phenolphthalein solution R* and then *strong sodium hydroxide solution R* until a pale pink colour is obtained. Dilute to 25 ml with *water R*. 12 ml of the solution complies with limit test A for heavy metals (50 ppm). Prepare the standard using *lead standard solution (2 ppm Pb) R*.

ASSAY

To 0.500 g add 30 ml of *tetrahydrofuran R* and heat with stirring on a water-bath under a hood for 10 min. The material dissolves completely. Add 60 ml of *methanol R* dropwise with stirring. A granular precipitate of poly(vinyl chloride) is formed. Allow to stand for a few minutes. Continue addition of *methanol R* until no further precipitation is observed. Transfer to a sintered-glass filter (40), using three small quantities of *methanol R* to aid transfer and to wash the precipitate. Dry the filter and the precipitate to constant mass at 60 °C and weigh.

In addition, carry out the following tests on sterilised sets.

Solution S3. Make a closed circulation system from three sets and a 300 ml borosilicate-glass vessel. Fit to the vessel a thermostat device that maintains the temperature of the liquid in the vessel at 37 ± 1 °C. Circulate 250 ml of *water for injections R* through the system in the direction used for transfusion for 2 h at a rate of 1 litre per hour (for example using a peristaltic pump applied to as short a piece of suitable silicone tubing as possible). Collect the whole of the solution and allow to cool.

Appearance of solution. Solution S3 is clear (*2.2.1*) and colourless (*2.2.2, Method II*).

Acidity or alkalinity. To 25 ml of solution S3 add 0.15 ml of *BRP indicator solution R*. Not more than 0.5 ml of *0.01 M sodium hydroxide* is required to change the colour of the indicator to blue. To 25 ml of solution S3 add 0.2 ml of *methyl orange solution R*. Not more than 0.5 ml of *0.01 M hydrochloric acid* is required to initiate the colour change of the indicator from yellow to orange.

Absorbance (*2.2.25*). Examined from 230 nm to 250 nm, solution S3 shows no absorbance greater than 0.30. Examined from 251 nm to 360 nm, solution S3 shows no absorbance greater than 0.15.

Reducing substances. Carry out the test within 4 h of preparation of solution S3. To 20.0 ml of solution S3 add 1 ml of *dilute sulphuric acid R* and 20.0 ml of *0.002 M potassium permanganate*. Boil for 3 min and cool immediately. Add 1 g of *potassium iodide R* and titrate with *0.01 M sodium thiosulphate* using 0.25 ml of *starch solution R* as indicator. Carry out a blank test using 20 ml of *water for injections R*. The difference between the titration volumes is not greater than 2.0 ml.

Water extractable substances. Evaporate 50.0 ml of solution S3 to dryness on a water-bath and dry to constant mass in an oven at 100 °C to 105 °C. Carry out a blank test using 50.0 ml of *water for injections R*. The residue obtained with solution S3 is not greater than 1.5 mg, taking account of the blank test.

01/2005:30103

3.1.3. POLYOLEFINES

DEFINITION

Polyolefines are obtained by polymerisation of ethylene or propylene or by copolymerisation of these substances with not more than 25 per cent of higher homologues (C_4 to C_{10}) or of carboxylic acids or of esters. Certain materials may be mixtures of polyolefines.

PRODUCTION

A certain number of additives are added to the polymer in order to optimise their chemical, physical and mechanical properties in order to adapt them for the intended use. All of these additives are chosen from the appended list which specifies for each product the maximum allowable content.

They may contain at most 3 antioxidants, one or several lubricants or antiblocking agents as well as titanium dioxide as an opacifying agent when the material must provide protection from light.

- butylhydroxytoluene (plastic additive 07) (not more than 0.125 per cent),
- pentaerythrityl tetrakis[3-(3,5-di-*tert*-butyl-4-hydroxyphenyl)propionate] (plastic additive 09) (not more than 0.3 per cent),
- 1,3,5-tris(3,5-di-*tert*-butyl-4-hydroxybenzyl)-*s*-triazine-2,4,6(1*H*,3*H*,5*H*)-trione, (plastic additive 13) (not more than 0.3 per cent),
- octadecyl 3-(3,5-di-*tert*-butyl-4-hydroxyphenyl)propionate (plastic additive 11) (not more than 0.3 per cent),
- ethylene bis[3,3-bis[3-(1,1-dimethylethyl)-4-hydroxyphenyl]butanoate] (plastic additive 08) (not more than 0.3 per cent),
- dioctadecyl disulphide (plastic additive 15) (not more than 0.3 per cent),
- 4,4′,4″-(2,4,6-trimethylbenzene-1,3,5-triyltrismethylene)trio[2,6-bis(1,1-dimethylethyl)phenol] (plastic additive 10) (not more than 0.3 per cent),
- 2,2′-bis(octadecyloxy)-5,5′-spirobi[1,3,2-dioxaphosphinane] (plastic additive 14) (not more than 0.3 per cent),
- didodecyl 3,3′-thiodipropionate (plastic additive 16) (not more than 0.3 per cent),
- dioctadecyl 3,3′-thiodipropionate (plastic additive 17) (not more than 0.3 per cent),
- tris[2,4-bis(1,1-dimethylethyl)phenyl] phosphite (plastic additive 12) (not more than 0.3 per cent),
- plastic additive 18 (not more than 0.1 per cent),
- copolymer of dimethyl succinate and (4-hydroxy-2,2,6,6-tetramethylpiperidin-1-yl)ethanol (plastic additive 22) (not more than 0.3 per cent).

The total of antioxidant additives listed above does not exceed 0.3 per cent.

- hydrotalcite (not more than 0.5 per cent),
- alkanamides (not more than 0.5 per cent),
- alkenamides (not more than 0.5 per cent),
- sodium silico-aluminate (not more than 0.5 per cent),
- silica (not more than 0.5 per cent),
- sodium benzoate (not more than 0.5 per cent),
- fatty acid esters or salts (not more than 0.5 per cent),
- trisodium phosphate (not more than 0.5 per cent),
- liquid paraffin (not more than 0.5 per cent),
- zinc oxide (not more than 0.5 per cent),

– talc (not more than 0.5 per cent),
– magnesium oxide (not more than 0.2 per cent),
– calcium stearate or zinc stearate or a mixture of both (not more than 0.5 per cent),
– titanium dioxide (not more than 4 per cent).

The supplier of the material must be able to demonstrate that the qualitative and quantitative composition of the type sample is satisfactory for each production batch.

CHARACTERS

Powder, beads, granules or, after transformation, sheets of varying thickness or containers. They are practically insoluble in water, soluble in hot aromatic hydrocarbons, practically insoluble in ethanol, in hexane and in methanol. They soften at temperatures between 65 °C and 165 °C. They burn with a blue flame.

IDENTIFICATION

If necessary, cut samples of the material to be examined into pieces of maximum dimension on a side of not greater than 1 cm.

A. To 0.25 g add 10 ml of *toluene R* and boil under a reflux condenser for about 15 min. Place a few drops of the solution obtained on a sodium chloride slide and evaporate the solvent in an oven at 80 °C. Examine by infrared absorption spectrophotometry (*2.2.24*). The spectrum of the material to be examined shows maxima in particular at some of the following wave-numbers: 2920 cm^{-1}, 2850 cm^{-1}, 1475 cm^{-1}, 1465 cm^{-1}, 1380 cm^{-1}, 1170 cm^{-1}, 735 cm^{-1}, 720 cm^{-1}; the spectrum obtained is identical to the spectrum obtained with the material selected for the type sample. If the material to be examined is in the form of sheets, the identification may be determined directly on a cut piece of suitable size.

B. It complies with the supplementary tests corresponding to the additives present.

C. In a platinum crucible, mix about 20 mg with 1 g of *potassium hydrogen sulphate R* and heat until completely melted. Allow to cool and add 20 ml of *dilute sulphuric acid R*. Heat gently. Filter the resulting solution. To the filtrate add 1 ml of *phosphoric acid R* and 1 ml of *strong hydrogen peroxide solution R*. If the substance is opacified with titanium dioxide, an orange-yellow colour develops.

TESTS

If necessary, cut samples of the material to be examined into pieces of maximum dimension on a side of not greater than 1 cm.

Solution S1. *Use solution S1 within 4 h of preparation.* Place 25 g in a borosilicate-glass flask with a ground-glass neck. Add 500 ml of *water for injections R* and boil under a reflux condenser for 5 h. Allow to cool and decant. Reserve a portion of the solution for the test for appearance of solution S1 and filter the rest through a sintered-glass filter (16).

Solution S2. Place 2.0 g in a conical borosilicate-glass flask with a ground-glass neck. Add 80 ml of *toluene R* and boil under a reflux condenser with constant stirring for 90 min. Allow to cool to 60 °C and add with continued stirring 120 ml of *methanol R*. Filter the solution through a sintered-glass filter (16). Rinse the flask and the filter with 25 ml of a mixture of 40 ml of *toluene R* and 60 ml of *methanol R*, add the rinsings to the filtrate and dilute to 250 ml with the same mixture of solvents. Prepare a blank solution.

Solution S3. Place 100 g in a conical borosilicate-glass flask with a ground-glass neck. Add 250 ml of *0.1 M hydrochloric acid* and boil under a reflux condenser with constant stirring for 1 h. Allow to cool and decant the solution.

Appearance of solution S1. Solution S1 is clear (*2.2.1*) and colourless (*2.2.2, Method II*).

Acidity or alkalinity. To 100 ml of solution S1, add 0.15 ml of *BRP indicator solution R*. Not more than 1.5 ml of *0.01 M sodium hydroxide* is required to change the colour of the indicator to blue. To 100 ml of solution S1 add 0.2 ml of *methyl orange solution R*. Not more than 1 ml of *0.01 M hydrochloric acid* is required to initiate the colour change of the indicator from yellow to orange.

Absorbance (*2.2.25*). At wavelengths from 220 nm to 340 nm, the absorbance of solution S1 is not greater than 0.2.

Reducing substances. To 20 ml of solution S1 add 1 ml of *dilute sulphuric acid R* and 20 ml of *0.002 M potassium permanganate*. Boil under a reflux condenser for 3 min and cool immediately. Add 1 g of *potassium iodide R* and titrate immediately with *0.01 M sodium thiosulphate*, using 0.25 ml of *starch solution R* as indicator. Carry out a blank titration. The difference between the titration volumes is not more than 3.0 ml.

Substances soluble in hexane. Place 10 g in a 250 ml conical borosilicate-glass flask with a ground-glass neck. Add 100 ml of *hexane R* and boil under a reflux condenser for 4 h, stirring constantly. Cool in iced water and filter rapidly (the filtration time must be less than 5 min; if necessary the filtration may be accelerated by applying pressure to the solution) through a sintered-glass filter (16) maintaining the solution at about 0 °C. Evaporate 20 ml of the filtrate in a tared borosilicate-glass dish on a water-bath. Dry the residue in an oven at 100-105 °C for 1 h. The mass of the residue obtained must be within 10 per cent of that of the residue obtained with the type sample and does not exceed 5 per cent.

Extractable aluminium. Not more than 1 ppm of extractable Al, determined by atomic emission spectrometry in an argon plasma (*2.2.22, Method I*).

Test solution. Use solution S3.

Reference solutions. Prepare the reference solutions using *aluminium standard solution (200 ppm Al) R*, diluted with *0.1 M hydrochloric acid.*

Carry out the determination using the emission of aluminium at 396.15 nm, the spectral background being taken as 396.25 nm.

Verify the absence of aluminium in the hydrochloric acid used.

Extractable titanium. Not more than 1 ppm of extractable Ti, determined by atomic emission spectrometry in an argon plasma (*2.2.22, Method I*).

Test solution. Use solution S3.

Reference solutions. Prepare the reference solutions using *titanium standard solution (100 ppm Ti) R*, diluted with *0.1 M hydrochloric acid.*

Carry out the determination using the emission of titanium at 336.12 nm, the spectral background being taken as 336.16 nm.

Verify the absence of titanium in the hydrochloric acid used.

Extractable zinc. Not more than 1 ppm of extractable Zn, determined by atomic absorption spectrometry (*2.2.23, Method I*).

Test solution. Use solution S3.

Reference solutions. Prepare the reference solutions using *zinc standard solution (10 ppm Zn) R*, diluted with *0.1 M hydrochloric acid*.

Measure the absorbance at 213.9 nm using a zinc hollow-cathode lamp as a source of radiation and an air-acetylene flame.

Verify the absence of zinc in the hydrochloric acid used.

Extractable heavy metals (*2.4.8*). Evaporate 50 ml of solution S3 to about 5 ml on a water-bath and dilute to 20.0 ml with *water R*. 12 ml of the solution complies with limit test A for heavy metals (2.5 ppm). Prepare the standard using 2.5 ml of *lead standard solution (10 ppm Pb) R*.

Sulphated ash (*2.4.14*). Not more than 1.0 per cent, determined on 5.0 g. This limit does not apply to material that has been opacified with titanium dioxide.

SUPPLEMENTARY TESTS

These tests are to be carried out, in whole or in part, only if required by the stated composition or the use of the material.

Phenolic antioxidants. Examine by liquid chromatography (*2.2.29*).

The chromatographic procedure may be carried out using:

- a stainless steel column 0.25 m long and 4.6 mm in internal diameter packed with *octadecylsilyl silica gel for chromatography R* (5 µm),
- as mobile phase one of the 4 following mixtures:

  Mobile phase 1 at a flow rate of 2 ml/min: 30 volumes of *water R*, 70 volumes of *acetonitrile R*,

  Mobile phase 2 at a flow rate of 1.5 ml/min: 10 volumes of *water R*, 30 volumes of *tetrahydrofuran R*, 60 volumes of *acetonitrile R*,

  Mobile phase 3 at a flow rate of 1.5 ml/min: 5 volumes of *water R*, 45 volumes of *2-propanol R*, 50 volumes of *methanol R*,

  Mobile phase 4 at a flow rate of 1.5 ml/min: 20 volumes of *tetrahydrofuran R*, 80 volumes of *acetonitrile R*,
- as detector a spectrophotometer set at 280 nm for mobile phases 1 to 3, and set at 270 nm for mobile phase 4.

The chromatographic system must ensure the following:

- a resolution of not less than 8.0 between the peaks corresponding to plastic additive 07 and plastic additive 08, with mobile phase 1,
- a resolution of not less than 2.0 between the peaks corresponding to plastic additive 09 and plastic additive 10, with mobile phase 2,
- a resolution of not less than 2.0 between the peaks corresponding to plastic additive 11 and plastic additive 12, with mobile phase 3,
- a resolution of not less than 6.0 between the 2 principal peaks (approximate retention times of 3.5 and 5.8) in the chromatogram obtained with plastic additive 18, with mobile phase 4.

Test solution S21. Evaporate 50 ml of solution S2 to dryness *in vacuo* at 45 °C. Dissolve the residue in 5.0 ml of a mixture of equal volumes of *acetonitrile R* and *tetrahydrofuran R*. Prepare a blank solution from the blank solution corresponding to solution S2.

Test solution S22. Evaporate 50 ml of solution S2 to dryness *in vacuo* at 45 °C. Dissolve the residue with 5.0 ml of *methylene chloride R*. Prepare a blank solution from the blank solution corresponding to solution S2.

Test solution S23. Evaporate 50 ml of solution S2 to dryness *in vacuo* at 45 °C. Dissolve the residue in 5.0 ml of a mixture of equal volumes of *acetonitrile R* and a 10 g/l solution of *tert-butylhydroperoxide R* in *tetrahydrofuran R*. Close the flask and allow to stand for 1 h. Prepare a blank solution using the blank of solution S2.

Of the following reference solutions, prepare only those that are necessary for the analysis of the phenolic antioxidants stated in the composition of the substance to be examined.

Reference solution (a). Dissolve 25.0 mg of *butylhydroxytoluene CRS* (plastic additive 07) and 60.0 mg of *plastic additive 08 CRS* in 10.0 ml of a mixture of equal volumes of *acetonitrile R* and *tetrahydrofuran R*. Dilute 2.0 ml to 50.0 ml with a mixture of equal volumes of *acetonitrile R* and *tetrahydrofuran R*.

Reference solution (b). Dissolve 60.0 mg of *plastic additive 09 CRS* and 60.0 mg of *plastic additive 10 CRS* in 10.0 ml of a mixture of equal volumes of *acetonitrile R* and *tetrahydrofuran R*. Dilute 2.0 ml to 50.0 ml with a mixture of equal volumes of *acetonitrile R* and *tetrahydrofuran R*.

Reference solution (c). Dissolve 60.0 mg of *plastic additive 11 CRS* and 60.0 mg of *plastic additive 12 CRS* in 10.0 ml of *methylene chloride R*. Dilute 2.0 ml to 50.0 ml with *methylene chloride R*.

Reference solution (d). Dissolve 25.0 mg of *plastic additive 07 CRS* in 10.0 ml of a mixture of equal volumes of *acetonitrile R* and *tetrahydrofuran R*. Dilute 2.0 ml to 50.0 ml with a mixture of equal volumes of *acetonitrile R* and *tetrahydrofuran R*.

Reference solution (e). Dissolve 60.0 mg of *plastic additive 08 CRS* in 10.0 ml of a mixture of equal volumes of *acetonitrile R* and *tetrahydrofuran R*. Dilute 2.0 ml to 50.0 ml with a mixture of equal volumes of *acetonitrile R* and *tetrahydrofuran R*.

Reference solution (f). Dissolve 60.0 mg of *plastic additive 13 CRS* in 10.0 ml of a mixture of equal volumes of *acetonitrile R* and *tetrahydrofuran R*. Dilute 2.0 ml to 50.0 ml with a mixture of equal volumes of *acetonitrile R* and *tetrahydrofuran R*.

Reference solution (g). Dissolve 60.0 mg of *plastic additive 09 CRS* in 10.0 ml of a mixture of equal volumes of *acetonitrile R* and *tetrahydrofuran R*. Dilute 2.0 ml to 50.0 ml with a mixture of equal volumes of *acetonitrile R* and *tetrahydrofuran R*.

Reference solution (h). Dissolve 60.0 mg of *plastic additive 10 CRS* in 10.0 ml of a mixture of equal volumes of *acetonitrile R* and *tetrahydrofuran R*. Dilute 2.0 ml to 50.0 ml with a mixture of equal volumes of *acetonitrile R* and *tetrahydrofuran R*.

Reference solution (i). Dissolve 60.0 mg of *plastic additive 11 CRS* in 10.0 ml of *methylene chloride R*. Dilute 2.0 ml to 50.0 ml with *methylene chloride R*.

Reference solution (j). Dissolve 60.0 mg of *plastic additive 12 CRS* in 10.0 ml of *methylene chloride R*. Dilute 2.0 ml to 50.0 ml with *methylene chloride R*.

Reference solution (k). Dissolve 20.0 mg of *plastic additive 18 CRS* in 10.0 ml of a mixture of equal volumes of *acetonitrile R* and a 10 g/l solution of *tert-butylhydroperoxide R* in *tetrahydrofuran R*. Allow to stand in a closed container for 1 h. Dilute 2.0 ml of the solution to 50.0 ml with a mixture of equal volumes of *acetonitrile R* and *tetrahydrofuran R*.

If the substance to be examined contains plastic additive 07 and/or plastic additive 08, use mobile phase 1 and inject 20 µl of test solution S21, 20 µl of the corresponding blank solution, 20 µl of reference solution (a), and either 20 µl each of reference solutions (d) or (e) or 20 µl each of reference solutions (d) and (e).

If the substance to be examined contains one or more of the following antioxidants:

- plastic additive 09,
- plastic additive 10,
- plastic additive 11,
- plastic additive 12,
- plastic additive 13,

use mobile phase 2 and inject 20 µl of test solution S21, 20 µl of the corresponding blank solution, 20 µl of reference solution (b) and 20 µl of each of the reference solutions of the antioxidants on the list above that are stated in the composition.

If the substance to be examined contains plastic additive 11 and/or plastic additive 12, use mobile phase 3 and inject 20 µl of test solution S22, 20 µl of the corresponding blank solution, 20 µl of reference solution (c), and either 20 µl of reference solution (i) or (j) or 20 µl of reference solutions (i) and (j).

If the substance to be examined contains plastic additive 18, use mobile phase 4 and inject 20 µl of test solution S23, 20 µl of the corresponding blank solution, and 20 µl of reference solution (k).

In all cases, record the chromatogram for 30 min; the chromatograms corresponding to test solutions S21, S22 and S23 only show peaks due to antioxidants stated in the composition and minor peaks that also appear in the chromatograms corresponding to the blank solutions. The areas of the peaks corresponding to test solutions S21, S22 and S23 are less than the corresponding areas of the peaks in the chromatograms obtained with reference solutions (d) to (k).

Non-phenolic antioxidants. Examine by thin-layer chromatography (*2.2.27*), using a *TLC silica gel GF_{254} plate R*.

Test solution S24. Evaporate 100 ml of solution S2 to dryness *in vacuo* at 45 °C. Dissolve the residue in 2 ml of *acidified methylene chloride R*.

Reference solution (l). Dissolve 60 mg of *plastic additive 14 CRS* in 10 ml of *methylene chloride R*. Dilute 2 ml of the solution to 10 ml with *acidified methylene chloride R*.

Reference solution (m). Dissolve 60 mg of *plastic additive 15 CRS* in 10 ml of *methylene chloride R*. Dilute 2 ml of the solution to 10 ml with *acidified methylene chloride R*.

Reference solution (n). Dissolve 60 mg of *plastic additive 16 CRS* in 10 ml of *methylene chloride R*. Dilute 2 ml of the solution to 10 ml with *acidified methylene chloride R*.

Reference solution (o). Dissolve 60 mg of *plastic additive 17 CRS* in 10 ml of *methylene chloride R*. Dilute 2 ml of the solution to 10 ml with *acidified methylene chloride R*.

Reference solution (p). Dissolve 60 mg of *plastic additive 16 CRS* and 60 mg of *plastic additive 17 CRS* in 10 ml of *methylene chloride R*. Dilute 2 ml of the solution to 10 ml with *acidified methylene chloride R*.

Apply separately to the plate 20 µl of test solution S24, 20 µl of reference solution (p) and 20 µl of each of the reference solutions corresponding to all the phenolic and non-phenolic antioxidants mentioned in the type composition of the material to be examined.

Develop over a path of 18 cm using *hexane R*. Allow the plate to dry. Develop a second time over a path of 17 cm using *methylene chloride R*. Allow the plate to dry and examine in ultraviolet light at 254 nm. Spray with *alcoholic iodine solution R* and examine in ultraviolet light at 254 nm after 10-15 min. Any spots in the chromatogram obtained with test solution S24 are not more intense than the spots in the corresponding positions in the chromatograms obtained with the reference solutions. The test is not valid unless the chromatogram obtained with reference solution (p) shows 2 clearly separated spots.

Plastic additive 22. Examine by liquid chromatography (*2.2.29*).

Test solution. Evaporate 25 ml of solution S2 to dryness *in vacuo* at 45 °C. Dissolve the residue in 10 ml of *toluene R* and 10 ml of a 10 g/l solution of *tetrabutylammonium hydroxide R* in a mixture of 35 volumes of *toluene R* and 65 volumes of *ethanol R*. Boil under a reflux condenser for 3 h. Allow to cool and filter if necessary.

Reference solution. Dissolve 30 mg of *plastic additive 22 CRS* in 50 ml of *toluene R*. Add 1 ml of this solution to 25 ml of blank solution S2 and evaporate to dryness *in vacuo* at 45 °C. Dissolve the residue in 10 ml of *toluene R* and 10 ml of a 10 g/l solution of *tetrabutylammonium hydroxide R* in a mixture of 35 volumes of *toluene R* and 65 volumes of *ethanol R*. Boil under a reflux condenser for 3 h. Allow to cool and filter if necessary.

The chromatographic procedure may be carried out using:

- a stainless steel column 0.25 m long and 4.6 mm in internal diameter packed with *aminopropylsilyl silica gel for chromatography R* (5 µm),
- as mobile phase at a flow rate of 2 ml/min a mixture of 11 volumes of *ethanol R* and 89 volumes of *hexane R*,
- as detector a spectrophotometer set at 227 nm.

Inject 20 µl of each solution. Record the chromatograms for 10 min. When the chromatograms are recorded in the prescribed conditions the resolution between the peaks corresponding respectively to the "diol" and diluent of the reference solution is at least 7.

In the chromatogram obtained with the test solution, the area of the peak corresponding to the "diol" component from plastic additive 22 is less than the corresponding peak in the chromatogram obtained with the reference solution.

Amides and stearates. Examine by thin-layer chromatography (*2.2.27*), using 2 plates of the *TLC silica gel GF_{254} plate R* type.

Test solution. Use test solution S24 described in the test for non-phenolic antioxidants.

Reference solution (q). Dissolve 20 mg of stearic acid (*plastic additive 19 CRS*) in 10 ml of *methylene chloride R*.

Reference solution (r). Dissolve 40 mg of oleamide (*plastic additive 20 CRS*) in 20 ml of *methylene chloride R*.

Reference solution (s). Dissolve 40 mg of erucamide (*plastic additive 21 CRS*) in 20 ml of *methylene chloride R*.

Apply to the 2 plates 10 µl of test solution S24. Apply 10 µl of reference solution (q) to the first plate and 10 µl each of reference solutions (r) and (s) to the second plate.

Develop the first plate over a path of 10 cm using a mixture of 25 volumes of *ethanol R* and 75 volumes of *trimethylpentane R*. Allow the plate to dry in air. Spray with a 2 g/l solution of *dichlorophenolindophenol, sodium salt R* in *ethanol R* and heat in an oven at 120 °C for a few minutes to intensify the spots. Any spot corresponding to plastic additive 19 in the chromatogram obtained with test solution S24 is identical in position to (R_f about 0.5) but not more intense than the spot in the chromatogram obtained with reference solution (q).

Develop the second plate over a path of 13 cm using *hexane R*. Allow the plate to dry in air. Develop a second time over a path of 10 cm using a mixture of 5 volumes of *methanol R* and 95 volumes of *methylene chloride R*. Allow the plate to dry. Spray with a 40 g/l solution of *phosphomolybdic acid R* in *ethanol R*. Heat in an oven at 120 °C until spots appear. Any spots corresponding to plastic additive 20 or plastic additive 21 in the chromatogram obtained with test solution S24 are identical in position to (R_f about 0.2) but not more intense than the corresponding spots in the chromatograms obtained with reference solutions (r) and (s).

01/2005:30104

3.1.4. POLYETHYLENE WITHOUT ADDITIVES FOR CONTAINERS FOR PARENTERAL PREPARATIONS AND FOR OPHTHALMIC PREPARATIONS

DEFINITION

Polyethylene without additives is obtained by the polymerisation of ethylene under high pressure in the presence of oxygen or free-radical-forming initiators as catalyst.

CHARACTERS

Beads, granules, powder or, after transformation, translucent sheets of varying thickness or containers, practically insoluble in water, soluble in hot aromatic hydrocarbons, practically insoluble in ethanol, in hexane and in methanol. It softens at temperatures above 65 °C.

The relative density (*2.2.5*) of the material is 0.910 to 0.937.

IDENTIFICATION

If necessary, cut the material to be examined into pieces of maximum dimension on a side of not greater than 1 cm.

A. To 0.25 g add 10 ml of *toluene R* and boil under a reflux condenser for about 15 min. Place a few drops of the solution on a sodium chloride disc and evaporate the solvent in an oven at 80 °C. Examine by infrared absorption spectrophotometry (*2.2.24*). The spectrum of the substance to be examined shows maxima in particular at some of the following wave-numbers: 2920 cm^{-1}, 2850 cm^{-1}, 1465 cm^{-1}, 730 cm^{-1}, 720 cm^{-1}; the spectrum obtained is identical to that obtained with the material selected for the type sample. If the material to be examined is in the form of sheets, the identification may be performed directly on a cut piece of suitable size.

B. The substance to be examined complies with the test for additives (see Tests).

TESTS

If necessary, cut the material to be examined into pieces of maximum dimension on a side of not greater than 1 cm.

Solution S1. Place 25 g in a borosilicate-glass flask with a ground-glass neck. Add 500 ml of *water for injections R* and heat under a reflux condenser for 5 h. Allow to cool and decant. Keep part of the solution for the test for appearance of solution. Filter the rest through a sintered glass filter (16). *Use solution S1 within 4 h of preparation.*

Solution S2. Place 2.0 g in a conical borosilicate-glass flask with a ground-glass neck. Add 80 ml of *toluene R* and boil under a reflux condenser with constant stirring for 1 h 30 min. Allow to cool to 60 °C and add with continued stirring 120 ml of *methanol R*. Filter the solution through a sintered-glass filter (16). Rinse the flask and the filter with 25 ml of a mixture of 40 ml of *toluene R* and 60 ml of *methanol R*, add the rinsings to the filtrate and dilute to 250 ml with the same mixture of solvents. Prepare a blank solution.

Solution S3. Place 100 g in a conical borosilicate-glass flask with a ground-glass neck. Add 250 ml of *0.1 M hydrochloric acid* and boil under a reflux condenser with constant stirring for 1 h. Allow to cool and decant the solution.

Appearance of solution. Solution S1 is clear (*2.2.1*) and colourless (*2.2.2, Method II*).

Acidity or alkalinity. To 100 ml of solution S1 add 0.15 ml of *BRP indicator solution R*. Not more than 1.5 ml of *0.01 M sodium hydroxide* is required to change the colour of the indicator to blue. To 100 ml of solution S1 add 0.2 ml of *methyl orange solution R*. Not more than 1.0 ml of *0.01 M hydrochloric acid* is required to reach the beginning of the colour change of the indicator from yellow to orange.

Absorbance (*2.2.25*). At wavelengths from 220 nm to 340 nm, the absorbance of solution S1 is not greater than 0.2.

Reducing substances. To 20 ml of solution S1 add 1 ml of *dilute sulphuric acid R* and 20 ml of *0.002 M potassium permanganate*. Boil under a reflux condenser for 3 min and cool immediately. Add 1 g of *potassium iodide R* and titrate immediately with *0.01 M sodium thiosulphate*, using 0.25 ml of *starch solution R* as indicator. Carry out a blank titration. The difference between the titration volumes is not more than 0.5 ml.

Substances soluble in hexane. Place 10 g in a 250 ml conical borosilicate-glass flask with a ground-glass neck. Add 100 ml of *hexane R* and boil under a reflux condenser for 4 h, stirring constantly. Cool in iced water and filter rapidly through a sintered-glass filter (16) maintaining the solution at 0 °C (the filtration time must be less than 5 min; if necessary the filtration may be accelerated by applying pressure to the solution). Evaporate 20 ml of the filtrate in a tared glass dish on a water-bath. Dry the residue in an oven at 100-105 °C for 1 h. The mass of the residue obtained is within 10 per cent of the residue obtained with the type sample and does not exceed 5 per cent.

Additives. Examine by thin-layer chromatography (*2.2.27*), using a *TLC silica gel G plate R*.

Test solution. Evaporate 50 ml of solution S2 to dryness *in vacuo* at 45 °C. Dissolve the evaporation residue with 5 ml of *methylene chloride R*. Prepare a blank solution from the blank solution corresponding to solution S2.

Reference solution. Dissolve 20 mg of *plastic additive 15 CRS* and 20 mg of *plastic additive 08 CRS* in *methylene chloride R* and dilute to 10 ml with the same solvent.

Apply to the plate 10 µl of each solution. Develop over a path of 13 cm using *hexane R*. Allow the plate to dry in air. Carry out a second development over a path of 10 cm using a mixture of 5 volumes of *methanol R* and 95 volumes of *methylene chloride R*. Allow the plate to dry in air, spray with a 40 g/l solution of *phosphomolybdic acid R* in *alcohol R* and heat at 120 °C until the spots appear in the chromatogram obtained with the reference solution. No spot appears in the chromatogram obtained with the test solution, except for a spot which may be at the solvent front from the first development and which corresponds to oligomers. Disregard any spots corresponding to those obtained in the chromatogram with the blank solution. The chromatogram obtained with the reference solution shows two distinct spots.

Extractable heavy metals (*2.4.8*). Evaporate 50 ml of solution S3 to about 5 ml on a water-bath and dilute to 20 ml with *water R*. 12 ml of solution complies with limit test A for heavy metals (2.5 ppm). Prepare the standard using 2.5 ml of *lead standard solution (10 ppm Pb) R*.

Sulphated ash (*2.4.14*). Not more than 0.02 per cent, determined on 5.0 g.

01/2005:30105

3.1.5. POLYETHYLENE WITH ADDITIVES FOR CONTAINERS FOR PARENTERAL PREPARATIONS AND FOR OPHTHALMIC PREPARATIONS

DEFINITION

Polyethylene with additives is obtained by the polymerisation of ethylene under pressure in the presence of a catalyst or by copolymerisation of ethylene with not more than 25 per cent of higher alkene homologues (C_3 to C_{10}).

PRODUCTION

A certain number of additives are added to the polymer in order to optimise their chemical, physical and mechanical properties in order to adapt them for the intended use. All these additives are chosen from the appended list which specifies for each product the maximum allowable content.

They may contain at most three antioxidants, one or several lubricants or antiblocking agents as well as titanium dioxide as an opacifying agent when the material must provide protection from light.

- butylhydroxytoluene (plastic additive 07) (not more than 0.125 per cent),
- pentaerythrityl tetrakis[3-(3,5-di-*tert*-butyl-4-hydroxyphenyl)propionate] (plastic additive 09) (not more than 0.3 per cent),
- 1,3,5-tris(3,5-di-*tert*-butyl-4-hydroxybenzyl)-*s*-triazine-2,4,6(1*H*,3*H*,5*H*)-trione (plastic additive 13) (not more than 0.3 per cent),
- octadecyl 3-(3,5-di-*tert*-butyl-4-hydroxyphenyl)propionate, (plastic additive 11) (not more than 0.3 per cent),
- ethylene bis[3,3-bis[3-(1,1-dimethylethyl)-4-hydroxyphenyl]butanoate] (plastic additive 08) (not more than 0.3 per cent),
- dioctadecyl disulphide (plastic additive 15) (not more than 0.3 per cent),
- 4,4′,4″-(2,4,6-trimethylbenzene-1,3,5-triyltrismethylene)tris[2,6-bis(1,1-dimethylethyl)phenol] (plastic additive 10) (not more than 0.3 per cent),
- 2,2′-bis(octadecyloxy)-5,5′-spirobi[1,3,2-dioxaphosphinane] (plastic additive 14) (not more than 0.3 per cent),
- didodecyl 3,3′-thiodipropionate (plastic additive 16) (not more than 0.3 per cent),
- dioctadecyl 3,3′-thiodipropionate (plastic additive 17) (not more than 0.3 per cent),
- tris [2,4-bis(1,1-dimethylethyl)phenyl] phosphite (plastic additive 12) (not more than 0.3 per cent).

The total of antioxidant additives listed above does not exceed 0.3 per cent.

- hydrotalcite (not more than 0.5 per cent),
- alkanamides (not more than 0.5 per cent),
- alkenamides (not more than 0.5 per cent),
- sodium silico-aluminate (not more than 0.5 per cent),
- silica (not more than 0.5 per cent),
- sodium benzoate (not more than 0.5 per cent),
- fatty acid esters or salts (not more than 0.5 per cent),
- trisodium phosphate (not more than 0.5 per cent),
- liquid paraffin (not more than 0.5 per cent),
- zinc oxide (not more than 0.5 per cent),
- magnesium oxide (not more than 0.2 per cent),
- calcium stearate or zinc stearate or a mixture of both (not more than 0.5 per cent),
- titanium dioxide (not more than 4 per cent) only for materials for containers for ophthalmic use.

The supplier of the material must be able to demonstrate that the qualitative and quantitative composition of the type sample is satisfactory for each production batch.

CHARACTERS

Powder, beads, granules or, after transformation, translucent sheets of varying thicknesses or containers. It is practically insoluble in water, soluble in hot aromatic hydrocarbons, practically insoluble in ethanol, in hexane and in methanol. It softens at temperatures between 70 °C and 140 °C.

The relative density (*2.2.5*) of the material is 0.890 to 0.965.

IDENTIFICATION

If necessary, cut the material to be examined into pieces of maximum dimension on a side of not greater than 1 cm.

A. To 0.25 g add 10 ml of *toluene R* and boil under a reflux condenser for about 15 min. Place a few drops of the solution on a sodium chloride disc and evaporate the solvent in an oven at 80 °C. Examine by infrared absorption spectrophotometry (*2.2.24*). The spectrum of the material to be examined shows maxima in particular at some of the following wave-numbers: 2920 cm^{-1}, 2850 cm^{-1}, 1465 cm^{-1}, 1375 cm^{-1}, 1170 cm^{-1}, 730 cm^{-1}, 720 cm^{-1}; the spectrum obtained is identical to the spectrum obtained with the material selected for the type sample. If the material to be examined is in the form of sheets, the identification may be performed directly on a cut piece of suitable size.

B. It complies with the supplementary tests corresponding to the additives present (see Tests).

C. In a platinum crucible, mix about 20 mg with 1 g of *potassium hydrogen sulphate R* and heat until completely melted. Allow to cool and add 20 ml of *dilute sulphuric acid R*. Heat gently. Filter the resulting solution. To the filtrate add 1 ml of *phosphoric acid R* and 1 ml of *strong hydrogen peroxide solution R*. If the substance is opacified with titanium dioxide, an orange-yellow colour develops.

TESTS

If necessary, cut the material to be examined into pieces of maximum dimension on a side of not greater than 1 cm.

Solution S1. Place 25 g in a borosilicate-glass flask with a ground-glass neck. Add 500 ml of *water for injections R* and boil under a reflux condenser for 5 h. Allow to cool and decant. Reserve a portion of the solution for the test for appearance of solution and filter the rest through a sintered-glass filter (16). *Use within 4 h of preparation.*

Solution S2. Place 2.0 g in a conical borosilicate-glass flask with a ground-glass neck. Add 80 ml of *toluene R* and boil under a reflux condenser with constant stirring for 90 min. Allow to cool to 60 °C and add with continued stirring 120 ml of *methanol R*. Filter the solution through a sintered-glass filter (16). Rinse the flask and the filter with 25 ml of a mixture of 40 ml of *toluene R* and 60 ml of *methanol R*, add the rinsings to the filtrate and dilute to 250.0 ml with the same mixture of solvents. Prepare a blank solution.

Solution S3. Place 100 g in a conical borosilicate-glass flask with a ground-glass neck. Add 250 ml of *0.1 M hydrochloric acid* and boil under a reflux condenser with constant stirring for 1 h. Allow to cool and decant the solution.

Appearance of solution. Solution S1 is clear (*2.2.1*) and colourless (*2.2.2, Method II*).

Acidity or alkalinity. To 100 ml of solution S1 add 0.15 ml of *BRP indicator solution R*. Not more than 1.5 ml of *0.01 M sodium hydroxide* is required to change the colour of the indicator to blue. To 100 ml of solution S1 add 0.2 ml of *methyl orange solution R*. Not more than 1.0 ml of *0.01 M hydrochloric acid* is required to reach the beginning of the colour change of the indicator from yellow to orange.

Absorbance (*2.2.25*). At wavelengths from 220 nm to 340 nm, the absorbance of solution S1 is not greater than 0.2.

Reducing substances. To 20 ml of solution S1 add 1 ml of *dilute sulphuric acid R* and 20 ml of *0.002 M potassium permanganate*. Boil under a reflux condenser for 3 min and cool immediately. Add 1 g of *potassium iodide R* and titrate immediately with *0.01 M sodium thiosulphate*, using 0.25 ml of *starch solution R* as indicator. Carry out a blank titration. The difference between the titration volumes is not more than 0.5 ml.

Substances soluble in hexane. Place 10 g in a 250 ml conical borosilicate-glass flask with a ground-glass neck. Add 100 ml of *hexane R* and boil under a reflux condenser for 4 h, stirring constantly. Cool in iced water and filter rapidly through a sintered-glass filter (16) maintaining the solution at 0 °C (the filtration time must be less than 5 min; if necessary the filtration may be accelerated by applying pressure to the solution). Evaporate 20 ml of the filtrate in a tared borosilicate-glass dish on a water-bath. Dry the residue in an oven at 100-105 °C for 1 h. The mass of the residue obtained must be within 10 per cent of the residue obtained with the type sample and does not exceed 5 per cent.

Extractable aluminium. Not more than 1 ppm of extractable Al, determined by atomic emission spectrometry in an argon plasma (*2.2.22, Method I*).

Test solution. Use solution S3.

Reference solutions. Prepare the reference solutions using *aluminium standard solution (200 ppm Al) R*, diluted with *0.1 M hydrochloric acid*.

Carry out the determination using the emission of aluminium at 396.15 nm, the spectral background being taken as 396.25 nm.

Verify the absence of aluminium in the hydrochloric acid used.

Extractable chromium. Not more than 0.05 ppm of extractable Cr, determined by atomic emission spectrometry in an argon plasma (*2.2.22, Method I*).

Test solution. Use solution S3.

Reference solutions. Prepare the reference solutions using *chromium standard solution (100 ppm Cr) R*, diluted with a mixture of 2 volumes of *hydrochloric acid R* and 8 volumes of *water R*.

Carry out the determination using the emission of chromium at 205.55 nm, the spectral background being taken as 205.50 nm.

Verify the absence of chromium in the hydrochloric acid used.

Extractable titanium. Not more than 1 ppm of extractable Ti, determined by atomic emission spectrometry in an argon plasma (*2.2.22, Method I*).

Test solution. Use solution S3.

Reference solutions. Prepare the reference solutions using *titanium standard solution (100 ppm Ti) R*, diluted with *0.1 M hydrochloric acid*.

Carry out the determination using the emission of titanium at 336.12 nm, the spectral background being taken as 336.16 nm.

Verify the absence of titanium in the hydrochloric acid used.

Extractable vanadium. Not more than 0.1 ppm of extractable V, determined by atomic emission spectrometry in an argon plasma (*2.2.22, Method I*).

Test solution. Use solution S3.

Reference solutions. Prepare the reference solutions using *vanadium standard solution (1 g/l V) R*, diluting with a mixture of 2 volumes of *hydrochloric acid R* and 8 volumes of *water R*.

Carry out the determination using the emission of vanadium at 292.40 nm, the spectral background being taken as 292.35 nm.

Verify the absence of vanadium in the hydrochloric acid used.

Extractable zinc. Not more than 1 ppm of extractable Zn, determined by atomic absorption spectrometry (*2.2.23, Method I*).

Test solution. Use solution S3.

Reference solutions. Prepare the reference solutions using *zinc standard solution (10 ppm Zn) R*, diluted with *0.1 M hydrochloric acid*.

Measure the absorbance at 213.9 nm using a zinc hollow-cathode lamp as a source of radiation and an air-acetylene flame.

Extractable zirconium. Not more than 0.1 ppm of extractable Zr, determined by atomic emission spectrometry in an argon plasma (*2.2.22, Method I*).

Test solution. Use solution S3.

Reference solutions. Prepare the reference solutions using *zirconium standard solution (1 g/l Zr) R*, diluted with a mixture of 2 volumes of *hydrochloric acid R* and 8 volumes of *water R*.

Carry out the determination using the emission of zirconium at 343.82 nm, the spectral background being taken as 343.92 nm.

Verify the absence of zirconium in the hydrochloric acid used.

Extractable heavy metals (*2.4.8*). Evaporate 50 ml of solution S3 to about 5 ml on a water-bath and dilute to 20.0 ml with *water R*. 12 ml of solution complies with limit test A for heavy metals (2.5 ppm). Prepare the standard using 2.5 ml of *lead standard solution (10 ppm Pb) R*.

Sulphated ash (*2.4.14*). Not more than 1.0 per cent, determined on 5.0 g. This limit does not apply to material opacified with titanium dioxide.

SUPPLEMENTARY TESTS

These tests are to be carried out, in whole or in part, only if required by the stated composition of the material.

Phenolic antioxidants. Examine by liquid chromatography (*2.2.29*).

The chromatographic procedure may be carried out using:

– a stainless steel column 0.25 m long and 4.6 mm in internal diameter packed with *octadecylsilyl silica gel for chromatography R* (5 μm),

- as mobile phase one of the 3 following mixtures:

  Mobile phase 1 at a flow rate of 2 ml/min: 30 volumes of *water R*, 70 volumes of *acetonitrile R*,

  Mobile phase 2 at a flow rate of 1.5 ml/min: 10 volumes of *water R*, 30 volumes of *tetrahydrofuran R*, 60 volumes of *acetonitrile R*,

  Mobile phase 3 at a flow rate of 1.5 ml/min: 5 volumes of *water R*, 45 volumes of *2-propanol R*, 50 volumes of *methanol R*,

- as detector a spectrophotometer set at 280 nm.

The chromatographic system must ensure the following:

- a resolution of not less than 8.0 between the peaks corresponding respectively to plastic additive 07 and plastic additive 08, with mobile phase 1,
- a resolution of not less than 2.0 between the peaks corresponding respectively to plastic additive 09 and plastic additive 10, with mobile phase 2,
- a resolution of not less than 2.0 between the peaks corresponding respectively to plastic additive 11 and plastic additive 12, with mobile phase 3.

Test solution S21. Evaporate 50 ml of solution S2 to dryness in vacuo at 45 °C. Dissolve the residue with 5.0 ml of a mixture of equal volumes of *acetonitrile R* and *tetrahydrofuran R*. Prepare a blank solution from the blank solution corresponding to solution S2.

Test solution S22. Evaporate 50 ml of solution S2 to dryness in vacuo at 45 °C. Dissolve the residue with 5.0 ml of *methylene chloride R*. Prepare a blank solution from the blank solution corresponding to solution S2.

Of the following reference solutions, only prepare those that are necessary for the analysis of the phenolic antioxidants stated in the composition of the substance to be examined.

Reference solution (a). Dissolve 25.0 mg of *butylhydroxytoluene CRS* (plastic additive 07) and 60.0 mg of *plastic additive 08 CRS* in 10.0 ml of a mixture of equal volumes of *acetonitrile R* and *tetrahydrofuran R*. Dilute 2.0 ml of the solution to 50.0 ml with a mixture of equal volumes of *acetonitrile R* and *tetrahydrofuran R*.

Reference solution (b). Dissolve 60.0 mg of *plastic additive 09 CRS* and 60.0 mg of *plastic additive 10 CRS* in 10.0 ml of a mixture of equal volumes of *acetonitrile R* and *tetrahydrofuran R*. Dilute 2.0 ml of the solution to 50.0 ml with a mixture of equal volumes of *acetonitrile R* and *tetrahydrofuran R*.

Reference solution (c). Dissolve 60.0 mg of *plastic additive 11 CRS* and 60.0 mg of *plastic additive 12 CRS* in 10.0 ml of *methylene chloride R*. Dilute 2.0 ml of the solution to 50.0 ml with *methylene chloride R*.

Reference solution (d). Dissolve 25.0 mg of *butylhydroxytoluene CRS* (plastic additive 07) in 10.0 ml of a mixture of equal volumes of *acetonitrile R* and *tetrahydrofuran R*. Dilute 2.0 ml of the solution to 50.0 ml with a mixture of equal volumes of *acetonitrile R* and *tetrahydrofuran R*.

Reference solution (e). Dissolve 60.0 mg of *plastic additive 08 CRS* in 10.0 ml of a mixture of equal volumes of *acetonitrile R* and *tetrahydrofuran R*. Dilute 2.0 ml of the solution to 50.0 ml with a mixture of equal volumes of *acetonitrile R* and *tetrahydrofuran R*.

Reference solution (f). Dissolve 60.0 mg of *plastic additive 13 CRS* in 10.0 ml of a mixture of equal volumes of *acetonitrile R* and *tetrahydrofuran R*. Dilute 2.0 ml of the solution to 50.0 ml with a mixture of equal volumes of *acetonitrile R* and *tetrahydrofuran R*.

Reference solution (g). Dissolve 60.0 mg of *plastic additive 09 CRS* in 10.0 ml of a mixture of equal volumes of *acetonitrile R* and *tetrahydrofuran R*. Dilute 2.0 ml of the solution to 50.0 ml with a mixture of equal volumes of *acetonitrile R* and *tetrahydrofuran R*.

Reference solution (h). Dissolve 60.0 mg of *plastic additive 10 CRS* in 10.0 ml of a mixture of equal volumes of *acetonitrile R* and *tetrahydrofuran R*. Dilute 2.0 ml of the solution to 50.0 ml with a mixture of equal volumes of *acetonitrile R* and *tetrahydrofuran R*.

Reference solution (i). Dissolve 60.0 mg of *plastic additive 11 CRS* in 10.0 ml of *methylene chloride R*. Dilute 2.0 ml of the solution to 50.0 ml with *methylene chloride R*.

Reference solution (j). Dissolve 60.0 mg of *plastic additive 12 CRS* in 10.0 ml of *methylene chloride R*. Dilute 2.0 ml of the solution to 50.0 ml with *methylene chloride R*.

If the substance to be examined contains plastic additive 07 and/or plastic additive 08, use mobile phase 1 and inject 20 µl of test solution S21, 20 µl of the corresponding blank solution, 20 µl of reference solution (a), and either 20 µl of reference solution (d) or (e), or 20 µl of reference solutions (d) and (e).

If the substance to be examined contains one or more of the following antioxidants:

- plastic additive 09,
- plastic additive 10,
- plastic additive 11,
- plastic additive 12,
- plastic additive 13,

use mobile phase 2 and inject 20 µl of test solution S21, 20 µl of the corresponding blank solution, 20 µl of reference solution (b) and 20 µl of the reference solutions of the antioxidants on the list above that are stated in the composition.

If the substance to be examined contains plastic additive 11 and/or plastic additive 12, use mobile phase 3 and inject 20 µl of test solution S22, 20 µl of the corresponding blank solution, 20 µl of reference solution (c), and either 20 µl of reference solution (i) or (j), or 20 µl of reference solutions (i) and (j).

In all cases record the chromatograms for 30 min; the chromatograms corresponding to test solutions S21 and S22 only show peaks due to antioxidants stated in the composition and minor peaks that also appear in the chromatograms corresponding to the blank solutions. The areas of the peaks of test solutions S21 and S22 are less than the areas of the corresponding peaks in the chromatograms obtained with reference solutions (d) to (j).

Non-phenolic antioxidants. Examine by thin-layer chromatography (*2.2.27*), using a *TLC silica gel* GF_{254} *plate R*.

Test solution S23. Evaporate 100 ml of solution S2 to dryness *in vacuo* at 45 °C. Dissolve the residue in 2 ml of *acidified methylene chloride R*.

Reference solution (k). Dissolve 60 mg of *plastic additive 14 CRS* in *methylene chloride R* and dilute to 10 ml with the same solvent. Dilute 2 ml of the solution to 10 ml with *acidified methylene chloride R*.

Reference solution (l). Dissolve 60 mg of *plastic additive 15 CRS* in *methylene chloride R* and dilute to 10 ml with the same solvent. Dilute 2 ml of the solution to 10 ml with *acidified methylene chloride R*.

Reference solution (m). Dissolve 60 mg of *plastic additive 16 CRS* in *methylene chloride R* and dilute to 10 ml with the same solvent. Dilute 2 ml of the solution to 10 ml with *acidified methylene chloride R.*

Reference solution (n). Dissolve 60 mg of *plastic additive 17 CRS* in *methylene chloride R* and dilute to 10 ml with the same solvent. Dilute 2 ml of the solution to 10 ml with *acidified methylene chloride R.*

Reference solution (o). Dissolve 60 mg of *plastic additive 16 CRS* and 60 mg of *plastic additive 17 CRS* in *methylene chloride R* and dilute to 10 ml with the same solvent. Dilute 2 ml of the solution to 10 ml with *acidified methylene chloride R.*

Apply separately to the plate 20 µl of test solution S23, 20 µl of reference solution (o) and 20 µl of the reference solutions corresponding to all the phenolic and non-phenolic antioxidants mentioned in the type composition of the material to be examined.

Develop over a path of 18 cm using *hexane R.* Allow the plate to dry. Develop a second time over a path of 17 cm using *methylene chloride R.* Allow the plate to dry and examine in ultraviolet light at 254 nm. Spray with *alcoholic iodine solution R* and examine in ultraviolet light at 254 nm after 10-15 min. Any spots in the chromatogram obtained with test solution S23 are not more intense than the spots in the same locations in the chromatograms obtained with the reference solutions. The test is not valid unless the chromatogram obtained with reference solution (o) shows two clearly separated spots.

Amides and stearates. Examine by thin-layer chromatography (*2.2.27*), using 2 plates of the *TLC silica gel GF_{254} plates R* type.

Test solution. Use test solution S23 described in the test for non-phenolic antioxidants.

Reference solution (p). Dissolve 20 mg of *stearic acid CRS* (plastic additive 19) in *methylene chloride R* and dilute to 10 ml with the same solvent.

Reference solution (q). Dissolve 40 mg of *plastic additive 20 CRS* in *methylene chloride R* and dilute to 20 ml with the same solvent.

Reference solution (r). Dissolve 40 mg of *plastic additive 21 CRS* in *methylene chloride R* and dilute to 20 ml with the same solvent.

Apply to each of the 2 plates 10 µl of test solution S23. Apply 10 µl of reference solution (p) to the first and 10 µl of reference solutions (q) and (r) to the second. Develop the first plate over a path of 10 cm using a mixture of 25 volumes of *ethanol R* and 75 volumes of *trimethylpentane R.* Allow the plate to dry in air. Spray with a 2 g/l solution of *dichlorophenolindophenol sodium salt R* in *ethanol R* and heat in an oven at 120 °C for a few minutes to intensify the spots. Any spot corresponding to plastic additive 19 in the chromatogram obtained with test solution S23 is identical in position (R_f about 0.5) but not more intense than the spot in the same location in the chromatogram obtained with reference solution (p).

Develop the second plate over a path of 13 cm using *hexane R.* Allow the plate to dry in air. Develop a second time over a path of 10 cm using a mixture of 5 volumes of *methanol R* and 95 volumes of *methylene chloride R.* Allow the plate to dry. Spray with a 40 g/l solution of *phosphomolybdic acid R* in *ethanol R.* Heat in an oven at 120 °C until spots appear. Any spots corresponding to plastic additive 20 or plastic additive 21 in the chromatogram obtained with test solution S23 are identical in position (R_f about 0.2) but not more intense than the corresponding spots in the chromatograms obtained with reference solutions (q) and (r).

01/2005:30106

3.1.6. POLYPROPYLENE FOR CONTAINERS AND CLOSURES FOR PARENTERAL PREPARATIONS AND OPHTHALMIC PREPARATIONS

DEFINITION

Polypropylene consists of the homopolymer of propylene or of a copolymer of propylene with not more than 25 per cent of ethylene or of a mixture (alloy) of polypropylene with not more than 25 per cent of polyethylene. It may contain additives.

PRODUCTION

A certain number of additives are added to the polymer in order to optimise their chemical, physical and mechanical properties in order to adapt them for the intended use. All these additives are chosen from the appended list which specifies for each product the maximum allowable content. They may contain at most three antioxidants, one or several lubricants or antiblocking agents as well as titanium dioxide as opacifying agent when the material must provide protection from light.

- butylhydroxytoluene (plastic additive 07) (not more than 0.125 per cent),
- pentaerythrityl tetrakis[3-(3,5-di-*tert*-butyl-4-hydroxyphenyl)propionate] (plastic additive 09) (not more than 0.3 per cent),
- 1,3,5-tris(3,5-di-*tert*-butyl-4-hydroxybenzyl)-*s*-triazine-2,4,6(1*H*,3*H*,5*H*)-trione (plastic additive 13) (not more than 0.3 per cent),
- octadecyl 3-(3,5-di-*tert*-butyl-4-hydroxyphenyl)propionate, (plastic additive 11) (not more than 0.3 per cent),
- ethylene bis[3,3-bis[3-(1,1-dimethylethyl)-4-hydroxyphenyl]butanoate] (plastic additive 08) (not more than 0.3 per cent),
- dioctadecyl disulphide (plastic additive 15) (not more than 0.3 per cent),
- 2,2′,2″,6,6′,6″-hexa-*tert*-butyl-4,4′,4″-[(2,4,6-trimethyl-1,3,5-benzenetriyl)trismethylene]triphenol (plastic additive 10) (not more than 0.3 per cent),
- 2,2′-bis(octadecyloxy)-5,5′-spirobi[1,3,2-dioxaphosphinane] (plastic additive 14) (not more than 0.3 per cent),
- didodecyl 3,3′-thiodipropionate (plastic additive 16) (not more than 0.3 per cent),
- dioctadecyl 3,3′-thiodipropionate (plastic additive 17) (not more than 0.3 per cent),
- tris(2,4-di-*tert*-butylphenyl) phosphite (plastic additive 12) (not more than 0.3 per cent),

The total of antioxidant additives listed above does not exceed 0.3 per cent.

- hydrotalcite (not more than 0.5 per cent),
- alkanamides (not more than 0.5 per cent),
- alkenamides (not more than 0.5 per cent),
- sodium silico-aluminate (not more than 0.5 per cent),
- silica (not more than 0.5 per cent),
- sodium benzoate (not more than 0.5 per cent),
- fatty acid esters or salts (not more than 0.5 per cent),

- trisodium phosphate (not more than 0.5 per cent),
- liquid paraffin (not more than 0.5 per cent),
- zinc oxide (not more than 0.5 per cent),
- talc (not more than 0.5 per cent),
- magnesium oxide (not more than 0.2 per cent),
- calcium stearate or zinc stearate or a mixture of both (not more than 0.5 per cent),
- titanium dioxide (not more than 4 per cent) only for materials for containers for ophthalmic use.

The supplier of the material must be able to demonstrate that the qualitative and quantitative composition of the type sample is satisfactory for each production batch.

CHARACTERS

Powder, beads, granules or, after transformation, translucent sheets of varying thicknesses or containers. It is practically insoluble in water, soluble in hot aromatic hydrocarbons, practically insoluble in ethanol, in hexane and in methanol. It softens at temperatures above about 120 °C.

IDENTIFICATION

If necessary, cut the material to be examined into pieces of maximum dimension on a side of not greater than 1 cm.

A. To 0.25 g add 10 ml of *toluene R* and boil under a reflux condenser for about 15 min. Place a few drops of the hot solution on a sodium chloride disc and evaporate the solvent in an oven at 80 °C. Examine by infrared absorption spectrophotometry (*2.2.24*). The spectrum obtained with the material to be examined presents a certain number of maxima, in particular at 1375 cm^{-1}, 1170 cm^{-1}, 995 cm^{-1} and 970 cm^{-1}. The spectrum obtained is identical to the spectrum obtained with the material selected for the type sample. If the material to be examined is in the form of sheets, the identification may be performed directly on a cut piece of suitable size.

B. It complies with the supplementary tests corresponding to the additives present (see Tests).

C. In a platinum crucible, mix about 20 mg with 1 g of *potassium hydrogen sulphate R* and heat until completely melted. Allow to cool and add 20 ml of *dilute sulphuric acid R*. Heat gently. Filter the resulting solution. To the filtrate add 1 ml of *phosphoric acid R* and 1 ml of *strong hydrogen peroxide solution R*. If the substance is opacified with titanium dioxide, an orange-yellow colour develops.

TESTS

If necessary, cut the material to be examined into pieces of maximum dimension on a side of not greater than 1 cm.

Solution S1. *Use solution S1 within 4 h of preparation.* Place 25 g in a borosilicate-glass flask with a ground-glass neck. Add 500 ml of *water for injections R* and boil under a reflux condenser for 5 h. Allow to cool and decant. Reserve a portion of the solution for the test for appearance of solution and filter the rest through a sintered-glass filter (16).

Solution S2. Place 2.0 g in a conical borosilicate-glass flask with a ground-glass neck. Add 80 ml of *toluene R* and boil under a reflux condenser with constant stirring for 1 h 30 min. Allow to cool to 60 °C and add with continued stirring 120 ml of *methanol R*. Filter the solution through a sintered-glass filter (16). Rinse the flask and the filter with 25 ml of a mixture of 40 ml of *toluene R* and 60 ml of *methanol R*, add the rinsings to the filtrate and dilute to 250.0 ml with the same mixture of solvents. Prepare a blank solution.

Solution S3. Place 100 g in a conical borosilicate-glass flask with a ground-glass neck. Add 250 ml of *0.1 M hydrochloric acid* and boil under a reflux condenser with constant stirring for 1 h. Allow to cool and decant the solution.

Appearance of solution. Solution S1 is not more opalescent than reference suspension II (*2.2.1*) and is colourless (*2.2.2, Method II*).

Acidity or alkalinity. To 100 ml of solution S1 add 0.15 ml of *BRP indicator solution R*. Not more than 1.5 ml of *0.01 M sodium hydroxide* is required to change the colour of the indicator to blue. To 100 ml of solution S1 add 0.2 ml of *methyl orange solution R*. Not more than 1.0 ml of *0.01 M hydrochloric acid* is required to reach the beginning of the colour change of the indicator from yellow to orange.

Absorbance (*2.2.25*). At wavelengths from 220 nm to 340 nm, the absorbance of solution S1 is not greater than 0.2.

Reducing substances. To 20 ml of solution S1 add 1 ml of *dilute sulphuric acid R* and 20 ml of *0.002 M potassium permanganate*. Boil under a reflux condenser for 3 min and cool immediately. Add 1 g of *potassium iodide R* and titrate immediately with *0.01 M sodium thiosulphate*, using 0.25 ml of *starch solution R* as indicator. Carry out a blank titration. The difference between the titration volumes is not more than 0.5 ml.

Substances soluble in hexane. Place 10 g in a 250 ml conical borosilicate-glass flask with a ground-glass neck. Add 100 ml of *hexane R* and boil under a reflux condenser for 4 h, stirring constantly. Cool in iced water and filter rapidly through a sintered-glass filter (16) maintaining the solution at 0 °C (the filtration time must be less than 5 min; if necessary the filtration may be accelerated by applying pressure to the solution). Evaporate 20 ml of the filtrate in a tared glass dish on a water-bath. Dry the residue in an oven at 100 °C to 105 °C for 1 h. The mass of the residue obtained must be within 10 per cent of the residue obtained with the type sample and does not exceed 5 per cent.

Extractable aluminium. Not more than 1 ppm of extractable Al, determined by atomic emission spectrometry in an argon plasma (*2.2.22, Method I*).

Test solution. Use solution S3.

Reference solutions. Prepare the reference solutions using *aluminium standard solution (200 ppm Al) R*, diluted with *0.1 M hydrochloric acid.*

Carry out the determination using the emission of aluminium at 396.15 nm, the spectral background being taken as 396.25 nm.

Verify the absence of aluminium in the hydrochloric acid used.

Extractable chromium. Not more than 0.05 ppm of extractable Cr, determined by atomic emission spectrometry in an argon plasma (*2.2.22, Method I*).

Test solution. Use solution S3.

Reference solutions. Prepare the reference solutions using *chromium standard solution (100 ppm Cr) R*, diluting with a mixture of 2 volumes of *hydrochloric acid R* and 8 volumes of *water R*.

Carry out the determination using the emission of chromium at 205.55 nm, the spectral background being taken as 205.50 nm.

Verify the absence of chromium in the hydrochloric acid used.

Extractable titanium. Not more than 1 ppm of extractable Ti, determined by atomic emission spectrometry in an argon plasma (*2.2.22, Method I*).

Test solution. Use solution S3.

Reference solutions. Prepare the reference solutions using *titanium standard solution (100 ppm Ti) R*, diluted with *0.1 M hydrochloric acid.*

Carry out the determination using the emission of titanium at 336.12 nm, the spectral background being taken as 336.16 nm.

Verify the absence of titanium in the hydrochloric acid used.

Extractable vanadium. Not more than 0.1 ppm of extractable V, determined by atomic emission spectrometry in an argon plasma (*2.2.22, Method I*).

Test solution. Use solution S3.

Reference solutions. Prepare the reference solutions using *vanadium standard solution (1 g/l V) R*, diluted with a mixture of 2 volumes of *hydrochloric acid R* and 8 volumes of *water R*.

Carry out the determination using the emission of vanadium at 292.40 nm, the spectral background being taken as 292.35 nm.

Verify the absence of vanadium in the hydrochloric acid used.

Extractable zinc. Not more than 1 ppm of extractable Zn, determined by atomic absorption spectrometry (*2.2.23, Method I*).

Test solution. Use solution S3.

Reference solutions. Prepare the reference solutions using *zinc standard solution (10 ppm Zn) R*, diluted with *0.1 M hydrochloric acid.*

Measure the absorbance at 213.9 nm using a zinc hollow-cathode lamp as a source of radiation and an air-acetylene flame.

Verify the absence of zinc in the hydrochloric acid used.

Extractable heavy metals (*2.4.8*). Concentrate 50 ml of solution S3 to about 5 ml on a water-bath and dilute to 20.0 ml with *water R*. 12 ml of the solution complies with limit test A for heavy metals (2.5 ppm). Prepare the standard using 2.5 ml of *lead standard solution (10 ppm Pb) R*.

Sulphated ash (*2.4.14*). Not more than 1.0 per cent, determined on 5.0 g. This limit does not apply to material that has been opacified with titanium dioxide.

SUPPLEMENTARY TESTS

These tests are to be carried out, in whole or in part, only if required by the stated composition of the material.

Phenolic antioxidants. Examine by liquid chromatography (*2.2.29*).

The chromatographic procedure may be carried out using:

- a stainless steel column 0.25 m long and 4.6 mm in internal diameter packed with *octadecylsilyl silica gel for chromatography R* (5 μm),
- as mobile phase one of the three following mixtures:

  Mobile phase 1 at a flow rate of 2 ml/min: 30 volumes of *water R*, 70 volumes of *acetonitrile R*,

  Mobile phase 2 at a flow rate of 1.5 ml/min: 10 volumes of *water R*, 30 volumes of *tetrahydrofuran R*, 60 volumes of *acetonitrile R*,

  Mobile phase 3 at a flow rate of 1.5 ml/min: 5 volumes of *water R*, 45 volumes of *2-propanol R*, 50 volumes of *methanol R*,
- as detector a spectrophotometer set at 280 nm.

The chromatographic system must ensure the following:

- a resolution of not less than 8.0 between the peaks corresponding respectively to plastic additive 07 and plastic additive 08, with mobile phase 1,
- a resolution of not less than 2.0 between the peaks corresponding respectively to plastic additive 09 and plastic additive 10, with mobile phase 2,
- a resolution of not less than 2.0 between the peaks corresponding respectively to plastic additive 11 and plastic additive 12, with mobile phase 3.

Test solution S21. Evaporate 50 ml of solution S2 to dryness *in vacuo* at 45 °C. Dissolve the residue with 5.0 ml of a mixture of equal volumes of *acetonitrile R* and *tetrahydrofuran R*. Prepare a blank solution from the blank solution corresponding to solution S2.

Test solution S22. Evaporate 50 ml of solution S2 to dryness *in vacuo* at 45 °C. Dissolve the residue with 5.0 ml of *methylene chloride R*. Prepare a blank solution from the blank solution corresponding to solution S2.

Of the following reference solutions, only prepare those that are necessary for the analysis of the phenolic antioxidants stated in the composition of the substance to be examined.

Reference solution (a). Dissolve 25.0 mg of *butylhydroxytoluene CRS* (plastic additive 07) and 60.0 mg of *plastic additive 08 CRS* in 10.0 ml of a mixture of equal volumes of *acetonitrile R* and *tetrahydrofuran R*. Dilute 2.0 ml of the solution to 50.0 ml with a mixture of equal volumes of *acetonitrile R* and *tetrahydrofuran R*.

Reference solution (b). Dissolve 60.0 mg of *plastic additive 09 CRS* and 60.0 mg of *plastic additive 10 CRS* in 10.0 ml of a mixture of equal volumes of *acetonitrile R* and *tetrahydrofuran R*. Dilute 2.0 ml of the solution to 50.0 ml with a mixture of equal volumes of *acetonitrile R* and *tetrahydrofuran R*.

Reference solution (c). Dissolve 60.0 mg of *plastic additive 11 CRS* and 60.0 mg of *plastic additive 12 CRS* in 10 ml of *methylene chloride R*. Dilute 2.0 ml of the solution to 50.0 ml with *methylene chloride R*.

Reference solution (d). Dissolve 25.0 mg of *butylhydroxytoluene CRS* (plastic additive 07) in 10.0 ml of a mixture of equal volumes of *acetonitrile R* and *tetrahydrofuran R*. Dilute 2.0 ml of the solution to 50.0 ml with a mixture of equal volumes of *acetonitrile R* and *tetrahydrofuran R*.

Reference solution (e). Dissolve 60.0 mg of *plastic additive 08 CRS* in 10.0 ml of a mixture of equal volumes of *acetonitrile R* and *tetrahydrofuran R*. Dilute 2.0 ml of the solution to 50.0 ml with a mixture of equal volumes of *acetonitrile R* and *tetrahydrofuran R*.

Reference solution (f). Dissolve 60.0 mg of *plastic additive 13 CRS* in 10.0 ml of a mixture of equal volumes of *acetonitrile R* and *tetrahydrofuran R*. Dilute 2.0 ml of the solution to 50.0 ml with a mixture of equal volumes of *acetonitrile R* and *tetrahydrofuran R*.

Reference solution (g). Dissolve 60.0 mg of *plastic additive 09 CRS* in 10.0 ml of a mixture of equal volumes of *acetonitrile R* and *tetrahydrofuran R*. Dilute 2.0 ml of the solution to 50.0 ml with a mixture of equal volumes of *acetonitrile R* and *tetrahydrofuran R*.

Reference solution (h). Dissolve 60.0 mg of *plastic additive 10 CRS* in 10.0 ml of a mixture of equal volumes of *acetonitrile R* and *tetrahydrofuran R*. Dilute 2.0 ml of the solution to 50.0 ml with a mixture of equal volumes of *acetonitrile R* and *tetrahydrofuran R*.

Reference solution (i). Dissolve 60.0 mg of *plastic additive 11 CRS* in 10.0 ml of *methylene chloride R*. Dilute 2.0 ml of the solution to 50.0 ml with *methylene chloride R*.

Reference solution (j). Dissolve 60.0 mg of *plastic additive 12 CRS* in 10.0 ml of *methylene chloride R*. Dilute 2.0 ml of the solution to 50.0 ml with *methylene chloride R*.

If the substance to be examined contains plastic additive 07 and/or plastic additive 08, use mobile phase 1 and inject 20 µl of test solution S21, 20 µl of the corresponding blank solution and 20 µl of reference solution (a), and either 20 µl of reference solution (d) or (e), or 20 µl of reference solutions (d) and (e).

If the substance to be examined contains one or more of the following antioxidants:

- plastic additive 09,
- plastic additive 10,
- plastic additive 11,
- plastic additive 12,
- plastic additive 13,

use mobile phase 2 and inject 20 µl of test solution S21, 20 µl of the corresponding blank solution, 20 µl of reference solution (b) and 20 µl of the reference solutions of the antioxidants on the list above that are stated in the composition.

If the substance to be examined contains plastic additive 11 and/or plastic additive 12, use mobile phase 3 and inject 20 µl of test solution S22, 20 µl of the corresponding blank solution, 20 µl of reference solution (c), and either 20 µl of reference solution (i) or (j), or 20 µl of reference solutions (i) and (j).

In all cases record the chromatogram for 30 min; the chromatograms corresponding to test solutions S21 and S22 only show peaks due to antioxidants stated in the composition and minor peaks that also appear in the chromatograms corresponding to the blank solutions. The areas of the peaks of test solutions S21 and S22 are less than the areas of the corresponding peaks in the chromatograms obtained with reference solutions (d) to (j).

Non-phenolic antioxidants. Examine by thin-layer chromatography (*2.2.27*), using a *TLC silica gel GF_{254} plate R*.

Test solution S23. Evaporate 100 ml of solution S2 to dryness *in vacuo* at 45 °C. Dissolve the residue with 2 ml of *acidified methylene chloride R*.

Reference solution (k). Dissolve 60 mg of *plastic additive 14 CRS* in *methylene chloride R* and dilute to 10 ml with the same solvent. Dilute 2 ml of the solution to 10 ml with *acidified methylene chloride R*.

Reference solution (l). Dissolve 60 mg of *plastic additive 15 CRS* in *methylene chloride R* and dilute to 10 ml with the same solvent. Dilute 2 ml of the solution to 10 ml with *acidified methylene chloride R*.

Reference solution (m). Dissolve 60 mg of *plastic additive 16 CRS* in *methylene chloride R* and dilute to 10 ml with the same solvent. Dilute 2 ml of the solution to 10 ml with *acidified methylene chloride R*.

Reference solution (n). Dissolve 60 mg of *plastic additive 17 CRS* in *methylene chloride R* and dilute to 10 ml with the same solvent. Dilute 2 ml of the solution to 10 ml with *acidified methylene chloride R*.

Reference solution (o). Dissolve 60 mg of *plastic additive 16 CRS* and 60 mg of *plastic additive 17 CRS* in *methylene chloride R* and dilute to 10 ml with the same solvent. Dilute 2 ml of the solution to 10 ml with *acidified methylene chloride R*.

Apply separately to the plate 20 µl of test solution S23, 20 µl of reference solution (o) and 20 µl of the reference solutions corresponding to all the phenolic and non-phenolic antioxidants mentioned in the type composition of the material to be examined. Develop over a path of 18 cm using *hexane R*. Allow the plate to dry. Develop a second time over a path of 17 cm using *methylene chloride R*. Allow the plate to dry and examine in ultraviolet light at 254 nm. Spray with *alcoholic iodine solution R* and examine in ultraviolet light at 254 nm after 10 min to 15 min. Any spots in the chromatogram obtained with test solution S23 are not more intense than the spots in the same locations in the chromatograms obtained with the reference solutions. The test is not valid unless the chromatogram obtained with reference solution (o) shows two clearly separated spots.

Amides and stearates. Examine by thin-layer chromatography (*2.2.27*), using 2 plates of the *TLC silica gel GF_{254} plate R* type.

Test solution. Use solution S23 described in the test for non-phenolic antioxidants.

Reference solution (p). Dissolve 20 mg of *stearic acid CRS* (plastic additive 19) in *methylene chloride R* and dilute to 10 ml with the same solvent.

Reference solution (q). Dissolve 40 mg of *plastic additive 20 CRS* in *methylene chloride R* and dilute to 20 ml with the same solvent.

Reference solution (r). Dissolve 40 mg of *plastic additive 21 CRS* in *methylene chloride R* and dilute to 20 ml with the same solvent.

Apply to each of the two plates 10 µl of solution S23. Apply 10 µl of reference solution (p) to the first and 10 µl each of reference solutions (q) and (r) to the second. Develop the first plate over a path of 10 cm using a mixture of 25 volumes of *ethanol R* and 75 volumes of *trimethylpentane R*. Allow the plate to dry in air. Spray with a 2 g/l solution of *dichlorophenolindophenol sodium salt R* in *ethanol R* and heat in an oven at 120 °C for a few minutes to intensify the spots. Any spot corresponding to plastic additive 19 in the chromatogram obtained with test solution S23 is identical in position (R_f about 0.5) but not more intense than the spot in the same position in the chromatogram obtained with reference solution (p).

Develop the second plate over a path of 13 cm using *hexane R*. Allow the plate to dry in air. Develop a second time over a path of 10 cm using a mixture of 5 volumes of *methanol R* and 95 volumes of *methylene chloride R*. Allow the plate to dry.

Spray with a 40 g/l solution of *phosphomolybdic acid R* in *ethanol R*. Heat in an oven at 120 °C until spots appear. Any spots corresponding to plastic additive 20 or plastic additive 21 in the chromatogram obtained with test solution S23 are identical in position (R_f about 0.2) but not more intense than the corresponding spots in the chromatograms obtained with reference solutions (q) and (r).

01/2005:30107

3.1.7. POLY(ETHYLENE - VINYL ACETATE) FOR CONTAINERS AND TUBING FOR TOTAL PARENTERAL NUTRITION PREPARATIONS

DEFINITION

Poly(ethylene - vinyl acetate), complying with the following requirements, is suitable for the manufacture of containers and tubing for total parenteral nutrition preparations.

3. Materials/ Containers

Poly(ethylene - vinyl acetate) is obtained by copolymerisation of mixtures of ethylene and vinyl acetate. This copolymer contains a defined quantity of not more than 25 per cent of vinyl acetate for material to be used for containers and not more than 30 per cent for material to be used for tubing.

PRODUCTION

A certain number of additives are added to the polymer in order to optimise their chemical, physical and mechanical properties in order to adapt them for the intended use. All these additives are chosen from the appended list which specifies for each product the maximum allowable content.

Poly(ethylene - vinyl acetate) may contain not more than three of the following antioxidants:

- butylhydroxytoluene (plastic additive 07) (not more than 0.125 per cent),
- pentaerythrityl tetrakis[3-(3,5-di-*tert*-butyl-4-hydroxyphenyl)propionate] (plastic additive 09) (not more than 0.2 per cent),
- octadecyl 3-(3,5-di-*tert*-butyl-4-hydroxyphenyl)propionate (plastic additive 11) (not more than 0.2 per cent),
- tris(2,4-di-*tert*-butylphenyl) phosphite (plastic additive 12) (not more than 0.2 per cent),
- 2,2′,2″,6,6′,6″-hexa-*tert*-butyl-4,4′,4″-[(2,4,6-trimethyl-1,3,5-benzenetriyl)trismethylene]triphenol (plastic additive 10) (not more than 0.2 per cent).

It may also contain:

- oleamide (plastic additive 20) (not more than 0.5 per cent),
- erucamide (plastic additive 21) (not more than 0.5 per cent),
- calcium stearate or zinc stearate or a mixture of both (not more than 0.5 per cent),
- calcium carbonate or potassium hydroxide (not more than 0.5 per cent of each),
- colloidal silica (not more than 0.2 per cent).

The supplier of the material must be able to demonstrate that the qualitative and quantitative composition of the type sample is satisfactory for each production batch.

CHARACTERS

Beads, granules or, after transformation, translucent sheets or tubing of varying thickness or samples of finished objects, practically insoluble in water, soluble in hot aromatic hydrocarbons, practically insoluble in ethanol, in methanol and in hexane, which dissolves, however, low molecular mass polymers. It burns with a blue flame. The temperature at which the substance softens changes with the vinyl acetate content; it decreases from about 100 °C for contents of a few per cent to about 70 °C for contents of 30 per cent.

IDENTIFICATION

If necessary, cut the material to be examined into pieces of maximum dimension on a side of not greater than 1 cm.

To 0.25 g add 10 ml of *toluene R* and boil under a reflux condenser for about 15 min. Place a few drops of the solution obtained on a disc of sodium chloride and evaporate the solvent in an oven at 80 °C. Examine by infrared absorption spectrophotometry (*2.2.24*). The spectrum obtained shows absorption maxima corresponding to vinyl acetate at the following positions: 1740 cm^{-1}, 1375 cm^{-1}, 1240 cm^{-1}, 1020 cm^{-1}, 610 cm^{-1}, and maxima corresponding to ethylene at the following positions: 2920 cm^{-1} to 2850 cm^{-1}, 1470 cm^{-1}, 1460 cm^{-1}, 1375 cm^{-1}, 730 cm^{-1}, 720 cm^{-1}. The spectrum obtained is, in addition, identical to the spectrum obtained with the type sample provided by the manufacturer. If the material to be examined is in the form of sheets, the spectrum may be determined directly on a cut piece of suitable size.

TESTS

If necessary, cut the material to be examined into pieces of maximum dimension on a side of not greater than 1 cm.

Solution S1. Place 2.0 g in a borosilicate-glass flask with a ground-glass neck. Add 80 ml of *toluene R* and heat under a reflux condenser with constant agitation for 90 min. Allow to cool to 60 °C and add 120 ml of *methanol R* to the flask with constant stirring. Filter the solution through a sintered-glass filter (16). Rinse the flask and the filter with 25 ml of a mixture of 40 ml of *toluene R* and 60 ml of *methanol R*, add the rinsing mixture to the filtrate and dilute to 250 ml with the same mixture of solvents.

Solution S2. *Use within 4 h of preparation.* Place 25 g in a borosilicate-glass flask with a ground-glass neck. Add 500 ml of *water for injections R* and boil under a reflux condenser for 5 h. Allow to cool and decant. Reserve a portion of the solution for the test for appearance of solution S2 and filter the rest through a sintered-glass filter (16).

Appearance of solution S2. Solution S2 is clear (*2.2.1*) and colourless (*2.2.2, Method II*).

Acidity or alkalinity. To 100 ml of solution S2 add 0.15 ml of *BRP indicator solution R*. Not more than 1.0 ml of *0.01 M sodium hydroxide* is required to change the colour of the indicator to blue. To 100 ml of solution S2 add 0.2 ml of *methyl orange solution R*. Not more than 1.5 ml of *0.01 M hydrochloric acid* is required to reach the beginning of the colour change of the indicator from yellow to orange.

Absorbance (*2.2.25*). At wavelengths from 220 nm to 340 nm, the absorbance of solution S2 is not greater than 0.2.

Reducing substances. To 20 ml of solution S2 add 1 ml of *dilute sulphuric acid R* and 20 ml of *0.002 M potassium permanganate*. Boil under a reflux condenser for 3 min and cool immediately. Add 1 g of *potassium iodide R* and titrate immediately with *0.01 M sodium thiosulphate*, using 0.25 ml of *starch solution R* as indicator. Carry out a blank titration. The difference between the titration volumes is not more than 0.5 ml.

Amides and stearic acid. Examine by thin-layer chromatography (*2.2.27*), using 2 plates of the *TLC silica gel GF_{254} plate R* type.

Test solution. Evaporate 100 ml of solution S1 to dryness *in vacuo* at 45 °C. Dissolve the residue in 2 ml of *acidified methylene chloride R*.

Reference solution (a). Dissolve 20 mg of *stearic acid CRS* (plastic additive 19) in 10 ml of *methylene chloride R*.

Reference solution (b). Dissolve 40 mg of *plastic additive 20 CRS* in 10 ml of *methylene chloride R*. Dilute 1 ml of the solution to 5 ml with *methylene chloride R*.

Reference solution (c). Dissolve 40 mg of *plastic additive 21 CRS* in 10 ml of *methylene chloride R*. Dilute 1 ml of the solution to 5 ml with *methylene chloride R*.

Apply separately 10 µl of each solution to the two plates. Develop the first plate over a path of 10 cm using a mixture of 25 volumes of *ethanol R* and 75 volumes of *trimethylpentane R*. Allow the plate to dry. Spray with a 2 g/l solution of *dichlorophenolindophenol sodium salt R* in *ethanol R* and heat in an oven at 120 °C for a few minutes to intensify the spots. Any spot corresponding to plastic additive 19 in the chromatogram obtained with the test solution is not more intense than the spot in the chromatogram obtained with reference solution (a).

Develop the second plate over a path of 13 cm using *hexane R*. Allow the plate to dry. Develop a second time over a path of 10 cm using a mixture of 5 volumes of *methanol R* and 95 volumes of *methylene chloride R*. Allow the plate to dry. Spray with a 40 g/l solution of *phosphomolybdic acid R* in *ethanol R*. Heat in an oven at 120 °C until spots appear. Any spots corresponding to plastic additive 21 or plastic additive 20 in the chromatogram obtained with the test solution are not more intense than the spots in the chromatograms obtained with reference solutions (b) and (c) respectively.

Phenolic antioxidants. Examine by liquid chromatography (*2.2.29*).

Test solution (a). Evaporate 50 ml of solution S1 to dryness *in vacuo* at 45 °C. Dissolve the residue in 5.0 ml of a mixture of equal volumes of *acetonitrile R* and *tetrahydrofuran R.*

Test solution (b). Evaporate 50 ml of solution S1 to dryness *in vacuo* at 45 °C. Dissolve the residue in 5.0 ml of *methylene chloride R.*

Reference solution (a). Dissolve 25 mg of *butylhydroxytoluene CRS* (plastic additive 07), 40 mg of *plastic additive 10 CRS,* 40 mg of *plastic additive 09 CRS* and 40 mg of *plastic additive 11 CRS* in 10 ml of a mixture of equal volumes of *acetonitrile R* and *tetrahydrofuran R.* Dilute 2 ml to 50.0 ml with a mixture of equal volumes of *acetonitrile R* and *tetrahydrofuran R.*

Reference solution (b). Dissolve 40 mg of *plastic additive 11 CRS* and 40 mg of *plastic additive 12 CRS* in 10 ml of *methylene chloride R.* Dilute 2 ml to 50.0 ml with *methylene chloride R.*

The chromatographic procedure may be carried out using:

- a stainless steel column 0.25 m long and 4.6 mm in internal diameter packed with *octadecylsilyl silica gel for chromatography R* (5 µm),
- as mobile phase at a flow rate of 1.5 ml/min one of the two following mixtures:

  Mobile phase 1: 10 volumes of *water R,* 30 volumes of *tetrahydrofuran R,* 60 volumes of *acetonitrile R,*

  Mobile phase 2: 5 volumes of *water R,* 45 volumes of *2-propanol R,* 50 volumes of *methanol R,*
- as detector a spectrophotometer set at 280 nm.

Using mobile phase 1, inject 20 µl of test solution (a) and 20 µl of reference solution (a). The chromatogram obtained with test solution (a) shows only principal peaks corresponding to the peaks in the chromatogram obtained with reference solution (a) with a retention time greater than 2 min.

The areas of the peaks in the chromatogram obtained with test solution (a) are not greater than those of the corresponding peaks in the chromatogram obtained with reference solution (a), except for the last peak eluted in the chromatogram obtained with reference solution (a).

The test is not valid unless, with mobile phase 1, the number of theoretical plates calculated for the peak corresponding to plastic additive 07 is at least 2500 and the resolution between the peaks corresponding to plastic additive 09 and plastic additive 10 is not less than 2.0.

If the chromatogram obtained with test solution (a) shows a peak with the same retention time as the last antioxidant eluted from reference solution (a), use mobile phase 2 as follows.

Inject 20 µl of test solution (b) and 20 µl of reference solution (b). The chromatogram obtained with test solution (b) shows only principal peaks corresponding to the peaks in the chromatogram obtained with reference solution (b) with a retention time greater than 3 min.

The areas of the peaks in the chromatogram obtained with test solution (b) are not greater than those of the corresponding peaks in the chromatogram obtained with reference solution (b).

The test is not valid unless the resolution between the peaks corresponding to plastic additive 11 and plastic additive 12 is at least 2.0.

Substances soluble in hexane. Place 5 g in a borosilicate-glass flask with a ground-glass neck. Add 50 ml of *hexane R,* fit a condenser and boil under reflux on a water-bath with constant stirring for 4 h. Cool in iced-water; a gel may form. Adapt a cooling jacket filled with iced water to a sintered-glass filter (16) fitted with a device allowing pressure to be applied during filtration. Allow the filter to cool for 15 min. Filter the hexane solution applying a gauge pressure of 27 kPa and without washing the residue; the filtration time must not exceed 5 min. Evaporate 20 ml of the solution to dryness on a water-bath. Dry at 100 °C for 1 h. The mass of the residue is not greater than 40 mg (2 per cent) for copolymer to be used for containers and not greater than 0.1 g (5 per cent) for copolymer to be used for tubing.

Sulphated ash (*2.4.14*). Not more than 1.2 per cent, determined on 5.0 g.

ASSAY

Introduce 0.250 g to 1.000 g of the substance to be examined, according to the vinyl acetate content of the copolymer to be examined, into a 300 ml conical flask with a ground-glass neck containing a magnetic stirrer. Add 40 ml of *xylene R.* Boil under a reflux condenser with stirring for 4 h. Stirring continuously, allow to cool until precipitation begins before slowly adding 25.0 ml of *alcoholic potassium hydroxide solution R1.* Boil again under a reflux condenser with stirring for 3 h. Allow to cool with continued stirring, rinse the condenser with 50 ml of *water R* and add 30.0 ml of *0.05 M sulphuric acid* to the flask. Transfer the contents of the flask into a 400 ml beaker; rinse the flask with two quantities, each of 50 ml, of a 200 g/l solution of *anhydrous sodium sulphate R* and three quantities, each of 20 ml, of *water R* and add all the rinsings to the beaker containing the initial solution. Titrate the excess sulphuric acid with *0.1 M sodium hydroxide,* determining the end-point potentiometrically (*2.2.20*). Carry out a blank titration.

1 ml of *0.05 M sulphuric acid* is equivalent to 8.609 mg of vinyl acetate.

01/2005:30108

3.1.8. SILICONE OIL USED AS A LUBRICANT

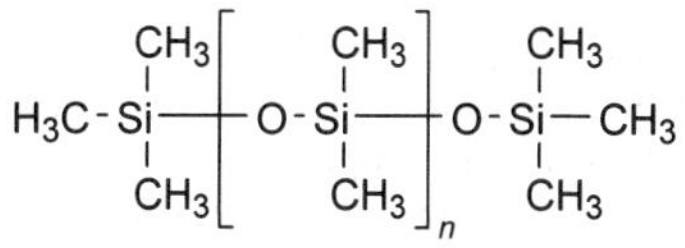

DEFINITION

Silicone oil used as a lubricant is a poly(dimethylsiloxane) obtained by hydrolysis and polycondensation of dichlorodimethylsilane and chlorotrimethylsilane. Different grades exist which are characterised by a number indicating the nominal viscosity placed after the name.

Silicone oil used as lubricants have a degree of polymerisation (n = 400 to 1200) such that their kinematic viscosities are nominally between 1000 $mm^2 \cdot s^{-1}$ and 30 000 $mm^2 \cdot s^{-1}$.

CHARACTERS

Clear, colourless liquids of various viscosities, practically insoluble in water and in methanol, miscible with ethyl acetate, with methyl ethyl ketone and with toluene, very slightly soluble in ethanol.

IDENTIFICATION

A. It is identified by its kinematic viscosity at 25 °C (see Tests).

B. Examine by infrared absorption spectrophotometry (*2.2.24*), comparing with the spectrum obtained with *silicone oil CRS*. The region of the spectrum from 850 cm^{-1} to 750 cm^{-1} is not taken into account since it may show slight differences depending on the degree of polymerisation.

C. Heat 0.5 g in a test-tube over a small flame until white fumes begin to appear. Invert the tube over a second tube containing 1 ml of a 1 g/l solution of *chromotropic acid, sodium salt R* in *sulphuric acid R* so that the fumes reach the solution. Shake the second tube for about 10 s and heat on a water-bath for 5 min. The solution is violet.

D. In a platinum crucible, prepare the sulphated ash (*2.4.14*) using 50 mg. The residue is a white powder that gives the reaction of silicates (*2.3.1*).

TESTS

Acidity. To 2.0 g add 25 ml of a mixture of equal volumes of *ethanol R* and *ether R*, previously neutralised to 0.2 ml of *bromothymol blue solution R1* and shake. Not more than 0.15 ml of *0.01 M sodium hydroxide* is required to change the colour of the solution to blue.

Viscosity (*2.2.10*). Determine the dynamic viscosity at 25 °C. Calculate the kinematic viscosity taking the relative density to be 0.97. The kinematic viscosity is not less than 95 per cent and not more than 105 per cent of the nominal viscosity stated on the label.

Mineral oils. Place 2 ml in a test-tube and examine in ultraviolet light at 365 nm. The fluorescence is not more intense than that of a solution containing 0.1 ppm of *quinine sulphate R* in *0.005 M sulphuric acid* examined in the same conditions.

Phenylated compounds. The refractive index (*2.2.6*) is not greater than 1.410.

Heavy metals. Mix 1.0 g with *methylene chloride R* and dilute to 20 ml with the same solvent. Add 1.0 ml of a freshly prepared 0.02 g/l solution of *dithizone R* in *methylene chloride R*, 0.5 ml of *water R* and 0.5 ml of a mixture of 1 volume of *dilute ammonia R2* and 9 volumes of a 2 g/l solution of *hydroxylamine hydrochloride R*. At the same time, prepare a standard as follows: to 20 ml of *methylene chloride R* add 1.0 ml of a freshly prepared 0.02 g/l solution of *dithizone R* in *methylene chloride R*, 0.5 ml of *lead standard solution (10 ppm Pb) R* and 0.5 ml of a mixture of 1 volume of *dilute ammonia R2* and 9 volumes of a 2 g/l solution of *hydroxylamine hydrochloride R*. Immediately shake each solution vigorously for 1 min. Any red colour in the test solution is not more intense than that in the standard (5 ppm).

Volatile matter. Not more than 2.0 per cent, determined on 2.00 g by heating in an oven at 150 °C for 24 h. Carry out the test using a dish 60 mm in diameter and 10 mm deep.

LABELLING

The label indicates the nominal viscosity by a number placed after the name of the product. The label also states that the contents are to be used as a lubricant.

01/2005:30109

3.1.9. SILICONE ELASTOMER FOR CLOSURES AND TUBING

DEFINITION

Silicone elastomer complying with the following requirements is suitable for the manufacture of closures and tubing.

Silicone elastomer is obtained by cross-linking a linear polysiloxane constructed mainly of dimethylsiloxy units with small quantities of methylvinylsiloxy groups; the chain ends are blocked by trimethylsiloxy or dimethylvinylsiloxy groups.

The general formula of the polysiloxane is:

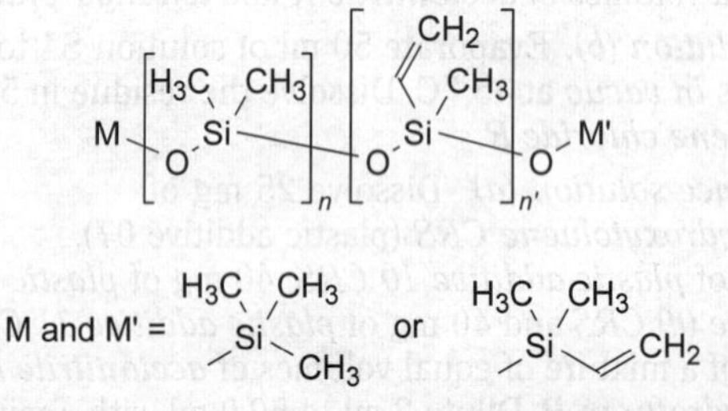

The cross-linking is carried out in the hot state either with:

– 2,4-dichlorobenzoyl peroxide for extruded products,

– 2,4-dichlorobenzoyl peroxide or dicumyl peroxide or *OO*-(1,1-dimethylethyl) *O*-isopropyl monoperoxycarbonate or 2,5-bis[(1,1-dimethylethyl)dioxy]-2,5-dimethylhexane for moulded products,

or

– by hydrosilylation by means of polysiloxane with -SiH groups using platinum as a catalyst.

In all cases, appropriate additives are used such as silica and sometimes small quantities of organosilicon additives (α,ω-dihydroxypolydimethylsiloxane).

CHARACTERS

A transparent or translucent material, practically insoluble in organic solvents, some of which, for example cyclohexane, hexane and methylene chloride, cause a reversible swelling of the material.

IDENTIFICATION

A. Examine by infrared absorption spectrophotometry recording the spectrum by the multiple reflection method for solids (*2.2.24*), comparing with the spectrum obtained with *silicone elastomer CRS*.

B. Heat 1.0 g in a test-tube over a small flame until white fumes begin to appear. Invert the tube over a second tube containing 1 ml of a 1 g/l solution of *chromotropic acid, sodium salt R* in *sulphuric acid R* so that the fumes reach the solution. Shake the second tube for about 10 s and heat on a water-bath for 5 min. The solution is violet.

C. 50 mg of the residue of combustion gives the reaction of silicates (*2.3.1*).

TESTS

If necessary, cut the material into pieces of maximum dimension on a side of not greater than 1 cm.

Solution S. Place 25 g in a borosilicate-glass flask with a ground-glass neck. Add 500 ml of *water R* and boil under a reflux condenser for 5 h. Allow to cool and decant the solution.

Appearance of solution. Solution S is clear (*2.2.1*).

Acidity or alkalinity. To 100 ml of solution S add 0.15 ml of *bromothymol blue solution R1*. Not more than 2.5 ml of *0.01 M sodium hydroxide* is required to change the colour of the indicator to blue. To a further 100 ml of solution S, add 0.2 ml of *methyl orange solution R*. Not more than 1.0 ml of *0.01 M hydrochloric acid* is required to reach the beginning of the colour change of the indicator from yellow to orange.

Relative density (*2.2.5*). 1.05 to 1.25, determined using a density bottle with *ethanol R* as the immersion liquid.

Reducing substances. To 20 ml of solution S add 1 ml of *dilute sulphuric acid R* and 20 ml of *0.002 M potassium permanganate*. Allow to stand for 15 min. Add 1 g of *potassium iodide R* and titrate immediately with *0.01 M sodium thiosulphate* using 0.25 ml of *starch solution R* as indicator. Carry out a blank titration using 20 ml of *water R* instead of solution S. The difference between the titration volumes is not more than 1.0 ml.

Substances soluble in hexane. Evaporate 25 ml of the solution obtained in the test for phenylated compounds in a glass evaporating dish on a water-bath and dry in an oven at 100 °C to 105 °C for 1 h. The residue weighs not more than 15 mg (3 per cent).

Phenylated compounds. Place 2.0 g in a borosilicate-glass flask with a ground-glass neck and add 100 ml of *hexane R*. Boil under a reflux condenser for 4 h. Cool, then filter rapidly through a sintered-glass filter (16). Collect the filtrate and close the container immediately to avoid evaporation. At wavelengths from 250 nm to 340 nm, the absorbance (*2.2.25*) is not greater than 0.4.

Mineral oils. Place 2 g in a 100 ml conical flask containing 30 ml of a mixture of 5 volumes of *ammonia R* and 95 volumes of *pyridine R*. Allow to stand for 2 h, shaking frequently. Decant the pyridine solution and examine in ultraviolet light at 365 nm. The fluorescence is not greater than that of a solution containing 1 ppm of *quinine sulphate R* in *0.005 M sulphuric acid* examined in the same conditions.

Volatile matter. Weigh 10.0 g of the substance previously stored for 48 h in a desiccator over *anhydrous calcium chloride R*. Heat in an oven at 200 °C for 4 h, allow to cool in a desiccator and weigh again. For silicone elastomer prepared using peroxides, the volatile matter is not greater than 0.5 per cent. For silicone elastomer prepared using platinum, the volatile matter is not greater than 2.0 per cent.

Silicone elastomer prepared using peroxides complies with the following additional test:

Residual peroxides. Place 5 g in a borosilicate-glass flask, add 150 ml of *methylene chloride R* and close the flask. Stir with a mechanical stirrer for 16 h. Filter rapidly, collecting the filtrate in a flask with a ground-glass neck. Replace the air in the container with *oxygen-free nitrogen R*, introduce 1 ml of a 200 g/l solution of *sodium iodide R* in *anhydrous acetic acid R*, close the flask, shake thoroughly and allow to stand protected from light for 30 min. Add 50 ml of *water R* and titrate immediately with *0.01 M sodium thiosulphate*, using 0.25 ml of *starch solution R* as indicator. Carry out a blank titration. The difference between the titration volumes is not greater than 2.0 ml (0.08 per cent calculated as dichlorobenzoyl peroxide).

Silicone elastomer prepared using platinum complies with the following additional test:

Platinum. In a quartz crucible, ignite 1.0 g of the material to be examined, raising the temperature gradually until a white residue is obtained. Transfer the residue to a graphite crucible. To the quartz crucible add 10 ml of a freshly prepared mixture of 1 volume of *nitric acid R* and 3 volumes of *hydrochloric acid R*, heat on a water-bath for 1 min to 2 min and transfer to the graphite crucible. Add 5 mg of *potassium chloride R* and 5 ml of *hydrofluoric acid R* and evaporate to dryness on a water-bath. Add 5 ml of *hydrofluoric acid R* and evaporate to dryness again; repeat this operation twice. Dissolve the residue in 5 ml of *1 M hydrochloric acid*, warming on a water-bath. Allow to cool and add the solution to 1 ml of a 250 g/l solution of *stannous chloride R* in *1 M hydrochloric acid*, rinse the graphite crucible with a few millilitres of *1 M hydrochloric acid* and dilute to 10.0 ml with the same acid. Prepare simultaneously a standard as follows: to 1 ml of a 250 g/l solution of *stannous chloride R* in *1 M hydrochloric acid* add 1.0 ml of *platinum standard solution (30 ppm Pt) R* and dilute to 10.0 ml with *1 M hydrochloric acid*. The colour of the test solution is not more intense than that of the standard (30 ppm).

LABELLING

The label states whether the material was prepared using peroxides or platinum.

01/2005:30110

3.1.10. MATERIALS BASED ON NON-PLASTICISED POLY(VINYL CHLORIDE) FOR CONTAINERS FOR NON-INJECTABLE, AQUEOUS SOLUTIONS

DEFINITION

Materials based on non-plasticised poly(vinyl chloride) that comply with the following specifications are suitable for the manufacture of containers for non-injectable aqueous solutions. They may also be used for solid forms for oral administration and in some cases, subject to special studies on the compatibility of the container with its contents, these materials may be suitable for the preparation of containers for suppositories. They consist of one or more poly(vinyl chloride/vinyl acetate) or of a mixture of poly(vinyl chloride) and poly(vinyl acetate) or of poly(vinyl chloride).

They contain not more than 1 ppm of vinyl chloride.

The chlorine content expressed in poly(vinyl chloride) is not less than 80 per cent.

They may contain not more than 15 per cent of copolymers based on acrylic and/or methacrylic acids and/or their esters, and/or on styrene and/or butadiene.

PRODUCTION

Materials based on non-plasticised poly(vinyl chloride) are produced by polymerisation methods which guarantee a residual vinyl chloride content of less than 1 ppm. The production method used is validated in order to demonstrate that the product complies with the following test:

Vinyl chloride. Not more than 1 ppm, determined by head-space gas chromatography (*2.2.28*), using *ether R* as the internal standard.

Internal standard solution. Using a microsyringe, inject 10 µl of *ether R* into 20.0 ml of *dimethylacetamide R*, immersing the tip of the needle in the solvent. Immediately before use, dilute the solution to 1000 times its volume with *dimethylacetamide R*.

Test solution. Place 1.000 g of the material to be examined in a 50 ml vial and add 10.0 ml of the internal standard solution. Close the vial and secure the stopper. Shake, avoiding contact between the stopper and the liquid. Place the vial in a water-bath at 60 ± 1 °C for 2 h.

Vinyl chloride primary solution. Prepare under a ventilated hood. Place 50.0 ml of *dimethylacetamide R* in a 50 ml vial, stopper the vial, secure the stopper and weigh to the nearest 0.1 mg. Fill a 50 ml polyethylene or polypropylene syringe with gaseous *vinyl chloride R*, allow the gas to remain in contact with the syringe for about 3 min, empty the syringe and fill again with 50 ml of gaseous *vinyl chloride R*. Fit a hypodermic needle to the syringe and reduce the volume of gas in the syringe from 50 ml to 25 ml. Inject these 25 ml of vinyl chloride slowly into the vial, shaking gently and avoiding contact between the liquid and the needle. Weigh the vial again; the increase in mass is about 60 mg (1 µl of the solution thus obtained contains about 1.2 µg of vinyl chloride). Allow to stand for 2 h. Keep the primary solution in a refrigerator.

Vinyl chloride standard solution. To 1 volume of the vinyl chloride primary solution add 3 volumes of *dimethylacetamide R*.

Reference solutions. Place 10.0 ml of the internal standard solution in each of six 50 ml vials. Close the vials and secure the stoppers. Inject 1 µl, 2 µl, 3 µl, 5 µl and 10 µl, respectively, of the vinyl chloride standard solution into five of the vials. The six solutions thus obtained contain respectively, 0 µg, about 0.3 µg, 0.6 µg, 0.9 µg, 1.5 µg and 3 µg of vinyl chloride. Shake, avoiding contact between the stopper and the liquid. Place the vials in a water-bath at 60 ± 1 °C for 2 h.

The chromatographic procedure may be carried out using:

- a stainless steel column 3 m long and 3 mm in internal diameter packed with *silanised diatomaceous earth for gas chromatography R* impregnated with 5 per cent *m/m* of *dimethylstearylamide R* and 5 per cent *m/m* of *macrogol 400 R*,
- *nitrogen for chromatography R* as the carrier gas at a flow rate of 30 ml/min,
- a flame-ionisation detector,

maintaining the temperature of the column at 45 °C, that of the injection port at 100 °C and that of the detector at 150 °C.

Inject 1 ml of the head-space of each vial. Calculate the content of vinyl chloride.

In order to obtain the required mechanical and stability characteristics, materials based on non-plasticised poly(vinyl chloride) may contain:

- not more than 8 per cent of epoxidised soya oil of which the oxiran oxygen content is 6 per cent to 8 per cent and the iodine value is not greater than 6,
- not more than 1.5 per cent of calcium salt or zinc salts of aliphatic fatty acids with more than seven carbon atoms or not more than 1.5 per cent of their mixture,
- not more than 1.5 per cent of liquid paraffin,
- not more than 1.5 per cent of waxes,
- not more than 2 per cent of hydrogenated oils or esters of aliphatic fatty acids,
- not more than 1.5 per cent of macrogol esters,
- not more than 1.5 per cent of sorbitol,
- not more than 1 per cent of 2,4-dinonylphenyl phosphite, or di(4-nonylphenyl) phosphite or tris(nonylphenyl) phosphite.

They may contain one of the following groups of stabilisers:

- not more than 0.25 per cent of tin as di(isooctyl) 2,2′-[(dioctylstannylene)bis(thio)]diacetate containing about 27 per cent of tri(isooctyl) 2,2′,2″-[(monooctylstannylidyne)tris(thio)]triacetate,
- not more than 0.25 per cent of tin as a mixture containing not more than 76 per cent of di(isooctyl) 2,2′-[(dimethylstannylene)bis(thio)]diacetate and not more than 85 per cent of tri(isooctyl) 2,2′,2″-[(monomethylstannylidyne)tris(thio)]triacetate; (isooctyl is e.g. 2-ethylhexyl),
- not more than 1 per cent of 1-phenyleicosane-1,3-dione (benzoylstearoylmethane) or 2-(4-dodecylphenyl)indole or didodecyl 1,4-dihydropyridine-2,6-dimethyl-3,5-dicarboxylate or 1 per cent of a mixture of two of these.

They may contain a colorant or pigment.

They may be opacified by titanium dioxide.

The supplier of the material must be able to demonstrate that the qualitative and quantitative composition of the type sample is satisfactory for each production batch.

CHARACTERS

Powder, beads, granules, sheets of varying thicknesses or samples taken from finished objects, insoluble in water, soluble in tetrahydrofuran, slightly soluble in methylene chloride, insoluble in ethanol. They burn with an orange-yellow flame edged with green, giving off thick black smoke.

IDENTIFICATION

Dissolve the residue (A) (see Tests: solution S2) in 5 ml of *tetrahydrofuran R*. Apply a few drops of the solution to a sodium chloride plate and evaporate to dryness in an oven at 100 °C to 105 °C. Examine by infrared absorption spectrophotometry (*2.2.24*). The material to be examined shows absorption maxima at 2975 cm^{-1}, 2910 cm^{-1}, 2865 cm^{-1}, 1430 cm^{-1}, 1330 cm^{-1}, 1255 cm^{-1}, 690 cm^{-1}, 615 cm^{-1}. In addition, the spectrum obtained is identical to that of the material selected for the type sample.

TESTS

If necessary, cut the material into pieces with a maximum dimension on a side of not greater than 1 cm.

Solution S1. Place 25 g in a borosilicate-glass flask. Add 500 ml of *water R* and cover the neck of the flask with aluminium foil or a borosilicate-glass beaker. Heat in an autoclave for 121 ± 2 °C for 20 min. Allow to cool and allow the solids to settle.

Solution S2. Dissolve 5.0 g in 80 ml of *tetrahydrofuran R* and dilute to 100 ml with the same solvent. Filter if necessary (the solution may remain opalescent). Dilute 20 ml of the solution and add dropwise with gentle shaking 70 ml of *alcohol R*. Cool in ice for 1 h. Filter or centrifuge. Wash the residue A with *alcohol R* and add the washings to the filtrate or the centrifugation liquid. Dilute to 100 ml with *alcohol R*.

Solution S3. Place 5 g in a borosilicate-glass flask with a ground-glass neck. Add 100 ml of *0.1 M hydrochloric acid* and boil under a reflux condenser for 1 h. Allow to cool and allow the solids to settle.

Appearance of solution S1. Solution S1 is not more opalescent than reference suspension II (*2.2.1*) and is colourless (*2.2.2, Method II*).

Absorbance of solution S1 (*2.2.25*). Evaporate to dryness 100 ml of solution S1. Dissolve the residue in 5 ml of *hexane R*. Filter if necessary through a filter previously rinsed with *hexane R*. At wavelengths from 250 nm to 310 nm, the absorbance of the filtrate is not greater than 0.25.

Absorbance of solution S2 (*2.2.25*). At wavelengths from 250 nm to 330 nm, the absorbance of solution S2 is not greater than 0.2 for tin-stabilised materials or 0.4 for other materials.

Extractable barium. Examine by atomic emission spectrometry in an argon plasma (*2.2.22, Method I*).

Test solution. Solution S3.

Reference solution. A solution containing 0.1 ppm of barium prepared by dilution of *barium standard solution (50 ppm Ba) R* with *0.1 M hydrochloric acid*.

Carry out the determination using the emission of barium at 455.40 nm, the spectral background being taken at 455.30 nm.

Verify the absence of barium in the hydrochloric acid used.

Examined at 455.40 nm, the emission of the test solution is not greater than that of the reference solution (2 ppm).

Extractable cadmium. Examine by atomic absorption spectrometry (*2.2.23, Method I*).

Test solution. Solution S3.

Reference solution. A solution containing 0.03 ppm of cadmium prepared by diluting *cadmium standard solution (0.1 per cent Cd) R* with *0.1 M hydrochloric acid*.

Verify the absence of cadmium in the hydrochloric acid used.

Examined at 228.8 nm, the absorbance of the test solution is not greater than that of the reference solution (0.6 ppm).

Tin-stabilised materials. To 0.10 ml of solution S2 in a test tube add 0.05 ml of *1 M hydrochloric acid*, 0.5 ml of *potassium iodide solution R* and 5 ml of *alcohol R*. Mix thoroughly and wait for 5 min. Add 9 ml of *water R* and 0.1 ml of a 5 g/l solution of *sodium sulphite R* and mix thoroughly. Add 1.5 ml of *dithizone solution R* freshly diluted one-hundred-fold with *methylene chloride R*, shake for 15 s and allow to stand for 2 min. At the same time prepare a reference solution in the same manner using 0.1 ml of tin standard solution.

Any violet colour in the lower layer obtained with solution S2 is not more intense than that obtained with the reference solution (0.25 per cent of Sn). The greenish-blue colour of dithizone solution turns pink in the presence of tin.

Tin stock solution. Dilute 81 mg of *plastic additive 23 CRS* in a 100 ml volumetric flask to 100 ml with *tetrahydrofuran R*.

Tin standard solution. Dilute 20 ml of tin stock solution in a 100 ml volumetric flask to 100 ml with *alcohol R*.

Non-tin stabilised materials. To 5 ml of solution S2 in a test tube add 0.05 ml of *1 M hydrochloric acid* and 0.5 ml of *potassium iodide solution R*. Mix thoroughly and wait for 5 min. Add 9 ml of *water R* and 0.1 ml of a 5 g/l solution of *sodium sulphite R* and mix thoroughly. If the solution obtained is not colourless, add the sodium sulphite solution in 0.05 ml fractions. Add 1.5 ml of *dithizone solution R* freshly diluted one hundred times with *methylene chloride R*, shake for 15 s and allow to stand for 2 min. At the same time prepare a standard in the same manner using 0.05 ml of tin standard solution.

Any violet colour in the lower layer obtained with solution S2 is not more intense than that obtained with the reference solution (25 ppm of Sn).

Extractable heavy metals (*2.4.8*). 12 ml of solution S3 complies with limit test A for heavy metals (20 ppm). Prepare the standard using 10 ml of *lead standard solution (1 ppm Pb) R*.

Extractable zinc. Examine by atomic absorption spectrometry (*2.2.23, Method I*).

Test solution. Solution S3 diluted ten times with *water R*.

Reference solution. A solution containing 0.50 ppm of zinc prepared by dilution of *zinc standard solution (5 mg/ml Zn) R* with *0.01 M hydrochloric acid*.

Verify the absence of zinc in the hydrochloric acid used.

Examined at 214.0 nm, the absorbance of the test solution is not greater than that of the reference solution (100 ppm).

Sulphated ash (*2.4.14*). Not more than 1.0 per cent, determined on 1.0 g. When the materials are opacified using titanium dioxide, the content of sulphated ash does not exceed 4.0 per cent.

ASSAY

Carry out the oxygen-flask method (*2.5.10*) using 50.0 mg of the substance to be examined. Absorb the combustion products in 20 ml of *1 M sodium hydroxide*. To the solution obtained add 2.5 ml of *nitric acid R*, 10.0 ml of *0.1 M silver nitrate*, 5 ml of *ferric ammonium sulphate solution R2* and 1 ml of *dibutyl phthalate R*. Titrate with *0.05 M ammonium thiocyanate* until a reddish-yellow colour is obtained. Carry out a blank titration.

1 ml of *0.1 M silver nitrate* is equivalent to 6.25 mg of poly(vinyl chloride).

01/2005:30111

3.1.11. MATERIALS BASED ON NON-PLASTICISED POLY(VINYL CHLORIDE) FOR CONTAINERS FOR DRY DOSAGE FORMS FOR ORAL ADMINISTRATION

DEFINITION

Materials based on non-plasticised poly(vinyl chloride) for containers for dry dosage forms for oral administration are suitable for the manufacture of sheets or containers.

They consist of one or more poly(vinyl chloride/vinyl acetate) or of a mixture of poly(vinyl chloride) and poly(vinyl acetate) or of poly(vinyl chloride).

They contain not more than 1 ppm of vinyl chloride.

The chlorine content expressed in poly(vinyl chloride) is not less than 80 per cent.

They may contain not more than 15 per cent of copolymers based on acrylic and/or methacrylic acids and/or their esters, and/or on styrene and/or butadiene.

PRODUCTION

Materials based on non-plasticised poly(vinyl chloride) are produced by polymerisation methods which guarantee a residual vinyl chloride content of less than 1 ppm. The production method used is validated in order to demonstrate that the product complies with the following test for vinyl chloride.

Vinyl chloride. Not more than 1 ppm, determined by head-space gas chromatography (*2.2.28*), using *ether R* as the internal standard.

Internal standard solution. Using a microsyringe, inject 10 µl of *ether R* into 20.0 ml of *dimethylacetamide R*, immersing the tip of the needle in the solvent. Immediately before use, dilute the solution to 1000 times its volume with *dimethylacetamide R*.

Test solution. Place 1.000 g of the material to be examined in a 50 ml vial and add 10.0 ml of the internal standard solution. Close the vial and secure the stopper. Shake, avoiding contact between the stopper and the liquid. Place the vial in a water-bath at 60 ± 1 °C for 2 h.

Vinyl chloride primary solution. Prepare under a ventilated hood. Place 50.0 ml of *dimethylacetamide R* in a 50 ml vial, stopper the vial, secure the stopper and weigh to the nearest 0.1 mg. Fill a 50 ml polyethylene or polypropylene syringe with gaseous *vinyl chloride R,* allow the gas to remain in contact with the syringe for about 3 min, empty the syringe and fill again with 50 ml of gaseous *vinyl chloride R.* Fit a hypodermic needle to the syringe and reduce the volume of gas in the syringe from 50 ml to 25 ml. Inject these 25 ml of vinyl chloride slowly into the vial, shaking gently and avoiding contact between the liquid and the needle. Weigh the vial again; the increase in mass is about 60 mg (1 µl of the solution thus obtained contains about 1.2 µg of vinyl chloride). Allow to stand for 2 h. Keep the primary solution in a refrigerator.

Vinyl chloride standard solution. To 1 volume of the vinyl chloride primary solution add 3 volumes of *dimethylacetamide R.*

Reference solutions. Place 10.0 ml of the internal standard solution in each of six 50 ml vials. Close the vials and secure the stoppers. Inject 1 µl, 2 µl, 3 µl, 5 µl and 10 µl, respectively, of the vinyl chloride standard solution into 5 of the vials. The 6 solutions thus obtained contain respectively, 0 µg, about 0.3 µg, 0.6 µg, 0.9 µg, 1.5 µg and 3 µg of vinyl chloride. Shake, avoiding contact between the stopper and the liquid. Place the vials in a water-bath at 60 ± 1 °C for 2 h.

The chromatographic procedure may be carried out using:

- a stainless steel column 3 m long and 3 mm in internal diameter packed with *silanised diatomaceous earth for gas chromatography R* impregnated with 5 per cent *m/m* of *dimethylstearylamide R* and 5 per cent *m/m* of *macrogol 400 R,*
- *nitrogen for chromatography R* as the carrier gas at a flow rate of 30 ml/min,
- a flame-ionisation detector,

maintaining the temperature of the column at 45 °C, that of the injection port at 100 °C and that of the detector at 150 °C.

Inject 1 ml of the head-space of each vial. Calculate the content of vinyl chloride.

Additives

In order to obtain the required mechanical and stability characteristics, materials based on non-plasticised poly(vinyl chloride) may contain:

- not more than 2 per cent of epoxidised soya oil of which the oxiran oxygen content is 6 per cent to 8 per cent and the iodine value is not greater than 6 for tin-stabilised materials,
- not more than 3 per cent of epoxidised soya oil of which the oxiran oxygen content is 6 per cent to 8 per cent and the iodine value is not greater than 6 for non-tin-stabilised materials,
- not more than 1.5 per cent of calcium, magnesium or zinc salts of aliphatic fatty acids with more than 7 carbon atoms or not more than 1.5 per cent of their mixture,
- not more than 4 per cent of waxes,
- not more than 1.5 per cent of liquid paraffin,
- not more than 2 per cent of hydrogenated oils or esters of aliphatic fatty acids,
- not more than 4 per cent for the percentage sum of the 3 lubricants above,
- not more than 1.5 per cent of macrogol esters,
- not more than 1.5 per cent of sorbitol,
- not more than 1 per cent of 2,4-dinonylphenyl phosphite, or di(4-nonylphenyl) phosphite or tris(nonylphenyl) phosphite,
- not more than 1 per cent of calcium carbonate,
- not more than 1 per cent of silica.

They may contain one of the following groups of stabilisers:

- not more than 0.25 per cent of tin as di(isooctyl) 2,2′-[(dioctylstannylene)bis(thio)]diacetate containing about 27 per cent of tri(isooctyl) 2,2′2″-[(monooctylstannylidyne)tris(thio)]triacetate,
- not more than 0.25 per cent of tin as a mixture containing not more than 76 per cent of di(isooctyl) 2,2′-[(dimethylstannylene)bis(thio)]diacetate and not more than 85 per cent of tri(isooctyl) 2,2′,2″-[(monomethylstannylidyne)tris(thio)]triacetate; (isooctyl is e.g. 2-ethylhexyl),
- not more than 1 per cent of 1-phenyleicosane-1,3-dione (benzoylstearoylmethane).

They may contain a colorant or pigment.

They may be opacified by titanium dioxide.

The supplier of the material must be able to demonstrate that the qualitative and quantitative composition of the type sample is satisfactory for each production batch.

CHARACTERS

Powder, beads, granules, sheets of varying thicknesses or samples taken from finished objects, insoluble in water, soluble in tetrahydrofuran, slightly soluble in methylene chloride, insoluble in ethanol. They burn with an orange-yellow flame edged with green, giving off thick black smoke.

IDENTIFICATION

Dissolve residue A (see Tests: solution S2) in 5 ml of *tetrahydrofuran R.* Apply a few drops of the solution to a sodium chloride plate and evaporate to dryness in an oven at 100-105 °C. Examine by infrared absorption spectrophotometry (*2.2.24*). The material to be examined shows absorption maxima at 2975 cm^{-1}, 2910 cm^{-1}, 2865 cm^{-1}, 1430 cm^{-1}, 1330 cm^{-1}, 1255 cm^{-1}, 690 cm^{-1}, 615 cm^{-1}. In addition, the spectrum obtained is identical to that of the material selected for the type sample.

TESTS

If necessary, cut the material into pieces with a maximum dimension on a side of not greater than 1 cm.

Solution S1. Place 25 g in a borosilicate glass flask. Add 500 ml of *water R* and cover the neck of the flask with aluminium foil or a borosilicate glass beaker. Heat in an autoclave for 121 ± 2 °C for 20 min. Allow to cool and allow the solids to settle.

Solution S2. Dissolve 5.0 g in 80 ml of *tetrahydrofuran R* and dilute to 100 ml with the same solvent. Filter if necessary (the solution may remain opalescent). Dilute 20 ml of the solution and add dropwise with gentle shaking 70 ml of *alcohol R.* Cool in ice for 1 h. Filter or centrifuge (residue A). Wash residue A with *alcohol R* and add the washings to the filtrate or the centrifugation liquid. Dilute to 100 ml with *alcohol R.*

Solution S3. Place 5 g in a borosilicate-glass flask with a ground-glass neck. Add 100 ml of *0.1 M hydrochloric acid* and boil under a reflux condenser for 1 h. Allow to cool and allow the solids to settle.

Appearance of solution S1. Solution S1 is not more opalescent than reference suspension II (*2.2.1*) and is colourless (*2.2.2, Method II*).

Absorbance of solution S1 (*2.2.25*). Evaporate to dryness 100 ml of solution S1. Dissolve the residue in 5 ml of *hexane R*. Filter if necessary through a filter previously rinsed with *hexane R*. At wavelengths from 250 nm to 310 nm, the absorbance of the filtrate is not greater than 0.3.

Absorbance of solution S2 (*2.2.25*). For material that does not contain 1-phenyleicosane-1,3-dione, at wavelengths from 250 nm to 330 nm, the absorbance of solution S2 is not greater than 0.5. For material that contains 1-phenyleicosane-1,3-dione, at wavelengths from 250 nm to 330 nm, the absorbance of a tenfold dilution of solution S2 in *alcohol R* is not greater than 0.4.

Tin-stabilised materials. To 0.10 ml of solution S2 in a test tube add 0.05 ml of *1 M hydrochloric acid*, 0.5 ml of *potassium iodide solution R* and 5 ml of *alcohol R*. Mix thoroughly and wait for 5 min. Add 9 ml of *water R* and 0.1 ml of a 5 g/l solution of *sodium sulphite R* and mix thoroughly. Add 1.5 ml of *dithizone solution R* freshly diluted one-hundred-fold with *methylene chloride R*, shake for 15 s and allow to stand for 2 min. At the same time prepare a reference solution in the same manner using 0.1 ml of tin standard solution.

Any violet colour in the lower layer obtained with solution S2 is not more intense than that obtained with the reference solution (0.25 per cent Sn). The greenish-blue colour of dithizone solution turns pink in the presence of tin.

Tin stock solution. Dilute 81 mg of *plastic additive 23 CRS* in a 100 ml volumetric flask to 100 ml with *tetrahydrofuran R*.

Tin standard solution. Dilute 20 ml of tin stock solution in a 100 ml volumetric flask to 100 ml with *alcohol R*.

Non tin-stabilised materials. To 5 ml of solution S2 in a test tube add 0.05 ml of *1 M hydrochloric acid* and 0.5 ml of *potassium iodide solution R*. Mix thoroughly and wait for 5 min. Add 9 ml of *water R* and 0.1 ml of a 5 g/l solution of *sodium sulphite R* and mix thoroughly. If the solution obtained is not colourless, add the sodium sulphite solution in 0.05 ml fractions. Add 1.5 ml of *dithizone solution R* freshly diluted 100 times with *methylene chloride R*, shake for 15 s and allow to stand for 2 min. At the same time prepare a standard in the same manner using 0.05 ml of tin standard solution.

Any violet colour in the lower layer obtained with solution S2 is not more intense than that obtained with the reference solution (25 ppm of Sn).

Extractable heavy metals (*2.4.8*). 12 ml of solution S3 complies with limit test A (20 ppm). Prepare the standard using 10 ml of *lead standard solution (1 ppm Pb) R*.

Extractable zinc. Examine by atomic absorption spectrometry (*2.2.23, Method I*).

Test solution. Solution S3 diluted 10 times with *water R*.

Reference solution. A solution containing 0.50 ppm of zinc prepared by dilution of *zinc standard solution (5 mg/ml Zn) R* with *0.01 M hydrochloric acid*.

Verify the absence of zinc in the hydrochloric acid used.

Examined at 214.0 nm, the absorbance of the test solution is not greater than that of the reference solution (100 ppm).

Sulphated ash (*2.4.14*). Not more than 1.0 per cent, determined on 1.0 g. When the materials are opacified using titanium dioxide, the content of sulphated ash does not exceed 4.0 per cent.

ASSAY

Carry out the oxygen-flask method (*2.5.10*) using 50.0 mg of the substance to be examined. Absorb the combustion products in 20 ml of *1 M sodium hydroxide*. To the solution obtained add 2.5 ml of *nitric acid R*, 10.0 ml of *0.1 M silver nitrate*, 5 ml of *ferric ammonium sulphate solution R2* and 1 ml of *dibutyl phthalate R*. Titrate with *0.05 M ammonium thiocyanate* until a reddish-yellow colour is obtained. Carry out a blank titration.

1 ml of *0.1 M silver nitrate* is equivalent to 6.25 mg of poly(vinyl chloride).

3. Materials/ Containers

01/2005:30113

3.1.13. PLASTIC ADDITIVES

NOTE: the nomenclature given first is according to the IUPAC rules. The synonym given in bold corresponds to the name given in the texts of Chapter 3. The synonym corresponding to the rules of the texts of "Chemical Abstracts" is also given.

add01. $C_{24}H_{38}O_4$. [117-81-7]. PM RN 74640.

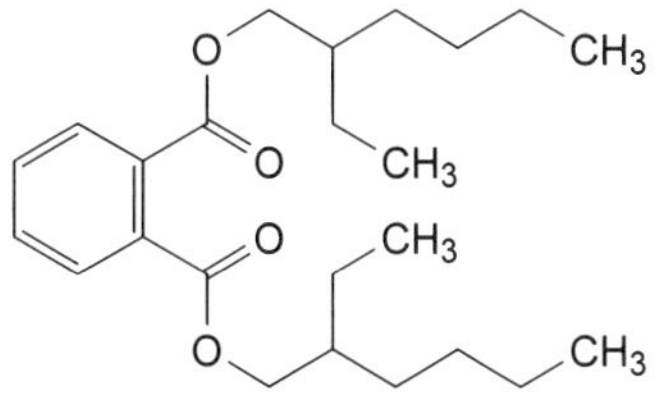

(2*RS*)-2-ethylhexyl benzene-1,2-dicarboxylate

synonyms: – **di(2-ethylhexyl) phthalate,**

– 1,2-benzenedicarboxylic acid, bis(2-ethylhexyl) ester.

add02. $C_{16}H_{30}O_4Zn$. [136-53-8]. PM RN 54120.

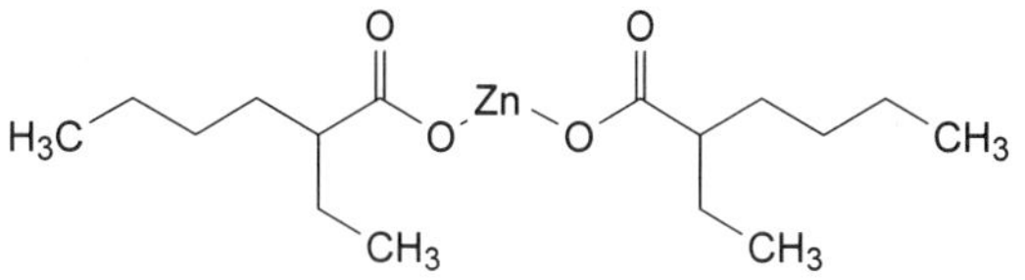

zinc (2*RS*)-2-ethylhexanoate

synonyms: – **zinc octanoate,**

– 2-ethylhexanoic acid, zinc salt (2:1),

– zinc 2-ethylcaproate.

add03. [05518-18-3]/[00110-30-5]. PM RN 53440/53520.

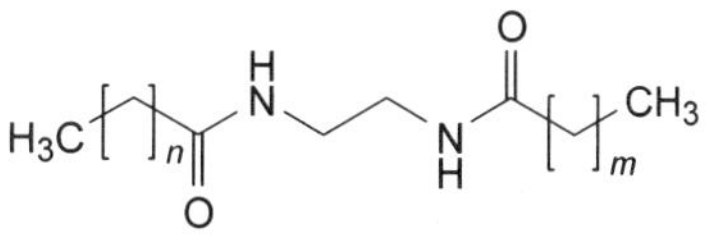

N,N'-ethylenedialcanamide (with *n* and *m* = 14 or 16)

synonyms: – ***N,N'*-diacylethylenediamines,**

– *N,N'*-diacylethylenediamine (in this context acyl means in particular palmitoyl and stearoyl).

add04. [8013-07-8]. PM RN 88640.

epoxidised soya oil

add05. [8016-11-3]. PM RN 64240.

epoxidised linseed oil

add06. [57455-37-5](TSCA)/[101357-30-6] (EINECS)/Pigment blue 29 (CI 77007)

ultramarine blue

add07. $C_{15}H_{24}O$. [128-37-0] PM RN 46640.

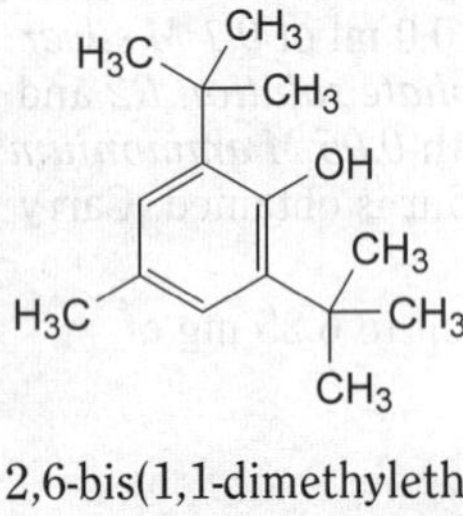

2,6-bis(1,1-dimethylethyl)-4-methylphenol

synonyms: – **butylhydroxytoluene,**

– 2,6-bis(1,1-dimethylethyl)-4-methylphenol,

– 2,6-di-*tert*-butyl-4-methylphenol.

add08. $C_{50}H_{66}O_8$. [32509-66-3]. PM RN 53670.

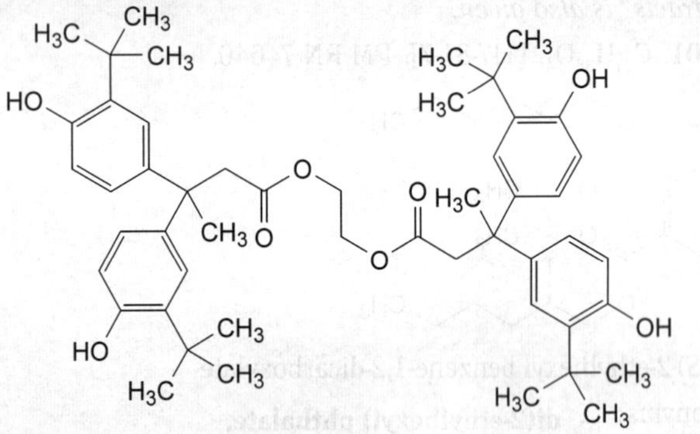

ethylene bis[3,3-bis[3-(1,1-dimethylethyl)-4-hydroxyphenyl]butanoate]

synonyms: – **ethylene bis[3,3-bis[3-(1,1-dimethylethyl)-4-hydroxyphenyl]butanoate],**

– butanoic acid, 3,3-bis[3-(1,1-dimethylethyl)-4-hydroxyphenyl]-, 1,2-ethanediyl ester,

– ethylene bis[3,3-bis(3-*tert*-butyl-4-hydroxyphenyl)butyrate].

add09. $C_{73}H_{108}O_{12}$. [6683-19-8]. PM RN 71680.

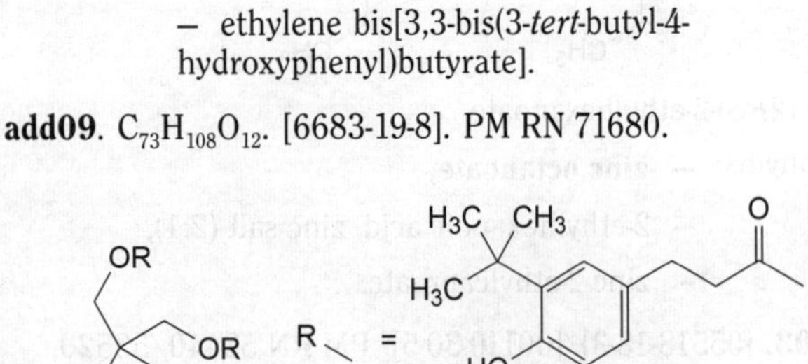

methanetetryltetramethyl tetrakis[3-[3,5-bis(1,1-dimethylethyl)-4-hydroxyphenyl]propanoate]

synonyms: – **pentaerythrityl tetrakis[3-(3,5-di-*tert*-butyl-4-hydroxyphenyl)propionate],**

– 2,2-bis[[[3-[3,5-bis(1,1-dimethylethyl)-4-hydroxyphenyl]propanoyl]oxy]methyl]propane-1,3-diyl 3-[3,5-bis(1,1-dimethylethyl)-4-hydroxyphenyl]propanoate,

– benzenepropanoic acid, 3,5-bis(1,1-dimethylethyl)-4-hydroxy-2,2-bis(hydroxymethyl)propane-1,3-diol ester (4:1),

– 2,2-bis(hydroxymethyl)propane-1,3-diol tetrakis[3-(3,5-di-*tert*-butyl-4-hydroxyphenyl)propionate].

add10. $C_{54}H_{78}O_3$. [1709-70-2]. PM RN 95200.

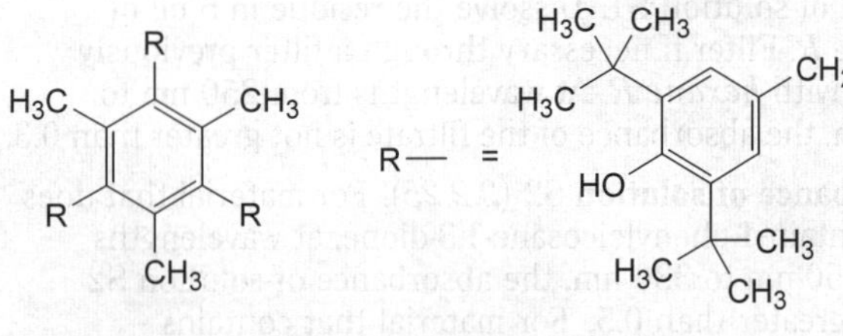

4,4′,4″-[(2,4,6-trimethylbenzene-1,3,5-triyl)tris(methylene)]tris[2,6-bis(1,1-dimethylethyl)phenol]

synonyms: – **2,2′,2″,6,6′,6″-hexa-*tert*-butyl-4,4′,4″-[(2,4,6-trimethyl- 1,3,5-benzenetriyl)trismethylene]triphenol,**

– 1,3,5-tris[3,5-di-*tert*-butyl-4-hydroxybenzyl]-2,4,6-trimethylbenzene,

– phenol,4,4′,4″-[(2,4,6-trimethyl-1,3,5-benzenetriyl)tris(methylene)]tris[2,6-bis(1,1-dimethylethyl)-.

add11. $C_{35}H_{62}O_3$. [2082-79-3]. PM RN 68320.

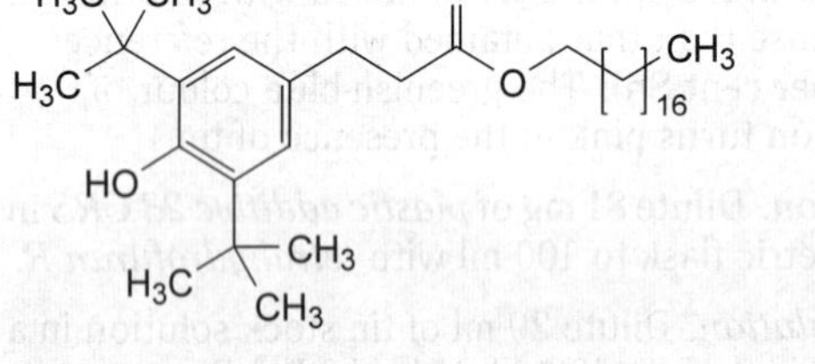

octadecyl 3-[3,5-bis(1,1-dimethylethyl)-4-hydroxyphenyl]propanoate

synonyms: – **octadecyl 3-(3,5-di-*tert*-butyl-4-hydroxyphenyl)propionate,**

– propanoic acid, 3-[3,5-bis(1,1-dimethylethyl)-4-hydroxyphenyl]-, octadecyl ester.

add12. $C_{42}H_{63}O_3P$. [31570-04-4]. PM RN 74240.

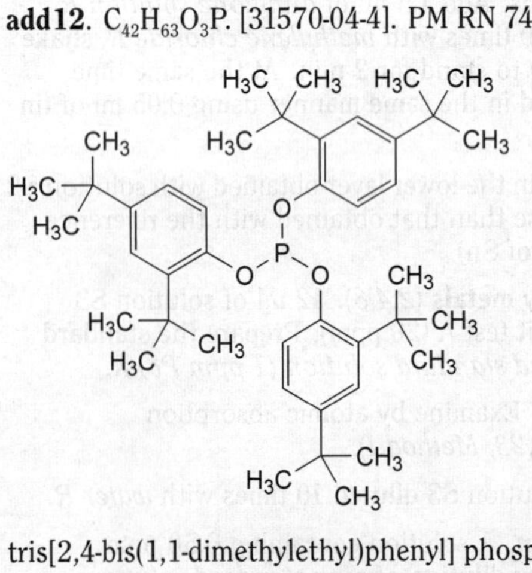

tris[2,4-bis(1,1-dimethylethyl)phenyl] phosphite

synonyms: – **tris(2,4-di-*tert*-butylphenyl) phosphite,**

– phenol, 2,4-bis(1,1-dimethylethyl)-, phosphite (3:1),

– 2,4-bis(1,1-dimethylethyl)phenyl, phosphite.

add13. $C_{48}H_{69}N_3O_6$. [27676-62-6]. PM RN 95360.

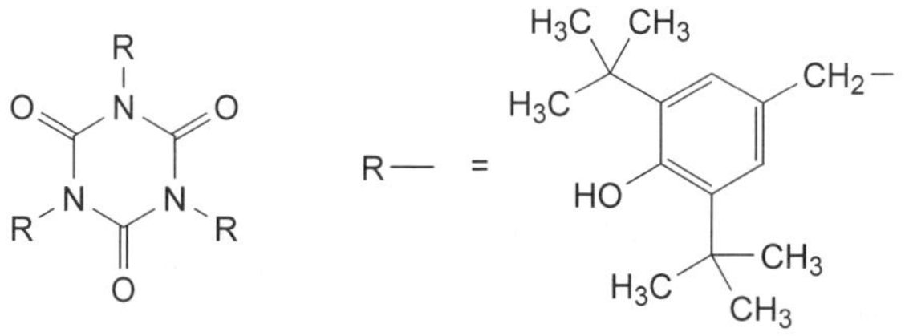

1,3,5-tris[3,5-bis(1,1-dimethylethyl)-4-hydroxybenzyl]-1,3,5-triazine-2,4,6(1*H*,3*H*,5*H*)-trione

synonyms: – **1,3,5-tris(3,5-di-*tert*-butyl-4-hydroxybenzyl)-*s*-triazine-2,4,6(1*H*,3*H*,5*H*)-trione,**

– 1,3,5-triazine-2,4,6(1*H*,3*H*,5*H*)-trione, 1,3,5-tris[[3,5-bis(1,1-dimethylethyl)-4-hydroxyphenyl]methyl]-.

add14. $C_{41}H_{82}O_6P_2$. [3806-34-6]. PM RN 50080.

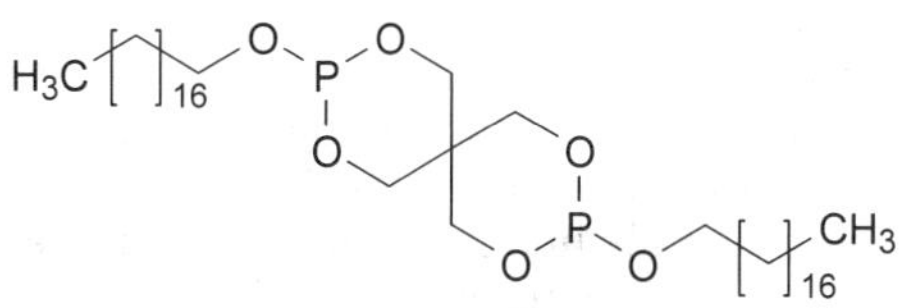

3,9-bis(octadecyloxy)-2,4,8,10-tetraoxa-3,9-diphosphaspiro[5.5]undecane

synonyms: – **2,2′-bis(octadecyloxy)-5,5′-spirobi[1,3,2-dioxaphosphinane],**

– 2,4,8,10-tetraoxa-3,9-diphosphaspiro[5.5]undecane, 3,9-bis(octadecyloxy)-.

add15. $C_{36}H_{74}S_2$. [2500-88-1]. PM RN 49840.

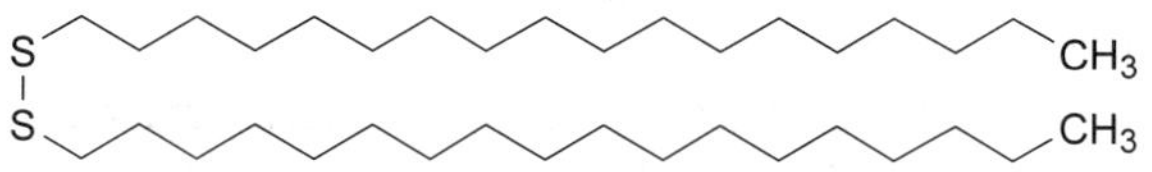

1,1′-disulphanediyldioctadecane

synonyms: – **dioctadecyl disulphide,**

– octadecane, 1,1′-dithio-.

add16. $C_{30}H_{58}O_4S$. [123-28-4]. PM RN 93120.

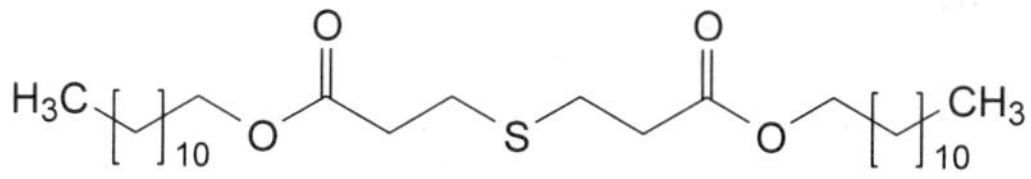

didodecyl 3,3′-sulphanediyldipropanoate

synonyms: – **didodecyl 3,3′-thiodipropionate,**

– didodecyl 3,3′-sulfanediyldipropanoate,

– propanoic acid, 3,3′-thiobis-, dodecyl diester,

– lauryl thiodipropionate.

add17. $C_{42}H_{82}O_4S$. [693-36-7]. PM RN 93280.

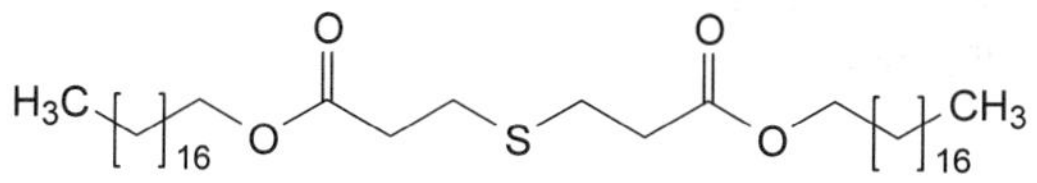

dioctadecyl 3,3′-sulphanediyldipropanoate

synonyms: – **dioctadecyl 3,3′-thiodipropionate,**

– dioctadecyl 3,3′-sulfanediyldipropanoate,

– propanoic acid, 3,3′-thiobis-, octadecyl diester,

– stearyl thiodipropionate.

add18. [119345-01-6]. PM RN 92560.

mixture of seven products corresponding to reaction product of di-*tert*-butyl phosphonite with biphosphorous trichloride, reaction products with biphenyl and 2,4-bis(1,1-dimethylethyl)phenol:

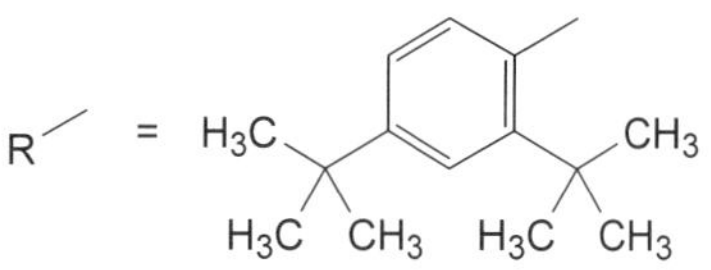

component I

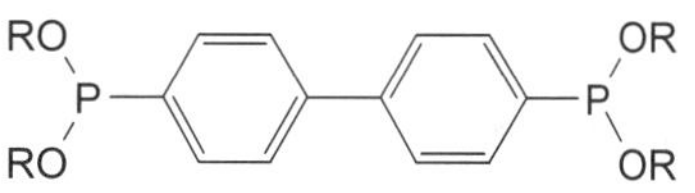

2,4-bis(1,1-dimethylethyl)phenyl biphenyl-4,4′-diyldiphosphonite

component II

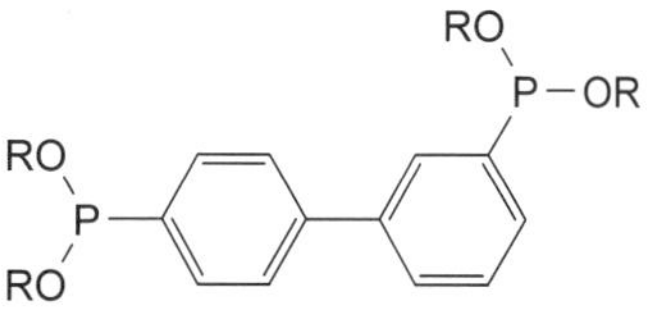

2,4-bis(1,1-dimethylethyl)phenyl biphenyl-3,4′-diyldiphosphonite

component III

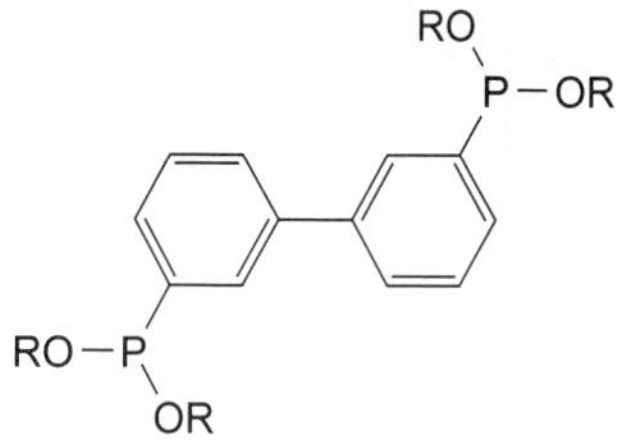

2,4-bis(1,1-dimethylethyl)phenyl biphenyl-3,3′-diyldiphosphonite

component IV

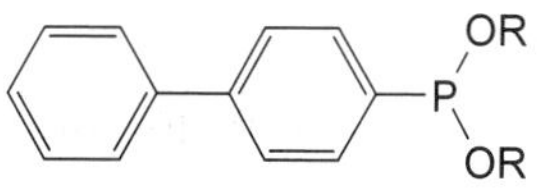

2,4-bis(1,1-dimethylethyl)phenyl biphenyl-4-ylphosphonite

component V

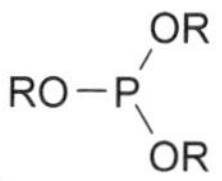

2,4-bis(1,1-dimethylethyl)phenyl phosphite

component VI

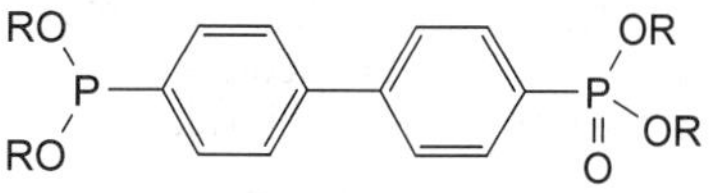

2,4-bis(1,1-dimethylethyl)phenyl 4′-[bis[2,4-bis(1,1-dimethylethyl)phenoxy]phosphanyl]biphenyl-4-ylphosphonate *component VII*

R-OH: 2,4-bis(1,1-dimethylethyl)phenol

add19. $C_{18}H_{36}O_2$. [57-11-4]. PM RN 24550.

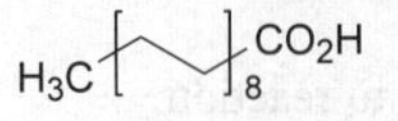

octadecanoic acid

synonyms: – **stearic acid,**
– octadecanoic acid.

add20. $C_{18}H_{35}NO$. [301-02-0]. PM RN 68960.

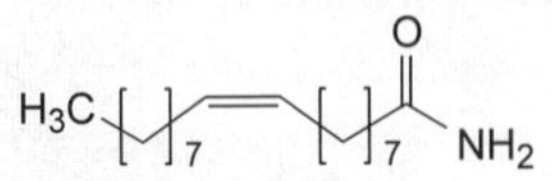

(*Z*)-octadec-9-enamide

synonyms: – **oleamide,**
– 9-octadecenamide, (*Z*)-,
– 9-*cis*-oleamide.

add21. $C_{22}H_{43}NO$. [112-84-5]. PM RN 52720.

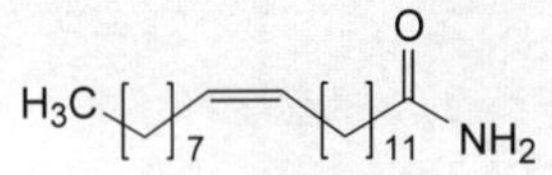

(*Z*)-docos-13-enamide

synonyms: – **erucamide,**
– 13-docosenamide, (*Z*)-,
– 13-*cis*-docosenamide.

add22. [65447-77-0]. PM RN 60800.

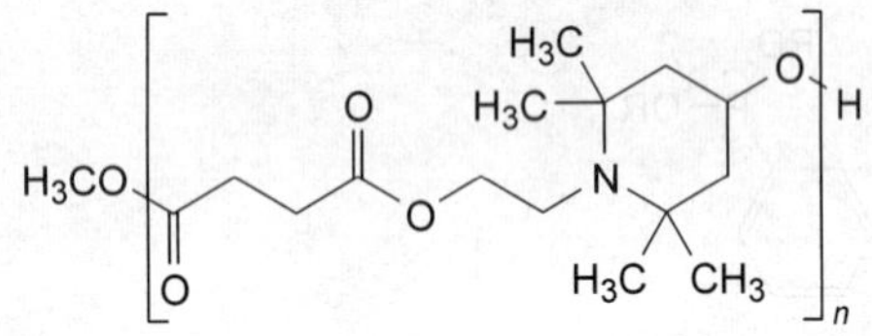

copolymer of dimethyl butanedioate and 1-(2-hydroxyethyl)-2,2,6,6-tetramethylpiperidin-4-ol

synonyms: – **copolymer of dimethyl succinate and (4-hydroxy-2,2,6,6-tetramethylpiperidin-1-yl)ethanol.**

01/2005:30114

3.1.14. MATERIALS BASED ON PLASTICISED POLY(VINYL CHLORIDE) FOR CONTAINERS FOR AQUEOUS SOLUTIONS FOR INTRAVENOUS INFUSION

DEFINITION

Materials based on plasticised poly(vinyl chloride) contain not less than 55 per cent of poly(vinyl chloride) and contain various additives, in addition to the high-molecular-mass polymer obtained by polymerisation of vinyl chloride.

Materials based on plasticised poly(vinyl chloride) for containers for aqueous solutions for intravenous infusion are defined by the nature and the proportions of the substances used in their manufacture.

PRODUCTION

Materials based on plasticised poly(vinyl chloride) are produced by polymerisation methods which guarantee a residual vinyl chloride content of less than 1 ppm. The production method used is validated in order to demonstrate that the product complies with the following test:

Vinyl chloride. Not more than 1 ppm, determined by head-space gas chromatography (*2.2.28*), using *ether R* as the internal standard.

Internal standard solution. Using a microsyringe, inject 10 µl of *ether R* into 20.0 ml of *dimethylacetamide R*, immersing the tip of the needle in the solvent. Immediately before use, dilute the solution to 1000 times its volume with *dimethylacetamide R*.

Test solution. Place 1.000 g of the material to be examined in a 50 ml vial and add 10.0 ml of the internal standard solution. Close the vial and secure the stopper. Shake, avoiding contact between the stopper and the liquid. Place the vial in a water-bath at 60 ± 1 °C for 2 h.

Vinyl chloride primary solution. Prepare under a ventilated hood. Place 50.0 ml of *dimethylacetamide R* in a 50 ml vial, stopper the vial, secure the stopper and weigh to the nearest 0.1 mg. Fill a 50 ml polyethylene or polypropylene syringe with gaseous *vinyl chloride R*, allow the gas to remain in contact with the syringe for about 3 min, empty the syringe and fill again with 50 ml of gaseous *vinyl chloride R*. Fit a hypodermic needle to the syringe and reduce the volume of gas in the syringe from 50 ml to 25 ml. Inject the remaining 25 ml of vinyl chloride slowly into the vial shaking gently and avoiding contact between the liquid and the needle. Weigh the vial again; the increase in mass is about 60 mg (1 µl of the solution thus obtained contains about 1.2 µg of vinyl chloride). Allow to stand for 2 h. Keep the primary solution in a refrigerator.

Vinyl chloride standard solution. To 1 volume of the vinyl chloride primary solution add 3 volumes of *dimethylacetamide R*.

Reference solutions. Place 10.0 ml of the internal standard solution in each of six 50 ml vials. Close the vials and secure the stoppers. Inject 1 µl, 2 µl, 3 µl, 5 µl and 10 µl, respectively, of the vinyl chloride standard solution into five of the vials. The six solutions thus obtained contain, respectively, 0 µg, about 0.3 µg, 0.6 µg, 0.9 µg, 1.5 µg and 3 µg of vinyl chloride. Shake, avoiding contact between the stopper and the liquid. Place the vials in a water-bath at 60 ± 1 °C for 2 h.

The chromatographic procedure may be carried out using:

- a stainless steel column 3 m long and 3 mm in internal diameter packed with *silanised diatomaceous earth for gas chromatography R* impregnated with 5 per cent *m/m* of *dimethylstearylamide R* and 5 per cent *m/m* of *macrogol 400 R*,
- *nitrogen for chromatography R* as the carrier gas at a flow rate of 30 ml/min,
- a flame-ionisation detector,

maintaining the temperature of the column at 45 °C, that of the injection port at 100 °C and that of the detector at 150 °C.

Inject 1 ml of the head-space of each vial. Calculate the content of vinyl chloride.

Additives

A certain number of additives is added to the polymers to optimise their chemical, physical and mechanical properties in order to adapt them for the intended use. All these additives are chosen from the following list which specifies for each product the maximum allowable content:

- not more than 40 per cent of di(2-ethylhexyl)phthalate (plastic additive 01),
- not more than 1 per cent of zinc octanoate (zinc 2-ethylhexanoate) (plastic additive 02),
- not more than 1 per cent of calcium stearate or zinc stearate or 1 per cent of a mixture of the two,
- not more than 1 per cent of *N,N'*-diacylethylenediamines (plastic additive 03),
- not more than 10 per cent of one of the following epoxidised oils or 10 per cent of a mixture of the two:
  - epoxidised soya oil (plastic additive 04) of which the oxiran oxygen content is 6 per cent to 8 per cent and the iodine value is not greater than 6,
  - epoxidised linseed oil (plastic additive 05) of which the oxiran oxygen content is not greater than 10 per cent and the iodine value is not greater than 7.

When colouring materials are added, ultramarine blue is used. Other inorganic pigments may be added, provided the safety of the material is demonstrated to the satisfaction of the competent authority. Very low amounts of antioxidants added to the vinyl chloride monomer used may be detected in the polymer.

The supplier of the material must be able to demonstrate that the qualitative and quantitative composition of the type sample is satisfactory for each production batch.

CHARACTERS

Colourless or pale yellow material in the form of powder, beads, granules or, after transformation, translucent sheets of varying thicknesses, with a slight odour. On combustion it gives off dense, black smoke.

IDENTIFICATION

If necessary, before use, cut the samples of the material to be examined into pieces of maximum dimension on a side of not greater than 1 cm.

To 2.0 g of the material to be examined add 200 ml of *peroxide-free ether R* and heat under a reflux condenser for 8 h. Separate the residue B and the solution A by filtration.

Evaporate solution A to dryness under reduced pressure in a water-bath at 30 °C. Dissolve the residue in 10 ml of *toluene R* (solution A1). Dissolve the residue B in 60 ml of *ethylene chloride R*, heating on a water-bath under a reflux condenser. Filter. Add the solution dropwise and with vigorous shaking to 600 ml of *heptane R* heated almost to boiling. Separate by filtration the coagulum B1 and the organic solution. Allow the latter to cool; separate the precipitate B2 that forms and filter through a tared sintered-glass filter (40).

A. Dissolve the coagulum B1 in 30 ml of *tetrahydrofuran R* and add, in small volumes with shaking, 40 ml of *ethanol R*. Separate the precipitate B3 by filtration and dry in vacuo at a temperature not exceeding 50 °C over *diphosphorus pentoxide R*. Dissolve a few milligrams of precipitate B3 in 1 ml of *tetrahydrofuran R*, place a few drops of the solution obtained on a sodium chloride plate and evaporate to dryness in an oven at 100 °C to 105 °C. Examine by infrared absorption spectrophotometry (*2.2.24*), comparing with the spectrum obtained with *poly(vinyl chloride) CRS*.

B. Examine the residue C obtained in the test for plastic additives 01, 04 and 05 by infrared absorption spectrophotometry (*2.2.24*), comparing with the spectrum obtained with *plastic additive 01 CRS*.

TESTS

If necessary, before use, cut the samples of the material to be examined into pieces of maximum dimension on a side of not greater than 1 cm.

Solution S1. Place 5.0 g in a combustion flask. Add 30 ml of *sulphuric acid R* and heat until a black, syrupy mass is obtained. Cool and add carefully 10 ml of *strong hydrogen peroxide solution R*. Heat gently. Allow to cool and add 1 ml of *strong hydrogen peroxide solution R*; repeat by alternating evaporation and addition of hydrogen peroxide solution until a colourless liquid is obtained. Reduce the volume to about 10 ml. Cool and dilute to 50.0 ml with *water R*.

Solution S2. Place 25 g in a borosilicate-glass flask. Add 500 ml of *water for injections R* and cover the neck of the flask with aluminium foil or a borosilicate-glass beaker. Heat in an autoclave at 121 ± 2 °C for 20 min. Allow to cool and decant the solution.

Appearance of solution S2. Solution S2 is clear (*2.2.1*) and colourless (*2.2.2, Method II*).

Acidity or alkalinity. To 100 ml of solution S2, add 0.15 ml of *BRP indicator solution R*. Not more than 1.5 ml of *0.01 M sodium hydroxide* is required to change the colour of the indicator to blue. To 100 ml of solution S2 add 0.2 ml of *methyl orange solution R*. Not more than 1.0 ml of *0.01 M hydrochloric acid* is required to initiate the colour change of the indicator from yellow to orange.

Absorbance (*2.2.25*). Evaporate 100.0 ml of solution S2 to dryness. Dissolve the residue in 5.0 ml of *hexane R*. From 250 nm to 310 nm the absorbance is not greater than 0.25.

Reducing substances. *Carry out the test within 4 h of preparation of solution S2.* To 20.0 ml of solution S2 add 1 ml of *dilute sulphuric acid R* and 20.0 ml of *0.002 M potassium permanganate*. Boil under a reflux condenser for 3 min and cool immediately. Add 1 g of *potassium iodide R* and titrate immediately with *0.01 M sodium thiosulphate*, using 0.25 ml of *starch solution R* as indicator. Carry out a blank titration using 20 ml of *water for injections R*. The difference between the titration volumes is not more than 2.0 ml.

Primary aromatic amines. To 2.5 ml of solution A1 obtained during the identification, add 6 ml of *water R* and 4 ml of *0.1 M hydrochloric acid*. Shake vigorously and discard the upper layer. To the aqueous layer add 0.4 ml of a freshly prepared 10 g/l solution of *sodium nitrite R*. Mix and allow to stand for 1 min. Add 0.8 ml of a 25 g/l solution of *ammonium sulphamate R*, allow to stand for 1 min and add 2 ml of a 5 g/l solution of *naphthylethylenediamine dihydrochloride R*. After 30 min, any colour in the solution is not more intense than that in a standard prepared at the same time in the same manner using a mixture of 1 ml of a 0.01 g/l solution of *naphthylamine R* in *0.1 M hydrochloric acid*, 5 ml of *water R* and 4 ml of *0.1 M hydrochloric acid* instead of the aqueous layer (20 ppm).

Plastic additives 01, 04 and 05. Examine by thin-layer chromatography (*2.2.27*), using a *TLC silica gel GF_{254} plate R* (1 mm thick).

Reference solutions. Prepare 0.1 mg/ml solutions of *plastic additive 01 CRS, plastic additive 04 CRS* and *plastic additive 05 CRS*, respectively, in *toluene R*.

Apply to the plate as a band 30 mm by 3 mm, 0.5 ml of solution A1 obtained during the identification. Apply to the plate 5 µl of each reference solution. Develop over a path of 15 cm using *toluene R*. Dry the plate carefully. Examine in ultraviolet light at 254 nm and locate the zone corresponding to plastic additive 01 (R_f about 0.4). Remove the area of silica gel corresponding to this zone and shake with 40 ml of *ether R* for 1 min. Filter, rinse with two quantities, each of 10 ml of *ether R*, add the rinsings to the filtrate and evaporate to dryness. The residue C weighs not more than 40 mg.

Expose the plate to iodine vapour for 5 min. Examine the chromatogram and locate the band corresponding to plastic additives 04 and 05 (R_f = 0). Remove the area of silica gel corresponding to this zone. Similarly remove a corresponding area of silica gel as a blank reference. Separately shake both samples for 15 min with 40 ml of *methanol R*. Filter, rinse with two quantities, each of 10 ml of *methanol R*, add the rinsings to the filtrate and evaporate to dryness. The difference between the masses of both residues is not more than 10 mg.

Plastic additive 03. Wash precipitate B2 obtained during the identification and contained in the tared sintered-glass filter (40) with *ethanol R*. Dry to constant mass over *diphosphorus pentoxide R* and weigh the filter. The precipitate weighs not more than 20 mg.

Examine the residue by infrared absorption spectrophotometry (*2.2.24*) comparing with the spectrum obtained with *plastic additive 03 CRS*.

Barium. Not more than 5 ppm of Ba, examined by atomic emission spectrometry in an argon plasma (*2.2.22, Method I*).

Test solution. Ignite 1.0 g of the substance to be examined in a silica crucible. Take up the residue with 10 ml of *hydrochloric acid R* and evaporate to dryness on a water-bath. Take up the residue with 20 ml of *0.1 M hydrochloric acid*.

Reference solution. A solution containing 0.25 ppm of barium prepared by dilution of *barium standard solution (50 ppm Ba) R* with *0.1 M hydrochloric acid*.

Carry out the determination using the emission of barium at 455.40 nm, the spectral background being taken at 455.30 nm.

Verify the absence of barium in the hydrochloric acid used.

Cadmium. Not more than 0.6 ppm of Cd, determined by atomic absorption spectrometry (*2.2.23, Method I*).

Test solution. Evaporate 10 ml of solution S1 to dryness. Take up the residue using 5 ml of a 1 per cent *V/V* solution of *hydrochloric acid R*, filter and dilute the filtrate to 10.0 ml with the same acid.

Reference solutions. Prepare the reference solutions using *cadmium standard solution (0.1 per cent Cd) R*, diluted with a l per cent *V/V* solution of *hydrochloric acid R*.

Measure the absorbance at 228.8 nm using a cadmium hollow-cathode lamp as the source of radiation and an air-acetylene flame.

Verify the absence of cadmium in the hydrochloric acid used.

Calcium. Not more than 0.07 per cent of Ca, examined by atomic emission spectrometry in an argon plasma (*2.2.22, Method I*).

Test solution. Use the test solution prepared for the determination of barium.

Reference solution. A solution containing 50.0 ppm of calcium prepared by dilution of *calcium standard solution (400 ppm Ca) R* with *0.1 M hydrochloric acid*.

Carry out the determination using the emission of calcium at 315.89 nm, the spectral background being taken at 315.60 nm.

Verify the absence of calcium in the hydrochloric acid used.

Tin. Not more than 20 ppm of Sn, examined by atomic emission spectrometry in an argon plasma (*2.2.22, Method I*).

Test solution. Dilute solution S1 ten times with *water R* immediately before use.

Reference solution. Introduce 2 ml of *tin standard solution (5 ppm (Sn) R)* into a 50 ml flask containing 5 ml of a 20 per cent *V/V* solution of *sulphuric acid R* and dilute to 50 ml with *water R* immediately before use.

Carry out the determination using the emission of tin at 189.99 nm, the spectral background being taken at 190.10 nm.

Verify the absence of tin in the hydrochloric acid used.

Zinc. Not more than 0.2 per cent of Zn, determined by atomic absorption spectrometry (*2.2.23, Method I*).

Test solution. Dilute solution S1 100 times with *0.1 M hydrochloric acid*.

Reference solutions. Prepare the reference solutions using *zinc standard solution (100 ppm Zn) R*, diluted with *0.1 M hydrochloric acid*.

Measure the absorbance at 213.9 nm using a zinc hollow-cathode lamp as the source of radiation and an air-acetylene flame.

Verify the absence of zinc in the hydrochloric acid used.

Heavy metals (*2.4.8*). To 10 ml of solution S1 add 0.5 ml of *phenolphthalein solution R* and then *strong sodium hydroxide solution R* until a pale pink colour is obtained. Dilute to 25 ml with *water R*. 12 ml of the solution complies with limit test A for heavy metals (50 ppm). Prepare the standard using *lead standard solution (2 ppm Pb) R*.

Water extractable substances. Evaporate 50 ml of solution S2 to dryness on a water-bath and dry at 100 °C to 105 °C until constant mass. Carry out a blank titration with 50.0 ml of *water for injections R*. The residue weighs not more than 7.5 mg (0.3 per cent) taking into account the blank test.

ASSAY

Carry out the oxygen-flask method (*2.5.10*) using 50.0 mg. Absorb the combustion products in 20 ml of *1 M sodium hydroxide*. To the solution obtained add 2.5 ml of *nitric acid R*, 10.0 ml of *0.1 M silver nitrate*, 5 ml of *ferric ammonium sulphate solution R2* and 1 ml of *dibutyl phthalate R*. Titrate with *0.05 M ammonium thiocyanate* until a reddish-yellow colour is obtained. Carry out a blank test.

1 ml of *0.1 M silver nitrate* is equivalent to 6.25 mg of poly(vinyl chloride).

01/2005:30115

3.1.15. POLYETHYLENE TEREPHTHALATE FOR CONTAINERS FOR PREPARATIONS NOT FOR PARENTERAL USE

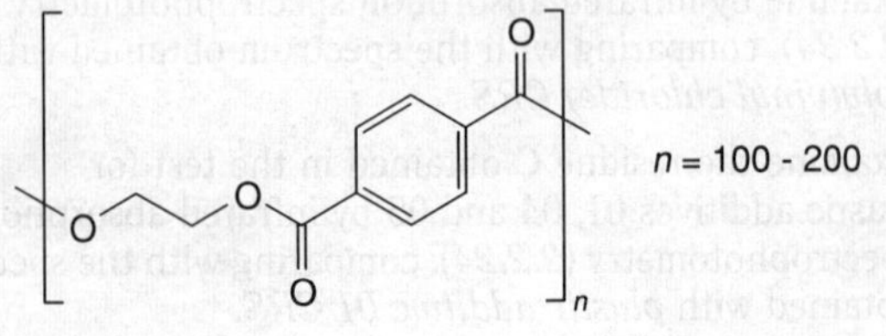

DEFINITION

Polyethylene terephthalate is obtained from the polymerisation of terephthalic acid or dimethyl terephthalate with ethylene glycol. Isophthalic acid, dimethyl isophthalate, 1,4-bis(hydroxymethyl)cyclohexane (cyclohexane-1,4-dimethanol) or diethylene glycol may be used in the polymerisation. It may contain not more than 0.5 per cent of silica or silicates and colouring matter approved by the competent authority.

PRODUCTION

The manufacturing process is validated to demonstrate that the residual acetaldehyde content is not greater than 10 ppm in the granules.

CHARACTERS

Appearance: clear or opaque granules.

Solubility: practically insoluble in water, in alcohol and in methylene chloride. It is hydrolysed by strong bases.

IDENTIFICATION

A. Place 0.10 g of the material to be examined into a borosilicate glass flask with a ground-glass neck. Add 25 ml of a 200 g/l solution of *potassium hydroxide R* in a 50 per cent *V/V* solution of *ethanol R*. Reflux for 30 min. Allow to cool and dilute to 100 ml with *water R*. Filter if necessary. Dilute 1.0 ml of the filtrate to 100 ml with *water R*. Examined between 210 nm and 330 nm (*2.2.25*), the solution shows an absorption maximum at 240 nm.

B. Dissolve 0.05 g of the material to be examined in 2 ml of *1,1,1,3,3,3-hexafluoropropan-2-ol R*. Apply to a glass plate on a water-bath in a fume-cupboard several drops of the solution to produce a film of about 15 mm by 15 mm. Allow the solvent to evaporate and remove the film using a stream of water and a scraper. Dry in an oven at 100-105 °C for 1-2 h. Examine the film by infrared absorption spectrophotometry (*2.2.24*). The spectrum of the material to be examined shows maxima in particular at 1725 cm^{-1}, 1410 cm^{-1}, 1265 cm^{-1}, 1120 cm^{-1}, 1100 cm^{-1}, 1020 cm^{-1}, 875 cm^{-1}, 725 cm^{-1}. The spectrum obtained, in addition, is identical to that of the material selected for the type sample.

TESTS

If necessary, cut out samples for testing to a maximum size of 1 cm per side.

Solution S1. Place 10.0 g of the material to be examined in a borosilicate glass flask with a ground-glass neck. Add 200 ml of *water R* and heat at 50 °C for 5 h. Allow to cool and decant the solution. *Use solution S1 within 4 h of its preparation.*

Solution S2. Place 10 g of the material to be examined in a borosilicate glass flask with a ground-glass neck. Add 100 ml of *alcohol R* and heat at 50 °C for 5 h. Allow to cool and decant the solution. *Use solution S2 within 4 h of its preparation.*

Solution S3. Place 20 g of the material to be examined in a borosilicate glass flask with a ground-glass neck. Add 50 ml of *0.1 M hydrochloric acid* and heat at 50 °C for 5 h. Allow to cool and decant the solution. *Use solution S3 within 4 h of its preparation.*

Solution S4. Place 20 g of the material to be examined into a borosilicate glass flask with a ground-glass neck. Add 50 ml of *0.01 M sodium hydroxide* and heat at 50 °C for 5 h. Allow to cool and decant. *Use solution S4 within 4 h of its preparation.*

Appearance of solution S1. Solution S1 is clear (*2.2.1*).

Appearance of solution S2. Solution S2 is clear (*2.2.1*) and colourless (*2.2.2, Method II*).

Acidity or alkalinity. To 50 ml of solution S1 add 0.15 ml of *BRP indicator solution R*. The solution turns yellow. Not more than 0.5 ml of *0.01 M sodium hydroxide* is required to change the colour of the indicator to blue. To another 50 ml of solution S1 add 0.2 ml of *methyl orange solution R*. The solution turns yellow. Not more than 0.5 ml of *0.01 M hydrochloric acid* is required to reach the beginning of the colour change of the indicator to orange.

Absorbance of solution S1 (*2.2.25*): maximum 0.20 between 220 nm and 340 nm. In addition, for coloured polyethylene terephthalate: maximum 0.05 between 400 nm to 800 nm.

Absorbance of solution S2 (*2.2.25*): maximum 0.05 between 400 nm and 800 nm.

Reducing substances. Add 2 ml of *0.5 M sulphuric acid* and 20.0 ml of *0.002 M potassium permanganate* to 20.0 ml of solution S1. Boil for 3 min. Cool immediately to ambient temperature. Add 1 g of *potassium iodide R*, 0.25 ml of *starch solution R* as indicator and titrate with *0.01 M sodium thiosulphate*. Perform a blank titration using 20.0 ml of *water R*. The difference in volume used in the 2 titrations is not greater than 0.5 ml.

Substances soluble in dioxan: maximum 3 per cent.

Place 2 g of the material to be examined in a borosilicate glass flask with a ground-glass neck. Add 20 ml of *dioxan R* and heat under reflux for 2 h. Evaporate 10 ml of the solution to dryness on a water-bath and then dry the residue at 100-105 °C. The residue weighs a maximum of 30 mg.

Extractable aluminium: maximum 1 ppm.

Atomic emission spectrometry in an argon plasma (*2.2.22, Method I*).

Test solution. Solution S3.

Reference solutions. Prepare the reference solutions using *aluminium standard solution (200 ppm Al) R*, diluted with *0.1 M hydrochloric acid.*

Wavelength: 396.15 nm, the spectral background being taken at 396.25 nm.

Verify the absence of aluminium in the *0.1 M hydrochloric acid* used.

Extractable antimony: maximum 1 ppm.

Atomic emission spectrometry in an argon plasma (*2.2.22, Method I*).

Test solution. Solution S4.

Reference solutions. Prepare the reference solutions using *antimony standard solution (100 ppm Sb) R*, diluted with *0.01 M sodium hydroxide.*

Wavelength: 231.15 nm or 217.58 nm, the spectral background being taken at 231.05 nm.

Extractable barium: maximum 1 ppm.

Atomic emission spectrometry in an argon plasma (*2.2.22, Method I*).

Test solution. Solution S3.

Reference solutions. Prepare the reference solutions using *barium standard solution (50 ppm Ba) R*, diluted with *0.1 M hydrochloric acid.*

Wavelength: 455.40 nm, the spectral background being taken at 455.30 nm.

Verify the absence of barium in the *0.1 M hydrochloric acid* used.

Extractable cobalt: maximum 1 ppm.

Atomic emission spectrometry in an argon plasma (*2.2.22, Method I*).

Test solution. Solution S3.

Reference solutions. Prepare the reference solutions using *cobalt standard solution (100 ppm Co) R*, diluted with *0.1 M hydrochloric acid*.

Wavelength: 228.62 nm, the spectral background being taken at 228.50 nm.

Verify the absence of cobalt in the *0.1 M hydrochloric acid* used.

Extractable germanium: maximum 1 ppm.

Atomic emission spectrometry in an argon plasma (*2.2.22, Method I*).

Test solution. Solution S4.

Reference solutions. Prepare the reference solutions using *germanium standard solution (100 ppm Ge) R*, diluted with *0.01 M sodium hydroxide*.

Wavelength: 206.87 nm or 265.12 nm, the spectral background being taken at 206.75 nm.

Extractable manganese: maximum 1 ppm.

Atomic emission spectrometry in an argon plasma (*2.2.22, Method I*).

Test solution. Solution S3.

Reference solutions. Prepare the reference solutions using *manganese standard solution (100 ppm Mn) R*, diluted with *0.1 M hydrochloric acid*.

Wavelength: 257.61 nm, the spectral background being taken at 257.50 nm.

Verify the absence of manganese in the *0.1 M hydrochloric acid* used.

Extractable titanium: maximum 1 ppm.

Atomic emission spectrometry in an argon plasma (*2.2.22, Method I*).

Test solution. Solution S3.

Reference solutions. Prepare the reference solutions using *titanium standard solution (100 ppm Ti) R*, diluted with *0.1 M hydrochloric acid*.

Wavelength: 323.45 nm or 334.94 nm, the spectral background being taken at 323.35 nm.

Verify the absence of titanium in the 0.1M hydrochloric acid used.

Extractable zinc: maximum 1 ppm.

Atomic emission spectrometry in an argon plasma (*2.2.22, Method I*).

Test solution. Solution S3.

Reference solutions. Prepare the reference solutions using *zinc standard solution (100 ppm Zn) R*, diluted with *0.1 M hydrochloric acid*.

Wavelength: 213.86 nm, the spectral background being taken at 213.75 nm.

Verify the absence of zinc in the *0.1 M hydrochloric acid* used.

Sulphated ash (*2.4.14*): maximum 0.5 per cent determined on 1.0 g.

3.2. CONTAINERS

01/2005:30200

3.2. CONTAINERS

A container for pharmaceutical use is an article which contains or is intended to contain a product and is, or may be, in direct contact with it. The closure is a part of the container.

The container (see *1.3. General Chapters*) is so designed that the contents may be removed in a manner appropriate to the intended use of the preparation. It provides a varying degree of protection depending on the nature of the product and the hazards of the environment, and minimises the loss of constituents. The container does not interact physically or chemically with the contents in a way that alters their quality beyond the limits tolerated by official requirements.

Single-dose container. A single-dose container holds a quantity of the preparation intended for total or partial use as a single administration.

Multidose container. A multidose container holds a quantity of the preparation suitable for two or more doses.

Well-closed container. A well-closed container protects the contents from contamination with extraneous solids and liquids and from loss of contents under ordinary conditions of handling, storage and transport.

Airtight container. An airtight container is impermeable to solids, liquids and gases under ordinary conditions of handling, storage and transport. If the container is intended to be opened on more than one occasion, it must be so designed that it remains airtight after re-closure.

Sealed container. A sealed container is a container closed by fusion of the material of the container.

Tamper-proof container. A tamper-proof container is a closed container fitted with a device that reveals irreversibly whether the container has been opened.

Child-proof container. A container that is fitted with a closure that prevents opening by children.

01/2005:30201

3.2.1. GLASS CONTAINERS FOR PHARMACEUTICAL USE

Glass containers for pharmaceutical use are glass articles intended to come into direct contact with pharmaceutical preparations.

Colourless glass is highly transparent in the visible spectrum.

Coloured glass is obtained by the addition of small amounts of metal oxides, chosen according to the desired spectral absorbance.

Neutral glass is a borosilicate glass containing significant amounts of boric oxide, aluminium oxide alkali and/or alkaline earth oxides. Due to its composition neutral glass has a high hydrolytic resistance and a high thermal shock resistance.

Soda-lime-silica glass is a silica glass containing alkali metal oxides, mainly sodium oxide and alkaline earth oxides, mainly calcium oxide. Due to its composition soda-lime-silica glass has only a moderate hydrolytic resistance.

The hydrolytic stability of glass containers for pharmaceutical use is expressed by the resistance to the release of soluble mineral substances into water under the prescribed conditions of contact between the inner surface of the container or glass grains and water. The hydrolytic resistance is evaluated by titrating released alkali. According to their hydrolytic resistance, glass containers are classified as follows:

- Type I glass containers: neutral glass, with a high hydrolytic resistance due to the chemical composition of the glass itself,
- Type II glass containers: usually of soda-lime-silica glass with a high hydrolytic resistance resulting from suitable treatment of the surface,
- Type III glass containers: usually of soda-lime-silica glass with only moderate hydrolytic resistance.

The following italicised statements constitute general recommendations concerning the type of glass container that may be used for different types of pharmaceutical preparations. The manufacturer of a pharmaceutical product is responsible for ensuring the suitability of the chosen container.

Type I glass containers are suitable for most preparations whether or not for parenteral use.

Type II glass containers are suitable for most acidic and neutral, aqueous preparations whether or not for parenteral use.

Type III glass containers are in general suitable for non-aqueous preparations for parenteral use, for powders for parenteral use (except for freeze-dried preparations) and for preparations not for parenteral use.

Glass containers with a hydrolytic resistance higher than that recommended above for a particular type of preparation may generally also be used.

The container chosen for a given preparation shall be such that the glass material does not release substances in quantities sufficient to affect the stability of the preparation or to present a risk of toxicity. In justified cases, it may be necessary to have detailed information on the glass composition, so that the potential hazards can be assessed.

Preparations for parenteral use are normally presented in colourless glass, but coloured glass may be used for substances known to be light-sensitive. Colourless or coloured glass is used for the other pharmaceutical preparations. It is recommended that all glass containers for liquid preparations and for powders for parenteral use permit the visual inspection of the contents.

The inner surface of glass containers may be specially treated to improve hydrolytic resistance, to confer water-repellancy, etc. The outer surface may also be treated, for example to reduce friction and to improve resistance to abrasion. The outer treatment is such that it does not contaminate the inner surface of the container.

Except for type I glass containers, glass containers for pharmaceutical preparations are not to be re-used. Containers for human blood and blood components must not be re-used.

Glass containers for pharmaceutical use comply with the relevant test or tests for hydrolytic resistance. When glass containers have non-glass components, the tests apply only to the glass part of the container.

To define the quality of glass containers according to the intended use, one or more of the following tests are necessary.

Tests for hydrolytic resistance are carried out to define the type of glass (I, II or III) and to control its hydrolytic resistance.

In addition, containers for aqueous parenteral preparations are tested for arsenic release and coloured glass containers are tested for spectral transmission.

HYDROLYTIC RESISTANCE

Table 3.2.1.-1. – *Types of glass*

Type of container	Test to be performed
Type I and Type II glass containers (to distinguish from Type III glass containers)	Test A (surface test)
Type I glass containers (to distinguish from Type II and Type III glass containers)	Test B (glass grains test) or test C (etching test)
Type I and Type II glass containers where it is necessary to determine whether the high hydrolytic resistance is due to the chemical composition or to the surface treatment	Tests A and B, or tests A and C

The test is carried out by titration of the extract solutions obtained under the conditions described for tests A, B and C.

EQUIPMENT

- an autoclave capable of maintaining a temperature of 121 °C ± 1 °C, equipped with a thermometer or a calibrated thermocouple recorder, a pressure gauge, a vent cock and a tray, of sufficient capacity to accommodate above the water level the number of containers needed to carry out the test; *clean the autoclave vessel and all ancillary equipment thoroughly before use with water R;*
- burettes with a suitable capacity;
- one-mark volumetric flasks, with a capacity of 1000 ml;
- pipettes and beakers;
- conical flasks with a capacity of 100 ml and 250 ml;
- a water-bath;
- a metal foil (e.g. aluminium, stainless steel).

Flasks and beakers shall have been already used for the test or have been filled with *water R* and kept in an autoclave at 121 °C at least for 1 h before being used.

DETERMINATION OF THE FILLING VOLUME

The filling volume is the volume of water to be filled in the container for the purpose of the test. For vials and bottles the filling volume is 90 per cent of the brimful capacity. For ampoules it is the volume up to the height of the shoulder.

Vials and bottles. Select, at random, 6 containers from the sample lot, or 3 if their capacity exceeds 100 ml, and remove any dirt or debris. Weigh the empty containers with an accuracy of 0.1 g. Place the containers on a horizontal surface and fill them with *distilled water R* until about the rim edge, avoiding overflow and introduction of air bubbles. Adjust the liquid levels to the brimful line. Weigh the filled containers to obtain the mass of the water expressed to 2 decimal places for containers having a nominal volume less or equal to 30 ml, and expressed to 1 decimal place for containers having a nominal volume greater than 30 ml. Calculate the mean value of the brimful capacity in millilitres and multiply it by 0.9. This volume, expressed to 1 decimal place, is the filling volume for the particular container lot.

Ampoules. Place at least 6 dry ampoules on a flat, horizontal surface and fill them with *distilled water R* from a burette, until the water reaches point A, where the body of the ampoule declines to the shoulder (see Figure 3.2.1.-1). Read the capacities (expressed to 2 decimal places) and calculate the mean value. This volume, expressed to 1 decimal place, is the filling volume for the particular ampoule lot. The filling volume may also be determined by weighing.

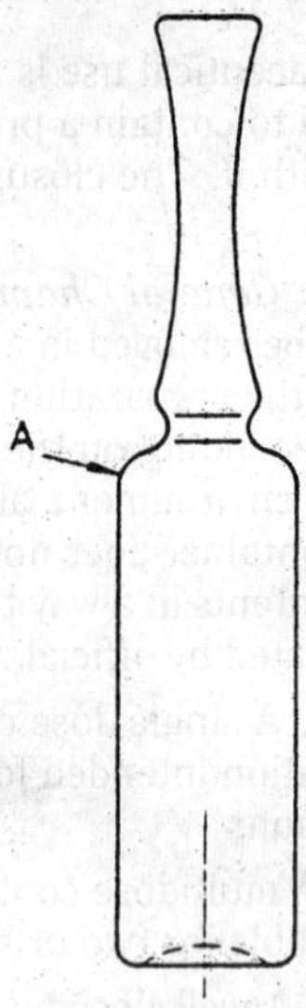

Figure 3.2.1.-1. – *Filling volume of ampoules (up to point A)*

TEST A. HYDROLYTIC RESISTANCE OF THE INNER SURFACES OF GLASS CONTAINERS (SURFACE TEST)

The determination is carried out on unused containers. The volumes of the test liquid necessary for the final determination are indicated in Table 3.2.1.-2.

Table 3.2.1.-2. – *Volume of test liquid and number of titrations*

Filling volume (ml)	Volume of test liquid for one titration (ml)	Number of titrations
Up to 3	25.0	1
Above 3 and up to 30	50.0	2
Above 30 and up to 100	100.0	2
Above 100	100.0	3

Cleaning. Remove any debris or dust. Shortly before the test, rinse each container carefully at least twice with *water R* and allow to stand. Immediately before testing empty the containers, rinse once with *water R* then with *water R1* and allow to drain. Complete the cleaning procedure from the first rinsing in not less than 20 min and not more than 25 min.

Heat closed ampoules on a water-bath or in an air-oven at about 50 °C for approximately 2 min before opening; do not rinse before testing.

Filling and heating. The containers are filled with *water R1* up to the filling volume. Containers in the form of cartridges or prefilled syringes are closed in a suitable manner with material that does not interfere with the test. Each container including ampoules shall be loosely capped with an inert material such as a dish of neutral glass or aluminium foil previously rinsed with *water R*. Place the containers on the tray of the autoclave. Place the tray in the autoclave containing a quantity of *water R* such that the tray remains clear of the water. Close the autoclave and carry out the following operations:

- heat the autoclave to 100 °C and allow the steam to issue from the vent cock for 10 min;
- close the ventcock and raise the temperature from 100 °C to 121 °C at a rate of 1 °C per min;
- maintain the temperature at 121 ± 1 °C for 60 ± 1 min;

- lower the temperature from 121 °C to 100 °C at a rate of 0.5 °C per min, venting to prevent vacuum;
- do not open the autoclave before it has cooled down to 95 °C;
- remove the containers from the autoclave using normal precautions, place them in a water-bath at 80 °C, and run cold tap water, taking care that the water does not contact the loose foil caps to avoid contamination of the extraction solution;
- cooling time does not exceed 30 min.

The extraction solutions are analysed by titration according to the method described below.

Method. Carry out the titration within 1 h of removal of the containers from the autoclave. Combine the liquids obtained from the containers and mix. Introduce the prescribed volume (Table 3.2.1.-2) into a conical flask. Place the same volume of *water R1* into a second similar flask as a blank. Add to each flask 0.05 ml of *methyl red solution R* for each 25 ml of liquid. Titrate the blank with *0.01 M hydrochloric acid.* Titrate the test liquid with the same acid until the colour of the resulting solution is the same as that obtained for the blank. Subtract the value found for the blank titration from that found for the test liquid and express the results in millilitres of *0.01 M hydrochloric acid* per 100 ml. Express titration values of less than 1.0 ml to 2 decimal places and titration values of more than or equal to 1.0 ml to 1 decimal place.

Limits. The results, or the average of the results if more than one titration is performed, is not greater than the values stated in Table 3.2.1.-3.

Table 3.2.1.-3. – *Limit values in the test for surface hydrolytic resistance*

	Maximum volume of 0.01 M HCl per 100 ml of test liquid (ml)	
	Glass containers	
Filling volume (ml)	**Types I and II**	**Type III**
Up to 1	2.0	20.0
Above 1 and up to 2	1.8	17.6
Above 2 and up to 5	1.3	13.2
Above 5 and up to 10	1.0	10.2
Above 10 and up to 20	0.80	8.1
Above 20 and up to 50	0.60	6.1
Above 50 and up to 100	0.50	4.8
Above 100 and up to 200	0.40	3.8
Above 200 and up to 500	0.30	2.9
Above 500	0.20	2.2

TEST B. HYDROLYTIC RESISTANCE OF GLASS GRAINS (GLASS GRAINS TEST)

Check that the articles as received have been annealed to a commercially acceptable quality.

The test may be performed on the canes used for the manufacture of tubing glass containers or on the containers.

Equipment

- a mortar, pestle (see Figure 3.2.1.-2) and hammer in tempered, magnetic steel,
- a set of 3 square-mesh sieves of stainless steel, mounted on frames of the same material and consisting of the following:

  (a) sieve no. 710,

  (b) sieve no. 425,

  (c) sieve no. 300;
- a permanent magnet;
- a metal foil (e.g. aluminium, stainless steel);
- a hot-air oven, capable of maintaining a temperature of 140 ± 5 °C;
- a balance, capable of weighing up to 500 g with an accuracy of 0.005 g;
- a desiccator;
- an ultrasonic bath.

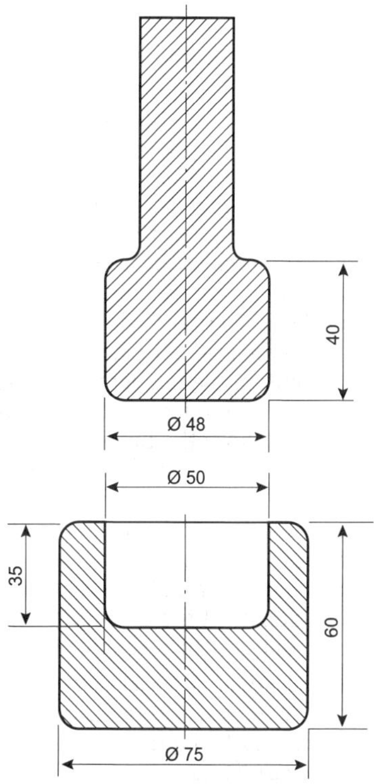

Figure 3.2.1.-2. – *Apparatus for glass grains method (dimensions in millimetres)*

Method. Rinse the containers to be tested with *water R* and dry in the oven. Wrap at least 3 of the glass articles in clean paper and crush to produce 2 samples of about 100 g each in pieces not more than 30 mm across. Place 30-40 g of the pieces between 10-30 mm across taken from 1 of the samples in the mortar, insert the pestle and strike it heavily once only with the hammer. Transfer the contents of the mortar, to the coarsest sieve (a) of the set. Repeat the operation until all fragments have been transferred to the sieve. Shake the set of sieves a short time by hand and remove the glass which remains on sieves (a) and (b). Submit these portions to further fracture, repeating the operation until about 10 g of glass remains on sieve (a). Reject this portion and the portion which passes through sieve (c). Reassemble the set of sieves and shake for 5 min. Transfer to a weighing bottle those glass grains which passed through sieve (b) and are retained on sieve (c). Repeat the crushing and sieving procedure with the other glass sample and thus 2 samples of grains, each of which shall be in excess of 10 g, are obtained. Spread each sample on a piece of clean glazed paper and remove any iron particles by passing the magnet over them. Transfer each sample into a beaker for cleaning. Add to the grains in each beaker 30 ml of *acetone R* and scour the grains by suitable means, such as a rubber or plastic-coated glass rod. After scouring the grains, allow to settle and decant as much acetone as possible. Add another 30 ml of *acetone R,* swirl, decant again and add a new portion of *acetone R.*

Fill the bath of the ultrasonic vessel with water at room temperature, then place the beaker in the rack and immerse it until the level of the acetone is at the level of the water; apply the ultrasound for 1 min. Swirl the beaker, allow to settle and decant the acetone as completely as possible and then repeat the ultrasonic cleaning operation. If a fine turbidity persists, repeat the ultrasonic cleaning and acetone washing until the solution remains clear. Swirl and decant the acetone then dry the grains, first by putting the beaker on a warm plate to remove excess acetone and then by heating at 140 °C for 20 min in the drying oven. Transfer the dried grains from each beaker into separate weighing bottles, insert the stoppers and cool in the desiccator. Weigh 10.00 g of the cleaned and dried grains into 2 separate conical flasks. Add 50 ml of *water R1* into each by means of a pipette (test solutions). Pipette 50 ml of *water R1* into a third conical flask which will serve as a blank. Distribute the grains evenly over the flat bases of the flasks by gentle shaking. Close the flasks with neutral glass dishes or aluminium foil rinsed with *water R* or with inverted beakers so that the inner surface of the beakers fit snugly down onto the top rims of the flasks. Place all 3 flasks in the rack in the autoclave containing the water at ambient temperature, and ensure that they are held above the level of the water in the vessel. Carry out the autoclaving procedure in a similar manner to that described under test A, but maintain the temperature of 121 ± 1 °C only for 30 ± 1 min. Do not open the autoclave until it has cooled to 95 °C. Remove the hot samples from the autoclave and cool the flasks in running tap water as soon as possible, avoiding thermal shock. To each of the 3 flasks add 0.05 ml of *methyl red solution R*. Titrate the blank solution immediately with *0.02 M hydrochloric acid* then titrate the test solutions until the colour matches that obtained with the blank solution. Substract the titration volume for the blank solution from that for the test solutions.

NOTE: where necessary to obtain a sharp end-point, the clear solution is to be decanted into a separate 250 ml flask. Rinse the grains with 3 quantities, each of 15 ml, of water R1 by swirling and add the washings to the main solution. Add 0.05 ml of the methyl red solution R. Titrate and calculate as described below. In this case also add 45 ml of water R1 and 0.05 ml of methyl red solution R to the blank solution.

Calculate the mean value of the results in millilitres of *0.02 M hydrochloric acid* per gram of the sample and if required its equivalent in alkali extracted, calculated as micrograms of sodium oxide per gram of glass grains.

1 ml of *0.02 M hydrochloric acid* is equivalent to 620 µg of sodium oxide.

Repeat the test if the highest and lowest observed values differ by more than 20 per cent.

Limits. Type I glass containers require not more than 1.0 ml of *0.02 M hydrochloric acid* (equivalent to 62 µg of Na_2O per gram of glass), Type II and Type III glass containers require not more than 8.5 ml of *0.02 M hydrochloric acid* (equivalent to 527 µg of Na_2O per gram of glass).

TEST C. TO DETERMINE WHETHER THE CONTAINERS HAVE BEEN SURFACE-TREATED (ETCHING TEST)

When it is necessary to determine if a container has been surface-treated, and/or distinguish between Type I and Type II glass containers, test C is used in addition to test A. Alternatively, test A and B may be used. Test C may be carried out either on unused samples or on samples previously tested for test A.

Vials and bottles. The volumes of test liquid required are shown in Table 3.2.1.-2.

Rinse the containers twice with *water R* and fill to the brimful point with a mixture of 1 volume of *hydrofluoric acid R* and 9 volumes of *hydrochloric acid R* and allow to stand for 10 min. Empty the containers and rinse carefully 5 times with *water R*. Immediately before the test, rinse once again with *water R*. Submit the containers thus prepared to the same autoclaving and determination procedure as described in test A for surface hydrolytic resistance. If the results are considerably higher than those obtained from the original surfaces (by about a factor of 5 to 10), the samples have been surface-treated.

Ampoules

NOTE: ampoules made from glass tubing are not normally subjected to internal surface treatment because their high chemical resistance is dependent upon the chemical composition of the glass as a material.

Apply the test method as described above for vials and bottles. If the ampoules are not surface-treated, the new values are slightly lower than those obtained in previous tests.

Distinction between Type I and Type II glass containers

The results obtained in Test C are compared to those obtained in Test A. The interpretation of the result is shown in Table 3.2.1.-4.

Table 3.2.1.-4. – *Distinction between Types I and II glass containers*

Type I	Type II
The values are closely similar to those found in the test for surface hydrolytic resistance for Type I glass containers.	The values greatly exceed those found in the test for surface hydrolytic resistance and are similar but not larger than those for Type III glass containers.

ARSENIC

The test applies to glass containers for aqueous parenteral preparations.

Hydride generation atomic absorption spectrometry (*2.2.23, Method I*).

Test solution. Use the extract solution obtained from containers of Types I and II, after autoclaving at 121 °C for 1 h as described under test A for surface hydrolytic resistance. Transfer 10.0 ml to a 100 ml volumetric flask. Add 10 ml of *hydrochloric acid R* and 5 ml of a 200 g/l solution of *potassium iodide R*. Heat on a water-bath at 80 °C for 20 min, allow to cool and dilute to 100.0 ml with *water R*.

Reference solutions. Prepare the reference solutions using *arsenic standard solution (1 ppm As) R*. Add 10 ml of *hydrochloric acid R* and 5 ml of a 200 g/l solution of *potassium iodide R*. Heat on a water-bath at 80 °C for 20 min, allow to cool and dilute to 100.0 ml with *water R*. The concentration range of the reference solutions is typically 0.005 ppm to 0.015 ppm of As.

Acid reservoir. Hydrochloric acid R.

Reducing reservoir. Sodium tetrahydroborate reducing solution R.

Use a hydride generation device to introduce the test solution into the cuvette of an atomic absorption spectrometer. Establish and standardise instrumental operating conditions according to the manufacturer's instructions, optimise the uptake rate of the peristaltic pump tubings, then connect tubings to the acid reservoir, the reducing reservoir and the test solution.

Source: hollow-cathode lamp.

Wavelength: 193.7 nm.

Atomisation device: air-acetylene flame.

Limit: maximum 0.1 ppm of As.

SPECTRAL TRANSMISSION FOR COLOURED GLASS CONTAINERS

Equipment. A UV-VIS spectrophotometer, equipped with a photodiode detector or equipped with a photomultiplier tube coupled with an integrating sphere.

Preparation of the specimen. Break the glass container or cut it with a circular saw fitted with a wet abrasive wheel, such as a carborundum or a bonded-diamond wheel. Select sections representative of the wall thickness and trim them as suitable for mounting in a spectrophotometer. If the specimen is too small to cover the opening in the specimen holder, mask the uncovered portion with opaque paper or tape, provided that the length of the specimen is greater than that of the slit. Before placing in the holder, wash, dry and wipe the specimen with lens tissue. Mount the specimen with the aid of wax, or by other convenient means, taking care to avoid leaving fingerprints or other marks.

Method. Place the specimen in the spectrophotometer with its cylindrical axis parallel to the slit and in such a way that the light beam is perpendicular to the surface of the section and that the losses due to reflection are at a minimum. Measure the transmission of the specimen with reference to air in the spectral region of 290-450 nm, continuously or at intervals of 20 nm.

Limits. The observed spectral transmission for coloured glass containers for preparations that are not for parenteral use does not exceed 10 per cent at any wavelength in the range of 290 nm to 450 nm, irrespective of the type and the capacity of the glass container. The observed spectral transmission in coloured glass containers for parenteral preparations does not exceed the limits given in Table 3.2.1.-5.

Table 3.2.1.-5. – *Limits of spectral transmission for coloured glass containers for parenteral preparations*

	Maximum percentage of spectral transmission at any wavelength between 290 nm and 450 nm	
Filling volume (ml)	**Flame-sealed containers**	**Containers with closures**
Up to 1	50	25
Above 1 and up to 2	45	20
Above 2 and up to 5	40	15
Above 5 and up to 10	35	13
Above 10 and up to 20	30	12
Above 20	25	10

Annex - test for surface hydrolytic resistance - determination by flame atomic absorption spectrometry (faas)

The surface hydrolytic resistance of glass of Types I and II may be determined by analysis of the leaching solution by flame atomic absorption spectrometry. A number of elements that, when present as oxides in glass, contribute to the alkalinity of the solution, are determined and used to express an alkali equivalent. The spectrometric method has the advantage of allowing the use of a much smaller sample of extract so that it can be applied to small individual containers. This enables an evaluation of the uniformity of the containers in a given batch where this is critical. The results of this measurement are not equivalent to those of titrimetry and the 2 methods cannot be considered interchangeable. A correlation between the 2 is dependent on the type of glass and the size and shape of the container.

The titrimetric method is the reference method of the Pharmacopoeia; the spectrometric method may be used in justified and authorised cases.

A method suitable for this type of analysis is shown below.

The determination is carried out on unused containers. The number of containers to be examined is indicated in Table 3.2.1.-6.

Table 3.2.1.-6. - *Number of containers to be examined for the spectrometric method*

Filling volume (ml)	Number of containers to be measured separately	Additional containers for preliminary measurements
Up to 2	20	2
Above 2 and up to 5	15	2
Above 5 and up to 30	10	2
Above 30 and up to 100	5	1
Above 100	3	1

Instructions on determination of the filling volume, cleaning of the containers, filling and heating are given above under Hydrolytic resistance and Test A. Hydrolytic resistance of the inner surfaces of glass containers.

SOLUTIONS

Spectrochemical buffer solution. Dissolve 80 g of *caesium chloride R* in about 300 ml of *water R1*, add 10 ml of *6 M hydrochloric acid* and transfer to a 1000 ml volumetric flask. Dilute to volume with *water R1* and mix.

Stock solutions:

- sodium oxide, $c(Na_2O)$ = 1 mg/ml,
- potassium oxide, $c(K_2O)$ = 1 mg/ml,
- calcium oxide, $c(CaO)$ = 1 mg/ml.

Commercially available stock solutions may also be used.

Standard solutions. Prepare standard solutions by diluting the stock solutions with *water R1* to obtain concentrations suitable for establishing the reference solutions in appropriate manner, e.g. with concentrations of 20 µg/ml of sodium oxide, potassium oxide and calcium oxide, respectively. Commercially available standard solutions may also be used.

Reference solutions. Prepare the reference solutions for establishing the calibration graph (set of calibration solutions) by diluting suitable concentrated standard solutions with *water R1*, so that the normal working ranges of the specific elements are covered, taking into account the instrument used for the measurement. Typical concentration ranges of the reference solutions are:

- for determination by atomic emission spectrometry of sodium oxide and potassium oxide: up to 10 µg/ml,
- for determination by atomic absorption spectrometry of sodium oxide and potassium oxide: up to 3 µg/ml,
- for determination by atomic absorption spectrometry of calcium oxide: up to 7 µg/ml.

Use reference solutions containing 5 per cent *V/V* of the spectrochemical buffer solution.

METHOD

Carry out preliminary measurements of the potassium oxide and calcium oxide concentrations on one of the extraction solutions. If, for one container type, the concentration of potassium oxide is less than 0.2 µg/ml and if the concentration of calcium oxide is less than 0.1 µg/ml, the remaining extraction solutions of this container type need not be analysed for these ions. Aspirate the extraction solution from each sample directly into the flame of the atomic absorption or atomic emission instrument and determine the approximate concentrations of sodium oxide (and potassium oxide and calcium oxide, if present) by reference to calibration graphs produced from the reference solutions of suitable concentration.

FINAL DETERMINATION

If dilution is unnecessary add to each container a volume of the spectrochemical buffer solution equivalent to 5 per cent of the filling volume, mix well and determine sodium oxide, calcium oxide and potassium oxide, if present, by reference to calibration graphs. For the determination of the calcium oxide concentration by flame atomic spectrometry, the nitrous oxide/acetylene flame shall be used.

If dilution is necessary, determine sodium oxide, calcium oxide and potassium oxide, if present, following the procedures as described above. The measuring solutions shall contain 5 per cent *V/V* of the spectrochemical buffer solution. Concentration values less than 1.0 μg/ml are expressed to 2 decimal places, values greater than or equal to 1.0 μg/ml to 1 decimal place. Correct the result for the buffer addition and for dilution, if any.

CALCULATION

Calculate the mean value of the concentration of individual oxides found in each of the samples tested, in micrograms of the oxide per millilitre of the extraction solution and calculate the sum of the individual oxides, expressed as micrograms of sodium oxide per millilitre of the extraction solution using the following mass conversion factors:

- 1 μg of potassium oxide corresponds to 0.658 μg of sodium oxide,
- 1 μg of calcium oxide corresponds to 1.105 μg of sodium oxide.

Limits. For each container tested, the result is not greater than the value given in Table 3.2.1.-7.

Table 3.2.1.-7. – *Limit values in the test for surface hydrolytic resistance by flame atomic absorption spectrometry*

Filling volume (ml)	Maximum values for the concentration of oxides, expressed as sodium oxide (μg/ml) — Glass containers — Types I and II
Up to 1	5.00
Above 1 and up to 2	4.50
Above 2 and up to 5	3.20
Above 5 and up to 10	2.50
Above 10 and up to 20	2.00
Above 20 and up to 50	1.50
Above 50 and up to 100	1.20
Above 100 and up to 200	1.00
Above 200 and up to 500	0.75
Above 500	0.50

01/2005:30202

3.2.2. PLASTIC CONTAINERS AND CLOSURES FOR PHARMACEUTICAL USE

A plastic container for pharmaceutical use is a plastic article which contains or is intended to contain a pharmaceutical product and is, or may be, in direct contact with it. The closure is a part of the container.

Plastic containers and closures for pharmaceutical use are made of materials in which may be included certain additives; these materials do not include in their composition any substance that can be extracted by the contents in such quantities as to alter the efficacy or the stability of the product or to present a risk of toxicity.

The most commonly used polymers are polyethylene (with and without additives), polypropylene, poly(vinyl chloride), poly(ethylene terephthalate) and poly(ethylene-vinyl acetate).

The nature and amount of the additives are determined by the type of the polymer, the process used to convert the polymer into the container and the intended purpose of the container. Additives may consist of antioxidants, stabilisers, plasticisers, lubricants, colouring matter and impact modifiers. Antistatic agents and mould-release agents may be used only for containers for preparations for oral use or for external use for which they are authorised. Acceptable additives are indicated in the type specification for each material described in the Pharmacopoeia. Other additives may be used provided they are approved in each case by the competent authority responsible for the licensing for sale of the preparation.

For selection of a suitable plastic container, it is necessary to know the full manufacturing formula of the plastic, including all materials added during formation of the container so that the potential hazards can be assessed. The plastic container chosen for any particular preparation should be such that:

- the ingredients of the preparation in contact with the plastic material are not significantly adsorbed on its surface and do not significantly migrate into or through the plastic,
- the plastic material does not release substances in quantities sufficient to affect the stability of the preparation or to present a risk of toxicity.

Using material or materials selected to satisfy these criteria, a number of identical type samples of the container are made by a well-defined procedure and submitted to practical testing in conditions that reproduce those of the intended use, including, where appropriate, sterilisation. In order to confirm the compatibility of the container and the contents and to ensure that there are no changes detrimental to the quality of the preparation, various tests are carried out such as verification of the absence of changes in physical characteristics, assessment of any loss or gain through permeation, detection of pH changes, assessment of changes caused by light, chemical tests and, where appropriate, biological tests.

The method of manufacture is such as to ensure reproducibility for subsequent bulk manufacture and the conditions of manufacture are chosen so as to preclude the possibility of contamination with other plastic materials or their ingredients. The manufacturer of the product must ensure that containers made in production are similar in every respect to the type samples.

For the results of the testing on type samples to remain valid, it is important that:

- there is no change in the composition of the material as defined for the type samples,
- there is no change in the manufacturing process as defined for the type samples, especially as regards the temperatures to which the plastic material is exposed during conversion or subsequent procedures such as sterilisation,
- scrap material is not used.

Recycling of excess material of well-defined nature and proportions may be permitted after appropriate validation.

Subject to satisfactory testing for compatibility of each different combination of container and contents, the materials described in the Pharmacopoeia are recognised as being suitable for the specific purposes indicated, as defined above.

01/2005:90003

3.2.2.1. PLASTIC CONTAINERS FOR AQUEOUS SOLUTIONS FOR PARENTERAL INFUSION

DEFINITION

Plastic containers for aqueous solutions for parenteral infusion are manufactured from one or more polymers, if necessary with additives. The containers described in this section are not necessarily suitable for emulsions. The polymers most commonly used are polyethylene, polypropylene and poly(vinyl chloride). The specifications of this text are to be read in conjunction with section *3.2.2. Plastic containers and closures for pharmaceutical use.*

The containers may be bags or bottles. They have a site suitable for the attachment of an infusion set designed to ensure a secure connection. They may have a site that allows an injection to be made at the time of use. They usually have a part that allows them to be suspended and which will withstand the tension occurring during use. The containers must withstand the sterilisation conditions to which they will be submitted. The design of the container and the method of sterilisation chosen are such that all parts of the containers that may be in contact with the infusion are sterilised. The containers are impermeable to micro-organisms after closure. The containers are such that after filling they are resistant to damage from accidental freezing which may occur during transport of the final preparation. The containers are and remain sufficiently transparent to allow the appearance of the contents to be examined at any time, unless otherwise justified and authorised.

The empty containers display no defects that may lead to leakage and the filled and closed containers show no leakage.

For satisfactory storage of some preparations, the container has to be enclosed in a protective envelope. The initial evaluation of storage has then to be carried out using the container enclosed in the envelope.

TESTS

Solution S. *Use solution S within 4 h of preparation.* Fill a container to its nominal capacity with *water R* and close it, if possible using the usual means of closure; otherwise close using a sheet of pure aluminium. Heat in an autoclave so that a temperature of 121 ± 2 °C is reached within 20 min to 30 min and maintain at this temperature for 30 min. If heating at 121 °C leads to deterioration of the container, heat at 100 °C for 2 h.

Blank. Prepare a blank by heating *water R* in a borosilicate-glass flask closed by a sheet of pure aluminium at the temperature and for the time used for the preparation of solution S.

Appearance of solution S. Solution S is clear (*2.2.1*) and colourless (*2.2.2, Method II*).

Acidity or alkalinity. To a volume of solution S corresponding to 4 per cent of the nominal capacity of the container add 0.1 ml of *phenolphthalein solution R.* The solution is colourless. Add 0.4 ml of *0.01 M sodium hydroxide.* The solution is pink. Add 0.8 ml of *0.01 M hydrochloric acid* and 0.1 ml of *methyl red solution R.* The solution is orange-red or red.

Absorbance (*2.2.25*). Measure the absorbance of solution S from 230 nm to 360 nm, using the blank (see solution S) as the compensation liquid. At these wavelengths, the absorbance is not greater than 0.20.

Reducing substances. To 20.0 ml of solution S add 1 ml of *dilute sulphuric acid R* and 20.0 ml of *0.002 M potassium permanganate.* Boil for 3 min. Cool immediately. Add 1 g of *potassium iodide R* and titrate immediately with *0.01 M sodium thiosulphate,* using 0.25 ml of *starch solution R* as indicator. Carry out a titration using 20.0 ml of the blank. The difference between the titration volumes is not greater than 1.5 ml.

Transparency. Fill a container previously used for the preparation of solution S with a volume equal to the nominal capacity of the primary opalescent suspension (*2.2.1*) diluted 1 in 200 for a container made from polyethylene or polypropylene and 1 in 400 for other containers. The cloudiness of the suspension is perceptible when viewed through the container and compared with a similar container filled with *water R.*

LABELLING

The label accompanying a batch of empty containers includes a statement of:

- the name and address of the manufacturer,
- a batch number which enables the history of the container and of the plastic material of which it is manufactured to be traced.

01/2005:30203

3.2.3. STERILE PLASTIC CONTAINERS FOR HUMAN BLOOD AND BLOOD COMPONENTS

Plastic containers for the collection, storage, processing and administration of blood and its components are manufactured from one or more polymers, if necessary with additives. The composition and the conditions of manufacture of the containers are registered by the appropriate competent authorities in accordance with the relevant national legislation and international agreements.

When the composition of the materials of the different parts of the containers correspond to the appropriate specifications, their quality is controlled by the methods indicated in those specifications (see *3.1. Materials used for the manufacture of containers* and subsections).

Materials other than those described in the Pharmacopoeia may be used provided that their composition is authorised by the competent authority and that the containers

3. Materials/ Containers

manufactured from them comply with the requirements prescribed for Sterile Plastic Containers for Human Blood and Blood Components.

In normal conditions of use the materials do not release monomers, or other substances, in amounts likely to be harmful nor do they lead to any abnormal modifications of the blood.

The containers may contain anticoagulant solutions, depending on their intended use, and are supplied sterile.

Each container is fitted with attachments suitable for the intended use. The container may be in the form of a single unit or the collecting container may be connected by one or more tubes to one or more secondary containers to allow separation of the blood components to be effected within a closed system.

The outlets are of a shape and size allowing for adequate connection of the container with the blood-giving equipment. The protective coverings on the blood-taking needle and on the appendages must be such as to ensure the maintenance of sterility. They must be easily removable but must be tamper-proof.

The capacity of the containers is related to the nominal capacity prescribed by the national authorities and to the appropriate volume of anticoagulant solution. The nominal capacity is the volume of blood to be collected in the container. The containers are of a shape such that when filled they may be centrifuged.

The containers are fitted with a suitable device for suspending or fixing which does not hinder the collection, storage, processing or administration of the blood.

The containers are enclosed in sealed, protective envelopes.

CHARACTERS

The container is sufficiently transparent to allow adequate visual examination of its contents before and after the taking of the blood and is sufficiently flexible to offer minimum resistance during filling and emptying under normal conditions of use. The container contains not more than 5 ml of air.

TESTS

Solution S_1. Fill the container with 100 ml of a sterile, pyrogen-free 9 g/l solution of *sodium chloride R*. Close the container and heat it in an autoclave so that the contents are maintained at 110 °C for 30 min.

If the container to be examined contains an anticoagulant solution, first empty it, rinse the container with 250 ml of *water for injections R* at 20 ± 1 °C and discard the rinsings.

Solution S_2. Introduce into the container a volume of *water for injections R* corresponding to the intended volume of anticoagulant solution. Close the container and heat it in an autoclave so that the contents are maintained at 110 °C for 30 min. After cooling, add sufficient *water for injections R* to fill the container to its nominal capacity.

If the container to be examined contains an anticoagulant solution, first empty it and rinse it as indicated above.

Resistance to centrifugation. Introduce into the container a volume of *water R*, acidified by the addition of 1 ml of *dilute hydrochloric acid R*, sufficient to fill it to its nominal capacity. Envelop the container with absorbent paper impregnated with a 1 in 5 dilution of *bromophenol blue solution R1* or other suitable indicator and then dried. Centrifuge at 5000 *g* for 10 min. No leakage perceptible on the indicator paper and no permanent distortion occur.

Resistance to stretch. Introduce into the container a volume of *water R*, acidified by the addition of 1 ml of *dilute hydrochloric acid R*, sufficient to fill it to its nominal capacity. Suspend the container by the suspending device at the opposite end from the blood-taking tube and apply along the axis of this tube an immediate force of 20 N (2.05 kgf). Maintain the traction for 5 s. Repeat the test with the force applied to each of the parts for filling and emptying. No break and no deterioration occur.

Leakage. Place the container which has been submitted to the stretch test between two plates covered with absorbent paper impregnated with a 1 in 5 dilution of *bromophenol blue solution R1* or other suitable indicator and then dried. Progressively apply force to the plates to press the container so that its internal pressure (i.e. the difference between the applied pressure and atmospheric pressure) reaches 67 kPa within 1 min. Maintain the pressure for 10 min. No signs of leakage are detectable on the indicator paper or at any point of attachment (seals, joints, etc.).

Vapour permeability. For a container containing an anticoagulant solution, fill with a volume of a 9 g/l solution of *sodium chloride R* equal to the volume of blood for which the container is intended.

For an empty container, fill with the same mixture of anticoagulant solution and sodium chloride solution. Close the container, weigh it and store it at 5 ± 1 °C in an atmosphere with a relative humidity of (50 ± 5) per cent for 21 days. At the end of this period the loss in mass is not greater than 1 per cent.

Emptying under pressure. Fill the container with a volume of *water R* at 5 ± 1 °C equal to the nominal capacity. Attach a transfusion set without an intravenous cannula to one of the connectors. Compress the container so as to maintain throughout the emptying an internal pressure (i.e the difference between the applied pressure and atmospheric pressure) of 40 kPa. The container empties in less than 2 min.

Speed of filling. Attach the container by means of the blood-taking tube fitted with the needle to a reservoir containing a suitable solution having a viscosity equal to that of blood, such as a 335 g/l solution of *sucrose R* at 37 °C. Maintain the internal pressure of the reservoir (i.e. the difference between the applied pressure and atmospheric pressure) at 9.3 kPa with the base of the reservoir and the upper part of the container at the same level. The volume of liquid which flows into the container in 8 min is not less than the nominal capacity of the container.

Resistance to temperature variations. Place the container in a suitable chamber having an initial temperature of 20 °C to 23 °C. Cool it rapidly in a deep-freeze to −80 °C and maintain it at this temperature for 24 h. Raise the temperature to 50 °C and maintain for 12 h. Allow to cool to room temperature. The container complies with the tests for resistance to centrifugation, resistance to stretch, leakage, vapour permeability emptying under pressure and speed of filling prescribed above.

Transparency. Fill the empty container with a volume equal to its nominal capacity of the primary opalescent suspension (*2.2.1*) diluted so as to have an absorbance (*2.2.25*) at 640 nm of 0.37 to 0.43 (dilution factor about 1 in 16). The cloudiness of the suspension must be perceptible when viewed through the bag, as compared with a similar container filled with *water R*.

Extractable matter. Tests are carried out by methods designed to simulate as far as possible the conditions of contact between the container and its contents which occur in conditions of use.

The conditions of contact and the tests to be carried out on the eluates are prescribed, according to the nature of the constituent materials, in the particular requirements for each type of container.

Haemolytic effects in buffered systems

Stock buffer solution. Dissolve 90.0 g of *sodium chloride R*, 34.6 g of *disodium hydrogen phosphate R* and 2.43 g of *sodium dihydrogen phosphate R* in *water R* and dilute to 1000 ml with the same solvent.

Buffer solution A_0. To 30.0 ml of stock buffer solution add 10.0 ml of *water R*.

Buffer solution B_0. To 30.0 ml of stock buffer solution add 20.0 ml of *water R*.

Buffer solution C_0. To 15.0 ml of stock buffer solution add 85.0 ml of *water R*.

Introduce 1.4 ml of solution S_2 into each of three centrifuge tubes. To tube I add 0.1 ml of buffer solution A_0, to tube II add 0.1 ml of buffer solution B_0 and to tube III add 0.1 ml of buffer solution C_0. To each tube add 0.02 ml of fresh, heparinised human blood, mix well and warm on a water-bath at 30 ± 1 °C for 40 min. Use blood collected less than 3 h previously or blood collected into an anticoagulant citrate-phosphate-dextrose solution (CPD) less than 24 h previously.

Prepare three solutions containing, respectively:

3.0 ml of buffer solution A_0 and 12.0 ml of *water R* (solution A_1),

4.0 ml of buffer solution B_0 and 11.0 ml of *water R* (solution B_1),

4.75 ml of buffer solution B_0 and 10.25 ml of *water R* (solution C_1).

To tubes I, II and III add, respectively, 1.5 ml of solution A_1, 1.5 ml of solution B_1 and 1.5 ml of solution C_1. At the same time and in the same manner, prepare three other tubes, replacing solution S_2 by *water R*. Centrifuge simultaneously the tubes to be examined and the control tubes at exactly 2500 *g* in the same horizontal centrifuge for 5 min. After centrifuging, measure the absorbances (*2.2.25*) of the liquids at 540 nm using the stock buffer solution as compensation liquid. Calculate the haemolytic value as a percentage from the expression:

$$\frac{A_{exp}}{A_{100}} \times 100$$

A_{100} = absorbance of tube III,

A_{exp} = absorbance of tube I or II or of the corresponding control tubes.

The solution in tube I gives a haemolytic value not greater than 10 per cent and the haemolytic value of the solution in tube II does not differ by more than 10 per cent from that of the corresponding control tube.

Sterility (*2.6.1*). The containers comply with the test for sterility. Introduce aseptically into the container 100 ml of a sterile 9 g/l solution of sodium chloride and shake the container to ensure that the internal surfaces have been entirely wetted. Filter the contents of the container through a membrane filter and place the membrane in the appropriate culture medium, as prescribed in the test for sterility.

Pyrogens (*2.6.8*). Solution S_1 complies with the test for pyrogens. Inject 10 ml of the solution per kilogram of the rabbit's mass.

Abnormal toxicity (*2.6.9*). Solution S_1 complies with the test for abnormal toxicity. Inject 0.5 ml of the solution into each mouse.

PACKAGING

The containers are packed in protective envelopes.

On removal from its protective envelope the container shows no leakage and no growth of micro-organisms. The protective envelope is sufficiently robust to withstand normal handling.

The protective envelope is sealed in such a manner that it cannot be opened and re-closed without leaving visible traces that the seal has been broken.

LABELLING

The labelling complies with the relevant national legislation and international agreements. The label states:

– the name and address of the manufacturer,
– a batch number which enables the history of the container and of the plastic material of which it is manufactured to be traced.

A part of the label is reserved for:

– the statement of the blood group, the reference number and all other information required by national legislation or international agreements, and an empty space is provided for the insertion of supplementary labelling.

The label of the *protective envelope* or the *label* on the container, visible through the envelope, states:

– the expiry date,
– that, once withdrawn from its protective envelope, the container must be used within 10 days.

The ink or other substance used to print the labels or the writing must not diffuse into the plastic material of the container and must remain legible up to the time of use.

01/2005:30204

3.2.4. EMPTY STERILE CONTAINERS OF PLASTICISED POLY(VINYL CHLORIDE) FOR HUMAN BLOOD AND BLOOD COMPONENTS

Unless otherwise authorised as described under *Sterile Plastic Containers for Human Blood and Blood Components* (*3.2.3*), the nature and composition of the material from which the containers are made comply with the requirements for *Materials based on Plasticised Poly(vinyl chloride) for Containers for Human Blood and Blood Components and for Containers for aqueous solutions for intravenous infusion* (*3.1.1*).

TESTS

They comply with the tests prescribed for *Sterile Plastic Containers for Human Blood and Blood Components* (*3.2.3*) and with the following tests to detect extractable matter.

Reference solution. Heat *water for injections R* in a borosilicate-glass flask in an autoclave at 110 °C for 30 min.

Oxidisable substances. Immediately after preparation of solution S_2 (see *3.2.3*), transfer to a borosilicate-glass flask a quantity corresponding to 8 per cent of the nominal capacity of the container. At the same time, prepare a blank using an equal volume of the freshly prepared reference solution in another borosilicate-glass flask. To each solution add

20.0 ml of *0.002 M potassium permanganate* and 1 ml of *dilute sulphuric acid R*. Allow to stand protected from light for 15 min. To each solution add 0.1 g of *potassium iodide R*. Allow to stand protected from light for 5 min and titrate immediately with *0.01 M sodium thiosulphate*, using 0.25 ml of *starch solution R* as indicator. The difference between the two titrations is not more than 2.0 ml.

Acidity or alkalinity. To a volume of solution S_2 corresponding to 4 per cent of the nominal capacity of the container add 0.1 ml of *phenolphthalein solution R*. The solution remains colourless. Add 0.4 ml of *0.01 M sodium hydroxide*. The solution is pink. Add 0.8 ml of *0.01 M hydrochloric acid* and 0.1 ml of *methyl red solution R*. The solution is orange-red or red.

Chlorides (*2.4.4*). 15 ml of solution S_2 complies with the limit test for chlorides (0.4 ppm). Prepare the standard using a mixture of 1.2 ml of *chloride standard solution (5 ppm Cl) R* and 13.8 ml of *water R*.

Ammonium (*2.4.1*). Dilute 5 ml of solution S_2 to 14 ml with *water R*. The solution complies with the limit test for ammonium (2 ppm).

Residue on evaporation. Evaporate to dryness 100 ml of solution S_2 in a borosilicate-glass beaker of appropriate capacity, previously heated to 105 °C. Evaporate to dryness in the same conditions 100 ml of the reference solution (blank test). Dry to constant mass at 100 °C to 105 °C. The residue from solution S_2 weighs not more than 3 mg, allowing for the blank test.

Absorbance (*2.2.25*). Measure the absorbance of solution S_2 from 230 nm to 360 nm, using the reference solution as compensation liquid. At wavelengths from 230 nm to 250 nm, the absorbance is not greater than 0.30. At wavelengths from 251 nm to 360 nm, the absorbance is not greater than 0.10.

Extractable di(2-ethylhexyl) phthalate. Extraction solvent, *alcohol R* diluted with *water R* to have a relative density (*2.2.5*) of 0.9389 to 0.9395, measured with a pycnometer.

Stock solution. Dissolve 0.100 g of *di(2-ethylhexyl) phthalate R* in the extraction solvent and dilute to 100.0 ml with the same solvent.

Standard solutions

(a) Dilute 20.0 ml of stock solution to 100.0 ml with extraction solvent.

(b) Dilute 10.0 ml of stock solution to 100.0 ml with extraction solvent.

(c) Dilute 5.0 ml of stock solution to 100.0 ml with extraction solvent.

(d) Dilute 2.0 ml of stock solution to 100.0 ml with extraction solvent.

(e) Dilute 1.0 ml of stock solution to 100.0 ml with extraction solvent.

Measure the absorbances (*2.2.25*) of the standard solutions at the maximum at 272 nm, using the extraction solvent as compensation liquid and plot a curve of absorbance against the concentration of di(2-ethylhexyl) phthalate.

Extraction procedure. Using the donor tubing and the needle or adaptor, fill the empty container with a volume equal to half the nominal volume with the extraction solvent, previously heated to 37 °C in a well-stoppered flask. Expel the air completely from the container and seal the donor tube. Immerse the filled container in a horizontal position in a water-bath maintained at 37 ± 1 °C for 60 ± 1 min without shaking. Remove the container from the water-bath, invert it gently ten times and transfer the contents to a glass flask. Immediately measure the absorbance at the maximum at 272 nm, using the extraction solvent as compensation liquid. Determine the concentration of di(2-ethylhexyl) phthalate in milligrams per 100 ml of extract from the calibration curve. The concentration does not exceed:

– 10 mg per 100 ml for containers of nominal volume greater than 300 ml but not greater than 500 ml;
– 13 mg per 100 ml for containers of nominal volume greater than 150 ml but not greater than 300 ml;
– 14 mg per 100 ml for containers of nominal volume up to 150 ml.

PACKAGING

See *Sterile Plastic Containers for Human Blood and Blood Components* (*3.2.3*).

LABELLING

See *Sterile Plastic Containers for Human Blood and Blood Components* (*3.2.3*).

01/2005:30205

3.2.5. STERILE CONTAINERS OF PLASTICISED POLY (VINYL CHLORIDE) FOR HUMAN BLOOD CONTAINING ANTICOAGULANT SOLUTION

Sterile plastic containers containing an anticoagulant solution complying with the monograph on *Anticoagulant and Preservative Solutions for Human Blood (0209)* are used for the collection, storage and administration of blood. Before filling they comply with the description and characters given under *Empty Sterile Containers of Plasticised Poly (vinyl chloride) for Human Blood and Blood Components* (*3.2.4*).

Unless otherwise authorised as described under *Sterile Plastic Containers for Human Blood and Blood Components* (*3.2.3*), the nature and composition of the material from which the containers are made should comply with the requirements prescribed for *Materials based on Plasticised Poly (vinyl chloride) for Containers for Human Blood and Blood Components and for containers for aqueous solutions for intravenous infusion* (*3.1.1*).

TESTS

They comply with the tests prescribed for *Sterile Plastic Containers for Human Blood and Blood Components* (*3.2.3*) and with the following tests to measure the volume of anticoagulant solution and to detect extractable matter.

Volume of anticoagulant solution. Empty the container, collecting the anticoagulant solution in a graduated cylinder. The volume does not differ by more than ± 10 per cent from the stated volume.

Spectrophotometric examination (*2.2.25*). Measure the absorbance of the anticoagulant solution from the container between 250 nm and 350 nm, using as the compensation liquid an anticoagulant solution of the same composition that has not been in contact with a plastic material. The absorbance at the maximum at 280 nm is not greater than 0.5.

Extractable di(2-ethylhexyl) phthalate. Carefully remove the anticoagulant solution by means of the flexible transfer tube. Using a funnel fitted to the tube, completely fill the container with *water R*, leave in contact for 1 min squeezing the container gently, then empty completely. Repeat the rinsing.

The container, so emptied and rinsed, complies with the test for extractable di(2-ethylhexyl) phthalate prescribed for *Empty Sterile Plastic Containers of Plasticised Poly (vinyl chloride) for Human Blood and Blood Components* (*3.2.4*).

PACKAGING AND LABELLING

See *Sterile Plastic Containers for Human Blood and Blood Components* (*3.2.3*).

01/2005:30206

3.2.6. SETS FOR THE TRANSFUSION OF BLOOD AND BLOOD COMPONENTS

Sets for the transfusion of blood and blood components consist principally of plastic tubing to which are fitted the parts necessary to enable the set to be used for transfusion in the appropriate manner. Sets include a closure-piercing device, a blood filter, a drip chamber, a flow regulator, a Luer connector and, usually, a site that allows an injection to be made at the time of use. When the sets are to be used with containers requiring an air-filter, this may be incorporated in the closure-piercing device or a separate air-inlet device may be used. The chamber enclosing the blood filter, the drip chamber and the main tubing are transparent. The materials chosen and the design of the set are such as to ensure absence of haemolytic effects. The sets comply with current standards regarding dimensions and performance.

All parts of the set that may be in contact with blood and blood components are sterile and pyrogen-free. Each set is presented in an individual package that maintains the sterility of the contents. The sets are not to be re-sterilised or re-used.

Sets for the transfusion of blood and blood components are manufactured in accordance with the rules of good manufacturing practice for medical devices and any relevant national regulations.

TESTS

Carry out the tests on sterilised sets.

Solution S. Make a closed circulation system from three sets and a 300 ml borosilicate-glass vessel. Fit to the vessel a thermostat device that maintains the temperature of the liquid in the vessel at 37 ± 1 °C. Circulate 250 ml of *water for injections R* through the system in the direction used for transfusion for 2 h at a rate of 1 litre/h (for example using a peristaltic pump applied to as short a piece of suitable silicone tubing as possible). Collect the whole of the solution and allow to cool.

Appearance of solution S. Solution S is clear (*2.2.1*) and colourless (*2.2.2, Method II*).

Acidity or alkalinity. To 25 ml of solution S add 0.15 ml of *BRP indicator solution R*. Not more than 0.5 ml of *0.01 M sodium hydroxide* is required to change the colour of the indicator to blue. To 25 ml of solution S add 0.2 ml of *methyl orange solution R*. Not more than 0.5 ml of *0.01 M hydrochloric acid* is required to reach the beginning of the colour change of the indicator.

Absorbance (*2.2.25*). Examined from 230 nm to 250 nm, solution S shows no absorbance greater than 0.30. Examined from 251 nm to 360 nm, solution S shows no absorbance greater than 0.15.

Ethylene oxide. If the label states that ethylene oxide has been used for sterilisation, the content of ethylene oxide, determined by the method prescribed below, is not greater than 10 ppm. Examine by gas chromatography (*2.2.28*).

The chromatographic procedure may be carried out using:

– a stainless steel column 1.5 m long and 6.4 mm in internal diameter packed with *silanised diatomaceous earth for gas chromatography R* impregnated with *macrogol 1500 R* (3 g per 10 g),

– *helium for chromatography R* as the carrier gas at a flow rate of 20 ml/min,

– a flame-ionisation detector,

maintaining the temperature of the column at 40 °C, that of the injector at 100 °C and that of the detector at 150 °C.

Verify the absence of peaks interfering with the ethylene oxide peak by carrying out the test using an unsterilised set or using a different chromatographic system such as:

– a stainless steel column 3 m long and 3.2 mm in internal diameter packed with *silanised diatomaceous earth for gas chromatography R* impregnated with *triscyanoethoxypropane R* (2 g per 10 g),

– *helium for chromatography R* as the carrier gas at a flow rate of 20 ml/min,

– a flame-ionisation detector,

maintaining the temperature of the column at 60 °C, that of the injector at 100 °C and that of the detector at 150 °C.

Ethylene oxide solution. Prepare under a ventilated hood. Place 50.0 ml of *dimethylacetamide R* in a 50 ml vial, stopper, secure the stopper and weigh to the nearest 0.1 mg. Fill a 50 ml polyethylene or polypropylene syringe with gaseous *ethylene oxide R*, allow the gas to remain in contact with the syringe for about 3 min, empty the syringe and fill again with 50 ml of gaseous *ethylene oxide R*. Fit a hypodermic needle to the syringe and reduce the volume of gas in the syringe from 50 ml to 25 ml. Inject these 25 ml of ethylene oxide slowly into the vial, shaking gently and avoiding contact between the needle and the liquid. Weigh the vial again: the increase in mass is 45 mg to 60 mg and is used to calculate the exact concentration of the solution (about 1 g/l).

Test. Weigh the set after removing the package. Cut the set into pieces of maximum dimension 1 cm and place the pieces in a 250 ml to 500 ml vial containing 150 ml of *dimethylacetamide R*. Close the vial with a suitable stopper and secure the stopper. Place the vial in an oven at 70 ± 1 °C for 16 h. Remove 1 ml of the hot gas from the vial and inject it onto the column. From the calibration curve and the height of the peak obtained, calculate the mass of ethylene oxide in the vial.

Calibration curve. In a series of seven vials of the same type as that used for the test and each containing 150 ml of *dimethylacetamide R*, place respectively 0 ml, 0.05 ml, 0.10 ml, 0.20 ml, 0.50 ml, 1.00 ml and 2.00 ml of the ethylene oxide solution, i.e. about 0 µg, 50 µg, 100 µg, 200 µg, 500 µg, 1000 µg and 2000 µg of ethylene oxide. Stopper the vials, secure the stoppers and place the vials in an oven at 70 ± 1 °C for 16 h. Inject 1 ml of the hot gas from each vial onto the column and draw a calibration curve from the heights of the peaks and the mass of ethylene oxide in each flask.

Reducing substances. *Carry out the test within 4 h of preparation of solution S.* To 20.0 ml of solution S add 1 ml of *dilute sulphuric acid R* and 20.0 ml of *0.002 M potassium permanganate*. Boil for 3 min and cool immediately. Add 1 g of *potassium iodide R* and titrate with *0.01 M sodium thiosulphate* using 0.25 ml of *starch solution R* as indicator.

Carry out a blank test using 20 ml of *water for injections R*. The difference between the titration volumes is not greater than 2.0 ml.

Extraneous particles. Fill the set via the normal inlet with a 0.1 g/l solution of *sodium laurilsulfate R*, previously filtered through a sintered-glass filter (16) and heated to 37 °C. Collect the liquid via the normal outlet. When examined under suitable conditions of visibility, the liquid is clear and practically free from visible particles and filaments (it is assumed that particles and filaments with a diameter equal to or greater than 50 μm are visible to the naked eye).

Flow rate. Pass through a complete set with the flow regulator fully open 50 ml of a solution having a viscosity of 3 mPa·s (3 cP) (for example a 33 g/l solution of *macrogol 4000 R* at 20 °C) under a static head of 1 m. The time required for passage of 50 ml of the solution is not greater than 90 s.

Resistance to pressure. Make tight the extremities of the set and any air-inlet device. Connect the set to a compressed air outlet fitted with a pressure regulator. Immerse the set in a tank of water at 20 °C to 23 °C. Apply progressively an excess pressure of 100 kPa and maintain for 1 min. No air bubble escapes from the set.

Transparency. Use as reference suspension the primary opalescent suspension (*2.2.1*) diluted 1 in 8 for sets having tubing with an external diameter less than 5 mm and diluted 1 in 16 for sets having tubing with an external diameter of 5 mm or greater. Circulate the reference suspension through the set and compare with a set from the same batch filled with *water R*. The opalescence and presence of bubbles are discernible.

Residue on evaporation. Evaporate 50.0 ml of solution S to dryness on a water-bath and dry to constant mass in an oven at 100 °C to 105 °C. Carry out a blank test using 50.0 ml of *water for injections R*. The difference between the masses of the residues is not greater than 1.5 mg.

Sterility (*2.6.1*). The sets comply with the test for sterility. If the sets are stated to be sterile only internally, pass 50 ml of buffered sodium chloride-peptone solution pH 7.0 (*2.6.12*) through the set and use to carry out the test by the membrane-filtration method.

If the sets are stated to be sterile both internally and externally, open the package with the necessary aseptic precautions and:

– for the direct inoculation method, place the set or its components in a suitable container containing a sufficient quantity of the culture medium to ensure complete immersion;

– for the membrane filtration method, place the set or its components in a suitable container containing a sufficient quantity of buffered sodium chloride-peptone solution pH 7.0 (*2.6.12*) to allow total rinsing for 10 min.

Pyrogens (*2.6.8*). Connect together five sets and pass through the assembly at a flow rate not exceeding 10 ml/min 250 ml of a sterile, pyrogen-free 9 g/l solution of *sodium chloride R*. Collect the solution aseptically in a pyrogen-free container. The solution complies with the test for pyrogens. Inject 10 ml per kilogram of the rabbit's mass.

LABELLING

The label states, where applicable, that the set has been sterilised using ethylene oxide.

01/2005:30208

3.2.8. STERILE SINGLE-USE PLASTIC SYRINGES

Sterile single-use plastic syringes are medical devices intended for immediate use for the administration of injectable preparations. They are supplied sterile and pyrogen-free and are not to be re-sterilised or re-used. They consist of a syringe barrel and a piston which may have an elastomer sealing ring; they may be fitted with a needle which may be non-detachable. Each syringe is presented with individual protection for maintaining sterility.

The barrel of the syringe is sufficiently transparent to permit dosages to be read without difficulty and allow air bubbles and foreign particles to be discerned.

The plastics and elastomer materials of which the barrel and piston are made comply with the appropriate specification or with the requirements of the competent authority. The most commonly used materials are polypropylene and polyethylene. The syringes comply with current standards regarding dimensions and performance.

Silicone oil (*3.1.8*) may be applied to the internal wall of the barrel to assist in the smooth operation of the syringe but there remains no excess capable of contaminating the contents at the time of use.

The inks, glues and adhesives for the marking on the syringe or on the package and, where necessary, the assembly of the syringe and its package, do not migrate across the walls.

TESTS

Solution S. Prepare the solution in a manner that avoids contamination by foreign particles. Using a sufficient number of syringes to produce 50 ml of solution, fill the syringes to their nominal volume with *water for injections R* and maintain at 37 °C for 24 h. Combine the contents of the syringes in a suitable borosilicate-glass container.

Appearance of solution. Solution S is clear (*2.2.1*) and colourless (*2.2.2, Method II*) and is practically free from foreign solid particles.

Acidity or alkalinity. To 20 ml of solution S add 0.1 ml of *bromothymol blue solution R1*. Not more than 0.3 ml of *0.01 M sodium hydroxide* or *0.01 M hydrochloric acid* is required to change the colour of the indicator.

Absorbance (*2.2.25*). Measure the absorbance of solution S from 220 nm to 360 nm. The absorbance does not exceed 0.40.

Ethylene oxide. If the label states that ethylene oxide has been used for sterilisation, the content of ethylene oxide, determined by the method described below, is not greater than 10 ppm. Examine by gas chromatography (*2.2.28*).

The chromatographic procedure may be carried out using:

– a stainless steel column 1.5 m long and 6.4 mm in internal diameter packed with *silanised diatomaceous earth for gas chromatography R* impregnated with *macrogol 1500 R* (3 g per 10 g),

– *helium for chromatography R* as the carrier gas at a flow rate of 20 ml/min,

– a flame-ionisation detector,

maintaining the temperature of the column at 40 °C, that of the injector at 100 °C and that of the detector at 150 °C. Verify the absence of peaks interfering with the ethylene oxide peak, either by carrying out the test using an unsterilised syringe or using a different chromatographic system such as:

- a stainless-steel column 3 m long and 3.2 mm in internal diameter packed with *silanised diatomaceous earth for gas chromatography R* impregnated with *triscyanoethoxypropane R* (2 g per 10 g),
- *helium for chromatography R* as carrier gas at a flow rate of 20 ml/min,
- a flame-ionisation detector,

maintaining the temperature of the column at 60 °C, that of the injector at 100 °C and that of the detector at 150 °C.

Ethylene oxide solution. Prepare under a ventilated hood. Place 50.0 ml of *dimethylacetamide R* in a 50 ml vial, stopper, secure the stopper and weigh to the nearest 0.1 mg. Fill a 50 ml polyethylene or polypropylene syringe with gaseous *ethylene oxide R*, allow the gas to remain in contact with the syringe for about 3 min, empty the syringe and fill again with 50 ml of gaseous *ethylene oxide R*. Fit a hypodermic needle to the syringe and reduce the volume of gas in the syringe from 50 ml to 25 ml. Inject these 25 ml of ethylene oxide slowly into the vial, shaking gently and avoiding contact between the needle and the liquid. Weigh the vial again: the increase in mass is 45 mg to 60 mg and is used to calculate the exact concentration of the solution (about 1 g/l).

Calibration curve. In a series of seven vials of the same type as that used for the test and each containing 150 ml of *dimethylacetamide R*, place respectively 0 ml, 0.05 ml, 0.10 ml, 0.20 ml, 0.50 ml, 1.00 ml and 2.00 ml of the ethylene oxide solution, i.e. about 0 µg, 50 µg, 100 µg, 200 µg, 500 µg, 1000 µg and 2000 µg of ethylene oxide. Stopper the vials, secure the stoppers and place the vials in an oven at 70 ± 1 °C for 16 h. Inject 1 ml of the hot gas from each vial onto the column and draw a calibration curve from the heights of the peaks and the mass of ethylene oxide in each flask.

Test. Weigh the syringe after removing the package. Cut the syringe into pieces of maximum dimension 1 cm and place the pieces in a 250 ml to 500 ml vial containing 150 ml of *dimethylacetamide R*. Close the vial with a suitable stopper and secure the stopper. Place the vial in an oven at 70 ± 1 °C for 16 h. Remove 1 ml of the hot gas from the vial and inject it onto the column. From the calibration curve and the height of the peak obtained, calculate the mass of ethylene oxide in the vial.

Silicone oil. Calculate the internal surface area of a syringe in square centimetres using the expression:

$$2\sqrt{V \cdot \pi \cdot h}$$

V = nominal volume of the syringe, in cubic centimetres,

h = height of the graduation, in centimetres.

Take a sufficient number of syringes to give an internal surface area of 100 cm^2 to 200 cm^2. Aspirate into each syringe a volume of *methylene chloride R* equal to half the nominal volume and make up to the nominal volume with air. Rinse the internal surface corresponding to the nominal volume with the solvent by inverting the syringe ten times in succession with the needle fitting closed by a finger covered by a plastic film inert to methylene chloride. Expel the extracts into a tared dish and repeat the operation. Evaporate the combined extracts to dryness on a water-bath. Dry at 100 °C to 105 °C for 1 h. The residue weighs not more than 0.25 mg per square centimetre of internal surface area.

Examine the residue by infrared absorption spectrophotometry (*2.2.24*). It shows absorption bands typical of silicone oil at 805 cm^{-1}, 1020 cm^{-1}, 1095 cm^{-1}, 1260 cm^{-1} and 2960 cm^{-1}.

Reducing substances. To 20.0 ml of solution S add 2 ml of *sulphuric acid R* and 20.0 ml of *0.002 M potassium permanganate*. Boil for 3 min. Cool immediately. Add 1 g of *potassium iodide R* and titrate immediately with *0.01 M sodium thiosulphate* using 0.25 ml of *starch solution R* as indicator. Carry out a blank titration using 20.0 ml of *water for injections R*. The difference between the titration volumes is not greater than 3.0 ml.

Transparency. Fill a syringe with *water R* (blank) and fill another with a 1 in 10 dilution of primary opalescent suspension (*2.2.1*). Use primary opalescent suspension that has been allowed to stand at 20 ± 2 °C for 24 h before use. Compare with the naked eye in diffused light against a dark background. The opalescence of the suspension is detectable when compared with the blank.

Sterility (*2.6.1*). *Syringes stated to be sterile comply with the test for sterility carried out as follows.* Using aseptic technique, open the package, withdraw the syringe, separate the components and place each in a suitable container containing sufficient culture media to cover the part completely. Use both the recommended media (*2.6.1*).

Syringes stated to be sterile only internally comply with the test for sterility carried out as follows. Use 50 ml of inoculation medium for each test syringe. Using aseptic technique, remove the needle protector and submerge the needle in the culture medium. Flush the syringe five times by withdrawing the plunger to its fullest extent.

Pyrogens (*2.6.8*). Syringes with a nominal volume equal to or greater than 15 ml comply with the test for pyrogens. Fill a minimum of three syringes to their nominal volume with a pyrogen-free 9 g/l solution of *sodium chloride R* and maintain at a temperature of 37 °C for 2 h. Combine the solutions aseptically in a pyrogen-free container and carry out the test immediately using for each rabbit 10 ml of the solution per kilogram of body mass.

LABELLING

The label on the *package* states:

- the batch number,
- a description of the syringe,
- that the syringe is for single-use only.

The label on the outer *package* states:

- the method of sterilisation,
- that the syringe is sterile or that it is sterile only internally,
- the identity of the manufacturer,
- that the syringe is not to be used if the packaging is damaged or the sterility protector is loose.

01/2005:30209

3.2.9. RUBBER CLOSURES FOR CONTAINERS FOR AQUEOUS PARENTERAL PREPARATIONS, FOR POWDERS AND FOR FREEZE-DRIED POWDERS

Rubber closures for containers for aqueous parenteral preparations for powders and for freeze-dried powders are made of materials obtained by vulcanisation (cross-linking) of macromolecular organic substances (elastomers), with appropriate additives. The specification also applies to closures for containers for powders and freeze-dried products to be dissolved in water immediately before use. The specification does not apply to closures made from silicone elastomer (which are dealt with in *3.1.9. Silicone elastomer for closures and tubing*), to laminated closures or to lacquered closures. The elastomers are produced from natural or synthetic substances by polymerisation, polyaddition or polycondensation. The nature of the principal components and of the various additives (for example vulcanisers, accelerators, stabilisers, pigments) depends on the properties required for the finished article.

Rubber closures may be classified in 2 types: type I closures are those which meet the strictest requirements and which are to be preferred; type II closures are those which, having mechanical properties suitable for special uses (for example, multiple piercing), cannot meet requirements as severe as those for the first category because of their chemical composition.

The closures chosen for use with a particular preparation are such that:

- the components of the preparation in contact with the closure are not adsorbed onto the surface of the closure and do not migrate into or through the closure to an extent sufficient to affect the preparation adversely,
- the closure does not yield to the preparation substances in quantities sufficient to affect its stability or to present a risk of toxicity.

The closures are compatible with the preparation for which they are used throughout its period of validity.

The manufacturer of the preparation must obtain from the supplier an assurance that the composition of the closure does not vary and that it is identical to that of the closure used during compatibility testing. When the supplier informs the manufacturer of the preparation of changes in the composition, compatibility testing must be repeated, totally or partly, depending on the nature of the changes.

The closures are washed and may be sterilised before use.

CHARACTERS

Rubber closures are elastic; they are translucent or opaque and have no characteristic colour, the latter depending on the additives used. They are practically insoluble in tetrahydrofuran, in which, however, a considerable reversible swelling may occur. They are homogeneous and practically free from flash and adventitious materials (for example fibres, foreign particles, waste rubber).

Identification of the type of rubber used for the closures is not within the scope of this specification. The identification test given below distinguishes elastomer and non-elastomer closures but does not differentiate the various types of rubber. Other identity tests may be carried out with the aim of detecting differences in a batch compared to the closures used for compatibility testing. One or more of the following analytical methods may be applied for this purpose: determination of relative density, determination of sulphated ash, determination of sulphur content, thin-layer chromatography carried out on an extract, ultraviolet absorption spectrophotometry of an extract, infrared absorption spectrophotometry of a pyrolysate.

IDENTIFICATION

A. The elasticity is such that a strip of material with a cross-section of 1 mm^2 to 5 mm^2 can be stretched by hand to at least twice its original length. Having been stretched to twice its length for 1 min, it contracts to less than 1.2 times its original length within 30 s.

B. Heat 1 g to 2 g in a heat-resistant test-tube over an open flame to dry the sample and continue heating until pyrolysate vapours are condensed near the top edge of the test-tube. Deposit a few drops of the pyrolysate on a potassium bromide disc and examine by infrared absorption spectrophotometry (*2.2.24*), comparing with the spectrum obtained with the type sample.

C. The total ash (*2.4.16*) is within ± 10 per cent of the result obtained with the type sample.

TESTS

The samples to be analysed may be washed and sterilised before use.

Solution S. Introduce a number of uncut closures corresponding to a surface area of about 100 cm^2 in a suitable glass container, cover with *water for injections R*, boil for 5 min and rinse 5 times with cold *water for injections R*. Place the washed closures in a wide-necked flask (glass type I, *3.2.1*), add 200 ml of *water for injections R* and weigh. Cover the mouth of the flask with a borosilicate-glass beaker. Heat in an autoclave so that a temperature of 121 ± 2 °C is reached within 20 min to 30 min and maintain at this temperature for 30 min. Cool to room temperature over about 30 min. Make up to the original mass with *water for injections R*. Shake and immediately separate the solution from the rubber by decantation. Shake solution S before each test

Blank. Prepare a blank in the same manner using 200 ml of *water for injections R*.

Appearance of solution. Solution S is not more opalescent than reference suspension II for type I closures and is not more opalescent than reference suspension III for type II closures (*2.2.1*). Solution S is not more intensely coloured than reference solution GY_5 (*2.2.2, Method II*).

Acidity or alkalinity. To 20 ml of solution S add 0.1 ml of *bromothymol blue solution R1*. Not more than 0.3 ml of *0.01 M sodium hydroxide* or 0.8 ml of *0.01 M hydrochloric acid* is required to obtain either a blue or a yellow colour, respectively.

Absorbance. *Carry out the test within 5 h of preparation of solution S.* Filter solution S on a membrane filter having approximately 0.45 μm pores rejecting the first few millilitres of filtrate. Measure the absorbance (*2.2.25*) of the filtrate at wavelengths from 220 nm to 360 nm using the blank (see solution S) as compensation liquid. At these wavelengths, the absorbance does not exceed 0.2 for type I closures or 4.0 for type II closures. If necessary, dilute the filtrate before measurement of the absorbance and correct the result for the dilution.

Reducing substances. *Carry out the test within 4 h of preparation of solution S.* To 20.0 ml of solution S add 1 ml of *dilute sulphuric acid R* and 20.0 ml of *0.002 M*

potassium permanganate. Boil for 3 min. Cool. Add 1 g of *potassium iodide R* and titrate immediately with *0.01 M sodium thiosulphate,* using 0.25 ml of *starch solution R* as indicator. Carry out a titration using 20.0 ml of the blank. The difference between the titration volumes is not greater than 3.0 ml for type I closures and 7.0 ml for type II closures.

Ammonium (*2.4.1*): maximum 2 ppm.

Dilute 5 ml of solution S to 14 ml with *water R.* The solution complies with limit test A.

Extractable zinc: maximum of 5 µg of extractable Zn per millilitre of solution S.

Atomic absorption spectrophotometry (*2.2.23, Method I*).

Test solution. Dilute 10.0 ml of solution S to 100 ml with *0.1 M hydrochloric acid.*

Reference solutions. Prepare the reference solutions using *zinc standard solution (10 ppm Zn) R* diluted with *0.1 M hydrochloric acid.*

Source: zinc hollow-cathode lamp.

Wavelength: 213.9 nm.

Flame: air-acetylene.

Extractable heavy metals (*2.4.8*): maximum 2 ppm.

Solution S complies with limit test A. Prepare the standard using *lead standard solution (2 ppm Pb) R.*

Residue on evaporation. Evaporate 50.0 ml of solution S to dryness on a water-bath and dry at 100 °C to 105 °C. The residue weighs not more than 2.0 mg for type I rubber and not more than 4.0 mg for type II rubber.

Volatile sulphides. Place closures, cut if necessary, with a total surface area of 20 ± 2 cm^2 in a 100 ml conical flask and add 50 ml of a 20 g/l solution of *citric acid R.* Place a piece of *lead acetate paper R* over the mouth of the flask and maintain the paper in position by placing over it an inverted weighing bottle. Heat in an autoclave at 121 ± 2 °C for 30 min. Any black stain on the paper is not more intense than that of a standard prepared at the same time in the same manner using 0.154 mg of *sodium sulphide R* and 50 ml of a 20 g/l solution of *citric acid R.*

For the tests for penetrability, fragmentation and self-sealing, use the closures treated as described for the preparation of solution S and allowed to dry.

Penetrability. For closures intended to be pierced by a hypodermic needle, carry out the following test. Fill 10 suitable vials to the nominal volume with *water R,* fit the closures to be examined and secure with a cap. Using for each closure a new, lubricated long-bevel[(1)] (bevel angle 12 ± 2°) hypodermic needle with an external diameter of 0.8 mm, pierce the closures with the needle perpendicular to the surface. The force required for piercing, determined with an accuracy of ± 0.25 N (25 gf), is not greater than 10 N (1 kgf) for each closure.

Fragmentation. For closures intended to be pierced by a hypodermic needle, carry out the following test. If the closures are to be used for aqueous preparations, place in 12 clean vials a volume of *water R* corresponding to the nominal volume minus 4 ml, close the vials with the closures to be examined, secure with a cap and allow to stand for 16 h. If the closures are to be used with dry preparations, close 12 clean vials with the closures to be examined. Using a lubricated long-bevel[(1)] (bevel angle 12 ± 2°) hypodermic needle with an external diameter of 0.8 mm fitted to a clean syringe, inject into the vial 1 ml of *water R* and remove 1 ml of air; carry out this operation 4 times for each closure, piercing each time at a different site. Use a new needle for each closure and check that the needle is not blunted during the test. Pass the liquid in the vials through a filter having approximately 0.5 µm pores. Count the fragments of rubber visible to the naked eye. The total number of fragments does not exceed 5. This limit is based on the assumption that fragments with a diameter equal to or greater than 50 µm are visible to the naked eye; in cases of doubt or dispute, the fragments are examined with a microscope to verify their nature and size.

Self-sealing test. For closures intended to be used with multidose containers, carry out the following test. Fill 10 suitable vials to the nominal volume with *water R,* fit the closures to be examined and secure with a cap. Using for each closure a new hypodermic needle with an external diameter of 0.8 mm, pierce each closure 10 times, piercing each time at a different site. Immerse the vials upright in a 1 g/l solution of *methylene blue R* and reduce the external pressure by 27 kPa for 10 min. Restore atmospheric pressure and leave the vials immersed for 30 min. Rinse the outside of the vials. None of the vials contains any trace of coloured solution.

(1) See ISO 7864 "Sterile hypodermic needles for single use".

4. REAGENTS

01/2005:40000

4. REAGENTS

Additional information for reagents that can only be fully identified by a trademark or whose availability is limited may be found on the EDQM website at the following address: http://www.pheur.org/knowledge.htm. This information is given only to make it easier to obtain such reagents and this does not suggest in any way that the mentioned suppliers are especially recommended or certified by the European Pharmacopoeia Commission or the Council of Europe. It is therefore acceptable to use reagents from another source provided that they comply with the standards of the Pharmacopoeia.

01/2005:40100

4.1. REAGENTS, STANDARD SOLUTIONS, BUFFER SOLUTIONS

Where the name of substance or a solution is followed by the letter R (the whole in italics), this indicates a reagent included in the following list. The specifications given for reagents do not necessarily guarantee their quality for use in medicines.

Within the description of each reagent there is a seven-figure reference code in italics (for example, 1002501). This number, which will remain unchanged for a given reagent during subsequent revisions of the list, is used for identification purposes by the Secretariat, and users of the Pharmacopoeia may also find it useful, for example in the management of reagent stocks. The description may also include a CAS number (Chemical Abstract Service Registry Number) recognisable by its typical format, for example 9002-93-1.

Some of the reagents included in the list are toxic and should be handled in conformity with good quality control laboratory practice.

Reagents in aqueous solution are prepared using *water R*. Where a reagent solution is described using an expression such as "hydrochloric acid (10 g/l HCl)", the solution is prepared by an appropriate dilution with *water R* of a more concentrated reagent solution specified in this chapter. Reagent solutions used in the limit tests for barium, calcium and sulphates are prepared using *distilled water R*. Where the name of the solvent is not stated, an aqueous solution is intended.

The reagents and reagent solutions are to be stored in well-closed containers. The labelling should comply with the relevant national legislation and international agreements.

01/2005:40101

4.1.1. REAGENTS

Acacia. *1000100.*

See *Acacia (0307).*

Acacia solution. *1000101.*

Dissolve 100 g of *acacia R* in 1000 ml of *water R*. Stir with a mechanical stirrer for 2 h. Centrifuge at about 2000 *g* for 30 min to obtain a clear solution.

Storage: in polyethylene containers of about 250 ml capacity at 0 °C to − 20 °C.

Acebutolol hydrochloride. *1148900.* [34381-68-5].

See *Acebutolol hydrochloride (0871).*

Acetal. $C_6H_{14}O_2$. (M_r 118.2). *1112300.* [105-57-7].
Acetaldehyde diethyl acetal. 1,1-Diethoxyethane.

A clear, colourless, volatile liquid, miscible with water and with alcohol.

d_{20}^{20}: about 0.824.

n_D^{20}: about 1.382.

bp: about 103 °C.

Acetaldehyde. C_2H_4O. (M_r 44.1). *1000200.* [75-07-0].
Ethanal.

A clear, colourless flammable liquid, miscible with water and with alcohol.

d_{20}^{20}: about 0.788.

n_D^{20}: about 1.332.

bp: about 21 °C.

Acetaldehyde ammonia trimer trihydrate.
$C_6H_{15}N_3,3H_2O$. (M_r 183.3). *1133500.* [76231-37-3].
2,4,6-Trimethylhexahydro-1,3,5-triazine trihydrate.

mp: 95 °C to 97 °C.

Acetic acid, anhydrous. $C_2H_4O_2$. (M_r 60.1). *1000300.* [64-19-7].

Content: minimum 99.6 per cent *m/m* of $C_2H_4O_2$.

A colourless liquid or white, shining, fern-like crystals, miscible with or very soluble in water, in alcohol, in glycerol (85 per cent), and in most fatty and essential oils.

d_{20}^{20}: 1.052 to 1.053.

bp: 117 °C to 119 °C.

A 100 g/l solution is strongly acid (*2.2.4*).

A 5 g/l solution neutralised with *dilute ammonia R2* gives reaction (b) of acetates (*2.3.1*).

Freezing point (*2.2.18*): minimum 15.8 °C.

Water (*2.5.12*): maximum 0.4 per cent. If the water content is more than 0.4 per cent it may be adjusted by adding the calculated amount of *acetic anhydride R*.

Storage: protected from light.

Acetic acid, glacial. $C_2H_4O_2$. (M_r 60.1). *1000400.* [64-19-7].

See *Acetic acid, glacial (0590).*

Acetic acid. *1000401.*

Content: 290 g/l to 310 g/l of $C_2H_4O_2$ (M_r 60.1).

Dilute 30 g of *glacial acetic acid R* to 100 ml with *water R*.

Acetic acid, dilute. *1000402.*

Content: 115 g/l to 125 g/l of $C_2H_4O_2$ (M_r 60.1).

Dilute 12 g of *glacial acetic acid R* to 100 ml with *water R*.

Acetic anhydride. $C_4H_6O_3$. (M_r 102.1). *1000500.* [108-24-7].

Content: minimum 97.0 per cent *m/m* of $C_4H_6O_3$.

A clear, colourless liquid.

bp: 136 °C to 142 °C.

Assay. Dissolve 2.00 g in 50.0 ml of *1 M sodium hydroxide* in a ground-glass-stoppered flask and boil under a reflux condenser for 1 h. Titrate with *1 M hydrochloric acid*, using 0.5 ml of *phenolphthalein solution R* as indicator. Calculate the number of millilitres of *1 M sodium hydroxide* required for 1 g (n_1). Dissolve 2.00 g in 20 ml of *cyclohexane R* in a ground-glass-stoppered flask, cool in ice and add a cold mixture of 10 ml of *aniline R* and 20 ml of *cyclohexane R*. Boil the mixture under a reflux condenser for 1 h, add 50.0 ml of *1 M sodium hydroxide* and shake vigorously. Titrate with *1 M hydrochloric acid*, using 0.5 ml of *phenolphthalein solution R* as indicator. Calculate the number of millilitres of *1 M sodium hydroxide* required for 1 g (n_2). Calculate the percentage of $C_4H_6O_3$ from the expression:

$$10.2\,(n_1 - n_2)$$

Acetic anhydride solution R1. *1000501.*

Dissolve 25.0 ml of *acetic anhydride R* in *anhydrous pyridine R* and dilute to 100.0 ml with the same solvent.

Storage: protected from light and air.

Acetic anhydride - sulphuric acid solution. *1000502.*

Carefully mix 5 ml of *acetic anhydride R* with 5 ml of *sulphuric acid R*. Add dropwise and with cooling to 50 ml of *ethanol R*.

Prepare immediately before use.

Acetone. *1000600.* [67-64-1].

See *Acetone (0872).*

Acetonitrile. C_2H_3N. (M_r 41.05). *1000700.* [75-05-8]. Methyl cyanide. Ethanenitrile.

A clear, colourless liquid, miscible with water, with acetone and with methanol.

d_{20}^{20}: about 0.78.

n_D^{20}: about 1.344.

A 100 g/l solution is neutral to litmus paper.

Distillation range (2.2.11). Not less than 95 per cent distils between 80 °C and 82 °C.

Acetonitrile used in spectrophotometry complies with the following additional requirement.

Minimum transmittance (2.2.25): 98 per cent from 255 nm to 420 nm, using *water R* as compensation liquid.

Acetonitrile for chromatography. *1000701.*

See *Acetonitrile R.*

Acetonitrile used in chromatography complies with the following additional requirements.

Minimum transmittance (2.2.25): 98 per cent from 240 nm, using *water R* as compensation liquid.

Minimum purity (2.2.28): 99.8 per cent.

Acetonitrile R1. *1000702.*

Complies with the requirements prescribed for *acetonitrile R* and with the following additional requirements.

Content: minimum 99.9 per cent of C_2H_3N.

Absorbance (2.2.25). The absorbance at 200 nm using *water R* as the compensation liquid is not more than 0.10.

Acetylacetamide. $C_4H_7NO_2$. (M_r 101.1). *1102600.* [5977-14-0]. 3-Oxobutanamide.

mp: 53 °C to 56 °C.

Acetylacetone. $C_5H_8O_2$. (M_r 100.1). *1000900.* [123-54-6]. 2,4-Pentanedione.

A colourless or slightly yellow, easily flammable liquid, freely soluble in water, miscible with acetone, with alcohol and with glacial acetic acid.

n_D^{20}: 1.452 to 1.453.

bp: 138 °C to 140 °C.

Acetylacetone reagent R1. *1000901.*

To 100 ml of *ammonium acetate solution R* add 0.2 ml of *acetylacetone R.*

***N*-Acetyl-ε-caprolactam.** $C_8H_{13}NO_2$. (M_r 155.2). *1102700.* [1888-91-1]. *N*-Acetylhexane-6-lactam.

Colourless liquid, miscible with ethanol.

d_{20}^{20}: about 1.100.

n_D^{20}: about 1.489.

bp: about 135 °C.

Acetyl chloride. C_2H_3ClO. (M_r 78.5). *1000800.* [75-36-5].

A clear, colourless liquid, flammable, decomposes in contact with water and with alcohol, miscible with ethylene chloride.

d_{20}^{20}: about 1.10.

Distillation range (2.2.11). Not less than 95 per cent distils between 49 °C and 53 °C.

Acetylcholine chloride. $C_7H_{16}ClNO_2$. (M_r 181.7). *1001000.* [60-31-1].

A crystalline powder, very soluble in cold water and in alcohol ; it decomposes in hot water and in alkalis.

Storage: at − 20 °C.

Acetyleugenol. $C_{12}H_{14}O_3$. (M_r 206.2). *1100700.* [93-28-7]. 2-Methoxy-4-(2-propenyl)phenylacetate.

A yellow coloured, oily liquid, freely soluble in alcohol, practically insoluble in water.

n_D^{20}: about 1.521.

bp: 281 °C to 282 °C.

Acetyleugenol used in gas chromatography complies with the following additional test.

Assay. Examine by gas chromatography (*2.2.28*) as prescribed in the monograph on *Clove oil (1091)* using the substance to be examined as the test solution.

The area of the principal peak is not less than 98.0 per cent of the total area of the peaks.

***N*-Acetylglucosamine.** $C_8H_{15}NO_6$. (M_r 221.2). *1133600.* [7512-17-6]. 2-(Acetylamino)-2-deoxy-D-glucopyranose.

mp: about 202 °C.

***N*-Acetylneuraminic acid.** $C_{11}H_{19}NO_9$. (M_r 309.3). *1001100.* [131-48-6]. *O*-Sialic acid.

White acicular crystals, soluble in water and in methanol, slightly soluble in ethanol, practically insoluble in acetone.

$[\alpha]_D^{20}$: about − 36, determined on a 10 g/l solution.

mp: about 186 °C, with decomposition.

***N*-Acetyltryptophan.** $C_{13}H_{14}N_2O_3$. (M_r 246.3). *1102800.* [1218-34-4]. 2-Acetylamino-3-(indol-3-yl)propanoic acid.

A white or almost white powder or colourless crystals, slightly soluble in water. It dissolves in dilute solutions of alkali hydroxides.

mp: about 205 °C.

Assay. Dissolve 10.0 mg in a mixture of 10 volumes of *acetonitrile R* and 90 volumes of *water R* and dilute to 100.0 ml with the same mixture of solvents. Examine as prescribed in the monograph on *Tryptophan (1272)* under "1,1′-Ethylidenebis(tryptophan) and other related substances". The area of the principal peak in the chromatogram obtained is not less than 99.0 per cent of the areas of all the peaks.

Acetyltyrosine ethyl ester. $C_{13}H_{17}NO_4,H_2O$. (M_r 269.3). *1001200.* [36546-50-6]. *N*-Acetyl-L-tyrosine ethyl ester monohydrate. Ethyl (*S*)-2-acetamido-3-(4-hydroxyphenyl)propionate monohydrate.

A white, crystalline powder suitable for the assay of chymotrypsin.

$[\alpha]_D^{20}$: + 21 to + 25, determined on a 10 g/l solution in *alcohol R*.

$A_{1\,cm}^{1\%}$: 60 to 68, determined at 278 nm in *alcohol R*.

Acetyltyrosine ethyl ester 0.2 M. *1001201.*

Dissolve 0.54 g of *acetyltyrosine ethyl ester R* in *alcohol R* and dilute to 10.0 ml with the same solvent.

Acid blue 83. $C_{45}H_{44}N_3NaO_7S_2$. (M_r 826). *1012200.* [6104-59-2].

Colour Index No. 42660.
Brilliant blue R. Coomassie brilliant blue R 250.

Brown powder insoluble in cold water, slightly soluble in boiling water and in ethanol, soluble in sulphuric acid, glacial acetic acid and in dilute solutions of alkali hydroxides.

Acid blue 90. $C_{47}H_{48}N_3NaO_7S_2$. (M_r 854). *1001300.* [6104-58-1].

Colour Index No. 42655.
Sodium [4-[[4-[(4-ethoxyphenyl)amino]phenyl][[4-(ethyl)(3-sulphonatobenzyl)amino]phenyl]methylene]cyclo-hexa-2,5-dien-1-ylidene](ethyl)-(3-sulphonatobenzyl)ammonium.

A dark brown powder, with a violet sheen and some particles having a metallic lustre, soluble in water and in ethanol.

$A_{1\,cm}^{1\%}$: greater than 500, determined at 577 nm using a 0.01 g/l solution in buffer solution pH 7.0 and calculated with reference to the dried substance.

Loss on drying (2.2.32): maximum 5.0 per cent, determined on 0.500 g by drying in an oven at 100-105 °C.

Acid blue 92. $C_{26}H_{16}N_3Na_3O_{10}S_3$. ($M_r$ 696). *1001400.* [3861-73-2].

Colour Index No. 13390.
Coomassie blue. Anazolene sodium. Trisodium 8-hydroxy-4′-(phenylamino)azonaphthalene-3,5′,6-trisulphonate.

Dark blue crystals slightly soluble in alcohol, soluble in water, in acetone and in ethylene glycol monoethylether.

Acid blue 92 solution. *1001401.*

Dissolve 0.5 g of *acid blue 92 R* in a mixture of 10 ml of *glacial acetic acid R*, 45 ml of *alcohol R* and 45 ml of *water R*.

Acid blue 93. $C_{37}H_{27}N_3Na_2O_9S_3$. ($M_r$ 800). *1134200.* [28983-56-4].

Colour Index No. 42780.
Methyl blue. Poirrier blue.

Mixture of triphenylrosaniline di- and trisulfonate and of triphenylpararosaniline.

Dark blue powder.

Colour change: pH 9.4 to pH 14.0.

Acid blue 93 solution. *1134201.*

Dissolve 0.2 g of *acid blue 93 R* in *water R* and dilute to 100 ml with the same solvent.

Acrylamide. C_3H_5NO. (M_r 71.1). *1001500.* [79-06-1].
Propenamide.

Colourless or white flakes or a white or almost white, crystalline powder, very soluble in water and in methanol, freely soluble in ethanol.

mp: about 84 °C.

30 per cent acrylamide/bisacrylamide (29:1) solution. *1001501.*

Prepare a solution containing 290 g of *acrylamide R* and 10 g of *methylenebisacrylamide R* per litre of *water R*. Filter.

30 per cent acrylamide/bisacrylamide (36.5:1) solution. *1001502.*

Prepare a solution containing 292 g of *acrylamide R* and 8 g of *methylenebisacrylamide R* per litre of *water R*. Filter.

Acrylic acid. $C_3H_4O_2$. (M_r 72.1). *1133700.* [79-10-7].
Prop-2-enoic acid. Vinylformic acid.

Content: minimum 99 per cent of $C_3H_4O_2$.

It is stabilised with 0.02 per cent of hydroquinone monomethyl ether.

Corrosive liquid, miscible with water and alcohol. It polymerises readily in the presence of oxygen.

d_{20}^{20} : about 1.05.

n_D^{20} : about 1.421.

bp: about 141 °C.

mp: 12 °C to 15 °C.

Acteoside. $C_{29}H_{36}O_{15}$. (M_r 624.6). *1145100.* [61276-17-3]. 2-(3,4-Dihydroxyphenyl)ethyl 3-*O*-(6-deoxy-α-L-mannopyranosyl)-4-*O*-[(2*E*)-3-(3,4-dihydroxyphenyl)prop-2-enoyl]-β-D-glucopyranoside.

Light yellowish powder, freely soluble in water and in methanol.

mp: about 140 °C, with decomposition.

Adenosine. $C_{10}H_{13}N_5O_4$. (M_r 267.2). *1001600.* [58-61-7].
6-Amino-9-β-D-ribofuranosyl-9*H*-purine.

A white, crystalline powder, slightly soluble in water, practically insoluble in acetone and in alcohol. It dissolves in dilute solutions of acids.

mp: about 234 °C.

Adipic acid. $C_6H_{10}O_4$. (M_r 146.1). *1095600.* [124-04-9].

Prisms, freely soluble in methanol, soluble in acetone, practically insoluble in light petroleum.

mp: about 152 °C.

Adrenaline. $C_9H_{13}NO_3$. (M_r 183.2). *1155000.* [51-43-4].
(1*R*)-1-(3,4-Dihydroxyphenyl)-2-(methylamino)ethanol.
4-[(1*R*)-1-hydroxy-2-(methylamino)ethyl]benzene-1,2-diol.

White or almost white powder, gradually becoming brown on exposure to light and air, very slightly soluble in water and in ethanol (96 per cent), insoluble in acetone. It dissolves in dilute solutions of mineral acids and alkali hydroxides.

mp: about 215 °C.

Adrenalone hydrochloride. $C_9H_{12}ClNO_3$. (M_r 217.7). *1155100.* [62-13-5]. 1-(3,4-Dihydroxyphenyl)-2-(methylamino)ethanone hydrochloride. 3′,4′-Dihydroxy-2-(methylamino)acetophenone hydrochloride.

Pale yellow crystals, freely soluble in water, soluble in ethanol (96 per cent).

mp: about 244 °C.

Aescin. *1001700.* [11072-93-8].

A mixture of related saponins obtained from the seeds of *Aesculus hippocastanum* L.

A fine, almost white or slightly reddish or yellowish, amorphous powder.

Chromatography. Examine as prescribed in the monograph on *Senega root (0202)* but apply 20 µl of the solution. After spraying with *anisaldehyde solution R* and heating, the chromatogram shows a principal band with an R_f of about 0.4.

4. Reagents

Agarose/cross-linked polyacrylamide. *1002200.*

Agarose trapped within a cross-linked polyacrylamide network; it is used for the separation of globular proteins with relative molecular masses of 2×10^4 to 35×10^4.

Agarose-DEAE for ion-exchange chromatography. *1002100.* [57407-08-6].

Cross-linked agarose substituted with diethylaminoethyl groups, presented as beads.

Agarose for chromatography. *1001800.* [9012-36-6].

Swollen beads 60 µm to 140 µm in diameter presented as a 4 per cent suspension in *water R*. It is used in size-exclusion chromatography for the separation of proteins with relative molecular masses of 6×10^4 to 20×10^6 and of polysaccharides with relative molecular masses of 3×10^3 to 5×10^6.

Agarose for chromatography, cross-linked. *1001900.* [61970-08-9].

Prepared from agarose by reaction with 2,3-dibromopropanol in strongly alkaline conditions.

It occurs as swollen beads 60 µm to 140 µm in diameter and is presented as a 4 per cent suspension in *water R*. It is used in size-exclusion chromatography for the separation of proteins with relative molecular masses of 6×10^4 to 20×10^6 and of polysaccharides with relative molecular masses of 3×10^3 to 5×10^6.

Agarose for chromatography, cross-linked R1. *1001901.* [65099-79-8].

Prepared for agarose by reaction with 2,3-dibromopropanol in strongly alkaline conditions.

It occurs as swollen beads 60 µm to 140 µm in diameter and is presented as a 4 per cent suspension in *water R*. It is used in size-exclusion chromatography for the separation of proteins with relative molecular masses of 7×10^4 to 40×10^6 and of polysaccharides with relative molecular masses of 1×10^5 to 2×10^7.

Agarose for electrophoresis. *1002000.* [9012-36-6].

A neutral, linear polysaccharide, the main component of which is derived from agar.

A white or almost white powder, practically insoluble in cold water, very slightly soluble in hot water.

Alanine. *1102900.* [56-41-7].

See *Alanine (0752).*

β-Alanine. *1004500.* [107-95-9].

See *3-aminopropionic acid R.*

Albumin, bovine. *1002300.* [9048-46-8].

Bovine serum albumin containing about 96 per cent of protein.

A white to light-yellowish-brown powder.

Water (*2.5.12*): maximum 3.0 per cent, determined on 0.800 g.

Bovine albumin used in the assay of tetracosactide should be pyrogen-free, free from proteolytic activity, when examined by a suitable means, for example using chromogenic substrate, and free from corticosteroid activity determined by measurement of fluorescence as described in the biological assay of Tetracosactide (0644).

Albumin, human. *1133800.*

Human serum albumin containing not less than 96 per cent of albumin.

Albumin solution, human. *1002400.* [9048-46-8].

See *Human albumin solution (0255).*

Albumin solution, human R1. *1002401.*

Dilute *human albumin solution R* with a 9 g/l solution of *sodium chloride R* to a concentration of 1 g/l of protein. Adjust the pH to 3.5-4.5 with *glacial acetic acid R.*

Alcohol. *1002500.* [64-17-5].

See *Ethanol (96 per cent) R.*

Alcohol (*x* per cent *V/V*). *1002502.*

See *Ethanol (x per cent V/V) R.*

Alcohol, aldehyde-free. *1002501.*

Mix 1200 ml of *alcohol R* with 5 ml of a 400 g/l solution of *silver nitrate R* and 10 ml of a cooled 500 g/l solution of *potassium hydroxide R*. Shake, allow to stand for a few days and filter. Distil the filtrate immediately before use.

Aldehyde dehydrogenase. *1103000.*

Enzyme obtained from baker's yeast which oxidises acetaldehyde to acetic acid in the presence of nicotinamide-adenine dinucleotide, potassium salts and thiols, at pH 8.0.

Aldehyde dehydrogenase solution. *1103001.*

Dissolve in *water R* a quantity of *aldehyde dehydrogenase R*, equivalent to 70 units and dilute to 10 ml with the same solvent. This solution is stable for 8 h at 4 °C.

Aldrin. $C_{12}H_8Cl_6$. (M_r 364.9). *1123100.* [309-00-2].

bp: about 145 °C.

mp: about 104 °C.

A suitable certified reference solution (10 ng/µl in cyclohexane) may be used.

Aleuritic acid. $C_{16}H_{32}O_5$. (M_r 304.4). *1095700.* [533-87-9].

(9*RS*,10*SR*)-9,10,16-Trihydroxyhexadecanoic acid.

A white powder, greasy to the touch, soluble in methanol.

mp: about 101 °C.

Alizarin S. $C_{14}H_7NaO_7S,H_2O$. (M_r 360.3). *1002600.* [130-22-3].

Schultz No. 1145.

Colour Index No. 58005.

Sodium 1,2-dihydroxyanthraquinone-3-sulphonate monohydrate. Sodium 3,4-dihydroxy-9,10-dioxo-9,10-dihydroanthracene-2-sulphonate monohydrate.

An orange-yellow powder, freely soluble in water and in alcohol.

Alizarin S solution. *1002601.*

A 1 g/l solution.

Test for sensitivity. If alizarin S solution is used for the standardisation of *0.05 M barium perchlorate*, it shows a colour change from yellow to orange-red when it is tested according to the standardisation of *0.05 M barium perchlorate* (*4.2.2*).

Colour change: pH 3.7 (yellow) to pH 5.2 (violet).

Aluminium. Al. (A_r 26.98). *1118200.* [7429-90-5].

A white, malleable, flexible, bluish metal, available as bars, sheets, powder, strips or wire. In moist air an oxide film forms which protects the metal from corrosion.

Analytical grade.

4. Reagents

Aluminium chloride. $AlCl_3,6H_2O$. (M_r 241.4). *1002700.* [7784-13-6]. Aluminium chloride hexahydrate.

Content: minimum 98.0 per cent of $AlCl_3,6H_2O$.

A white to slightly yellowish, crystalline powder, hygroscopic, freely soluble in water and in alcohol.

Storage: in an airtight container.

Aluminium chloride reagent. *1002702.*

Dissolve 2.0 g of *aluminium chloride R* in 100 ml of a 5 per cent *V/V* solution of *glacial acetic acid R* in *methanol R.*

Aluminium chloride solution. *1002701.*

Dissolve 65.0 g of *aluminium chloride R* in *water R* and dilute to 100 ml with the same solvent. Add 0.5 g of *activated charcoal R,* stir for 10 min, filter and add to the filtrate, with continuous stirring, sufficient of a 10 g/l solution of *sodium hydroxide R* (about 60 ml) to adjust the pH to about 1.5.

Aluminium nitrate. $Al(NO_3)_3,9H_2O$. (M_r 375.1). *1002800.* [7784-27-2]. Aluminium nitrate nonahydrate.

Crystals, deliquescent, very soluble in water and alcohol, very slightly soluble in acetone.

Storage: in an airtight container.

Aluminium oxide, anhydrous. *1002900.* [1344-28-1].

An aluminium oxide, consisting of γ-Al_2O_3, dehydrated and activated by heat treatment. Particle size 75 µm to 150 µm.

Aluminium oxide, basic. *1118300.*

A basic grade of *anhydrous aluminium oxide R* suitable for column chromatography.

pH (2.2.3). Shake 1 g with 10 ml of *carbon dioxide-free water R* for 5 min. The pH of the suspension is 9 to 10.

Aluminium oxide, neutral. Al_2O_3. (M_r 102.0). *1118400.*

See *Aluminium oxide, hydrated (0311).*

Aluminium potassium sulphate. *1003000.* [7784-24-9].

See *Alum (0006).*

Amido black 10B. $C_{22}H_{14}N_6Na_2O_9S_2$. ($M_r$ 617). *1003100.* [1064-48-8].

Schultz No. 299.

Colour Index No. 20470.
Disodium 5-amino-4-hydroxy-6-[(4-nitrophenyl)azo]-3-(phenylazo)naphthalene-2,7-disulphonate.

A dark-brown to black powder, sparingly soluble in water, soluble in alcohol.

Amido black 10B solution. *1003101.*

A 5 g/l solution of *amido black 10B R* in a mixture of 10 volumes of *acetic acid R* and 90 volumes of *methanol R.*

Aminoazobenzene. $C_{12}H_{11}N_3$. (M_r 197.2). *1003200.* [60-09-3].

Colour Index No. 11000.
4-(Phenylazo)aniline.

Brownish-yellow needles with a bluish tinge, slightly soluble in water, freely soluble in alcohol.

mp: about 128 °C.

2-Aminobenzoic acid. $C_7H_7NO_2$. (M_r 137.1). *1003400.* [118-92-3]. Anthranilic acid.

A white to pale-yellow, crystalline powder, sparingly soluble in cold water, freely soluble in hot water, in alcohol and in glycerol. Solutions in alcohol or in ether and, particularly, in glycerol show a violet fluorescence.

mp: about 145 °C.

3-Aminobenzoic acid. $C_7H_7NO_2$. (M_r 137.1). *1147400.* [99-05-8].

White or almost white crystals. An aqueous solution turns brown on standing in air.

mp: about 174 °C.

Storage: in an airtight container, protected from light.

4-Aminobenzoic acid. $C_7H_7NO_2$. (M_r 137.1). *1003300.* [150-13-0].

A white, crystalline powder, slightly soluble in water, freely soluble in alcohol, practically insoluble in light petroleum.

mp: about 187 °C.

Chromatography. Examine as prescribed in the monograph on *Procaine hydrochloride (0050)*; the chromatogram shows only one principal spot.

Storage: protected from light.

4-Aminobenzoic acid solution. *1003301.*

Dissolve 1 g of *4-aminobenzoic acid R* in a mixture of 18 ml of *anhydrous acetic acid R,* 20 ml of *water R* and 1 ml of *phosphoric acid R.* Immediately before use, mix 2 volumes of the solution with 3 volumes of *acetone R.*

***N*-(4-Aminobenzoyl)-L-glutamic acid.** $C_{12}H_{14}N_2O_5$. (M_r 266.3). *1141700.* [4271-30-1]. ABGA. (2*S*)-2-[(4-Aminobenzoyl)amino]pentanedioic acid.

White or almost white, crystalline powder.

mp: about 175 °C, with decomposition.

4-Aminobutanoic acid. $C_4H_9NO_2$. (M_r 103.1). *1123200.* [56-12-2]. γ-Aminobutyric acid. GABA.

Leaflets from methanol and ether, needles from water and alcohol. Freely soluble in water, practically insoluble or slightly soluble in other solvents.

mp: about 202 °C (decreases on rapid heating).

Aminobutanol. $C_4H_{11}NO$. (M_r 89.1). *1003500.* [5856-63-3]. 2-Aminobutanol.

Oily liquid, miscible with water, soluble in alcohol.

d_{20}^{20}: about 0.94.

n_D^{20}: about 1.453.

bp: about 180 °C.

Aminochlorobenzophenone. $C_{13}H_{10}ClNO$. (M_r 231.7). *1003600.* [719-59-5]. 2-Amino-5-chlorobenzophenone.

A yellow, crystalline powder, practically insoluble in water, freely soluble in acetone, soluble in alcohol.

mp: about 97 °C.

Chromatography. Examine as prescribed in the monograph on *Chlordiazepoxide hydrochloride (0474)* but apply 5 µl of a 0.5 g/l solution in *methanol R*; the chromatogram shows only one principal spot, at an R_f of about 0.9.

Storage: protected from light.

6-Aminohexanoic acid. $C_6H_{13}NO_2$. (M_r 131.2). *1103100.* [60-32-2].

Colourless crystals, freely soluble in water, sparingly soluble in methanol, practically insoluble in ethanol.

mp: about 205 °C.

Aminohippuric acid. $C_9H_{10}N_2O_3$. (M_r 194.2). *1003700.* [61-78-9]. (4-Aminobenzamido)acetic acid.

A white or almost white powder, sparingly soluble in water, soluble in alcohol.

mp: about 200 °C.

Aminohippuric acid reagent. *1003701.*

Dissolve 3 g of *phthalic acid R* and 0.3 g of *aminohippuric acid R* in *alcohol R* and dilute to 100 ml with the same solvent.

Aminohydroxynaphthalenesulphonic acid. $C_{10}H_9NO_4S$. (M_r 239.3). *1112400.* [116-63-2]. 4-Amino-3-hydroxynaphthalene-1-sulphonic acid.

White or grey needles, turning pink on exposure to light, especially when moist, practically insoluble in water and in alcohol, soluble in solutions of alkali hydroxides and in hot solutions of sodium metabisulphite.

Storage: protected from light.

Aminohydroxynaphthalenesulphonic acid solution. *1112401.*

Mix 5.0 g of *anhydrous sodium sulphite R* with 94.3 g of *sodium hydrogensulphite R* and 0.7 g of *aminohydroxynaphthalenesulphonic acid R*. Dissolve 1.5 g of the mixture in *water R* and dilute to 10.0 ml with the same solvent. Prepare the solution daily.

Aminomethylalizarindiacetic acid. $C_{19}H_{15}NO_8,2H_2O$. (M_r 421.4). *1003900.* [3952-78-1]. 2,2′-[(3,4-dihydroxy-anthraquinon-3-yl)methylenenitrilo]diacetic acid dihydrate. Alizarin complexone dihydrate.

A fine, pale brownish-yellow to orange-brown powder, practically insoluble in water, soluble in solutions of alkali hydroxides.

mp: about 185 °C.

Loss on drying (*2.2.32*): maximum 10.0 per cent, determined on 1.000 g.

Aminomethylalizarindiacetic acid reagent. *1003901.*

Solution I. Dissolve 0.36 g of *cerous nitrate R* in *water R* and dilute to 50 ml with the same solvent.

Solution II. Suspend 0.7 g of *aminomethylalizarindiacetic acid R* in 50 ml of *water R*. Dissolve with the aid of about 0.25 ml of *concentrated ammonia R*, add 0.25 ml of *glacial acetic acid R* and dilute to 100 ml with *water R*.

Solution III. Dissolve 6 g of *sodium acetate R* in 50 ml of *water R*, add 11.5 ml of *glacial acetic acid R* and dilute to 100 ml with *water R*.

To 33 ml of *acetone R* add 6.8 ml of solution III, 1.0 ml of solution II and 1.0 ml of solution I and dilute to 50 ml with *water R*.

Test for sensitivity. To 1.0 ml of *fluoride standard solution (10 ppm F) R* add 19.0 ml of *water R* and 5.0 ml of the aminomethylalizarindiacetic acid reagent. After 20 min, the solution assumes a blue colour.

Storage: use within 5 days.

Aminomethylalizarindiacetic acid solution. *1003902.*

Dissolve 0.192 g of *aminomethylalizarindiacetic acid R* in 6 ml of freshly prepared *1 M sodium hydroxide*. Add 750 ml of *water R*, 25 ml of *succinate buffer solution pH 4.6 R* and, dropwise, *0.5 M hydrochloric acid* until the colour changes from violet-red to yellow (pH 4.5 to 5). Add 100 ml of *acetone R* and dilute to 1000 ml with *water R*.

Aminonitrobenzophenone. $C_{13}H_{10}N_2O_3$. (M_r 242.2). *1004000.* [1775-95-7]. 2-Amino-5-nitrobenzophenone.

A yellow, crystalline powder, practically insoluble in water, soluble in tetrahydrofuran, slightly soluble in methanol.

mp: about 160 °C.

$A_{1\,cm}^{1\%}$: 690 to 720, determined at 233 nm using a 0.01 g/l solution in *methanol R*.

Aminophenazone. $C_{13}H_{17}N_3O$. (231.3). *1133900.* [58-15-1]. 4-(Dimethylamino)-1,5-dimethyl-2-phenyl-1,2-dihydro-3*H*-pyrazol-3-one.

White, crystalline powder or colourless crystals, soluble in water, freely soluble in alcohol.

mp: about 108 °C.

2-Aminophenol. C_6H_7NO. (M_r 109.1). *1147500.* [95-55-6].

Pale yellowish-brown crystals which rapidly become brown, sparingly soluble in water, soluble in alcohol.

mp: about 172 °C.

Storage: in an airtight container, protected from light.

3-Aminophenol. C_6H_7NO. (M_r 109.1). *1147600.* [591-27-5].

Pale yellowish-brown crystals, sparingly soluble in water.

mp: about 122 °C.

4-Aminophenol. C_6H_7NO. (M_r 109.1). *1004300.* [123-30-8].

Content: minimum 95 per cent of C_6H_7NO.

A white or slightly coloured, crystalline powder, becoming coloured on exposure to air and light, sparingly soluble in water, soluble in ethanol.

mp: about 186 °C, with decomposition.

Storage: protected from light.

Aminopolyether. $C_{18}H_{36}N_2O_6$. (M_r 376.5). *1112500.* [23978-09-8]. 4,7,13,16,21,24-hexaoxa-1,10-diazabicyclo[8,8,8]hexacosane.

mp: 70 °C to 73 °C.

3-Aminopropanol. C_3H_9NO. (M_r 75.1). *1004400.* [156-87-6]. 3-Aminopropan-1-ol. Propanolamine.

A clear, colourless, viscous liquid.

d_{20}^{20}: about 0.99.

n_D^{20}: about 1.461.

mp: about 11 °C.

3-Aminopropionic acid. $C_3H_7NO_2$. (M_r 89.1). *1004500.* [107-95-9]. β-Alanine.

Content: minimum 99 per cent of $C_3H_7NO_2$.

A white, crystalline powder, freely soluble in water, slightly soluble in alcohol, practically insoluble in acetone.

mp: about 200 °C, with decomposition.

Aminopyrazolone. $C_{11}H_{13}N_3O$. (M_r 203.2). *1004600.* [83-07-8]. 4-Amino-2,3-dimethyl-1-phenylpyrazolin-5-one.

Light-yellow needles or powder, sparingly soluble in water, freely soluble in alcohol.

mp: about 108 °C.

Aminopyrazolone solution. *1004601.*

A 1 g/l solution in *buffer solution pH 9.0 R*.

Ammonia, concentrated. *1004700.*

See *Concentrated ammonia solution (0877)*.

Ammonia. *1004701.*

Content: 170 g/l to 180 g/l of NH_3 (M_r 17.03).

Dilute 67 g of *concentrated ammonia R* to 100 ml with *water R*.

d_{20}^{20}: 0.931 to 0.934.

When used in the limit test for iron, *ammonia R* complies with the following additional requirement. Evaporate 5 ml of ammonia to dryness on a water-bath, add 10 ml of *water R*, 2 ml of a 200 g/l solution of *citric acid R* and 0.1 ml of *thioglycollic acid R*. Make alkaline by adding *ammonia R* and dilute to 20 ml with *water R*. No pink colour develops.

Storage: protected from atmospheric carbon dioxide, at a temperature below 20 °C.

Ammonia, dilute R1. *1004702.*

Content: 100 g/l to 104 g/l of NH_3 (M_r 17.03).

Dilute 41 g of *concentrated ammonia R* to 100 ml with *water R*.

Ammonia, dilute R2. *1004703.*

Content: 33 g/l to 35 g/l of NH_3 (M_r 17.03).

Dilute 14 g of *concentrated ammonia R* to 100 ml with *water R*.

Ammonia, dilute R3. *1004704.*

Content: 1.6 g/l to 1.8 g/l of NH_3 (M_r 17.03).

Dilute 0.7 g of *concentrated ammonia R* to 100 ml with *water R*.

Ammonia, lead-free. *1004705.*

Complies with the requirements prescribed for *dilute ammonia R1* and with the following additional test: to 20 ml of lead-free ammonia, add 1 ml of *lead-free potassium cyanide solution R*, dilute to 50 ml with *water R* and add 0.10 ml of *sodium sulphide solution R*. The solution is not more intensely coloured than a reference solution prepared without sodium sulphide.

Ammonia, concentrated R1. *1004800.*

Content: minimum 32.0 per cent *m/m* of NH_3 (M_r 17.03).

A clear, colourless liquid.

d_{20}^{20}: 0.883 to 0.889.

Assay. Weigh accurately a ground-glass-stoppered flask containing 50.0 ml of *1 M hydrochloric acid*. Introduce 2 ml of the concentrated ammonia and weigh again. Titrate the solution with *1 M sodium hydroxide*, using 0.5 ml of *methyl red mixed solution R* as indicator.

1 ml of *1 M hydrochloric acid* is equivalent to 17.03 mg of NH_3.

Storage: protected from atmospheric carbon dioxide, at a temperature below 20 °C.

Ammonium acetate. $C_2H_7NO_2$. (M_r 77.1). *1004900.* [631-61-8].

Colourless crystals, very deliquescent, very soluble in water and in alcohol.

Storage: in an airtight container.

Ammonium acetate solution. *1004901.*

Dissolve 150 g of *ammonium acetate R* in *water R*. Add 3 ml of *glacial acetic acid R* and dilute to 1000 ml with *water R*.

Storage: use within 1 week.

Ammonium and cerium nitrate. $(NH_4)_2Ce(NO_3)_6$. (M_r 548.2). *1005000.* [16774-21-3].

An orange-yellow, crystalline powder, or orange transparent crystals, soluble in water.

Ammonium and cerium sulphate. $(NH_4)_4Ce(SO_4)_4,2H_2O$. (M_r 633). *1005100.* [10378-47-9].

Orange-yellow, crystalline powder or crystals, slowly soluble in water.

(1*R*)-(–)-Ammonium 10-camphorsulphonate. $C_{10}H_{19}NO_4S$. (M_r 249.3). *1103200.*

Content: minimum 97.0 per cent of (1*R*)-(–)-ammonium 10-camphorsulphonate.

$[\alpha]_D^{20}$: – 18 ± 2 (50 g/l solution in *water R*).

Ammonium carbonate. *1005200.* [506-87-6]. A mixture of varying proportions of ammonium hydrogen carbonate (NH_4HCO_3, M_r 79.1) and ammonium carbamate (NH_2COONH_4, M_r 78.1).

A white translucent mass, slowly soluble in about 4 parts of water. It is decomposed by boiling water. Ammonium carbonate liberates not less than 30 per cent *m/m* of NH_3 (M_r 17.03).

Assay. Dissolve 2.00 g in 25 ml of *water R*. Slowly add 50.0 ml of *1 M hydrochloric acid*, titrate with *1 M sodium hydroxide*, using 0.1 ml of *methyl orange solution R* as indicator.

1 ml of *1 M hydrochloric acid* is equivalent to 17.03 mg of NH_3.

Storage: at a temperature below 20 °C.

Ammonium carbonate solution. *1005201.*

A 158 g/l solution.

Ammonium chloride. *1005300.* [12125-02-9].

See *Ammonium chloride (0007)*.

Ammonium chloride solution. *1005301.*

A 107 g/l solution.

Ammonium citrate. $C_6H_{14}N_2O_7$. (M_r 226.2). *1103300.* [3012-65-5]. Diammonium hydrogen citrate.

A white, crystalline powder or colourless crystals, freely soluble in water, slightly soluble in alcohol.

pH (2.2.3): about 4.3 for a 22.6 g/l solution.

Ammonium dihydrogen phosphate. $(NH_4)H_2PO_4$. (M_r 115.0). *1005400.* [7722-76-1]. Monobasic ammonium phosphate.

A white, crystalline powder or colourless crystals, freely soluble in water.

pH (2.2.3): about 4.2 for a 23 g/l solution.

Ammonium formate. CH_5NO_2. (M_r 63.1). *1112600.* [540-69-2].

Deliquescent crystals or granules, very soluble in water, soluble in alcohol.

mp: 119 °C to 121 °C.

Storage: in an airtight container.

Ammonium hexafluorogermanate (IV). $(NH_4)_2GeF_6$. (M_r 222.7). *1134000.* [16962-47-3].

White crystals, freely soluble in water.

Ammonium hydrogen carbonate. NH_4HCO_3. (M_r 79.1). *1005500.* [1066-33-7].

Content: minimum 99 per cent of NH_4HCO_3.

Ammonium molybdate. $(NH_4)_6Mo_7O_{24},4H_2O$. (M_r 1236). *1005700.* [12054-85-2].

Colourless or slightly yellow or greenish crystals, soluble in water, practically insoluble in alcohol.

Ammonium molybdate reagent. *1005701.*

Mix, in the given order, 1 volume of a 25 g/l solution of *ammonium molybdate R*, 1 volume of a 100 g/l solution of *ascorbic acid R* and 1 volume of *sulphuric acid R* (294.5 g/l H_2SO_4). Add 2 volumes of *water R*.

Storage: use within 1 day.

Ammonium molybdate reagent R1. *1005706.*

Mix 10 ml of a 60 g/l solution of *disodium arsenate R*, 50 ml of *ammonium molybdate solution R*, 90 ml of *dilute sulphuric acid R* and dilute to 200 ml in *water R*.

Storage: in amber flasks at 37 °C for 24 h.

Ammonium molybdate reagent R2. *1005708.*

Dissolve 50 g of *ammonium molybdate R* in 600 ml of *water R*. To 250 ml of cold *water R* add 150 ml of *sulphuric acid R* and cool. Mix the 2 solutions together.

Storage: use within 1 day.

Ammonium molybdate solution. *1005702.*

A 100 g/l solution.

Ammonium molybdate solution R2. *1005703.*

Dissolve 5.0 g of *ammonium molybdate R* with heating in 30 ml of *water R*. Cool, adjust the pH to 7.0 with *dilute ammonia R2* and dilute to 50 ml with *water R*.

Ammonium molybdate solution R3. *1005704.*

Solution I. Dissolve 5 g of *ammonium molybdate R* in 20 ml of *water R* with heating.

Solution II. Mix 150 ml of *alcohol R* with 150 ml of *water R*. Add with cooling 100 ml of *sulphuric acid R*.

Immediately before use add 80 volumes of solution II to 20 volumes of solution I.

Ammonium molybdate solution R4. *1005705.*

Dissolve 1.0 g of *ammonium molybdate R* in *water R* and dilute to 40 ml with the same solvent. Add 3 ml of *hydrochloric acid R* and 5 ml of *perchloric acid R* and dilute to 100 ml with *acetone R*.

Storage: protected from light; use within 1 month.

Ammonium molybdate solution R5. *1005707.*

Dissolve 1.0 g of *ammonium molybdate R* in 40.0 ml of a 15 per cent *V/V* solution of *sulphuric acid R*. Prepare the solution daily.

Ammonium molybdate solution R6. *1005709.*

Slowly add 10 ml of *sulphuric acid R* to about 40 ml of *water R*. Mix and allow to cool. Dilute to 100 ml with *water R* and mix. Add 2.5 g of *ammonium molybdate R* and 1 g of *cerium sulphate R*, and shake for 15 min to dissolve.

Ammonium nitrate. NH_4NO_3. (M_r 80.0). *1005800.* [6484-52-2].

A white, crystalline powder or colourless crystals, hygroscopic, very soluble in water, freely soluble in methanol, soluble in alcohol.

Storage: in an airtight container.

Ammonium nitrate R1. *1005801.* [6484-52-2].

Complies with the requirements prescribed for *ammonium nitrate R* and with the following additional requirements.

Acidity. The solution of the substance is faintly acid (*2.2.4*).

Chlorides (*2.4.4*). 0.50 g complies with the limit test for chlorides (100 ppm).

Sulphates (*2.4.13*). 1.0 g complies with the limit test for sulphates (150 ppm).

Sulphated ash (*2.4.14*): maximum 0.05 per cent, determined on 1.0 g.

Ammonium oxalate. $C_2H_8N_2O_4,H_2O$. (M_r 142.1). *1005900.* [6009-70-7].

Colourless crystals, soluble in water.

Ammonium oxalate solution. *1005901.*

A 40 g/l solution.

Ammonium persulphate. $(NH_4)_2S_2O_8$. (M_r 228.2). *1006000.* [7727-54-0].

White, crystalline powder or granular crystals, freely soluble in water.

Ammonium phosphate. $(NH_4)_2HPO_4$. (M_r 132.1). *1006100.* [7783-28-0]. Diammonium hydrogen phosphate.

White crystals or granules, hygroscopic, very soluble in water, practically insoluble in alcohol.

pH (*2.2.3*): about 8 for a 200 g/l solution.

Storage: in an airtight container.

Ammonium pyrrolidinedithiocarbamate. $C_5H_{12}N_2S_2$. (M_r 164.3). *1006200.* [5108-96-3]. Ammonium 1-pyrrolidinyl-dithioformate.

A white to pale yellow, crystalline powder, sparingly soluble in water, very slightly soluble in alcohol.

Storage: in a bottle containing a piece of ammonium carbonate in a muslin bag.

Ammonium reineckate. $NH_4[Cr(NCS)_4(NH_3)_2],H_2O$. ($M_r$ 354.4). *1006300.* [13573-16-5]. Ammonium diamine-tetrakis(isothiocyanato)chromate(III) monohydrate.

Red powder or crystals, sparingly soluble in cold water, soluble in hot water and in alcohol.

Ammonium reineckate solution. *1006301.*

A 10 g/l solution. Prepare immediately before use.

Ammonium sulphamate. $NH_2SO_3NH_4$. (M_r 114.1). *1006400.* [7773-06-0].

A white, crystalline powder or colourless crystals, hygroscopic, very soluble in water, slightly soluble in alcohol.

mp: about 130 °C.

Storage: in an airtight container.

Ammonium sulphate. $(NH_4)_2SO_4$. (M_r 132.1). *1006500.* [7783-20-2].

Colourless crystals or white granules, very soluble in water, practically insoluble in acetone and in alcohol.

pH (*2.2.3*): 4.5 to 6.0 for a 50 g/l solution in *carbon dioxide-free water R*.

Sulphated ash (*2.4.14*): maximum 0.1 per cent.

Ammonium sulphide solution. *1123300.*

Saturate 120 ml of *dilute ammonia R1* with *hydrogen sulphide R* and add 80 ml of *dilute ammonia R1*. Prepare immediately before use.

Ammonium thiocyanate. NH_4SCN. (M_r 76.1). *1006700.* [1762-95-4].

Colourless crystals, deliquescent, very soluble in water, soluble in alcohol.

Storage: in an airtight container.

Ammonium thiocyanate solution. *1006701.*

A 76 g/l solution.

Ammonium vanadate. NH_4VO_3. (M_r 117.0). *1006800.* [7803-55-6]. Ammonium trioxovanadate(V).

A white to slightly yellowish, crystalline powder, slightly soluble in water, soluble in *dilute ammonia R1.*

Ammonium vanadate solution. *1006801.*

Dissolve 1.2 g of *ammonium vanadate R* in 95 ml of *water R* and dilute to 100 ml with *sulphuric acid R.*

Amoxicillin trihydrate. *1103400.*

See *Amoxicillin trihydrate (0260).*

α-Amylase. *1100800.* 1,4-α-D-glucane-glucanohydrolase (EC *3.2.1.1*).

A white to light brown powder.

α-Amylase solution. *1100801.*

A solution of *α-amylase R* with an activity of 800 FAU/g.

β-Amyrin. $C_{30}H_{50}O$. (M_r 426.7). *1141800.* [559-70-6]. Olean-12-en-3β-ol.

White or almost white powder.

mp: 187 °C to 190 °C.

Anethole. $C_{10}H_{12}O$. (M_r 148.2). *1006900.* [4180-23-8]. 1-Methoxy-4-(propen-1-yl)benzene.

A white, crystalline mass up to 20 °C to 21 °C, liquid above 23 °C, practically insoluble in water, freely soluble in ethanol, soluble in ethyl acetate and in light petroleum.

n_D^{25}: about 1.56.

bp: about 230 °C.

Anethole used in gas chromatography complies with the following test.

Assay. Examine by gas chromatography (*2.2.28*) under the conditions described in the monograph on *Anise oil (0804)* using the substance to be examined as the test solution.

The area of the principal peak, corresponding to *trans*-anethole, with a retention time of about 41 min, is not less than 99.0 per cent of the total area of the peaks.

***cis*-Anethole.** $C_{10}H_{12}O$. (M_r 148.2). *1007000.* (*Z*)-1-Methoxy-4-(propen-1-yl)benzene.

A white, crystalline mass up to 20 °C to 21 °C, liquid above 23 °C, practically insoluble in water, freely soluble in ethanol, soluble in ethyl acetate and in light petroleum.

n_D^{25}: about 1.56.

bp: about 230 °C.

cis-Anethole used in gas chromatography complies with the following test.

Assay. Examine by gas chromatography (*2.2.28*) in the conditions described in the monograph on *Anise oil (0804)* using the substance to be examined as the test solution.

The area of the principal peak is not less than 92.0 per cent of the total area of the peaks.

Aniline. C_6H_7N. (M_r 93.1). *1007100.* [62-53-3]. Benzeneamine.

A colourless or slightly yellowish liquid, soluble in water, miscible with alcohol.

d_{20}^{20}: about 1.02.

bp: 183 °C to 186 °C.

Storage: protected from light.

Aniline hydrochloride. C_6H_8ClN. (M_r 129.6). *1147700.* [142-04-1]. Benzenamine hydrochloride.

Crystals. It darkens on exposure to air and light.

mp: about 198 °C.

Storage: protected from light.

Anion exchange resin. *1007200.*

A resin in chlorinated form containing quaternary ammonium groups [$CH_2N^+(CH_3)_3$] attached to a polymer lattice consisting of polystyrene cross-linked with 2 per cent of divinylbenzene. It is available as spherical beads and the particle size is specified in the monograph.

Wash the resin with *1 M sodium hydroxide* on a sintered-glass filter (40) until the washings are free from chloride, then wash with *water R* until the washings are neutral. Suspend in freshly prepared *ammonium-free water R* and protect from atmospheric carbon dioxide.

Anion exchange resin R1. *1123400.*

A resin containing quaternary ammonium groups [$CH_2N^+(CH_3)_3$] attached to a lattice consisting of methacrylate.

Anion exchange resin R2. *1141900.*

A conjugate of homogeneous 10 µm hydrophilic polyether particles, and a quaternary ammonium salt, providing a matrix suitable for strong anion-exchange chromatography of proteins.

Anion exchange resin for chromatography, strongly basic. *1112700.*

A resin with quaternary amine groups attached to a lattice of latex cross linked with divinylbenzene.

Anion exchange resin, strongly basic. *1026600.*

A gel-type resin in hydroxide form containing quaternary ammonium groups [$CH_2N^+(CH_3)_3$, type 1] attached to a polymer lattice consisting of polystyrene cross-linked with 8 per cent of divinylbenzene.

Brown transparent beads.

Particle size: 0.2-1.0 mm.

Moisture content: about 50 per cent.

Total exchange capacity: minimum 1.2 meq/ml.

Anion exchange resin, weak. *1146700.*

A resin with diethylaminoethyl groups attached to a lattice consisting of poly(methyl methacrylate).

Anisaldehyde. $C_8H_8O_2$. (M_r 136.1). *1007300.* [123-11-5]. 4-Methoxybenzaldehyde.

An oily liquid, very slightly soluble in water, miscible with alcohol.

bp: about 248 °C.

Anisaldehyde used in gas chromatography complies with the following test.

Assay. Examine by gas chromatography (*2.2.28*) in the conditions described in the monograph on *Anise oil (0804)* the substance to be examined as the test solution.

The area of the principal peak is not less than 99.0 per cent of the total area of the peaks.

Anisaldehyde solution. *1007301.*

Mix in the following order, 0.5 ml of *anisaldehyde R*, 10 ml of *glacial acetic acid R*, 85 ml of *methanol R* and 5 ml of *sulphuric acid R.*

Anisaldehyde solution R1. *1007302.*

To 10 ml of *anisaldehyde R* add 90 ml of *alcohol R*, mix, add 10 ml of *sulphuric acid R* and mix again.

***p*-Anisidine.** C_7H_9NO. (M_r 123.2). *1103500.* [104-94-9]. 4-Methoxyaniline.

White crystals, sparingly soluble in water, soluble in ethanol.

Content: minimum 97.0 per cent of C_7H_9NO.

Caution: skin irritant, sensitiser.

4. Reagents

Storage: protected from light, at 0 °C to 4 °C.

On storage, *p*-anisidine tends to darken as a result of oxidation. A discoloured reagent can be reduced and decolorised in the following way: dissolve 20 g of *p-anisidine R* in 500 ml of *water R* at 75 °C. Add 1 g of *sodium sulphite R* and 10 g of *activated charcoal R* and stir for 5 min. Filter, cool the filtrate to about 0 °C and allow to stand at this temperature for at least 4 h. Filter, wash the crystals with a small quantity of *water R* at about 0 °C and dry the crystals in vacuum over *diphosphorus pentoxide R*.

Anolyte for isoelectric focusing pH 3 to 5. *1112800.*

0.1 M Glutamic acid, 0.5 M phosphoric acid.

Dissolve 14.71 g of *glutamic acid R* in *water R*. Add 33 ml of *phosphoric acid R* and dilute to 1000 ml with *water R*

Anthracene. $C_{14}H_{10}$. (M_r 178.2). *1007400.* [120-12-7].

A white, crystalline powder, practically insoluble in water, slightly soluble in chloroform.

mp: about 218 °C.

Anthrone. $C_{14}H_{10}O$. (M_r 194.2). *1007500.* [90-44-8]. 9(10*H*)-Anthracenone.

A pale yellow, crystalline powder.

mp: about 155 °C.

Antimony potassium tartrate. $C_4H_4KO_7Sb,{}^1/_2H_2O$. (M_r 333.9). *1007600.* Potassium aqua[tartrato(4−)-O^1,O^2,O^3]-antimoniate(III) hemihydrate.

A white, granular powder or colourless, transparent crystals, soluble in water and in glycerol, freely soluble in boiling water, practically insoluble in alcohol. The aqueous solution is slightly acid.

Antimony trichloride. $SbCl_3$. (M_r 228.1). *1007700.* [10025-91-9].

Colourless crystals or a transparent crystalline mass, hygroscopic, freely soluble in ethanol. Antimony trichloride is hydrolysed by water.

Storage: in an airtight container, protected from moisture.

Antimony trichloride solution. *1007701.*

Rapidly wash 30 g of *antimony trichloride R* with two quantities, each of 15 ml, of *ethanol-free chloroform R*, drain off the washings, and dissolve the washed crystals immediately in 100 ml of *ethanol-free chloroform R*, warming slightly.

Storage: over a few grams of *anhydrous sodium sulphate R*.

Antimony trichloride solution R1. *1007702.*

Solution I. Dissolve 110 g of *antimony trichloride R* in 400 ml of *ethylene chloride R*. Add 2 g of *anhydrous aluminium oxide R*, mix and filter through a sintered-glass filter (40). Dilute to 500.0 ml with *ethylene chloride R* and mix. The absorbance (*2.2.25*) of the solution, determined at 500 nm in a 2 cm cell, is not greater than 0.07.

Solution II. Under a hood, mix 100 ml of freshly distilled *acetyl chloride R* and 400 ml of *ethylene chloride R*.

Mix 90 ml of solution I and 10 ml of solution II.

Storage: in brown ground-glass-stoppered bottle for 7 days. Discard any reagent in which colour develops.

Antithrombin III. *1007800.* [90170-80-2].

Antithrombin III is purified from human plasma by heparin agarose chromatography and should have a specific activity of at least 6 IU/mg.

Antithrombin III solution R1. *1007801.*

Reconstitute *antithrombin III R* as directed by the manufacturer and dilute with *tris(hydroxymethyl)aminomethane sodium chloride buffer solution pH 7.4 R* to 1 IU/ml.

Antithrombin III solution R2. *1007802.*

Reconstitute *antithrombin III R* as directed by the manufacturer and dilute with *tris(hydroxymethyl)aminomethane sodium chloride buffer solution pH 7.4 R* to 0.5 IU/ml.

Apigenin. $C_{15}H_{10}O_5$. (M_r 270.2). *1095800.* [520-36-5]. 4′,5,7-Trihydroxyflavone.

Light yellowish powder; practically insoluble in water, sparingly soluble in alcohol.

mp: about 310 °C, with decomposition.

Chromatography. Examine as prescribed in the monograph on *Roman chamomile flower (0380)*, applying 10 µl of a 0.25 g/l solution in *methanol R*. The chromatogram shows in the upper third a principal zone of yellowish-green fluorescence.

Apigenin 7-glucoside. $C_{21}H_{20}O_{10}$. (M_r 432.4). *1095900.* [578-74-5]. Apigetrin. 7-(β-D-Glucopyranosyloxy)-5-hydroxy-2-(4-hydroxyphenyl)-4*H*-1-benzopyran-4-one.

Light yellowish powder, practically insoluble in water, sparingly soluble in alcohol.

mp: 198 °C to 201 °C.

Chromatography. Examine as prescribed in the monograph on *Roman chamomile flower (0380)*, applying 10 µl of a 0.25 g/l solution in *methanol R*. The chromatogram shows in the middle third a principal zone of yellowish fluorescence.

Apigenin-7-glucoside used in liquid chromatography complies with the following additional test.

Assay. Examine by liquid chromatography (*2.2.29*) as prescribed in the monograph on *Matricaria flower (0404)*.

Test solution. Dissolve 10.0 mg in *methanol R* and dilute to 100.0 ml with the same solvent.

The content of apigenin-7-glucoside is not less than 95.0 per cent, calculated by the normalisation procedure.

Aprotinin. *1007900.* [9087-70-1].

See *Aprotinin (0580)*.

Arabinose. $C_5H_{10}O_5$. (M_r 150.1). *1008000.* [87-72-9]. L-(+)-Arabinose.

A white, crystalline powder, freely soluble in water.

$[\alpha]_D^{20}$: + 103 to + 105, determined on a 50 g/l solution in *water R* containing about 0.05 per cent of NH_3.

Arachidyl alcohol. $C_{20}H_{42}O$. (M_r 298.5). *1156300.* [629-96-9]. 1-Eicosanol.

mp: about 65 °C.

Content: minimum 96 per cent of $C_{20}H_{42}O$.

Arbutin. $C_{12}H_{16}O_7$. (M_r 272.3). *1008100.* [497-76-7]. Arbutoside. 4-Hydroxyphenyl-β-D-glucopyranoside.

Fine, white, shiny needles, freely soluble in water, very soluble in hot water, soluble in alcohol.

$[\alpha]_D^{20}$: about − 64, determined on a 20 g/l solution.

mp: about 200 °C.

Chromatography. Examine by thin-layer chromatography (*2.2.27*) as prescribed in the monograph *Bearberry leaf (1054)*; the chromatogram shows only one principal spot.

Arbutin used in the arbutin assay in the monograph Bearberry leaf (1054) complies with the following additional requirement.

Assay. Examine by liquid chromatography (*2.2.29*) as prescribed in the monograph *Bearberry leaf (1054).*

The content of arbutin is not less than 95 per cent, calculated by the normalisation procedure.

Arginine. *1103600.* [74-79-3].

See *Arginine (0806).*

Argon. Ar. (A_r 39.95). *1008200.* [7440-37-1].

Content: minimum 99.995 per cent *V/V* of Ar.

Carbon monoxide. When used as described in the test for *carbon monoxide in medicinal gases* (*Method I, 2.5.25*), after passage of 10 litres of *argon R* at a flow rate of 4 litres per hour, not more than 0.05 ml of *0.002 M sodium thiosulphate* is required for the titration (0.6 ppm *V/V*).

Aromadendrene. $C_{15}H_{24}$. (M_r 204.4). *1139100.* [489-39-4]. (1*R*,2*S*,4*R*,8*R*,11*R*)-3,3,11-Trimethyl-7-methylenetricyclo-[6.3.0.0^{2,4}]undecane.

Clear, almost colourless liquid.

d_4^{20}: about 0.911.

n_D^{20}: about 1.497.

$[\alpha]_D^{20}$: about + 12.

bp: : about 263 °C.

Aromadendrene used in gas chromatography complies with the following additional test.

Assay. Examine by gas chromatography (*2.2.28*) as prescribed in the monograph on *Tea tree oil (1837).*

The content is not less than 92 per cent, calculated by the normalisation procedure.

Arsenious trioxide. As_2O_3. (M_r 197.8). *1008300.* [1327-53-3]. Arsenious anhydride. Diarsenic trioxide.

A crystalline powder or a white mass, slightly soluble in water, soluble in boiling water.

Arsenite solution. *1008301.*

Dissolve 0.50 g of *arsenious trioxide R* in 5 ml of *dilute sodium hydroxide solution R*, add 2.0 g of *sodium hydrogen carbonate R* and dilute to 100.0 ml with *water R.*

Ascorbic acid. *1008400.* [50-81-7].

See *Ascorbic acid (0253).*

Ascorbic acid solution. *1008401.*

Dissolve 50 mg in 0.5 ml of *water R* and dilute to 50 ml with *dimethylformamide R.*

Asiaticoside. $C_{48}H_{78}O_{19}$. (M_r 959). *1123500.* [16830-15-2]. *O*-6-Deoxy-α-L-mannopyranosyl-(1→4)-*O*-β-D-glucopyranosyl-(1→6)-β-D-glucopyranosyl 2α,3β,23-trihydroxy-4α-urs-12-en-28-oate.

A white powder, hygroscopic, soluble in methanol, slightly soluble in ethanol, insoluble in acetonitrile.

mp: about 232 °C, with decomposition.

Water (*2.5.12*): 6.0 per cent.

Storage: protected from humidity.

Asiaticoside used in liquid chromatography complies with the following additional test.

Assay. Examine by liquid chromatography (*2.2.29*) as prescribed in the monograph on *Centella (1498).*

The content is not less than 97.0 per cent calculated by the normalisation procedure.

Aspartic acid. *1134100.* [56-84-8].

See *Aspartic acid (0797).*

L-Aspartyl-L-phenylalanine. $C_{13}H_{16}N_2O_5$. (M_r 280.3). *1008500.* [13433-09-5]. (*S*)-3-Amino-*N*-[(*S*)-1-carboxy-2-phenylethyl]-succinamic acid.

A white powder.

mp: about 210 °C, with decomposition.

Aucubin. $C_{15}H_{22}O_9$. (M_r 346.3). *1145200.* [479-98-1]. [1*S*,4a*R*,5*S*,7a*S*)-5-Hydroxy-7-(hydroxymethyl)-1,4a,5,7a-tetrahydrocyclopenta[*c*]pyran-1-yl β-D-glucopyranoside.

Crystals, soluble in water, in alcohol and in methanol, practically insoluble in light petroleum.

$[\alpha]_D^{20}$: about − 163.

mp: about 181 °C.

Azomethine H. $C_{17}H_{12}NNaO_8S_2$. (M_r 445.4). *1008700.* [5941-07-1]. Sodium hydrogeno-4-hydroxy-5-(2-hydroxybenzylideneamino)-2,7-naphthalenedisulphonate.

Azomethine H solution. *1008701.*

Dissolve 0.45 g of *azomethine H R* and 1 g of *ascorbic acid R* with gentle heating in *water R* and dilute to 100 ml with the same solvent.

Barbaloin. $C_{21}H_{22}O_9,H_2O$. (M_r 436.4). *1008800.* [1415-73-2]. Aloin. 1,8-Dihydroxy-3-hydroxymethyl-10-β-D-glucopyranosyl-10*H*-anthracen-9-one.

A yellow to dark-yellow, crystalline powder, or yellow needles, darkening on exposure to air and light, sparingly soluble in water and in alcohol, soluble in acetone, in ammonia and in solutions of alkali hydroxides.

$A_{1\,cm}^{1\%}$: about 192 at 269 nm, about 226 at 296.5 nm, about 259 at 354 nm, determined on a solution in *methanol R* and calculated with reference to the anhydrous substance.

Chromatography. Examine as prescribed in the monograph on *Frangula bark (0025)*; the chromatogram shows only one principal spot.

Barbital. *1008900.* [57-44-3].

See *Barbital (0170).*

Barbital sodium. $C_8H_{11}N_2NaO_3$. (M_r 206.2). *1009000.* [144-02-5].

Content: minimum 98.0 per cent of the sodium derivative of 5,5-diethyl-1*H*,3*H*,5*H*-pyrimidine-2,4,6-trione.

A white, crystalline powder or colourless crystals, freely soluble in water, slightly soluble in alcohol.

Barbituric acid. $C_4H_4N_2O_3$. (M_r 128.1). *1009100.* [67-52-7]. 1*H*,3*H*,5*H*-Pyrimidine-2,4,6-trione.

A white or almost white powder, slightly soluble in water, freely soluble in boiling water and in dilute acids.

mp: about 253 °C.

Barium carbonate. $BaCO_3$. (M_r 197.3). *1009200.* [513-77-9].

A white powder or friable masses, practically insoluble in water.

Barium chloride. $BaCl_2,2H_2O$. (M_r 244.3). *1009300.* [10326-27-9]. Barium dichloride.

Colourless crystals, freely soluble in water, slightly soluble in alcohol.

Barium chloride solution R1. *1009301.*

A 61 g/l solution.

Barium chloride solution R2. *1009302.*

A 36.5 g/l solution.

Barium hydroxide. $Ba(OH)_2,8H_2O$. (M_r 315.5). *1009400.* [12230-71-6]. Barium dihydroxide.

Colourless crystals, soluble in water.

Barium hydroxide solution. *1009401.*

A 47.3 g/l solution.

Barium sulphate. *1009500.* [7727-43-7].

See *Barium sulphate (0010).*

Benzaldehyde. C_7H_6O. (M_r 106.1). *1009600.* [100-52-7].

A colourless or slightly yellow liquid, slightly soluble in water, miscible with alcohol.

d_{20}^{20}: about 1.05.

n_D^{20}: about 1.545.

Distillation range (*2.2.11*). Not less than 95 per cent distils between 177 °C and 180 °C.

Storage: protected from light.

Benzene. C_6H_6. (M_r 78.1). *1009800.* [71-43-2].

A clear, colourless, flammable liquid, practically insoluble in water, miscible with alcohol.

bp: about 80 °C.

Benzethonium chloride. $C_{27}H_{42}ClNO_2,H_2O$. (M_r 466.1). *1009900.* [121-54-0]. Benzyldimethyl[2-[2-[4-(1,1,3,3-tetramethylbutyl)phenoxy]ethoxy]ethyl]ammonium chloride monohydrate.

A fine, white powder or colourless crystals, soluble in water and in alcohol.

mp: about 163 °C.

Storage: protected from light.

Benzidine. $C_{12}H_{12}N_2$. (M_r 184.2). *1145300.* [92-87-5]. Biphenyl-4,4′-diamine.

Content: minimum 95 per cent of $C_{12}H_{12}N_2$.

White or slightly yellowish or reddish powder, darkening on exposure to air and light.

mp: about 120 °C.

Storage: protected from light.

Benzil. $C_{14}H_{10}O_2$. (M_r 210.2). *1117800.* [134-81-6]. Diphenylethanedione.

A yellow, crystalline powder, practically insoluble in water, soluble in alcohol, ethyl acetate and toluene.

mp: 95 °C.

Benzocaine. $C_9H_{11}NO_2$. (M_r 165.2). *1123600.* [94-09-7].

See *Benzocaine (0011).*

Benzoic acid. *1010100.* [65-85-0].

See *Benzoic acid (0066).*

Benzoin. $C_{14}H_{12}O_2$. (M_r 212.3). *1010200.* [579-44-2]. 2-Hydroxy-1,2-diphenylethanone.

Slightly yellowish crystals, very slightly soluble in water, freely soluble in acetone, soluble in hot alcohol.

mp: about 137 °C.

Benzophenone. $C_{13}H_{10}O$. (M_r 182.2). *1010300.* [119-61-9]. Diphenylmethanone.

Prismatic crystals, practically insoluble in water, freely soluble in alcohol.

mp: about 48 °C.

1,4-Benzoquinone. $C_6H_4O_2$. (M_r 108.1). *1118500.* [106-51-4]. Cyclohexa-2,5-diene-1,4-dione.

Content: minimum 98.0 per cent of $C_6H_4O_2$.

Benzoylarginine ethyl ester hydrochloride. $C_{15}H_{23}ClN_4O_3$. (M_r 342.8). *1010500.* [2645-08-1]. *N*-Benzoyl-L-arginine ethyl ester hydrochloride. Ethyl (*S*)-2-benzamido-5-guanidinovalerate hydrochloride.

A white, crystalline powder, very soluble in water and in ethanol.

$[\alpha]_D^{20}$: − 15 to − 18, determined on a 10 g/l solution.

mp: about 129 °C.

$A_{1\,cm}^{1\%}$: 310 to 340, determined at 227 nm using a 0.01 g/l solution.

Benzoyl chloride. C_7H_5ClO. (M_r 140.6). *1010400.* [98-88-4].

A colourless, lachrymatory liquid, decomposed by water and by alcohol.

d_{20}^{20}: about 1.21.

bp: about 197 °C.

***N*-Benzoyl-L-prolyl-L-phenylalanyl-L-arginine 4-nitroanilide acetate.** $C_{35}H_{42}N_8O_8$. (M_r 703). *1010600.*

2-Benzoylpyridine. $C_{12}H_9NO$. (M_r 183.2). *1134300.* [91-02-1]. Phenyl(pyridin-2-yl)methanone.

Colourless crystals, soluble in alcohol.

mp: about 43 °C.

Benzyl alcohol. *1010700.* [100-51-6].

See *Benzyl alcohol (0256).*

Benzyl benzoate. *1010800.* [120-51-4].

See *Benzyl benzoate (0705).*

Chromatography. Examine as prescribed in the monograph on *Peru balsam (0754)* applying 20 µl of a 0.3 per cent *V/V* solution in *ethyl acetate R*. After spraying and heating, the chromatogram shows a principal band with an R_f of about 0.8.

Benzyl cinnamate. $C_{16}H_{14}O_2$. (M_r 238.3). *1010900.* [103-41-3]. Benzyl 3-phenylprop-2-enoate.

Colourless or yellowish crystals, practically insoluble in water, soluble in alcohol.

mp: about 39 °C.

Chromatography. Examine as prescribed in the monograph on *Peru balsam (0754)* applying 20 µl of a 3 g/l solution in *ethyl acetate R*. After spraying and heating, the chromatogram shows a principal band with an R_f of about 0.6.

Benzyl ether. $C_{14}H_{14}O$. (M_r 198.3). *1140900.* [103-50-4]. Dibenzyl ether.

Clear, colourless liquid, practically insoluble in water, miscible with acetone and with ethanol.

d_{20}^{20}: about 1.043.

n_D^{20}: about 1.562.

bp: about 296 °C, with decomposition.

Benzylpenicillin sodium. *1011000.* [69-57-8].

See *Benzylpenicillin sodium (0114).*

2-Benzylpyridine. $C_{12}H_{11}N$. (M_r 169.2). *1112900.* [101-82-6].

Content: minimum 98.0 per cent of $C_{12}H_{11}N$.

A yellow liquid.

mp: 13 °C to 16 °C.

Benzyltrimethylammonium chloride. $C_{10}H_{16}ClN$. (M_r 185.7). *1155700.* [56-93-9]. *N,N,N*-Trimethylphenylmethanaminium chloride. *N,N,N*-Trimethylbenzenemethanaminium chloride.

White powder, soluble in water.

mp: about 230 °C, with decomposition.

Berberine chloride. $C_{20}H_{18}ClNO_4,2H_2O$. (*M*r 407.8). *1153400.* [5956-60-5]. 9,10-Dimethoxy-5,6-dihydrobenzo[*g*]-1,3-benzodioxolo[5,6-*a*]quinolizinium chloride.

Yellow crystals, slightly soluble in water, practically insoluble in alcohol.

mp: 204 °C to 206 °C.

Berberine chloride used in liquid chromatography complies with the following additional requirement.

Assay. Examine by liquid chromatography (*2.2.29*) as prescribed in the monograph on *Goldenseal rhizome (1831)*. The content is not less than 95 per cent, calculated by the normalisation procedure.

Bergapten. $C_{12}H_8O_4$. (*M*r 216.2). *1103700.* [484-20-8]. 5-Methoxypsoralen.

Colourless crystals, practically insoluble in water, sparingly soluble in alcohol and slightly soluble in glacial acetic acid.

mp: about 188 °C.

Betulin. $C_{30}H_{50}O_2$. (*M*r 442.7). *1011100.* [473-98-3]. Lup-20(39)-ene-3β,28-diol.

A white, crystalline powder.

mp: 248 °C to 251 °C.

Bibenzyl. $C_{14}H_{14}$. (*M*r 182.3). *1011200.* [103-29-7]. 1,2-Diphenylethane.

A white, crystalline powder, practically insoluble in water, very soluble in methylene chloride, freely soluble in acetone, soluble in alcohol.

mp: 50 °C to 53 °C.

Biphenyl-4-ol. $C_{12}H_{10}O$. (*M*r 170.2). *1011300.* [90-43-7]. 4-Phenylphenol.

A white, crystalline powder, practically insoluble in water.

mp: 164 °C to 167 °C.

Bisbenzimide. $C_{25}H_{27}Cl_3N_6O,5H_2O$. (*M*r 624). *1103800.* [23491-44-3]. 4-[5-[5-(4-Methylpiperazin-1-yl)benzimidazol-2-yl]benzimidazol-2-yl]phenol trihydrochloride pentahydrate.

Bisbenzimide stock solution. *1103801.*

Dissolve 5 mg of *bisbenzimide R* in *water R* and dilute to 100 ml with the same solvent.

Storage: in the dark.

Bisbenzimide working solution. *1103802.*

Immediately before use, dilute 100 µl of *bisbenzimide stock solution R* to 100 ml with *phosphate-buffered saline pH 7.4 R*.

Bismuth subnitrate. $[4BiNO_3(OH)_2,BiO(OH)]$. (*M*r 1462). *1011500.* [1304-85-4].

A white powder, practically insoluble in water.

Bismuth subnitrate R1. *1011501.*

Content: 71.5 per cent to 74.0 per cent of bismuth (Bi), and 14.5 per cent to 16.5 per cent of nitrate, calculated as nitrogen pentoxide (N_2O_5).

Bismuth subnitrate solution. *1011502.*

Dissolve 5 g of *bismuth subnitrate R1* in a mixture of 8.4 ml of *nitric acid R* and 50 ml of *water R* and dilute to 250 ml with *water R*. Filter if necessary.

Acidity. To 10 ml add 0.05 ml of *methyl orange solution R*. 5.0 ml to 6.25 ml of *1 M sodium hydroxide* is required to change the colour of the indicator.

Biuret. $C_2H_5N_3O_2$. (*M*r 103.1). *1011600.* [108-19-0].

White crystals, hygroscopic, soluble in water, sparingly soluble in alcohol.

mp: 188 °C to 190 °C, with decomposition.

Storage: in an airtight container.

Biuret reagent. *1011601.*

Dissolve 1.5 g of *copper sulphate R* and 6.0 g of *sodium potassium tartrate R* in 500 ml of *water R*. Add 300 ml of a carbonate-free 100 g/l solution of *sodium hydroxide R*, dilute to 1000 ml with the same solution and mix.

Blocking solution. *1122400.*

A 10 per cent *V/V* solution of *acetic acid R*.

Blue dextran 2000. *1011700.* [9049-32-5].

Prepared from dextran having an average relative molecular mass of 2 × 10^6 by introduction of a polycyclic chromophore that colours the substance blue. The degree of substitution is 0.017. It is freeze-dried and dissolves rapidly and completely in water and aqueous saline solutions.

A 1 g/l solution in a *phosphate buffer solution pH 7.0 R* shows an absorption maximum (*2.2.25*) at 280 nm.

Boldine. $C_{19}H_{21}NO_4$. (*M*r 327.3). *1118800.* [476-70-0]. 1,10-Dimethoxy-6aα-aporphine-2,9-diol.

A white crystalline powder, very slightly soluble in water, soluble in alcohol and in dilute solutions of acids.

$[\alpha]_D^{25}$: about + 127, determined on a 1 g/l solution in *ethanol R*.

mp: about 163 °C.

Chromatography. Examined as prescribed in the monograph on *Boldo leaf (1396)* the chromatogram shows a single principal spot.

Assay. Examine by liquid chromatography (*2.2.29*) under the conditions described in the monograph on *Boldo leaf (1396)* using the substance to be examined as the test solution.

The area of the principal peak is not less than 99.0 per cent of the total area of the peaks.

Boric acid. *1011800.* [10043-35-3].

See *Boric acid (0001)*.

Boric acid solution, saturated, cold. *1011801.*

To 3 g of *boric acid R* add 50 ml of *water R* and shake for 10 min. Place the solution for 2 h in the refrigerator.

Borneol. $C_{10}H_{18}O$. (*M*r 154.3). *1011900.* [507-70-0]. *endo*-1,7,7-Trimethylbicyclo[2.2.1]heptan-2-ol.

Colourless crystals, readily sublimes, practically insoluble in water, freely soluble in alcohol and in light petroleum.

mp: about 208 °C.

Chromatography. Examine by thin-layer chromatography (*2.2.27*), using *silica gel G R* as the coating substance. Apply to the plate 10 µl of a 1 g/l solution in *toluene R*. Develop over a path of 10 cm using *chloroform R*. Allow the plate to dry in air, spray with *anisaldehyde solution R*, using 10 ml for a plate 200 mm square, and heat at 100 °C to 105 °C for 10 min. The chromatogram obtained shows only one principal spot.

Bornyl acetate. $C_{12}H_{20}O_2$. (M_r 196.3). *1012000.* [5655-61-8]. *endo*-1,7,7-Trimethylbicyclo[2.2.1]hept-2-yl acetate.

Colourless crystals or a colourless liquid, very slightly soluble in water, soluble in alcohol.

mp: about 28 °C.

Chromatography. Examine by thin-layer chromatography (*2.2.27*), using *silica gel G R* as the coating substance. Apply to the plate 10 µl of a 2 g/l solution in *toluene R*. Develop over a path of 10 cm using *chloroform R*. Allow the plate to dry in air, spray with *anisaldehyde solution R*, using 10 ml for a plate 200 mm square, and heat at 100 °C to 105 °C for 10 min. The chromatogram obtained shows only one principal spot.

Boron trichloride. BCl_3. (M_r 117.2). *1112000.* [10294-34-5].

Colourless gas. Reacts violently with water. Available as solutions in suitable solvents (2-chloroethanol, methylene chloride, hexane, heptane, methanol).

n_D^{20}: about 1.420.

bp: about 12.6 °C.

Caution: toxic, corrosive.

Boron trichloride-methanol solution. *1112001.*

A 120 g/l solution of BCl_3 in *methanol R*.

Storage: protected from light at − 20 °C, preferably in sealed tubes.

Boron trifluoride. BF_3. (M_r 67.8). *1012100.* [7637-07-2].

Colourless gas.

Boron trifluoride-methanol solution. *1012101.*

A 140 g/l solution of *boron trifluoride R* in *methanol R*.

Brilliant blue. *1012200.* [6104-59-2].

See *acid blue 83 R*.

Bromelains. *1012300.* [37189-34-7].

A concentrate of proteolytic enzymes derived from *Ananas comosus* Merr.

A dull-yellow powder.

Activity. 1 g liberates about 1.2 g of amino-nitrogen from a solution of *gelatin R* in 20 min at 45 °C and pH 4.5.

Bromelains solution. *1012301.*

A 10 g/l solution of *bromelains R* in a mixture of 1 volume of *phosphate buffer solution pH 5.5 R* and 9 volumes of a 9 g/l solution of *sodium chloride R*.

Bromine. Br_2. (M_r 159.8). *1012400.* [7726-95-6].

A brownish-red fuming liquid, slightly soluble in water, soluble in alcohol.

d_{20}^{20}: about 3.1.

Bromine solution. *1012401.*

Dissolve 30 g of *bromine R* and 30 g of *potassium bromide R* in *water R* and dilute to 100 ml with the same solvent.

Bromine water. *1012402.*

Shake 3 ml of *bromine R* with 100 ml of *water R* to saturation.

Storage: over an excess of *bromine R*, protected from light.

Bromine water R1. *1012403.*

Shake 0.5 ml of *bromine R* with 100 ml of *water R*.

Storage: protected from light; use within 1 week.

Bromocresol green. $C_{21}H_{14}Br_4O_5S$. (M_r 698). *1012600.* [76-60-8]. 3′,3″,5′,5″-Tetrabromo-*m*-cresol-sulfonphthalein. 4,4′-(3*H*-2,1-Benzoxathiol-3-ylidene)bis(2,6-dibromo-3-methylphenol)-*S,S*-dioxide.

A brownish-white powder, slightly soluble in water, soluble in alcohol and in dilute solutions of alkali hydroxides.

Bromocresol green-methyl red solution. *1012602.*

Dissolve 0.15 g of *bromocresol green R* and 0.1 g of *methyl red R* in 180 ml of *ethanol R* and dilute to 200 ml with *water R*.

Bromocresol green solution. *1012601.*

Dissolve 50 mg of *bromocresol green R* in 0.72 ml of *0.1 M sodium hydroxide* and 20 ml of *alcohol R* and dilute to 100 ml with *water R*.

Test for sensitivity. To 0.2 ml of the bromocresol green solution add 100 ml of *carbon dioxide-free water R*. The solution is blue. Not more than 0.2 ml of *0.02 M hydrochloric acid* is required to change the colour to yellow.

Colour change: pH 3.6 (yellow) to pH 5.2 (blue).

Bromocresol purple. $C_{21}H_{16}Br_2O_5S$. (M_r 540.2). *1012700.* [115-40-2]. 3′,3″-Dibromo-*o*-cresolsulfonphthalein. 4,4′-(3*H*-2,1-Benzoxathiol-3-ylidene)bis(2-bromo-6-methylphenol)-*S,S*-dioxide.

A pinkish powder, practically insoluble in water, soluble in alcohol and in dilute solutions of alkali hydroxides.

Bromocresol purple solution. *1012701.*

Dissolve 50 mg of *bromocresol purple R* in 0.92 ml of *0.1 M sodium hydroxide* and 20 ml of *alcohol R* and dilute to 100 ml with *water R*.

Test for sensitivity. To 0.2 ml of the bromocresol purple solution add 100 ml of *carbon dioxide-free water R* and 0.05 ml of *0.02 M sodium hydroxide*. The solution is bluish-violet. Not more than 0.2 ml of *0.02 M hydrochloric acid* is required to change the colour to yellow.

Colour change: pH 5.2 (yellow) to pH 6.8 (bluish-violet).

5-Bromo-2′-deoxyuridine. $C_9H_{11}BrN_2O_5$. (M_r 307.1). *1012500.* [59-14-3]. 5-Bromo-1-(2-deoxy-β-d-*erythro*-pentofuranosyl)-1*H*,3*H*-pyrimidine-2,4-dione.

mp: about 194 °C.

Chromatography. Examine as prescribed in the monograph on *Idoxuridine (0669)*, applying 5 µl of a 0.25 g/l solution. The chromatogram obtained shows only one principal spot.

Bromophenol blue. $C_{19}H_{10}Br_4O_5S$. (M_r 670). *1012800.* [115-39-9]. 3′,3″,5′,5″-Tetrabromophenolsulfonphthalein. 4,4′-(3*H*-2,1-Benzoxathiol-3-ylidene)bis(2,6-dibromophenol) *S,S*-dioxide.

A light orange-yellow powder, very slightly soluble in water, slightly soluble in alcohol, freely soluble in solutions of alkali hydroxides.

Bromophenol blue solution. *1012801.*

Dissolve 0.1 g of *bromophenol blue R* in 1.5 ml of *0.1 M sodium hydroxide* and 20 ml of *alcohol R* and dilute to 100 ml with *water R*.

Test for sensitivity. To 0.05 ml of the bromophenol blue solution add 20 ml of *carbon dioxide-free water R* and 0.05 ml of *0.1 M hydrochloric acid*. The solution is yellow. Not more than 0.1 ml of *0.1 M sodium hydroxide* is required to change the colour to bluish-violet.

Colour change: pH 2.8 (yellow) to pH 4.4 (bluish-violet).

Bromophenol blue solution R1. *1012802.*

Dissolve 50 mg of *bromophenol blue R* with gentle heating in 3.73 ml of *0.02 M sodium hydroxide* and dilute to 100 ml with *water R.*

Bromophenol blue solution R2. *1012803.*

Dissolve with heating 0.2 g of *bromophenol blue R* in 3 ml of *0.1 M sodium hydroxide* and 10 ml of *alcohol R.* After solution is effected, allow to cool and dilute to 100 ml with *alcohol R.*

Bromophos. $C_8H_8BrCl_2O_3PS$. (M_r 366.0). *1123700.* [2104-96-3].

A suitable certified reference solution (10 ng/μl in iso-octane) may be used.

Bromophos-ethyl. $C_{10}H_{12}BrCl_2O_3PS$. (M_r 394.0). *1123800.* [4824-78-6].

A suitable certified reference solution (10 ng/μl in iso-octane) may be used.

Bromothymol blue. $C_{27}H_{28}Br_2O_5S$. (M_r 624). *1012900.* [76-59-5]. 3′,3″-Dibromothymolsulfonphthalein. 4,4′-(3*H*-2,1-Benzoxathiol-3-ylidene)bis(2-bromo-6-isopropyl-3-methylphenol) *S,S*-dioxide.

A reddish-pink or brownish powder, practically insoluble in water, soluble in alcohol and in dilute solutions of alkali hydroxides.

Bromothymol blue solution R1. *1012901.*

Dissolve 50 mg of *bromothymol blue R* in a mixture of 4 ml of *0.02 M sodium hydroxide* and 20 ml of *alcohol R* and dilute to 100 ml with *water R.*

Test for sensitivity. To 0.3 ml of *bromothymol blue solution R1* add 100 ml of *carbon dioxide-free water R.* The solution is yellow. Not more than 0.1 ml of *0.02 M sodium hydroxide* is required to change the colour to blue.

Colour change: pH 5.8 (yellow) to pH 7.4 (blue).

Bromothymol blue solution R2. *1012902.*

A 10 g/l solution in *dimethylformamide R.*

Bromothymol blue solution R3. *1012903.*

Warm 0.1 g of *bromothymol blue R* with 3.2 ml of *0.05 M sodium hydroxide* and 5 ml of *alcohol (90 per cent V/V) R.* After solution is effected, dilute to 250 ml with *alcohol (90 per cent V/V) R.*

BRP indicator solution. *1013000.*

Dissolve 0.1 g of *bromothymol blue R,* 20 mg of *methyl red R* and 0.2 g of *phenolphthalein R* in *alcohol R* and dilute to 100 ml with the same solvent. Filter.

Brucine. $C_{23}H_{26}N_2O_4,2H_2O$. (M_r 430.5). *1013100.* [357-57-3]. 10,11-Dimethoxystrychnine.

Colourless crystals, slightly soluble in water, freely soluble in alcohol.

mp: about 178 °C.

Butanal. C_4H_8O. (M_r 72.1). *1134400.* [123-72-8]. Butyraldehyde.

d_{20}^{20}: 0.806.

n_D^{20}: 1.380.

bp: 75 °C.

Butanol. $C_4H_{10}O$. (M_r 74.1). *1013200.* [71-36-3]. *n*-Butanol. 1-Butanol.

A clear, colourless liquid, miscible with alcohol.

d_{20}^{20}: about 0.81.

bp: 116 °C to 119 °C.

2-Butanol R1. $C_4H_{10}O$. (M_r 74.1). *1013301.* [78-92-2]. *sec*-Butyl alcohol.

Content: minimum 99.0 per cent of $C_4H_{10}O$.

A clear, colourless liquid, soluble in water, miscible with alcohol.

d_{20}^{20}: about 0.81.

Distillation range (*2.2.11*). Not less than 95 per cent distils between 99 °C and 100 °C.

Assay. By gas chromatography as described in the monograph on *Isopropyl alcohol (0970).*

Butyl acetate. $C_6H_{12}O_2$. (M_r 116.2). *1013400.* [123-86-4].

A clear, colourless liquid, flammable, slightly soluble in water, miscible with alcohol.

d_{20}^{20}: about 0.88.

n_D^{20}: about 1.395.

Distillation range (*2.2.11*). Not less than 95 per cent distils between 123 °C and 126 °C.

Butyl acetate R1. *1013401.*

A clear, colourless liquid, flammable, slightly soluble in water, miscible with alcohol.

d_{20}^{20}: about 0.883.

n_D^{20}: about 1.395.

Butanol: maximum 0.2 per cent, determined by gas chromatography.

n-Butyl formate: maximum 0.1 per cent, determined by gas chromatography.

n-Butyl propionate: maximum 0.1 per cent, determined by gas chromatography.

Water: maximum 0.1 per cent.

Assay: minimum 99.5 per cent of $C_6H_{12}O_2$, determined by gas chromatography.

Butylamine. $C_4H_{11}N$. (M_r 73.1). *1013600.* [109-73-9]. 1-Butanamine.

Distil and use within one month.

A colourless liquid, miscible with water, with alcohol.

n_D^{20}: about 1.401.

bp: about 78 °C.

***tert*-Butylamine.** *1100900.* [75-64-9].

See *1,1-dimethylethylamine R.*

Butylated hydroxytoluene. *1013800.* [128-37-0].

See *Butylhydroxytoluene R.*

Butylboronic acid. $C_4H_{11}BO_2$. (M_r 101.9). *1013700.* [4426-47-5].

Content: minimum 98 per cent of $C_4H_{11}BO_2$.

mp: 90 °C to 92 °C.

***tert*-Butylhydroperoxide.** $C_4H_{10}O_2$. (M_r 90.1). *1118000.* [75-91-2]. 1,1-Dimethylethylhydroperoxide.

Flammable liquid, soluble in organic solvents.

d_{20}^{20}: 0.898.

n_D^{20}: 1.401.

bp: 35 °C.

Butylhydroxytoluene. *1013800.* [128-37-0].

See *Butylhydroxytoluene (0581).*

Butyl methacrylate. $C_8H_{14}O_2$. (M_r 142.2). *1145400.* [97-88-1]. Butyl 2-methylpropenoate.

Clear, colourless solution.

d_4^{20}: about 0.894.

n_D^{20}: about 1.424.

bp: about 163 °C.

***tert*-Butyl methyl ether.** *1013900.* [1634-04-4].

See *1,1-dimethylethyl methyl ether R.*

Butyl parahydroxybenzoate. *1103900.* [94-26-8].

See *Butyl parahydroxybenzoate (0881).*

Butyric acid. $C_4H_8O_2$. (M_r 88.1). *1014000.* [107-92-6]. Butanoic acid.

Content: minimum 99.0 per cent of $C_4H_8O_2$.

An oily liquid, miscible with water and with alcohol.

d_{20}^{20}: about 0.96.

n_D^{20}: about 1.398.

bp: about 163 °C.

Butyrolactone. $C_4H_6O_2$. (M_r 86.1). *1104000.* [96-48-0]. Dihydro-2(3*H*)-furanone. γ-Butyrolactone.

Oily liquid, miscible with water, soluble in methanol.

n_D^{25}: about 1.435.

bp: about 204 °C.

Cadmium. Cd. (A_r 112.4). *1014100.* [10108-64-2].

A silvery-white, lustrous metal, practically insoluble in water, freely soluble in nitric acid and in hot hydrochloric acid.

Caesium chloride. CsCl. (M_r 168.4). *1014200.* [7647-17-8].

A white powder, very soluble in water, freely soluble in methanol, practically insoluble in acetone.

Caffeic acid. $C_9H_8O_4$. (M_r 180.2). *1014300.* [331-39-5]. (*E*)-3-(3,4-Dihydroxyphenyl)propenoic acid.

White or almost white crystals or plates, freely soluble in hot water and in alcohol, sparingly soluble in cold water.

mp: about 225 °C, with decomposition.

A freshly prepared solution at pH 7.6 shows 2 absorption maxima (*2.2.25*), at 293 nm and 329 nm.

Caffeine. *1014400.* [58-08-2].

See *Caffeine (0267).*

Calcium carbonate. *1014500.* [471-34-1].

See *Calcium carbonate (0014).*

Calcium carbonate R1. *1014501.*

It complies with the requirements of *calcium carbonate R* and with the following additional requirement:

Chlorides (*2.4.4*): maximum 50 ppm.

Calcium chloride. *1014600.* [10035-04-8].

See *Calcium chloride (0015).*

Calcium chloride solution. *1014601.*

A 73.5 g/l solution.

Calcium chloride solution 0.01 M. *1014602.*

Dissolve 0.147 g of *calcium chloride R* in *water R* and dilute to 100.0 ml with the same solvent.

Calcium chloride solution 0.02 M. *1014603.*

Dissolve 2.94 g of *calcium chloride R* in 900 ml of *water R*, adjust to pH 6.0 to 6.2 and dilute to 1000.0 ml with *water R*.

Storage: at 2 °C to 8 °C.

Calcium chloride R1. $CaCl_2,4H_2O$. (M_r 183.1). *1014700.* Calcium chloride tetrahydrate.

Content: maximum 0.05 ppm of Fe.

Calcium chloride, anhydrous. $CaCl_2$. (M_r 111.0). *1014800.* [10043-52-4].

Content: minimum 98.0 per cent of $CaCl_2$, calculated with reference to the dried substance.

White granules, deliquescent, very soluble in water, freely soluble in alcohol and in methanol.

Loss on drying (2.2.32): maximum 5.0 per cent, determined by drying in an oven at 200 °C.

Storage: in an airtight container, protected from moisture.

Calcium hydroxide. $Ca(OH)_2$. (M_r 74.1). *1015000.* [1305-62-0]. Calcium dihydroxide.

A white powder, almost completely soluble in 600 parts of water.

Calcium hydroxide solution. *1015001.*

A freshly prepared saturated solution.

Calcium lactate. *1015100.* [41372-22-9].

See *Calcium lactate pentahydrate (0468).*

Calcium sulphate. $CaSO_4,{}^1/_2H_2O$. (M_r 145.1). *1015200.* [10034-76-1]. Calcium sulphate hemihydrate.

A white powder, soluble in about 1500 parts of water, practically insoluble in alcohol. When mixed with half its mass of water it rapidly solidifies to a hard and porous mass.

Calcium sulphate solution. *1015201.*

Shake 5 g of *calcium sulphate R* with 100 ml of *water R* for 1 h and filter.

Calconecarboxylic acid. $C_{21}H_{14}N_2O_7S,3H_2O$. ($M_r$ 492.5). *1015300.* [3737-95-9]. 2-Hydroxy-1-(2-hydroxy-4-sulpho-1-naphthylazo)naphthalene-3-carboxylic acid.

A brownish-black powder, slightly soluble in water, very slightly soluble in acetone and in alcohol, sparingly soluble in dilute solutions of sodium hydroxide.

Calconecarboxylic acid triturate. *1015301.*

Mix 1 part of *calconecarboxylic acid R* with 99 parts of *sodium chloride R*.

Test for sensitivity. Dissolve 50 mg of calconecarboxylic acid triturate in a mixture of 2 ml of *strong sodium hydroxide solution R* and 100 ml of *water R*. The solution is blue but becomes violet on addition of 1 ml of a 10 g/l solution of *magnesium sulphate R* and 0.1 ml of a 1.5 g/l solution of *calcium chloride R* and turns pure blue on addition of 0.15 ml of *0.01 M sodium edetate*.

Camphene. $C_{10}H_{16}$. (M_r 136.2). *1139200.* [79-92-5]. 2,2-Dimethyl-3-methylenebicyclo[2.2.1]heptane.

Camphene used in gas chromatography complies with the following additional test.

Assay. Examine by gas chromatography (*2.2.28*) as prescribed in the monograph on *Rosemary Oil (1846)*.

The content is not less than 90 per cent calculated by the normalisation procedure.

Camphor. *1113000.* [76-22-2]. See *Camphor, racemic (0655).*

Camphor used in gas chromatography complies with the following additional test.

Assay. Examine by gas chromatography (*2.2.28*) as prescribed in the monograph on *Lavender oil (1338)*.

Test solution. A 10 g/l solution of the substance to be examined in *hexane R*.

The area of the principal peak is not less than 98.0 per cent of the area of all the peaks in the chromatogram obtained. Disregard the peak due to hexane.

(1*S*)-(+)-10-Camphorsulphonic acid. $C_{10}H_{16}O_4S$. (M_r 232.3). *1104100.* [3144-16-9]. (1*S*,4*R*)-(+)-2-Oxo-10-bornenesulphonic acid. [(1*S*)-7,7-Dimethyl-2-oxobicyclo[2.2.1]heptan-1-yl]methanesulphonic acid. Reychler's acid.

Prismatic crystals, hygroscopic, soluble in water.

Content: minimum 99.0 per cent of (1*S*)-(+)-10-camphorsulphonic acid.

$[\alpha]_D^{20}$: +20 ± 1 (43 g/l solution in *water R*).

mp: about 194 °C, with decomposition.

ΔA (*2.2.41*): 10.2 × 10^3 determined at 290.5 nm on a 1.0 g/l solution.

Capric acid. $C_{10}H_{20}O_2$. (M_r 172.3). *1142000.* [334-48-5]. Decanoic acid.

Crystalline solid, very slightly soluble in water, soluble in ethanol.

bp: about 270 °C.

mp: about 31.4 °C.

Capric acid used in the assay of total fatty acids in Saw palmetto fruit (1848) complies with the following additional requirement.

Assay. Examine by gas chromatography (*2.2.28*) as prescribed in the monograph on *Saw palmetto fruit (1848).*

The content of capric acid is not less than 98 per cent, calculated by the normalisation procedure.

Capric alcohol. *1024700.*

See *Decanol R.*

Caproic acid. $C_6H_{12}O_2$. (M_r 116.2). *1142100.* [142-62-1]. Hexanoic acid.

Oily liquid, sparingly soluble in water.

d_4^{20} : about 0.926.

n_D^{20} : about 1.417.

bp: about 205 °C.

Caproic acid used in the assay of total fatty acids in Saw palmetto fruit (1848) complies with the following additional requirement.

Assay. Examine by gas chromatography (*2.2.28*) as prescribed in the monograph on *Saw palmetto fruit (1848).*

The content of caproic acid is not less than 98 per cent, calculated by the normalisation procedure.

ε-Caprolactam. $C_6H_{11}NO$. (M_r 113.2). *1104200.* [105-60-2]. Hexane-6-lactam.

Hygroscopic flakes, freely soluble in water, in ethanol and in methanol.

mp: about 70 °C.

Caprylic acid. $C_8H_{16}O_2$. (M_r 144.2). *1142200.* [124-07-2]. Octanoic acid.

Slightly yellow, oily liquid.

d_4^{20} : about 0.910.

n_D^{20} : about 1.428.

bp: about 239.7 °C.

mp: about 16.7 °C.

Caprylic acid used in the assay of total fatty acids in Saw palmetto fruit (1848) complies with the following additional requirement.

Assay. Examine by gas chromatography (*2.2.28*) as prescribed in the monograph on *Saw palmetto fruit (1848).*

The content of caprylic acid is not less than 98 per cent, calculated by the normalisation procedure.

Capsaicin. $C_{18}H_{27}NO_3$. (M_r 305.4). *1147900.* [404-86-4]. (*E*)-*N*-[(4-Hydroxy-3-methoxyphenyl)methyl]-8-methylnon-6-enamide.

White, crystalline powder, practically insoluble in water, freely soluble in ethanol.

mp: about 65 °C.

Capsaicin used in the assay in Capsicum (1859) complies with the following additional requirement.

Assay. Examine by liquid chromatography (*2.2.29*) as prescribed in the monograph on *Capsicum (1859).* The content of capsaicin is not less than 95.0 per cent, calculated by the normalisation procedure.

Carbazole. $C_{12}H_9N$. (M_r 167.2). *1015400.* [86-74-8]. Dibenzopyrrole.

Crystals, practically insoluble in water, freely soluble in acetone, slightly soluble in ethanol.

mp: about 245 °C.

Carbomer. *1015500.* [9007-20-9].

A cross-linked polymer of acrylic acid; it contains a large proportion (56 per cent to 68 per cent) of carboxylic acid (CO_2H) groups after drying at 80 °C for 1 h. Average relative molecular mass about 3 × 10^6.

pH (*2.2.3*): about 3 for a 10 g/l suspension.

Carbon dioxide. *1015600.* [124-38-9].

See *Carbon dioxide (0375).*

Carbon dioxide R1. CO_2. (M_r 44.01). *1015700.*

Content: minimum 99.995 per cent *V/V* of CO_2.

Carbon monoxide: less than 5 ppm.

Oxygen: less than 25 ppm.

Nitric oxide: less than 1 ppm.

Carbon dioxide R2. CO_2. (M_r 44.01). *1134500.*

Content: minimum 99 per cent *V/V* of CO_2.

Carbon disulphide. CS_2. (M_r 76.1). *1015800.* [75-15-0].

A colourless or yellowish, flammable liquid, practically insoluble in water, miscible with ethanol.

d_{20}^{20} : about 1.26.

bp: 46 °C to 47 °C.

Carbon for chromatography, graphitised. *1015900.*

Carbon chains having a length greater than C_9 with a particle size of 400 μm to 850 μm.

Relative density: 0.72.

Surface area: 10 m^2/g.

Do not use at a temperature higher than 400 °C.

Carbon for chromatography, graphitised R1. *1153500.*

Porous spherical carbon particles comprised of flat sheets of hexagonally arranged carbon atoms.

Particle size: 5-7 μm.

Pore volume: 0.7 cm^3/g.

Carbon monoxide. CO. (M_r 28.01). *1016000.* [630-08-0].

Content: minimum 99.97 per cent *V/V* of CO.

Carbon monoxide R1. CO. (M_r 28.01). *1134600.* [630-08-0].

Content: minimum 99 per cent *V/V* of CO.

Carbon tetrachloride. CCl_4. (M_r 153.8). *1016100.* [56-23-5]. Tetrachloromethane.

A clear, colourless liquid, practically insoluble in water, miscible with alcohol.

d_{20}^{20}: 1.595 to 1.598.

bp: 76 °C to 77 °C.

Carbophenothion. $C_{11}H_{16}ClO_2PS_3$. (M_r 342.9). *1016200.* [786-19-6]. *O,O*-Diethyl *S*-[[(4-chlorophenyl)thio]methyl]-phosphorodithioate.

Yellowish liquid, practically insoluble in water, miscible with organic solvents.

d_4^{25}: about 1.27.

For the monograph *Wool Fat (0134)*, a suitable certified reference solution (10 ng/µl in iso-octane) may be used.

Car-3-ene. $C_{10}H_{16}$. (M_r 136.2). *1124000.* [498-15-7]. 3,7,7-Trimethylbicyclo[4.1.0]hept-3-ene. 4,7,7-Trimethyl-3-norcarene.

A liquid with a pungent odour, slightly soluble in water, soluble in organic solvents.

d_{20}^{20}: about 0.864.

n_D^{20}: 1.473 to 1.474.

$[\alpha]_D^{20}$: + 15 to + 17.

bp: 170 °C to 172 °C.

Car-3-ene used in gas chromatography complies with the following additional test.

Assay. Examine by gas chromatography (*2.2.28*) as prescribed in the monograph on *Nutmeg oil (1552).*

The content is not less than 95.0 per cent, calculated by the normalisation procedure.

Carminic acid. $C_{22}H_{20}O_{13}$. (M_r 492.4). *1156700.* [1260-17-9]. 7-α-D-Glucopyranosyl-3,5,6,8-tetrahydroxy-1-methyl-9,10-dioxo-9,10-dihydroanthracene-2-carboxylic acid.

Dark red powder, very slightly soluble in water, soluble in dimethyl sulphoxide, very slightly soluble in ethanol (96 per cent).

Carob bean gum. *1104500.*

The ground endosperm of the fruit kernels of *Ceratonia siliqua* L. Taub.

A white powder containing 70 per cent to 80 per cent of a water-soluble gum consisting mainly of galactomannoglycone.

Carvacrol. $C_{10}H_{14}O$. (M_r 150.2). *1016400.* [499-75-2]. 5-Isopropyl-2-methylphenol.

Brownish liquid, practically insoluble in water, very soluble in alcohol.

d_{20}^{20}: about 0.975.

n_D^{20}: about 1.523.

bp: about 237 °C.

Carvacrol used in gas chromatography complies with the following additional test.

Assay. Examine by gas chromatography (*2.2.28*) as prescribed in the monograph on *Peppermint oil (0405).*

Test solution. Dissolve 0.1 g in about 10 ml of *acetone R*.

The area of the principal peak is not less than 95.0 per cent of the area of all the peaks in the chromatogram obtained. Disregard the peak due to acetone.

Carvone. $C_{10}H_{14}O$. (M_r 150.2). *1016500.* [2244-16-8]. (*S*)-*p*-Mentha-6,8-dien-2-one. (+)-2-Methyl-5-(1-methylethenyl)-cyclohex-2-enone.

A liquid, practically insoluble in water, miscible with alcohol.

d_{20}^{20}: about 0.965

n_D^{20}: about 1.500.

$[\alpha]_D^{20}$: about + 61.

bp: about 230 °C.

Carvone used in gas chromatography complies with the following additional test.

Assay. Examine by gas chromatography (*2.2.28*) as prescribed in the monograph on *Peppermint oil (0405)* using the substance to be examined as the test solution.

The area of the principal peak is not less than 98.0 per cent of the total area of the peaks.

β-Caryophyllene. $C_{15}H_{24}$. (M_r 204.4). *1101000.* [87-44-5]. (*E*)-(1*R*,9*S*)-4,11,11-Trimethyl-8-methylenebicyclo[7.2.0]undec-4-ene.

An oily liquid, practically insoluble in water, miscible with alcohol.

d_4^{17}: about 0.905.

n_D^{20}: about 1.492.

$[\alpha]_D^{15}$: about −5.2.

bp_{14}: 129 °C to 130 °C.

β-Caryophyllene used in gas chromatography complies with the following additional test.

Assay. Examine by gas chromatography (*2.2.28*) as prescribed in the monograph on *Clove oil (1091)* using the substance to be examined as the test solution.

The area of the principal peak is not less than 98.5 per cent of the total area of the peaks.

Caryophyllene oxide. $C_{15}H_{24}O$. (M_r 220.4). *1149000.* [1139-30-6]. (-)-β-Caryophyllene epoxide. (1*R*,4*R*,6*R*,10*S*)-4,12,12-Trimethyl-9-methylene-5-oxatricyclo[8.2.0.0^{4,6}]dodecane.

Colourless, fine crystals with lumps.

mp: 62 °C to 63 °C.

Caryophyllene oxide used in gas chromatography complies with the following additional test.

Assay. Examine by gas chromatography (*2.2.28*) as prescribed in the monograph on *Turpentine oil, Pinus pinaster type (1627).*

The content is not less than 99.0 per cent, calculated by the normalisation procedure.

Casein. *1016600.* [9000-71-9].

A mixture of related phosphoproteins obtained from milk.

White, amorphous powder or granules, very slightly soluble in water and in non-polar organic solvents. It dissolves in concentrated hydrochloric acid giving a pale-violet solution. It forms salts with acids and bases. Its isoelectric point is at about pH 4.7. Alkaline solutions are laevorotatory.

Catalpol. $C_{15}H_{22}O_{10}$. (M_r 362.3). *1142300.* [2415-24-9]. (1a*S*,1b*S*,2*S*,5a*R*,6*S*,6a*S*)-6-Hydroxy-1a-(hydroxymethyl)-1a,1b,2,5a,6,6a-hexahydrooxireno[4,5]cyclopenta[1,2-*c*]pyran-2-yl β-D-glucopyranoside.

mp: 203 °C to 205 °C.

Catechin. $C_{15}H_{14}O_6,xH_2O$. (M_r 290.3 for the anhydrous substance). *1119000.* [154-23-4]. (+)-(2*R*,3*S*)-2-(3,4-Dihydroxyphenyl)-3,4-dihydro-2*H*-chromene-3,5,7-triol. Catechol. Cianidanol. Cyanidol.

Catholyte for isoelectric focusing pH 3 to 5. *113100.* 0.1 M β-Alanine.

Dissolve 8.9 g of *β-alanine R* in *water R* and dilute to 1000 ml with the same solvent.

Cation exchange resin. *1016700.*

A resin in protonated form with sulphonic acid groups attached to a polymer lattice consisting of polystyrene cross-linked with 8 per cent of divinylbenzene. It is available as beads and the particle size is specified after the name of the reagent in the tests where it is used.

Cation exchange resin R1. *1121900.*

A resin in protonated form with sulphonic acid groups attached to a polymer lattice consisting of polystyrene cross-linked with 4 per cent of divinylbenzene. It is available as beads and the particle size is specified after the name of the reagent in the tests where it is used.

Cation-exchange resin, strong. *1156800.*

A strong cation-exchange resin in protonated form with sulphonic acid groups attached to a polymer lattice consisting of polystyrene cross-linked with divinylbenzene. The particle size is specified after the name of the reagent in the tests where it is used.

Cation exchange resin (calcium form), strong. *1104600.*

A resin in calcium form with sulphonic acid groups attached to a polymer lattice consisting of polystyrene cross-linked with 8 per cent of divinylbenzene. The particle size is specified after the name of the reagent in the tests where it is used.

Cellulose for chromatography. *1016800.* [9004-34-6].

A fine, white, homogeneous powder with an average particle size less than 30 µm.

Preparation of a thin layer. Suspend 15 g in 100 ml of *water R* and homogenise in an electric mixer for 60 s. Coat carefully cleaned plates with a layer 0.1 mm thick using a spreading device. Allow to dry in air.

Cellulose for chromatography R1. *1016900.*

Microcrystalline cellulose. A fine, white homogeneous powder with an average particle size less than 30 µm.

Preparation of a thin layer. Suspend 25 g in 90 ml of *water R* and homogenise in an electric mixer for 60 s. Coat carefully cleaned plates with a layer 0.1 mm thick using a spreading device. Allow to dry in air.

Cellulose for chromatography F_{254}. *1017000.*

Microcrystalline cellulose F_{254}. A fine, white, homogeneous powder with an average particle size less than 30 µm, containing a fluorescent indicator having an optimal intensity at 254 nm.

Preparation of a thin layer. Suspend 25 g in 100 ml of *water R* and homogenise using an electric mixer for 60 s. Coat carefully cleaned plates with a layer 0.1 mm thick using a spreading device. Allow to dry in air.

Cephalin. *1017200.*

To 0.5 g to 1 g of *acetone-dried ox brain R* add 20 ml of *acetone R* and allow to stand for 2 h. Centrifuge at 500 *g* for 2 min and decant the supernatant liquid. Dry the residue under reduced pressure and, to the dried material, add 20 ml of *chloroform R* and allow to stand for 2 h, shaking frequently. Remove the solid material by filtration or centrifugation and evaporate the chloroform under reduced pressure. Suspend the residue in 5 ml to 10 ml of a 9 g/l solution of *sodium chloride R.*

Solvents used to prepare the reagent should contain a suitable antioxidant, for example, 0.02 g/l of butylated hydroxyanisole.

Storage: frozen or freeze-dried for 3 months.

Cerium sulphate. $Ce(SO_4)_2,4H_2O$. (M_r 404.3). *1017300.* [123333-60-8]. Cerium(IV) sulphate. Ceric sulphate.

Yellow or orange-yellow, crystalline powder or crystals, very slightly soluble in water, slowly soluble in dilute acids.

Cerous nitrate. $Ce(NO_3)_3,6H_2O$. (M_r 434.3). *1017400.* [10294-41-4]. Cerium trinitrate hexahydrate.

A colourless or pale yellow, crystalline powder, freely soluble in water and in alcohol.

Cetostearyl alcohol. *1017500.* [67762-27-0].

See *Cetostearyl alcohol (0702).*

Cetrimide. *1017600.* [8044-71-1].

See *Cetrimide (0378).*

Cetyltrimethylammonium bromide. $C_{19}H_{42}BrN$. (M_r 364.5). *1017700.* [57-09-0]. Cetrimonium bromide. *N*-Hexadecyl-*N,N,N*-trimethylammonium bromide.

A white, crystalline powder, soluble in water, freely soluble in alcohol.

mp: about 240 °C.

Chamazulene. $C_{14}H_{16}$. (M_r 184.3). *1148000.* [529-05-5]. 7-Ethyl-1,4-dimethylazulene.

A blue liquid, very slightly soluble in water, soluble in alcohol, miscible with fatty oils, with essential oils and with liquid paraffin, soluble with discolouration in phosphoric acid (85 per cent *m/m*) and sulphuric acid (50 per cent *V/V*).

Appearance of solution. 50 mg is soluble in 2.5 ml of *hexane R.* The blue solution is clear in a thin-layer obtained by tilting the test-tube.

Chamazulene used for gas chromatography complies with the following additional test.

Assay. Examine by gas chromatography (*2.2.28*) as prescribed in the monograph on *Matricaria oil (1836),* using a 4 g/l solution in *cyclohexane R.*

The content of chamazulene is not less than 95.0 per cent, calculated by the normalisation procedure.

Charcoal, activated. *1017800.* [64365-11-3].

See *Activated charcoal (0313).*

Chloral hydrate. *1017900.* [302-17-0].

See *Choral hydrate (0265).*

Chloral hydrate solution. *1017901.*

A solution of 80 g in 20 ml of *water R.*

Chloramine. *1018000.* [7080-50-4].

See *Chloramine (0381).*

Chloramine solution. *1018001.*

A 20 g/l solution. Prepare immediately before use.

Chloramine solution R1. *1018002.*

A 0.1 g/l solution of *chloramine R.* Prepare immediately before use.

Chloramine solution R2. *1018003.*

A 0.2 g/l solution. Prepare immediately before use.

Chlordane. $C_{10}H_6Cl_8$. (M_r 409.8). *1124100.* [12789-03-6].

bp: about 175 °C.

mp: about 106 °C.

A suitable certified reference solution of technical grade (10 ng/µl in iso-octane) may be used.

Chlordiazepoxide. *1113200.* [58-25-3].

See *Chlordiazepoxide (0656).*

Chlorfenvinphos. $C_{12}H_{14}Cl_3O_4P$. (M_r 359.6). *1124200.* [470-90-6].

A suitable certified reference solution (10 ng/μl in cyclohexane) may be used.

Chloroacetanilide. C_8H_8ClNO. (M_r 169.6). *1018100.* [539-03-7]. 4′-Chloroacetanilide.

Content: minimum 95 per cent of C_8H_8ClNO.

A crystalline powder, practically insoluble in water, soluble in alcohol.

mp: about 178 °C.

Chloroacetic acid. $C_2H_3ClO_2$. (M_r 94.5). *1018200.* [79-11-8].

Colourless or white crystals, deliquescent, very soluble in water, soluble in alcohol.

Storage: in an airtight container.

Chloroaniline. C_6H_6ClN. (M_r 127.6). *1018300.* [106-47-8]. 4-Chloroaniline.

Crystals, soluble in hot water, freely soluble in alcohol.

mp: about 71 °C.

4-Chlorobenzenesulphonamide. $C_6H_6ClNO_2S$. (M_r 191.6). *1097400.* [98-64-6].

White powder.

mp: about 145 °C.

2-Chlorobenzoic acid. $C_7H_5ClO_2$. (M_r 156.6). *1139300.* [118-91-2].

Soluble in water, slightly soluble in ethanol.

bp: about 285 °C.

mp: about 140 °C.

Chlorobutanol. *1018400.* [57-15-8].

See *Anhydrous chlorobutanol (0382)*.

2-Chloro-2-deoxy-D-glucose. $C_6H_{11}ClO_5$. (M_r 198.6). *1134700.* [14685-79-1].

A white crystalline, very hygroscopic powder, soluble in water and in dimethyl sulphoxide, practically insoluble in alcohol.

2-Chloroethanol. C_2H_5ClO. (M_r 80.5). *1097500.* [107-07-3].

Colourless liquid, soluble in alcohol.

d_{20}^{20}: about 1.197.

n_D^{20}: about 1.442.

bp: about 130 °C.

mp: about −89 °C.

2-Chloroethanol solution. *1097501.*

Dissolve 125 mg of *2-chloroethanol R* in *2-propanol R* and dilute to 50 ml with the same solvent. Dilute 5 ml of the solution to 50 ml with *2-propanol R*.

Chloroethylamine hydrochloride. $C_2H_7Cl_2N$. (M_r 116.0). *1124300.* [870-24-6]. 2-Chloroethanamine hydrochloride.

mp: about 145 °C.

(2-Chloroethyl)diethylamine hydrochloride. $C_6H_{15}Cl_2N$. (M_r 172.1). *1018500.* [869-24-9].

A white, crystalline powder, very soluble in water and in methanol, freely soluble in methylene chloride, practically insoluble in hexane.

mp: about 211 °C.

Chloroform. $CHCl_3$. (M_r 119.4). *1018600.* [67-66-3]. Trichloromethane.

A clear, colourless liquid, slightly soluble in water, miscible with alcohol.

d_{20}^{20}: 1.475 to 1.481.

bp: about 60 °C.

Chloroform contains 0.4 per cent *m/m* to 1.0 per cent *m/m* of ethanol.

Ethanol. Introduce 1.00 g (*m* g) into a ground-glass-stoppered flask. Add 15.0 ml of *nitrochromic reagent R*, close the flask, shake vigorously for 2 min and allow to stand for 15 min. Add 100 ml of *water R* and 5 ml of a 200 g/l solution of *potassium iodide R*. After 2 min titrate with *0.1 M sodium thiosulphate*, using 1 ml of *starch solution R* as indicator, until a light green colour is obtained (n_1 ml of *0.1 M sodium thiosulphate*). Carry out a blank assay (n_2 ml of *0.1 M sodium thiosulphate*). Calculate the percentage of ethanol using the expression:

$$\frac{(n_2 - n_1)\,0.115}{m}$$

Chloroform, acidified. *1018601.*

To 100 ml of *chloroform R* add 10 ml of *hydrochloric acid R*. Shake, allow to stand and separate the 2 layers.

Chloroform, ethanol-free. *1018602.*

Shake 200 ml of *chloroform R* with four quantities, each of 100 ml, of *water R*. Dry over 20 g of *anhydrous sodium sulphate R* for 24 h. Distil the filtrate over 10 g of *anhydrous sodium sulphate R*. Discard the first 20 ml of distillate. Prepare immediately before use.

Chloroform stabilised with amylene. $CHCl_3$. (M_r 119.4). *1018700.*

A clear, colourless liquid, slightly soluble in water, miscible with alcohol.

Water: maximum 0.05 per cent.

Residue on evaporation: maximum 0.001 per cent.

Minimum transmittance (*2.2.25*), determined using *water R* as compensation liquid: 50 per cent at 255 nm, 80 per cent at 260 nm, 98 per cent at 300 nm.

Assay: minimum 99.8 per cent of $CHCl_3$, determined by gas chromatography.

Chlorogenic acid. $C_{16}H_{18}O_9$. (M_r 354.3). *1104700.* [327-97-9]. (1*S*,3*R*,4*R*,5*R*)-3-[(3,4-Dihydroxycinnamoyl)oxy]-1,4,5-trihydroxycyclohexanecarboxylic acid.

A white, crystalline powder or white needles, freely soluble in boiling water, in acetone and in ethanol.

$[\alpha]_D^{26}$: about −35.2.

mp: about 208 °C.

Chromatography. Examined under the conditions described on Identification A in the monograph on *Belladonna leaf dry extract, standardised (1294)*, the chromatogram shows only one principal zone.

3-Chloro-2-methylaniline. C_7H_8ClN. (M_r 141.6). *1139400.* [87-60-5]. 6-Chloro-2-toluidine.

Not miscible with water, slightly soluble in ethanol.

d_{20}^{20}: : about 1.171.

n_D^{20}: : about 1.587.

bp: about 115 °C.

mp: about 2 °C.

2-Chloro-4-nitroaniline. $C_6H_5ClN_2O_2$. (M_r 172.6). *1018800.* [121-87-9].

A yellow, crystalline powder, freely soluble in methanol.

mp: about 107 °C.

Storage: protected from light.

Chlorophenol. C_6H_5ClO. (M_r 128.6). *1018900.* [106-48-9]. 4-Chlorophenol.

Colourless or almost colourless crystals, slightly soluble in water, very soluble in alcohol and in solutions of alkali hydroxides.

mp: about 42 °C.

Chloroplatinic acid. $H_2Cl_6Pt,6H_2O$. (M_r 517.9). *1019000.* [18497-13-7]. Hydrogen hexachloroplatinate(IV) hexahydrate.

Content: minimum 37.0 per cent *m/m* of platinum (A_r 195.1).

Brownish-red crystals or a crystalline mass, very soluble in water, soluble in alcohol.

Assay. Ignite 0.200 g to constant mass at 900 °C and weigh the residue (platinum).

Storage: protected from light.

3-Chloropropane-1,2-diol. $C_3H_7ClO_2$. (M_r 110.5). *1097600.* [96-24-2].

Colourless liquid, soluble in water and alcohol.

d_{20}^{20}: about 1.322.

n_D^{20}: about 1.480

bp: about 213 °C.

5-Chloroquinolin-8-ol. C_9H_6ClNO. (M_r 179.6). *1156900.* [130-16-5]. 5-Chlorooxine.

Sparingly soluble in cold dilute hydrochloric acid.

mp: about 123 °C.

Content: minimum 95.0 per cent of C_9H_6ClNO.

5-Chlorosalicylic acid. $C_7H_5ClO_3$. (M_r 172.6). *1019100.* [321-14-2].

A white or almost white, crystalline powder, soluble in methanol.

mp: about 173 °C.

Chlorothiazide. *1112100.* [58-94-6].

See *Chlorothiazide (0385).*

Chlorotrimethylsilane. C_3H_9ClSi. (M_r 108.6). *1019300.* [75-77-4].

A clear, colourless liquid, fuming in air.

d_{20}^{20}: about 0.86.

n_D^{20}: about 1.388.

bp: about 57 °C.

Chlorpyriphos. $C_9H_{11}Cl_3NO_3PS$. (M_r 350.6). *1124400.* [2921-88-2].

bp: about 200 °C.

mp: 42 °C to 44 °C.

A suitable certified reference solution (10 ng/μl in cyclohexane) may be used.

Chlorpyriphos-methyl. $C_7H_7Cl_3NO_3PS$. (M_r 322.5). *1124500.* [5598-13-0].

mp: 45 °C to 47 °C.

A suitable certified reference solution (10 ng/μl in cyclohexane) may be used.

Chlortetracycline hydrochloride. *1145500.*

See *Chlortetracycline hydrochloride (0173).*

Cholesterol. *1019400.* [57-88-5].

See *Cholesterol (0993).*

Choline chloride. $C_5H_{14}ClNO$. (M_r 139.6). *1019500.* [67-48-1]. (2-Hydroxyethyl)trimethylammonium chloride.

Deliquescent crystals, very soluble in water and in alcohol.

Chromatography. Examine as prescribed in the monograph *Suxamethonium chloride (0248),* applying 5 μl of a 0.2 g/l solution in *methanol R*. The chromatogram shows one principal spot.

Storage: in an airtight container.

Chromazurol S. $C_{23}H_{13}Cl_2Na_3O_9S$. (M_r 605). *1019600.* [1667-99-8].

Schultz No. 841.

Colour Index No. 43825.

Trisodium 5-[(3-carboxylato-5-methyl-4-oxocyclohexa-2,5-dien-1-ylidene)(2,6-dichloro-3-sulphonatophenyl)methyl]-2-hydroxy-3-methylbenzoate.

A brownish-black powder, soluble in water, slightly soluble in alcohol.

Chromic acid cleansing mixture. *1019700.*

A saturated solution of *chromium trioxide R* in *sulphuric acid R.*

Chromic potassium sulphate. $CrK(SO_4)_2,12H_2O$. (M_r 499.4). *1019800.* [7788-99-0]. Chrome alum.

Large, violet-red to black crystals, freely soluble in water, practically insoluble in alcohol.

Chromium(III) trichloride hexahydrate. $[Cr(H_2O)_4Cl_2]Cl,2H_2O$. (M_r 266.5). *1104800.* [10060-12-5].

A dark green crystalline powder, hygroscopic.

Storage: protected from humidity and oxidising agents.

Chromium trioxide. CrO_3. (M_r 100.0). *1019900.* [1333-82-0].

Dark brownish-red needles or granules, deliquescent, very soluble in water.

Storage: in an airtight glass container.

Chromophore substrate R1. *1020000.*

Dissolve *N*-α-benzyloxycarbonyl-D-arginyl-L-glycyl-L-arginine-4-nitroanilide dihydrochloride in *water R* to give a 0.003 M solution. Dilute in *tris(hydroxymethyl)aminomethane-EDTA buffer solution pH 8.4 R* to 0.0005 M before use.

Chromophore substrate R2. *1020100.*

Dissolve D-phenylalanyl-L-pipecolyl-L-arginine-4-nitroanilide dihydrochloride in *water R* to give a 0.003 M solution. Dilute before use in titrating in *tris(hydroxymethyl)aminomethane-EDTA buffer solution pH 8.4 R* to give a 0.0005 M solution.

Chromophore substrate R3. *1149100.*

Dissolve D-valyl-leucyl-lysyl-4-nitroanilide dihydrochloride in *water R* to give a 0.003 M solution.

Chromotrope II B. $C_{16}H_9N_3Na_2O_{10}S_2$. ($M_r$ 513.4). *1020200.* [548-80-1].

Schultz No. 67.

Colour Index No. 16575.

Disodium 4,5-dihydroxy-3-(4-nitrophenylazo)naphthalene-2,7-disulphonate.

A reddish-brown powder, soluble in water giving a yellowish-red colour, practically insoluble in alcohol.

Chromotrope II B solution. *1020201.*

A 0.05 g/l solution in *sulphuric acid R.*

Chromotropic acid, sodium salt. $C_{10}H_6Na_2O_8S_2,2H_2O$. ($M_r$ 400.3). *1020300.* [5808-22-0].

Schultz No. 1136.

Disodium 4,5-dihydroxynaphthalene-2,7-disulphonate dihydrate. Disodium 1,8-dihydroxynaphthalene-3,6-disulphonate dihydrate.

A yellowish-white powder, soluble in water, practically insoluble in alcohol.

Chromotropic acid, sodium salt solution. *1020301.*

Dissolve 0.60 g of *chromotropic acid, sodium salt R* in about 80 ml of *water R* and dilute to 100 ml with the same solvent. Use this solution within 24 h.

Chrysanthemin. $C_{21}H_{21}ClO_{11}$. (M_r 485.5). *1134800.* [7084-24-4]. Kuromanin chloride. 2-(3,4-Dihydroxyphenyl)-3-(β-D-glucopyranosyl)oxy-5,7-dihydroxy-1-benzopyrylium chloride.

A reddish-brown crystalline powder, soluble in water and in alcohol.

Absorbance (*2.2.25*). A 0.01 g/l solution in a mixture of 1 volume of *hydrochloric acid R* and 999 volumes of *methanol R* shows a maximum at 528 nm.

α-Chymotrypsin for peptide mapping. *1142400.*

α-Chymotrypsin of high purity, treated to eliminate tryptic activity.

Cinchonidine. $C_{19}H_{22}N_2O$. (M_r 294.4). *1020400.* [485-71-2]. (*R*)-(Quinol-4-yl)[(2*S*,4*S*,5*R*)-5-vinylquinuclidin-2-yl]methanol.

A white, crystalline powder, very slightly soluble in water and in light petroleum, soluble in alcohol.

$[\alpha]_D^{20}$: − 105 to − 110, determined on a 50 g/l solution in *alcohol R*.

mp: about 208 °C, with decomposition.

Storage: protected from light.

Cinchonine. $C_{19}H_{22}N_2O$. (M_r 294.4). *1020500.* [118-10-5]. (*S*)-(Quinol-4-yl)[(2*R*,4*S*,5*R*)-5-vinylquinuclidin-2-yl]methanol.

A white, crystalline powder, very slightly soluble in water, sparingly soluble in alcohol and in methanol.

$[\alpha]_D^{20}$: + 225 to + 230, determined on a 50 g/l solution in *alcohol R*.

mp: about 263 °C.

Storage: protected from light.

Cineole. $C_{10}H_{18}O$. (M_r 154.3). *1020600.* [470-82-6]. 1,8-Cineole. Eucalyptol. 1,8-Epoxy-*p*-menthane.

A colourless liquid, practically insoluble in water, miscible with ethanol.

d_{20}^{20}: 0.922 to 0.927.

n_D^{20} : 1.456 to 1.459.

Freezing point (*2.2.18*): 0 °C to 1 °C.

Distillation range (*2.2.11*): 174 °C to 177 °C.

Phenol. Shake 1 g with 20 ml of *water R*. Allow to separate and add to 10 ml of the aqueous layer 0.1 ml of *ferric chloride solution R1*. No violet colour develops.

Turpentine oil. Dissolve 1 g in 5 ml of *alcohol (90 per cent V/V) R*. Add dropwise freshly prepared *bromine water R*. Not more than 0.5 ml is required to give a yellow colour lasting for 30 min.

Residue on evaporation: maximum 0.05 per cent. To 10.0 ml add 25 ml of *water R*, evaporate on a water-bath and dry the residue to constant mass at 100-105 °C.

Cineole used in gas chromatography complies with the following additional test.

Assay. Examine by gas chromatography (*2.2.28*) as prescribed in the monograph on *Peppermint oil (0405)* using the substance to be examined as the test solution. The area of the principal peak is not less than 98.0 per cent of the total area of the peaks.

1,4-Cineole. $C_{10}H_{18}O$. (M_r 154.3). *1142500.* [470-67-7]. 1-Methyl-4-(1-methylethyl)-7-oxabicyclo[2.2.1]heptane. 1-Isopropyl-4-methyl-7-oxabicyclo[2.2.1]heptane.

A colourless liquid.

d_4^{20} : about 0.900.

n_D^{20} : about 1.445.

bp: about 173 °C.

Cinnamamide. C_9H_9NO. (M_r 147.2). *1154800.* [621-79-4]. (*E*)-3-Phenylprop-2-enamide.

White or almost white powder.

mp: about 149 °C.

Cinnamic aldehyde. C_9H_8O. (M_r 132.2). *1020700.* [104-55-2]. 3-Phenylpropenal.

A yellowish to greenish-yellow, oily liquid, slightly soluble in water, very soluble in alcohol.

d_{20}^{20}: 1.048 to 1.051.

n_D^{20} : about 1.620.

Storage: protected from light.

***trans*-Cinnamic aldehyde.** C_9H_8O. (M_r 132.2). *1124600.* [14371-10-9]. *(E)*-3-Phenylprop-2-enal.

trans-Cinnamic aldehyde used in gas chromatography complies with the following additional test.

Assay. Examine by gas chromatography (*2.2.28*) as prescribed in the monograph on *Cassia oil (1496)*.

The content is not less than 99.0 per cent, calculated by the normalisation procedure.

Cinnamyl acetate. $C_{11}H_{12}O_2$. (M_r 176.2). *1124700.* [103-54-8]. 3-Phenylprop-2-en-1-yl acetate.

n_D^{20} : about 1.542.

bp: about 262 °C.

Cinnamyl acetate used in gas chromatography complies with the following additional test.

Assay. Examine by gas chromatography (*2.2.28*) as prescribed in the monograph on *Cassia oil (1496)*.

The content is not less than 99.0 per cent, calculated by the normalisation procedure.

Citral. $C_{10}H_{16}O$. (M_r 152.2). *1020800.* [5392-40-5]. Mixture of (2*E*)- and (2*Z*)-3,7-Dimethylocta-2,6-dienal.

A light yellow liquid, practically insoluble in water, miscible with alcohol and with glycerol.

Chromatography. Examine by thin-layer chromatography (*2.2.27*), using *silica gel GF_{254} R* as the coating substance. Apply to the plate 10 µl of a 1 g/l solution in *toluene R*. Develop over a path of 15 cm using a mixture of 15 volumes of *ethyl acetate R* and 85 volumes of *toluene R*. Allow the plate to dry in air and examine in ultraviolet light at 254 nm. The chromatogram obtained shows only one principal spot.

Citral used in gas chromatography complies with the following additional test.

Assay. Examine by gas chromatography (*2.2.28*) as prescribed in the monograph on *Citronella oil (1609)*.

The content of citral (neral + geranial) is not less than 95.0 per cent calculated by the normalisation procedure.

Citrated rabbit plasma. *1020900.*

Collect blood by intracardiac puncture from a rabbit kept fasting for 12 h, using a plastic syringe with a No. 1 needle containing a suitable volume of 38 g/l solution of *sodium citrate R* so that the final volume ratio of citrate solution to blood is 1: 9. Separate the plasma by centrifugation at 1500 *g* to 1800 *g* at 15 °C to 20 °C for 30 min.

Storage: at 0 °C to 6 °C; use within 4 h of collection.

Citric acid. *1021000.* [5949-29-1]. See *Citric acid monohydrate (0456).*

When used in the limit test for iron, it complies with the following additional requirement.

Dissolve 0.5 g in 10 ml of *water R*, add 0.1 ml of *thioglycollic acid R*, mix and make alkaline with *ammonia R*. Dilute to 20 ml with *water R*. No pink colour appears in the solution.

Citric acid, anhydrous. *1021200.* [77-92-9].

See *Anhydrous citric acid (0455).*

Citronellal. $C_{10}H_{18}O$. (M_r 154.3). *1113300.* [106-23-0]. 3,7-Dimethyl-6-octenal.

Very slightly soluble in water, soluble in alcohols.

d_{20}^{20}: 0.848 to 0.856.

n_D^{20}: about 1.446.

$[\alpha]_D^{25}$: about + 11.50.

Citronellal used in gas chromatography complies with the following additional test.

Assay. Examine by gas chromatography (*2.2.28*) as prescribed in the monograph on *Citronella oil (1609).*

The content is not less than 95.0 per cent calculated by the normalisation procedure.

Citronellol. $C_{10}H_{20}O$. (M_r 156.3). *1134900.* [106-22-9]. 3,7-Dimethyloct-6-en-1-ol.

A clear, colourless liquid, practically insoluble in water, miscible with alcohol.

d_{20}^{20}: 0.857.

n_D^{20}: 1.456.

bp: 220 °C to 222 °C.

Citronellol used in gas chromatography complies with the following additional test.

Assay. Examine by gas chromatography (*2.2.28*) as prescribed in the monograph on *Citronella oil (1609).*

The content is not less than 95.0 per cent calculated by the normalisation procedure.

Storage: in an airtight container, protected from light.

Citronellyl acetate. $C_{12}H_{22}O_2$. (M_r 198.3). *1135000.* [150-84-5]. 3,7-Dimethyl-6-octen-1-yl acetate.

d_{20}^{20}: 0.890.

n_D^{20}: 1.443.

bp: 229 °C.

Citronellyl acetate used in gas chromatography complies with the following additional test.

Assay. Examine by gas chromatography (*2.2.28*) as prescribed in the monograph on *Citronella oil (1609).*

The content is not less than 97.0 per cent calculated by the normalisation procedure.

Storage: in an airtight container, protected from light.

Citropten. $C_{11}H_{10}O_4$. (M_r 206.2). *1021300.* [487-06-9]. Limettin. 5,7-Dimethoxy-2*H*-1-benzopyran-2-one.

Needle-shaped crystals, practically insoluble in water and in light petroleum, freely soluble in acetone and in alcohol.

mp: about 145 °C.

Chromatography. Examine by thin-layer chromatography (*2.2.27*), using *silica gel GF₂₅₄R* as the coating substance. Apply to the plate 10 µl of a 1 g/l solution in *toluene R*. Develop over a path of 15 cm using a mixture of 15 volumes of *ethyl acetate R* and 85 volumes of *toluene R*. Allow the plate to dry in air and examine in ultraviolet light at 254 nm. The chromatogram obtained shows only one principal spot.

Clobetasol propionate. $C_{25}H_{32}ClFO_5$. (M_r 467.0). *1097700.* [25122-46-7]. 21-Chloro-9-fluoro-11β,17-dihydroxy-16β-methylpregna-1,4-diene-3,20-dione 17-propionate.

A white crystalline powder, insoluble in water, soluble in alcohol and in acetone.

$[\alpha]_D^{20}$: about + 104 (in dioxan).

mp: about 196 °C.

Coagulation factor V solution. *1021400.*

Coagulation factor V solution may be prepared by the following method or by any other method which excludes factor VIII.

Prepare the factor V reagent from fresh oxalated bovine plasma, by fractionation at 4 °C with a saturated solution of *ammonium sulphate R* prepared at 4 °C. Separate the fraction which precipitates between 38 per cent and 50 per cent of saturation, which contains factor V without significant contamination with factor VIII. Remove the ammonium sulphate by dialysis and dilute the solution with a 9 g/l solution of *sodium chloride R* to give a solution containing between 10 per cent and 20 per cent of the quantity of factor V present in fresh human normal plasma.

Determination of factor V content. Prepare two dilutions of the preparation of factor V in *imidazole buffer solution pH 7.3 R* containing 1 volume of the preparation in 10 volumes and in 20 volumes of the buffer solution respectively. Test each dilution as follows: mix 0.1 ml of *plasma substrate deficient in factor V R*, 0.1 ml of the solution to be examined, 0.1 ml of *thromboplastin R* and 0.1 ml of a 3.5 g/l solution of *calcium chloride R* and measure the coagulation times, i.e. the interval between the moment at which the calcium chloride solution is added and the first indication of the formation of fibrin, which may be observed visually or by means of a suitable apparatus.

In the same manner, determine the coagulation time (in duplicate) of four dilutions of human normal plasma in *imidazole buffer solution pH 7.3 R*, containing respectively, 1 volume in 10 (equivalent to 100 per cent of factor V), 1 volume in 50 (20 per cent), 1 volume in 100 (10 per cent), and 1 volume in 1000 (1 per cent). Using two-way logarithmic paper plot the average coagulation times for each dilution of human plasma against the equivalent percentage of factor V and read the percentage of factor V for the two dilutions of the factor V solution by interpolation. The mean of the two results gives the percentage of factor V in the solution to be examined.

Storage: in the frozen state at a temperature not higher than − 20 °C.

Cobalt chloride. $CoCl_2,6H_2O$. (M_r 237.9). *1021600.* [7791-13-1].

A red, crystalline powder or deep-red crystals, very soluble in water, soluble in alcohol.

4. Reagents

Cobalt nitrate. $Co(NO_3)_2,6H_2O$. (M_r 291.0). *1021700.* [10026-22-9].

Small garnet-red crystals, very soluble in water.

Codeine. *1021800.* [6059-47-8].

See *Codeine (0076).*

Codeine phosphate. *1021900.* [52-28-8].

See *Codeine phosphate hemihydrate (0074).*

Congo red. $C_{32}H_{22}N_6Na_2O_6S_2$. ($M_r$ 697). *1022000.* [573-58-0]. Schultz No. 360.

Colour Index No. 22120.

Disodium (biphenyl-4,4′-diyl-bis-2,2′-azo)bis(1-aminonaphthalene-4-sulphonate).

A brownish-red powder, soluble in water.

Congo red paper. *1022002.*

Immerse strips of filter paper for a few minutes in *congo red solution R.* Allow to dry.

Congo red solution. *1022001.*

Dissolve 0.1 g of *congo red R* in a mixture of 20 ml of *alcohol R* and *water R* and dilute to 100 ml with *water R.*

Test for sensitivity. To 0.2 ml of the congo red solution add 100 ml of *carbon dioxide-free water R* and 0.3 ml of *0.1 M hydrochloric acid.* The solution is blue. Not more than 0.3 ml of *0.1 M sodium hydroxide* is required to change the colour to pink.

Colour change: pH 3.0 (blue) to pH 5.0 (pink).

Coomassie blue. *1001400.* [3861-73-2].

See *acid blue 92 R.*

Coomassie blue solution. *1001401.*

See *acid blue 92 solution R.*

Coomassie staining solution. *1012201.*

A 1.25 g/l solution of *acid blue 83 R* in a mixture consisting of 1 volume of *glacial acetic acid R,* 4 volumes of *methanol R* and 5 volumes of *water R.* Filter.

Copper. Cu. (A_r 63.55). *1022100.* [7440-50-8].

Cleaned foil, turnings, wire or powder of the pure metal of electrolytic grade.

Copper acetate. $C_4H_6CuO_4,H_2O$. (M_r 199.7). *1022200.* [142-71-2].

Blue-green crystals or powder, freely soluble in boiling water, soluble in water and in alcohol, slightly soluble in glycerol (85 per cent).

Copper edetate solution. *1022300.*

To 2 ml of a 20 g/l solution of *copper acetate R* add 2 ml of *0.1 M sodium edetate* and dilute to 50 ml with *water R.*

Copper nitrate. $Cu(NO_3)_2,3H_2O$. (M_r 241.6). *1022400.* [10031-43-3]. Chloride dinitrate trihydrate.

Dark blue crystals, hygroscopic, very soluble in water giving a strongly acid reaction, freely soluble in alcohol and in dilute nitric acid.

Storage: in an airtight container.

Copper sulphate. $CuSO_4,5H_2O$. (M_r 249.7). *1022500.* [7758-99-8].

A blue powder or deep-blue crystals, slowly efflorescent, very soluble in water, slightly soluble in alcohol.

Copper sulphate solution. *1022501.*

A 125 g/l solution.

Copper tetrammine, ammoniacal solution of. *1022600.*

Dissolve 34.5 g of *copper sulphate R* in 100 ml of *water R* and, whilst stirring, add dropwise *concentrated ammonia R* until the precipitate which forms dissolves completely. Keeping the temperature below 20 °C, add dropwise with continuous shaking 30 ml of *strong sodium hydroxide solution R.* Filter through a sintered-glass filter (40), wash with *water R* until the filtrate is clear and take up the precipitate with 200 ml of *concentrated ammonia R.* Filter through a sintered-glass filter and repeat the filtration to reduce the residue to a minimum.

Cortisone acetate. *1097800.* [50-04-4].

See *Cortisone acetate (0321).*

Coumaphos. $C_{14}H_{16}ClO_5PS$. (M_r 362.8). *1124800.* [56-72-4].

mp: 91 °C to 92 °C.

A suitable certified reference solution (10 ng/µl in iso-octane) may be used.

Coumarin. $C_9H_6O_2$. (M_r 146.1). *1124900.* [91-64-5]. 2*H*-Chromen-2-one. 2*H*-1-Benzopyran-2-one.

A colourless, crystalline powder or orthorhombic or rectangular crystals, very soluble in boiling water, soluble in alcohol. It dissolves in solutions of alkali hydroxides.

mp: 68 °C to 70 °C.

Coumarin used in gas chromatography complies with the following additional test.

Assay. Examine by gas chromatography (*2.2.28*) as prescribed in the monograph on *Cassia oil (1496).*

The content is not less than 98.0 per cent, calculated by the normalisation procedure.

Cresol. C_7H_8O. (M_r 108.1). *1022700.* [95-48-7]. *o*-Cresol. 2-Methylphenol.

Crystals or a super-cooled liquid becoming dark on exposure to light and air, miscible with ethanol, soluble in about 50 parts of water and soluble in solutions of alkali hydroxides.

d_{20}^{20}: about 1.05.

n_D^{20}: 1.540 to 1.550.

bp: about 190 °C.

Freezing point (*2.2.18*): minimum 30.5 °C.

Residue on evaporation: maximum 0.1 per cent *m/m*, determined by evaporating on a water-bath and drying in an oven at 100-105 °C.

Storage: protected from light, moisture and oxygen.

Distil before use.

***p*-Cresol.** C_7H_8O. (M_r 108.1). *1153100.* [106-44-5]. 4-Methylphenol.

Colourless or white crystals or crystalline mass.

d_{20}^{20}: about 1.02.

bp: about 202 °C.

***m*-Cresol purple.** $C_{21}H_{18}O_5S$. (M_r 382.44). *1121700.* [2303-01-7]. *m*-Cresolsulphonphthalein.

An olive-green, crystalline powder, slightly soluble in water, soluble in alcohol, in glacial acetic acid and in methanol.

***m*-Cresol purple solution.** *1121701.*

Dissolve 0.1 g of *m-cresol purple R* in 13 ml of *0.01 M sodium hydroxide,* dilute to 100 ml with *water R* and mix.

Colour change: pH 1.2 (red) to pH 2.8 (yellow); pH 7.4 (yellow) to pH 9.0 (purple).

Cresol red. $C_{21}H_{18}O_5S$. (M_r 382.4). *1022800.* [1733-12-6]. Cresolsulfonphthalein. 4,4′-(3*H*-2,1-Benzoxathiol-3-ylidene)bis-(2-methylphenol) *S,S*-dioxide.

A reddish-brown crystalline powder, slightly soluble in water, soluble in alcohol and in dilute solutions of alkali hydroxides.

Cresol red solution. *1022801.*

Dissolve 0.1 g of *cresol red R* in a mixture of 2.65 ml of *0.1 M sodium hydroxide* and 20 ml of *alcohol R* and dilute to 100 ml with *water R.*

Test for sensitivity. A mixture of 0.1 ml of the cresol red solution and 100 ml of *carbon dioxide-free water R* to which 0.15 ml of *0.02 M sodium hydroxide* has been added is purple-red. Not more than 0.15 ml of *0.02 M hydrochloric acid* is required to change the colour to yellow.

Colour change: pH 7.0 (yellow) to pH 8.6 (red).

Crystal violet. $C_{25}H_{30}ClN_3$. (M_r 408.0). *1022900.* [548-62-9].

Schultz No. 78.

Colour Index No. 42555.

Hexamethyl-pararosanilinium chloride.

Dark-green powder or crystals, soluble in water and in alcohol.

Crystal violet solution. *1022901.*

Dissolve 0.5 g of *crystal violet R* in *anhydrous acetic acid R* and dilute to 100 ml with the same solvent.

Test for sensitivity. To 50 ml of *anhydrous acetic acid R* add 0.1 ml of the crystal violet solution. On addition of 0.1 ml of *0.1 M perchloric acid* the bluish-purple solution turns bluish-green.

Cupric chloride. $CuCl_2,2H_2O$. (M_r 170.5). *1023000.* [10125-13-0]. Cupric chloride dihydrate.

Greenish-blue powder or crystals, deliquescent in moist air, efflorescent in dry air, freely soluble in water, in alcohol and in methanol, sparingly soluble in acetone.

Storage: in an airtight container.

Cupri-citric solution. *1023100.*

Dissolve 25 g of *copper sulphate R,* 50 g of *citric acid R* and 144 g of *anhydrous sodium carbonate R* in *water R* and dilute to 1000 ml with the same solvent.

Cupri-citric solution R1. *1023200.*

Dissolve 25 g of *copper sulphate R,* 50 g of *citric acid R* and 144 g of *anhydrous sodium carbonate R* in *water R* and dilute to 1000 ml with the same solvent.

Adjust the solution so that it complies with the following requirements.

a) To 25.0 ml add 3 g of *potassium iodide R.* Add 25 ml of a 25 per cent *m/m* solution of *sulphuric acid R* with precaution and in small quantities. Titrate with *0.1 M sodium thiosulphate* using 0.5 ml of *starch solution R,* added towards the end of the titration, as indicator.

24.5 ml to 25.5 ml of *0.1 M sodium thiosulphate* is used in the titration.

b) Dilute 10.0 ml to 100.0 ml with *water R* and mix. To 10.0 ml of the solution, add 25.0 ml of *0.1 M hydrochloric acid* and heat for 1 h on a water-bath. Cool, adjust with *water R* to the initial volume and titrate with *0.1 M sodium hydroxide,* using 0.1 ml of *phenolphthalein solution R1* as indicator.

5.7 ml to 6.3 ml of *0.1 M sodium hydroxide* is used in the titration.

c) Dilute 10.0 ml to 100.0 ml with *water R* and mix. Titrate 10.0 ml of the solution with *0.1 M hydrochloric acid,* using 0.1 ml of *phenolphthalein solution R1* as indicator.

6.0 ml to 7.5 ml of *0.1 M hydrochloric acid* is used in the titration.

Cupriethylenediamine hydroxide solution. *3008700.* [14552-35-3].

The molar ratio of ethylenediamine to copper is 2.00 ± 0.04.

This solution is commercially available.

Cupri-tartaric solution. *1023300.*

Solution I. Dissolve 34.6 g of *copper sulphate R* in *water R* and dilute to 500 ml with the same solvent.

Solution II. Dissolve 173 g of *sodium potassium tartrate R* and 50 g of *sodium hydroxide R* in 400 ml of *water R.* Heat to boiling, allow to cool and dilute to 500 ml with *carbon dioxide-free water R.*

Mix equal volumes of the 2 solutions immediately before use.

Cupri-tartaric solution R2. *1023302.*

Add 1 ml of a solution containing 5 g/l of *copper sulphate R* and 10 g/l of *potassium tartrate R* to 50 ml of *sodium carbonate solution R1.* Prepare immediately before use.

Cupri-tartaric solution R3. *1023303.*

Prepare a solution containing 10 g/l of *copper sulphate R* and 20 g/l of *sodium tartrate R.* To 1.0 ml of the solution add 50 ml of *sodium carbonate solution R2.* Prepare immediately before use.

Cupri-tartaric solution R4. *1023304.*

Solution I. 150 g/l *copper sulphate R.*

Solution II. Dissolve 2.5 g of *anhydrous sodium carbonate R,* 2.5 g of *potassium sodium tartrate R,* 2.0 g of *sodium hydrogen carbonate R,* and 20.0 g of *anhydrous sodium sulphate R* in *water R* and dilute to 100 ml with the same solvent.

Mix 1 part of solution I with 25 parts of solution II immediately before use.

Curcumin. $C_{21}H_{20}O_6$. (M_r 368.4). *1023500.* [458-37-7]. 1,7-bis(4-Hydroxy-3-methoxyphenyl)hepta-1,6-diene-3,5-dione.

An orange-brown, crystalline powder, practically insoluble in water, soluble in glacial acetic acid.

mp: about 183 °C.

Cyanoacetic acid. $C_3H_3NO_2$. (M_r 85.1). *1097900.* [372-09-8].

White to yellowish-white, hygroscopic crystals, very soluble in water.

Storage: in an airtight container.

Cyanocobalamin. *1023600.* [68-19-9].

See *Cyanocobalamin (0547).*

Cyanogen bromide solution. *1023700.* [506-68-3].

Add dropwise, with cooling *0.1 M ammonium thiocyanate* to *bromine water R* until the yellow colour disappears. Prepare immediately before use.

β-Cyclodextrin for chiral chromatography, modified. *1154600.*

30 per cent of 2,3-di-*O*-ethyl-6-*O*-*tert*-butyldimethylsilyl-β-cyclodextrin dissolved in *poly(dimethyl)(85)(diphenyl)(15)siloxane R.*

4. Reagents

Cyanoguanidine. $C_2H_4N_4$. (M_r 84.1). *1023800.* [461-58-5]. Dicyandiamide. 1-Cyanoguanidine.

A white, crystalline powder, sparingly soluble in water and in alcohol, practically insoluble in methylene chloride.

mp: about 210 °C.

Cyclohexane. C_6H_{12}. (M_r 84.2). *1023900.* [110-82-7].

A clear, colourless, flammable liquid, practically insoluble in water, miscible with organic solvents.

d_{20}^{20}: about 0.78.

bp: about 80.5 °C.

Cyclohexane used in spectrophotometry complies with the following additional requirements.

Minimum transmittance (*2.2.25*), determined using *water R* as compensation liquid: 45 per cent at 220 nm, 70 per cent at 235 nm, 90 per cent at 240 nm, 98 per cent at 250 nm.

Cyclohexane R1. *1023901.*

Complies with the requirements prescribed for *cyclohexane R* and with the following additional requirement.

The fluorescence, measured at 460 nm, under illumination with an excitant light beam at 365 nm, is not more intense than that of a solution containing 0.002 ppm of *quinine R* in *0.05 M sulphuric acid.*

Cyclohexylamine. $C_6H_{13}N$. (M_r 99.2). *1024000.* [108-91-8].

A colourless liquid, soluble in water, miscible with usual organic solvents.

n_D^{20}: about 1.460.

bp: 134 °C to 135 °C.

Cyclohexylenedinitrilotetra-acetic acid. $C_{14}H_{22}N_2O_8,H_2O$. (M_r 364.4). *1024100.* *trans*-Cyclohexylene-1,2-dinitrilo-*N,N,N',N'*-tetra-acetic acid.

A white, crystalline powder.

mp: about 204 °C.

Cyclohexylmethanol. $C_7H_{14}O$. (M_r 114.2). *1135200.* [100-49-2]. Cyclohexylcarbinol.

A liquid with a slight odour of camphor, soluble in alcohol.

n_D^{25}: about 1.464.

bp: about 185 °C.

3-Cyclohexylpropionic acid. $C_9H_{16}O_2$. (M_r 156.2). *1119200.* [701-97-3].

A clear liquid.

d_{20}^{20}: about 0.998.

n_D^{20}: about 1.4648.

bp: about 130 °C.

Cyhalothrin. $C_{23}H_{19}ClF_3NO_3$. (M_r 449.9). *1125000.* [91465-08-6].

bp: 187 °C to 190 °C.

mp: about 49 °C.

A suitable certified reference solution (10 ng/µl in cyclohexane) may be used.

***p*-Cymene.** $C_{10}H_{14}$. (M_r 134.2). *1113400.* [99-87-6]. 1-Isopropyl-4-methylbenzene.

A colourless liquid, practically insoluble in water, soluble in alcohol.

d_{20}^{20}: about 0.858.

n_D^{20}: about 1.4895.

bp: 175 °C to 178 °C.

p-Cymene used in gas chromatography complies with the following additional test.

Assay. Examine by gas chromatography (*2.2.28*) as prescribed in the monograph *Peppermint oil (0405).*

Test solution. The substance to be examined.

The area of the principal peak is not less than 96.0 per cent of the area of all the peaks in the chromatogram obtained.

Cypermethrin. $C_{22}H_{19}Cl_2NO_3$. (M_r 416.3). *1125100.* [52315-07-8].

bp: 170 °C to 195 °C.

mp: 60 °C to 80 °C.

A suitable certified reference solution (10 ng/µl in cyclohexane) may be used.

L-Cysteine. $C_3H_7NO_2S$. (M_r 121.1). *1024200.* [52-90-4].

A powder, freely soluble in water, in alcohol and in acetic acid, practically insoluble in acetone.

Cysteine hydrochloride. *1024300.* [7048-04-6].

See *Cysteine hydrochloride monohydrate (0895).*

L-Cystine. $C_6H_{12}N_2O_4S_2$. (M_r 240.3). *1024400.* [56-89-3].

A white, crystalline powder, practically insoluble in water and in alcohol. It dissolves in dilute solutions of alkali hydroxides. It decomposes at 250 °C.

$[\alpha]_D^{20}$: − 218 to − 224, determined in *1 M hydrochloric acid.*

Dantron. $C_{14}H_8O_4$. (M_r 240.2). *1024500.* [117-10-2]. 1,8-Dihydroxyanthraquinone. 1,8-Dihydroxyanthracene-9,10-dione.

A crystalline orange powder, practically insoluble in water, slightly soluble in alcohol, soluble in solutions of alkali hydroxides.

mp: about 195 °C.

Dantron used in the sesquiterpenic acids assay in Valerian root (0453) complies with the following additional requirements.

$A_{1\,cm}^{1\%}$: 355 to 375, determined at 500 nm in *1 M potassium hydroxide.*

Assay. Examine by liquid chromatography (*2.2.29*) as prescribed in the monograph on *Valerian Root (0453)* at the concentration of the reference solution. The content of dantron is not less than 95 per cent calculated by the normalisation procedure

***o,p'*-DDD.** $C_{14}H_{10}Cl_4$. (M_r 320.0). *1125200.* [53-19-0]. 1-(2-Chlorophenyl)-1-(4-chlorophenyl)-2,2-dichloroethane.

A suitable certified reference solution (10 ng/µl in cyclohexane) may be used.

***p,p'*-DDD.** $C_{14}H_{10}Cl_4$. (M_r 320.0). *1125300.* [72-54-8]. 1,1-bis(4-Chlorophenyl)-2,2-dichloroethane.

bp: about 193 °C.

mp: about 109 °C.

A suitable certified reference solution (10 ng/µl in cyclohexane) may be used.

***o,p'*-DDE.** $C_{14}H_8Cl_4$. (M_r 318.0). *1125400.* [3424-82-6]. 1-(2-Chlorophenyl)-1-(4-chlorophenyl)-2,2-dichloroethylene.

A suitable certified reference solution (10 ng/µl in cyclohexane) may be used.

***p,p'*-DDE.** $C_{14}H_8Cl_4$. (M_r 318.0). *1125500.* [72-55-9]. 1,1-bis(4-Chlorophenyl)-2,2-dichloroethylene.

bp: 316 °C to 317 °C.

mp: 88 °C to 89 °C.

A suitable certified reference solution (10 ng/µl in cyclohexane) may be used.

***o,p'*-DDT.** $C_{14}H_9Cl_5$. (M_r 354.5). *1125600.* [789-02-6]. 1-(2-Chlorophenyl)-1-(4-chlorophenyl)-2,2,2-trichloroethane.

A suitable certified reference solution (10 ng/µl in cyclohexane) may be used.

***p,p'*-DDT.** $C_{14}H_9Cl_5$. (M_r 354.5). *1125700.* [50-29-3]. 1,1-bis(4-Chlorophenyl)-2,2,2-trichloroethane.

bp: about 260 °C.

mp: 108 °C to 109 °C.

A suitable certified reference solution (10 ng/µl in cyclohexane) may be used.

Decanal. $C_{10}H_{20}O$. (M_r 156.3). *1149200.* [112-31-2]. Decyl aldehyde.

Oily, colourless liquid, with a characteristic odour of orange, practically insoluble in water, soluble in chloroform.

d_4^{20}: 0.825 to 0.829.

n_D^{20}: 1.420 to 1.430.

bp: 207 °C to 209 °C.

Decanal used in gas chromatography complies with the following additional test.

Assay. Examine by gas chromatography (*2.2.28*) as prescribed in the monograph on *Sweet orange oil (1811)*.

The content is not less than 99 per cent, calculated by the normalisation procedure.

Decane. $C_{10}H_{22}$. (M_r 142.3). *1024600.* [124-18-5].

A colourless liquid, practically insoluble in water.

n_D^{20}: about 1.411.

bp: about 174 °C.

Decanol. $C_{10}H_{22}O$. (M_r 158.3). *1024700.* [112-30-1]. *n*-Decyl alcohol.

A viscous liquid, solidifying at about 6 °C, practically insoluble in water, soluble in alcohol.

n_D^{20}: about 1.436.

bp: about 230 °C.

Deltamethrin. $C_{22}H_{19}Br_2NO_3$. (M_r 505.2). *1125800.* [52918-63-5].

bp: about 300 °C.

mp: about 98 °C.

A suitable certified reference solution (10 ng/µl in cyclohexane) may be used.

Demeclocycline hydrochloride. *1145600.*

See *Demeclocycline hydrochloride (0176)*.

Demethylflumazenil. $C_{14}H_{12}FN_3O_3$. (M_r 289.3). *1149300.* [79089-72-8].

Ethyl 8-fluoro-6-oxo-5,6-dihydro-4*H*-imidazo[1,5-*a*][1, 4]benzodiazepine-3-carboxylate.

mp: about 288 °C.

Colourless needles, soluble in dimethyl sulphoxide and in hot methanol.

2'-Deoxyuridine. $C_9H_{12}N_2O_5$. (M_r 228.2). *1024800.* [951-78-0]. 1-(2-Deoxy-β-d-*erythro*-pentofuranosyl)-1*H*,3*H*-pyrimidine-2,4-dione.

mp: about 165 °C.

Chromatography. Examine as prescribed in the monograph on *Idoxuridine (0669)*, applying 5 µl of a 0.25 g/l solution. The chromatogram obtained shows only one principal spot.

Destaining solution. *1012202.*

A mixture consisting of 1 volume of *glacial acetic acid R*, 4 volumes of *methanol R* and 5 volumes of *water R*.

Deuterated acetic acid. $C_2{}^2H_4O_2$. (M_r 64.1). *1101100.* [1186-52-3]. Tetradeuteroacetic acid. Acetic-d_3 acid-*d*.

The degree of deuteration is not less than 99.7 per cent.

d_{20}^{20}: about 1.12.

n_D^{20}: about 1.368.

bp: about 115 °C.

mp: about 16 °C.

Deuterated acetone. $C_3{}^2H_6O$. (M_r 64.1). *1024900.* [666-52-4]. Acetone-d_6. ($^2H_6$)-Acetone.

The degree of deuteration is not less than 99.5 per cent.

A clear, colourless liquid, miscible with water, with dimethylformamide, with ethanol and with methanol.

d_{20}^{20}: about 0.87.

n_D^{20}: about 1.357.

bp: about 55 °C.

Water and deuterium oxide. Not more than 0.1 per cent.

Deuterated chloroform. C^2HCl_3. (M_r 120.4). *1025000.* [865-49-6]. (^2H)-Chloroform. Chloroform-*d*.

The degree of deuteration is not less than 99.7 per cent.

A clear, colourless liquid, practically insoluble in water, miscible with acetone and with alcohol. It may be stabilised over silver foil.

d_{20}^{20}: about 1.51.

n_D^{20}: about 1.445.

bp: about 60 °C.

Water and deuterium oxide: maximum 0.05 per cent.

Deuterated dimethyl sulphoxide. $C_2{}^2H_6OS$. (M_r 84.2). *1025100.* [2206-27-1]. ($^2H_6$)-Dimethyl sulphoxide. Dimethyl sulphoxide-d_6.

The degree of deuteration is not less than 99.8 per cent.

A very hygroscopic liquid, practically colourless, viscous, soluble in water, in acetone and in ethanol.

d_{20}^{20}: about 1.18.

mp: about 20 °C.

Water and deuterium oxide: maximum 0.1 per cent.

Storage: in an airtight container.

Deuterated methanol. C^2H_4O. (M_r 36.1). *1025200.* [811-98-3]. (^2H)-Methanol. Methanol-*d*.

The degree of deuteriation is not less than 99.8 per cent.

Clear, colourless liquid miscible with water, with alcohol and with methylene chloride.

d_{20}^{20}: about 0.888.

n_D^{20}: about 1.326.

bp: 65.4 °C.

Deuterium oxide. ^2H_2O. (M_r 20.03). *1025300.* [7789-20-0]. Deuterated water.

The degree of deuteration is not less than 99.7 per cent.

d_{20}^{20}: about 1.11.

n_D^{20}: about 1.328.

bp: about 101 °C.

Deuterium oxide R1. ^2H_2O. (M_r 20.03). *1025301.* [7789-20-0]. Deuterated water.

The degree of deuteration is not less than 99.95 per cent.

Developer solution. *1122500.*

Dilute 2.5 ml of a 20 g/l solution of *citric acid R* and 0.27 ml of *formaldehyde R* to 500.0 ml with *water R*.

4. Reagents

Dextran for chromatography, cross-linked R2. *1025500.*

A bead-form dextran with a fraction range suitable for the separation of peptides and proteins with relative molecular masses of 15 × 10^2 to 30 × 10^3. When dry, the beads have a diameter of 20 µm to 80 µm.

Dextran for chromatography, cross-linked R3. *1025600.*

A bead-form dextran with a fraction range suitable for the separation of peptides and proteins with relative molecular masses of 4 × 10^3 to 15 × 10^4. When dry, the beads have a diameter of 40 µm to 120 µm.

Dextrose. *1025700.* [50-99-7].

See *glucose R.*

3,3′-Diaminobenzidine tetrahydrochloride. $C_{12}H_{18}Cl_4N_4, 2H_2O$. ($M_r$ 396.1). *1098000.* [7411-49-6].

3,3′,4,4′-Biphenyl-tetramine.

An almost white or slightly pink powder, soluble in water.

mp: about 280 °C, with decomposition.

Diatomaceous earth. *1025900.* [91053-39-3].

A white or almost white, fine granular powder, made up of siliceous frustules of fossil diatoms or of debris of fossil diatoms, practically insoluble in water and in alcohol.

The substance may be identified by microscopic examination with a magnification of × 500.

Diatomaceous earth for gas chromatography. *1026000.*

A white or almost white, fine granular powder, made up of siliceous frustules of fossil diatoms or of debris of fossil diatoms, practically insoluble in water and in alcohol. The substance may be identified by microscopic examination with a magnification of × 500. The substance is purified by treating with *hydrochloric acid R* and washing with *water R.*

Particle size. Not more than 5 per cent is retained on a sieve No. 180. Not more than 10 per cent passes a sieve No. 125.

Diatomaceous earth for gas chromatography R1. *1026100.*

A white or almost white, fine granular powder, made up of siliceous frustules of fossil diatoms or of debris of fossil diatoms, practically insoluble in water and in alcohol. The substance may be identified by microscopic examination with a magnification of × 500. The substance is purified by treating with *hydrochloric acid R* and washing with *water R.*

Particle size. Not more than 5 per cent is retained on a sieve No. 250. Not more than 10 per cent passes a sieve No. 180.

Diatomaceous earth for gas chromatography R2. *1026200.*

A white or almost white, fine granular powder with a specific surface area of about 0.5 m^2/g, made up of siliceous frustules of fossil diatoms or of debris of fossil diatoms, practically insoluble in water and in alcohol. The substance may be identified by microscopic examination with a magnification of × 500. The substance is purified by treating with *hydrochloric acid R* and washing with *water R.*

Particle size. Not more than 5 per cent is retained on a sieve No. 180. Not more than 10 per cent passes a sieve No. 125.

Diatomaceous earth for gas chromatography, silanised. *1026300.*

Diatomaceous earth for gas chromatography R silanised with dimethyldichlorosilane or other suitable silanising agents.

Diatomaceous earth for gas chromatography, silanised R1. *1026400.*

Prepared from crushed pink firebrick and silanised with dimethyldichlorosilane or other suitable silanising agents. The substance is purified by treating with *hydrochloric acid R* and washing with *water R.*

Diazinon. $C_{12}H_{21}N_2O_3PS$. (M_r 304.3). *1125900.* [333-41-5].

bp: about 306 °C.

A suitable certified reference solution (10 ng/µl in iso-octane) may be used.

Diazobenzenesulphonic acid solution R1. *1026500.*

Dissolve 0.9 g of *sulphanilic acid R* in a mixture of 30 ml of *dilute hydrochloric acid R* and 70 ml of *water R.* To 3 ml of the solution add 3 ml of a 50 g/l solution of *sodium nitrite R.* Cool in an ice-bath for 5 min, add 12 ml of the sodium nitrite solution and cool again. Dilute to 100 ml with *water R* and keep the reagent in an ice-bath. Prepare extemporaneously but allow to stand for 15 min before use.

Dibutylamine. $C_8H_{19}N$. (M_r 129.3). *1126000.* [111-92-2].

N-Butylbutan-1-amine.

Colourless liquid.

n_D^{20}: about 1.417.

bp: about 159 °C.

Dibutyl ether. $C_8H_{18}O$. (M_r 130.2). *1026700.* [142-96-1].

A colourless, flammable liquid, practically insoluble in water, miscible with ethanol.

d_{20}^{20}: about 0.77.

n_D^{20}: about 1.399.

Do not distil if the dibutyl ether does not comply with the test for peroxides.

Peroxides. Place 8 ml of *potassium iodide and starch solution R* in a 12 ml ground-glass-stoppered cylinder about 1.5 cm in diameter. Fill completely with the substance to be examined, shake vigorously and allow to stand protected from light for 30 min. No colour is produced.

The name and concentration of any added stabiliser are stated on the label.

Dibutyl phthalate. $C_{16}H_{22}O_4$. (M_r 278.3). *1026800.* [84-74-2].

Dibutyl benzene-1,2-dicarboxylate.

A clear, colourless or faintly coloured, oily liquid, very slightly soluble in water, miscible with acetone and with alcohol.

d_{20}^{20}: 1.043 to 1.048.

n_D^{20}: 1.490 to 1.495.

Dicarboxidine hydrochloride. $C_{20}H_{26}Cl_2N_2O_6$. (M_r 461.3). *1026900.* [56455-90-4]. 4,4′-[(4,4′-Diaminobiphenyl-3,3′-diyl)dioxy]dibutanoic acid dihydrochloride.

Dichlofenthion. $C_{10}H_{13}Cl_2O_3PS$. (M_r 315.2). *1126100.* [97-17-6].

A suitable certified reference solution (10 ng/µl in cyclohexane) may be used.

Dichloroacetic acid. $C_2H_2Cl_2O_2$. (M_r 128.9). *1027000.* [79-43-6].

Colourless liquid, miscible with water and alcohol.

d_{20}^{20}: about 1.566.

n_D^{20}: about 1.466.

bp: about 193 °C.

Dichloroacetic acid solution. *1027001.*

Dilute 67 ml of *dichloroacetic acid R* to 300 ml with *water R* and neutralise to *blue litmus paper R* using *ammonia R*. Cool, add 33 ml of *dichloroacetic acid R* and dilute to 600 ml with *water R*.

Dichlorobenzene. $C_6H_4Cl_2$. (M_r 147.0). *1027100.* [95-50-1]. 1,2-Dichlorobenzene.

A colourless, oily liquid, practically insoluble in water, soluble in ethanol.

d_{20}^{20}: about 1.31.

bp: about 180 °C.

2,3-Dichloro-5,6-dicyanobenzoquinone. $C_8Cl_2N_2O_2$. (M_r 227.0). *1153600.* [84-58-2]. 4,5-Dichloro-3,6-dioxo-cyclohexa-1,4-diene-1,2-dicarbonitrile.

Yellow or orange crystals, soluble in dioxan and in acetic acid, slightly soluble in methylene chloride. It decomposes in water.

mp: about 214 °C.

Storage: at a temperature of 2 °C to 8 °C.

(S)-3,5-Dichloro-2,6-dihydroxy-*N*-[(1-ethylpyrrolidin-2-yl)methyl]benzamide hydrobromide. $C_{14}H_{19}BrCl_2N_2O_3$. (M_r 414.1). *1142600.* [113310-88-6].

White, crystalline powder.

$[\alpha]_D^{22}$: + 11.4, determined on a 15.0 g/l solution in *ethanol R*.

mp: about 212 °C.

Dichlorofluorescein. $C_{20}H_{10}Cl_2O_5$. (M_r 401.2). *1027200.* [76-54-0]. 2,7-Dichlorofluorescein. 2-(2,7-Dichloro-6-hydroxy-3-oxo-3*H*-xanthen-9-yl)benzoic acid.

A yellowish-brown to yellow-orange powder, slightly soluble in water, freely soluble in alcohol and in dilute solutions of alkali hydroxides giving a solution showing a yellowish-green fluorescence.

Dichlorophenolindophenol, sodium salt. $C_{12}H_6Cl_2NNaO_2,2H_2O$. ($M_r$ 326.1). *1027300.* [620-45-1]. The sodium derivative of 2,6-dichloro-*N*-(4-hydroxyphenyl)-1,4-benzoquinone monoimine dihydrate.

A dark-green powder, freely soluble in water and in ethanol. The aqueous solution is dark blue; when acidified it becomes pink.

Dichlorophenolindophenol standard solution. *1027301.*

Dissolve 50.0 mg of *dichlorophenolindophenol, sodium salt R* in 100.0 ml of *water R* and filter.

Standardisation. Dissolve 20.0 mg of *ascorbic acid R* in 10 ml of a freshly prepared 200 g/l solution of *metaphosphoric acid R* and dilute to 250.0 ml with *water R*. Titrate 5.0 ml rapidly with the dichloro-phenolindophenol standard solution, added from a microburette graduated in 0.01 ml, until the pink colour persists for 10 s, the titration occupying not more than 2 min. Dilute the dichlorophenolindophenol solution with *water R* to make 1 ml of the solution equivalent to 0.1 mg of ascorbic acid ($C_6H_8O_6$).

Storage: use within 3 days.

Standardise immediately before use.

5,7-Dichloroquinolin-8-ol. $C_9H_5Cl_2NO$. (M_r 214.1). *1157000.* [773-76-2]. 5,7-Dichlorooxine.

Yellow, crystalline powder, soluble in acetone, slightly soluble in ethanol (96 per cent).

mp: about 179 °C.

Content: minimum 95.0 per cent of $C_9H_5Cl_2NO$.

Dichloroquinonechlorimide. $C_6H_2Cl_3NO$. (M_r 210.4). *1027400.* [101-38-2]. 2,6-Dichloro-*N*-chloro-1,4-benzoquinone mono-imine.

A pale yellow or greenish-yellow crystalline powder, practically insoluble in water, soluble in alcohol and in dilute alkaline solutions.

mp: about 66 °C.

Dichlorvos. $C_4H_7Cl_2O_4P$. (M_r 221). *1101200.* [62-73-7]. 2,2-Dichlorovinyl dimethyl phosphate.

Colourless or brownish-yellow liquid, soluble in water, miscible with most organic solvents.

n_D^{25}: about 1.452.

Dicyclohexyl. $C_{12}H_{22}$. (M_r 166.3). *1135300.* [92-51-3]. Bicyclohexyl.

d_{20}^{20}: about 0.864.

bp: about 227 °C.

mp: about 4 °C.

Dicyclohexylamine. $C_{12}H_{23}N$. (M_r 181.3). *1027500.* [101-83-7]. *N,N*-Dicyclohexylamine.

Colourless liquid, sparingly soluble in water, miscible with the usual organic solvents.

n_D^{20}: about 1.484.

bp: about 256 °C.

Freezing point (2.2.18): 0 °C to 1 °C.

Dicyclohexylurea. $C_{13}H_{24}N_2O$. (M_r 224.4). *1027600.* [2387-23-7]. 1,3-Dicyclohexylurea.

A white, crystalline powder.

mp: about 232 °C.

Didocosahexaenoin. $C_{47}H_{68}O_5$. (M_r 713.0). *1142700.* [88315-12-2]. Diglyceride of docosahexaenoic acid (C22:6). Glycerol didocosahexaenoate. (*all-Z*)-Docosahexaenoic acid, diester with propane-1,2,3-triol.

Didodecyl 3,3′-thiodipropionate. $C_{30}H_{58}O_4S$. (M_r 514.8). *1027700.* [123-28-4].

A white, crystalline powder, practically insoluble in water, freely soluble in acetone and in light petroleum, slightly soluble in alcohol.

mp: about 39 °C.

Dieldrin. $C_{12}H_8Cl_6O$. (M_r 380.9). *1126200.* [60-57-1].

bp: about 385 °C.

mp: about 176 °C.

A suitable certified reference solution (10 ng/μl in cyclohexane) may be used.

Diethanolamine. $C_4H_{11}NO_2$. (M_r 105.1). *1027800.* [111-42-2]. 2,2′-Iminobisethanol.

A viscous, clear, slightly yellow liquid or deliquescent crystals melting at about 28 °C, very soluble in water, in acetone and in methanol.

d_{20}^{20}: about 1.09.

pH (2.2.3): 10.0 to 11.5 for a 50 g/l solution.

Diethanolamine used in the test for alkaline phosphatase complies with the following additional test.

Ethanolamine: maximum 1.0 per cent. Examine by gas chromatography (*2.2.28*), using *3-aminopropanol R* as the internal standard.

Internal standard solution. Dissolve 1.00 g of *3-aminopropanol R* in *acetone R* and dilute to 10.0 ml with the same solvent.

4. Reagents

Test solution (a). Dissolve 5.00 g of the substance to be examined in *acetone R* and dilute to 10.0 ml with the same solvent.

Test solution (b). Dissolve 5.00 g of the substance to be examined in *acetone R*, add 1.0 ml of the internal standard solution and dilute to 10.0 ml with the same solvent.

Reference solutions. Dissolve 0.50 g of *ethanolamine R* in *acetone R* and dilute to 10.0 ml with the same solvent. To 0.5 ml, 1.0 ml and 2.0 ml of this solution, add 1.0 ml of the internal standard solution and dilute to 10.0 ml with *acetone R*.

The chromatographic procedure may be carried out using:

- a column 1 m long and 4 mm in internal diameter packed with *diphenylphenylene oxide polymer R* (180 μm to 250 μm),
- *nitrogen for chromatography R* as the carrier gas at a flow rate of 40 ml/min,
- a flame-ionisation detector.

Maintain the temperature of the column at 125 °C for 3 min and then raise to 300 °C at a rate of 12 °C/min. Maintain the temperature of the injection port at 250 °C and that of the detector at 280 °C. Inject 1.0 μl of each test solution and 1.0 μl of each reference solution.

Storage: in an airtight container.

Diethoxytetrahydrofuran. $C_8H_{16}O_3$. (M_r 160.2). *1027900.* [3320-90-9]. 2,5-Diethoxytetrahydrofuran. A mixture of the *cis* and *trans* isomers.

A clear, colourless or slightly yellowish liquid, practically insoluble in water, soluble in alcohol and in most other organic solvents.

d_{20}^{20}: about 0.98.

n_D^{20}: about 1.418.

Diethylamine. $C_4H_{11}N$. (M_r 73.1). *1028000.* [109-89-7].

A clear, colourless, flammable liquid, strongly alkaline, miscible with water and with alcohol.

d_{20}^{20}: about 0.71.

bp: about 55 °C.

Diethylaminoethyldextran. *1028200.*

Anion exchange resin presented as the hydrochloride.

A powder forming gels with water.

***N,N*-Diethylaniline.** $C_{10}H_{15}N$. (M_r 149.2). *1028400.* [91-66-7].

d_{20}^{20}: about 0.938.

bp: about 217 °C.

mp: about −38 °C.

Diethylene glycol. $C_4H_{10}O_3$. (M_r 106.1). *1028300.* [111-46-6]. 2,2′-Oxydiethanol.

Content: minimum 99.5 per cent *m/m* of $C_4H_{10}O_3$.

A clear, colourless liquid, hygroscopic, miscible with water, with acetone and with alcohol.

d_{20}^{20}: about 1.118.

n_D^{20}: about 1.447.

bp: 244 °C to 246 °C.

Storage: in an airtight container.

***N,N*-Diethylethane-1,2-diamine.** *1028500.* [100-36-7].

See *N,N-diethylethylenediamine R.*

***N,N*-Diethylethylenediamine.** $C_6H_{16}N_2$. (M_r 116.2). *1028500.* [100-36-7].

Content: minimum 98.0 per cent of $C_6H_{16}N_2$.

A slightly oily liquid, colourless or slightly yellow, strong odour of ammonia, irritant to the skin, eyes and mucous membranes.

d_{20}^{20}: 0.827.

bp: 145 °C to 147 °C.

Water (2.5.12): maximum 1.0 per cent, determined on 0.500 g.

Di(2-ethylhexyl) phthalate. $C_{24}H_{38}O_4$. (M_r 390.5). *1028100.* Di(2-ethylhexyl) benzene-1,2-dicarboxylate.

A colourless, oily liquid, practically insoluble in water, soluble in organic solvents.

d_{20}^{20}: about 0.98.

n_D^{20}: about 1.486.

Viscosity (2.2.9): about 80 mPa·s.

Diethylphenylenediamine sulphate. $C_{10}H_{18}N_2O_4S$. (M_r 262.3). *1028600.* [6283-63-2]. *N,N′*-Diethyl-*p*-phenylenediamine sulphate. *N,N′*-Diethylbenzene-1,4-diamine sulphate.

A white or slightly yellow powder, soluble in water.

mp: about 185 °C, with decomposition.

Storage: protected from light.

Diethylphenylenediamine sulphate solution. *1028601.*

To 250 ml of *water R* add 2 ml of *sulphuric acid R* and 25 ml of *0.02 M sodium edetate*. Dissolve in this solution 1.1 g of *diethylphenylenediamine sulphate R* and dilute to 1000 ml with *water R*.

Do not use if the solution is not colourless.

Storage: protected from light and heat for 1 month.

Digitonin. $C_{56}H_{92}O_{29}$. (M_r 1229). *1028700.* [11024-24-1]. 3β-[*O*-β-D-Glucopyranosyl-(1→3)-*O*-β-D-galactopyranosyl-(1→2)-*O*-[β-D-xylopyranosyl-(1→3)]-*O*-β-D-galactopyranosyl-(1→4)-*O*-β-D-galactopyranosyloxy]-(25*R*)-5α-spirostan-2α, 15β-diol.

Crystals, practically insoluble in water, sparingly soluble in ethanol, slightly soluble in alcohol.

Digitoxin. *1028800.* [71-63-6].

See *Digitoxin (0078).*

Diammonium 2,2′-azinobis(3-ethylbenzothiazoline-6-sulphonate). $C_{18}H_{24}N_6O_6S_4$. (M_r 548.7). *1153000.* [30931-67-0]. ABTS. Diammonium 2,2′-(diazanediylidene)bis[3-ethyl-2,3-dihydrobenzothiazole-6-sulphonate].

Chromogenic substrate suitable for use in ELISA procedures.

Green tablets, freely soluble in water.

pH *(2.2.3)*: 4.2 to 5.8 for a 0.1 g/l solution.

Dihydrocapsaicin. $C_{18}H_{29}NO_3$. (M_r 307.4). *1148100.* [19408-84-5]. *N*-[(4-Hydroxy-3-methoxyphenyl)methyl]-8-methylnonanamide.

White, crystalline powder, practically insoluble in cold water, freely soluble in ethanol.

10,11-Dihydrocarbamazepine. $C_{15}H_{14}N_2O$. (M_r 238.3). *1028900.* [3564-73-6]. 10,11-Dihydro-5*H*-dibenzo[*b,f*]azepine-5-carboxamide.

mp: 205 °C to 210 °C.

2,5-Dihydroxybenzoic acid. $C_7H_6O_4$. (M_r 154.1). *1148200.* [490-79-9]. Gentisic acid.

Light yellow crystals.

mp: about 200 °C.

5,7-Dihydroxy-4-methylcoumarin. $C_{10}H_8O_4$. (M_r 192.2). *1149400.* [2107-76-8]. 5,7-Dihydroxy-4-methyl-2*H*-1-benzopyran-2-one.

Light yellowish powder, practically insoluble in water, sparingly soluble in alcohol.

mp: 295 °C to 303 °C.

Dihydroxynaphthalene. *1029000.* [132-86-5].

See *1,3-dihydroxynaphthalene R.*

1,3-Dihydroxynaphthalene. $C_{10}H_8O_2$. (M_r 160.2). *1029000.* [132-86-5]. Naphthalene-1,3-diol.

A crystalline, generally brownish-violet powder, freely soluble in water and in alcohol.

mp: about 125 °C.

2,7-Dihydroxynaphthalene. $C_{10}H_8O_2$. (M_r 160.2). *1029100.* [582-17-2]. Naphthalene-2,7-diol.

Needles, soluble in water and in alcohol.

mp: about 190 °C.

2,7-Dihydroxynaphthalene solution. *1029101.*

Dissolve 10 mg of *2,7-dihydroxynaphthalene R* in 100 ml of *sulphuric acid R* and allow to stand until decolorised.

Storage: use within 2 days.

5,7-Diiodoquinolin-8-ol. $C_9H_5I_2NO$. (M_r 397.0). *1157100.* [83-73-8]. 5,7-Diiodooxine.

Yellowish-brown powder, sparingly soluble in acetone and in ethanol (96 per cent).

Content: minimum 95.0 per cent of $C_9H_5I_2NO$.

Di-isobutyl ketone. $C_9H_{18}O$. (M_r 142.2). *1029200.* [108-83-8].

A clear, colourless liquid, slightly soluble in water, miscible with most organic solvents.

n_D^{20}: about 1.414

bp: about 168 °C.

Di-isopropyl ether. $C_6H_{14}O$. (M_r 102.2). *1029300.* [108-20-3].

A clear, colourless liquid, very slightly soluble in water, miscible with alcohol.

d_{20}^{20}: 0.723 to 0.728.

bp: 67 °C to 69 °C.

Do not distil if the di-isopropyl ether does not comply with the test for peroxides.

Peroxides. Place 8 ml of *potassium iodide and starch solution R* in a 12 ml ground-glass-stoppered cylinder about 1.5 cm in diameter. Fill completely with the substance to be examined, shake vigorously and allow to stand protected from light for 30 min. No colour is produced.

The name and concentration of any added stabiliser are stated on the label.

Storage: protected from light.

***N,N'*-Diisopropylethylenediamine.** $C_8H_{20}N_2$. (M_r 144.3). *1140600.* [4013-94-9]. *N,N'*-bis(1-Methylethyl)-1,2-ethanediamine.

Colourless to yellowish, corrosive, flammable, hygroscopic liquid.

d_{20}^{20}: about 0.798.

n_D^{20}: about 1.429.

bp: about 170 °C.

4,4'-Dimethoxybenzophenone. $C_{15}H_{14}O_3$. (M_r 242.3). *1126300.* [90-96-0]. bis(4-Methoxyphenyl)methanone.

A white powder, practically insoluble in water and slightly soluble in alcohol.

mp: about 142 °C.

Dimethoxypropane. $C_5H_{12}O_2$. (M_r 104.1). *1105200.* [77-76-9]. 2,2-Dimethoxypropane.

A colourless liquid, decomposing on exposure to moist air or water.

d_{20}^{20}: about 0.847.

n_D^{20}: about 1.378.

bp: about 83 °C.

Dimethylacetamide. C_4H_9NO. (M_r 87.1). *1029700.* [127-19-5]. *N,N*-Dimethylacetamide.

Content: minimum 99.5 per cent of C_4H_9NO.

A colourless liquid, miscible with water and with many organic solvents.

d_{20}^{20}: about 0.94.

n_D^{20}: about 1.437.

bp: about 165 °C.

Dimethylaminobenzaldehyde. $C_9H_{11}NO$. (M_r 149.2). *1029800.* [100-10-7]. 4-Dimethylaminobenzaldehyde.

White or yellowish-white crystals, soluble in alcohol and in dilute acids.

mp: about 74 °C.

Dimethylaminobenzaldehyde solution R1. *1029801.*

Dissolve 0.2 g of *dimethylaminobenzaldehyde R* in 20 ml of *alcohol R* and add 0.5 ml of *hydrochloric acid R.* Shake the solution with *activated charcoal R* and filter. The colour of the reagent is less intense than that of *iodine solution R3.* Prepare immediately before use.

Dimethylaminobenzaldehyde solution R2. *1029802.*

Dissolve 0.2 g of *dimethylaminobenzaldehyde R,* without heating, in a mixture of 4.5 ml of *water R* and 5.5 ml of *hydrochloric acid R.* Prepare immediately before use.

Dimethylaminobenzaldehyde solution R6. *1029803.*

Dissolve 0.125 g of *dimethylaminobenzaldehyde R* in a cooled mixture of 35 ml of *water R* and 65 ml of *sulphuric acid R.* Add 0.1 ml of a 50 g/l solution of *ferric chloride R.* Before use allow to stand for 24 h, protected from light.

Storage: when stored at room temperature it must be used within 1 week; when kept in a refrigerator, it may be stored for several months.

Dimethylaminobenzaldehyde solution R7. *1029804.*

Dissolve 1.0 g of *dimethylaminobenzaldehyde R* in 50 ml of *hydrochloric acid R* and add 50 ml of *alcohol R.*

Storage: protected from light; use within 4 weeks.

Dimethylaminobenzaldehyde solution R8. *1029805.*

Dissolve 0.25 g of *dimethylaminobenzaldehyde R* in a mixture of 5 g of *phosphoric acid R,* 45 g of *water R* and 50 g of *anhydrous acetic acid R.* Prepare immediately before use.

4-Dimethylaminocinnamaldehyde. $C_{11}H_{13}NO$. (M_r 175.2). *1029900.* [6203-18-5]. 3-(4-Dimethylaminophenyl)prop-2-enal.

Orange to orange-brown crystals or powder. Sensitive to light.

mp: about 138 °C.

4-Dimethylaminocinnamaldehyde solution. *1029901.*

Dissolve 2 g of *4-dimethylaminocinnamaldehyde R* in a mixture of 100 ml of *hydrochloric acid R1* and 100 ml of *ethanol R.* Dilute the solution to four times its volume with *ethanol R* immediately before use.

2-(Dimethylamino)ethyl methacrylate. $C_8H_{15}NO_2$. (M_r 157.2). *1147200*. [2867-47-2]. 2-(Dimethylamino)ethyl 2-methylpropenoate.

d_4^{20}: about 0.930.

bp: about 187 °C.

Dimethylaminonaphthalenesulphonyl chloride. $C_{12}H_{12}ClNO_2S$. (M_r 269.8). *1030000*. [605-65-2]. 5-Dimethyl-amino-1-naphthalenesulphonyl chloride.

A yellow, crystalline powder, slightly soluble in water, soluble in methanol.

mp: about 70 °C.

3-Dimethylaminophenol. $C_8H_{11}NO$. (M_r 137.2). *1156500*. [99-07-0]. 3-(Dimethylamino)phenol.

Grey powder, slightly soluble in water.

mp: about 80 °C.

Dimethylaniline. $C_8H_{11}N$. (M_r 121.2). *1030100*. [121-69-7]. *N,N*-Dimethylaniline.

A clear, oily liquid, almost colourless when freshly distilled, darkening on storage to reddish-brown, practically insoluble in water, freely soluble in alcohol.

n_D^{20}: about 1.558.

Distillation range (*2.2.11*). Not less than 95 per cent distils between 192 °C and 194 °C.

***N,N*-Dimethylaniline.** *1030100*. [121-69-7].

See *Dimethylaniline R*.

2,3-Dimethylaniline. $C_8H_{11}N$. (M_r 121.2). *1105300*. [87-59-2]. 2,3-Xylidine.

A yellowish liquid, sparingly soluble in water, soluble in alcohol.

d_{20}^{20}: 0.993 to 0.995.

n_D^{20}: about 1.569.

bp: about 224 °C.

2,6-Dimethylaniline. $C_8H_{11}N$. (M_r 121.2). *1030200*. [87-62-7]. 2,6-Xylidine.

A colourless liquid, sparingly soluble in water, soluble in alcohol.

d_{20}^{20}: about 0.98.

2,4-Dimethyl-6-*tert*-butylphenol. $C_{12}H_{18}O$. (M_r 178.3). *1126500*. [1879-09-0].

Dimethyl carbonate. $C_3H_6O_3$. (M_r 90.1). *1119300*. [616-38-6]. Carbonic acid dimethyl ester.

Liquid, insoluble in water, miscible with alcohol.

d_4^{17}: 1.065.

n_D^{20}: 1.368.

bp: about 90 °C.

Dimethyldecylamine. $C_{12}H_{27}N$. (M_r 185.4). *1113500*. [1120-24-7]. *N,N*-dimethyldecylamine.

Content: minimum 98.0 per cent *m/m* of $C_{12}H_{27}N$.

bp: about 234 °C.

1,1-Dimethylethylamine. $C_4H_{11}N$. (M_r 73.1). *1100900*. [75-64-9]. 2-Amino-2-methylpropane. *tert*-Butylamine.

Liquid, miscible with alcohol.

d_{20}^{20}: about 0.694.

n_D^{20}: about 1.378.

bp: about 46 °C.

1,1-Dimethylethyl methyl ether. $C_5H_{12}O$. (M_r 88.1). *1013900*. [1634-04-4]. 2-Methoxy-2-methylpropane. *tert*-Butyl methyl ether.

A colourless, clear, flammable liquid.

n_D^{20}: about 1.376.

Minimum transmittance (*2.2.25*), determined using *water R* as compensation liquid: 50 per cent at 240 nm, 80 per cent at 255 nm, 98 per cent at 280 nm.

1,1-Dimethylethyl methyl ether R1. *1126400*.

Content: minimum 99.5 per cent of $C_5H_{12}O$.

d_{20}^{20}: about 0.741.

n_D^{20}: about 1.369.

bp: about 55 °C.

Dimethylformamide. C_3H_7NO. (M_r 73.1). *1030300*. [68-12-2].

A clear, colourless neutral liquid, miscible with water and with alcohol.

d_{20}^{20}: 0.949 to 0.952.

bp: about 153 °C.

Water (*2.5.12*): maximum 0.1 per cent.

Dimethylformamide diethylacetal. $C_7H_{17}NO_2$. (M_r 147.2). *1113600*. [1188-33-6]. *N,N*-Dimethylformamide diethylacetal.

n_D^{20}: about 1.40.

bp: 128 °C to 130 °C.

***N,N*-Dimethylformamide dimethylacetal.** $C_5H_{13}NO_2$. (M_r 119.2). *1140700*. [4637-24-5]. 1,1-Dimethoxytrimethylamine.

Clear, colourless liquid.

d_{20}^{20}: about 0.896.

n_D^{20}: about 1.396.

bp: about 103 °C.

Dimethylglyoxime. $C_4H_8N_2O_2$. (M_r 116.1). *1030400*. [95-45-4]. 2,3-Butanedione dioxime.

A white, crystalline powder or colourless crystals, practically insoluble in cold water, very slightly soluble in boiling water, soluble in alcohol.

mp: about 240 °C, with decomposition.

Sulphated ash (*2.4.14*): maximum 0.05 per cent.

1,3-Dimethyl-2-imidazolidinone. $C_5H_{10}N_2O$. (M_r 114.2). *1135400*. [80-73-9]. *N,N'*-Dimethylethylene urea. 1,3-Dimethyl-2-imidazolidone.

n_D^{20}: 1.4720.

bp: about 224 °C.

***N,N*-Dimethyloctylamine.** $C_{10}H_{23}N$. (M_r 157.3). *1030500*. [7378-99-6]. Octyldimethylamine.

Colourless liquid.

d_{20}^{20}: about 0.765.

n_D^{20}: about 1.424.

bp: about 195 °C.

2,6-Dimethylphenol. $C_8H_{10}O$. (M_r 122.2). *1030600*. [576-26-1].

Colourless needles, slightly soluble in water, very soluble in alcohol.

bp: about 203 °C.

mp: 46 °C to 48 °C.

3,4-Dimethylphenol. $C_8H_{10}O$. (M_r 122.2). *1098100.* [95-65-8].

White or almost white crystals, slightly soluble in water, freely soluble in alcohol.

bp: about 226 °C.

mp: 25 °C to 27 °C.

Dimethylpiperazine. $C_6H_{14}N_2$. (M_r 114.2). *1030700.* [106-58-1]. 1,4-Dimethylpiperazine.

A colourless liquid, miscible with water and with alcohol.

d_{20}^{20}: about 0.85.

n_D^{20}: about 1.446.

bp: about 131 °C.

Dimethylstearamide. $C_{20}H_{41}NO$. (M_r 311.6). *1030800.* *N,N*-Dimethylstearamide.

A white or almost white solid mass, soluble in many organic solvents, including acetone.

mp: about 51 °C.

Dimethylstearylamide. *1030800.*

See *dimethylstearamide R.*

Dimethyl sulphone. $C_2H_6O_2S$. (M_r 94.1). *1030900.* [67-71-0].

A white, crystalline powder, freely soluble in water, soluble in acetone and alcohol.

mp: 108 °C to 110 °C.

Dimethyl sulphoxide. *1029500.* [67-68-5].

See *Dimethyl sulphoxide (0763).*

Dimethyl sulphoxide used in spectrophotometry complies with the following additional test.

Minimum transmittance (2.2.25), determined using *water R* as compensation liquid: 10 per cent at 262 nm, 35 per cent at 270 nm, 70 per cent at 290 nm, 98 per cent at 340 nm and at higher wavelengths.

Dimethyl sulphoxide R1. *1029501.*

Content: minimum 99.7 per cent of C_2H_6OS, determined by gas chromatography.

Dimeticone. *1105400.* [9016-00-6].

See *Dimeticone (0138).*

Dimidium bromide. $C_{20}H_{18}BrN_3$. (M_r 380.3). *1031100.* [518-67-2]. 3,8-Diamino-5-methyl-6-phenylphenanthridinium bromide.

Dark-red crystals, slightly soluble in water at 20 °C, sparingly soluble in water at 60 °C and in alcohol.

Dimidium bromide-sulphan blue mixed solution. *1031101.*

Dissolve separately 0.5 g of *dimidium bromide R* and 0.25 g of *sulphan blue R* in 30 ml of a hot mixture of 1 volume of *ethanol R* and 9 volumes of *water R*, stir, mix the two solutions, and dilute to 250 ml with the same mixture of solvents. Mix 20 ml of this solution with 20 ml of a 14.0 per cent *V/V* solution of *sulphuric acid R* previously diluted with about 250 ml of *water R* and dilute to 500 ml with *water R.*

Storage: protected from light.

Dinitrobenzene. $C_6H_4N_2O_4$. (M_r 168.1). *1031200.* [528-29-0]. 1,3-Dinitrobenzene.

Yellowish crystalline powder or crystals, practically insoluble in water, slightly soluble in alcohol.

mp: about 90 °C.

Dinitrobenzene solution. *1031201.*

A 10 g/l solution in *alcohol R.*

Dinitrobenzoic acid. $C_7H_4N_2O_6$. (M_r 212.1). *1031300.* [99-34-3]. 3,5-Dinitrobenzoic acid.

Almost colourless crystals, slightly soluble in water, very soluble in alcohol.

mp: about 206 °C.

Dinitrobenzoic acid solution. *1031301.*

A 20 g/l solution in *alcohol R.*

Dinitrobenzoyl chloride. $C_7H_3ClN_2O_5$. (M_r 230.6). *1031400.* [99-33-2]. 3,5-Dinitrobenzoyl chloride.

Translucent, yellow or greenish-yellow powder or yellowish crystals, soluble in acetone and in toluene.

mp: about 68 °C.

Suitability test. To 1 ml of *ethanol R* and 0.1 g of *dinitrobenzoyl chloride R* add 0.05 ml of *dilute sulphuric acid R* and boil under a reflux condenser for 30 min. After evaporation on a water-bath add 5 ml of *heptane R* to the residue and heat to boiling. Filter the hot solution. Wash the crystals formed on cooling to room temperature with a small quantity of *heptane R* and dry in a desiccator. The crystals melt *(2.2.14)* at 94 °C to 95 °C.

Dinitrophenylhydrazine. $C_6H_6N_4O_4$. (M_r 198.1). *1031500.* [119-26-6]. 2,4-Dinitrophenylhydrazine.

Reddish-orange crystals, very slightly soluble in water, slightly soluble in alcohol.

mp: about 203 °C (instantaneous method).

Dinitrophenylhydrazine-aceto-hydrochloric solution. *1031501.*

Dissolve 0.2 g of *dinitrophenylhydrazine R* in 20 ml of *methanol R* and add 80 ml of a mixture of equal volumes of *acetic acid R* and *hydrochloric acid R1.* Prepare immediately before use.

Dinitrophenylhydrazine-hydrochloric solution. *1031502.*

Dissolve by heating 0.50 g of *dinitrophenylhydrazine R* in *dilute hydrochloric acid R* and complete to 100 ml with the same solvent. Allow to cool and filter. Prepare immediately before use.

Dinitrophenylhydrazine-sulphuric acid solution. *1031503.*

Dissolve 1.5 g of *dinitrophenylhydrazine R* in 50 ml of a 20 per cent *V/V* solution of *sulphuric acid R.* Prepare immediately before use.

Dinonyl phthalate. $C_{26}H_{42}O_4$. (M_r 418.6). *1031600.* [28553-12-0].

A colourless to pale yellow, viscous liquid.

d_{20}^{20}: 0.97 to 0.98.

n_D^{20}: 1.482 to 1.489.

Acidity. Shake 5.0 g with 25 ml of *water R* for 1 min. Allow to stand, filter the separated aqueous layer and add 0.1 ml of *phenolphthalein solution R.* Not more than 0.3 ml of *0.1 M sodium hydroxide* is required to change the colour of the solution (0.05 per cent, calculated as phthalic acid).

Water (2.5.12): maximum 0.1 per cent.

Dioctadecyl disulphide. $C_{36}H_{74}S_2$. (M_r 571.1). *1031700.* [1844-09-3].

A white powder, practically insoluble in water.

mp: 53 °C to 58 °C.

4. Reagents

2,2′-Di(octadecyloxy)-5,5′-spirobi(1,3,2-dioxaphosphorinane). $C_{41}H_{82}O_6P_2$. (M_r 733). *1031800.*

White, waxy solid, practically insoluble in water, soluble in hydrocarbons.

mp: 40 °C to 70 °C.

Dioctadecyl 3,3′-thiodipropionate. $C_{42}H_{82}O_4S$. (M_r 683). *1031900.* [693-36-7].

A white, crystalline powder, practically insoluble in water, freely soluble in methylene chloride, sparingly soluble in acetone, in alcohol and in light petroleum.

mp: 58 °C to 67 °C.

Dioxan. $C_4H_8O_2$. (M_r 88.1). *1032000.* [123-91-1]. 1,4-Dioxan.

A clear, colourless liquid, miscible with water and with most organic solvents.

d_{20}^{20}: about 1.03.

Freezing-point (2.2.18): 9 °C to 11 °C.

Water (2.5.12): maximum 0.5 per cent.

Do not distil if the dioxan does not comply with the test for peroxides.

Peroxides. Place 8 ml of *potassium iodide and starch solution R* in a 12 ml ground-glass-stoppered cylinder about 1.5 cm in diameter. Fill completely with the substance to be examined, shake vigorously and allow to stand in the dark for 30 min. No colour is produced.

Dioxan used for liquid scintillation is of a suitable analytical grade.

Dioxan solution. *1032002.*

Dilute 50.0 ml of *dioxan stock solution R* to 100.0 ml with *water R*. (0.5 mg/ml of dioxan).

Dioxan solution R1. *1032003.*

Dilute 10.0 ml of *dioxan solution R* to 50.0 ml with *water R*. (0.1 mg/ml of dioxan).

Dioxan stock solution. *1032001.*

Dissolve 1.00 g of *dioxan R* in *water R* and dilute to 100.0 ml with the same solvent. Dilute 5.0 ml of this solution to 50.0 ml with *water R* (1.0 mg/ml).

Diphenylamine. $C_{12}H_{11}N$. (M_r 169.2). *1032100.* [122-39-4].

White crystals, slightly soluble in water, soluble in alcohol.

mp: about 55 °C.

Storage: protected from light.

Diphenylamine solution. *1032101.*

A 1 g/l solution in *sulphuric acid R*.

Storage: protected from light.

Diphenylamine solution R1. *1032102.*

A 10 g/l solution in *sulphuric acid R*. The solution is colourless.

Diphenylamine solution R2. *1032103.*

Dissolve 1 g of *diphenylamine R* in 100 ml of *glacial acetic acid R* and add 2.75 ml of *sulphuric acid R*. Use immediately.

Diphenylanthracene. $C_{26}H_{18}$. (M_r 330.4). *1032200.* [1499-10-1]. 9,10-Diphenylanthracene.

Yellowish to yellow, crystalline powder, practically insoluble in water.

mp: about 248 °C.

Diphenylbenzidine. $C_{24}H_{20}N_2$. (M_r 336.4). *1032300.* [531-91-9]. *N,N′*-Diphenylbenzidine. *N,N′*-Diphenylbiphenyl-4,4′-diamine.

A white or faintly grey, crystalline powder, practically insoluble in water, slightly soluble in acetone and in alcohol.

mp: about 248 °C.

Nitrates. Dissolve 8 mg in a cooled mixture of 5 ml of *water R* and 45 ml of *nitrogen-free sulphuric acid R*. The solution is colourless or very pale blue.

Sulphated ash (2.4.14): maximum 0.1 per cent.

Storage: protected from light.

Diphenylboric acid aminoethyl ester. $C_{14}H_{16}BNO$. (M_r 225.1). *1032400.* [524-95-8].

A white or slightly yellow, crystalline powder, practically insoluble in water, soluble in alcohol.

mp: about 193 °C.

Diphenylcarbazide. $C_{13}H_{14}N_4O$. (M_r 242.3). *1032500.* [140-22-7]. 1,5-Diphenylcarbonodihydrazide.

A white, crystalline powder which gradually becomes pink on exposure to air, very slightly soluble in water, soluble in acetone, in alcohol and in glacial acetic acid.

mp: about 170 °C.

Sulphated ash (2.4.14): maximum 0.1 per cent.

Storage: protected from light.

Diphenylcarbazide solution. *1032501.*

Dissolve 0.2 g of *diphenylcarbazide R* in 10 ml of *glacial acetic acid R* and dilute to 100 ml with *ethanol R*. Prepare immediately before use.

Diphenylcarbazone. $C_{13}H_{12}N_4O$. (M_r 240.3). *1032600.* [538-62-5]. 1,5-Diphenylcarbazone.

An orange-yellow, crystalline powder, practically insoluble in water, freely soluble in alcohol.

mp: about 157 °C, with decomposition.

Diphenylcarbazone mercuric reagent. *1032601.*

Solution I. Dissolve 0.1 g of *diphenylcarbazone R* in *ethanol R* and dilute to 50 ml with the same solvent.

Solution II. Dissolve 1 g of *mercuric chloride R* in *ethanol R* and dilute to 50 ml with the same solvent.

Mix equal volumes of the two solutions.

1,2-Diphenylhydrazine. $C_{12}H_{12}N_2$. (M_r 184.3). *1140800.* [122-66-7]. Hydrazobenzene. 1,2-Diphenyldiazane.

Orange powder.

mp: about 125 °C.

Diphenylmethanol. $C_{13}H_{12}O$. (M_r 184.2). *1145700.* [91-01-0]. Benzhydrol.

A white, crystalline powder.

mp: about 66 °C.

Diphenyloxazole. $C_{15}H_{11}NO$. (M_r 221.3). *1032700.* [92-71-7]. 2,5-Diphenyloxazole.

A white powder, practically insoluble in water, soluble in methanol, sparingly soluble in dioxan and in glacial acetic acid.

mp: about 70 °C.

$A_{1\,cm}^{1\%}$: about 1260 determined at 305 nm in *methanol R*.

Diphenyloxazole used for liquid scintillation is of a suitable analytical grade.

Diphenylphenylene oxide polymer. *1032800.* 2,6-Diphenyl-*p*-phenylene oxide polymer.

White or almost white, porous beads. The size range of the beads is specified after the name of the reagent in the tests where it is used.

Diphosphorus pentoxide. P_2O_5. (M_r 141.9). *1032900.* [1314-56-3]. Phosphorus pentoxide. Phosphoric anhydride.

A white powder, amorphous, deliquescent. It is hydrated by water with the evolution of heat.

Storage: in an airtight container.

Dipotassium hydrogen phosphate. K_2HPO_4. (M_r 174.2). *1033000.* [7758-11-4].

A white, crystalline powder, hygroscopic, very soluble in water, slightly soluble in alcohol.

Storage: in an airtight container.

Dipotassium sulphate. K_2SO_4. (M_r 174.3). *1033100.* [7778-80-5].

Colourless crystals, soluble in water.

Disodium arsenate. $Na_2HAsO_4,7H_2O$. (M_r 312.0). *1102500.* [10048-95-0]. Disodium hydrogen arsenate heptahydrate. Dibasic sodium arsenate.

Crystals, efflorescent in warm air, freely soluble in water, soluble in glycerol, slightly soluble in alcohol. The aqueous solution is alcaline to litmus.

d_{20}^{20}: about 1.87.

mp: about 57 °C when rapidly heated.

Disodium bicinchoninate. $C_{20}H_{10}N_2Na_2O_4$. (M_r 388.3). *1126600.* [979-88-4]. Disodium 2,2′-biquinoline-4-4′-dicarboxylate.

Disodium hydrogen citrate. $C_6H_6Na_2O_7,1^1/_2H_2O$. (M_r 263.1). *1033200.* [144-33-2]. Sodium acid citrate. Disodium hydrogen 2-hydroxypropane-1,2,3-tricarboxylate sesquihydrate.

A white powder, soluble in less than 2 parts of water, practically insoluble in alcohol.

Disodium hydrogen phosphate. *1033300.* [10039-32-4].

See *Disodium phosphate dodecahydrate (0118).*

Disodium hydrogen phosphate solution. *1033301.*

A 90 g/l solution.

Disodium hydrogen phosphate, anhydrous. Na_2HPO_4. (M_r 142.0). *1033400.* [7558-79-4].

Disodium hydrogen phosphate dihydrate. *1033500.* [10028-24-7].

See *Disodium phosphate dihydrate (0602).*

Disodium tetraborate. *1033600.* [1303-96-4].

See *Borax (0013).*

Borate solution. *1033601.*

Dissolve 9.55 g of *disodium tetraborate R* in *sulphuric acid R,* heating on a water-bath, and dilute to 1 litre with the same acid.

Ditalimphos. $C_{12}H_{14}NO_4PS$. (M_r 299.3). *1126700.* [5131-24-8]. *O,O*-Diethyl (1,3-dihydro-1,3-dioxo-2*H*-isoindol-2-yl)phosphonothioate.

Very slightly soluble in water, in ethyl acetate and in ethanol.

A suitable certified reference solution may be used.

5,5′-Dithiobis(2-nitrobenzoic acid). $C_{14}H_8N_2O_8S_2$. (M_r 396.4). *1097300.* [69-78-3]. 3-Carboxy-4-nitrophenyldisulphide. Ellman's reagent. DTNB.

Yellow powder sparingly soluble in alcohol.

mp: about 242 °C.

Dithiol. $C_7H_8S_2$. (M_r 156.3). *1033800.* [496-74-2]. Toluene-3,4-dithiol. 4-Methylbenzene-1,2-dithiol.

White crystals, hygroscopic, soluble in methanol and in solutions of alkali hydroxides.

mp: about 30 °C.

Storage: in an airtight container.

Dithiol reagent. *1033801.*

To 1 g of *dithiol R* add 2 ml of *thioglycollic acid R* and dilute to 250 ml with a 20 g/l solution of *sodium hydroxide R.* Prepare immediately before use.

Dithiothreitol. $C_4H_{10}O_2S_2$. (M_r 154.2). *1098200.* [27565-41-9]. *threo*-1,4-Dimercaptobutane-2,3-diol.

Slightly hygroscopic needles, freely soluble in water, in acetone and in ethanol.

Storage: in an airtight container.

Dithizone. $C_{13}H_{12}N_4S$. (M_r 256.3). *1033900.* [60-10-6]. 1,5-Diphenylthiocarbazone.

A bluish-black, brownish-black or black powder, practically insoluble in water, soluble in alcohol.

Storage: protected from light.

Dithizone solution. *1033901.*

A 0.5 g/l solution in *chloroform R.* Prepare immediately before use.

Dithizone solution R2. *1033903.*

Dissolve 40.0 mg of *dithizone R* in *chloroform R* and dilute to 1000.0 ml with the same solvent. Dilute 30.0 ml of the solution to 100.0 ml with *chloroform R.*

Standardisation. Dissolve a quantity of *mercuric chloride R* equivalent to 0.1354 g of $HgCl_2$ in a mixture of equal volumes of *dilute sulphuric acid R* and *water R* and dilute to 100.0 ml with the same mixture of solvents. Dilute 2.0 ml of this solution to 100.0 ml with a mixture of equal volumes of *dilute sulphuric acid R* and *water R.* (This solution contains 20 ppm of Hg). Transfer 1.0 ml of the solution to a separating funnel and add 50 ml of *dilute sulphuric acid R,* 140 ml of *water R* and 10 ml of a 200 g/l solution of *hydroxylamine hydrochloride R.* Titrate with the dithizone solution; after each addition, shake the mixture twenty times and towards the end of the titration allow to separate and discard the chloroform layer. Titrate until a bluish-green colour is obtained. Calculate the equivalent in micrograms of mercury per millilitre of the dithizone solution from the expression $20/V$, where V is the volume in millilitres of the dithizone solution used in the titration.

Dithizone R1. $C_{13}H_{12}N_4S$. (M_r 256.3). *1105500.* [60-10-6]. 1,5-Diphenylthiocarbazone.

Content: minimum 98.0 per cent of $C_{13}H_{12}N_4S$.

A bluish-black, brownish-black or black powder, practically insoluble in water, soluble in alcohol.

Storage: protected from light.

Divanadium pentoxide. V_2O_5. (M_r 181.9). *1034000.* [1314-62-1]. Vanadic anhydride.

Content: minimum 98.5 per cent of V_2O_5.

A yellow-brown to rust-brown powder, slightly soluble in water, soluble in strong mineral acids and in solutions of alkali hydroxides with formation of salts.

Appearance of solution. Heat 1 g for 30 min with 10 ml of *sulphuric acid R.* Allow to cool and dilute to 10 ml with the same acid. The solution is clear (*2.2.1*).

Sensitivity to hydrogen peroxide. Dilute 1.0 ml of the solution prepared for the test for appearance of solution cautiously to 50.0 ml with *water R.* To 0.5 ml of the solution add 0.1 ml of a solution of *hydrogen peroxide R* (0.1 g/l of H_2O_2). The solution has a distinct orange colour compared with a blank prepared from 0.5 ml of the solution to be examined and 0.1 ml of *water R.* After the addition of 0.4 ml of hydrogen peroxide solution (0.1 g/l H_2O_2), the orange solution becomes orange-yellow.

Loss on ignition: maximum 1.0 per cent, determined on 1.00 g at 700 °C.

Assay. Dissolve 0.200 g with heating in 20 ml of a 70 per cent *m/m* solution of *sulphuric acid R.* Add 100 ml of *water R* and *0.02 M potassium permanganate* until a reddish colour is obtained. Decolorise the excess of potassium permanganate by the addition of a 30 g/l solution of *sodium nitrite R.* Add 5 g of *urea R* and 80 ml of a 70 per cent *m/m* solution of *sulphuric acid R.* Cool. Using 0.1 ml of *ferroin R* as indicator, titrate the solution immediately with *0.1 M ferrous sulphate* until a greenish-red colour is obtained.

1 ml of *0.1 M ferrous sulphate* is equivalent to 9.095 mg of V_2O_5.

Divanadium pentoxide solution in sulphuric acid. *1034001.*

Dissolve 0.2 g of *divanadium pentoxide R* in 4 ml of *sulphuric acid R* and dilute to 100 ml with *water R.*

Docosahexaenoic acid methyl ester. $C_{23}H_{34}O_2$. (M_r 342.5). *1142800.* [301-01-9]. DHA methyl ester. Cervonic acid methyl ester. (all-*Z*)-Docosa-4,7,10,13,16,19-hexaenoic acid methyl ester.

Content: minimum 90.0 per cent of $C_{23}H_{34}O_2$, determined by gas chromatography.

Docusate sodium. *1034100.* [577-11-7].

See *Docusate sodium (1418).*

Dodecyltrimethylammonium bromide. $C_{15}H_{34}BrN$. (M_r 308.4). *1135500.* [1119-94-4]. *N,N,N*-Trimethyldodecan-1-aminium bromide.

White crystals.

mp: about 246 °C.

Dotriacontane. $C_{32}H_{66}$. (M_r 450.9). *1034200.* [544-85-4]. *n*-Dotriacontane.

White plates, practically insoluble in water, sparingly soluble in hexane.

mp: about 69 °C.

Impurities. Not more than 0.1 per cent of impurities with the same t_R value as α-tocopherol acetate, determined by the gas chromatographic method prescribed in the monograph on *α-Tocopherol acetate (0439).*

Doxycycline. *1145800.*

See *Doxycycline monohydrate (0820).*

Electrolyte reagent for the micro determination of water. *1113700.*

Commercially available anhydrous reagent or a combination of anhydrous reagents for the coulometric titration of water, containing suitable organic bases, sulphur dioxide and iodide dissolved in a suitable solvent.

Elementary standard solution for atomic spectrometry (1.000 g/l). *5004000.*

This solution is prepared, generally in acid conditions, from the element or a salt of the element whose minimum content is not less than 99.0 per cent. The quantity per litre of solution is greater than 0.995 g throughout the guaranteed period, as long as the vial has not been opened. The starting material (element or salt) and the characteristics of the final solvent (nature and acidity, etc.) are mentioned on the label.

Emetine dihydrochloride. *1034300.* [316-42-7].

See *Emetine hydrochloride pentahydrate (0081).*

Emodin. $C_{15}H_{10}O_5$. (M_r 270.2). *1034400.* [518-82-1]. 1,3,8-Trihydroxy-6-methylanthraquinone.

Orange-red needles, practically insoluble in water, soluble in alcohol and in solutions of alkali hydroxides.

Chromatography. Examine as prescribed in the monograph on *Rhubarb (0291)*; the chromatogram shows only one principal spot.

α-Endosulphan. $C_9H_6Cl_6O_3S$. (M_r 406.9). *1126800.* [959-98-8].

bp: about 200 °C.

mp: about 108 °C.

A suitable certified reference solution (10 ng/μl in cyclohexane) may be used.

β-Endosulphan. $C_9H_6Cl_6O_3S$. (M_r 406.9). *1126900.* [33213-65-9].

bp: about 390 °C.

mp: about 207 °C.

A suitable certified reference solution (10 ng/μl in cyclohexane) may be used.

Endrin. $C_{12}H_8Cl_6O$. (M_r 380.9). *1127000.* [72-20-8].

A suitable certified reference solution (10 ng/μl in cyclohexane) may be used.

Erucamide. $C_{22}H_{43}NO$. (M_r 337.6). *1034500.* [112-84-5]. (*Z*)-Docos-13-enoamide.

Yellowish or white powder or granules, practically insoluble in water, very soluble in methylene chloride, soluble in ethanol.

mp: about 70 °C.

Erythritol. *1113800.* [149-32-6].

See *Erythritol (1803).*

Esculin. $C_{15}H_{16}O_9,1^1/_2H_2O$. ($M_r$ 367.3). *1119400.* [531-75-9]. 6-(β-D-Glucopyranosyloxy)-7-hydroxy-2*H*-chromen-2-one.

A white to almost white powder or colourless crystals, sparingly soluble in water and in alcohol, freely soluble in hot water and in hot alcohol.

Chromatography (*2.2.27*). Examine as prescribed in the monograph on *Eleutherococcus (1419).* The chromatogram shows only one principal spot.

Estradiol. $C_{18}H_{24}O_2$. (M_r 272.4). *1135600.* [50-28-2]. Estra-1,3,5(10)-triène-3,17β-diol. β-Estradiol.

Prisms stable in air, practically insoluble in water, freely soluble in alcohol, soluble in acetone and in dioxane, sparingly soluble in vegetable oils.

mp: 173 °C to 179 °C.

17α-Estradiol. $C_{18}H_{24}O_2$. (M_r 272.4). *1034600.* [57-91-0].

A white or almost white, crystalline powder or colourless crystals.

mp: 220 °C to 223 °C.

Estragole. $C_{10}H_{12}O$. (M_r 148.2). *1034700.* [140-67-0]. 1-Methoxy-4-prop-2-enylbenzene.

Liquid, miscible with alcohol.

n_D^{20}: about 1.52.

bp: about 216 °C.

Estragole used in gas chromatography complies with the following test.

Assay. Examine by gas chromatography (*2.2.28*) under the conditions described in the monograph on *Anise oil (0804)* using the substance to be examined as the test solution.

The area of the principal peak is not less than 98.0 per cent of the total area of the peaks.

Ethanol. *1034800.* [64-17-5].

See *Ethanol, anhydrous R.*

Ethanol, anhydrous. *1034800.* [64-17-5].

See *Ethanol, anhydrous (1318).*

Ethanol R1. *1034801.*

Complies with the requirements prescribed for the monograph *Ethanol, anhydrous (1318)* and with the following requirement.

Methanol: maximum 0.005 per cent *V/V*, determined by gas chromatography (*2.2.28*).

Test solution. Use the substance to be examined.

Reference solution. Dilute 0.50 ml of *anhydrous methanol R* to 100.0 ml with the substance to be examined. Dilute 1.0 ml of this solution to 100.0 ml with the substance to be examined.

The chromatographic procedure may be carried out using:

- a glass column 2 m long and 2 mm in internal diameter packed with *ethylvinylbenzene-divinyl-benzene copolymer R* (75 µm to 100 µm),
- *nitrogen for chromatography R* as the carrier gas at a flow rate of 30 ml/min,
- a flame-ionisation detector.

Maintain the temperature of the column at 130 °C, that of the injection port at 150 °C and that of the detector at 200 °C.

Inject 1 µl of the test solution and 1 µl of the reference solution, alternately, three times. After each chromatography, heat the column to 230 °C for 8 min. Integrate the methanol peak. Calculate the percentage methanol content from the expression:

$$\frac{a \times b}{c - b}$$

a = percentage *V/V* content of methanol in the reference solution,

b = area of the methanol peak in the chromatogram obtained with the test solution,

c = area of the methanol peak in the chromatogram obtained with the reference solution.

Ethanol (96 per cent). *1002500.* [64-17-5].

See *Ethanol (96 per cent) (1317).*

Ethanol (*x* per cent *V/V*). *1002502.*

Mix appropriate volumes of *water R* and *ethanol (96 per cent) R*, allowing for the effects of warming and volume contraction inherent to the preparation of such a mixture, to obtain a solution whose final content of ethanol corresponds to the value of *x*.

Ethanolamine. C_2H_7NO. (M_r 61.1). *1034900.* [141-43-5]. 2-Aminoethanol.

A clear, colourless, viscous, hygroscopic liquid, miscible with water and with methanol.

d_{20}^{20}: about 1.04.

n_D^{20}: about 1.454.

mp: about 11 °C.

Storage: in an airtight container.

Ether. $C_4H_{10}O$. (M_r 74.1). *1035000.* [60-29-7].

A clear, colourless, volatile and very mobile liquid, very flammable, hygroscopic, soluble in water, miscible with alcohol.

d_{20}^{20}: 0.713 to 0.715.

bp: 34 °C to 35 °C.

Do not distil if the ether does not comply with the test for peroxides.

Peroxides. Place 8 ml of *potassium iodide and starch solution R* in a 12 ml ground-glass-stoppered cylinder about 1.5 cm in diameter. Fill completely with the substance to be examined, shake vigorously and allow to stand in the dark for 30 min. No colour is produced.

The name and concentration of any added stabilisers are stated on the label.

Storage: in an airtight container, protected from light, at a temperature not exceeding 15 °C.

Ether, peroxide-free. *1035100.*

See *Anaesthetic ether (0367).*

Ethion. $C_9H_{22}O_4P_2S_4$. (M_r 384.5). *1127100.* [563-12-2].

mp: −24 °C to −25 °C.

A suitable certified reference solution (10 ng/µl in cyclohexane) may be used.

Ethoxychrysoidine hydrochloride. $C_{14}H_{17}ClN_4O$. (M_r 292.8). *1035200.* [2313-87-3]. 4-[(4-Ethoxyphenyl)diazenyl]phenylene-1,3-diamine hydrochloride.

A reddish powder, soluble in alcohol.

Ethoxychrysoidine solution. *1035201.*

A 1 g/l solution in *alcohol R.*

Test for sensitivity. To a mixture of 5 ml of *dilute hydrochloric acid R* and 0.05 ml of the ethoxy-chrysoidine solution add 0.05 ml of *0.0167 M bromide-bromate.* The colour changes from red to light yellow within 2 min.

Ethyl acetate. $C_4H_8O_2$. (M_r 88.1). *1035300.* [141-78-6].

A clear, colourless liquid, soluble in water, miscible with alcohol.

d_{20}^{20}: 0.901 to 0.904.

bp: 76 °C to 78 °C.

Ethyl acetate, treated. *1035301.*

Disperse 200 g of *sulphamic acid R* in *ethyl acetate R* and make up to 1000 ml with the same solvent. Stir the suspension obtained for three days and filter through a filter paper.

Storage: use within 1 month.

Ethyl acrylate. $C_5H_8O_2$. (M_r 100.1). *1035400.* [140-88-5]. Ethyl prop-2-enoate.

A colourless liquid.

d_{20}^{20}: about 0.924.

n_D^{20}: about 1.406.

bp: about 99 °C.

mp: about −71 °C.

4-[(Ethylamino)methyl]pyridine. $C_8H_{12}N_2$. (M_r 136.2). *1101300.* [33403-97-3].

A pale yellow liquid.

d_{20}^{20}: about 0.98.

n_D^{20}: about 1.516.

bp: about 98 °C.

Ethylbenzene. C_8H_{10}. (M_r 106.2). *1035800.* [100-41-4].

Content: minimum 99.5 per cent *m/m* of C_8H_{10}, determined by gas chromatography. A clear, colourless liquid, practically insoluble in water, soluble in acetone, and in alcohol.

d_{20}^{20}: about 0.87.

n_D^{20}: about 1.496.

bp: about 135 °C.

Ethyl benzoate. $C_9H_{10}O_2$. (M_r 150.2). *1135700.* [93-89-0].

A clear, colourless, refractive liquid, practically insoluble in water, miscible with alcohol and with light petroleum.

d_4^{25}: about 1.050.

n_D^{20}: about 1.506.

bp: 211 °C to 213 °C.

Ethyl 5-bromovalerate. $C_7H_{13}BrO_2$. (M_r 209.1). *1142900.* [14660-52-7]. Ethyl 5-bromopentanoate.

Clear, colourless liquid.

d_{20}^{20}: about 1.321.

bp: 104 °C to 109 °C.

Ethyl cyanoacetate. $C_5H_7NO_2$. (M_r 113.1). *1035500.* [105-56-6].

A colourless to pale yellow liquid, slightly soluble in water, miscible with alcohol.

bp: 205 °C to 209 °C, with decomposition.

Ethylene chloride. $C_2H_4Cl_2$. (M_r 99.0). *1036000.* [107-06-2]. 1,2-Dichloroethane.

A clear, colourless liquid, soluble in about 120 parts of water and in 2 parts of alcohol.

d_{20}^{20}: about 1.25.

Distillation range (*2.2.11*). Not less than 95 per cent distils between 82 °C and 84 °C.

Ethylenediamine. $C_2H_8N_2$. (M_r 60.1). *1036500.* [107-15-3]. Ethane-1,2-diamine.

A clear, colourless, fuming liquid, strongly alkaline, miscible with water and with alcohol.

bp: about 116 °C.

Ethylene bis[3,3-di(3-*tert*-butyl-4-hydroxyphenyl)butyrate]. *1035900.* [32509-66-3].

See *ethylene bis[3,3-di(3-(1,1-dimethylethyl)-4-hydroxyphenyl)butyrate] R*.

Ethylene bis[3,3-di(3-(1,1-dimethylethyl)-4-hydroxyphenyl)butyrate]. $C_{50}H_{66}O_8$. (M_r 795). *1035900.* [32509-66-3]. Ethylene bis[3,3-di(3-*tert*-butyl-4-hydroxyphenyl)butyrate].

A crystalline powder, practically insoluble in water and in light petroleum, very soluble in acetone and in methanol.

mp: about 165 °C.

(Ethylenedinitrilo)tetra-acetic acid. $C_{10}H_{16}N_2O_8$. (M_r 292.2). *1105800.* [60-00-4]. *N,N'*-1,2-Ethanediylbis[*N*-(carboxymethyl)glycine]. Edetic acid.

A white crystalline powder, very slightly soluble in water.

mp: about 250 °C, with decomposition.

Ethylene glycol. $C_2H_6O_2$. (M_r 62.1). *1036100.* [107-21-1]. Ethane-1,2-diol.

A colourless, slightly viscous liquid, hygroscopic, miscible with water and with alcohol.

d_{20}^{20}: 1.113 to 1.115.

n_D^{20}: about 1.432.

bp: about 198 °C.

mp: about −12 °C.

Acidity. To 10 ml add 20 ml of *water R* and 1 ml of *phenolphthalein solution R*. Not more than 0.15 ml of *0.02 M sodium hydroxide* is required to change the colour of the indicator to pink.

Water (*2.5.12*): maximum 0.2 per cent

Ethylene glycol monoethyl ether. $C_4H_{10}O_2$. (M_r 90.1). *1036200.* [110-80-5]. 2-Ethoxyethanol.

A clear, colourless liquid, miscible with water, with acetone and with alcohol.

d_{20}^{20}: about 0.93.

n_D^{25}: about 1.406

bp: about 135 °C.

Ethylene glycol monomethyl ether. $C_3H_8O_2$. (M_r 76.1). *1036300.* [109-86-4]. 2-Methoxyethanol.

A clear, colourless liquid, miscible with water, with acetone and with alcohol.

d_{20}^{20}: about 0.97.

n_D^{20}: about 1.403.

bp: about 125 °C.

Ethylene oxide. C_2H_4O. (M_r 44.05). *1036400.* [75-21-8]. Oxirane.

Colourless, flammable gas, very soluble in water and in ethanol.

Liquefaction point: about 12 °C.

Ethylene oxide solution. *1036402.*

Weigh a quantity of cool *ethylene oxide stock solution R* equivalent to 2.5 mg of ethylene oxide into a cool flask and dilute to 50.0 g with *macrogol 200 R1*. Mix well and dilute 2.5 g of this solution to 25.0 ml with *macrogol 200 R1* (5 µg of ethylene oxide per gram of solution). Prepare immediately before use.

Ethylene oxide solution R1. *1036403.*

Dilute 1.0 ml of cooled *ethylene oxide stock solution R* (check the exact volume by weighing) to 50.0 ml with *macrogol 200 R1.* Mix well and dilute 2.5 g of this solution to 25.0 ml with *macrogol 200 R1.* Calculate the exact amount of ethylene oxide in ppm from the volume determined by weighing and taking the density of *macrogol 200 R1* as 1.127. Prepare immediately before use.

Ethylene oxide solution R2. *1036404.*

Weigh 1.00 g of cold *ethylene oxide stock solution R* (equivalent to 2.5 mg of ethylene oxide) into a cold flask containing 40.0 g of cold *macrogol 200 R1.* Mix and determine the exact mass and dilute to a calculated mass to obtain a solution containing 50 µg of ethylene oxide per gram of solution. Weigh 10.00 g into a flask containing about 30 ml of *water R,* mix and dilute to 50.0 ml with *water R* (10 µg/ml of ethylene oxide). Prepare immediately before use.

Ethylene oxide solution R3. *1036405.*

Dilute 10.0 ml of *ethylene oxide solution R2* to 50.0 ml with *water R* (2 µg/ml of ethylene oxide). Prepare immediately before use.

Ethylene oxide solution R4. *1036407.*

Dilute 1.0 ml of *ethylene oxide stock solution R1* to 100.0 ml with *water R.* Dilute 1.0 ml of this solution to 25.0 ml with *water R.*

Ethylene oxide solution R5. *1036408.*

A 50 g/l solution of *ethylene oxide R* in *methylene chloride R.*

Either use a commercially available reagent or prepare the solution corresponding to the above-mentioned composition.

Ethylene oxide stock solution. *1036401.*

All operations carried out in the preparation of these solutions must be conducted in a fume-hood. The operator must protect both hands and face by wearing polyethylene protective gloves and an appropriate face mask.

Store all solutions in an airtight container in a refrigerator at 4 °C to 8 °C. Carry out all determinations three times.

Into a dry, clean test-tube, cooled in a mixture of 1 part of *sodium chloride R* and 3 parts of crushed ice, introduce a slow current of *ethylene oxide R* gas, allowing condensation onto the inner wall of the test-tube. Using a glass syringe, previously cooled to − 10 °C, inject about 300 µl (corresponding to about 0.25 g) of liquid *ethylene oxide R* into 50 ml of *macrogol 200 R1.* Determine the absorbed quantity of ethylene oxide by weighing before and after absorption (M_{eo}). Dilute to 100.0 ml with *macrogol 200 R1.* Mix well before use.

Assay. To 10 ml of a 500 g/l suspension of *magnesium chloride R* in *ethanol R* add 20.0 ml of *0.1 M alcoholic hydrochloric acid* in a flask. Stopper and shake to obtain a saturated solution and allow to stand overnight to equilibrate. Weigh 5.00 g of *ethylene oxide stock solution (2.5 g/l) R* into the flask and allow to stand for 30 min. Titrate with *0.1 M alcoholic potassium hydroxide* determining the end-point potentiometrically (*2.2.20*).

Carry out a blank titration, replacing the substance to be examined with the same quantity of *macrogol 200 R1.*

Ethylene oxide content in milligrams per gram is given by:

$$\frac{(V_0 - V_1) \times f \times 4.404}{m}$$

Where V_0 and V_1 are the volumes of alcoholic potassium hydroxide used respectively for the blank titration and the assay,

f = factor of the alcoholic potassium hydroxide solution,

m = mass of the sample taken (g).

Ethylene oxide stock solution R1. *1036406.*

A 50 mg/ml solution of *ethylene oxide R* in *methanol R.*

Ethyl formate. $C_3H_6O_2$. (M_r 74.1). *1035600.* [109-94-4].

Ethyl methanoate.

A clear, colourless, flammable liquid, freely soluble in water, miscible with alcohol.

d_{20}^{20}: about 0.919.

n_D^{20}: about 1.36.

bp: about 54 °C.

2-Ethylhexane-1,3-diol. $C_8H_{18}O_2$. (M_r 146.2). *1105900.* [94-96-2].

A slightly oily liquid, soluble in ethanol, 2-propanol, propylene glycol and castor oil.

d_{20}^{20}: about 0.942.

n_D^{20}: about 1.451.

bp: about 244 °C.

2-Ethylhexanoic acid. $C_8H_{16}O_2$. (M_r 144.2). *1036600.* [149-57-5].

A colourless liquid.

d_{20}^{20}: about 0.91.

n_D^{20}: about 1.425.

Related substances. Examine by gas chromatography (*2.2.28*). Inject 1 µl of a solution prepared as follows: suspend 0.2 g of the 2-ethylhexanoic acid in 5 ml of *water R,* add 3 ml of *dilute hydrochloric acid R* and 5 ml of *hexane R,* shake for 1 min, allow the layers to separate and use the upper layer. Carry out the chromatographic procedure as prescribed in the test for 2-ethylhexanoic acid in the monograph on *Amoxicillin sodium (0577).* The sum of the area of any peaks, apart from the principal peak and the peak due to the solvent, is not greater than 2.5 per cent of the area of the principal peak.

***N*-Ethylmaleimide.** $C_6H_7NO_2$. (M_r 125.1). *1036700.* [128-53-0]. 1-Ethyl-1*H*-pyrrole-2,5-dione.

Colourless crystals, sparingly soluble in water, freely soluble in alcohol.

mp: 41 °C to 45 °C.

Storage: at a temperature of 2 °C to 8 °C.

Ethyl methyl ketone. *1054100.* [78-93-3].

See *methyl ethyl ketone R.*

2-Ethyl-2-methylsuccinic acid. $C_7H_{12}O_4$. (M_r 160.2). *1036800.* [631-31-2]. 2-Ethyl-2-methylbutanedioic acid.

mp: 104 °C to 107 °C.

Ethyl parahydroxybenzoate. *1035700.* [120-47-8].

See *Ethyl parahydroxybenzoate (0900).*

2-Ethylpyridine. C_7H_9N. (M_r 107.2). *1133400.* [100-71-0].

Colourless or brownish liquid.

d_{20}^{20}: about 0.939.

4. Reagents

n_D^{20}: about 1.496.
bp: about 149 °C.

Ethylvinylbenzene-divinylbenzene copolymer. *1036900.*

Porous, rigid, cross-linked polymer beads. Several grades are available with different sizes of bead. The size range of the beads is specified after the name of the reagent in the tests where it is used.

Ethylvinylbenzene-divinylbenzene copolymer R1. *1036901.*

Porous, rigid, cross-linked polymer beads, with a nominal specific surface area of 500 m^2/g to 600 m^2/g and having pores with a mean diameter of 7.5 nm. Several grades are available with different sizes of beads. The size range of the beads is specified after the name of the reagent in the tests where it is used.

Eugenol. $C_{10}H_{12}O_2$. (M_r 164.2). *1037000.* [97-53-0].
4-Allyl-2-methoxyphenol.

A colourless or pale yellow, oily liquid, darkening on exposure to air and light and becoming more viscous, practically insoluble in water, miscible with alcohol and with fatty and essential oils.

d_{20}^{20}: about 1.07.
bp: about 250 °C.

Eugenol used in gas chromatography complies with the following additional test.

Assay. Examine by gas chromatography (*2.2.28*) as prescribed in the monograph on *Clove oil (1091)* using the substance to be examined as the test solution.

The area of the principal peak is not less than 98.0 per cent of the total area of the peaks.

Storage: protected from light.

Euglobulins, bovine. *1037100.*

Use fresh bovine blood collected into an anticoagulant solution (for example, sodium citrate solution). Discard any haemolysed blood. Centrifuge at 1500 *g* to 1800 *g* at 15 °C to 20 °C to obtain a supernatant plasma poor in platelets.

To 1 litre of bovine plasma add 75 g of *barium sulphate R* and shake for 30 min. Centrifuge at not less than 1500 *g* to 1800 *g* at 15 °C to 20 °C and draw off the clear supernatant liquid. Add 10 ml of a 0.2 mg/ml solution of *aprotinin R* and shake to ensure mixing. In a container with a minimum capacity of 30 litres in a chamber at 4 °C introduce 25 litres of *distilled water R* at 4 °C and add about 500 g of solid carbon dioxide. Immediately add, while stirring, the supernatant liquid obtained from the plasma. A white precipitate is formed. Allow to settle at 4 °C for 10 h to 15 h. Remove the clear supernatant solution by siphoning. Collect the precipitate by centrifuging at 4 °C. Suspend the precipitate by dispersing mechanically in 500 ml of *distilled water R* at 4 °C, shake for 5 min and collect the precipitate by centrifuging at 4 °C. Disperse the precipitate mechanically in 60 ml of a solution containing 9 g/l of *sodium chloride R* and 0.9 g/l *sodium citrate R* and adjust to pH 7.2 to 7.4 by adding a 10 g/l solution of *sodium hydroxide R*. Filter through a sintered glass filter; to facilitate the dissolution of the precipitate crush the particles of the precipitate with a suitable instrument. Wash the filter and the instrument with 40 ml of the chloride-citrate solution described above and dilute to 100 ml with the same solution. Freeze-dry the solution. The yields are generally 6 g to 8 g of euglobulins per litre of bovine plasma.

Test for suitability. For this test, prepare the solutions using *phosphate buffer solution pH 7.4 R* containing 30 g/l of *bovine albumin R*.

Into a test-tube 8 mm in diameter placed in a water-bath at 37 °C introduce 0.2 ml of a solution of a reference preparation of urokinase containing 100 IU/ml and 0.1 ml of a solution of *human thrombin R* containing 20 IU/ml. Add rapidly 0.5 ml of a solution containing 10 mg of bovine euglobulins per millilitre. A firm clot forms in less than 10 s. Note the time that elapses between the addition of the solution of bovine euglobulins and the lysis of the clot. The lysis time does not exceed 15 min.

Storage: protected from moisture at 4 °C; use within 1 year.

Euglobulins, human. *1037200.*

For the preparation, use fresh human blood collected into an anticoagulant solution (for example sodium citrate solution) or human blood for transfusion that has been collected in plastic blood bags and which has just reached its expiry date. Discard any haemolysed blood. Centrifuge at 1500 *g* to 1800 *g* at 15 °C to obtain a supernatant plasma poor in platelets. Iso-group plasmas may be mixed.

To 1 litre of the plasma add 75 g of *barium sulphate R* and shake for 30 min. Centrifuge at not less than 15 000 *g* at 15 °C and draw off the clear supernatant liquid. Add 10 ml of a solution of *aprotinin R* containing 0.2 mg/ml and shake to ensure mixing. In a container with a minimum capacity of 30 litres in a chamber at 4 °C introduce 25 litres of *distilled water R* at 4 °C and add about 500 g of solid carbon dioxide. Immediately add while stirring the supernatant liquid obtained from the plasma. A white precipitate is formed. Allow to settle at 4 °C for 10 h to 15 h. Remove the clear supernatant solution by siphoning. Collect the precipitate by centrifuging at 4 °C. Suspend the precipitate by dispersing mechanically in 500 ml of *distilled water R* at 4 °C, shake for 5 min and collect the precipitate by centrifuging at 4 °C. Disperse the precipitate mechanically in 60 ml of a solution containing 9 g/l of *sodium chloride R* and 0.9 g/l of *sodium citrate R*, and adjust the pH to 7.2 to 7.4 by adding a 10 g/l solution of *sodium hydroxide R*. Filter through a sintered-glass filter; to facilitate the dissolution of the precipitate crush the particles of the precipitate with a suitable instrument. Wash the filter and the instrument with 40 ml of the chloride-citrate solution described above and dilute to 100 ml with the same solution. Freeze-dry the solution. The yields are generally 6 g to 8 g of euglobulins per litre of human plasma.

Test for suitability. For this test, prepare the solutions using *phosphate buffer solution pH 7.2 R* containing 30 g/l of *bovine albumin R*. Into a test-tube 8 mm in diameter placed in a water-bath at 37 °C introduce 0.1 ml of a solution of a reference preparation of streptokinase containing 10 IU of streptokinase activity per millilitre and 0.1 ml of a solution of *human thrombin R* containing 20 IU/ml. Add rapidly 1 ml of a solution containing 10 mg of human euglobulins per millilitre. A firm clot forms in less than 10 s. Note the time that elapses between the addition of the solution of human euglobulins and the lysis of the clot. The lysis time does not exceed 15 min.

Storage: in an airtight container at 4 °C; use within 1 year.

Factor Xa, bovine, coagulation. *1037300.* [9002-05-5].

An enzyme which converts prothrombin to thrombin. The semi-purified preparation is obtained from liquid bovine plasma and it may be prepared by activation of the zymogen factor X with a suitable activator such as Russell's viper venom.

Store freeze-dried preparation at − 20 °C and frozen solution at a temperature lower than − 20 °C.

Factor Xa solution, bovine. *1037301.*

Reconstitute as directed by the manufacturer and dilute with *tris(hydroxymethyl)aminomethane sodium chloride buffer solution pH 7.4 R.*

Any change in the absorbance of the solution, measured at 405 nm (*2.2.25*) against *tris(hydroxymethyl)aminomethane sodium chloride buffer solution pH 7.4 R* as the blank is not more than 0.15 to 0.20 per minute.

Fast blue B salt. $C_{14}H_{12}Cl_2N_4O_2$. (M_r 339.2). *1037400.* [84633-94-3].

Schultz No. 490.

Colour Index No. 37235.
3,3′-Dimethoxy(biphenyl)-4,4′-bisdiazonium dichloride.

A dark green powder, soluble in water. It is stabilised by addition of zinc chloride.

Storage: in an airtight container, at a temperature between 2 °C and 8 °C.

Fast red B salt. $C_{17}H_{13}N_3O_9S_2$. (M_r 467.4). *1037500.* [56315-29-8].

Schultz No. 155.

Colour Index No. 37125.
2-Methoxy-4-nitrobenzenediazonium hydrogen naphthalene-1,5-disulphonate.

An orange-yellow powder, soluble in water, slightly soluble in alcohol.

Storage: in an airtight container, protected from light, at 2 °C to 8 °C.

Fenchlorphos. $C_8H_8Cl_3O_3PS$. (M_r 321.5). *1127200.* [299-84-3].

mp: about 35 °C.

A suitable certified reference solution (10 ng/μl in cyclohexane) may be used.

Fenchone. $C_{10}H_{16}O$. (M_r 152.2). *1037600.* [7787-20-4].
1,3,3-Trimethylbicyclo[2.2.1]heptan-2-one.

An oily liquid, miscible with alcohol, practically insoluble in water.

n_D^{20}: about 1.46.

bp_{15mm}: about 66 °C.

Fenchone used in gas chromatography complies with the following test.

Assay. Examine by gas chromatography (*2.2.28*) under the conditions described in the monograph on *Bitter fennel (0824)* using the substance to be examined as the test solution.

The area of the principal peak is not less than 98.0 per cent of the total area of the peaks.

Fenvalerate. $C_{25}H_{22}ClNO_3$. (M_r 419.9). *1127300.* [51630-58-1].

bp: about 300 °C.

A suitable certified reference solution (10 ng/μl in cyclohexane) may be used.

Ferric ammonium sulphate. $FeNH_4(SO_4)_2,12H_2O$. (M_r 482.2). *1037700.* [7783-83-7]. Ammonium iron disulphate dodecahydrate.

Pale-violet crystals, efflorescent, very soluble in water, practically insoluble in alcohol.

Ferric ammonium sulphate solution R2. *1037702.*

A 100 g/l solution. If necessary filter before use.

Ferric ammonium sulphate solution R5. *1037704.*

Shake 30.0 g of *ferric ammonium sulphate R* with 40 ml of *nitric acid R* and dilute to 100 ml with *water R*. If the solution is turbid, centrifuge or filter it.

Storage: protected from light.

Ferric ammonium sulphate solution R6. *1037705.*

Dissolve 20 g of *ferric ammonium sulphate R* in 75 ml of *water R*, add 10 ml of a 2.8 per cent *V/V* solution of *sulphuric acid R* and dilute to 100 ml with *water R*.

Ferric chloride. $FeCl_3,6H_2O$. (M_r 270.3). *1037800.* [10025-77-1]. Iron trichloride hexahydrate.

Yellowish-orange or brownish crystalline masses, deliquescent, very soluble in water, soluble in alcohol. On exposure to light, ferric chloride and its solutions are partly reduced.

Storage: in an airtight container.

Ferric chloride solution R1. *1037801.*

A 105 g/l solution.

Ferric chloride solution R2. *1037802.*

A 13 g/l solution.

Ferric sulphate pentahydrate. $Fe_2(SO_4)_3,5H_2O$. (M_r 489.9). *1153700.* [142906-29-4].

White or yellowish powder.

Ferric chloride solution R3. *1037803.*

Dissolve 2.0 g of *ferric chloride R* in *ethanol R* and dilute to 100.0 ml with the same solvent.

Ferric chloride-sulphamic acid reagent. *1037804.*

A solution containing 10 g/l of *ferric chloride R* and 16 g/l of *sulphamic acid R*.

Ferric nitrate. $Fe(NO_3)_3,9H_2O$. (M_r 404). *1106100.* [7782-61-8].

Content: minimum 99.0 per cent *m/m* of $Fe(NO_3)_3,9H_2O$.

Light-purple crystals or crystalline mass, very soluble in water.

Free acid: not more than 0.3 per cent (as HNO_3).

Ferric sulphate. $Fe_2(SO_4)_3,xH_2O$. *1037900.* [10028-22-5]. Iron(III) trisulphate hydrated.

A yellowish-white powder, very hygroscopic, decomposes in air, slightly soluble in water and in alcohol.

Storage: in an airtight container, protected from light.

Ferrocyphene. $C_{26}H_{16}FeN_6$. (M_r 468.3). *1038000.* [14768-11-7]. Dicyanobis(1,10-phenanthroline)iron(II).

A violet-bronze, crystalline powder, practically insoluble in water and in alcohol.

Storage: protected from light and moisture.

Ferroin. *1038100.* [14634-91-4].

Dissolve 0.7 g of *ferrous sulphate R* and 1.76 g of *phenanthroline hydrochloride R* in 70 ml of *water R* and dilute to 100 ml with the same solvent.

Test for sensitivity. To 50 ml of *dilute sulphuric acid R* add 0.15 ml of *osmium tetroxide solution R* and 0.1 ml of the ferroin. After the addition of 0.1 ml of *0.1 M ammonium and cerium nitrate* the colour changes from red to light blue.

Ferrous ammonium sulphate. $Fe(NH_4)_2(SO_4)_2,6H_2O$. (*M*r 392.2). *1038200.* [7783-85-9]. Diammonium iron disulphate hexahydrate.

Pale bluish-green crystals or granules, freely soluble in water, practically insoluble in alcohol.

Storage: protected from light.

Ferrous sulphate. *1038300.* [7782-63-0].

See *Ferrous sulphate (0083).*

Ferrous sulphate solution R2. *1038301.*

Dissolve 0.45 g of *ferrous sulphate R* in 50 ml of *0.1 M hydrochloric acid* and dilute to 100 ml with *carbon dioxide-free water R*. Prepare immediately before use.

Ferulic acid. $C_{10}H_{10}O_4$. (*M*r 194.2). *1149500.* [1135-24-6]. 4-Hydroxy-3-methoxycinnamic acid. 3-(4-Hydroxy-3-methoxyphenyl)propenoic acid.

Faint yellow powder, freely soluble in methanol.

mp: 172.9 °C to 173.9 °C.

Ferulic acid used in the assay of eleutherosides in Eleutherococcus (1419) complies with the following additional requirement.

Assay. Examine by liquid chromatography (*2.2.29*) as prescribed in the monograph on *Eleutherococcus (1419).*

The content is not less than 99 per cent, calculated by the normalisation procedure.

Fibrin blue. *1101400.*

Mix 1.5 g of fibrin with 30 ml of a 5 g/l solution of *indigo carmine R* in 1 per cent *V/V dilute hydrochloric acid R*. Heat the mixture to 80 °C and maintain at this temperature whilst stirring for about 30 min. Allow to cool. Filter. Wash extensively by resuspension in 1 per cent *V/V dilute hydrochloric acid R* and mixing for about 30 min; filter. Repeat the washing operation three times. Dry at 50 °C. Grind.

Fibrin congo red. *1038400.*

Take 1.5 g of fibrin and leave overnight in 50 ml of a 20 g/l solution of *congo red R* in *alcohol (90 per cent V/V) R*. Filter, rinse the fibrin with *water R* and store under *ether R*.

Fibrinogen. *1038500.* [9001-32-5].

See *Human fibrinogen, freeze-dried (0024).*

Fixing solution. *1122600.*

To 250 ml of *methanol R*, add 0.27 ml of *formaldehyde R* and dilute to 500.0 ml with *water R*.

Fixing solution for isoelectric focusing in polyacrylamide gel. *1138700.*

A solution containing 35 g of *sulphosalicylic acid R* and 100 g of *trichloroacetic acid R* per litre of *water R*.

Flufenamic acid. $C_{14}H_{10}F_3NO_2$. (*M*r 281.2). *1106200.* [530-78-9]. 2-[[3-(Trifluoromethyl)phenyl]amino]benzoic acid.

Pale yellow, crystalline powder or needles, practically insoluble in water, freely soluble in alcohol.

mp: 132 °C to 135 °C.

Flumazenil. *1149600.* [78755-81-4].

See *Flumazenil (1326).*

Flunitrazepam. *1153800.* [1622-62-4].

See *Flunitrazepam (0717).*

Fluoranthene. $C_{16}H_{10}$. (*M*r 202.3). *1038600.* [206-44-0]. 1,2-(1,8-Naphtylene)benzene. 1,2-Benzacenaphtene.

Yellow or yellowish-brown crystals.

bp: about 384 °C.

mp: 109 °C to 110 °C.

Fluorene. $C_{13}H_{10}$. (*M*r 166.2). *1127400.* [86-73-7]. Diphenylenemethane.

White crystals, freely soluble in anhydrous acetic acid, soluble in hot alcohol.

mp: 113 °C to 115 °C.

Fluorescamine. $C_{17}H_{10}O_4$. (*M*r 278.3). *1135800.* [38183-12-9]. 4-Phenylspiro[furan-2(3*H*),1'(3'*H*)-isobenzofuran]-3,3'-dione.

mp: 154 °C to 155 °C.

Fluorescein. $C_{20}H_{12}O_5$. (*M*r 332.3). *1106300.* [2321-07-5]. 3′,6′-Dihydroxyspiro[isobenzofurane-1(3*H*),9′-[9*H*]xanthen]-3-one.

An orange-red powder, practically insoluble in water, soluble in warm alcohol, soluble in alkaline solutions. In solution, fluorescein displays a green fluorescence.

mp: about 315 °C.

Fluorescein-conjugated rabies antiserum. *1038700.*

Immunoglobulin fraction with a high rabies antibody titre, prepared from the sera of suitable animals that have been immunised with inactivated rabies virus; the immunoglobulin is conjugated with fluorescein isothiocyanate.

2-Fluoro-2-deoxy-D-glucose. $C_6H_{11}FO_5$. (*M*r 182.2). *1113900.* [86783-82-6].

A white crystalline powder.

mp: 174 °C to 176 °C.

Fluorodinitrobenzene. $C_6H_3FN_2O_4$. (*M*r 186.1). *1038800.* [70-34-8]. 1-Fluoro-2,4-dinitrobenzene.

Pale yellow crystals, soluble in propylene glycol.

mp: about 29 °C.

1-Fluoro-2-nitro-4-(trifluoromethyl)benzene. $C_7H_3F_4NO_2$. (*M*r 209.1). *1038900.* [367-86-2].

mp: about 197 °C.

Folic acid. *1039000.* [75708-92-8].

See *Folic acid (0067).*

Formaldehyde. *1039100.* [50-00-0].

See *Formaldehyde solution R.*

Formaldehyde solution. *1039101.*

See *Formaldehyde solution (35 per cent) (0826).*

Formamide. CH_3NO. (*M*r 45.0). *1039200.* [75-12-7].

A clear, colourless, oily liquid, hygroscopic, miscible with water and with alcohol. It is hydrolysed by water.

bp: about 103 °C, determined at a pressure of 2 kPa.

Storage: in an airtight container.

Formamide R1. *1039202.*

Complies with the requirements prescribed for *formamide R* and with the following additional test.

Water (*2.5.12*): maximum 0.1 per cent determined with an equal volume of *anhydrous methanol R*.

Formamide, treated. *1039201.*

Disperse 1.0 g of *sulphamic acid R* in 20.0 ml of *formamide R* containing 5 per cent *V/V* of *water R*.

Formic acid, anhydrous. CH_2O_2. (M_r 46.03). *1039300.* [64-18-6].

Content: minimum 98.0 per cent *m/m* of CH_2O_2.

A colourless liquid, corrosive, miscible with water and with alcohol.

d_{20}^{20}: about 1.22.

Assay. Weigh accurately a conical flask containing 10 ml of *water R*, quickly add about 1 ml of the acid and weigh again. Add 50 ml of *water R* and titrate with *1 M sodium hydroxide*, using 0.5 ml of *phenolphthalein solution R* as indicator.

1 ml of *1 M sodium hydroxide* is equivalent to 46.03 mg of CH_2O_2.

Fructose. *1106400.* [57-48-7].

See *Fructose (0188).*

Fuchsin, basic. *1039400.* [632-99-5].

A mixture of rosaniline hydrochloride ($C_{20}H_{20}ClN_3$; M_r 337.9; Colour Index No. 42510; Schultz No. 780) and *para*-rosaniline hydrochloride ($C_{19}H_{18}ClN_3$; M_r 323.8; Colour Index No. 42500; Schultz No. 779).

If necessary, purify in the following manner. Dissolve 1 g in 250 ml of *dilute hydrochloric acid R*. Allow to stand for 2 h at room temperature, filter and neutralise with *dilute sodium hydroxide solution R* and add 1 ml to 2 ml in excess. Filter the precipitate through a sintered-glass filter (40) and wash with *water R*. Dissolve the precipitate in 70 ml of *methanol R*, previously heated to boiling, and add 300 ml of *water R* at 80 °C. Allow to cool to room temperature, filter and dry the crystals *in vacuo*.

Crystals with a greenish-bronze sheen, soluble in water and in alcohol.

Storage: protected from light.

Fuchsin solution, decolorised. *1039401.*

Dissolve 0.1 g of *basic fuchsin R* in 60 ml of *water R*. Add a solution containing 1 g of *anhydrous sodium sulphite R* or 2 g of *sodium sulphite R* in 10 ml of *water R*. Slowly and with continuous shaking add 2 ml of *hydrochloric acid R*. Dilute to 100 ml with *water R*. Allow to stand protected from light for at least 12 h, decolorise with *activated charcoal R* and filter. If the solution becomes cloudy, filter before use. If on standing the solution becomes violet, decolorise again by adding *activated charcoal R*.

Test for sensitivity. To 1.0 ml add 1.0 ml of *water R* and 0.1 ml of *aldehyde-free alcohol R*. Add 0.2 ml of a solution containing 0.1 g/l of formaldehyde (CH_2O, M_r 30.0). A pale-pink colour develops within 5 min.

Storage: protected from light.

Fuchsin solution, decolorised R1. *1039402.*

To 1 g of *basic fuchsin R* add 100 ml of *water R*. Heat to 50 °C and allow to cool with occasional shaking. Allow to stand for 48 h, shake and filter. To 4 ml of the filtrate add 6 ml of *hydrochloric acid R*, mix and dilute to 100 ml with *water R*. Allow to stand for at least 1 h before use.

Fucose. $C_6H_{12}O_5$. (M_r 164.2). *1039500.* [6696-41-9]. 6-Deoxy-L-galactose.

A white powder, soluble in water and in alcohol.

$[\alpha]_D^{20}$: about −76, determined on a 90 g/l solution 24 h after dissolution.

mp: about 140 °C.

Fumaric acid. $C_4H_4O_4$. (M_r 116.1). *1153200.* [110-17-8]. (*E*)-Butenedioic acid.

White crystals, slightly soluble in water, soluble in alcohol, slightly soluble in acetone.

mp: about 300 °C.

Furfural. $C_5H_4O_2$. (M_r 96.1). *1039600.* [98-01-1]. 2-Furaldehyde. 2-Furanecarbaldehyde.

A clear, colourless to brownish-yellow, oily liquid, miscible in 11 parts of water, miscible with alcohol.

d_{20}^{20}: 1.155 to 1.161.

Distillation range (*2.2.11*). Not less than 95 per cent distils between 159 °C and 163 °C.

Storage: in a dark place.

Galactose. $C_6H_{12}O_6$. (M_r 180.2). *1039700.* [59-23-4]. D-(+)-Galactose.

A white, crystalline powder, freely soluble in water.

$[\alpha]_D^{20}$: + 79 to + 81, determined on a 100 g/l solution in *water R* containing about 0.05 per cent of NH_3.

Gallic acid. $C_7H_6O_5,H_2O$. (M_r 188.1). *1039800.* [5995-86-8]. 3,4,5-Trihydroxybenzoic acid monohydrate.

A crystalline powder or long needles, colourless or slightly yellow, soluble in water, freely soluble in hot water, in alcohol and in glycerol.

It loses its water of crystallisation at 120 °C and it melts at about 260 °C, with decomposition.

Chromatography. Examine as prescribed in the monograph on *Bearberry leaf (1054)*; the chromatogram shows only one principal spot.

Gastric juice, artificial. *1039900.*

Dissolve 2.0 g of *sodium chloride R* and 3.2 g of *pepsin powder R* in *water R*. Add 80 ml of *1 M hydrochloric acid* and dilute to 1000 ml with *water R*.

GC concentrical column. *1135100.*

A commercially available system consisting of 2 concentrically arranged tubes. The outer tube is packed with molecular sieves and the inner tube is packed with a porous polymer mixture. The main application is the separation of gases.

Gelatin. *1040000.* [9000-70-8].

See *Gelatin (0330).*

Gelatin, hydrolysed. *1040100.*

Dissolve 50 g of *gelatin R* in 1000 ml of *water R*. Autoclave in saturated steam at 121 °C for 90 min and freeze dry.

Geraniol. $C_{10}H_{18}O$. (M_r 154.2). *1135900.* [106-24-1]. (*E*)-3,7-Dimethylocta-2,6-dien-1-ol.

An oily liquid, slight odour of rose, practically insoluble in water, miscible with alcohol.

d_{20}^{20}: 0.890.

n_D^{20}: 1.477.

bp: 229 °C to 230 °C.

Geraniol used in gas chromatography complies with the following additional test.

Assay. Examine by gas chromatography (*2.2.28*) as prescribed in the monograph on *Citronella oil (1609).*

The content is not less than 98.5 per cent calculated by the normalisation procedure.

Storage: in an airtight container, protected from light

Geranyl acetate. $C_{12}H_{20}O_2$. (M_r 196.3). *1106500.* [105-87-3]. (*E*)-3,7-Dimethylocta-2,6-dien-1-yl acetate.

A colourless or slightly yellow liquid, slight odour of rose and lavender.

d_{25}^{25}: 0.896 to 0.913.

n_D^{15}: about 1.463.

bp_{25}: about 138 °C.

Geranyl acetate used in gas chromatography complies with the following additional test.

Assay. Examine by gas chromatography (*2.2.28*) as prescribed in the monograph on *Bitter-orange-flower oil (1175)*, using the substance to be examined as the test solution. The area of the principal peak is not less than 99.0 per cent of the total area of the peaks.

Ginsenoside Rb1. $C_{54}H_{92}O_{23},3H_2O$. (M_r 1163). *1127500.* [41753-43-9]. (20*S*)-3β-di-D-Glucopyranosyl-20-di-D-glucopyranosylprotopanaxadiol. (20*S*)-3β-[(2-*O*-β-D-Glucopyranosyl-β-D-glucopyranosyl)oxy]-20-[(6-*O*-β-D-glucopyranosyl-β-D-glucopyranosyl)oxy]-5α-dammar-24-en-12β-ol. (20*S*)-3β-[(2-*O*-β-D-Glucopyranosyl-β-D-glucopyranosyl)oxy]-20-[(6-*O*-β-D-glucopyranosyl-β-D-glucopyranosyl)oxy]-4,4,8,14-tetramethyl-18-nor-5α-cholest-24-en-12β-ol.

A colourless solid, soluble in water, in ethanol and in methanol.

$[\alpha]_D^{20}$: + 11.3 determined on a 10 g/l solution in *methanol R.*

mp: about 199 °C.

Water (2.5.12): maximum 6.8 per cent.

Assay. Examined by liquid chromatography (*2.2.29*) as prescribed in the monograph on *Ginseng (1523).*

Test solution. Dissolve 3.0 mg, accurately weighted, of *ginsenoside Rb1* in 10 ml of *methanol R.*

The content is not less than 95.0 per cent calculated by the normalisation procedure.

Ginsenoside Rf. $C_{42}H_{72}O_{14},2H_2O$. (M_r 837). *1127700.* [52286-58-5]. (20*S*)-6-*O*-[β-D-Glucopyranosyl-(1→2)-β-D-glycopyranoside]-dammar-24-ene-3β,6α,12β,20-tetrol.

A colourless solid, soluble in water, in ethanol and in methanol.

$[\alpha]_D^{20}$: + 12.8 determined on a 10 g/l solution in *methanol R.*

mp: about 198 °C.

Ginsenoside Rg1. $C_{42}H_{72}O_{14},2H_2O$. (M_r 837). *1127600.* [22427-39-0]. (20*S*)-6β-D-Glucopyranosyl-D-glucopyranosylprotopanaxatriol. (20*S*)-6α,20-bis(β-D-Glucopyranosyloxy)-5α-dammar-24-ene-3β,12β-diol. (20*S*)-6α,20-bis(β-D-Glucopyranosyloxy)-4,4,8,14-tetramethyl-18-nor-5α-cholest-24-ene-3β,12β-diol.

A colourless solid, soluble in water, in ethanol and in methanol.

$[\alpha]_D^{20}$: + 31.2 determined on a 10 g/l solution in *methanol R.*

mp: 188 °C to 191 °C.

Water (2.5.12): maximum 4.8 per cent.

Assay. Examined by liquid chromatography (*2.2.29*) as prescribed in the monograph on *Ginseng (1523).*

Test solution. Dissolve 3.0 mg, accurately weighted, of *ginsenoside Rg1* in 10 ml of *methanol R.*

The content is not less than 95.0 per cent calculated by the normalisation procedure.

Gitoxin. $C_{41}H_{64}O_{14}$. (M_r 781). *1040200.* [4562-36-1]. Glycoside of *Digitalis purpurea* L. 3β-(*O*-2,6-Dideoxy-β-d-*ribo*-hexopyranosyl-(1→4)-*O*-2,6-dideoxy-β-d-*ribo*-hexopyranosyl-(1→4)-2,6-dideoxy-β-d-*ribo*-hexopyranosyloxy)-14,16β-dihydroxy-5β,14β-card-20(22)-enolide.

A white, crystalline powder, practically insoluble in water and in most common organic solvents, soluble in pyridine.

$[\alpha]_D^{20}$: + 20 to + 24, determined on a 5 g/l solution in a mixture of equal volumes of *chloroform R* and *methanol R.*

Chromatography. Examine as prescribed in the monograph on *Digitalis leaf (0117)*; the chromatogram shows only one principal spot.

Glucosamine hydrochloride. $C_6H_{14}ClNO_5$. (M_r 215.6). *1040300.* [66-84-2]. D-Glucosamine hydrochloride.

Crystals, soluble in water.

$[\alpha]_D^{20}$: + 100, decreasing to + 47.5 after 30 min, determined on a 100 g/l solution in *water R.*

Glucose. *1025700.* [50-99-7].

See *Anhydrous glucose (0177).*

D-Glucuronic acid. $C_6H_{10}O_7$. (M_r 194.1). *1119700.* [6556-12-3].

Content: minimum 96.0 per cent of $C_6H_{10}O_7$, calculated with reference to the substance dried *in vacuo* (*2.2.32*).

Soluble in water and in alcohol.

Shows mutarotation: $[\alpha]_D^{24}$: + 11.7 → + 36.3

Assay. Dissolve 0.150 g in 50 ml of *anhydrous methanol R* while stirring under nitrogen. Titrate with *0.1 M tetrabutylammonium hydroxide,* protecting the solution from atmospheric carbon dioxide throughout solubilisation and titration. Determine the end-point potentiometrically (*2.2.20*).

1 ml of *0.1 M tetrabutylammonium hydroxide* is equivalent to 19.41 mg of $C_6H_{10}O_7$.

Glutamic acid. *1040400.* [56-86-0].

See *Glutamic acid (0750).*

Glutaraldehyde. $C_5H_8O_2$. (M_r 100.1). *1098300.* [111-30-8].

An oily liquid, soluble in water.

n_D^{25}: about 1.434.

bp: about 188 °C.

Glutaric acid. $C_5H_8O_4$. (M_r 132.1). *1149700.* [110-94-1]. Pentanedioic acid.

White, crystalline powder.

Glycerol. *1040500.* [56-81-5].

See *Glycerol (0496).*

Glycerol R1. *1040501.*

Glycerol complying with the monograph *Glycerol (0496)* and free from diethylene glycol when examined as described in the test for Impurity A and related substances in that monograph.

Glycerol (85 per cent). *1040600.*

See *Glycerol (85 per cent) (0497).*

Glycerol (85 per cent) R1. *1040601.*

Glycerol complying with the monograph *Glycerol 85 per cent (0497)* and free from diethylene glycol when examined as described in the test for Impurity A and related substances in that monograph.

Glycidol. $C_3H_6O_2$. (M_r 74.1). *1127800.* [556-52-5].

A slightly viscous liquid, miscible with water.

d_4^{20} : about 1.115.

n_D^{20} : about 1.432.

Glycine. *1040700.* [56-40-6].

See *Glycine (0614).*

Glycollic acid. $C_2H_4O_3$. (M_r 76.0). *1040800.* [79-14-1]. 2-Hydroxyacetic acid.

Crystals, soluble in water, in acetone, in alcohol and in methanol.

mp: about 80 °C.

Glycyrrhetic acid. $C_{30}H_{46}O_4$. (M_r 470.7). *1040900.* [471-53-4]. Glycyrrhetinic acid. 12,13-Didehydro-3β-hydroxy-11-oxo-olean-30-oic acid.

A mixture of α- and β-glycyrrhetic acids in which the β-isomer is predominant.

A white or yellowish-brown powder, practically insoluble in water, soluble in ethanol and in glacial acetic acid.

$[\alpha]_D^{20}$: + 145 to + 155, determined on a 10.0 g/l solution in *ethanol R*.

Chromatography. Examine by thin-layer chromatography (*2.2.27*) using *silica gel GF_{254} R* as the coating substance; prepare the slurry using a 0.25 per cent *V/V* solution of *phosphoric acid R*. Apply to the plate 5 µl of a 5 g/l solution of the glycyrrhetic acid in a mixture of equal volumes of *chloroform R* and *methanol R*. Develop over a path of 10 cm using a mixture of 5 volumes of *methanol R* and 95 volumes of *chloroform R*. Examine the chromatogram in ultraviolet light at 254 nm. The chromatogram shows a dark spot (R_f about 0.3) corresponding to β-glycyrrhetic acid and a smaller spot (R_f about 0.5) corresponding to α-glycyrrhetic acid. Spray with *anisaldehyde solution R* and heat at 100 °C to 105 °C for 10 min. Both spots are coloured bluish-violet. Between them a smaller bluish-violet spot may be present.

18α-Glycyrrhetinic acid. $C_{30}H_{46}O_4$. (M_r 470.7). *1127900.* [1449-05-4]. (20β)-3β-Hydroxy-11-oxo-18α-olean-12-en-29-oic acid.

A white or almost white powder, practically insoluble in water, soluble in ethanol, sparingly soluble in methylene chloride.

Glyoxalhydroxyanil. $C_{14}H_{12}N_2O_2$. (M_r 240.3). *1041000.* [1149-16-2]. Glyoxal bis(2-hydroxyanil).

White crystals, soluble in hot alcohol.

mp: about 200 °C.

Glyoxal solution. *1098400.* [107-22-2].

Contains about 40 per cent (*m/m*) glyoxal.

Assay. In a ground-glass stoppered flask place 1.000 g of glyoxal solution, 20 ml of a 70 g/l solution of *hydroxylamine hydrochloride R* and 50 ml of *water R*. Allow to stand for 30 min and add 1 ml of *methyl red mixed solution R* and titrate with *1 M sodium hydroxide* until the colour changes from red to green. Carry out a blank titration.

1 ml of *1 M sodium hydroxide* is equivalent to 29.02 mg of glyoxal ($C_2H_2O_2$).

Gonadotrophin, chorionic. *1041100.* [9002-61-3].

See *Chorionic gonadotrophin (0498).*

Gonadotrophin, serum. *1041200.*

See *Equine serum gonadotrophin for veterinary use (0719).*

Guaiacol. $C_7H_8O_2$. (M_r 124.1). *1148300.* [90-05-1]. 2-Methoxyphenol. 1-Hydroxy-2-methoxybenzene.

Crystalline mass or colourless or yellowish liquid, hygroscopic, slightly soluble in water, very soluble in methylene chloride, freely soluble in alcohol.

bp: about 205 °C.

mp: about 28 °C.

Guaiacum resin. *1041400.*

Resin obtained from the heartwood of *Guaiacum officinale* L. and *Guaiacum sanctum* L.

Reddish-brown or greenish-brown, hard, glassy fragments; fracture shiny.

Guaiazulene. $C_{15}H_{18}$. (M_r 198.3). *1041500.* [489-84-9]. 1,4-Dimethyl-7-isopropylazulene.

Dark-blue crystals or blue liquid, very slightly soluble in water, miscible with fatty and essential oils and with liquid paraffin, sparingly soluble in alcohol, soluble in 500 g/l sulphuric acid and 80 per cent *m/m* phosphoric acid, giving a colourless solution.

mp: about 30 °C.

Storage: protected from light and air.

Guanidine hydrochloride. CH_5N_3HCl. (M_r 95.5). *1098500.* [50-01-1].

Crystalline powder, freely soluble in water and in alcohol.

Guanine. $C_5H_5N_5O$. (M_r 151.1). *1041600.* [73-40-5]. 2-Amino-1,7-dihydro-6*H*-purin-6-one.

An amorphous white powder, practically insoluble in water, slightly soluble in alcohol. It dissolves in ammonia and in dilute solutions of alkali hydroxides.

Haemoglobin. *1041700.* [9008-02-0].

Nitrogen: 15 per cent to 16 per cent.

Iron: 0.2 per cent to 0.3 per cent.

Loss on drying (*2.2.32*): maximum 2 per cent.

Sulphated ash (*2.4.14*): maximum 1.5 per cent.

Haemoglobin solution. *1041701.*

Transfer 2 g of *haemoglobin R* to a 250 ml beaker and add 75 ml of *dilute hydrochloric acid R2*. Stir until solution is complete. Adjust the pH to 1.6 ± 0.1 (*2.2.3*) using *1 M hydrochloric acid*. Transfer to a 100 ml flask with the aid of *dilute hydrochloric acid R2*. Add 25 mg of *thiomersal R*. Prepare daily, store at 5 ± 3 °C and readjust to pH 1.6 before use.

Storage: at 2 °C to 8 °C.

Harpagoside. $C_{24}H_{30}O_{11}$. (M_r 494.5). *1098600.*

A white, crystalline powder, very hygroscopic, soluble in water and in alcohol.

mp: 117 °C to 121 °C.

Storage: in an airtight container.

Helium for chromatography. He. (A_r 4.003). *1041800.* [7440-59-7].

Content: minimum 99.995 per cent *V/V* of He.

Heparin. *1041900.* [9041-08-1].

See *Heparin sodium (0333).*

Heptachlor. $C_{10}H_5Cl_7$. (M_r 373.3). *1128000.* [76-44-8].

bp: about 135 °C.

mp: about 95 °C.

A suitable certified reference solution (10 ng/µl in cyclohexane) may be used.

Heptachlor epoxide. $C_{10}H_5Cl_7O$. (M_r 389.3). *1128100.* [1024-57-3].

bp: about 200 °C.

mp: about 160 °C.

A suitable certified reference solution (10 ng/μl in cyclohexane) may be used.

Heptafluoro-*N*-methyl-*N*-(trimethylsilyl)butanamide. $C_8H_{12}F_7NOSi$. (M_r 299.3). *1139500.* [53296-64-3]. 2,2,3,3,4,4,4-Heptafluoro-*N*-methyl-*N*-(trimethylsilyl)butyramide.

Clear, colourless liquid, flammable.

n_D^{20}: about 1.351.

bp: about 148 °C.

Heptane. C_7H_{16}. (M_r 100.2). *1042000.* [142-82-5].

A colourless, flammable liquid, practically insoluble in water, miscible with ethanol.

d_{20}^{20}: 0.683 to 0.686.

n_D^{20}: 1.387 to 1.388.

Distillation range (*2.2.11*). Not less than 95 per cent distils between 97 °C and 98 °C.

Hesperidin. $C_{28}H_{34}O_{15}$. (M_r 611). *1139000.* [520-26-3]. (*S*)-7-[[6-*O*-(6-Deoxy–α-L-mannopyranosyl)-β-D-glucopyranosyl]oxy]-5-hydroxy-2-(3-hydroxy-4-methoxyphenyl)-2,3-dihydro-4*H*-1-benzopyran-4-one.

Hygroscopic powder, slightly soluble in water and in methanol.

mp: 258 °C to 262 °C.

Hexachlorobenzene. C_6Cl_6. (M_r 284.8). *1128200.* [118-74-1].

bp: about 332 °C.

mp: about 230 °C.

A suitable certified reference solution (10 ng/μl in cyclohexane) may be used.

α-Hexachlorocyclohexane. $C_6H_6Cl_6$. (M_r 290.8). *1128300.* [319-84-6].

bp: about 288 °C.

mp: about 158 °C.

A suitable certified reference solution (10 ng/μl in cyclohexane) may be used.

β-Hexachlorocyclohexane. $C_6H_6Cl_6$. (M_r 290.8). *1128400.* [319-85-7].

A suitable certified reference solution (10 ng/μl in cyclohexane) may be used.

δ-Hexachlorocyclohexane. $C_6H_6Cl_6$. (M_r 290.8). *1128500.* [319-86-8].

A suitable certified reference solution (10 ng/μl in cyclohexane) may be used.

Hexacosane. $C_{26}H_{54}$. (M_r 366.7). *1042200.* [630-01-3].

Colourless or white flakes.

mp: about 57 °C.

Hexadimethrine bromide. $(C_{13}H_{30}Br_2N_2)_n$. *1042300.* [28728-55-4]. 1,5-Dimethyl-1,5-diazaundecamethylene polymethobromide. Poly(1,1,5,5-tetramethyl-1,5-azoniaundecamethylene dibromide).

A white, amorphous powder, hygroscopic, soluble in water.

Storage: in an airtight container.

2,2′,2″,6,6′,6″-Hexa(1,1-dimethylethyl)-4,4′,4″-[(2,4,6-trimethyl-1,3,5-benzenetriyl)trismethylene]triphenol. $C_{54}H_{78}O_3$. (M_r 775). *1042100.* 2,2′,2″,6,6′,6″-Hexa-*tert*-butyl-4,4′,4″-[(2,4,6-trimethyl-1,3,5-benzenetriyl)trismethylene]triphenol.

A crystalline powder, practically insoluble in water, soluble in acetone, slightly soluble in alcohol.

mp: about 244 °C.

1,1,1,3,3,3-Hexafluoropropan-2-ol. $C_3H_2F_6O$. (M_r 168.0). *1136000.* [920-66-1].

Content: minimum 99.0 per cent of $C_3H_2F_6O$, determined by gas chromatography.

A clear, colourless liquid, miscible with water and with ethanol.

d_{20}^{20}: about 1.596.

bp: about 59 °C.

Hexamethyldisilazane. $C_6H_{19}NSi_2$. (M_r 161.4). *1042400.* [999-97-3].

A clear, colourless liquid.

d_{20}^{20}: about 0.78.

n_D^{20}: about 1.408.

bp: about 125 °C.

Storage: in an airtight container.

Hexamethylenetetramine. $C_6H_{12}N_4$. (M_r 140.2). *1042500.* [100-97-0]. Hexamine. 1,3,5,7-Tetra-azatricyclo [3.3.1.1^{3,7}]decane.

A colourless, crystalline powder, very soluble in water.

Hexane. C_6H_{14}. (M_r 86.2). *1042600.* [110-54-3].

A colourless, flammable liquid, practically insoluble in water, miscible with ethanol.

d_{20}^{20}: 0.659 to 0.663.

n_D^{20}: 1.375 to 1.376.

Distillation range (*2.2.11*). Not less than 95 per cent distils between 67 °C and 69 °C.

Hexane used in spectrophotometry complies with the following additional test.

Minimum transmittance (*2.2.25*), determined using *water R* as compensation liquid: 97 per cent from 260 nm to 420 nm.

Hexylamine. $C_6H_{15}N$. (M_r 101.2). *1042700.* [111-26-2]. Hexanamine.

A colourless liquid, slightly soluble in water, soluble in alcohol.

d_{20}^{20}: about 0.766.

n_D^{20}: about 1.418.

bp: 127 °C to 131 °C.

Histamine dihydrochloride. *1042800.* [56-92-8].

See *Histamine dihydrochloride (0143)*.

Histamine phosphate. *1042900.* [23297-93-0].

See *Histamine phosphate (0144)*.

Histamine solution. *1042901.*

A 9 g/l solution of *sodium chloride R* containing 0.1 μg per millilitre of histamine base (as the phosphate or dihydrochloride).

Histidine monohydrochloride. $C_6H_{10}ClN_3O_2,H_2O$. (M_r 209.6). *1043000.* [123333-71-1]. (*RS*)-2-Amino-3-(imidazol-4-yl)propionic acid hydrochloride monohydrate.

A crystalline powder or colourless crystals, soluble in water.

mp: about 250 °C, with decomposition.

Chromatography. Examine as prescribed in the monograph on *Histamine dihydrochloride (0143)*; the chromatogram shows only one principal spot.

Holmium oxide. Ho_2O_3. (M_r 377.9). *1043100.* [12055-62-8]. Diholmium trioxide.

A yellowish powder, practically insoluble in water.

Holmium perchlorate solution. *1043101.*

A 40 g/l solution of *holmium oxide R* in a solution of *perchloric acid R* containing 141 g/l of $HClO_4$.

DL-Homocysteine. $C_4H_9NO_2S$. (M_r 135.2). *1136100.* [454-29-5]. (2*RS*)-2-Amino-4-sulphanylbutanoic acid.

A white, crystalline powder.

mp: about 232 °C.

L-Homocysteine thiolactone hydrochloride. C_4H_8ClNOS. (M_r 153.6). *1136200.* [31828-68-9]. (3*S*)-3-Aminodihydrothiophen-2(3*H*)-one hydrochloride.

A white, crystalline powder.

mp: about 202 °C.

Hyaluronidase diluent. *1043300.*

Mix 100 ml of *phosphate buffer solution pH 6.4 R* with 100 ml of *water R*. Dissolve 0.140 g of *hydrolysed gelatin R* in the solution at 37 °C.

Storage: use within 2 h.

Hydrastine hydrochloride. $C_{21}H_{22}ClNO_6$. (M_r 419.9). *1154000.* [5936-28-7]. (3*S*)-6,7-Dimethoxy-3-[(5*R*)-6-methyl-5,6,7,8-tetrahydro-1,3-dioxolo[4,5-*g*]isoquinolin-5-yl]isobenzofuran-1(3*H*)-one hydrochloride.

A white powder, hygroscopic, very soluble in water and in alcohol.

$[\alpha]_D^{17}$: about + 127.

mp: about 116 °C.

Hydrastine hydrochloride used in liquid chromatography complies with the following additional test.

Assay. Examine by liquid chromatography (*2.2.29*) as prescribed in the monograph on *Goldenseal rhizome (1831)*. The content is not less than 98 per cent, calculated by the normalisation procedure.

Hydrazine. H_4N_2. (M_r 32.05). *1136300.* [302-01-2]. Diazane.

A slightly oily liquid, colourless, with a strong odour of ammonia, miscible with water. Dilute solutions in water are commercially available.

Caution: toxic and corrosive.

n_D^{20} : about 1.470.

bp: about 113 °C.

mp: about 1.5 °C.

Hydrazine sulphate. $H_6N_2O_4S$. (M_r 130.1). *1043400.* [10034-93-2].

Colourless crystals, sparingly soluble in cold water, soluble in hot water (50 °C) and freely soluble in boiling water, practically insoluble in alcohol.

Arsenic (*2.4.2*). 1.0 g complies with limit test A (1 ppm).

Sulphated ash (*2.4.14*): maximum 0.1 per cent.

Hydriodic acid. HI. (M_r 127.9). *1098900.* [10034-85-2].

Prepare by distilling hydriodic acid over red phosphorus, passing *carbon dioxide R* or *nitrogen R* through the apparatus during the distillation. Use the colourless or almost colourless, constant-boiling mixture (55 per cent to 58 per cent of HI) distilling between 126 °C and 127 °C.

Place the acid in small, amber, glass-stoppered bottles previously flushed with *carbon dioxide R* or *nitrogen R*, seal with paraffin.

Storage: in a dark place.

Hydrobromic acid, 30 per cent. *1098700.* [10035-10-6].

30 per cent hydrobromic acid in *glacial acetic acid R*.

Degas with caution the contents before opening.

Hydrobromic acid, dilute. *1098701.*

Place 5.0 ml of *30 per cent hydrobromic acid R* in amber vials equipped with polyethylene stoppers. Seal under *argon R* and store in the dark. Add 5.0 ml of *glacial acetic acid R* immediately before use. Shake.

Storage: in the dark.

Hydrobromic acid, 47 per cent. *1118900.*

A 47 per cent *m/m* solution of hydrobromic acid in *water R*.

Hydrobromic acid, dilute R1. *1118901.*

Contains 7,9 g/l of HBr.

Dissolve 16.81 g of *47 per cent hydrobromic acid R* in *water R* and dilute to 1000 ml with the same solvent.

Hydrochloric acid. *1043500.* [7647-01-0].

See *Concentrated hydrochloric acid (0002)*.

Hydrochloric acid R1. *1043501.*

Contains 250 g/l of HCl.

Dilute 70 g of *hydrochloric acid R* to 100 ml with *water R*.

Hydrochloric acid, brominated. *1043507.*

To 1 ml of *bromine solution R* add 100 ml of *hydrochloric acid R*.

Hydrochloric acid, dilute. *1043503.*

Contains 73 g/l of HCl.

Dilute 20 g of *hydrochloric acid R* to 100 ml with *water R*.

Hydrochloric acid, dilute, heavy metal-free. *1043509.*

Complies with the requirements prescribed for *dilute hydrochloric acid R* and with the following maximum contents of heavy metals:

As: 0.005 ppm;

Cd: 0.003 ppm;

Cu: 0.003 ppm;

Fe: 0.05 ppm;

Hg: 0.005 ppm;

Ni: 0.004 ppm;

Pb: 0.001 ppm;

Zn: 0.005 ppm.

Hydrochloric acid, dilute R1. *1043504.*

Contains 0.37 g/l of HCl.

Dilute 1.0 ml of *dilute hydrochloric acid R* to 200.0 ml with *water R*.

Hydrochloric acid, dilute R2. *1043505.*

Dilute 30 ml of *1 M hydrochloric acid* to 1000 ml with *water R*; adjust to pH 1.6 ± 0.1.

4. Reagents

Hydrochloric acid, ethanolic. *1043506.*

Dilute 5.0 ml of *1 M hydrochloric acid* to 500.0 ml with *alcohol R.*

Hydrochloric acid, heavy metal-free. *1043510.*

Complies with the requirements prescribed for *hydrochloric acid R* and with the following maximum contents of heavy metals:

As: 0.005 ppm;

Cd: 0.003 ppm;

Cu: 0.003 ppm;

Fe: 0.05 ppm;

Hg: 0.005 ppm;

Ni: 0.004 ppm;

Pb: 0.001 ppm;

Zn: 0.005 ppm.

Hydrochloric acid, lead-free. *1043508.*

Complies with the requirements prescribed for *hydrochloric acid R* and with the following additional test.

Lead: maximum 20 ppb of Pb determined by atomic emission spectrometry (*2.2.22, Method I*).

Test solution. In a quartz crucible evaporate 200 g of the acid to be examined almost to dryness. Take up the residue in 5 ml of nitric acid prepared by sub-boiling distillation of *nitric acid R* and evaporate to dryness. Take up the residue in 5 ml of nitric acid prepared by sub-boiling distillation of *nitric acid R.*

Reference solutions. Prepare the reference solutions using *lead standard solution (0.1 ppm Pb) R* diluted with nitric acid prepared by sub-boiling distillation of *nitric acid R.* Measure the emission intensity at 220.35 nm.

Hydrocortisone acetate. *1098800.* [50-03-3].

See *Hydrocortisone acetate (0334).*

Hydrofluoric acid. HF. (M_r 20.01). *1043600.* [7664-39-3].

Content: minimum 40.0 per cent *m/m* of HF.

A clear, colourless liquid.

Residue on ignition. Not more than 0.05 per cent *m/m.* Evaporate the hydrofluoric acid in a platinum crucible and gently ignite the residue to constant mass.

Assay. Weigh accurately a glass-stoppered flask containing 50.0 ml of *1 M sodium hydroxide.* Introduce 2 g of the hydrofluoric acid and weigh again. Titrate the solution with *0.5 M sulphuric acid,* using 0.5 ml of *phenolphthalein solution R* as indicator.

1 ml of *1 M sodium hydroxide* is equivalent to 20.01 mg of HF.

Storage: in a polyethylene container.

Hydrogen for chromatography. H_2. (M_r 2.016). *1043700.* [1333-74-0].

Content: minimum 99.95 per cent *V/V* of H_2.

Hydrogen peroxide solution, dilute. *1043800.* [7722-84-1].

See *Hydrogen peroxide solution (3 per cent) (0395).*

Hydrogen peroxide solution, strong. *1043900.* [7722-84-1].

See *Hydrogen peroxide solution (30 per cent) (0396).*

Hydrogen sulphide. H_2S. (M_r 34.08). *1044000.* [7783-06-4].

A gas, slightly soluble in water.

Hydrogen sulphide solution. *1136400.*

A recently prepared solution of *hydrogen sulphide R* in *water R.* The saturated solution contains about 0.4 per cent to 0.5 per cent of H_2S at 20 °C.

Hydrogen sulphide R1. H_2S. (M_r 34.08). *1106600.*

Content: minimum 99.7 per cent *V/V* of H_2S.

Hydroquinone. $C_6H_6O_2$. (M_r 110.1). *1044100.* [123-31-9].

Benzene-1,4-diol.

Fine, colourless or white needles, darkening on exposure to air and light, soluble in water and in alcohol.

mp: about 173 °C.

Storage: protected from light and air.

Hydroquinone solution. *1044101.*

Dissolve 0.5 g of *hydroquinone R* in *water R,* add 20 µl of *sulphuric acid R* and dilute to 50 ml with *water R.*

4-Hydroxybenzohydrazide. $C_7H_8N_2O_2$. (M_r 152.2). *1145900.* [5351-23-5]. *p*-Hydroxybenzohydrazide.

4-Hydroxybenzoic acid. $C_7H_6O_3$. (M_r 138.1). *1106700.* [99-96-7].

Crystals, slightly soluble in water, very soluble in alcohol, soluble in acetone.

mp: 214 °C to 215 °C.

2-[4-(2-Hydroxyethyl)piperazin-1-yl]ethanesulphonic acid. $C_8H_{18}N_2O_4S$. (M_r 238.3). *1106800.* [7365-45-9]. HEPES.

A white powder.

mp: about 236 °C, with decomposition

4-Hydroxyisophthalic acid. $C_8H_6O_5$. (M_r 182.1). *1106900.* [636-46-4]. 4-Hydroxybenzene-1,3-dicarboxylic acid.

Needles or platelets, very slightly soluble in water, freely soluble in alcohol.

mp: about 314 °C, with decomposition.

Hydroxylamine hydrochloride. NH_4ClO. (M_r 69.5). *1044300.* [5470-11-1].

A white, crystalline powder, very soluble in water, soluble in alcohol.

Hydroxylamine hydrochloride solution R2. *1044304.*

Dissolve 2.5 g of *hydroxylamine hydrochloride R* in 4.5 ml of hot *water R* and add 40 ml of *alcohol R* and 0.4 ml of *bromophenol blue solution R2.* Add *0.5 M alcoholic potassium hydroxide* until a greenish-yellow colour is obtained. Dilute to 50.0 ml with *alcohol R.*

Hydroxylamine solution, alcoholic. *1044301.*

Dissolve 3.5 g of *hydroxylamine hydrochloride R* in 95 ml of *alcohol (60 per cent V/V) R,* add 0.5 ml of a 2 g/l solution of *methyl orange R* in *alcohol (60 per cent V/V) R* and sufficient *0.5 M potassium hydroxide in alcohol (60 per cent V/V)* to give a pure yellow colour. Dilute to 100 ml with *alcohol (60 per cent V/V) R.*

Hydroxylamine solution, alkaline. *1044302.*

Immediately before use, mix equal volumes of a 139 g/l solution of *hydroxylamine hydrochloride R* and a 150 g/l solution of *sodium hydroxide R.*

Hydroxylamine solution, alkaline R1. *1044303.*

Solution A. Dissolve 12.5 g of *hydroxylamine hydrochloride R* in *methanol R* and dilute to 100 ml with the same solvent.

Solution B. Dissolve 12.5 g of *sodium hydroxide R* in *methanol R* and dilute to 100 ml with the same solvent.

Mix equal volumes of solution A and solution B immediately before use.

Hydroxymethylfurfural. $C_6H_6O_3$. (M_r 126.1). *1044400.* [67-47-0]. 5-Hydroxymethylfurfural.

Acicular crystals, freely soluble in water, in acetone and in alcohol.

mp: about 32 °C.

Hydroxynaphthol blue, sodium salt. $C_{20}H_{11}N_2Na_3O_{11}S_3$. ($M_r$ 620). *1044500.* [63451-35-4]. Trisodium 2,2′-dihydroxy-1,1′-azonaphthalene-3′,4,6′-trisulphonate.

2-Hydroxypropylbetadex for chromatography R. *1146000.* Betacyclodextrin modified by the bonding of (*R*) or (*RS*) propylene oxide groups on the hydroxyl groups.

Hydroxypropyl-β-cyclodextrin. *1128600.* [94035-02-6].

See *Hydroxypropylbetadex (1804).*

pH (*2.2.3*): 5.0-7.5 (20 g/l solution).

Hydroxyquinoline. C_9H_7NO. (M_r 145.2). *1044600.* [148-24-3]. 8-Hydroxyquinoline. Quinolin-8-ol.

A white or slightly yellowish, crystalline powder, slightly soluble in water, freely soluble in acetone, in alcohol and in dilute mineral acids.

mp: about 75 °C.

Sulphated ash (*2.4.14*): maximum 0.05 per cent.

12-Hydroxystearic acid. $C_{18}H_{36}O_3$. (M_r 300.5). *1099000.* [106-14-9]. 12-Hydroxyoctadecanoic acid.

White powder.

mp: 71 °C to 74 °C.

5-Hydroxyuracil. $C_4H_4N_2O_3$. (M_r 128.1). *1044700.* [496-76-4]. Isobarbituric acid. Pyrimidine-2,4,5-triol.

A white, crystalline powder.

mp: about 310 °C, with decomposition.

Chromatography. Examined as prescribed in the monograph on *Fluorouracil (0611),* the chromatogram shows a principal spot with an R_f of about 0.3.

Storage: in an airtight container.

Hyoscine hydrobromide. *1044800.* [6533-68-2].

See *Hyoscine hydrobromide (0106).*

Hyoscyamine sulphate. *1044900.* [620-61-1].

See *Hyoscyamine sulphate (0501).*

Hypericin. $C_{30}H_{16}O_8$. (M_r 504.4). *1149800.* [548-04-9]. 1,3,4,6,8,13-Hexahydroxy-10,11-dimethylphenanthro[1,10,9,8-*opqra*]perylene-7,14-dione.

Content: minimum 85 per cent of $C_{30}H_{16}O_8$.

Hyperoside. $C_{21}H_{20}O_{12}$. (M_r 464.4). *1045000.* 2-(3,4-Dihydroxyphenyl)-3-β-D-galactopyranosyloxy-5,7-dihydroxy-chromen-4-one.

Faint yellow needles, soluble in methanol.

$[\alpha]_D^{20}$: − 8.3, determined on a 2 g/l solution in *pyridine R*.

mp: about 240 °C, with decomposition.

A solution in *methanol R* shows two absorption maxima (*2.2.25*), at 259 nm and at 364 nm.

Hypophosphorous reagent. *1045200.*

Dissolve with the aid of gentle heat, 10 g of *sodium hypophosphite R* in 20 ml of *water R* and dilute to 100 ml with *hydrochloric acid R.* Allow to settle and decant or filter through glass wool.

Hypoxanthine. $C_5H_4N_4O$. (M_r 136.1). *1045300.* [68-94-0]. 1*H*-Purin-6-one.

A white, crystalline powder, very slightly soluble in water, sparingly soluble in boiling water, soluble in dilute acids and in dilute alkali hydroxide solutions, decomposes without melting at about 150 °C.

Chromatography. Examine as prescribed in the monograph on *Mercaptopurine (0096)*; the chromatogram shows only one principal spot.

Imidazole. $C_3H_4N_2$. (M_r 68.1). *1045400.* [288-32-4].

A white, crystalline powder, soluble in water and in alcohol.

mp: about 90 °C.

Iminodibenzyl. $C_{14}H_{13}N$. (M_r 195.3). *1045500.* [494-19-9]. 10,11-Dihydrodibenz[*b,f*]azepine.

A pale yellow, crystalline powder, practically insoluble in water, freely soluble in acetone.

mp: about 106 °C.

Indigo carmine. $C_{16}H_8N_2Na_2O_8S_2$. (M_r 466.3). *1045600.* [860-22-0].

Schultz No. 1309.

Colour Index No. 73015.

3,3′-Dioxo-2,2′-bisindolylidene-5,5′-disulphonate disodium. E 132.

It usually contains sodium chloride.

A blue or violet-blue powder or blue granules with a coppery lustre, sparingly soluble in water, practically insoluble in alcohol. It is precipitated from an aqueous solution by sodium chloride.

Indigo carmine solution. *1045601.*

To a mixture of 10 ml of *hydrochloric acid R* and 990 ml of 200 g/l *nitrogen-free sulphuric acid R* add 0.2 g of *indigo carmine R.*

The solution complies with the following test.

Add 10 ml to a solution of 1.0 mg of *potassium nitrate R* in 10 ml of *water R*, rapidly add 20 ml of *nitrogen-free sulphuric acid R* and heat to boiling. The blue colour is discharged within 1 min.

Indigo carmine solution R1. *1045602.*

Dissolve 4 g of *indigo carmine R* in about 900 ml of *water R* added in several portions. Add 2 ml of *sulphuric acid R* and dilute to 1000 ml with *water R.*

Standardisation. Place in a 100 ml conical flask with a wide neck 10.0 ml of *nitrate standard solution (100 ppm NO_3) R*, 10 ml of *water R*, 0.05 ml of the *indigo carmine solution R1*, and then in a single addition, but with caution, 30 ml of *sulphuric acid R.* Titrate the solution immediately, using the *indigo carmine solution R1*, until a stable blue colour is obtained.

The number of millilitres used, *n*, is equivalent to 1 mg of NO_3.

Indometacin. *1101500.* [53-86-1].

See *Indometacin (0092).*

Iodine. *1045800.* [7553-56-2].

See *Iodine (0031).*

Iodine solution R1. *1045801.*

To 10.0 ml of *0.05 M iodine* add 0.6 g of *potassium iodide R* and dilute to 100.0 ml with *water R.* Prepare immediately before use.

4. Reagents

Iodine solution R2. *1045802.*

To 10.0 ml of *0.05 M iodine* add 0.6 g of *potassium iodide R* and dilute to 1000.0 ml with *water R*. Prepare immediately before use.

Iodine solution R3. *1045803.*

Dilute 2.0 ml of *iodine solution R1* to 100.0 ml with *water R*. Prepare immediately before use.

Iodine solution R4. *1045806.*

Dissolve 14 g of *iodine R* in 100 ml of a 400 g/l solution of *potassium iodide R*, add 1 ml of *dilute hydrochloric acid R* and dilute to 1000 ml with *water R*.

Storage: protected from light.

Iodine solution, alcoholic. *1045804.*

A 10 g/l solution in *alcohol R*.

Storage: protected from light.

Iodine solution, chloroformic. *1045805.*

A 5 g/l solution in *chloroform R*.

Storage: protected from light.

4. Reagents

Iodine bromide. IBr. (M_r 206.8). *1045900.* [7789-33-5].

Bluish-black or brownish-black crystals, freely soluble in water, in alcohol and in glacial acetic acid.

bp: about 116 °C.

mp: about 40 °C.

Storage: protected from light.

Iodine bromide solution. *1045901.*

Dissolve 20 g of *iodine bromide R* in *glacial acetic acid R* and dilute to 1000 ml with the same solvent.

Storage: protected from light.

Iodine chloride. ICl. (M_r 162.4). *1143000.* [7790-99-0].

Black crystals, soluble in water, in acetic acid and in alcohol.

bp: about 97.4 °C.

Iodine chloride solution. *1143001.*

Dissolve 1.4 g of *iodine chloride R* in *glacial acetic acid R* and dilute to 100 ml with the same acid.

Storage: protected from light.

Iodine pentoxide, recrystallised. I_2O_5. (M_r 333.8). *1046000.* [12029-98-0]. Di-iodine pentoxide. Iodic anhydride.

Content: minimum 99.5 per cent of I_2O_5.

A white, crystalline powder, or white or greyish-white granules, hygroscopic, very soluble in water forming HIO_3.

Stability on heating. Dissolve 2 g, previously heated for 1 h at 200 °C, in 50 ml of *water R*. A colourless solution is obtained.

Assay. Dissolve 0.100 g in 50 ml of *water R*, add 3 g of *potassium iodide R* and 10 ml of *dilute hydrochloric acid R*. Titrate the liberated iodine with *0.1 M sodium thiosulphate*, using 1 ml of *starch solution R* as indicator.

1 ml of *0.1 M sodium thiosulphate* is equivalent to 2.782 mg of I_2O_5.

Storage: in an airtight container, protected from light.

Iodoacetic acid. $C_2H_3IO_2$. (M_r 185.9). *1107000.* [64-69-7].

Colourless or white crystals, soluble in water and in alcohol.

mp: 82 °C to 83 °C.

2-Iodobenzoic acid. $C_7H_5IO_2$. (M_r 248.0). *1046100.* [88-67-5].

A white or slightly yellow, crystalline powder, slightly soluble in water, soluble in alcohol.

mp: about 160 °C.

Chromatography. Examine by thin-layer chromatography (*2.2.27*), using cellulose for chromatography f_{254} R as the coating substance. Apply to the plate 20 µl of a solution of the 2-iodobenzoic acid, prepared by dissolving 40 mg in 4 ml of *0.1 M sodium hydroxide* and diluting to 10 ml with *water R*. Develop over a path of about 12 cm using as the mobile phase the upper layer obtained by shaking together 20 volumes of *water R*, 40 volumes of *glacial acetic acid R* and 40 volumes of *toluene R*. Allow the plate to dry in air and examine in ultraviolet light at 254 nm. The chromatogram shows only one principal spot.

Iodoethane. C_2H_5I. (M_r 155.9). *1099100.* [75-03-6].

Colourless to slightly yellowish liquid, darkening on exposure to air and light, miscible with alcohol and most organic solvents.

d_{20}^{20}: about 1.95.

n_D^{20}: about 1.513.

bp: about 72 °C.

Storage: in an airtight container.

2-Iodohippuric acid. $C_9H_8INO_3,2H_2O$. (M_r 341.1). *1046200.* [147-58-0]. 2-(2-Iodobenzamido)acetic acid.

A white or almost white, crystalline powder, sparingly soluble in water.

mp: about 170 °C.

Water (*2.5.12*): 9 per cent to 13 per cent, determined on 1.000 g.

Chromatography. Examine by thin-layer chromatography (*2.2.27*), using *cellulose for chromatography F_{254} R* as the coating substance. Apply to the plate 20 µl of a solution of the 2-iodohippuric acid, prepared by dissolving 40 mg in 4 ml of *0.1 M sodium hydroxide* and diluting to 10 ml with *water R*. Develop over a path of about 12 cm using as the mobile phase the upper layer obtained by shaking together 20 volumes of *water R*, 40 volumes of *glacial acetic acid R* and 40 volumes of *toluene R*. Allow the plate to dry in air and examine in ultraviolet light at 254 nm. The chromatogram shows only one principal spot.

Iodoplatinate reagent. *1046300.*

To 3 ml of a 100 g/l solution of *chloroplatinic acid R* add 97 ml of *water R* and 100 ml of a 60 g/l solution of *potassium iodide R*.

Storage: protected from light.

Iodosulphurous reagent. *1046400.*

The apparatus, which must be kept closed and dry during the preparation, consists of a 3000 ml to 4000 ml round-bottomed flask with three inlets for a stirrer and a thermometer and fitted with a drying tube. To 700 ml of *anhydrous pyridine R* and 700 ml of *ethyleneglycol monomethyl ether R* add, with constant stirring, 220 g of finely powdered *iodine R*, previously dried over *diphosphorus pentoxide R*. Continue stirring until the iodine has completely dissolved (about 30 min). Cool to − 10 °C, and add quickly, still stirring, 190 g of *sulphur dioxide R*. Do not allow the temperature to exceed 30 °C. Cool.

Standardisation. Add about 20 ml of *anhydrous methanol R* to a titration vessel and titrate to the end-point with the iodosulphurous reagent (*2.5.12*). Introduce in an appropriate form a suitable amount of *water R*, accurately weighed, and repeat the determination of water. Calculate the water equivalent in milligrams per millilitre of iodosulphurous reagent.

The minimum water equivalent is 3.5 mg of water per millilitre of reagent.

Work protected from humidity. Standardise immediately before use.

Storage: in a dry container.

5-Iodouracil. $C_4H_3IN_2O_2$. (M_r 238.0). *1046500.* [696-07-1]. 5-Iodo-1*H*,3*H*-pyrimidine-2,4-dione.

mp: about 276 °C, with decomposition.

Chromatography. Examine as prescribed in the monograph on *Idoxuridine (0669)*, applying 5 µl of a 0.25 g/l solution. The chromatogram obtained shows only one principal spot.

Ion-exclusion resin for chromatography. *1131000.*

A resin with sulphonic acid groups attached to a polymer lattice consisting of polystyrene cross-linked with divinylbenzene.

Ion-exchange resin, strongly acidic. *1085400.*

A resin in protonated form with sulphonic acid groups attached to a lattice consisting of polystyrene cross-linked with 8 per cent of divinylbenzene. It is available as spherical beads; unless otherwise prescribed, the particle size is 0.3 mm to 1.2 mm.

Capacity. 4.5 mmol to 5 mmol per gram, with a water content of 50 per cent to 60 per cent.

Preparation of a column. Unless otherwise prescribed, use a tube with a fused-in sintered glass disc having a length of 400 mm, an internal diameter of 20 mm and a filling height of about 200 mm. Introduce the resin, mixing it with *water R* and pouring the slurry into the tube, ensuring that no air bubbles are trapped between the particles. When in use, the liquid must not be allowed to fall below the surface of the resin. If the resin is in its protonated form, wash with *water R* until 50 ml requires not more than 0.05 ml of *0.1 M sodium hydroxide* for neutralisation, using 0.1 ml of *methyl orange solution R* as indicator.

If the resin is in its sodium form or if it requires regeneration, pass about 100 ml of a mixture of equal volumes of *hydrochloric acid R1* and *water R* slowly through the column and then wash with *water R* as described above.

Iron. Fe. (A_r 55.85). *1046600.* [7439-89-6].

Grey powder or wire, soluble in dilute mineral acids.

Iron salicylate solution. *1046700.*

Dissolve 0.1 g of *ferric ammonium sulphate R* in a mixture of 2 ml of *dilute sulphuric acid R* and 48 ml of *water R* and dilute to 100 ml with *water R*. Add 50 ml of a 11.5 g/l solution of *sodium salicylate R*, 10 ml of *dilute acetic acid R*, 80 ml of a 136 g/l solution of *sodium acetate R* and dilute to 500 ml with *water R*. The solution should be recently prepared.

Storage: in an airtight container, protected from light.

Isatin. $C_8H_5NO_2$. (M_r 147.1). *1046800.* [91-56-5]. Indoline-2,3-dione.

Small, yellowish-red crystals, slightly soluble in water, soluble in hot water and in alcohol, soluble in solutions of alkali hydroxides giving a violet colour becoming yellow on standing.

mp: about 200 °C, with partial sublimation.

Sulphated ash (*2.4.14*): maximum 0.2 per cent.

Isatin reagent. *1046801.*

Dissolve 6 mg of *ferric sulphate R* in 8 ml of *water R* and add cautiously 50 ml of *sulphuric acid R*. Add 6 mg of *isatin R* and stir until dissolved.

The reagent should be pale yellow, but not orange or red.

Isoamyl alcohol. $C_5H_{12}O$. (M_r 88.1). *1046900.* [123-51-3]. 3-Methylbutan-1-ol.

A colourless liquid, slightly soluble in water, miscible with alcohol.

bp: about 130 °C.

Isoandrosterone. $C_{19}H_{30}O_2$. (M_r 290.4). *1107100.* [481-29-8]. Epiandrosterone. 3β-Hydroxy-5α-androstan-17-one.

A white powder, practically insoluble in water, soluble in organic solvents.

$[\alpha]_D^{20}$: + 88, determined on 20 g/l solution in *methanol R*.

mp: 172 °C to 174 °C.

Δ*A* (*2.2.41*): 14.24 × 10^3, determined at 304 nm on a 1.25 g/l solution.

Isodrin. $C_{12}H_8Cl_6$. (M_r 364.9). *1128700.* [465-73-6]. 1,2,3,4,10,10-Hexachloro-1,4,4a,5,8,8a-hexahydro-*endo,endo*-1,4:5,8-dimethanonaphthalene.

Practically insoluble in water, soluble in common organic solvents such as acetone.

A suitable certified reference solution may be used.

Isomenthol. $C_{10}H_{20}O$. (M_r 156.3). *1047000.* [23283-97-8]. (+)-*Isomenthol:* (1*S*,2*R*,5*R*)-2-isopropyl-5-methylcyclohexanol. (±)-*Isomenthol:* a mixture of equal parts of (1*S*,2*R*,5*R*)- and (1*R*,2*S*,5*S*)-2-isopropyl-5-methylcyclohexanol.

Colourless crystals, practically insoluble in water, very soluble in alcohol.

$[\alpha]_D^{20}$: (+)-*Isomenthol*: about + 24, determined on a 100 g/l solution in *alcohol R*.

bp: (+)-*Isomenthol*: about 218 °C. (±)-*Isomenthol*: about 218 °C.

mp: (+)-*Isomenthol*: about 80 °C. (±)-*Isomenthol*: about 53 °C.

(+)-Isomenthone. $C_{10}H_{18}O$. (M_r 154.2). *1047100.* (1*R*)-*cis*-*p*-Menthan-3-one. (1*R*)-*cis*-2-Isopropyl-5-methylcyclohexanone.

Contains variable amounts of menthone. A colourless liquid, very slightly soluble in water, soluble in alcohol.

d_{20}^{20}: about 0.904.

n_D^{20}: about 1.453.

$[\alpha]_D^{20}$: about + 93.2.

Isomenthone used in gas chromatography complies with the following additional test.

Assay. Examine by gas chromatography (*2.2.28*) as prescribed in the monograph on *Peppermint oil (0405)* using the substance to be examined as the test solution.

The area of the principal peak is not less than 80.0 per cent of the total area of the peaks.

Isopropylamine. C_3H_9N. (M_r 59.1). *1119800.* [75-31-0]. Propan-2-amine.

A colourless, highly volatile, flammable liquid.

n_D^{20}: about 1.374.

bp: 32 °C to 34 °C.

Isopropyl myristate. *1047200.* [110-27-0].

See *Isopropyl myristate (0725)*.

4-Isopropylphenol. $C_9H_{12}O$. (M_r 136.2). *1047300.* [99-89-8].

Content: minimum 98 per cent of $C_9H_{12}O$.

bp: about 212 °C.

mp: 59 °C to 61 °C.

Isopulegol. $C_{10}H_{18}O$. (M_r 154.2). *1139600.* [89-79-2]. (−)-Isopulegol. (1*R*,2*S*,5*R*)-2-Isopropenyl-5-methylcyclohexanol.

d_4^{20}: about 0.911.

n_D^{20}: about 1.472.

bp: about 91 °C.

Isopulegol used in gas chromatography complies with the following additional test.

Assay. Examine by gas chromatography (*2.2.28*) as prescribed in the monograph on *Mint oil, partly dementholised (1838).*

The content is not less than 99 per cent, calculated by the normalisation procedure.

Isoquercitroside. $C_{21}H_{20}O_{12}$. (M_r 464.4). *1136500.* [21637-25-2]. Isoquercitrin. 2-(3,4-Dihydroxyphenyl)-3-(β-D-glucofuranosyloxy)-5,7-dihydroxy-4*H*-1-benzopyran-4-one. 3,3′,4′,5,7-Pentahydroxyflavone-3-glucoside.

Isosilibinin. $C_{25}H_{22}O_{10}$. (M_r 482.4). *1149900.* [72581-71-6]. 3,5,7-Trihydroxy-2-[2-(4-hydroxy-3-methoxyphenyl)-3-hydroxymethyl-2,3-dihydro-1,4-benzodioxin-6-yl]chroman-4-one.

White to yellowish powder, practically insoluble in water, soluble in acetone and in methanol.

Kaolin, light. *1047400.* [1332-58-7].

A purified native hydrated aluminium silicate. It contains a suitable dispersing agent.

A light, white powder free from gritty particles, unctuous to the touch, practically insoluble in water and in mineral acids.

Coarse particles. Place 5.0 g in a ground-glass-stoppered cylinder about 160 mm long and 35 mm in diameter and add 60 ml of a 10 g/l solution of *sodium pyrophosphate R.* Shake vigorously and allow to stand for 5 min. Using a pipette, remove 50 ml of the liquid from a point about 5 cm below the surface. To the remaining liquid add 50 ml of *water R*, shake, allow to stand for 5 min and remove 50 ml as before. Repeat the operations until a total of 400 ml has been removed. Transfer the remaining suspension to an evaporating dish. Evaporate to dryness on a water-bath and dry the residue to constant mass at 100 °C to 105 °C. The residue weighs not more than 25 mg (0.5 per cent).

Fine particles. Disperse 5.0 g in 250 ml of *water R* by shaking vigorously for 2 min. Immediately pour into a glass cylinder 50 mm in diameter and, using a pipette, transfer 20 ml to a glass dish, evaporate to dryness on a water-bath and dry to constant mass at 100 °C to 105 °C. Allow the remainder of the suspension to stand at 20 °C for 4 h and, using a pipette with its tip exactly 5 cm below the surface, withdraw a further 20 ml without disturbing the sediment, place in a glass dish, evaporate to dryness on a water-bath and dry to constant mass at 100 °C to 105 °C. The mass of the second residue is not less than 70 per cent of that of the first residue.

Kieselguhr for chromatography. *1047500.*

A white or yellowish-white, light powder, practically insoluble in water, in dilute acids and in organic solvents.

Filtration rate. Use a chromatography column 0.25 m long and 10 mm in internal diameter with a sintered-glass (100) plate and two marks at 0.10 m and 0.20 m above the plate. Place sufficient of the substance to be examined in the column to reach the first mark and fill to the second mark with *water R*. When the first drops begin to flow from the column, fill to the second mark again with *water R* and measure the time required for the first 5 ml to flow from the column. The flow rate is not less than 1 ml/min.

Appearance of the eluate. The eluate obtained in the test for filtration rate is colourless (*Method I, 2.2.2*).

Acidity or alkalinity. To 1.00 g add 10 ml of *water R*, shake vigorously and allow to stand for 5 min. Filter the suspension on a filter previously washed with hot *water R* until the washings are neutral. To 2.0 ml of the filtrate add 0.05 ml of *methyl red solution R*; the solution is yellow. To 2.0 ml of the filtrate add 0.05 ml of *phenolphthalein solution R1*; the solution is at most slightly pink.

Water-soluble substances. Place 10.0 g in a chromatography column 0.25 m long and 10 mm in internal diameter and elute with *water R*. Collect the first 20 ml of eluate, evaporate to dryness and dry the residue at 100 °C to 105 °C. The residue weighs not more than 10 mg.

Iron (*2.4.9*). To 0.50 g add 10 ml of a mixture of equal volumes of *hydrochloric acid R1* and *water R*, shake vigorously, allow to stand for 5 min and filter. 1.0 ml of the filtrate complies with the limit test for iron (200 ppm).

Loss on ignition: maximum 0.5 per cent. During heating to red heat (600 °C) the substance does not become brown or black.

Kieselguhr G. *1047600.*

Consists of kieselguhr treated with hydrochloric acid and calcined, to which is added about 15 per cent of calcium sulphate hemihydrate.

A fine greyish-white powder; the grey colour becomes more pronounced on triturating with water. The average particle size is 10 µm to 40 µm.

Calcium sulphate content. Determine by the method prescribed for *silica gel G R.*

pH (*2.2.3*). Shake 1 g with 10 ml of *carbon dioxide-free water R* for 5 min. The pH of the suspension is 7 to 8.

Chromatographic separation. Examine by thin-layer chromatography (*2.2.27*). Prepare plates using a slurry of the kieselguhr G with a 2.7 g/l solution of *sodium acetate R.* Apply 5 µl of a solution containing 0.1 g/l of lactose, sucrose, glucose and fructose in *pyridine R.* Develop over a path of 14 cm using a mixture of 12 volumes of *water R*, 23 volumes of *2-propanol R* and 65 volumes of *ethyl acetate R.* The migration time of the solvent is about 40 min. Dry, spray onto the plate about 10 ml of *anisaldehyde solution R* and heat for 5 min to 10 min at 100 °C to 105 °C. The chromatogram shows four well-defined spots without tailing and well separated from each other.

Lactic acid. *1047800.* [50-21-5].

See *Lactic acid (0458).*

Lactic reagent. *1047801.*

Solution A. To 60 ml of *lactic acid R* add 45 ml of previously filtered *lactic acid R* saturated without heating with *Sudan red G R*; as lactic acid saturates slowly without heating, an excess of colorant is always necessary.

Solution B. Prepare 10 ml of a saturated solution of *aniline R.* Filter.

Solution C. Dissolve 75 mg of *potassium iodide R* in water and dilute to 70 ml with the same solvent. Add 10 ml of *alcohol R* and 0.1 g of *iodine R.* Shake.

Mix solutions A and B. Add solution C.

4. Reagents

Lactobionic acid. $C_{12}H_{22}O_{12}$. (M_r 358.3). *1101600.* [96-82-2].

A white, crystalline powder, freely soluble in water, practically insoluble in alcohol.

mp: about 115 °C.

Lactose. *1047900.* [5989-81-1].

See *Lactose (0187).*

β-Lactose. $C_{12}H_{22}O_{11}$. (M_r 342.3). *1150100.* [5965-66-2]. β-D-Lactose.

White or slightly yellowish powder.

The α-D-lactose content is not greater than 35 per cent.

Assay. Gas chromatography (*2.2.28*): use the normalisation procedure.

Inject an appropriate derivatised sample.

Column:

- *size*: *l* = 30 m, Ø = 0.25 mm,
- *stationary phase*: *poly[(cyanopropyl)(phenyl)][dimethyl] siloxane R* (film thickness 1 µm).

Carrier gas: *helium for chromatography R.*

Temperature:

	Time (min)	Temperature (°C)
Column	0 - 32.5	20 → 280
Injection port		250
Detector		250

Detection: flame ionisation.

The area of the peak due to β-lactose is not less than 99 per cent of the total peak area.

α-Lactose monohydrate. $C_{12}H_{22}O_{11},H_2O$. (M_r 360.3). *1150000.* [5989-81-1]. α-D-Lactose monohydrate.

White powder.

The β-D-lactose content is less than 3 per cent.

Assay. Gas chromatography (*2.2.28*): use the normalisation procedure.

Inject an appropriate derivatised sample.

Column:

- *size*: *l* = 30 m, Ø = 0.25 mm,
- *stationary phase*: *poly(dimethyl)siloxane R* (film thickness 1 µm).

Carrier gas: *helium for chromatography R.*

Temperature:

	Time (min)	Temperature (°C)
Column	0 - 12.5	230 → 280
Injection port		250
Detector		280

Detection: flame ionisation.

The area of the peak due to α-lactose is not less than 97 per cent of the total peak area.

Lanthanum nitrate. $La(NO_3)_3,6H_2O$. (M_r 433.0). *1048000.* [10277-43-7]. Lanthanum trinitrate hexahydrate.

Colourless crystals, deliquescent, freely soluble in water.

Storage: in an airtight container.

Lanthanum nitrate solution. *1048001.*

A 50 g/l solution.

Lanthanum trioxide. La_2O_3. (M_r 325.8). *1114000.* [1312-81-8].

An almost white, amorphous powder, practically insoluble in *water R*. It dissolves in dilute solutions of mineral acids and absorbs atmospheric carbon dioxide.

Calcium: maximum 5 ppm.

Lanthanum chloride solution. *1114001.*

To 58.65 g of *lanthanum trioxide R* slowly add 100 ml of *hydrochloric acid R*. Heat to boiling. Allow to cool and dilute to 1000.0 ml with *water R*.

Lauric acid. $C_{12}H_{24}O_2$. (M_r 200.3). *1143100.* [143-07-7]. Dodecanoic acid.

White, crystalline powder, practically insoluble in water, freely soluble in alcohol.

mp: about 44 °C.

Lauric acid used in the assay of total fatty acids in Saw palmetto fruit (1848) complies with the following additional requirement.

Assay. Examine by gas chromatography (*2.2.28*) as prescribed in the monograph on *Saw palmetto fruit (1848).*

The content of lauric acid is not less than 98 per cent, calculated by the normalisation procedure.

Lauryl alcohol. $C_{12}H_{26}O$. (M_r 186.3). *1119900.* [112-53-8]. 1-Dodecanol.

d_{20}^{20}: about 0.820.

mp: 24 °C to 27 °C.

Lavandulol. $C_{10}H_{18}O$. (M_r 154.2). *1114100.* [498-16-8]. (*R*)-5-Methyl-2-(1-methylethenyl)-4-hexen-1-ol.

An oily liquid with a characteristic odour.

d_{20}^{20}: about 0.875.

n_D^{20}: about 1.407.

$[\alpha]_D^{20}$: about − 10.2.

bp_{13}: about 94 °C.

Lavandulol used in gas chromatography complies with the following additional test.

Assay. Examine by gas chromatography (*2.2.28*) as prescribed in the monograph on *Lavender oil (1338).*

Test solution. The substance to be examined.

The area of the principal peak is not less than 98.0 per cent of the area of all the peaks in the chromatogram obtained.

Lavandulyl acetate. $C_{12}H_{20}O_2$. (M_r 196.3). *1114200.* [50373-59-6]. 2-Isopropenyl-5-methylhex-4-en-1-yl acetate.

A colourless liquid with a characteristic odour.

d_{20}^{20}: about 0.911.

n_D^{20}: about 1.454.

bp_{13}: 106 °C to 107 °C.

Lavandulyl acetate used in gas chromatography complies with the following additional test.

Assay. Examine by gas chromatography (*2.2.28*) as prescribed in the monograph on *Lavender oil (1338).*

Test solution. The substance to be examined.

The area of the principal peak is not less than 93.0 per cent of the area of all the peaks in the chromatogram obtained.

Lead acetate. $C_4H_6O_4Pb,3H_2O$. (M_r 379.3). *1048100.* [6080-56-4]. Lead di-acetate.

Colourless crystals, efflorescent, freely soluble in water, soluble in alcohol.

Lead acetate cotton. *1048101.*

Immerse absorbent cotton in a mixture of 1 volume of *dilute acetic acid R* and 10 volumes of *lead acetate solution R*. Drain off the excess of liquid, without squeezing the cotton, by placing it on several layers of filter paper. Allow to dry in air.

Storage: in an airtight container.

Lead acetate paper. *1048102.*

Immerse filter paper weighing about 80 g/m^2 in a mixture of 1 volume of *dilute acetic acid R* and 10 volumes of *lead acetate solution R*. After drying, cut the paper into strips 15 mm by 40 mm.

Lead acetate solution. *1048103.*

A 95 g/l solution in *carbon dioxide-free water R*.

Lead dioxide. PbO_2. (M_r 239.2). *1048200.* [1309-60-0].

A dark brown powder, evolving oxygen when heated, practically insoluble in water, soluble in hydrochloric acid with evolution of chlorine, soluble in dilute nitric acid in the presence of hydrogen peroxide, oxalic acid or other reducing agents, soluble in hot, concentrated alkali hydroxide solutions.

Lead nitrate. $Pb(NO_3)_2$. (M_r 331.2). *1048300.* [10099-74-8]. Lead dinitrate.

A white, crystalline powder or colourless crystals, freely soluble in water.

Lead nitrate solution. *1048301.*

A 33 g/l solution.

Lead subacetate solution. *1048400.* [1335-32-6]. Basic lead acetate solution.

Content: 16.7 per cent *m/m* to 17.4 per cent *m/m* of Pb (A_r 207.2) in a form corresponding approximately to the formula $C_8H_{14}O_{10}Pb_3$.

Dissolve 40.0 g of *lead acetate R* in 90 ml of *carbon dioxide-free water R*. Adjust the pH to 7.5 with *strong sodium hydroxide solution R*. Centrifuge and use the clear colourless supernatant solution.

The solution remains clear when stored in a well-closed container.

Leiocarposide. $C_{27}H_{34}O_{16}$. (M_r 614.5). *1150200.* [71953-77-0]. 2-(β-D-Glucopyranosyloxy)benzyl 3-(β-D-glucopyranosyloxy)-6-hydroxy-2-methoxybenzoate. 2-[[[3-(β-D-Glucopyranosyloxy)-6-hydroxy-2-methoxybenzoyl]oxy]methyl]phenyl-β-D-glucopyranoside.

White powder, soluble in water, freely soluble in methanol, slightly soluble in alcohol.

mp: 190 °C to 193 °C.

Lemon oil. *1101700.*

See *Lemon oil (0620).*

Leucine. *1048500.* [61-90-5].

See *Leucine (0771).*

Levomenol. $C_{15}H_{26}O$. (M_r 222.4). *1128800.* [23089-26-1]. (2*S*)-6-Methyl-2-[(1*S*)-4-methylcyclohex-3-enyl]hept-5-en-2-ol. (-)-α-Bisabolol.

Colourless, viscous liquid with a slight, characteristic odour, practically insoluble in water, freely soluble in alcohol, in methanol, in toluene, in fatty oils and in essential oils.

d_{20}^{20}: 0.925 to 0.935.

n_D^{20}: 1.492 to 1.500.

$[\alpha]_D^{20}$: −54.5 to −58.0, determined on a 50 mg/ml solution in *alcohol R*.

Levomenol used for gas chromatography complies with the following additional test.

Assay. Examine by gas chromatography (*2.2.28*) as prescribed in the monograph on *Matricaria oil (1836)*, using a 4 g/l solution in *cyclohexane R*.

The content of levomenol is not less than 95.0 per cent, calculated by the normalisation procedure.

Limonene. $C_{10}H_{16}$. (M_r 136.2). *1048600.* [5989-27-5]. D-Limonene. (+)-*p*-Mentha-1,8-diene. (*R*)-4-Isopropenyl-1-methylcyclohex-1-ene.

A colourless liquid, practically insoluble in water, soluble in alcohol.

d_{20}^{20}: about 0.84.

n_D^{20}: 1.471 to 1.474.

$[\alpha]_D^{20}$: + 96 to + 106.

bp: 175 °C to 177 °C.

Limonene used in gas chromatography complies with the following additional test.

Assay. Examine by gas chromatography (*2.2.28*) as prescribed in the monograph on *Peppermint oil (0405)* using the substance to be examined as the test solution.

The area of the principal peak is not less than 99.0 per cent of the total area of the peaks.

Linalol. $C_{10}H_{18}O$. (M_r 154.2). *1048700.* [78-70-6]. (*RS*)-3,7-Dimethylocta-1,6-dien-3-ol.

Mixture of two stereoisomers (licareol and coriandrol).

Liquid, practically insoluble in water.

d_{20}^{20}: about 0.860.

n_D^{20}: about 1.462.

bp: about 200 °C.

Linalol used in gas chromatography complies with the following test.

Assay. Examine by gas chromatography (*2.2.28*) under the conditions described in the monograph on *Anise oil (0804)* using the substance to be examined as the test solution.

The area of the principal peak is not less than 98.0 per cent of the total area of the peaks.

Linalyl acetate. $C_{12}H_{20}O_2$. (M_r 196.3). *1107200.* [115-95-7]. (*RS*)-1,5-Dimethyl-1-vinylhex-4-enyl acetate.

A colourless or slightly yellow liquid with a strong odour of bergamot and lavender.

d_{25}^{25}: : 0.895 to 0.912.

n_D^{20}: 1.448 to 1.451.

bp: about 215 °C.

Linalyl acetate used in gas chromatography complies with the following additional test.

Assay. Examine by gas chromatography (*2.2.28*) as prescribed in the monograph on *Bitter-orange-flower oil (1175)*, using the substance to be examined as the test solution.

The area of the principal peak is not less than 95.0 per cent of the total area of the peaks.

Lindane. $C_6H_6Cl_6$. (M_r 290.8). *1128900.* [58-89-9]. γ-Hexachlorocyclohexane.

See *Lindane (0772).*

For the monograph *Wool fat (0134)*, a suitable certified reference solution (10 ng/µl in cyclohexane) may be used.

Linoleic acid. $C_{18}H_{32}O_2$. (M_r 280.5). *1143200.* [60-33-3]. (9*Z*,12*Z*)-Octadeca-9,12-dienoic acid.

Colourless, oily liquid.

d_4^{20}: about 0.903.

n_D^{20}: about 1.470.

Linoleic acid used in the assay of total fatty acids in Saw palmetto fruit (1848) complies with the following additional requirement.

Assay. Examine by gas chromatography (*2.2.28*) as prescribed in the monograph on *Saw palmetto fruit (1848).*

The content of linoleic acid is not less than 98 per cent, calculated by the normalisation procedure.

Linolenic acid. $C_{18}H_{30}O_2$. (M_r 278.4). *1143300.* [463-40-1]. (9*Z*,12*Z*,15*Z*)-Octadeca-9,12,15-trienoic acid.

Colourless liquid, practically insoluble in water, soluble in organic solvents.

d_4^{20}: about 0.915.

n_D^{20}: about 1.480.

Linolenic acid used in the assay of total fatty acids in Saw palmetto fruit (1848) complies with the following additional requirement.

Assay. Examine by gas chromatography (*2.2.28*) as prescribed in the monograph on *Saw palmetto fruit (1848).*

The content of linolenic acid is not less than 98 per cent, calculated by the normalisation procedure.

Linolenyl alcohol. $C_{18}H_{32}O$. (M_r 264.4). *1156200.* [24149-05-1]. (9*Z*,12*Z*,15*Z*)-octadeca-9,12,15-trien-1-ol.

Content: minimum 96 per cent of $C_{18}H_{32}O$.

Linoleyl alcohol. $C_{18}H_{34}O$. (M_r 266.5). *1155900.* [506-43-4]. (9*Z*,12*Z*)-octadeca-9,12-dien-1-ol.

Relative density: 0.830.

Content: minimum 85 per cent of $C_{18}H_{34}O$.

Lithium. Li. (A_r 6.94). *1048800.* [7439-93-2].

A soft metal whose freshly cut surface is silvery-grey. It rapidly tarnishes in contact with air. It reacts violently with water, yielding hydrogen and giving a solution of lithium hydroxide; soluble in methanol, yielding hydrogen and a solution of lithium methoxide; practically insoluble in light petroleum.

Storage: under light petroleum or liquid paraffin.

Lithium carbonate. Li_2CO_3. (M_r 73.9). *1048900.* [554-13-2]. Dilithium carbonate.

A white, light powder, sparingly soluble in water, very slightly soluble in alcohol. A saturated solution at 20 °C contains about 13 g/l of Li_2CO_3.

Lithium chloride. LiCl. (M_r 42.39). *1049000.* [7447-41-8].

Crystalline powder or granules or cubic crystals, deliquescent, freely soluble in water, soluble in acetone and in alcohol. Aqueous solutions are neutral or slightly alkaline.

Storage: in an airtight container.

Lithium hydroxide. $LiOH,H_2O$. (M_r 41.96). *1049100.* [1310-66-3]. Lithium hydroxide monohydrate.

A white, granular powder, strongly alkaline, it rapidly absorbs water and carbon dioxide, soluble in water, sparingly soluble in alcohol.

Storage: in an airtight container.

Lithium metaborate, anhydrous. $LiBO_2$. (M_r 49.75). *1120000.* [13453-69-5].

Lithium sulphate. Li_2SO_4,H_2O. (M_r 128.0). *1049200.* [10102-25-7]. Dilithium sulphate monohydrate.

Colourless crystals, freely soluble in water, practically insoluble in alcohol.

Litmus. *1049300.* [1393-92-6].

Schultz No. 1386.

Indigo-blue fragments prepared from various species of Rocella, Lecanora or other lichens, soluble in water, practically insoluble in alcohol.

Colour change: pH 5 (red) to pH 8 (blue).

Litmus paper, blue. *1049301.*

Boil 10 parts of coarsely powdered *litmus R* for 1 h with 100 parts of *alcohol R*. Decant the alcohol and add to the residue a mixture of 45 parts of *alcohol R* and 55 parts of *water R*. After 2 days decant the clear liquid. Impregnate strips of filter paper with the solution and allow to dry.

Test for sensitivity. Immerse a strip measuring 10 mm by 60 mm in a mixture of 10 ml of *0.02 M hydrochloric acid* and 90 ml of *water R*. On shaking the paper turns red within 45 s.

Litmus paper, red. *1049302.*

To the blue litmus extract, add *dilute hydrochloric acid R* dropwise until the blue colour becomes red. Impregnate strips of filter paper with the solution and allow to dry.

Test for sensitivity. Immerse a strip measuring 10 mm by 60 mm in a mixture of 10 ml of *0.02 M sodium hydroxide* and 90 ml of *water R*. On shaking the paper turns blue within 45 s.

Loganin. $C_{17}H_{26}O_{10}$. (M_r 390.4). *1136700.* [18524-94-2]. Methyl (1*S*,4a*S*,6*S*,7*R*,7a*S*)-1-(β-D-glucopyranosyloxy)-6-hydroxy-7-methyl-1,4a,5,6,7,7a-hexahydrocyclopenta[*c*]pyran-4-carboxylate.

mp: 220 °C to 221 °C.

Longifolene. $C_{15}H_{24}$. (M_r 204.4). *1150300.* [475-20-7]. (1*S*,3a*R*,4*S*,8a*S*)-4,8,8-Trimethyl-9-methylenedecahydro-1,4-methanoazulene.

Oily, colourless liquid, practically insoluble in water, miscible with alcohol.

d_4^{18}: 0.9319.

n_D^{20}: 1.5050.

$[\alpha]_D^{20}$: + 42.7.

bp: 254 °C to 256 °C.

Longifolene used in gas chromatography complies with the following additional test.

Assay. Examine by gas chromatography (*2.2.28*) as prescribed in the monograph on *Turpentine oil, Pinus pinaster type (1627).*

The content is not less than 98.0 per cent, calculated by the normalisation procedure.

Low-vapour-pressure hydrocarbons (type L). *1049400.*

Unctuous mass, soluble in benzene and in toluene.

Lumiflavine. $C_{13}H_{12}N_4O_2$. (M_r 256.3). *1141000.* [1088-56-8]. 7,8,10-Trimethylbenzo[*g*]pteridine-2,4(3*H*,10*H*)-dione.

Yellow powder or orange crystals, very slightly soluble in water, freely soluble in methylene chloride.

Macrogol 23 lauryl ether. *1129000.*

Complies with the monograph *Macrogol lauryl ether (1124)*, the nominal value for the amount of ethylene oxide reacted with lauryl alcohol being 23.

Macrogol 200. *1099200.* [25322-68-3]. Polyethyleneglycol 200.

A clear, colourless or almost colourless viscous liquid, very soluble in acetone and in ethanol, practically insoluble in fatty oils.

d_{20}^{20}: about 1.127.

n_D^{20}: about 1.450.

Macrogol 200 R1. *1099201.*

Introduce 500 ml of *macrogol 200 R* into a 1000 ml round bottom flask. Using a rotation evaporator remove any volatile components applying for 6 h a temperature of 60 °C and a vacuum with a pressure of 1.5 kPa to 2.5 kPa.

Macrogol 300. *1067100.* [25322-68-3]. Polyethyleneglycol 300.

See *Macrogols (1444).*

Macrogol 400. *1067200.* [25322-68-3]. Polyethyleneglycol 400.

See *Macrogols (1444).*

Macrogol 1000. *1067300.* [25322-68-3]. Polyethyleneglycol 1000.

See *Macrogols (1444).*

Macrogol 1500. *1067400.* [25322-68-3]. Polyethyleneglycol 1500.

See *Macrogols (1444).*

Macrogol 20 000. *1067600.* Polyethyleneglycol 20 000.

See *Macrogols (1444).*

Macrogol 20 000 2-nitroterephthalate. *1067601.* Polyethyleneglycol 20 000 2-nitroterephthalate.

Macrogol 20 000 R modified by treating with 2-nitroterephthalate acid.

A hard, white or almost white, waxy solid, soluble in acetone.

Magnesium. Mg. (A_r 24.30). *1049500.* [7439-95-4].

Silver-white ribbon, turnings or wire, or a grey powder.

Magnesium acetate. $C_4H_6MgO_4,4H_2O$. (M_r 214.5). *1049600.* [16674-78-5]. Magnesium diacetate tetrahydrate.

Colourless crystals, deliquescent, freely soluble in water and in alcohol.

Storage: in an airtight container.

Magnesium chloride. *1049700.* [7791-18-6].

See *Magnesium chloride hexahydrate (0402).*

Magnesium nitrate. $Mg(NO_3)_2,6H_2O$. (M_r 256.4). *1049800.* [13446-18-9]. Magnesium nitrate hexahydrate.

Colourless, clear crystals, deliquescent, very soluble in water, freely soluble in alcohol.

Storage: in an airtight container.

Magnesium nitrate solution. *1049801.*

Dissolve 17.3 g of *magnesium nitrate R* in 5 ml of *water R* warming gently and add 80 ml of *alcohol R*. Cool and dilute to 100.0 ml with the same solvent.

Magnesium nitrate solution R1. *1049802.*

Dissolve 20 g of *magnesium nitrate R* ($Mg(NO_3)_2,6H_2O$) in *deionised distilled water R* and dilute to 100 ml with the same solvent. Immediately before use, dilute 10 ml to 100 ml with *deionised distilled water R*. A volume of 5 µl will provide 0.06 mg of Mg $(NO_3)_2$.

Magnesium oxide. *1049900.* [1309-48-4].

See *Light magnesium oxide (0040).*

Magnesium oxide R1. *1049901.*

Complies with the requirements prescribed for *magnesium oxide R* with the following modifications.

Arsenic (*2.4.2*). Dissolve 0.5 g in a mixture of 5 ml of *water R* and 5 ml of *hydrochloric acid R1*. The solution complies with limit test A for arsenic (2 ppm).

Heavy metals (*2.4.8*). Dissolve 1.0 g in a mixture of 3 ml of *water R* and 7 ml of *hydrochloric acid R1*. Add 0.05 ml of *phenolphthalein solution R* and *concentrated ammonia R* until a pink colour is obtained. Neutralise the excess of ammonia by the addition of *glacial acetic acid R*. Add 0.5 ml in excess and dilute to 20 ml with *water R*. Filter, if necessary. 12 ml of the solution complies with limit test A for heavy metals (10 ppm). Prepare the standard using a mixture of 5 ml of *lead standard solution (1 ppm Pb) R* and 5 ml of *water R*.

Iron (*2.4.9*). Dissolve 0.2 g in 6 ml of *dilute hydrochloric acid R* and dilute to 10 ml with *water R*. The solution complies with the limit test for iron (50 ppm).

Magnesium oxide, heavy. *1050000.* [1309-48-4].

See *Heavy magnesium oxide (0041).*

Magnesium silicate for pesticide residue analysis. *1129100.* [1343-88-0].

Magnesium silicate for chromatography (60-100 mesh).

Magnesium sulphate. *1050200.* [10034-99-8].

See *Magnesium sulphate heptahydrate (0044).*

Maize oil. *1050400.*

See *Maize oil, refined (1342).*

Malachite green. $C_{23}H_{25}ClN_2$. (M_r 364.9). *1050500.* [123333-61-9].

Schultz No. 754.

Colour Index No. 42000.

[4-[[4-(Dimethylamino)phenyl]phenylmethylene]cyclohexa-2, 5-dien-1-ylidene]dimethylammonium chloride.

Green crystals with a metallic lustre, very soluble in water giving a bluish-green solution, soluble in alcohol and in methanol.

A 0.01 g/l solution in *alcohol R* shows an absorption maximum (*2.2.25*) at 617 nm.

Malachite green solution. *1050501.*

A 5 g/l solution in *anhydrous acetic acid R*.

Malathion. $C_{10}H_{19}O_6PS_2$. (M_r 330.3). *1129200.* [121-75-5].

bp: about 156 °C.

A suitable certified reference solution (10 ng/µl in iso-octane) may be used.

Maleic acid. *1050600.* [110-16-7].

See *Maleic acid (0365).*

Maleic anhydride. $C_4H_2O_3$. (M_r 98.1). *1050700.* [108-31-6]. Butenedioic anhydride. 2,5-Furandione.

White crystals, soluble in water forming maleic acid, very soluble in acetone and in ethyl acetate, freely soluble in toluene, soluble in alcohol with ester formation, very slightly soluble in light petroleum.

mp: about 52 °C.

Any residue insoluble in toluene does not exceed 5 per cent (maleic acid).

Maleic anhydride solution. *1050701.*

Dissolve 5 g of *maleic anhydride R* in *toluene R* and dilute to 100 ml with the same solvent. Use within one month. If the solution becomes turbid, filter.

Maltitol. *1136800.* [585-88-6].

See *Maltitol (1235).*

Manganese sulphate. $MnSO_4,H_2O$. (M_r 169.0). *1050900.* [10034-96-5]. Manganese sulphate monohydrate.

Pale-pink, crystalline powder or crystals, freely soluble in water, practically insoluble in alcohol.

Loss on ignition: 10.0 per cent to 12.0 per cent, determined on 1.000 g at 500 °C.

Mannitol. *1051000.* [69-65-8].

See *Mannitol (0559).*

Mannose. $C_6H_{12}O_6$. (M_r 180.2). *1051100.* [3458-28-4]. D-(+)-Mannose.

A white, crystalline powder or small, white crystals, very soluble in water, slightly soluble in ethanol.

$[\alpha]_D^{20}$: + 13.7 + 14.7, determined on a 200 g/l solution in *water R* containing about 0.05 per cent of NH_3.

mp: about 132 °C, with decomposition.

Meclozine hydrochloride. *1051200.* [1104-22-9].

See *Meclozine hydrochloride (0622).*

Melamine. $C_3H_6N_6$. (M_r 126.1). *1051300.* [108-78-1]. 1,3,5-Triazine-2,4,6-triamine.

A white, amorphous powder, very slightly soluble in water and in alcohol.

Menadione. *1051400.* [58-27-5].

See *Menadione (0507).*

Menthofuran. $C_{10}H_{14}O$. (M_r 150.2). *1051500.* [17957-94-7]. 3,9-Epoxy-*p*-mentha-3,8-diene. 3,6-Dimethyl-4,5,6,7-tetrahydro-benzofuran.

A slightly bluish liquid, very slightly soluble in water, soluble in alcohol.

d_{15}^{20}: about 0.965.

n_D^{20}: about 1.480.

$[\alpha]_D^{20}$: about + 93.

bp: 196 °C.

Menthofuran used in gas chromatography complies with the following additional test.

Assay. Examine by gas chromatography (*2.2.28*) as prescribed in the monograph on *Peppermint oil (0405)* using the substance to be examined as the test solution.

The area of the principal peak is not less than 97.0 per cent of the total area of the peaks.

Menthol. *1051600.* [2216-51-5]. See *Levomenthol (0619)* and *Racemic menthol (0623).*

Menthol used in gas chromatography complies with the following additional test.

Assay. Examine by gas chromatography (*2.2.28*) as prescribed in the Related substances test included in the monograph on *Racemic menthol (0623).*

The area of the principal peak is not less than 98.0 per cent of the total area of the peaks, disregarding any peak due to the solvent.

Menthone. $C_{10}H_{18}O$. (M_r 154.2). *1051700.* [14073-97-3]. (2*S*,5*R*)-2-Isopropyl-5-methylcyclohexanone. (−)-*trans*-*p*-Menthan-3-one.

Contains variable amounts of isomenthone.

A colourless liquid, very slightly soluble in water, very soluble in alcohol.

d_{20}^{20}: about 0.897.

n_D^{20}: about 1.450.

Menthone used in gas chromatography complies with the following additional test.

Assay. Examine by gas chromatography (*2.2.28*) as prescribed in the monograph on *Peppermint oil (0405)* using the substance to be examined as the test solution.

The area of the principal peak is not less than 90.0 per cent of the total area of the peaks.

Menthyl acetate. $C_{12}H_{22}O_2$. (M_r 198.3). *1051800.* [2623-23-6]. 2-Isopropyl-5-methylcyclohexyl acetate.

A colourless liquid, slightly soluble in water, miscible with alcohol.

d_{20}^{20}: about 0.92.

n_D^{20}: about 1.447.

bp: about 228 °C.

Menthyl acetate used in gas chromatography complies with the following additional test.

Assay. Examine by gas chromatography (*2.2.28*) as prescribed in the monograph on *Peppermint oil (0405)* using the substance to be examined as the test solution.

The area of the principal peak is not less than 97.0 per cent of the total area of the peaks.

2-Mercaptoethanol. C_2H_6OS. (M_r 78.1). *1099300.* [60-24-2].

A liquid, miscible with water.

d_{20}^{20}: about 1.116.

bp: about 157 °C.

Mercaptopurine. *1051900.* [6112-76-1].

See *Mercaptopurine (0096).*

Mercuric acetate. $C_4H_6HgO_4$. (M_r 318.7). *1052000.* [1600-27-7]. Mercury diacetate.

White crystals, freely soluble in water, soluble in alcohol.

Mercuric acetate solution. *1052001.*

Dissolve 3.19 g of *mercuric acetate R* in *anhydrous acetic acid R* and dilute to 100 ml with the same acid. If necessary, neutralise the solution with *0.1 M perchloric acid* using 0.05 ml of *crystal violet solution R* as indicator.

Mercuric bromide. $HgBr_2$. (M_r 360.4). *1052100.* [7789-47-1]. Mercury dibromide.

White or faintly yellow crystals or a crystalline powder, slightly soluble in water, soluble in alcohol.

4. Reagents

Mercuric bromide paper. *1052101.*

In a rectangular dish place a 50 g/l solution of *mercuric bromide R* in *ethanol R* and immerse in it pieces of white filter paper weighing 80 g per square metre (speed of filtration = filtration time expressed in seconds for 100 ml of water at 20 °C with a filter surface of 10 cm^2 and constant pressure of 6.7 kPa: 40 s to 60 s), each measuring 1.5 cm by 20 cm and folded in two. Allow the excess liquid to drain and allow the paper to dry, protected from light, suspended over a non-metallic thread. Discard 1 cm from each end of each strip and cut the remainder into 1.5 cm squares or discs of 1.5 cm diameter.

Storage: in a glass-stoppered container wrapped with black paper.

Mercuric chloride. *1052200.* [7487-94-7].

See *Mercuric chloride (0120).*

Mercuric chloride solution. *1052201.*

A 54 g/l solution.

Mercuric iodide. HgI_2. (M_r 454.4). *1052300.* [7774-29-0].

Mercury di-iodide.

A dense, scarlet, crystalline powder, slightly soluble in water, sparingly soluble in acetone and in alcohol, soluble in an excess of *potassium iodide solution R.*

Storage: protected from light.

Mercuric nitrate. $Hg(NO_3)_2,H_2O$. (M_r 342.6). *1052400.* [7782-86-7]. Mercury dinitrate monohydrate.

Colourless or slightly coloured crystals, hygroscopic, soluble in water in the presence of a small quantity of nitric acid.

Storage: in an airtight container, protected from light.

Mercuric oxide. HgO. (M_r 216.6). *1052500.* [21908-53-2].

Yellow mercuric oxide. Mercury oxide.

A yellow to orange-yellow powder, practically insoluble in water and in alcohol.

Storage: protected from light.

Mercuric sulphate solution. *1052600.* [7783-35-9].

Dissolve 1 g of *mercuric oxide R* in a mixture of 20 ml of *water R* and 4 ml of *sulphuric acid R.*

Mercuric thiocyanate. $Hg(SCN)_2$. (M_r 316.7). *1052700.* [592-85-8]. Mercury di(thiocyanate).

A white, crystalline powder, very slightly soluble in water, slightly soluble in alcohol, soluble in solutions of sodium chloride.

Mercuric thiocyanate solution. *1052701.*

Dissolve 0.3 g of *mercuric thiocyanate R* in *ethanol R* and dilute to 100 ml with the same solvent.

Storage: use within 1 week.

Mercury. Hg. (A_r 200.6). *1052800.* [7439-97-6].

A silver-white liquid, breaking into spherical globules which do not leave a metallic trace when rubbed on paper.

d_{20}^{20}: about 13.5.

bp: about 357 °C.

Mercury, nitric acid solution of. *1052801.*

Carefully dissolve 3 ml of *mercury R* in 27 ml of *fuming nitric acid R*. Dilute the solution with an equal volume of *water R.*

Storage: protected from light; use within 2 months.

Mesityl oxide. $C_6H_{10}O$. (M_r 98.1). *1120100.* [141-79-7].

4-Methylpent-3-en-2-one.

Colourless, oily liquid, soluble in 30 parts of water, miscible with most organic solvents.

d_{20}^{20}: about 0.858.

bp: 129 °C to 130 °C.

Metanil yellow. $C_{18}H_{14}N_3NaO_3S$. (M_r 375.4). *1052900.* [587-98-4].

Schultz No. 169.

Colour Index No. 13065.

Sodium 3-[4-(phenylamino)phenylazo]benzenesulphonate.

A brownish-yellow powder, soluble in water and in alcohol.

Metanil yellow solution. *1052901.*

A 1 g/l solution in *methanol R.*

Test for sensitivity. To 50 ml of *anhydrous acetic acid R* add 0.1 ml of the metanil yellow solution. Add 0.05 ml of *0.1 M perchloric acid*; the colour changes from pinkish-red to violet.

Colour change: pH 1.2 (red) to pH 2.3 (orange-yellow).

Metaphosphoric acid. $(HPO_3)_x$. *1053000.* [37267-86-0].

Glassy lumps or sticks containing a proportion of sodium metaphosphate, hygroscopic, very soluble in water.

Nitrates. Boil 1.0 g with 10 ml of *water R*, cool, add 1 ml of *indigo carmine solution R*, 10 ml of *nitrogen-free sulphuric acid R* and heat to boiling. The blue colour is not entirely discharged.

Reducing substances: maximum 0.01 per cent, calculated as H_3PO_3. Dissolve 35.0 g in 50 ml of *water R*. Add 5 ml of a 200 g/l solution of *sulphuric acid R*, 50 mg of *potassium bromide R* and 5.0 ml of *0.02 M potassium bromate* and heat on a water-bath for 30 min. Allow to cool and add 0.5 g of *potassium iodide R*. Titrate the liberated iodine with *0.1 M sodium thiosulphate*, using 1 ml of *starch solution R* as indicator. Carry out a blank test.

1 ml of *0.02 M potassium bromate* is equivalent to 4.10 mg of H_3PO_3.

Storage: in an airtight container.

Methacrylic acid. $C_4H_6O_2$. (M_r 86.1). *1101800.* [79-41-4].

2-Methylprop-2-enoic acid.

A colourless liquid.

n_D^{20}: about 1.431.

bp: about 160 °C.

mp: about 16 °C.

Methanesulphonic acid. CH_4O_3S. (M_r 96.1). *1053100.* [75-75-2].

A clear, colourless liquid, solidifying at about 20 °C, miscible with water, slightly soluble in toluene, practically insoluble in hexane.

d_{20}^{20}: about 1.48.

n_D^{20}: about 1.430.

Methanol. CH_4O. (M_r 32.04). *1053200.* [67-56-1].

A clear, colourless, flammable liquid, miscible with water and with alcohol.

d_{20}^{20}: 0.791 to 0.793.

bp: 64 °C to 65 °C.

Methanol R1. *1053201.*

Complies with the requirements prescribed for *methanol R* and the following additional requirement.

Minimum transmittance (*2.2.25*), determined using *water R* as compensation liquid: 20 per cent at 210 nm, 50 per cent at 220 nm, 75 per cent at 230 nm, 95 per cent at 250 nm, 98 per cent at 260 nm and at higher wavelengths.

Methanol R2. *1053202.*

Methanol R2 used in liquid chromatography complies with the following additional requirements.

Content: minimum 99.8 per cent of CH_4O (M_r 32.04).

Absorbance (2.2.25). The absorbance at 225 nm using *water R* as the compensation liquid is not more than 0.17.

Methanol, hydrochloric. *1053203.*

Dilute 1.0 ml of *hydrochloric acid R1* to 100.0 ml with *methanol R*.

Methanol, aldehyde-free. *1053300.*

Dissolve 25 g of *iodine R* in 1 litre of *methanol R* and pour the solution, with constant stirring, into 400 ml of *1 M sodium hydroxide*. Add 150 ml of *water R* and allow to stand for 16h. Filter. Boil under a reflux condenser until the odour of iodoform disappears. Distil the solution by fractional distillation.

Content: maximum 0.001 per cent of aldehydes and ketones.

Methanol, anhydrous. *1053400.* [67-56-1].

Treat 1000 ml of *methanol R* with 5 g of *magnesium R*. If necessary initiate the reaction by adding 0.1 ml of *mercuric chloride solution R*. When the evolution of gas has ceased, distil the liquid and collect the distillate in a dry container protected from moisture.

Water (*2.5.12*): maximum 0.3 g/l.

DL-Methionine. *1129400.* [59-51-8].

See *DL-Methionine (0624)*.

L-Methionine. *1053500.* [63-68-3].

See *Methionine (1027)*.

***(RS)*-Methotrexate.** *1120200.* [60388-53-6]. (*RS*)-2-[4-[[(2,4-diaminopteridin-6-yl)methyl]methylamino]benzoylamino]pentanedioic acid.

Content: minimum 96.0 per cent of $C_{20}H_{22}N_8O_5$.

mp: about 195 °C.

Methoxychlor. $C_{16}H_{15}Cl_3O_2$. (M_r 345.7). *1129300.* [72-43-5]. 1,1-(2,2,2-Trichloroethylidene)-bis(4-methoxybenzene).

Practically insoluble in water, freely soluble in most organic solvents.

bp: about 346 °C.

mp: 78 °C to 86 °C.

A suitable certified reference solution (10 ng/µl in iso-octane) may be used.

***trans*-2-Methoxycinnamaldehyde.** $C_{10}H_{10}O_2$. (M_r 162.2). *1129500.* [60125-24-8].

mp: 44 °C to 46 °C.

trans-2-Methoxycinnamaldehyde used in gas chromatography complies with the following additional test.

Assay. Examine by gas chromatography (*2.2.28*) as prescribed in the monograph on *Cassia oil (1496)*.

The content is not less than 96.0 per cent, calculated by the normalisation procedure.

Methoxyphenylacetic acid. $C_9H_{10}O_3$. (M_r 166.2). *1053600.* [7021-09-2]. (*RS*)-2-Methoxy-2-phenylacetic acid.

A white, crystalline powder or white or almost white crystals, sparingly soluble in water, freely soluble in alcohol.

mp: about 70 °C.

Methoxyphenylacetic reagent. *1053601.*

Dissolve 2.7 g of *methoxyphenylacetic acid R* in 6 ml of *tetramethylammonium hydroxide solution R* and add 20 ml of *ethanol R*.

Storage: in a polyethylene container.

Methyl acetate. $C_3H_6O_2$. (M_r 74.1). *1053700.* [79-20-9].

A clear, colourless liquid, soluble in water, miscible with alcohol.

d_{20}^{20}: about 0.933.

n_D^{20}: about 1.361

bp: 56 °C to 58 °C.

Methyl 4-acetylbenzoate. $C_{10}H_{10}O_3$. (M_r 178.2). *1154100.* [3609-53-8].

mp: about 94 °C.

Methyl 4-acetylbenzoate reagent. *1154101.*

Dissolve 0.25 g of *methyl 4-acetylbenzoate R* in a mixture of 5 ml of *sulphuric acid R* and 85 ml of cooled *methanol R*.

4-Methylaminophenol sulphate. $C_{14}H_{20}N_2O_6S$. (M_r 344.4). *1053800.* [55-55-0].

Colourless crystals, very soluble in water, slightly soluble in alcohol.

mp: about 260 °C.

Methyl anthranilate. $C_8H_9NO_2$. (M_r 151.2). *1107300.* [134-20-3]. Methyl 2-aminobenzoate.

Colourless crystals or a colourless or yellowish liquid, soluble in water, freely soluble in alcohol.

bp: 134 °C to 136 °C.

mp: 24 °C to 25 °C.

Methyl anthranilate used in gas chromatography complies with the following additional test.

Assay. Examine by gas chromatography (*2.2.28*) as prescribed in the monograph on *Bitter-orange-flower oil (1175)*, using the substance to be examined as the test solution. The area of the principal peak is not less than 95.0 per cent of the total area of the peaks.

Methyl arachidate. $C_{21}H_{42}O_2$. (M_r 326.6). *1053900.* [1120-28-1]. Methyl eicosanoate.

Content: minimum 98.0 per cent of $C_{21}H_{42}O_2$, determined by gas chromatography (*2.4.22*).

A white or yellow, crystalline mass, soluble in alcohol and in light petroleum.

mp: about 46 °C.

Methyl behenate. $C_{23}H_{46}O_2$. (M_r 354.6). *1107500.* [929-77-1]. Methyl docosanoate.

mp: 54 °C to 55 °C.

Methylbenzothiazolone hydrazone hydrochloride. $C_8H_{10}ClN_3S,H_2O$. (M_r 233.7). *1055300.* [38894-11-0]. 3-Methylbenzothiazol-2(3*H*)-one hydrazone hydrochloride monohydrate.

An almost white or yellowish, crystalline powder.

mp: about 270 °C.

Suitability for determination of aldehydes. To 2 ml of *aldehyde-free methanol R* add 60 µl of a 1 g/l solution of *propionaldehyde R* in *aldehyde-free methanol R* and 5 ml of a 4 g/l solution of methylbenzothiazolone hydrazone hydrochloride. Mix. Allow to stand for 30 min. Prepare a blank omitting the propionaldehyde solution. Add 25.0 ml of a 2 g/l solution of *ferric chloride R* to the test solution and to the blank, dilute to 100.0 ml with *acetone R* and mix. The absorbance (*2.2.25*) of the test solution, measured at 660 nm using the blank as compensation liquid, is not less than 0.62.

2-Methylbutane. C_5H_{12}. (M_r 72.2). *1099500.* [78-78-4]. Isopentane.

Content: minimum 99.5 per cent of C_5H_{12}.

A very flammable colourless liquid.

d_{20}^{20}: about 0.621.

n_D^{20}: about 1.354.

bp: about 29 °C.

Water (2.5.12): maximum 0.02 per cent.

Residue on evaporation: maximum 0.0003 per cent.

Minimum transmittance (2.2.25), determined using *water R* as compensation liquid: 50 per cent at 210 nm, 85 per cent at 220 nm, 98 per cent at 240 nm and at higher wavelengths.

2-Methylbut-2-ene. C_5H_{10}. (M_r 70.1). *1055400.* [513-35-9].

A very flammable liquid, practically insoluble in water, miscible with alcohol.

bp: 37.5 °C to 38.5 °C.

Methyl caprate. *1054000.*

See *Methyl decanoate R.*

Methyl caproate. $C_7H_{14}O_2$. (M_r 130.2). *1120300.* [106-70-7]. Methyl hexanoate.

d_{20}^{20}: about 0.885.

n_D^{20}: about 1.405.

bp: 150 °C to 151 °C.

Methyl caprylate. $C_9H_{18}O_2$. (M_r 158.2). *1120400.* [111-11-5]. Methyl octanoate.

d_{20}^{20}: about 0.876.

n_D^{20}: about 1.417.

bp: 193 °C to 194 °C.

Methylcellulose 450. *1055500.* [9004-67-5].

See *Methylcellulose (0345).*

The nominal viscosity is 450 mPa·s

Methyl cinnamate. $C_{10}H_{10}O_2$. (M_r 162.2). *1099400.* [103-26-4].

Colourless crystals practically insoluble in water, soluble in alcohol.

n_D^{20}: about 1.56.

bp: about 260 °C.

mp: 34 °C to 36 °C.

Methyl decanoate. $C_{11}H_{22}O_2$. (M_r 186.3). *1054000.* [110-42-9]. Methyl *n*-decanoate.

Content: minimum 99.0 per cent of $C_{11}H_{22}O_2$.

A clear, colourless or yellow liquid, soluble in light petroleum.

d_{20}^{20}: 0.871 to 0.876.

n_D^{20}: 1.425 to 1.426.

Foreign substances. Examine by gas chromatography (*2.2.28*), injecting equal volumes of each of the following: (I) a 0.02 g/l solution of the substance to be examined in *carbon disulphide R,* (II) a 2 g/l solution of the substance to be examined in *carbon disulphide R,* and (III) *carbon disulphide R.* Carry out the chromatographic procedure under the conditions of the test for butylated hydroxytoluene prescribed in the monograph on *Wool fat (0134).* The total area of any peaks, apart from the solvent peak and the principal peak, in the chromatogram obtained with solution (II) is less than the area of the principal peak in the chromatogram obtained with solution (I).

3-*O*-Methyldopamine hydrochloride. $C_9H_{14}ClNO_2$. (M_r 203.7). *1055600.* [1477-68-5]. 4-(2-Aminoethyl)-2-methoxyphenol hydrochloride.

mp: 213 °C to 215 °C.

Chromatography. Examine as prescribed in the monograph on *Dopamine hydrochloride (0664),* applying 10 µl of a 0.075 g/l solution in *methanol R.* The chromatogram obtained shows only one principal spot.

4-*O*-Methyldopamine hydrochloride. $C_9H_{14}ClNO_2$. (M_r 203.7). *1055700.* [645-33-0]. 5-(2-Aminoethyl)-2-methoxyphenol hydrochloride.

mp: 207 °C to 208 °C.

Chromatography. Examine as prescribed in the monograph on *Dopamine hydrochloride (0664),* applying 10 µl of a 0.075 g/l solution in *methanol R.* The chromatogram obtained shows only one principal spot.

Methylenebisacrylamide. $C_7H_{10}N_2O_2$. (M_r 154.2). *1056000.* [110-26-9]. *N,N'*-Methylenebispropenamide.

A fine, white or almost white powder, slightly soluble in water, soluble in alcohol.

mp: It melts with decomposition at a temperature above 300 °C.

Methylene blue. $C_{16}H_{18}ClN_3S,xH_2O$. (M_r 319.9 for the anhydrous substance). *1055800.* [7220-79-3].

Schultz No. 1038.

Colour Index No. 52015.

3,7-Dimethylaminophenothiazin-5-ium chloride.

It occurs in different hydrated forms and may contain up to 22 per cent of water. A dark-green or bronze, crystalline powder, freely soluble in water, soluble in alcohol.

Methylene chloride. CH_2Cl_2. (M_r 84.9). *1055900.* [75-09-2]. Dichloromethane.

A colourless liquid, sparingly soluble in water, miscible with alcohol.

bp: 39 °C to 42 °C.

Methylene chloride used in fluorimetry complies with the following additional requirement.

Fluorescence. Under irradiation at 365 nm, the fluorescence (*2.2.21*) measured at 460 nm in a 1 cm cell is not more intense than that of a solution containing 0.002 ppm of *quinine R* in *0.5 M sulphuric acid* measured in the same conditions.

Methylene chloride, acidified. *1055901.*

To 100 ml of *methylene chloride R* add 10 ml of *hydrochloric acid R,* shake, allow to stand and separate the two layers. Use the lower layer.

Methyl eicosenoate. $C_{21}H_{40}O_2$. (M_r 324.5). *1120500.* [2390-09-2]. (11*Z*)-eicos-11-enoate.

Methyl erucate. $C_{23}H_{44}O_2$. (M_r 352.6). *1146100.* [1120-34-9]. Methyl *cis*-13-docosenoate.

d_{20}^{20}: about 0.871.

n_D^{20}: about 1.456.

3-*O*-Methylestrone. $C_{19}H_{24}O_2$. (M_r 284.4). *1137000.* [1624-62-0]. 3-Methoxy-1,3,5(10)-estratrien-17-one.

White to yellowish-white powder.

$[\alpha]_D^{20}$: about + 157.

mp: about 173 °C.

Methyl ethyl ketone. C_4H_8O. (M_r 72.1). *1054100.* [78-93-3]. Ethyl methyl ketone. 2-Butanone.

A clear, colourless, flammable liquid, very soluble in water, miscible with alcohol.

d_{20}^{20}: about 0.81.

bp: 79 °C to 80 °C.

Methyl green. $C_{26}H_{33}Cl_2N_3$. (M_r 458.5). *1054200.* [7114-03-6].

Schultz No. 788.

Colour Index No. 42585.

4-[[4-(Dimethyl-amino)phenyl][4-(dimethyliminio)cyclohexa-2,5-dienylidene]-methylphenyl]trimethylammonium dichloride.

Green powder, soluble in water, soluble in sulphuric acid giving a yellow solution turning green on dilution with water.

Methyl green-iodomercurate paper. *1054201.*

Immerse thin strips of suitable filter paper in a 40 g/l solution of *methyl green R* and allow to dry in air. Immerse the strips for 1 h in a solution containing 140 g/l of *potassium iodide R* and 200 g/l of *mercuric iodide R*. Wash with *distilled water R* until the washings are practically colourless and allow to dry in air.

Storage: protected from light; use within 48 h.

1-Methylimidazole. $C_4H_6N_2$. (M_r 82.1). *1139700.* [616-47-7]. 1-Methyl-1*H*-imidazole.

Colourless or slightly yellowish liquid.

n_D^{20}: about 1.495.

bp: 195 °C to 197 °C.

Storage: in an airtight container, protected from light.

1-Methylimidazole R1. *1139701.*

Complies with the requirements described for *1-methylimidazole R* with the following additional requirement.

Content: minimum 95.0 per cent.

2-Methylimidazole. $C_4H_6N_2$. (M_r 82.1). *1143400.* [693-98-1].

White, crystalline powder.

mp: about 145 °C.

Methyl isobutyl ketone. $C_6H_{12}O$. (M_r 100.2). *1054300.* [108-10-1]. 4-Methyl-2-pentanone.

A clear, colourless liquid, slightly soluble in water, miscible with most organic solvents.

d_{20}^{20}: about 0.80.

bp: about 115 °C.

Distillation range (*2.2.11*). Distil 100 ml. The range of temperature of distillation from 1 ml to 95 ml of distillate does not exceed 4.0 °C.

Residue on evaporation: maximum 0.01 per cent, determined by evaporating on a water-bath and drying at 100-105 °C.

Methyl isobutyl ketone R1. *1054301.*

Shake 50 ml of freshly distilled *methyl isobutyl ketone R* with 0.5 ml of *hydrochloric acid R1* for 1 min. Allow the phases to separate and discard the lower phase. Prepare immediately before use.

Methyl isobutyl ketone R3. *1054302.*

Complies with the requirements for *methyl isobutyl ketone R* and with the following limits:

Chromium: maximum 0.02 ppm.

Copper: maximum 0.02 ppm.

Lead: maximum 0.1 ppm.

Nickel: maximum 0.02 ppm.

Tin: maximum 0.1 ppm.

Methyl laurate. $C_{13}H_{26}O_2$. (M_r 214.4). *1054400.* [111-82-0]. Methyl dodecanoate.

Content: minimum 98.0 per cent of $C_{13}H_{26}O_2$, determined by gas chromatography (*2.4.22*).

A colourless or yellow liquid, soluble in alcohol and in light petroleum.

d_{20}^{20}: about 0.87.

n_D^{20}: about 1.431.

mp: about 5 °C.

Methyl lignocerate. $C_{25}H_{50}O_2$. (M_r 382.7). *1120600.* [2442-49-1]. Methyl tetracosanoate.

Flakes.

mp: about 58 °C.

Methyl linoleate. $C_{19}H_{34}O_2$. (M_r 294.5). *1120700.* [112-63-0]. Methyl (9*Z*,12*Z*)-octadeca-9,12-dienoate.

d_{20}^{20}: about 0.888.

n_D^{20}: about 1.466.

bp: 207 °C to 208 °C.

Methyl linolenate. $C_{19}H_{32}O_2$. (M_r 292.5). *1120800.* [301-00-8]. Methyl (9*Z*,12*Z*,15*Z*)-octadeca-9,12,15-trienoate.

d_{20}^{20}: about 0.901.

n_D^{20}: about 1.471.

bp: about 207 °C.

Methyl margarate. $C_{18}H_{36}O_2$. (M_r 284.5). *1120900.* [1731-92-6]. Methyl heptadecanoate.

White or almost white powder.

mp: 32 °C to 34 °C.

Methyl margarate used in the assay of total fatty acids in Saw palmetto fruit (1848) complies with the following additional requirement.

Assay. Examine by gas chromatography (*2.2.28*) as prescribed in the monograph on *Saw palmetto fruit (1848)*.

The content of methyl margarate is not less than 97 per cent, calculated by the normalisation procedure.

Methyl methacrylate. $C_5H_8O_2$. (M_r 100.1). *1054500.* [80-62-6]. Methyl 2-methylprop-2-enoate.

A colourless liquid.

n_D^{20}: about 1.414.

bp: about 100 °C.

mp: about −48 °C.

It contains a suitable stabilising reagent.

Methyl myristate. $C_{15}H_{30}O_2$. (M_r 242.4). *1054600.* [124-10-7]. Methyl tetradecanoate.

Content: minimum 98.0 per cent of $C_{15}H_{30}O_2$, determined by gas chromatography (*2.4.22*).

4. Reagents

A colourless or slightly yellow liquid, soluble in alcohol and in light petroleum.

d_{20}^{20}: about 0.87.

n_D^{20}: about 1.437.

mp: about 20 °C.

2-Methyl-5-nitroimidazole. $C_4H_5N_3O_2$. (M_r 127.1). *1056100.* [88054-22-2].

White to light yellow powder.

mp: 252 °C to 254 °C.

Content: minimum 98.0 per cent of $C_4H_5N_3O_2$.

Methyl oleate. $C_{19}H_{36}O_2$. (M_r 296.4). *1054700.* [112-62-9]. Methyl (*Z*)-octadec-9-enoate.

Content: minimum 98.0 per cent of $C_{19}H_{36}O_2$, determined by gas chromatography (*2.4.22*).

A colourless or slightly yellow liquid, soluble in alcohol and in light petroleum.

d_{20}^{20}: about 0.88.

n_D^{20}: about 1.452.

Methyl orange. $C_{14}H_{14}N_3NaO_3S$. (M_r 327.3). *1054800.* [547-58-0].

Schultz No. 176.

Colour Index No. 13025.

Sodium 4′-(dimethylamino)azobenzene-4-sulphonate.

An orange-yellow, crystalline powder, slightly soluble in water, practically insoluble in alcohol.

Methyl orange mixed solution. *1054801.*

Dissolve 20 mg of *methyl orange R* and 0.1 g of *bromocresol green R* in 1 ml of *0.2 M sodium hydroxide* and dilute to 100 ml with *water R.*

Colour change: pH 3.0 (orange) to pH 4.4 (olive-green).

Methyl orange solution. *1054802.*

Dissolve 0.1 g of *methyl orange R* in 80 ml of *water R* and dilute to 100 ml with *alcohol R.*

Test for sensitivity. A mixture of 0.1 ml of the methyl orange solution and 100 ml of *carbon dioxide-free water R* is yellow. Not more than 0.1 ml of *1 M hydrochloric acid* is required to change the colour to red.

Colour change: pH 3.0 (red) to pH 4.4 (yellow).

Methyl palmitate. $C_{17}H_{34}O_2$. (M_r 270.5). *1054900.* [112-39-0]. Methyl hexadecanoate.

Content: minimum 98.0 per cent of $C_{17}H_{34}O_2$, determined by gas chromatography (*2.4.22*).

A white or yellow, crystalline mass, soluble in alcohol and in light petroleum.

mp: about 30 °C.

Methyl palmitoleate. $C_{17}H_{32}O_2$. (M_r 268.4). *1121000.* [1120-25-8]. Methyl (9*Z*)-hexadec-9-enoate.

d_{20}^{20}: about 0.876.

n_D^{20}: about 1.451.

Methyl parahydroxybenzoate. *1055000.* [99-76-3].

See *Methyl parahydroxybenzoate (0409).*

Methyl pelargonate. $C_{10}H_{20}O_2$. (M_r 172.3). *1143500.* [1731-84-6]. Methyl nonanoate.

Clear, colourless liquid.

d_4^{20}: about 0.873.

n_D^{20}: about 1.422.

bp: 91 °C to 92 °C.

Methyl pelargonate used in the assay of total fatty acids in Saw palmetto fruit (1848) complies with the following additional requirement.

Assay. Examine by gas chromatography (*2.2.28*) as prescribed in the monograph on *Saw palmetto fruit (1848).*

The content of methyl pelargonate is not less than 98 per cent, calculated by the normalisation procedure.

3-Methylpentan-2-one. $C_6H_{12}O$. (M_r 100.2). *1141100.* [565-61-7].

Colourless, flammable liquid.

d_{20}^{20}: about 0.815.

n_D^{20}: about 1.400.

bp: about 118 °C

4-Methylpentan-2-ol. $C_6H_{14}O$. (M_r 102.2). *1114300.* [108-11-2].

A clear, colourless, volatile liquid.

d_4^{20}: : about 0.802.

n_D^{20}: about 1.411.

bp: about 132 °C.

Methylphenyloxazolylbenzene. $C_{26}H_{20}N_2O_2$. (M_r 392.5). *1056200.* [3073-87-8]. 1,4-Bis[2-(4-methyl-5-phenyl)oxazolyl]benzene.

A fine, greenish-yellow powder with a blue fluorescence or small crystals, soluble in alcohol, sparingly soluble in xylene.

mp: about 233 °C.

Methylphenyloxazolylbenzene used for liquid scintillation is of a suitable analytical grade.

1-Methyl-4-phenyl-1,2,3,6-tetrahydropyridine. $C_{12}H_{15}N$. (173.3). *1137100.* [28289-54-5]. MPTP.

A white or almost white, crystalline powder, slightly soluble in water.

mp: about 41 °C.

Methylpiperazine. $C_5H_{12}N_2$. (M_r 100.2). *1056300.* [74879-18-8]. 1-Methylpiperazine.

A colourless liquid, miscible with water and with alcohol.

d_{20}^{20}: about 0.90.

n_D^{20}: about 1.466.

bp: about 138 °C.

4-(4-Methylpiperidino)pyridine. $C_{11}H_{16}N_2$. (M_r 176.3). *1114400.* [80965-30-6].

A clear liquid.

n_D^{20}: about 1.565.

2-Methylpropanol. $C_4H_{10}O$. (M_r 74.1). *1056400.* [78-83-1]. Isobutyl alcohol. 2-Methylpropan-1-ol.

A clear colourless liquid, soluble in water, miscible with alcohol.

d_{20}^{20}: about 0.80.

n_D^{15}: 1.397 to 1.399.

bp: about 107 °C.

Distillation range (*2.2.11*). Not less than 96 per cent distils between 107 °C and 109 °C.

2-Methyl-2-propanol. $C_4H_{10}O$. (M_r 74.1). *1056500.* [75-65-0]. 1,1-Dimethyl ethyl alcohol. *tert*-Butyl alcohol.

A clear, colourless liquid or crystalline mass, soluble in water, miscible with alcohol.

Freezing point (*2.2.18*): about 25 °C.

Distillation range (*2.2.11*). Not less than 95 per cent distils between 81 °C and 83 °C.

Methyl red. $C_{15}H_{15}N_3O_2$. (M_r 269.3). *1055100.* [493-52-7].
Schultz No. 250.

Colour Index No. 13020.
2-(4-Dimethylamino-phenylazo)benzoic acid.

A dark-red powder or violet crystals, practically insoluble in water, soluble in alcohol.

Methyl red mixed solution. *1055101.*

Dissolve 0.1 g of *methyl red R* and 50 mg of *methylene blue R* in 100 ml of *alcohol R*.

Colour change: pH 5.2 (red-violet) to pH 5.6 (green).

Methyl red solution. *1055102.*

Dissolve 50 mg in a mixture of 1.86 ml of *0.1 M sodium hydroxide* and 50 ml of *alcohol R* and dilute to 100 ml with *water R*.

Test for sensitivity. To 0.1 ml of the methyl red solution add 100 ml of *carbon dioxide-free water R* and 0.05 ml of *0.02 M hydrochloric acid.* The solution is red. Not more than 0.1 ml of *0.02 M sodium hydroxide* is required to change the colour to yellow.

Colour change: pH 4.4 (red) to pH 6.0 (yellow).

Methyl salicylate. *1146200.* [119-36-8].

See *Methyl salicylate (0230)*

Methyl stearate. $C_{19}H_{38}O_2$. (M_r 298.5). *1055200.* [112-61-8]. Methyl octadecanoate.

Content: minimum 98.0 per cent of $C_{19}H_{38}O_2$, determined by gas chromatography (*2.4.22*).

A white or yellow, crystalline mass, soluble in alcohol and in light petroleum.

mp: about 38 °C.

Methyl tricosanoate. $C_{24}H_{48}O_2$. (M_r 368.6). *1111500.* [2433-97-8]. Tricosanoic acid methyl ester.

Content: minimum 99.0 per cent of $C_{24}H_{48}O_2$.

White crystals, practically insoluble in water, soluble in hexane.

mp: 55 °C to 56 °C.

Methyl tridecanoate. $C_{14}H_{28}O_2$. (M_r 228.4). *1121100.* [1731-88-0].

A colourless or slightly yellow liquid, soluble in alcohol and in light petroleum.

d_{20}^{20}: about 0.86.

n_D^{20}: about 1.441.

mp: about 6 °C.

***N*-Methyltrimethylsilyl-trifluoroacetamide.** $C_6H_{12}F_3NOSi$. (M_r 199.3). *1129600.* [24589-78-4]. 2,2,2-Trifluoro-*N*-methyl-*N*-(trimethylsilyl)acetamide.

n_D^{20}: about 1.380.

bp: 130 °C to 132 °C.

Minocycline hydrochloride. *1146300.*

See *Minocycline hydrochloride (1030).*

Molecular sieve. *1056600.*

Molecular sieve composed of sodium aluminosilicate. It is available as beads with a pore size of 0.4 nm and with a diameter of 2 mm.

Molecular sieve for chromatography. *1129700.*

A molecular sieve composed of sodium aluminosilicate. The pore size is indicated after the name of the reagent in the tests where it is used. If necessary, the particle size is also indicated.

Molybdovanadic reagent. *1056700.*

In a 150 ml beaker, mix 4 g of finely powdered *ammonium molybdate R* and 0.1 g of finely powdered *ammonium vanadate R*. Add 70 ml of *water R* and grind the particles using a glass rod. A clear solution is obtained within a few minutes. Add 20 ml of *nitric acid R* and dilute to 100 ml with *water R*.

Monodocosahexaenoin. $C_{25}H_{38}O_4$. (M_r 402.6). *1143600.* [124516-13-8]. Monoglyceride of docosahexaenoic acid (C22:6). Glycerol monodocosahexaenoate. (*all-Z*)-Docosa-4,7,10,13,16,19-hexaenoic acid, monoester with propane-1,2,3-triol.

Mordant black 11. $C_{20}H_{12}N_3NaO_7S$. (M_r 461.4). *1056800.* [1787-61-7].

Schultz No. 241.

Colour Index No. 14645.
Sodium 2-hydroxy-1-[(1-hydroxynaphth-2-yl)azo]-6-nitronaphthalene-4-sulphonate. Eriochrome black.

A brownish-black powder, soluble in water and in alcohol.

Storage: in an airtight container, protected from light.

Mordant black 11 triturate. *1056801.*

Mix 1 g of *mordant black 11 R* with 99 g of *sodium chloride R*.

Test for sensitivity. Dissolve 50 mg in 100 ml of *water R*. The solution is brownish-violet. On addition of 0.3 ml of *dilute ammonia R1* the solution turns blue. On the subsequent addition of 0.1 ml of a 10 g/l solution of *magnesium sulphate R*, it turns violet.

Storage: in an airtight container, protected from light.

Morphine hydrochloride. *1056900.*

See *Morphine hydrochloride (0097).*

Morpholine. C_4H_9NO. (M_r 87.1). *1057000.* [110-91-8]. Tetrahydro-1,4-oxazine.

A colourless, hygroscopic liquid, flammable, soluble in water and in alcohol.

d_{20}^{20}: about 1.01.

Distillation range (*2.2.11*). Not less than 95 per cent distils between 126 °C and 130 °C.

Storage: in an airtight container.

Morpholine for chromatography. *1057001.*

It complies with the requirements of *morpholine R* and with the following requirement.

Content: minimum 99.5 per cent of C_4H_9NO.

Murexide. $C_8H_8N_6O_6,H_2O$. (M_r 302.2). *1137200.* 5,5′-Nitrilobis(pyrimidine-2,4,6(1*H*,3*H*,5*H*)-trione) monoammonium salt.

Brownish-red crystalline powder, sparingly soluble in cold water, soluble in hot water, practically insoluble in alcohol, soluble in solutions of potassium hydroxide or sodium hydroxide giving a blue colour.

Myosmine. $C_9H_{10}N_2$. (M_r 146.2). *1121200.* [532-12-7]. 3-(4,5-Dihydro-3*H*-pyrrol-2-yl)pyridine.

Colourless crystals.

mp: about 45 °C.

4. Reagents

β-Myrcene. $C_{10}H_{16}$. (M_r 136.2). *1114500.* [123-35-3]. 7-Methyl-3-methylenocta-1,6-diene.

An oily liquid with a pleasant odour, practically insoluble in water, miscible with alcohol, soluble in glacial acetic acid. It dissolves in solutions of alkali hydroxides.

d_4^{20}: about 0.794.

n_D^{20}: about 1.470.

β-Myrcene used in gas chromatography complies with the following additional test.

Assay. Examine by gas chromatography (*2.2.28*) as prescribed in the monograph on *Peppermint oil (0405)*.

Test solution. The substance to be examined.

The area of the principal peak is not less than 90.0 per cent of the area of all the peaks in the chromatogram obtained.

Myristic acid. $C_{14}H_{28}O_2$. (M_r 228.4). *1143700.* [544-63-8]. Tetradecanoic acid.

Colourless or white flakes.

mp: about 58.5 °C.

Myristic acid used in the assay of total fatty acids in Saw palmetto fruit (1848) complies with the following additional requirement.

Assay. Examine by gas chromatography (*2.2.28*) as prescribed in the monograph on *Saw palmetto fruit (1848)*.

The content of myristic acid is not less than 97 per cent, calculated by the normalisation procedure.

Myristicine. $C_{11}H_{12}O_3$. (M_r 192.2). *1099600.* [607-91-0]. 5-Allyl-1-methoxy-2,3-methylenedioxybenzene. 4-Methoxy-6-(prop-2-enyl)-1,3-benzodioxole.

An oily colourless liquid, practically insoluble in water, slightly soluble in ethanol, miscible with toluene and with xylene.

d_{20}^{20}: about 1.144.

n_D^{20}: about 1.540.

bp: 276 °C to 277 °C.

mp: about 173 °C.

Chromatography. Examined as prescribed in the monograph on *Star anise (1153)*, the chromatogram obtained shows only one principal spot.

Myristicine used in gas chromatography complies with the following additional test.

Assay. Examine by gas chromatography (*2.2.28*) under the conditions prescribed in the monograph on *Nutmeg oil (1552)*.

The content is not less than 95.0 per cent, calculated by the normalisation procedure.

Storage: protected from light.

Myristyl alcohol. $C_{14}H_{30}O$. (M_r 214.4). *1121300.* [112-72-1]. 1-Tetradecanol.

d_{20}^{20}: about 0.823.

mp: 38 °C to 40 °C.

Naphthalene. $C_{10}H_8$. (M_r 128.2). *1057100.* [91-20-3].

White crystals, practically insoluble in water, soluble in alcohol.

mp: about 80 °C.

Naphthalene used for liquid scintillation is of a suitable analytical grade.

Naphtharson. $C_{16}H_{11}AsN_2Na_2O_{10}S_2$. ($M_r$ 576.3). *1121400.* [132-33-2]. Thorin. Disodium 4-[(2-arsonophenyl)azo]-3-hydroxynaphthalene-2,7-disulphonate.

A red powder, soluble in water.

Naphtharson solution. *1121401.*

A 0.58 g/l solution.

Test for sensitivity. To 50 ml of *alcohol R*, add 20 ml of *water R*, 1 ml of *0.05 M sulphuric acid* and 1 ml of the naphtharson solution. Titrate with *0.025 M barium perchlorate*; the colour changes from orange-yellow to orange-pink.

Storage: protected from light; use within 1 week.

α-Naphthol. $C_{10}H_8O$. (M_r 144.2). *1057300.* [90-15-3]. 1-Naphthol.

A white, crystalline powder or colourless or white crystals, darkening on exposure to light, slightly soluble in water, freely soluble in alcohol.

mp: about 95 °C.

Storage: protected from light.

α-Naphthol solution. *1057301.*

Dissolve 0.10 g of α-naphthol R in 3 ml of a 150 g/l solution of *sodium hydroxide R* and dilute to 100 ml with *water R*. Prepare immediately before use.

β-Naphthol. $C_{10}H_8O$. (M_r 144.2). *1057400.* [135-19-3]. 2-Naphthol.

White or slightly pink plates or crystals, very slightly soluble in water, very soluble in alcohol.

mp: about 122 °C.

Storage: protected from light.

β-Naphthol solution. *1057401.*

Dissolve 5 g of freshly recrystallised β-naphthol R in 40 ml of *dilute sodium hydroxide solution R* and dilute to 100 ml with *water R*. Prepare immediately before use.

β-Naphthol solution R1. *1057402.*

Dissolve 3.0 mg of *β-naphthol R* in 50 ml of *sulphuric acid R* and dilute to 100.0 ml with the same acid. Use the recently prepared solution.

Naphtholbenzein. $C_{27}H_{20}O_3$. (M_r 392.5). *1057600.* [6948-88-5]. α-Naphtholbenzein. Phenylbis(4-hydroxy-naphthyl)methanol.

A brownish-red powder or shiny brownish-black crystals, practically insoluble in water, soluble in alcohol and in glacial acetic acid.

Naphtholbenzein solution. *1057601.*

A 2 g/l solution in *anhydrous acetic acid R*.

Test for sensitivity. To 50 ml of *glacial acetic acid R* add 0.25 ml of the naphtholbenzein solution. The solution is brownish-yellow. Not more than 0.05 ml of *0.1 M perchloric acid* is required to change the colour to green.

Naphthol yellow. $C_{10}H_5N_2NaO_5$. (M_r 256.2). *1136600.* 2,4-Dinitro-1-naphthol, sodium salt.

Orange-yellow powder or crystals, freely soluble in water, slightly soluble in ethanol.

Naphthol yellow S. $C_{10}H_4N_2Na_2O_8S$. (M_r 358.2). *1143800.* [846-70-8].

Colour Index No. 10316.

8-Hydroxy-5,7-dinitro-2-naphthalenesulphonic acid disodium salt. Disodium 5,7-dinitro-8-oxidonaphthalene-2-sulphonate.

Yellow or orange-yellow powder, freely soluble in water.

1-Naphthylacetic acid. $C_{12}H_{10}O_2$. (M_r 186.2). *1148400.* [86-87-3]. (Naphthalen-1-yl)acetic acid.

White to yellow crystalline powder, very slightly soluble in water, freely soluble in acetone.

mp: about 135 °C.

Naphthylamine. $C_{10}H_9N$. (M_r 143.2). *1057700.* [134-32-7]. 1-Naphthylamine.

A white, crystalline powder, turning pink on exposure to light and air, slightly soluble in water, freely soluble in alcohol.

mp: about 51 °C.

Storage: protected from light.

Naphthylethylenediamine dihydrochloride. $C_{12}H_{16}Cl_2N_2$. (M_r 259.2). *1057800.* [1465-25-4]. *N*-(1-Naphthyl)ethylene-diamine dihydrochloride.

It may contain methanol of crystallisation.

A white to yellowish-white powder, soluble in water, slightly soluble in alcohol.

Naphthylethylenediamine dihydrochloride solution. *1057801.*

Dissolve 0.1 g of *naphthylethylenediamine dihydrochloride R* in *water R* and dilute to 100 ml with the same solvent. Prepare immediately before use.

Naringin. $C_{27}H_{32}O_{14}$. (M_r 580.5). *1137300.* [10236-47-2]. 7-[[2-*O*-(6-Deoxy-α-L-mannopyranosyl)-β-D-glucopyranosyl]oxy]-5-hydroxy-2-(4-hydroxyphenyl)-2,3-dihydro-4*H*-chromen-4-one.

A white or almost white crystalline powder, slightly soluble in water, soluble in methanol and in dimethylformamide.

mp: about 171 °C.

Absorbance (*2.2.25*). Naringin dissolved in a 5 g/l solution of *dimethylformamide R* in *methanol R* shows an absorption maximum at 283 nm.

***trans*-Nerolidol.** $C_{15}H_{26}O$. (M_r 222.4). *1107900.* [40716-66-3]. 3,7,11-Trimethyldodeca-1,6,10-trien-3-ol.

A slightly yellow liquid, slight odour of lily and lily of the valley, practically insoluble in water and in glycerol, miscible with alcohol.

d_{20}^{20}: about 0.876.

n_D^{20}: about 1.479.

bp_{12}: 145 °C to 146 °C.

trans-Nerolidol used in gas chromatography complies with the following additional test.

Assay. Examine by gas chromatography (*2.2.28*) as prescribed in the monograph on *Bitter-orange-flower oil (1175)*, using the substance to be examined as the test solution. The area of the principal peak is not less than 90.0 per cent of the total area of the peaks.

Neryl acetate. $C_{12}H_{20}O_2$. (M_r 196.3). *1108000.* [141-12-8]. (*Z*)-3,7-Dimethylocta-2,6-dienyl acetate.

A colourless, oily liquid.

d_{20}^{20}: about 0.907.

n_D^{20}: about 1.460.

bp_{25}: 134 °C.

Neryl acetate used in gas chromatography complies with the following additional test.

Assay. Examine by gas chromatography (*2.2.28*) as prescribed in the monograph on *Bitter-orange-flower oil (1175)*, using the substance to be examined as the test solution. The area of the principal peak is not less than 93.0 per cent of the total area of the peaks.

Nickel-aluminium alloy. *1058100.*

Contains 48 per cent to 52 per cent of aluminium (Al; A_r 26.98) and 48 per cent to 52 per cent of nickel (Ni; A_r 58.70).

Before use, reduce to a fine powder (180).

It is practically insoluble in water and soluble in mineral acids.

Nickel-aluminium alloy (halogen-free). *1118100.*

Contains 48 per cent to 52 per cent of aluminium (Al; A_r 26.98) and 48 per cent to 52 per cent of nickel (Ni; A_r 58.71).

Fine, grey powder, practically insoluble in water, soluble in mineral acids with formation of salts.

Chlorides: maximum 10 ppm.

Dissolve 0.400 g in 40 ml of a mixture of 67 volumes of *sulphuric acid R* and 33 volumes of *dilute nitric acid R.* Evaporate the solution nearly to dryness, dissolve the residue in *water R* and dilute to 20.0 ml with the same solvent. To one half-aliquot of the solution, add 1.0 ml of *0.1 M silver nitrate.* Filter after 15 min and add 0.2 ml of sodium chloride solution (containing 10 µg of chlorides per millilitre) to the filtrate. After 5 min the solution is more opalescent than a mixture of the second half-aliquot of the solution with 1.0 ml of *0.1 M silver nitrate.*

Nickel chloride. $NiCl_2$. (M_r 129.6). *1057900.* [7718-54-9]. Nickel chloride, anhydrous.

A yellow, crystalline powder, very soluble in water, soluble in alcohol. It sublimes in the absence of air and readily absorbs ammonia. The aqueous solution is acid.

Nickel sulphate. $NiSO_4,7H_2O$. (M_r 280.9). *1058000.* [10101-98-1]. Nickel sulphate heptahydrate.

A green, crystalline powder or crystals, freely soluble in water, slightly soluble in alcohol.

Nicotinamide-adenine dinucleotide. $C_{21}H_{27}N_7O_{14}P_2$. (M_r 663). *1108100.* [53-84-9]. NAD^+.

A white powder, very hygroscopic, freely soluble in water.

Nicotinamide-adenine dinucleotide solution. *1108101.*

Dissolve 40 mg of *nicotinamide-adenine dinucleotide R* in *water R* and dilute to 10 ml with the same solvent. Prepare immediately before use.

Nile blue A. $C_{20}H_{21}N_3O_5S$. (M_r 415.5). *1058200.* [3625-57-8]. Schultz No. 1029.

Colour Index No. 51180.

5-Amino-9-(diethylamino)benzo[*a*]phenoxazinylium hydrogen sulphate.

A green, crystalline powder with a bronze lustre, sparingly soluble in alcohol, in glacial acetic acid and in pyridine.

A 0.005 g/l solution in *alcohol (50 per cent V/V) R* shows an absorption maximum (*2.2.25*) at 640 nm.

Nile blue A solution. *1058201.*

A 10 g/l solution in *anhydrous acetic acid R.*

Test for sensitivity. To 50 ml of *anhydrous acetic acid R* add 0.25 ml of the Nile blue A solution. The solution is blue. On the addition of 0.1 ml of *0.1 M perchloric acid,* the colour changes to blue-green.

Colour change: pH 9.0 (blue) to pH 13.0 (red).

Ninhydrin. $C_9H_4O_3,H_2O$. (M_r 178.1). *1058300.* [485-47-2]. 1,2,3-Indanetrione monohydrate.

A white or very pale yellow, crystalline powder, soluble in water and in alcohol.

Storage: protected from light.

4. Reagents

Ninhydrin and stannous chloride reagent. *1058301.*

Dissolve 0.2 g of *ninhydrin R* in 4 ml of hot *water R,* add 5 ml of a 1.6 g/l solution of *stannous chloride R,* allow to stand for 30 min, then filter and store at a temperature of 2 °C to 8 °C. Immediately before use dilute 2.5 ml of the solution with 5 ml of *water R* and 45 ml of *2-propanol R.*

Ninhydrin and stannous chloride reagent R1. *1058302.*

Dissolve 4 g of *ninhydrin R* in 100 ml of *ethylene glycol monomethyl ether R.* Shake gently with 1 g of *cation exchange resin R* (300 µm to 840 µm) and filter (solution a). Dissolve 0.16 g of *stannous chloride R* in 100 ml of *buffer solution pH 5.5 R* (solution b). Immediately before use, mix equal volumes of each solution.

Ninhydrin solution. *1058303.*

A 2 g/l solution of *Ninhydrin R* in a mixture of 5 volumes of *dilute acetic acid R* and 95 volumes of *butanol R.*

Ninhydrin solution R1. *1058304.*

Dissolve 1.0 g of *ninhydrin R* in 50 ml of *alcohol R* and add 10 ml of *glacial acetic acid R.*

Ninhydrin solution R2. *1058305.*

Dissolve 3 g of *ninhydrin R* in 100 ml of a 45.5 g/l solution of *sodium metabisulphite R.*

Ninhydrin solution R3. *1058306.*

A 4 g/l solution in a mixture of 5 volumes of *anhydrous acetic acid R* and 95 volumes of *butanol R.*

Nitrazepam. *1143900.* [146-22-5].

See *Nitrazepam (0415).*

Nitric acid. HNO_3. (M_r 63.0). *1058400.* [7697-37-2].

Content: 63.0 per cent *m/m* to 70.0 per cent *m/m* of HNO_3.

A clear, colourless or almost colourless liquid, miscible with water.

d_{20}^{20}: 1.384 to 1.416.

A 10 g/l solution is strongly acid and gives the reaction of nitrates (*2.3.1*).

Appearance. Nitric acid is clear (*2.2.1*) and not more intensely coloured than reference solution Y_6 (*Method II, 2.2.2*).

Chlorides (*2.4.4*). To 5 g add 10 ml of *water R* and 0.3 ml of *silver nitrate solution R2* and allow to stand for 2 min protected from light. Any opalescence is not more intense than that of a standard prepared in the same manner using 13 ml of *water R,* 0.5 ml of *nitric acid R,* 0.5 ml of *chloride standard solution (5 ppm Cl) R* and 0.3 ml of *silver nitrate solution R2* (0.5 ppm).

Sulphates (*2.4.13*). Evaporate 10 g to dryness with 0.2 g of *sodium carbonate R.* Dissolve the residue in 15 ml of *distilled water R.* The solution complies with the limit test for sulphates (2 ppm). Prepare the standard using a mixture of 2 ml of *sulphate standard solution (10 ppm SO_4) R* and 13 ml of *distilled water R.*

Arsenic (*2.4.2*). Gently heat 50 g with 0.5 ml of *sulphuric acid R* until white fumes begin to evolve. To the residue add 1 ml of a 100 g/l solution of *hydroxylamine hydrochloride R* and dilute to 2 ml with *water R.* The solution complies with limit test A for arsenic (0.02 ppm). Prepare the standard using 1.0 ml of *arsenic standard solution (1 ppm As) R.*

Heavy metals (*2.4.8*). Dilute 10 ml of the solution prepared for the limit test for iron to 20 ml with *water R.* 12 ml of the solution complies with limit test A for heavy metals (2 ppm). Prepare the standard using *lead standard solution (2 ppm Pb) R.*

Iron (*2.4.9*). Dissolve the residue from the determination of sulphated ash in 1 ml of *dilute hydrochloric acid R* and dilute to 50 ml with *water R.* 5 ml of the solution diluted to 10 ml with *water R* complies with the limit test for iron (1 ppm).

Sulphated ash. Carefully evaporate 100 g to dryness. Moisten the residue with a few drops of *sulphuric acid R* and heat to dull red. The residue does not exceed 0.001 per cent.

Assay. To 1.50 g add about 50 ml of *water R* and titrate with *1 M sodium hydroxide,* using 0.1 ml of *methyl red solution R* as indicator.

1 ml of *1 M sodium hydroxide* is equivalent to 63.0 mg of HNO_3.

Storage: protected from light.

Nitric acid, cadmium- and lead-free. *1058401.*

Complies with the requirements prescribed for Nitric acid R and with the following additional test.

Test solution. To 100 g add 0.1 g of *anhydrous sodium carbonate R* and evaporate to dryness. Dissolve the residue in *water R* heating slightly, and dilute to 50.0 ml with the same solvent.

Cadmium: maximum 0.1 ppm of cadmium (Cd) determined by atomic absorption spectrometry (*Method II, 2.2.23*) measuring the absorbance at 228.8 nm using a cadmium hollow-cathode lamp and an air-acetylene or air-propane flame.

Lead: maximum 0.1 ppm of lead (Pb) determined by atomic absorption spectrometry (*Method II, 2.2.23*) measuring the absorbance at 283.3 nm or 217.0 nm using a lead hollow-cathode lamp and an air-acetylene flame.

Nitric acid, dilute. *1058402.*

Contains about 125 g/l of HNO_3 (M_r 63.0).

Dilute 20 g of *nitric acid R* to 100 ml with *water R.*

Nitric acid, heavy metal-free. *1058404.*

Complies with the requirements prescribed for *nitric acid R* and with the following maximum contents of heavy metals:

As: 0.005 ppm;

Cd: 0.005 ppm;

Cu: 0.001 ppm;

Fe: 0.02 ppm;

Hg: 0.002 ppm;

Ni: 0.005 ppm;

Pb: 0.001 ppm;

Zn: 0.01 ppm.

Nitric acid, lead-free. *1058403.*

Complies with the requirements prescribed for *Nitric acid R* and with the following additional test:

To 100 g add 0.1 g of *anhydrous sodium carbonate R* and evaporate to dryness. Dissolve the residue in *water R,* heating slightly, and dilute to 50.0 ml with the same solvent. Determine the lead content by atomic absorption spectrometry (*Method II, 2.2.23*) measuring the absorbance at 283.3 nm or 217.0 nm using a lead hollow-cathode lamp and an air-acetylene flame. It contains not more than 0.1 ppm of lead (Pb).

Nitric acid, lead-free R1. *1058405.*

Nitric acid R containing not more than 1 µg/kg of lead.

Nitric acid, lead-free, dilute. *1058406.*

Dilute 5 g of *lead-free nitric acid R1* to 100 ml with *deionised distilled water R.*

Nitric acid, fuming. *1058500.* [52583-42-3].

A clear, slightly yellowish liquid, fuming on contact with air.

d_{20}^{20}: about 1.5.

Nitrilotriacetic acid. $C_6H_9NO_6$. (M_r 191.1). *1137400.* [139-13-9].

White crystalline powder, practically insoluble in water and in most organic solvents.

mp: about 240 °C, with decomposition.

Nitroaniline. $C_6H_6N_2O_2$. (M_r 138.1). *1058600.* [100-01-6]. 4-Nitroaniline.

A bright yellow, crystalline powder, very slightly soluble in water, sparingly soluble in boiling water, soluble in alcohol, forms water-soluble salts with strong mineral acids.

mp: about 147 °C.

Nitrobenzaldehyde. $C_7H_5NO_3$. (M_r 151.1). *1058700.* [552-89-6]. 2-Nitrobenzaldehyde.

Yellow needles, slightly soluble in water, freely soluble in alcohol, volatile in steam.

mp: about 42 °C.

Nitrobenzaldehyde paper. *1058701.*

Dissolve 0.2 g of *nitrobenzaldehyde R* in 10 ml of a 200 g/l solution of *sodium hydroxide R*. Use the solution within 1 h. Immerse the lower half of a slow filter paper strip 10 cm long and 0.8 cm to 1 cm wide. Absorb the excess reagent between two sheets of filter paper. Use within a few minutes of preparation.

Nitrobenzaldehyde solution. *1058702.*

Add 0.12 g of powdered *nitrobenzaldehyde R* to 10 ml of *dilute sodium hydroxide solution R*; allow to stand for 10 min shaking frequently and filter. Prepare immediately before use.

Nitrobenzene. $C_6H_5NO_2$. (M_r 123.1). *1058800.* [98-95-3].

A colourless or very slightly yellow liquid, practically insoluble in water, miscible with alcohol.

bp: about 211 °C.

Dinitrobenzene. To 0.1 ml add 5 ml of *acetone R*, 5 ml of *water R* and 5 ml of *strong sodium hydroxide solution R*. Shake and allow to stand. The upper layer is almost colourless.

4-Nitrobenzoic acid. $C_7H_5NO_4$. (M_r 167.1). *1144000.* [62-23-7].

Yellow crystals.

mp: about 240 °C.

Nitrobenzoyl chloride. $C_7H_4ClNO_3$. (M_r 185.6). *1058900.* [122-04-3]. 4-Nitrobenzoyl chloride.

Yellow crystals or a crystalline mass, decomposing in moist air, completely soluble in sodium hydroxide solution giving a yellowish-orange colour.

mp: about 72 °C.

Nitrobenzyl chloride. $C_7H_6ClNO_2$. (M_r 171.6). *1059000.* [100-14-1]. 4-Nitrobenzyl chloride.

Pale-yellow crystals, lachrymatory, practically insoluble in water, very soluble in alcohol.

4-(4-Nitrobenzyl)pyridine. $C_{12}H_{10}N_2O_2$. (M_r 214.2). *1101900.* [1083-48-3].

Yellow powder.

mp: about 70 °C.

Nitrochromic reagent. *1059100.*

Dissolve 0.7 g of *potassium dichromate R* in *nitric acid R* and dilute to 100 ml with the same acid.

Nitroethane. $C_2H_5NO_2$. (M_r 75.1). *1059200.* [79-24-3].

A clear, oily, colourless liquid.

bp: about 114 °C.

Nitrofurantoin. *1099700.* [67-20-9].

See *Nitrofurantoin (0101).*

(5-Nitro-2-furyl)methylene diacetate. $C_9H_9NO_7$. (M_r 243.2). *1099800.* [92-55-7]. Nitrofurfural diacetate. 5-Nitrofurfurylidene diacetate.

Yellow crystals.

mp: about 90 °C.

Nitrogen. N_2. (M_r 28.01). *1059300.* [7727-37-9].

Nitrogen, washed and dried.

Nitrogen R1. *1059400.*

Content: minimum 99.999 per cent *V/V* of N_2.

Carbon monoxide: less than 5 ppm.

Oxygen: less than 5 ppm.

Nitrogen for chromatography. *1059500.*

Content: minimum 99.95 per cent *V/V* of N_2.

Nitrogen gas mixture. *1136900.*

Nitrogen R containing 1 per cent *V/V* of each of the following gases: *carbon dioxide R2, carbon monoxide R1* and *oxygen R1.*

Nitrogen monoxide. NO. (M_r 30.01). *1108300.*

Content: minimum 98.0 per cent *V/V* of NO.

Nitrogen, oxygen-free. *1059600.*

Nitrogen R which has been freed from oxygen by passing it through *alkaline pyrogallol solution R.*

Nitromethane. CH_3NO_2. (M_r 61.0). *1059700.* [75-52-5].

A clear, colourless, oily liquid, slightly soluble in water, miscible with alcohol.

d_{20}^{20}: 1.132 to 1.134.

n_D^{20}: 1.381 to 1.383.

Distillation range (*2.2.11*). Not less than 95 per cent distils between 100 °C and 103 °C.

Nitro-molybdovanadic reagent. *1060100.*

Solution I. Dissolve 10 g of *ammonium molybdate R* in *water R*, add 1 ml of *ammonia R* and dilute to 100 ml with *water R.*

Solution II. Dissolve 2.5 g of *ammonium vanadate R* in hot *water R*, add 14 ml of *nitric acid R* and dilute to 500 ml with *water R.*

To 96 ml of *nitric acid R* add 100 ml of solution I and 100 ml of solution II and dilute to 500 ml with *water R.*

4-Nitrophenol. $C_6H_5NO_3$. (M_r 139.1). *1146400.* [100-02-7]. *p*-Nitrophenol.

Content: minimum 95 per cent of $C_6H_5NO_3$.

Colourless or slightly yellow powder, sparingly soluble in water and in methanol.

mp: about 114 °C.

***N*-Nitrosodiethanolamine.** $C_4H_{10}N_2O_3$. (M_r 134.1). *1129800.* [1116-54-7]. 2,2′-(Nitrosoimino)diethanol.

A yellow liquid, miscible with ethanol.

n_D^{20}: about 1.485.
bp: about 125 °C.

Nitrosodipropylamine. $C_6H_{14}N_2O$. (M_r 130.2). *1099900.* [621-64-7]. Dipropylnitrosamine.
Liquid, soluble in ethanol and in strong acids.
d_{20}^{20}: about 0.915.
bp: about 78 °C.
Appropriate grade for chemiluminescence determination.

Nitrosodipropylamine solution. *1099901.*
Inject 78.62 g of *ethanol R* through the septum of a vial containing *nitrosodipropylamine R.* Dilute 1/100 in *ethanol R* and place 0.5 ml aliquots in crimp-sealed vials.
Storage: in the dark at 5 °C.

Nitrotetrazolium blue. $C_{40}H_{30}Cl_2N_{10}O_6$. ($M_r$ 818). *1060000.* [298-83-9]. 3,3′-(3,3′-Dimethoxy-4,4′-diphenylene)di[2-(4-nitrophenyl)-5-phenyl-2*H*-tetrazolium] dichloride. *p*-Nitro-tetrazolium blue.
Crystals, soluble in methanol, giving a clear, yellow solution.
mp: about 189 °C, with decomposition.

Nitrous oxide. N_2O. (M_r 44.01). *1108500.*
Content: minimum 99.99 per cent *V/V* of N_2O.
Nitrogen monoxide: less than 1 ppm.
Carbon monoxide: less than 1 ppm.

Nonivamide. $C_{17}H_{27}NO_3$. (M_r 293.4). *1148500.* [2444-46-4]. *N*-[(4-Hydroxy-3-methoxyphenyl)methyl]nonanamide.
White, crystalline powder, practically insoluble in cold water, freely soluble in ethanol.
Nonivamide used in the test for nonivamide in Capsicum (1859) complies with the following additional requirement.
Assay. Examine by liquid chromatography (*2.2.29*) as prescribed in the monograph on *Capsicum (1859).* The content of nonivamide is not less than 98.0 per cent, calculated by the normalisation procedure.

Nonylamine. $C_9H_{21}N$. (M_r 143.3). *1139800.* [112-20-9]. 1-Aminononane.
Corrosive, colourless, clear liquid.
d_4^{20}: about 0.788.
n_D^{20}: about 1.433.

Nordazepam. $C_{15}H_{11}ClN_2O$. (M_r 270.7). *1060200.* [340-57-8]. 7-Chloro-2,3-dihydro-5-phenyl-1*H*-1,4-benzodiazepin-2-one.
A white or pale yellow, crystalline powder, practically insoluble in water, slightly soluble in alcohol.
mp: about 216 °C.

DL-Norleucine. $C_6H_{13}NO_2$. (M_r 131.2). *1060300.* [616-06-8]. (*RS*)-2-Aminohexanoic acid.
Shiny crystals, sparingly soluble in water and in alcohol, soluble in acids.

Noscapine hydrochloride. *1060500.* [912-60-7].
See *Noscapine hydrochloride (0515).*

Octadecyl [3-[3,5-bis(1,1-dimethylethyl)-4-hydroxyphenyl]-propionate]. $C_{35}H_{62}O_3$. (M_r 530.9). *1060600.* [2082-79-3]. Octadecyl 3-(3,5-di-*tert*-butyl-4-hydroxyphenyl)propionate.
A white or slightly yellowish, crystalline powder, practically insoluble in water, very soluble in acetone and in hexane, slightly soluble in methanol.
mp: 49 °C to 55 °C.

Octanal. $C_8H_{16}O$. (M_r 128.2). *1150400.* [124-13-0]. Octyl aldehyde.
Oily, colourless liquid. Practically insoluble in water.
d_4^{20}: 0.822.
n_D^{20}: 1.419.
bp: 171 °C.
Octanal used in gas chromatography complies with the following additional test.
Assay. Examine by gas chromatography (*2.2.28*) as prescribed in the monograph on *Sweet orange oil (1811).*
The content is not less than 99 per cent, calculated by the normalisation procedure.

Octanol. $C_8H_{18}O$. (M_r 130.2). *1060700.* [111-87-5]. 1-Octanol. Caprylic alcohol.
A colourless liquid, practically insoluble in water, miscible with alcohol.
d_{20}^{20}: about 0.828.
bp: about 195 °C.

3-Octanone. $C_8H_{16}O$. (M_r 128.2). *1114600.* [106-68-3]. Ethylpentylketone.
A colourless liquid with a characteristic odour.
d_{20}^{20}: about 0.822.
n_D^{20}: about 1.415.
bp: about 167 °C.
3-Octanone used in gas chromatography complies with the following additional test.
Assay. Examine by gas chromatography (*2.2.28*) as prescribed in the monograph on *Lavender oil (1338).*
Test solution. The substance to be examined.
The area of the principal peak is not less than 98.0 per cent of the area of all the peaks in the chromatogram obtained.

Octoxinol 10. $C_{34}H_{62}O_{11}$ (average). (M_r 647). *1060800.* [9002-93-1]. α-[4-(1,1,3,3-Tetramethylbutyl)phenyl]-ω-hydroxypoly-(oxyethylene).
A clear, pale-yellow, viscous liquid, miscible with water, with acetone and with alcohol, soluble in toluene.
Storage: in an airtight container.

Octylamine. $C_8H_{19}N$. (M_r 129.2). *1150500.* [111-86-4]. Octan-1-amine.
Colourless liquid.
d_{20}^{20}: about 0.782.
bp: 175 °C to 179 °C.

Oleamide. $C_{18}H_{35}NO$. (M_r 281.5). *1060900.* (*Z*)-Octadec-9-enoamide.
Yellowish or white powder or granules, practically insoluble in water, very soluble in methylene chloride, soluble in ethanol.
mp: about 80 °C.

Oleic acid. $C_{18}H_{34}O_2$. (M_r 282.5). *1144100.* [112-80-1]. (9*Z*)-Octadec-9-enoic acid.
Clear, colourless liquid, practically insoluble in water.
d_4^{20}: about 0.891.
n_D^{20}: about 1.459.
mp: 13 °C to 14 °C.
Oleic acid used in the assay of total fatty acids in Saw palmetto fruit (1848) complies with the following additional requirement.
Assay. Examine by gas chromatography (*2.2.28*) as prescribed in the monograph on *Saw palmetto fruit (1848).*

The content of oleic acid is not less than 98 per cent, calculated by the normalisation procedure.

Oleuropein. $C_{25}H_{32}O_{13}$. (M_r 540.5). *1152900.* [32619-42-4]. 2-(3,4-Dihydroxyphenyl)ethyl[(2*S*,3*E*,4*S*)-3-ethylidene-2-(b-d-glucopyranosyloxy)-5-(methoxycarbonyl)-3,4-dihydro-2*H*-pyran-4-yl]acetate.

Powder, soluble in methanol.

Oleuropein used in Olive leaf (1878) complies with the following requirement.

Assay. Examine by liquid chromatography (*2.2.29*) as prescribed in the monograph on *Olive leaf (1878)*.

The content of oleuropein is not less than 80 per cent, calculated by the normalisation procedure.

Oleyl alcohol. $C_{18}H_{36}O$. (M_r 268.5). *1156000.* [143-28-2]. (9*Z*)-octadec-9-en-1-ol.

bp: about 207 °C.

n_D^{20}: 1.460.

Content: minimum 85 per cent of $C_{18}H_{36}O$.

Olive oil. *1061000.* [8001-25-0].

See *Olive oil, virgin (0518).*

Oracet blue 2R. $C_{20}H_{14}N_2O_2$. (M_r 314.3). *1061100.* [4395-65-7].

Colour Index No. 61110.

1-Amino-4-(phenylamino)anthracene-9,10-dione.

mp: about 194 °C.

Orcinol. $C_7H_8O_2,H_2O$. (M_r 142.2). *1108700.* [6153-39-5]. 5-Methylbenzene-1,3-diol monohydrate.

A crystalline powder, sensitive to light.

bp: about 290 °C.

mp: 58 °C to 61 °C.

Organosilica polymer, amorphous, octadecylsilyl. *1144200.*

Synthetic, spherical hybrid particles, containing both inorganic (silica) and organic (organosiloxanes) components, chemically modified at the surface by trifunctionally bonded octadecylsilyl groups.

Organosilica polymer, amorphous, polar-embedded octadecylsilyl, end-capped. *1150600.*

Synthetic, spherical hybrid particles containing both inorganic (silica) and organic (organosiloxanes) components, chemically modified at the surface by the bonding of polar embedded octadecylsilyl groups.

To minimise any interaction with basic compounds, it is carefully end-capped to cover most of the remaining silanol groups. The particle size is indicated after the name of the reagent in the tests where it is used.

Osmium tetroxide. OsO_4. (M_r 254.2). *1061200.* [20816-12-0].

Light-yellow needles or a yellow, crystalline mass, hygroscopic, light sensitive, soluble in water and in alcohol.

Storage: in an airtight container.

Osmium tetroxide solution. *1061201.*

A 2.5 g/l solution in *0.05 M sulphuric acid.*

Oxalic acid. $C_2H_2O_4,2H_2O$. (M_r 126.1). *1061400.* [6153-56-6]. Ethanedioic acid dihydrate.

White crystals, soluble in water, freely soluble in alcohol.

Oxalic acid and sulphuric acid solution. *1061401.*

A 50 g/l solution of *oxalic acid R* in a cooled mixture of equal volumes of *sulphuric acid R* and *water R.*

Oxazepam. *1144300.* [604-75-1].

See *Oxazepam (0778).*

Ox brain, acetone-dried. *1061300.*

Cut into small pieces a fresh ox brain previously freed from vascular and connective tissue. Place in *acetone R* for preliminary dehydration. Complete the dehydration by pounding in a mortar 30 g of this material with successive quantities, each of 75 ml, of *acetone R* until a dry powder is obtained after filtration. Dry at 37 °C for 2 h or until the odour of acetone is no longer present.

2,2′-Oxybis(*N,N*-dimethylethylamine). $C_8H_{20}N_2O$. (M_r 160.3). *1141200.* [3033-62-3]. bis(2-Dimethylaminoethyl) ether.

Colourless, corrosive liquid.

d_{20}^{20}: about 0.85.

n_D^{20}: about 1.430.

Oxygen. O_2. (M_r 32.00). *1108800.*

Content: minimum 99.99 per cent *V/V* of O_2.

Nitrogen and argon: less than 100 ppm.

Carbon dioxide: less than 10 ppm.

Carbon monoxide: less than 5 ppm.

Oxygen R1. O_2. (M_r 32.00). *1137600.*

Content: minimum 99 per cent *V/V* of O_2.

Oxytetracycline hydrochloride. *1146500.*

See *Oxytetracycline hydrochloride (0198).*

Palladium. Pd. (A_r 106.4). *1114700.* [7440-05-3].

Grey white metal, soluble in hydrochloric acid.

Palladium chloride. $PdCl_2$. (M_r 177.3). *1061500.* [7647-10-1].

Red crystals.

mp: 678 °C to 680 °C.

Palladium chloride solution. *1061501.*

Dissolve 1 g of *palladium chloride R* in 10 ml of warm *hydrochloric acid R*. Dilute the solution to 250 ml with a mixture of equal volumes of *dilute hydrochloric acid R* and *water R*. Dilute this solution immediately before use with 2 volumes of *water R*.

Palmitic acid. $C_{16}H_{32}O_2$. (M_r 256.4). *1061600.* [57-10-3]. Hexadecanoic acid.

White, crystalline scales, practically insoluble in water, freely soluble in hot alcohol.

mp: about 63 °C.

Chromatography. Examine as prescribed in the monograph on *Chloramphenicol palmitate (0473)*. The chromatogram shows only one principal spot.

Palmitic acid used in the assay of total fatty acids in Saw palmetto fruit (1848) complies with the following additional requirement.

Assay. Examine by gas chromatography (*2.2.28*) as prescribed in the monograph on *Saw palmetto fruit (1848)*.

The content of palmitic acid is not less than 98 per cent, calculated by the normalisation procedure.

Palmitoleic acid. $C_{16}H_{30}O_2$. (M_r 254.4). *1144400.* [373-49-9]. (9*Z*)-Hexadec-9-enoic acid.

Clear, colourless liquid.

bp: about 162 °C.

Palmitoleic acid used in the assay of total fatty acids in Saw palmetto fruit (1848) complies with the following additional requirement.

4. Reagents

Assay. Examine by gas chromatography (*2.2.28*) as prescribed in the monograph on *Saw palmetto fruit (1848)*. The content of palmitoleic acid is not less than 98 per cent, calculated by the normalisation procedure.

Palmityl alcohol. $C_{16}H_{34}O$. (M_r 242.4). *1156100.* [36653-82-4]. Cetyl alcohol. 1-Hexadecanol.

mp: about 48 °C.

Content: minimum 96 per cent of $C_{16}H_{34}O$.

Pancreas powder. *1061700.*

See *Pancreas powder (0350).*

Papain. *1150700.* [9001-73-4].

A proteolytic enzyme obtained from the latex of the green fruit and leaves of *Carica papaya* L.

Papaverine hydrochloride. *1061800.* [61-25-6].

See *Papaverine hydrochloride (0102).*

Paper chromatography performance test solutions. *1150800.*

Test solution (a). Sodium pertechnetate (^{99m}Tc) injection (fission) (0124) or *Sodium pertechnetate (^{99m}Tc) injection (non-fission) (0283).*

Test solution (b). In a closed vial mix 100 µl of a 5 g/l solution of *stannous chloride R* in *0.05 M hydrochloric acid* and 100 MBq to 200 MBq of *Sodium pertechnetate (^{99m}Tc) injection (fission) (0124)* or *Sodium pertechnetate (^{99m}Tc) injection (non-fission) (0283)* in a volume not exceeding 2 ml.

Paper for chromatography. *1150900.*

Pure cellulose grade thin paper with a smooth surface and a thickness of about 0.2 mm.

Chromatographic separation. To 2 strips of *paper for chromatography R* apply separately 2-5 µl of test solution (a) and test solution (b) of *paper chromatography performance test solutions R*. Develop over a pathlength of 3/4 of the paper height, using a mixture of equal volumes of *methanol R* and *water R*. Allow to dry and determine the distribution of radioactivity using a suitable detector. The paper is not satisfactory, unless the chromatogram obtained with test solution (a) shows a single radioactivity spot with an R_f value in the range 0.8-1.0 and the chromatogram obtained with test solution (b) shows a single radioactivity spot at the application point (R_f value in the range 0.0-0.1).

Paracetamol. *1061900.* [103-90-2].

See *Paracetamol (0049).*

Paracetamol, 4-aminophenol-free. *1061901.*

Recrystallise *paracetamol R* from *water R* and dry *in vacuo* at 70 °C; repeat the procedure until the product complies with the following test: dissolve 5 g of the dried substance in a mixture of equal volumes of *methanol R* and *water R* and dilute to 100 ml with the same mixture of solvents. Add 1 ml of a freshly prepared solution containing 10 g/l of *sodium nitroprusside R* and 10 g/l of *anhydrous sodium carbonate R*, mix and allow to stand for 30 min protected from light. No blue or green colour is produced.

Paraffin, liquid. *1062000.* [8042-47-5].

See *Liquid paraffin (0239).*

Paraffin, white soft. *1062100.*

A semi-liquid mixture of hydrocarbons obtained from petroleum and bleached, practically insoluble in water and in alcohol, soluble in *light petroleum R1*, the solution sometimes showing a slight opalescence.

Paraldehyde. *1151000.* [123-63-7].

See *Paraldehyde (0351).*

Pararosaniline hydrochloride. $C_{19}H_{18}ClN_3$. (M_r 323.8). *1062200.* [569-61-9].

Schultz No. 779.

Colour Index No. 42500.

4-[bis(4-Aminophenyl)methylene]cyclohexa-2,5-dieniminium chloride.

A bluish-red, crystalline powder, slightly soluble in water, soluble in ethanol. Solutions in water and ethanol are deep-red; solutions in sulphuric acid and in hydrochloric acid are yellow.

mp: about 270 °C, with decomposition.

Decolorised pararosaniline solution. *1062201.*

To 0.1 g of *pararosaniline hydrochloride R* in a ground-glass-stoppered flask add 60 ml of *water R* and a solution of 1.0 g of *anhydrous sodium sulphite R* or 2.0 g of *sodium sulphite R* or 0.75 g of *sodium metabisulphite R* in 10 ml of *water R*. Slowly and with stirring add 6 ml of *dilute hydrochloric acid R*, stopper the flask and continue stirring until dissolution is complete. Dilute to 100 ml with *water R*. Allow to stand for 12 h before use.

Storage: protected from light.

Parthenolide. $C_{15}H_{20}O_3$. (M_r 248.3). *1129900.* [20554-84-1]. (4*E*)-(1a*R*,7a*S*,10a*S*,10b*S*)-1a,5-Dimethyl-8-methylene-2,3,6,7,7a,8,10a,10b-octahydro-oxireno[9,10]cyclodeca[1,2-*b*]furan-9(1a*H*)-one. (*E*)-(5*S*,6*S*)-4,5-Epoxygermacra-1(10),11(13)-dieno-12(6)-lactone.

A white, crystalline powder, very slightly soluble in water, very soluble in methylene chloride, soluble in methanol.

$[\alpha]_D^{22}$: −71.4, determined on a 2.2 g/l solution in *methylene chloride R*.

mp: 115 °C to 116 °C.

Absorbance (*2.2.25*). A 0.01 g/l solution in *alcohol R* shows an absorption maximum at 214 nm.

Assay. Examine by liquid chromatography (*2.2.29*), as prescribed in the monograph on *Feverfew (1516)*, at the concentration of the reference solution. The content of parthenolide is not less than 90 per cent calculated by the normalisation procedure.

Penicillinase solution. *1062300.*

Dissolve 10 g of casein hydrolysate, 2.72 g of *potassium dihydrogen phosphate R* and 5.88 g of *sodium citrate R* in 200 ml of *water R*, adjust to pH 7.2 with a 200 g/l solution of *sodium hydroxide R* and dilute to 1000 ml with *water R*. Dissolve 0.41 g of *magnesium sulphate R* in 5 ml of *water R* and add 1 ml of a 1.6 g/l solution of *ferrous ammonium sulphate R* and sufficient *water R* to produce 10 ml. Sterilise both solutions by heating in an autoclave, cool, mix, distribute in shallow layers in conical flasks and inoculate with *Bacillus cereus* (NCTC 9946). Allow the flasks to stand at 18 °C to 37 °C until growth is apparent and then maintain at 35 °C to 37 °C for 16 h, shaking constantly to ensure maximum aeration. Centrifuge and sterilise the supernatant liquid by filtration through a membrane filter. 1.0 ml of penicillinase solution contains not less than 0.4 microkatals (corresponding to the hydrolysis of not less than 500 mg of benzylpenicillin to benzylpenicilloic acid per hour) at 30 °C and pH 7, provided that the concentration of benzylpenicillin does not fall below the level necessary for enzyme saturation. The Michaelis constant for benzylpenicillin of the penicillinase in penicillinase solution is approximately 12 µg/ml.

Sterility (*2.6.1*). It complies with the test for sterility.

Storage: at a temperature between 0 °C and 2 °C for 2 to 3 days. When freeze-dried and kept in sealed ampoules, it may be stored for several months.

Pentaerythrityl tetrakis[3-(3,5-di(1,1-dimethylethyl)-4-hydroxyphenyl)propionate]. $C_{73}H_{108}O_{12}$. (M_r 1178). *1062400.* [6683-19-8]. Pentaerythrityl tetrakis[3-(3,5-di-*tert*-butyl-4-hydroxyphenyl) propionate]. 2,2′-bis(Hydroxymethyl)propane-1,3-diol tetrakis[3-[3,5-di(1, 1-dimethylethyl)-4-hydroxyphenyl]]propionate.

A white to slightly yellow, crystalline powder, practically insoluble in water, very soluble in acetone, soluble in methanol, slightly soluble in hexane.

mp: 110 °C to 125 °C.

α-form: 120 °C to 125 °C.

β-form: 110 °C to 115 °C.

Pentafluoropropanoic acid. $C_3HF_5O_2$. (M_r 164.0). *1151100.* [422-64-0].

Clear, colourless liquid.

d_{20}^{20}: about 1.561.

n_D^{20}: about 1.284.

bp: about 97 °C.

Pentane. C_5H_{12}. (M_r 72.2). *1062500.* [109-66-0].

A clear, colourless, flammable liquid, very slightly soluble in water, miscible with acetone and with ethanol.

d_{20}^{20}: about 0.63.

n_D^{20}: about 1.359.

bp: about 36 °C.

Pentane used in spectrophotometry complies with the following additional requirement.

Minimum transmittance (*2.2.25*), determined using *water R* as compensation liquid: 20 per cent at 200 nm, 50 per cent at 210 nm, 85 per cent at 220 nm, 93 per cent at 230 nm, 98 per cent at 240 nm.

1,2-Pentanediol. $C_5H_{12}O_2$. (M_r 104.2). *1155800.* [5343-92-0]. (2*RS*)-Pentane-1,2-diol.

d_4^{20}: about 0.971.

n_D^{20}: about 1.439.

bp: about 201 °C.

Pentanol. $C_5H_{12}O$. (M_r 88.1). *1062600.* [71-41-0]. 1-Pentanol.

Colourless liquid, sparingly soluble in water, miscible with alcohol.

n_D^{20}: about 1.410.

bp: about 137 °C.

***tert*-Pentyl alcohol.** $C_5H_{12}O$. (M_r 88.1). *1062700.* [75-85-4]. *tert*-Amyl alcohol. 2-Methyl-2-butanol.

A volatile, flammable liquid, freely soluble in water, miscible with alcohol and with glycerol.

d_{20}^{20}: about 0.81.

Distillation range (*2.2.11*). Not less than 95 per cent distils between 100 °C and 104 °C.

Storage: protected from light.

Pepsin powder. *1062800.* [9001-75-6].

See *Pepsin powder (0682)*.

Perchloric acid. $HClO_4$. (M_r 100.5). *1062900.* [7601-90-3].

Content: 70.0 per cent *m/m* to 73.0 per cent *m/m* of $HClO_4$.

A clear, colourless liquid, miscible with water.

d_{20}^{20}: about 1.7.

Assay. To 2.50 g add 50 ml of *water R* and titrate with *1 M sodium hydroxide*, using 0.1 ml of *methyl red solution R* as indicator.

1 ml of *1 M sodium hydroxide* is equivalent to 100.5 mg of $HClO_4$.

Perchloric acid solution. *1062901.*

Dilute 8.5 ml of *perchloric acid R* to 100 ml with *water R*.

Periodic acetic acid solution. *1063000.*

Dissolve 0.446 g of *sodium periodate R* in 2.5 ml of a 25 per cent *V/V* solution of *sulphuric acid R*. Dilute to 100.0 ml with *glacial acetic acid R*.

Periodic acid. H_5IO_6. (M_r 227.9). *1108900.* [10450-60-9].

Crystals, freely soluble in water and soluble in alcohol.

mp: about 122 °C.

Permethrin. $C_{21}H_{20}Cl_2O_3$. (M_r 391.3). *1130000.* [52645-53-1].

mp: 34 °C to 35 °C.

A suitable certified reference solution (10 ng/µl in cyclohexane) may be used.

Peroxide test strips. *1147800.*

Use commercial test strips with a suitable scale in the range from 0 ppm to 25 ppm peroxide.

Perylene. $C_{20}H_{12}$. (M_r 252.3). *1130100.* [198-55-0]. Dibenz(de,kl)anthracene.

Orange powder.

mp: about 279 °C.

Petroleum, light. *1063100.* [8032-32-4].

A clear, colourless, flammable liquid without fluorescence, practically insoluble in water, miscible with alcohol.

d_{20}^{20}: 0.661 to 0.664.

Distillation range (*2.2.11*): 50 °C to 70 °C.

Petroleum, light R1. *1063101.*

Complies with the requirements prescribed for *light petroleum R*, with the following modifications:

d_{20}^{20}: 0.630 to 0.656.

Distillation range (*2.2.11*): 40 °C to 60 °C.

It does not become cloudy at 0 °C.

Petroleum, light R2. *1063102.*

Complies with the requirements prescribed for *light petroleum R*, with the following modifications:

d_{20}^{20}: 0.620 to 0.630.

Distillation range (*2.2.11*): 30 °C to 40 °C.

It does not become cloudy at 0 °C.

α-Phellandrene. $C_{10}H_{16}$. (M_r 136.2). *1130400.* [4221-98-1]. (*R*)-5-Isopropyl-2-methyl-cyclohexa-1,3-diene. (−)-p-Mentha-1,5-diene.

d_{20}^{20}: about 0.839.

n_D^{20}: about 1.471.

$[\alpha]_D^{20}$: about −217.

bp: 171 °C to 174 °C.

α-Phellandrene used in gas chromatography complies with the following additional test.

Assay. Examine by gas chromatography (*2.2.28*) as prescribed in the monograph on *Eucalyptus oil (0390)* using the substance to be examined as the test solution.

The area of the principal peak is not less than 98.0 per cent of the total area of the peaks.

4. Reagents

Phenanthrene. $C_{14}H_{10}$. (M_r 178.2). *1063200.* [85-01-8].

White crystals, practically insoluble in water, sparingly soluble in alcohol.

mp: about 100 °C.

Phenanthroline hydrochloride. $C_{12}H_9ClN_2,H_2O$. (M_r 234.7). *1063300.* [3829-86-5]. 1,10-Phenanthroline hydrochloride monohydrate.

A white or almost white, crystalline powder, freely soluble in water, soluble in alcohol.

mp: about 215 °C, with decomposition.

Phenazone. *1063400.* [60-80-0].

See *Phenazone (0421).*

Phenol. *1063500.* [108-95-2].

See *Phenol (0631).*

Phenolphthalein. $C_{20}H_{14}O_4$. (M_r 318.3). *1063700.* [77-09-8]. 3,3-bis(4-Hydroxyphenyl)-3*H*-isobenzofuran-1-one.

A white to yellowish-white powder, practically insoluble in water, soluble in alcohol.

Phenolphthalein paper. *1063704.*

Immerse strips of filter paper for a few minutes in *phenolphthalein solution R*. Allow to dry.

Phenolphthalein solution. *1063702.*

Dissolve 0.1 g of *phenolphthalein R* in 80 ml of *alcohol R* and dilute to 100 ml with *water R.*

Test for sensitivity. To 0.1 ml of the phenolphthalein solution add 100 ml of *carbon dioxide-free water R*. The solution is colourless. Not more than 0.2 ml of *0.02 M sodium hydroxide* is required to change the colour to pink.

Colour change: pH 8.2 (colourless) to pH 10.0 (red).

Phenolphthalein solution R1. *1063703.*

A 10 g/l solution in *alcohol R.*

Phenol red. *1063600.* [143-74-8].

Bright red or dark red, crystalline powder, very slightly soluble in water, slightly soluble in alcohol.

Phenol red solution. *1063601.*

Dissolve 0.1 g of *phenol red R* in a mixture of 2.82 ml of *0.1 M sodium hydroxide* and 20 ml of *alcohol R* and dilute to 100 ml with *water R.*

Test for sensitivity. Add 0.1 ml of the phenol red solution to 100 ml of *carbon dioxide-free water R*. The solution is yellow. Not more than 0.1 ml of *0.02 M sodium hydroxide* is required to change the colour to reddish-violet.

Colour change: pH 6.8 (yellow) to pH 8.4 (reddish-violet).

Phenol red solution R2. *1063603.*

Solution I. Dissolve 33 mg of *phenol red R* in 1.5 ml of *dilute sodium hydroxide solution R* and dilute to 100 ml with *water R.*

Solution II. Dissolve 25 mg of *ammonium sulphate R* in 235 ml of *water R*; add 105 ml of *dilute sodium hydroxide solution R* and 135 ml of *dilute acetic acid R.*

Add 25 ml of solution I to solution II. If necessary, adjust the pH of the mixture to 4.7.

Phenol red solution R3. *1063604.*

Solution I. Dissolve 33 mg of *phenol red R* in 1.5 ml of *dilute sodium hydroxide solution R* and dilute to 50 ml with *water R.*

Solution II. Dissolve 50 mg of *ammonium sulphate R* in 235 ml of *water R*; add 105 ml of *dilute sodium hydroxide solution R* and 135 ml of *dilute acetic acid R.*

Add 25 ml of solution I to solution II; if necessary, adjust the pH of the mixture to 4.7.

Phenoxyacetic acid. $C_8H_8O_3$. (M_r 152.1). *1063800.* [122-59-8]. 2-Phenoxyethanoic acid.

Almost white crystals, sparingly soluble in water, freely soluble in alcohol, and in glacial acetic acid.

mp: about 98 °C.

Chromatography. Examine as prescribed in the monograph on *Phenoxymethylpenicillin (0148)*; the chromatogram shows only one principal spot.

Phenoxybenzamine hydrochloride. $C_{18}H_{23}Cl_2NO$. (M_r 340.3). *1063900.* *N*-(2-Chloroethyl)-*N*-(1-methyl-2-phenoxyethyl)-benzylamine hydrochloride.

Content: 97.0 per cent to the equivalent of 103.0 per cent of $C_{18}H_{23}Cl_2NO$, calculated with reference to the dried substance.

A white or almost white, crystalline powder, sparingly soluble in water, freely soluble in alcohol.

mp: about 138 °C.

Loss on drying (*2.2.32*): maximum 0.5 per cent, determined by drying over *diphosphorus pentoxide R* at a pressure not exceeding 670 Pa for 24 h.

Assay. Dissolve 0.500 g in 50.0 ml of *ethanol-free chloroform R* and extract with three quantities, each of 20 ml, of *0.01 M hydrochloric acid.* Discard the acid extracts, filter the chloroform layer through cotton and dilute 5.0 ml of the filtrate to 500.0 ml with *ethanol-free chloroform R.* Measure the absorbance of the resulting solution in a closed cell at the maximum at 272 nm.

Calculate the content of $C_{18}H_{23}Cl_2NO$, taking the specific absorbance to be 56.3.

Storage: protected from light.

Phenoxyethanol. $C_8H_{10}O_2$. (M_r 138.2). *1064000.* [122-99-6]. 2-Phenoxyethanol.

A clear, colourless, oily liquid, slightly soluble in water, freely soluble in alcohol.

d_{20}^{20}: about 1.11.

n_D^{20}: about 1.537.

Freezing point (*2.2.18*): minimum 12 °C.

Phenylalanine. *1064100.* [63-91-2].

See *Phenylalanine (0782).*

***p*-Phenylenediamine dihydrochloride.** $C_6H_{10}Cl_2N_2$. (M_r 181.1). *1064200.* [615-28-1]. 1,4-Diaminobenzene dihydrochloride.

A crystalline powder or white or slightly coloured crystals, turning reddish on exposure to air, freely soluble in water, slightly soluble in alcohol.

α-Phenylglycine. $C_8H_9NO_2$. (M_r 151.2). *1064300.* [2835-06-5]. (*RS*)-2-Amino-2-phenylacetic acid.

D-Phenylglycine. $C_8H_9NO_2$. (M_r 151.2). *1144500.* [875-74-1]. (2*R*)-2-Amino-2-phenylacetic acid.

Content: minimum 99 per cent of $C_8H_9NO_2$.

White or almost white, crystalline powder.

Phenylhydrazine hydrochloride. $C_6H_9ClN_2$. (M_r 144.6). *1064500.* [59-88-1].

A white or almost white, crystalline powder, becoming brown on exposure to air, soluble in water and in alcohol.

mp: about 245 °C, with decomposition.

Storage: protected from light.

Phenylhydrazine hydrochloride solution. *1064501.*

Dissolve 0.9 g of *phenylhydrazine hydrochloride R* in 50 ml of *water R*. Decolorise with *activated charcoal R* and filter. To the filtrate add 30 ml of *hydrochloric acid R* and dilute to 250 ml with *water R*.

Phenylhydrazine-sulphuric acid solution. *1064502.*

Dissolve 65 mg of *phenylhydrazine hydrochloride R*, previously recrystallised from *alcohol (85 per cent V/V) R*, in a mixture of 80 volumes of *water R* and 170 volumes of *sulphuric acid R* and dilute to 100 ml with the same mixture of solvents. Prepare immediately before use.

Phenyl isothiocyanate. C_7H_5NS. (M_r 135.2). *1121500.* [103-72-0].

A liquid, insoluble in water, soluble in alcohol.

d_{20}^{20}: about 1.13.

n_D^{20}: about 1.65.

bp: about 221 °C.

mp: about −21 °C.

Use a grade suitable for protein sequencing.

1-Phenylpiperazine. $C_{10}H_{14}N_2$. (M_r 162.2). *1130500.* [92-54-6].

Slightly viscous, yellow liquid, not miscible with water.

d_4^{20}: about 1.07.

n_D^{20}: about 1.588.

Phloroglucinol. $C_6H_6O_3,2H_2O$. (M_r 162.1). *1064600.* [6099-90-7]. Benzene-1,3,5-triol.

White or yellowish crystals, slightly soluble in water, soluble in alcohol.

mp: about 223 °C (instantaneous method).

Phloroglucinol solution. *1064601.*

To 1 ml of a 100 g/l solution of *phloroglucinol R* in *alcohol R*, add 9 ml of *hydrochloric acid R*.

Storage: protected from light.

Phosalone. $C_{12}H_{15}ClNO_4PS_2$. (M_r 367.8). *1130200.* [2310-17-0].

mp: 45 °C to 48 °C

A suitable certified reference solution (10 ng/µl in iso-octane) may be used.

Phospholipids. *1064800.*

Wash a quantity of human or bovine brain, well separated from the meninges and blood vessels and liquidise in a suitable apparatus. Weigh 1000 g to 1300 g of the liquidised substance and measure the volume (*V* ml). Extract with three quantities, each of 4*V* ml, of *acetone R*, filter under reduced pressure and dry the residue at 37 °C for 18 h. Extract the residue with two quantities, each of 2*V* ml, of a mixture of 2 volumes of *light petroleum R2* and 3 volumes of *light petroleum R1*, filtering each extract on a filter paper previously moistened with the mixture of solvents. Combine the extracts and evaporate to dryness at 45 °C at a pressure not exceeding 670 Pa. Dissolve the residue in 0.2*V* ml of *ether R* and allow to stand at 4 °C until a deposit forms. Centrifuge and evaporate the clear supernatant liquid under low pressure to a volume of 100 ml per kilogram of the liquidised substance and weigh. Allow to stand at 4 °C until a precipitate forms (12 h to 24 h) and centrifuge. Add to the clear supernatant liquid five times its volume of *acetone R*, centrifuge and reject the supernatant liquid. Dry the precipitate.

Storage: in a desiccator under vacuum, protected from light.

Phosphomolybdic acid. $12MoO_3,H_3PO_4,xH_2O$. *1064900.* [51429-74-4].

Orange-yellow, fine crystals, freely soluble in water, soluble in alcohol.

Phosphomolybdic acid solution. *1064901.*

Dissolve 4 g of *phosphomolybdic acid R* in *water R* and dilute to 40 ml with the same solvent. Add cautiously and with cooling 60 ml of *sulphuric acid R*. Prepare immediately before use.

Phosphomolybdotungstic reagent. *1065000.*

Dissolve 100 g of *sodium tungstate R* and 25 g of *sodium molybdate R* in 700 ml of *water R*. Add 100 ml of *hydrochloric acid R* and 50 ml of *phosphoric acid R*. Heat the mixture under a reflux condenser in a glass apparatus for 10 h. Add 150 g of *lithium sulphate R*, 50 ml of *water R* and a few drops of *bromine R*. Boil to remove the excess of bromine (15 min), allow to cool, dilute to 1000 ml with *water R* and filter. The reagent should be yellow in colour. If it acquires a greenish tint, it is unsatisfactory for use but may be regenerated by boiling with a few drops of *bromine R*. Care must be taken to remove the excess of bromine by boiling.

Storage: at 2 °C to 8 °C.

Phosphomolybdotungstic reagent, dilute. *1065001.*

To 1 volume of *phosphomolybdotungstic reagent R* add 2 volumes of *water R*.

Phosphoric acid. *1065100.* [7664-38-2].

See *Concentrated phosphoric acid (0004)*.

Phosphoric acid, dilute. *1065101.*

See *Dilute phosphoric acid (0005)*.

Phosphoric acid, dilute R1. *1065102.*

Dilute 93 ml of *dilute phosphoric acid R* to 1000 ml with *water R*.

Phosphorous acid. H_3PO_3. (M_r 82.0). *1130600.* [13598-36-2].

White, very hygroscopic and deliquescent crystalline mass; slowly oxidised by oxygen (air) to H_3PO_4.

Unstable, orthorhombic crystals, soluble in water, in alcohol and in a mixture of 3 volumes of ether and 1 volume of alcohol.

d_4^{21}: 1.651.

mp: about 73 °C.

Phosphotungstic acid solution. *1065200.*

Heat under a reflux condenser for 3 h, 10 g of *sodium tungstate R* with 8 ml of *phosphoric acid R* and 75 ml of *water R*. Allow to cool and dilute to 100 ml with *water R*.

Phthalaldehyde. $C_8H_6O_2$. (M_r 134.1). *1065300.* [643-79-8]. Benzene-1,2-dicarboxaldehyde.

A yellow, crystalline powder.

mp: about 55 °C.

Storage: protected from light and air.

Phthalaldehyde reagent. *1065301.*

Dissolve 2.47 g of *boric acid R* in 75 ml of *water R*, adjust to pH 10.4 using a 450 g/l solution of *potassium hydroxide R* and dilute to 100 ml with *water R*. Dissolve 1.0 g of *phthalaldehyde R* in 5 ml of *methanol R*, add 95 ml of the boric acid solution and 2 ml of *thioglycollic acid R* and adjust to pH 10.4 with a 450 g/l solution of *potassium hydroxide R*.

Storage: protected from light; use within 3 days.

Phthalazine. $C_8H_6N_2$. (M_r 130.1). *1065400.* [253-52-1].

Pale yellow crystals, freely soluble in water, soluble in ethanol, in ethyl acetate and in methanol.

mp: 89 °C to 92 °C.

Phthalein purple. $C_{32}H_{32}N_2O_{12},xH_2O$. ($M_r$ 637, anhydrous substance). *1065500.* [2411-89-4]. Metalphthalein. 2,2′,2″,2‴-[*o*-Cresolphthalein-3′,3″-bis(methylenenitrilo)]tetra-acetic acid. (1,3-Dihydro-3-oxo-isobenzofuran-1-ylidene)bis[(6-hydroxy-5-methyl-3,1-phenylene)bis(methyleneimino)diacetic acid].

A yellowish-white to brownish powder, practically insoluble in water, soluble in alcohol. The product may be found in commerce in the form of the sodium salt: a yellowish-white to pink powder, soluble in water, practically insoluble in alcohol.

Test for sensitivity. Dissolve 10 mg in 1 ml of *concentrated ammonia R* and dilute to 100 ml with *water R*. To 5 ml of the solution add 95 ml of *water R*, 4 ml of *concentrated ammonia R*, 50 ml of *alcohol R* and 0.1 ml of *0.1 M barium chloride*. The solution is blue-violet. Add 0.15 ml of *0.1 M sodium edetate*. The solution becomes colourless.

Phthalic acid. $C_8H_6O_4$. (M_r 166.1). *1065600.* [88-99-3]. Benzene-1,2-dicarboxylic acid.

A white, crystalline powder, soluble in hot water and in alcohol.

Phthalic anhydride. $C_8H_4O_3$. (M_r 148.1). *1065700.* [85-44-9]. Isobenzofuran-1,3-dione.

Content: minimum 99.0 per cent of $C_8H_4O_3$.

White flakes.

mp: 130 °C to 132 °C.

Assay. Dissolve 2.000 g in 100 ml of *water R* and boil under a reflux condenser for 30 min. Cool and titrate with *1 M sodium hydroxide*, using *phenolphthalein solution R* as indicator.

1 ml of *1 M sodium hydroxide* is equivalent to 74.05 mg of $C_8H_4O_3$.

Phthalic anhydride solution. *1065701.*

Dissolve 42 g of *phthalic anhydride R* in 300 ml of *anhydrous pyridine R*. Allow to stand for 16 h.

Storage: protected from light; use within 1 week.

Picein. $C_{14}H_{18}O_7$. (M_r 298.3). *1130700.* [530-14-3]. 1-[4-(β-D-Glucopyranosyloxy)phenyl]ethanone. *p*-(Acetylphenyl)-β-D-glucopyranoside.

mp: 194 °C to 195 °C.

Picric acid. $C_6H_3N_3O_7$. (M_r 229.1). *1065800.* [88-89-1]. 2,4,6-Trinitrophenol.

Yellow prisms or plates, soluble in water and in alcohol.

Storage: moistened with *water R*.

Picric acid solution. *1065801.*

A 10 g/l solution.

Picric acid solution R1. *1065802.*

Prepare 100 ml of a saturated solution of *picric acid R* and add 0.25 ml of *strong sodium hydroxide solution R*.

α-Pinene. $C_{10}H_{16}$. (M_r 136.2). *1130800.* [7785-70-8]. (1*R*,5*R*)-2,6,6-Trimethylbicyclo[3.1.1]hept-2-ene.

A liquid not miscible with water.

d_{20}^{20}: about 0.859.

n_D^{20}: about 1.466.

bp: 154 °C to 156 °C.

α-Pinene used in gas chromatography complies with the following additional test.

Assay. Examine by gas chromatography (*2.2.28*) as prescribed in the monograph on *Bitter-orange-flower oil (1175)* using the substance to be examined as the test solution.

The area of the principal peak is not less than 99.0 per cent of the total area of the peaks.

β-Pinene. $C_{10}H_{16}$. (M_r 136.2). *1109000.* [18172-67-3]. 6,6-Dimethyl-2-methylenebicyclo[*3.1.1*]heptane.

A colourless, oily liquid, odour reminiscent of turpentine, practically insoluble in water, miscible with alcohol.

d_{20}^{20}: about 0.867.

n_D^{20}: about 1.474.

bp: 164 °C to 166 °C.

β-Pinene used in gas chromatography complies with the following additional test.

Assay. Examine by gas chromatography (*2.2.28*) as prescribed in the monograph on *Bitter-orange-flower oil (1175)*, using the substance to be examined as the test solution. The area of the principal peak is not less than 99.0 per cent of the total area of the peaks.

Piperazine hydrate. *1065900.* [142-63-2].

See *Piperazine hydrate (0425)*.

Piperidine. $C_5H_{11}N$. (M_r 85.2). *1066000.* [110-89-4]. Hexahydropyridine.

A colourless to slightly yellow, alkaline liquid, miscible with water, with alcohol and with light petroleum.

bp: about 106 °C.

Piperitone. $C_{10}H_{16}O$. (M_r 152.2). *1151200.* [89-81-6]. 6-Isopropyl-3-methyl-cyclohex-2-en-1-one.

Pirimiphos-ethyl. $C_{13}H_{24}N_3O_3PS$. (M_r 333.4). *1130300.* [23505-41-1].

mp: 15 °C to 18 °C.

A suitable certified reference solution (10 ng/μl in cyclohexane) may be used.

Plasma, platelet-poor. *1066100.*

Withdraw 45 ml of human blood into a 50 ml plastic syringe containing 5 ml of a sterile 38 g/l solution of *sodium citrate R*. Without delay, centrifuge at 1500 *g* at 4 °C for 30 min. Remove the upper two-thirds of the supernatant plasma using a plastic syringe and without delay centrifuge at 3500 *g* at 4 °C for 30 min. Remove the upper two-thirds of the liquid and freeze it rapidly in suitable amounts in plastic tubes at or below − 40 °C. Use plastic or silicone-treated equipment.

Plasma substrate. *1066200.*

Separate the plasma from human or bovine blood collected into one-ninth its volume of a 38 g/l solution of *sodium citrate R*, or into two-sevenths its volume of a solution containing 20 g/l of *disodium hydrogen citrate R* and

25 g/l of *glucose R*. With the former, prepare the substrate on the day of collection of the blood. With the latter, prepare within two days of collection of the blood.

Storage: at − 20 °C.

Plasma substrate R1. *1066201.*

Use water-repellent equipment (made from materials such as suitable plastics or suitably silicone-treated glass) for taking and handling blood.

Collect a suitable volume of blood from each of at least five sheep; a 285 ml volume of blood collected into 15 ml of anticoagulant solution is suitable but smaller volumes may be collected, taking the blood, either from a live animal or at the time of slaughter, using a needle attached to a suitable cannula which is long enough to reach the bottom of the collecting vessel. Discarding the first few millilitres and collecting only free-flowing blood, collect the blood in a sufficient quantity of an anticoagulant solution containing 8.7 g of *sodium citrate R* and 4 mg of *aprotinin R* per 100 ml of *water R* to give a final ratio of blood to anticoagulant solution of 19 to 1. During and immediately after collection, swirl the flask gently to ensure mixing but do not allow frothing to occur. When collection is complete, close the flask and cool to 10 °C to 15 °C. When cold, pool the contents of all the flasks with the exception of any that show obvious haemolysis or clots and keep the pooled blood at 10 °C to 15 °C.

As soon as possible and within 4 h of collection, centrifuge the pooled blood at 1000 *g* to 2000 *g* at 10 °C to 15 °C for 30 min. Separate the supernatant liquid and centrifuge it at 5000 *g* for 30 min. (Faster centrifugation, for example 20 000 *g* for 30 min, may be used if necessary to clarify the plasma, but filtration procedures should not be used.) Separate the supernatant liquid and, without delay, mix thoroughly and distribute the plasma substrate into small stoppered containers in portions sufficient for a complete heparin assay (for example 10 ml to 30 ml). Without delay, rapidly cool to a temperature below − 70 °C (for example by immersing the containers into liquid nitrogen) and store at a temperature below − 30 °C.

The plasma is suitable for use as plasma substrate in the assay for heparin if, under the conditions of the assay, it gives a clotting time appropriate to the method of detection used and if it provides reproducible, steep log dose-response curves.

When required for use, thaw a portion of the plasma substrate in a water-bath at 37 °C, gently swirling until thawing is complete; once thawed it should be kept at 10 °C to 20 °C and used without delay. The thawed plasma substrate may be lightly centrifuged if necessary; filtration procedures should not be used.

Plasma substrate R2. *1066202.*

Prepare from human blood containing less than 1 per cent of the normal amount of factor IX. Collect the blood into one-ninth its volume of a 38 g/l solution of *sodium citrate R*.

Storage: in small amounts in plastic tubes at a temperature of − 30 °C or lower.

Plasma substrate R3. *1066203.*

Prepare from human blood containing less than 1 per cent of the normal amount of factor XI. Collect the blood into one-ninth its volume of a 38 g/l solution of *sodium citrate R*.

Storage: in small amounts in plastic tubes at a temperature of − 30 °C or lower.

Plasma substrate deficient in factor V. *1066300.*

Use preferably a plasma which is congenitally deficient, or prepare it as follows: separate the plasma from human blood collected into one tenth of its volume of a 13.4 g/l solution of *sodium oxalate R*. Incubate at 37 °C for 24 h to 36 h. The coagulation time determined by the method described for *coagulation factor V solution R* should be 70 s to 100 s. If the coagulation time is less than 70 s, incubate again for 12 h to 24 h.

Storage: in small quantities at a temperature of − 20 °C or lower.

Plasminogen, human. *1109100.* [9001-91-6].

A substance present in blood that may be activated to plasmin, an enzyme that lyses fibrin in blood clots.

Platelet substitute. *1066400.*

To 0.5 g to 1 g of *phospholipid R* add 20 ml of *acetone R* and allow to stand for 2 h with frequent shaking. Centrifuge for 2 min and discard the supernatant liquid. Dry the residue using a water pump, mix with 20 ml of *chloroform R* and shake for 2 h. Filter under vacuum and suspend the residue obtained in 5 ml to 10 ml of a 9 g/l solution of *sodium chloride R*.

For use in the assay of factor IX, prepare a dilution in a 9 g/l solution of *sodium chloride R* that will give coagulation time differences between consecutive dilutions of the reference preparation of about 10 s.

Storage of the diluted suspensions: at − 30 °C; use within 6 weeks.

Poly[(cyanopropyl)methylphenylmethylsiloxane]. *1066500.*

See *poly[(cyanopropyl)(methyl)][(phenyl)(methyl)]siloxane R*.

Poly[(cyanopropyl)(methyl)][(phenyl)(methyl)]siloxane. *1066500.*

Contains 25 per cent of cyanopropyl groups, 25 per cent of phenyl groups and 50 per cent of methyl groups. (Average relative molecular mass 8000).

A very viscous liquid (viscosity about 9000 mPa·s).

d_{25}^{25}: about 1.10.

n_D^{25}: about 1.502.

Poly[(cyanopropyl)(phenyl)][dimethyl]siloxane. *1114800.*

Stationary phase for gas chromatography.

Contains 6 per cent of (cyanopropyl)(phenyl) groups and 94 per cent of dimethyl groups.

Poly(cyanopropyl)(phenylmethyl)siloxane. *1066600.*

Stationary phase for gas chromatography.

Contains 90 per cent of cyanopropylgroups and 10 per cent of phenylmethyl groups.

Poly(cyanopropyl)(7)(phenyl)(7)(methyl)(86)siloxane. *1109200.*

Stationary phase for gas chromatography.

Polysiloxane substituted with 7 per cent of cyanopropyl groups, 7 per cent of phenyl groups and 86 per cent of dimethyl groups.

Poly(cyanopropyl)siloxane. *1066700.*

Polysiloxane substituted with 100 per cent of cyanopropyl groups.

Poly(dimethyl)(diphenyl)(divinyl)siloxane. *1100000.*

Stationary phase for gas chromatography.

Contains 94 per cent of methyl groups, 5 per cent of phenyl groups and 1 per cent of vinyl groups. SE54.

Poly(dimethyl)(diphenyl)siloxane. *1066900.*
Stationary phase for gas chromatography.
Contains 95 per cent of methyl groups and 5 per cent of phenyl groups. DB-5, SE52.

Poly(dimethyl)(85)(diphenyl)(15)siloxane. *1154700.*
Stationary phase for chromatography.
Contains 85 per cent of methyl groups and 15 per cent of phenyl groups. PS086.

Poly(dimethyl)siloxane. *1066800.*
Silicone gum rubber (methyl). Organosilicon polymer with the appearance of a semi-liquid, colourless gum.
The intrinsic viscosity, determined as follows is about 115 ml·g^{-1}. Weigh 1.5 g, 1 g and 0.3 g of the substance to be examined to the nearest 0.1 mg, into 100 ml volumetric flasks. Add 40 ml to 50 ml of *toluene R*, shake until the substance is completely dissolved and dilute to 100.0 ml with the same solvent. Determine the viscosity (*2.2.9*) of each solution. Determine the viscosity of *toluene R* under the same conditions. Reduce the concentration of each solution by half by diluting with *toluene R*. Determine the viscosity of these solutions.

c = concentration in grams per 100 ml,
t_1 = flow time of the solution to be examined,
t_2 = flow time of toluene,
η_1 = viscosity of the solution to be examined in millipascal seconds,
η_2 = viscosity of toluene in millipascal seconds,
d_1 = relative density of the solution to be examined,
d_2 = relative density of toluene.

To obtain the relative densities use the following data.

Concentration (g/100 ml)	Relative density (d_1)
0 - 0.5	1.000
0.5 - 1.25	1.001
1.25 - 2.20	1.002
2.20 - 2.75	1.003
2.75 - 3.20	1.004
3.20 - 3.75	1.005
3.75 - 4.50	1.006

The specific viscosity is obtained from the equation:

$$\eta_{sp} = \frac{\eta_1 - \eta_2}{\eta_2} = \frac{t_1 d_1}{t_2 d_2} - 1$$

and the reduced viscosity from:

$$\eta_{red} = \frac{\eta_{sp}}{c}$$

The intrinsic viscosity (η) is obtained by extrapolating the preceding equation to $c = 0$. This is done by plotting the curve η_{sp}/c or $\log \eta_{sp}/c$ as a function of c. Extrapolation to $c = 0$ gives η. The intrinsic viscosity is expressed in millilitres per gram; the value obtained must therefore be multiplied by 100.
The infrared absorption spectrum (*2.2.24*) obtained by applying the substance, if necessary dispersed in a few drops of *carbon tetrachloride R*, to a sodium chloride plate, does not show absorption at 3053 cm^{-1}, corresponding to vinyl groups.

Loss on drying (*2.2.32*): maximum 2.0 per cent, determined on 1.000 g by drying *in vacuo* at 350 °C for 15 min; maximum 0.8 per cent, determined on 2.000 g by drying at 200 °C for 2 h.

Polyether hydroxylated gel for chromatography. *1067000.*
Gel with a small particle size having a hydrophilic surface with hydroxyl groups. It has an exclusion limit for dextran of relative molecular mass 2×10^5 to 2.5×10^6.

Polyethyleneglycol adipate. $(C_8H_{12}O_4)_n$. (M_r $(172.2)_n$). *1067700.*
A white, wax-like mass, practically insoluble in water.
mp: about 43 °C.

Polyethyleneglycol succinate. $(C_6H_8O_4)_n$. (M_r $(144.1)_n$). *1067800.*
A white, crystalline powder, practically insoluble in water.
mp: about 102 °C.

Polymethacrylate gel, hydroxylated. *1151300.*
Stationary phase for size-exclusion chromatography.
Gel based on hydroxylated methacrylic acid polymer.

Polymethylphenylsiloxane. *1067900.*
Stationary phase for gas chromatography.
Contains 50 per cent of methyl groups and 50 per cent of phenyl groups. (Average relative molecular mass 4000).
A very viscous liquid (viscosity about 1300 mPa·s).
d_{25}^{25}: about 1.09.
n_D^{25}: about 1.540.

Poly[methyl(95)phenyl(5)]siloxane. *1068000.*
See *Poly(dimethyl)(diphenyl)siloxane R.*

Poly[methyl(94)phenyl(5)vinyl(1)]siloxane. *1068100.*
See *Poly(dimethyl)(diphenyl)(divinyl)siloxane R.*

Polyoxyethylated castor oil. *1068200.*
A light yellow liquid. It becomes clear above 26 °C.

Polysorbate 20. *1068300.* [9005-64-5].
See *Polysorbate 20 (0426).*

Polysorbate 80. *1068400.* [9005-65-6].
See *Polysorbate 80 (0428).*

Polystyrene 900-1000. *1112200.* [9003-53-6].
Organic standard used for calibration in gas chromatography.
M_w: about 950.
M_w/M_n: 1.10.

Potassium bicarbonate. *1069900.* [298-14-6].
See *potassium hydrogen carbonate R.*

Potassium bicarbonate solution, saturated methanolic. *1069901.*
See *potassium hydrogen carbonate solution, saturated methanolic R.*

Potassium bromate. $KBrO_3$. (M_r 167.0). *1068700.* [7758-01-2].
White granular powder or crystals, soluble in water, slightly soluble in alcohol.

Potassium bromide. *1068800.* [7758-02-3]. See *Potassium bromide (0184).*

Potassium bromide used for infrared absorption spectrophotometry (2.2.24) also complies with the following requirement.

A disc 2 mm thick prepared from the substance previously dried at 250 °C for 1 h, has a substantially flat baseline over the range 4000 cm^{-1} to 620 cm^{-1}. It exhibits no maxima with absorbance greater than 0.02 above the baseline, except maxima for water at 3440 cm^{-1} and 1630 cm^{-1}.

Potassium carbonate. K_2CO_3. (M_r 138.2). *1068900.* [584-08-7]. Dipotassium carbonate.

A white, granular powder, hygroscopic, very soluble in water, practically insoluble in ethanol.

Storage: in an airtight container.

Potassium chlorate. $KClO_3$. (M_r 122.6). *1069000.* [3811-04-9].

A white powder, granules or crystals, soluble in water.

Potassium chloride. *1069100.* [7447-40-7]. See *Potassium chloride (0185).*

Potassium chloride used for infrared absorption spectrophotometry (2.2.24) also complies with the following requirement.

A disc 2 mm thick, prepared from the substance previously dried at 250 °C for 1 h, has a substantially flat baseline over the range 4000 cm^{-1} to 620 cm^{-1}. It exhibits no maxima with absorbance greater than 0.02 above the baseline, except maxima for water at 3440 cm^{-1} and 1630 cm^{-1}.

Potassium chloride, 0.1 M. *1069101.*

A solution of *potassium chloride R* containing the equivalent of 7.46 g of KCl in 1000.0 ml.

Potassium chromate. K_2CrO_4. (M_r 194.2). *1069200.* [7789-00-6]. Dipotassium chromate.

Yellow crystals, freely soluble in water.

Potassium chromate solution. *1069201.*

A 50 g/l solution.

Potassium citrate. *1069300.* [6100-05-6].

See *Potassium citrate (0400).*

Potassium cyanide. KCN. (M_r 65.1). *1069400.* [151-50-8].

A white, crystalline powder or white mass or granules, freely soluble in water, slightly soluble in alcohol.

Potassium cyanide solution. *1069401.*

A 100 g/l solution.

Potassium cyanide solution, lead-free. *1069402.*

Dissolve 10 g of *potassium cyanide R* in 90 ml of *water R,* add 2 ml of *strong hydrogen peroxide solution R* diluted 1 to 5. Allow to stand for 24 h, dilute to 100 ml with *water R* and filter.

The solution complies with the following test: take 10 ml of the solution, add 10 ml of *water R* and 10 ml of *hydrogen sulphide solution R.* No colour is evolved even after addition of 5 ml of *dilute hydrochloric acid R.*

Potassium dichromate. $K_2Cr_2O_7$. (M_r 294.2). *1069500.* [7778-50-9]. Dipotassium dichromate.

Potassium dichromate used for the calibration of spectrophotometers (*2.2.25*) contains not less than 99.9 per cent of $K_2Cr_2O_7$, calculated with reference to the substance dried at 130 °C.

Orange-red crystals, soluble in water, practically insoluble in alcohol.

Assay. Dissolve 1.000 g in *water R* and dilute to 250.0 ml with the same solvent. To 50.0 ml of this solution add a freshly prepared solution of 4 g of *potassium iodide R,* 2 g of *sodium hydrogen carbonate R* and 6 ml of *hydrochloric acid R* in 100 ml of *water R* in a 500 ml flask. Stopper the flask and allow to stand protected from light for 5 min. Titrate with *0.1 M sodium thiosulphate,* using 1 ml of *iodide-free starch solution R* as indicator.

1 ml of *0.1 M sodium thiosulphate* is equivalent to 4.903 mg of $K_2Cr_2O_7$.

Potassium dichromate solution. *1069501.*

A 106 g/l solution.

Potassium dichromate solution R1. *1069502.*

A 5 g/l solution.

Potassium dihydrogen phosphate. *1069600.* [7778-77-0]. See *Potassium dihydrogen phosphate (0920).*

Potassium dihydrogen phosphate, 0.2 M. *1069601.*

A solution of *potassium dihydrogen phosphate R* containing the equivalent of 27.22 g of KH_2PO_4 in 1000.0 ml.

Potassium ferricyanide. $K_3[Fe(CN)_6]$. (M_r 329.3). *1069700.* [13746-66-2]. Potassium hexacyanoferrate(III).

Red crystals, freely soluble in water.

Potassium ferricyanide solution. *1069701.*

Wash 5 g of *potassium ferricyanide R* with a little *water R,* dissolve and dilute to 100 ml with *water R.* Prepare immediately before use.

Potassium ferrocyanide. $K_4[Fe(CN)_6],3H_2O$. (M_r 422.4). *1069800.* [14459-95-1]. Potassium hexacyanoferrate(II).

Transparent yellow crystals, freely soluble in water, practically insoluble in alcohol.

Potassium ferrocyanide solution. *1069801.*

A 53 g/l solution.

Potassium fluoride. KF. (M_r 58.1). *1137800.* [7789-23-3].

Colourless crystals or white crystalline powder, deliquescent, soluble in water, practically insoluble in alcohol.

Potassium hydrogen carbonate. $KHCO_3$. (M_r 100.1). *1069900.* [298-14-6]. Potassium bicarbonate.

Transparent, colourless crystals, freely soluble in water, practically insoluble in alcohol.

Potassium hydrogen carbonate solution, saturated methanolic. *1069901.*

Dissolve 0.1 g of *potassium hydrogen carbonate R* in 0.4 ml of *water R,* heating on water-bath. Add 25 ml of *methanol R* and swirl, keeping the solution on the water-bath until dissolution is complete. Use a freshly prepared solution.

Potassium hydrogen phthalate. $C_8H_5KO_4$. (M_r 204.2). *1070000.* [877-24-7]. Potassium hydrogen benzene-1,2-dicarboxylate.

White crystals, soluble in water, slightly soluble in alcohol.

Potassium hydrogen phthalate, 0.2 M. *1070001.*

A solution of *potassium hydrogen phthalate R* containing the equivalent of 40.84 g of $C_8H_5KO_4$ in 1000.0 ml.

Potassium hydrogen sulphate. $KHSO_4$. (M_r 136.2). *1070100.* [7646-93-7].

Colourless, transparent, hygroscopic crystals, freely soluble in water giving a strongly acid solution.

Storage: in an airtight container.

Potassium hydrogen tartrate. $C_4H_5KO_6$. (M_r 188.2). *1070200.* [868-14-4]. Potassium hydrogen (2*R*,3*R*)-2,3-dihydroxybutane-1,4-dioate.

A white, crystalline powder or colourless, slightly opaque crystals, slightly soluble in water, soluble in boiling water, practically insoluble in alcohol.

Potassium hydroxide. *1070300.* [1310-58-3].

See *Potassium hydroxide (0840).*

Potassium hydroxide, alcoholic, 2 M. *1070301.*

Dissolve 12 g of *potassium hydroxide R* in 10 ml of *water R* and dilute to 100 ml with *alcohol R*.

Potassium hydroxide in alcohol (10 per cent *V/V*), 0.5 M. *1070302.*

Dissolve 28 g of *potassium hydroxide R* in 100 ml of *alcohol R* and dilute to 1000 ml with *water R*.

Potassium hydroxide solution, alcoholic. *1070303.*

Dissolve 3 g of *potassium hydroxide R* in 5 ml of *water R* and dilute to 100 ml with *aldehyde-free alcohol R*. Decant the clear solution. The solution should be almost colourless.

Potassium hydroxide solution, alcoholic R1. *1070304.*

Dissolve 6.6 g of *potassium hydroxide R* in 50 ml of *water R* and dilute to 1000 ml with *ethanol R*.

Potassium iodate. KIO_3. (M_r 214.0). *1070400.* [7758-05-6].

A white, crystalline powder, soluble in water.

Potassium iodide. *1070500.* [7681-11-0].

See *Potassium iodide (0186).*

Potassium iodide and starch solution. *1070501.*

Dissolve 0.75 g of *potassium iodide R* in 100 ml of *water R*. Heat to boiling and add whilst stirring a solution of 0.5 g of *soluble starch R* in 35 ml of *water R*. Boil for 2 min and allow to cool.

Test for sensitivity. A mixture of 15 ml of the potassium iodide and starch solution, 0.05 ml of *glacial acetic acid R* and 0.3 ml of *iodine solution R2* is blue.

Potassium iodide solution. *1070502.*

A 166 g/l solution.

Potassium iodide solution, iodinated. *1070503.*

Dissolve 2 g of *iodine R* and 4 g of *potassium iodide R* in 10 ml of *water R*. When solution is complete dilute to 100 ml with *water R*.

Potassium iodide solution, saturated. *1070504.*

A saturated solution of *potassium iodide R* in *carbon dioxide-free water R*. Make sure the solution remains saturated as indicated by the presence of undissolved crystals.

Test by adding to 0.5 ml of the saturated potassium iodide solution 30 ml of a mixture of 2 volumes of *chloroform R* and 3 volumes of *glacial acetic acid R,* as well as 0.1 ml of *starch solution R* . Any blue colour formed should be discharged by the addition of 0.05 ml of *0.1 M sodium thiosulphate.*

Storage: protected from light.

Potassium iodobismuthate solution. *1070600.*

To 0.85 g of *bismuth subnitrate R* add 40 ml of *water R,* 10 ml of *glacial acetic acid R* and 20 ml of a 400 g/l solution of *potassium iodide R.*

Potassium iodobismuthate solution R1. *1070601.*

Dissolve 100 g of *tartaric acid R* in 400 ml of *water R* and add 8.5 g of *bismuth subnitrate R.* Shake for 1 h, add 200 ml of a 400 g/l solution of *potassium iodide R* and shake well. Allow to stand for 24 h and filter.

Storage: protected from light.

Potassium iodobismuthate solution R2. *1070602.*

Stock solution. Suspend 1.7 g of *bismuth subnitrate R* and 20 g of *tartaric acid R* in 40 ml of *water R.* To the suspension add 40 ml of a 400 g/l solution of *potassium iodide R* and stir for 1 h. Filter. The solution may be kept for several days in brown bottles.

Spray solution. Mix immediately before use 5 ml of the stock solution with 15 ml of *water R.*

Potassium iodobismuthate solution R3. *1070604.*

Dissolve 0.17 g of *bismuth subnitrate R* in a mixture of 2 ml of *glacial acetic acid R* and 18 ml of *water R.* Add 4 g of *potassium iodide R,* 1 g of *iodine R* and dilute to 100 ml with *dilute sulphuric acid R.*

Potassium iodobismuthate solution R4. *1070605.*

Dissolve 1.7 g of *bismuth subnitrate R* in 20 ml of *glacial acetic acid R.* Add 80 ml of *distilled water R,* 100 ml of a 400 g/l solution of *potassium iodide R,* 200 ml of *glacial acetic acid R* and dilute to 1000 ml with *distilled water R.* Mix 2 volumes of this solution with 1 volume of a 200 g/l solution of *barium chloride R.*

Potassium iodobismuthate solution, dilute. *1070603.*

Dissolve 100 g of *tartaric acid R* in 500 ml of *water R* and add 50 ml of *potassium iodobismuthate solution R1.*

Storage: protected from light.

Potassium nitrate. KNO_3. (M_r 101.1). *1070700.* [7757-79-1].

Colourless crystals, very soluble in water.

Potassium periodate. KIO_4. (M_r 230.0). *1070800.* [7790-21-8].

A white, crystalline powder or colourless crystals, soluble in water.

Potassium ferriperiodate solution. *1070801.*

Dissolve 1 g of *potassium periodate R* in 5 ml of a freshly prepared 120 g/l solution of *potassium hydroxide R.* Add 20 ml of *water R* and 1.5 ml of *ferric chloride solution R1.* Dilute to 50 ml with a freshly prepared 120 g/l solution of *potassium hydroxide R.*

Potassium permanganate. *1070900.* [7722-64-7].

See *Potassium permanganate (0121).*

Potassium permanganate and phosphoric acid solution. *1070901.*

Dissolve 3 g of *potassium permanganate R* in a mixture of 15 ml of *phosphoric acid R* and 70 ml of *water R.* Dilute to 100 ml with *water R.*

Potassium permanganate solution. *1070902.*

A 30 g/l solution.

Potassium perrhenate. $KReO_4$. (M_r 289.3). *1071000.* [10466-65-6].

A white, crystalline powder, soluble in water, slightly soluble in alcohol, in methanol and in propylene glycol.

Potassium persulphate. $K_2S_2O_8$. (M_r 270.3). *1071100.* [7727-21-1]. Dipotassium peroxodisulphate.

Colourless crystals or a white, crystalline powder, sparingly soluble in water, practically insoluble in alcohol. Aqueous solutions decompose at room temperature and more rapidly on warming.

Potassium plumbite solution. *1071200.*

Dissolve 1.7 g of *lead acetate R*, 3.4 g of *potassium citrate R* and 50 g of *potassium hydroxide R* in *water R* and dilute to 100 ml with the same solvent.

Potassium pyroantimonate. $KSb(OH)_6$. (M_r 262.9). *1071300.* [12208-13-8]. Potassium hexahydroxoantimoniate.

White crystals or a white, crystalline powder, sparingly soluble in water.

Potassium pyroantimonate solution. *1071301.*

Dissolve 2 g of *potassium pyroantimonate R* in 95 ml of hot *water R*. Cool quickly and add a solution containing 2.5 g of *potassium hydroxide R* in 50 ml of *water R* and 1 ml of *dilute sodium hydroxide solution R*. Allow to stand for 24 h, filter and dilute to 150 ml with *water R*.

Potassium tartrate. $C_4H_4K_2O_6,{}^1/_2H_2O$. (M_r 235.3). *1071400.* [921-53-9]. Dipotassium (2*R*,3*R*)-2,3-dihydroxybutane-1,4-dioate hemihydrate.

White, granular powder or crystals, very soluble in water, very slightly soluble in alcohol.

Potassium tetraiodomercurate solution. *1071500.*

Dissolve 1.35 g of *mercuric chloride R* in 50 ml of *water R*. Add 5 g of *potassium iodide R* and dilute to 100 ml with *water R*.

Potassium tetraiodomercurate solution, alkaline. *1071600.*

Dissolve 11 g of *potassium iodide R* and 15 g of *mercuric iodide R* in *water R* and dilute to 100 ml with the same solvent. Immediately before use, mix 1 volume of this solution with an equal volume of a 250 g/l solution of *sodium hydroxide R*.

Potassium tetroxalate. $C_4H_3KO_8,2H_2O$. (M_r 254.2). *1071700.* [6100-20-5].

A white, crystalline powder, sparingly soluble in water, soluble in boiling water, slightly soluble in alcohol.

Potassium thiocyanate. KSCN. (M_r 97.2). *1071800.* [333-20-0].

Colourless crystals, deliquescent, very soluble in water and in alcohol.

Storage: in an airtight container.

Potassium thiocyanate solution. *1071801.*

A 97 g/l solution.

Povidone. *1068500.* [9003-39-8].

See *Povidone (0685).*

Procaine hydrochloride. *1109400.*

See *Procaine hydrochloride (0050).*

Proline. $C_5H_9NO_2$. (M_r 115.1). *1152200.* [147-85-3]. L-Proline. (*S*)-Pyrrolidine-2-carboxylic acid.

White or almost white, finely crystallised powder, freely soluble in water and in mineral acids, soluble in alcohol.

Content: minimum 99.0 per cent of $C_5H_9NO_2$.

$[\alpha]_D^{22}$: − 51 to − 53, determined on a 5.0 per cent *m/V* solution in *1 M hydrochloric acid.*

Propanol. C_3H_8O. (M_r 60.1). *1072000.* [71-23-8]. 1-Propanol.

A clear colourless liquid, miscible with water and with alcohol.

d_{20}^{20}: about 0.802 to 0.806.

bp: about 97.2 °C.

Distillation range (2.2.11). Not less than 95 per cent distils between 96 °C and 99 °C.

2-Propanol. C_3H_8O. (M_r 60.1). *1072100.* [67-63-0]. Isopropyl alcohol.

A clear, colourless, flammable liquid, miscible with water and with alcohol.

d_{20}^{20}: about 0.785.

bp: 81 °C to 83 °C.

2-Propanol R1. *1072101.*

Complies with the requirements prescribed for *2-propanol R* and with the following requirements:

n_D^{20}: about 1.378.

Water (2.5.12): maximum 0.05 per cent, determined on 10 g.

Minimum transmittance (2.2.25), determined using *water R* as compensation liquid: 25 per cent at 210 nm, 55 per cent at 220 nm, 75 per cent at 230 nm, 95 per cent at 250 nm, 98 per cent at 260 nm.

Propetamphos. $C_{10}H_{20}NO_4PS$. (M_r 281.3). *1130900.* [31218-83-4].

A suitable certified reference solution (10 ng/μl in cyclohexane) may be used.

Propidium iodide. $C_{27}H_{34}I_2N_4$. (M_r 668.4). *1154200.* [25535-16-4]. 3,8-Diamino-5-[3(diethylmethylammonio)propyl]-6-phenylphenanthridinium diiodide.

Dark red solid.

Propionaldehyde. C_3H_6O. (M_r 58.1). *1072300.* [123-38-6]. Propanal.

A liquid freely soluble in water, miscible with alcohol.

d_{20}^{20}: about 0.81.

n_D^{20}: about 1.365.

bp: about 49 °C.

mp: about − 81 °C.

Propionic acid. $C_3H_6O_2$. (M_r 74.1). *1072400.* [79-09-4].

An oily liquid, soluble in alcohol, miscible with water.

d_{20}^{20}: about 0.993.

n_D^{20}: about 1.387.

bp: about 141 °C.

mp: about − 21 °C.

Propionic anhydride. $C_6H_{10}O_3$. (M_r 130.1). *1072500.* [123-62-6].

A clear, colourless liquid, soluble in alcohol.

d_{20}^{20}: about 1.01.

bp: about 167 °C.

Propionic anhydride reagent. *1072501.*

Dissolve 1 g of *toluenesulphonic acid R* in 30 ml of *glacial acetic acid R*, add 5 ml of *propionic anhydride R* and allow to stand for at least 15 min before use.

Storage: use within 24 h.

Propyl acetate. $C_5H_{10}O_2$. (M_r 102.1). *1072600.* [109-60-4].

d_{20}^{20}: about 0.888.

bp: about 102 °C.

mp: about − 95 °C.

Propyl parahydroxybenzoate. *1072700.* [94-13-3].

See *Propyl parahydroxybenzoate (0431).*

D-Prolyl-L-phenylalanyl-L-arginine 4-nitroanilide dihydrochloride. $C_{26}H_{36}Cl_2N_8O_5$. (M_r 612). *1072800.*

Propylene glycol. *1072900.* [57-55-6].

See *Propylene glycol (0430).*

Propylene oxide. C_3H_6O. (M_r 58.1). *1121800.* [75-56-9].

Colourless liquid, miscible with alcohol.

Protamine sulphate. *1073000.* [53597-25-4 (salmine) 9007-31-2 (clupeine)].

See *Protamine sulphate (0569).*

Pteroic acid. $C_{14}H_{12}N_6O_3$. (M_r 312.3). *1144600.* [119-24-4]. 4-[[(2-Amino-4-oxo-1,4-dihydropteridin-6-yl)methyl]amino]benzoic acid.

Crystals, soluble in solutions of alkali hydroxides.

Pulegone. $C_{10}H_{16}O$. (M_r 152.2). *1073100.* [89-82-7]. (*R*)-2-Isopropylidene-5-methylcyclohexanone. (+)-*p*-Menth-4-en-3-one.

An oily, colourless liquid, practically insoluble in water, miscible with alcohol.

d_{15}^{20}: about 0.936.

n_D^{20}: 1.485 to 1.489.

$[\alpha]_D^{20}$: + 19.5 to + 22.5.

bp: 222 °C to 224 °C.

Pulegone used in gas chromatography complies with the following additional test.

Assay. Examine by gas chromatography (*2.2.28*) as prescribed in the monograph on *Peppermint oil (0405)* using the substance to be examined as the test solution.

The area of the principal peak is not less than 98.0 per cent of the total area of the peaks.

Putrescine. $C_4H_{12}N_2$. (M_r 88.15). *1137900.* [110–60–1]. 1,4-Butanediamine. Tetramethylenediamine.

A colourless oily liquid, very soluble in water. Strong piperidine-like odour.

bp: about 159 °C.

mp: about 23 °C.

Pyridine. C_5H_5N. (M_r 79.1). *1073200.* [110-86-1].

A clear, colourless liquid, hygroscopic, miscible with water and with alcohol.

bp: about 115 °C.

Storage: in an airtight container.

Pyridine, anhydrous. *1073300.* [110-86-1].

Dry *pyridine R* over *anhydrous sodium carbonate R.* Filter and distil.

Water (*2.5.12*): maximum 0.01 per cent *m/m.*

Pyrid-2-ylamine. $C_5H_6N_2$. (M_r 94.1). *1073400.* [504-29-0]. 2-Aminopyridine.

Large crystals soluble in water and in alcohol.

bp: about 210 °C.

mp: about 58 °C.

Pyridylazonaphthol. $C_{15}H_{11}N_3O$. (M_r 249.3). *1073500.* [85-85-8]. 1-(2-Pyridylazo)-2-naphthol.

A brick-red powder, practically insoluble in water, soluble in alcohol, in methanol and in hot dilute alkali solutions.

mp: about 138 °C.

Pyridylazonaphthol solution. *1073501.*

A 1 g/l solution in *ethanol R.*

Test for sensitivity. To 50 ml of *water R* add 10 ml of *acetate buffer solution pH 4.4 R,* 0.10 ml of *0.02 M sodium edetate* and 0.25 ml of the pyridylazonaphthol solution. After addition of 0.15 ml of a 5 g/l solution of *copper sulphate R,* the colour changes from light yellow to violet.

4-(2-Pyridylazo)resorcinol monosodium salt. $C_{11}H_8N_3NaO_2,H_2O$. (M_r 255.2). *1131500.* [16593-81-0].

Orange crystalline powder.

Pyrocatechol. $C_6H_6O_2$. (M_r 110.1). *1073600.* [120-80-9]. Benzene-1,2-diol.

Colourless or slightly yellow crystals, soluble in water, in acetone and in alcohol.

mp: about 102 °C.

Storage: protected from light.

Pyrogallol. $C_6H_6O_3$. (M_r 126.1). *1073700.* [87-66-1]. Benzene-1,2,3-triol.

White crystals, becoming brownish on exposure to air and light, very soluble in water and in alcohol, slightly soluble in carbon disulphide. On exposure to air, aqueous solutions, and more rapidly alkaline solutions, become brown owing to the absorption of oxygen.

mp: about 131 °C.

Storage: protected from light.

Pyrogallol solution, alkaline. *1073701.*

Dissolve 0.5 g of *pyrogallol R* in 2 ml of *carbon dioxide-free water R.* Dissolve 12 g of *potassium hydroxide R* in 8 ml of *carbon dioxide-free water R.* Mix the two solutions immediately before use.

2-Pyrrolidone. C_4H_7NO. (M_r 85.1). *1138000.* [616-45-5]. Pyrrolidin-2-one.

Liquid above 25 °C, miscible with water, with ethanol and with ethyl acetate.

d_4^{25}: 1.116.

Pyruvic acid. $C_3H_4O_3$. (M_r 88.1). *1109300.* [127-17-3]. 2-Oxopropanoic acid.

A yellowish liquid, miscible with water and with ethanol.

d_{20}^{20}: about 1.267.

n_D^{20}: about 1.413.

bp: about 165 °C.

Quercetin dihydrate. $C_{15}H_{10}O_7,2H_2O$. (M_r 338.2). *1138100.* 2-(3,4-Dihydroxyphenyl)-3,5,7-trihydroxy-*4H*-1-benzopyran-4-one.

Yellow crystals or yellowish powder, practically insoluble in water, soluble in acetone and in methanol.

Water (*2.5.12*): maximum 12.0 per cent, determined on 0.100 g.

Assay. Examine by liquid chromatography (*2.2.29*) as prescribed in the monograph on *Ginkgo leaf (1828).*

The content is not less than 90 per cent (anhydrous substance) calculated by the normalisation procedure.

Storage: protected from light.

Quercitrin. $C_{21}H_{20}O_{11}$. (M_r 448.4). *1138200.* [522-12-3]. Quercetin 3-L-rhamnopyranoside. 3-[(6-Deoxy-α-L-mannopyranosyl)oxy]-2-(3,4-dihydroxyphenyl)-5,7-dihydroxy-4*H*-1-benzopyran-4-one. Quercitroside.

Yellow crystals, practically insoluble in cold water, soluble in alcohol.

mp: 176 °C to 179 °C.

Chromatography. Examine as prescribed in the monograph on *Goldenrod (1892)* applying 20 µl of the solution. After spraying, the chromatogram shows a yellowish-brown fluorescent zone with an R_f of about 0.6.

Storage: at a temperature of 2 °C to 8 °C.

Quinaldine red. $C_{21}H_{23}IN_2$. (M_r 430.3). *1073800.* [117-92-0]. 2-[2-[4-(Dimethylamino)phenyl]ethenyl]-1-ethylquinolinium iodide.

Dark bluish-black powder, sparingly soluble in water, freely soluble in alcohol.

Quinaldine red solution. *1073801.*

Dissolve 0.1 g of *quinaldine red R* in *methanol R* and dilute to 100 ml with the same solvent.

Colour change: pH 1.4 (colourless) to pH 3.2 (red).

Quinhydrone. $C_{12}H_{10}O_4$. (M_r 218.2). *1073900.* [106-34-3]. Equimolecular compound of 1,4-benzoquinone and hydroquinone.

Dark green, lustrous crystals or a crystalline powder, slightly soluble in water, sparingly soluble in hot water, soluble in alcohol and in concentrated ammonia.

mp: about 170 °C.

Quinidine. $C_{20}H_{24}N_2O_2$. (M_r 324.4). *1074000.* [56-54-2]. (*S*)-(6-Methoxyquinol-4-yl)[(2*R*,4*S*,5*R*)-5-vinylquinuclidin-2-yl]methanol.

White crystals, very slightly soluble in water, sparingly soluble in alcohol, slightly soluble in methanol.

$[\alpha]_D^{20}$: about + 260, determined on a 10 g/l solution in *ethanol R*.

mp: about 172 °C.

Storage: protected from light.

Quinidine sulphate. *1109500.* [6591-63-5].

See *Quinidine sulphate (0017).*

Quinine. $C_{20}H_{24}N_2O_2$. (M_r 324.4). *1074100.* [130-95-0]. (*R*)-(6-Methoxyquinol-4-yl)[(2*S*,4*S*,5*R*)-5-vinylquinuclidin-2-yl]methanol.

A white, microcrystalline powder, very slightly soluble in water, slightly soluble in boiling water, very soluble in ethanol.

$[\alpha]_D^{20}$: about − 167, determined on a 10 g/l solution in *ethanol R*.

mp: about 175 °C.

Storage: protected from light.

Quinine hydrochloride. *1074200.* [6119-47-7].

See *Quinine hydrochloride (0018).*

Quinine sulphate. *1074300.* [6119-70-6].

See *Quinine sulphate (0019).*

Rabbit erythrocyte suspension. *1074500.*

Prepare a 1.6 per cent *V/V* suspension of rabbit erythrocytes as follows: defibrinate 15 ml of freshly drawn rabbit blood by shaking with glass beads, centrifuge at 2000 *g* for 10 min and wash the erythrocytes with three quantities, each of 30 ml, of a 9 g/l solution of *sodium chloride R*. Dilute 1.6 ml of the suspension of erythrocytes to 100 ml with a mixture of 1 volume of *phosphate buffer solution pH 7.2 R* and 9 volumes of a 9 g/l solution of *sodium chloride R*.

Raclopride tartrate. $C_{19}H_{26}Cl_2N_2O_9$. (M_r 497.3). *1144700.* [98185-20-7]. Raclopride L-tartrate.

A white solid, sensitive to light, soluble in water.

$[\alpha]_D^{25}$: + 0.3, determined on a 3 g/l solution.

mp: about 141 °C.

Rapeseed oil. *1074600.*

See *Rapeseed oil, refined (1369).*

Reducing mixture. *1074700.*

Grind the substances added in the following order to obtain a homogeneous mixture: 20 mg of *potassium bromide R*, 0.5 g of *hydrazine sulphate R* and 5 g of *sodium chloride R*.

Resin for reversed-phase ion chromatography. *1131100.*

A neutral, macroporous, high specific surface area with a non-polar character resin consisting of polymer lattice of polystyrene cross-linked with divinylbenzene.

Resin, weak cationic. *1096000.*

See *weak cationic resin R.*

Resorcinol. *1074800.* [108-46-3].

See *Resorcinol (0290).*

Resorcinol reagent. *1074801.*

To 80 ml of *hydrochloric acid R1* add 10 ml of a 20 g/l solution of *resorcinol R* and 0.25 ml of a 25 g/l solution of *copper sulphate R* and dilute to 100.0 ml with *water R*. Prepare the solution at least 4 h before use.

Storage: at 2 °C to 8 °C for 1 week.

Rhamnose. $C_6H_{12}O_5,H_2O$. (M_r 182.2). *1074900.* [6155-35-7]. L-(+)-Rhamnose. 6-Deoxy-L-mannose.

A white, crystalline powder, freely soluble in water.

$[\alpha]_D^{20}$: + 7.8 to + 8.3, determined on a 50 g/l solution in *water R* containing about 0.05 per cent of NH_3.

Rhaponticin. $C_{21}H_{24}O_9$. (M_r 420.4). *1075000.* [155-58-8]. 3-Hydroxy-5-[2-(3-hydroxy-4-methoxyphenyl)ethenyl]phenyl β-D-glucopyranoside.

A yellowish-grey, crystalline powder, soluble in alcohol and in methanol.

Chromatography. Examine as prescribed in the monograph on *Rhubarb (0291)*; the chromatogram shows only one principal spot.

Rhodamine 6 G. $C_{28}H_{31}ClN_2O_3$. (M_r 479.0). *1153300.* [989-38-8].

Colour Index No. 45160.

9-[2-(Ethoxycarbonyl)phenyl]-3,6-bis(ethylamino)-2,7-dimethylxanthenylium chloride.

Brownish-red powder.

Rhodamine B. $C_{28}H_{31}ClN_2O_3$. (M_r 479.0). *1075100.* [81-88-9].

Schultz No. 864.

Colour Index No. 45170.

[9-(2-Carboxyphen-yl)-6-(diethylamino)-3*H*-xanthen-3-ylidene]diethylammonium chloride.

Green crystals or reddish-violet powder, very soluble in water and in alcohol.

Ribose. $C_5H_{10}O_5$. (M_r 150.1). *1109600.* [50-69-1]. D-Ribose.

Soluble in water, slightly soluble in alcohol.

mp: 88 °C to 92 °C.

Ricinoleic acid. $C_{18}H_{34}O_3$. (M_r 298.5). *1100100.* [141-22-0]. 12-Hydroxyoleic acid.

A yellow or yellowish-brown viscous liquid, consisting of a mixture of fatty acids obtained by the hydrolysis of castor oil, practically insoluble in water, very soluble in ethanol.

d_{20}^{20}: about 0.942.

n_D^{20}: about 1.472.

mp: about 285 °C, with decomposition.

Rosmarinic acid. $C_{18}H_{16}O_8$. (M_r 360.3). *1138300.* [20283-92-5].

mp: 170 °C to 174 °C.

Ruscogenins. *1141300.*
Mixture of neoruscogenin ($C_{27}H_{40}O_4$; M_r 428.6) and ruscogenin ($C_{27}H_{42}O_4$; M_r 430.6).

White powder, very slightly soluble in water, soluble in alcohol.

Ruscogenins used in liquid chromatography complies with the following additional requirement.

Assay. Examine by liquid chromatography (*2.2.29*) as prescribed in the monograph on *Butcher's broom (1847).* The content is not less than 90 per cent of ruscogenins of which at least 60 per cent consists of neoruscogenin, calculated by the normalisation procedure.

Ruthenium red. $[(NH_3)_5RuORu(NH_3)_4ORu(NH_3)_5]Cl_6,4H_2O$. ($M_r$ 858). *1075200.* [11103-72-3].

A brownish-red powder, soluble in water.

Ruthenium red solution. *1075201.*

A 0.8 g/l solution in *lead acetate solution R.*

Rutin. $C_{27}H_{30}O_{16},3H_2O$. (M_r 665). *1075300.* [153-18-4]. Rutoside. 3-(*O*-6-Deoxy-α-L-mannopyranosyl-(1→6)-β-D-glucopyranosyloxy)-2-(3,4-dihydroxyphenyl)-5,7-dihydroxy-4*H*-chromen-4-one.

A yellow, crystalline powder, darkening in light, very slightly soluble in water, soluble in about 400 parts of boiling water, slightly soluble in alcohol, soluble in solutions of the alkali hydroxides and in ammonia.

mp: about 210 °C, with decomposition.

A solution in *alcohol R* shows two absorption maxima (*2.2.25*), at 259 nm and 362 nm.

Storage: protected from light.

Sabinene. $C_{10}H_{16}$. (M_r 136.2). *1109700.* [2009-00-9]. Thuj-4(10)-ene. 4-Methylene-1-isopropylbicyclo[3.1.0]hexane.

A colourless, oily liquid.

d_{25}^{25}: about 0.843.

n_D^{20}: about 1.468.

bp: 163 °C to 165 °C.

Sabinene used in gas chromatography complies with the following additional test.

Assay. Examine by gas chromatography (*2.2.28*) as prescribed in the monograph on *Bitter-orange-flower oil (1175),* using the substance to be examined as the test solution.

The area of the principal peak is not less than 99.0 per cent of the total area of the peaks.

Saccharin sodium. *1131400.* [128-44-9].

See *Saccharin sodium (0787).*

Safrole. $C_{10}H_{10}O_2$. (M_r 162.2). *1131200.* [94-59-7]. 5-(Prop-2-enyl)-1,3-benzodioxole. 4-Allyl-1,2-(methylenedioxy)benzene.

A colourless or slightly yellow, oily liquid, with the odour of sassafras, insoluble in water, very soluble in alcohol, miscible with hexane.

d_{20}^{20}: 1.095 to 1.096.

n_D^{20}: 1.537 to 1.538.

bp: 232 °C to 234 °C.

Freezing point: about 11 °C.

Safrole used in gas chromatography complies with the following additional test.

Assay. Examine by gas chromatography (*2.2.28*) as prescribed in the monograph on *Cinnamon bark oil, Ceylon (1501).*

The content is not less than 96.0 per cent, calculated by the normalisation procedure.

Salicin. $C_{13}H_{18}O_7$. (M_r 286.3). *1131300.* [138-52-3]. 2-(Hydroxymethyl)phenyl-β-D-glucopyranoside. Salicoside.

$[\alpha]_D^{20}$: − 62.5 ± 2.

mp: 199 °C to 201 °C.

Assay. Examine by liquid chromatography (*2.2.29*) as prescribed in the monograph on *Willow bark (1583)* at the concentration of the reference solution. The content is not less than 99.0 per cent calculated by the normalisation procedure.

Salicylaldehyde. $C_7H_6O_2$. (M_r 122.1). *1075400.* [959-36-4]. 2-Hydroxybenzaldehyde.

A clear, colourless, oily liquid.

d_{20}^{20}: about 1.167.

n_D^{20}: about 1.574.

bp: about 196 °C.

mp: about − 7 °C.

Salicylaldehyde azine. $C_{14}H_{12}N_2O_2$. (M_r 240.3). *1075500.* [959-36-4]. 2,2′-Azinodimethyldiphenol.

Dissolve 0.30 g of *hydrazine sulphate R* in 5 ml of *water R,* add 1 ml of *glacial acetic acid R* and 2 ml of a freshly prepared 20 per cent *V/V* solution of *salicylaldehyde R* in *2-propanol R.* Mix, allow to stand until a yellow precipate is formed. Shake with two quantities, each of 15 ml, of *methylene chloride R.* Combine the organic layers and dry over *anhydrous sodium sulphate R.* Decant or filter the solution and evaporate to dryness. Recrystallise from a mixture of 40 volumes of *methanol R* and 60 volumes of *toluene R* with cooling. Dry the crystals *in vacuo.*

mp: about 213 °C.

Chromatography. Examine as prescribed in the test for hydrazine in the monograph on *Povidone (0685)*; the chromatogram shows only one principal spot.

Salicylic acid. *1075600.* [69-72-7].

See *Salicylic acid (0366).*

Sand. *1075800.*

White or slightly greyish grains of silica with a particle size between 150 μm and 300 μm.

Santonin. $C_{15}H_{18}O_3$. (M_r 246.3). *1122000.* [481-06-1]. (−)-α-Santonin. 3,5a,9-Trimethyl-3a,5,5a,9b-tetrahydro-3*H*,4*H*-naphtho[1,2]furan-2,8-dione.

Colourless, shiny crystals colouring yellow in light, very slightly soluble in water, freely soluble in hot ethanol, sparingly soluble in ethanol.

$[\alpha]_D^{18}$: − 173 in ethanol.

mp: 174 °C to 176 °C.

Chromatography. Examine as prescribed in identification test C in the monograph on *Arnica flower (1391)*, the chromatogram obtained with 10 µl of the solution shows a quenching zone with an R_f value of about 0.5. Spray with *anisaldehyde solution R* and examine while heating at 105 °C for 5 min to 10 min. In daylight the quenching zone is at first a yellow zone that quickly changes to a violet-red zone.

Sclareol. $C_{20}H_{36}O_2$. (M_r 308.5). *1139900.* [515-03-7]. (1*R*,2*R*,4a*S*,8a*S*)-1-[(3*R*)-3-Hydroxy-3-methylpent-4-enyl]-2,5, 5,8a-tetramethyldecahydronaphthalen-2-ol.

Odourless crystals.

$[\alpha]_D^{20}$: 6.7, in solution in ethanol.

$bp_{19\ mm}$: 218 °C to 220 °C.

mp: 96 °C to 98 °C.

Sclareol used in the chromatographic profile test in the monograph on Clary sage oil (1850) complies with the following additional test.

Assay. Examine by gas chromatography (*2.2.28*) as prescribed in the monograph on *Clary sage oil (1850)*.

The content of sclareol is not less than 97 per cent, calculated by the normalisation procedure.

SDS-PAGE running buffer. *1114900.*

Dissolve 151.4 g of *tris(hydroxymethyl)aminomethane R*, 721.0 g of *glycine R* and 50.0 g of *sodium lauryl sulphate R* in *water R* and dilute to 5000 ml with the same solvent. Immediately before use, dilute to 10 times its volume with *water R* and mix. Measure the pH (*2.2.3*) of the diluted solution. The pH is between 8.1 and 8.8.

SDS-PAGE sample buffer (concentrated). *1115000.*

Dissolve 1.89 g of *tris(hydroxymethyl)aminomethane R*, 5.0 g of *sodium lauryl sulphate R* and 50 mg of *bromophenol blue R* in *water R*. Add 25.0 ml of *glycerol R* and dilute to 100 ml with *water R*. Adjust the pH to 6.8 with *hydrochloric acid R*, and dilute to 125 ml with *water R*.

SDS-PAGE sample buffer for reducing conditions (concentrated). *1122100.*

Dissolve 3.78 g of *tris(hydroxymethyl)aminomethane R*, 10.0 g of *sodium dodecyl sulphate R* and 100 mg of *bromophenol blue R* in *water R*. Add 50.0 ml of *glycerol R* and dilute to 200 ml with *water R*. Add 25.0 ml of *2-mercaptoethanol R*. Adjust to pH 6.8 (*2.2.3*) with *hydrochloric acid R*, and dilute to 250.0 ml with *water R*.

Alternatively, dithiothreitol may be used as reducing agent instead of 2-mercaptoethanol. In this case prepare the sample buffer as follows: dissolve 3.78 g of *tris(hydroxymethyl)aminomethane R*, 10.0 g of *sodium dodecyl sulphate R* and 100 mg of *bromophenol blue R* in *water R*. Add 50.0 ml of *glycerol R* and dilute to 200 ml with *water R*. Adjust to pH 6.8 (*2.2.3*) with *hydrochloric acid R*, and dilute to 250.0 ml with *water R*. Immediately before use, add *dithiothreitol R* to a final concentration of 100 mM.

Selenious acid. H_2SeO_3. (M_r 129.0). *1100200.* [7783-00-8].

Deliquescent crystals, freely soluble in water.

Storage: in an airtight container.

Selenium. Se. (A_r 79.0). *1075900.* [7782-49-2].

A brown-red to black powder or granules, practically insoluble in water and in alcohol, soluble in nitric acid.

mp: about 220 °C.

Serine. *1076000.* [56-45-1].

See *Serine (0788)*.

Sialic acid. *1001100.* [131-48-6].

See *N-acetylneuraminic acid R*.

Silibinin. $C_{25}H_{22}O_{10}$. (M_r 482.4). *1151400.* [22888-70-6]. Silybin. (2*R*,3*R*)-3,5,7-Trihydroxy-2-[(2*R*,3*R*)-3-(4-hydroxy-3-methoxyphenyl)-2-(hydroxymethyl)-2,3-dihydro-1,4-benzodioxin-6-yl]-2,3-dihydro-4*H*-1-benzopyran-4-one.

White to yellowish powder, practically insoluble in water, soluble in acetone and in methanol.

Silibinin used in the assay of Milk-thistle fruit (1860) complies with the following requirement.

Assay. Examine by liquid chromatography (*2.2.29*) as prescribed in the monograph on *Milk-thistle fruit (1860)*.

Test solution. Dissolve 5.0 mg of silibinin, dried *in vacuo*, in *methanol R* and dilute to 50.0 ml with the same solvent.

The silibinin A and silibinin B content is not less than 95.0 per cent, calculated by the normalisation procedure.

Silica gel AGP for chiral chromatography. *1148700.*

A very finely divided silica gel for chromatography consisting of spherical particles coated with α1- acid glycoprotein. The particle size is indicated after the name of the reagent in the tests where it is used.

Silica gel, anhydrous. *1076100.* [112926-00-8].

Partly dehydrated polymerised, amorphous silicic acid, absorbing at 20 °C about 30 per cent of its mass of water. It contains cobalt chloride as indicator. Practically insoluble in water, partly soluble in solutions of sodium hydroxide.

Silica gel for chromatography. *1076900.*

A very finely divided (3 µm-10 µm) silica gel. The particle size is indicated after the name of the reagent in the tests where it is used.

A fine, white, homogeneous powder, practically insoluble in water and in alcohol.

Silica gel for chromatography, aminohexadecylsilyl. *1138400.*

A very finely divided (3-10 µm) silica gel with a fine particle size chemically modified at the surface by the bonding of aminohexadecylsilyl groups. The particle size is indicated after the name of the reagent in the test where it is used.

A fine, white, homogeneous powder, practically insoluble in water and in alcohol.

Silica gel for chromatography, aminopropylmethylsilyl. *1102400.*

Silica gel with a fine particle size (between 3 µm and 10 µm), chemically modified by bonding aminopropylmethylsilyl groups on the surface. The particle size is indicated after the name of the reagent in the tests where it is used.

A fine, white, homogeneous powder, practically insoluble in water and in alcohol.

Silica gel for chromatography, aminopropylsilyl. *1077000.*

Silica gel with a fine particle size (between 3 µm and 10 µm), chemically modified by bonding aminopropylsilyl groups on the surface. The particle size is indicated after the name of the reagent in the tests where it is used.

A fine, white, homogeneous powder, practically insoluble in water and in alcohol.

Silica gel for chromatography, amylose derivative of. *1109800.*

A very finely divided (10 µm) silica gel, chemically modified at the surface by the bonding of an amylose derivative. The particle size is indicated after the name of the reagent in the test where it is used.

A fine, white, homogenous powder, practically insoluble in water and in alcohol.

Silica gel for chromatography, butylsilyl. *1076200.*

A very finely divided silica gel (3 µm-10 µm), chemically modified at the surface by the bonding of butylsilyl groups. The particle size is indicated after the name of the reagent in the tests where it is used.

A fine, white, homogeneous powder, practically insoluble in water and in alcohol.

Spheroidal silica: 30 nm.

Pore volume: 0.6 cm^3/g.

Specific surface area: 80 m^2/g.

Silica gel for chromatography, cyanosilyl. *1109900.*

A very finely divided silica gel chemically modified at the surface by the bonding of cyanosilyl groups. The particle size is indicated after the name of the reagent in the tests where it is used.

A fine, white, homogeneous powder, practically insoluble in water and in alcohol.

Silica gel for chromatography, di-isobutyloctadecylsilyl. *1140000.*

A very finely divided silica gel chemically modified at the surface by the bonding of di-isobutyloctadecylsilyl groups. The particle size is indicated after the name of the reagent in the tests where it is used.

Silica gel for chromatography, dimethyloctadecylsilyl. *1115100.*

A very finely divided silica gel (3 µm-10 µm), chemically modified at the surface by the bonding of dimethyloctadecylsilyl groups. The particle size is indicated after the name of the reagent in the tests where it is used.

A fine, white, homogeneous powder, practically insoluble in water and in alcohol. Irregular particle size.

Specific surface area: 300 m^2/g.

Silica gel for chromatography, diol. *1110000.*

Spherical silica particles to which dihydroxypropyl groups are bonded. Pore size 10 nm.

Silica gel for chromatography, hexylsilyl. *1077100.*

A very finely divided (3 µm-10 µm) silica gel, chemically modified at the surface by the bonding of hexylsilyl groups. The particle size is indicated after the name of the reagent in the tests where it is used.

A fine, white, homogeneous powder, practically insoluble in water and in alcohol.

Silica gel for chromatography, human albumin coated. *1138500.*

A very finely divided (3 µm to 10 µm) silica gel, chemically modified at the surface by the bonding of human albumin. The particle size is indicated after the name of the reagent in the tests where it is used.

A white, fine, homogeneous powder.

Silica gel for chromatography, hydrophilic. *1077200.*

A very finely divided (3 µm-10 µm) silica gel whose surface has been modified to provide hydrophilic characteristics. The particle size may be stated after the name of the reagent in the tests where it is used.

Silica gel for chromatography, nitrile. *1077300.*

A very finely divided silica gel, chemically modified at the surface by the bonding of cyanopropylsilyl groups. The particle size is indicated after the name of the reagent in the test where it is used.

A fine white, homogenous powder, practically insoluble in water and in alcohol.

Silica gel for chromatography, nitrile R1. *1077400.*

A very finely divided silica gel consisting of porous, spherical particles with chemically bonded nitrile groups. The particle size is indicated after the name of the reagent in the test where it is used.

A fine, white, homogeneous powder, practically insoluble in water and in alcohol.

Silica gel for chromatography, nitrile R2. *1119500.*

Ultrapure silica gel, chemically modified at the surface by the introduction of cyanopropylsilyl groups. Less than 20 ppm of metals. The particle size is indicated after the name of the reagent in the tests where it is used.

A fine white, homogenous powder, practically insoluble in water and in alcohol.

Silica gel for chromatography, octadecanoylaminopropylsilyl. *1115200.*

A very finely divided (3 µm-10 µm) silica gel, chemically modified at the surface by the bonding of aminopropylsilyl groups which are acylated with octadecanoyl groups. The particle size is indicated after the name of the reagent in the tests where it is used.

A fine, white, homogeneous powder, practically insoluble in water and in alcohol.

Silica gel for chromatography, octadecylsilyl. *1077500.*

A very finely divided (3 µm-10 µm) silica gel, chemically modified at the surface by the bonding of octadecylsilyl groups. The particle size is indicated after the name of the reagent in the tests where it is used.

A fine, white, homogeneous powder, practically insoluble in water and in alcohol.

Silica gel for chromatography, octadecylsilyl R1. *1110100.*

A very finely divided ultrapure silica gel, chemically modified at the surface by the bonding of octadecylsilyl groups. The particle size, the pore size and the carbon loading are indicated after the name of the reagent in the tests where it is used. Less than 20 ppm of metals.

Silica gel for chromatography, octadecylsilyl R2. *1115300.*

A very finely divided (15 nm pore size) ultrapure silica gel, chemically modified at the surface by the bonding of octadecylsilyl groups (20 per cent carbon load), optimised for the analysis of polycyclic aromatic hydrocarbons. The particle size is indicated after the name of the reagent in the tests where it is used.

A fine, white, homogeneous powder, practically insoluble in water and in alcohol.

Silica gel for chromatography, octadecylsilyl, base-deactivated. *1077600.*

A very finely divided (3 µm-10 µm) silica gel, pretreated before the bonding of octadecylsilyl groups by careful washing and hydrolysing most of the superficial siloxane bridges to minimise the interaction with basic components. The particle size is indicated after the name of the reagent in the tests where it is used.

A fine, white, homogeneous powder, practically insoluble in water and in alcohol.

Silica gel for chromatography, octadecylsilyl, end-capped. *1115400.*

A very finely divided (3 µm-10 µm) silica gel, chemically modified at the surface by the bonding of octadecylsilyl groups. To minimise any interaction with basic compounds it is carefully end-capped to cover most of the remaining silanol groups. The particle size is indicated after the name of the reagent in the tests where it is used.

A fine, white, homogenous powder, practically insoluble in water and in alcohol.

Silica gel for chromatography, octadecylsilyl, end-capped, base-deactivated. *1108600.*

A very finely divided (3 µm-10 µm) silica gel with a pore size of 10 nm and a carbon loading of 16 per cent, pre-treated before the bonding of octadecylsilyl groups by washing and hydrolysing most of the superficial siloxane bridges. To further minimise any interaction with basic compounds it is carefully end-capped to cover most of the remaining silanol groups. The particle size is indicated after the name of the reagent in the test where it is used.

A fine, white, homogeneous powder, practically insoluble in water and in alcohol.

Silica gel for chromatography, octadecylsilyl, monolithic. *1154500.*

Monolithic rods of highly porous (greater than 80 per cent) metal-free silica with a bimodal pore structure, modified at the surface by the bonding of octadecylsilyl groups.

Silica gel for chromatography, octylsilyl. *1077700.*

A very finely divided (3 µm-10 µm) silica gel, chemically modified at the surface by the bonding of octylsilyl groups. The particle size is indicated after the name of the reagent in the tests where it is used.

A fine, white, homogeneous powder, practically insoluble in water and in alcohol.

Silica gel for chromatography, octylsilyl R1. *1077701.*

A very finely divided (3 µm-10 µm) silica gel, chemically modified at the surface by the bonding of octylsilyl and methyl groups (double bonded phase). The particle size is indicated after the name of the reagent in the tests where it is used.

A fine, white, homogeneous powder, practically insoluble in water and in alcohol.

Silica gel for chromatography, octylsilyl R2. *1077702.*

Ultrapure very finely divided (10 nm pore size) silica gel, chemically modified at the surface by the bonding of octylsilyl groups (19 per cent carbon load). Less than 20 ppm of metals.

Silica gel for chromatography, octylsilyl R3. *1155200.*

A very finely divided ultrapure silica gel, chemically modified at the surface by the bonding of octylsilyl groups and sterically protected with branched hydrocarbons at the silanes. The particle size is indicated after the name of the reagent in the tests where it is used.

Silica gel for chromatography, octylsilyl, base-deactivated. *1131600.*

A very finely divided (3 µm-10 µm) silica gel, pretreated before the bonding of octylsilyl groups by careful washing and hydrolysing most of the superficial siloxane bridges to minimise the interaction with basic components. The particle size is indicated after the name of the reagent in the tests where it is used.

A fine, white, homogeneous powder, practically insoluble in water and in alcohol.

Silica gel for chromatography, octylsilyl, end-capped. *1119600.*

A very finely divided (3 µm-10 µm) silica gel, chemically modified at the surface by the bonding of octylsilyl groups. To minimise any interaction with basic compounds, it is carefully end-capped to cover most of the remaining silanol groups. The particle size is indicated after the name of the reagent in the tests where it is used.

A fine, white, homogeneous powder, practically insoluble in water and in alcohol.

Silica gel for chromatography, octylsilyl, end-capped, base-deactivated. *1148800.*

A very finely divided (3 µm-10 µm) silica gel, pre-treated before the bonding of octylsilyl groups by washing and hydrolysing most of the superficial siloxane bridges. To further minimise any interaction with basic compounds it is carefully end-capped to cover most of the remaining silanol groups. The particle size is indicated after the name of the reagent in the test where it is used.

A fine, white, homogeneous powder, practically insoluble in water and in alcohol.

Silica gel for chromatography, octylsilyl, with polar incorporated groups, end-capped. *1152600.*

A very finely divided silica gel (3-10 µm). The particles are based on silica, chemically modified with a reagent providing a surface with chains having polar incorporated groups and terminating octyl groups. Furthermore, the packing material is end-capped. The particle size is indicated after the name of the reagent in the tests where it is used.

A fine, white, homogeneous powder.

Silica gel for chromatography, palmitamidopropylsilyl, end-capped. *1115200.*

A very finely divided (3 µm-10 µm) silica gel, chemically modified at the surface by the bonding of palmitamidopropyl groups and end-capped with acetamidopropyl groups. The particle size is indicated after the name of the reagent in the tests where it is used.

A fine, white, homogeneous powder, practically insoluble in water and in alcohol.

Silica gel for chromatography, phenylhexylsilyl. *1153900.*

A very finely divided silica gel, chemically modified at the surface by the bonding of phenylhexyl groups. The particle size is indicated after the name of the reagent in the tests where it is used.

Silica gel for chromatography, phenylsilyl. *1110200.*

A very finely divided (5 µm-10 µm) silica gel, chemically modified at the surface by the bonding of phenyl groups.

Silica gel for chromatography, phenylsilyl R1. *1075700.*

A very finely divided silica gel (5 µm), chemically modified at the surface by the bonding of phenyl groups. The particle size is indicated after the name of the reagent in the tests where it is used.

A fine, white, homogeneous powder, practically insoluble in water, in alcohol and in methylene chloride.

Spheroidal silica: 8 nm.

Specific surface area: 180 m^2/g.

Carbon loading: 5.5 per cent.

Silica gel for chromatography, phenylsilyl, end-capped. *1154900.*

A very finely divided (5-10 µm) silica gel, chemically modified at the surface by the bounding of phenyl groups. To minimise any interaction with basic compounds it is carefully end-capped to cover most of the remaining silanol groups. The particle size is indicated after the name of the reagent in the tests where it is used.

Silica gel for chromatography, strong-anion-exchange. *1077800.*

A very finely divided (3 µm-10 µm) silica gel, chemically modified at the surface by the bonding of quaternary ammonium groups. The particle size is indicated after the name of the reagent in the tests where it is used.

A fine, white, homogeneous powder, practically insoluble in water and in alcohol.

pH limit of use: 2 to 8.

Silica gel for chromatography, trimethylsilyl. *1115500.*

A very finely divided (3 µm-10 µm) silica gel, chemically modified at the surface by the bonding of trimethylsilyl groups. The particle size is indicated after the name of the reagent in the tests where it is used.

A fine, white, homogeneous powder, practically insoluble in water and in alcohol.

Silica gel for size-exclusion chromatography. *1077900.*

A very finely divided silica gel (10 µm) with a very hydrophilic surface. The average diameter of the pores is about 30 nm. It is compatible with aqueous solutions between pH 2 and 8 and with organic solvents. It is suitable for the separation of proteins with relative molecular masses of 1×10^3 to 3×10^5.

Silica gel G. *1076300.* [112926-00-8].

Contains about 13 per cent of calcium sulphate hemihydrate.

A fine, white, homogeneous powder with a particle size of about 15 µm.

Calcium sulphate content. Place 0.25 g in a ground-glass stoppered flask, add 3 ml of *dilute hydrochloric acid R* and 100 ml of *water R* and shake vigorously for 30 min. Filter through a sintered-glass filter and wash the residue. Carry out on the combined filtrate and washings the complexometric assay of calcium (*2.5.11*).

1 ml of *0.1 M sodium edetate* is equivalent to 14.51 mg of $CaSO_4,{}^1/_2H_2O$.

pH (*2.2.3*). Shake 1 g for 5 min with 10 ml of *carbon dioxide-free water R*. The pH of the suspension is about 7.

Silica gel GF$_{254}$. *1076400.* [112926-00-8].

Contains about 13 per cent of calcium sulphate hemihydrate and about 1.5 per cent of a fluorescent indicator having an optimal intensity at 254 nm.

A fine, white, homogeneous powder with a particle size of about 15 µm.

Calcium sulphate content. Determine by the method prescribed for *silica gel G R*.

pH (2.2.3). Complies with the test prescribed for *silica gel G R*.

Fluorescence. Examine by thin-layer chromatography (*2.2.27*) using *silica gel GF$_{254}$ R* as the coating substance. Apply separately to the plate at ten points increasing volumes from 1 µl to 10 µl of a 1 g/l solution of *benzoic acid R* in a mixture of 10 volumes of *anhydrous formic acid R* and 90 volumes of *2-propanol R*. Develop over a path of 10 cm with the same mixture of solvents. After evaporating the solvents examine the chromatogram in ultraviolet light at 254 nm. The benzoic acid appears as dark spots on a fluorescent background in the upper third of the chromatogram for quantities of 2 µg and greater.

Silica gel H. *1076500.* [112926-00-8].

A fine, white, homogeneous powder with a particle size of about 15 µm.

pH (2.2.3). Complies with the test prescribed for *silica gel G R*.

Silica gel H, silanised. *1076600.*

Preparation of a thin layer. See *silanised silica gel HF$_{254}$ R*.

A fine, white homogeneous powder which, after being shaken with water, floats on the surface because of its water-repellent properties.

Chromatographic separation. Complies with the test prescribed for *silanised silica gel HF$_{254}$ R*.

Silica gel HF$_{254}$. *1076700.*

Contains about 1.5 per cent of a fluorescent indicator having an optimal intensity at 254 nm.

A fine, white, homogeneous powder with a particle size of about 15 µm.

pH (2.3.3). Complies with the test prescribed for *silica gel G R*.

Fluorescence. Complies with the test prescribed for *silica gel GF$_{254}$ R*.

Silica gel HF$_{254}$, silanised. *1076800.*

Contains about 1.5 per cent of a fluorescent indicator having an optimal intensity at 254 nm.

A fine, white, homogeneous powder which, after shaking with water, floats on the surface because of its water-repellent properties.

Preparation of a thin layer. Vigorously shake 30 g for 2 min with 60 ml of a mixture of 1 volume of *methanol R* and 2 volumes of *water R*. Coat carefully cleaned plates with a layer 0.25 mm thick using a spreading device. Allow the coated plates to dry in air and then heat in an oven at 100 °C to 105 °C for 30 min.

Chromatographic separation. Introduce 0.1 g each of *methyl laurate R, methyl myristate R, methyl palmitate R* and *methyl stearate R* into a 250 ml conical flask. Add 40 ml of *alcoholic potassium hydroxide solution R* and heat under a reflux condenser on a water-bath for 1 h. Allow to cool, transfer the solution to a separating funnel by means of 100 ml of *water R*, acidify (pH 2 to 3) with *dilute hydrochloric acid R* and shake with three quantities, each of 10 ml of *chloroform R*. Dry the combined chloroform extracts over *anhydrous sodium sulphate R*, filter and evaporate to dryness on a water-bath. Dissolve the residue in 50 ml of *chloroform R*. Examine by thin-layer chromatography (*2.2.27*), using silanised silica gel HF_{254} as the coating substance. Apply to the plate at each of three separate points 10 µl of the chloroformic solution. Develop over a path of 14 cm with a mixture of 10 volumes of *glacial acetic acid R*, 25 volumes of *water R* and 65 volumes of *dioxan R*. Dry the plate at 120 °C for 30 min. Allow to cool, spray with a 35 g/l solution of *phosphomolybdic acid R* in *2-propanol R* and heat at 150 °C until the spots become visible. Treat the plate with ammonia vapour until the background is white. The chromatograms show four clearly separated, well-defined spots.

Silica gel OC for chiral separations. *1146800.*

A very finely divided silica gel for chromatography (5 μm) coated with the following derivative:

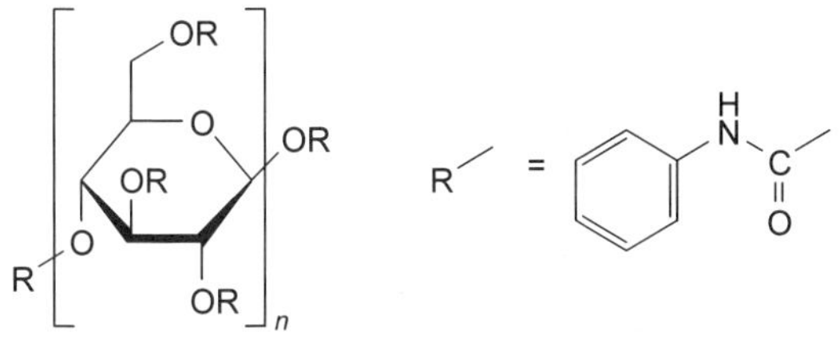

Silica gel OD for chiral separations. *1110300.*

A very finely divided silica gel for chromatography (5 μm) coated with the following derivative:

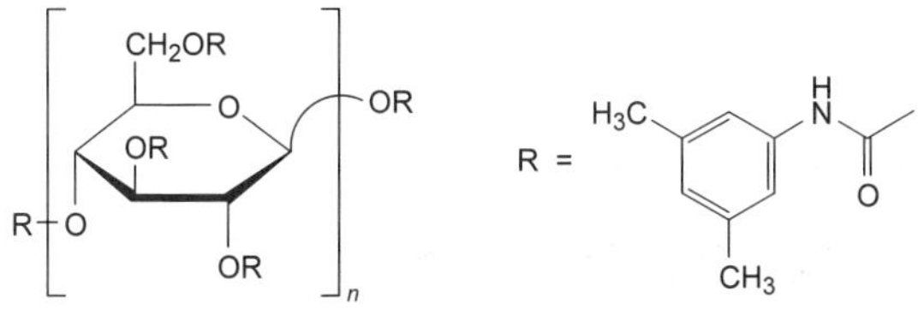

Silicotungstic acid. $H_4SiW_{12}O_{40},xH_2O$. *1078000.* [11130-20-4].

White or yellowish-white crystals, deliquescent, very soluble in water and in alcohol.

Storage: in an airtight container.

Silicristin. $C_{25}H_{22}O_{10}$. (M_r 482.4). *1151500.* [33889-69-9]. (2*R*,3*R*)-3,5,7-Trihydroxy-2-[(2*R*,3*S*)-7-hydroxy-2-(4-hydroxy-3-methoxyphenyl)-3-hydroxymethyl-2,3-dihydro-1-benzofuran-5-yl]chroman-4-one.

White to yellowish powder, practically insoluble in water, soluble in acetone and in methanol.

Silidianin. $C_{25}H_{22}O_{10}$. (M_r 482.4). *1151600.* [29782-68-1]. (3*R*,3a*R*,6*R*,7a*R*,8*R*)-7a-Hydroxy-8-(4-hydroxy-3-methoxyphenyl)-4-[(2*R*, 3*R*)-3,5,7-trihydroxy-4-oxochroman-2-yl]-2,3,3a,7a-tetrahydro-3,6-methano-1-benzofuran-7(6a*H*)-one.

White to yellowish powder, practically insoluble in water, soluble in acetone and in methanol.

Silver diethyldithiocarbamate. $C_5H_{10}AgNS_2$. (M_r 256.1). *1110400.* [1470-61-7].

A pale-yellow or greyish-yellow powder, practically insoluble in water, soluble in pyridine.

It may be prepared as follows. Dissolve 1.7 g of *silver nitrate R* in 100 ml of *water R*. Separately dissolve 2.3 g of *sodium diethyldithiocarbamate R* in 100 ml of *water R*. Cool both solutions to 10 °C, then mix and while stirring collect the yellow precipitate on a sintered-glass filter and wash with 200 ml of cold *water R*. Dry the precipitate *in vacuo* for 2-3 h.

Silver diethyldithiocarbamate may be used provided it has not changed in colour or developed a strong odour.

Silver manganese paper. *1078200.*

Immerse strips of slow filter paper into a solution containing 8.5 g/l of *manganese sulphate R* and 8.5 g/l of *silver nitrate R*. Maintain for a few minutes and allow to dry over *diphosphorus pentoxide R* protected from acid and alkaline vapours.

Silver nitrate. *1078300.* [7761-88-8].

See *Silver nitrate (0009).*

Silver nitrate reagent. *1078305.*

To a mixture of 3 ml of *concentrated ammonia R* and 40 ml of *1 M sodium hydroxide*, add 8 ml of a 200 g/l solution of *silver nitrate R*, dropwise, with stirring. Dilute to 200 ml with *water R*.

Silver nitrate solution R1. *1078301.*

A 42.5 g/l solution.

Storage: protected from light.

Silver nitrate solution R2. *1078302.*

A 17 g/l solution.

Storage: protected from light.

Silver nitrate solution, ammoniacal. *1078303.*

Dissolve 2.5 g of *silver nitrate R* in 80 ml of *water R* and add *dilute ammonia R1* dropwise until the precipitate has dissolved. Dilute to 100 ml with *water R*. Prepare immediately before use.

Silver nitrate solution in pyridine. *1078304.*

An 85 g/l solution in *pyridine R*.

Storage: protected from light.

Silver oxide. Ag_2O. (M_r 231.7). *1078400.* [20667-12-3]. Disilver oxide.

A brownish-black powder, practically insoluble in water and in alcohol, freely soluble in dilute nitric acid and in ammonia.

Storage: protected from light.

Sinensetin. $C_{20}H_{20}O_7$. (M_r 372.4). *1110500.* [2306-27-6]. 3′,4′,5,6,7-Pentamethoxyflavone.

A white, crystalline powder, practically insoluble in water, soluble in alcohol.

mp: about 177 °C.

Absorbance (*2.2.25*). A solution in *methanol R* shows 3 absorption maxima, at 243 nm, 268 nm and 330 nm.

Assay. Examine by liquid chromatography (*2.2.29*) as prescribed in the monograph on *Java tea (1229).*

The content is not less than 95 per cent, calculated by the normalisation procedure.

Sitostanol. $C_{29}H_{52}O$. (M_r 416.7). *1140100.* [19466-47-8]. Dihydro-β-sitosterol.

Content: minimum 95.0 per cent of $C_{29}H_{52}O$.

β-Sitosterol. $C_{29}H_{50}O$. (M_r 414.7). *1140200.* [83-46-5]. Stigmast-5-en-3β-ol. 22,23-Dihydrostigmasterol.

A white powder, practically insoluble in water, sparingly soluble in tetrahydrofuran.

Content: minimum 75.0 per cent *m/m* of $C_{29}H_{50}O$, calculated with reference to the dried substance.

Assay. Gas chromatography (*2.2.28*), as prescribed in the monograph on *Phytosterol (1911).*

Test solution. Dissolve 0.100 g of the substance to be examined in *tetrahydrofuran R* and dilute to 10.0 ml with the same solvent. Introduce 100 μl of this solution into a suitable 3 ml flask and evaporate to dryness under *nitrogen R*. To the residue add 100 μl of a freshly prepared mixture of 50 μl of *1-methylimidazole R* and 1.0 ml of *heptafluoro-N-methyl-N-(trimethylsilyl)butanamide R*. Close the flask tightly and heat at 100 °C for 15 min. Allow to cool.

Inject 1 μl of the test solution.

Sodium. Na. (A_r 22.99). *1078500.* [7440-23-5].

A metal whose freshly cut surface is bright silver-grey. It rapidly tarnishes in contact with air and is oxidised completely to sodium hydroxide and converted to sodium carbonate. It reacts violently with water, yielding hydrogen and a solution of sodium hydroxide; soluble in anhydrous methanol, yielding hydrogen and a solution of sodium methoxide; practically insoluble in light petroleum.

Storage: under light petroleum or liquid paraffin.

Sodium acetate. *1078600.* [6131-90-4].

See *Sodium acetate (0411).*

Sodium acetate, anhydrous. $C_2H_3NaO_2$. (M_r 82.0). *1078700.* [127-09-3].

Colourless crystals or granules, very soluble in water, sparingly soluble in alcohol.

Loss on drying (*2.2.32*). Not more than 2.0 per cent, determined by drying in an oven at 100 °C to 105 °C.

Sodium ascorbate solution. *1078800.* [134-03-2].

Dissolve 3.5 g of *ascorbic acid R* in 20 ml of *1 M sodium hydroxide.* Prepare immediately before use.

Sodium azide. NaN_3. (M_r 65.0). *1078900.* [26628-22-8].

A white, crystalline powder or crystals, freely soluble in water, slightly soluble in alcohol.

Sodium bicarbonate. *1081300.* [144-55-8].

See *sodium hydrogen carbonate R.*

Sodium bismuthate. $NaBiO_3$. (M_r 280.0). *1079000.* [12232-99-4].

Content: minimum 85.0 per cent of $NaBiO_3$.

A yellow or yellowish-brown powder, slowly decomposing when moist or at a high temperature, practically insoluble in cold water.

Assay. Suspend 0.200 g in 10 ml of a 200 g/l solution of *potassium iodide R* and add 20 ml of *dilute sulphuric acid R.* Using 1 ml of *starch solution R* as indicator, titrate with *0.1 M sodium thiosulphate* until an orange colour is obtained.

1 ml of *0.1 M sodium thiosulphate* is equivalent to 14.00 mg of $NaBiO_3$.

Sodium bromide. *1154300.* [7647-15-6].

See *Sodium bromide (0190).*

Sodium butanesulphonate. $C_4H_9NaO_3S$. (M_r 160.2). *1115600.* [2386-54-1].

A white, crystalline powder, soluble in water.

mp: greater than 300 °C.

Sodium carbonate. *1079200.* [6132-02-1].

See *Sodium carbonate decahydrate (0191).*

Sodium carbonate, anhydrous. Na_2CO_3. (M_r 106.0). *1079300.* [497-19-8]. Disodium carbonate.

A white powder, hygroscopic, freely soluble in water.

When heated to about 300 °C it loses not more than 1 per cent of its mass.

Storage: in an airtight container.

Sodium carbonate solution. *1079301.*

A 106 g/l solution of *anhydrous sodium carbonate R.*

Sodium carbonate solution R1. *1079302.*

A 20 g/l solution of *anhydrous sodium carbonate R* in *0.1 M sodium hydroxide.*

Sodium carbonate solution R2. *1079303.*

A 40 g/l solution of *anhydrous sodium carbonate R* in *0.2 M sodium hydroxide.*

Sodium carbonate monohydrate. Na_2CO_3,H_2O. *1131700.* [5968-11-6].

See *Sodium carbonate monohydrate (0192).*

Sodium cetostearyl sulphate. *1079400.*

See *Sodium cetostearyl sulphate (0847).*

Sodium chloride. *1079500.* [7647-14-5].

See *Sodium chloride (0193).*

Sodium chloride solution. *1079502.*

A 20 per cent *m/m* solution.

Sodium chloride solution, saturated. *1079503.*

Mix 1 part of *sodium chloride R* with 2 parts of *water R,* shake from time to time and allow to stand. Before use, decant the solution from any undissolved substance and filter, if necessary.

Sodium citrate. *1079600.* [6132-04-3].

See *Sodium citrate (0412).*

Sodium cobaltinitrite. $Na_3[Co(NO_2)_6]$. (M_r 403.9). *1079700.* [13600-98-1]. Trisodium hexanitrocobaltate(III).

Orange-yellow powder, freely soluble in water, slightly soluble in alcohol.

Sodium cobaltinitrite solution. *1079701.*

A 100 g/l solution. Prepare immediately before use.

Sodium decanesulphonate. $C_{10}H_{21}NaO_3S$. (M_r 244.3). *1079800.* [13419-61-9].

Crystalline powder or flakes, white or almost white, freely soluble in water, soluble in methanol.

Sodium decyl sulphate. $C_{10}H_{21}NaO_4S$. (M_r 260.3). *1138600.* [142-87-0].

Content: minimum 95.0 per cent of $C_{10}H_{21}NaO_4S$.

White or almost white powder, freely soluble in water.

Sodium deoxycholate. $C_{24}H_{39}NaO_4$. (M_r 414.6). *1131800.* [302-95-4]. Sodium 3α,12α-dihydroxy-5β-cholan-24-oate.

Sodium deoxyribonucleate. (About 85 per cent has a relative molecular mass of 2 × 10^7 or greater). *1079900.* [73049-39-5].

A white, fibrous preparation obtained from calf thymus.

Test for suitability. Dissolve 10 mg in *imidazole buffer solution pH 6.5 R* and dilute to 10.0 ml with the same buffer solution (solution a). Dilute 2.0 ml of solution (a) to 50.0 ml with *imidazole buffer solution pH 6.5 R.* The absorbance (*2.2.25*) of the solution, measured at 260 nm, is 0.4 to 0.8.

To 0.5 ml of solution (a) add 0.5 ml of *imidazole buffer solution pH 6.5 R* and 3 ml of perchloric acid (25 g/l $HClO_4$). A precipitate is formed. Centrifuge. The absorbance of the supernatant liquid, measured at 260 nm using a mixture of 1 ml of *imidazole buffer solution pH 6.5 R* and 3 ml of perchloric acid (25 g/l $HClO_4$) as compensation liquid, is not greater than 0.3.

In each of two tubes, place 0.5 ml of solution (a) and 0.5 ml of a solution of a reference preparation of streptodornase containing 10 IU/ml in *imidazole buffer solution pH 6.5 R.* To one tube add immediately 3 ml of perchloric acid (25 g/l $HClO_4$). A precipitate is formed. Centrifuge and collect the supernatant liquid (a). Heat the other tube at 37 °C for 15 min and add 3 ml of perchloric acid (25 g/l $HClO_4$). Centrifuge and collect the supernatant liquid (b). The absorbance of supernatant liquid (b), measured at 260 nm with reference to supernatant liquid (a) is not less than 0.15.

Sodium diethyldithiocarbamate. $C_5H_{10}NNaS_2,3H_2O$. (M_r 225.3). *1080000.* [20624-25-3].

White or colourless crystals, freely soluble in water, soluble in alcohol. The aqueous solution is colourless.

Sodium dihydrogen phosphate. *1080100.* [13472-35-0].

See *Sodium dihydrogen phosphate dihydrate (0194).*

Sodium dihydrogen phosphate, anhydrous. NaH_2PO_4. (M_r 120.0). *1080200.* [7558-80-7].

White powder, hygroscopic.

Storage: in an airtight container.

Sodium dihydrogen phosphate monohydrate. NaH_2PO4,H_2O. (M_r 138.0). *1080300.* [10049-21-5].

White, slightly deliquescent crystals or granules, freely soluble in water, practically insoluble in alcohol.

Storage: in an airtight container.

Sodium dithionite. $Na_2S_2O_4$. (M_r 174.1). *1080400.* [7775-14-6].

White or greyish-white, crystalline powder, oxidises in air, very soluble in water, slightly soluble in alcohol.

Storage: in an airtight container.

Sodium dodecyl sulphate. *1080500.* [151-21-3].

See *Sodium laurilsulfate (0098)* except for the content which should be not less than 99.0 per cent.

Sodium edetate. *1080600.* [6381-92-6].

See *Disodium edetate (0232).*

Sodium fluoresceinate. $C_{20}H_{10}Na_2O_5$. (M_r 376.3). *1080700.* [518-47-8].

Schultz No. 880.

Colour Index No. 45350.

Fluorescein sodium. Disodium 2-(3-oxo-6-oxido-3H-xanthen-9-yl)benzoate.

An orange-red powder, freely soluble in water. Aqueous solutions display an intense yellowish-green fluorescence.

Sodium fluoride. *1080800.* [7681-49-4].

See *Sodium fluoride (0514).*

Sodium formate. $CHNaO_2$. (M_r 68.0). *1122200.* [141-53-7]. Sodium methanoate.

White, crystalline powder or deliquescent granules, soluble in water and in glycerol, slightly soluble in alcohol.

mp: about 253 °C.

Sodium glucuronate. $C_6H_9NaO_7,H_2O$. (M_r 234.1). *1080900.* Sodium D-glucuronate monohydrate.

$[\alpha]_D^{20}$: about + 21.5, determined on a 20 g/l solution.

Sodium glycocholate. $C_{26}H_{42}NNaO_6,2H_2O$. (M_r 523.6). *1155500.* [207300-80-9]. Sodium [(3,7,12-trihydroxy-5-cholan-24-oyl)amino]acetate dihydrate. *N*-[(3,5,7,12)-3,7,12-Trihydroxy-24-oxocholan-24-yl]glycine monosodium salt dihydrate.

Content: minimum 99 per cent of $C_{26}H_{42}NNaO_6,2H_2O$.

Sodium heptanesulphonate. $C_7H_{15}NaO_3S$. (M_r 202.3). *1081000.* [22767-50-6].

A white or almost white, crystalline mass, freely soluble in water, soluble in methanol.

Sodium heptanesulphonate monohydrate. $C_7H_{15}NaO_3S,H_2O$. (M_r 220.3). *1081100.*

Content: minimum 96 per cent of $C_7H_{15}NaO_3S$, calculated with reference to the anhydrous substance.

A white, crystalline powder, soluble in water, very slightly soluble in ethanol.

Water (*2.5.12*): maximum 8 per cent, determined on 0.300 g.

Assay. Dissolve 0.150 g in 50 ml of *anhydrous acetic acid R*. Titrate with *0.1 M perchloric acid*, determining the end-point potentiometrically (*2.2.20*).

1 ml of *0.1 M perchloric acid* is equivalent to 20.22 mg of $C_7H_{15}NaO_3S$.

Sodium hexanesulphonate. $C_6H_{13}NaO_3S$. (M_r 188.2). *1081200.* [2832-45-3].

A white or almost white powder, freely soluble in water.

Sodium hydrogen carbonate. *1081300.* [144-55-8].

See *Sodium hydrogen carbonate (0195).*

Sodium hydrogen carbonate solution. *1081301.*

A 42 g/l solution.

Sodium hydrogen sulphate. $NaHSO_4$. (M_r 120.1). *1131900.* [7681-38-1]. Sodium bisulphate.

Freely soluble in water, very soluble in boiling water. It decomposes in alcohol into sodium sulphate and free sulphuric acid.

mp: about 315 °C.

Sodium hydrogensulphite. $NaHO_3S$. (M_r 104.1). *1115700.* [7631-90-5].

A white, crystalline powder, freely soluble in water, sparingly soluble in alcohol.

On exposure to air, some sulphur dioxide is lost and the substance is gradually oxidated to sulphate.

Sodium hydroxide. *1081400.* [1310-73-2].

See *Sodium hydroxide (0677).*

Sodium hydroxide solution. *1081401.*

Dissolve 20.0 g of *sodium hydroxide R* in *water R* and dilute to 100.0 ml with the same solvent. Verify the concentration by titration with *1 M hydrochloric acid,* using *methyl orange solution R* as indicator, and adjust if necessary to 200 g/l.

Sodium hydroxide solution, carbonate-free. *1081406.*

Dissolve *sodium hydroxide R* in *carbon dioxide-free water R* to give a concentration of 500 g/l and allow to stand. Decant the clear supernatant liquid, taking precautions to avoid the introduction of carbon dioxide.

Sodium hydroxide solution, dilute. *1081402.*

Dissolve 8.5 g of *sodium hydroxide R* in *water R* and dilute to 100 ml with the same solvent.

Sodium hydroxide solution, methanolic. *1081403.*

Dissolve 40 mg of *sodium hydroxide R* in 50 ml of *water R*. Cool and add 50 ml of *methanol R*.

Sodium hydroxide solution, methanolic R1. *1081405.*

Dissolve 200 mg of *sodium hydroxide R* in 50 ml of *water R*. Cool and add 50 ml of *methanol R*.

Sodium hydroxide solution, strong. *1081404.*

Dissolve 42 g of *sodium hydroxide R* in *water R* and dilute to 100 ml with the same solvent.

Sodium hypobromite solution. *1081500.*

In a bath of iced water mix 20 ml of *strong sodium hydroxide solution R* and 500 ml of *water R*, add 5 ml of *bromine solution R* and stir gently until solution is complete. Prepare immediately before use.

Sodium hypochlorite solution, strong. *1081600.*

Content: 25 g/l to 30 g/l of active chlorine.

A yellowish liquid with an alkaline reaction.

Assay. Introduce into a flask, successively, 50 ml of *water R*, 1 g of *potassium iodide R* and 12.5 ml of *dilute acetic acid R*. Dilute 10.0 ml of the substance to be examined to 100.0 ml with *water R*. Introduce 10.0 ml of this solution into the flask and titrate with *0.1 M sodium thiosulphate*, using 1 ml of *starch solution R* as indicator.

1 ml of *0.1 M sodium thiosulphate* is equivalent to 3.546 mg of active chlorine.

Storage: protected from light.

Sodium hypophosphite. NaH_2PO_2,H_2O. (M_r 106.0). *1081700.* [10039-56-2]. Sodium phosphinate monohydrate.

A white, crystalline powder or colourless crystals, hygroscopic, freely soluble in water, soluble in alcohol.

Storage: in an airtight container.

Sodium iodide. *1081800.* [7681-82-5].

See *Sodium iodide (0196).*

Sodium laurilsulfate. *1081900.* [151-21-3].

See *Sodium laurilsulfate (0098).*

Sodium lauryl sulphate. *1081900.* [151-21-3].

See *Sodium laurilsulfate R.*

Sodium laurylsulphonate for chromatography. $C_{12}H_{25}NaO_3S$. (M_r 272.4). *1132000.* [2386-53-0].

White or almost white powder or crystals, freely soluble in water.

Absorbance $A^{5\%}_{1\,cm}$ (*2.2.25*), determined in *water R*:

about 0.05 at 210 nm,

about 0.03 at 220 nm,

about 0.02 at 230 nm,

about 0.02 at 500 nm.

Sodium metabisulphite. *1082000.* [7681-57-4].

See *Sodium metabisulphite (0849).*

Sodium methanesulphonate. CH_3SO_3Na. (M_r 118.1). *1082100.* [2386-57-4].

A white, crystalline powder, hygroscopic.

Storage: in an airtight container.

Sodium molybdate. $Na_2MoO_4,2H_2O$. (M_r 242.0). *1082200.* [10102-40-6]. Disodium molybdate dihydrate.

A white, crystalline powder or colourless crystals, freely soluble in water.

Sodium naphthoquinonesulphonate. $C_{10}H_5NaO_5S$. (M_r 260.2). *1082300.* [521-24-4]. Sodium 1,2-naphthoquinone-4-sulphonate.

A yellow to orange-yellow, crystalline powder, freely soluble in water, practically insoluble in alcohol.

Sodium nitrate. $NaNO_3$. (M_r 85.0). *1082400.* [7631-99-4].

White powder or granules or colourless, transparent crystals, deliquescent in moist air, freely soluble in water, slightly soluble in alcohol.

Storage: in an airtight container.

Sodium nitrite. $NaNO_2$. (M_r 69.0). *1082500.* [7632-00-0].

Content: minimum 97.0 per cent of $NaNO_2$.

A white, granular powder or a slightly yellow, crystalline powder, freely soluble in water.

Assay. Dissolve 0.100 g in 50 ml of *water R*. Add 50.0 ml of *0.02 M potassium permanganate* and 15 ml of *dilute sulphuric acid R*. Add 3 g of *potassium iodide R*. Titrate with *0.1 M sodium thiosulphate*, using 1.0 ml of *starch solution R* added towards the end of the titration as indicator.

1 ml of *0.02 M potassium permanganate* is equivalent to 3.450 mg of $NaNO_2$.

Sodium nitrite solution. *1082501.*

A 100 g/l solution. Prepare immediately before use.

Sodium nitroprusside. $Na_2[Fe(CN)_5(NO)],2H_2O$. (M_r 298.0). *1082600.* [13755-38-9]. Sodium pentacyano-nitrosylferrate(III) dihydrate.

Reddish-brown powder or crystals, freely soluble in water, slightly soluble in alcohol.

Sodium octanesulphonate. $C_8H_{17}NaO_3S$. (M_r 216.3). *1082700.* [5324-84-5].

Content: minimum 98.0 per cent of $C_8H_{17}NaO_3S$.

White or almost white, crystalline powder or flakes, freely soluble in water, soluble in methanol.

Absorbance. The absorbance (*2.2.25*) of a 54 g/l solution measured at 200 nm is not greater than 0.10 and that measured at 250 nm is not greater than 0.01.

Sodium octyl sulphate. $C_8H_{17}NaO_4S$. (M_r 232.3). *1082800.* [142-31-4].

White or almost white, crystalline powder or flakes, freely soluble in water, soluble in methanol.

Sodium oxalate. $C_2Na_2O_4$. (M_r 134.0). *1082900.* [62-76-0].

A white, crystalline powder, soluble in water, practically insoluble in alcohol.

Sodium pentanesulphonate. $C_5H_{11}NaO_3S$. (M_r 174.2). *1083000.* [22767-49-3].

A white, crystalline solid, soluble in water.

Sodium pentanesulphonate monohydrate. $C_5H_{11}NaO_3S,H_2O$. (M_r 192.2). *1132100.*

A white crystalline solid, soluble in water.

Sodium perchlorate. $NaClO_4,H_2O$. (M_r 140.5). *1083100.* [7791-07-3].

Content: minimum 99.0 per cent of $NaClO_4,H_2O$.

White, deliquescent crystals, very soluble in water.

Storage: in a well-closed container.

Sodium periodate. $NaIO_4$. (M_r 213.9). *1083200.* [7790-28-5]. Sodium metaperiodate.

Content: minimum 99.0 per cent of $NaIO_4$.

A white, crystalline powder or white crystals, soluble in water and in mineral acids.

Sodium periodate solution. *1083201.*

Dissolve 1.07 g of *sodium periodate R* in *water R*, add 5 ml of *dilute sulphuric acid R* and dilute to 100.0 ml with *water R*. Use a freshly prepared solution.

Sodium phosphite pentahydrate. $Na_2HPO_3,5H_2O$. (M_r 216.0). *1132200.* [13517-23-2].

A white, crystalline powder, hygroscopic, freely soluble in water.

Storage: in an airtight container.

Sodium picrate solution, alkaline. *1083300.*

Mix 20 ml of *picric acid solution R* and 10 ml of a 50 g/l solution of *sodium hydroxide R* and dilute to 100 ml with *water R.*

Storage: use within 2 days.

Sodium potassium tartrate. $C_4H_4KNaO_6,4H_2O$. (M_r 282.2). *1083500.* [6381-59-5].

Colourless, prismatic crystals, very soluble in water.

Sodium pyrophosphate. $Na_4P_2O_7,10H_2O$. (M_r 446.1). *1083600.* [13472-36-1]. Tetrasodium diphosphate decahydrate.

Colourless, slightly efflorescent crystals, freely soluble in water.

Sodium rhodizonate. $C_6Na_2O_6$. (M_r 214.0). *1122300.* [523-21-7]. [(3,4,5,6-Tetraoxocyclohex-1-en-1,2-ylene)dioxy]disodium.

Violet crystals, soluble in water with an orange-yellow colour. Solutions are unstable and must be prepared on the day of use.

Sodium salicylate. *1083700.* [54-21-7].

See *Sodium salicylate (0413).*

Sodium sulphate, anhydrous. *1083800.* [7757-82-6].

Ignite at 600 °C to 700 °C anhydrous sodium sulphate complying with the requirements prescribed in the monograph on *Anhydrous sodium sulphate (0099).*

Loss on drying (2.2.32): maximum 0.5 per cent, determined by drying in an oven at 130 °C.

Sodium sulphate decahydrate. $Na_2SO_4,10H_2O$. (M_r 322.2). *1132300.* [7727-73-3].

See *Sodium sulphate decahydrate (0100).*

Sodium sulphide. $Na_2S,9H_2O$. (M_r 240.2). *1083900.* [1313-84-4]. Disodium sulphide nonahydrate.

Colourless, rapidly yellowing crystals, deliquescent, very soluble in water.

Storage: in an airtight container.

Sodium sulphide solution. *1083901.*

Dissolve 12 g of *sodium sulphide R* with heating in 45 ml of a mixture of 10 volumes of *water R* and 29 volumes of *glycerol (85 per cent) R,* allow to cool and dilute to 100 ml with the same mixture of solvents.

The solution should be colourless.

Sodium sulphide solution R1. *1083902.*

Prepare by one of the following methods.

- Dissolve 5 g of *sodium sulphide R* in a mixture of 10 ml of *water R* and 30 ml of *glycerol R.*
- Dissolve 5 g of *sodium hydroxide R* in a mixture of 30 ml of *water R* and 90 ml of *glycerol R.* Divide the solution into 2 equal portions. Saturate 1 portion with *hydrogen sulphide R,* with cooling. Mix the 2 portions.

Storage: in a well-filled container, protected from light; use within 3 months.

Sodium sulphite. *1084000.* [10102-15-5].

See *Sodium sulphite heptahydrate (0776).*

Sodium sulphite, anhydrous. *1084100.* [7757-83-7].

See *Anhydrous sodium sulphite (0775).*

Sodium tartrate. $C_4H_4Na_2O_6,2H_2O$. (M_r 230.1). *1084200.* [6106-24-7]. Disodium (2*R*,3*R*)-2,3-dihydroxybutanedioate dihydrate.

White crystals or granules, very soluble in water, practically insoluble in alcohol.

Sodium taurodeoxycholate. $C_{26}H_{44}NNaO_6S,H_2O$. (M_r 539.7). *1155600.* [110026-03-4]. Sodium 2-[(3,12-dihydroxy-5-cholan-24-oyl)amino]ethanesulphonate monohydrate. 2-[[(3,5,12)-3,12-Dihydroxy-24-oxocholan-24-yl]amino]ethanesulphonic acid monosodium salt monohydrate.

Content: minimum 94 per cent of $C_{26}H_{44}NNaO_6S,H_2O$.

Sodium tetradeuteriodimethylsilapentanoate. $C_6H_9{}^2H_4NaO_2Si$. (M_r 172.3). *1084300.* TSP. Sodium (2,2,3,3-tetradeuterio)-4,4-dimethyl-4-silapentanoate.

The degree of deuteration is not less than 99 per cent.

A white, crystalline powder, freely soluble in water, in ethanol and in methanol.

mp: about 300 °C.

Water and deuterium oxide: maximum 0.5 per cent.

Sodium tetrahydroborate. $NaBH_4$. (M_r 37.8). *1146900.* [16940-66-2]. Sodium borohydride.

Colourless, hygroscopic crystals, freely soluble in water, soluble in anhydrous ethanol, decomposing at higher temperature or in the presence of acids or certain metal salts forming borax and hydrogen.

Storage: in an airtight container.

Sodium tetrahydroborate reducing solution. *1146901.*

Introduce about 100 ml of *water R* into a 500 ml volumetric flask containing a stirring bar. Add 5.0 g of *sodium hydroxide R* in pellets and 2.5 g of *sodium tetrahydroborate R.* Stir until complete dissolution, dilute to 500.0 ml with *water R* and mix. Prepare immediately before use.

Sodium tetraphenylborate. $NaB(C_6H_5)_4$. (M_r 342.2). *1084400.* [143-66-8].

A white or slightly yellowish, bulky powder, freely soluble in water and in acetone.

Sodium tetraphenylborate solution. *1084401.*

Filter before use if necessary.

A 10 g/l solution.

Storage: use within 1 week.

Sodium thioglycollate. $C_2H_3NaO_2S$. (M_r 114.1). *1084500.* [367-51-1]. Sodium mercaptoacetate.

White, granular powder or crystals, hygroscopic, freely soluble in water and in methanol, slightly soluble in alcohol.

Storage: in an airtight container.

Sodium thiosulphate. *1084600.* [10102-17-7].

See *Sodium thiosulphate (0414).*

Sodium tungstate. $Na_2WO_4,2H_2O$. (M_r 329.9). *1084700.* [10213-10-2]. Disodium tungstate dihydrate.

A white, crystalline powder or colourless crystals, freely soluble in water forming a clear solution, practically insoluble in alcohol.

Sorbitol. *1084800.* [50-70-4].

See *Sorbitol (0435).*

Squalane. $C_{30}H_{62}$. (M_r 422.8). *1084900.* [111-01-3].
2,6,10,15,19,23-Hexamethyltetracosane.

A colourless, oily liquid, freely soluble in fatty oils, slightly soluble in acetone, in alcohol, in glacial acetic acid and in methanol.

d_{20}^{20}: 0.811 to 0.813.

n_D^{20}: 1.451 to 1.453.

Stannous chloride. $SnCl_2,2H_2O$. (M_r 225.6). *1085000.* [10025-69-1]. Tin dichloride dihydrate.

Content: minimum 97.0 per cent of $SnCl_2,2H_2O$.

Colourless crystals, very soluble in water, freely soluble in alcohol, in glacial acetic acid and in dilute and concentrated hydrochloric acid.

Assay. Dissolve 0.500 g in 15 ml of *hydrochloric acid R* in a ground-glass-stoppered flask. Add 10 ml of *water R* and 5 ml of *chloroform R.* Titrate rapidly with *0.05 M potassium iodate* until the chloroform layer is colourless.

1 ml of *0.05 M potassium iodate* is equivalent to 22.56 mg of $SnCl_2,2H_2O$.

Stannous chloride solution. *1085001.*

Heat 20 g of *tin R* with 85 ml of *hydrochloric acid R* until no more hydrogen is released. Allow to cool.

Storage: over an excess of *tin R,* protected from air.

Stannous chloride solution R1. *1085002.*

Immediately before use, dilute 1 volume of *stannous chloride solution R* with 10 volumes of *dilute hydrochloric acid R.*

Stannous chloride solution R2. *1085003.*

To 8 g of *stannous chloride R* add 100 ml of a 20 per cent *V/V* solution of *hydrochloric acid R.* Shake until dissolved, heating, if necessary, on a water-bath at 50 °C. Pass a current of *nitrogen R* for 15 min. Prepare immediately before use.

Stanolone. $C_{19}H_{30}O_2$. (M_r 290.4). *1154400.* [521-18-6].
17β-Hydroxy-5α-androstan-3-one.

White or almost white powder.

mp: about 180 °C.

Standard solution for the micro determination of water. *1147300.*

Commercially available standard solution for the coulometric titration of water, containing a certified content of water in a suitable solvent.

***Staphylococcus aureus* strain V8 protease. Type XVII-B.** *1115800.* [66676-43-5].

Microbial extracellular proteolytic enzyme. A lyophilised powder containing 500 units to 1000 units per milligram of solid.

Starch, soluble. *1085100.* [9005-84-9].

A white powder.

Prepare a 20 g/l solution in hot *water R.* The solution is at most slightly opalescent and remains fluid on cooling.

Starch iodate paper. *1085101.*

Immerse strips of filter paper in 100 ml of *iodide-free starch solution R* containing 0.1 g of *potassium iodate R.* Drain and allow to dry protected from light.

Starch iodide paper. *1085106.*

Immerse strips of filter paper in 100 ml of *starch solution R* containing 0.5 g of *potassium iodide R.* Drain and allow to dry protected from light.

Test for sensitivity. Mix 0.05 ml of *0.1 M sodium nitrite* with 4 ml of *hydrochloric acid R* and dilute to 100 ml with *water R.* Apply one drop of the solution to starch iodide paper; a blue spot appears.

Starch solution. *1085103.*

Triturate 1.0 g of *soluble starch R* with 5 ml of *water R* and whilst stirring pour the mixture into 100 ml of boiling *water R* containing 10 mg of *mercuric iodide R.*

Carry out the test for sensitivity each time the reagent is used.

Test for sensitivity. To a mixture of 1 ml of the starch solution and 20 ml of *water R,* add about 50 mg of *potassium iodide R* and 0.05 ml of *iodine solution R1.* The solution is blue.

Starch solution, iodide-free. *1085104.*

Prepare the solution as prescribed for *starch solution R* omitting the mercuric iodide. Prepare immediately before use.

Starch solution R1. *1085105.*

Mix 1 g of *soluble starch R* and a small amount of cold *water R.* Add this mixture, while stirring, to 200 ml of boiling *water R.* Add 250 mg of *salicylic acid R* and boil for 3 min. Immediately remove from the heat and cool.

Storage: long storage is required, the solution shall be stored at 4 °C to 10 °C. A fresh starch solution shall be prepared when the end-point of the titration from blue to colourless fails to be sharp. If stored under refrigeration, the starch solution is stable for about 2 to 3 weeks.

Test for sensitivity. A mixture of 2 ml of *starch solution R1,* 20 ml of *water R,* about 50 mg of *potassium iodide R* and 0.05 ml of *iodine solution R1* is blue.

Starch solution R2. *1085107.*

Triturate 1.0 g of *soluble starch R* with 5 ml of *water R* and whilst stirring pour the mixture into 100 ml of boiling *water R.* Use a freshly prepared solution.

Test for sensitivity. To a mixture of 1 ml of the starch solution and 20 ml of *water R,* add about 50 mg of *potassium iodide R* and 0.05 ml of *iodine solution R1.* The solution is blue.

Stearic acid. $C_{18}H_{36}O_2$. (M_r 284.5). *1085200.* [57-11-4].
Octadecanoic acid.

White powder or flakes, greasy to the touch, practically insoluble in water, soluble in hot alcohol.

mp: about 70 °C.

Stearic acid used in the assay of total fatty acids in Saw palmetto fruit (1848) complies with the following additional requirement.

Assay. Examine by gas chromatography (*2.2.28*) as prescribed in the monograph on *Saw palmetto fruit (1848).*

The content of stearic acid is not less than 98 per cent, calculated by the normalisation procedure.

Stearyl alcohol. $C_{18}H_{38}O$. (M_r 270.5). *1156400.* [112-92-5].
1-Octadecanol.

mp: about 60 °C.

Content: minimum 95 per cent of $C_{18}H_{38}O$.

Stigmasterol. $C_{29}H_{48}O$. (M_r 412.7). *1141400.* [83-48-7]. (22*E*)-Stigmasta-5,22-dien-3β-ol. (22*E*)-24-Ethylcholesta-5,22-dien-3β-ol.

White powder, insoluble in water.

mp: about 170 °C.

$[\alpha]_D^{22}$: about − 51 (*c* = 2 in chloroform).

Streptomycin sulphate. *1085300.* [3810-74-0].

See *Streptomycin sulphate (0053).*

Strongly acidic ion-exchange resin. *1085400.*

See *ion-exchange resin, strongly acidic R.*

Strontium carbonate. $SrCO_3$. (M_r 147.6). *1122700.* [1633-05-2].

A white, crystalline powder.

Content: minimum 99.5 per cent of $SrCO_3$.

Styrene. C_8H_8. (M_r 104.2). *1151700.* [100-42-5]. Ethenylbenzene.

bp: about 145 °C.

Colourless, oily liquid, very slightly soluble in water.

Styrene-divinylbenzene copolymer. *1085500.*

Porous, rigid, cross-linked polymer beads. Several grades are available with different sizes of beads. The size range of the beads is specified after the name of the reagent in the tests where it is used.

Succinic acid. $C_4H_6O_4$. (M_r 118.1). *1085600.* [110-15-6]. Butanedioic acid.

A white, crystalline powder or colourless crystals, soluble in water and in alcohol.

mp: 184 °C to 187 °C.

Sucrose. *1085700.* [57-50-1].

See *Sucrose (0204).*

When sucrose is used for controlling the polarimeter, it must be kept dry in a sealed ampoule.

Sudan orange. $C_{16}H_{12}N_2O$. (M_r 248.3). *1110700.* [842-07-9].

Colour Index No. 12055.

1-(Phenylazo)naphthalen-2-ol. Sudan I.

An orange-red powder, practically insoluble in water, soluble in methylene chloride.

mp: about 131 °C.

Sudan red G. $C_{17}H_{14}N_2O_2$. (M_r 278.3). *1085800.*

Schultz No. 149.

Colour Index No. 12150.

Solvent Red 1. 1-[(2-Methoxyphenyl)azo]naphtalen-2-ol.

A reddish-brown powder, practically insoluble in water.

Chromatography. Examine by thin-layer chromatography (*2.2.27*) using *silica gel G R* as the coating substance. Apply 10 µl of a 0.1 g/l solution in *methylene chloride R* and develop over a path of 10 cm with the same solvent. The chromatogram shows only one principal spot.

Sulfanilamide. $C_6H_8N_2O_2S$. (M_r 172.2). *1086100.* [63-74-1]. 4-Aminobenzenesulphonamide.

A white powder, slightly soluble in water, freely soluble in boiling water, in acetone, in dilute acids and in solutions of the alkali hydroxides, sparingly soluble in alcohol and in light petroleum.

mp: about 165 °C.

Sulphamic acid. H_3NO_3S. (M_r 97.1). *1085900.* [5329-14-6].

White crystalline powder or crystals, freely soluble in water, sparingly soluble in acetone, in alcohol and in methanol.

mp: about 205 °C, with decomposition.

Sulphan blue. $C_{27}H_{31}N_2NaO_6S_2$. (M_r 566.6). *1086000.* [129-17-9].

Schultz No. 769.

Colour Index No. 42045.

Acid Blue 1. Patent Blue VF. Disulphine blue.

Blue VS. Sodium [[[(4-diethylamino)phenyl](2,4-disulphonatophenyl)methylene]cyclohexa-2,5-dien-1-ylidene]diethylammonium.

A violet powder, soluble in water. Dilute solutions are blue and turn yellow on the addition of concentrated hydrochloric acid.

Sulphanilic acid. $C_6H_7NO_3S$. (M_r 173.2). *1086200.* [121-57-3]. 4-Aminobenzenesulphonic acid.

Colourless crystals, sparingly soluble in water, practically insoluble in alcohol.

Sulphanilic acid solution. *1086203.*

Dissolve 0.33 g of *sulphanilic acid R* in 75 ml of *water R* heating gently if necessary and dilute to 100 ml with *glacial acetic acid R.*

Sulphanilic acid solution R1. *1086201.*

Dissolve 0.5 g of *sulphanilic acid R* in a mixture of 75 ml of *dilute acetic acid R* and 75 ml of *water R.*

Sulphanilic acid solution, diazotised. *1086202.*

Dissolve, with warming, 0.9 g of *sulphanilic acid R* in 9 ml of *hydrochloric acid R,* and dilute to 100 ml with *water R.* Cool 10 ml of this solution in iced water and add 10 ml of an ice-cold 4.5 per cent *m/V* solution of *sodium nitrite R.* Allow to stand at 0 °C for 15 min (if stored at this temperature, the solution is stable for 3 days) and immediately before use add 20 ml of a 10 per cent *m/V* solution of *sodium carbonate R.*

Sulfathiazole. $C_9H_9N_3O_2S_2$. (M_r 255.3). *1086300.* [72-14-0]. 4-Amino-*N*-(thiazol-2-yl)benzenesulphonamide.

White or yellowish-white powder or crystals, very slightly soluble in water, soluble in acetone, slightly soluble in alcohol. It dissolves in dilute mineral acids and in solutions of alkali hydroxides and carbonates.

mp: about 200 °C.

Sulphomolybdic reagent R2. *1086400.*

Dissolve about 50 mg of *ammonium molybdate R* in 10 ml of *sulphuric acid R.*

Sulphomolybdic reagent R3. *1086500.*

Dissolve with heating 2.5 g of *ammonium molybdate R* in 20 ml of *water R.* Dilute 28 ml of *sulphuric acid R* in 50 ml of *water R,* then cool. Mix the two solutions and dilute to 100 ml with *water R.*

Storage: in a polyethylene container.

Sulphosalicylic acid. $C_7H_6O_6S,2H_2O$. (M_r 254.2). *1086600.* [5965-83-3]. 2-Hydroxy-5-sulphobenzoic acid.

A white, crystalline powder or crystals, very soluble in water and in alcohol.

mp: about 109 °C.

Sulphur. *1110800.* [7704-34-9].

See *Sulphur for external use (0953).*

Sulphur dioxide. SO_2. (M_r 64.1). *1086700.* [7446-09-5]. Sulphurous anhydride.

A colourless gas. When compressed it is a colourless liquid.

Sulphur dioxide R1. SO_2. (M_r 64.1). *1110900.*

Content: minimum 99.9 per cent *V/V* of SO_2.

Sulphuric acid. H_2SO_4. (M_r 98.1). *1086800.* [7664-93-9].

Content: 95.0 per cent *m/m* to 97.0 per cent *m/m* of H_2SO_4.

A colourless, caustic liquid with an oily consistency, highly hygroscopic, miscible with water and with alcohol producing intense heat.

d_{20}^{20}: 1.834 to 1.837.

A 10 g/l solution is strongly acid and gives the reactions of sulphates (*2.3.1*).

Appearance. It is clear (*2.2.1*) and colourless (*2.2.2, Method II*).

Oxidisable substances. Pour 20 g cautiously, with cooling, into 40 ml of *water R*. Add 0.5 ml of *0.002 M potassium permanganate*. The violet colour persists for at least 5 min.

Chlorides. Pour 10 g, carefully and while cooling, into 10 ml of *water R* and after cooling dilute to 20 ml with the same solvent. Add 0.5 ml of *silver nitrate solution R2*. Allow to stand for 2 min protected from bright light. The solution is not more opalescent than a standard prepared at the same time using a mixture of 1 ml of *chloride standard solution (5 ppm Cl) R*, 19 ml of *water R* and 0.5 ml of *silver nitrate solution R2* (0.5 ppm).

Nitrates. Pour 50 g or 27.2 ml, carefully and while cooling, into 15 ml of *water R*. Add 0.2 ml of a freshly prepared 50 g/l solution of *brucine R* in *glacial acetic acid R*. After 5 min any colour is less intense than that of a reference mixture prepared in the same manner and containing 12.5 ml of *water R*, 50 g of *nitrogen-free sulphuric acid R*, 2.5 ml of *nitrate standard solution (10 ppm NO_3) R* and 0.2 ml of a 50 g/l solution of *brucine R* in *glacial acetic acid R* (0.5 ppm).

Ammonium. Pour 2.5 g, carefully and while cooling, into *water R* and dilute to 20 ml with the same solvent. Cool, and add dropwise 10 ml of a 200 g/l solution of *sodium hydroxide R*, followed by 1 ml of *alkaline potassium tetraiodomercurate solution R*. The colour of the solution is less intense than that of a mixture of 5 ml of *ammonium standard solution (1 ppm NH_4) R*, 15 ml of *water R*, 10 ml of a 200 g/l solution of *sodium hydroxide R* and 1 ml of *alkaline potassium tetraiodomercurate solution R* (2 ppm).

Arsenic (*2.4.2*). To 50 g add 3 ml of *nitric acid R* and evaporate carefully until the volume is reduced to about 10 ml. Cool, add to the residue 20 ml of *water R* and concentrate to 5 ml. The solution complies with limit test A for arsenic (0.02 ppm). Prepare the standard using 1.0 ml of *arsenic standard solution (1 ppm As) R*.

Heavy metals (*2.4.8*). Dilute 10 ml of the solution obtained in the test for iron to 20 ml with *water R*. 12 ml of the solution complies with limit test A for heavy metals (2 ppm). Prepare the standard using *lead standard solution (2 ppm Pb) R*.

Iron (*2.4.9*). Dissolve the residue on ignition with slight heating in 1 ml of *dilute hydrochloric acid R* and dilute to 50.0 ml with *water R*. 5 ml of the solution diluted to 10 ml with *water R* complies with the limit test for iron (1 ppm).

Residue on ignition: maximum 0.001 per cent, determined on 100 g by evaporating cautiously in a small crucible over a naked flame and igniting the residue to redness.

Assay. Weigh accurately a ground-glass-stoppered flask containing 30 ml of *water R*, introduce 0.8 ml of the sulphuric acid, cool and weigh again. Titrate with *1 M sodium hydroxide*, using 0.1 ml of *methyl red solution R* as indicator.

1 ml of *1 M sodium hydroxide* is equivalent to 49.04 mg of H_2SO_4.

Storage: in a ground-glass-stoppered container made of glass or other inert material.

Sulphuric acid, alcoholic, 2.5 M. *1086801.*

Carefully and with constant cooling, stir 14 ml of *sulphuric acid R* into 60 ml of *ethanol R*. Allow to cool and dilute to 100 ml with *ethanol R*. Prepare immediately before use.

Sulphuric acid, alcoholic, 0.25 M. *1086802.*

Dilute 10 ml of *2.5 M alcoholic sulphuric acid R* to 100 ml with *ethanol R*. Prepare immediately before use.

Sulphuric acid, alcoholic solution of. *1086803.*

Carefully and with constant cooling, stir 20 ml of *sulphuric acid R* into 60 ml of *alcohol R*. Allow to cool and dilute to 100 ml with *alcohol R*. Prepare immediately before use.

Sulphuric acid, dilute. *1086804.*

Contains 98 g/l of H_2SO_4.

Add 5.5 ml of *sulphuric acid R* to 60 ml of *water R*, allow to cool and dilute to 100 ml with the same solvent.

Assay. Into a ground-glass-stoppered flask containing 30 ml of *water R*, introduce 10.0 ml of the dilute sulphuric acid. Titrate with *1 M sodium hydroxide*, using 0.1 ml of *methyl red solution R* as indicator.

1 ml of *1 M sodium hydroxide* is equivalent to 49.04 mg of H_2SO_4.

Sulphuric acid-formaldehyde reagent. *1086805.*

Mix 2 ml of *formaldehyde solution R* with 100 ml of *sulphuric acid R*.

Sulphuric acid, heavy metal-free. *1086807.*

Complies with the requirements prescribed for *sulphuric acid R* and with the following maximum contents of heavy metals:

As: 0.005 ppm;

Cd: 0.002 ppm;

Cu: 0.001 ppm;

Fe: 0.05 ppm;

Hg: 0.005 ppm;

Ni: 0.002 ppm;

Pb: 0.001 ppm;

Zn: 0.005 ppm.

Sulphuric acid, nitrogen-free. *1086806.*

Complies with the requirements prescribed for *sulphuric acid R* and with the following additional test.

Nitrates. To 5 ml of *water R* add carefully 45 ml of the sulphuric acid, allow to cool to 40 °C and add 8 mg of *diphenylbenzidine R*. The solution is faint pink or very pale blue.

Sulphuric acid, nitrogen-free R1. *1086808.*

Nitrogen-free sulphuric acid R containing 95.0 per cent *m/m* to 95.5 per cent *m/m* of H_2SO_4.

Sunflower oil. *1086900.*

See *Sunflower oil, refined (1371).*

Tagatose. $C_6H_{12}O_6$. (M_r 180.16). *1111000.* [87-81-0].

D-*lyxo*-Hexulose.

White powder.

$[\alpha]_D^{20}$: −2.3 (21.9 g/l solution in *water R*).

mp: 134 °C to 135 °C.

Talc. *1087000.* [14807-96-6].

See *Talc (0438).*

Tannic acid. *1087100.* [1401-55-4].

Yellowish to light-brown, glistening scales or amorphous powder, very soluble in water, freely soluble in alcohol, soluble in acetone.

Storage: protected from light.

Tartaric acid. *1087200.* [87-69-4].

See *Tartaric acid (0460).*

Taxifolin. $C_{15}H_{12}O_7$. (M_r 304.3). *1151800.* [480-18-2]. (2*R*,3*R*)-2-(3,4-Dihydroxyphenyl)-3,5,7-trihydroxy-2,3-dihydro-4*H*-1-benzopyran-4-one.

White or almost white powder, slightly soluble in ethanol.

A solution in *ethanol R* shows an absorption maximum (*2.2.25*) at 290 nm.

Tecnazene. $C_6HCl_4NO_2$. (M_r 260.9). *1132400.* [117-18-0].

bp: about 304 °C.

mp: 99 °C to 100 °C.

A suitable certified reference solution (10 ng/μl in cyclohexane) may be used.

α-Terpinene. $C_{10}H_{16}$. (M_r 136.2). *1140300.* [99-86-5]. 1-Isopropyl-4-methylcyclohexa-1,3-diene.

Clear, almost colourless liquid.

d_4^{20}: about 0.837.

n_D^{20}: about 1.478.

bp: about 174 °C.

α-Terpinene used in gas chromatography complies with the following additional test.

Assay. Examine by gas chromatography (*2.2.28*) as prescribed in the monograph on *Tea tree oil (1837).*

The content is not less than 95 per cent, calculated by the normalisation procedure.

γ-Terpinene. $C_{10}H_{16}$. (M_r 136.2). *1115900.* [99-85-4]. 1-Isopropyl-4-methylcyclohexa-1,4-diene.

An oily liquid.

d_4^{15}: about 0.850.

n_D^{15}: 1.474 to 1.475.

bp: 183 °C to 186 °C.

γ-Terpinene used in gas chromatography complies with the following additional test.

Assay. Examine by gas chromatography (*2.2.28*) as prescribed in the monograph *Peppermint oil (0405).*

Test solution. The substance to be examined.

The area of the principal peak is not less than 93.0 per cent of the area of all the peaks in the chromatogram obtained.

Terpinen-4-ol. $C_{10}H_{18}O$. (M_r 154.2). *1116000.* [562-74-3]. 4-Methyl-1-(1-methylethyl)cyclohex-3-en-1-ol. *p*-Menth-1-en-4-ol.

An oily, colourless liquid.

d_{20}^{20}: about 0.934.

n_D^{20}: about 1.477.

bp: 209 °C to 212 °C.

Terpinen-4-ol used in gas chromatography complies with the following additional test.

Assay. Examine by gas chromatography (*2.2.28*) as prescribed in the monograph on *Lavender oil (1338).*

Test solution. The substance to be examined.

The area of the principal peak is not less than 98.0 per cent of the area of all the peaks in the chromatogram obtained.

α-Terpineol. $C_{10}H_{18}O$. (M_r 154.2). *1087300.* [98-55-5]. (*RS*)-2-(4-Methylcyclohex-3-enyl)-2-propanol.

Colourless crystals, practically insoluble in water, soluble in alcohol.

d_{20}^{20}: about 0.935.

n_D^{20}: about 1.483.

$[\alpha]_D^{20}$: about 92.5.

mp: about 35 °C.

It may contain 1 to 3 per cent of β-terpineol.

α-Terpineol used in gas chromatography complies with the following test.

Assay. Examine by gas chromatography (*2.2.28*) under the conditions described in the monograph on *Anise oil (0804).*

Test solution. A 100 g/l solution in *hexane R.*

The area of the principal peak is not less than 97.0 per cent of the total area of the peaks. Disregard the peak due to hexane.

Terpinolene. $C_{10}H_{16}$. (M_r 136.2). *1140400.* [586-62-9]. *p*-Mentha-1,4(8)-diene. 4-Isopropylidene-1-methylcyclohexene.

Clear, almost colourless liquid.

d_4^{20}: about 0.863.

n_D^{20}: about 1.488.

bp: about 184 °C.

Terpinolene used in gas chromatography complies with the following additional test.

Assay. Examine by gas chromatography (*2.2.28*) as prescribed in the monograph on *Tea tree oil (1837).*

The content is not less than 90 per cent, calculated by the normalisation procedure.

Testosterone. *1116100.* [58-22-0].

See *Testosterone (1373).*

Testosterone propionate. *1087400.* [57-85-2].

See *Testosterone propionate (0297).*

Tetrabutylammonium bromide. $C_{16}H_{36}BrN$. (M_r 322.4). *1087500.* [1643-19-2].

White or almost white crystals.

mp: 102 °C to 104 °C.

Tetrabutylammonium dihydrogen phosphate. $C_{16}H_{38}NO_4P$. (M_r 339.5). *1087600.* [5574-97-0].

White powder, hygroscopic.

pH (2.2.3): about 7.5 for a 170 g/l solution.

Absorbance (*2.2.25*): about 0.10 determined at 210 nm using a 170 g/l solution.

Storage: in an airtight container.

Tetrabutylammonium hydrogen sulphate. $C_{16}H_{37}NO_4S$. (M_r 339.5). *1087700.* [32503-27-8].

A crystalline powder or colourless crystals, freely soluble in water and in methanol.

mp: 169 °C to 173 °C.

Absorbance (*2.2.25*). The absorbance of a 50 g/l solution, at wavelengths from 240 nm to 300 nm, is not greater than 0.05.

Tetrabutylammonium hydrogen sulphate R1. *1087701.*

Complies with the requirements prescribed for *tetrabutylammonium hydrogen sulphate R* and with the following additional requirement:

Absorbance (*2.2.25*). The absorbance of a 50 g/l solution, at wavelengths from 215 nm to 300 nm, is not greater than 0.02.

Tetrabutylammonium hydroxide. $C_{16}H_{37}NO,30H_2O$. (M_r 800). *1087800.* [2052-49-5].

Content: minimum 98.0 per cent of $C_{16}H_{37}NO,30H_2O$.

White or almost white crystals, soluble in water.

Assay. Dissolve 1.000 g in 100 ml of *water R*. Titrate immediately with *0.1 M hydrochloric acid* determining the end-point potentiometrically (*2.2.20*). Carry out a blank titration.

1 ml of *0.1 M hydrochloric acid* is equivalent to 80.0 mg $C_{16}H_{37}NO,30H_2O$.

Tetrabutylammonium hydroxide solution (104 g/l). *1087801.* [2052-49-5].

A solution containing 104 g/l of $C_{16}H_{37}NO$ (M_r 259.5), prepared by dilution of a suitable reagent grade.

Tetrabutylammonium hydroxide solution (400 g/l). *1087802.* [2052-49-5].

A solution containing 400 g/l of $C_{16}H_{37}NO$ M_r 259.5) of a suitable grade.

Tetrabutylammonium iodide. $C_{16}H_{36}IN$. (M_r 369.4). *1087900.* [311-28-4].

Content: minimum 98.0 per cent of $C_{16}H_{36}IN$.

White or slightly coloured, crystalline powder or crystals, soluble in alcohol.

Sulphated ash (*2.4.14*): maximum 0.02 per cent.

Assay. Dissolve 1.200 g in 30 ml of *water R*. Add 50.0 ml of *0.1 M silver nitrate* and 5 ml of *dilute nitric acid R*. Titrate the excess of silver nitrate with *0.1 M ammonium thiocyanate*, using 2 ml of *ferric ammonium sulphate solution R2* as indicator.

1 ml of *0.1 M silver nitrate* is equivalent to 36.94 mg of $C_{16}H_{36}IN$.

Tetrachloroethane. $C_2H_2Cl_4$. (M_r 167.9). *1088000.* [79-34-5]. 1,1,2,2-Tetrachloroethane.

A clear, colourless liquid, slightly soluble in water, miscible with alcohol.

d_{20}^{20}: about 1.59.

n_D^{20}: about 1.495.

Distillation range (*2.2.11*). Not less than 95 per cent distils between 145 °C and 147 °C.

Tetrachlorvinphos. $C_{10}H_9Cl_4O_4P$. (M_r 366.0). *1132500.* [22248-79-9].

mp: about 95 °C.

A suitable certified reference solution (10 ng/µl in iso-octane) may be used.

Tetracos-15-enoic acid methyl ester. $C_{25}H_{48}O_2$. (M_r 380.7). *1144800.* [2733-88-2]. 15-Tetracosaenoic acid methyl ester. Methyl tetracos-15-enoate. Nervonic acid methyl ester.

Content: minimum 99.0 per cent of $C_{25}H_{48}O_2$, determined by gas chromatography.

Liquid.

Tetracycline hydrochloride. *1147000.*

See *Tetracycline hydrochloride (0210)*.

Tetradecane. $C_{14}H_{30}$. (M_r 198.4). *1088200.* [629-59-4]. *n*-Tetradecane.

Content: minimum 99.5 per cent *m/m* of $C_{14}H_{30}$.

A colourless liquid.

d_{20}^{20}: about 0.76.

n_D^{20}: about 1.429.

bp: about 252 °C.

mp: about −5 °C.

Tetradecylammonium bromide. $C_{40}H_{84}BrN$. (M_r 659). *1088300.* [14937-42-9]. Tetrakis(decyl)ammonium bromide.

A white or slightly coloured, crystalline powder or crystals.

mp: 88 °C to 89 °C.

Tetraethylammonium hydrogen sulphate. $C_8H_{21}NO_4S$. (M_r 227.3). *1116200.* [16873-13-5].

Hygroscopic powder.

mp: about 245 °C.

Tetraethylammonium hydroxide solution. $C_8H_{21}NO$. (M_r 147.3). *1100300.* [77-98-5].

A 200 g/l aqueous solution, colourless liquid, strongly alkaline.

d_{20}^{20}: about 1.01.

n_D^{20}: about 1.372.

HPLC grade.

Tetraethylene pentamine. $C_8H_{23}N_5$. (M_r 189.3). *1102000.* [112-57-2]. 3,6,9-Triazaundecan-1,11-diamine.

Colourless liquid, soluble in acetone.

n_D^{20}: about1.506.

Storage: protected from humidity and heat.

Tetraheptylammonium bromide. $C_{28}H_{60}BrN$. (M_r 490.7). *1088400.* [4368-51-8].

A white or slightly coloured, crystalline powder or crystals.

mp: 89 °C to 91 °C.

Tetrahexylammonium bromide. $C_{24}H_{52}BrN$. (M_r 434.6). *1152500.* [4328-13-6]. *N,N,N*-Trihexylhexan-1-aminium bromide.

White, crystalline powder, hygroscopic.

mp: about 100 °C.

Tetrahexylammonium hydrogen sulphate. $C_{24}H_{53}NO_4S$. (M_r 451.8). *1116300.* [32503-34-7]. *N,N,N*-Trihexylhexan-1-aminium hydrogen sulphate.

White crystals.

mp: 100 °C to 102 °C.

Tetrahydrofuran. C_4H_8O. (M_r 72.1). *1088500.* [109-99-9]. Tetramethylene oxide.

A clear, colourless, flammable liquid, miscible with water, with alcohol.

d_{20}^{20}: about 0.89.

Do not distil if the tetrahydrofuran does not comply with the test for peroxides.

Peroxides. Place 8 ml of *potassium iodide and starch solution R* in a 12 ml ground-glass-stoppered cylinder about 1.5 cm in diameter. Fill completely with the substance to be examined, shake vigorously and allow to stand protected from light for 30 min. No colour is produced.

Tetrahydrofuran used in spectrophotometry complies with the following additional requirement.

Minimum transmittance (*2.2.25*), determined using *water R* as compensation liquid: 20 per cent at 255 nm, 80 per cent at 270 nm, 98 per cent at 310 nm.

Tetrahydrofuran for chromatography R. *1147100.*

It complies with the requirements of *tetrahydrofuran R* and with the following requirements:

d_{4}^{20} = 0.8892.

bp: about 66 °C.

Content: minimum 99.8 per cent of C_4H_8O.

Tetramethylammonium bromide. $C_4H_{12}BrN$. (M_r 154.1). *1156600.* [64-20-0]. *N,N,N*-Trimethylmethanaminium bromide.

White or slightly yellow crystals, freely soluble in water.

mp: about 285 °C, with decomposition.

Tetramethylammonium chloride. $C_4H_{12}ClN$. (M_r 109.6). *1100400.* [75-57-0].

Colourless crystals, soluble in water and in alcohol.

mp: about 300 °C, with decomposition.

Tetramethylammonium hydrogen sulphate. $C_4H_{13}NO_4S$. (M_r 171.2). *1116400.* [80526-82-5].

Hygroscopic powder.

mp: about 295 °C.

Tetramethylammonium hydroxide. $C_4H_{13}NO,5H_2O$. (M_r 181.2). *1122800.* [10424-65-4]. Tetramethylammonium hydroxide pentahydrate.

Suitable grade for HPLC.

Tetramethylammonium hydroxide solution. *1088600.* [75-59-2].

Content: minimum 10.0 per cent *m/m* of $C_4H_{13}NO$. (M_r 91.2).

A clear, colourless or very pale yellow liquid, miscible with water and with alcohol.

Assay. To 1.000 g add 50 ml of *water R* and titrate with *0.05 M sulphuric acid,* using 0.1 ml of *methyl red solution R* as indicator.

1 ml of *0.05 M sulphuric acid* is equivalent to 9.12 mg of $C_4H_{13}NO$.

Tetramethylammonium hydroxide solution, dilute. *1088601.*

Dilute 10 ml of *tetramethylammonium hydroxide solution R* to 100 ml with *aldehyde-free alcohol R.* Prepare immediately before use.

Tetramethylbenzidine. $C_{16}H_{20}N_2$. (M_r 240.3). *1132600.* [54827-17-7]. 3,3′,5,5′-Tetramethylbiphenyl-4,4′-diamine.

A powder, practically insoluble in water, very soluble in methanol.

mp: about 169 °C.

1,1,3,3-Tetramethylbutylamine. $C_8H_{19}N$. (M_r 129.3). *1141500.* [107-45-9]. 2-Amino-2,4,4-trimethylpentane.

Clear, colourless liquid.

d_{20}^{20}: about 0.805.

n_{D}^{20}: about 1.424.

bp: about 140 °C.

Tetramethyldiaminodiphenylmethane. $C_{17}H_{22}N_2$. (M_r 254.4). *1088700.* [101-61-1]. 4,4′-Methylenebis-(*N,N*-dimethylaniline).

White to bluish-white crystals or leaflets, practically insoluble in water, slightly soluble in alcohol, soluble in mineral acids.

mp: about 90 °C.

Tetramethyldiaminodiphenylmethane reagent. *1088701.*

Solution A. Dissolve 2.5 g of *tetramethyldiaminodiphenylmethane R* in 10 ml of *glacial acetic acid R* and add 50 ml of *water R.*

Solution B. Dissolve 5 g of *potassium iodide R* in 100 ml of *water R.*

Solution C. Dissolve 0.30 g of *ninhydrin R* in 10 ml of *glacial acetic acid R* and add 90 ml of *water R.*

Mix solution A, solution B and 1.5 ml of solution C.

Tetramethylethylenediamine. $C_6H_{16}N_2$. (M_r 116.2). *1088800.* [110-18-9]. *N,N,N′,N′*-Tetramethylethylenediamine.

A colourless liquid, miscible with water and with alcohol.

d_{20}^{20}: about 0.78.

n_{D}^{20}: about 1.418.

bp: about 121 °C.

Tetramethylsilane. $C_4H_{12}Si$. (M_r 88.2). *1088900.* [75-76-3]. TMS.

A clear, colourless liquid, very slightly soluble in water, soluble in acetone and in alcohol.

d_{20}^{20}: about 0.64.

n_{D}^{20}: about 1.358.

bp: about 26 °C.

Tetramethylsilane used in nuclear magnetic resonance spectrometry complies with the following additional requirement.

In the nuclear magnetic resonance spectrum of an approximately 10 per cent *V/V* solution of the tetramethylsilane in *deuterated chloroform R*, the intensity of any foreign signal, excluding those due to spinning side bands and to chloroform, is not greater than the intensity of the C-13 satellite signals located at a distance of 59.1 Hz on each side of the principal signal of tetramethylsilane.

Tetrapropylammonium chloride. $C_{12}H_{28}ClN$. (M_r 221.8). *1151900.* [5810-42-4].

White, crystalline powder, sparingly soluble in water.

mp: about 241 °C.

Tetrazolium blue. $C_{40}H_{32}Cl_2N_8O_2$. (M_r 728). *1089000.* [1871-22-3]. 3,3′-(3,3′-Dimethoxy[1,1′-biphenyl]-4,4′-diyl)bis[2,5-diphenyl-2*H*-tetrazolium] dichloride.

Yellow crystals, slightly soluble in water, freely soluble in alcohol and in methanol, practically insoluble in acetone.

mp: about 245 °C, with decomposition.

Tetrazolium bromide. $C_{18}H_{16}BrN_5S$. (M_r 414.3). *1152700.* [298-93-1]. 3-(4,5-Dimethylthiazol-2-yl)-2,5-diphenyltetrazolium bromide. MTT.

Thallous sulphate. Tl_2SO_4. (M_r 504.8). *1089100.* [7446-18-6]. Dithallium sulphate.

White, rhomboid prisms, slightly soluble in water, practically insoluble in alcohol.

Thebaine. $C_{19}H_{21}NO_3$. (M_r 311.4). *1089200.* [115-37-7]. (5*R*,9*R*,13*S*)-4,5-Epoxy-3,6-dimethoxy-9a-methylmorphina-6,8-diene.

A white or pale yellow, crystalline powder, very slightly soluble in water, soluble in hot ethanol and in toluene.

mp: about 193 °C.

Chromatography (2.2.27). Examine as prescribed in identification test B in the monograph on *Raw opium (0777),* applying to the plate as a band (20 mm × 3 mm) 20 µl of a 0.5 g/l solution. The chromatogram obtained shows an orange-red or red principal band with an R_f of about 0.5.

Theobromine. *1138800.* [83-67-0].

See *Theobromine (0298).*

Theophylline. *1089300.* [58-55-9].

See *Theophylline (0299).*

Thiamazole. $C_4H_6N_2S$. (M_r 114.2). *1089400.* [60-56-0]. Methimazole. 1-Methyl-1*H*-imidazole-2-thiol.

A white or almost white, crystalline powder, freely soluble in water, soluble in alcohol and in methylene chloride.

mp: about 145 °C.

2-(2-Thienyl)acetic acid. $C_6H_6O_2S$. (M_r 142.1). *1089500.* [1918-77-0].

A brown powder.

mp: about 65 °C.

Thioacetamide. C_2H_5NS. (M_r 75.1). *1089600.* [62-55-5].

A crystalline powder or colourless crystals, freely soluble in water and in alcohol.

mp: about 113 °C.

Thioacetamide reagent. *1089601.*

To 0.2 ml of *thioacetamide solution R* add 1 ml of a mixture of 5 ml of *water R*, 15 ml of *1 M sodium hydroxide* and 20 ml of *glycerol (85 per cent) R*. Heat in a water-bath for 20 s. Prepare immediately before use.

Thioacetamide solution. *1089602.*

A 40 g/l solution.

Thiobarbituric acid. $C_4H_4N_2O_2S$. (M_r 144.2). *1111200.* [504-17-6]. 4,6-Dihydroxy-2-sulfanylpyrimidine.

Thiodiethylene glycol. $C_4H_{10}O_2S$. (M_r 122.2). *1122900.* [111-48-8]. Di(2-hydroxyethyl) sulphide.

A colourless or yellow, viscous liquid. It contains at least 99.0 per cent of $C_4H_{10}O_2S$.

d_{20}^{20}: about 1.18.

Thioglycollic acid. $C_2H_4O_2S$. (M_r 92.1). *1089700.* [68-11-1]. 2-Mercaptoacetic acid.

A colourless liquid, miscible with water, soluble in alcohol.

Thiomersal. $C_9H_9HgNaO_2S$. (M_r 404.8). *1089800.* [54-64-8]. Sodium mercurothiolate. Sodium 2-[(ethylmercurio)thio]benzoate.

A light, yellowish-white, crystalline powder, very soluble in water, freely soluble in alcohol.

Thiourea. CH_4N_2S. (M_r 76.1). *1089900.* [62-56-6].

White, crystalline powder or crystals, soluble in water and in alcohol.

mp: about 178 °C.

Threonine. *1090000.* [72-19-5].

See *Threonine (1049).*

Thrombin, bovine. *1090200.* [9002-04-4].

A preparation of the enzyme, obtained from bovine plasma, that converts fibrinogen into fibrin.

A yellowish-white powder.

Storage: at a temperature below 0 °C.

Thrombin, human. *1090100.* [9002-04-4].

Dried human thrombin. A preparation of the enzyme which converts human fibrinogen into fibrin. It is obtained from liquid human plasma and may be prepared by precipitation with suitable salts and organic solvents under controlled conditions of pH, ionic strength and temperature.

A yellowish-white powder, freely soluble in a 9 g/l solution of sodium chloride forming a cloudy, pale yellow solution.

Storage: in a sealed, sterile container under nitrogen, protected from light, at a temperature below 25 °C.

Thrombin solution, human. *1090101.*

Reconstitute *human thrombin R* as directed by the manufacturer and dilute with *tris(hydroxymethyl)aminomethane sodium chloride buffer solution pH 7.4 R* to 5 IU/ml.

Thromboplastin. *1090300.*

Extract 1.5 g of *acetone-dried ox brain R* with 60 ml of *water R* at 50 °C for 10 min to 15 min, centrifuge at 1500 r/min for 2 min and decant the supernatant liquid. The extract retains its activity for several days when stored in a refrigerator. It may contain 3 g/l of *cresol R* as an antimicrobial preservative.

Thujone. $C_{10}H_{16}O$. (M_r 152.2). *1116500.* [546-80-5]. 4-Methyl-1-(1-methylethyl)bicyclo[3.1.0]hexan-3-one.

A colourless or almost colourless liquid, practically insoluble in water, soluble in alcohol and in many other organic solvents.

d_{20}^{20}: about 0.925.

n_D^{20}: about 1.455.

$[\alpha]_D^{20}$: about − 15.

bp: about 200 °C.

Thymine. $C_5H_6N_2O_2$. (M_r 126.1). *1090400.* [65-71-4]. 5-Methylpyrimidine-2,4(1*H*,3*H*)-dione.

Short needles or plates, slightly soluble in cold water, soluble in hot water. It dissolves in dilute solution of alkali hydroxides.

Thymol. *1090500.* [89-83-8]. See *Thymol (0791).*

Thymol used in gas chromatography complies with the following additional test.

Assay. Examine by gas chromatography (*2.2.28*) as prescribed in the monograph *Peppermint oil (0405)*.

Test solution. Dissolve 0.1 g in about 10 ml of *acetone R*.

The area of the principal peak is not less than 95.0 per cent of the area of all the peaks in the chromatogram obtained. Disregard the peak due to acetone.

Thymol blue. $C_{27}H_{30}O_5S$. (M_r 466.6). *1090600.* [76-61-9]. Thymolsulphonphthalein. 4,4′-(3*H*-2,1-Benzoxathiol-3-ylidene)bis(2-isopropyl-5-methylphenol) *S,S*-dioxide.

A brownish-green to greenish-blue, crystalline powder, slightly soluble in water, soluble in alcohol and in dilute solutions of alkali hydroxides.

Thymol blue solution. *1090601.*

Dissolve 0.1 g of *thymol blue R* in a mixture of 2.15 ml of *0.1 M sodium hydroxide* and 20 ml of *alcohol R* and dilute to 100 ml with *water R*.

Test for sensitivity. To 0.1 ml of the thymol blue solution add 100 ml of *carbon dioxide-free water R* and 0.2 ml of *0.02 M sodium hydroxide*. The solution is blue. Not more than 0.15 ml of *0.02 M hydrochloric acid* is required to change the colour to yellow.

Colour change: pH 1.2 (red) to pH 2.8 (yellow); pH 8.0 (olive-green) to pH 9.6 (blue).

Thymolphthalein. $C_{28}H_{30}O_4$. (M_r 430.5). *1090700.* [125-20-2]. 3,3-bis(4-Hydroxy-5-isopropyl-2-methylphenyl)-3*H*-isobenzo-furan-1-one.

A white or yellowish-white powder, practically insoluble in water, soluble in alcohol and in dilute solutions of alkali hydroxides.

Thymolphthalein solution. *1090701.*

A 1 g/l solution in *alcohol R*.

Test for sensitivity. To 0.2 ml of the thymolphthalein solution add 100 ml of *carbon dioxide-free water R*. The solution is colourless. Not more than 0.05 ml of *0.1 M sodium hydroxide* is required to change the colour to blue.

Colour change: pH 9.3 (colourless) to pH 10.5 (blue).

Tin. Sn. (A_r 118.7). *1090800.* [7440-31-5].

Silvery-white granules, soluble in hydrochloric acid with release of hydrogen.

Arsenic (2.4.2). 0.1 g complies with limit test A (10 ppm).

Titan yellow. $C_{28}H_{19}N_5Na_2O_6S_4$. ($M_r$ 696). *1090900.* [1829-00-1].

Schultz No. 280.

Colour Index No. 19540.

Thiazol yellow. Disodium 2,2′-[(1-triazene-1,3-diyl)di-4,1-phenylene]bis-[6-methylbenzothiazole-7-sulphonate].

A yellowish-brown powder, freely soluble in water and in alcohol.

Titan yellow paper. *1090901.*

Immerse strips of filter paper in *titan yellow solution R* and leave for a few minutes. Allow to dry at room temperature.

Titan yellow solution. *1090902.*

A 0.5 g/l solution.

Test for sensitivity. To 0.1 ml of the titan yellow solution add 10 ml of *water R*, 0.2 ml of *magnesium standard solution (10 ppm Mg) R* and 1.0 ml of *1 M sodium hydroxide*. A distinct pink colour is visible by comparison with a reference solution prepared in a similar manner omitting the magnesium.

Titanium. Ti. (A_r 47.88). *1091000.* [7440-32-6].

Content: minimum 99 per cent of Ti.

Metal powder, fine wire (diameter not more than 0.5 mm), sponge.

mp: about 1668 °C.

Density: about 4.507 g/cm^3.

Titanium dioxide. *1117900.* [13463-67-7].

See *Titanium dioxide (0150).*

Titanium trichloride. $TiCl_3$. (M_r 154.3). *1091200.* [7705-07-9]. Titanium(III) chloride.

Reddish-violet crystals, deliquescent, soluble in water and in alcohol.

mp: about 440 °C.

Storage: in an airtight container.

Titanium trichloride solution. *1091201.*

d_{20}^{20}: about 1.19.

A 150 g/l solution in hydrochloric acid (100 g/l HCl).

Titanium trichloride-sulphuric acid reagent. *1091202.*

Carefully mix 20 ml of *titanium trichloride solution R* with 13 ml of *sulphuric acid R*. Add sufficient *strong hydrogen peroxide solution R* to give a yellow colour. Heat until white fumes are evolved. Allow to cool. Dilute with *water R* and repeat the evaporation and addition of *water R* until a colourless solution is obtained. Dilute to 100 ml with *water R*.

TLC octadecylsilyl silica gel plate. *1148600.*

Support of glass, metal or plastic coated with a layer of octadecylsilyl silica gel. The plate may contain an organic binder.

TLC octadecylsilyl silica gel F_{254} plate R. *1146600.*

Support of glass, metal or plastic coated with a layer of octadecylsilyl silica gel.

It contains a fluorescent indicator having a maximum absorbance in ultraviolet light at 254 nm.

TLC performance test solution. *1116600.*

Prepare a mixture of 1.0 ml of each of the following solutions and dilute to 10.0 ml with *acetone R*: a 0.5 g/l solution of *Sudan red G R* in *toluene R*, a 0.5 g/l solution of *methyl orange R* in *ethanol R* prepared immediately before use, a 0.5 g/l solution of *bromocresol green R* in *acetone R* and a 0.25 g/l solution of *methyl red R* in *acetone R*.

TLC silica gel plate. *1116700.*

Support of glass, metal or plastic, coated with a layer of silica gel of a suitable thickness and particle size (usually 2 µm to 10 µm for fine particle size (High Performance Thin-Layer Chromatography, HPTLC) plates and 5 µm to 40 µm for normal TLC plates). If necessary, the particle size is indicated after the name of the reagent in the tests where it is used.

The plate may contain an organic binder.

Chromatographic separation. Apply to the plate an appropriate volume (10 µl for a normal TLC plate and 1 µl to 2 µl for a fine particle size plate) of *TLC performance test solution R*. Develop over a pathlength two-thirds of the plate height, using a mixture of 20 volumes of *methanol R* and 80 volumes of *toluene R*. The plate is not satisfactory, unless the chromatogram shows four clearly separated spots, the spot of bromocresol green with an R_f value less than 0.15, the spot of methyl orange with an R_f value in the range of 0.1 to 0.25, the spot of methyl red with an R_f value in the range of 0.35 to 0.55 and the spot of Sudan red G with an R_f value in the range of 0.75 to 0.98.

TLC silica gel F_{254} plate. *1116800.*

It complies with the requirements prescribed for *TLC silica gel plate R* with the following modification.

It contains a fluorescent indicator having a maximum absorbance at 254 nm.

Fluorescence suppression. Apply separately to the plate at five points increasing volumes (1 µl to 10 µl for normal TLC plates and 0.2 µl to 2 µl for fine particle size plates) of a 1 g/l solution of *benzoic acid R* in a mixture of 15 volumes of *ethanol R* and 85 volumes of *cyclohexane R*. Develop over a pathlength half of the plate height with the same mixture of solvents. After evaporating the solvents examine the chromatogram in ultraviolet light at 254 nm. For normal TLC plates the benzoic acid appears as dark spots on a fluorescent background approximately in the middle of the chromatogram for quantities of 2 µg and greater. For fine particle size plates the benzoic acid appears as dark spots on a fluorescent background approximately in the middle of the chromatogram for quantities of 0.2 µg and greater.

TLC silica gel F_{254}, silanised plate. *1117200.*

It complies with the requirements prescribed for *TLC silica gel silanised plate R* with the following modification.

It contains a fluorescent indicator having a maximum absorbance at 254 nm.

TLC silica gel G plate. *1116900.*

It complies with the requirements prescribed for *TLC silica gel plate R* with the following modification.

It contains calcium sulphate hemihydrate as binder.

TLC silica gel GF_{254} plate. *1117000.*

It complies with the requirements prescribed for *TLC silica gel plate R* with the following modifications.

It contains calcium sulphate hemihydrate as binder and a fluorescent indicator having a maximum absorbance at 254 nm.

Fluorescence suppression. Complies with the test prescribed for *TLC silica gel F_{254} plate R*.

TLC silica gel plate for chiral separations, octadecylsilyl. *1137700.*

Support of glass, metal or plastic, coated with a layer of octadecylsilyl silica gel, impregnated with Cu^{2+} ions and enantiomerically pure hydroxyproline. The plate may contain an organic binder.

TLC silica gel, silanised plate. *1117100.*

Support of glass, metal or plastic, coated with a layer of silanised silica gel of a suitable thickness and particle size (usually 2 µm to 10 µm for fine particle size (High Performance Thin-Layer Chromatography, HPTLC) plates and 5 µm to 40 µm for normal TLC plates). If necessary, the particle size is indicated after the name of the reagent in the tests where it is used.

The plate may contain an organic binder.

Chromatographic separation. Introduce 0.1 g each of *methyl laurate R, methyl myristate R, methyl palmitate R* and *methyl stearate R* into a 250 ml conical flask. Add 40 ml of *alcoholic potassium hydroxide solution R* and heat under a reflux condenser on a water-bath for 1 h. Allow to cool, transfer the solution to a separating funnel by means of 100 ml of *water R*, acidify (pH 2 to 3) with *dilute hydrochloric acid R* and shake with three quantitites each of 10 ml of *methylene chloride R*. Dry the combined methylene chloride extracts over *anhydrous sodium sulphate R*, filter and evaporate to dryness on a water-bath. Dissolve the residue in 50 ml of *methylene chloride R*. Examine by thin-layer chromatography (*2.2.27*), using *silanised TLC silica gel plate R*. Apply an appropriate quantity (about 10 µl for normal TLC plates and about 1 µl to 2 µl for fine particle size plates) of the methylene chloride solution at each of three separate points. Develop over a pathlength two-thirds of the plate height with a mixture of 10 volumes of *glacial acetic acid R*, 25 volumes of *water R* and 65 volumes of *dioxan R*. Dry the plate at 120 °C for 30 min. Allow to cool, spray with a 35 g/l solution of *phosphomolybdic acid R* in *2-propanol R* and heat at 150 °C until the spots become visible. Treat the plate with ammonia vapour until the background is white. The chromatograms show four clearly separated, well-defined spots.

α-Tocopherol. *1152300.* [10191-41-0].

See *all-rac-α-Tocopherol (0692)*.

α-Tocopheryl acetate. *1152400.* [7695-91-2].

See *all-rac-α-Tocopheryl acetate (0439)*.

o-Tolidine. $C_{14}H_{16}N_2$. (M_r 212.3). *1123000.* [119-93-7]. 3,3′-Dimethylbenzidine.

Content: minimum 97.0 per cent of $C_{14}H_{16}N_2$.

A light brownish, crystalline power.

mp: about 130 °C.

o-Tolidine solution. *1123001.*

Dissolve 0.16 g of *o-tolidine R* in 30.0 ml of *glacial acetic acid R*, add 1.0 g of *potassium iodide R* and dilute to 500.0 ml with *water R*.

Toluene. C_7H_8. (M_r 92.1). *1091300.* [108-88-3]. Methylbenzene.

A clear, colourless, flammable liquid, very slightly soluble in water, miscible with alcohol.

d_{20}^{20}: 0.865 to 0.870.

bp: about 110 °C.

Toluene, sulphur-free. *1091301.*

Complies with the requirements prescribed for *toluene R* and with the following additional requirements:

Sulphur compounds. To 10 ml add 1 ml of *ethanol R* and 3 ml of *potassium plumbite solution R* and boil under a reflux condenser for 15 min. Allow to stand for 5 min. No darkening is produced in the aqueous layer.

Thiophen-related substances. Shake 2 ml with 5 ml of *isatin reagent R* for 5 min and allow to stand for 15 min. No blue colour is produced in the lower layer.

Toluenesulphonamide. $C_7H_9NO_2S$. (M_r 171.2). *1091500.* [70-55-3]. 4-Methylbenzenesulphonamide. *p*-Toluenesulphonamide.

A white, crystalline powder, slightly soluble in water, soluble in alcohol and in solutions of alkali hydroxides.

mp: about 136 °C.

Chromatography. Examine as prescribed in the monograph on *Tolbutamide (0304)*; the chromatogram shows only one principal spot.

o-Toluenesulphonamide. $C_7H_9NO_2S$. (M_r 171.2). *1091400.* [88-19-7]. 2-Methylbenzenesulphonamide.

A white, crystalline powder, slightly soluble in water, soluble in alcohol and in solutions of alkali hydroxides.

mp: about 156 °C.

p-Toluenesulphonamide. *1091500.* [70-55-3].

See *toluenesulphonamide R*.

Toluenesulphonic acid. $C_7H_8O_3S,H_2O$. (M_r 190.2). *1091600.* [6192-52-5]. 4-Methylbenzenesulphonic acid.

Content: minimum 87.0 per cent of $C_7H_8O_3S$.

A white, crystalline powder or crystals, freely soluble in water, soluble in alcohol.

o-Toluidine. C_7H_9N. (M_r 107.2). *1091700.* [95-53-4]. 2-Methylaniline.

A pale-yellow liquid becoming reddish-brown on exposure to air and light, slightly soluble in water, soluble in alcohol and in dilute acids.

d_{20}^{20}: about 1.01.

n_D^{20}: about 1.569.

bp: about 200 °C.

Storage: in an airtight container, protected from light.

o-Toluidine hydrochloride. $C_7H_{10}ClN$. (M_r 143.6). *1117300.* [636-21-5]. 2-Methylaniline hydrochloride. 2-Methylbenzenamine hydrochloride.

Content: minimum 98.0 per cent of $C_7H_{10}ClN$.

mp: 215 °C to 217 °C.

p-Toluidine. C_7H_9N. (M_r 107.2). *1091800.* [106-49-0]. 4-Methylaniline.

Lustrous plates or flakes, slightly soluble in water, freely soluble in acetone and in alcohol.

mp: about 44 °C.

Toluidine blue. $C_{15}H_{16}ClN_3S$. (M_r 305.8). *1091900.* [92-31-9].

Schultz No. 1041.

Colour Index No. 52040.

Toluidine Blue O. 3-Amino-7-dimethylamino-2-methylphenothiazin-5-ium chloride.

A dark-green powder, soluble in water, slightly soluble in alcohol.

Tosylarginine methyl ester hydrochloride. $C_{14}H_{23}ClN_4O_4S$. (M_r 378.9). *1092000.* [1784-03-8]. *N*-Tosyl-L-arginine methyl ester hydrochloride. Methyl (*S*)-5-guanidino-2-(4-methylbenzenesulphonamido)valerate hydrochloride.

$[\alpha]_D^{20}$: − 12 to − 16, determined on a 40 g/l solution.

mp: about 145 °C.

Tosylarginine methyl ester hydrochloride solution. *1092001.*

To 98.5 mg of *tosylarginine methyl ester hydrochloride R* add 5 ml of *tris(hydroxymethyl)aminomethane buffer solution pH 8.1 R* and shake to dissolve. Add 2.5 ml of *methyl red mixed solution R* and dilute to 25.0 ml with *water R*.

Tosyl-lysyl-chloromethane hydrochloride. $C_{14}H_{22}Cl_2N_2O_3S$. (M_r 369.3). *1092100.* [4238-41-9]. *N*-Tosyl-L-lysyl-chloromethane hydrochloride. (3*S*)-7-Amino-1-chloro-3-(4-methylbenzenesulphonamido)heptan-2-one hydrochloride.

$[\alpha]_D^{20}$: − 7 to − 9, determined on a 20 g/l solution.

mp: about 155 °C, with decomposition.

$A_{1\,cm}^{1\%}$: 310 to 340, determined at 230 nm in *water R*.

Tosylphenylalanylchloromethane. $C_{17}H_{18}ClNO_3S$. (M_r 351.9). *1092200.* [402-71-1]. *N*-Tosyl-L-phenylalanylchloromethane.

$[\alpha]_D^{20}$: − 85 to − 89, determined on a 10 g/l solution in *alcohol R*.

mp: about 105 °C.

$A_{1\,cm}^{1\%}$: 290 to 320, determined at 228.5 nm in *alcohol R*.

Toxaphene. *1132800.* [8001-35-2].

A mixture of polychloro derivatives.

mp: 65 °C to 90 °C.

A suitable certified reference solution (10 ng/μl in iso-octane) may be used.

Tragacanth. *1092300.* [9000-65-1].

See *Tragacanth (0532)*.

Triacetin. $C_9H_{14}O_6$. (M_r 218.2). *1092400.* [102-76-1]. Propane-1,2,3-triyl triacetate.

An almost clear, colourless to yellowish liquid, soluble in water, miscible with alcohol.

d_{20}^{20} : about 1.16.

n_D^{20} : about 1.43.

bp: about 260 °C.

Triamcinolone. $C_{21}H_{27}FO_6$. (M_r 394.4). *1111300.* [124-94-7]. 9-Fluoro-11β,16α,17,21-tetrahydroxypregna-1,4-diene-3,20-dione.

A crystalline powder.

mp: 262 °C to 263 °C.

Triamcinolone acetonide. *1133100.* [76-25-5].

See *Triamcinolone acetonide (0533)*.

Tributyl citrate. $C_{18}H_{32}O_7$. (M_r 360.4). *1152800.* [77-94-1]. Tributyl 2-hydroxypropane-1,2,3-tricarboxylate.

d_4^{20} : about 1.043.

n_D^{20} : about 1.445.

Trichlorethylene. *1102100.*

See *Trichloroethylene R*.

Trichloroacetic acid. $C_2HCl_3O_2$. (M_r 163.4). *1092500.* [76-03-9].

Colourless crystals or a crystalline mass, very deliquescent, very soluble in water and in alcohol.

Storage: in an airtight container.

Trichloroacetic acid solution. *1092501.*

Dissolve 40.0 g of *trichloroacetic acid R* in *water R* and dilute to 1000.0 ml with the same solvent. Verify the concentration by titration with *0.1 M sodium hydroxide* and adjust if necessary to 40 ± 1 g/l.

1,1,1-Trichloroethane. $C_2H_3Cl_3$. (M_r 133.4). *1092600.* [71-55-6]. Methylchloroform.

A non-flammable liquid, practically insoluble in water, soluble in acetone and in methanol.

d_{20}^{20} : about 1.34.

n_D^{20} : about 1.438.

bp: about 74 °C.

Trichloroethylene. C_2HCl_3. (M_r 131.4). *1102100.* [79-01-6].

A colourless liquid, practically insoluble in water, miscible with alcohol.

d_{20}^{20} : about 1.46.

n_D^{20} : about 1.477.

Trichlorotrifluoroethane. $C_2Cl_3F_3$. (M_r 187.4). *1092700.* [76-13-1]. 1,1,2-Trichloro-1,2,2-trifluoroethane.

A colourless, volatile liquid, practically insoluble in water, miscible with acetone.

d_{20}^{20} : about 1.58.

Distillation range (*2.2.11*). Not less than 98 per cent distils between 47 °C and 48 °C.

Tricine. $C_6H_{13}NO_5$. (M_r 179.2). *1138900.* [5704−04−1]. *N*-[2-Hydroxy-1,1-bis(hydroxymethyl)ethyl]glycine.

Use electrophoresis-grade reagent.

mp: about 183 °C.

Tricosane. $C_{23}H_{48}$. (M_r 324.6). *1092800.* [638-67-5].

White crystals, practically insoluble in water, soluble in hexane.

n_D^{20} : about 1.447.

mp: about 48 °C.

Tridocosahexaenoin. $C_{69}H_{98}O_6$. (M_r 1023.5). *1144900.* [124596-98-1]. Triglyceride of docosahexaenoic acid (C22:6). Glycerol tridocosahexaenoate. Propane-1,2,3-triyl tri-(*all-Z*)-docosa-4,7,10,13,16,19-hexaenoate.

The reagent from Nu-Chek Prep, Inc. has been found suitable.

Triethanolamine. *1092900.* [102-71-6].

See *Trolamine (1577)*.

Triethylamine. $C_6H_{15}N$. (M_r 101.2). *1093000.* [121-44-8]. *N,N*-Diethylethanamine.

A colourless liquid, slightly soluble in water at a temperature below 18.7 °C, miscible with alcohol.

d_{20}^{20} : about 0.727.

n_D^{20} : about 1.401.

bp: about 90 °C.

Triethylenediamine. $C_6H_{12}N_2$. (M_r 112.2). *1093100.* 1,4-Diazabicyclo[2.2.2]octane.

Crystals, very hygroscopic, sublimes readily at room temperature, freely soluble in water, in acetone and in ethanol.

bp: about 174 °C.

mp: about 158 °C.

Storage: in an airtight container.

Triethyl phosphonoformate. $C_7H_{15}O_5P$. (M_r 210.2). *1132900.* [1474-78-8]. Ethyl (diethoxyphosphoryl)formate.

Colourless liquid.

$bp_{12\ mm}$: about 135 °C.

Trifluoroacetic acid. $C_2HF_3O_2$. (M_r 114.0). *1093200.* [76-05-1].

Content: minimum 99 per cent of $C_2HF_3O_2$.

Liquid, miscible with acetone and with alcohol.

d_{20}^{20}: about 1.53.

bp: about 72 °C.

Use a grade suitable for protein sequencing.

Storage: in an airtight container.

Trifluoroacetic anhydride. $C_4F_6O_3$. (M_r 210.0). *1093300.* [407-25-0].

Colourless liquid.

d_{20}^{20}: about 1.5.

Trigonelline hydrochloride. $C_7H_8ClNO_2$. (M_r 173.6). *1117400.* [6138-41-6]. 3-Carboxy-1-methylpyridinium chloride. Nicotinic acid *N*-methylbetaine hydrochloride.

A crystalline powder, very soluble in water, soluble in alcohol.

mp: about 258 °C.

Trimethylpentane. C_8H_{18}. (M_r 114.2). *1093400.* [540-84-1]. Iso-octane. 2,2,4-Trimethylpentane.

A colourless, flammable liquid, practically insoluble in water, soluble in ethanol.

d_{20}^{20}: 0.691 to 0.696.

n_D^{20}: 1.391 to 1.393.

Distillation range (*2.2.11*). Not less than 95 per cent distils between 98 °C and 100 °C.

Trimethylpentane used in spectrophotometry complies with the following additional requirement.

Minimum transmittance (*2.2.25*), determined using *water R* as compensation liquid: 98 per cent from 250 nm to 420 nm.

Trimethylpentane R1. *1093401.*

Complies with the requirements prescribed for *trimethylpentane R* with the following modification.

Absorbance (2.2.25). Not more than 0.07 from 220 nm to 360 nm, determined using *water R* as the compensation liquid.

***N,O*-bis(Trimethylsilyl)acetamide.** $C_8H_{21}NOSi_2$. (M_r 203.4). *1093600.* [10416-59-8].

Colourless liquid.

d_{20}^{20}: about 0.83.

***N*-Trimethylsilylimidazole.** $C_6H_{12}N_2Si$. (M_r 140.3). *1100500.* [18156-74-6]. 1-Trimethylsilylimidazole.

A colourless, hygroscopic liquid.

d_{20}^{20}: about 0.96.

n_D^{20}: about 1.48.

Storage: in an airtight container.

***N,O*-bis(Trimethylsilyl)trifluoroacetamide.** $C_8H_{18}F_3NOSi_2$. (M_r 257.4). *1133200.* [25561-30-2]. BSTFA.

Colourless liquid.

d_{20}^{20}: about 0.97.

n_D^{20}: about 1.38.

bp_{12mm}: about 40 °C

Trimethylsulphonium hydroxide. $C_3H_{10}OS$. (M_r 94.2). *1145000.* [17287-03-5].

d_4^{20}: about 0.81.

2,4,6-Trinitrobenzene sulphonic acid. $C_6H_3N_3O_9S,3H_2O$. (M_r 347.2). *1117500.* [2508-19-2].

A white, crystalline powder, soluble in water.

mp: 190 °C to 195 °C.

Triphenylmethanol. $C_{19}H_{16}O$. (M_r 260.3). *1093700.* [76-84-6]. Triphenylcarbinol.

Colourless crystals, practically insoluble in water, freely soluble in alcohol.

Triphenyltetrazolium chloride. $C_{19}H_{15}ClN_4$. (M_r 334.8). *1093800.* [298-96-4]. 2,3,5-Triphenyl-2*H*-tetrazolium chloride.

Content: minimum 98.0 per cent of $C_{19}H_{15}ClN_4$. A pale or dull-yellow powder, soluble in water, in acetone and in alcohol.

mp: about 240 °C, with decomposition.

Assay. Dissolve 1.000 g in a mixture of 5 ml of *dilute nitric acid R* and 45 ml of *water R*. Add 50.0 ml of *0.1 M silver nitrate* and heat to boiling. Allow to cool, add 3 ml of *dibutyl phthalate R*, shake vigorously and titrate with *0.1 M ammonium thiocyanate*, using 2 ml of *ferric ammonium sulphate solution R2* as indicator.

1 ml of *0.1 M silver nitrate* is equivalent to 33.48 mg of $C_{19}H_{15}ClN_4$.

Storage: protected from light.

Triphenyltetrazolium chloride solution. *1093801.*

A 5 g/l solution in *aldehyde-free alcohol R*.

Storage: protected from light.

Triscyanoethoxypropane. $C_{12}H_{17}N_3O_3$. (M_r 251.3). *1093900.* 1,2,3-Tris(2-cyanoethoxy)propane.

A viscous, brown-yellow liquid, soluble in methanol. Used as a stationary phase in gas chromatography.

d_{20}^{20}: about 1.11.

Viscosity (*2.2.9*): about 172 mPa·s.

1,3,5-Tris[3,5-di(1,1-dimethylethyl)-4-hydroxybenzyl]-1,3,5-triazine-2,4,6(1*H*,3*H*,5*H*)-trione. $C_{48}H_{69}O_6N_3$. (M_r 784.1). *1094000.* [27676-62-6].

A white, crystalline powder.

mp: 218 °C to 222 °C.

Tris[2,4-di(1,1-dimethylethyl)phenyl] phosphite. $C_{42}H_{63}O_3P$. (M_r 647). *1094100.* [31570-04-4].

White powder.

mp: 182 °C to 186 °C.

Tris(hydroxymethyl)aminomethane. *1094200.* [77-86-1]. See *Trometamol (1053).*

Tris(hydroxymethyl)aminomethane solution. *1094201.*

A solution containing the equivalent of 24.22 g of $C_4H_{11}NO_3$ in 1000.0 ml.

Tris(hydroxymethyl)aminomethane solution R1. *1094202.*

Dissolve 60.6 mg of *tris(hydroxymethyl)aminomethane R* and 0.234 g of *sodium chloride R* in *water R* and dilute to 100 ml with the same solvent.

Storage: at 2 °C to 8 °C; use within 3 days.

Tripotassium phosphate trihydrate. $K_3PO_4,3H_2O$. (M_r 266.3). *1155300.* [22763-03-7].

White or almost white crystalline powder, freely soluble in water.

Trisodium phosphate dodecahydrate. $Na_3PO_4,12H_2O$. (M_r 380.1). *1094300.* [10101-89-0].

Colourless or white crystals, freely soluble in water.

Trypsin. *1094500.* [9002-07-7].

A proteolytic enzyme obtained by activation of trypsinogen extracted from the pancreas of beef (*Bos taurus* L.).

A white, crystalline or amorphous powder, sparingly soluble in water.

Trypsin for peptide mapping. *1094600.* [9002-07-7].

Trypsin of high purity treated to eliminate chymotryptic activity.

Tryptophan. $C_{11}H_{12}N_2O_2$. (M_r 204.2). *1094700.* [73-22-3].

A white or yellowish-white, crystalline powder or colourless crystals, slightly soluble in water, very slightly soluble in alcohol.

$[\alpha]_D^{20}$: about −30, determined on a 10 g/l solution.

Tyramine. $C_8H_{11}NO$. (M_r 137.2). *1117600.* [51-67-2].
4-(2-Aminoethyl)phenol.

Crystals, sparingly soluble in water, soluble in boiling ethanol.

mp: 164 °C to 165 °C.

Tyrosine. $C_9H_{11}NO_3$. (M_r 181.2). *1094800.* [60-18-4].
2-Amino-3-(4-hydroxyphenyl)propionic acid.

A white, crystalline powder or colourless or white crystals, slightly soluble in water, practically insoluble in acetone and in ethanol, soluble in dilute hydrochloric acid and in solutions of alkali hydroxides.

Chromatography. Examine as prescribed in the monograph on *Levodopa (0038)*; the chromatogram shows only one principal spot.

Umbelliferone. $C_9H_6O_3$. (M_r 162.1). *1137500.* [93-35-6].
7-Hydroxycoumarin. 7-Hydroxy-2*H*-1-benzopyran-2-one.

Needles from water.

mp: 225 °C to 228 °C.

Urea. *1095000.* [57-13-6].
See *Urea (0743).*

Uridine. $C_9H_{12}N_2O_6$. (M_r 244.2). *1095100.* [58-96-8].
1-β-D-Ribofuranosyluracil.

A white or almost white, crystalline powder, soluble in water.

mp: about 165 °C.

Ursolic acid. $C_{30}H_{48}O_3$. (M_r 456.7). *1141600.* [77-52-1].
(3β)-3-Hydroxyurs-12-en-28-oic acid.

White powder, practically insoluble in water, sparingly soluble in methanol, slightly soluble in alcohol.

$[\alpha]_D^{21}$: about 67.50 (10 g/l solution in a 56.1 g/l solution of *potassium hydroxide R* in *alcohol R*).

mp: 285 °C to 288 °C.

Valencene. $C_{15}H_{24}$. (M_r 204.4). *1152100.*
[4630-07-3]. 4β*H*,5α-Eremophila-1(10),11-diene.
(1*R*,7*R*,8a*S*)-1,8a-Dimethyl-7-(1-methylethenyl)-1,2,3,5,6,7,8,8a-octahydronaphthalene.

Oily, colourless to pale yellow liquid, with a characteristic odour, practically insoluble in water, soluble in alcohol.

d_4^{20} : about 0.918.

n_D^{20} : about 1.508.

bp: about 123 °C.

Valencene used in gas chromatography complies with the following additional test.

Assay. Examine by gas chromatography (*2.2.28*) as prescribed in the monograph on *Sweet orange oil (1811).*

The content is not less than 90 per cent, calculated by the normalisation procedure.

Valeric acid. $C_5H_{10}O_2$. (M_r 102.1). *1095200.* [109-52-4].
Pentanoic acid.

A colourless liquid, soluble in water, freely soluble in alcohol.

d_{20}^{20} : about 0.94.

n_D^{20} : about 1.409.

bp: about 186 °C.

Vanillin. *1095300.* [121-33-5].
See *Vanillin (0747).*

Vanillin reagent. *1095301.*

Carefully add, dropwise, 2 ml of *sulphuric acid R* to 100 ml of a 10 g/l solution of *vanillin R* in *alcohol R.*

Storage: use within 48 h.

Vanillin solution, phosphoric. *1095302.*

Dissolve 1.0 g of *vanillin R* in 25 ml of *alcohol R.* Add 25 ml of *water R* and 35 ml of *phosphoric acid R.*

Verbenone. $C_{10}H_{14}O$. (M_r 150.2). *1140500.* [1196-01-6].
(1*S*,5*S*)-4,6,6-Trimethylbicyclo[3.1.1]hept-3-en-2-one.

Oil with a characteristic odour, practically insoluble in water, miscible with organic solvents.

d_{20}^{20} : about 0.978.

n_D^{18} : about 1.49.

$[\alpha]_D^{18}$: about + 249.6.

bp: 227 °C to 228 °C.

mp: about 6.5 °C.

Verbenone used in gas chromatography complies with the following additional test.

Assay. Examine by gas chromatography (*2.2.28*) as prescribed in the monograph on *Rosemary oil (1846).*

The content is not less than 99 per cent, calculated by the normalisation procedure.

Vinyl acetate. $C_4H_6O_2$. (M_r 86,10). *1111800.* [108-05-4].
Ethenyl acetate.

d_{20}^{20} : about 0.930.

bp: about 72 °C.

Vinyl chloride. C_2H_3Cl. (M_r 62.5). *1095400.* [75-01-4].

A colourless gas, slightly soluble in organic solvents.

Vinyl polymer for chromatography, octadecyl. *1155400.*

Spherical particles (5 μm) of a vinyl alcohol copolymer chemically modified by bonding of octadecyl groups on the hydroxyl groups.

Vinyl polymer for chromatography, octadecylsilyl. *1121600.*

Spherical particles (5 µm) of a vinyl alcohol copolymer bonded to an octadecylsilane. Carbon content of 17 per cent.

2-Vinylpyridine. C_7H_7N. (M_r 105.1). *1102200.* [100-69-6].

A yellow liquid, miscible in water.

d_{20}^{20}: about 0.97.

n_D^{20}: about 1.549.

1-Vinylpyrrolidin-2-one. C_6H_9NO. (M_r 111.1). *1111900.* [88-12-0]. 1-Ethenylpyrrolidin-2-one.

Content: minimum 99.0 per cent of C_6H_9NO.

A clear colourless liquid.

Water (*2.5.12*): maximum 0.1 per cent, determined on 2.5 g. Use as the solvent, a mixture of 50 ml of *anhydrous methanol R* and 10 ml of *butyrolactone R*.

Assay. Examine by gas chromatography (*2.2.28*).

The chromatography may be carried out using

- a fused-silica column 30 m long and 0.5 mm in internal diameter the inner wall of which is coated with a 1.0 µm layer of *macrogol 20 000 R*,
- *helium for chromatography R* as the carrier gas,
- a flame-ionisation detector,

maintaining the temperature of the injection port at 190 °C and programming the temperature of the column as follows: maintain the temperature at 80 °C for 1 min and then increase it to 190 °C at a rate of 10 °C per minute. Maintain at 190 °C for 15 min. Inject 0.3 µl of the substance to be examined and adjust the flow rate of the carrier gas so that the retention time of the peak corresponding to 1-vinylpyrrolidin-2-one is about 17 min. Determine the content of C_6H_9NO by internal normalisation.

Vitexin. $C_{21}H_{20}O_{10}$. (M_r 448.4). *1133300.* [3681-93-4]. Apigenin 8-glucoside.

Yellow powder.

Storage: in an airtight container, protected from light.

Water. *1095500.* [7732-18-5].

See *Purified water (0008)*.

Water R1. *1095508.*

Prepared from *distilled water R* by multiple distillation. Remove carbon dioxide by boiling for at least 15 min before use in a boiling flask of fused silica or borosilicate glass and cool. Any other suitable method may be used. The boiling flask has been already used for the test or has been filled with *water R* and kept in an autoclave at 121 °C for at least 1 h prior to first use. When tested immediately before use, *water R1* is neutral to *methyl red solution R*, i.e. it shall produce an orange-red (not a violet-red or yellow) colour corresponding to pH 5.5 ± 0.1 when 0.05 ml of *methyl red solution R* is added to 50 ml of the water to be examined.

Conductivity: maximum 1 µS·cm^{-1}, determined at 25 °C by an in-line conductivity meter (see *Purified water (0008)*).

Water, ammonium-free. *1095501.* [7732-18-5].

To 100 ml of *water R* add 0.1 ml of *sulphuric acid R*. Distil using the apparatus described for the determination of *Distillation range* (*2.2.11*). Reject the first 10 ml and collect the following 50 ml.

Water, carbon dioxide-free. *1095502.* [7732-18-5].

Water R which has been boiled for a few minutes and protected from the atmosphere during cooling and storage.

Water for chromatography. *1095503.* [7732-18-5].

Deionised *water R* with a resistivity of not less than 0.18 Mohm·m.

Water, distilled. *1095504.* [7732-18-5].

Water R prepared by distillation.

Water, distilled, deionised. *1095508.*

Deionised *water R* prepared by distillation with a resistivity of not less than 18 Mohm·m.

Water for injections. *1095505.* [7732-18-5].

See *Water for injections (0169)*.

Water, nitrate-free. *1095506.* [7732-18-5].

To 100 ml of *water R* add a few milligrams of *potassium permanganate R* and of *barium hydroxide R*. Distil using the apparatus described for the determination of *Distillation range* (*2.2.11*). Reject the first 10 ml and collect the following 50 ml.

Water, particle-free. *1095507.* [7732-18-5].

Filter *water R* through a membrane with a pore size of 0.22 µm.

Weak cationic resin. *1096000.*

Polymethacrylic resin, slightly acid, with carboxyl groups present in a protonated form.

Particle size: 75 µm to 160 µm.

pH limits of use: 5 to 14.

Maximum temperature of use: 120 °C.

Xanthydrol. $C_{13}H_{10}O_2$. (M_r 198.2). *1096100.* [90-46-0]. 9-Xanthenol.

Content: minimum 90.0 per cent of $C_{13}H_{10}O_2$.

A white to pale-yellow powder, very slightly soluble in water, soluble in alcohol and in glacial acetic acid.

It is also available as a methanolic solution containing 90 g/l to 110 g/l of xanthydrol.

mp: about 123 °C.

Assay. In a 250 ml flask dissolve 0.300 g in 3 ml of *methanol R* or use 3.0 ml of solution. Add 50 ml of *glacial acetic acid R* and, dropwise with shaking, 25 ml of a 20 g/l solution of *urea R*. Allow to stand for 12 h, collect the precipitate on a sintered-glass filter (16), wash with 20 ml of *alcohol R*, dry in an oven at 100 °C to 105 °C and weigh.

1 g of precipitate is equivalent to 0.9429 g of xanthydrol.

Storage: protected from light. If a methanolic solution is used, store in small sealed ampoules and filter before use if necessary.

Xanthydrol R1. *1096101.*

Complies with the requirements prescribed for *xanthydrol R* and with the following requirement.

Content: minimum 98.0 per cent of $C_{13}H_{10}O_2$.

Xanthydrol solution. *1096102.*

To 0.1 ml of a 100 g/l solution of *xanthydrol R* in *methanol R* add 100 ml of *anhydrous acetic acid R* and 1 ml of *hydrochloric acid R*. Allow to stand for 24 h before using.

Xylene. C_8H_{10}. (M_r 106.2). *1096200.* [1330-20-7].

Mixture of isomers. A clear, colourless, flammable liquid, practically insoluble in water, miscible with alcohol.

d_{20}^{20}: about 0.867.

n_D^{20}: about 1.497.

bp: about 138 °C.

***m*-Xylene.** C_8H_{10}. (M_r 106.2). *1117700.* [108-38-3]. 1,3-Dimethylbenzene.

A clear, colourless, flammable liquid, practically insoluble in water, miscible with alcohol.

d_{20}^{20}: about 0.884.

n_D^{20}: about 1.497.

bp: about 139 °C.

mp: about −47 °C.

***o*-Xylene.** C_8H_{10}. (M_r 106.2). *1100600.* [95-47-6]. 1,2-Dimethylbenzene.

A clear, colourless, flammable liquid, practically insoluble in water, miscible with alcohol.

d_{20}^{20}: about 0.881.

n_D^{20}: about 1.505.

bp: about 144 °C.

mp: about −25 °C.

Xylenol orange. $C_{31}H_{28}N_2Na_4O_{13}S$. ($M_r$ 761). *1096300.* [3618-43-7]. Tetrasodium 3,3′-(3*H*-2,1-benzoxathiol-3-ylidene)bis[(6-hydroxy-5-methyl-3,1-phenylene)methyleneiminobisacetate] *S,S*-dioxide.

A reddish-brown crystalline powder, soluble in water.

Xylenol orange triturate. *1096301.*

Triturate 1 part of *xylenol orange R* with 99 parts of *potassium nitrate R.*

Test for sensitivity. To 50 ml of *water R* add 1 ml of *dilute acetic acid R*, 50 mg of the xylenol orange triturate and 0.05 ml of *lead nitrate solution R.* Add *hexamethylenetetramine R* until the colour changes from yellow to violet-red. After addition of 0.1 ml of *0.1 M sodium edetate* the colour changes to yellow.

Xylose. *1096400.* [58-86-6].

See *Xylose (1278).*

Zinc. Zn. (A_r 65.4). *1096500.* [7440-66-6].

Content: minimum 99.5 per cent of Zn.

Silver-white cylinders, granules, pellets or filings with a blue sheen.

Arsenic (2.4.2). 5.0 g complies with limit test A (0.2 ppm). Dissolve in a mixture of the 15 ml of *hydrochloric acid R* and 25 ml of *water R* prescribed.

Zinc, activated. *1096501.*

Place the zinc cylinders or pellets to be activated in a conical flask and add a sufficient quantity of a 50 ppm solution of *chloroplatinic acid R* to cover the metal. Allow the metal to remain in contact with the solution for 10 min, wash, drain and dry immediately.

Arsenic. To 5 g of the activated zinc add 15 ml of *hydrochloric acid R,* 25 ml of *water R,* 0.1 ml of *stannous chloride solution R* and 5 ml of *potassium iodide solution R.* Treat as described in limit test A for arsenic *(2.4.2).* No stain is produced on the *mercuric bromide paper R.*

Activity. Repeat the test for arsenic using the same reagents and adding a solution containing 1 µg of arsenic. An appreciable stain appears on the *mercuric bromide paper R.*

Zinc acetate. $(C_2H_3O_2)_2Zn,2H_2O$. (M_r 219.5). *1102300.* [5970-45-6]. Zinc acetate dihydrate.

Bright white crystals, slightly efflorescent, freely soluble in water, soluble in alcohol. It loses its crystallisation water at 100 °C.

d_{20}^{20}: about 1.735.

mp: about 237 °C.

Zinc acetate solution. *1102301.*

Mix 600 ml of *water R* with 150 ml of *glacial acetic acid R,* 54.9 g of *zinc acetate R* and stir to dissolve. Continue stirring while adding 150 ml of *concentrated ammonia R.* Cool to room temperature and adjust with *ammonia R* to pH 6.4. Dilute the mixture to 1 litre with *water R.*

Zinc chloride. *1096600.* [7646-85-7].

See *Zinc chloride (0110).*

Zinc chloride-formic acid solution. *1096601.*

Dissolve 20 g of *zinc chloride R* in 80 g of an 850 g/l solution of *anhydrous formic acid R.*

Zinc chloride solution, iodinated. *1096602.*

Dissolve 20 g of *zinc chloride R* and 6.5 g of *potassium iodide R* in 10.5 ml of *water R.* Add 0.5 g of *iodine R* and shake for 15 min. Filter if necessary.

Storage: protected from light.

Zinc iodide and starch solution. *1096502.*

To a solution of 2 g of *zinc chloride R* in 10 ml of *water R* add 0.4 g of *soluble starch R* and heat until the starch has dissolved. After cooling to room temperature add 1.0 ml of a colourless solution containing 0.10 g *zinc R* as filings and 0.2 g of *iodine R* in *water R.* Dilute the solution to 100 ml with *water R* and filter.

Storage: protected from light.

Test for sensitivity. Dilute 0.05 ml of *sodium nitrite solution R* to 50 ml with *water R.* To 5 ml of this solution add 0.1 ml of *dilute sulphuric acid R* and 0.05 ml of the zinc iodide and starch solution and mix. The solution becomes blue.

Zinc oxide. *1096700.* [1314-13-2].

See *Zinc oxide (0252).*

Zinc powder. Zn. (A_r 65.4). *1096800.* [7440-66-6].

Content: minimum 90.0 per cent of Zn (A_r 65.4).

A very fine, grey powder, soluble in *dilute hydrochloric acid R.*

Zinc sulphate. *1097000.* [7446-20-0].

See *Zinc sulphate (0111).*

Zirconyl chloride. A basic salt corresponding approximately to the formula $ZrCl_2O, 8H_2O$. *1097100.* [15461-27-5].

Content: minimum 96.0 per cent of $ZrCl_2O,8H_2O$.

White or almost white, crystalline powder or crystals, freely soluble in water and in alcohol.

Assay. Dissolve 0.600 g in a mixture of 5 ml of *nitric acid R* and 50 ml of *water R.* Add 50.0 ml of *0.1 M silver nitrate* and 3 ml of *dibutyl phthalate R* and shake. Using 2 ml of *ferric ammonium sulphate solution R2* as indicator, titrate with *0.1 M ammonium thiocyanate* until a reddish-yellow colour is obtained.

1 ml of *0.1 M silver nitrate* is equivalent to 16.11 mg of $ZrCl_2O,8H_2O$.

Zirconyl nitrate. A basic salt corresponding approximately to the formula $ZrO(NO_3)_2,2H_2O$. *1097200*. [14985-18-3].

A white powder or crystals, hygroscopic, soluble in water. The aqueous solution is a clear or at most slightly opalescent liquid.

Storage: in an airtight container.

Zirconyl nitrate solution. *1097201.*

A 1 g/l solution in a mixture of 40 ml of *water R* and 60 ml of *hydrochloric acid R*.

01/2005:40102

4.1.2. STANDARD SOLUTIONS FOR LIMIT TESTS

Acetaldehyde standard solution (100 ppm C_2H_4O). *5000100.*

Dissolve 1.0 g of *acetaldehyde R* in *2-propanol R* and dilute to 100.0 ml with the same solvent. Dilute 5.0 ml of the solution to 500.0 ml with *2-propanol R*. Prepare immediately before use.

Acetaldehyde standard solution (100 ppm C_2H_4O) R1. *5000101.*

Dissolve 1.0 g of *acetaldehyde R* in *water R* and dilute to 100.0 ml with the same solvent. Dilute 5.0 ml of the solution to 500.0 ml with *water R*. Prepare immediately before use.

Aluminium standard solution (200 ppm Al). *5000200.*

Dissolve in *water R* a quantity of *aluminium potassium sulphate R* equivalent to 0.352 g of $AlK(SO_4)_2,12H_2O$. Add 10 ml of *dilute sulphuric acid R* and dilute to 100.0 ml with *water R*.

Aluminium standard solution (100 ppm Al). *5000203.*

Immediately before use, dilute with *water R* to 10 times its volume a solution containing 8.947 g of *aluminium chloride R* in 1000.0 ml of *water R*.

Aluminium standard solution (10 ppm Al). *5000201.*

Immediately before use, dilute with *water R* to 100 times its volume in a solution containing *aluminium nitrate R* equivalent to 1.39 g of $Al(NO_3)_3,9H_2O$ in 100.0 ml.

Aluminium standard solution (2 ppm Al). *5000202.*

Immediately before use, dilute with *water R* to 100 times its volume a solution containing *aluminium potassium sulphate R* equivalent to 0.352 g of $AlK(SO_4)_2,12H_2O$ and 10 ml of *dilute sulphuric acid R* in 100.0 ml.

Ammonium standard solution (100 ppm NH_4). *5000300.*

Immediately before use, dilute to 25 ml with *water R* 10 ml of a solution containing *ammonium chloride R* equivalent to 0.741 g of NH_4Cl in 1000 ml.

Ammonium standard solution (2.5 ppm NH_4). *5000301.*

Immediately before use, dilute with *water R* to 100 times its volume a solution containing *ammonium chloride R* equivalent to 0.741 g of NH_4Cl in 1000.0 ml.

Ammonium standard solution (1 ppm NH_4). *5000302.*

Immediately before use, dilute ammonium standard solution (2.5 ppm NH_4) R to 2.5 times its volume with *water R*.

Antimony standard solution (100 ppm Sb). *5000401.*

Dissolve *antimony potassium tartrate R* equivalent to 0.274 g of $C_4H_4KO_7Sb,{}^1/_2H_2O$ in 500 ml of *1M hydrochloric acid* and dilute the clear solution to 1000 ml with *water R*.

Antimony standard solution (1 ppm Sb). *5000400.*

Dissolve *antimony potassium tartrate R* equivalent to 0.274 g of $C_4H_4KO_7Sb,{}^1/_2H_2O$ in 20 ml of *hydrochloric acid R1* and dilute the clear solution to 100.0 ml with *water R*. To 10.0 ml of this solution add 200 ml of *hydrochloric acid R1* and dilute to 1000.0 ml with *water R*. To 100.0 ml of this solution add 300 ml of *hydrochloric acid R1* and dilute to 1000.0 ml with *water R*. Prepare the dilute solutions immediately before use.

Arsenic standard solution (10 ppm As). *5000500.*

Immediately before use, dilute with *water R* to 100 times its volume a solution prepared by dissolving *arsenious trioxide R* equivalent to 0.330 g of As_2O_3 in 5 ml of *dilute sodium hydroxide solution R* and diluting to 250.0 ml with *water R*.

Arsenic standard solution (1 ppm As). *5000501.*

Immediately before use, dilute *arsenic standard solution (10 ppm As) R* to 10 times its volume with *water R*.

Arsenic standard solution (0.1 ppm As). *5000502.*

Immediately before use, dilute *arsenic standard solution (1 ppm As) R* to 10 times its volume with *water R*.

Barium standard solution (50 ppm Ba). *5000600.*

Immediately before use, dilute with *distilled water R* to 20 times its volume a solution in *distilled water R* containing *barium chloride R* equivalent to 0.178 g of $BaCl_2,2H_2O$ in 100.0 ml.

Bismuth standard solution (100 ppm Bi). *5005300.*

Dissolve *bismuth R* equivalent to 0.500 g of Bi in 50 ml of *nitric acid R* and dilute to 500.0 ml with *water R*. Dilute the solution to 10 times its volume with *dilute nitric acid R* immediately before use.

Cadmium standard solution (0.1 per cent Cd). *5000700.*

Dissolve *cadmium R* equivalent to 0.100 g of Cd in the smallest necessary amount of a mixture of equal volumes of *hydrochloric acid R* and *water R* and dilute to 100.0 ml with a 1 per cent *V/V* solution of *hydrochloric acid R*.

Cadmium standard solution (10 ppm Cd) . *5000701.*

Immediately before use, dilute *cadmium standard solution (0.1 per cent Cd) R* to 100 times its volume with a 1 per cent *V/V* solution of *hydrochloric acid R*.

Calcium standard solution (400 ppm Ca). *5000800.*

Immediately before use, dilute with *distilled water R* to 10 times its volume a solution in *distilled water R* containing *calcium carbonate R* equivalent to 1.000 g of $CaCO_3$ and 23 ml of *1 M hydrochloric acid* in 100.0 ml.

Calcium standard solution (100 ppm Ca). *5000801.*

Immediately before use, dilute with *distilled water R* to 10 times its volume a solution in *distilled water R* containing *calcium carbonate R* equivalent to 0.624 g of $CaCO_3$ and 3 ml of *acetic acid R* in 250.0 ml.

Calcium standard solution (100 ppm Ca) R1. *5000804.*

Immediately before use, dilute with *water R* to 10 times its volume a solution containing *anhydrous calcium chloride R* equivalent to 2.769 g of $CaCl_2$ in 1000.0 ml of *dilute hydrochloric acid R*.

Calcium standard solution (100 ppm Ca), alcoholic. *5000802.*

Immediately before use, dilute with *alcohol R* to 10 times its volume a solution in *distilled water R* containing *calcium carbonate R* equivalent to 2.50 g of $CaCO_3$ and 12 ml of *acetic acid R* in 1000.0 ml.

Calcium standard solution (10 ppm Ca). *5000803.*

Immediately before use, dilute with *distilled water R* to 100 times its volume a solution in *distilled water R* containing *calcium carbonate R* equivalent to 0.624 g of $CaCO_3$ and 3 ml of *acetic acid R* in 250.0 ml.

Chloride standard solution (50 ppm Cl). *5004100.*

Immediately before use, dilute with *water R* to 10 times its volume a solution containing *sodium chloride R* equivalent to 0.824 g of NaCl in 1000.0 ml.

Chloride standard solution (8 ppm Cl). *5000900.*

Immediately before use, dilute with *water R* to 100 times its volume a solution containing *sodium chloride R* equivalent to 1.32 g of NaCl in 1000.0 ml.

Chloride standard solution (5 ppm Cl). *5000901.*

Immediately before use, dilute with *water R* to 100 times its volume a solution containing *sodium chloride R* equivalent to 0.824 g of NaCl in 1000.0 ml.

Chromium liposoluble standard solution (1000 ppm Cr). *5004600.*

A chromium (metal) organic compound in an oil.

Chromium standard solution (0.1 per cent Cr). *5001002.*

Dissolve *potassium dichromate R* equivalent to 2.83 g of $K_2Cr_2O_7$ in *water R* and dilute to 1000.0 ml with the same solvent.

Chromium standard solution (100 ppm Cr). *5001000.*

Dissolve *potassium dichromate R* equivalent to 0.283 g of $K_2Cr_2O_7$ in *water R* and dilute to 1000.0 ml with the same solvent.

Chromium standard solution (0.1 ppm Cr). *5001001.*

Immediately before use, dilute *chromium standard solution (100 ppm Cr) R* to 1000 times its volume with *water R.*

Cobalt standard solution (100 ppm Co). *5004300.*

Dissolve *cobalt nitrate R* equivalent to 0.494 g of $Co(NO_3)_2,6H_2O$ in 500 ml of *1M nitric acid* and dilute the clear solution to 1000 ml with *water R.*

Copper liposoluble standard solution (1000 ppm Cu). *5004700.*

A copper (metal) organic compound in an oil.

Copper standard solution (0.1 per cent Cu). *5001100.*

Dissolve *copper sulphate R* equivalent to 0.393 g of $CuSO_4,5H_2O$ in *water R* and dilute to 100.0 ml with the same solvent.

Copper standard solution (10 ppm Cu). *5001101.*

Immediately before use, dilute *copper standard solution (0.1 per cent Cu) R* to 100 times its volume with *water R.*

Copper standard solution (0.1 ppm Cu). *5001102.*

Immediately before use, dilute *copper standard solution (10 ppm Cu) R* to 100 times its volume with *water R.*

Ferrocyanide standard solution (100 ppm $Fe(CN)_6$). *5001200.*

Immediately before use, dilute with *water R* to 10 times its volume a solution containing *potassium ferrocyanide R* equivalent to 0.20 g of $K_4Fe(CN)_6,3H_2O$ in 100.0 ml.

Ferricyanide standard solution (50 ppm $Fe(CN)_6$). *5001300.*

Immediately before use, dilute with *water R* to 100 times its volume a solution containing *potassium ferricyanide R* equivalent to 0.78 g of $K_3Fe(CN)_6$ in 100.0 ml.

Fluoride standard solution (10 ppm F). *5001400.*

Dissolve in *water R sodium fluoride R* previously dried at 300 °C for 12 h, equivalent to 0.442 g of NaF, and dilute to 1000.0 ml with the same solvent (1 ml = 0.2 mg F). Store in a polyethylene container. Immediately before use, dilute the solution to 20 times its volume with *water R.*

Fluoride standard solution (1 ppm F). *5001401.*

Immediately before use, dilute *fluoride standard solution (10 ppm F) R* to 10 times its volume with *water R.*

Formaldehyde standard solution (5 ppm CH_2O). *5001500.*

Immediately before use, dilute with *water R* to 200 times its volume a solution containing 1.0 g of CH_2O per litre prepared from *formaldehyde solution R.*

Germanium standard solution (100 ppm Ge). *5004400.*

Dissolve *ammonium hexafluorogermanate (IV) R* equivalent to 0.307 g of $(NH_4)_2GeF_6$ in a 0.01 per cent *V/V* solution of *hydrofluoric acid R.* Dilute the clear solution to 1000 ml with *water R.*

Glyoxal standard solution (20 ppm $C_2H_2O_2$). *5003700.*

In a 100 ml graduated flask weigh a quantity of *glyoxal solution R* corresponding to 0.200 g of $C_2H_2O_2$ and make up to volume with *ethanol R.* Immediately before use dilute the solution to 100 times its volume with the same solvent.

Glyoxal standard solution (2 ppm $C_2H_2O_2$). *5003701.*

Immediately before use, dilute *glyoxal standard solution (20 ppm $C_2H_2O_2$) R* to 10 times its volume with *ethanol R.*

Hydrogen peroxide standard solution (10 ppm H_2O_2). *5005200.*

Dilute 10.0 ml of *dilute hydrogen peroxide solution R* to 300.0 ml with *water R.* Dilute 10.0 ml of this solution to 1000.0 ml with *water R.* Prepare immediately before use.

Iodide standard solution (10 ppm I). *5003800.*

Immediately before use, dilute with *water R* to 100 times its volume a solution containing *potassium iodide R* equivalent to 0.131 g of KI in 100.0 ml.

Iron standard solution (0.1 per cent Fe). *5001605.*

Dissolve 0.100 g of Fe in the smallest amount necessary of a mixture of equal volumes of *hydrochloric acid R* and *water R* and dilute to 100.0 ml with *water R.*

Iron standard solution (250 ppm Fe). *5001606.*

Immediately before use, dilute with *water R* to 40 times its volume a solution containing 4.840 g of *ferric chloride R* in a 150 g/l solution of *hydrochloric acid R* diluted to 100.0 ml.

Iron standard solution (20 ppm Fe). *5001600.*

Immediately before use, dilute with *water R* to 10 times its volume a solution containing *ferric ammonium sulphate R* equivalent to 0.863 g of $FeNH_4(SO_4)_2,12H_2O$ and 25 ml of *dilute sulphuric acid R* in 500.0 ml.

Iron standard solution (10 ppm Fe). *5001601.*
Immediately before use, dilute with *water R* to 100 times its volume a solution containing *ferrous ammonium sulphate R* equivalent to 7.022 g of $Fe(NH_4)_2(SO_4)_2,6H_2O$ and 25 ml of *dilute sulphuric acid R* in 1000.0 ml.

Iron standard solution (8 ppm Fe). *5001602.*
Immediately before use, dilute with *water R* to 10 times its volume a solution containing 80 mg of *iron R* and 50 ml of *hydrochloric acid R* (220 g/l HCl) in 1000.0 ml.

Iron standard solution (2 ppm Fe). *5001603.*
Immediately before use, dilute *iron standard solution (20 ppm Fe) R* to 10 times its volume with *water R.*

Iron standard solution (1 ppm Fe). *5001604.*
Immediately before use, dilute *iron standard solution (20 ppm Fe) R* to 20 times its volume with *water R.*

Lead liposoluble standard solution (1000 ppm Pb). *5004800.*
A lead (metal) organic compound in an oil.

Lead standard solution (0.1 per cent Pb). *5001700.*
Dissolve *lead nitrate R* equivalent to 0.400 g of $Pb(NO_3)_2$ in *water R* and dilute to 250.0 ml with the same solvent.

Lead standard solution (0.1 per cent Pb) R1. *5005400.*
Dissolve in *dilute lead-free nitric acid R* a quantity of *lead nitrate R* equivalent to 0.400 g of Pb $(NO_3)_2$ and dilute to 250.0 ml with the same solvent.

Lead standard solution (100 ppm Pb). *5001701.*
Immediately before use, dilute *lead standard solution (0.1 per cent Pb) R* to 10 times its volume with *water R.*

Lead standard solution (10 ppm Pb). *5001702.*
Immediately before use, dilute *lead standard solution (100 ppm Pb) R* to 10 times its volume with *water R.*

Lead standard solution (10 ppm Pb) R1. *5001706.*
Immediately before use, dilute with *water R* to 10 times its volume a solution containing 0.160 g of *lead nitrate R* in 100 ml of *water R*, to which is added 1 ml of *lead-free nitric acid R* and dilute to 1000.0 ml.

Lead standard solution (10 ppm Pb) R2. *5005401.*
Dilute *lead standard solution (0.1 per cent Pb) R1* to 100 times its volume with *dilute lead-free nitric acid R*. Use within 1 week.

Lead standard solution (2 ppm Pb). *5001703.*
Immediately before use, dilute *lead standard solution (10 ppm Pb) R* to 5 times its volume with *water R.*

Lead standard solution (1 ppm Pb). *5001704.*
Immediately before use, dilute *lead standard solution (10 ppm Pb) R* to 10 times its volume with *water R.*

Lead standard solution (0.5 ppm Pb). *5005402.*
Dilute *lead standard solution (10 ppm Pb) R2* to 20 times its volume with *dilute lead-free nitric acid R*. Use within 1 day.

Lead standard solution (0.1 ppm Pb). *5001705.*
Immediately before use, dilute *lead standard solution (1 ppm Pb) R* to 10 times its volume with *water R.*

Magnesium standard solution (100 ppm Mg). *5001800.*
Immediately before use, dilute with *water R* to 10 times its volume a solution containing *magnesium sulphate R* equivalent to 1.010 g of $MgSO_4,7H_2O$ in 100.0 ml.

Magnesium standard solution (10 ppm Mg). *5001801.*
Immediately before use, dilute magnesium standard solution (100 ppm Mg) R to 10 times its volume with *water R.*

Magnesium standard solution (10 ppm Mg) R1. *5001802.*
Immediately before use, dilute with *water R* to 100 times its volume a solution containing 8.365 g of *magnesium chloride R* in 1000.0 ml of *dilute hydrochloric acid R.*

Manganese standard solution (100 ppm Mn). *5004500.*
Dissolve *manganese sulphate R* equivalent to 0.308 g of $MnSO_4,H_2O$ in 500 ml of *1M nitric acid* and dilute the clear solution to 1000 ml with *water R.*

Mercury standard solution (1000 ppm Hg). *5001900.*
Dissolve *mercuric chloride R* equivalent to 1.354 g of $HgCl_2$ in 50 ml of *dilute nitric acid R* and dilute to 1000.0 ml with *water R.*

Mercury standard solution (10 ppm Hg). *5001901.*
Immediately before use, dilute with water to 100 times its volume a solution containing *mercuric chloride R* equivalent to 0.338 g of $HgCl_2$ in 250.0 ml.

Nickel liposoluble standard solution (1000 ppm Ni). *5004900.*
A nickel (metal) organic compound in an oil.

Nickel standard solution (10 ppm Ni). *5002000.*
Immediately before use, dilute with *water R* to 100 times its volume a solution containing *nickel sulphate R* equivalent to 4.78 g of $NiSO_4,7H_2O$ in 1000.0 ml.

Nickel standard solution (0.2 ppm Ni). *5002002.*
Immediately before use, dilute *nickel standard solution (10 ppm Ni) R* to 50 times its volume with *water R.*

Nickel standard solution (0.1 ppm Ni). *5002001.*
Immediately before use, dilute *nickel standard solution (10 ppm Ni) R* to 100 times its volume with *water R.*

Nitrate standard solution (100 ppm NO_3). *5002100.*
Immediately before use, dilute with *water R* to 10 times its volume a solution containing *potassium nitrate R* equivalent to 0.815 g of KNO_3 in 500.0 ml.

Nitrate standard solution (10 ppm NO_3). *5002101.*
Immediately before use, dilute *nitrate standard solution (100 ppm NO_3) R* to 10 times its volume with *water R.*

Nitrate standard solution (2 ppm NO_3). *5002102.*
Immediately before use, dilute *nitrate standard solution (10 ppm NO_3) R* to 5 times its volume with *water R.*

Palladium standard solution (500 ppm Pd). *5003600.*
Dissolve 50.0 mg of *palladium R* in 9 ml of *hydrochloric acid R* and dilute to 100.0 ml with *water R.*

Palladium standard solution (20 ppm Pd). *5003602.*
Dissolve 0.333 g of *palladium chloride R* in 2 ml of warm *hydrochloric acid R*. Dilute the solution to 1000.0 ml with a mixture of equal volumes of *dilute hydrochloric acid R* and *water R*. Immediately before use dilute to 10 times its volume with *water R.*

Palladium standard solution (0.5 ppm Pd). *5003601.*
Dilute 1 ml of *palladium standard solution (500 ppm Pd) R* to 1000 ml with a mixture of 0.3 volumes of *nitric acid R* and 99.7 volumes of *water R.*

Phosphate standard solution (200 ppm PO_4). *5004200.*
Dissolve *potassium dihydrogen phosphate R* equivalent to 0.286 g of KH_2PO_4 in *water R* and dilute to 1000.0 ml with the same solvent.

Phosphate standard solution (5 ppm PO_4). *5002200.*
Immediately before use, dilute with *water R* to 100 times its volume a solution containing *potassium dihydrogen phosphate R* equivalent to 0.716 g of KH_2PO_4 in 1000.0 ml.

Platinum standard solution (30 ppm Pt). *5002300.*
Immediately before use, dilute with *1 M hydrochloric acid* to 10 times its volume a solution containing 80 mg of *chloroplatinic acid R* in 100.0 ml of *1 M hydrochloric acid.*

Potassium standard solution (600 ppm K). *5005100.*
Immediately before use, dilute with *water R* to 20 times its volume a solution containing *dipotassium sulphate R* equivalent to 2.676 g of K_2SO_4 in 100.0 ml.

Potassium standard solution (100 ppm K). *5002400.*
Immediately before use, dilute with *water R* to 20 times its volume a solution containing *dipotassium sulphate R* equivalent to 0.446 g of K_2SO_4 in 100.0 ml.

Potassium standard solution (20 ppm K). *5002401.*
Immediately before use, dilute *potassium standard solution (100 ppm K) R* to 5 times its volume with *water R.*

Selenium standard solution (100 ppm Se). *5002500.*
Dissolve 0.100 g of *selenium R* in 2 ml of *nitric acid R.* Evaporate to dryness. Take up the residue in 2 ml of *water R* and evaporate to dryness; carry out three times. Dissolve the residue in 50 ml of *dilute hydrochloric acid R* and dilute to 1000.0 ml with the same acid.

Selenium standard solution (1 ppm Se). *5002501.*
Immediately before use, dilute with *water R* to 40 times its volume a solution containing *selenious acid R* equivalent to 6.54 mg of H_2SeO_3 in 100.0 ml.

Silver standard solution (5 ppm Ag). *5002600.*
Immediately before use, dilute with *water R* to 100 times its volume a solution containing *silver nitrate R* equivalent to 0.790 g of $AgNO_3$ in 1000.0 ml.

Sodium standard solution (200 ppm Na). *5002700.*
Immediately before use, dilute with *water R* to 10 times its volume a solution containing *sodium chloride R* equivalent to 0.509 g of NaCl in 100.0 ml.

Sodium standard solution (50 ppm Na). *5002701.*
Dilute the *sodium standard solution (200 ppm Na) R* to four times its volume with *water R.*

Strontium standard solution (1.0 per cent Sr). *5003900.*
Cover with *water R, strontium carbonate R* equivalent to 1.6849 g of $SrCO_3$. Cautiously add *hydrochloric acid R* until all the solid has dissolved and there is no sign of further effervescence. Dilute to 100.0 ml with *water R.*

Sulphate standard solution (100 ppm SO_4). *5002802.*
Immediately before use, dilute with *distilled water R* to 10 times its volume a solution in *distilled water R* containing *dipotassium sulphate R* equivalent to 0.181 g of K_2SO_4 in 100.0 ml.

Sulphate standard solution (10 ppm SO_4). *5002800.*
Immediately before use, dilute with *distilled water R* to 100 times its volume a solution in *distilled water R* containing *dipotassium sulphate R* equivalent to 0.181 g of K_2SO_4 in 100.0 ml.

Sulphate standard solution (10 ppm SO_4) R1. *5002801.*
Immediately before use, dilute with *alcohol (30 per cent V/V) R* to 100 times its volume a solution containing *dipotassium sulphate R* equivalent to 0.181 g of K_2SO_4 in 100.0 ml of *alcohol (30 per cent V/V) R.*

Sulphite standard solution (80 ppm SO_2). *5005500.*
Dissolve 3.150 g of *anhydrous sodium sulphite R* in freshly prepared *distilled water R* and dilute to 100.0 ml with the same solvent. Dilute 0.5 ml to 100.0 ml with freshly prepared *distilled water R.*

Sulphite standard solution (1.5 ppm SO_2). *5002900.*
Dissolve *sodium metabisulphite R* equivalent to 0.152 g of $Na_2S_2O_5$ in *water R* and dilute to 100.0 ml with the same solvent. Dilute 5.0 ml of this solution to 100.0 ml with *water R.* To 3.0 ml of the resulting solution, add 4.0 ml of *0.1 M sodium hydroxide* and dilute to 100.0 ml with *water R.*

Thallium standard solution (10 ppm Tl). *5003000.*
Dissolve *thallous sulphate R* equivalent to 0.1235 g of Tl_2SO_4 in a 9 g/l solution of *sodium chloride R* and dilute to 1000.0 ml with the same solution. Dilute 10.0 ml of the solution to 100.0 ml with the 9 g/l solution of *sodium chloride R.*

Tin liposoluble standard solution (1000 ppm Sn). *5005000.*
A tin metal organic compound in an oil.

Tin standard solution (5 ppm Sn). *5003100.*
Dissolve *tin R* equivalent to 0.500 g of Sn in a mixture of 5 ml of *water R* and 25 ml of *hydrochloric acid R* and dilute to 1000.0 ml with *water R.* Dilute the solution to 100 times its volume with a 2.5 per cent *V/V* solution of *hydrochloric acid R* immediately before use.

Tin standard solution (0.1 ppm Sn). *5003101.*
Immediately before use, dilute *tin standard solution (5 ppm Sn) R* to 50 times its volume with *water R.*

Titanium standard solution (100 ppm Ti). *5003200.*
Dissolve 100.0 mg of *titanium R* in 100 ml of *hydrochloric acid R* diluted to 150 ml with *water R,* heating if necessary. Allow to cool and dilute to 1000 ml with *water R.*

Vanadium standard solution (1 g/l V). *5003300.*
Dissolve in *water R ammonium vanadate R* equivalent to 0.230 g of NH_4VO_3 and dilute to 100.0 ml with the same solvent.

Zinc standard solution (5 mg/ml Zn). *5003400.*
Dissolve 3.15 g of *zinc oxide R* in 15 ml of *hydrochloric acid R* and dilute to 500.0 ml with *water R.*

Zinc standard solution (100 ppm Zn). *5003401.*
Immediately before use, dilute with *water R* to 10 times its volume a solution containing *zinc sulphate R* equivalent to 0.440 g of $ZnSO_4,7H_2O$ and 1 ml of *acetic acid R* in 100.0 ml.

Zinc standard solution (10 ppm Zn). *5003402.*
Immediately before use, dilute *zinc standard solution (100 ppm Zn) R* to 10 times its volume with *water R.*

Zinc standard solution (5 ppm Zn). *5003403.*
Immediately before use, dilute *zinc standard solution (100 ppm Zn) R* to 20 times its volume with *water R.*

Zirconium standard solution (1 g/l Zr). *5003500.*
Dissolve *zirconyl nitrate R* equivalent to 0.293 g of $ZrO(NO_3)_2,2H_2O$ in a mixture of 2 volumes of *hydrochloric acid R* and 8 volumes of *water R* and dilute to 100.0 ml with the same mixture of solvents.

01/2005:40103

4.1.3. BUFFER SOLUTIONS

Buffered acetone solution. *4000100.*

Dissolve 8.15 g of *sodium acetate R* and 42 g of *sodium chloride R* in *water R*, add 68 ml of *0.1 M hydrochloric acid* and 150 ml of *acetone R* and dilute to 500 ml with *water R*.

Buffer solution pH 2.0. *4000200.*

Dissolve 6.57 g of *potassium chloride R* in *water R* and add 119.0 ml of *0.1 M hydrochloric acid.* Dilute to 1000.0 ml with *water R*.

Phosphate buffer solution pH 2.0. *4007900.*

Dissolve 8.95 g of *disodium hydrogen phosphate R* and 3.40 g of *potassium dihydrogen phosphate R* in *water R* and dilute to 1000.0 ml with the same solvent. If necessary adjust the pH (*2.2.3*) with *phosphoric acid R*.

Sulphate buffer solution pH 2.0. *4008900.*

Dissolve 132.1 g of *ammonium sulphate R* in *water R* and dilute to 500.0 ml with the same solvent (Solution I). Carefully and with constant cooling stir 14 ml of sulphuric acid R into about 400 ml of *water R*; allow to cool and dilute to 500.0 ml with *water R* (Solution II). Mix equal volumes of solutions I and II. Adjust the pH (*2.2.3*) if necessary.

Buffer solution pH 2.2. *4010500.*

Mix of 6.7 ml of *phosphoric acid R* with 50.0 ml of a 4 per cent solution of *dilute sodium hydroxide solution R* and dilute to 1000.0 ml with *water R*.

Buffer solution pH 2.5. *4000300.*

Dissolve 100 g of *potassium dihydrogen phosphate R* in 800 ml of *water R*; adjust to pH 2.5 (*2.2.3*) with *hydrochloric acid R* and dilute to 1000.0 ml with *water R*.

Buffer solution pH 2.5 R1. *4000400.*

To 4.9 g of *dilute phosphoric acid R* add 250 ml of *water R*. Adjust the pH (*2.2.3*) with *dilute sodium hydroxide solution R* and dilute to 500.0 ml with *water R*.

Phosphate buffer solution pH 2.8. *4010600.*

Dissolve 7.8 g of *sodium dihydrogen phosphate R* in 900 ml of *water R*, adjust to pH 2.8 (*2.2.3*) with *phosphoric acid R* and dilute to 1000 ml with the same solvent.

Buffer solution pH 3.0. *4008000.*

Dissolve 21.0 g of *citric acid R* in 200 ml of *1 M sodium hydroxide* and dilute to 1000 ml with *water R*. Dilute 40.3 ml of this solution to 100.0 ml with *0.1 M hydrochloric acid.*

Phosphate buffer solution pH 3.0. *4000500.*

Mix 0.7 ml of *phosphoric acid R* with 100 ml of *water R*. Dilute to 900 ml with the same solvent. Adjust to pH 3.0 (*2.2.3*) with *strong sodium hydroxide solution R* and dilute to 1000 ml with *water R*.

0.1 M Phosphate buffer solution pH 3.0. *4011500.*

Dissolve 12.0 g of *anhydrous sodium dihydrogen phosphate R* in *water R*, adjust the pH (*2.2.3*) with *dilute phosphoric acid R1* and dilute to 1000 ml with *water R*.

Phosphate buffer solution pH 3.0 R1. *4010000.*

Dissolve 3.40 g of *potassium dihydrogen phosphate R* in 900 ml of *water R*. Adjust to pH 3.0 (*2.2.3*) with *phosphoric acid R* and dilute to 1000.0 ml with *water R*.

Phosphate buffer solution pH 3.2. *4008100.*

To 900 ml of a 4 g/l solution of *sodium dihydrogen phosphate R*, add 100 ml of a 2.5 g/l solution of *phosphoric acid R*. Adjust the pH (*2.2.3*) if necessary.

Phosphate buffer solution pH 3.2 R1. *4008500.*

Adjust a 35.8 g/l solution of *disodium hydrogen phosphate R* to pH 3.2 (*2.2.3*) with *dilute phosphoric acid R*. Dilute 100.0 ml of the solution to 2000.0 ml with *water R*.

Buffer solution pH 3.5. *4000600.*

Dissolve 25.0 g of *ammonium acetate R* in 25 ml of *water R* and add 38.0 ml of *hydrochloric acid R1*. Adjust the pH (*2.2.3*) if necessary with *dilute hydrochloric acid R* or *dilute ammonia R1*. Dilute to 100.0 ml with *water R*.

Phosphate buffer solution pH 3.5. *4000700.*

Dissolve 68.0 g of *potassium dihydrogen phosphate R* in *water R* and dilute to 1000.0 ml with the same solvent. Adjust the pH (*2.2.3*) with *phosphoric acid R*.

Buffer solution pH 3.6. *4000800.*

To 250.0 ml of *0.2 M potassium hydrogen phthalate R* add 11.94 ml of *0.2 M hydrochloric acid.* Dilute to 1000.0 ml with *water R*.

Buffer solution pH 3.7. *4000900.*

To 15.0 ml of *acetic acid R* add 60 ml of *alcohol R* and 20 ml of *water R*. Adjust to pH 3.7 (*2.2.3*) by the addition of *ammonia R*. Dilute to 100.0 ml with *water R*.

Buffered copper sulphate solution pH 4.0. *4001000.*

Dissolve 0.25 g of *copper sulphate R* and 4.5 g of *ammonium acetate R* in *dilute acetic acid R* and dilute to 100.0 ml with the same solvent.

Acetate buffer solution pH 4.4. *4001100.*

Dissolve 136 g of *sodium acetate R* and 77 g of *ammonium acetate R* in *water R* and dilute to 1000.0 ml with the same solvent; add 250.0 ml of *glacial acetic acid R* and mix.

Phthalate buffer solution pH 4.4. *4001200.*

Dissolve 2.042 g of *potassium hydrogen phthalate R* in 50 ml of *water R*, add 7.5 ml of *0.2 M sodium hydroxide* and dilute to 200.0 ml with *water R*.

Acetate buffer solution pH 4.5. *4012500.*

Dissolve 77.1 g of *ammonium acetate R* in *water R*. Add 70 ml of *glacial acetic acid R* and dilute to 1000.0 ml with *water R*.

0.05 M Phosphate buffer solution pH 4.5. *4009000.*

Dissolve 6.80 g of *potassium dihydrogen phosphate R* in 1000.0 ml of *water R*. The pH (*2.2.3*) of the solution is 4.5.

Sodium acetate buffer solution pH 4.5. *4010100.*

Dissolve 63 g of *anhydrous sodium acetate R* in *water R*, add 90 ml *acetic acid R* and adjust to pH 4.5, and dilute to 1000 ml with *water R*.

Acetate buffer solution pH 4.6. *4001400.*

Dissolve 5.4 g of *sodium acetate R* in 50 ml of *water R*, add 2.4 g of *glacial acetic acid R* and dilute to 100.0 ml with *water R*. Adjust the pH (*2.2.3*) if necessary.

Succinate buffer solution pH 4.6. *4001500.*

Disssolve 11.8 g of *succinic acid R* in a mixture of 600 ml of *water R* and 82 ml of *1 M sodium hydroxide* and dilute to 1000.0 ml with *water R*.

4. Reagents

Acetate buffer solution pH 4.7. *4001600.*

Dissolve 136.1 g of *sodium acetate R* in 500 ml of *water R*. Mix 250 ml of this solution with 250 ml of *dilute acetic acid R*. Shake twice with a freshly prepared, filtered, 0.1 g/l solution of *dithizone R* in *chloroform R*. Shake with *carbon tetrachloride R* until the extract is colourless. Filter the aqueous layer to remove traces of carbon tetrachloride.

Acetate buffer solution pH 5.0. *4009100.*

To 120 ml of a 6 g/l solution of *glacial acetic acid R* add 100 ml of *0.1 M potassium hydroxide* and about 250 ml of *water R*. Mix. Adjust the pH to 5.0 with a 6 g/l solution of *acetic acid R* or with *0.1 M potassium hydroxide* and dilute to 1000.0 ml with *water R*.

Citrate buffer solution pH 5.0. *4010700.*

Prepare a solution containing 20.1 g/l of *citric acid R* and 8.0 g/l of *sodium hydroxide R*. Adjust the pH with *dilute hydrochloric acid R*.

Phosphate buffer solution pH 5.0. *4011300.*

Dissolve 2.72 g of *potassium dihydrogen phosphate R* in 800 ml of *water R*. Adjust the pH (*2.2.3*) with *1 M potassium hydroxide* and dilute to 1000 ml with *water R*.

Buffer solution pH 5.2. *4001700.*

Dissolve 1.02 g of *potassium hydrogen phthalate R* in 30.0 ml of *0.1 M sodium hydroxide*. Dilute to 100.0 ml with *water R*.

0.067 M Phosphate buffer solution pH 5.4. *4012000.*

Mix appropriate volumes of a 23.99 g/l solution of *disodium hydrogen phosphate R* with a 9.12 g/l solution of *sodium dihydrogen phosphate monohydrate R* to obtain pH 5.4 (*2.2.3*).

Acetate-edetate buffer solution pH 5.5. *4001900.*

Dissolve 250 g of *ammonium acetate R* and 15 g *sodium edetate R* in 400 ml of *water R* and add 125 ml of *glacial acetic acid R*.

Buffer solution pH 5.5. *4001800.*

Dissolve 54.4 g of *sodium acetate R* in 50 ml of *water R*, heating to 35 °C if necessary. After cooling, slowly add 10 ml of *anhydrous acetic acid R*. Shake and dilute to 100.0 ml with *water R*.

Phosphate buffer solution pH 5.5. *4002000.*

Solution I. Dissolve 13.61 g of *potassium dihydrogen phosphate R* in *water R* and dilute to 1000.0 ml with the same solvent.

Solution II. Dissolve 35.81 g of *disodium hydrogen phosphate R* in *water R* and dilute to 1000.0 ml with the same solvent.

Mix 96.4 ml of solution I and 3.6 ml of solution II.

Phosphate-citrate buffer solution pH 5.5. *4008700.*

Mix 56.85 ml of a 28.4 g/l solution of *anhydrous disodium hydrogen phosphate R* and 43.15 ml of a 21 g/l solution of *citric acid R*.

Phosphate buffer solution pH 5.6. *4011200.*

Solution I. Dissolve 0.908 g of *potassium dihydrogen phosphate R* in *water R* and dilute to 100.0 ml with the same solvent.

Solution II. Dissolve 1.161 g of *dipotassium hydrogen phosphate R* in *water R* and dilute to 100.0 ml with the same solvent.

Mix 94.4 ml of solution I and 5.6 ml of solution II. If necessary, adjust to pH 5.6 (*2.2.3*) using solution I or solution II.

Phosphate buffer solution pH 5.8. *4002100.*

Dissolve 1.19 g of *disodium hydrogen phosphate dihydrate R* and 8.25 g of *potassium dihydrogen phosphate R* in *water R* and dilute to 1000.0 ml with the same solvent.

Acetate buffer solution pH 6.0. *4002200.*

Dissolve 100 g of *ammonium acetate R* in 300 ml of *water R*, add 4.1 ml of *glacial acetic acid R*, adjust the pH (*2.2.3*) if necessary using *ammonia R* or *acetic acid R* and dilute to 500.0 ml with *water R*.

Diethylammonium phosphate buffer solution pH 6.0. *4002300.*

Dilute 68 ml of *phosphoric acid R* to 500 ml with *water R*. To 25 ml of this solution add 450 ml of *water R* and 6 ml of *diethylamine R*, adjust to pH 6 ± 0.05 (*2.2.3*), if necessary, using *diethylamine R* or *phosphoric acid R* and dilute to 500.0 ml with *water R*.

Phosphate buffer solution pH 6.0. *4002400.*

Mix 63.2 ml of a 71.5 g/l solution of *disodium hydrogen phosphate R* and 36.8 ml of a 21 g/l solution of *citric acid R*.

Phosphate buffer solution pH 6.0 R1. *4002500.*

Dissolve 6.8 g of *sodium dihydrogen phosphate R* in *water R* and dilute to 1000.0 ml with *water R*. Adjust the pH (*2.2.3*) with *strong sodium hydroxide solution R*.

Phosphate buffer solution pH 6.0 R2. *4002600.*

To 250.0 ml of *0.2 M potassium dihydrogen phosphate R* add 28.5 ml of *0.2 M sodium hydroxide* and dilute to 1000.0 ml with *water R*.

Phosphate buffer solution pH 6.4. *4002800.*

Dissolve 2.5 g of *disodium hydrogen phosphate R*, 2.5 g of *sodium dihydrogen phosphate R* and 8.2 g of *sodium chloride R* in 950 ml of *water R*. Adjust the pH (*2.2.3*) of the solution to 6.4 with *1 M sodium hydroxide* or *1 M hydrochloric acid*, if necessary. Dilute to 1000.0 ml with *water R*.

0.5 M Phthalate buffer solution pH 6.4. *4009200.*

Dissolve 100 g of *potassium hydrogen phthalate R* in *water R* and dilute to 1000.0 ml with the same solvent. Adjust the pH (*2.2.3*) if necessary, using *strong sodium hydroxide solution R*.

Buffer solution pH 6.5. *4002900.*

Dissolve 60.5 g of *disodium hydrogen phosphate R* and 46 g of *potassium dihydrogen phosphate R* in *water R*. Add 100 ml of *0.02 M sodium edetate* and 20 mg of *mercuric chloride R* and dilute to 1000.0 ml with *water R*.

Imidazole buffer solution pH 6.5. *4003000.*

Dissolve 6.81 g of *imidazole R*, 1.23 g of *magnesium sulphate R* and 0.73 g of *calcium sulphate R* in 752 ml of *0.1 M hydrochloric acid*. Adjust the pH (*2.2.3*) if necessary and dilute to 1000.0 ml with *water R*.

0.1 M phosphate buffer solution pH 6.5. *4010800.*

Dissolve 13.80 g of *sodium dihydrogen phosphate monohydrate R* in 900 ml of *distilled water R*. Adjust the pH (*2.2.3*) using a 400 g/l solution of *sodium hydroxide R*. Dilute to 1000 ml with *distilled water R*.

Buffer solution pH 6.6. *4003100.*

To 250.0 ml of *0.2 M potassium dihydrogen phosphate R* add 89.0 ml of *0.2 M sodium hydroxide*. Dilute to 1000.0 ml with *water R*.

Phosphate buffered saline pH 6.8. *4003200.*

Dissolve 1.0 g of *potassium dihydrogen phosphate R*, 2.0 g of *dipotassium hydrogen phosphate R* and 8.5 g of *sodium chloride R* in 900 ml of *water R*, adjust the pH (*2.2.3*) if necessary and dilute to 1000.0 ml with the same solvent.

Phosphate buffer solution pH 6.8. *4003300.*

Mix 77.3 ml of a 71.5 g/l solution of *disodium hydrogen phosphate R* with 22.7 ml of a 21 g/l solution of *citric acid R*.

Phosphate buffer solution pH 6.8 R1. *4003400.*

To 51.0 ml of a 27.2 g/l solution of *potassium dihydrogen phosphate R* add 49.0 ml of a 71.6 g/l solution of *disodium hydrogen phosphate R*. Adjust the pH (*2.2.3*) if necessary.

Storage: at 2 °C to 8 °C.

1 M tris-hydrochloride buffer solution pH 6.8. *4009300.*

Dissolve 60.6 g of *tris(hydroxymethyl)aminomethane R* in 400 ml of *water R*. Adjust the pH (*2.2.3*) with *hydrochloric acid R* and dilute to 500.0 ml with *water R*.

Buffer solution pH 7.0. *4003500.*

To 1000 ml of a solution containing 18 g/l of *disodium hydrogen phosphate R* and 23 g/l of *sodium chloride R* add sufficient (about 280 ml) of a solution containing 7.8 g/l of *sodium dihydrogen phosphate R* and 23 g/l of *sodium chloride R* to adjust the pH (*2.2.3*). Dissolve in the solution sufficient *sodium azide R* to give a 0.2 g/l solution.

Maleate buffer solution pH 7.0. *4003600.*

Dissolve 10.0 g of *sodium chloride R*, 6.06 g of *tris(hydroxymethyl)aminomethane R* and 4.90 g of *maleic anhydride R* in 900 ml of *water R*. Adjust the pH (*2.2.3*) using a 170 g/l solution of *sodium hydroxide R*. Dilute to 1000.0 ml with *water R*.

Storage: at 2 °C to 8 °C; use within 3 days.

0.025 M Phosphate buffer solution pH 7.0. *4009400.*

Mix 1 volume of *0.063 M phosphate buffer solution pH 7.0 R* with 1.5 volumes of *water R*.

0.03 M Phosphate buffer solution pH 7.0. *4010300.*

Dissolve 5.2 g of *dipotassium hydrogen phosphate R* in 900 ml of *water for chromatography R*. Adjust the solution to pH 7.0 ± 0.1 using *phosphoric acid R* and dilute to 1000 ml with *water for chromatography R*.

0.05 M Phosphate buffer solution pH 7.0. *4012400.*

Mix 34 ml of *water R* and 100 ml of *0.067 M phosphate buffer solution pH 7.0 R*.

0.063 M Phosphate buffer solution pH 7.0. *4009500.*

Dissolve 5.18 g of *anhydrous disodium hydrogen phosphate R* and 3.65 g of *sodium dihydrogen phosphate monohydrate R* in 950 ml of *water R* and adjust the pH (*2.2.3*) with *phosphoric acid R*; dilute to 1000.0 ml with *water R*.

0.067 M Phosphate buffer solution pH 7.0. *4003800.*

Solution I. Dissolve 0.908 g of *potassium dihydrogen phosphate R* in *water R* and dilute to 100.0 ml with the same solvent.

Solution II. Dissolve 2.38 g of *disodium hydrogen phosphate R* in *water R* and dilute to 100.0 ml with the same solvent.

Mix 38.9 ml of solution I and 61.1 ml of solution II. Adjust the pH (*2.2.3*) if necessary.

0.1 M Phosphate buffer solution pH 7.0. *4008200.*

Dissolve 1.361 g of *potassium dihydrogen phosphate R* in *water R* and dilute to 100.0 ml with the same solvent. Adjust the pH (*2.2.3*) using a 35 g/l solution of *disodium hydrogen phosphate R*.

Phosphate buffer solution pH 7.0. *4003700.*

Mix 82.4 ml of a 71.5 g/l solution of *disodium hydrogen phosphate R* with 17.6 ml of a 21 g/l solution of *citric acid R*.

Phosphate buffer solution pH 7.0 R1. *4003900.*

Mix 250.0 ml of *0.2 M potassium dihydrogen phosphate R* and 148.2 ml of a 8 g/l solution of *sodium hydroxide R*, adjust the pH (*2.2.3*) if necessary. Dilute to 1000.0 ml with *water R*.

Phosphate buffer solution pH 7.0 R2. *4004000.*

Mix 50.0 ml of a 136 g/l solution of *potassium dihydrogen phosphate R* with 29.5 ml of *1 M sodium hydroxide* and dilute to 100.0 ml with *water R*. Adjust the pH (*2.2.3*) to 7.0 ± 0.1.

Phosphate buffer solution pH 7.0 R3. *4008600.*

Dissolve 5 g of *potassium dihydrogen phosphate R* and 11 g of *dipotassium hydrogen phosphate R* in 900 ml of *water R*. Adjust to pH 7.0 (*2.2.3*) with *dilute phosphoric acid R* or *dilute sodium hydroxide solution R*. Dilute to 1000 ml with *water R* and mix.

Phosphate buffer solution pH 7.0 R4. *4010200.*

Dissolve 28.4 g of *anhydrous disodium hydrogen phosphate R* and 18.2 g of *potassium dihydrogen phosphate R* in *water R* and dilute to 500 ml with the same solvent.

Phosphate buffer solution pH 7.0 R5. *4011400.*

Dissolve 28.4 g of *anhydrous disodium hydrogen phosphate R* in 800 ml of *water R*. Adjust the pH (*2.2.3*) using a 30 per cent *m/m* solution of *phosphoric acid R* and dilute to 1000 ml with *water R*.

Tetrabutylammonium buffer solution pH 7.0. *4010900.*

Dissolve 6.16 g of *ammonium acetate R* in a mixture of 15 ml of *tetrabutylammonium hydroxide solution (400 g/l) R* and 185 ml of *water R*. Adjust the pH (*2.2.3*) with *nitric acid R*.

Buffered salt solution pH 7.2. *4004300.*

Dissolve in *water R* 8.0 g of *sodium chloride R*, 0.2 g of *potassium chloride R*, 0.1 g of *anhydrous calcium chloride R*, 0.1 g of *magnesium chloride R*, 3.18 g of *disodium hydrogen phosphate R* and 0.2 g of *potassium dihydrogen phosphate R* and dilute to 1000.0 ml with *water R*.

Buffer solution pH 7.2. *4004100.*

To 250.0 ml of *0.2 M potassium dihydrogen phosphate R* add 175.0 ml of *0.2 M sodium hydroxide*. Dilute to 1000.0 ml with *water R*. Adjust the pH (*2.2.3*) if necessary.

Phosphate-albumin buffered saline pH 7.2. *4004400.*

Dissolve 10.75 g of *disodium hydrogen phosphate R*, 7.6 g of *sodium chloride R* and 10 g of *bovine albumin R* in *water R* and dilute to 1000.0 ml with the same solvent. Immediately before use adjust the pH (*2.2.3*) using *dilute sodium hydroxide solution R* or *dilute phosphoric acid R*.

Phosphate-albumin buffered saline pH 7.2 R1. *4009600.*

Dissolve 10.75 g of *disodium hydrogen phosphate R*, 7.6 g of *sodium chloride R* and 1 g of *bovine albumin R* in *water R* and dilute to 1000.0 ml with the same solvent. Immediately before use adjust the pH (*2.2.3*) using *dilute sodium hydroxide solution R* or *dilute phosphoric acid R*.

Phosphate buffer solution pH 7.2. *4004200.*

Mix 87.0 ml of a 71.5 g/l solution of *disodium hydrogen phosphate R* with 13.0 ml of a 21 g/l solution of *citric acid R*.

Imidazole buffer solution pH 7.3. *4004500.*

Dissolve 3.4 g of *imidazole R* and 5.8 g of *sodium chloride R* in *water R*, add 18.6 ml of *1 M hydrochloric acid* and dilute to 1000.0 ml with *water R*. Adjust the pH (*2.2.3*) if necessary.

Barbital buffer solution pH 7.4. *4004700.*

Mix 50 ml of a solution in *water R* containing 19.44 g/l of *sodium acetate R* and 29.46 g/l of *barbital sodium R* with 50.5 ml of *0.1 M hydrochloric acid*, add 20 ml of an 85 g/l of *sodium chloride R* and dilute to 250 ml with *water R*.

Buffer solution pH 7.4. *4004600.*

Dissolve 0.6 g of *potassium dihydrogen phosphate R*, 6.4 g of *disodium hydrogen phosphate R* and 5.85 g of *sodium chloride R* in *water R*, and dilute to 1000.0 ml with the same solvent. Adjust the pH (*2.2.3*) if necessary.

Phosphate buffered saline pH 7.4. *4005000.*

Dissolve 2.38 g of *disodium hydrogen phosphate R*, 0.19 g of *potassium dihydrogen phosphate R* and 8.0 g of *sodium chloride R* in water. Dilute to 1000.0 ml with the same solvent. Adjust the pH (*2.2.3*) if necessary.

Phosphate buffer solution pH 7.4. *4004800.*

Add 250.0 ml of *0.2 M potassium dihydrogen phosphate R* to 393.4 ml of *0.1 M sodium hydroxide*.

Tris(hydroxymethyl)aminomethane buffer solution pH 7.4. *4012100.*

Dissolve 30.3 g of *tris(hydroxymethyl)aminomethane R* in approximately 200 ml of *water R*. Add 183 ml of *1 M hydrochloric acid*. Dilute to 500.0 ml with *water R*. *Note: the pH is 7.7-7.8 at room temperature and 7.4 at 37 °C. This solution is stable for several months at 4 °C.*

Tris(hydroxymethyl)aminomethane sodium chloride buffer solution pH 7.4. *4004900.*

Dissolve 6.08 g of *tris(hydroxymethyl)aminomethane R*, 8.77 g of *sodium chloride R* in 500 ml of *distilled water R*. Add 10.0 g of *bovine albumin R*. Adjust the pH (*2.2.3*) using *hydrochloric acid R*. Dilute to 1000.0 ml with *distilled water R*.

Tris(hydroxymethyl)aminomethane sodium chloride buffer solution pH 7.4 R1. *4012200.*

Dissolve 0.1 g of *bovine albumin R* in a mixture containing 2 ml of *tris(hydroxymethyl)aminomethane buffer solution pH 7.4 R* and 50 ml of a 5.84 mg/ml solution of *sodium chloride R*. Dilute to 100.0 ml with *water R*.

Borate buffer solution pH 7.5. *4005200.*

Dissolve 2.5 g of *sodium chloride R*, 2.85 g of *disodium tetraborate R* and 10.5 g of *boric acid R* in *water R* and dilute to 1000.0 ml with the same solvent. Adjust the pH (*2.2.3*) if necessary.

Storage: at 2 °C to 8 °C.

Buffer (HEPES) solution pH 7.5. *4009700.*

Dissolve 2.38 g of *2-[4-(2-hydroxyethyl)piperazin-1-yl]ethanesulphonic acid R* in about 90 ml of *water R*. Adjust the pH to 7.5 with *sodium hydroxide solution R*. Dilute to 100 ml with *water R*.

0.2 M Phosphate buffer solution pH 7.5. *4005400.*

Dissolve 27.22 g of *potassium dihydrogen phosphate R* in 930 ml of *water R*, adjust to pH 7.5 (*2.2.3*) with a 300 g/l solution of *potassium hydroxide R* and dilute to 1000.0 ml with *water R*.

0.33 M Phosphate buffer solution pH 7.5. *4005300.*

Solution I. Dissolve 119.31 g of *disodium hydrogen phosphate R* in *water R* and dilute to 1000.0 ml with the same solvent.

Solution II. Dissolve 45.36 g of *potassium dihydrogen phosphate R* in *water R* and dilute to 1000.0 ml with the same solvent.

Mix 85 ml of solution I and 15 ml of solution II. Adjust the pH (*2.2.3*) if necessary.

0.05 M Tris-hydrochloride buffer solution pH 7.5. *4005600.*

Dissolve 6.057 g of *tris(hydroxymethyl)aminomethane R* in *water R* and adjust the pH (*2.2.3*) with *hydrochloric acid R*. Dilute to 1000.0 ml with *water R*.

Tris(hydroxymethyl)aminomethane buffer solution pH 7.5. *4005500.*

Dissolve 7.27 g of *tris(hydroxymethyl)aminomethane R* and 5.27 g of *sodium chloride R* in *water R*, and adjust the pH (*2.2.3*) if necessary. Dilute to 1000.0 ml with *water R*.

Sodium citrate buffer solution pH 7.8 (0.034 M sodium citrate, 0.101 M sodium chloride). *4009800.*

Dissolve 10.0 g of *sodium citrate R* and 5.90 g of *sodium chloride R* in 900 ml of *water R*. Adjust the pH (*2.2.3*) by addition of *hydrochloric acid R* and dilute to 1000 ml with *water R*.

0.0015 M Borate buffer solution pH 8.0. *4006000.*

Dissolve 0.572 g of *disodium tetraborate R* and 2.94 g of *calcium chloride R* in 800 ml of *water R*. Adjust the pH (*2.2.3*) with *1 M hydrochloric acid*. Dilute to 1000.0 ml with *water R*.

Buffer solution pH 8.0. *4005900.*

To 50.0 ml of *0.2 M potassium dihydrogen phosphate R* add 46.8 ml of *0.2 M sodium hydroxide*. Dilute to 200.0 ml with *water R*.

Buffer solution pH 8.0 R1. *4010400.*

Dissolve 20 g of *dipotassium hydrogen phosphate R* in 900 ml of *water R*. Adjust the pH (*2.2.3*) with *phosphoric acid R*. Dilute to 1000 ml with *water R*.

0.02 M Phosphate buffer solution pH 8.0. *4006100.*

To 50.0 ml of *0.2 M potassium dihydrogen phosphate R* add 46.8 ml of *0.2 M sodium hydroxide*. Dilute to 500.0 ml with *water R*.

0.1 M Phosphate buffer solution pH 8.0. *4008400.*

Dissolve 0.523 g of *potassium dihydrogen phosphate R* and 16.73 g of *dipotassium hydrogen phosphate R* in *water R* and dilute to 1000.0 ml with the same solvent.

1 M Phosphate buffer solution pH 8.0. *4007800.*

Dissolve 136.1 g of *potassium dihydrogen phosphate R* in *water R*, adjust the pH (*2.2.3*) with *1 M sodium hydroxide*. Dilute to 1000.0 ml with *water R*.

Tris-hydrochloride buffer solution pH 8.0. *4012300.*

Dissolve 1.21 g of *tris(hydroxymethyl)aminomethane R* and 29.4 mg of *calcium chloride R* in *water R*. Adjust the pH (*2.2.3*) with *1 M hydrochloric acid* and dilute to 100.0 ml with *water R*.

Tris(hydroxymethyl)aminomethane buffer solution pH 8.1. *4006200.*

Dissolve 0.294 g of *calcium chloride R* in 40 ml of *tris(hydroxymethyl)aminomethane solution R* and adjust the pH (*2.2.3*) with *1 M hydrochloric acid*. Dilute to 100.0 ml with *water R*.

Tris-glycine buffer solution pH 8.3. *4006300.*

Dissolve 6.0 g of *tris(hydroxymethyl)aminomethane R* and 28.8 g of *glycine R* in *water R* and dilute to 1000.0 ml with the same solvent. Dilute 1 volume to 10 volumes with *water R* immediately before use.

Tris-hydrochloride buffer solution pH 8.3. *4011800.*

Dissolve 9.0 g of *tris(hydroxymethyl)aminomethane R* in 2.9 litres of *water R*. Adjust the pH (*2.2.3*) with *1 M hydrochloric acid*. Adjust the volume to 3 litres with *water R*.

Barbital buffer solution pH 8.4. *4006400.*

Dissolve 8.25 g of *barbital sodium R* in *water R* and dilute to 1000.0 ml with the same solvent.

Tris-EDTA BSA buffer solution pH 8.4. *4006500.*

Dissolve 6.1 g of *tris(hydroxymethyl)aminomethane R*, 2.8 g of *sodium edetate R*, 10.2 g of *sodium chloride R* and 10 g of *bovine albumin R* in *water R*, adjust to pH 8.4 (*2.2.3*) using *1 M hydrochloric acid* and dilute to 1000.0 ml with *water R*.

Tris(hydroxymethyl)aminomethane EDTA buffer solution pH 8.4. *4006600.*

Dissolve 5.12 g of *sodium chloride R*, 3.03 g of *tris(hydroxymethyl)aminomethane R* and 1.40 g of *sodium edetate R* in 250 ml of *distilled water R*. Adjust the pH (*2.2.3*) to 8.4 using *hydrochloric acid R*. Dilute to 500.0 ml with *distilled water R*.

Tris acetate buffer solution pH 8.5. *4006700.*

Dissolve 0.294 g of *calcium chloride R* and 12.11 g of *tris(hydroxymethyl)aminomethane R* in *water R*. Adjust the pH (*2.2.3*) with *acetic acid R*. Dilute to 1000.0 ml with *water R*.

Barbital buffer solution pH 8.6 R1. *4006900.*

Dissolve in *water R* 1.38 g of *barbital R*, 8.76 g of *barbital sodium R* and 0.38 g of *calcium lactate R* and dilute to 1000.0 ml with the same solvent.

1.5 M tris-hydrochloride buffer solution pH 8.8. *4009900.*

Dissolve 90.8 g of *tris(hydroxymethyl)aminomethane R* in 400 ml of *water R*. Adjust the pH (*2.2.3*) with *hydrochloric acid R* and dilute to 500.0 ml with *water R*.

Buffer (phosphate) solution pH 9.0. *4008300.*

Dissolve 1.74 g of *potassium dihydrogen phosphate R* in 80 ml of *water R*, adjust the pH (*2.2.3*) with *1 M potassium hydroxide* and dilute to 100.0 ml with *water R*.

Buffer solution pH 9.0. *4007000.*

Solution I. Dissolve 6.18 g of *boric acid R* in *0.1 M potassium chloride R* and dilute to 1000.0 ml with the same solvent.

Solution II. 0.1 M sodium hydroxide.

Mix 1000.0 ml of solution I and 420.0 ml of solution II.

Buffer solution pH 9.0 R1. *4007100.*

Dissolve 6.20 g of *boric acid R* in 500 ml of *water R* and adjust the pH (*2.2.3*) with *1 M sodium hydroxide* (about 41.5 ml). Dilute to 1000.0 ml with *water R*.

Ammonium chloride buffer solution pH 9.5. *4007200.*

Dissolve 33.5 g of *ammonium chloride R* in 150 ml of *water R*, add 42.0 ml of *concentrated ammonia R* and dilute to 250.0 ml with *water R*.

Storage: in a polyethylene container.

Ammonium chloride buffer solution pH 10.0. *4007300.*

Dissolve 5.4 g of *ammonium chloride R* in 20 ml of *water R*, add 35.0 ml of *ammonia R* and dilute to 100.0 ml with *water R*.

Diethanolamine buffer solution pH 10.0. *4007500.*

Dissolve 96.4 g of *diethanolamine R* in *water R* and dilute to 400 ml with the same solvent. Add 0.5 ml of an 186 g/l solution of *magnesium chloride R* and adjust the pH (*2.2.3*) with *1 M hydrochloric acid*. Dilute to 500.0 ml with *water R*.

0.1 M Ammonium carbonate buffer solution pH 10.3. *4011900.*

Dissolve 7.91 g of *ammonium carbonate R* in 800 ml of *water R*. Adjust the pH (*2.2.3*) with *dilute sodium hydroxide solution R*. Dilute to 1000.0 ml with *water R*.

Ammonium chloride buffer solution pH 10.4. *4011000.*

Dissolve 70 g of *ammonium chloride R* in 200 ml of *water R*, add 330 ml of *concentrated ammonia R* and dilute to 1000.0 ml with *water R*. If necessary, adjust to pH 10.4 with *ammonia R*.

Borate buffer solution pH 10.4. *4011100.*

Dissolve 24.64 g of *boric acid R* in 900 ml of *distilled water R*. Adjust the pH (*2.2.3*) using a 400 g/l solution of *sodium hydroxide R*. Dilute to 1000 ml with *distilled water R*.

Buffer solution pH 10.9. *4007600.*

Dissolve 6.75 g of *ammonium chloride R* in *ammonia R* and dilute to 100.0 ml with the same solvent.

Total-ionic-strength-adjustment buffer. *4007700.*

Dissolve 58.5 g of *sodium chloride R*, 57.0 ml of *glacial acetic acid R*, 61.5 g of *sodium acetate R* and 5.0 g of *cyclohexylene-dinitrilotetra-acetic acid R* in *water R* and dilute to 500.0 ml with the same solvent. Adjust to pH 5.0 to 5.5 with a 335 g/l solution of *sodium hydroxide R* and dilute to 1000.0 ml with *distilled water R*.

Total-ionic-strength-adjustment buffer R1. *4008800.*

Solution (a). Dissolve 210 g of *citric acid R* in 400 ml of *distilled water R*. Adjust to pH 7.0 (*2.2.3*) with *concentrated ammonia R*. Dilute to 1000.0 ml with *distilled water R*.

Solution (b). Dissolve 132 g of *ammonium phosphate R* in *distilled water R* and dilute to 1000.0 ml with the same solvent.

Solution (c). To a suspension of 292 g of (ethylenedinitrilo)tetra-*acetic acid R* in about 500 ml of *distilled water R*, add about 200 ml of *concentrated ammonia R* to dissolve. Adjust the pH to 6 to 7 (*2.2.3*) with *concentrated ammonia R*. Dilute to 1000.0 ml with *distilled water R*.

Mix equal volumes of solution (a), (b), and (c) and adjust to pH 7.5 with *concentrated ammonia R*.

4.2. VOLUMETRIC ANALYSIS

01/2005:40201

4.2.1. PRIMARY STANDARDS FOR VOLUMETRIC SOLUTIONS

Primary standards for volumetric solutions are indicated by the suffix RV. Primary standards of suitable quality may be obtained from commercial sources or prepared by the following methods.

Benzoic acid. $C_7H_6O_2$. (M_r 122.1). *2000200.* [65-85-0].

Sublime *benzoic acid R* in a suitable apparatus.

Potassium bromate. $KBrO_3$. (M_r 167.0). *2000300.* [7758-01-2].

Crystallise *potassium bromate R* from boiling *water R*. Collect the crystals and dry to constant mass at 180 °C.

Potassium hydrogen phthalate. $C_8H_5KO_4$. (M_r 204.2). *2000400.* [877-24-7].

Recrystallise *potassium hydrogen phthalate R* from boiling *water R*, collect the crystals at a temperature above 35 °C and dry to constant mass at 110 °C.

Sodium carbonate. Na_2CO_3 . (M_r 106.0). *2000500.* [497-19-8].

Filter at room temperature a saturated solution of *sodium carbonate R*. Introduce slowly into the filtrate a stream of *carbon dioxide R* with constant cooling and stirring. After about 2 h, collect the precipitate on a sintered-glass filter. Wash the filter with iced *water R* containing carbon dioxide. After drying at 100 °C to 105 °C, heat to constant mass at 270 °C to 300 °C, stirring from time to time.

Sodium chloride. NaCl. (M_r 58.44). *2000600.* [7647-14-5].

To 1 volume of a saturated solution of *sodium chloride R* add 2 volumes of *hydrochloric acid R*. Collect the crystals formed and wash with *hydrochloric acid R1*. Remove the hydrochloric acid by heating on a water-bath and dry the crystals to constant mass at 300 °C.

Sulphanilic acid. $C_6H_7NO_3S$. (M_r 173.2). *2000700.* [121-57-3].

Recrystallise *sulphanilic acid R* from boiling *water R*. Filter and dry to constant mass at 100 °C to 105 °C.

Zinc. Zn. (M_r 65.4). *2000800.* [7440-66-6].

Use a quality containing not less than 99.9 per cent of Zn.

01/2005:40202

4.2.2. VOLUMETRIC SOLUTIONS

Volumetric solutions are prepared according to the usual chemical analytical methods. The accuracy of the apparatus used is verified to ensure that it is appropriate for the intended use.

The concentration of volumetric solutions is indicated in terms of molarity. Molarity expresses, as the number of moles, the amount of substance dissolved in 1 litre of solution. A solution which contains *x* moles of substance per litre is said to be *x* M.

Volumetric solutions do not differ from the prescribed strength by more than 10 per cent. The molarity of the volumetric solutions is determined by an appropriate number of titrations. The repeatability does not exceed 0.2 per cent (relative standard deviation).

Volumetric solutions are standardised by the methods described below. When a volumetric solution is to be used in an assay in which the end-point is determined by an electrochemical process (for example, amperometry or potentiometry) the solution is standardised by the same method. The composition of the medium in which a volumetric solution is standardised should be the same as that in which it is to be used.

Solutions more dilute than those described are obtained by diluting the latter with *carbon dioxide-free water R*. The correction factors of these solutions are the same as those from which the dilutions were prepared.

0.1 M Acetic acid. *3008900.*

Dilute 6.0 g of *glacial acetic acid R* to 1000.0 ml with *water R*.

Standardisation. To 25.0 ml of acetic acid add 0.5 ml of *phenolphthalein solution R* and titrate with *0.1 M sodium hydroxide*.

0.1 M Ammonium and cerium nitrate. *3000100.*

Shake for 2 min a solution containing 56 ml of sulphuric acid R and 54.82 g of *ammonium and cerium nitrate R*, add five successive quantities, each of 100 ml, of *water R*, shaking after each addition. Dilute the clear solution to 1000.0 ml with *water R*. Standardise the solution after 10 days.

Standardisation. To 25.0 ml of the ammonium and cerium nitrate solution add 2.0 g of *potassium iodide R* and 150 ml of *water R*. Titrate immediately with *0.1 M sodium thiosulphate*, using 1 ml of *starch solution R* as indicator.

Storage: protected from light.

0.01 M Ammonium and cerium nitrate. *3000200.*

To 100.0 ml of *0.1 M ammonium and cerium nitrate* add, with cooling, 30 ml of sulphuric acid R and dilute to 1000.0 ml with *water R*.

0.1 M Ammonium and cerium sulphate. *3000300.*

Dissolve 65.0 g of *ammonium and cerium sulphate R* in a mixture of 500 ml of *water R* and 30 ml of sulphuric acid R. Allow to cool and dilute to 1000.0 ml with *water R*.

Standardisation. To 25.0 ml of the ammonium and cerium sulphate solution add 2.0 g of *potassium iodide R* and 150 ml of *water R*. Titrate immediately with *0.1 M sodium thiosulphate*, using 1 ml of *starch solution R* as indicator.

0.01 M Ammonium and cerium sulphate. *3000400.*

To 100.0 ml of *0.1 M ammonium and cerium sulphate* add, with cooling, 30 ml of sulphuric acid R and dilute to 1000.0 ml with *water R*.

0.1 M Ammonium thiocyanate. *3000500.*

Dissolve 7.612 g of *ammonium thiocyanate R* in *water R* and dilute to 1000.0 ml with the same solvent.

Standardisation. To 20.0 ml of *0.1 M silver nitrate* add 25 ml of *water R*, 2 ml of *dilute nitric acid R* and 2 ml of *ferric ammonium sulphate solution R2*. Titrate with the ammonium thiocyanate solution until a reddish-yellow colour is obtained.

0.1 M Barium chloride. *3000600.*

Dissolve 24.4 g of *barium chloride R* in *water R* and dilute to 1000.0 ml with the same solvent.

Standardisation. To 10.0 ml of the barium chloride solution add 60 ml of *water R*, 3 ml of *concentrated ammonia R* and 0.5 mg to 1 mg of *phthalein purple R*. Titrate with *0.1 M sodium edetate*. When the solution begins to decolorise, add 50 ml of *alcohol R* and continue the titration until the blue-violet colour disappears.

0.05 M Barium perchlorate. *3000700.*

Dissolve 15.8 g of *barium hydroxide R* in a mixture of 7.5 ml of *perchloric acid R* and 75 ml of *water R* , adjust the solution to pH 3 by adding *perchloric acid R* and filter if necessary. Add 150 ml of *alcohol R* and dilute to 250 ml with *water R*. Dilute to 1000.0 ml with *buffer solution pH 3.7 R*.

Standardisation. To 5.0 ml of *0.05 M sulphuric acid* add 5 ml of *water R*, 50 ml of *buffer solution pH 3.7 R* and 0.5 ml of *alizarin s solution R*. Titrate with the barium perchlorate solution until an orange-red colour appears. Standardise immediately before use.

0.025 M Barium perchlorate. *3009600.*

Dilute 500.0 ml of *0.05 M barium perchlorate* to 1000.0 ml with *buffer solution pH 3.7 R*.

0.004 M Benzethonium chloride. *3000900.*

Dissolve in *water R* 1.792 g of *benzethonium chloride R*, previously dried to constant mass at 100 °C to 105 °C, and dilute to 1000.0 ml with the same solvent.

Standardisation. Calculate the molarity of the solution from the content of $C_{27}H_{42}ClNO_2$ in the dried benzethonium chloride determined as follows. Dissolve 0.350 g of the dried substance in 30 ml of *anhydrous acetic acid R* and add 6 ml of *mercuric acetate solution R*. Titrate with *0.1 M perchloric acid*, using 0.05 ml of *crystal violet solution R* as indicator. Carry out a blank titration.

1 ml of *0.1 M perchloric acid* is equivalent to 44.81 mg of $C_{27}H_{42}ClNO_2$.

0.0167 M Bromide-bromate. *3001000.*

Dissolve 2.7835 g of *potassium bromate RV* and 13 g of *potassium bromide R* in *water R* and dilute to 1000.0 ml with the same solvent.

0.1 M Cerium sulphate. *3001100.*

Dissolve 40.4 g of *cerium sulphate R* in a mixture of 500 ml of *water R* and 50 ml of sulphuric acid R. Allow to cool and dilute to 1000.0 ml with *water R*.

Standardisation. To 25.0 ml of the cerium sulphate solution, add 2.0 g of *potassium iodide R* and 150 ml of *water R*. Titrate immediately with *0.1 M sodium thiosulphate* using 1 ml of *starch solution R* as indicator.

0.02 M Copper sulphate. *3001200.*

Dissolve 5.0 g of *copper sulphate R* in *water R* and dilute to 1000.0 ml with the same solvent.

Standardisation. To 20.0 ml of the copper sulphate solution add 2 g of *sodium acetate R* and 0.1 ml of *pyridylazonaphthol solution R*. Titrate with *0.02 M sodium edetate* until the colour changes from violet-blue to bright green. Titrate slowly towards the end of the titration.

0.1 M Ferric ammonium sulphate. *3001300.*

Dissolve 50.0 g of *ferric ammonium sulphate R* in a mixture of 6 ml of sulphuric acid R and 300 ml of *water R* and dilute to 1000.0 ml with *water R*.

Standardisation. To 25.0 ml of the ferric ammonium sulphate solution, add 3 ml of *hydrochloric acid R* and 2 g of *potassium iodide R*. Allow to stand for 10 min. Titrate with *0.1 M sodium thiosulphate*, using 1 ml of *starch solution R* as indicator.

1 ml of *0.1 M sodium thiosulphate* is equivalent to 48.22 mg of $FeNH_4(SO_4)_2,12H_2O$.

0.1 M Ferrous sulphate. *3001400.*

Dissolve 27.80 g of *ferrous sulphate R* in 500 ml of *dilute sulphuric acid R* and dilute to 1000.0 ml with *water R*.

Standardisation. To 25.0 ml of the ferrous sulphate solution add 3 ml of *phosphoric acid R* and titrate immediately with *0.02 M potassium permanganate*. Standardise immediately before use.

6 M Hydrochloric acid. *3001500.*

Dilute 618.0 g of *hydrochloric acid R* to 1000.0 ml with *water R*.

3 M Hydrochloric acid. *3001600.*

Dilute 309.0 g of *hydrochloric acid R* to 1000.0 ml with *water R*.

2 M Hydrochloric acid. *3001700.*

Dilute 206.0 g of *hydrochloric acid R* to 1000.0 ml with *water R*.

1 M Hydrochloric acid. *3001800.*

Dilute 103.0 g of *hydrochloric acid R* to 1000.0 ml with *water R*.

Standardisation. Dissolve 1.000 g of *sodium carbonate RV* in 50 ml of *water R*, add 0.1 ml of *methyl orange solution R* and titrate with the hydrochloric acid until the solution just becomes yellowish-red. Boil for 2 min. The solution reverts to yellow. Cool and continue the titration until a yellowish-red colour is obtained.

1 ml of *1 M hydrochloric acid* is equivalent to 53.00 mg of Na_2CO_3.

0.1 M Hydrochloric acid. *3002100.*

Dilute 100.0 ml of *1 M hydrochloric acid* to 1000.0 ml with *water R*.

Standardisation. Carry out the titration described for *1 M hydrochloric acid* using 0.100 g of *sodium carbonate RV* dissolved in 20 ml of *water R*.

1 ml of *0.1 M hydrochloric acid* is equivalent to 5.30 mg of Na_2CO_3.

0.1 M Hydrochloric acid, alcoholic. *3008800.*

Dilute 9.0 ml of *hydrochloric acid R* to 1000.0 ml with *aldehyde-free alcohol R*.

0.5 M Iodine. *3009400.*

Dissolve 127 g of *iodine R* and 200 g of *potassium iodide R* in *water R* and dilute to 1000.0 ml with the same solvent.

Standardisation. To 2.0 ml of the iodine solution add 1 ml of *dilute acetic acid R* and 50 ml of *water R*. Titrate with *0.1 M sodium thiosulphate*, using *starch solution R* as indicator.

Storage: protected from light.

0.05 M Iodine. *3002700.*

Dissolve 12.7 g of *iodine R* and 20 g of *potassium iodide R* in *water R* and dilute to 1000.0 ml with the same solvent.

Standardisation. To 20.0 ml of the iodine solution add 1 ml of *dilute acetic acid R* and 30 ml of *water R*. Titrate with *0.1 M sodium thiosulphate*, using *starch solution R* as indicator.

Storage: protected from light.

0.01 M Iodine. *3002900.*

Add 0.3 g of *potassium iodide R* to 20.0 ml of *0.05 M iodine* and dilute to 100.0 ml with *water R.*

0.1 M Lead nitrate. *3003100.*

Dissolve 33 g of *lead nitrate R* in *water R* and dilute to 1000.0 ml with the same solvent.

Standardisation. Take 20.0 ml of the lead nitrate solution and carry out the determination of lead by complexometry (*2.5.11*).

0.05 M Lead nitrate. *3009700.*

Dilute 50.0 ml of *0.1 M Lead nitrate* to 100.0 ml with *water R.*

0.1 M Lithium methoxide. *3003300.*

Dissolve 0.694 g of *lithium R* in 150 ml of *anhydrous methanol R* and dilute to 1000.0 ml with *toluene R.*

Standardisation. To 10 ml of *dimethylformamide R* add 0.05 ml of a 3 g/l solution of *thymol blue R* in *methanol R* and titrate with the lithium methoxide solution until a pure blue colour is obtained. Immediately add 0.200 g of *benzoic acid RV.* Stir to effect solution and titrate with the lithium methoxide solution until the pure blue colour is again obtained. Protect the solution from atmospheric carbon dioxide throughout the titration. From the volume of titrant used in the second titration ascertain the exact strength of the lithium methoxide solution. Standardise immediately before use.

1 ml of *0.1 M lithium methoxide* is equivalent to 12.21 mg of $C_7H_6O_2$.

0.1 M Magnesium chloride. *3003400.*

Dissolve 20.33 g of *magnesium chloride R* in *water R* and dilute to 1000.0 ml with the same solvent.

Standardisation. Carry out the determination of magnesium by complexometry (*2.5.11*).

1 M Nitric acid. *3003600.*

Dilute 96.6 g of *nitric acid R* to 1000.0 ml with *water R.*

Standardisation. Dissolve 1.000 g of *sodium carbonate RV* in 50 ml of *water R,* add 0.1 ml of *methyl orange solution R* and titrate with the nitric acid until the solution just becomes reddish-yellow; boil for 2 min. The solution reverts to yellow. Cool and continue the titration until a reddish-yellow colour is obtained.

1 ml of *1 M nitric acid* is equivalent to 53.00 mg of Na_2CO_3.

0.1 M Perchloric acid. *3003900.*

Place 8.5 ml of *perchloric acid R* in a volumetric flask containing about 900 ml of *glacial acetic acid R* and mix. Add 30 ml of *acetic anhydride R,* dilute to 1000.0 ml with *glacial acetic acid R,* mix and allow to stand for 24 h. Determine the water content (*2.5.12*) without addition of methanol and, if necessary, adjust the water content to between 0.1 per cent and 0.2 per cent by adding either *acetic anhydride R* or *water R.* Allow to stand for 24 h.

Standardisation. Dissolve 0.350 g of *potassium hydrogen phthalate RV* in 50 ml of *anhydrous acetic acid R,* warming gently if necessary. Allow to cool protected from the air, and titrate with the perchloric acid solution, using 0.05 ml of *crystal violet solution R* as indicator. Note the temperature of the perchloric acid solution at the time of the titration.

If the temperature at which an assay is carried out is different from that at which the *perchloric acid R* has been standardised the volume used in the assay becomes:

$$V_c = V\,[1 + (t_1 - t_2)\,0.0011]$$

where t_1 is the temperature during standardisation, and t_2 is the temperature during the assay, V_c is the corrected volume and V the observed volume.

1 ml of *0.1 M perchloric acid* is equivalent to 20.42 mg of $C_8H_5KO_4$.

0.05 M Perchloric acid. *3004000.*

Dilute 50.0 ml of *0.1 M perchloric acid* to 100.0 ml with *anhydrous acetic acid R.*

0.033 M Potassium bromate. *3004200.*

Dissolve 5.5670 g of *potassium bromate RV* in *water R* and dilute to 1000.0 ml with the same solvent.

0.02 M Potassium bromate. *3004300.*

Dissolve 3.340 g of *potassium bromate RV* in *water R* and dilute to 1000.0 ml with the same solvent.

0.0167 M Potassium bromate. *3004400.*

Prepare by diluting *0.033 M Potassium bromate.*

0.0083 M Potassium bromate. *3004500.*

Prepare by diluting *0.033 M Potassium bromate.*

0.0167 M Potassium dichromate. *3004600.*

Dissolve 4.90 g of *potassium dichromate R* in *water R* and dilute to 1000.0 ml with the same solvent.

Standardisation. To 20.0 ml of the potassium dichromate solution add 1 g of *potassium iodide R* and 7 ml of *dilute hydrochloric acid R.* Add 250 ml of *water R* and titrate with *0.1 M sodium thiosulphate,* using 3 ml of *starch solution R* as indicator, until the colour changes from blue to light green.

0.1 M Potassium hydrogen phthalate. *3004700.*

In a conical flask containing about 800 ml of *anhydrous acetic acid R,* dissolve 20.42 g of *potassium hydrogen phthalate RV.* Heat on a water-bath until completely dissolved, protected from humidity. Cool to 20 °C and dilute to 1000.0 ml with *anhydrous acetic acid R.*

1 M Potassium hydroxide. *3009100.*

Dissolve 60 g of *potassium hydroxide R* in *carbon dioxide-free water R* and dilute to 1000.0 ml with the same solvent.

Standardisation. Titrate 20.0 ml of the potassium hydroxide solution with *1 M hydrochloric acid,* using 0.5 ml of *phenolphthalein solution R* as indicator.

0.1 M Potassium hydroxide. *3004800.*

Dissolve 6 g of *potassium hydroxide R* in *carbon dioxide-free water R* and dilute to 1000.0 ml with the same solvent.

Standardisation. Titrate 20.0 ml of the potassium hydroxide solution with *0.1 M hydrochloric acid,* using 0.5 ml of *phenolphthalein solution R* as indicator.

0.5 M Potassium hydroxide in alcohol (60 per cent *V/V*). *3004900.*

Dissolve 3 g of *potassium hydroxide R* in *aldehyde-free alcohol R* (60 per cent *V/V*) and dilute to 100.0 ml with the same solvent.

Standardisation. Titrate 20.0 ml of the alcoholic potassium hydroxide solution (60 per cent *V/V*) with *0.5 M hydrochloric acid,* using 0.5 ml of *phenolphthalein solution R* as indicator.

0.5 M Potassium hydroxide, alcoholic. *3005000.*

Dissolve 3 g of *potassium hydroxide R* in 5 ml of *water R* and dilute to 100.0 ml with *aldehyde-free alcohol R.*

Standardisation. Titrate 20.0 ml of the alcoholic potassium hydroxide solution with *0.5 M hydrochloric acid,* using 0.5 ml of *phenolphthalein solution R* as indicator.

0.1 M Potassium hydroxide, alcoholic. *3005100.*

Dilute 20.0 ml of *0.5 M alcoholic potassium hydroxide* to 100.0 ml with *aldehyde-free alcohol R.*

0.01 M Potassium hydroxide, alcoholic. *3009000.*

Dilute 2.0 ml of *0.5 M alcoholic potassium hydroxide* to 100.0 ml with *aldehyde-free alcohol R.*

0.05 M Potassium iodate. *3005200.*

Dissolve 10.70 g of *potassium iodate R* in *water R* and dilute to 1000.0 ml with the same solvent.

Standardisation. Dilute 25.0 ml of the potassium iodate solution to 100.0 ml with *water R.* To 20.0 ml of this solution add 2 g of *potassium iodide R* and 10 ml of *dilute sulphuric acid R.* Titrate with *0.1 M sodium thiosulphate,* using 1 ml of *starch solution R,* added towards the end of the titration, as indicator.

0.001 M Potassium iodide. *3009200.*

Dilute 10.0 ml of *potassium iodide solution R* (166 g/l) to 100.0 ml with *water R.* Dilute 5.0 ml of this solution to 500.0 ml with *water R.*

0.02 M Potassium permanganate. *3005300.*

Dissolve 3.2 g of *potassium permanganate R* in *water R* and dilute to 1000.0 ml with the same solvent. Heat the solution for 1 h on a water-bath, allow to cool and filter through a sintered-glass filter.

Standardisation. To 20.0 ml of the potassium permanganate solution, add 2 g of *potassium iodide R* and 10 ml of *dilute sulphuric acid R.* Titrate with *0.1 M sodium thiosulphate,* using 1 ml of *starch solution R,* added towards the end of the titration, as indicator. Standardise immediately before use.

Storage: protected from light.

0.1 M Silver nitrate. *3005600.*

Dissolve 17.0 g of *silver nitrate R* in *water R* and dilute to 1000.0 ml with the same solvent.

Standardisation. Dissolve 0.100 g of *sodium chloride RV* in 30 ml of *water R.* Titrate with the silver nitrate solution, determining the end-point potentiometrically (*2.2.20*).

1 ml of *0.1 M silver nitrate* is equivalent to 5.844 mg of NaCl.

Storage: protected from light.

0.001 M Silver nitrate. *3009300.*

Dilute 5.0 ml of silver nitrate 0.1 M to 500.0 ml with *water R.*

0.1 M Sodium edetate. *3005900.*

Dissolve 37.5 g of *sodium edetate R* in 500 ml of *water R,* add 100 ml of *1 M sodium hydroxide* and dilute to 1000.0 ml with *water R.*

Standardisation. Dissolve 0.120 g of *zinc RV* in 4 ml of *hydrochloric acid R1* and add 0.1 ml of *bromine water R.* Drive off the excess of bromine by boiling, add *dilute sodium hydroxide solution R* until the solution is weakly acid or neutral and carry out the assay of zinc by complexometry (*2.5.11*).

1 ml of *0.1 M sodium edetate* is equivalent to 6.54 mg of Zn.

Storage: in a polyethylene container.

0.02 M Sodium edetate. *3006000.*

Dissolve 7.444 g of *sodium edetate R* in *water R* and dilute to 1000.0 ml with the same solvent.

Standardisation. Dissolve 0.100 g of *zinc RV* in 4 ml of *hydrochloric acid R1* and add 0.1 ml of *bromine water R.* Drive off the excess of bromine by boiling. Transfer the solution to a volumetric flask and dilute to 100.0 ml with *water R.* Transfer 25.0 ml of the solution to a 500 ml conical flask and dilute to 200 ml with *water R.* Add about 50 mg of *xylenol orange triturate R* and *hexamethylenetetramine R* until the solution becomes violet-pink. Add 2 g of *hexamethylenetetramine R* in excess. Titrate with the sodium edetate solution until the violet-pink colour changes to yellow.

1 ml of *0.02 M sodium edetate* is equivalent to 1.308 mg of Zn.

1 M Sodium hydroxide. *3006300.*

Dissolve 42 g of *sodium hydroxide R* in *carbon dioxide-free water R* and dilute to 1000.0 ml with the same solvent.

Standardisation. Titrate 20.0 ml of the sodium hydroxide solution with *1 M hydrochloric acid* using the indicator prescribed in the assay in which *1 M sodium hydroxide* is used.

If sodium hydroxide free from carbonate is prescribed, prepare it as follows. Dissolve *sodium hydroxide R* in *water R* to give a concentration of 400 g/l to 600 g/l and allow to stand. Decant the clear supernatant liquid, taking precautions to avoid the introduction of carbon dioxide, and dilute with *carbon dioxide-free water R* to the required molarity. The solution complies with the following test. Titrate 20.0 ml of hydrochloric acid of the same molarity with the solution of sodium hydroxide, using 0.5 ml of *phenolphthalein solution R* as indicator. At the end-point add just sufficient of the acid to discharge the pink colour and concentrate the solution to 20 ml by boiling. During boiling add just sufficient acid to discharge the pink colour, which should not reappear after prolonged boiling. The volume of acid used does not exceed 0.1 ml.

0.1 M Sodium hydroxide. *3006600.*

Dilute 100.0 ml of *1 M sodium hydroxide* to 1000.0 ml with *carbon dioxide-free water R.*

Standardisation. Titrate 20.0 ml of the sodium hydroxide solution with *0.1 M hydrochloric acid,* using the end-point detection prescribed for the assay in which the *0.1 M sodium hydroxide* is used.

Standardisation (for use in the assay of halide salts of organic bases). Dissolve 0.100 g of *benzoic acid RV* in a mixture of 5 ml of *0.01 M hydrochloric acid* and 50 ml of *alcohol R.* Carry out the titration (*2.2.20*), using the sodium hydroxide solution. Note the volume added between the 2 points of inflexion.

1 ml of *0.1 M sodium hydroxide* is equivalent to 12.21 mg of $C_7H_6O_2$.

2 M Sodium hydroxide. *3009800.*

Dissolve 84 g of *sodium hydroxide R* in *carbon dioxide-free water R* and dilute to 1000.0 ml with the same solvent.

0.1 M Sodium hydroxide, ethanolic. *3007000.*

To 250 ml of *ethanol R* add 3.3 g of *strong sodium hydroxide solution R.*

Standardisation. Dissolve 0.100 g of *benzoic acid RV* in 2 ml of *water R* and 10 ml of *alcohol R.* Titrate with the ethanolic sodium hydroxide solution, using 0.2 ml of *thymolphthalein solution R* as indicator. Standardise immediately before use.

1 ml of *0.1 M ethanolic sodium hydroxide* is equivalent to 12.21 mg of $C_7H_6O_2$.

0.1 M Sodium methoxide. *3007100.*

Cool 175 ml of *anhydrous methanol R* in iced *water R* and add, in small portions, about 2.5 g of freshly cut *sodium R*. When the metal has dissolved, dilute to 1000.0 ml with *toluene R*.

Standardisation. To 10 ml of *dimethylformamide R* add 0.05 ml of a 3 g/l solution of *thymol blue R* in *methanol R*, and titrate with the sodium methoxide solution until a pure blue colour is obtained. Immediately add 0.200 g of *benzoic acid RV*. Stir to effect solution and titrate with the sodium methoxide solution until the pure blue colour is again obtained. Protect the solution from atmospheric carbon dioxide throughout the titration. From the volume of titrant used in the second titration ascertain the exact strength of the sodium methoxide solution. Standardise immediately before use.

1 ml of *0.1 M sodium methoxide* is equivalent to 12.21 mg of $C_7H_6O_2$.

0.1 M Sodium nitrite. *3007200.*

Dissolve 7.5 g of *sodium nitrite R* in *water R* and dilute to 1000.0 ml with the same solvent.

Standardisation. Dissolve 0.300 g of *sulphanilic acid RV* in 50 ml of *dilute hydrochloric acid R* and carry out the determination of primary aromatic amino-nitrogen (*2.5.8*), using the sodium nitrite solution and determining the end-point electrometrically. Standardise immediately before use.

1 ml of *0.1 M sodium nitrite* is equivalent to 17.32 mg of $C_6H_7NO_3S$.

0.1 M Sodium periodate. *3009500.*

Dissolve 21.4 g of *sodium periodate R* in about 500 ml of *water R* and dilute to 1000.0 ml with the same solvent.

Standardisation. In a stoppered flask, introduce 20.0 ml of the sodium periodate solution and add 5 ml of *perchloric acid R*. Close the flask and shake. Adjust the solution to pH 6.4 (*2.2.3*) using a saturated solution of *sodium hydrogen carbonate R*. Add 10 ml of *potassium iodide solution R*, close, shake and allow to stand for 2 min. Titrate with *0.025 M sodium arsenite* until the yellow colour almost disappears. Add 2 ml of *starch solution R* and titrate slowly until the colour is completely discharged.

0.1 M Sodium thiosulphate. *3007300.*

Dissolve 25 g of *sodium thiosulphate R* and 0.2 g of *sodium carbonate R* in *carbon dioxide-free water R* and dilute to 1000.0 ml with the same solvent.

Standardisation. To 10.0 ml of *0.033 M potassium bromate*, add 40 ml of *water R*, 10 ml of *potassium iodide solution R* and 5 ml of *hydrochloric acid R1*. Titrate with the sodium thiosulphate solution, using 1 ml of *starch solution R*, added towards the end of the titration, as indicator.

0.5 M Sulphuric acid. *3007800.*

Dissolve 28 ml of sulphuric acid R in *water R* and dilute to 1000.0 ml with the same solvent.

Standardisation. Dissolve 1.000 g of *sodium carbonate RV* in 50 ml of *water R*, add 0.1 ml of *methyl orange solution R*, and titrate with the sulphuric acid until the solution begins to turn reddish-yellow. Boil for about 2 min. The colour of the solutions reverts to yellow. Cool and titrate again until the reddish-yellow colour reappears.

1 ml of *0.5 M sulphuric acid* is equivalent to 53.00 mg of Na_2CO_3.

0.05 M Sulphuric acid. *3008000.*

Dilute 100.0 ml of *0.5 M sulphuric acid* to 1000.0 ml with *water R*.

Standardisation. Carry out the titration described for *0.5 M sulphuric acid*, using 0.100 g of *sodium carbonate RV*, dissolved in 20 ml of *water R*.

1 ml of *0.05 M sulphuric acid* is equivalent to 5.30 mg of Na_2CO_3.

0.1 M Tetrabutylammonium hydroxide. *3008300.*

Dissolve 40 g of *tetrabutylammonium iodide R* in 90 ml of *anhydrous methanol R*, add 20 g of finely powdered *silver oxide R* and shake vigorously for 1 h. Centrifuge a few millilitres of the mixture and test the supernatant liquid for iodides. If a positive reaction is obtained, add an additional 2 g of *silver oxide R* and shake for a further 30 min. Repeat this procedure until the liquid is free from iodides, filter the mixture through a fine sintered-glass filter and rinse the reaction vessel and filter with three quantities, each of 50 ml, of *toluene R*. Add the washings to the filtrate and dilute to 1000.0 ml with *toluene R*. Pass dry carbon dioxide-free nitrogen through the solution for 5 min.

Standardisation. To 10 ml of *dimethylformamide R* add 0.05 ml of a 3 g/l solution of *thymol blue R* in *methanol R* and titrate with the tetrabutylammonium hydroxide solution until a pure blue colour is obtained. Immediately add 0.200 g of *benzoic acid RV*. Stir to effect solution, and titrate with the tetrabutylammonium hydroxide solution until the pure blue colour is again obtained. Protect the solution from atmospheric carbon dioxide throughout the titration. From the volume of titrant used in the second titration ascertain the exact strength of the tetrabutylammonium hydroxide solution. Standardise immediately before use.

1 ml of *0.1 M tetrabutylammonium hydroxide* is equivalent to 12.21 mg of $C_7H_6O_2$.

0.1 M Tetrabutylammonium hydroxide in 2-propanol. *3008400.*

Prepare as described for *0.1 M tetrabutylammonium hydroxide* using *2-propanol R* instead of *toluene R* and standardise as described.

0.05 M Zinc chloride. *3008500.*

Dissolve 6.82 g of *zinc chloride R*, weighed with appropriate precautions, in *water R*. If necessary, add dropwise *dilute hydrochloric acid R* until the opalescence disappears. Dilute to 1000.0 ml with *water R*.

Standardisation. To 20.0 ml of the zinc chloride solution add 5 ml of *dilute acetic acid R* and carry out the determination of zinc by complexometry (*2.5.11*).

0.1 M Zinc sulphate. *3008600.*

Dissolve 29 g of *zinc sulphate R* in *water R* and dilute to 1000.0 ml with the same solvent.

Standardisation. To 20.0 ml of the zinc sulphate solution add 5 ml of *dilute acetic acid R* and carry out the determination of zinc by complexometry (*2.5.11*).

5. GENERAL TEXTS

5.1. GENERAL TEXTS ON STERILITY

5.1. GENERAL TEXTS ON STERILITY

01/2005:50101

5.1.1. METHODS OF PREPARATION OF STERILE PRODUCTS

Sterility is the absence of viable micro-organisms. The sterility of a product cannot be guaranteed by testing; it has to be assured by the application of a suitably validated production process. It is essential that the effect of the chosen sterilisation procedure on the product (including its final container or package) is investigated to ensure effectiveness and the integrity of the product and that the procedure is validated before being applied in practice. It is recommended that the choice of the container is such as to allow the optimum sterilisation to be applied. Failure to follow meticulously a validated process involves the risk of a non-sterile product or of a deteriorated product. Revalidation is carried out whenever major changes in the sterilisation procedure, including changes in the load, take place. It is expected that the principles of good manufacturing practice (as described in, for example, the European Community Guide to GMP) will have been observed in the design of the process including, in particular, the use of:

- qualified personnel with appropriate training,
- adequate premises,
- suitable production equipment, designed for easy cleaning and sterilisation,
- adequate precautions to minimise the bioburden prior to sterilisation,
- validated procedures for all critical production steps,
- environmental monitoring and in-process testing procedures.

The precautions necessary to minimise the pre-sterilisation bioburden include the use of components with an acceptable low degree of microbial contamination. Microbiological monitoring and setting of suitable action limits may be advisable for ingredients which are liable to be contaminated because of their origin, nature or method of preparation.

The methods described here apply mainly to the inactivation or removal of bacteria, yeasts and moulds. For biological products of animal or human origin or in cases where such material has been used in the production process, it is necessary during validation to demonstrate that the process is capable of the removal or inactivation of relevant viral contamination. Guidance on this aspect is provided in, for example, the appropriate European Community Notes for Guidance.

Wherever possible, a process in which the product is sterilised in its final container (terminal sterilisation) is chosen. When a fully validated terminal sterilisation method by steam, dry heat or ionising radiation is used, parametric release, that is the release of a batch of sterilised items based on process data rather than on the basis of submitting a sample of the items to sterility testing, may be carried out, subject to the approval of the competent authority.

If terminal sterilisation is not possible, filtration through a bacteria-retentative filter or aseptic processing is used; wherever possible, appropriate additional treatment of the product (for example, heating of the product) in its final container is applied. In all cases, the container and closure are required to maintain the sterility of the product throughout its shelf-life.

Sterility Assurance Level (SAL)

Where appropriate reference is made within the methods described below, to a "sterility assurance level" or "SAL". The achievement of sterility within any one item in a population of items submitted to a sterilisation process cannot be guaranteed nor can it be demonstrated. The inactivation of micro-organisms by physical or chemical means follows an exponential law; thus there is always a finite statistical probability that a micro-organism may survive the sterilising process. For a given process, the probability of survival is determined by the number, types and resistance of the micro-organisms present and by the environment in which the organisms exist during treatment. The SAL of a sterilising process is the degree of assurance with which the process in question renders a population of items sterile. The SAL for a given process is expressed as the probability of a non-sterile item in that population. An SAL of 10^{-6}, for example, denotes a probability of not more than one viable micro-organism in 1×10^6 sterilised items of the final product. The SAL of a process for a given product is established by appropriate validation studies.

METHODS AND CONDITIONS OF STERILISATION

Sterilisation may be carried out by one of the methods described below. Modifications to, or combinations of, these methods may be used provided that the chosen procedure is validated both with respect to its effectiveness and the integrity of the product including its container or package.

For all methods of sterilisation the critical conditions of the operation are monitored in order to confirm that the previously determined required conditions are achieved throughout the batch during the whole sterilisation process This applies in all cases including those where the reference conditions are used.

TERMINAL STERILISATION

For terminal sterilisation it is essential to take into account the non-uniformity of the physical and, where relevant, chemical conditions within the sterilising chamber. The location within the sterilising chamber that is least accessible to the sterilising agent is determined for each loading configuration of each type and size of container or package (for example, the coolest location in an autoclave). The minimum lethality delivered by the sterilising cycle and the reproducibility of the cycle are also determined in order to ensure that all loads will consistently receive the specified treatment.

Having established a terminal sterilisation process, knowledge of its performance in routine use is gained wherever possible, by monitoring and suitably recording the physical and, where relevant, chemical conditions achieved within the load in the chamber throughout each sterilising cycle.

Steam sterilisation (Heating in an autoclave). Sterilisation by saturated steam under pressure is preferred, wherever applicable, especially for aqueous preparations. For this method of terminal sterilisation the reference conditions for aqueous preparations are heating at a minimum of 121 °C for 15 min. Other combinations of time and temperature may be used provided that it has been satisfactorily demonstrated that the process chosen delivers an adequate and reproducible level of lethality when operating routinely within the established tolerances. The procedures and precautions employed are such, as to give an SAL of 10^{-6} or better. Guidance concerning validation by means of the F_0 concept is provided below (*5.1.5*).

Knowledge of the physical conditions (temperature and pressure) within the autoclave chamber during the sterilisation procedure is obtained. The temperature is usually measured by means of temperature-sensing elements inserted into representative containers together with additional elements at the previously established coolest part of the loaded chamber. The conditions throughout each cycle are suitably recorded, for example, as a temperature-time chart, or by any other suitable means.

Where a biological assessment is carried out, this is obtained using a suitable biological indicator (*5.1.2*).

Dry heat sterilisation. For this method of terminal sterilisation the reference conditions are a minimum of 160 °C for at least 2 h. Other combinations of time and temperature may be used provided that it has been satisfactorily demonstrated that the process chosen delivers an adequate and reproducible level of lethality when operated routinely within the established tolerances. The procedures and precautions employed are such as to give an SAL of 10^{-6} or better.

Dry heat sterilisation is carried out in an oven equipped with forced air circulation or other equipment specially designed for the purpose. The steriliser is loaded in such a way that a uniform temperature is achieved throughout the load. Knowledge of the temperature within the steriliser during the sterilisation procedure is usually obtained by means of temperature-sensing elements inserted into representative containers together with additional elements at the previously established coolest part of the loaded steriliser. The temperature throughout each cycle is suitably recorded.

Where a biological assessment is carried out, this is obtained using a suitable biological indicator (*5.1.2*).

Dry heat at temperatures greater than 220 °C is frequently used for sterilisation and depyrogenation of glassware. In this case demonstration of a 3-log reduction in heat resistant endotoxin can be used as a replacement for biological indicators (*5.1.2*).

Ionising radiation sterilisation. Sterilisation by this method is achieved by exposure of the product to ionising radiation in the form of gamma radiation from a suitable radioisotopic source (such as cobalt 60) or of a beam of electrons energised by a suitable electron accelerator.

In some countries there are regulations that lay down rules for the use of ionising radiation for sterilisation purposes, for example, in the appropriate European Community Notes for Guidance.

For this method of terminal sterilisation the reference absorbed dose is 25 kGy. Other doses may be used provided that it has satisfactorily been demonstrated that the dose chosen delivers an adequate and reproducible level of lethality when the process is operated routinely within the established tolerances. The procedures and precautions employed are such as to give an SAL of 10^{-6} or better.

During the sterilisation procedure the radiation absorbed by the product is monitored regularly by means of established dosimetry procedures that are independent of dose rate. Dosimeters are calibrated against a standard source at a reference radiation plant on receipt from the supplier and at suitable intervals of not longer than one year thereafter.

Where a biological assessment is carried out, this is obtained using a suitable biological indicator (*5.1.2*).

Gas sterilisation. This method of sterilisation is only to be used where there is no suitable alternative. It is essential that penetration by gas and moisture into the material to be sterilised is ensured and that it is followed by a process of elimination of the gas under conditions that have been previously established to ensure that any residue of gas or its transformation products in the sterilised product is below the concentration that could give rise to toxic effects during use of the product. Guidance on this aspect with respect to the use of ethylene oxide is provided, for example, in the appropriate European Community Notes for Guidance.

Wherever possible, the gas concentration, relative humidity, temperature and duration of the process are measured and recorded. Measurements are made where sterilisation conditions are least likely to be achieved, as determined at validation.

The effectiveness of the process applied to each sterilisation load is checked using a suitable biological indicator (*5.1.2*).

A suitable sample of each batch is tested for sterility (*2.6.1*) before the batch is released.

FILTRATION

Certain active ingredients and products that cannot be terminally sterilised may be subjected to a filtration procedure using a filter of a type that has been demonstrated to be satisfactory by means of a microbial challenge test using a suitable test micro-organism. A suspension of *Pseudomonas diminuta* (ATCC 19146, NCIMB 11091 or CIP 103020) may be suitable. It is recommended that a challenge of at least 10^7 CFU per cm^2 of active filter surface is used and that the suspension is prepared in tryptone soya broth which, after passage throug the filter, is collected aseptically and incubated aerobically at 32 °C. Such products need special precautions. The production process and environment are designed to minimise microbial contamination and are regularly subjected to appropriate monitoring procedures. The equipment, containers and closures and, wherever possible, the ingredients are subjected to an appropriate sterilisation process. It is recommended that the filtration process is carried out as close as possible to the filling point. The operations following filtration are carried out under aseptic conditions.

Solutions are passed through a bacteria-retentive membrane with a nominal pore size of 0.22 μm or less or any other type of filter known to have equivalent properties of bacteria retention. Appropriate measures are taken to avoid loss of solute by adsorption on to the filter and to avoid the release of contaminants from the filter. Attention is given to the bioburden prior to filtration, filter capacity, batch size and duration of filtration. The filter is not used for a longer period than has been approved by validation of the combination of the filter and the product in question.

The integrity of an assembled sterilising filter is verified before use and confirmed after use by carrying out tests appropriate to the type of filter used and the stage of testing, for example bubble-point, pressure hold or diffusion rate tests.

Due to the potential additional risks of the filtration method as compared with other sterilisation processes, a prefiltration through a bacteria-retentative filter may be advisable in cases where a low bioburden cannot be ensured by other means.

ASEPTIC PREPARATION

The objective of aseptic processing is to maintain the sterility of a product that is assembled from components, each of which has been sterilised by one of the above methods. This is achieved by using conditions and facilities designed to prevent microbial contamination. Aseptic processing may include aseptic filling of products into container/closure systems, aseptic blending of formulations followed by aseptic filling and aseptic packaging.

In order to maintain the sterility of the components and the product during processing, careful attention needs to be given to:

– environment,
– personnel,

Table 5.1.3.-2. - *Topical preparations*

		Log reduction			
		2 d	**7 d**	**14 d**	**28 d**
Bacteria	A	2	3	-	NI
	B	-	-	3	NI
Fungi	A	-	-	2	NI
	B	-	-	1	NI

The A criteria express the recommended efficacy to be achieved. In justified cases where the A criteria cannot be attained, for example for reasons of an increased risk of adverse reactions, the B criteria must be satisfied.

Table 5.1.3.-3. - *Oral preparations*

	Log reduction	
	14 d	**28 d**
Bacteria	3	NI
Fungi	1	NI

The above criteria express the recommended efficacy to be achieved.

01/2005:50104

5.1.4. MICROBIOLOGICAL QUALITY OF PHARMACEUTICAL PREPARATIONS

The following chapter is published for information.

In the manufacture, packaging, storage and distribution of pharmaceutical preparations, suitable means must be taken to ensure their microbiological quality. The pharmaceutical preparations should comply with the criteria given below.

Category 1

Preparations required to be sterile by the relevant monograph on the dosage form and other preparations labelled sterile.

- Test for sterility (*2.6.1*).

Category 2

Preparations for topical use and for use in the respiratory tract except where required to be sterile and transdermal patches.

- Total viable aerobic count (*2.6.12*). Not more than 10^2 micro-organisms (aerobic bacteria plus fungi) per gram, per millilitre or per patch (including the adhesive and backing layer).
- Transdermal patches: absence of enterobacteria and certain other gram-negative bacteria, determined on 1 patch (including the adhesive and backing layer). Other preparations: not more than 10^1 enterobacteria and certain other gram-negative bacteria per gram or per millilitre (*2.6.13*).
- Absence of *Pseudomonas aeruginosa,* determined on 1 g, 1 ml or one patch (including the adhesive and backing layer) (*2.6.13*).
- Absence of *Staphylococcus aureus,* determined on 1 g, 1 ml or one patch (including the adhesive and backing layer) (*2.6.13*).

Category 3

A. *Preparations for oral and rectal administration.*
   - Total viable aerobic count (*2.6.12*). Not more than 10^3 bacteria and not more than 10^2 fungi per gram or per millilitre.
   - Absence of *Escherichia coli* (1 g or 1 ml) (*2.6.13*).

B. *Preparations for oral administration containing raw materials of natural (animal, vegetable or mineral) origin for which antimicrobial pretreatment is not feasible and for which the competent authority accepts microbial contamination of the raw material exceeding 10^3 viable micro-organisms per gram or per millilitre. Herbal medicinal products described in category 4 are excluded.*
   - Total viable aerobic count (*2.6.12*). Not more than 10^4 bacteria and not more than 10^2 fungi per gram or per millilitre.
   - Not more than 10^2 enterobacteria and certain other gram-negative bacteria per gram or per millilitre (*2.6.13*).
   - Absence of *Salmonella* (10 g or 10 ml) (*2.6.13*).
   - Absence of *Escherichia coli* (1 g or 1 ml) (*2.6.13*).
   - Absence of *Staphylococcus aureus* (1 g or 1 ml) (*2.6.13*).

Category 4

Herbal medicinal products consisting solely of one or more herbal drugs (whole, reduced or powdered).

A. *Herbal medicinal products to which boiling water is added before use.*
   - Total viable aerobic count (*2.6.12*). Not more than 10^7 bacteria and not more than 10^5 fungi per gram or per millilitre.
   - Not more than 10^2 *Escherichia coli* per gram or per millilitre (*2.6.13*, using suitable dilutions).

B. *Herbal medicinal products to which boiling water is not added before use.*
   - Total viable aerobic count (*2.6.12*). Not more than 10^5 bacteria and not more than 10^4 fungi per gram or per millilitre.
   - Not more than 10^3 enterobacteria and certain other gram-negative bacteria per gram or per millilitre (*2.6.13*).
   - Absence of *Escherichia coli* (1 g or 1 ml) (*2.6.13*).
   - Absence of *Salmonella* (10 g or 10 ml) (*2.6.13*).

01/2005:50105

5.1.5. APPLICATION OF THE F_0 CONCEPT TO STEAM STERILISATION OF AQUEOUS PREPARATIONS

The following chapter is published for information.

The F_0 value of a saturated steam sterilisation process is the lethality expressed in terms of the equivalent time in minutes at a temperature of 121 °C delivered by the process to the product in its final container with reference to micro-organisms possessing a *Z*-value of 10.

The total F_0 of a process takes account of the heating up and cooling down phases of the cycle and can be calculated by integration of lethal rates with respect to time at discrete temperature intervals.

When a steam sterilisation cycle is chosen on the basis of the F_0 concept, great care must be taken to ensure that an adequate assurance of sterility is consistently

5. General texts

achieved. In addition to validating the process, it may also be necessary to perform continuous, rigorous microbiological monitoring during routine production to demonstrate that the microbiological parameters are within the established tolerances so as to give an SAL of 10^{-6} or better.

In connection with sterilisation by steam, the *Z*-value relates the heat resistance of a micro-organism to changes in temperature. The *Z*-value is the change in temperature required to alter the *D*-value by a factor of 10.

The *D*-value (or decimal reduction value) is the value of a parameter of sterilisation (duration or absorbed dose) required to reduce the number of viable organisms to 10 per cent of the original number. It is only of significance under precisely defined experimental conditions.

The following mathematical relationships apply:

$$F_0 = D_{121} (\log N_0 - \log N) = D_{121} \log IF$$

D_{121} = *D*-value of the reference spores (*5.1.2*) at 121 °C,

N_0 = initial number of viable micro-organisms,

N = final number of viable micro-organisms,

IF = inactivation factor.

$$Z = \frac{T_2 - T_1}{\log D_1 - \log D_2}$$

D_1 = *D*-value of the micro-organism at temperature T_1,

D_2 = *D*-value of the micro-organism at temperature T_2.

$$IF = N_0 - N = 10^{t/D}$$

t = exposure time,

D = *D*-value of micro-organism in the exposure conditions.

5. General texts

5.2. GENERAL TEXTS ON VACCINES

5.2. GENERAL TEXTS ON VACCINES

01/2005:50201

5.2.1. TERMINOLOGY USED IN MONOGRAPHS ON VACCINES

For some items, alternative terms commonly used in connection with veterinary vaccines are shown in parenthesis.

Seed-lot system. A seed-lot system is a system according to which successive batches of a product are derived from the same master seed lot. For routine production, a working seed lot may be prepared from the master seed lot. The origin and the passage history of the master seed lot and the working seed lot are recorded.

Master seed lot. A culture of a micro-organism distributed from a single bulk into containers and processed together in a single operation in such a manner as to ensure uniformity and stability and to prevent contamination. A master seed lot in liquid form is usually stored at or below − 70 °C. A freeze-dried master seed lot is stored at a temperature known to ensure stability.

Working seed lot. A culture of a micro-organism derived from the master seed lot and intended for use in production. Working seed lots are distributed into containers and stored as described above for master seed lots.

Cell-bank system (Cell-seed system). A system whereby successive final lots (batches) of a product are manufactured by culture in cells derived from the same master cell bank (master cell seed). A number of containers from the master cell bank (master cell seed) are used to prepare a working cell bank (working cell seed). The cell-bank system (cell-seed system) is validated for the highest passage level achieved during routine production.

Master cell bank (Master cell seed). A culture of cells distributed into containers in a single operation, processed together and stored in such a manner as to ensure uniformity and stability and to prevent contamination. A master cell bank (master cell seed) is usually stored at − 70 °C or lower.

Working cell bank (Working cell seed). A culture of cells derived from the master cell bank (master cell seed) and intended for use in the preparation of production cell cultures. The working cell bank (working cell seed) is distributed into containers, processed and stored as described for the master cell bank (master cell seed).

Primary cell cultures. Cultures of cells obtained by trypsination of a suitable tissue or organ. The cells are essentially identical to those of the tissue of origin and are no more than 5 *in vitro* passages from the initial preparation from the animal tissue.

Cell lines. Cultures of cells that have a high capacity for multiplication *in vitro*. In diploid cell lines, the cells have essentially the same characteristics as those of the tissue of origin. In continuous cell lines, the cells are able to multiply indefinitely in culture and may be obtained from healthy or tumoral tissue. Some continuous cell lines have oncogenic potential under certain conditions.

Production cell culture. A culture of cells intended for use in production; it may be derived from one or more containers of the working cell bank (working cell seed) or it may be a primary cell culture.

Control cells. A quantity of cells set aside, at the time of virus inoculation, as uninfected cell cultures. The uninfected cells are incubated under similar conditions to those used for the production cell cultures.

Single harvest. Material derived on one or more occasions from a single production cell culture inoculated with the same working seed lot or a suspension derived from the working seed lot, incubated, and harvested in a single production run.

Monovalent pooled harvest. Pooled material containing a single strain or type of micro-organism or antigen and derived from a number of eggs, cell culture containers etc. that are processed at the same time.

Final bulk vaccine. Material that has undergone all the steps of production except for the final filling. It consists of one or more monovalent pooled harvests from cultures of one or more species or types of micro-organism, after clarification, dilution or addition of any adjuvant or other auxiliary substance. It is treated to ensure its homogeneity and is used for filling the containers of one or more final lots (batches).

Final lot (Batch). A collection of closed, final containers or other final dosage units that are expected to be homogeneous and equivalent with respect to risk of contamination during filling or preparation of the final product. The dosage units are filled, or otherwise prepared, from the same final bulk vaccine, freeze-dried together (if applicable) and closed in one continuous working session. They bear a distinctive number or code identifying the final lot (batch). Where a final bulk vaccine is filled and/or freeze-dried on several separate sessions, there results a related set of final lots (batches) that are usually identified by the use of a common part in the distinctive number or code; these related final lots (batches) are sometimes referred to as sub-batches, sub-lots or filling lots.

Combined vaccine. A multicomponent preparation formulated so that different antigens are administered simultaneously. The different antigenic components are intended to protect against different strains or types of the same organism and/or different organisms. A combined vaccine may be supplied by the manufacturer either as a single liquid or freeze-dried preparation or as several constituents with directions for admixture before use.

01/2005:50202

5.2.2. CHICKEN FLOCKS FREE FROM SPECIFIED PATHOGENS FOR THE PRODUCTION AND QUALITY CONTROL OF VACCINES

INTRODUCTION

Where specified in a monograph, chickens, embryos or cell cultures used for the production or quality control of vaccines are derived from eggs produced by chicken flocks free from specified pathogens (SPF). The SPF status of a flock is ensured by means of the system described below. The list of micro-organisms given is based on current knowledge and will be updated as necessary.

GENERAL PRINCIPLES AND PROCEDURES

A flock is defined as a group of birds sharing a common environment and having their own caretakers who have no contact with non-SPF flocks. Once a flock is defined, no non-SPF birds are added to it.

5. General texts

For SPF flocks established on a rolling basis, all replacements are hatched and reared in the controlled environment house. Subject to the agreement of the competent authorities, SPF embryos derived from a tested SPF flock from another house on the same site may be introduced. From 8 weeks of age, these replacement birds are regarded as a flock and monitored monthly in accordance with the Subsequent Testing requirements. At point of lay, all these replacement birds are tested in accordance with the Initial Testing requirements.

The flock is housed so as to minimise the chance of contamination. It is not sited near to non-SPF flocks of birds and is housed in an isolator or on wire in a building with filtered air under positive pressure. Appropriate measures are taken to prevent access of rodents, wild birds, insects and unauthorised people.

Personnel authorised to enter must have no contact with other birds or with agents likely to infect the flock. It is advisable for personnel to shower and change clothing or to wear protective clothing before entering the chicken house.

Items taken into the flock are sterilised. The feed is suitably treated to avoid the introduction of undesirable micro-organisms and water is obtained from a chlorinated supply. No medication is given that could interfere with detection of disease in the flock.

A permanent record is kept of the general health of the flock and any abnormality is investigated. Factors to be monitored include morbidity, mortality, general physical condition, feed consumption, daily egg production and egg quality, fertility and hatchability. Dirty eggs are discarded; clean eggs may be surface-disinfected whilst warm.

The flock originates from chickens shown to be free from vertically-transmitted agents. In particular, each chicken from which the flock is derived is tested repeatedly to ensure freedom from leucosis viruses and their antibodies. In order to establish the SPF status of a flock, it is kept under SPF conditions for a test period of not less than 4 months. Each bird in the entire flock is shown to be free from evidence of infection with the agents listed below under Initial Testing after 6 weeks and at the end of the test period.

For each new generation in an established flock, all of the birds in the flock are tested at not later than 20 weeks of age, using the tests prescribed below under Initial Testing. After the initial test, monthly tests are carried out on a representative 5 per cent sample (but not less than ten and not more than two hundred birds), using the tests prescribed below under Subsequent Testing, with a final test at 4 weeks after the last collection of eggs.

For all tests, blood samples are collected from an appropriate number of birds at the specified time. The resultant serum samples are examined for antibodies against the relevant agents. Serum-neutralisation tests are done on pools of not more than five sera. All other tests are done on each individual serum. Positive and negative controls are used in all tests. The reagents used in the tests are standardised against international or European standard reagents where these are available. For avian leucosis virus, in addition to tests for antibodies carried out on serum samples, appropriate samples are taken for testing for the virus.

In addition to serological tests, clinical examination is carried out at least once per week to verify that the birds are free from fowl-pox and signs of other infections. Necropsy and, where necessary to confirm diagnosis, histopathological examination are carried out on any bird that dies to verify that there is no sign of infection. The absence of *Salmonella* spp. is determined by cultural examination of faecal samples at least once every 4 weeks; a pool of up to ten samples may be used for the tests.

If a positive result is obtained in any test carried out to establish the SPF status of a flock, the flock may not be designated as an SPF flock. If a positive result is obtained in any test carried out on an established flock, the flock loses its SPF status. Special provisions apply to chick anaemia agent (CAA) as described below. Any chickens, embryos or cell cultures collected since the previous negative test are not suitable for use: any product made from them must be discarded and any quality control tests done with them are invalid and must be repeated.

In order to regain SPF status, the flock is maintained under SPF conditions and routine 5 per cent monthly testing shall continue except that every bird in the entire flock is tested every month for infection with the particular agent that gave the positive result. Infected birds and their progeny are removed from the flock. SPF status is regained after two such consecutive tests have yielded completely negative results.

A positive result for CAA does not necessarily exclude use of material derived from the flock, but live vaccines for use in birds less than 7 days old must be produced using material from CAA-negative flocks. Inactivated vaccines for use in birds less than 7 days old may be produced using material from flocks that have not been shown to be free from CAA, provided it has been demonstrated that the inactivation process inactivates CAA.

Permanent records of mortality and of results of flock testing are kept for a minimum of five years. Details of any deterioration in egg production or hatchability, except for accidental cases identified as being of non-infectious origin, and of any test results indicating infection with a specified agent, are immediately submitted to the user of the eggs.

INITIAL TESTING

Subject to agreement by the competent authority, other types of test may be used provided they are at least as sensitive as those indicated and of appropriate specificity.

Micro-organism	Type of test
Avian adenoviruses	Enzyme-linked immuno-sorbent assay
Avian encephalomyelitis virus	Enzyme-linked immuno-sorbent assay
Avian infectious bronchitis virus	Enzyme-linked immuno-sorbent assay
Avian infectious laryngotracheitis virus	Serum neutralisation
Avian leucosis viruses	Enzyme-linked immuno-sorbent assay for virus and serum neutralisation for antibody
Avian nephritis virus	Fluorescent antibody
Avian reoviruses	Enzyme-linked immuno-sorbent assay
Avian reticuloendotheliosis virus	Fluorescent antibody
Chick anaemia agent	Fluorescent antibody
Haemagglutinating avian adenovirus (Egg drop syndrome 76- EDS 76 virus)	Haemagglutination inhibition
Infectious bursal disease virus	Serum neutralisation against each serotype present in the country of origin
Influenza A virus	Enzyme-linked immuno-sorbent assay
Marek's disease virus	Enzyme-linked immuno-sorbent assay

Micro-organism	Type of test
Newcastle disease virus	Haemagglutination inhibition
Turkey rhinotracheitis virus	Enzyme-linked immuno-sorbent assay
Mycoplasma gallisepticum	Agglutination and, to confirm a positive test, haemagglutination inhibition
Mycoplasma synoviae	Agglutination and, to confirm a positive test, haemagglutination inhibition
Salmonella pullorum	Agglutination

SUBSEQUENT TESTING

Subject to agreement by the competent authority, other types of test may be used provided they are at least as sensitive as those indicated and of appropriate specificity.

Micro-organism	Type of test
Avian adenoviruses	Enzyme-linked immuno-sorbent assay
Avian encephalomyelitis virus	Enzyme-linked immuno-sorbent assay
Avian infectious bronchitis virus	Enzyme-linked immuno-sorbent assay
Avian infectious laryngotracheitis virus	Serum neutralisation
Avian leucosis viruses	Enzyme-linked immuno-sorbent assay for the antibody
Avian nephritis virus	Fluorescent antibody
Avian reoviruses	Fluorescent antibody
Avian reticuloendotheliosis virus	Fluorescent antibody
Chick anaemia agent	Fluorescent antibody
Haemagglutinating avian adenovirus	Haemagglutination inhibition
Infectious bursal disease virus	Immunodiffusion against each serotype present in the country of origin
Influenza A virus	Enzyme-linked immuno-sorbent assay
Marek's disease virus	Enzyme-linked immuno-sorbent assay
Newcastle disease virus	Haemagglutination inhibition
Turkey rhinotracheitis virus	Enzyme-linked immuno-sorbent assay
Mycoplasma gallisepticum	Agglutination and, to confirm a positive test, haemagglutination inhibition
Mycoplasma synoviae	Agglutination and, to confirm a positive test, haemagglutination inhibition
Salmonella pullorum	Agglutination

01/2005:50203

5.2.3. CELL SUBSTRATES FOR THE PRODUCTION OF VACCINES FOR HUMAN USE

This general chapter deals with diploid cell lines and continuous cell lines used for the production of vaccines for human use; specific issues relating to vaccines prepared by recombinant DNA technology are covered by the monograph on *Products of recombinant DNA technology (0784)*. Testing to be carried out at various stages (cell seed, master cell bank, working cell bank, cells at or beyond the maximum population doubling level used for production) is indicated in Table 5.2.3.-1. General provisions for the use of cell lines and test methods are given below. Where primary cells or cells that have undergone a few passages without constitution of a cell bank are used for vaccine production, requirements are given in the individual monograph for the vaccine concerned.

Diploid cell lines. A diploid cell line has a high but finite capacity for multiplication *in vitro*.

Continuous cell lines. A continuous cell line has the capacity to multiply indefinitely *in vitro*; the cells often have differences in karyotype compared to the original cells; they may be obtained from healthy or tumoral tissue.

For injectable vaccines produced in continuous cell lines, the purification process is validated to demonstrate removal of substrate-cell DNA to a level equivalent to not more than 10 ng per single human dose, unless otherwise prescribed.

Cell-bank system. Production of vaccines in diploid and continuous cell lines is based on a cell-bank system. The *in vitro* age of the cells is counted from the master cell bank. Each working cell bank is prepared from one or more containers of the master cell bank. The use, identity and inventory control of the containers is carefully documented.

Media and substances of animal and human origin. The composition of media used for isolation and all subsequent culture is recorded in detail and if substances of animal origin are used they must be free from extraneous agents.

If human albumin is used, it complies with the monograph on *Human albumin solution (0255)*.

Bovine serum used for the preparation and maintenance of cell cultures is tested and shown to be sterile and free from bovine viruses, notably bovine diarrhoea virus and mycoplasmas.

Trypsin used for the preparation of cell cultures is examined by suitable methods and shown to be sterile and free from mycoplasmas and viruses, notably pestiviruses and parvoviruses.

Cell seed. The data used to assess the suitability of the cell seed comprise information, where available, on source, history and characterisation.

Source of the cell seed. For human cell lines, the following information concerning the donor is recorded: ethnic and geographical origin, age, sex, general physiological condition, tissue or organ used, results of any tests for pathogens.

For animal cell lines, the following information is recorded concerning the source of the cells: species, strain, breeding conditions, geographical origin, age, sex, general physiological condition, tissue or organ used, results of any tests for pathogens.

Cells of neural origin, such as neuroblastoma and P12 cell lines, may contain substances that concentrate agents of spongiform encephalopathies and such cells are not used for vaccine production.

History of the cell seed. The following information is recorded: the method used to isolate the cell seed, culture methods and any other procedures used to establish the master cell bank, notably any that might expose the cells to extraneous agents.

Full information may not be available on the ingredients of media used in the past for cultivation of cells, for example on the source of substances of animal origin; where justified and authorised, cell banks already established using such media may be used for vaccine production.

Characterisation of the cell seed. The following properties are investigated:

(1) the identity of the cells (for example, isoenzymes, serology, nucleic acid fingerprinting);

Table 5.2.3.-1 – *Testing of cell lines*

Test	Cell seed	Master cell bank (MCB)	Working cell bank (WCB)	Cells at or beyond the maximum population doubling level used for production
1. IDENTITY AND PURITY				
Morphology	+	+	+	+
Relevant selection of the following tests: biochemical (e.g. isoenzymes), immunological (e.g. histocompatibility), cytogenetic markers, nucleic acid fingerprinting	+	+	+	+
Karyotype (diploid cell lines)	+	+	+(1)	+(1)
Life span (diploid cell lines)	−	+	+	−
2. EXTRANEOUS AGENTS				
Bacterial and fungal contamination	−	+	+	−
Mycoplasmas	−	+	+	−
Tests in cell cultures	−	−	+	−
Co-cultivation	−	−	+(2)	+(2)
Tests in animals and eggs	−	−	+(2)	+(2)
Specific tests for possible contaminants depending on the origin of the cells (see above under Infectious extraneous agents)	−	−	+(2)	+(2)
Retroviruses	−	+(3)	−	+(3)
3. TUMORIGENICITY				
Tumorigenicity	−	−	−	+(4)

(1) The diploid character is established for each working cell bank but using cells at or beyond the maximum population doubling level used for production.

(2) Testing is carried out for each working cell bank, but using cells at or beyond the maximum population doubling level used for production.

(3) Testing is carried out for the master cell bank, but using cells at or beyond the maximum population doubling level used for production.

(4) The MRC-5 cell line, the WI-38 cell line and the FRhL-2 cell line are recognised as being non-tumorigenic and they need not be tested. Tests are not carried out on cell lines that are known or assumed to be tumorigenic.

(2) the growth characteristics of the cells and their morphological properties (light and electron microscopes);

(3) for diploid cell lines, karyotype;

(4) for diploid cell lines, the *in vitro* life span in terms of population doubling level.

Cell substrate stability. Suitable viability of the cell line in the intended storage conditions must be demonstrated. For a given product to be prepared in the cell line, it is necessary to demonstrate that consistent production can be obtained with cells at passage levels at the beginning and end of the intended span of use.

Infectious extraneous agents. Cell lines for vaccine production shall be free from infectious extraneous agents. Tests for extraneous agents are carried out as shown in Table 5.2.3.-1.

Depending on the origin and culture history of the cell line, it may be necessary to carry out tests for selected, specific potential contaminants, particularly those that are known to infect latently the species of origin, for example simian virus 40 in rhesus monkeys. For cell lines of rodent origin, antibody-production tests are carried out in mice, rats and hamsters to detect species-specific viruses.

Cell lines are examined for the presence of retroviruses as described below. Cell lines that show the presence of retroviruses capable of replication are not acceptable for production of vaccines.

Tumorigenicity. For the preparation of live vaccines, the cell line must not be tumorigenic at any population doubling level used for vaccine production. Where a tumorigenic cell line is used for the production of other types of vaccine, the purification process is validated to demonstrate that residual substrate-cell DNA is reduced to less than 10 ng per single human dose of the vaccine, unless otherwise prescribed, and that substrate-cell protein is reduced to an acceptable level.

A cell line which is known to have tumorigenic potential does not have to be tested further. If a cell line is of unknown tumorigenic potential, it is either regarded as being tumorigenic or it is tested for tumorigenicity using an *in vitro* test as described below; if the result of the *in vitro* test is negative or not clearly positive, an *in vivo* test as described below is carried out. The tests are carried out using cells at or beyond the maximum population doubling level that will be used for vaccine production.

The MRC-5, the WI-38 and the FRhL-2 cell lines are recognised as being non-tumorigenic and further testing is not necessary.

Chromosomal characterisation. Diploid cell lines shall be shown to be diploid. More extensive characterisation of a diploid cell line by karyotype analysis is required if the removal of intact cells during processing after harvest has not been validated. Samples from four passage levels evenly spaced over the life-span of the cell line are examined. A minimum of 200 cells in metaphase are examined for exact count of chromosomes and for frequency of hyperploidy, hypoploidy, polyploidy, breaks and structural abnormalities.

The MRC-5, the WI-38 and the FRhL-2 cell lines are recognised as being diploid and well characterised; where they are not genetically modified, further characterisation is not necessary.

TEST METHODS FOR CELL CULTURES

Identification. Nucleic-acid-fingerprint analysis and a relevant selection of the following are used to establish the identity of the cells:

(1) biochemical characteristics (isoenzyme analysis),

(2) immunological characteristics (histocompatibility antigens),

(3) cytogenetic markers.

Contaminating cells. The nucleic-acid-fingerprint analysis carried out for identification also serves to demonstrate freedom from contaminating cells.

Bacterial and fungal contamination. The master cell bank and each working cell bank comply with the test for sterility (*2.6.1*), carried out using for each medium 10 ml of supernatant fluid from cell cultures. Carry out the test on 1 per cent of the containers with a minimum of two containers.

Mycoplasmas (*2.6.7*). The master cell bank and each working cell bank comply with the test for mycoplasmas by the culture method and the indicator cell culture method. Use one or more containers for the test.

Test for extraneous agents in cell cultures. The cells comply with the test for haemadsorbing viruses and with the tests in cell cultures for other extraneous agents given in chapter *2.6.16* under Production cell culture: control cells. If the cells are of simian origin, they are also inoculated into rabbit kidney cell cultures to test for herpesvirus B (cercopithecid herpesvirus 1).

Co-cultivation. Co-cultivate intact and disrupted cells separately with other cell systems including human cells and simian cells. Carry out examinations to detect possible morphological changes. Carry out tests on the cell culture fluids to detect haemagglutinating viruses. The cells comply with the test if no evidence of any extraneous agent is found.

Retroviruses. Examine for the presence of retroviruses using:

(1) infectivity assays,

(2) transmission electron microscopy,

(3) if tests (1) and (2) give negative results, reverse transcriptase assays (in the presence of magnesium and manganese) carried out on pellets obtained by high-speed centrifugation.

Tests in animals. Inject intramuscularly (or, for suckling mice, subcutaneously) into each of the following groups of animals 10^7 viable cells divided equally between the animals in each group:

(1) two litters of suckling mice less than 24 h old, comprising not fewer than ten animals,

(2) ten adult mice.

Inject intracerebrally into each of ten adult mice 10^6 viable cells to detect the possible presence of lymphocytic choriomeningitis virus.

Observe the animals for at least 4 weeks. Investigate animals that become sick or show any abnormality to establish the cause of illness. The cells comply with the test if no evidence of any extraneous agent is found. The test is invalid if fewer than 80 per cent of the animals in each group remain healthy and survive to the end of the observation period.

For cells obtained from a rodent species (for example, Chinese hamster ovary cells or baby hamster kidney cells), tests for antibodies against likely viral contaminants of the species in question are carried out on animals that have received injections of the cells.

Tests in eggs. Using an inoculum of 10^6 viable cells per egg, inoculate the cells into the allantoic cavity of ten SPF embryonated hens' eggs (*5.2.2*) 9 to 11 days old and into the yolk sac of ten SPF embryonated hens' eggs 5 to 6 days old. Incubate for not less than 5 days. Test the allantoic fluids for the presence of haemagglutinins using mammalian and avian red blood cells; carry out the test at 5 ± 3 °C and 20-25 °C and read the results after 30 min and 60 min. The cells comply with the test if no evidence of any extraneous agent is found. The test is invalid if fewer than 80 per cent of the embryos remain healthy and survive to the end of the observation period.

Tests for tumorigenicity *in vitro*. The following test systems may be used:

(1) colony formation in soft agar gels,

(2) production of invasive cell growth following inoculation into organ cultures,

(3) study of transformation activity using, for example, the 3T3 assay system for active oncogenes.

Tests for tumorigenicity *in vivo*. The test consists in establishing a comparison between the cell line and a suitable positive control (for example, HeLa or Hep2 cells).

Animal systems that have been shown to be suitable for this test include:

(1) athymic mice (Nu/Nu genotype),

(2) newborn mice, rats or hamsters that have been treated with antithymocyte serum or globulin,

(3) thymectomised and irradiated mice that have been reconstituted (T^-, B^+) with bone marrow from healthy mice.

Whichever animal system is selected, the cell line and the reference cells are injected into separate groups of 10 animals each. In both cases, the inoculum for each animal is 10^7 cells suspended in a volume of 0.2 ml, and the injection may be by either the intramuscular or subcutaneous route. Newborn animals are treated with 0.1 ml of antithymocyte serum or globulin on days 0, 2, 7 and 14 after birth. A potent serum or globulin is one that suppresses the immune mechanisms of growing animals to the extent that the subsequent inoculum of 10^7 positive reference cells regularly produces tumours and metastases. Severely affected animals showing evident progressively growing tumours are killed before the end of the test to avoid unnecessary suffering.

At the end of the observation period all animals, including the reference group(s), are killed and examined for gross and microscopic evidence of the proliferation of inoculated cells at the site of injection and in other organs (for example lymph nodes, lungs, kidneys and liver).

In all test systems, the animals are observed and palpated at regular intervals for the formation of nodules at the sites of injection. Any nodules formed are measured in two perpendicular dimensions, the measurements being recorded regularly to determine whether there is progressive growth of the nodule. Animals showing nodules which begin to regress during the period of observation are killed before the nodules are no longer palpable, and processed for histological examination. Animals with progressively growing nodules are observed for 1-2 weeks. Among those without nodule formation, half are observed for 3 weeks and half for 12 weeks before they are killed and processed for histological examination. A necropsy is performed on each animal and includes examination for gross evidence of tumour formation at the site of injection and in other organs such as lymph nodes, lungs, brain, spleen, kidneys and liver. All tumour-like lesions and the site of injection are examined histologically. In addition, since some cell lines may give rise to metastases without evidence of local tumour growth, any detectable regional lymph nodes and the lungs of all animals are examined histologically.

The test is invalid if fewer than nine of ten animals injected with the positive reference cells show progressively growing tumours.

01/2005:50204

5.2.4. CELL CULTURES FOR THE PRODUCTION OF VETERINARY VACCINES

Cell cultures for the production of vaccines for veterinary use comply with the requirements of this section. It may also be necessary that cell cultures used for testing of vaccines for veterinary use also comply with some or all of these requirements.

For most mammalian viruses, propagation in cell lines is possible and the use of primary cells is then not acceptable.

Permanently infected cells used for production of veterinary vaccines comply with the appropriate requirements described below. The cells shall be shown to be infected only with the agent stated.

CELL LINES

Cell lines are normally handled according to a cell-seed system. Each master cell seed is assigned a specific code for identification purposes. The master cell seed is stored in aliquots at − 70 °C or lower. Production of vaccine is not normally undertaken on cells more than twenty passages from the master cell seed. Where suspension cultures are used, an increase in cell numbers equivalent to approximately three population doublings is considered equivalent to one passage. If cells beyond twenty passage levels are to be used for production, it shall be demonstrated, by validation or further testing, that the production cell cultures are essentially similar to the master cell seed with regard to their biological characteristics and purity and that the use of such cells has no deleterious effect on vaccine production.

The history of the cell line shall be known and recorded in detail (for example, origin, number of passages and media used for multiplication, storage conditions).

The method of storing and using the cells, including details of how it is ensured that the maximum number of passages permitted is not exceeded during product manufacture, are recorded. A sufficient quantity of the master cell seed and each working cell seed are kept for analytical purposes.

The tests described below are carried out (as prescribed in Table 5.2.4.-1) on a culture of the master cell seed and the working cell seed or on cell cultures from the working cell seed at the highest passage level used for production and derived from a homogeneous sample demonstrated to be representative.

Characteristics of culture. The appearance of cell monolayers, before and after histological staining, is described. Information, if possible numerical data, is provided especially on the speed and rate of growth. Similarly, the presence or absence of contact inhibition, polynucleated cells and any other cellular abnormalities are specified.

Karyotype. A chromosomal examination is made of not fewer than fifty cells undergoing mitosis in the master cell seed and at a passage level at least as high as that to be used in production. Any chromosomal marker present in the master cell seed must also be found in the high passage cells and the modal number of chromosomes in these cells must not be more than 15 per cent higher than of cells of the master cell seed. The karyotypes must be identical. If the modal number exceeds the level stated, if the chromosomal markers are not found in the working cell seed at the highest level used for production or if the karyotype differs, the cell line shall not be used for manufacture.

Table 5.2.4.-1. – *Cell culture stage at which tests are carried out*

	Master cell seed	Working cell seed	Cell from working cell seed at highest passage level
General microscopy	+	+	+
Bacteria and fungi	+	+	−
Mycoplasmas	+	+	−
Viruses	+	+	−
Identification of species	+	−	+
Karyotype	+	−	+
Tumorigenicity	+	−	−

Identification of the species. It shall be shown, by one validated method, that the master cell seed and the cells from the working cell seed at the highest passage level used for production come from the species of origin specified. When a fluorescence test is carried out and the corresponding serum to the species of origin of cells is used and shows that all the tested cells are fluorescent, it is not necessary to carry out other tests with reagents able to detect contamination by cells of other species.

Bacterial and fungal contamination. The cells comply with the test for sterility (*2.6.1*). The sample of cells to be examined consists of not less than the number of cells in a monolayer with an area of 70 cm² or, for cells grown in suspension, an approximately equivalent number of cells. The cells are maintained in culture for at least 15 days without antibiotics before carrying out the test.

Mycoplasmas (*2.6.7*). The cells comply with the test for mycoplasmas. The cells are maintained in culture for at least 15 days without antibiotics before carrying out the test.

Absence of contaminating viruses. The cells must not be contaminated by viruses; suitably sensitive tests, including those prescribed below, are carried out.

The monolayers tested shall have an area of at least 70 cm², and shall be prepared and maintained using medium and additives, and grown under similar conditions to those used for the preparation of the vaccine. The monolayers are maintained in culture for a total of at least 28 days. Subcultures are made at 7-day intervals, unless the cells do not survive for this length of time, when the subcultures are made on the latest day possible. Sufficient cells, in suitable containers, are produced for the final subculture to carry out the tests specified below.

The monolayers are examined regularly throughout the incubation period for the possible presence of cytopathic effects and at the end of the observation period for cytopathic effects, haemadsorbent viruses and specific viruses by immuno-fluorescence and other suitable tests as indicated below.

Detection of cytopathic viruses. Two monolayers of at least 6 cm² each are stained with an appropriate cytological stain. The entire area of each stained monolayer is examined for any inclusion bodies, abnormal numbers of giant cells or any other lesion indicative of a cellular abnormality which might be attributable to a contaminant.

Detection of haemadsorbent viruses. Monolayers totalling at least 70 cm^2 are washed several times with an appropriate buffer and a sufficient volume of a suspension of suitable red blood cells added to cover the surface of the monolayer evenly. After different incubation times cells are examined for the presence of haemadsorption.

Detection of specified viruses. Tests are carried out for freedom from contaminants specific for the species of origin of the cell line and for the species for which the product is intended. Sufficient cells on suitable supports are prepared to carry out tests for the agents specified. Suitable positive controls are included in each test. The cells are subjected to suitable tests, for example using fluorescein-conjugated antibodies or similar reagents.

Tests in other cell cultures. Monolayers totalling at least 140 cm^2 are required. The cells are frozen and thawed at least three times and then centrifuged to remove cellular debris. Inoculate aliquots onto the following cells at any time up to 70 per cent confluency:

- primary cells of the source species;
- cells sensitive to viruses pathogenic for the species for which the vaccine is intended;
- cells sensitive to pestiviruses.

The inoculated cells are maintained in culture for at least 7 days, after which freeze-thawed extracts are prepared as above and inoculated onto sufficient fresh cultures of the same cell types to allow for the testing as described below. The cells are incubated for at least a further 7 days. The cultures are examined regularly for the presence of any cytopathic changes indicative of living organisms.

At the end of this period of 14 days, the inoculated cells are subjected to the following checks:

- freedom from cytopathic and haemadsorbent organisms, using the methods specified in the relevant paragraphs above,
- absence of pestiviruses and other specific contaminants by immunofluorescence or other validated methods as indicated in the paragraph above on Detection of Specified Viruses.

Tumorigenicity. The risk of a cell line for the target species must be evaluated and, if necessary, tests are carried out.

PRIMARY CELLS

For most mammalian vaccines, the use of primary cells is not acceptable for the manufacture of vaccines since cell lines can be used. If there is no alternative to the use of primary cells, the cells are obtained from a herd or flock free from specified pathogens, with complete protection from introduction of diseases (for example, disease barriers, filters on air inlets, suitable quarantine before introduction of animals). Chicken flocks comply with the requirements prescribed under *Chicken Flocks Free from Specified Pathogens for the Production and Quality Control of Vaccines* (*5.2.2*). For all other species, the herd or flock is shown to be free from relevant specified pathogens. All the breeding stock in the herd or flock intended to be used to produce primary cells for vaccine manufacture is subject to a suitable monitoring procedure including regular serological checks carried out at least twice a year and two supplementary serological examinations performed in 15 per cent of the breeding stock in the herd between the two checks mentioned above.

Wherever possible, particularly for mammalian cells, a seed-lot system is used with, for example, a master cell seed formed after less than five passages, the working cell seed being no more than five passages from the initial preparation of the cell suspension from the animal tissues.

Each master cell seed, working cell seed and cells of the highest passage of primary cells are checked in accordance with Table 5.2.4.-2 and the procedure described below. The sample tested shall cover all the sources of cells used for the manufacture of the batch. No batches of vaccine manufactured using the cells may be released if any one of the checks performed produces unsatisfactory results.

Table 5.2.4.-2. – *Cell culture stage at which tests are carried out*

	Master cell seed	Working cell seed	Highest passage level
General microscopy	+	+	+
Bacteria and fungi	+	+	–
Mycoplasmas	+	+	–
Viruses	+	+	–
Identification of species	+	–	–

Characteristics of cultures. The appearance of cell monolayers, before and after histological staining, is described. Information, if possible numerical data, is recorded, especially on the speed and rate of growth. Similarly, the presence or absence of contact inhibition, polynucleated cells and any other cellular abnormalities are specified.

Identification of species. It shall be demonstrated by one validated test that the master cell seed comes from the specified species of origin.

When a fluorescence test is carried out and the corresponding serum to the species of origin of cells is used and shows that all the tested cells are fluorescent, it is not necessary to carry out other tests with reagents able to detect contamination by cells of other species.

Bacterial and fungal sterility. The cells comply with the test for sterility (*2.6.1*). The sample of cells to be examined consists of not less than the number of cells in a monolayer with an area of 70 cm^2 or for cells grown in suspension an approximately equivalent number of cells. The cells are maintained in culture for at least 15 days without antibiotics before carrying out the test.

Mycoplasmas (*2.6.7*). The cells comply with the test for mycoplasmas. The cells are maintained in culture for at least 15 days without antibiotics before carrying out the test.

Absence of contaminating viruses. The cells must not be contaminated by viruses; suitably sensitive tests, including those prescribed below are carried out.

The monolayers tested shall be at least 70 cm^2, and shall be prepared and maintained in culture using the same medium and additives, and under similar conditions to those used for the preparation of the vaccine.

The monolayers are maintained in culture for a total of at least 28 days or for the longest period possible if culture for 28 days is impossible. Subcultures are made at 7-day intervals, unless the cells do not survive for this length of time when the subcultures are made on the latest day possible. Sufficient cells, in suitable containers are produced for the final subculture to carry out the tests specified below.

The monolayers are examined regularly throughout the incubation period for the possible presence of cytopathic effects and at the end of the observation period for cytopathic effects, haemadsorbent viruses and specific viruses by immunofluorescence and other suitable tests as indicated below.

Detection of cytopathic viruses. Two monolayers of at least 6 cm^2 each are stained with an appropriate cytological stain. Examine the entire area of each stained monolayer for any inclusion bodies, abnormal numbers of giant cells or any other lesion indicative of a cellular abnormality that might be attributable to a contaminant.

Detection of haemadsorbent viruses. Monolayers totalling at least 70 cm^2 are washed several times with a suitable buffer solution and a sufficient volume of a suspension of suitable red blood cells added to cover the surface of the monolayer evenly. After different incubation times, examine cells for the presence of haemadsorption.

Detection of specified viruses. Tests are be carried out for freedom of contaminants specific for the species of origin of the cells and for the species for which the product is intended.

Sufficient cells on suitable supports are prepared to carry out tests for the agents specified. Suitable positive controls are included in each test. The cells are subjected to suitable tests using fluorescein-conjugated antibodies or similar reagents.

Tests in other cell cultures. Monolayers totalling at least 140 cm^2 are required. The cells are frozen and thawed at least three times and then centrifuged to remove cellular debris. Aliquots are inoculated onto the following cells at any time up to 70 per cent confluency:

- primary cells of the source species;
- cells sensitive to viruses pathogenic for the species for which the vaccine is intended;
- cells sensitive to pestiviruses.

The inoculated cells are maintained in culture for at least 7 days, after which freeze-thawed extracts are prepared as above, and inoculated onto sufficient fresh cultures of the same cell types to allow for the testing as described below. The cells are incubated for at least a further 7 days. All cultures are regularly examined for the presence of any cytopathic changes indicative of living organisms.

At the end of this period of 14 days, the inoculated cells are subjected to the following checks:

- freedom from cytopathic and haemadsorbent organisms is demonstrated using the methods specified in the relevant paragraphs above;
- relevant substrates are tested for the absence of pestiviruses and other specific contaminants by immunofluorescence or other validated methods as indicated in the paragraph above on Detection of Specified Viruses.

01/2005:50205

5.2.5. SUBSTANCES OF ANIMAL ORIGIN FOR THE PRODUCTION OF VETERINARY VACCINES

Substances of animal origin (for example, serum, trypsin and serum albumin) may be used during the manufacture of veterinary immunological products, as ingredients of culture media etc. or as added constituents of vaccines or diluents. It is recommended to reduce, wherever practicable, the use of such substances.

Certain restrictions are placed upon the use of such substances to minimise the risk associated with pathogens that may be present in them.

- The use of substances of animal origin as constituents of vaccines or diluents is not generally acceptable except where such substances are sterilised by a suitable, validated method. Where the use of such substances has been shown to be essential and sterilisation is not possible, the criteria described under Requirements apply.
- Substances of animal origin used during production are either subjected to a suitable, validated sterilisation or inactivation procedure or the substance is tested for the absence of extraneous organisms in accordance with the Requirements below. For inactivated vaccines, the method used for inactivation of the vaccine strain may also be validated for inactivation of possible contaminants from substances of animal origin.

In addition to the restrictions described below, manufacturers must consider restrictions on the handling of substances of animal origin in the vaccine manufacturing premises.

The restrictions imposed by these sections may need to be varied in accordance with changes in the incidence of disease in the country of origin and in Europe.

REQUIREMENTS

Substances of animal origin comply with the requirements of the Pharmacopoeia (where a relevant monograph exists).

Source. The risk related to the animal diseases occurring in the country of origin of the substance and to the potential infectious diseases occurring in the source species, in relation to the proposed recipient species must be carefully evaluated. The strictest possible selection criteria must be applied, in particular for substances for use in products intended for the same species and for substances of bovine, caprine, ovine and porcine origin.

Preparation. Substances of animal origin are prepared from a homogeneous bulk designated with a batch number. A batch may contain substances derived from as many animals as desired but once defined and given a batch number, the batch is not added to or contaminated in any way.

All batches of substances shall be shown to be free from contaminants as described below and/or are subject to a validated inactivation procedure.

Inactivation. The inactivation procedure chosen shall have been shown to be capable of reducing the titre of certain potential contaminants in the substance concerned by at least 10^6. If this reduction in titre cannot be shown experimentally, kinetic studies for the inactivation procedure must be carried out and shown to be satisfactory, taking into account the possible level of contamination.

The list of potential contaminating organisms that the procedure must be shown to be capable of inactivating must be appropriate to the particular species of origin of the substance. The evidence for the efficacy of the procedure, which must relate to the current circumstances, may take the form of references to published literature or experimental data generated by the manufacturer.

Tests. For examination of the substance for freedom from contaminants, any solids are dissolved or suspended in a suitable medium in such a way as to create a solution or suspension containing at least 300 g/l of the substance to be examined. If the substance is not soluble or where cytotoxic reactions occur, a lower concentration may be used.

Any batch of substance found to contain living organisms of any kind is unsatisfactory and is either discarded or repro-cessed and shown to be satisfactory.

Freedom from extraneous viruses. The solution or suspension of the solid substance or the undiluted liquid substance is tested for contaminants by suitably sensitive methods. These methods shall include tests in suitably

5. General texts

sensitive cell cultures, including primary cells from the same species as the substances to be examined. A proportion of the cells is passaged at least twice.

The cells are observed regularly for 21 days for cytopathic effects. At the end of each 7 day period, a proportion of the original cultures is fixed, stained and examined for cytopathic effects; a proportion is tested for haemadsorbing agents; and a proportion is tested for specific agents by appropriate serodiagnostic tests.

Bacterial and fungal contamination. Before use, substances are tested for sterility (*2.6.1*) and freedom from mycoplasmas (*2.6.7*) or sterilised to inactivate any bacterial, fungal or mycoplasmal contaminants.

01/2005:50206

5.2.6. EVALUATION OF SAFETY OF VETERINARY VACCINES

During the development of the vaccine, safety tests are carried out in the target species to show the risks from use of the vaccine. Live vaccines are prepared only from strains of organisms that have been shown to be safe.

In the tests, "dose" means that quantity of the product to be recommended for use and containing the maximum titre or potency likely to be contained in production batches. For live vaccines, a batch or batches of vaccine prepared from the least attenuated passage to be used for production shall be used in the tests.

The safety of each of the components of combined vaccines and the safety of the combined product shall be demonstrated. For inactivated vaccines, safety tests carried out on the combined vaccine may be regarded as sufficient to demonstrate the safety of the individual components.

The tests described below, modified or supplemented by tests described in the Production section of a specific monograph may be carried out as part of the tests necessary during development to demonstrate the safety of a vaccine.

A. LABORATORY TESTS

Safety of the administration of one dose. For each of the recommended routes of administration, administer one dose of vaccine to susceptible animals of each species and category for which use of the vaccine is to be recommended. This must include animals of the youngest recommended age and pregnant animals, if appropriate. The animals are observed and examined for signs of abnormal local and systemic reactions. Where appropriate, these studies shall include detailed post-mortem macroscopic and microscopic examinations of the injection site; such examinations are not usually necessary for non-food animals. Other objective criteria are recorded, such as rectal temperature (for mammals) and performance measurements. The rectal temperatures are recorded on at least the day before vaccination, at the time of vaccination, 4 h after vaccination and on the following 4 days. The animals are observed and examined until reactions may no longer be expected but, in all cases, the observation and examination period extends at least until 14 days after administration.

As part of these studies, examination of reproductive performance must also be considered when data suggest that the starting material from which the product is derived may be a risk factor. Where prescribed in a monograph, reproductive performance of males and non-pregnant and pregnant females and harmful effects on the progeny, including teratogenic and abortifacient effects, are investigated.

Safety of one administration of an overdose. An overdose of the product is administered by each recommended route of administration to animals of the most sensitive categories of the target species, including animals of the youngest age and pregnant animals, if appropriate. The overdose normally consists of 10 doses of a live vaccine or 2 doses of an inactivated product. The animals are observed and examined for signs of local and systemic reactions. Other objective criteria are recorded, such as rectal temperature (for mammals) and performance measurements. The animals are observed and examined for at least 14 days after administration.

Safety of the repeated administration of one dose. Repeated administration of one dose may be required to reveal any adverse effects induced by such administration. These tests are carried out on the most sensitive categories of the target species, using the recommended route of administration. The animals are observed and examined for at least 14 days after the last administration for signs of systemic and local reactions. Other objective criteria are recorded, such as rectal temperature (for mammals) and performance measurements.

Residues. It is not normally necessary to undertake a study of residues. However, where adjuvants and/or preservatives are used in the manufacture of veterinary vaccines, consideration shall be given to the possibility of any residue remaining in the foodstuffs. If necessary, the effects of such residues are investigated. Moreover, in the case of live vaccines for well established zoonotic diseases, the determination of residual vaccine organisms at the injection site may be required, in addition to the studies of dissemination described below.

Adverse effects on immunological functions. Where the vaccine might adversely affect the immune response of the vaccinated animal or of its progeny, suitable tests on the immunological functions are carried out.

Special requirements for live vaccines. The following laboratory tests must also be carried out with live vaccines.

a) Spread of the vaccine strain. Spread of the vaccine strain from vaccinated to unvaccinated target animals is investigated using the recommended route of administration most likely to result in spread. Moreover, it may be necessary to investigate the safety of spread to non-target species that could be highly susceptible to a live vaccine strain. An assessment must be made of how many animal-to-animal passages are likely to be sustainable under normal circumstances together with an assessment of the likely consequences.

b) Dissemination in vaccinated animal. Faeces, urine, milk, eggs, oral, nasal and other secretions shall be tested for the presence of the organism. Moreover, studies may be required of the dissemination of the vaccine strain in the body, with particular attention being paid to the predilection sites for replication of the organism. In the case of live vaccines for well-established zoonotic diseases for food-producing animals, these studies are obligatory.

c) Reversion to or increase in virulence. For attenuated vaccines, use material from the passage level that is least attenuated for the target species between the master seed lot and the final product. For other live vaccines, use material from the passage likely to have maximum virulence for the target species. The initial vaccination is carried out using the recommended route of administration most likely to lead to reversion to virulence. After this, not fewer than 5 further serial passages through animals of the target species are undertaken. Where this is not technically possible due to failure of the organism to replicate adequately, the test is repeated and as many passages as possible are carried out in the target species. If necessary, *in vitro* propagation of the organism may be carried out between two passages *in vivo*. The passages are undertaken by the route of administration most likely to lead to reversion to virulence. Not fewer than two fully susceptible animals are used for each passage. At each passage, the presence of living vaccine-derived organisms in the material used for passage is demonstrated. The safety of material from the highest successful passage is compared with that of unpassaged material.

For particular viruses, a monograph may require more passages in more animals if there is an indication from available data that this is relevant. At least the final passage is done using animals most appropriate to the potential risk being assessed.

d) Biological properties of the vaccine strain. Other tests may be necessary to determine as precisely as possible the intrinsic biological properties of the vaccine strain (for example, neurotropism). For vector vaccines, evaluation is made of the risk of changing the tropism or virulence of the strain and where necessary specific tests are carried out. Such tests are systematically carried out where the product of a foreign gene is incorporated into the strain as a structural protein.

e) Recombination or genomic reassortment of strain. The probability of recombination or genomic reassortment with field or other strains shall be considered.

B. FIELD STUDIES

Results from laboratory studies shall normally be supplemented with supportive data from field studies.

For food-producing mammals, the studies include measurement of the rectal temperatures of a sufficient number of animals, before and after vaccination; for other mammals, such measurements are carried out if the laboratory studies indicate that there might be a problem. The size and persistence of any local reaction and the proportion of animals showing local or systemic reactions are recorded. Performance measurements are made, where appropriate.

C. ECOTOXICITY

An assessment is made of the potential harmful effects of the vaccine for the environment and any necessary precautionary measures to reduce such risks are identified. The likely degree of exposure of the environment to the vaccine is assessed taking into account: the target species and mode of administration; excretion of the product; disposal of unused vaccine. If these factors indicate that there will be significant exposure of the environment to the product, the potential ecotoxicity is evaluated taking into account the properties of the vaccine as determined, for example, in the tests described in this section.

01/2005:50207

5.2.7. EVALUATION OF EFFICACY OF VETERINARY VACCINES

During development of a vaccine, tests are carried out to demonstrate that the vaccine is efficacious when administered by each of the recommended routes and methods of vaccination and using the recommended schedule to animals of each species and category for which use of the vaccine is to be recommended. The type of efficacy testing to be carried out varies considerably depending on the particular type of vaccine.

As part of or in addition to tests carried out during development to establish efficacy, the tests described in the Production section of a specific monograph may be carried out; the following must be taken into account.

The dose to be used is that quantity of the product to be recommended for use and containing the minimum titre or potency expected at the end of the period of validity.

For live vaccines, vaccine prepared from the most attenuated passage to be used for production is used.

The efficacy evidence must support all the claims being made. For example, claims for protection against respiratory disease must be supported by at least evidence of protection from clinical signs of respiratory disease. Where it is claimed that there is protection from infection this must be demonstrated using re-isolation techniques. If more than one claim is made, supporting evidence for each claim is required.

The influence of passively acquired and maternally derived antibodies on the efficacy of a vaccine is adequately evaluated. Any claims, stated or implied, regarding onset and duration of protection shall be supported by data from trials.

The efficacy of each of the components of multivalent and combined products shall be demonstrated using the combined vaccine.

Studies of immunological compatibility are undertaken when simultaneous administration is recommended or where it is a part of a usual vaccination schedule. Wherever a product is to recommended as part of a vaccination scheme, the priming or booster effect or the contribution of the product to the efficacy of the scheme as a whole shall be demonstrated.

LABORATORY TESTS

In principle, demonstration of efficacy is undertaken under well-controlled laboratory conditions by challenge after administration of the product to the target animal under the recommended conditions of use. Challenge is carried out using a strain different from the one used in the production of the vaccine. In so far as possible, the conditions under which the challenge is carried out shall mimic the natural conditions for infection, for example with regard to the amount of challenge organism and the route of administration of the challenge.

If possible, the immune mechanism (cell-mediated/humoral, local/general, classes of immunoglobulin) that is initiated after the administration of the vaccine to target animals shall be determined.

FIELD TRIALS

In general, results from laboratory tests are supplemented with data from field trials, carried out with untreated control animals. Where laboratory trials cannot be supportive of efficacy, the performance of field trials alone may be acceptable.

01/2005:50208

5.2.8. MINIMISING THE RISK OF TRANSMITTING ANIMAL SPONGIFORM ENCEPHALOPATHY AGENTS VIA HUMAN AND VETERINARY MEDICINAL PRODUCTS

This chapter is identical with the Note for Guidance on Minimising the Risk of Transmitting Animal Spongiform Encephalopathy Agents via Human and Veterinary Medicinal Products - Revision 2, October 2003 [Committee for Proprietary Medicinal Products (CPMP), Committee for Veterinary Medicinal Products (CVMP), European Agency for the Evaluation of Medicinal Products].

Contents

1. INTRODUCTION

1-1. *SCIENTIFIC BACKGROUND*

Transmissible Spongiform Encephalopathies (TSEs) are chronic degenerative nervous diseases characterised by the accumulation of an abnormal isoform of a cellular glycoprotein known as PrP (or prion protein). The abnormal isoform of PrP (PrP^{Sc}) differs from normal PrP (PrP^{c}) in being highly resistant to protease and heat denaturation treatments. PrP^{Sc} is considered to be the infective agent responsible for transmitting TSE disease.

TSE diseases in animals include:

- bovine spongiform encephalopathy (BSE) in cattle,
- scrapie in sheep and goats,
- chronic wasting disease (CWD) in cervids (deer and elk),
- transmissible mink encephalopathy (TME) in farmed mink,
- feline spongiform encephalopathy (FSE) in felidae (specifically domestic cats and captive large cats), and
- spongiform encephalopathy of exotic ungulates in zoos.

In humans, spongiform encephalopathies include different forms of Creutzfeldt-Jakob Disease (CJD), Kuru, Gerstmann-Sträussler-Scheinker Syndrome (GSS), and Fatal Familial Insomnia (FFI).

Iatrogenic transmission of spongiform encephalopathies has been reported. In sheep, scrapie has been accidentally transmitted by the use of Louping Ill vaccine prepared from pooled, formaldehyde treated ovine brain and spleen in which material from scrapie-infected sheep had been inadvertently incorporated. In man, cases of transmission of CJD have been reported which have been attributed to the parenteral administration of growth hormone and gonadotropin derived from human cadaveric pituitary glands. Cases of CJD have also been attributed to the use of contaminated instruments in brain surgery and with the transplantation of human dura mater and cornea.

Interspecies TSE transmission is restricted by a number of natural barriers, transmissibility being affected by the species of origin, the prion strain, dose, route of exposure and, in some species, the host allele of the PrP gene. Species barriers can be crossed under appropriate conditions.

Bovine spongiform encephalopathy (BSE) was first recognised in the United Kingdom in 1986 and a large number of cattle and individual herds have been affected. It is clear that BSE is a food borne disease associated with feeding meat and bone meal derived from TSE affected animals. Other countries have experienced cases of BSE, either in animals imported from the United Kingdom or in indigenous animals. There is convincing evidence to show that the variant form of CJD (vCJD) is caused by the agent which is responsible for BSE in cattle. Therefore, a cautious approach continues to be warranted if biological materials from species naturally affected by TSE diseases, especially bovine species, are used for the manufacture of medicinal products.

Scrapie occurs worldwide and has been reported in most European countries. It has the highest incidence in the United Kingdom. While humans have been exposed to naturally occurring scrapie for over 200 years, there is no epidemiological evidence directly linking scrapie to spongiform encephalopathies in humans. However, there remains a theoretical and currently unquantifiable risk that some BSE-contaminated protein supplement may have been fed to sheep. If such feed causes a recurrent BSE infection in sheep, it may be diagnosed as scrapie and might as such pose a risk of human TSEs. Further, it should also be assumed that any BSE agent introduced into the small ruminant population via contaminated feed is likely to be recycled and amplified.

1-2. *REGULATORY COMPLIANCE*

Risk assessment. Since the use of animal-derived materials is unavoidable for the production of some medicinal products and that complete elimination of risk at source is rarely possible, the measures taken to manage the risk of transmitting animal TSEs via medicinal products represent risk minimisation rather than risk elimination. Consequently, the basis for regulatory compliance should be based on a risk assessment, taking into consideration all pertinent factors as identified in this chapter (see below).

Legal Aspects. The note for guidance has been given the force of law by virtue of Annex I to European Parliament and Council Directives 2001/82/EC and 2001/83/EC

5. General texts

(as amended by Commission Directive 2003/63/EC[1]), governing the veterinary and human medicinal products, respectively. These directives require that applicants for marketing authorisation for human and veterinary medicinal products must demonstrate that medicinal products are manufactured in accordance with the latest version of this note for guidance published in the *Official Journal of the European Union*. This is a continuing obligation after the marketing authorisation has been granted.

By definition, the principle of Specified Risk Materials as defined in Regulation (EC) No 999/2001 of the European Parliament and of the Council[2] does not apply to medicinal products. The use of substances derived from high infectivity tissues must be fully justified following an appropriate benefit/risk evaluation (see further below).

The note for guidance should be read in conjunction with the various European Community legal instruments including Commission decisions progressively implemented since 1991. Where appropriate, references to these decisions are given in the text. Position statements and explanatory notes made by the Committee for Proprietary Medicinal Products (CPMP) and Committee for Veterinary Medicinal Products (CVMP) are still applicable for the purpose of regulatory compliance unless otherwise superseded by the note for guidance.

The general monograph *Products with risk of transmitting agents of animal spongiform encephalopathies* of the European Pharmacopoeia refers to this chapter, which is identical with the note for guidance. The monograph forms the basis for issuing Certificates of Suitability as a procedure for demonstrating TSE compliance for substances and materials used in the manufacture of human and veterinary medicinal products.

Clarification of note for guidance. As the scientific understanding of TSEs, especially the pathogenesis of the diseases, is evolving, from time to time CPMP and its Biotechnology Working Party in collaboration with CVMP and its Immunologicals Working Party may be required in the future to develop supplementary guidance in the form of position statements or explanatory notes for the purpose of clarifying the note for guidance. The supplementary guidance shall be published by the Commission and on the website of the European Agency for the Evaluation of Medicinal Products (EMEA) and taken into consideration accordingly in the scope of the certification of the European Directorate for the Quality of Medicines (EDQM).

Implementation of the revised note for guidance. All authorised medicinal products in the European Union have demonstrated compliance with the note for guidance on minimising the risk of transmitting animal spongiform encephalopathy agents via human and veterinary medicinal products (EMEA/410/01-Rev.1) in line with the legal requirement as inscribed in Annex I to Directive 2001/82/EC (veterinary medicines) or Directive 2001/83/EC as amended by Directive 2003/63/EC (medicines for human use). The revised note for guidance is to be applied prospectively, i.e. for all medicinal products that will be authorised or whose marketing authorisation will be renewed after the time of coming into operation of the revised note for guidance.

2. SCOPE OF THE CHAPTER

TSE-RELEVANT ANIMAL SPECIES

Cattle, sheep, goats and animals that are naturally susceptible to infection with transmissible spongiform encephalopathy agents or susceptible to infection through the oral route other than humans[3] and non-human primates are defined as "TSE-relevant animal species"[4].

MATERIALS

This chapter is concerned with materials derived from "TSE-relevant animal species" that are used for the preparation of:

- active substances,
- excipients and adjuvants,
- raw and starting materials and reagents used in production (e.g. bovine serum albumin; enzymes; culture media including those used to prepare working cell banks, or new master cell banks for medicinal products which are subject to a new marketing authorisation).

This chapter is also applicable to materials that come into direct contact with the equipment used in manufacture of the medicinal product or that come in contact with the medicinal product and therefore have the potential for contamination.

Materials used in the qualification of plant and equipment, such as culture media used in media fill experiments to validate the aseptic filling process, shall be considered in compliance with this chapter provided that the constituent or constituents are derived from tissues with no detectable infectivity (category C tissues), where the risk of cross-contamination with potentially infective tissues has been considered (see section 3-3) and where the materials are sourced from a GBR I/II country (see section 3-2). Such information shall be provided in the dossier for a marketing authorisation and verified during routine inspection for compliance with Good Manufacturing Practice (GMP).

Other materials such as cleaning agents, softeners and lubricants that come into contact with the medicinal product during its routine manufacture or in the finishing stage or in the primary packaging are considered in compliance with this chapter if they are derived from tallow under the conditions described in section 6.

SEED LOTS, CELL BANKS AND ROUTINE FERMENTATION/PRODUCTION[5]

For the purpose of regulatory compliance, master seeds or master cell banks in marketing authorisation applications lodged after 1 July 2000 (for human medicinal products) or 1 October 2000 (for veterinary medicinal products) are covered by the note for guidance.

Master seeds and master cell banks,

- for vaccine antigens;
- for a biotechnology-derived medicinal product within the meaning of Part A of the Annex to Council Regulation (EC) No 2309/93; and
- for other medicinal products using seed lots or cell banking systems in their manufacture,

that have already been approved for the manufacture of a constituent of an authorised medicinal product shall be considered in compliance with the note for guidance even if they are incorporated in marketing authorisation

(1) O.J. L 159, 27.06.2003, p. 46
(2) O.J. L 147, 31.05.2001, p. 1
(3) Regulatory guidance and position papers have been issued by the Committee for Proprietary Medicinal Products and its Biotechnology Working Party on human tissue derived medicinal products in relation with CJD and vCJD. Such guidance can be found on http://www.emea.eu.int.
(4) Pigs and birds, which are animal species of particular interest for the production of medicinal products, are not naturally susceptible to infection via the oral route. Therefore they are not TSE-relevant animal species within the meaning of this chapter. Also dogs, rabbits and fish are non TSE-relevant animal species within the meaning of this chapter.
(5) See also: Position paper on the assessment of the risk of transmission of animal spongiform encephalopathy agents by master seed materials used in the production of veterinary vaccines (EMEA/CVMP/019/01-February 2001 adopted by the Committee for Veterinary Medicinal products (CVMP) in July 2001, Official Journal of the European Communities C 286 of 12 October 2001, p.12.

applications lodged after 1 July 2000 (for human medicinal products) or 1 October 2000 (for veterinary medicinal products).

Master cell banks and master seeds established before 1 July 2000 (for human medicinal products) or 1 October 2000 (for veterinary medicinal products), but not yet approved as a constituent of an authorised medicinal product shall demonstrate that they fulfil the requirements of the note for guidance. If, for some raw or starting materials or reagents used for the establishment of these cell banks or seeds, full documentary evidence is not/no longer available, the applicant should present a risk assessment as described in Section 4 of the note for guidance.

Established working seeds or cell banks used in the manufacture of medicinal products authorised before 1 July 2000 (human medicines) or 1 October 2000 (veterinary medicines), which have been subjected to a properly conducted risk assessment by a competent authority of the Member States or the EMEA and declared to be acceptable, shall also be considered compliant.

However, where materials derived from the "TSE-relevant animal species" are used in fermentation/routine production processes or in the establishment of working seeds and working cell banks, the applicant must demonstrate that they fulfil the requirements of the note for guidance.

3. GENERAL CONSIDERATIONS

3-1. *SCIENTIFIC PRINCIPLES FOR MINIMISING RISK*

When manufacturers have a choice, the use of materials from "non TSE-relevant animal species" or non-animal origin is preferred. The rationale for using materials derived from "TSE-relevant animal species" instead of materials from "non-TSE-relevant species" or of non-animal origin should be given. If materials from "TSE-relevant animal species" have to be used, consideration should be given to all the necessary measures to minimise the risk of transmission of TSE.

Readily applicable diagnostic tests for TSE infectivity *in vivo* are not yet available. Diagnosis is based on post-mortem confirmation of characteristic brain lesions by histopathology and/or detection of PrP^{Sc} by Western blot or immunoassay. The demonstration of infectivity by the inoculation of suspect tissue into target species or laboratory animals is also used for confirmation. However, due to the long incubation periods of all TSEs, results of *in vivo* tests are available only after months or years.

Several *in vitro* diagnostic tests capable of detecting PrP^{Sc} in brain samples from infected animals have been approved for use but in the main they are less sensitive than *in vivo* infectivity assays. Nonetheless, screening of source animals by *in vitro* tests may prevent the use of animals at late stages of incubation of the disease and may provide information about the epidemiological status of a given country or region.

Minimising the risks of transmission of TSE is based upon three complementary parameters:

- the source animals and their geographical origin,
- nature of animal material used in manufacture and any procedures in place to avoid cross-contamination with higher risk materials,
- production process(es) including the quality assurance system in place to ensure product consistency and traceability.

3-2. *SOURCE ANIMALS*

The source materials used for the production of materials for the manufacture of medicinal products shall be derived from animals fit for human consumption following ante- and post-mortem inspection in accordance with Community or equivalent (third country) conditions, except for materials derived from live animals, which should be found healthy after clinical examination.

3-2-1. **Geographical sourcing**

3-2-1-1. *Bovine materials*

There are currently two organisations involved in the assessment of the BSE status of a specified country or zone. Firstly, the Organisation Internationale des Epizooties (OIE)[(6)] lays down the criteria for the assessment of the status of countries in the chapter of the International Animal Health Code on bovine spongiform encephalopathy. OIE also provides a list of notified BSE cases worldwide. Secondly, the European Commission Scientific Steering Committee (SSC)[(7)] has established a system for classifying the countries according to their geographical BSE risk (GBR).

Regulation (EC) No 999/2001 of the European Parliament and of the Council laying down rules for the prevention, control and eradication of certain transmissible spongiform encephalopathies (TSE Regulation)[(2)] entered into force on 1 July 2001. While medicinal products, medical devices and cosmetics are excluded from the scope of this Regulation, the principles for the determination of BSE status should be taken into account in the categorisation of the BSE status of a given country or region.

For the purposes of this chapter, the SSC GBR classification should be used as the indicator of the status of a given country. However, when countries are categorised according to Regulation (EC) No 999/2001, this categorisation should be used.

European Commission Scientific Steering Committee Classification

The European Scientific Steering Committee classification for geographical BSE risk (GBR) gives an indication of the level of likelihood of the presence of one or more cattle clinically or pre-clinically infected with BSE in a given country or region. A definition of the four categories is provided in the following Table.

GBR level	Presence of one or more cattle clinically or pre-clinically infected with BSE in a geographical region/country
I	Highly unlikely
II	Unlikely but not excluded
III	Likely but not confirmed or confirmed at a lower level
IV	Confirmed at a higher level[(1)]

(1) ≥ 100 cases/1 Million adult cattle per year

Reports of the GBR assessment of the countries are available on the SSC website[(8)]. If the BSE status of a country has not been classified by the SSC, a risk assessment shall be submitted taking into account the SSC criteria for the GBR classification.

Where there is a choice, animals should be sourced from countries with the lowest possible GBR level unless the use of material from higher GBR countries is justified. Some of the materials identified in Section 6, "Specific Conditions" can be sourced from GBR category III and, in some cases, category IV countries, provided that the controls and

(6) http://www.oie.int
(7) The Scientific Steering Committee established by Commission Decision 97/404/EC shall assist the Commission to obtain the best scientific advice available on matters relating to consumer health. Since May 2003, its tasks have been taken over by the European Food Safety Agency (EFSA): http://www.efsa.eu.int
(8) http://europa.eu.int/comm/food/fs/sc/ssc/outcome_en.html

requirements as specified in the relevant sections below are applied. Apart from these exceptions, animals must not be sourced from category IV countries, and justifications for the use of animals from category III countries must always be provided.

3-2-1-2. Sheep and goats (small ruminants)

Naturally occurring clinical scrapie cases have been reported in a number of countries worldwide. As BSE in sheep could possibly be mistaken for scrapie, as a precautionary measure, sourcing of materials derived from small ruminants shall take into account the prevalence of both BSE and scrapie in the country and the tissues from which the materials are derived.

The principles related to "BSE Negligible risk (closed) bovine herds" (see section 3-2-2) could equally be applied in the context of small ruminants in order to develop a framework to define the TSE status of a flock of small ruminants. For sheep, because of the concern over the possibility of BSE in sheep, the use of (a) genotype(s) shown to be resistant to BSE/scrapie infection shall be considered in establishing TSE free flocks. However, goats have not been studied sufficiently with regard to a genotype specific sensitivity.

Material of small ruminant origin should preferably be sourced from countries with a long history of absence of scrapie, such as New Zealand or Australia or from proven TSE-free flocks. Justification shall be required if the material is sourced from some other origin.

3-2-2. **BSE negligible risk (closed) bovine herds**. The safest sourcing is from countries where the presence of BSE is highly unlikely i.e. GBR I. Other countries may have or have had cases of BSE at some point in time and the practical concept of "Negligible risk (closed) bovine herds" has been developed by the SSC and endorsed by the CPMP and CVMP. Criteria for establishing and maintaining a "BSE negligible risk (closed) bovine herd" can be found in the SSC opinion of 22-23 July 1999[(9)].

For the time being it is not possible to quantify the reduction of the geographical BSE risk for cattle from BSE negligible risk (closed) bovine herds. However, it is expected that this risk reduction is substantial. Therefore, sourcing from such closed bovine herds shall be considered in the risk assessment in conjunction with the GBR classification of the country.

3-3. *ANIMAL PARTS, BODY FLUIDS AND SECRETIONS AS STARTING MATERIALS*

In a TSE infected animal, different organs and secretions have different levels of infectivity[(10)]. The tables in the Annex of this chapter[(11)] summarise current data about the distribution of infectivity and PrP^{Sc} in cattle with BSE, and in sheep and goats with scrapie.

The information in the tables is based exclusively upon observations of naturally occurring disease or primary experimental infection by the oral route (in cattle) but does not include data on models using strains of TSE that have been adapted to experimental animals, because passaged strain phenotypes can differ significantly and unpredictably from those of naturally occurring disease. Because immunohistochemical and/or Western blot detection of misfolded host protein (PrP^{Sc}) have proven to be a surrogate marker of infectivity, PrP^{Sc} testing results have been presented in parallel with bioassay data. Tissues are grouped into three major infectivity categories, irrespective of the stage of disease:

Category A	**High-infectivity tissues** central nervous system (CNS) tissues that attain a high titre of infectivity in the later stages of all TSEs, and certain tissues that are anatomically associated with the CNS
Category B	**Lower-infectivity tissues** peripheral tissues that have tested positive for infectivity and/or PrP^{Sc} in at least one form of TSE
Category C	**Tissues with no detectable infectivity** tissues that have been examined for infectivity, without any infectivity detected, and/or PrP^{Sc}, with negative results

Category A tissues and substances derived from them shall not be used in the manufacture of medicinal products, unless justified (see Section 5).

Although the category of lower risk tissues (category B tissues) almost certainly includes some (e.g. blood) with a lower risk than others (e.g. lymphoreticular tissues), the data about infectivity levels in these tissues are too limited to subdivide the category into different levels of risk. It is also evident that the placement of a given tissue in one or another category can be disease and species specific, and subject to revision as new data emerges.

For the risk assessment (see section 4), manufacturers and/or marketing authorisation holders/applicants shall take into account the tissue classification tables in the Annex to this chapter[(12)].

The categories in the tables are only indicative and it is important to note the following points.

- In certain situations there could be cross-contamination of tissues of different categories of infectivity. The potential risk will be influenced by the circumstances in which tissues were removed, especially by contact of tissues with lower-infectivity tissues or no detectable infectivity (categories B and C tissues) with high-infectivity tissues (category A tissues). Thus, cross-contamination of some tissues may be increased if infected animals are slaughtered by penetrative brain stunning or if the brain and/or spinal cord is sawed. The risk of cross-contamination will be decreased if body fluids are collected with minimal damage to tissue and cellular components are removed, and if foetal blood is collected without contamination from other maternal or foetal tissues including placenta, amniotic and allantoic fluids. For certain tissues, it is very difficult or impossible to prevent cross-contamination with category A tissues (e.g. skull). This has to be considered in the risk assessment.
- For certain classes of substances the stunning/slaughtering techniques used may be important in minimising the potential risk[(13)] because of the likelihood of disseminating the brain particles into the peripheral organs, particularly to the lungs. Stunning/slaughtering techniques should be described as well as the procedures to remove high infectivity tissues. The procedures to collect the animal tissues/organs to be used and the measures in place to avoid cross-contamination with a higher risk material must also be described in detail.

(9) SSC Scientific Opinion on the conditions related to "BSE Negligible Risk (Closed) Bovine Herds" adopted at the meeting of 22-23 July 1999. http://europa.eu.int/comm/food/fs/sc/ssc/out56_en.html
(10) If materials from "TSE-relevant animal species" have to be used, consideration should be given to use of materials of the lowest category of risk.
(11) The tissue classification tables are based upon the most recent *WHO guidelines on transmissible spongiform encephalopathies in relation to biological and pharmaceutical products* (February 2003) WHO/BCT/QSD/03.01.
(12) The introduction of the 3-category tissue classification system does not invalidate the risk-assessments based on the previously used 4-category tissue classification, performed for authorised medicinal products.
(13) SSC opinion on stunning methods and BSE risk (the risk of dissemination of brain particles into the blood and carcass when applying certain stunning methods), adopted at the meeting of 10-11 January 2002. http://europa.eu.int/comm/food/fs/sc/ssc/out245_en.pdf

- The risk of contamination of tissues and organs with BSE-infectivity potentially harboured in central nervous material as a consequence of the stunning method used for cattle slaughtering depends on the following factors:
  - the amount of BSE-infectivity in the brain of the slaughtered animal,
  - the extent of brain damage,
  - the dissemination of brain particles in the animal body.

  These factors must be considered in conjunction with the GBR classification of the source animals, the age of the animals in the case of cattle and the post-mortem testing of the cattle using a validated method.

  The underlying principles indicated above would be equally applicable to sheep and goats.

The risk posed by cross-contamination will be dependent on several complementary factors including:

- measures adopted to avoid contamination during collection of tissues (see above),
- level of contamination (amount of the contaminating tissue),
- amount and type of materials collected at the same time.

Manufacturers or the marketing authorisation holders/applicants should take into account the risk with respect to cross-contamination.

3-4. *AGE OF ANIMALS*

As the TSE infectivity accumulates in bovine animals over an incubation period of several years, it is prudent to source from young animals.

3-5. *MANUFACTURING PROCESS*

The assessment of the overall TSE risk reduction of a medicinal product shall take into account the control measures instituted with respect to:

- sourcing of the raw/starting materials, and
- the manufacturing process.

Controlled sourcing is a very important criterion in achieving acceptable safety of the product, due to the documented resistance of TSE agents to most inactivation procedures.

A quality assurance system, such as ISO 9000 certification, HACCP(14) or GMP, must be put in place for monitoring the production process and for batch delineation (i.e. definition of batch, separation of batches, cleaning between batches). Procedures shall be put in place to ensure traceability as well as self-auditing and to auditing suppliers of raw/starting materials.

Certain production procedures may contribute considerably to the reduction of the risk of TSE contamination, e.g. procedures used in the manufacture of tallow derivatives (see section 6). As such rigorous processing cannot be applied to many products, processes involving physical removal, such as precipitation and filtration to remove prion-rich material, are likely to be more appropriate than chemical treatments. A description of the manufacturing process, including in-process controls applied, shall be presented and the steps that might contribute to reduction or elimination of TSE contamination should be discussed. Whenever different manufacturing sites are involved, the steps performed at each site shall be clearly identified. The measures in place in order to ensure traceability of every production batch to the source material should be described.

Cleaning process. Cleaning of process equipment may be difficult to validate for the elimination of TSE agents. It is reported that after exposure to high titre preparations of TSE agent, detectable infectivity can remain bound to the surface of stainless steel. The removal of all adsorbed protein by the use of sodium hydroxide or chlorine releasing disinfectants (e.g. 20 000 ppm chlorine for 1 h) have been considered acceptable approaches where equipment that cannot be replaced has been exposed to potentially contaminated material. In the case of using category A materials in the manufacture of a product, dedicated equipment shall be used, unless otherwise justified.

If risk materials are used in the manufacture of a product, cleaning procedures, including control measures, shall be put in place in order to minimise the risk of cross-contamination between production batches. This is especially important if materials from different risk categories are handled in the same plant with the same equipment.

Removal/Inactivation validation. Validation studies of removal/inactivation procedures for TSEs are difficult to interpret. It is necessary to take into consideration the nature of the spiked material and its relevance to the natural situation, the design of the study (including scaling-down of processes) and the method of detection of the agent (*in vitro* or *in vivo* assay). Further research is needed to develop an understanding of the most appropriate "spike preparation" for validation studies. Therefore, validation studies are currently not generally required. However, if claims are made for the safety of the product with respect to TSEs based on the ability of manufacturing processes to remove or inactivate TSE agents, they must be substantiated by appropriate validation studies.

In addition to appropriate sourcing, manufacturers are encouraged to continue their investigations into removal and inactivation methods to identify steps/processes that would have benefit in assuring the removal or inactivation of TSE agents. In any event, a production process wherever possible shall be designed taking account of available information on methods which are thought to inactivate or remove TSE agents.

4. RISK ASSESSMENT OF MATERIALS OR SUBSTANCES USED IN THE MANUFACTURE AND PREPARATION OF A MEDICINAL PRODUCT IN THE CONTEXT OF REGULATORY COMPLIANCE

The assessment of the risk associated with TSE needs careful consideration of all of the parameters as outlined in section 3-1 (Scientific Principles for Minimising Risk).

As indicated in the introduction to this chapter, regulatory compliance is based on a favourable outcome from a risk assessment. The risk assessments, conducted by the manufacturers and/or the marketing authorisation holders or applicants for the different materials or substances from "TSE-relevant animal species" used in the manufacture of a medicinal product shall show that all TSE risk factors have been taken into account and, where possible, risk has been minimised by application of the principles described in this chapter. TSE Certificates of suitability issued by the EDQM may be used by the marketing authorisation holders or applicants as the basis of the risk assessments.

An overall risk assessment for the medicinal product, conducted by the marketing authorisation holders or applicants, shall take into account the risk assessments for all the different materials from "TSE-relevant animal species" and, where appropriate, TSE reduction or inactivation by the manufacturing steps of the active substance and/or finished product.

The final determination of regulatory compliance rests with the competent authority.

(14) Hazard Analysis Critical Control Point.

It is incumbent upon the manufacturers and/or the marketing authorisation holders or applicants for both human and veterinary medicinal products to select and justify the control measures for a given "TSE-relevant animal species" derivative, taking into account the state of the art of science and technology.

5. BENEFIT/RISK EVALUATION

In addition to the parameters as mentioned in sections 3 and 4, the acceptability of a particular medicinal product containing materials derived from a "TSE-relevant animal species", or which as a result of manufacture could contain these materials, shall take into account the following factors:

- route of administration of the medicinal product,
- quantity of animal material used in the medicinal product,
- maximum therapeutic dosage (daily dose and duration of treatment),
- intended use of the medicinal product and its clinical benefit.

High-infectivity tissues (category A tissues) and substances derived thereof shall not be used in manufacture of medicinal products, their starting materials and intermediate products (including active substances, excipients and reagents), unless justified. A justification why no other materials can be used shall be provided. In these exceptional and justified circumstances, the use of high-infectivity tissues could be envisaged for the manufacture of active substances, when, after performing the risk assessment as described in Section 4 of this chapter, and taking into account the intended clinical use, a positive benefit/risk assessment can be presented by the marketing authorisation applicant. Substances from category A materials, if their use is justified, must be produced from animals of GBR I countries.

6. SPECIFIC CONSIDERATIONS

The following materials prepared from "TSE-relevant animal species" are considered in compliance with this chapter provided that they meet at least the conditions specified below. The relevant information or a certificate of suitability granted by the EDQM shall be provided by the marketing authorisation applicant/holder.

6-1. *COLLAGEN*

Collagen is a fibrous protein component of mammalian connective tissue.

For collagen, documentation to demonstrate compliance with this chapter needs to be provided taking into account the provisions listed in sections 3 to 5. In addition, consideration should be given to the following.

- For collagen produced from bones, the conditions specified for gelatin are applicable (see below).
- Collagen produced from tissues such as hides and skins do not usually present a measurable TSE risk provided that contamination with potentially infected materials, for example spillage of blood and/or central nervous tissues, is avoided during their procurement.

6-2. *GELATIN*

Gelatin is a natural, soluble protein, gelling or non-gelling, obtained by the partial hydrolysis of collagen produced from bones, hides and skins, tendons and sinews of animals.

For gelatin, documentation to demonstrate compliance with this chapter needs to be provided taking into account the provisions listed in sections 3 to 5. In addition, consideration should be given to the following.

The source material used

Gelatin used in medicinal products can be manufactured from bones or hides.

Hides as the starting material. On the basis of current knowledge, hides used for gelatin production represent a much safer source material as compared to bones. However, it is highly recommended that measures should be put in place to avoid cross-contamination with potentially infected materials during procurement.

Bones as the starting material. Where bones are used to manufacture gelatin, more stringent production conditions shall be applied (see below). In any case, the removal of skulls and spinal cords from the starting material is considered as a first precautionary measure which largely affects the safety of the product. As far as practicable, bones should be sourced from countries classified as GBR I and II. Bones from category GBR III countries can be used if the gelatin is manufactured under defined conditions as indicated below and if vertebrae from cattle over 12 months of age are removed from the raw/starting materials[15].

Manufacturing methods

No specific measures with regard to the processing conditions are required for gelatin produced from hides provided that control measures are put in place to avoid cross-contamination both during the procurement of the hides and during the manufacturing process.

However, the mode of manufacture must be taken into account where bones are used as the starting material.

- Bones (including vertebrae) for the production of gelatin using acid treatment shall be sourced only from GBR category I or II countries. An additional alkaline treatment (pH 13, 1 h) of the bones/ossein may further increase the TSE safety of acid-derived bone gelatin.

  For bones sourced from a GBR category III country, the alkaline process shall be applied. However, this manufacturing method is optional for bones coming from GBR category I and II countries.
- For a typical alkaline manufacturing process, bones are finely crushed, degreased with hot water and demineralised with dilute hydrochloric acid (at a minimum of 4 per cent and pH < 1.5) over a period of at least 2 days to produce the ossein. This is followed by an alkaline treatment with saturated lime solution (pH at least 12.5) for a period of at least 20 days. The gelatin is extracted, washed, filtered and concentrated. A "flash" heat treatment (sterilisation) step using 138-140 °C for 4 s is applied. Bovine hide gelatin can also be produced by the alkaline process. Bovine bones may also be treated by an acid process. The liming step is then replaced by an acid pre-treatment where the ossein is soaked overnight at pH < 4.

6-3. *BOVINE BLOOD DERIVATIVES*

Foetal bovine serum is commonly used in cell cultures. Foetal bovine serum should be obtained from foetuses harvested in abattoirs from healthy dams fit for human consumption and the womb should be completely removed and the foetal blood harvested in dedicated space or area by cardiac puncture into a closed collection system using aseptic technique.

New born calf serum is obtained from calves under 20 days old and calf serum from animals under the age of 12 months. In the case of donor bovine serum, given that it may be derived from animals less than 36 months old, the TSE status

(15) Regulation (EC) No 1774/2002 of the European Parliament and of the Council laying down health rules concerning animal by-products not intended for human consumption shall apply unless justified. Regarding the manufacturing of gelatin and collagen or import of raw material for such manufacturing for use in pharmaceutical products, only material from animals fit for human consumption shall be used. The use of vertebrae from such animals from category II countries, which according to the risk assessment is safe, shall continue to be allowed.

of the donor herd shall be well defined and documented. In all cases, serum shall be collected according to specified protocols by personnel trained in these procedures to avoid cross-contamination with higher risk tissues.

For bovine blood derivatives, documentation to demonstrate compliance with this chapter needs to be provided taking into account the provisions listed in sections 3 to 5. In addition, consideration should be given to the following.

Traceability

Traceability to the slaughterhouse must be assured for each batch of serum or plasma. Slaughterhouses must have available lists of farms from which the animals are originated. If serum is produced from living animals, records must be available for each serum batch which assures the traceability to the farms.

Geographical origin

Whilst tissue infectivity of BSE in cattle is more restricted than scrapie, as a precautionary measure bovine blood must be sourced from countries classified GBR I and II, unless otherwise justified.

Stunning methods

If it is sampled from slaughtered animals, the method of slaughter is of importance to assure the safety of the material. It has been demonstrated that stunning by captive bolt stunner with or without pithing as well as by pneumatic stunner, especially if it injects air, can destroy the brain and disseminate brain material into the blood stream. Negligible risk can be expected from a non-penetrative stunner and from electro-narcosis[16]. The stunning methods must therefore be described for the bovine blood collection process.

If sourcing is allowed from countries where cases of BSE have been detected (GBR III) a non-penetrative stunner shall be used for slaughter.

6-4. *TALLOW DERIVATIVES*

Tallow is fat obtained from tissues including subcutaneous, abdominal and inter-muscular areas and bones. Tallow used as the starting material for the manufacture of tallow derivatives shall be category 3 material or equivalent, as defined in Regulation (EC) No 1774/2002[17] of the European Parliament and of the Council of 3 October 2002 laying down health rules concerning animal by-products not intended for human consumption.

Tallow derivatives, such as glycerol and fatty acids, manufactured from tallow by rigorous processes are thought unlikely to be infectious and they have been the subject of specific consideration by CPMP and CVMP. For this reason, such materials manufactured under the conditions at least as rigorous as those given below shall be considered in compliance for this chapter, irrespective of the geographical origin and the nature of the tissues from which tallow derivatives are derived. Examples of rigorous processes are:

- trans-esterification or hydrolysis at not less than 200 °C for not less than 20 min under pressure (glycerol, fatty acids and fatty acid esters production),
- saponification with 12 M NaOH (glycerol and soap production):
  - batch process: at not less than 95 °C for not less than 3 h,
  - continuous process: at not less than 140 °C, under pressure for not less than 8 min, or equivalent,
- distillation at 200 °C.

Tallow derivatives manufactured according to these conditions are unlikely to present any TSE risk and shall therefore be considered compliant with this chapter.

Tallow derivatives produced using other conditions must demonstrate compliance with this chapter.

6-5. *ANIMAL CHARCOAL*

Animal charcoal is prepared by carbonisation of animal tissues, such as bones, using high temperature at > 800 °C. Unless otherwise justified, the starting material for the manufacture of animal charcoal shall be category 3 material or equivalent, as defined in Regulation (EC) No 1774/2002 of the European Parliament and of the Council of 3 October 2002 laying down health rules concerning animal by-products not intended for human consumption. Irrespective of the geographical origin and the nature of the tissue, for the purpose of regulatory compliance, animal charcoal shall be considered in compliance with this chapter.

Charcoal manufactured according to these conditions is unlikely to present any TSE risk and shall therefore be considered compliant with this chapter. Charcoal produced using other conditions must demonstrate compliance with this chapter.

6-6. *MILK AND MILK DERIVATIVES*

In the light of the current scientific knowledge and irrespective of the geographical origin, milk is unlikely to present any risk of TSE contamination.

Certain materials, including lactose, are extracted from whey, the spent liquid from cheese production following coagulation. Coagulation can involve the use of calf rennet, an extract from abomasum, or rennet derived from other ruminants. The CPMP/CVMP have performed a risk assessment for lactose and other whey derivatives produced using calf rennet and concluded that the TSE risk is negligible if the calf rennet is produced in accordance with the process described in the risk assessment report[18]. The conclusion was endorsed by the SSC[19] which has also performed an assessment of the TSE risk of rennet in general[20].

Milk derivatives manufactured according to the conditions below are unlikely to present any TSE risk and shall therefore be considered compliant with this chapter.

- The milk is sourced from healthy animals in the same conditions as milk collected for human consumption, and
- no other ruminant materials, with the exception of calf rennet, are used in the preparation of such derivatives (e.g. pancreatic enzyme digests of casein).

Milk derivatives produced using other processes or rennet derived from other ruminant species must demonstrate compliance with this chapter.

6-7. *WOOL DERIVATIVES*

Derivatives of wool and hair of ruminants, such as lanolin and wool alcohols derived from hair shall be considered in compliance with this chapter, provided the wool and hair are sourced from live animals.

(16) SSC Opinion on stunning methods and BSE risk (The risk of dissemination of brain particles into the blood and carcass when applying certain stunning methods) adopted at the meeting on 10-11 January 2002. http://europa.eu.int/comm/food/fs/sc/ssc/out245_en.pdf
(17) OJ L 273, 10.10.2002, p. 1
(18) Committee for Proprietary Medicinal Products and its Biotechnology Working Party conducted a risk and regulatory assessment of lactose prepared using calf rennet. The risk assessment included the source of the animals, the excision of the abomasums and the availability of well-defined quality assurance procedures. The quality of any milk replacers used as feed for the animals from which abomasums are obtained is particularly important. The report can be found on http://www.emea.eu.int
(19) Provisional statement on the safety of calf-derived rennet for the manufacture of lactose. Adopted by the SSC at its meeting of 4-5 April 2002. (http://europa.eu.int/comm/food/fs/sc/ssc/out255_en.pdf)
(20) The SSC issued an opinion on the safety of animal rennet in regard to risks from animal TSE and BSE in particular, adopted at its meeting of 16 May 2002. (http://europa.eu.int/comm/food/fs/sc/ssc/out265_en.pdf)

Wool derivatives produced from wool which is sourced from slaughtered animals declared "fit for human consumption" and the manufacturing process in relation to pH, temperature and duration of treatment meets at least one of the stipulated processing conditions listed below are unlikely to present any TSE risk and shall therefore be considered compliant with this chapter.

- Treatment at pH ≥ 13 (initial; corresponding to a NaOH concentration of at least 0.1 M NaOH) at ≥ 60 °C for at least 1 h. This occurs normally during the reflux stage of the organic-alkaline treatment.
- Molecular distillation at ≥ 220 °C under reduced pressure.

Wool derivatives produced using other conditions must demonstrate compliance with this chapter.

6-8. *AMINO ACIDS*

Amino acids can be obtained by hydrolysis of materials from various sources.

Unless otherwise justified, the starting material for the manufacture of amino acids shall be category 3 material or equivalent, as defined in Regulation (EC) No 1774/2002 of the European Parliament and of the Council of 3 October 2002 laying down health rules concerning animal by-products not intended for human consumption.

Amino acids prepared using the following processing conditions, in accordance with Commission Decision 98/256/EC[21] and Commission Decision 2001/376/EC[22], are unlikely to present any TSE risk and shall be considered compliant with this chapter:

- amino acids produced from hides and skins by a process which involves exposure of the material to a pH of 1 to 2, followed by a pH of > 11, followed by heat treatment at 140 °C for 30 min at 3 bar,
- the resulting amino acids or peptides must be filtered after production, and
- analysis is performed using a validated and sensitive method to control any residual intact macromolecules, with an appropriate limit set.

Amino acids prepared using other conditions must demonstrate compliance with this chapter.

Annex: major categories of infectivity

The tables below are adapted from the *WHO Guideline on Transmissible Spongiform Encephalopathies in Relation to Biological and Pharmaceutical Products* (February 2003).

Data entries are shown as follows:

+	=	presence of infectivity or PrP^{TSE}[23],
–	=	absence of detectable infectivity or PrP^{TSE},
NT	=	not tested,
?	=	controversial or uncertain results.

Category A: High-infectivity tissues

Tissues	Cattle BSE		Sheep and goats Scrapie	
	Infectivity[1]	PrP^{TSE}	Infectivity[1]	PrP^{TSE}
Brain	+	+	+	+
Spinal cord	+	+	+	+
Retina, Optic nerve	+	NT	NT	+
Spinal ganglia	+	NT	NT	+
Trigeminal ganglia	+	NT	NT	+
Pituitary gland[2]	–	NT	+	NT
Dura mater[2]	NT	NT	NT	NT

1. Infectivity bioassays of cattle tissues have been conducted in either cattle or mice (or both); and most bioassays of sheep and/or goat tissues have been conducted only in mice. In regard to sheep and goats not all results are consistent for both species.

2. No experimental data about infectivity in human pituitary gland or dura mater have been reported, but cadaveric dura mater patches, and growth hormone derived from cadaveric pituitaries have transmitted disease to scores of people and therefore must be included in the category of high-risk tissues.

Category B: Lower-infectivity tissues

Tissues	Cattle BSE		Sheep and goats Scrapie	
	Infectivity	PrP^{TSE}	Infectivity	PrP^{TSE}
Peripheral Nervous system				
Peripheral nerves	–	NT	+	NT
Enteric plexuses[1]	NT	+	NT	+
Lymphoreticular tissues				
Spleen	–	–	+	+
Lymph nodes	–	–	+	+
Tonsil	+	NT	+	+
Nictitating membrane	NT	–	NT	+
Thymus	–	NT	+	NT
Alimentary tract				
Esophagus	–	NT	NT	+
Fore-stomach[2] (ruminants only)	–	NT	NT	+
Stomach/ abomasum[2]	–	NT	NT	+
Duodenum	–	NT	NT	+
Jejunum	–	NT	NT	+
Ileum[3]	+	+	+	+
Large intestine	–	NT	+	+
Reproductive tissues				
Placenta	–	NT	+	+
Other tissues				
Lung*	–	NT	–	NT
Liver	–	NT	+	NT

(21) OJ L 113, 15.4.1998, p. 32
(22) OJ L 132, 15.5.2001, p. 17
(23) In the main body of this chapter the abnormal isoform of the prion protein is referred to as PrP^{Sc}. However, as these tables are transcribed directly from the WHO guideline mentioned above, the WHO nomenclature for the abnormal prion protein (PrP^{TSE}) has been maintained.

Tissues	Cattle BSE		Sheep and goats Scrapie	
	Infectivity	PrP^TSE	Infectivity	PrP^TSE
Kidney*	–	–	–	–
Adrenal	NT	NT	+	NT
Pancreas	–	NT	+	NT
Bone marrow	+	NT	+	NT
Blood vessels	–	NT	NT	+
Olfactory mucosa	–	NT	+	NT
Gingival tissue*	NT	NT	NT	NT
Salivary gland	–	NT	+	NT
Cornea[4]*	NT	NT	NT	NT
Body fluids				
CSF	–	NT	+	NT
Blood[5]	–	NT	+	–

1. In cattle, limited to the distal ileum.

2. Ruminant forestomachs (reticulum, rumen, and omasum) are widely consumed, as is the true stomach (abomasum). The abomasum of cattle (and sometimes sheep) is also a source of rennet.

3. In cattle and sheep, only the distal ileum has been bioassayed for infectivity.

4. Because only one or two cases of CJD have been plausibly attributed to corneal transplants among hundreds of thousands of recipients, cornea is categorised as a lower-risk tissue; other anterior chamber tissues (lens, aqueous humor, iris, conjunctiva) have been tested with a negative result both in vCJD and other human TSEs, and there is no epidemiological evidence that they have been associated with iatrogenic disease transmission.

5. Early reports on the transmission of disease to rodents from the blood of patients with sCJD have not been confirmed, and evaluation of the ensemble of experimental and epidemiological data relevant to TSE transmission through blood, blood components, and therapeutic plasma products fails to suggest transmission from blood of patients with any form of "classical" TSE. Not enough data has accumulated to be able to make the same statement about blood from patients with vCJD. Foetal calf blood contains no detectable infectivity, but in genotypically susceptible sheep with natural scrapie or experimentally induced BSE, transfusion of large blood volumes has transmitted disease to healthy sheep. Infectivity has also been demonstrated in studies of rodent-adapted strains of TSE.

* These tissues have been classified under category B: Lower-infectivity tissues, because infectivity and/or PrP^TSE have been found in human CJD (vCJD or other).

Category C: Tissues with no detected infectivity

Tissues	Cattle BSE		Sheep and goats Scrapie	
	Infectivity	PrP^TSE	Infectivity	PrP^TSE
Reproductive tissues				
Testis	–	NT	–	NT
Prostate/Epididymis/Seminal vesicle	–	NT	–	NT
Semen	–	NT	NT	NT
Ovary	–	NT	–	NT
Uterus (Non-gravid)	–	NT	–	NT
Placenta fluids	–	NT	NT	NT
Foetus[1]	–	NT	–	NT
Embryos[1]	–	NT	?	NT
Musculo-skeletal tissues				
Bone	–	NT	NT	NT
Skeletal muscle[2]	–	NT	–	NT
Tongue	–	NT	NT	NT
Heart/pericardium	–	NT	–	NT
Tendon	–	NT	NT	NT
Other tissues				
Trachea	–	NT	NT	NT
Skin	–	NT	–	NT
Adipose tissue	–	NT	NT	NT
Thyroid gland	NT	NT	–	NT
Mammary gland/udder	–	NT	–	NT
Body fluids, secretions and excretions				
Milk[3]	–	NT	–	NT
Colostrum[4]	NT	NT	–	NT
Cord blood[4]	–	NT	NT	NT
Saliva	NT	NT	–	NT
Sweat	NT	NT	NT	NT
Tears	NT	NT	NT	NT
Nasal mucus	NT	NT	NT	NT
Urine[4,5]	–	NT	NT	NT
Faeces	–	NT	–	NT

1. Embryos from BSE-affected cattle have not transmitted disease to mice, but no infectivity measurements have been made on foetal calf tissues other than blood (negative mouse bioassay). Calves born of dams that received embryos from BSE-affected cattle have survived for observations periods of up to seven years, and examination of the brains of both the unaffected dams and their calves revealed no spongiform encephalopathy or PrP^TSE.

2. Intracerebral inoculation of muscle homogenates has not transmitted disease to 1) primates from humans with sCJD; 2) mice or cattle from cattle with BSE; and 3) mice from sheep and goats with natural or experimentally-induced scrapie. However, older reports described single instances of transmission from goat and hamster muscle, and a more recent report described transmission from the muscle of wild type and transgenic mice, but as each of these studies were conducted with passaged strains of TSE, their relevance to natural disease remains undetermined. A recent human case report described a patient with CJD and inclusion body myositis with abundant PrP^TSE in diseased muscle. After much deliberation, the committee nevertheless elected to retain muscle in the 'no detected infectivity' tissue category until more information about uncomplicated natural infections becomes available.

3. Evidence that infectivity is not present in milk includes temporo-spatial epidemiologic observations failing to detect maternal transmission; clinical observations of over a hundred calves nursed by infected cows that have not developed BSE; and experimental observations that milk from infected cows has not transmitted disease when administered intracerebrally or orally to mice. Experiments are in progress in which large volumes of milk from experimentally infected cows are concentrated and tested for the presence of PrP^TSE.

4. Single reports of transmission of CJD infectivity from human cord blood, colostrum, and urine have never been confirmed and are considered improbable.

5. A previously unreported PrP type, termed PrP^u, has been identified in the urine of sporadic and familial CJD patients, but its significance for transmission risk remains to be determined.

5.3. STATISTICAL ANALYSIS OF RESULTS OF BIOLOGICAL ASSAYS AND TESTS

01/2005:50300

1. INTRODUCTION

This chapter provides guidance for the design of bioassays prescribed in the European Pharmacopoeia (Ph. Eur.) and for analysis of their results. It is intended for use by those whose primary training and responsibilities are not in statistics, but who have responsibility for analysis or interpretation of the results of these assays, often without the help and advice of a statistician. The methods of calculation described in this annex are not mandatory for the bioassays which themselves constitute a mandatory part of the Ph. Eur. Alternative methods may be used, provided that they are not less reliable than those described here. A wide range of computer software is available and may be useful depending on the facilities available to, and the expertise of, the analyst.

Professional advice should be obtained in situations where: a comprehensive treatment of design and analysis suitable for research or development of new products is required; the restrictions imposed on the assay design by this chapter are not satisfied, for example particular laboratory constraints may require customized assay designs, or equal numbers of equally spaced doses may not be suitable; analysis is required for extended non-linear dose-response curves, for example as may be encountered in immunoassays. An outline of extended dose-response curve analysis for one widely used model is nevertheless included in Section 3.4 and a simple example is given in Section 5.4.

1.1. GENERAL DESIGN AND PRECISION

Biological methods are described for the assay of certain substances and preparations whose potency cannot be adequately assured by chemical or physical analysis. The principle applied wherever possible throughout these assays is that of comparison with a standard preparation so as to determine how much of the substance to be examined produces the same biological effect as a given quantity, the *Unit*, of the standard preparation. It is an essential condition of such methods of biological assay that the tests on the standard preparation and on the substance to be examined be carried out at the same time and under identical conditions.

For certain assays (determination of virus titre for example) the potency of the test sample is not expressed relative to a standard. This type of assay is dealt with in Section 4.5.

Any estimate of potency derived from a biological assay is subject to random error due to the inherent variability of biological responses and calculations of error should be made, if possible, from the results of each assay, even when the official method of assay is used. Methods for the design of assays and the calculation of their errors are, therefore, described below. In every case, before a statistical method is adopted, a preliminary test is to be carried out with an appropriate number of assays, in order to ascertain the applicability of this method.

The confidence interval for the potency gives an indication of the precision with which the potency has been estimated in the assay. It is calculated with due regard to the experimental design and the sample size. The 95 per cent confidence interval is usually chosen in biological assays. Mathematical statistical methods are used to calculate these limits so as to warrant the statement that there is a 95 per cent probability that these limits include the true potency. Whether this precision is acceptable to the European Pharmacopoeia depends on the requirements set in the monograph for the preparation concerned.

The terms "mean" and "standard deviation" are used here as defined in most current textbooks of biometry.

The terms "stated potency" or "labelled potency", "assigned potency", "assumed potency", "potency ratio" and "estimated potency" are used in this section to indicate the following concepts:

- "stated potency" or "labelled potency": in the case of a formulated product a nominal value assigned from knowledge of the potency of the bulk material; in the case of bulk material the potency estimated by the manufacturer;
- "assigned potency": the potency of the standard preparation;
- "assumed potency": the provisionally assigned potency of a preparation to be examined which forms the basis of calculating the doses that would be equipotent with the doses to be used of the standard preparation;
- "potency ratio" of an unknown preparation; the ratio of equipotent doses of the standard preparation and the unknown preparation under the conditions of the assay;
- "estimated potency": the potency calculated from assay data.

Section 9 (Glossary of symbols) is a tabulation of the more important uses of symbols throughout this annex. Where the text refers to a symbol not shown in this section or uses a symbol to denote a different concept, this is defined in that part of the text.

2. RANDOMISATION AND INDEPENDENCE OF INDIVIDUAL TREATMENTS

The allocation of the different treatments to different experimental units (animals, tubes, etc.) should be made by some strictly random process. Any other choice of experimental conditions that is not deliberately allowed for in the experimental design should also be made randomly. Examples are the choice of positions for cages in a laboratory and the order in which treatments are administered. In particular, a group of animals receiving the same dose of any preparation should not be treated together (at the same time or in the same position) unless there is strong evidence that the relevant source of variation (for example, between times, or between positions) is negligible. Random allocations may be obtained from computers by using the built-in randomisation function. The analyst must check whether a different series of numbers is produced every time the function is started.

The preparations allocated to each experimental unit should be as independent as possible. Within each experimental group, the dilutions allocated to each treatment are not normally divisions of the same dose, but should be prepared individually. Without this precaution, the variability inherent in the preparation will not be fully represented in the experimental error variance. The result will be an under-estimation of the residual error leading to:

1) an unjustified increase in the stringency of the test for the analysis of variance (see Sections 3.2.3 and 3.2.4),

2) an under-estimation of the true confidence limits for the test which, as shown in Section 3.2.5, are calculated from the estimate of s^2, the residual error mean square.

3. ASSAYS DEPENDING UPON QUANTITATIVE RESPONSES

3.1. STATISTICAL MODELS

3.1.1. GENERAL PRINCIPLES

The bioassays included in the Ph. Eur. have been conceived as "dilution assays", which means that the unknown preparation to be assayed is supposed to contain the same active principle as the standard preparation, but in a different ratio of active and inert components. In such a case the unknown preparation may in theory be derived from the standard preparation by dilution with inert components. To check whether any particular assay may be regarded as a dilution assay, it is necessary to compare the dose-response relationships of the standard and unknown preparations. If these dose-response relationships differ significantly, then the theoretical dilution assay model is not valid. Significant differences in the dose-response relationships for the standard and unknown preparations may suggest that one of the preparations contains, in addition to the active principle, other components which are not inert but which influence the measured responses.

To make the effect of dilution in the theoretical model apparent, it is useful to transform the dose-response relationship to a linear function on the widest possible range of doses. 2 statistical models are of interest as models for the bioassays prescribed: the parallel-line model and the slope-ratio model.

The application of either is dependent on the fulfilment of the following conditions:

1) the different treatments have been randomly assigned to the experimental units,

2) the responses to each treatment are normally distributed,

3) the standard deviations of the responses within each treatment group of both standard and unknown preparations do not differ significantly from one another.

When an assay is being developed for use, the analyst has to determine that the data collected from many assays meet these theoretical conditions.

- Condition 1 can be fulfilled by an efficient use of Section 2.
- Condition 2 is an assumption which in practice is almost always fulfilled. Minor deviations from this assumption will in general not introduce serious flaws in the analysis as long as several replicates per treatment are included. In case of doubt, a test for deviations from normality (e.g. the Shapiro-Wilk(1) test) may be performed.
- Condition 3 can be checked with a test for homogeneity of variances (e.g. Bartlett's(2) test, Cochran's(3) test). Inspection of graphical representations of the data can also be very instructive for this purpose (see examples in Section 5).

When conditions 2 and/or 3 are not met, a transformation of the responses may bring a better fulfilment of these conditions. Examples are $\ln y$, $\sqrt{y}$, y^2.

- Logarithmic transformation of the responses y to $\ln y$ can be useful when the homogeneity of variances is not satisfactory. It can also improve the normality if the distribution is skewed to the right.
- The transformation of y to $\sqrt{y}$ is useful when the observations follow a Poisson distribution i.e. when they are obtained by counting.
- The square transformation of y to y^2 can be useful if, for example, the dose is more likely to be proportional to the area of an inhibition zone rather than the measured diameter of that zone.

For some assays depending on quantitative responses, such as immunoassays or cell-based *in vitro* assays, a large number of doses is used. These doses give responses that completely span the possible response range and produce an extended non-linear dose-response curve. Such curves are typical for all bioassays, but for many assays the use of a large number of doses is not ethical (for example, *in vivo* assays) or practical, and the aims of the assay may be achieved with a limited number of doses. It is therefore customary to restrict doses to that part of the dose-response range which is linear under suitable transformation, so that the methods of Sections 3.2 or 3.3 apply. However, in some cases analysis of extended dose-response curves may be desirable. An outline of one model which may be used for such analysis is given in Section 3.4 and a simple example is shown in Section 5.4.

There is another category of assays in which the response cannot be measured in each experimental unit, but in which only the fraction of units responding to each treatment can be counted. This category is dealt with in Section 4.

3.1.2. ROUTINE ASSAYS

When an assay is in routine use, it is seldom possible to check systematically for conditions 1 to 3, because the limited number of observations per assay is likely to influence the sensitivity of the statistical tests. Fortunately, statisticians have shown that, in symmetrical balanced assays, small deviations from homogeneity of variance and normality do not seriously affect the assay results. The applicability of the statistical model needs to be questioned only if a series of assays shows doubtful validity. It may then be necessary to perform a new series of preliminary investigations as discussed in Section 3.1.1.

2 other necessary conditions depend on the statistical model to be used:

- for the parallel-line model:

  4A) the relationship between the logarithm of the dose and the response can be represented by a straight line over the range of doses used,

  5A) for any unknown preparation in the assay the straight line is parallel to that for the standard.

- for the slope-ratio model:

  4B) the relationship between the dose and the response can be represented by a straight line for each preparation in the assay over the range of doses used,

  5B) for any unknown preparation in the assay the straight line intersects the y-axis (at zero dose) at the same point as the straight line of the standard preparation (i.e. the response functions of all preparations in the assay must have the same intercept as the response function of the standard).

Conditions 4A and 4B can be verified only in assays in which at least 3 dilutions of each preparation have been tested. The use of an assay with only 1 or 2 dilutions may be justified when experience has shown that linearity and parallelism or equal intercept are regularly fulfilled.

(1) Wilk, M.B. and Shapiro, S.S. (1968). The joint assessment of normality of several independent samples, *Technometrics* 10, 825-839.
(2) Bartlett, M.S. (1937). Properties of sufficiency and statistical tests, *Proc. Roy. Soc. London*, Series A 160, 280-282.
(3) Cochran, W.G. (1951). Testing a linear relation among variances, *Biometrics* 7, 17-32.

After having collected the results of an assay, and before calculating the relative potency of each test sample, an analysis of variance is performed, in order to check whether conditions 4A and 5A (or 4B and 5B) are fulfilled. For this, the total sum of squares is subdivided into a certain number of sum of squares corresponding to each condition which has to be fulfilled. The remaining sum of squares represents the residual experimental error to which the absence or existence of the relevant sources of variation can be compared by a series of *F*-ratios.

When validity is established, the potency of each unknown relative to the standard may be calculated and expressed as a potency ratio or converted to some unit relevant to the preparation under test e.g. an International Unit. Confidence limits may also be estimated from each set of assay data.

Assays based on the parallel-line model are discussed in Section 3.2 and those based on the slope-ratio model in Section 3.3.

If any of the 5 conditions (1, 2, 3, 4A, 5A or 1, 2, 3, 4B, 5B) are not fulfilled, the methods of calculation described here are invalid and an investigation of the assay technique should be made.

The analyst should not adopt another transformation unless it is shown that non-fulfilment of the requirements is not incidental but is due to a systematic change in the experimental conditions. In this case, testing as described in Section 3.1.1 should be repeated before a new transformation is adopted for the routine assays.

Excess numbers of invalid assays due to non-parallelism or non-linearity, in a routine assay carried out to compare similar materials, are likely to reflect assay designs with inadequate replication. This inadequacy commonly results from incomplete recognition of all sources of variability affecting the assay, which can result in underestimation of the residual error leading to large *F*-ratios.

It is not always feasible to take account of all possible sources of variation within one single assay (e.g. day-to-day variation). In such a case, the confidence intervals from repeated assays on the same sample may not satisfactorily overlap, and care should be exercised in the interpretation of the individual confidence intervals. In order to obtain a more reliable estimate of the confidence interval it may be necessary to perform several independent assays and to combine these into one single potency estimate and confidence interval (see Section 6).

For the purpose of quality control of routine assays it is recommended to keep record of the estimates of the slope of regression and of the estimate of the residual error in control charts.

- An exceptionally high residual error may indicate some technical problem. This should be investigated and, if it can be made evident that something went wrong during the assay procedure, the assay should be repeated. An unusually high residual error may also indicate the presence of an occasional outlying or aberrant observation. A response that is questionable because of failure to comply with the procedure during the course of an assay is rejected. If an aberrant value is discovered after the responses have been recorded, but can then be traced to assay irregularities, omission may be justified. The arbitrary rejection or retention of an apparently aberrant response can be a serious source of bias. In general, the rejection of observations solely because a test for outliers is significant, is discouraged.
- An exceptionally low residual error may once in a while occur and cause the *F*-ratios to exceed the critical values. In such a case it may be justified to replace the residual error estimated from the individual assay, by an average residual error based on historical data recorded in the control charts.

3.1.3. CALCULATIONS AND RESTRICTIONS

According to general principles of good design the following 3 restrictions are normally imposed on the assay design. They have advantages both for ease of computation and for precision.

a) Each preparation in the assay must be tested with the same number of dilutions.

b) In the parallel-line model, the ratio of adjacent doses must be constant for all treatments in the assay; in the slope-ratio model, the interval between adjacent doses must be constant for all treatments in the assay.

c) There must be an equal number of experimental units to each treatment.

If a design is used which meets these restrictions, the calculations are simple. The formulae are given in Sections 3.2 and 3.3. It is recommended to use software which has been developed for this special purpose. There are several programs in existence which can easily deal with all assay-designs described in the monographs. Not all programs may use the same formulae and algorithms, but they should all lead to the same results.

Assay designs not meeting the above mentioned restrictions may be both possible and correct, but the necessary formulae are too complicated to describe in this text. A brief description of methods for calculation is given in Section 7.1. These methods can also be used for the restricted designs, in which case they are equivalent with the simple formulae.

The formulae for the restricted designs given in this text may be used, for example, to create *ad hoc* programs in a spreadsheet. The examples in Section 5 can be used to clarify the statistics and to check whether such a program gives correct results.

3.2. THE PARALLEL-LINE MODEL

3.2.1. INTRODUCTION

The parallel-line model is illustrated in Figure 3.2.1.-I. The logarithm of the doses are represented on the horizontal axis with the lowest concentration on the left and the highest concentration on the right. The responses are indicated on the vertical axis. The individual responses to each treatment are indicated with black dots. The 2 lines are the calculated ln(dose)-response relationship for the standard and the unknown.

Note: the natural logarithm (ln or $\log_e$) is used throughout this text. Wherever the term "antilogarithm" is used, the quantity e^x is meant. However, the Briggs or "common" logarithm (log or $\log_{10}$) can equally well be used. In this case the corresponding antilogarithm is 10^x.

For a satisfactory assay the assumed potency of the test sample must be close to the true potency. On the basis of this assumed potency and the assigned potency of the standard, equipotent dilutions (if feasible) are prepared, i.e. corresponding doses of standard and unknown are expected to give the same response. If no information on the assumed potency is available, preliminary assays are carried out over a wide range of doses to determine the range where the curve is linear.

5. General texts

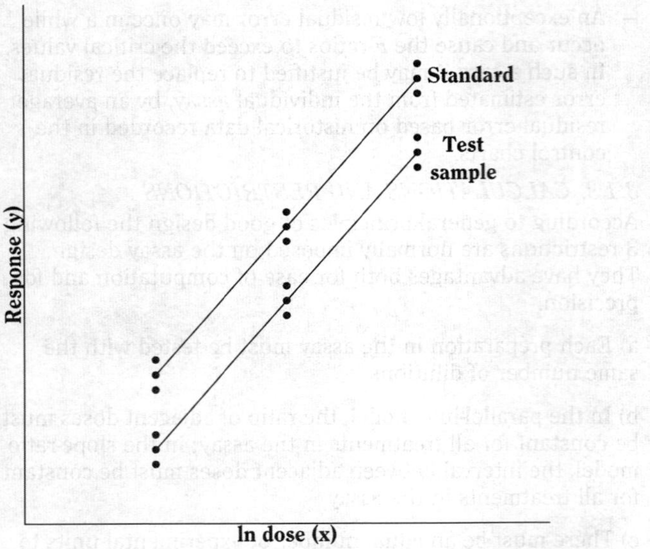

Figure 3.2.1.-I. – *The parallel-line model for a 3 + 3 assay*

The more nearly correct the assumed potency of the unknown, the closer the 2 lines will be together, for they should give equal responses at equal doses. The horizontal distance between the lines represents the "true" potency of the unknown, relative to its assumed potency. The greater the distance between the 2 lines, the poorer the assumed potency of the unknown. If the line of the unknown is situated to the right of the standard, the assumed potency was overestimated, and the calculations will indicate an estimated potency lower than the assumed potency. Similarly, if the line of the unknown is situated to the left of the standard, the assumed potency was underestimated, and the calculations will indicate an estimated potency higher than the assumed potency.

3.2.2. ASSAY DESIGN

The following considerations will be useful in optimising the precision of the assay design:

1) the ratio between the slope and the residual error should be as large as possible,

2) the range of doses should be as large as possible,

3) the lines should be as close together as possible, i.e. the assumed potency should be a good estimate of the true potency.

The allocation of experimental units (animals, tubes, etc.) to different treatments may be made in various ways.

3.2.2.1. Completely randomised design

If the totality of experimental units appears to be reasonably homogeneous with no indication that variability in response will be smaller within certain recognisable sub-groups, the allocation of the units to the different treatments should be made randomly.

If units in sub-groups such as physical positions or experimental days are likely to be more homogeneous than the totality of the units, the precision of the assay may be increased by introducing one or more restrictions into the design. A careful distribution of the units over these restrictions permits irrelevant sources of variation to be eliminated.

3.2.2.2. Randomised block design

In this design it is possible to segregate an identifiable source of variation, such as the sensitivity variation between litters of experimental animals or the variation between Petri dishes in a diffusion microbiological assay. The design requires that every treatment be applied an equal number of times in every block (litter or Petri dish) and is suitable only when the block is large enough to accommodate all treatments once. This is illustrated in Section 5.1.3. It is also possible to use a randomised design with repetitions. The treatments should be allocated randomly within each block. An algorithm to obtain random permutations is given in Section 8.5.

3.2.2.3. Latin square design

This design is appropriate when the response may be affected by two different sources of variation each of which can assume k different levels or positions. For example, in a plate assay of an antibiotic the treatments may be arranged in a $k \times k$ array on a large plate, each treatment occurring once in each row and each column. The design is suitable when the number of rows, the number of columns and the number of treatments are equal. Responses are recorded in a square format known as a Latin square. Variations due to differences in response among the k rows and among the k columns may be segregated, thus reducing the error. An example of a Latin square design is given in Section 5.1.2. An algorithm to obtain Latin squares is given in Section 8.6.

3.2.2.4. Cross-over design

This design is useful when the experiment can be sub-divided into blocks but it is possible to apply only 2 treatments to each block. For example, a block may be a single unit that can be tested on 2 occasions. The design is intended to increase precision by eliminating the effects of differences between units while balancing the effect of any difference between general levels of response at the 2 occasions. If 2 doses of a standard and of an unknown preparation are tested, this is known as a twin cross-over test.

The experiment is divided into 2 parts separated by a suitable time interval. Units are divided into 4 groups and each group receives 1 of the 4 treatments in the first part of the test. Units that received one preparation in the first part of the test receive the other preparation on the second occasion, and units receiving small doses in one part of the test receive large doses in the other. The arrangement of doses is shown in Table 3.2.2.-I. An example can be found in Section 5.1.5.

Table 3.2.2.-I. – *Arrangement of doses in cross-over design*

Group of units	Time I	Time II
1	S_1	T_2
2	S_2	T_1
3	T_1	S_2
4	T_2	S_1

3.2.3. ANALYSIS OF VARIANCE

This section gives formulae that are required to carry out the analysis of variance and will be more easily understood by reference to the worked examples in Section 5.1. Reference should also be made to the glossary of symbols (Section 9).

The formulae are appropriate for symmetrical assays where one or more preparations to be examined (T, U, etc.) are compared with a standard preparation (S). It is stressed that the formulae can only be used if the doses are equally spaced, if equal numbers of treatments per preparation are applied, and each treatment is applied an equal number of times. It should not be attempted to use the formulae in any other situation.

Apart from some adjustments to the error term, the basic analysis of data derived from an assay is the same for completely randomised, randomised block and Latin square designs. The formulae for cross-over tests do not entirely fit this scheme and these are incorporated into Example 5.1.5.

Having considered the points discussed in Section 3.1 and transformed the responses, if necessary, the values should be averaged over each treatment and each preparation, as shown in Table 3.2.3.-I. The linear contrasts, which relate to the slopes of the ln(dose)-response lines, should also be formed. 3 additional formulae, which are necessary for the construction of the analysis of variance, are shown in Table 3.2.3.-II.

The total variation in response caused by the different treatments is now partitioned as shown in Table 3.2.3.-III the sums of squares being derived from the values obtained in Tables 3.2.3.-I and 3.2.3.-II. The sum of squares due to non-linearity can only be calculated if at least 3 doses per preparation are included in the assay.

The residual error of the assay is obtained by subtracting the variations allowed for in the design from the total variation in response (Table 3.2.3.-IV). In this table $\bar{y}$ represents the mean of all responses recorded in the assay. It should be noted that for a Latin square the number of replicate responses (n) is equal to the number of rows, columns or treatments (dh).

The analysis of variance is now completed as follows. Each sum of squares is divided by the corresponding number of degrees of freedom to give mean squares. The mean square for each variable to be tested is now expressed as a ratio to the residual error (s^2) and the significance of these values (known as F-ratios) are assessed by use of Table 8.1 or a suitable sub-routine of a computer program.

3.2.4. *TESTS OF VALIDITY*

Assay results are said to be "statistically valid" if the outcome of the analysis of variance is as follows.

1) The linear regression term is significant, i.e. the calculated probability is less than 0.05. If this criterion is not met, it is not possible to calculate 95 per cent confidence limits.

2) The term for non-parallelism is not significant, i.e. the calculated probability is not less than 0.05. This indicates that condition 5A, Section 3.1, is satisfied;

3) The term for non-linearity is not significant, i.e. the calculated probability is not less than 0.05. This indicates that condition 4A, Section 3.1, is satisfied.

A significant deviation from parallelism in a multiple assay may be due to the inclusion in the assay-design of a preparation to be examined that gives an ln(dose)-response line with a slope different from those for the other preparations. Instead of declaring the whole assay invalid, it may then be decided to eliminate all data relating to that preparation and to restart the analysis from the beginning.

When statistical validity is established, potencies and confidence limits may be estimated by the methods described in the next section.

Table 3.2.3.-I. – *Formulae for parallel-line assays with d doses of each preparation*

	Standard (S)	**1st Test sample (T)**	**2nd Test sample (U, etc.)**
Mean response lowest dose	S_1	T_1	U_1
Mean response 2nd dose	S_2	T_2	U_2
...	...	...	...
Mean response highest dose	S_d	T_d	U_d
Total preparation	$P_S = S_1 + S_2 + ... + S_d$	$P_T = T_1 + T_2 + ... + T_d$	$P_U = ...\text{etc.}$
Linear contrast	$L_S = 1S_1{+}2S_2{+}...{+}dS_d{+}{-}\frac{1}{2}(d+1)P_S$	$L_T = 1T_1{+}2T_2{+}...{+}dT_d{+}{-}\frac{1}{2}(d+1)P_T$	$L_U = ...\text{etc.}$

Table 3.2.3.-II. – *Additional formulae for the construction of the analysis of variance*

$H_P = \frac{n}{d}$	$H_L = \frac{12n}{d^3 - d}$	$K = \frac{n(P_S + P_T + ...)^2}{hd}$

Table 3.2.3.-III. – *Formulae to calculate the sum of squares and degrees of freedom*

Source of variation	**Degrees of freedom (f)**	**Sum of squares**
Preparations	$h - 1$	$SS_{\text{prep}} = H_P(P_S^2 + P_T^2 + ...) - K$
Linear regression	1	$SS_{\text{reg}} = \frac{1}{h} H_L (L_S + L_T + ...)^2$
Non-parallelism	$h - 1$	$SS_{\text{par}} = H_L(L_S^2 + L_T^2 + ...) - SS_{\text{reg}}$
Non-linearity(*)	$h(d - 2)$	$SS_{\text{lin}} = SS_{\text{treat}} - SS_{\text{prep}} - SS_{\text{reg}} - SS_{\text{par}}$
Treatments	$hd - 1$	$SS_{\text{treat}} = n(S_1^2 + ... + S_d^2 + T_1^2 + ... + T_d^2 + ...) - K$

(*) Not calculated for two-dose assays

Table 3.2.3.-IV. – *Estimation of the residual error*

Source of variation		Degrees of freedom	Sum of squares
Blocks (rows)(*)		$n - 1$	$SS_{\text{block}} = hd\,(R_1^2 + ... + R_n^2) - K$
Columns(**)		$n - 1$	$SS_{\text{col}} = hd\,(C_1^2 + ... + C_n^2) - K$
Residual error(***)	Completely randomised	$hd\,(n - 1)$	$SS_{\text{res}} = SS_{\text{tot}} - SS_{\text{treat}}$
	Randomised block	$(hd - 1)\,(n - 1)$	$SS_{\text{res}} = SS_{\text{tot}} - SS_{\text{treat}} - SS_{\text{block}}$
	Latin square	$(hd - 2)\,(n - 1)$	$SS_{\text{res}} = SS_{\text{tot}} - SS_{\text{treat}} - SS_{\text{block}} - SS_{\text{col}}$
Total		$nhd - 1$	$SS_{\text{tot}} = \sum (y - \bar{y})^2$

(*) Not calculated for completely randomised designs
(**) Only calculated for Latin square designs
(***) Depends on the type of design

3.2.5. ESTIMATION OF POTENCY AND CONFIDENCE LIMITS

If *I* is the ln of the ratio between adjacent doses of any preparation, the common slope (*b*) for assays with *d* doses of each preparation is obtained from:

$$b = \frac{H_L\,(L_S + L_T + ...)}{Inh} \qquad (3.2.5.\text{-}1)$$

and the logarithm of the potency ratio of a test preparation, for example *T*, is:

$$M'_T = \frac{P_T - P_S}{db} \qquad (3.2.5.\text{-}2)$$

The calculated potency is an estimate of the "true potency" of each unknown. Confidence limits may be calculated as the antilogarithms of:

$$CM'_T \pm \sqrt{(C-1)\,(CM'^2_T + 2V)} \qquad (3.2.5.\text{-}3)$$

$$\text{where } C = \frac{SS_{\text{reg}}}{SS_{\text{reg}} - s^2t^2} \quad \text{and} \quad V = \frac{SS_{\text{reg}}}{b^2dn}$$

The value of *t* may be obtained from Table 8.2 for $p = 0.05$ and degrees of freedom equal to the number of the degrees of freedom of the residual error. The estimated potency (R_T) and associated confidence limits are obtained by multiplying the values obtained by A_T after antilogarithms have been taken. If the stock solutions are not exactly equipotent on the basis of assigned and assumed potencies, a correction factor is necessary (See Examples 5.1.2 and 5.1.3).

3.2.6. MISSING VALUES

In a balanced assay, an accident totally unconnected with the applied treatments may lead to the loss of one or more responses, for example because an animal dies. If it is considered that the accident is in no way connected with the composition of the preparation administered, the exact calculations can still be performed but the formulae are necessarily more complicated and can only be given within the framework of general linear models (see Section 7.1). However, there exists an approximate method which keeps the simplicity of the balanced design by replacing the missing response by a calculated value. The loss of information is taken into account by diminishing the degrees of freedom for the total sum of squares and for the residual error by the number of missing values and using one of the formulae below for the missing values. It should be borne in mind that this is only an approximate method, and that the exact method is to be preferred.

If more than one observation is missing, the same formulae can be used. The procedure is to make a rough guess at all the missing values except one, and to use the proper formula for this one, using all the remaining values including the rough guesses. Fill in the calculated value. Continue by similarly calculating a value for the first rough guess. After calculating all the missing values in this way the whole cycle is repeated from the beginning, each calculation using the most recent guessed or calculated value for every response to which the formula is being applied. This continues until 2 consecutive cycles give the same values; convergence is usually rapid.

Provided that the number of values replaced is small relative to the total number of observations in the full experiment (say less than 5 per cent), the approximation implied in this replacement and reduction of degrees of freedom by the number of missing values so replaced is usually fairly satisfactory. The analysis should be interpreted with great care however, especially if there is a preponderance of missing values in one treatment or block, and a biometrician should be consulted if any unusual features are encountered. Replacing missing values in a test without replication is a particularly delicate operation.

Completely randomised design

In a completely randomised assay the missing value can be replaced by the arithmetic mean of the other responses to the same treatment.

Randomised block design

The missing value is obtained using the equation:

$$y' = \frac{nB' + kT' - G'}{(n-1)\,(k-1)} \qquad (3.2.6.\text{-}1)$$

where B' is the sum of the responses in the block containing the missing value, T' the corresponding treatment total and G' is the sum of all responses recorded in the assay.

Latin square design

The missing value y' is obtained from:

$$y' = \frac{k\,(B' + C' + T') - 2G'}{(k-1)\,(k-2)} \qquad (3.2.6.\text{-}2)$$

where B' and C' are the sums of the responses in the row and column containing the missing value. In this case $k = n$.

Cross-over design

If an accident leading to loss of values occurs in a cross-over design, a book on statistics should be consulted (e.g. D.J. Finney, see Section 10), because the appropriate formulae depend upon the particular treatment combinations.

3.3. THE SLOPE-RATIO MODEL

3.3.1. INTRODUCTION

This model is suitable, for example, for some microbiological assays when the independent variable is the concentration of an essential growth factor below the optimal concentration of the medium. The slope-ratio model is illustrated in Figure 3.3.1.-I.

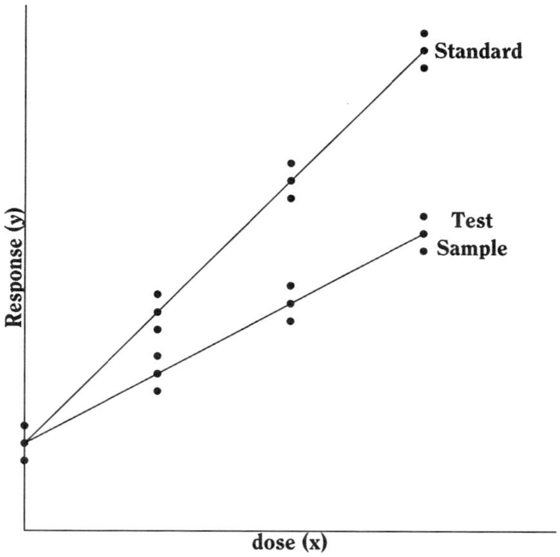

Figure 3.3.1.-I. – *The slope-ratio model for a 2 × 3 + 1 assay*

The doses are represented on the horizontal axis with zero concentration on the left and the highest concentration on the right. The responses are indicated on the vertical axis. The individual responses to each treatment are indicated with black dots. The 2 lines are the calculated dose-response relationship for the standard and the unknown under the assumption that they intersect each other at zero-dose. Unlike the parallel-line model, the doses are not transformed to logarithms.

Just as in the case of an assay based on the parallel-line model, it is important that the assumed potency is close to the true potency, and to prepare equipotent dilutions of the test preparations and the standard (if feasible). The more nearly correct the assumed potency, the closer the 2 lines will be together. The ratio of the slopes represents the "true" potency of the unknown, relative to its assumed potency. If the slope of the unknown preparation is steeper than that of the standard, the potency was underestimated and the calculations will indicate an estimated potency higher than the assumed potency. Similarly, if the slope of the unknown is less steep than that of the standard, the potency was overestimated and the calculations will result in an estimated potency lower than the assumed potency.

In setting up an experiment, all responses should be examined for the fulfilment of the conditions 1, 2 and 3 in Section 3.1. The analysis of variance to be performed in routine is described in Section 3.3.3 so that compliance with conditions 4B and 5B of Section 3.1 may be examined.

3.3.2. ASSAY DESIGN

The use of the statistical analysis presented below imposes the following restrictions on the assay:

a) the standard and the test preparations must be tested with the same number of equally spaced dilutions,

b) an extra group of experimental units receiving no treatment may be tested (the blanks),

c) there must be an equal number of experimental units to each treatment.

As already remarked in Section 3.1.3, assay designs not meeting these restrictions may be both possible and correct, but the simple statistical analyses presented here are no longer applicable and either expert advice should be sought or suitable software should be used.

A design with 2 doses per preparation and 1 blank, the "common zero (2*h* + 1)-design", is usually preferred, since it gives the highest precision combined with the possibility to check validity within the constraints mentioned above. However, a linear relationship cannot always be assumed to be valid down to zero-dose. With a slight loss of precision a design without blanks may be adopted. In this case 3 doses per preparation, the "common zero (3*h*)-design", are preferred to 2 doses per preparation. The doses are thus given as follows:

1) the standard is given in a high dose, near to but not exceeding the highest dose giving a mean response on the straight portion of the dose-response line,

2) the other doses are uniformly spaced between the highest dose and zero dose,

3) the test preparations are given in corresponding doses based on the assumed potency of the material.

A completely randomised, a randomised block or a Latin square design may be used, such as described in Section 3.2.2. The use of any of these designs necessitates an adjustment to the error sum of squares as described for assays based on the parallel-line model. The analysis of an assay of one or more test preparations against a standard is described below.

3.3.3. ANALYSIS OF VARIANCE

3.3.3.1. The (*hd* + 1)-design

The responses are verified as described in Section 3.1 and, if necessary, transformed. The responses are then averaged over each treatment and each preparation as shown in Table 3.3.3.1.-I. Additionally, the mean response for blanks (B) is calculated.

The sums of squares in the analysis of variance are calculated as shown in Tables 3.3.3.1.-I to 3.3.3.1.-III. The sum of squares due to non-linearity can only be calculated if at least 3 doses of each preparation have been included in the assay. The residual error is obtained by subtracting the variations allowed for in the design from the total variation in response (Table 3.3.3.1.-IV).

The analysis of variance is now completed as follows. Each sum of squares is divided by the corresponding number of degrees of freedom to give mean squares. The mean square for each variable to be tested is now expressed as a ratio to the residual error (s^2) and the significance of these values (known as *F*-ratios) are assessed by use of Table 8.1 or a suitable sub-routine of a computer program.

3.3.3.2. The (*hd*)-design

The formulae are basically the same as those for the (*hd* + 1)-design, but there are some slight differences.

– B is discarded from all formulae.

– $K = \dfrac{n\,(P_S + P_T + ...)^2}{hd}$

– SS_{blank} is removed from the analysis of variance.

– The number of degrees of freedom for treatments becomes $hd - 1$.

– The number of degrees of freedom of the residual error and the total variance is calculated as described for the parallel-line model (see Table 3.2.3.-IV).

Validity of the assay, potency and confidence interval are found as described in Sections 3.3.4 and 3.3.5.

Table 3.3.3.1.-I. – *Formulae for slope-ratio assays with d doses of each preparation and a blank*

	Standard (S)	**1st Test sample (T)**	**2nd Test sample (U, etc.)**
Mean response lowest dose	S_1	T_1	U_1
Mean response 2nd dose	S_2	T_2	U_2
...	...	...	...
Mean response highest dose	S_d	T_d	U_d
Total preparation	$P_S = S_1 + S_2 + ... + S_d$	$P_T = T_1 + T_2 + ... + T_d$	$P_U = ...$
Linear product	$L_S = 1S_1 + 2S_2 + ... + dS_d$	$L_T = 1T_1 + 2T_2 + ... + dT_d$	$L_U = ...$
Intercept value	$a_S = (4d+2)P_S - 6L_S$	$a_T = (4d+2)P_T - 6L_T$	$a_U = ...$
Slope value	$b_S = 2L_S - (d+1)P_S$	$b_T = 2L_T - (d+1)P_T$	$b_U = ...$
Treatment value	$G_S = S_1^2 + ... + S_d^2$	$G_T = T_1^2 + ... + T_d^2$	$G_U = ...$
Non-linearity(*)	$J_S = G_S - \frac{P_S^2}{d} - \frac{3b_S^2}{d^3 - d}$	$J_T = G_T - \frac{P_T^2}{d} - \frac{3b_T^2}{d^3 - d}$	$J_U = ...$

(*) Not calculated for two-dose assays

Table 3.3.3.1.-II. – *Additional formulae for the construction of the analysis of variance*

$H_B = \frac{nhd^2 - nhd}{hd^2 - hd + 4d + 2}$	$H_I = \frac{n}{4d^3 - 2d^2 - 2d}$	$a = \frac{a_S + a_T + ...}{h(d^2 - d)}$	$K = \frac{n(B + P_S + P_T + ...)^2}{hd + 1}$

Table 3.3.3.1.-III. – *Formulae to calculate the sum of squares and degrees of freedom*

Source of variation	**Degrees of freedom (f)**	**Sum of squares**
Regression	h	$SS_{\mathrm{reg}} = SS_{\mathrm{treat}} - SS_{\mathrm{blank}} - SS_{\mathrm{int}} - SS_{\mathrm{lin}}$
Blanks	1	$SS_{\mathrm{blank}} = H_B (B - a)^2$
Intersection	$h - 1$	$SS_{\mathrm{int}} = H_I \left((a_S^2 + a_T^2 + ...) - h(d^2 - d)^2 a^2\right)$
Non-linearity(*)	$h(d - 2)$	$SS_{\mathrm{lin}} = n(J_S + J_T + ...)$
Treatments	hd	$SS_{\mathrm{treat}} = n(B^2 + G_S + G_T + ...) - K$

(*) Not calculated for two-dose assays

3.3.4. TESTS OF VALIDITY

Assay results are said to be "statistically valid" if the outcome of the analysis of variance is as follows:

1) the variation due to blanks in (*hd* + 1)-designs is not significant, i.e. the calculated probability is not smaller than 0.05. This indicates that the responses of the blanks do not significantly differ from the common intercept and the linear relationship is valid down to zero dose;

2) the variation due to intersection is not significant, i.e. the calculated probability is not less than 0.05. This indicates that condition 5B, Section 3.1 is satisfied;

3) in assays including at least 3 doses per preparation, the variation due to non-linearity is not significant, i.e. the calculated probability is not less than 0.05. This indicates that condition 4B, Section 3.1 is satisfied.

A significant variation due to blanks indicates that the hypothesis of linearity is not valid near zero dose. If this is likely to be systematic rather than incidental for the type of assay, the (*hd*-design) is more appropriate. Any response to blanks should then be disregarded.

When these tests indicate that the assay is valid, the potency is calculated with its confidence limits as described in Section 3.3.5.

3.3.5. ESTIMATION OF POTENCY AND CONFIDENCE LIMITS

3.3.5.1. The (*hd* + 1)-design

The common intersection a' of the preparations can be calculated from:

$$a' = \frac{(2d+1)B + (2d-3)ha}{h(2d-3) + 2d + 1} \qquad (3.3.5.1.\text{-}1)$$

The slope of the standard, and similarly for each of the other preparations, is calculated from:

$$b'_S = \frac{6L_S - 3d(d+1)a'}{2d^3 + 3d^2 + d} \qquad (3.3.5.1.\text{-}2)$$

The potency ratio of each of the test preparations can now be calculated from:

Table 3.3.3.1.-IV. – *Estimation of the residual error*

Source of variation		Degrees of freedom	Sum of squares
Blocks (rows)(*)		$n - 1$	$SS_{block} = hd\,(R_1^2 + ... + R_n^2) - K$
Columns(**)		$n - 1$	$SS_{col} = hd\,(C_1^2 + ... + C_n^2) - K$
Residual error(***)	**Completely randomised**	$(hd + 1)\,(n - 1)$	$SS_{res} = SS_{tot} - SS_{treat}$
	Randomised block	$hd\,(n - 1)$	$SS_{res} = SS_{tot} - SS_{treat} - SS_{block}$
	Latin square	$(hd - 1)\,(n - 1)$	$SS_{res} = SS_{tot} - SS_{treat} - SS_{block} - SS_{col}$
Total		$nhd + n - 1$	$SS_{tot} = \sum (y - \overline{y})^2$

(*) Not calculated for completely randomised designs
(**) Only calculated for Latin square designs
(***) Depends on the type of design

$$R'_T = \frac{b'_T}{b'_S} \qquad (3.3.5.1.\text{-}3)$$

which has to be multiplied by A_T, the assumed potency of the test preparation, in order to find the estimated potency R_T. If the step between adjacent doses was not identical for the standard and the test preparation, the potency has to be multiplied by I_S/I_T. Note that, unlike the parallel-line analysis, no antilogarithms are calculated.

The confidence interval for R_T' is calculated from:

$$CR'_T - K' \pm \sqrt{(C-1)\,(CR'^2_T + 1) + K'\,(K' - 2CR'_T)} \qquad (3.3.5.1.\text{-}4)$$

$$\text{where } C = \frac{b'^2_S}{b'^2_S - s^2t^2V_1} \text{ and } K' = (C - 1)\,V_2$$

V_1 are V_2 are related to the variance and covariance of the numerator and denominator of R_T. They can be obtained from:

$$V_1 = \frac{6}{n\,(2d+1)}\left(\frac{1}{d\,(d+1)} + \frac{3}{2\,(2d+1) + hd\,(d-1)}\right) \qquad (3.3.5.1.\text{-}5)$$

$$V_2 = \frac{3d\,(d+1)}{(3d+1)\,(d+2) + hd\,(d-1)} \qquad (3.3.5.1.\text{-}6)$$

The confidence limits are multiplied by A_T, and if necessary by I_S/I_T.

3.3.5.2. The (*hd*)-design

The formulae are the same as for the (*hd* + 1)-design, with the following modifications:

$$a' = a \qquad (3.3.5.2.\text{-}1)$$

$$V_1 = \frac{6}{nd\,(2d+1)}\left(\frac{1}{d+1} + \frac{3}{h\,(d-1)}\right) \qquad (3.3.5.2.\text{-}2)$$

$$V_2 = \frac{3\,(d+1)}{3\,(d+1) + h\,(d-1)} \qquad (3.3.5.2.\text{-}3)$$

3.4. EXTENDED SIGMOID DOSE-RESPONSE CURVES

This model is suitable, for example, for some immunoassays when analysis is required of extended sigmoid dose-response curves. This model is illustrated in Figure 3.4.-I.

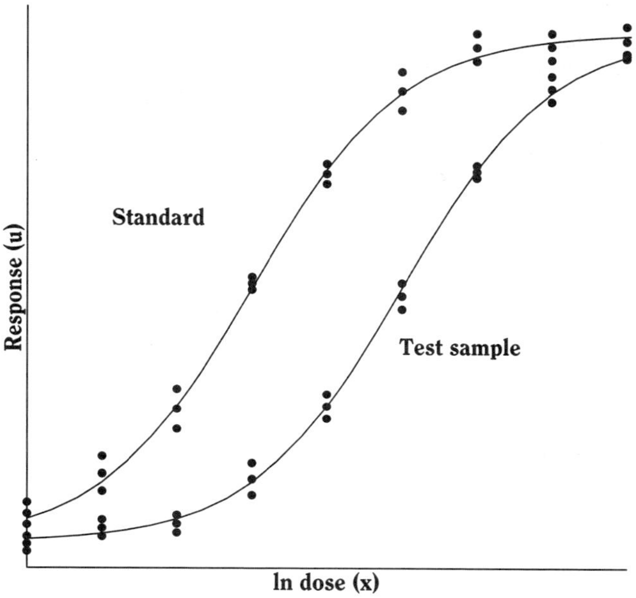

Figure 3.4.-I. – *The four-parameter logistic curve model*

The logarithms of the doses are represented on the horizontal axis with the lowest concentration on the left and the highest concentration on the right. The responses are indicated on the vertical axis. The individual responses to each treatment are indicated with black dots. The 2 curves are the calculated ln(dose)-response relationship for the standard and the test preparation.

The general shape of the curves can usually be described by a logistic function but other shapes are also possible. Each curve can be characterised by 4 parameters: The upper asymptote (α), the lower asymptote (δ), the slope-factor (β), and the horizontal location (γ). This model is therefore often referred to as a four-parameter model. A mathematical representation of the ln(dose)-response curve is:

$$u = \delta + \frac{\alpha - \delta}{1 + e^{-\beta(x-\gamma)}}$$

For a valid assay it is necessary that the curves of the standard and the test preparations have the same slope-factor, and the same maximum and minimum response level at the extreme parts. Only the horizontal location (γ) of the curves may be different. The horizontal distance between the curves is related to the "true" potency of the unknown. If the assay is used routinely, it may be sufficient to test the condition of equal upper and lower response levels when the assay is developed, and then to retest this condition directly only at suitable intervals or when there are changes in materials or assay conditions.

The maximum-likelihood estimates of the parameters and their confidence intervals can be obtained with suitable computer programs. These computer programs may include some statistical tests reflecting validity. For example, if the maximum likelihood estimation shows significant deviations from the fitted model under the assumed conditions of equal upper and lower asymptotes and slopes, then one or all of these conditions may not be satisfied.

The logistic model raises a number of statistical problems which may require different solutions for different types of assays, and no simple summary is possible. A wide variety of possible approaches is described in the relevant literature. Professional advice is therefore recommended for this type of analysis. A simple example is nevertheless included in Section 5.4 to illustrate a "possible" way to analyse the data presented. A short discussion of alternative approaches and other statistical considerations is given in Section 7.5.

If professional advice or suitable software is not available, alternative approaches are possible: 1) if "reasonable" estimates of the upper limit (α) and lower limit (δ) are available, select for all preparations the doses with mean of the responses (u) falling between approximately 20 per cent and 80 per cent of the limits, transform responses of the selected doses to $y = \ln\left(\frac{u-\delta}{\alpha-u}\right)$ and use the parallel line model (Section 3.2) for the analysis; 2) select a range of doses for which the responses (u) or suitably transformed responses, for example ln(u), are approximately linear when plotted against ln(dose); the parallel line model (Section 3.2) may then be used for analysis.

4. ASSAYS DEPENDING UPON QUANTAL RESPONSES

4.1. INTRODUCTION

In certain assays it is impossible or excessively laborious to measure the effect on each experimental unit on a quantitative scale. Instead, an effect such as death or hypoglycaemic symptoms may be observed as either occurring or not occurring in each unit, and the result depends on the number of units in which it occurs. Such assays are called quantal or all-or-none.

The situation is very similar to that described for quantitative assays in Section 3.1, but in place of n separate responses to each treatment a single value is recorded, i.e. the fraction of units in each treatment group showing a response. When these fractions are plotted against the logarithms of the doses the resulting curve will tend to be sigmoid (S-shaped) rather than linear. A mathematical function that represents this sigmoid curvature is used to estimate the dose-response curve. The most commonly used function is the cumulative normal distribution function. This function has some theoretical merit, and is perhaps the best choice if the response is a reflection of the tolerance of the units. If the response is more likely to depend upon a process of growth, the logistic distribution model is preferred, although the difference in outcome between the 2 models is usually very small.

The maximum likelihood estimators of the slope and location of the curves can be found only by applying an iterative procedure. There are many procedures which lead to the same outcome, but they differ in efficiency due to the speed of convergence. One of the most rapid methods is direct optimisation of the maximum-likelihood function (see Section 7.1), which can easily be performed with computer programs having a built-in procedure for this purpose. Unfortunately, most of these procedures do not yield an estimate of the confidence interval, and the technique to obtain it is too complicated to describe here. The technique described below is not the most rapid, but has been chosen for its simplicity compared to the alternatives. It can be used for assays in which one or more test preparations are compared to a standard. Furthermore, the following conditions must be fulfilled:

1) the relationship between the logarithm of the dose and the response can be represented by a cumulative normal distribution curve,

2) the curves for the standard and the test preparation are parallel, i.e. they are identically shaped and may only differ in their horizontal location,

3) in theory, there is no natural response to extremely low doses and no natural non-response to extremely high doses.

4.2. THE PROBIT METHOD

The sigmoid curve can be made linear by replacing each response, i.e. the fraction of positive responses per group, by the corresponding value of the cumulative standard normal distribution. This value, often referred to as "normit", ranges theoretically from $-\infty$ to $+\infty$. In the past it was proposed to add 5 to each normit to obtain "probits". This facilitated the hand-performed calculations because negative values were avoided. With the arrival of computers the need to add 5 to the normits has disappeared. The term "normit method" would therefore be better for the method described below. However, since the term "probit analysis" is so widely spread, the term will, for historical reasons, be maintained in this text.

Once the responses have been linearised, it should be possible to apply the parallel-line analysis as described in Section 3.2. Unfortunately, the validity condition of homogeneity of variance for each dose is not fulfilled. The variance is minimal at normit = 0 and increases for positive and negative values of the normit. It is therefore necessary to give more weight to responses in the middle part of the curve, and less weight to the more extreme parts of the curve. This method, the analysis of variance, and the estimation of the potency and confidence interval are described below.

4.2.1. TABULATION OF THE RESULTS

Table 4.2.1.-I is used to enter the data into the columns indicated by numbers:

(1) the dose of the standard or the test preparation,

(2) the number n of units submitted to that treatment,

(3) the number of units r giving a positive response to the treatment,

(4) the logarithm x of the dose,

(5) the fraction $p = r/n$ of positive responses per group.

The first cycle starts here.

(6) column Y is filled with zeros at the first iteration,

(7) the corresponding value $\Phi = \Phi(Y)$ of the cumulative standard normal distribution function (see also Table 8.4).

The columns (8) to (10) are calculated with the following formulae:

(8) $$Z = \frac{e^{-Y^2/2}}{\sqrt{2\pi}} \qquad (4.2.1.\text{-}1)$$

(9) $$y = Y + \frac{p-\Phi}{Z} \qquad (4.2.1.\text{-}2)$$

(10) $$w = \frac{nZ^2}{\Phi - \Phi^2} \qquad (4.2.1.\text{-}3)$$

5. General texts

The columns (11) to (15) can easily be calculated from columns (4), (9) and (10) as wx, wy, wx^2 , wy^2 and wxy respectively, and the sum (Σ) of each of the columns (10) to (15) is calculated separately for each of the preparations.

The sums calculated in Table 4.2.1.-I are transferred to columns (1) to (6) of Table 4.2.1.-II and 6 additional columns (7) to (12) are calculated as follows:

(7) $$S_{xx} = \sum wx^2 - \frac{(\sum wx)^2}{\sum w} \qquad (4.2.1.\text{-}4)$$

(8) $$S_{xy} = \sum wxy - \frac{(\sum wx)(\sum wy)}{\sum w} \qquad (4.2.1.\text{-}5)$$

(9) $$S_{yy} = \sum wy^2 - \frac{(\sum wy)^2}{\sum w} \qquad (4.2.1.\text{-}6)$$

(10) $$\overline{x} = \frac{\sum wx}{\sum w} \qquad (4.2.1.\text{-}7)$$

(11) $$\overline{y} = \frac{\sum wy}{\sum w} \qquad (4.2.1.\text{-}8)$$

The common slope b can now be obtained as:

$$b = \frac{\sum S_{xy}}{\sum S_{xx}} \qquad (4.2.1.\text{-}9)$$

and the intercept a of the standard, and similarly for the test preparations is obtained as:

(12) $$a = \overline{y} - b\overline{x} \qquad (4.2.1.\text{-}10)$$

Column (6) of the first working table can now be replaced by $Y = a + bx$ and the cycle is repeated until the difference between 2 cycles has become small (e.g. the maximum difference of Y between 2 consecutive cycles is smaller than 10^{-8}).

4.2.2. TESTS OF VALIDITY

Before calculating the potencies and confidence intervals, validity of the assay must be assessed. If at least 3 doses for each preparation have been included, the deviations from linearity can be measured as follows: add a 13th column to Table 4.2.1.-II and fill it with:

$$S_{yy} - \frac{S_{xy}^2}{S_{xx}} \qquad (4.2.2.\text{-}1)$$

The column total is a measure of deviations from linearity and is approximately χ^2 distributed with degrees of freedom equal to $N - 2h$. Significance of this value may be assessed with the aid of Table 8.3 or a suitable sub-routine in a computer program. If the value is significant at the 0.05 probability level, the assay must probably be rejected (see Section 4.2.4).

When the above test gives no indication of significant deviations from linear regression, the deviations from parallelism are tested at the 0.05 significance level with:

$$\chi^2 = \sum \frac{S_{xy}^2}{S_{xx}} - \frac{(\sum S_{xy})^2}{\sum S_{xx}} \qquad (4.2.2.\text{-}2)$$

with $h - 1$ degrees of freedom.

4.2.3. ESTIMATION OF POTENCY AND CONFIDENCE LIMITS

When there are no indications for a significant departure from parallelism and linearity the ln(potency ratio) M'_T is calculated as:

$$M'_T = \frac{a_T - a_S}{b} \qquad (4.2.3.\text{-}1)$$

and the antilogarithm is taken. Now let $t = 1.96$ and $s = 1$. Confidence limits are calculated as the antilogarithms of:

$$CM'_T - (C-1)(\overline{x}_S - \overline{x}_T) \pm \sqrt{(C-1)\left(V\sum S_{xx} + C(M'_T - \overline{x}_S + \overline{x}_T)^2\right)} \qquad (4.2.3.\text{-}2)$$

where $C = \dfrac{b^2 \sum S_{xx}}{b^2 \sum S_{xx} - s^2 t^2}$ and $V = \dfrac{1}{\sum_S w} + \dfrac{1}{\sum_T w}$

Table 4.2.1.-I. – *First working table*

	(1)	(2)	(3)	(4)	(5)	(6)	(7)	(8)	(9)	(10)	(11)	(12)	(13)	(14)	(15)
	dose	n	r	x	p	Y	Φ	Z	y	w	wx	wy	wx^2	wy^2	wxy
S	.	.	.	.	.	.	.	.	.	.	.	.	.	.	.
	.	.	.	.	.	.	.	.	.	.	.	.	.	.	.
	.	.	.	.	.	.	.	.	.	.	.	.	.	.	.
										Σ =	Σ =	Σ =	Σ =	Σ =	Σ =
T	.	.	.	.	.	.	.	.	.	.	.	.	.	.	.
	.	.	.	.	.	.	.	.	.	.	.	.	.	.	.
	.	.	.	.	.	.	.	.	.	.	.	.	.	.	.
										Σ =	Σ =	Σ =	Σ =	Σ =	Σ =
etc.															

Table 4.2.1.-II. – *Second working table*

	(1)	(2)	(3)	(4)	(5)	(6)	(7)	(8)	(9)	(10)	(11)	(12)
	Σw	Σwx	Σwy	Σwx^2	Σwy^2	Σwxy	S_{xx}	S_{xy}	S_{yy}	$\overline{x}$	$\overline{y}$	a
S	.	.	.	.	.	.	.	.	.	.	.	.
T	.	.	.	.	.	.	.	.	.	.	.	.
etc.	.	.	.	.	.	.	.	.	.	.	.	.
							Σ =	Σ =				

4.2.4. INVALID ASSAYS

If the test for deviations from linearity described in Section 4.2.2 is significant, the assay should normally be rejected. If there are reasons to retain the assay, the formulae are slightly modified. t becomes the t-value (p = 0.05) with the same number of degrees of freedom as used in the check for linearity and s^2 becomes the χ^2 value divided by the same number of degrees of freedom (and thus typically is greater than 1).

The test for parallelism is also slightly modified. The χ^2 value for non-parallelism is divided by its number of degrees of freedom. The resulting value is divided by s^2 calculated above to obtain an F-ratio with h - 1 and N - 2h degrees of freedom, which is evaluated in the usual way at the 0.05 significance level.

4.3. THE LOGIT METHOD

As indicated in Section 4.1 the logit method may sometimes be more appropriate. The name of the method is derived from the logit function which is the inverse of the logistic distribution. The procedure is similar to that described for the probit method with the following modifications in the formulae for Φ and Z.

$$\Phi = \frac{1}{1+e^{-Y}} \qquad (4.3.\text{-}1)$$

$$Z = \frac{e^{-Y}}{(1+e^{-Y})^2} \qquad (4.3.\text{-}2)$$

4.4. OTHER SHAPES OF THE CURVE

The probit and logit method are almost always adequate for the analysis of quantal responses called for in the European Pharmacopoeia. However, if it can be made evident that the ln(dose)-response curve has another shape than the 2 curves described above, another curve Φ may be adopted. Z is then taken to be the first derivative of Φ.

For example, if it can be shown that the curve is not symmetric, the Gompertz distribution may be appropriate (the gompit method) in which case $\Phi = 1 - e^{-e^Y}$ and $Z = e^{Y-e^Y}$.

4.5. THE MEDIAN EFFECTIVE DOSE

In some types of assay it is desirable to determine a median effective dose which is the dose that produces a response in 50 per cent of the units. The probit method can be used to determine this median effective dose (ED_{50}), but since there is no need to express this dose relative to a standard, the formulae are slightly different.

Note: a standard can optionally be included in order to validate the assay. Usually the assay is considered valid if the calculated ED_{50} of the standard is close enough to the assigned ED_{50}. What "close enough" in this context means depends on the requirements specified in the monograph.

The tabulation of the responses to the test samples, and optionally a standard, is as described in Section 4.2.1. The test for linearity is as described in Section 4.2.2. A test for parallelism is not necessary for this type of assay. The ED_{50} of test sample T, and similarly for the other samples, is obtained as described in Section 4.2.3, with the following modifications in formulae 4.2.3.-1 and 4.2.3.-2).

$$M'_T = \frac{-a_T}{b} \qquad (4.5.\text{-}1)$$

$$CM'_T-(C-1)\bar{x}_T \pm \sqrt{(C-1)\left(V\sum S_{xx}+C\left(M'_T+\bar{x}_T\right)^2\right)} \qquad (4.5.\text{-}2)$$

where $V = \dfrac{1}{\sum_T w}$ and C is left unchanged

5. EXAMPLES

This section consists of worked examples illustrating the application of the formulae. The examples have been selected primarily to illustrate the statistical method of calculation. They are not intended to reflect the most suitable method of assay, if alternatives are permitted in the individual monographs. To increase their value as program checks, more decimal places are given than would usually be necessary. It should also be noted that other, but equivalent methods of calculation exist. These methods should lead to exactly the same final results as those given in the examples.

5.1. PARALLEL-LINE MODEL

5.1.1. TWO-DOSE MULTIPLE ASSAY WITH COMPLETELY RANDOMISED DESIGN

An assay of corticotrophin by subcutaneous injection in rats

The standard preparation is administered at 0.25 and 1.0 unit per 100 g of body mass. 2 preparations to be examined are both assumed to have a potency of 1 unit per milligram and they are administered in the same quantities as the standard. The individual responses and means per treatment are given in Table 5.1.1.-I. A graphical presentation (Figure 5.1.1.I) gives no rise to doubt the homogeneity of variance and normality of the data, but suggests problems with parallelism for preparation U.

Table 5.1.1.-I. – *Response metameter y - mass of ascorbic acid (mg) per 100 g of adrenal gland*

	Standard *S*		**Preparation *T***		**Preparation *U***	
	S_1	S_2	T_1	T_2	U_1	U_2
	300	289	310	230	250	236
	310	221	290	210	268	213
	330	267	360	280	273	283
	290	236	341	261	240	269
	364	250	321	241	307	251
	328	231	370	290	270	294
	390	229	303	223	317	223
	360	269	334	254	312	250
	342	233	295	216	320	216
	306	259	315	235	265	265
Mean	332.0	248.4	323.9	244.0	282.2	250.0

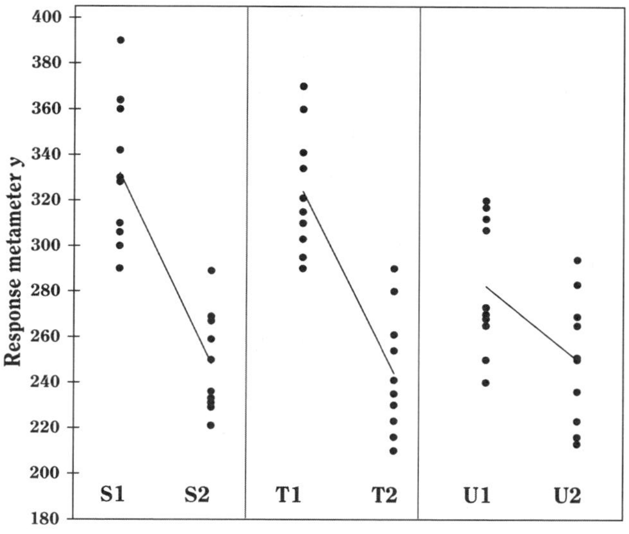

Figure 5.1.1.-I.

The formulae in Tables 3.2.3.-I and 3.2.3.-II lead to:

P_S = 580.4 L_S = −41.8

P_T = 567.9 L_T = −39.95

P_U = 532.2 L_U = −16.1

$H_P = \frac{10}{2} = 5$ $H_L = \frac{120}{6} = 20$

The analysis of variance can now be completed with the formulae in Tables 3.2.3-III and 3.2.3.-IV. This is shown in Table 5.1.1.-II.

Table 5.1.1.-II. – *Analysis of variance*

Source of variation	Degrees of freedom	Sum of squares	Mean square	F-ratio	Probability
Preparations	2	6256.6	3128.3		
Regression	1	63 830.8	63 830.8	83.38	0.000
Non-parallelism	2	8218.2	4109.1	5.37	0.007
Treatments	5	78 305.7			
Residual error	54	41 340.9	765.57		
Total	59	119 646.6			

The analysis confirms a highly significant linear regression. Departure from parallelism, however, is also significant (p = 0.0075) which was to be expected from the graphical observation that preparation U is not parallel to the standard. This preparation is therefore rejected and the analysis repeated using only preparation T and the standard.

Table 5.1.1.-III. – *Analysis of variance without sample U*

Source of variation	Degrees of freedom	Sum of squares	Mean square	F-ratio	Probability
Preparations	1	390.6	390.6		
Regression	1	66 830.6	66 830.6	90.5	0.000
Non-parallelism	1	34.2	34.2	0.05	0.831
Treatments	3	67 255.5			
Residual error	36	26 587.3	738.54		
Total	39	93 842.8			

The analysis without preparation U results in compliance with the requirements with respect to both regression and parallelism and so the potency can be calculated. The formulae in Section 3.2.5 give:

– for the common slope:

$$b = \frac{20\,(-41.8 - 39.95)}{\ln 4 \times 10 \times 2} = -58.970$$

– the ln(potency ratio) is:

$$M'_T = \frac{567.9 - 580.4}{2 \times (-58.970)} = 0.1060$$

$$C = \frac{66\,830.6}{66\,830.6 - 738.54 \times 2.028^2} = 1.0476$$

$$V = \frac{66\,830.6}{(-58.970)^2 \times 2 \times 10} = 0.9609$$

– and ln(confidence limits) are:

$$1.0476 \times 0.1060 \pm \sqrt{0.0476 \times (1.0476 \times 0.1060^2 + 2 \times 0.9609)}$$
$$= 0.1110 \pm 0.3034$$

By taking the antilogarithms we find a potency ratio of 1.11 with 95 per cent confidence limits from 0.82-1.51.

Multiplying by the assumed potency of preparation T yields a potency of 1.11 units/mg with 95 per cent confidence limits from 0.82 to 1.51 units/mg.

5.1.2. THREE-DOSE LATIN SQUARE DESIGN

Antibiotic agar diffusion assay using a rectangular tray

The standard has an assigned potency of 4855 IU/mg. The test preparation has an assumed potency of 5600 IU/mg. For the stock solutions 25.2 mg of the standard is dissolved in 24.5 ml of solvent and 21.4 mg of the test preparation is dissolved in 23.95 ml of solvent. The final solutions are prepared by first diluting both stock solutions to 1/20 and further using a dilution ratio of 1.5.

A Latin square is generated with the method described in Section 8.6 (see Table 5.1.2.-I). The responses of this routine assay are shown in Table 5.1.2.-II (inhibition zones in mm × 10). The treatment mean values are shown in Table 5.1.2.-III. A graphical representation of the data (see Figure 5.1.2.-I) gives no rise to doubt the normality or homogeneity of variance of the data.

The formulae in Tables 3.2.3.-I and 3.2.3.-II lead to:

P_S = 529.667 L_S = 35.833

P_T = 526.333 L_T = 39.333

$H_P = \frac{6}{3} = 2$ $H_L = \frac{72}{24} = 3$

The analysis of variance can now be completed with the formulae in Tables 3.2.3.-III and 3.2.3.-IV. The result is shown in Table 5.1.2.-IV.

The analysis shows significant differences between the rows. This indicates the increased precision achieved by using a Latin square design rather than a completely randomised design. A highly significant regression and no significant departure of the individual regression lines from parallelism and linearity confirms that the assay is satisfactory for potency calculations.

Table 5.1.2.-I. – *Distribution of treatments over the plate*

	1	2	3	4	5	6
1	S_1	T_1	T_2	S_3	S_2	T_3
2	T_1	T_3	S_1	S_2	T_2	S_3
3	T_2	S_3	S_2	S_1	T_3	T_1
4	S_3	S_2	T_3	T_1	S_1	T_2
5	S_2	T_2	S_3	T_3	T_1	S_1
6	T_3	S_1	T_1	T_2	S_3	S_2

Table 5.1.2.-II. – *Measured inhibition zones in mm × 10*

	1	2	3	4	5	6	Row mean
1	161	160	178	187	171	194	175.2 = R_1
2	151	192	150	172	170	192	171.2 = R_2
3	162	195	174	161	193	151	172.7 = R_3
4	194	184	199	160	163	171	178.5 = R_4
5	176	181	201	202	154	151	177.5 = R_5
6	193	166	161	186	198	182	181.0 = R_6
Col. Mean	172.8 = C_1	179.7 = C_2	177.2 = C_3	178.0 = C_4	174.8 = C_5	173.5 = C_6	

Table 5.1.2.-III. – *Means of the treatments*

	Standard *S*			Preparation *T*		
	S_1	S_2	S_3	T_1	T_2	T_3
Mean	158.67	176.50	194.50	156.17	174.67	195.50

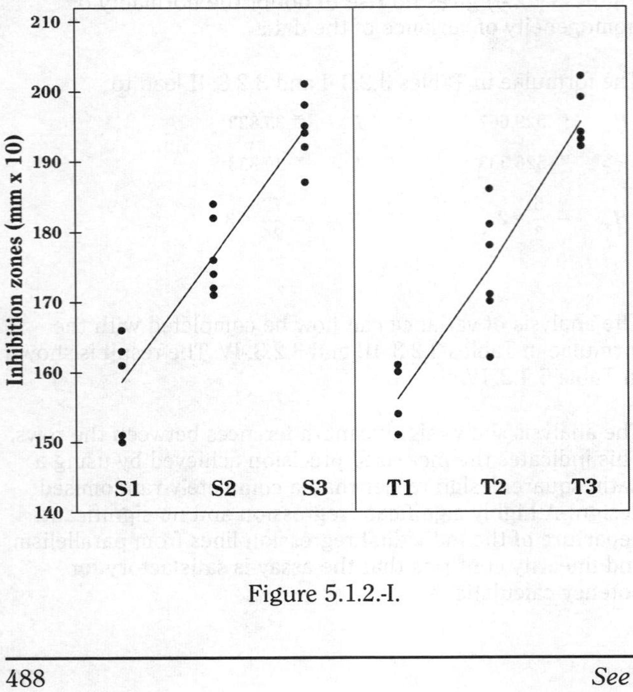

Figure 5.1.2.-I.

Table 5.1.2.-IV. – *Analysis of variance*

Source of variation	Degrees of freedom	Sum of squares	Mean square	*F*-ratio	Probability
Preparations	1	11.1111	11.1111		
Regression	1	8475.0417	8475.0417	408.1	0.000
Non-parallelism	1	18.3750	18.3750	0.885	0.358
Non-linearity	2	5.4722	2.7361	0.132	0.877
Treatments	5	8510			
Rows	5	412	82.40	3.968	0.012
Columns	5	218.6667	43.73	2.106	0.107
Residual error	20	415.3333	20.7667		
Total	35	9556			

The formulae in Section 3.2.5 give:

– for the common slope:

$$b = \frac{3 \times (35.833 + 39.333)}{\ln(1.5) \times 6 \times 2} = 46.346$$

– the ln(potency ratio) is:

$$M'_T = \frac{526.333 - 529.667}{3 \times 46.346} = -0.023974$$

$$C = \frac{8475.0417}{8475.0417 - 20.7667 \times 2.086^2} = 1.0108$$

$$V = \frac{8475.0417}{46.346^2 \times 3 \times 6} = 0.2192$$

– and ln(confidence limits) are:

$$1.0108 \times (-0.0240) \pm \sqrt{0.0108 \times (1.0108 \times (-0.0240)^2 + 2 \times 0.2192)} = -0.02423 \pm 0.06878$$

The potency ratio is found by taking the antilogarithms, resulting in 0.9763 with 95 per cent confidence limits from 0.9112-1.0456.

A correction factor of $\frac{4855 \times 25.2/24.5}{5600 \times 21.4/23.95} = 0.99799$ is necessary because the dilutions were not exactly equipotent on the basis of the assumed potency. Multiplying by this correction factor and the assumed potency of 5600 IU/mg yields a potency of 5456 IU/mg with 95 per cent confidence limits from 5092 to 5843 IU/mg.

5.1.3. FOUR-DOSE RANDOMISED BLOCK DESIGN

Antibiotic turbidimetric assay

This assay is designed to assign a potency in international units per vial. The standard has an assigned potency of 670 IU/mg. The test preparation has an assumed potency of 20 000 IU/vial. On the basis of this information the stock solutions are prepared as follows. 16.7 mg of the standard is dissolved in 25 ml solvent and the contents of one vial of the test preparation are dissolved in 40 ml solvent. The final solutions are prepared by first diluting to 1/40 and further using a dilution ratio of 1.5. The tubes are placed in a water-bath in a randomised block arrangement (see Section 8.5). The responses are listed in Table 5.1.3.-I.

Inspection of Figure 5.1.3.-I gives no rise to doubt the validity of the assumptions of normality and homogeneity of variance of the data. The standard deviation of S_3 is somewhat high but is no reason for concern.

The formulae in Tables 3.2.3.-I and 3.2.3.-II lead to:

P_S = 719.4 L_S = −229.1

P_T = 687.6 L_T = −222

$H_P = \frac{5}{4} = 1.25$ $H_L = \frac{60}{60} = 1$

The analysis of variance is constructed with the formulae in Tables 3.2.3.-III and 3.2.3.-IV. The result is shown in Table 5.1.3.-II.

Table 5.1.3.-I. – *Absorbances of the suspensions (× 1000)*

	Standard *S*				Preparation *T*				
Block	S_1	S_2	S_3	S_4	T_1	T_2	T_3	T_4	Mean
1	252	207	168	113	242	206	146	115	181.1
2	249	201	187	107	236	197	153	102	179.0
3	247	193	162	111	246	197	148	104	176.0
4	250	207	155	108	231	191	159	106	175.9
5	235	207	140	98	232	186	146	95	167.4
Mean	246.6	203.0	162.4	107.4	237.4	195.4	150.4	104.4	

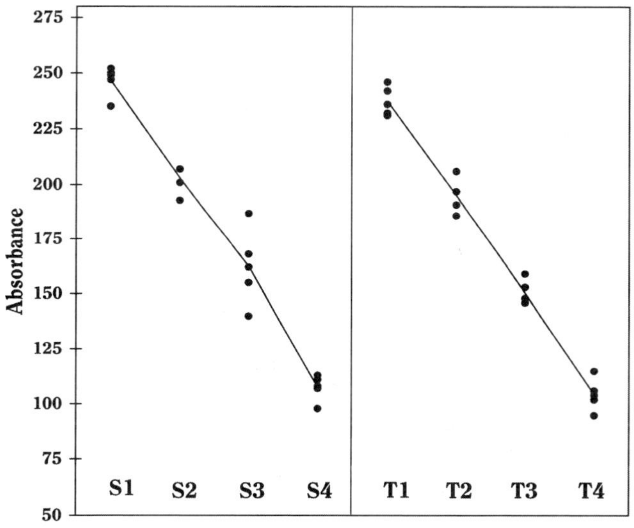

Figure 5.1.3.-I.

Table 5.1.3.-II. – *Analysis of variance*

Source of variation	Degrees of freedom	Sum of squares	Mean square	*F*-ratio	Probability
Preparations	1	632.025	632.025		
Regression	1	101 745.6	101 745.6	1887.1	0.000
Non-parallelism	1	25.205	25.205	0.467	0.500
Non-linearity	4	259.14	64.785	1.202	0.332
Treatments	7	102 662			
Blocks	4	876.75	219.188	4.065	0.010
Residual error	28	1509.65	53.916		
Total	39	105 048.4			

A significant difference is found between the blocks. This indicates the increased precision achieved by using a randomised block design. A highly significant regression and no significant departure from parallelism and linearity confirms that the assay is satisfactory for potency calculations. The formulae in Section 3.2.5 give:

– for the common slope:

$$b = \frac{1 \times (-229.1 - 222)}{\ln(1.5) \times 5 \times 2} = -111.255$$

– the ln(potency ratio) is:

$$M_T' = \frac{687.6 - 719.4}{4 \times (-111.255)} = 0.071457$$

$$C = \frac{101\,745.6}{101\,745.6 - 53.916 \times 2.048^2} = 1.00223$$

$$V = \frac{101\,745.6}{(-111.255)^2 \times 4 \times 5} = 0.4110$$

– and ln(confidence limits) are:

$$1.00223 \times 0.0715 \pm \sqrt{0.00223 \times (1.00223 \times 0.0715^2 + 2 \times 0.4110)} = 0.07162 \pm 0.04293$$

The potency ratio is found by taking the antilogarithms, resulting in 1.0741 with 95 per cent confidence limits from 1.0291 to 1.1214. A correction factor of $\frac{670 \times 16.7/25}{20\,000 \times 1/40} = 0.89512$ is necessary because the dilutions were not exactly equipotent on the basis of the assumed potency. Multiplying by this correction factor and the assumed potency of 20 000 IU/vial yields a potency of 19 228 IU/vial with 95 per cent confidence limits from 18 423-20 075 IU/vial.

5.1.4. FIVE-DOSE MULTIPLE ASSAY WITH COMPLETELY RANDOMISED DESIGN

An in-vitro assay of three hepatitis B vaccines against a standard

3 independent two-fold dilution series of 5 dilutions were prepared from each of the vaccines. After some additional steps in the assay procedure, absorbances were measured. They are shown in Table 5.1.4.-I.

Table 5.1.4.-I. – *Optical densities*

Dilution	Standard *S*			Preparation *T*		
1:16 000	0.043	0.045	0.051	0.097	0.097	0.094
1:8000	0.093	0.099	0.082	0.167	0.157	0.178
1:4000	0.159	0.154	0.166	0.327	0.355	0.345
1:2000	0.283	0.295	0.362	0.501	0.665	0.576
1:1000	0.514	0.531	0.545	1.140	1.386	1.051

Dilution	Preparation *U*			Preparation *V*		
1:16 000	0.086	0.071	0.073	0.082	0.082	0.086
1:8000	0.127	0.146	0.133	0.145	0.144	0.173
1:4000	0.277	0.268	0.269	0.318	0.306	0.316
1:2000	0.586	0.489	0.546	0.552	0.551	0.624
1:1000	0.957	0.866	1.045	1.037	1.039	1.068

The logarithms of the optical densities are known to have a linear relationship with the logarithms of the doses. The mean responses of the ln-transformed optical densities are listed in Table 5.1.4.-II. No unusual features are discovered in a graphical presentation of the data.

Table 5.1.4.-II. – *Means of the ln-transformed absorbances*

S_1	−3.075	T_1	−2.344	U_1	−2.572	V_1	−2.485
S_2	−2.396	T_2	−1.789	U_2	−2.002	V_2	−1.874
S_3	−1.835	T_3	−1.073	U_3	−1.305	V_3	−1.161
S_4	−1.166	T_4	−0.550	U_4	−0.618	V_4	−0.554
S_5	−0.635	T_5	0.169	U_5	−0.048	V_5	0.047

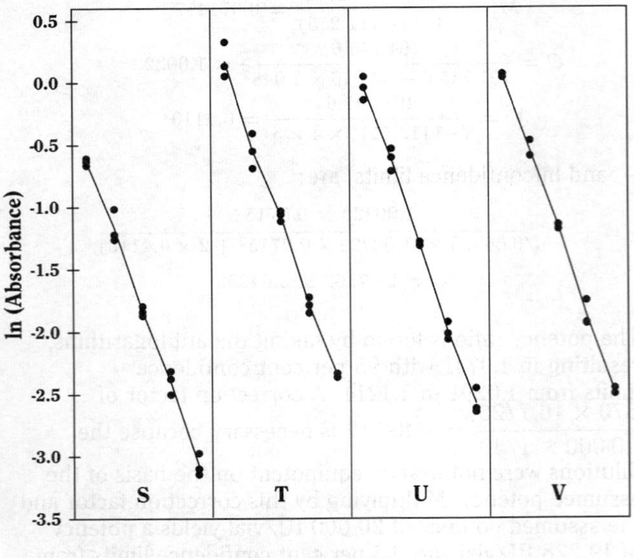

Figure 5.1.4.-I.

The formulae in Tables 3.2.3.-I and 3.2.3.-II give:

$P_S = -9.108$ $L_S = 6.109$

$P_T = -5.586$ $L_T = 6.264$

$P_U = -6.544$ $L_U = 6.431$

$P_V = -6.027$ $L_V = 6.384$

$H_P = \frac{3}{5} = 0.6$ $H_L = \frac{36}{120} = 0.3$

The analysis of variance is completed with the formulae in Tables 3.2.3.-III and 3.2.3.-IV. This is shown in Table 5.1.4.-III.

Table 5.1.4.-III. – *Analysis of variance*

Source of variation	Degrees of freedom	Sum of squares	Mean square	*F*-ratio	Probability
Preparations	3	4.475	1.492		
Regression	1	47.58	47.58	7126	0.000
Non-parallelism	3	0.0187	0.006	0.933	0.434
Non-linearity	12	0.0742	0.006	0.926	0.531
Treatments	19	52.152			
Residual error	40	0.267	0.0067		
Total	59	52.42			

A highly significant regression and a non-significant departure from parallelism and linearity confirm that the potencies can be safely calculated. The formulae in Section 3.2.5 give:

– for the common slope:

$$b = \frac{0.3 \times (6.109 + 6.264 + 6.431 + 6.384)}{\ln 2 \times 3 \times 4} = 0.90848$$

– the ln(potency ratio) for preparation *T* is:

$$M'_T = \frac{-5.586 - (-9.108)}{5 \times 0.90848} = 0.7752$$

$$C = \frac{47.58}{47.58 - 0.0067 \times 2.021^2} = 1.00057$$

$$V = \frac{47.58}{0.9085^2 \times 5 \times 3} = 3.8436$$

– and ln(confidence limits) for preparation *T* are:

$$1.00057 \times 0.7752 \pm \sqrt{0.00057 \times (1.00057 \times 0.7752^2 + 2 \times 3.8436)}$$

$$= 0.7756 \pm 0.0689$$

By taking the antilogarithms a potency ratio of 2.171 is found with 95 per cent confidence limits from 2.027 to 2.327. All samples have an assigned potency of 20 μg protein/ml and so a potency of 43.4 μg protein/ml is found for test preparation *T* with 95 per cent confidence limits from 40.5-46.5 μg protein/ml.

The same procedure is followed to estimate the potency and confidence interval of the other test preparations. The results are listed in Table 5.1.4.-IV.

Table 5.1.4.-IV. – *Final potency estimates and 95 per cent confidence intervals of the test vaccines (in μg protein/ml)*

	Lower limit	Estimate	Upper limit
Vaccine *T*	40.5	43.4	46.5
Vaccine *U*	32.9	35.2	37.6
Vaccine *V*	36.8	39.4	42.2

5.1.5. TWIN CROSS-OVER DESIGN

Assay of insulin by subcutaneous injection in rabbits

The standard preparation was administered at 1 unit and 2 units per millilitre. Equivalent doses of the unknown preparation were used based on an assumed potency of 40 units per millilitre. The rabbits received subcutaneously 0.5 ml of the appropriate solutions according to the design in Table 5.1.5.-I and responses obtained are shown in Table 5.1.5.-II. The large variance illustrates the variation between rabbits and the need to employ a cross-over design.

Table 5.1.5.-I. – *Arrangements of treatments*

	Group of rabbits			
	1	2	3	4
Day 1	S_1	S_2	T_1	T_2
Day 2	T_2	T_1	S_2	S_1

Table 5.1.5.-II. – *Response y: sum of blood glucose readings (mg/100 ml) at 1 hour and $2\frac{1}{2}$ hours*

	Group 1		Group 2		Group 3		Group 4	
	S_1	T_2	S_2	T_1	T_1	S_2	T_2	S_1
	112	104	65	72	105	91	118	144
	126	112	116	160	83	67	119	149
	62	58	73	72	125	67	42	51
	86	63	47	93	56	45	64	107
	52	53	88	113	92	84	93	117
	110	113	63	71	101	56	73	128
	116	91	50	65	66	55	39	87
	101	68	55	100	91	68	31	71
Mean	95.6	82.8	69.6	93.3	89.9	66.6	72.4	106.8

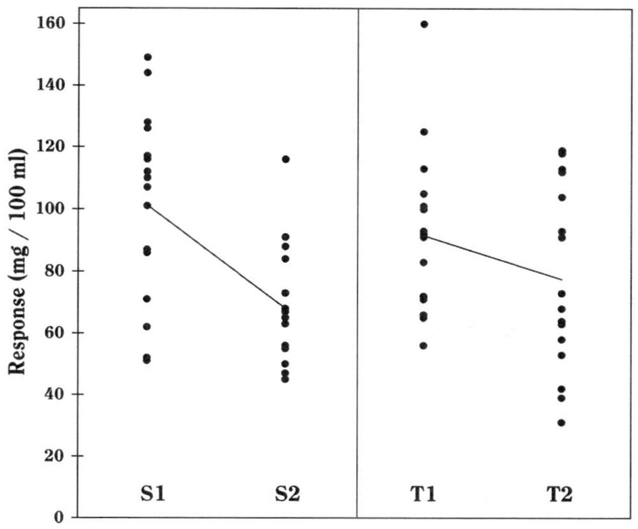

Figure 5.1.5.-I.

The analysis of variance is more complicated for this assay than for the other designs given because the component of the sum of squares due to parallelism is not independent of the component due to rabbit differences. Testing of the parallelism of the regression lines involves a second error-mean-square term obtained by subtracting the parallelism component and 2 "interaction" components from the component due to rabbit differences.

3 "interaction" components are present in the analysis of variance due to replication within each group:

days × preparation; days × regression; days × parallelism.

These terms indicate the tendency for the components (preparations, regression and parallelism) to vary from day to day. The corresponding *F*-ratios thus provide checks on these aspects of assay validity. If the values of *F* obtained are significantly high, care should be exercised in interpreting the results of the assay and, if possible, the assay should be repeated.

The analysis of variance is constructed by applying the formulae given in Tables 3.2.3.-I to 3.2.3.-III separately for both days and for the pooled set of data. The formulae in Tables 3.2.3.-I and 3.2.3.-II give:

Day 1:	$P_S = 165.25$	$L_S = -13$
	$P_T = 162.25$	$L_T = -8.75$
	$H_P = \frac{8}{2} = 4$	$H_L = \frac{96}{6} = 16$
Day 2:	$P_S = 173.38$	$L_S = -20.06$
	$P_T = 176.00$	$L_T = -5.25$
	$H_P = \frac{8}{2} = 4$	$H_L = \frac{96}{6} = 16$
Pooled:	$P_S = 169.31$	$L_S = -16.53$
	$P_T = 169.13$	$L_T = -7.00$
	$H_P = \frac{16}{2} = 8$	$H_L = \frac{192}{6} = 32$

and with the formulae in Table 3.2.3.-III this leads to:

Day 1	Day 2	Pooled
$SS_{prep} = 18.000$	$SS_{prep} = 13.781$	$SS_{prep} = 0.141$
$SS_{reg} = 3784.5$	$SS_{reg} = 5125.8$	$SS_{reg} = 8859.5$
$SS_{par} = 144.5$	$SS_{par} = 1755.3$	$SS_{par} = 1453.5$

The interaction terms are found as Day 1 + Day 2 - Pooled.

$$SS_{\text{days}\times\text{prep}} = 31.64$$

$$SS_{\text{days}\times\text{reg}} = 50.77$$

$$SS_{\text{days}\times\text{par}} = 446.27$$

In addition the sum of squares due to day-to-day variation is calculated as:

$$SS_{\text{days}} = \frac{1}{2}N\left(D_1^2 + D_2^2\right) - K = 478.52$$

and the sum of squares due to blocks (the variation between rabbits) as:

$$SS_{\text{block}} = 2\sum B_i^2 - K = 39\,794.7$$

where B_i is the mean response per rabbit.

The analysis of variance can now be completed as shown in Table 5.1.5.-III.

Table 5.1.5.-III. – *Analysis of variance*

Source of variation	Degrees of freedom	Sum of squares	Mean square	*F*-ratio	Probability
Non-parallelism	1	1453.5	1453.5	1.064	0.311
Days × Prep.	1	31.6	31.6	0.023	0.880
Days × Regr.	1	50.8	50.8	0.037	0.849
Residual error between rabbits	28	38 258.8	1366.4		
Rabbits	31	39 794.7	1283.7		
Preparations	1	0.14	0.14	0.001	0.975
Regression	1	8859.5	8859.5	64.532	0.000
Days	1	478.5	478.5	3.485	0.072
Days × non-par.	1	446.3	446.3	3.251	0.082
Residual error within rabbits	28	3844.1	137.3		
Total	63	53 423.2			

The analysis of variance confirms that the data fulfil the necessary conditions for a satisfactory assay: a highly significant regression, no significant departures from parallelism, and none of the three interaction components is significant.

The formulae in Section 3.2.5 give:

– for the common slope:

$$b = \frac{32 \times (-16.53 - 7)}{\ln 2 \times 16 \times 2} = -33.95$$

– the ln(potency ratio) is:

$$M'_T = \frac{169.13 - 169.31}{2 \times (-33.95)} = 0.00276$$

$$C = \frac{8859.5}{8859.5 - 137.3 \times 2.048^2} = 1.0695$$

$$V = \frac{8859.5}{(-33.95)^2 \times 2 \times 16} = 0.2402$$

– and ln(confidence limits) are:

$$1.0695 \times 0.00276 \pm \sqrt{0.0695 \times (1.0695 \times 0.00276^2 + 2 \times 0.2402)}$$
$$= 0.00295 \pm 0.18279$$

5. General texts

By taking the antilogarithms a potency ratio of 1.003 with 95 per cent confidence limits from 0.835 to 1.204 is found. Multiplying by $A_T = 40$ yields a potency of 40.1 units per millilitre with 95 per cent confidence limits from 33.4-48.2 units per millilitre.

5.2. SLOPE-RATIO MODEL

5.2.1. A COMPLETELY RANDOMISED (0,3,3)-DESIGN

An assay of factor VIII

A laboratory carries out a chromogenic assay of factor VIII activity in concentrates. The laboratory has no experience with the type of assay but is trying to make it operational. 3 equivalent dilutions are prepared of both the standard and the test preparation. In addition a blank is prepared, although a linear dose-response relationship is not expected for low doses. 8 replicates of each dilution are prepared, which is more than would be done in a routine assay.

A graphical presentation of the data shows clearly that the dose-response relationship is indeed not linear at low doses. The responses to blanks will therefore not be used in the calculations (further assays are of course needed to justify this decision). The formulae in Tables 3.3.3.1.-I and 3.3.3.1.-II yield.

P_S	= 0.6524	P_T	= 0.5651
L_S	= 1.4693	L_T	= 1.2656
a_S	= 0.318	a_T	= 0.318
b_S	= 0.329	b_T	= 0.271
G_S	= 0.1554	G_T	= 0.1156
J_S	= $4.17 \cdot 10^{-8}$	J_T	= $2.84 \cdot 10^{-6}$

and

$H_1 = 0.09524 \qquad a' = 0.05298 \qquad K = 1.9764$

and the analysis of variance is completed with the formulae in Tables 3.3.3.1.-III and 3.3.3.1.-IV.

A highly significant regression and no significant deviations from linearity and intersection indicate that the potency can be calculated.

Slope of standard:

$$b'_S = \frac{6 \times 1.469 - 36 \times 0.0530}{84} = 0.0822$$

Slope of test sample:

$$b'_T = \frac{6 \times 1.266 - 36 \times 0.0530}{84} = 0.0677$$

Formula 3.3.5.1.-3 gives:

$$R = \frac{0.0677}{0.0822} = 0.823$$

$$C = \frac{0.0822^2}{0.0822^2 - 3.86 \cdot 10^{-6} \times 2.018^2 \times 0.0357} = 1.000083$$

$$K' = 0.000083 \times 0.75 = 0.000062$$

and the 95 per cent confidence limits are:

$$0.823 \pm \sqrt{0.000083 \times 1.678 + 0.000062 \times (-1.646)}$$
$$= 0.823 \pm 0.006$$

The potency ratio is thus estimated as 0.823 with 95 per cent confidence limits from 0.817 to 0.829.

Table 5.2.1.-I. – *Absorbances*

	Blank	Standard *S* (in IU/ml)			Preparation *T* (in IU/ml)		
Conc.	*B*	S_1 0.01	S_2 0.02	S_3 0.03	T_1 0.01	T_2 0.02	T_3 0.03
	0.022	0.133	0.215	0.299	0.120	0.188	0.254
	0.024	0.133	0.215	0.299	0.119	0.188	0.253
	0.024	0.131	0.216	0.299	0.118	0.190	0.255
	0.026	0.136	0.218	0.297	0.120	0.190	0.258
	0.023	0.137	0.220	0.297	0.120	0.190	0.257
	0.022	0.136	0.220	0.305	0.121	0.191	0.257
	0.022	0.138	0.219	0.299	0.121	0.191	0.255
	0.023	0.137	0.218	0.302	0.121	0.190	0.254
Mean	0.0235	0.1351	0.2176	0.2996	0.1200	0.1898	0.2554

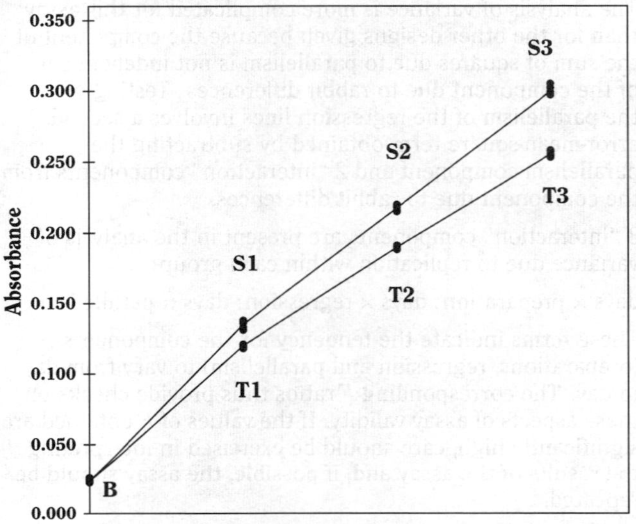

Figure 5.2.1.-I.

Table 5.2.1.-II. – *Analysis of variance*

Source of variation	Degrees of freedom	Sum of squares	Mean square	*F*-ratio	Probability
Regression	2	0.1917	0.0958	24 850	0.000
Intersection	1	$3 \cdot 10^{-9}$	$3 \cdot 10^{-9}$	$7 \cdot 10^{-4}$	0.978
Non-linearity	2	$2 \cdot 10^{-5}$	$1 \cdot 10^{-5}$	2.984	0.061
Treatments	5	0.1917			
Residual error	42	$1.62 \cdot 10^{-4}$	$3.86 \cdot 10^{-6}$		
Total	47	0.1919			

5.2.2. A COMPLETELY RANDOMISED (0,4,4,4)-DESIGN

An in-vitro assay of influenza vaccines

The haemagglutinin antigen (HA) content of 2 influenza vaccines is determined by single radial immunodiffusion. Both have a labelled potency of 15 µg HA per dose, which is equivalent with a content of 30 µg HA/ml. The standard has an assigned content of 39 µg HA/ml.

Standard and test vaccines are applied in 4 duplicate concentrations which are prepared on the basis of the assigned and the labelled contents. When the equilibrium between the external and the internal reactant is established, the zone of the annulus precipitation area is measured. The results are shown in Table 5.2.2.-I.

A graphical presentation of the data shows no unusual features. The formulae in Tables 3.3.3.1.-I and 3.3.3.1.-II yield

P_S = 108.2	P_T = 103.85	P_U = 85.8
L_S = 301.1	L_T = 292.1	L_U = 234.1
a_S = 141.0	a_T = 116.7	a_U = 139.8
b_S = 61.2	b_T = 64.95	b_U = 39.2
G_S = 3114.3	G_T = 2909.4	G_U = 1917.3
J_S = 0.223	J_T = 2.227	J_U = 0.083

and

H_I = 0.0093	a' = 11.04	K = 14 785.8

and the analysis of variance is completed with the formulae in Tables 3.3.3.1.-III and 3.3.3.1.-IV. This is shown in Table 5.2.2.-II.

A highly significant regression and no significant deviations from linearity and intersection indicate that the potency can be calculated.

Slope of standard:

$$b'_S = \frac{6 \times 301.1 - 60 \times 11.04}{180} = 6.356$$

Slope of T is:

$$b'_T = \frac{6 \times 292.1 - 60 \times 11.04}{180} = 6.056$$

Slope of U is:

$$b'_U = \frac{6 \times 234.1 - 60 \times 11.04}{180} = 4.123$$

This leads to a potency ratio of 6.056/6.356 = 0.953 for vaccine T and 4.123/6.356 = 0.649 for vaccine U.

$$C = \frac{6.356^2}{6.356^2 - 1.068 \times 2.179^2 \times 0.0444} = 1.0056$$

$$K' = 0.0056 \times 0.625 = 0.0035$$

And the confidence limits are found with formula 3.3.5.1.-4.

For vaccine T:

$$0.955 \pm \sqrt{0.0056 \times 1.913 + 0.0035 \times (-1.913)} = 0.955 \pm 0.063$$

For vaccine U:

$$0.649 \pm \sqrt{0.0056 \times 1.423 + 0.0035 \times (-1.301)} = 0.649 \pm 0.058$$

The HA content in µg/dose can be found by multiplying the potency ratios and confidence limits by the assumed content of 15 µg/dose. The results are given in Table 5.2.2.-III.

Table 5.2.2.-I. – *Zone of precipitation area (mm²)*

Conc. (µg/ml)	Standard *S* I	Standard *S* II	Preparation *T* I	Preparation *T* II	Preparation *U* I	Preparation *U* II
7.5	18.0	18.0	15.1	16.8	15.4	15.7
15.0	22.8	24.5	23.1	24.2	20.2	18.6
22.5	30.4	30.4	28.9	27.4	24.2	23.1
30.0	35.7	36.6	34.4	37.8	27.4	27.0

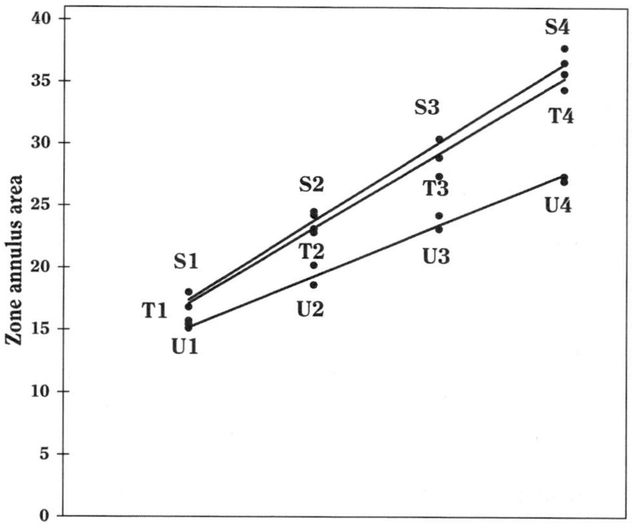

Figure 5.2.2.-I.

Table 5.2.2.-II. – *Analysis of variance*

Source of variation	Degrees of freedom	Sum of squares	Mean square	*F*-ratio	Probability
Regression	3	1087.7	362.6	339.5	0.000
Intersection	2	3.474	1.737	1.626	0.237
Non-linearity	6	5.066	0.844	0.791	0.594
Treatments	11	1096.2			
Residual error	12	12.815	1.068		
Total	23	1109.0			

Table 5.2.2.-III. – *Estimates of HA content* (µg/dose)

	Lower limit	Estimate	Upper limit
Vaccin *T*	13.4	14.3	15.3
Vaccin *U*	8.9	9.7	10.6

5.3. QUANTAL RESPONSES

5.3.1. PROBIT ANALYSIS OF A TEST PREPARATION AGAINST A REFERENCE

An in-vivo assay of a diphtheria vaccine

A diphtheria vaccine (assumed potency 140 IU/vial) is assayed against a standard (assigned potency 132 IU/vial). On the basis of this information, equivalent doses are prepared and randomly administered to groups of guinea-pigs. After a given period, the animals are challenged with diphtheria toxin and the number of surviving animals recorded as shown in Table 5.3.1.-I.

Table 5.3.1.-I. – *Raw data from a diphtheria assay in guinea-pigs*

Standard (*S*) Assigned potency 132 IU/vial			**Test preparation (*T*) Assumed potency 140 IU/vial**		
dose (IU/ml)	challenged	protected	dose (I.U./ml)	challenged	protected
1.0	12	0	1.0	11	0
1.6	12	3	1.6	12	4
2.5	12	6	2.5	11	8
4.0	11	10	4.0	11	10

The observations are transferred to the first working table and the subsequent columns are computed as described in Section 4.2.1. Table 5.3.1.-II shows the first cycle of this procedure.

The sums of the last 6 columns are then calculated per preparation and transferred to the second working table (see Table 5.3.1.-III). The results in the other columns are found with formulae 4.2.1.-4 to 4.2.1.-10. This yields a common slope *b* of 1.655.

The values for *Y* in the first working table are now replaced by *a* + *bx* and a second cycle is carried out (see Table 5.3.1.-IV).

The cycle is repeated until the difference between 2 consecutive cycles has become small. The second working table should then appear as shown in Table 5.3.1.-V.

Linearity is tested as described in Section 4.2.2. The χ^2-value with 4 degrees of freedom is 0.851 + 1.070 = 1.921 representing a *p*-value of 0.750 which is not significant.

Since there are no significant deviations from linearity, the test for parallelism can be carried out as described in the same section. The χ^2-value with 1 degree of freedom is $(16.71 + 17.27) - \frac{14.15^2}{5.89} = 0.001$ representing a *p*-value of 0.974 which is not significant.

The ln(potency ratio) can now be estimated as described in Section 4.2.3.

$$M'_T = \frac{-1.721 - (-2.050)}{2.401} = 0.137$$

Further:

$$C = \frac{2.401^2 \times 5.893}{2.401^2 \times 5.893 - 1^2 \times 1.960^2} = 1.127$$

$$V = \frac{1}{18.37} + \frac{1}{17.96} = 0.110$$

So ln confidence limits are:

$$0.155 - 0.013 \pm \sqrt{0.127\,(0.649 + 1.127 \times 0.036^2)} = 0.142 \pm 0.288$$

The potency and confidence limits can now be found by taking the antilogarithms and multiplying these by the assumed potency of 140 IU/vial. This yields an estimate of 160.6 IU/vial with 95 per cent confidence limits from 121.0-215.2 IU/vial.

Table 5.3.1.-II. – *First working table in the first cycle*

Vaccine	Dose	*n*	*r*	*x*	*p*	*Y*	*Φ*	*Z*	*y*	*w*	*wx*	*wy*	*wx²*	*wy²*	*wxy*
S	1.0	12	0	0.000	0.000	0	0.5	0.399	−1.253	7.64	0.00	−9.57	0.00	12.00	0.00
	1.6	12	3	0.470	0.250	0	0.5	0.399	−0.627	7.64	3.59	−4.79	1.69	3.00	−2.25
	2.5	12	6	0.916	0.500	0	0.5	0.399	0.000	7.64	7.00	0.00	6.41	0.00	0.00
	4.0	11	10	1.386	0.909	0	0.5	0.399	1.025	7.00	9.71	7.18	13.46	7.36	9.95
T	1.0	11	0	0.000	0.000	0	0.5	0.399	−1.253	7.00	0.00	−8.78	0.00	11.00	0.00
	1.6	12	4	0.470	0.333	0	0.5	0.399	−0.418	7.64	3.59	−3.19	1.69	1.33	−1.50
	2.5	11	8	0.916	0.727	0	0.5	0.399	0.570	7.00	6.42	3.99	5.88	2.27	3.66
	4.0	11	10	1.386	0.909	0	0.5	0.399	1.025	7.00	9.71	7.18	13.46	7.36	9.95

Table 5.3.1.-III. – *Second working table in the first cycle*

Vaccine	Σ*w*	Σ*wx*	Σ*wy*	Σ*wx²*	Σ*wy²*	Σ*wxy*	S_{xx}	S_{xy}	S_{yy}	$\bar{x}$	$\bar{y}$	*a*
S	29.92	20.30	−7.18	21.56	22.36	7.70	7.79	12.58	20.64	0.68	−0.24	−1.36
T	28.65	19.72	−0.80	21.03	21.97	12.11	7.46	12.66	21.95	0.69	−0.03	−1.17

Table 5.3.1.-IV. – *First working table in the second cycle*

Vaccine	Dose	*n*	*r*	*x*	*p*	*Y*	*Φ*	*Z*	*y*	*w*	*wx*	*wy*	*wx²*	*wy²*	*wxy*
S	1.0	12	0	0.000	0.000	−1.36	0.086	0.158	−1.911	3.77	0.00	−7.21	0.00	13.79	0.00
	1.6	12	3	0.470	0.250	−0.58	0.279	0.336	−0.672	6.74	3.17	−4.53	1.49	3.04	−2.13
	2.5	12	6	0.916	0.500	0.15	0.561	0.394	−0.001	7.57	6.94	−0.01	6.36	0.00	−0.01
	4.0	11	10	1.386	0.909	0.93	0.824	0.258	1.260	5.07	7.03	6.39	9.75	8.05	8.86
T	1.0	11	0	0.000	0.000	−1.17	0.122	0.202	−1.769	4.20	0.00	−7.43	0.00	13.14	0.00
	1.6	12	4	0.470	0.333	−0.39	0.349	0.370	−0.430	7.23	3.40	−3.11	1.60	1.34	−1.46
	2.5	11	8	0.916	0.727	0.35	0.637	0.375	0.591	6.70	6.14	3.96	5.62	2.34	3.63
	4.0	11	10	1.386	0.909	1.13	0.870	0.211	1.311	4.35	6.03	5.70	8.36	7.48	7.90

Table 5.3.1.-V. – *Second working table after sufficient cycles*

Vaccine	Σ*w*	Σ*wx*	Σ*wy*	Σ*wx²*	Σ*wy²*	Σ*wxy*	S_{xx}	S_{xy}	S_{yy}	$\bar{x}$	$\bar{y}$	*a*
S	18.37	14.80	−2.14	14.85	17.81	5.28	2.93	7.00	17.56	0.81	−0.12	−2.05
T	17.96	12.64	−0.55	11.86	18.35	6.76	2.96	7.15	18.34	0.70	−0.03	−1.72

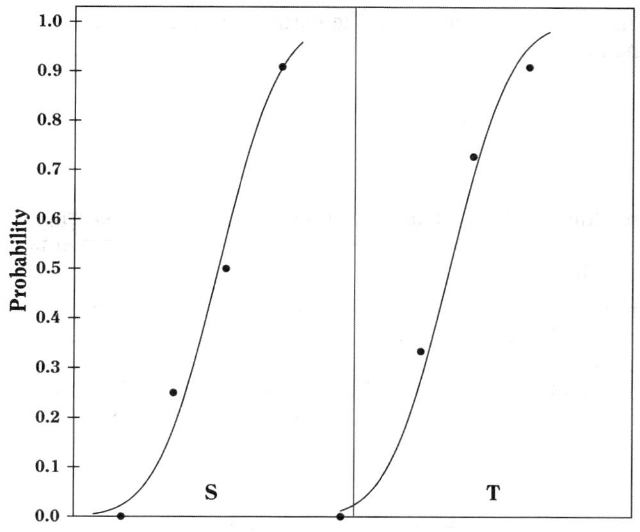

Figure 5.3.1.-I.

5.3.2. LOGIT ANALYSIS AND OTHER TYPES OF ANALYSES OF A TEST PREPARATION AGAINST A REFERENCE

Results will be given for the situation where the logit method and other "classical" methods of this family are applied to the data in Section 5.3.1. This should be regarded as an exercise rather than an alternative to the probit method in this specific case. Another shape of the curve may be adopted only if this is supported by experimental or theoretical evidence.

Table 5.3.2.-I. – *Results by using alternative curves*

	Logit	Gompit	Angle(*)
Φ	$\dfrac{1}{1+e^{-Y}}$	$1-e^{-e^{Y}}$	$\dfrac{1}{2}\sin Y+\dfrac{1}{2}$
Z	$\dfrac{e^{-Y}}{(1+e^{-Y})^2}$	$e^{Y-e^{Y}}$	$\dfrac{1}{2}\cos Y$
slope b	4.101	2.590	1.717
χ^2 lin	2.15	3.56	1.50
χ^2 par	0.0066	0.168	0.0010
Potency	162.9	158.3	155.8
Lower limit	121.1	118.7	122.6
Upper limit	221.1	213.3	200.7

(*) $\begin{cases} \text{If } Y < -\frac{1}{2}\pi \text{ then } \Phi = 0 \text{ and } Z = 0 \\ \text{If } Y > \frac{1}{2}\pi \text{ then } \Phi = 1 \text{ and } Z = 0 \end{cases}$

5.3.3. THE ED_{50} DETERMINATION OF A SUBSTANCE USING THE PROBIT METHOD

An in-vitro assay of oral poliomyelitis vaccine

In an ED_{50} assay of oral poliomyelitis vaccine with 10 different dilutions in 8 replicates of 50 µl on an ELISA-plate, results were obtained as shown in Table 5.3.3.-I.

The observations are transferred to the first working table and the subsequent columns are computed as described in Section 4.2.1. Table 5.3.3.-II shows the first cycle of this procedure.

Table 5.3.3.-I. – *Dilutions (10^x µl of the undiluted vaccine)*

−3.5	−4.0	−4.5	−5.0	−5.5	−6.0	−6.5	−7.0	−7.5	−8.0
+	+	+	+	−	−	−	−	−	−
+	+	+	+	−	−	−	−	−	−
+	+	−	−	−	−	−	−	−	−
+	+	+	+	−	−	−	−	−	−
+	+	+	−	−	−	−	−	−	−
+	+	+	+	+	−	−	−	−	−
+	+	+	+	+	−	+	−	−	−
+	+	+	+	−	+	−	−	−	−

The sums of the last 6 columns are calculated and transferred to the second working table (see Table 5.3.3.-III). The results in the other columns are found with formulae 4.2.1.-4 to 4.2.1.-10. This yields a common slope *b* of −0.295.

The values for *Y* in the first working table are now replaced by *a* + *bx* and a second cycle is carried out. The cycle is repeated until the difference between 2 consecutive cycles has become small. The second working table should then appear as shown in Table 5.3.3.-IV.

Linearity is tested as described in Section 4.2.2. The χ^2-value with 8 degrees of freedom is 2.711 representing a *p*-value of 0.951 which is not significant.

The potency ratio can now be estimated as described in Section 4.5.

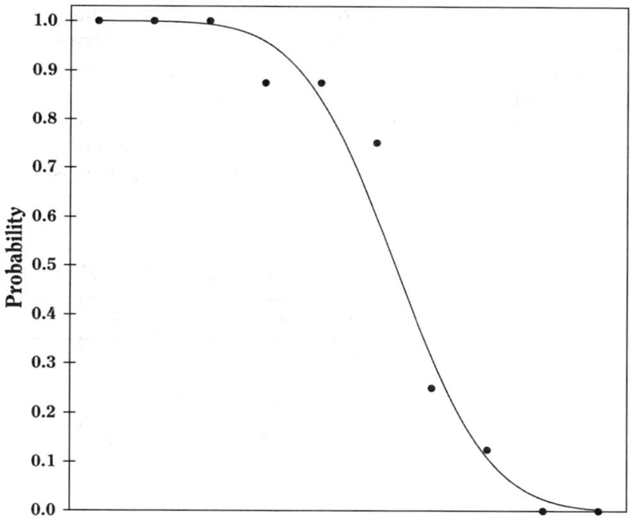

Figure 5.3.3.-I.

$$M'_T = \frac{-(-7.931)}{-0.646} = -12.273$$

Further:

$$C = \frac{(-0.646)^2 \times 55.883}{(-0.646)^2 \times 55.883 - 1^2 \times 1.960^2} = 1.197$$

$$V = \frac{1}{19.39} = 0.052$$

So ln confidence limits are:

$$-14.692-(-2.420)\pm\sqrt{0.197\times(2.882+1.197\times0.009^2)}$$
$$=-12.272\pm0.754$$

This estimate is still expressed in terms of the ln(dilutions). In order to obtain estimates expressed in $\ln(ED_{50})$/ml the values are transformed to $-M'_T+\ln\left(\frac{1000}{50}\right)$.

Since it has become common use to express the potency of this type of vaccine in terms of $\log_{10}(ED_{50})$/ml, the results have to be divided by ln(10). The potency is thus estimated as 6.63 $\log_{10}(ED_{50})$/ml with 95 per cent confidence limits from 6.30 to 6.96 $\log_{10}(ED_{50})$/ml.

5.4. EXTENDED SIGMOID DOSE-RESPONSE CURVES

5.4.1. FOUR-PARAMETER LOGISTIC CURVE ANALYSIS

A serological assay of tetanus sera

As already stated in Section 3.4, this example is intended to illustrate a "possible" way to analyse the data presented, but not necessarily to reflect the "only" or the "most appropriate" way. Many other approaches can be found in the literature, but in most cases they should not yield dramatically different outcomes. A short discussion of alternative approaches and other statistical considerations is given in Section 7.5.

A guinea-pig antiserum is assayed against a standard serum (0.4 IU/ml) using an enzyme-linked immunosorbent assay technique (ELISA). 10 two-fold dilutions of each serum were applied on a 96-well ELISA plate. Each dilution was applied twice. The observed responses are listed in Table 5.4.1.-I.

For this example, it will be assumed that the laboratory has validated conditions 1 to 3 in Section 3.1.1 when the assay was being developed for routine use. In addition, the laboratory has validated that the upper limit and lower limit of the samples can be assumed to be equal.

No unusual features are discovered in a graphical representation. A least squares method of a suitable computer program is used to fit the parameters of the logistic function, assuming that the residual error terms are independent and identically distributed normal random variables. In this case, 3 parameters (α, β and δ) are needed to describe the common slope-factor and the common lower and upper asymptotes. 2 additional parameters (γ_S and γ_T) are needed to describe the horizontal location of the 2 curves.

The following estimates of the parameters are returned by the program:

$$\alpha = 3.196 \qquad \gamma_S = -4.307$$

$$\beta = 1.125 \qquad \gamma_T = -4.684$$

$$\delta = 0.145$$

In addition, the estimated residual variance (s^2) is returned as 0.001429 with 20 degrees of freedom (within-treatments variation).

In order to obtain confidence limits, and also to check for parallelism and linearity, the observed responses (u) are linearised and submitted to a weighted parallel-line analysis by the program. This procedure is very similar to that described in Section 4.2 for probit analysis with the following modifications:

$$Y = \beta(x - \gamma) \qquad y = Y + \frac{\left(\frac{u-\delta}{\alpha-\delta}\right) - \Phi}{Z}$$

$$\Phi = \frac{1}{1+e^{-Y}} \qquad w = \frac{Z^2(\alpha-\delta)^2}{s^2}$$

$$Z = \frac{e^{-Y}}{(1+e^{-Y})^2}$$

The resulting weighted analysis of variance of the transformed responses (y) using weights (w) is as follows:

There are no significant deviations from parallelism and linearity and thus the assay is satisfactory for potency calculations. If the condition of equal upper and lower asymptotes is not fulfilled, significant deviations from linearity and/or parallelism are likely to occur because the tests for linearity and parallelism reflect the goodness of fit of the complete four-parameter model. The residual error in the analysis of variance is always equal to 1 as a result of the transformation. However, a heterogeneity factor (analogous to that for the probit model) can be computed.

Table 5.3.3.-II. – *First working table in the first cycle*

Vaccine	Dose	n	r	x	p	Y	Φ	Z	y	w	wx	wy	wx^2	wy^2	wxy
T	$10^{-3.5}$	8	0	−8.06	0.000	0.00	0.5	0.399	−1.253	5.09	−41.04	−6.38	330.8	8.00	51.4
	$10^{-4.0}$	8	0	−9.21	0.000	0.00	0.5	0.399	−1.253	5.09	−46.91	−6.38	432.0	8.00	58.8
	$10^{-4.5}$	8	1	−10.36	0.125	0.00	0.5	0.399	−0.940	5.09	−52.77	−4.79	546.8	4.50	49.6
	$10^{-5.0}$	8	2	−11.51	0.250	0.00	0.5	0.399	−0.627	5.09	−58.63	−3.19	675.1	2.00	36.7
	$10^{-5.5}$	8	6	−12.66	0.750	0.00	0.5	0.399	0.627	5.09	−64.50	3.19	816.8	2.00	−40.4
	$10^{-6.0}$	8	7	−13.82	0.875	0.00	0.5	0.399	0.940	5.09	−70.36	4.79	972.1	4.50	−66.1
	$10^{-6.5}$	8	7	−14.97	0.875	0.00	0.5	0.399	0.940	5.09	−76.23	4.79	1140.8	4.50	−71.7
	$10^{-7.0}$	8	8	−16.12	1.000	0.00	0.5	0.399	1.253	5.09	−82.09	6.38	1323.1	8.00	−102.9
	$10^{-7.5}$	8	8	−17.27	1.000	0.00	0.5	0.399	1.253	5.09	−87.95	6.38	1518.9	8.00	−110.2
	$10^{-8.0}$	8	8	−18.42	1.000	0.00	0.5	0.399	1.253	5.09	−93.82	6.38	1728.2	8.00	−117.6

Table 5.3.3.-III. – *Second working table in the first cycle*

Vaccine	Σw	Σwx	Σwy	Σwx^2	Σwy^2	Σwxy	S_{xx}	S_{xy}	S_{yy}	$\bar{x}$	$\bar{y}$	a
T	50.93	−674.3	11.17	9484.6	57.50	−312.32	556.92	−164.43	55.05	−13.24	0.219	−3.690

Table 5.3.3.-IV. – *Second working table after sufficient cycles*

Vaccine	Σw	Σwx	Σwy	Σwx^2	Σwy^2	Σwxy	S_{xx}	S_{xy}	S_{yy}	$\bar{x}$	$\bar{y}$	a
T	19.39	−238.2	0.11	2981.1	26.05	−37.45	55.88	−36.11	26.05	−12.28	0.006	−7.931

The relative potency of the test preparation can be obtained as the antilogarithm of $\gamma_S - \gamma_T$. Multiplying by the assigned potency of the standard yields an estimate of $1.459 \times 0.4 = 0.584$ IU/ml. Formula 4.2.3.-2 gives 95 per cent confidence limits from 0.557-0.612 IU/ml.

Table 5.4.1.-I. – *Observed responses*

Standard *S*			**Preparation to be examined *T***		
Dil.	Obs. 1	Obs. 2	Dil.	Obs. 1	Obs. 2
1/10	2.912	2.917	1/10	3.017	2.987
1/20	2.579	2.654	1/20	2.801	2.808
1/40	2.130	2.212	1/40	2.401	2.450
1/80	1.651	1.638	1/80	1.918	1.963
1/160	1.073	0.973	1/160	1.364	1.299
1/320	0.585	0.666	1/320	0.861	0.854
1/640	0.463	0.356	1/640	0.497	0.496
1/1280	0.266	0.234	1/1280	0.340	0.344
1/2560	0.228	0.197	1/2560	0.242	0.217
1/5120	0.176	0.215	1/5120	0.178	0.125

Table 5.4.1.-II – *Weighted analysis of variance*

Source of variation	**Degrees of freedom**	**Chi-square**	**Probability**
Preparations	1	0.529653	0.467
Regression	1	6599.51	0.000
Non-parallelism	1	0.0458738	0.830
Non-linearity	16	8.89337	0.918
Treatments	19	6608.98	0.000
Residual error	20	20.0000	
Total	39	6628.98	

6. COMBINATION OF ASSAY RESULTS

6.1. INTRODUCTION

Replication of independent assays and combination of their results is often needed to fulfil the requirements of the European Pharmacopoeia. The question then arises as to whether it is appropriate to combine the results of such assays and if so in what way.

2 assays may be regarded as mutually independent when the execution of either does not affect the probabilities of the possible outcomes of the other. This implies that the random errors in all essential factors influencing the result (for example, dilutions of the standard and of the preparation to be examined, the sensitivity of the biological indicator) in one assay must be independent of the corresponding random errors in the other one. Assays on successive days using the original and retained dilutions of the standard therefore are not independent assays.

There are several methods for combining the results of independent assays, the most theoretically acceptable being the most difficult to apply. 3 simple, approximate methods are described below; others may be used provided the necessary conditions are fulfilled.

Before potencies from assays based on the parallel-line or probit model are combined they must be expressed in logarithms; potencies derived from assays based on the slope-ratio model are used as such. As the former models are more common than those based on the slope-ratio model, the symbol M denoting ln potency is used in the formulae in this section; by reading R (slope-ratio) for M, the analyst may use the same formulae for potencies derived from assays based on the slope-ratio model. All estimates of potency must be corrected for the potency assigned to each preparation to be examined before they are combined.

6.2. WEIGHTED COMBINATION OF ASSAY RESULTS

This method can be used provided the following conditions are fulfilled:

1) the potency estimates are derived from independent assays;

2) for each assay C is close to 1 (say less than 1.1);

3) the number of degrees of freedom of the individual residual errors is not smaller than 6, but preferably larger than 15;

4) the individual potency estimates form a homogeneous set (see Section 6.2.2).

When these conditions are not fulfilled this method cannot be applied. The method described in Section 6.3 may then be used to obtain the best estimate of the mean potency to be adopted in further assays as an assumed potency.

6.2.1. CALCULATION OF WEIGHTING COEFFICIENTS

It is assumed that the results of each of the n' assays have been analysed to give n' values of M with associated confidence limits. For each assay the logarithmic confidence interval L is obtained by subtracting the lower limit from the upper. A weight W for each value of M is calculated from equation 6.2.1.-1, where t has the same value as that used in the calculation of confidence limits.

$$W = \frac{4t^2}{L^2} \qquad (6.2.1.\text{-}1)$$

6.2.2. HOMOGENEITY OF POTENCY ESTIMATES

By squaring the deviation of each value of M from the weighted mean, multiplying by the appropriate weight and summing over all assays, a statistic is obtained which is approximately distributed as χ^2 (see Table 8.3) and which may be used to test the homogeneity of a set of ln potency estimates:

$$\chi^2 \approx \sum_{n'} W\left(M - \overline{M}\right)^2 \quad \text{where } \overline{M} = \frac{\sum WM}{\sum W} \qquad (6.2.2.\text{-}1)$$

If the calculated χ^2 is smaller than the tabulated value corresponding to $(n' - 1)$ degrees of freedom the potencies are homogeneous and the mean potency and limits obtained in Section 6.2.3 will be meaningful.

If the calculated value of this statistic is greater than the tabulated value, the potencies are heterogeneous. This means that the variation between individual estimates of M is greater than would have been predicted from the estimates of the confidence limits, i.e. that there is a significant variability between the assays. Under these circumstances condition 4 is not fulfilled and the equations in Section 6.2.3 are no longer applicable. Instead, the formulae in Section 6.2.4 may be used.

6.2.3. CALCULATION OF THE WEIGHTED MEAN AND CONFIDENCE LIMITS

The products WM are formed for each assay and their sum divided by the total weight for all assays to give the logarithm of the weighted mean potency.

$$\overline{M} = \frac{\sum WM}{\sum W} \qquad (6.2.3.\text{-}1)$$

The standard error of the ln (mean potency) is taken to be the square root of the reciprocal of the total weight:

$$s_{\overline{M}} = \sqrt{\frac{1}{\sum W}} \qquad (6.2.3.\text{-}2)$$

and approximate confidence limits are obtained from the antilogarithms of the value given by

$$\overline{M} \pm t \times s_{\overline{M}} \qquad (6.2.3.\text{-}3)$$

where the number of degrees of freedom of t equals the sum of the number of degrees of freedom for the error mean squares in the individual assays.

6.2.4. *WEIGHTED MEAN AND CONFIDENCE LIMITS BASED ON THE INTRA- AND INTER-ASSAY VARIATION*

When results of several repeated assays are combined, the (χ^2-value may be significant. The observed variation is then considered to have two components:

– the intra-assay variation $s_M^2 = 1/W$,

– the inter-assay variation $s_{\overline{M}}^2 = \dfrac{\sum\left(M - \overline{M}\right)^2}{n'\left(n'-1\right)}$

where $\overline{M}$ is the unweighted mean. The former varies from assay to assay whereas the latter is common to all M.

For each M a weighting coefficient is then calculated as:

$$W' = \frac{1}{s_M^2 + s_{\overline{M}}^2}$$

which replaces W in Section 6.2.3. where t is taken to be approximately 2.

6.3. UNWEIGHTED COMBINATION OF ASSAY RESULTS

To combine the n' estimates of M from n' assays in the simplest way, the mean is calculated and an estimate of its standard deviation is obtained by calculating:

$$s_{\overline{M}}^2 = \frac{\sum\left(M - \overline{M}\right)^2}{n'\left(n'-1\right)} \qquad (6.3.\text{-}1)$$

and the limits are:

$$\overline{M} \pm t s_{\overline{M}} \qquad (6.3.\text{-}2)$$

where t has $(n' - 1)$ degrees of freedom. The number n' of estimates of M is usually small, and hence the value of t is quite large.

6.4. EXAMPLE OF A WEIGHTED MEAN POTENCY WITH CONFIDENCE LIMITS

Table 6.4.-I lists 6 independent potency estimates of the same preparation together with their 95 per cent confidence limits and the number of degrees of freedom of their error variances. Conditions 1, 2 and 3 in Section 6.2. are met. The ln potencies and the weights are calculated as described in Section 6.2.

Table 6.4.-I. – *Potency estimates and confidence intervals of 6 independent assays*

Potency estimate (I.U./vial)	Lower limit (I.U./vial)	Upper limit (I.U./vial)	Degrees of freedom	ln potency *M*	Weight *W*
18 367	17 755	19 002	20	9.8183	3777.7
18 003	17 415	18 610	20	9.7983	3951.5
18 064	17 319	18 838	20	9.8017	2462.5
17 832	17 253	18 429	20	9.7887	4003.0
18 635	17 959	19 339	20	9.8328	3175.6
18 269	17 722	18 834	20	9.8130	4699.5

Homogeneity of potency estimates is assessed with formula 6.2.2.-1 which gives a χ^2 of 4.42 with 5 degrees of freedom. This is not significant ($p = 0.49$) and thus all conditions are met.

A weighted mean potency is calculated with formula 6.2.3.-1 which yields 9.8085.

Formula 6.2.3.-2 gives a standard deviation of 0.00673 and approximate 95 per cent confidence limits of 9.7951 and 9.8218 are calculated with formula 6.2.3.-3 where t has 120 degrees of freedom.

By taking the antilogarithms a potency of 18 187 IU/vial is found with 95 per cent confidence limits from 17 946-18 431 IU/vial.

7. BEYOND THIS ANNEX

It is impossible to give a comprehensive treatise of statistical methods in a pharmacopoeial text. However, the methods described in this annex should suffice for most pharmacopoeial purposes. This section tries to give a more abstract survey of alternative or more general methods that have been developed. The interested reader is encouraged to further explore the existing literature in this area. The use of more specialised statistical methods should, in any case, be left to qualified personnel.

7.1. GENERAL LINEAR MODELS

The methods given in this annex can be described in terms of general linear models (or generalised linear models to include the probit and logit methods). The principle is to define a linear structure matrix X (or design matrix) in which each row represents an observation and each column a linear effect (preparation, block, column, dose). For example: the Latin square design in example 5.1.2 would involve a matrix with 36 rows and 13 columns. 1 column for each of the preparations, 1 column for the doses, 5 columns for each block except the first, and 5 columns for each row except the first. All columns, except the one for doses, are filled with 0 or 1 depending on whether or not the observation relates to the effect. A vector Y is filled with the (transformed) observations. The effects are estimated with the formula $(X'X)^{-1}X'Y$ from which the potency estimate m can easily be derived as a ratio of relevant effects. Confidence intervals are calculated from Fieller's theorem:

$$m_L, m_U = \frac{\left[m - \frac{g v_{12}}{v_{22}} \pm \frac{ts}{b}\sqrt{v_{11} - 2mv_{12} + m^2 v_{22} - g\left(v_{11} - \frac{v_{12}^2}{v_{22}}\right)}\right]}{(1-g)}$$

where $g = \dfrac{t^2 s^2 v_{22}}{b^2}$

and v_{11}, v_{22}, v_{12} represent the variance multipliers for the numerator, the denominator and their covariance multiplier respectively. These are taken directly from $(X'X)^{-1}$ or indirectly by noting that:

$$\mathrm{Var}(a_1 - a_2) = \mathrm{Var}(a_1) + \mathrm{Var}(a_2) - 2\mathrm{Cov}(a_1, a_2)$$

$$\text{and } \mathrm{Cov}(a_1 - a_2, b) = \mathrm{Cov}(a_1, b) - \mathrm{Cov}(a_2, b)$$

A full analysis of variance in which all components are partitioned is slightly more complicated as it involves a renewed definition of X with more columns to relax the assumptions of parallelism and linearity, after which the linear hypotheses can be tested. For assays depending upon quantal responses the linear effects (intercepts a_S, a_T etc. and the common slope b are found by maximising the sum over treatments of $n\ln\Phi(a_i + bx) + (n - r)\ln(1 - \Phi(a_i + bx))$ where x is the ln(dose), Φ denotes the shape of the distribution and $i \in \{S, T, ...\}$.

7.2. HETEROGENEITY OF VARIANCE

Heterogeneity of variance cannot always be solved by simply transforming the responses. A possible way to cope with this problem is to perform a weighted linear regression. In order to obtain an unbiased estimate, the weight of the observations is taken to be proportional to the reciprocal of the error variances. Since the true error variance is not always known, an iterative reweighted linear procedure may be followed. However, the calculation of the confidence interval involves new problems.

7.3. OUTLIERS AND ROBUST METHODS

The method of least squares described in this annex has the disadvantage of being very sensitive to outliers. A clear outlier may completely corrupt the calculations. This problem is often remedied by discarding the outlying result from the dataset. This policy can lead to arbitrary rejection of data and is not always without danger. It is not easy to give a general guideline on how to decide whether or not a specific observation is an outlier and it is for this reason that many robust methods have been developed. These methods are less sensitive to outliers because they give less weight to observations that are far away from the predicted value. New problems usually arise in computing confidence intervals or defining a satisfactory function to be minimised.

7.4. CORRELATED ERRORS

Absolute randomisation is not always feasible or very undesirable from a practical point of view. Thus, subsequent doses within a dilution series often exhibit correlated errors leading to confidence limits that are far too narrow. Some methods have been developed that take account of this autocorrelation effect.

7.5. EXTENDED NON-LINEAR DOSE-RESPONSE CURVES

Analysis of extended non-linear dose-response curves raises a number of statistical questions which require consideration, and for which professional advice is recommended. Some of these are indicated below.

1) An example using the four-parameter logistic function has been shown. However, models based on functions giving other sigmoid curves may also be used. Models incorporating additional asymmetry parameters have been suggested.

2) Heterogeneity of variance is common when responses cover a wide range. If the analysis ignores the heterogeneity, interpretation of results may not be correct and estimates may be biased. Use of the reciprocal of the error variances as weights is unlikely to be reliable with limited numbers of replicates. It may be appropriate to estimate a function which relates variance to mean response.

3) The statistical curve-fitting procedures may give different estimates depending on assumptions made about the homogeneity of the variance and on the range of responses used.

4) In principle, equality of upper and lower response limits for the different preparations included in an assay can be directly tested in each assay. However, interpretation of the results of these tests may not be straightforward. The tests for linearity and parallelism given by the simplified method of analysis (Example 5.4.1) indirectly incorporate tests for equality and accuracy of upper and lower limits.

5) Many assays include "controls" which are intended to identify the upper and/or lower response limits. However, these values may not be consistent with the statistically fitted upper and lower response limits based on the extended dose-response curve.

6) The simplified method of analysis given in Example 5.4.1 provides approximate confidence intervals. Other methods may also be used, for example intervals based on lack-of-fit of the completely specified model. For typical assay data, with responses covering the complete range for each preparation tested, all methods give similar results.

8. TABLES AND GENERATING PROCEDURES

The tables in this section list the critical values for the most frequently occurring numbers of degrees of freedom. If a critical value is not listed, reference should be made to more extensive tables. Many computer programs include statistical functions and their use is recommended instead of the tables in this section. Alternatively, the generating procedures given below each table can be used to compute the probability corresponding to a given statistic and number of degrees of freedom.

8.1. THE *F*-DISTRIBUTION

If an observed value is higher than the value in Table 8.1.-I, it is considered to be significant (upper lines, $p = 0.05$) and highly significant (lower lines, $p = 0.01$). *df*1 is the number of degrees of freedom of the numerator and *df*2 is the number of degrees of freedom of the denominator.

Generating procedure. Let `F` be the *F*-ratio and `df1` and `df2` as described above. Let `pi` = π = 3.14159265358979... The procedure in Table 8.1.-II will then generate the *p*-value.

8.2. THE *t*-DISTRIBUTION

If an observed value is higher than the value in Table 8.2.-I, it is considered to be significant ($p = 0.05$) and highly significant ($p = 0.01$).

Generating procedures. The *p*-value for a given *t* with df degrees of freedom can be found with the procedures in Section 8.1 where `F` = t^2, `df1` = 1 and `df2` = df.

The *t*-value ($p = 0.05$) for a given number of degrees of freedom df can be found with the procedure in Table 8.2.-II which should be accurate up to 6 decimal places.

Table 8.1.-I – *Critical values of the F-distribution*

df1 → **df2 ↓**	**1**	**2**	**3**	**4**	**5**	**6**	**8**	**10**	**12**	**15**	**20**	**∞**
10	4.965	4.103	3.708	3.478	3.326	3.217	3.072	2.978	2.913	2.845	2.774	2.538
	10.044	7.559	6.552	5.994	5.636	5.386	5.057	4.849	4.706	4.558	4.405	3.909
12	4.747	3.885	3.490	3.259	3.106	2.996	2.849	2.753	2.687	2.617	2.544	2.296
	9.330	6.927	5.953	5.412	5.064	4.821	4.499	4.296	4.155	4.010	3.858	3.361
15	4.543	3.682	3.287	3.056	2.901	2.790	2.641	2.544	2.475	2.403	2.328	2.066
	8.683	6.359	5.417	4.893	4.556	4.318	4.004	3.805	3.666	3.522	3.372	2.868
20	4.351	3.493	3.098	2.866	2.711	2.599	2.447	2.348	2.278	2.203	2.124	1.843
	8.096	5.849	4.938	4.431	4.103	3.871	3.564	3.368	3.231	3.088	2.938	2.421
25	4.242	3.385	2.991	2.759	2.603	2.490	2.337	2.236	2.165	2.089	2.007	1.711
	7.770	5.568	4.675	4.177	3.855	3.627	3.324	3.129	2.993	2.850	2.699	2.169
30	4.171	3.316	2.922	2.690	2.534	2.421	2.266	2.165	2.092	2.015	1.932	1.622
	7.562	5.390	4.510	4.018	3.699	3.473	3.173	2.979	2.843	2.700	2.549	2.006
50	4.034	3.183	2.790	2.557	2.400	2.286	2.130	2.026	1.952	1.871	1.784	1.438
	7.171	5.057	4.199	3.720	3.408	3.186	2.890	2.698	2.563	2.419	2.265	1.683
∞	3.841	2.996	2.605	2.372	2.214	2.099	1.938	1.831	1.752	1.666	1.571	1.000
	6.635	4.605	3.782	3.319	3.017	2.802	2.511	2.321	2.185	2.039	1.878	1.000

Table 8.1.-II – *Generating procedure for the F-distribution*

If df1 is even	If df1 is odd and df2 is even	If df1 and df2 are odd
`x=df1/(df1+df2/F)`	`x=df2/(df2+df1*F)`	`x=atn(sqr(df1*F/df2))`
`s=1`	`s=1`	`cs=cos(x)`
`t=1`	`t=1`	`sn=sin(x)`
`for i=2 to (df1-2) step 2`	`for i=2 to (df2-2) step 2`	`x=x/2`
`t=t*x*(df2+i-2)/i`	`t=t*x*(df1+i-2)/i`	`s=0`
`s=s+t`	`s=s+t`	`t=sn*cs/2`
`next i`	`next i`	`v=0`
`p=s*(1-x)^(df2/2)`	`p=1-s*(1-x)^(df1/2)`	`w=1`
		`for i=2 to (df2-1) step 2`
		`s=s+t`
		`t=t*i/(i+1)*cs*cs`
		`next i`
		`for i=1 to (df1-2) step 2`
		`v=v+w`
		`w=w*(df2+i)/(i+2)*sn*sn`
		`next i`
		`p=1+(t*df2*v-x-s)/pi*4`

Table 8.2.-I – *Critical values of the t-distribution*

df	$p = 0.05$	$p = 0.01$	df	$p = 0.05$	$p = 0.01$
1	12.706	63.656	22	2.074	2.819
2	4.303	9.925	24	2.064	2.797
3	3.182	5.841	26	2.056	2.779
4	2.776	4.604	28	2.048	2.763
5	2.571	4.032	30	2.042	2.750
6	2.447	3.707	35	2.030	2.724
7	2.365	3.499	40	2.021	2.704
8	2.306	3.355	45	2.014	2.690
9	2.262	3.250	50	2.009	2.678
10	2.228	3.169	60	2.000	2.660
12	2.179	3.055	70	1.994	2.648
14	2.145	2.977	80	1.990	2.639
16	2.120	2.921	90	1.987	2.632
18	2.101	2.878	100	1.984	2.626
20	2.086	2.845	∞	1.960	2.576

Table 8.2.-II – *Generating procedure for the t-distribution*

```
t = 1.959964+
    2.37228/df+
    2.82202/df^2+
    2.56449/df^3+
    1.51956/df^4+
    1.02579/df^5+
    0.44210/df^7
```

8.3. THE χ^2-DISTRIBUTION

Table 8.3.-I – *Critical values of the χ^2-distribution*

df	$p = 0.05$	$p = 0.01$	df	$p = 0.05$	$p = 0.01$
1	3.841	6.635	11	19.675	24.725
2	5.991	9.210	12	21.026	26.217
3	7.815	11.345	13	22.362	27.688
4	9.488	13.277	14	23.685	29.141
5	11.070	15.086	15	24.996	30.578
6	12.592	16.812	16	26.296	32.000
7	14.067	18.475	20	31.410	37.566
8	15.507	20.090	25	37.652	44.314
9	16.919	21.666	30	43.773	50.892
10	18.307	23.209	40	55.758	63.691

If an observed value is higher than the value in Table 8.3.-I, it is considered to be significant ($p = 0.05$) or highly significant ($p = 0.01$).

Generating procedure. Let X2 be the χ^2-value and df as described above. The procedure in Table 8.3.-II will then generate the *p*-value.

Table 8.3.-II – *Generating procedure for the χ^2-distribution*

If df is even	If df is odd
`s=0`	`x=sqr(x2)`
`t=exp(-x2/2)`	`s=0`
`for i=2 to df step 2`	`t=x*exp(-x2/2)/sqr(pi/2)`
`s=s+t`	`for i=3 to df step 2`
`t=t*x2/i`	`s=s+t`
`next i`	`t=t*x2/i`
`p=1-s`	`next i`
	`p=1-s-2*phi(x)`

In this procedure phi is the cumulative standard normal distribution function Φ (see Section 8.4).

8.4. THE Φ-DISTRIBUTION (THE CUMULATIVE STANDARD NORMAL DISTRIBUTION)

Table 8.4.-I – *Values of the Φ-distribution*

x	Φ	x	Φ	x	Φ
0.00	0.500	1.00	0.841	2.00	0.977
0.05	0.520	1.05	0.853	2.05	0.980
0.10	0.540	1.10	0.864	2.10	0.982
0.15	0.560	1.15	0.875	2.15	0.984
0.20	0.579	1.20	0.885	2.20	0.986
0.25	0.599	1.25	0.894	2.25	0.988
0.30	0.618	1.30	0.903	2.30	0.989
0.35	0.637	1.35	0.911	2.35	0.991
0.40	0.655	1.40	0.919	2.40	0.992
0.45	0.674	1.45	0.926	2.45	0.993
0.50	0.691	1.50	0.933	2.50	0.994
0.55	0.709	1.55	0.939	2.55	0.995
0.60	0.726	1.60	0.945	2.60	0.995
0.65	0.742	1.65	0.951	2.65	0.996
0.70	0.758	1.70	0.955	2.70	0.997
0.75	0.773	1.75	0.960	2.75	0.997
0.80	0.788	1.80	0.964	2.80	0.997
0.85	0.802	1.85	0.968	2.85	0.998
0.90	0.816	1.90	0.971	2.90	0.998
0.95	0.829	1.95	0.974	2.95	0.998

The Φ-value for negative *x* is found from table 8.4.-I as 1 - Φ(-*x*).

Generating procedure: Let x be the *x*-value. The procedure in Table 8.4.-II will generate the corresponding Φ-value if $0 \leq x \leq 8.15$. If *x* is greater than 8.15 the Φ-value can be set to 1. If *x* is negative, the formula given above can be used.

This procedure assumes that the computer can represent about 15 decimal places. If less digits or more digits can be represented, the procedure needs some trivial modifications.

Table 8.4.-II – *Generating procedure for the Φ-distribution*

```
s=0
t=x
i=1
repeat
s=s+t
i=i+2
t=t*x*x/i
until t<1E-16
phi=0.5+s*exp(-x*x/2)/sqr(2*pi)
```

8.5. RANDOM PERMUTATIONS

Random permutations are needed in randomised block designs. The following algorithm shows how the built-in random generator of a computer can be used to create random permutations of *N* treatments.

Step 1. Write the *N* possible treatments down in a row.

Step 2. Obtain a random integer *r* such that $1 \leq r \leq N$.

Step 3. Exchange the *r*-th treatment with the *N*-th treatment in the row.

Step 4. Let $N = N - 1$ and repeat steps 2 to 4 until $N = 1$.

An example with 6 treatments will illustrate this algorithm.

1.	$N = 6$	S_1	S_2	S_3	T_1	T_2	T_3
2.	$r = 2$		→				←
3.		S_1	T_3	S_3	T_1	T_2	S_2
4.	$N = 5$						
2.	$r = 4$				→	←	
3.		S_1	T_3	S_3	T_2	T_1	S_2
4.	$N = 4$						
2.	$r = 4$				↓		
3.		S_1	T_3	S_3	T_2	T_1	S_2
4.	$N = 3$						
2.	$r = 1$	→		←			
3.		S_3	T_3	S_1	T_2	T_1	S_2
4.	$N = 2$						
2.	$r = 1$	→	←				
3.		T_3	S_3	S_1	T_2	T_1	S_2
4.	$N = 1$						

8.6. LATIN SQUARES

The following example shows how 3 independent permutations can be used to obtain a Latin square.

1). Generate a random permutation of the *N* possible treatments (see Section 8.5):

T_3	S_3	S_1	T_2	T_1	S_2

2). A simple Latin square can now be constructed by "rotating" this permutation to the right. This can be done as follows. Write the permutation found in step 1 down on the first row. The second row consists of the same permutation, but with all treatments shifted to the right. The rightmost treatment is put on the empty place at the left. This is repeated for all the rows until all the treatments appear once in each column:

T_3	S_3	S_1	T_2	T_1	S_2
S_2	T_3	S_3	S_1	T_2	T_1
T_1	S_2	T_3	S_3	S_1	T_2
T_2	T_1	S_2	T_3	S_3	S_1
S_1	T_2	T_1	S_2	T_3	S_3
S_3	S_1	T_2	T_1	S_2	T_3

3). Generate 2 independent random permutations of the figures 1 to N:

– one for the rows:

2	**3**	**6**	**1**	**4**	**5**

– and one for the columns:

3	**4**	**6**	**2**	**5**	**1**

4). The Latin square can now be found by sorting the rows and columns of the simple Latin square according to the 2 permutations for the rows and columns:

	3	4	6	2	5	1
2	T_3	S_3	S_1	T_2	T_1	S_2
3	S_2	T_3	S_3	S_1	T_2	T_1
6	T_1	S_2	T_3	S_3	S_1	T_2
1	T_2	T_1	S_2	T_3	S_3	S_1
4	S_1	T_2	T_1	S_2	T_3	S_3
5	S_3	S_1	T_2	T_1	S_2	T_3

↓

	1	2	3	4	5	6
1	S_1	T_3	T_2	T_1	S_3	S_2
2	S_2	T_2	T_3	S_3	T_1	S_1
3	T_1	S_1	S_2	T_3	T_2	S_3
4	S_3	S_2	S_1	T_2	T_3	T_1
5	T_3	T_1	S_3	S_1	S_2	T_2
6	T_2	S_3	T_1	S_2	S_1	T_3

9. GLOSSARY OF SYMBOLS

Symbol	**Definition**
a	Intersection of linear regression of responses on dose or ln(dose)
b	Slope of linear regression of responses on dose or on ln(dose)
d	Number of dose levels for each preparation (excluding the blank in slope-ratio assays)
e	Base of natural logarithms (= 2.71828182845905...)
g	Statistic used in Fieller's theorem: $g = \frac{C-1}{C}$
h	Number of preparations in an assay, including the standard preparation
m	Potency estimate obtained as a ratio of effects in general linear models
n	Number of replicates for each treatment
p	Probability of a given statistic being larger than the observed value. Also used as the ratio r/n in probit analysis
r	The number of responding units per treatment group in assays depending upon quantal responses
s	Estimate of standard deviation ($= \sqrt{s^2}$)
s^2	Estimate of residual variance given by error mean square in analysis of variance
t	Student's statistic (Table 8.2.)
u	Observed response in four-parameter analysis
v_{11}, v_{12}, v_{22}	(Co)variance multipliers for numerator and denominator of ratio m in Fieller's theorem
w	Weighting coefficient
x	The ln(dose)
y	Individual response or transformed response
A	Assumed potencies of test preparations when making up doses
B	Mean response to blanks in slope-ratio assays
C	Statistic used in the calculation of confidence intervals: $C = \frac{1}{1-g}$
$C_1, \ldots, C_n$	Mean response to each column of a Latin square design
D_1, D_2	Mean response on time 1 or time 2 in the twin cross-over design
F	Ratio of 2 independent estimates of variance following an F-distribution (Table 8.1.)
$G_S, G_T, \ldots$	Treatment values used in the analysis of variance for slope-ratio assays
H_P, H_L	Multipliers used in the analysis of variance for parallel-line assays
H_B, H_I	Multipliers used in the analysis of variance for slope-ratio assays

5. General texts

Symbol	Definition
I	In parallel-line assays, the ln of the ratio between adjacent doses. In slope-ratio assays, the interval between adjacent doses
J_S, J_T ...	Linearity values used in the analysis of variance for slope-ratio assays
K	Correction term used in the calculation of sums of squares in the analysis of variance
L	Width of confidence interval in logarithms
L_S, L_T ...	Linear contrasts of standard and test preparations
M'	ln potency ratio of a given test preparation
N	Total number of treatments in the assay (= dh)
P_S, P_T ...	Sum of standard and test preparations
R	Estimated potency of a given test preparation
R'	Potency ratio of a given test preparation
R_1, ... , R_n	Mean response in each of rows 1 to n of a Latin square design, or in each block of a randomised block design
S	Standard preparation
S_1, ... , S_d	Mean response to the lowest dose 1 up to the highest dose d of the standard preparation S
SS	Sum of squares due to a given source of variation
T, U, V, ...	Test preparations
T_1, ... , T_d	Mean response to the lowest dose 1 up to the highest dose d of test preparation T
V	Variance coefficient in the calculation of confidence limits
W	Weighting factor in combination of assay results
X	Linear structure or design matrix used in general linear models

Symbol	Definition
Y	Vector representing the (transformed) responses in general linear models
Z	The first derivative of Φ
α	Upper asymptote of the ln(dose)-response curve in four-parameter analysis
β	Slope-factor of the ln(dose)-response curve in four-parameter analysis
γ	The ln(dose) giving 50 per cent response in the four-parameter analysis
δ	Lower asymptote of the ln(dose)-response curve in four-parameter analysis
π	3.141592653589793238...
Φ	Cumulative standard normal distribution function (Table 8.4.)
χ^2	Chi-square statistic (Table 8.3.)

10. LITERATURE

This section lists some recommended literature for further study.

Finney, D.J. (1971). *Probit Analysis,* 3rd Ed. Cambridge University Press, Cambridge.

Nelder, J.A. & Wedderburn, R.W.M. (1972). Generalized linear models, *Journal of the Royal Statistical Society, Series* A 135, 370-384.

DeLean, A., Munson, P.J., and Rodbard, D. (1978). *Simultaneous analysis of families of sigmoidal curves: Application to bioassay, radioligand assay, and physiological dose-response curves,* Am. J. Physiol. 235(2): E97-E102.

Finney, D.J. (1978). *Statistical Method in Biological Assay,* 3rd Ed. Griffin, London.

Sokal, R.R. & Rohlf, F.R. (1981). *Biometry: Principles and Practice of Statistics in Biological Research,* 2nd Ed. W.H. Freemann & CO, New York.

Peace, K.E. (1988). *Biopharmaceutical Statistics for Drug Development,* Marcel Dekker Inc., New York/Basel.

Bowerman, B.L. & O'Connell, R.T. (1990). *Linear Statistical Models an Applied Approach,* 2nd Ed. PWS-KENT Publishing Company, Boston.

Govindarajulu, Z. (2001). *Statistical Techniques in Bioassay,* 2nd revised and enlarged edition, Karger, New York.

5.4. RESIDUAL SOLVENTS

01/2005:50400

5.4. RESIDUAL SOLVENTS

LIMITING RESIDUAL SOLVENT LEVELS IN ACTIVE SUBSTANCES, EXCIPIENTS AND MEDICINAL PRODUCTS

The International Conference on Harmonisation of Technical Requirements for Registration of Pharmaceuticals for Human Use (ICH) has adopted Impurities Guidelines for Residual Solvents which prescribes limits for the content of solvents which may remain in active substances, excipients and medicinal products after processing. This guideline, the text of which is reproduced below, excludes existing marketed products. The European Pharmacopoeia is, however, applying the same principles enshrined in the guideline to existing active substances, excipients and medicinal products whether or not they are the subject of a monograph of the Pharmacopoeia. All substances and products are to be tested for the content of solvents likely to be present in a substance or product.

Where the limits to be applied comply with those given below, tests for residual solvents are not generally mentioned in specific monographs since the solvents employed may vary from one manufacturer to another and the requirements of this general chapter are applied via the general monograph on *Substances for Pharmaceutical Use (2034)*. The competent authority is to be informed of the solvents employed during the production process. This information is also given in the dossier submitted for a certificate of suitability of the monographs of the European Pharmacopoeia and is mentioned on the certificate.

Where only Class 3 solvents are used, a test for loss on drying may be applied or a specific determination of the solvent may be made. If for a Class 3 solvent a justified and authorised limit higher than 0.5 per cent is applied, a specific determination of the solvent is required.

When Class 1 residual solvents or Class 2 residual solvents (or Class 3 residual solvents which exceed the 0.5 per cent) are used, the methodology described in the general method (*2.4.24*) is to be applied wherever possible. Otherwise an appropriate validated method is to be employed.

When a quantitative determination of a residual solvent is carried out, the result is taken into account for the calculation of the content of the substance except where a test for drying is carried out.

IMPURITIES: GUIDELINES FOR RESIDUAL SOLVENTS (CPMP/ICH/283/95)

1. INTRODUCTION

The objective of this guideline is to recommend acceptable amounts of residual solvents in pharmaceuticals for the safety of the patient. The guideline recommends the use of less toxic solvents and describes levels considered to be toxicologically acceptable for some residual solvents.

Residual solvents in pharmaceuticals are defined here as organic volatile chemicals that are used or produced in the manufacture of active substances or excipients, or in the preparation of medicinal products. The solvents are not completely removed by practical manufacturing techniques. Appropriate selection of the solvent for the synthesis of active substance may enhance the yield, or determine characteristics such as crystal form, purity, and solubility. Therefore, the solvent may sometimes be a critical parameter in the synthetic process. This guideline does not address solvents deliberately used as excipients nor does it address solvates. However, the content of solvents in such products should be evaluated and justified.

Since there is no therapeutic benefit from residual solvents, all residual solvents should be removed to the extent possible to meet product specifications, good manufacturing practices, or other quality-based requirements. Medicinal products should contain no higher levels of residual solvents than can be supported by safety data. Some solvents that are known to cause unacceptable toxicities (Class 1, Table 1) should be avoided in the production of active substances, excipients, or medicinal products unless their use can be strongly justified in a risk-benefit assessment. Some solvents associated with less severe toxicity (Class 2, Table 2) should be limited in order to protect patients from potential adverse effects. Ideally, less toxic solvents (Class 3, Table 3) should be used where practical. The complete list of solvents included in this guideline is given in Appendix 1.

The lists are not exhaustive and other solvents can be used and later added to the lists. Recommended limits of Class 1 and 2 solvents or classification of solvents may change as new safety data becomes available. Supporting safety data in a marketing application for a new medicinal product containing a new solvent may be based on concepts in this guideline or the concept of qualification of impurities as expressed in the guideline for active substances (*Q3A*,

5. General texts

Impurities in New Active Substances) or medicinal products (*Q3B*, Impurities in New Medicinal Products), or all three guidelines.

2. SCOPE OF THE GUIDELINE

Residual solvents in active substances, excipients, and in medicinal products are within the scope of this guideline. Therefore, testing should be performed for residual solvents when production or purification processes are known to result in the presence of such solvents. It is only necessary to test for solvents that are used or produced in the manufacture or purification of active substances, excipients, or medicinal product. Although manufacturers may choose to test the medicinal product, a cumulative method may be used to calculate the residual solvent levels in the medicinal product from the levels in the ingredients used to produce the medicinal product. If the calculation results in a level equal to or below that recommended in this guideline, no testing of the medicinal product for residual solvents need be considered. If however, the calculated level is above the recommended level, the medicinal product should be tested to ascertain whether the formulation process has reduced the relevant solvent level to within the acceptable amount. Medicinal product should also be tested if a solvent is used during its manufacture.

This guideline does not apply to potential new active substances, excipients, or medicinal products used during the clinical research stages of development, nor does it apply to existing marketed medicinal products.

The guideline applies to all dosage forms and routes of administration. Higher levels of residual solvents may be acceptable in certain cases such as short term (30 days or less) or topical application. Justification for these levels should be made on a case by case basis.

See Appendix 2 for additional background information related to residual solvents.

3. GENERAL PRINCIPLES

3.1. CLASSIFICATION OF RESIDUAL SOLVENTS BY RISK ASSESSMENT

The term "tolerable daily intake" (TDI) is used by the International Program on Chemical Safety (IPCS) to describe exposure limits of toxic chemicals and "acceptable daily intake" (ADI) is used by the World Health Organisation (WHO) and other national and international health authorities and institutes. The new term "permitted daily exposure" (PDE) is defined in the present guideline as a pharmaceutically acceptable intake of residual solvents to avoid confusion of differing values for ADI's of the same substance.

Residual solvents assessed in this guideline are listed in Appendix 1 by common names and structures. They were evaluated for their possible risk to human health and placed into one of three classes as follows:

Class 1 solvents: Solvents to be avoided

Known human carcinogens, strongly suspected human carcinogens, and environmental hazards.

Class 2 solvents: Solvents to be limited

Non-genotoxic animal carcinogens or possible causative agents of other irreversible toxicity such as neurotoxicity or teratogenicity.

Solvents suspected of other significant but reversible toxicities.

Class 3 solvents: Solvents with low toxic potential

Solvents with low toxic potential to man; no health-based exposure limit is needed. Class 3 solvents have PDEs of 50 mg or more per day.

3.2. METHODS FOR ESTABLISHING EXPOSURE LIMITS

The method used to establish permitted daily exposures for residual solvents is presented in Appendix 3. Summaries of the toxicity data that were used to establish limits are published in *Pharmeuropa*, Vol. 9, No. 1, Supplement April 1997.

3.3. OPTIONS FOR DESCRIBING LIMITS OF CLASS 2 SOLVENTS

Two options are available when setting limits for Class 2 solvents.

Option 1: The concentration limits in ppm stated in Table 2 can be used. They were calculated using equation (1) below by assuming a product mass of 10 g administered daily.

$$\text{Concentration (ppm)} = \frac{1000 \times \text{PDE}}{\text{dose}} \qquad (1)$$

Here, PDE is given in terms of mg/day and dose is given in g/day.

These limits are considered acceptable for all substances, excipients, or products. Therefore this option may be applied if the daily dose is not known or fixed. If all excipients and active substances in a formulation meet the limits given in Option 1, then these components may be used in any proportion. No further calculation is necessary provided the daily dose does not exceed 10 g. Products that are administered in doses greater than 10 g per day should be considered under Option 2.

Option 2: It is not considered necessary for each component of the medicinal product to comply with the limits given in Option 1. The PDE in terms of mg/day as stated in Table 2 can be used with the known maximum daily dose and equation (1) above to determine the concentration of residual solvent allowed in a medicinal product. Such limits are considered acceptable provided that is has been demonstrated that the residual solvent has been reduced to the practical minimum. The limits should be realistic in relation to analytical precision, manufacturing capability, reasonable variation in the manufacturing process, and the limits should reflect contemporary manufacturing standards.

Option 2 may be applied by adding the amounts of a residual solvent present in each of the components of the medicinal product. The sum of the amounts of solvent per day should be less than that given by the PDE.

Consider an example of the use of Option l and Option 2 applied to acetonitrile in a medicinal product. The permitted daily exposure to acetonitrile is 4.1 mg per day; thus, the Option 1 limit is 410 ppm. The maximum administered daily mass of a medicinal product is 5.0 g, and the medicinal product contains two excipients. The composition of the medicinal product and the calculated maximum content of residual acetonitrile are given in the following table.

Component	Amount in formulation	Acetonitrile content	Daily exposure
Active substance	0.3 g	800 ppm	0.24 mg
Excipient 1	0.9 g	400 ppm	0.36 mg
Excipient 2	3.8 g	800 ppm	3.04 mg
Medicinal product	5.0 g	728 ppm	3.64 mg

Excipient l meets the Option l limit, but the drug substance, excipient 2, and medicinal product do not meet the Option l limit. Nevertheless, the product meets the Option 2 limit of 4.l mg per day and thus conforms to the recommendations in this guideline.

Consider another example using acetonitrile as residual solvent. The maximum administered daily mass of a medicinal product is 5.0 g, and the medicinal product contains two excipients. The composition of the medicinal product and the calculated maximum content of residual acetonitrile is given in the following table.

Component	Amount in formulation	Acetonitrile content	Daily exposure
Active substance	0.3 g	800 ppm	0.24 mg
Excipient 1	0.9 g	2000 ppm	1.80 mg
Excipient 2	3.8 g	800 ppm	3.04 mg
Medicinal product	5.0 g	1016 ppm	5.08 mg

In this example, the product meets neither the Option 1 nor the Option 2 limit according to this summation. The manufacturer could test the medicinal product to determine if the formulation process reduced the level of acetonitrile. If the level of acetonitrile was not reduced during formulation to the allowed limit, then the manufacturer of the medicinal product should take other steps to reduce the amount of acetonitrile in the medicinal product. If all of these steps fail to reduce the level of residual solvent, in exceptional cases the manufacturer could provide a summary of efforts made to reduce the solvent level to meet the guideline value, and provide a risk-benefit analysis to support allowing the product to be utilised containing residual solvent at a higher level.

3.4. ANALYTICAL PROCEDURES

Residual solvents are typically determined using chromatographic techniques such as gas chromatography. Any harmonised procedures for determining levels of residual solvents as described in the pharmacopoeias should be used, if feasible. Otherwise, manufacturers would be free to select the most appropriate validated analytical procedure for a particular application. If only Class 3 solvents are present, a non-specific method such as loss on drying may be used.

Validation of methods for residual solvents should conform to ICH guidelines "Text on Validation of Analytical Procedures" and "Extension of the ICH Text on Validation of Analytical Procedures".

3.5. REPORTING LEVELS OF RESIDUAL SOLVENTS

Manufacturers of pharmaceutical products need certain information about the content of residual solvents in excipients or active substances in order to meet the criteria of this guideline. The following statements are given as acceptable examples of the information that could be provided from a supplier of excipients or active substances to a pharmaceutical manufacturer. The supplier might choose one of the following as appropriate:

- Only Class 3 solvents are likely to be present. Loss on drying is less than 0.5 per cent.
- Only Class 2 solvents X, Y, ... are likely to be present. All are below the Option 1 limit

  (Here the supplier would name the Class 2 solvents represented by X, Y, ...)
- Only Class 2 solvents X, Y, ... and Class 3 solvents are likely to be present. Residual Class 2 solvents are below the Option 1 limit and residual Class 3 solvents are below 0.5 per cent.

If Class 1 solvents are likely to be present, they should be identified and quantified. "Likely to be present" refers to the solvent used in the final manufacturing step and to solvents that are used in earlier manufacturing steps and not removed consistently by a validated process.

If solvents of Class 2 or Class 3 are present at greater than their Option 1 limits or 0.5 per cent, respectively, they should be identified and quantified.

4. LIMITS OF RESIDUAL SOLVENTS

4.1. SOLVENTS TO BE AVOIDED

Solvents in Class 1 should not be employed in the manufacture of active substances, excipients, and medicinal products because of their unacceptable toxicity or their deleterious environmental effect. However, if their use is unavoidable in order to produce a medicinal product with a significant therapeutic advance, then their levels should be restricted as shown in Table 1, unless otherwise justified. 1,1,1-Trichloroethane is included in Table 1 because it is an environmental hazard. The stated limit of 1500 ppm is based on a review of the safety data.

Table 1. – *Class 1 solvents in pharmaceutical products (solvents that should be avoided)*

Solvent	Concentration limit (ppm)	Concern
Benzene	2	Carcinogen
Carbon tetrachloride	4	Toxic and environmental hazard
1,2-Dichloroethane	5	Toxic
1,1-Dichloroethene	8	Toxic
1,1,1-Trichloroethane	1500	Environmental hazard

4.2. SOLVENTS TO BE LIMITED

Solvents in Table 2 should be limited in pharmaceutical products because of their inherent toxicity. PDEs are given to the nearest 0.1 mg/day, and concentrations are given to the nearest 10 ppm. The stated values do not reflect the necessary analytical precision of determination. Precision should be determined as part of the validation of the method.

Table 2. – *Class 2 solvents in pharmaceutical products*

Solvent	PDE (mg/day)	Concentration limit (ppm)
Acetonitrile	4.1	410
Chlorobenzene	3.6	360
Chloroform	0.6	60
Cyclohexane	38.8	3880
1,2-Dichloroethene	18.7	1870
Dichloromethane	6.0	600
1,2-Dimethoxyethane	1.0	100
N,N-Dimethylacetamide	10.9	1090
N,N-Dimethylformamide	8.8	880
1,4-Dioxane	3.8	380
2-Ethoxyethanol	1.6	160
Ethyleneglycol	6.2	620
Formamide	2.2	220
Hexane	2.9	290
Methanol	30.0	3000
2-Methoxyethanol	0.5	50
Methylbutylketone	0.5	50
Methylcyclohexane	11.8	1180
N-Methylpyrrolidone	5.3	530
Nitromethane	0.5	50
Pyridine	2.0	200

Solvent	PDE (mg/day)	Concentration limit (ppm)
Sulfolane	1.6	160
Tetrahydrofuran	7.2	720
Tetralin	1.0	100
Toluene	8.9	890
1,1,2-Trichloroethene	0.8	80
Xylene*	21.7	2170

*usually 60 per cent *m*-xylene, 14 per cent *p*-xylene,9 per cent *o*-xylene with 17 per cent ethyl benzene

4.3. SOLVENTS WITH LOW TOXIC POTENTIAL

Solvents in Class 3 (shown in Table 3) may be regarded as less toxic and of lower risk to human health. Class 3 includes no solvent known as a human health hazard at levels normally accepted in pharmaceuticals. However, there are no long-term toxicity or carcinogenicity studies for many of the solvents in Class 3. Available data indicate that they are less toxic in acute or short-term studies and negative in genotoxicity studies. It is considered that amounts of these residual solvents of 50 mg per day or less (corresponding to 5000 ppm or 0.5 per cent under Option l) would be acceptable without justification. Higher amounts may also be acceptable provided they are realistic in relation to manufacturing capability and good manufacturing practice.

Table 3. – *Class 3 solvents which should be limited by GMP or other quality-based requirements*

Acetic acid	Heptane
Acetone	Isobutyl acetate
Anisole	Isopropyl acetate
1-Butanol	Methyl acetate
2-Butanol	3-Methyl-1-butanol
Butyl acetate	Methylethylketone
tert-Butylmethyl ether	Methylisobutylketone
Cumene	2-Methyl-l-propanol
Dimethyl sulphoxide	Pentane
Ethanol	1-Pentanol
Ethyl acetate	1-Propanol
Ethyl ether	2-Propanol
Ethyl formate	Propyl acetate
Formic acid	

4.4. SOLVENTS FOR WHICH NO ADEQUATE TOXICOLOGICAL DATA WAS FOUND

The following solvents (Table 4) may also be of interest to manufacturers of excipients, active substances, or medicinal products. However, no adequate toxicological data on which to base a PDE was found. Manufacturers should supply justification for residual levels of these solvents in pharmaceutical products.

Table 4. – *Solvents for which no adequate toxicological data was found*

1,1-Diethoxypropane	Methylisopropylketone
1,1-Dimethoxymethane	Methyltetrahydrofuran
2,2-Dimethoxypropane	Petroleum ether
Isooctane	Trichloroacetic acid
Isopropyl ether	Trifluoroacetic acid

GLOSSARY

Genotoxic carcinogens: Carcinogens which produce cancer by affecting genes or chromosomes.

LOEL: Abbreviation for lowest-observed effect level.

Lowest-observed effect level: The lowest dose of substance in a study or group of studies that produces biologically significant increases in frequency or severity of any effects in the exposed humans or animals.

Modifying factor: A factor determined by professional judgement of a toxicologist and applied to bioassay data to relate that data safely to humans.

Neurotoxicity: The ability of a substance to cause adverse effects on the nervous system.

NOEL: Abbreviation for *no-observed-effect level.*

No-observed-effect level: The highest dose of substance at which there are no biologically significant increases in frequency or severity of any effects in the exposed humans or animals.

PDE: Abbreviation for *permitted daily exposure.*

Permitted daily exposure: The maximum acceptable intake per day of residual solvent in pharmaceutical products.

Reversible toxicity: The occurrence of harmful effects that are caused by a substance and which disappear after exposure to the substance ends.

Strongly suspected human carcinogen: A substance for which there is no epidemiological evidence of carcinogenesis but there are positive genotoxicity data and clear evidence of carcinogenesis in rodents.

Teratogenicity: The occurrence of structural malformations in a developing foetus when a substance is administered during pregnancy.

APPENDIX 1. LIST OF SOLVENTS INCLUDED IN THE GUIDELINE

Solvent	Other Names	Structure	Class
Acetic acid	Ethanoic acid	CH_3COOH	Class 3
Acetone	2-Propanone Propan-2-one	CH_3COCH_3	Class 3
Acetonitrile		CH_3CN	Class 2
Anisole	Methoxybenzene	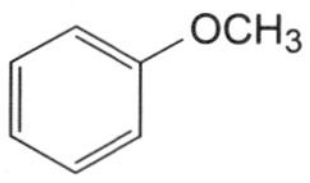	Class 3
Benzene	Benzol	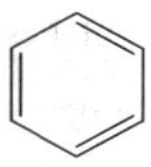	Class 1
1-Butanol	*n*-Butyl alcohol Butan-1-ol	$CH_3[CH_2]_3OH$	Class 3
2-Butanol	*sec*-Butyl alcohol Butan-2-ol	$CH_3CH_2CH(OH)CH_3$	Class 3
Butyl acetate	Acetic acid butyl ester	$CH_3COO[CH_2]_3CH_3$	Class 3
tert-Butylmethyl ether	2-Methoxy-2-methylpropane	$(CH_3)_3COCH_3$	Class 3
Carbon tetrachloride	Tetrachloromethane	CCl_4	Class 1
Chlorobenzene		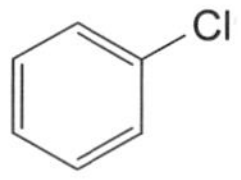	Class 2
Chloroform	Trichloromethane	$CHCl_3$	Class 2
Cumene	Isopropylbenzene (1-Methylethyl)benzene	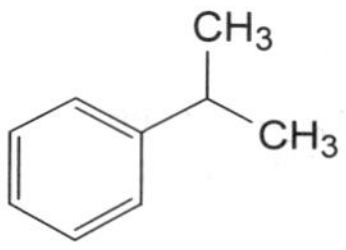	Class 3
Cyclohexane	Hexamethylene	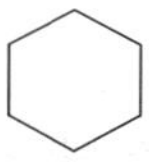	Class 2
1,2-Dichloroethane	*sym*-Dichloroethane Ethylene dichloride Ethylene chloride	CH_2ClCH_2Cl	Class 1
1,1-Dichloroethene	1,1-Dichloroethylene Vinylidene chloride	$H_2C=CCl_2$	Class 1
1,2-Dichloroethene	1,2-Dichloroethylene Acetylene dichloride	$ClHC=CHCl$	Class 2
Dichloromethane	Methylene chloride	CH_2Cl_2	Class 2
1,2-Dimethoxyethane	Ethyleneglycol dimethyl ether Monoglyme Dimethyl cellosolve	$H_3COCH_2CH_2OCH_3$	Class 2
N,N-Dimethylacetamide	DMA	$CH_3CON(CH_3)_2$	Class 2
N,N-Dimethylformamide	DMF	$HCON(CH_3)_2$	Class 2
Dimethyl sulphoxide	Methylsulphinylmethane Methyl sulphoxide DMSO	$(CH_3)_2SO$	Class 3
1,4-Dioxane	*p*-Dioxane [1,4]Dioxane	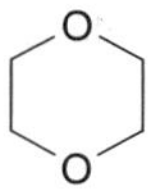	Class 2
Ethanol	Ethyl alcohol	CH_3CH_2OH	Class 3
2-Ethoxyethanol	Cellosolve	$CH_3CH_2OCH_2CH_2OH$	Class 2
Ethyl acetate	Acetic acid ethyl ester	$CH_3COOCH_2CH_3$	Class 3

Solvent	Other Names	Structure	Class
Ethyleneglycol	1,2-Dihydroxyethane 1,2-Ethanediol	$HOCH_2CH_2OH$	Class 2
Ethyl ether	Diethyl ether Ethoxyethane 1,1′-Oxybisethane	$CH_3CH_2OCH_2CH_3$	Class 3
Ethyl formate	Formic acid ethyl ester	$HCOOCH_2CH_3$	Class 3
Formamide	Methanamide	$HCONH_2$	Class 2
Formic acid		$HCOOH$	Class 3
Heptane	*n*-Heptane	$CH_3[CH_2]_5CH_3$	Class 3
Hexane	*n*-Hexane	$CH_3[CH_2]_4CH_3$	Class 2
Isobutyl acetate	Acetic acid isobutyl ester	$CH_3COOCH_2CH(CH_3)_2$	Class 3
Isopropyl acetate	Acetic acid isopropyl ester	$CH_3COOCH(CH_3)_2$	Class 3
Methanol	Methyl alcohol	CH_3OH	Class 2
2-Methoxyethanol	Methyl cellosolve	$CH_3OCH_2CH_2OH$	Class 2
Methyl acetate	Acetic acid methyl ester	CH_3COOCH_3	Class 3
3-Methyl-1-butanol	Isoamyl alcohol Isopentyl alcohol 3-Methylbutan-1-ol	$(CH_3)_2CHCH_2CH_2OH$	Class 3
Methylbutylketone	2-Hexanone Hexan-2-one	$CH_3[CH_2]_3COCH_3$	Class 2
Methylcyclohexane	Cyclohexylmethane	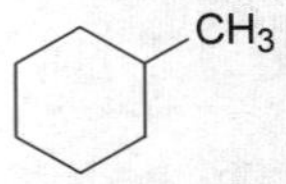	Class 2
Methylethylketone	2-Butanone MEK Butan-2-one	$CH_3CH_2COCH_3$	Class 3
Methylisobutylketone	4-Methylpentan-2-one 4-Methyl-2-pentanone MIBK	$CH_3COCH_2CH(CH_3)_2$	Class 3
2-Methyl-1-propanol	Isobutyl alcohol 2-Methylpropan-1-ol	$(CH_3)_2CHCH_2OH$	Class 3
N-Methylpyrrolidone	1-Methylpyrrolidin-2-one 1-Methyl-2-pyrrolidinone	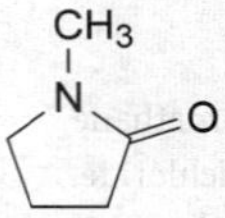	Class 2
Nitromethane		CH_3NO_2	Class 2
Pentane	*n*-Pentane	$CH_3[CH_2]_3CH_3$	Class 3
1-Pentanol	Amyl alcohol Pentan-1-ol Pentyl alcohol	$CH_3[CH_2]_3CH_2OH$	Class 3
1-Propanol	Propan-1-ol Propyl alcohol	$CH_3CH_2CH_2OH$	Class 3
2-Propanol	Propan-2-ol Isopropyl alcohol	$(CH_3)_2CHOH$	Class 3
Propyl acetate	Acetic acid propyl ester	$CH_3COOCH_2CH_2CH_3$	Class 3
Pyridine		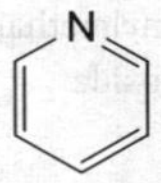	Class 2
Sulfonane	Tetrahydrothiophene 1,1-dioxide	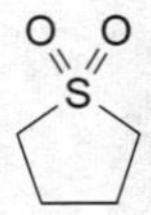	Class 2

Solvent	Other Names	Structure	Class
Tetrahydrofuran	Tetramethylene oxide Oxacyclopentane	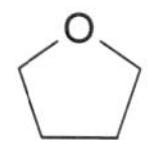	Class 2
Tetralin	1,2,3,4-Tetrahydronaphthalene	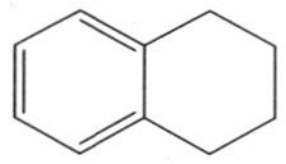	Class 2
Toluene	Methylbenzene	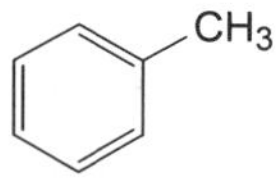	Class 2
1,1,1-Trichloroethane	Methylchloroform	CH_3CCl_3	Class 1
1,1,2-Trichloroethene	Trichloroethene	$HClC{=}CCl_2$	Class 2
Xylene*	Dimethybenzene Xylol	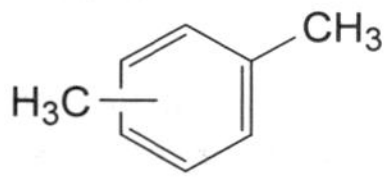	Class 2

*usually 60 per cent *m*-xylene, 14 per cent *p*-xylene, 9 per cent *o*-xylene with 17 per cent ethyl benzene.

APPENDIX 2. ADDITIONAL BACKGROUND

A2.1. ENVIRONMENTAL REGULATION OF ORGANIC VOLATILE SOLVENTS

Several of the residual solvents frequently used in the production of pharmaceuticals are listed as toxic chemicals in Environmental Health Criteria (EHC) monographs and the Integrated Risk Information System (IRIS). The objectives of such groups as the International Programme on Chemical Safety (IPCS), the United States Environmental Protection Agency (USEPA) and the United States Food and Drug Administration (USFDA) include the determination of acceptable exposure levels. The goal is protection of human health and maintenance of environmental integrity against the possible deleterious effects of chemicals resulting from long-term environmental exposure. The methods involved in the estimation of maximum safe exposure limits are usually based on long-term studies. When long-term study data are unavailable, shorter term study data can be used with modification of the approach such as use of larger safety factors. The approach described therein relates primarily to long-term or life-time exposure of the general population in the ambient environment, i.e. ambient air, food, drinking water and other media.

A2.2. RESIDUAL SOLVENTS IN PHARMACEUTICALS

Exposure limits in this guideline are established by referring to methodologies and toxicity data described in EHC and IRIS monographs. However, some specific assumptions about residual solvents to be used in the synthesis and formulation of pharmaceutical products should be taken into account in establishing exposure limits. They are:

1) Patients (not the general population) use pharmaceuticals to treat their diseases or for prophylaxis to prevent infection or disease.

2) The assumption of life-time patient exposure is not necessary for most pharmaceutical products but may be appropriate as a working hypothesis to reduce risk to human health.

3) Residual solvents are unavoidable components in pharmaceutical production and will often be a part of medicinal products.

4) Residual solvents should not exceed recommended levels except in exceptional circumstances.

5) Data from toxicological studies that are used to determine acceptable levels for residual solvents should have been generated using appropriate protocols such as those described for example, by OECD and the FDA Red Book.

APPENDIX 3. METHODS FOR ESTABLISHING EXPOSURE LIMITS

The Gaylor-Kodell method of risk assessment (Gaylor, D. W. and Kodell, R. L. Linear Interpolation algorithm for low dose assessment of toxic substance. J. Environ. Pathology, 4, 305, 1980) is appropriate for Class 1 carcinogenic solvents. Only in cases where reliable carcinogenicity data are available should extrapolation by the use of mathematical models be applied to setting exposure limits. Exposure limits for Class 1 solvents could be determined with the use of a large safety factor (i.e., 10 000 to 100 000) with respect to the no-observed-effect level (NOEL). Detection and quantification of these solvents should be by state-of-the-art analytical techniques.

Acceptable exposure levels in this guideline for Class 2 solvents were established by calculation of PDE values according to the procedures for setting exposure limits in pharmaceuticals (*Pharmacopeial Forum*, Nov-Dec 1989), and the method adopted by IPCS for Assessing Human Health Risk of Chemicals (*Environmental Health Criteria 170*, WHO, 1994). These methods are similar to those used by the USEPA (IRIS) and the USFDA (*Red Book*) and others. The method is outlined here to give a better understanding of the origin of the PDE values. It is not necessary to perform these calculations in order to use the PDE values tabulated in Section 4 of this document.

PDE is derived from the no-observed-effect level (NOEL), or the lowest-observed effect level (LOEL), in the most relevant animal study as follows:

$$\mathrm{PDE} = \frac{\mathrm{NOEL} \times \mathrm{Weight\ Adjustment}}{\mathrm{F1} \times \mathrm{F2} \times \mathrm{F3} \times \mathrm{F4} \times \mathrm{F5}}$$

The PDE is derived preferably from a NOEL. If no NOEL is obtained, the LOEL may be used. Modifying factors proposed here, for relating the data to humans, are the same kind of "uncertainty factors" used in Environmental Health Criteria (*Environmental Health Criteria* 170, World Health Organisation, Geneva, 1994), and "modifying factors" or "safety factors" in *Pharmacopoeial Forum*. The assumption of 100 per cent systemic exposure is used in all calculations regardless of route of administration.

The modifying factors are as follows:

F1 = A factor to account for extrapolation between species

F1 = 2 for extrapolation from dogs to humans

F1 = 2.5 for extrapolation from rabbits to humans

F1 = 3 for extrapolation from monkeys to humans

F1 = 5 for extrapolation from rats to humans

F1 = 10 for extrapolation from other animals to humans

F1 = 12 for extrapolation from mice to humans

F1 takes into account the comparative surface area: body weight ratios for the species concerned and for man. Surface area (*S*) is calculated as:

$$S = km^{0.67}$$

in which *m* = body mass, and the constant *k* has been taken to be 10. The body weight used in the equation are those shown below in Table A3.-1.

Table A3.-1. – *Values used in the calculations in this document*

Rat body weight	425 g
Pregnant rat body weight	330 g
Mouse body weight	28 g
Pregnant mouse body weight	30 g
Guinea-pig body weight	500 g
Rhesus monkey body weight	2.5 kg
Rabbit body weight (pregnant or not)	4 kg
Beagle dog body weight	11.5 kg
Rat respiratory volume	290 l/day
Mouse respiratory volume	43 l/day
Rabbit respiratory volume	1440 l/day
Guinea-pig respiratory volume	430 l/day
Human respiratory volume	28800 l/day
Dog respiratory volume	9000 l/day
Monkey respiratory volume	1150 l/day
Mouse water consumption	5 ml/day
Rat water consumption	30 ml/day
Rat food consumption	30 g/day

F2 = A factor of 10 to account for variability between individuals. A factor of 10 is generally given for all organic solvents, and 10 is used consistently in this guideline.

F3 = A variable factor to account for toxicity studies of short-term exposure.

F3 = 1 for studies that last at least one half-lifetime (1 year for rodents or rabbits; 7 years for cats, dogs and monkeys).

F3 = 1 for reproductive studies in which the whole period of organogenesis is covered.

F3 = 2 for a 6 month study in rodents, or a 3.5 year study in non-rodents.

F3 = 5 for a 3 month study in rodents, or a 2 year study in non-rodents.

F3 = 10 for studies of a shorter duration.

In all cases, the higher factor has been used for study durations between the time points, e.g. a factor of 2 for a 9 month rodent study.

F4 = A factor that may be applied in cases of severe toxicity, e.g. non-genotoxic carcinogenicity, neurotoxicity or teratogenicity. In studies of reproductive toxicity, the following factors are used:

F4 = 1 for foetal toxicity associated with maternal toxicity

F4 = 5 for foetal toxicity without maternal toxicity

F4 = 5 for a teratogenic effect with maternal toxicity

F4 = 10 for a teratogenic effect without maternal toxicity

F5 = A variable factor that may be applied if the no-effect level was not established.

When only a LOEL is available, a factor of up to 10 can be used depending on the severity of the toxicity.

The weight adjustment assumes an arbitrary adult human body weight for either sex of 50 kg. This relatively low weight provides an additional safety factor against the standard weights of 60 kg or 70 kg that are often used in this type of calculation. It is recognised that some adult patients weigh less than 50 kg; these patients are considered to be accommodated by the built-in safety factors used to determine a PDE. If the solvent was present in a formulation specifically intended for paediatric use, an adjustment for a lower body weight would be appropriate.

As an example of the application of this equation, consider the toxicity study of acetonitrile in mice that is summarised in *Pharmeuropa*, Vol. 9. No. 1, Supplement, April 1997, page S24. The NOEL is calculated to be 50.7 mg kg^{-1} day^{-1}. The PDE for acetonitrile in this study is calculated as follows:

$$\text{PDE} = \frac{50.7\text{mg kg}^{-1}\text{ day}^{-1} \times 50\text{ kg}}{12 \times 10 \times 5 \times 1 \times 1} = 4.22\text{ mg day}^{-1}$$

In this example,

F1 = 12 to account for the extrapolation from mice to humans

F2 = 10 to account for differences between individual humans

F3 = 5 because the duration of the study was only 13 weeks

F4 = 1 because no severe toxicity was encountered

F5 = 1 because the no-effect level was determined

The equation for an ideal gas, $PV = nRT$, is used to convert concentrations of gases used in inhalation studies from units of ppm to units of mg/l or mg/m³. Consider as an example the rat reproductive toxicity study by inhalation of carbon tetrachloride (molecular weight 153.84) summarised in *Pharmeuropa*, Vol. 9, No. 1, Supplement, April 1997, page S9.

$$\frac{n}{V} = \frac{P}{RT} = \frac{300 \times 10^{-6}\ \text{atm} \times 153\,840\ \text{mg mol}^{-1}}{0.082\,\text{l atm K}^{-1}\text{mol}^{-1} \times 298\ \text{K}}$$

$$= \frac{46.15\ \text{mg}}{24.45\ \text{l}} = 1.89\ \text{mg/l}$$

The relationship 1000 litres = 1 m³ is used to convert to mg/ m³.

5.5. ALCOHOLIMETRIC TABLES

01/2005:50500

5.5. ALCOHOLIMETRIC TABLES

The general formula agreed by the Council of the European Communities in its Directive of 27 July 1976 on alcoholimetry served as the basis for establishing the following tables.

% *V/V*	% *m/m*	ρ_{20} (kg/m^3)
0.0	0.0	998.20
0.1	0.08	998.05
0.2	0.16	997.90
0.3	0.24	997.75
0.4	0.32	997.59
0.5	0.40	997.44
0.6	0.47	997.29
0.7	0.55	997.14
0.8	0.63	996.99
0.9	0.71	996.85
1.0	0.79	996.70
1.1	0.87	996.55
1.2	0.95	996.40
1.3	1.03	996.25
1.4	1.11	996.11
1.5	1.19	995.96
1.6	1.27	995.81
1.7	1.35	995.67
1.8	1.43	995.52
1.9	1.51	995.38
2.0	1.59	995.23
2.1	1.67	995.09
2.2	1.75	994.94
2.3	1.82	994.80
2.4	1.90	994.66
2.5	1.98	994.51
2.6	2.06	994.37
2.7	2.14	994.23
2.8	2.22	994.09
2.9	2.30	993.95
3.0	2.38	993.81
3.1	2.46	993.66
3.2	2.54	993.52
3.3	2.62	993.38
3.4	2.70	993.24
3.5	2.78	993.11
3.6	2.86	992.97
3.7	2.94	992.83
3.8	3.02	992.69
3.9	3.10	992.55
4.0	3.18	992.41
4.1	3.26	992.28
4.2	3.34	992.14
4.3	3.42	992.00
4.4	3.50	991.87
4.5	3.58	991.73
4.6	3.66	991.59
4.7	3.74	991.46
4.8	3.82	991.32
4.9	3.90	991.19
5.0	3.98	991.06
5.1	4.06	990.92
5.2	4.14	990.79
5.3	4.22	990.65
5.4	4.30	990.52
5.5	4.38	990.39
5.6	4.46	990.26
5.7	4.54	990.12
5.8	4.62	989.99
5.9	4.70	989.86
6.0	4.78	989.73
6.1	4.86	989.60
6.2	4.95	989.47
6.3	5.03	989.34
6.4	5.11	989.21
6.5	5.19	989.08
6.6	5.27	988.95
6.7	5.35	988.82
6.8	5.43	988.69
6.9	5.51	988.56
7.0	5.59	988.43
7.1	5.67	988.30
7.2	5.75	988.18
7.3	5.83	988.05
7.4	5.91	987.92
7.5	5.99	987.79
7.6	6.07	987.67
7.7	6.15	987.54
7.8	6.23	987.42
7.9	6.32	987.29
8.0	6.40	987.16

% V/V	% m/m	ρ_{20} (kg/m³)
8.1	6.48	987.04
8.2	6.56	986.91
8.3	6.64	986.79
8.4	6.72	986.66
8.5	6.80	986.54
8.6	6.88	986.42
8.7	6.96	986.29
8.8	7.04	986.17
8.9	7.12	986.05
9.0	7.20	985.92
9.1	7.29	985.80
9.2	7.37	985.68
9.3	7.45	985.56
9.4	7.53	985.44
9.5	7.61	985.31
9.6	7.69	985.19
9.7	7.77	985.07
9.8	7.85	984.95
9.9	7.93	984.83
10.0	8.01	984.71
10.1	8.10	984.59
10.2	8.18	984.47
10.3	8.26	984.35
10.4	8.34	984.23
10.5	8.42	984.11
10.6	8.50	983.99
10.7	8.58	983.88
10.8	8.66	983.76
10.9	8.75	983.64
11.0	8.83	983.52
11.1	8.91	983.40
11.2	8.99	983.29
11.3	9.07	983.17
11.4	9.15	983.05
11.5	9.23	982.94
11.6	9.32	982.82
11.7	9.40	982.70
11.8	9.48	982.59
11.9	9.56	982.47
12.0	9.64	982.35
12.1	9.72	982.24
12.2	9.80	982.12
12.3	9.89	982.01

% V/V	% m/m	ρ_{20} (kg/m³)
12.4	9.97	981.89
12.5	10.05	981.78
12.6	10.13	981.67
12.7	10.21	981.55
12.8	10.29	981.44
12.9	10.37	981.32
13.0	10.46	981.21
13.1	10.54	981.10
13.2	10.62	980.98
13.3	10.70	980.87
13.4	10.78	980.76
13.5	10.87	980.64
13.6	10.95	980.53
13.7	11.03	980.42
13.8	11.11	980.31
13.9	11.19	980.19
14.0	11.27	980.08
14.1	11.36	979.97
14.2	11.44	979.86
14.3	11.52	979.75
14.4	11.60	979.64
14.5	11.68	979.52
14.6	11.77	979.41
14.7	11.85	979.30
14.8	11.93	979.19
14.9	12.01	979.08
15.0	12.09	978.97
15.1	12.17	978.86
15.2	12.26	978.75
15.3	12.34	978.64
15.4	12.42	978.53
15.5	12.50	978.42
15.6	12.59	978.31
15.7	12.67	978.20
15.8	12.75	978.09
15.9	12.83	977.98
16.0	12.91	977.87
16.1	13.00	977.76
16.2	13.08	977.65
16.3	13.16	977.55
16.4	13.24	977.44
16.5	13.32	977.33
16.6	13.41	977.22

% *V/V*	% *m/m*	ρ_{20} (kg/m³)
16.7	13.49	977.11
16.8	13.57	977.00
16.9	13.65	976.89
17.0	13.74	976.79
17.1	13.82	976.68
17.2	13.90	976.57
17.3	13.98	976.46
17.4	14.07	976.35
17.5	14.15	976.25
17.6	14.23	976.14
17.7	14.31	976.03
17.8	14.40	975.92
17.9	14.48	975.81
18.0	14.56	975.71
18.1	14.64	975.60
18.2	14.73	975.49
18.3	14.81	975.38
18.4	14.89	975.28
18.5	14.97	975.17
18.6	15.06	975.06
18.7	15.14	974.95
18.8	15.22	974.85
18.9	15.30	974.74
19.0	15.39	974.63
19.1	15.47	974.52
19.2	15.55	974.42
19.3	15.63	974.31
19.4	15.72	974.20
19.5	15.80	974.09
19.6	15.88	973.99
19.7	15.97	973.88
19.8	16.05	973.77
19.9	16.13	973.66
20.0	16.21	973.56
20.1	16.30	973.45
20.2	16.38	973.34
20.3	16.46	973.24
20.4	16.55	973.13
20.5	16.63	973.02
20.6	16.71	972.91
20.7	16.79	972.80
20.8	16.88	972.70
20.9	16.96	972.59
21.0	17.04	972.48
21.1	17.13	972.37
21.2	17.21	972.27
21.3	17.29	972.16
21.4	17.38	972.05
21.5	17.46	971.94
21.6	17.54	971.83
21.7	17.62	971.73
21.8	17.71	971.62
21.9	17.79	971.51
22.0	17.87	971.40
22.1	17.96	971.29
22.2	18.04	971.18
22.3	18.12	971.08
22.4	18.21	970.97
22.5	18.29	970.86
22.6	18.37	970.75
22.7	18.46	970.64
22.8	18.54	970.53
22.9	18.62	970.42
23.0	18.71	970.31
23.1	18.79	970.20
23.2	18.87	970.09
23.3	18.96	969.98
23.4	19.04	969.87
23.5	19.13	969.76
23.6	19.21	969.65
23.7	19.29	969.54
23.8	19.38	969.43
23.9	19.46	969.32
24.0	19.54	969.21
24.1	19.63	969.10
24.2	19.71	968.99
24.3	19.79	968.88
24.4	19.88	968.77
24.5	19.96	968.66
24.6	20.05	968.55
24.7	20.13	968.43
24.8	20.21	968.32
24.9	20.30	968.21
25.0	20.38	968.10
25.1	20.47	967.99

% V/V	% m/m	ρ_{20} (kg/m^3)
25.2	20.55	967.87
25.3	20.63	967.76
25.4	20.72	967.65
25.5	20.80	967.53
25.6	20.88	967.42
25.7	20.97	967.31
25.8	21.05	967.19
25.9	21.14	967.08
26.0	21.22	966.97
26.1	21.31	966.85
26.2	21.39	966.74
26.3	21.47	966.62
26.4	21.56	966.51
26.5	21.64	966.39
26.6	21.73	966.28
26.7	21.81	966.16
26.8	21.90	966.05
26.9	21.98	965.93
27.0	22.06	965.81
27.1	22.15	965.70
27.2	22.23	965.58
27.3	22.32	965.46
27.4	22.40	965.35
27.5	22.49	965.23
27.6	22.57	965.11
27.7	22.65	964.99
27.8	22.74	964.88
27.9	22.82	964.76
28.0	22.91	964.64
28.1	22.99	964.52
28.2	23.08	964.40
28.3	23.16	964.28
28.4	23.25	964.16
28.5	23.33	964.04
28.6	23.42	963.92
28.7	23.50	963.80
28.8	23.59	963.68
28.9	23.67	963.56
29.0	23.76	963.44
29.1	23.84	963.32
29.2	23.93	963.20
29.3	24.01	963.07
29.4	24.10	962.95

% V/V	% m/m	ρ_{20} (kg/m^3)
29.5	24.18	962.83
29.6	24.27	962.71
29.7	24.35	962.58
29.8	24.44	962.46
29.9	24.52	962.33
30.0	24.61	962.21
30.1	24.69	962.09
30.2	24.78	961.96
30.3	24.86	961.84
30.4	24.95	961.71
30.5	25.03	961.59
30.6	25.12	961.46
30.7	25.20	961.33
30.8	25.29	961.21
30.9	25.38	961.08
31.0	25.46	960.95
31.1	25.55	960.82
31.2	25.63	960.70
31.3	25.72	960.57
31.4	25.80	960.44
31.5	25.89	960.31
31.6	25.97	960.18
31.7	26.06	960.05
31.8	26.15	959.92
31.9	26.23	959.79
32.0	26.32	959.66
32.1	26.40	959.53
32.2	26.49	959.40
32.3	26.57	959.27
32.4	26.66	959.14
32.5	26.75	959.01
32.6	26.83	958.87
32.7	26.92	958.74
32.8	27.00	958.61
32.9	27.09	958.47
33.0	27.18	958.34
33.1	27.26	958.20
33.2	27.35	958.07
33.3	27.44	957.94
33.4	27.52	957.80
33.5	27.61	957.66
33.6	27.69	957.53
33.7	27.78	957.39

% *V/V*	% *m/m*	ρ_{20} (kg/m³)
33.8	27.87	957.26
33.9	27.95	957.12
34.0	28.04	956.98
34.1	28.13	956.84
34.2	28.21	956.70
34.3	28.30	956.57
34.4	28.39	956.43
34.5	28.47	956.29
34.6	28.56	956.15
34.7	28.65	956.01
34.8	28.73	955.87
34.9	28.82	955.73
35.0	28.91	955.59
35.1	28.99	955.45
35.2	29.08	955.30
35.3	29.17	955.16
35.4	29.26	955.02
35.5	29.34	954.88
35.6	29.43	954.73
35.7	29.52	954.59
35.8	29.60	954.44
35.9	29.69	954.30
36.0	29.78	954.15
36.1	29.87	954.01
36.2	29.95	953.86
36.3	30.04	953.72
36.4	30.13	953.57
36.5	30.21	953.42
36.6	30.30	953.28
36.7	30.39	953.13
36.8	30.48	952.98
36.9	30.56	952.83
37.0	30.65	952.69
37.1	30.74	952.54
37.2	30.83	952.39
37.3	30.92	952.24
37.4	31.00	952.09
37.5	31.09	951.94
37.6	31.18	951.79
37.7	31.27	951.63
37.8	31.35	951.48
37.9	31.44	951.33

% *V/V*	% *m/m*	ρ_{20} (kg/m³)
38.0	31.53	951.18
38.1	31.62	951.02
38.2	31.71	950.87
38.3	31.79	950.72
38.4	31.88	950.56
38.5	31.97	950.41
38.6	32.06	950.25
38.7	32.15	950.10
38.8	32.24	949.94
38.9	32.32	949.79
39.0	32.41	949.63
39.1	32.50	949.47
39.2	32.59	949.32
39.3	32.68	949.16
39.4	32.77	949.00
39.5	32.86	948.84
39.6	32.94	948.68
39.7	33.03	948.52
39.8	33.12	948.37
39.9	33.21	948.21
40.0	33.30	948.05
40.1	33.39	947.88
40.2	33.48	947.72
40.3	33.57	947.56
40.4	33.66	947.40
40.5	33.74	947.24
40.6	33.83	947.08
40.7	33.92	946.91
40.8	34.01	946.75
40.9	34.10	946.58
41.0	34.19	946.42
41.1	34.28	946.26
41.2	34.37	946.09
41.3	34.46	945.93
41.4	34.55	945.76
41.5	34.64	945.59
41.6	34.73	945.43
41.7	34.82	945.26
41.8	34.91	945.09
41.9	35.00	944.93
42.0	35.09	944.76
42.1	35.18	944.59
42.2	35.27	944.42

% *V/V*	% *m/m*	ρ_{20} (kg/m³)
42.3	35.36	944.25
42.4	35.45	944.08
42.5	35.54	943.91
42.6	35.63	943.74
42.7	35.72	943.57
42.8	35.81	943.40
42.9	35.90	943.23
43.0	35.99	943.06
43.1	36.08	942.88
43.2	36.17	942.71
43.3	36.26	942.54
43.4	36.35	942.37
43.5	36.44	942.19
43.6	36.53	942.02
43.7	36.62	941.84
43.8	36.71	941.67
43.9	36.80	941.49
44.0	36.89	941.32
44.1	36.98	941.14
44.2	37.07	940.97
44.3	37.16	940.79
44.4	37.25	940.61
44.5	37.35	940.43
44.6	37.44	940.26
44.7	37.53	940.08
44.8	37.62	939.90
44.9	37.71	939.72
45.0	37.80	939.54
45.1	37.89	939.36
45.2	37.98	939.18
45.3	38.08	939.00
45.4	38.17	938.82
45.5	38.26	938.64
45.6	38.35	938.46
45.7	38.44	938.28
45.8	38.53	938.10
45.9	38.62	937.91
46.0	38.72	937.73
46.1	38.81	937.55
46.2	38.90	937.36
46.3	38.99	937.18
46.4	39.08	937.00
46.5	39.18	936.81
46.6	39.27	936.63
46.7	39.36	936.44
46.8	39.45	936.26
46.9	39.54	936.07
47.0	39.64	935.88
47.1	39.73	935.70
47.2	39.82	935.51
47.3	39.91	935.32
47.4	40.00	935.14
47.5	40.10	934.95
47.6	40.19	934.76
47.7	40.28	934.57
47.8	40.37	934.38
47.9	40.47	934.19
48.0	40.56	934.00
48.1	40.65	933.81
48.2	40.75	933.62
48.3	40.84	933.43
48.4	40.93	933.24
48.5	41.02	933.05
48.6	41.12	932.86
48.7	41.21	932.67
48.8	41.30	932.47
48.9	41.40	932.28
49.0	41.49	932.09
49.1	41.58	931.90
49.2	41.68	931.70
49.3	41.77	931.51
49.4	41.86	931.31
49.5	41.96	931.12
49.6	42.05	930.92
49.7	42.14	930.73
49.8	42.24	930.53
49.9	42.33	930.34
50.0	42.43	930.14
50.1	42.52	929.95
50.2	42.61	929.75
50.3	42.71	929.55
50.4	42.80	929.35
50.5	42.90	929.16
50.6	42.99	928.96
50.7	43.08	928.76
50.8	43.18	928.56

5. General texts

% *V/V*	% *m/m*	ρ_{20} (kg/m³)
50.9	43.27	928.36
51.0	43.37	928.16
51.1	43.46	927.96
51.2	43.56	927.77
51.3	43.65	927.57
51.4	43.74	927.36
51.5	43.84	927.16
51.6	43.93	926.96
51.7	44.03	926.76
51.8	44.12	926.56
51.9	44.22	926.36
52.0	44.31	926.16
52.1	44.41	925.95
52.2	44.50	925.75
52.3	44.60	925.55
52.4	44.69	925.35
52.5	44.79	925.14
52.6	44.88	924.94
52.7	44.98	924.73
52.8	45.07	924.53
52.9	45.17	924.32
53.0	45.26	924.12
53.1	45.36	923.91
53.2	45.46	923.71
53.3	45.55	923.50
53.4	45.65	923.30
53.5	45.74	923.09
53.6	45.84	922.88
53.7	45.93	922.68
53.8	46.03	922.47
53.9	46.13	922.26
54.0	46.22	922.06
54.1	46.32	921.85
54.2	46.41	921.64
54.3	46.51	921.43
54.4	46.61	921.22
54.5	46.70	921.01
54.6	46.80	920.80
54.7	46.90	920.59
54.8	46.99	920.38
54.9	47.09	920.17
55.0	47.18	919.96

% *V/V*	% *m/m*	ρ_{20} (kg/m³)
55.1	47.28	919.75
55.2	47.38	919.54
55.3	47.47	919.33
55.4	47.57	919.12
55.5	47.67	918.91
55.6	47.77	918.69
55.7	47.86	918.48
55.8	47.96	918.27
55.9	48.06	918.06
56.0	48.15	917.84
56.1	48.25	917.63
56.2	48.35	917.42
56.3	48.45	917.20
56.4	48.54	916.99
56.5	48.64	916.77
56.6	48.74	916.56
56.7	48.84	916.35
56.8	48.93	916.13
56.9	49.03	915.91
57.0	49.13	915.70
57.1	49.23	915.48
57.2	49.32	915.27
57.3	49.42	915.05
57.4	49.52	914.83
57.5	49.62	914.62
57.6	49.72	914.40
57.7	49.81	914.18
57.8	49.91	913.97
57.9	50.01	913.75
58.0	50.11	913.53
58.1	50.21	913.31
58.2	50.31	913.09
58.3	50.40	912.87
58.4	50.50	912.65
58.5	50.60	912.43
58.6	50.70	912.22
58.7	50.80	912.00
58.8	50.90	911.78
58.9	51.00	911.55
59.0	51.10	911.33
59.1	51.19	911.11
59.2	51.29	910.89
59.3	51.39	910.67

% *V/V*	% *m/m*	ρ_{20} (kg/m^3)
59.4	51.49	910.45
59.5	51.59	910.23
59.6	51.69	910.01
59.7	51.79	909.78
59.8	51.89	909.56
59.9	51.99	909.34
60.0	52.09	909.11
60.1	52.19	908.89
60.2	52.29	908.67
60.3	52.39	908.44
60.4	52.49	908.22
60.5	52.59	908.00
60.6	52.69	907.77
60.7	52.79	907.55
60.8	52.89	907.32
60.9	52.99	907.10
61.0	53.09	906.87
61.1	53.19	906.64
61.2	53.29	906.42
61.3	53.39	906.19
61.4	53.49	905.97
61.5	53.59	905.74
61.6	53.69	905.51
61.7	53.79	905.29
61.8	53.89	905.06
61.9	53.99	904.83
62.0	54.09	904.60
62.1	54.19	904.37
62.2	54.30	904.15
62.3	54.40	903.92
62.4	54.50	903.69
62.5	54.60	903.46
62.6	54.70	903.23
62.7	54.80	903.00
62.8	54.90	902.77
62.9	55.00	902.54
63.0	55.11	902.31
63.1	55.21	902.08
63.2	55.31	901.85
63.3	55.41	901.62
63.4	55.51	901.39
63.5	55.61	901.15
63.6	55.72	900.92
63.7	55.82	900.69
63.8	55.92	900.46
63.9	56.02	900.23
64.0	56.12	899.99
64.1	56.23	899.76
64.2	56.33	899.53
64.3	56.43	899.29
64.4	56.53	899.06
64.5	56.64	898.83
64.6	56.74	898.59
64.7	56.84	898.36
64.8	56.94	898.12
64.9	57.05	897.89
65.0	57.15	897.65
65.1	57.25	897.42
65.2	57.36	897.18
65.3	57.46	896.94
65.4	57.56	896.71
65.5	57.67	896.47
65.6	57.77	896.23
65.7	57.87	896.00
65.8	57.98	895.76
65.9	58.08	895.52
66.0	58.18	895.28
66.1	58.29	895.05
66.2	58.39	894.81
66.3	58.49	894.57
66.4	58.60	894.33
66.5	58.70	894.09
66.6	58.81	893.85
66.7	58.91	893.61
66.8	59.01	893.37
66.9	59.12	893.13
67.0	59.22	892.89
67.1	59.33	892.65
67.2	59.43	892.41
67.3	59.54	892.17
67.4	59.64	891.93
67.5	59.74	891.69
67.6	59.85	891.45
67.7	59.95	891.20
67.8	60.06	890.96
67.9	60.16	890.72

% *V/V*	% *m/m*	ρ_{20} (kg/m³)
68.0	60.27	890.48
68.1	60.37	890.23
68.2	60.48	889.99
68.3	60.58	889.75
68.4	60.69	889.50
68.5	60.80	889.26
68.6	60.90	889.01
68.7	61.01	888.77
68.8	61.11	888.52
68.9	61.22	888.28
69.0	61.32	888.03
69.1	61.43	887.79
69.2	61.54	887.54
69.3	61.64	887.29
69.4	61.75	887.05
69.5	61.85	886.80
69.6	61.96	886.55
69.7	62.07	886.31
69.8	62.17	886.06
69.9	62.28	885.81
70.0	62.39	885.56
70.1	62.49	885.31
70.2	62.60	885.06
70.3	62.71	884.82
70.4	62.81	884.57
70.5	62.92	884.32
70.6	63.03	884.07
70.7	63.13	883.82
70.8	63.24	883.57
70.9	63.35	883.32
71.0	63.46	883.06
71.1	63.56	882.81
71.2	63.67	882.56
71.3	63.78	882.31
71.4	63.89	882.06
71.5	63.99	881.81
71.6	64.10	881.55
71.7	64.21	881.30
71.8	64.32	881.05
71.9	64.43	880.79
72.0	64.53	880.54
72.1	64.64	880.29

% *V/V*	% *m/m*	ρ_{20} (kg/m³)
72.2	64.75	880.03
72.3	64.86	879.78
72.4	64.97	879.52
72.5	65.08	879.27
72.6	65.19	879.01
72.7	65.29	878.75
72.8	65.40	878.50
72.9	65.51	878.24
73.0	65.62	877.99
73.1	65.73	877.73
73.2	65.84	877.47
73.3	65.95	877.21
73.4	66.06	876.96
73.5	66.17	876.70
73.6	66.28	876.44
73.7	66.39	876.18
73.8	66.50	875.92
73.9	66.61	875.66
74.0	66.72	875.40
74.1	66.83	875.14
74.2	66.94	874.88
74.3	67.05	874.62
74.4	67.16	874.36
74.5	67.27	874.10
74.6	67.38	873.84
74.7	67.49	873.58
74.8	67.60	873.32
74.9	67.71	873.06
75.0	67.82	872.79
75.1	67.93	872.53
75.2	68.04	872.27
75.3	68.15	872.00
75.4	68.26	871.74
75.5	68.38	871.48
75.6	68.49	871.21
75.7	68.60	870.95
75.8	68.71	870.68
75.9	68.82	870.42
76.0	68.93	870.15
76.1	69.04	869.89
76.2	69.16	869.62
76.3	69.27	869.35
76.4	69.38	869.09

% V/V	% m/m	ρ_{20} (kg/m^3)
76.5	69.49	868.82
76.6	69.61	868.55
76.7	69.72	868.28
76.8	69.83	868.02
76.9	69.94	867.75
77.0	70.06	867.48
77.1	70.17	867.21
77.2	70.28	866.94
77.3	70.39	866.67
77.4	70.51	866.40
77.5	70.62	866.13
77.6	70.73	865.86
77.7	70.85	865.59
77.8	70.96	865.32
77.9	71.07	865.05
78.0	71.19	864.78
78.1	71.30	864.50
78.2	71.41	864.23
78.3	71.53	863.96
78.4	71.64	863.69
78.5	71.76	863.41
78.6	71.87	863.14
78.7	71.98	862.86
78.8	72.10	862.59
78.9	72.21	862.31
79.0	72.33	862.04
79.1	72.44	861.76
79.2	72.56	861.49
79.3	72.67	861.21
79.4	72.79	860.94
79.5	72.90	860.66
79.6	73.02	860.38
79.7	73.13	860.10
79.8	73.25	859.83
79.9	73.36	859.55
80.0	73.48	859.27
80.1	73.60	858.99
80.2	73.71	858.71
80.3	73.83	858.43
80.4	73.94	858.15
80.5	74.06	857.87
80.6	74.18	857.59
80.7	74.29	857.31

% V/V	% m/m	ρ_{20} (kg/m^3)
80.8	74.41	857.03
80.9	74.53	856.75
81.0	74.64	856.46
81.1	74.76	856.18
81.2	74.88	855.90
81.3	74.99	855.62
81.4	75.11	855.33
81.5	75.23	855.05
81.6	75.34	854.76
81.7	75.46	854.48
81.8	75.58	854.19
81.9	75.70	853.91
82.0	75.82	853.62
82.1	75.93	853.34
82.2	76.05	853.05
82.3	76.17	852.76
82.4	76.29	852.48
82.5	76.41	852.19
82.6	76.52	851.90
82.7	76.64	851.61
82.8	76.76	851.32
82.9	76.88	851.03
83.0	77.00	850.74
83.1	77.12	850.45
83.2	77.24	850.16
83.3	77.36	849.87
83.4	77.48	849.58
83.5	77.60	849.29
83.6	77.72	848.99
83.7	77.84	848.70
83.8	77.96	848.41
83.9	78.08	848.11
84.0	78.20	847.82
84.1	78.32	847.53
84.2	78.44	847.23
84.3	78.56	846.93
84.4	78.68	846.64
84.5	78.80	846.34
84.6	78.92	846.05
84.7	79.04	845.75
84.8	79.16	845.45
84.9	79.28	845.15

% *V/V*	% *m/m*	ρ_{20} (kg/m^3)
85.0	79.40	844.85
85.1	79.53	844.55
85.2	79.65	844.25
85.3	79.77	843.95
85.4	79.89	843.65
85.5	80.01	843.35
85.6	80.14	843.05
85.7	80.26	842.75
85.8	80.38	842.44
85.9	80.50	842.14
86.0	80.63	841.84
86.1	80.75	841.53
86.2	80.87	841.23
86.3	81.00	840.92
86.4	81.12	840.62
86.5	81.24	840.31
86.6	81.37	840.00
86.7	81.49	839.70
86.8	81.61	839.39
86.9	81.74	839.08
87.0	81.86	838.77
87.1	81.99	838.46
87.2	82.11	838.15
87.3	82.24	837.84
87.4	82.36	837.52
87.5	82.49	837.21
87.6	82.61	836.90
87.7	82.74	836.59
87.8	82.86	836.27
87.9	82.99	835.96
88.0	83.11	835.64
88.1	83.24	835.32
88.2	83.37	835.01
88.3	83.49	834.69
88.4	83.62	834.37
88.5	83.74	834.05
88.6	83.87	833.73
88.7	84.00	833.41
88.8	84.13	833.09
88.9	84.25	832.77
89.0	84.38	832.45
89.1	84.51	832.12
89.2	84.64	831.80
89.3	84.76	831.48
89.4	84.89	831.15
89.5	85.02	830.82
89.6	85.15	830.50
89.7	85.28	830.17
89.8	85.41	829.84
89.9	85.54	829.51
90.0	85.66	829.18
90.1	85.79	828.85
90.2	85.92	828.52
90.3	86.05	828.19
90.4	86.18	827.85
90.5	86.31	827.52
90.6	86.44	827.18
90.7	86.57	826.85
90.8	86.71	826.51
90.9	86.84	826.17
91.0	86.97	825.83
91.1	87.10	825.49
91.2	87.23	825.15
91.3	87.36	824.81
91.4	87.49	824.47
91.5	87.63	824.13
91.6	87.76	823.78
91.7	87.89	823.44
91.8	88.02	823.09
91.9	88.16	822.74
92.0	88.29	822.39
92.1	88.42	822.04
92.2	88.56	821.69
92.3	88.69	821.34
92.4	88.83	820.99
92.5	88.96	820.63
92.6	89.10	820.28
92.7	89.23	819.92
92.8	89.37	819.57
92.9	89.50	819.21
93.0	89.64	818.85
93.1	89.77	818.49
93.2	89.91	818.12
93.3	90.05	817.76
93.4	90.18	817.40
93.5	90.32	817.03

% *V/V*	% *m/m*	ρ_{20} (kg/m^3)	% *V/V*	% *m/m*	ρ_{20} (kg/m^3)
93.6	90.46	816.66	96.9	95.16	803.70
93.7	90.59	816.30			
93.8	90.73	815.93	97.0	95.31	803.27
93.9	90.87	815.55	97.1	95.45	802.85
			97.2	95.60	802.42
94.0	91.01	815.18	97.3	95.75	801.99
94.1	91.15	814.81	97.4	95.90	801.55
94.2	91.29	814.43	97.5	96.05	801.12
94.3	91.43	814.06	97.6	96.21	800.68
94.4	91.56	813.68	97.7	96.36	800.24
94.5	91.70	813.30	97.8	96.51	799.80
94.6	91.84	812.92	97.9	96.66	799.35
94.7	91.98	812.54			
94.8	92.13	812.15	98.0	96.81	798.90
94.9	92.27	811.77	98.1	96.97	798.45
			98.2	97.12	798.00
95.0	92.41	811.38	98.3	97.28	797.54
95.1	92.55	810.99	98.4	97.43	797.08
95.2	92.69	810.60	98.5	97.59	796.62
95.3	92.83	810.21	98.6	97.74	796.15
95.4	92.98	809.82	98.7	97.90	795.68
95.5	93.12	809.42	98.8	98.06	795.21
95.6	93.26	809.02	98.9	98.22	794.73
95.7	93.41	808.63			
95.8	93.55	808.23	99.0	98.38	794.25
95.9	93.69	807.82	99.1	98.53	793.77
			99.2	98.69	793.28
96.0	93.84	807.42	99.3	98.86	792.79
96.1	93.98	807.01	99.4	99.02	792.30
96.2	94.13	806.61	99.5	99.18	791.80
96.3	94.27	806.20	99.6	99.34	791.29
96.4	94.42	805.78	99.7	99.50	790.79
96.5	94.57	805.37	99.8	99.67	790.28
96.6	94.71	804.96	99.9	99.83	789.76
96.7	94.86	804.54			
96.8	95.01	804.12	100.0	100.0	789.24

5.6. ASSAY OF INTERFERONS

01/2005:50600

5.6. ASSAY OF INTERFERONS

The following chapter is published for information.

1. INTRODUCTION

Monographs on human interferons generally contain a bioassay based on the inhibitory activity of the interferon on the cytopathic action of a virus on a cell line in culture. In most cases, however, the virus, cell line and the assay details are not specified, in order to allow the appropriate flexibility, where the monograph covers more than one sub-class of interferon.

The present text is intended to provide outline information for the analyst on how to design, optimise and validate such an assay once an appropriate combination of cell line and cytopathic virus has been identified. A detailed procedure for a particular cytopathic antiviral assay is described as an example of a suitable method, together with information on other virus-cell line combinations and guidance on how to adapt and validate the procedure for these other combinations.

2. ANTIVIRAL (CYTOPATHIC EFFECT REDUCTION) ASSAYS

The antiviral assay of human interferons is based on the induction of a cellular response in human cells, which prevents or reduces the cytopathic effect of an infectious virus. The potency of interferon is estimated by comparing its protective effect against a viral cytopathic effect with the same effect of the appropriate reference preparation calibrated in International Units.

3. INTERFERON ASSAY USING Hep2c CELLS AND INFECTIOUS ENCEPHALOMYOCARDITIS VIRUS

The antiviral assay of human interferons described is of the cytopathic effect reduction type. It uses human Hep2c cells infected by encephalomyocarditis virus (EMCV) to measure the potencies of different human interferon test preparations. This assay has been used in three World Health Organisation (WHO) international collaborative studies of candidate International Standards for human interferon alpha, human interferon beta and human interferon gamma and has repeatedly been demonstrated to be sensitive, reliable and reproducible for potency estimations of the different types of human interferon.

For the culture of mammalian cells, all procedures are carried out using standard operating procedures for the maintenance of such cell lines in culture. Volumes of reagents are indicated for cell cultures carried out in 75 cm^2 flasks. Other types of containers (flasks or plates) may be used but volumes must be adapted accordingly.

3.1. MAINTENANCE AND PREPARATION OF Her2c CELLS

Hep2c cells are maintained and passaged in culture medium A.

Cells are stored as frozen stocks using standard operating procedures. Growing cells may be maintained in culture up to a permitted passage number of 30, after which new cultures are established from frozen stocks.

At the beginning of the assay procedure, harvest the cells from the flasks showing 90 per cent confluent monolayers using the trypsin-treatment procedure described below.

- Remove the culture medium from the flasks.
- To each flask, add 5 ml of trypsin solution heated at 37 °C (a trypsin stock solution contains 4 mg/ml of *trypsin R* and 4 mg/ml of *sodium edetate R*; immediately before use, dilute 50 times with phosphate buffered saline). Swirl the capped flask to wash the cell monolayer. Remove the excess of trypsin solution.
- Incubate the flasks for 5 min to 10 min at 37 °C. Microscopically or visually observe the cells for signs of detachment. When viewed microscopically, the cells appear rounded up or detached and free-floating. Shake the flask vigorously to detach all the cells, add approximately 5 ml of culture medium A. Shake vigorously to yield a suspension of single cells.
- To prepare the cell suspensions for the assay procedure, carefully disperse the cells by pipetting up and down to disrupt cell aggregates, count the cells and resuspend at a concentration of 6×10^5 cells/ml.

3.2. PROPAGATION OF ENCEPHALOMYOCARDITIS VIRUS

Encephalomyocarditis virus is propagated in mouse L-929 cells in order to produce a stock of progeny virus. L-929 cells are maintained by trypsin treatment and passage as described for Hep2c cells (*NOTE: it may be necessary to substitute neonatal calf serum with foetal bovine serum if the cells show poor growth*).

Take several flasks containing confluent cultures of L-929 cells. Pour off the medium from the flasks. Inoculate with 2 ml of the EMCV suspension appropriately diluted in culture medium B so that it contains approximately 2.5×10^8 plaque forming units (PFU) per millilitre. Each flask will contain $4\text{-}6 \times 10^7$ L-929 cells and therefore the multiplicity of infection (m.o.i.) will be approximately 10 PFU/cell. Carefully swirl the virus suspension over the entire cell monolayer and return the flasks to the incubator for approximately 1 h. Maintain the medium at pH 7.4 to 7.8.

After adsorption of the EMCV, add approximately 40 ml of culture medium B to each flask and return the flasks to the incubator at 37 °C for about 30 h. Maintain the medium at pH 7.4 to 7.8 to obtain a maximum virus yield. Remove the culture fluid and store at approximately 40 °C.

Place the flasks at − 20 °C to freeze the cell monolayer. Then thaw to room temperature. Add approximately 5 ml of culture medium and shake the flask to disrupt the cell walls. Transfer the contents of each flask to the container of culture fluid. Transfer the culture fluid containing the EMCV to 50 ml plastic centrifuge tubes and centrifuge at approximately 500 *g* for about 10 min to remove cell debris. Dispense the clarified culture fluid into glass screw-capped bottles, in quantities of 20 ml, 10 ml, 5 ml, 1 ml, 0.5 ml or 0.2 ml, as appropriate. Store at − 70 °C. Larger volumes can be thawed, dispensed into smaller quantities and re-frozen when required. The EMCV stock will retain its original titre if stored permanently at approximately − 70 °C, but repeated freeze-thaw cycles or storage at higher temperatures, e.g. at approximately − 20 °C, results in progressive loss of titre.

3.3. ASSAY PROCEDURE

3.3.1. Determination of the dose-response range

Preparation of the solutions

Dilute the appropriate standard for interferon (for example a specific WHO sub-type interferon standard) in culture medium A, in 10-fold dose increments, to give doses covering the range of 1000 - 0.001 IU/ml. Carry out the assay procedure in 96-well microtitre plates. To each well add 100 µl of culture medium A. Add approximately 100 µl of each dilution of the reference preparation to each well except for those intended for virus controls. Using a multichannel pipette set at 100 µl, mix the contents of the wells.

Dispensing of the cell suspension

Pour the cell suspension of Hep2c cells, which has been adjusted to contain approximately 6 × 10^5 cells/ml of culture medium A, into a plastic Petri-dish. Dispense the cell suspension from the Petri-dish into each well of the microtitre plates, using a multichannel pipette set at 100 µl.

Incubate the plates for about 24 h in an incubator set at 37 °C and 5 per cent CO_2.

Viral infection

At this stage, using an inverted microscope, check that the monolayers of Hep2c cells are confluent, that they show a relatively even distribution of cells, that they have correct morphology and that they are healthy.

Remove most of the culture medium from the wells by inverting the plate and shaking it and blotting on a paper towel (proceed in an identical way when discarding fluids from micro-titre plates as described later). Dilute the EMCV stock with fresh culture medium A to a titre of approximately 3 × 10^7 PFU/ml (*NOTE: each plate requires approximately 20 ml of diluted virus, plus 5 per cent to 10 per cent of extra volume*). Dispense the diluted suspension from a 9 cm sterile Petri-dish using a multichannel pipette set at 200 µl to all wells including virus controls, but excluding cell controls. Add approximately 200 µl of culture medium A without virus to each of the cell control wells.

Return the plates to the incubator set at 37 °C and 5 per cent CO_2 for approximately 24 h.

Staining

Examine the plates microscopically to check that the EMCV has caused a cytopathic effect (c.p.e.) in the virus controls. The time interval for maximum c.p.e. may vary from one assay to the next because of inherent variation of Hep2c cells to virus challenge over a given period of continuous cultivation.

Remove most of the culture medium from the wells by discarding into an appropriate decontaminating solution (sodium hypochlorite is suitable). Dispense *phosphate buffered saline pH 7.4 R* into each well. Discard the *phosphate buffered saline pH 7.4 R* into a decontaminating solution. Dispense into each well 150 µl of staining solution. Stain the cells for approximately 30 min at room temperature. Discard the staining solution into a decontaminating solution. Dispense approximately 150 µl of fixing solution. Fix for 10 min at room temperature. Discard the fixing solution into a decontaminating solution and wash the cell monolayers by immersing the assay plates in a plastic box containing running water. Discard the water and superficially dry the plates with paper towels. Dry the assay plates at 20 °C to 37 °C until all moisture has evaporated.

Add 150 µl of *0.1 M sodium hydroxide* to each well. Elute the stain by gentle agitation of the plates or by hitting them against the palm of the hand. Make sure that the stain is evenly distributed in all wells before making spectrophotometric readings.

Read the absorbance at 610 nm to 620 nm, using a microtitre plate reader, taking as a blank a well or a column of wells containing no cells and approximately 150 µl of *0.1 M sodium hydroxide*.

Estimate the concentrations of interferon standard that give the maximum and minimum reduction of cytopathic effect. This is the dose response corresponding to the working range of the assay.

3.3.2. Assay procedure

Carry out the assay as described above, using:

- as test solutions, the substance to be examined, diluted in two-fold increments with culture medium A to give nominal concentrations covering the working range of the assay,
- as reference solutions, the appropriate standard for interferon (for example, a specific WHO sub-type interferon) in culture medium A, diluted in two-fold increments to give nominal concentrations covering the working range of the assay.

3.3.3. Data analysis

Results of the cytopathic effect reduction assay generally fit a sigmoidal dose-response curve, when the interferon concentration (the log of the reciprocal of the interferon dilution) is plotted versus stain absorbance.

Plot the interferon concentration (log reciprocal of dilution) versus the stain absorbance for the interferon reference preparation and for the interferon test solutions. Using the linear portion of the curve, calculate the concentration of interferon in the sample by comparing the responses for test and reference solutions, using the usual statistical methods for a parallel line assay.

4. VALIDATION OF OTHER PROCEDURES

4.1. CHOICE OF CELL LINE AND VIRUS

A number of other combinations of cell line and virus have been used in anti-viral assays for interferons. For example, EMCV has been used in combination with the A549 epithelial lung carcinoma cell line, Semliki Forest virus or Sindbis virus have been used with human fibroblasts, and vesicular stomatitis virus has been used with either human diploid fibroblasts, the human amnion WISH cell line or the Madin-Darby bovine kidney cell line. In each case the choice of the cell line/virus combination is usually based on that which gives the most sensitive response to the interferon preparation to be assayed, and gives parallel responses when comparing the test preparation and interferon standard.

4.2. CHOICE OF RESPONSE

The staining procedure described above measures remaining viable cells. A number of other responses have been used, including methyl violet or crystal violet staining, or the thiazolyl blue (MTT) conversion procedure. In each case, the method is selected on the basis of producing a suitably linear and sensitive relationship between response colour and viable cell count.

4.3. STATISTICAL VALIDATION

As with all parallel line bioassays, the assay must satisfy the usual statistical criteria of linearity of response, parallelism and variance.

4.4. VALIDATION OF ASSAY LAYOUT

As with all microtitre plate assay procedures, attention must be given to validating the assay layout. In particular, bias due to non-random pipetting order or plate edge effects must be investigated and eliminated, by randomising the assay layout, or by avoiding the use of edge wells.

REAGENTS AND CULTURE MEDIA

Culture medium A (10 per cent neonatal calf serum)

RPMI 1640 culture medium, supplemented with antibiotics if necessary (penicillin 10 000 IU/ml; streptomycin 10 ng/ml)	450 ml
L-Glutamine, 200 mM, sterile	5 ml
Neonatal calf serum	50 ml

Culture medium B (2 per cent foetal bovine serum)

RPMI 1640 culture medium, supplemented with antibiotics if necessary (penicillin 10 000 IU/ml; streptomycin 10 ng/ml)	490 ml
L-Glutamine, 200 mM, sterile	5 ml
Foetal bovine serum	10 ml

Staining solution

Naphthalene black	0.5 g
Acetic acid, glacial	90 ml
Sodium acetate, anhydrous	8.2 g
Water to produce	1000 ml

Fixing solution

Formaldehyde, 40 per cent	100 ml
Acetic acid, glacial	90 ml
Sodium acetate, anhydrous	8.2 g
Water to produce	1000 ml

5.7. TABLE OF PHYSICAL CHARACTERISTICS OF RADIONUCLIDES MENTIONED IN THE EUROPEAN PHARMACOPOEIA

01/2005:50700

5.7. TABLE OF PHYSICAL CHARACTERISTICS OF RADIONUCLIDES MENTIONED IN THE EUROPEAN PHARMACOPOEIA

The following table is given to complete the general monograph on *Radiopharmaceutical preparations (0125)*.

The values are obtained from the database of the National Nuclear Data Center (NNDC) at Brookhaven National Laboratory, Upton. N.Y., USA, directly accessible via Internet at the address: "http://www.nndc.bnl.gov/nndc/nudat/radform.html".

In case another source of information is preferred (more recent values), this source is explicitly mentioned.

Other data sources:

* DAMRI (Département des Applications et de la Métrologie des Rayonnements Ionisants, CEA Gif-sur-Yvette, France),

** PTB (Physikalisch-Technische Bundesanstalt, Braunschweig, Germany),

*** NPL (National Physical Laboratory, Teddington, Middlesex, UK).

The uncertainty of the half-lives are given in parentheses. In principle the digits in parentheses are the standard uncertainty of the corresponding last digits of the indicated numerical value "Guide to the Expression of Uncertainty in measurement", International Organisation for Standardisation (ISO), 1993, ISBN 92-67-10188-9).

The following abbreviations are used:

e_A = Auger electrons,

ce = conversion electrons,

β^- = electrons,

β^+ = positrons,

γ = gamma rays,

X = X-rays.

Radionuclide	Half-life	Electronic emission			Photon emission		
		Type	Energy (MeV)	Emission probability (per 100 disintegrations)	Type	Energy (MeV)	Emission probability (per 100 disintegrations)
Tritium (^3H)	*12.33 (6) years	*β^-	*0.006 (I) (max: 0.019)	*100			
Carbon-11 (^{11}C)	20.385 (20) min	β^+	0.386 (I) (max: 0.960)	99.8	γ	0.511	199.5 (II)
Nitrogen-13 (^{13}N)	9.965 (4) min	β^+	0.492 (I) (max: 1.198)	99.8	γ	0.511	199.6 (II)
Oxygen-15 (^{15}O)	122.24 (16) s	β^+	0.735 (I) (max: 1.732)	99.9	γ	0.511	199.8 (II)
Fluorine-18 (^{18}F)	109.77 (5) min	β^+	0.250 (I) (max: 0.633)	96.7	γ	0.511	193.5 (II)
Phosphorus-32 (^{32}P)	14.26 (4) days	β^-	0.695 (I) (max: 1.71)	100			
Phosphorus-33 (^{33}P)	25.34 (12) days	β^-	0.076 (I) (max: 0.249)	100			
Sulphur-35 (^{35}S)	87.51 (12) days	β^-	0.049 (I) (max: 0.167)	100			
Chromium-51 (^{51}Cr)	27.7025 (24) days	e_A	0.004	67	X	0.005	22.3
					γ	0.320	9.9

(I) Mean energy of the β spectrum.
(II) Maximum emission probability corresponding to a total annihilation in the source per 100 disintegrations.

5. General texts

Radionuclide	Half-life	Electronic emission			Photon emission		
		Type	Energy (MeV)	Emission probability (per 100 disintegrations)	Type	Energy (MeV)	Emission probability (per 100 disintegrations)
Cobalt-56 (^{56}Co)	77.27 (3) days	e_A	0.006	47	X	0.006-0.007	25
		β^+	0.179 (I)	0.9	γ	0.511	38.0 (II)
			0.631 (I)	18.1		0.847	100.0
						1.038	14.1
						1.175	2.2
						1.238	66.1
						1.360	4.3
						1.771	15.5
						2.015	3.0
						2.035	7.8
						2.598	17.0
						3.202	3.1
						3.253	7.6
Cobalt-57 (^{57}Co)	271.79 (9) days	e_A+ce	0.006-0.007	177.4	X	0.006-0.007	57
		ce	0.014	7.4	γ	0.014	9.2
			0.115	1.8		0.122	85.6
			0.129	1.3		0.136	10.7
						0.692	0.15
Cobalt-58 (^{58}Co)	70.86 (7) days	e_A	0.006	49.4	X	0.006-0.007	26.3
		β^+	0.201 (I)	14.9	γ	0.511	29.9 (II)
						0.811	99.4
						0.864	0.7
						1.675	0.5
Cobalt-60 (^{60}Co)	5.2714 (5) years	β^-	0.096 (I) (max: 0.318)	99.9	γ	1.173	100.0
						1.333	100.0

(I) Mean energy of the β spectrum.
(II) Maximum emission probability corresponding to a total annihilation in the source per 100 disintegrations.

5. General texts

Radionuclide	Half-life	Electronic emission			Photon emission		
		Type	Energy (MeV)	Emission probability (per 100 disintegrations)	Type	Energy (MeV)	Emission probability (per 100 disintegrations)
Gallium-66 (^{66}Ga)	9.49 (7) hours	e_A	0.008	21	X	0.009-0.010	19.1
		β^+	0.157 (I)	1	γ	0.511	112 (II)
			0.331 (I)	0.7		0.834	5.9
			0.397 (I)	3.8		1.039	37
			0.782 (I)	0.3		1.333	1.2
			1.90 (I)	50		1.919	2.1
						2.190	5.6
						2.423	1.9
						2.752	23.4
						3.229	1.5
						3.381	1.5
						3.792	1.1
						4.086	1.3
						4.295	4.1
						4.807	1.8
Gallium-67 (^{67}Ga)	3.2612 (6) days	e_A	0.008	62	X	0.008-0.010	57
		ce	0.082-0.084	30.4	γ	0.091-0.093	42.4
			0.090-0.092	3.6		0.185	21.2
			0.175	0.3		0.209	2.4
						0.300	16.8
						0.394	4.7
						0.888	0.15
Germanium-68 (^{68}Ge) in equilibrium with Gallium-68 (^{68}Ga)	270.82 (27) days	e_A	0.008	42.4	X	0.009-0.010	44.1
	(^{68}Ga: 67.629 (24) min)	β^+	0.353 (I)	1.2	γ	0.511	178.3
			0.836 (I)	88.0		1.077	3.0
Gallium-68 (^{68}Ga)	67.629 (24) min	e_A	0.008	5.1	X	0.009-0.010	4.7
		β^+	0.353 (I)	1.2	γ	0.511	178.3
			0.836 (I)	88.0		1.077	3.0
Krypton-81m (^{81m}Kr)	13.10 (3) s	ce	0.176	26.4	X	0.012-0.014	17.0
			0.189	4.6			
					γ	0.190	67.6

(I) Mean energy of the β spectrum.

(II) Maximum emission probability corresponding to a total annihilation in the source per 100 disintegrations.

Radionuclide	Half-life	Electronic emission: Type	Electronic emission: Energy (MeV)	Electronic emission: Emission probability (per 100 disintegrations)	Photon emission: Type	Photon emission: Energy (MeV)	Photon emission: Emission probability (per 100 disintegrations)
Rubidium-81 (^{81}Rb) in equilibrium with Krypton-81m (^{81m}Kr)	4.576 (5) hours	e_A	0.011	31.3	X	0.013-0.014	57.2
		ce	0.176	25.0	γ	0.190	64
			0.188	4.3		0.446	23.2
						0.457	3.0
		$β^+$	0.253 (I)	1.8		0.510	5.3
			0.447 (I)	25.0		0.511	54.2
	(^{81m}Kr:13.10 (3) s)					0.538	2.2
Strontium-89 (^{89}Sr) in equilibrium with Yttrium-89m (^{89m}Y)	50.53 (7) days (^{89m}Y:16.06 (4) s)	$β^-$	0.583 (I) (max: 1.492)	99.99	γ	0.909	0.01
Strontium-90 (^{90}Sr) in equilibrium with Yttrium-90 (^{90}Y)	28.74 (4) years (^{90}Y: 64.10 (8) hours)	$β^-$	0.196 (I) (max: 0.546)	100			
Yttrium-90 (^{90}Y)	64.10 (8) hours	$β^-$	0.934 (I) (max: 2.280)	100			
Molybdene-99 (^{99}Mo) in equilibrium with Technetium-99m (^{99m}Tc)	65.94 (1) hours	$β^-$	0.133 (I)	16.4	X	0.018-0.021	3.6
			0.290 (I)	1.1			
			0.443 (I)	82.4	γ	0.041	1.1
						0.141	4.5
						0.181	6
						0.366	1.2
	(^{99m}Tc: 6.01 (1) hours)					0.740	12.1
						0.778	4.3
Technetium-99m (^{99m}Tc)	6.01 (1) hours	ce	0.002	74	X	0.018-0.021	7.3
		e_A	0.015	2.1	γ	0.141	89.1
		ce	0.120	9.4			
			0.137-0.140	1.3			
Technetium-99 (^{99}Tc)	2.11 × 10^5 years	$β^-$	0.085 (I) (max: 0.294)	100			

(I) Mean energy of the β spectrum.
(II) Maximum emission probability corresponding to a total annihilation in the source per 100 disintegrations.

Radionuclide	Half-life	Electronic emission			Photon emission		
		Type	**Energy (MeV)**	**Emission probability (per 100 disintegrations)**	**Type**	**Energy (MeV)**	**Emission probability (per 100 disintegrations)**
	39.26 (2) days	e_A+ce	0.017	12	X	0.020-0.023	9.0
Ruthenium-103 (^{103}Ru) in equilibrium with Rhodium-103m (^{103m}Rh)		ce	0.030-0.039	88.3	γ	0.497	91
						0.610	5.8
		β^-	0.031 (I)	6.6			
	(^{103m}Rh: 56.114 (20) min)		0.064 (I)	92.2			
	4.9 (1) hours	e_A	0.019	13.4	X	0.023-0.026	70.5
					γ	0.642	25.9
Indium-110 (^{110}In)						0.658	98.3
						0.885	92.9
						0.938	68.4
						0.997	10.5
	69.1 (5) min	e_A	0.019	5.3	X	0.023-0.026	27.8
Indium-110m (^{110m}In)		β^+	1.015 (I)	61	γ	0.511	123.4 (II)
						0.658	97.8
						2.129	2.1
	2.8047 (5) days	e_A	0.019	15.6	X	0.003	6.9
						0.023-0.026	82.3
Indium-111 (^{111}In)		ce	0.145	7.8			
			0.167-0.171	1.3	γ	0.171	90.2
			0.219	4.9		0.245	94.0
			0.241-0.245	1.0			
	49.51 (1) days	ce	0.162	40	X	0.023-0.027	36.3
Indium-114m (^{114m}In) in equilibrium with Indium-114 (^{114}In)			0.186-0.190	40			
					γ	0.190	15.6
		˙β^-	0.777 (I) (max: 1.985)	95		0.558	3.2
	(^{114}In: 71.9 (1) s)					0.725	3.2
	154.0 (7) days	e_A	0.003	88.0	X	0.026-0.031	50.5
			0.022-0.023	7.4			
Tellurium-121m (^{121m}Te) in equilibrium with Tellure-121 (^{121}Te)					γ	0.212	81.4
		ce	0.050	33.2		1.102	2.5
	(^{121}Te: 19.16 (5) days)		0.077	40.0			
			0.180	6.1			

(I) Mean energy of the β spectrum.
(II) Maximum emission probability corresponding to a total annihilation in the source per 100 disintegrations.

5. General texts

Radionuclide	Half-life	Electronic emission: Type	Electronic emission: Energy (MeV)	Electronic emission: Emission probability (per 100 disintegrations)	Photon emission: Type	Photon emission: Energy (MeV)	Photon emission: Emission probability (per 100 disintegrations)
Tellurium-121 (^{121}Te)	19.16 (5) days	e_A	0.022	11.6	X	0.026-0.030	75.6
					γ	0.470	1.4
						0.508	17.7
						0.573	80.3
Iodine-123 (^{123}I)	13.27 (8) hours	e_A	0.023	12.3	X	0.004	9.3
						0.027-0.031	86.6
		ce	0.127	13.6			
			0.154	1.8	γ	0.159	83.3
			0.158	0.4		0.346	0.1
						0.440	0.4
						0.505	0.3
						0.529	1.4
						0.538	0.4
Iodine-125 (^{125}I)	59.402 (14) days	e_A+ce	0.004	80	X	0.004	15.5
			0.023-0.035	33		0.027	114
						0.031	26
					γ	0.035	6.7
Iodine-126 (^{126}I)	13.11 (5) days	e_A	0.023	6	X	0.027-0.031	42.2
		ce	0.354	0.5	γ	0.388	34
			0.634	0.1		0.491	2.9
						0.511	2.3 (II)
		β^-	0.109 (I)	3.6		0.666	33
			0.290 (I)	32.1		0.754	4.2
			0.459 (I)	8.0		0.880	0.8
						1.420	0.3
		β^+	0.530 (I)	1			

(I) Mean energy of the β spectrum.
(II) Maximum emission probability corresponding to a total annihilation in the source per 100 disintegrations.

Radionuclide	Half-life	Electronic emission			Photon emission		
		Type	Energy (MeV)	Emission probability (per 100 disintegrations)	Type	Energy (MeV)	Emission probability (per 100 disintegrations)
Iodine-131 (^{131}I)	8.02070 (11) days	ce	0.46	3.5	X	0.029-0.030	3.9
			0.330	1.6			
					γ	0.080	2.6
		β^-	0.069 (I)	2.1		0.284	6.1
			0.097 (I)	7.3		0.365	81.7
			0.192 (I)	89.9		0.637	7.2
						0.723	1.8
Xenon-131m (^{131m}Xe)	11.84 (7) days	e_A	0.025	6.8	X	0.004	8.3
						0.030	44.0
		ce	0.129	61		0.034	10.2
			0.159	28.5			
			0.163	8.3	γ	0.164	2.0
Iodine-133 (^{133}I) (decays to radioactive Xenon-133)	20.8 (1) hours	β^-	0.140 (I)	3.8	γ	0.530	87
			0.162 (I)	3.2		0.875	4.5
			0.299 (I)	4.2		1.298	2.4
			0.441 (I)	83			
Xenon-133 (^{133}Xe)	5.243 (1) days	e_A	0.026	5.8	X	0.004	6.3
						0.031	40.3
		ce	0.045	55.1		0.035	9.4
			0.075-0.080	9.9			
					γ	0.080	38.3
		β^-	0.101 (I)	99.0			
Xenon-133m (^{133m}Xe) (decays to radioactive Xenon-133)	2.19 (1) days	e_A	0.025	7	X	0.004	7.8
						0.030	45.9
		ce	0.199	64.0		0.034	10.6
			0.228	20.7			
			0.232	4.6	γ	0.233	10.0

(I) Mean energy of the β spectrum.
(II) Maximum emission probability corresponding to a total annihilation in the source per 100 disintegrations.

5. General texts

Radionuclide	Half-life	Electronic emission: Type	Electronic emission: Energy (MeV)	Electronic emission: Emission probability (per 100 disintegrations)	Photon emission: Type	Photon emission: Energy (MeV)	Photon emission: Emission probability (per 100 disintegrations)
Iodine-135 (^{135}I) (decays to radioactive Xenon-135)	6.57 (2) hours	β⁻	0.140 (I)	7.4	γ	0.527	13.8
			0.237 (I)	8		0.547	7.2
			0.307 (I)	8.8		0.837	6.7
			0.352 (I)	21.9		1.039	8.0
			0.399 (I)	8		1.132	22.7
			0.444 (I)	7.5		1.260	28.9
			0.529 (I)	23.8		1.458	8.7
						1.678	9.6
						1.791	7.8
Xenon-135 (^{135}Xe)	9.14 (2) hours	ce	0.214	5.5	X	0.031-0.035	5.0
		β⁻	0.171	3.1	γ	0.250	90.2
			0.308	96.0		0.608	2.9
Caesium-137 (^{137}Cs) in equilibrium with Barium-137m (^{137m}Ba)	30.04 (3) years	e_A	0.026	0.8	X	0.005	1
						0.032-0.036	7
		ce	0.624	8.0			
			0.656	1.4	γ	0.662	85.1
		β⁻	0.174 (I)	94.4			
	(^{137m}Ba: 2.552 (1) min)		0.416 (I)	5.6			
Thallium-200 (^{200}Tl)	26.1 (1) hours	ce	0.285	3.4	X	0.010	32.0
			0.353	1.4		0.069-0.071	63.3
						0.08	17.5
		β⁺	0.495 (I)	0.3			
					γ	0.368	87.2
						0.579	13.8
						0.828	10.8
						1.206	29.9
						1.226	3.4
						1.274	3.3
						1.363	3.4
						1.515	4.0

(I) Mean energy of the β spectrum.
(II) Maximum emission probability corresponding to a total annihilation in the source per 100 disintegrations.

Radionuclide	Half-life	Electronic emission			Photon emission		
		Type	**Energy (MeV)**	**Emission probability (per 100 disintegrations)**	**Type**	**Energy (MeV)**	**Emission probability (per 100 disintegrations)**
Lead-201 (^{201}Pb) (decays to radioactive Thallium-201)	9.33 (3) hours	e_A	0.055	3	X	0.070-0.073	69
						0.083	19
		ce	0.246	8.5			
			0.276	2	γ	0.331	79
			0.316	2.3		0.361	9.9
						0.406	2.0
						0.585	3.6
						0.692	4.3
						0.767	3.2
						0.826	2.4
						0.908	5.7
						0.946	7.9
						1.099	1.8
						1.277	1.6
Thallium-201 (^{201}Tl)	72.912 (17) hours	ce	0.016-0.017	17.7	X	0.010	46.0
			0.027-0.029	4.1		0.069-0.071	73.7
			0.052	7.2		0.080	20.4
			0.084	15.4			
			0.153	2.6	γ	0.135	2.6
						0,167	10.0
Thallium-202 (^{202}Tl)	12.23 (2) days	e_A	0.054	2.8	X	0.010	31.0
						0.069-0.071	61.6
		ce	0.357	2.4		0.080	17.1
					γ	0.440	91.4
Lead-203 (^{203}Pb)	51.873 (9) hours	e_A	0.055	3.0	X	0.010	37.0
						0.071-0.073	69.6
		ce	0.194	13.3		0.083	19.4
					γ	0.279	80.8
						0.401	3.4

(I) Mean energy of the β spectrum.
(II) Maximum emission probability corresponding to a total annihilation in the source per 100 disintegrations.

5.8. PHARMACOPOEIAL HARMONISATION

01/2005:50800

5.8. PHARMACOPOEIAL HARMONISATION

This general chapter is included for guidance of users. It provides information on the degree of harmonisation and consequently interchangeability of various general chapters and monographs of the European Pharmacopoeia and those of the Japanese Pharmacopoeia and United States Pharmacopoeia. The chapter does not affect in any way the status of the monographs and general chapters as the authoritative reference in any case of doubt or dispute where compliance with the European Pharmacopoeia is required.

The European Pharmacopoeia Commission recognises the utility of working with other pharmacopoeial bodies to develop harmonised monographs and general chapters. Such harmonisation is fully compatible with the declared aims of the Commission and has benefits of different kinds, notably the simplification and rationalisation of quality control methods and licensing procedures. Such harmonisation also enhances the benefits of the work of the International Conference on Harmonisation (ICH) and the Veterinary International Co-operation on Harmonisation (VICH) since some of the guidelines developed depend on pharmacopoeial general chapters for their application.

Work on harmonisation is carried out by a well-defined but informal process in the Pharmacopoeial Discussion Group (PDG), in which the European Pharmacopoeia, the Japanese Pharmacopoeia and the United States Pharmacopoeia are associated. Information will be given in subsequent revised versions of this general chapter on items that have been dealt with by the PDG.

Where harmonisation of general chapters is carried out, the aim is to arrive at interchangeable methods or requirements so that demonstration of compliance using a general chapter from one of the three pharmacopoeias implies that the same result would be obtained using the general chapter of either of the other pharmacopoeias. If residual differences remain in harmonised general chapters, information will be given in subsequent versions of this general chapter.

Where harmonisation of monographs is carried out, the aim is to arrive at identical requirements for all attributes of a product. For some products, it can be extremely difficult to achieve complete harmonisation, for example because of differences in legal status and interpretation. It has therefore appeared to the PDG worthwhile to approve and publish monographs in which as many attributes as possible are harmonised. Information on any non-harmonised attributes will be included in subsequent versions of this general chapter.

The three Pharmacopoeias have undertaken not to make unilateral changes to harmonised monographs and general chapters but rather to apply the agreed revision procedure whereby all partners adopt a revision simultaneously.

5.9. POLYMORPHISM

01/2005:50900

5.9. POLYMORPHISM

Polymorphism (or crystal polymorphism) is a phenomenon related to the solid state; it is the ability of a compound in the solid state to exist in different crystalline forms having the same chemical composition. Substances that exist in a non-crystalline solid state are said to be amorphous.

When this phenomenon is observed for a chemical element (for example, sulphur), the term allotropy is used instead of polymorphism.

The term pseudopolymorphism is used to describe solvates (including hydrates), where a solvent is present in the crystal matrix in stoichiometric proportions; the term may also be extended to include compounds where the solvent is trapped in the matrix in variable proportions. However the term pseudopolymorphism is ambiguous because of its use in different circumstances. It is therefore preferable to use only the terms "solvates" and "hydrates".

Where a monograph indicates that a substance shows polymorphism, this may be true crystal polymorphism, occurence of solvates, allotropy or occurrence of the amorphous form.

The identity of chemical composition implies that all crystalline and amorphous forms of a given species have the same chemical behaviour in solution or as a melt; in contrast, their physico-chemical and physical characteristics (solubility, hardness, compressibility, density, melting point, etc.), and therefore their reactivity and bioavailability may be different at the solid state.

When a compound shows polymorphism, the form for which the free enthalpy is lowest at a given temperature and pressure is the most thermodynamically stable. The other forms are said to be in a metastable state. At normal temperature and pressure, a metastable form may remain unchanged or may change to a thermodynamically more stable form.

If there are several crystalline forms, one form is thermodynamically more stable at a given temperature and pressure. A given crystalline form may constitute a phase that can reach equilibrium with other solid phases and with the liquid and gas phases.

If each crystalline form is the more stable within a given temperature range, the change from one form to another is reversible and is said to be enantiotropic. The change from one phase to another is a univariate equilibrium, so that at a given pressure this state is characterised by a transition temperature. However, if only one of the forms is stable over the entire temperature range, the change is irreversible or monotropic.

Different crystalline forms or solvates may be produced by varying the crystallisation conditions (temperature, pressure, solvent, concentration, rate of crystallisation, seeding of the crystallisation medium, presence and concentration of impurities, etc.).

The following techniques may be used to study polymorphism:

- X-ray diffraction of powders,
- X-ray diffraction of single crystals,
- thermal analysis (*2.2.34*) (differential scanning calorimetry, thermogravimetry, thermomicroscopy),
- microcalorimetry,
- moisture absorption analysis,
- optical and electronic microscopy,
- solid-state nuclear magnetic resonance,
- infrared absorption spectrophotometry (*2.2.24*),
- Raman spectrometry (*2.2.48*),
- measurement of solubility and intrinsic dissolution rate,
- density measurement.

These techniques are often complementary and it is indispensable to use several of them.

Pressure/temperature and energy/temperature diagrams based on analytical data are valuable tools for fully understanding the energetic relationship (enantiotropism, monotropism) and the thermodynamic stability of the individual modifications of a polymorphic compound.

For solvates, differential scanning calorimetry and thermogravimetry are preferable, combined with measurements of solubility, intrinsic dissolution rate and X-ray diffraction.

For hydrates, water sorption/desorption isotherms are determined to demonstrate the zones of relative stability.

In general, hydrates are less soluble in water than anhydrous forms, and likewise solvates are less soluble in their solvent than unsolvated forms.

5.10. CONTROL OF IMPURITIES IN SUBSTANCES FOR PHARMACEUTICAL USE

01/2005:51000

5.10. CONTROL OF IMPURITIES IN SUBSTANCES FOR PHARMACEUTICAL USE

Preamble

The monographs of the European Pharmacopoeia on substances for pharmaceutical use are designed to ensure acceptable quality for users. The role of the Pharmacopoeia in public health protection requires that adequate control of impurities be provided by monographs. The quality required is based on scientific, technical and regulatory considerations.

Requirements concerning impurities are given in specific monographs and in the general monograph *Substances for pharmaceutical use (2034)*. Specific monographs and the general monograph are complementary: specific monographs prescribe acceptance criteria for impurities whereas the general monograph deals with the need for qualification, identification and reporting of any organic impurities that occur in *active substances.*

The thresholds for reporting, identification and qualification contained in the general monograph *Substances for pharmaceutical use (2034)* apply to all related substances. However, if a monograph does not contain a related substances test based on a quantitative method, any new impurities occurring above a threshold may be overlooked since the test is not capable to detect those impurities.

The provisions of the Related substances section of the general monograph *Substances for pharmaceutical use (2034)*, notably those concerning thresholds, do not apply to excipients; also excluded from the provisions of this section are: biological and biotechnological products; peptides; oligonucleotides; radiopharmaceuticals; fermentation products and semisynthetic products derived therefrom; herbal products and crude products of animal and plant origin. Although the thresholds stated in the general monograph do not apply, the general concepts of reporting, identification (wherever possible) and qualification of impurities are equally valid for these classes.

Basis for the elaboration of monographs of the European Pharmacopoeia

European Pharmacopoeia monographs are elaborated on substances that are present in medicinal products that have been authorised by the competent authorities of Parties to the *European Pharmacopoeia Convention*. Consequently, these monographs do not necessarily cover all sources of substances for pharmaceutical use on the world market.

Organic and inorganic impurities present in those substances that have been evaluated by the competent authorities are qualified with respect to safety at the maximum authorised content (at the maximum daily dose) unless new safety data that become available following evaluation justify lower limits.

European Pharmacopoeia monographs on substances for pharmaceutical use are elaborated by groups of experts and working parties collaborating with national pharmacopoeia authorities, the competent authorities for marketing authorisation, national control laboratories and the European Pharmacopoeia laboratory; they are also assisted by the producers of the substances and/or the pharmaceutical manufacturers that use these substances.

Control of impurities in substances for pharmaceutical use

The quality with respect to impurities is controlled by a set of tests within a monograph. These tests are intended to cover organic and inorganic impurities that are relevant in view of the sources of active substances in authorised medicinal products.

Control of residual solvents is provided by the general monograph *Substances for pharmaceutical use (2034)* and general chapter *5.4. Residual solvents*. The certificate of suitability of a monograph of the European Pharmacopoeia for a given source of a substance indicates the residual solvents that are controlled together with the specified acceptance criteria and the validated control method where this differs from those described in general chapter *2.4.24. Identification and control of residual solvents.*

Monographs on organic chemicals usually have a test entitled "Related substances" that covers relevant organic impurities. This test may be supplemented by specific tests where the general test does not control a given impurity or where there are particular reasons (for example, safety reasons) for requiring special control.

Where a monograph has no Related substances (or equivalent) test but only specific tests, the user of a substance must nevertheless ensure that there is suitable control of organic impurities; those occurring above the identification threshold are to be identified (wherever possible) and, unless justified, those occurring above the qualification threshold are to be qualified (see also under Recommendations to users of monographs of active substances).

Where the monograph covers substances with different impurity profiles, it may have a single related substances test to cover all impurities mentioned in the Impurities section or several tests may be necessary to give control of all known profiles. Compliance may be established by carrying out only the tests relevant to the known impurity profile for the source of the substance.

Instructions for control of impurities may be included in the Production section of a monograph, for example where the only analytical method appropriate for the control of a given impurity is to be performed by the manufacturer since the method is too technically complex for general use or cannot be applied to the final drug substance and/or where validation of the production process (including the purification step) will give sufficient control.

Impurities section in monographs on active substances

The Impurities section in a monograph includes impurities (chemical structure and name wherever possible), which are usually organic, that are known to be detected by the tests prescribed in the monograph. It is based on information available at the time of elaboration or revision of the monograph and is not necessarily exhaustive. The section includes specified impurities and, where so indicated, other detectable impurities.

Specified impurities have an acceptance criterion not greater than that authorised by the competent authorities.

Other detectable impurities are potential impurities with a defined structure but not known to be normally present above the identification threshold in substances used in medicinal products that have been authorised by the competent authorities of Parties to the Convention. They are given in the Impurities section for information.

Where an impurity other than a specified impurity is found in an active substance it is the responsibility of the user of the substance to check whether it has to be identified/qualified, depending on its content, nature, maximum daily dose and relevant identification/qualification threshold, in accordance with the general monograph on *Substances for pharmaceutical use (2034)*, Related substances section.

It should be noted that specific thresholds are applied to substances exclusively for veterinary use.

Interpretation of the test for related substances in the monographs on active substances

A specific monograph on a substance for pharmaceutical use is to be read and interpreted in conjunction with the general monograph on *Substances for pharmaceutical use (2034)*.

Where a general acceptance criterion for impurities ("any other impurity", "other impurities", "any impurity") equivalent to a nominal content greater than the applicable identification threshold (see the general monograph on *Substances for pharmaceutical use (2034)*) is prescribed, this is valid only for specified impurities mentioned in the Impurities section. The need for identification (wherever possible), reporting, specification and qualification of other impurities that occur must be considered according to the requirements of the general monograph. It is the responsibility of the user of the substance to determine the validity of the acceptance criteria for impurities not mentioned in the Impurities section and for those indicated as other detectable impurities.

The following examples are given as an aid in the interpretation of acceptance criteria for impurities in specific monographs. The examples correspond to different styles currently used in monographs pending harmonisation in a future edition.

Example 1

Consider a monograph on a substance for human use where the Impurities section lists 8 impurities (A-H), 2 of which are indicated to be other detectable impurities (G, H) and there are the following acceptance criteria:

– *impurity A*: not more than the area of the principal peak in the chromatogram obtained with reference solution (b) (0.5 per cent),
– *any other impurity*: not more than the area of the principal peak in the chromatogram obtained with reference solution (c) (0.2 per cent),
– *total*: not more than twice the area of the principal peak in the chromatogram obtained with reference solution (b) (1.0 per cent),
– *disregard limit*: 0.25 times the area of the principal peak in the chromatogram obtained with reference solution (c) (0.05 per cent).

A substance complies with the test if:

– impurity A is present at a nominal concentration less than or equal to 0.5 per cent,
– impurities B, C, D, E, F are each present at a nominal concentration less than or equal to 0.2 per cent,
– any other impurity is present at a nominal concentration less than or equal to the identification threshold applicable for the active substance,
– the sum of nominal concentrations of impurities that are above the disregard limit is less than or equal to 1.0 per cent.

Example 2

Consider a monograph on a substance for human use where the Impurities section lists 6 impurities (A-F) with the following acceptance criteria.

In the chromatogram obtained with the test solution: the area of any peak, apart from the principal peak, is not greater than the area of the principal peak in the chromatogram obtained with reference solution (b) (0.5 per cent); the sum of the areas of all peaks, apart from the principal peak, is not greater than twice the area of the principal peak in the chromatogram obtained with reference solution (b) (1.0 per cent). Disregard any peak obtained with the blank and any peak with an area less than 0.1 times the area of the principal peak in the chromatogram obtained with reference solution (b).

A substance complies with the test if:

– impurities A, B, C, D, E, F are each present at a nominal concentration less than or equal to 0.5 per cent,
– any other impurity is present at a nominal concentration less than or equal to the identification threshold applicable for the active substance,
– the sum of nominal concentrations of impurities that are above the disregard limit is less than or equal to 1.0 per cent.

Example 3

Consider a monograph on a substance for human use (for which the maximum daily dose is not more than 2 g/day) in more explicit style where the Impurities section lists 7 impurities, 6 of which (A-F) are defined as *Specified impurities* and the seventh (G) is given under *Other detectable impurities*.

Limits:

– *correction factor*: for the calculation of content, multiply the peak area of impurity A by 2.3,
– *impurity B*: not more than 3 times the area of the principal peak in the chromatogram obtained with reference solution (a) (0.3 per cent),
– *impurity E*: not more than 4 times the area of the principal peak in the chromatogram obtained with reference solution (a) (0.4 per cent),
– *impurities A, C, D, F*: for each impurity, not more than twice the area of the principal peak in the chromatogram obtained with reference solution (a) (0.2 per cent),
– *any other impurity*: for each impurity, not more than the area of the principal peak in the chromatogram obtained with reference solution (a) (0.1 per cent),
– *total*: not more than the area of the principal peak in the chromatogram obtained with reference solution (b) (1.0 per cent),
– *disregard limit*: 0.5 times the area of the principal peak in the chromatogram obtained with reference solution (a) (0.05 per cent).

A substance complies with the test if:

– impurity B is present at a nominal concentration less than or equal to 0.3 per cent,
– impurity E is present at a nominal concentration less than or equal to 0.4 per cent,
– impurities A, C, D, F are each present at a nominal concentration less than or equal to 0.2 per cent; the peak area of impurity A has been multiplied by 2.3 for the calculation of content,
– any other impurity is present at a nominal concentration less than or equal to 0.10 per cent (identification threshold),
– the sum of nominal concentrations of impurities that are above the disregard limit is less than or equal to 1.0 per cent.

Recommendations to users of monographs of active substances

Monographs give a specification for suitable quality of substances with impurity profiles corresponding to those taken into account during elaboration and/or revision of the monograph. It is the responsibility of the user of the substance to check that the monograph provides adequate control of impurities for a substance for pharmaceutical use from a given source, notably by using the procedure for certification of suitability of the monographs of the European Pharmacopoeia.

A monograph with a related substances test based on a quantitative method (such as liquid chromatography, gas chromatography and capillary electrophoresis) provides adequate control of impurities for a substance from a given source if impurities present in amounts above the applicable identification threshold are specified impurities mentioned in the Impurities section.

If the substance contains impurities other than those mentioned in the Impurities section, it has to be verified that these impurities are detectable by the method described in the monograph, otherwise a new method must be developed and revision of the monograph must be requested. Depending on the contents found and the limits proposed, the identification and/or the qualification of these impurities must be considered.

Where a single related substances test covers different impurity profiles, only impurities for the known profile from a single source need to be reported in the certificate of analysis unless the marketing authorisation holder uses active substances with different impurity profiles.

Identification of impurities (peak assignment)

Where a monograph has an individual limit for an impurity, it is often necessary to define means of identification, for example using a reference substance, a representative chromatogram or relative retention. The user of the substance may find it necessary to identify impurities other than those for which the monograph provides a means of identification, for example to check the suitability of the specification for a given impurity profile by comparison with the Impurities section. The European Pharmacopoeia does not provide reference substances, representative chromatograms or information on relative retentions for this purpose, unless prescribed in the monograph. Users will therefore have to apply the available scientific techniques for identification.

New impurities/Specified impurities above the specified limit

Where a new manufacturing process or change in an established process leads to the occurrence of a new impurity, it is necessary to apply the provisions of the general monograph on *Substances for pharmaceutical use (2034)* regarding identification and qualification and to verify the suitability of the monograph for control of the impurity. A certificate of suitability is a means for confirming for a substance from a given source that the new impurity is adequately controlled or the certificate contains a method for control with a defined acceptance criterion. In the latter case revision of the monograph will be initiated.

Where a new manufacturing process or change in an established process leads to the occurrence of a specified impurity above the specified limit, it is necessary to apply the provisions of the general monograph on *Substances for pharmaceutical use (2034)* regarding qualification.

Chromatographic methods

General chapter *2.2.46. Chromatographic separation techniques* deals with various aspects of impurities control. Information is available via the EDQM web site (www.pheur.org) on commercial names for columns and other reagents and equipment found suitable during monograph development, where this is considered useful.

GLOSSARY

Disregard limit: in chromatographic tests, the nominal content at or below which peaks/signals are not taken into account for calculating a sum of impurities. The numerical values for the disregard limit and the reporting threshold are usually the same.

Identification threshold: a limit above which an impurity is to be identified.

Identified impurity: an impurity for which structural characterisation has been achieved.

Impurity: any component of a substance for pharmaceutical use that is not the chemical entity defined as the substance.

Nominal concentration: concentration calculated on the basis of the concentration of the prescribed reference and taking account of the prescribed correction factor.

Other detectable impurities: potential impurities with a defined structure that are known to be detected by the tests in a monograph but not known to be normally present above the identification threshold in substances used in medicinal products that have been authorised by the competent authorities of Parties to the Convention. They are unspecified impurities and are thus limited by a general acceptance criterion.

Potential impurity: an impurity that theoretically can arise during manufacture or storage. It may or may not actually appear in the substance. Where a potential impurity is known to be detected by the tests in a monograph but not known to be normally present in substances used in medicinal products that have been authorised by the competent authorities of Parties to the Convention, it will be included in the Impurities section under *Other detectable impurities* for information.

Qualification: the process of acquiring and evaluating data that establishes the biological safety of an individual impurity or a given impurity profile at the level(s) specified.

Qualification threshold: a limit above which an impurity is to be qualified.

Related substances: title used in monographs for general tests for organic impurities.

Reporting threshold: a limit above which an impurity is to be reported. Synonym: reporting level.

Specified impurity: an impurity that is individually listed and limited with a specific acceptance criterion in a monograph. A specified impurity can be either identified or unidentified.

Unidentified impurity: an impurity for which a structural characterisation has not been achieved and that is defined solely by qualitative analytical properties (for example, relative retention).

Unspecified impurity: an impurity that is limited by a general acceptance criterion and not individually listed with its own specific acceptance criterion.

5.11. CHARACTERS SECTION IN MONOGRAPHS

01/2005:51100

5.11. CHARACTERS SECTION IN MONOGRAPHS

The General Notices indicate that the statements included in the Characters section are not to be interpreted in a strict sense and are not requirements. For information of users, the methods recommended to authors of monographs as the basis for statements concerning hygroscopicity, crystallinity and solubility are given below.

HYGROSCOPICITY

This method is to be carried out on a substance that complies with the test for loss on drying or water content of the monograph. The method gives an indication of the degree of hygroscopicity rather than a true determination.

Use a glass weighing vessel 50 mm in external diameter and 15 mm high. Weigh the vessel and stopper (m_1). Place the amount of substance prescribed for the test for loss on drying or water in the vessel and weigh (m_2). Place the unstoppered vessel in a desiccator at 25 °C containing a saturated solution of ammonium chloride or ammonium sulphate or place it in a climatic cabinet set at 25 ± 1 °C and 80 ± 2 per cent relative humidity. Allow to stand for 24 h. Stopper the weighing vessel and weigh (m_3).

Calculate the percentage increase in mass using the expression:

$$\frac{m_3 - m_2}{m_2 - m_1} \times 100$$

The result is interpreted as follows:

- *deliquescent*: sufficient water is absorbed to form a liquid,
- *very hygroscopic*: increase in mass is equal to or greater than 15 per cent,
- *hygroscopic*: increase in mass is less than 15 per cent and equal to or greater than 2 per cent,
- *slightly hygroscopic*: increase in mass is less than 2 per cent and equal to or greater than 0.2 per cent.

CRYSTALLINITY

This method is employed to establish the crystalline or amorphous nature of a substance.

Mount a few particles of the substance to be examined in mineral oil on a clean glass slide. Examine under a polarising microscope. Crystalline particles exhibit birefringence and extinction positions when the microscope stage is revolved.

SOLUBILITY

For this test a maximum of 111 mg of substance (for each solvent) and a maximum of 30 ml of each solvent are necessary.

Dissolving procedure

Shake vigorously for 1 min and place in a constant temperature device, maintained at a temperature of 25.0 ± 0.5 °C for 15 min. If the substance is not completely dissolved, repeat the shaking for 1 min and place the tube in the constant temperature device for 15 min.

Method

Weigh 100 mg of finely powdered substance (90) in a stoppered tube (16 mm in internal diameter and 160 mm long), add 0.1 ml of the solvent and proceed as described under Dissolving Procedure. If the substance is completely dissolved, it is *very soluble*.

If the substance is not completely dissolved, add 0.9 ml of the solvent and proceed as described under Dissolving Procedure. If the substance is completely dissolved, it is *freely soluble*.

If the substance is not completely dissolved, add 2.0 ml of the solvent and proceed as described under Dissolving Procedure. If the substance is completely dissolved, it is *soluble*.

If the substance is not completely dissolved, add 7.0 ml of the solvent and proceed as described under Dissolving Procedure. If the substance is completely dissolved, it is *sparingly soluble*.

If the substance is not completely dissolved, weigh 10 mg of finely powdered substance (90) in a stoppered tube, add 10.0 ml of the solvent and proceed as described under Dissolving Procedure. If the substance is completely dissolved, it is *slightly soluble*.

If the substance is not completely dissolved, weigh 1 mg of finely powdered substance (90) in a stoppered tube, add 10.0 ml of the solvent and proceed as described under Dissolving Procedure. If the substance is completely dissolved, it is *very slightly soluble*.

GENERAL MONOGRAPHS

01/2005:1063

ALLERGEN PRODUCTS

Producta allergenica

DEFINITION

Allergen products are pharmaceutical preparations derived from extracts of naturally occurring source materials containing allergens, which are substances that cause or provoke allergic (hypersensitivity) disease. The allergenic components are most often of a proteinaceous nature. Allergen products are intended for *in vivo* diagnosis or treatment of allergic (hypersensitivity) diseases attributed to these allergens.

Allergen products are available as finished products, as bulk preparations in dried form, solutions or suspensions intended to be further concentrated or diluted prior to use or as final preparations in solutions, suspensions or freeze-dried. Allergen products intended for parenteral, bronchial and conjunctival administration are sterile.

For *diagnostic use*, allergen products are usually prepared as unmodified extracts in a 50 per cent *V/V* solution of glycerol for skin-prick testing. For intradermal diagnosis or for provocation tests by nasal, ocular or bronchial routes, suitable dilutions of allergen products may be prepared by dilution of aqueous or glycerinated extracts, or by reconstitution immediately before use of unmodified freeze-dried extracts.

For *immunotherapy*, allergen products may be either unmodified extracts or extracts modified chemically and/or by adsorption onto different carriers (for example, aluminium hydroxide, calcium phosphate or tyrosine).

This monograph does not apply: to chemicals that are used solely for diagnosis of contact dermatitis; to chemically synthesised products; to allergens derived by rDNA technology; to finished products used on a named-patient basis. It does not necessarily apply to allergen products for veterinary use.

PRODUCTION

Allergen products are derived from a wide range of allergenic source materials. They are often prepared as bulk products intended to be further diluted or concentrated prior to use. They may be treated to modify or reduce the allergenic activity or remain unmodified.

SOURCE MATERIALS

Source materials for the preparation of allergen products are mostly pollens, moulds, mites, animal epithelia, hymenoptera venoms and certain foods.

They are described by their origin, nature, method of collection or production and pretreatment, and are stored under defined conditions which minimise deterioration.

The collection or production, as well as the handling of the source materials are such that uniform qualitative and quantitative composition is ensured as far as possible from batch to batch.

Pollens. Potential chemical contaminants, such as pesticides and heavy metals, must be minimised. Pollens contain not more than 1 per cent of foreign pollens as determined by microscopic examination. Pollens contain not more than 1 per cent of mould spores as determined by microscopic examination.

Mites and moulds. Biologically active contaminants such as mycotoxins in moulds must be minimised and any presence justified. Care must be taken to minimise any allergenic constituents of the media used for the cultivation of mites and moulds as source materials. Culture media that contain substances of human or animal origin must be justified and, when required must be suitably treated to ensure the inactivation or elimination of possible transmissible agents of disease.

Animal epithelia. Animal epithelia must be obtained from healthy animals selected to avoid possible transmissible agents of disease.

MANUFACTURING PROCESS

Allergen products are generally obtained by extraction, and may be purified, from the source materials using appropriate methods shown to preserve the biological properties of the allergenic components. Allergen products are manufactured under conditions designed to minimise microbial growth and enzymatic degradation.

A purification procedure, if any, is designed to minimise the content of any potential irritant low-molecular-mass components or other non-allergenic components.

Allergen products may contain a suitable antimicrobial preservative. The nature and the concentration of the antimicrobial preservative have to be justified.

The manufacturing process comprises various stages.

Native allergen extracts result after separation from the extracted source materials.

Intermediate allergen products are obtained by further processing or modification of the native allergen extracts. The modification may be achieved by chemical processes (chemical conjugation) or physical processes (physical adsorption onto different carriers, for example, aluminium hydroxide, calcium phosphate or tyrosine). They may also be modified by inclusion into such vehicles as liposomes or microspheres, or by the addition of other biologically active agents to enhance efficacy or safety. Intermediate allergen products may be freeze-dried.

Bulk allergen preparations consist of products in solution or suspension which will not be further processed or modified, and are ready for dilution or filling into final containers.

IN-HOUSE REFERENCE PREPARATION

An appropriate representative preparation is selected as the In-House Reference Preparation (IHRP), characterised and used to verify batch-to-batch consistency. The IHRP is stored in suitably sized aliquots under conditions ensuring its stability, usually freeze-dried.

Characterisation of the In-House Reference Preparation. *The extent of characterisation of the IHRP depends on the nature of the allergenic source material, knowledge of the allergenic components and availability of suitable reagents, as well as the intended use. The characterised IHRP is used as reference in the batch control of native allergen extracts or intermediate allergen products and, if possible, in the batch control of final allergen preparations.*

The In-House Reference Preparation (IHRP) is characterised by the protein content determination and a protein profile using relevant methods (such as isoelectric focusing, polyacrylamide gel electrophoresis, immunoelectrophoresis or molecular-mass profiling). Allergenic components may be detected by appropriate methods (for example immunoblotting or crossed radio-immunoelectrophoresis). Characterisation of the allergenic components may include identification of relevant allergens based on serological or others techniques using a pool or individual sera from allergic patients, or allergen-specific polyclonal or monoclonal antibodies. When allergen reference substances are available determination of the content of individual allergens may be performed. Individual allergens are identified according to internationally established nomenclature whenever possible.

Where possible, the biological potency of the IHRP is established by *in vivo* techniques such as skin testing, and expressed in units of biological activity. If not, for certain extracts, potency may be established by suitable immunoassays (for example, those based on the inhibition of the binding capacity of specific immunoglobulin E antibodies) or by quantitative techniques for a single major component.

IDENTIFICATION

Identity is confirmed at the intermediate or other applicable stage by comparison with the IHRP using protein profiling by appropriate methods (for example, isoelectric focusing, sodium dodecyl sulphate-polyacrylamide gel electrophoresis or immunoelectrophoresis).

TESTS

Various biochemical and immunological tests have been developed in order to characterise allergens qualitatively and quantitatively. However, some of the methods, particularly for the determination of allergenic activity and allergen profile, are not applicable to all products at present. This is because knowledge of the allergenic components or the required reagents is not available. Accordingly, allergen products have been classified in different categories with increasing test requirements, according to quality and intended use.

Where possible the following tests are applied to the final preparations. If not, they must be performed on the extracts as late as possible in the manufacturing process, for example, at the stage immediately prior to that stage (modification, dilution etc.) which renders the test not feasible on the final preparation.

Water (*2.5.12*). Not more than 5 per cent for freeze-dried products.

Sterility (*2.6.1*). Allergen products intended for parenteral, bronchial and conjunctival administration comply with the test for sterility.

Protein content: 80 per cent to 120 per cent of the stated content of a given batch. If the biological potency can be determined then the test for protein content may be omitted.

Protein profile. The protein composition determined by suitable methods corresponds to that of the IHRP.

Abnormal toxicity (*2.6.9*). Allergen products obtained from moulds and intended for parenteral administration (except skin-prick tests) comply with the test for abnormal toxicity for immunosera and vaccines for human use.

Various additional tests, somewith increasing selectivity, depending on the allergen product concerned can be applied, but in any case for allergen products intended for therapeutic use a validated test measuring the potency (total allergenic activity, determination of individual allergens or any other justified tests) must be applied.

Aluminium (*2.5.13*). Not less than 80 per cent and not more than 120 per cent of the stated amount but in any case not more than 1.25 mg per human dose unless otherwise justified and authorised, when aluminium hydroxide or aluminium phosphate is used as adsorbent.

Calcium (*2.5.14*). Not less than 80 per cent and not more than 120 per cent of the stated amount when calcium phosphate is used as adsorbent.

Antigen profile. The antigens are identified by means of suitable techniques using antigen-specific animal antibodies.

Allergen profile. Relevant allergenic components are identified by means of suitable techniques using allergen-specific human antibodies.

Total allergenic activity. The activity is 50 per cent to 200 per cent of the stated amount as assayed by inhibition of the binding capacity of specific immunoglobulin E antibodies or a suitable equivalent *in vitro* method.

Individual allergens: 50 per cent to 200 per cent of the stated amount, determined by a suitable method.

STORAGE

Adsorbed allergen products should not be frozen.

LABELLING

The label states:

- the biological potency and/or the protein content and/or the extraction concentration;
- the route of administration and the intended use;
- the storage conditions;
- where applicable, the name and amount of added antimicrobial preservative;
- for freeze-dried preparations:
  - the name, composition and volume of the reconstituting liquid to be added
  - the period of time within which the preparation is to be used after reconstitution;
- where applicable, that the preparation is sterile;
- where applicable the name and amount of adsorbent.

01/2005:0765

EXTRACTS

Extracta

DEFINITION

Extracts are preparations of liquid (liquid extracts and tinctures), semi-solid (soft extracts) or solid (dry extracts) consistency, obtained from herbal drugs or animal matters, which are usually in a dry state.

Different types of extract may be distinguished. Standardised extracts are adjusted within an acceptable tolerance to a given content of constituents with known therapeutic activity; standardisation is achieved by adjustment of the extract with inert material or by blending batches of extracts. Quantified extracts are adjusted to a defined range of constituents; adjustments are made by blending batches of extracts. Other extracts are essentially defined by their production process (state of the herbal drug or animal matter to be extracted, solvent, extraction conditions) and their specifications.

PRODUCTION

Extracts are prepared by suitable methods using ethanol or other suitable solvents. Different batches of the herbal drug or animal matter may be blended prior to extraction. The herbal drug or animal matter to be extracted may undergo a preliminary treatment, for example, inactivation of enzymes, grinding or defatting. In addition, unwanted matter may be removed after extraction.

Herbal drugs, animal matters and organic solvents used for the preparation of extracts comply with any relevant monograph of the Pharmacopoeia. For soft and dry extracts where the organic solvent is removed by evaporation, recovered or recycled solvent may be used, provided that the recovery procedures are controlled and monitored to ensure that solvents meet appropriate standards before re-use or admixture with other approved materials. Water used for the preparation of extracts is of suitable quality. Except for the test for bacterial endotoxins, water complying with

General monographs

the section on Purified water in bulk of the monograph on *Purified water (0008)* is suitable. Potable water may be suitable if it complies with a defined specification that allows the consistent production of a suitable extract.

Where applicable, concentration to the intended consistency is carried out using suitable methods, usually under reduced pressure, and at a temperature at which deterioration of the constituents is reduced to a minimum. Essential oils that have been separated during processing may be restored to the extracts at an appropriate stage in the manufacturing process. Suitable excipients may be added at the various stages of the manufacturing process for example to improve technological qualities such as homogeneity or consistency. Suitable stabilisers and antimicrobial preservatives may also be added.

Extraction with a given solvent leads to typical proportions of characterised constituents in the extractable matter; during production of standardised and quantified extracts, purification procedures may be applied that increase these proportions with respect to the expected values; such extracts are referred to as "refined".

IDENTIFICATION

Extracts are identified using a suitable method.

TESTS

Where applicable, as a result of analysis of the herbal drug or animal matter used for production and in view of the production process, tests for microbiological quality (*5.1.4*), heavy metals, aflatoxins, pesticide residues (*2.8.13*) in the extracts may be necessary.

ASSAY

Wherever possible, extracts are assayed by a suitable method.

LABELLING

The label states:

- the herbal drug or animal matter used,
- whether the extract is liquid, soft or dry, or whether it is a tincture,
- for standardised extracts, the content of constituents with known therapeutic activity,
- for quantified extracts, the content of constituents (markers) used for quantification,
- the ratio of the starting material to the genuine extract (DER),
- the solvent or solvents used for extraction,
- where applicable, that a fresh herbal drug or fresh animal matter has been used,
- where applicable, that the extract is "refined",
- the name and amount of any excipient used including stabilisers and antimicrobial preservatives,
- where applicable, the percentage of dry residue.

Liquid extracts – extracta fluida

DEFINITION

Liquid extracts are liquid preparations of which, in general, 1 part by mass or volume is equivalent to 1 part by mass of the dried herbal drug or animal matter. These preparations are adjusted, if necessary, so that they satisfy the requirements for content of solvent, and, where applicable, for constituents.

PRODUCTION

Liquid extracts are prepared by using ethanol of suitable concentration or water to extract the herbal drug or animal matter, or by dissolving a soft or dry extract (which has been produced using the same strength of extraction solvent as is used in preparing the liquid extract by direct extraction) of the herbal drug or animal matter in either ethanol of suitable concentration or water. Liquid extracts may be filtered, if necessary.

A slight sediment may form on standing, which is acceptable as long as the composition of the liquid extract is not changed significantly.

TESTS

Relative density (*2.2.5*). Where applicable, the liquid extract complies with the limits prescribed in the monograph.

Ethanol (*2.9.10*). For alcoholic liquid extracts, carry out the determination of ethanol content. The ethanol content complies with that prescribed.

Methanol and 2-propanol (*2.9.11*): maximum 0.05 per cent *V/V* of methanol and maximum 0.05 per cent *V/V* of 2-propanol for alcoholic liquid extracts unless otherwise prescribed.

Dry residue (*2.8.16*). Where applicable, the liquid extract complies with the limits prescribed in the monograph, corrected if necessary, taking into account any excipient used.

STORAGE

Protected from light.

LABELLING

The label states in addition to the requirements listed above:

- where applicable, the ethanol content in per cent *V/V* in the final extract.

Tinctures – tincturae

DEFINITION

Tinctures are liquid preparations which are usually obtained using either 1 part of herbal drug or animal matter and 10 parts of extraction solvent or 1 part of herbal drug or animal matter and 5 parts of extraction solvent.

PRODUCTION

Tinctures are prepared by maceration or percolation (outline methodology is given below) using only ethanol of a suitable concentration for extraction of the herbal drug or animal matter, or by dissolving a soft or dry extract (which has been produced using the same strength of extraction solvent as is used in preparing the tincture by direct extraction) of the herbal drug or animal matter in ethanol of a suitable concentration. Tinctures are filtered, if necessary.

Tinctures are usually clear. A slight sediment may form on standing which is acceptable as long as the composition of the tincture is not changed significantly.

Production by maceration. Unless otherwise prescribed, reduce the herbal drug or animal matter to be extracted to pieces of suitable size, mix thoroughly with the prescribed extraction solvent and allow to stand in a closed container for an appropriate time. The residue is separated from the extraction solvent and, if necessary, pressed out. In the latter case, the 2 liquids obtained are combined.

Production by percolation. If necessary, reduce the herbal drug or animal matter to be extracted to pieces of suitable size. Mix thoroughly with a portion of the prescribed extraction solvent and allow to stand for an appropriate time. Transfer to a percolator and allow the percolate to flow at room temperature slowly making sure that the herbal drug or animal matter to be extracted is always covered with the remaining extraction solvent. The residue may be pressed out and the expressed liquid combined with the percolate.

TESTS

Relative density (*2.2.5*). Where applicable, the tincture complies with the limits prescribed in the monograph.

Ethanol (*2.9.10*). The ethanol content complies with that prescribed.

Methanol and 2-propanol (*2.9.11*): maximum 0.05 per cent *V/V* of methanol and maximum 0.05 per cent *V/V* of 2-propanol, unless otherwise prescribed.

Dry residue (*2.8.16*). Where applicable, the tincture complies with the limits prescribed in the monograph, corrected if necessary, taking into account any excipient used.

STORAGE

Protected from light.

LABELLING

The label states in addition to the requirements listed above:

- for tinctures other than standardised and quantified tinctures, the ratio of starting material to extraction liquid or of starting material to final tincture,
- the ethanol content in per cent *V/V* in the final tincture.

Soft extracts – extracta spissa

DEFINITION

Soft extracts are semi-solid preparations obtained by evaporation or partial evaporation of the solvent used for extraction.

TESTS

Dry residue (*2.8.16*). The soft extract complies with the limits prescribed in the monograph.

Solvents. Where applicable, a monograph on a soft extract prescribes a limit test for the solvent used for extraction.

STORAGE

Protected from light.

Dry extracts – extracta sicca

DEFINITION

Dry extracts are solid preparations obtained by evaporation of the solvent used for their production. Dry extracts usually have a loss on drying or a water content of not greater than 5 per cent *m/m*.

TESTS

Water (*2.2.13*). Where applicable, the dry extract complies with the limits prescribed in the monograph.

Loss on drying (*2.8.17*). Where applicable, the dry extract complies with the limits prescribed in the monograph.

Solvents. Where applicable, a monograph on a dry extract prescribes a limit test for the solvent used for extraction.

STORAGE

In an airtight container, protected from light.

01/2005:1434

HERBAL DRUG PREPARATIONS

Plantae medicinales praeparatore

DEFINITION

Herbal drug preparations are obtained by subjecting herbal drugs to treatments such as extraction, distillation, expression, fractionation, purification, concentration or fermentation. These include comminuted or powdered herbal drugs, tinctures, extracts, essential oils, expressed juices and processed exudates.

Herbal teas comply with the monograph on *Herbal teas (1435)*.

Instant herbal teas consist of powder or granules of one or more herbal drug preparation(s) intended for the preparation of an oral solution immediately before use.

01/2005:1433

HERBAL DRUGS

Plantae medicinales

DEFINITION

Herbal drugs are mainly whole, fragmented or cut, plants, parts of plants, algae, fungi, lichen in an unprocessed state, usually in dried form but sometimes fresh. Certain exudates that have not been subjected to a specific treatment are also considered to be herbal drugs. Herbal drugs are precisely defined by the botanical scientific name according to the binominal system (genus, species, variety and author).

PRODUCTION

Herbal drugs are obtained from cultivated or wild plants. Suitable collection, cultivation, harvesting, drying, fragmentation and storage conditions are essential to guarantee the quality of herbal drugs.

Herbal drugs are, as far as possible, free from impurities such as soil, dust, dirt and other contaminants such as fungal, insect and other animal contaminations. They are not rotten.

If a decontaminating treatment has been used, it is necessary to demonstrate that the constituents of the plant are not affected and that no harmful residues remain. The use of ethylene oxide is prohibited for the decontamination of herbal drugs.

IDENTIFICATION

Herbal drugs are identified using their macroscopic and microscopic descriptions and any further tests that may be required (for example, thin-layer chromatography).

TESTS

A test for foreign matter (*2.8.2*) is carried out, unless otherwise prescribed in the individual monographs.

A specific appropriate test may apply to herbal drugs liable to be falsified.

If appropriate, the herbal drugs comply with other tests, for example, total ash (*2.4.16*), ash insoluble in hydrochloric acid (*2.8.1*), extractable matter, swelling index (*2.8.4*) and bitterness value.

The test for loss on drying (*2.2.32*) is carried out on herbal drugs, unless otherwise prescribed in the individual monographs. A determination of water (*2.2.13*) is carried out for herbal drugs with a high essential oil content.

Herbal drugs comply with the requirements for pesticide residues (*2.8.13*). The requirements take into account the nature of the plant, where necessary the preparation in which the plant might be used, and where available the knowledge of the complete record of treatment of the batch of the plant. The content of pesticide residues may be determined by the method described in the annex to the general method.

The risk of contamination of herbal drugs by heavy metals must be considered. If an individual monograph does not prescribe limits for heavy metals or specific elements such limits may be required if justified.

Recommendations on the microbiological quality of products consisting solely of one or more herbal drugs are given in the text on *Microbiological quality of pharmaceutical preparations (5.1.4. – Category 4)*.

Where necessary limits for aflatoxins may be required.

In some specific circumstances, the risk of radioactive contamination is to be considered.

ASSAY

Unless otherwise justified and authorised herbal drugs are assayed by an appropriate method.

STORAGE

Store protected from light.

01/2005:1435

HERBAL TEAS

Plantae ad ptisanam

DEFINITION

Herbal teas consist exclusively of one or more herbal drugs intended for oral aqueous preparations by means of decoction, infusion or maceration. The preparation is prepared immediately before use.

Herbal teas are usually supplied in bulk form or in sachets.

The herbal drugs used comply with the appropriate individual European Pharmacopoeia monographs or in their absence to the general monograph on *Herbal drugs (1433)*.

Recommendations on the microbiological quality of herbal teas (*5.1.4. – Category 4*) take into account the prescribed preparation method (use of boiling or non-boiling water).

IDENTIFICATION

The identity of herbal drugs present in herbal teas is checked by botanical examinations.

TESTS

The proportion of herbal drugs present in herbal teas is checked by appropriate methods.

Herbal teas in sachets comply with the following test:

Uniformity of mass. Determine the average mass of twenty randomly chosen units as follows: weigh a single full sachet of herbal tea, open it without losing any fragments. Empty it completely using a brush. Weigh the empty sachet and calculate the mass of the contents by subtraction. Repeat the operation on the nineteen remaining sachets. Unless otherwise justified not more than two of the twenty individual masses of the contents deviate from the average mass of the contents by more than the percentage deviation shown in the table below and none deviates by more than twice that percentage.

Average mass	Percentage deviation
less than 1.5 g	15 per cent
1.5 g to 2.0 g included	10 per cent
more than 2.0 g	7.5 per cent

STORAGE

Store protected from light.

01/2005:0084

IMMUNOSERA FOR HUMAN USE, ANIMAL

Immunosera ex animale ad usum humanum

DEFINITION

Animal immunosera for human use are liquid or freeze-dried preparations containing purified immunoglobulins or immunoglobulin fragments obtained from serum or plasma of immunised animals of different species.

The immunoglobulins or immunoglobulin fragments have the power of specifically neutralising or binding to the antigen used for immunisation. The antigens include microbial or other toxins, human antigens, suspensions of bacterial and viral antigens and venoms of snakes, scorpions and spiders. The preparation is intended for intravenous or intramuscular administration, after dilution where applicable.

PRODUCTION

GENERAL PROVISIONS

The production method shall have been shown to yield consistently immunosera of acceptable safety, potency in man and stability.

Any reagent of biological origin used in the production of immunosera shall be free of contamination with bacteria, fungi and viruses. The method of preparation includes a step or steps that have been shown to remove or inactivate known agents of infection.

Methods used for production are validated, effective, reproducible and do not impair biological activity of the product.

The production method is validated to demonstrate that the product, if tested, would comply with the test for abnormal toxicity for immunosera and vaccines for human use (*2.6.9*).

Reference preparation. A batch shown to be suitable in clinical trials, or a batch representative thereof, is used as the reference preparation for the tests for high molecular mass proteins and purity.

ANIMALS

The animals used are of a species approved by the competent authority, are healthy and exclusively reserved for production of immunoserum. They are tested and shown to be free from a defined list of infectious agents. The introduction of animals into a closed herd follows specified procedures, including definition of quarantine measures. Where appropriate, additional specific agents are considered depending on the geographical localisation of the establishment used for the breeding and production of the animals. The feed originates from a controlled source and no animal proteins are added. The suppliers of animals are certified by the competent authority.

If the animals are treated with antibiotics, a suitable withdrawal period is allowed before collection of blood or plasma. The animals are not treated with penicillin antibiotics. If a live vaccine is administered, a suitable waiting period is imposed between vaccination and collection of serum or plasma for immunoserum production.

IMMUNISATION

The antigens used are identified and characterised, where appropriate; where relevant, they are shown to be free from extraneous infectious agents. They are identified by their names and a batch number; information on the source and preparation are recorded.

The selected animals are isolated for at least 1 week before being immunised according to a defined schedule with booster injections at suitable intervals. Adjuvants may be used.

Animals are kept under general health surveillance and specific antibody production is controlled at each cycle of immunisation.

Animals are thoroughly examined before collection of blood or plasma. If an animal shows any pathological lesion not related to the immunisation process, it is not used, nor are any other of the animals in the group concerned, unless it is evident that their use will not impair the safety of the product.

COLLECTION OF BLOOD OR PLASMA

Collection of blood is made by venepuncture or plasmapheresis. The puncture area is shaved, cleaned and disinfected. The animals may be anaesthetised under conditions that do not influence the quality of the product. Unless otherwise prescribed, an antimicrobial preservative may be added. The blood or plasma is collected in such a manner as to maintain sterility of the product. The blood or plasma collection is conducted at a site separate from the area where the animals are kept or bred and the area where the immunoserum is purified. If the serum or plasma is stored before further processing, precautions are taken to avoid microbial contamination.

Several single plasma or serum samples may be pooled before purification. The single or pooled samples are tested before purification for the following tests.

Tests for contaminating viruses. If an antimicrobial preservative is added, it must be neutralised before carrying out the tests or the tests carried out on a sample taken before addition of the antimicrobial preservative. Each pool is tested for contaminating viruses by suitable *in vitro* tests.

Each pool is tested for viruses by inoculation to cell cultures capable of detecting a wide range of viruses relevant for the particular product.

Potency. Carry out a biological assay as indicated in the monograph and express the result in International Units per millilitre, where applicable. A validated *in vitro* method may also be used.

Protein content. Dilute the product to be examined with a 9 g/l solution of *sodium chloride R* to obtain a solution containing about 15 mg of protein in 2 ml. To 2 ml of this solution in a round-bottomed centrifuge tube add 2 ml of a 75 g/l solution of *sodium molybdate R* and 2 ml of a mixture of 1 volume of *nitrogen-free sulphuric acid R* and 30 volumes of *water R*. Shake, centrifuge for 5 min, decant the supernatant liquid and allow the inverted tube to drain on filter paper. Determine the nitrogen in the residue by the method of sulphuric acid digestion (*2.5.9*) and calculate the content of protein by multiplying by 6.25. The protein content is within approved limits.

PURIFICATION AND VIRAL INACTIVATION

The immunoglobulins are concentrated and purified by fractional precipitation, chromatography, immunoadsorption or by other chemical or physical methods. They may be processed further by enzyme treatment. The methods are selected and validated to avoid contamination at all steps of processing and to avoid formation of protein aggregates that effect immunobiological characteristics of the product. For products intended to consist of immunoglobulin fragments, the methods are validated to guarantee total fragmentation. The methods of purification used are such that they do not generate additional components that compromise the quality and the safety of the product.

Unless otherwise justified and authorised, validated procedures are applied for removal and/or inactivation of viruses. The procedures are selected to avoid the formation of polymers or aggregates and, unless the product is intended to consist of Fab′ fragments, to minimise the splitting of F(ab′)2 into Fab′ fragments.

After purification and treatment for removal and/or inactivation of viruses, a stabiliser may be added to the intermediate product, which may be stored for a period defined in the light of stability data.

Only an intermediate product that complies with the following requirements may be used in the preparation of the final bulk.

Purity. Examine by non-reducing polyacrylamide gel electrophoresis (*2.2.31*), by comparison with the reference preparation, the bands are compared in intensity and no additional bands are found.

FINAL BULK

The final bulk is prepared from a single intermediate product or from a pool of intermediate products obtained from animals of the same species. Intermediate products with different specificities may be pooled.

An antimicrobial preservative and a stabiliser may be added. If an antimicrobial preservative has been added to the blood or plasma, the same substance is used as antimicrobial preservative in the final bulk.

Only a final bulk that complies with the following requirements may be used in the preparation of the final lot.

Antimicrobial preservative. Where applicable, determine the amount of antimicrobial preservative by a suitable physico-chemical method. It contains not less than 85 per cent and not more than 115 per cent of the amount stated on the label.

Sterility (*2.6.1*). It complies with the test for sterility.

FINAL LOT

The final bulk of immunoserum is distributed aseptically into sterile, tamper-proof containers. The containers are closed so as to prevent contamination.

Only a final lot that complies with the requirements prescribed below under Identification, Tests and Assay may be released for use. Provided that the tests for osmolality, protein content, molecular-size distribution, antimicrobial preservative, stabiliser, purity, foreign proteins and albumin and the assay have been carried out with satisfactory results on the final bulk, they may be omitted on the final lot.

Reconstitute the preparation to be examined as stated on the label immediately before carrying out the identification, tests (except those for solubility and water) and assay.

IDENTIFICATION

The identity is established by immunological tests and, where necessary, by determination of biological activity. The assay may also serve for identification.

CHARACTERS

Immunosera are clear to opalescent and colourless to very faintly yellow liquids. They are free from turbidity. Freeze-dried products are white or slightly yellow powders or solid friable masses. After reconstitution they show the same characteristics as liquid preparations.

TESTS

Solubility. To a container of the preparation to be examined, add the volume of the liquid for reconstitution stated on the label. The preparation dissolves completely within the time stated on the label.

Extractable volume (*2.9.17*). It complies with the requirement for extractable volume.

pH (*2.2.3*). The pH is within the limits approved for the particular product.

Osmolality (*2.2.35*): minimum 240 mosmol/kg after dilution, where applicable.

Protein content: 90 per cent to 110 per cent of the amount stated on the label, and not more than 100 g/l.

Dilute the preparation to be examined with a 9 g/l solution of *sodium chloride R* to obtain a solution containing about 15 mg of protein in 2 ml. To 2 ml of this solution in a round-bottomed centrifuge tube add 2 ml of 75 g/l solution of *sodium molybdate R* and 2 ml of a mixture of 1 volume of *nitrogen-free sulphuric acid R* and 30 volumes of *water R*. Shake, centrifuge for 5 min, decant the supernatant liquid and allow the inverted tube to drain on filter paper. Determine the nitrogen in the residue by the method of sulphuric acid digestion (*2.5.9*) and calculate the content of protein by multiplying by 6.25.

Molecular-size distribution. Examine by liquid chromatography (*2.2.29* or *2.2.30*). It complies with the specification approved for the particular product.

Antimicrobial preservative. Where applicable, determine the amount of antimicrobial preservative by a suitable physicochemical method. The amount is not less than the minimum amount shown to be effective and is not greater than 115 per cent of that stated on the label.

Phenol (*2.5.15*): maximum 2.5 g/l for preparations containing phenol.

Stabiliser. Determine the amount of stabiliser by a suitable physico-chemical method. The preparation contains not less than 80 per cent and not more than 120 per cent of the quantity stated on the label.

Purity. Examine by non-reducing polyacrylamide gel electrophoresis (*2.2.31*), by comparison with the reference preparation. No additional bands are found for the preparation to be examined.

Foreign proteins. When examined by precipitation tests with specific antisera, only protein from the declared animals species is shown to be present, unless otherwise prescribed, for example where material of human origin is used during production.

Albumin. Unless otherwise prescribed in the monograph, when examined electrophoretically, the content of albumin is not greater than the limit approved for the particular product and, in any case, not greater than 3 per cent.

Water (*2.5.12*): maximum 3 per cent.

Sterility (*2.6.1*). It complies with the test for sterility.

Pyrogens (*2.6.8*). Unless otherwise justified and authorised, it complies with the test for pyrogens. Unless otherwise prescribed, inject 1 ml per kilogram of the rabbit's body mass.

ASSAY

Carry out a biological assay as indicated in the monograph and express the result in International Units per millilitre, where appropriate. A validated *in vitro* method may also be used.

STORAGE

Store protected from light at the temperature stated on the label. Do not allow liquid preparations to freeze.

Expiry date. The expiry date is calculated from the beginning of the assay.

LABELLING

The label states:

- the number of International Units per millilitre, where applicable,
- the amount of protein per container,
- for freeze-dried preparations,
  - the name and volume of the reconstituting liquid to be added,
  - that the immunoserum is to be used immediately after reconstitution,
  - the time required for complete dissolution,
- the route of administration,
- the storage conditions,
- the expiry date, except for containers of less than 1 ml which are individually packed. The expiry date may be omitted from the label on the container, provided it is shown on the package and the label on the package states that the container must be kept in the package until required for use,
- the animal species of origin,
- the name and amount of any antimicrobial preservative, any stabiliser and any other substance added to the immunoserum.

01/2005:0030

IMMUNOSERA FOR VETERINARY USE

Immunosera ad usum veterinarium

DEFINITION

Immunosera for veterinary use are preparations containing immunoglobulins which have the power of specifically neutralising the toxins formed by or of specifically combining with the antigen used for their preparation. They may be crude or purified.

PRODUCTION

Immunosera are obtained from the serum of healthy animals immunised by injections of toxins or toxoids, venins of snakes, viruses, suspensions of micro-organisms or other suitable antigens. If a penicillin is used during immunisation, animals must not be bled until 8 days after the last administration. One or more suitable antimicrobial preservatives may be added and are invariably added if the preparations are issued in multidose containers.

For purified immunosera, the globulins containing the immune substances may be obtained from the crude immunoserum by enzyme treatment and fractional precipitation or by other chemical or physical methods. Purified immunosera are most stable at about pH 6.

General monographs

CHARACTERS

Immunosera are liquids that vary in colour according to the method of preparation. They are distributed aseptically in sterile containers which are then closed. When they are freeze-dried they consist of crusts or powders that are soluble in water.

TESTS

The following requirements refer to liquid immunosera and reconstituted freeze-dried immunosera.

pH (*2.2.3*). The pH of crude immunosera is 7.0 to 8.0. The pH of purified immunosera is 6.0 to 7.0.

Foreign proteins. When examined by precipitation with specific antisera, immunosera are shown to consist exclusively of proteins of the animal species used for the preparation.

Albumins. Purified immunosera comply with the test for albumins. Unless otherwise prescribed in the monograph, when examined electrophoretically, purified immunosera show not more than a trace of albumin.

Total protein Not more than 170 g/l. Carry out the determination of nitrogen by sulphuric acid digestion (*2.5.9*) and multiply the result by 6.25.

Phenol (*2.5.15*). When the immunoserum contains phenol, the concentration is not more than 5 g/l.

Sterility (*2.6.1*). Immunosera comply with the test for sterility. When the volume of liquid in a container is greater than 100 ml, the method of membrane filtration is used wherever possible. If this method is used, incubate the media for not less than 14 days. Where the method of membrane filtration cannot be used, the method of direct inoculation may be used.

Where the volume of liquid in each container is 20 ml or more, the minimum volume to be used for each culture medium is 10 per cent of the contents or 5 ml whichever is less.

The appropriate number of items to be tested (*2.6.1*) is 1 per cent of the batch with a minimum of 4 and a maximum of 10.

POTENCY

Carry out the biological assay prescribed in the monograph and express the result in International Units per millilitre when such exist.

STORAGE

Store protected from light at a temperature of 5 ± 3 °C. Liquid immunosera should not be allowed to freeze.

Expiry date. The expiry date is calculated from the beginning of the test for Potency. It applies to immunosera stored in the prescribed conditions.

LABELLING

The label states:

- the name of the preparation,
- "for veterinary use",
- the number of International Units per millilitre, where such exist,
- the batch number or other reference,
- the storage conditions,
- the expiry date,
- the animal species for which the immunoserum is intended,
- the name of the animal species of origin,
- the name and amount of any antimicrobial preservative or other substance added to the immunoserum,
- whether any substance is likely to cause an adverse reaction,
- any contra-indications to the use of the product,
- for freeze-dried immunosera:
  - the name or composition and the volume of the reconstituting liquid to be added,
  - that the immunoserum should be used immediately after reconstitution,
- the doses recommended for different species,
- the name and address of the manufacturer.

01/2005:1468

PRODUCTS OF FERMENTATION

Producta ab fermentatione

This monograph applies to indirect gene products obtained by fermentation. It is not applicable to:

- *monographs in the Pharmacopoeia concerning vaccines for human or veterinary use;*
- *products derived from continuous cell lines of human or animal origin;*
- *direct gene products that result from the transcription and translation from nucleic acid to protein, whether or not subject to post-translational modification;*
- *products obtained by semi-synthesis from a product of fermentation and those obtained by biocatalytic transformation;*
- *whole broth concentrates or raw fermentation products.*

This monograph provides general requirements for the development and manufacture of products of fermentation. These requirements are not necessarily comprehensive in a given case and requirements complementary or additional to those prescribed in this monograph may be imposed in an individual monograph or by the competent authority.

DEFINITION

For the purposes of this monograph, products of fermentation are active or inactive pharmaceutical substances produced by controlled fermentation as indirect gene products. They are primary or secondary metabolites of micro-organisms such as bacteria, yeasts, fungi and micro-algae, whether or not modified by traditional procedures or recombinant DNA (rDNA) technology. Such metabolites include vitamins, amino acids, antibiotics, alkaloids and polysaccharides.

They may be obtained by batch or continuous fermentation processes followed by procedures such as extraction, concentration, purification and isolation.

PRODUCTION

Production is based on a process that has been validated and shown to be suitable. The extent of validation depends on the critical nature of the respective process step.

CHARACTERISATION OF THE PRODUCER MICRO-ORGANISM

The history of the micro-organism used for production is documented. The micro-organism is adequately characterised. This may include determination of the phenotype of the micro-organism, macroscopic and microscopic methods and biochemical tests and, if appropriate, determination of the genotype of the micro-organism and molecular genetic tests.

General monographs

PROCESSES USING A SEED-LOT SYSTEM

The *master cell bank* is a homogeneous suspension or lyophilisate of the original cells distributed into individual containers for storage. The viability and productivity of the cells under the selected storage conditions and their suitability for initiating a satisfactory production process after storage must be demonstrated.

Propagation of the master cell bank may take place through a seed-lot system that uses a working cell bank.

The *working cell bank* is a homogeneous suspension or lyophilisate of the cell material derived from the master cell bank, distributed in equal volumes into individual containers for storage (for example, in liquid nitrogen).

Production may take place by batch or continuous culture and may be terminated under defined conditions.

All containers in a cell bank are stored under identical conditions. Once removed from storage, the individual ampoules, vials or culture straws are not returned to the cell bank.

PROCESSES USING STAGED GROWTH IN CULTURES

The contents of a container of the working cell bank are used, if necessary after resuspension, to prepare an inoculum in a suitable medium. After a suitable period of growth, the cultures are used to initiate the fermentation process, if necessary following preculture in a prefermentor. The conditions to be used at each stage of the process are defined and must be met with each production run.

CHANGE CONTROL

If the production process is altered in a way that causes a significant change in the impurity profile of the product, the critical steps associated with this change in impurity profile are revalidated.

If a significant change has taken place in the micro-organism used for production that causes a significant change in the impurity profile of the product, the critical steps of the production process associated with this change, particularly the procedure for purification and isolation, are revalidated.

Revalidation includes demonstration that new impurities present in the product as a result of the change are adequately controlled by the test procedures. If necessary, additional or alternative tests must be introduced with appropriate limits. If the change in the process or in the micro-organism results in an increase in the level of an impurity already present, the acceptability of such an increase is addressed.

When a master cell bank is replaced, the critical steps of the production process must be revalidated to the extent necessary to demonstrate that no adverse change has occurred in the quality and safety of the product. Particular attention must be given to possible changes in the impurity profile of the product if a modified or new micro-organism is introduced into the process.

RAW MATERIALS

The raw materials employed in the fermentation and/or down-stream processing are of suitable quality for the intended purpose. They are tested to ensure that they comply with written specifications.

Levels of bioburden in media or in the inlet air for aeration are reduced to an adequately low level to ensure that if microbiological contamination occurs, it does not adversely affect the quality, purity and safety of the product. Addition of components such as nutrients, precursors, and substrates during fermentation takes place aseptically.

IN-PROCESS CONTROLS

In-process controls are in place to ensure the consistency of the conditions during fermentation and down-stream processing and of the quality of the isolated product. Particular attention must be paid to ensure that any microbial contamination that adversely affects the quality, purity and safety of the product is detected by the controls applied.

Production conditions may be monitored, as appropriate, by suitable procedures for example to control and check:

- temperature,
- pH,
- rate of aeration,
- rate of agitation,
- pressure,

and to monitor the concentration of the required product.

DOWN-STREAM PROCESSING

At the end of fermentation, the producer micro-organism is inactivated or removed. Further processing is designed to reduce residues originating from the culture medium to an acceptable level and to ensure that the desired product is recovered with consistent quality.

Various purification processes may be used, for example, charcoal treatment, ultrafiltration and solvent extraction. It must be demonstrated that the process or processes chosen reduce to a minimum or remove:

- residues from the producer micro-organism, culture media, substrates and precursors,
- unwanted transformation products of substrates and precursors.

If necessary, suitable tests are performed either as in-process controls or on the isolated product of fermentation.

IDENTIFICATION, TESTS AND ASSAY

The requirements with which the product must comply throughout its period of validity, as well as specific test methods, are stated in the individual monographs.

STORAGE

See the individual monographs.

LABELLING

See the individual monographs.

General monographs

01/2005:1483

PRODUCTS WITH RISK OF TRANSMITTING AGENTS OF ANIMAL SPONGIFORM ENCEPHALOPATHIES

Producta cum possibili transmissione vectorium enkephalopathiarum spongiformium animalium

DEFINITION

Products with risk of transmitting agents of animal spongiform encephalopathies are those derived from tissues or secretions of animals susceptible to transmissible spongiform encephalopathies other than by experimental challenge. This monograph applies to all substances or preparations obtained from such animals and to all substances or preparations where products obtained from such animals are included as active substances or excipients or have been used during production, for example as raw or source materials, starting materials or reagents.

PRODUCTION

Production complies with chapter *Minimising the risk of transmitting animal spongiform encephalophathy agents via medicinal products* (*5.2.8*).

01/2005:0125

RADIOPHARMACEUTICAL PREPARATIONS

Radiopharmaceutica

DEFINITION

For the purposes of this general monograph, radiopharmaceutical preparations cover:

- radiopharmaceutical: any medicinal product which, when ready for use, contains one or more radionuclides (radioactive isotopes) included for a medicinal purpose,
- radionuclide generator: any system incorporating a fixed parent radionuclide from which is produced a daughter radionuclide which is to be removed by elution or by any other method and used in a radiopharmaceutical preparation,
- kit for radiopharmaceutical preparation: any preparation to be reconstituted and/or combined with radionuclides in the final radiopharmaceutical preparation, usually prior to its administration,
- radiopharmaceutical precursor: any other radionuclide produced for the radio-labelling of another substance prior to administration.

A nuclide is a species of atom characterised by the number of protons and neutrons in its nucleus (and hence by its atomic number Z, and mass number A) and also by its nuclear energy state. Isotopes of an element are nuclides with the same atomic number but different mass numbers. Nuclides containing an unstable arrangement of protons and neutrons will transform spontaneously to either a stable or another unstable combination of protons and neutrons with a constant statistical probability. Such nuclides are said to be radioactive and are called radionuclides. The initial unstable nuclide is referred to as the parent radionuclide and the resulting nuclide as the daughter nuclide.

The radioactive decay or transformation may involve the emission of charged particles, electron capture (EC) or isomeric transition (IT). The charged particles emitted from the nucleus may be alpha particles (helium nucleus of mass number 4) or beta particles (negatively charged, generally called electrons or positively charged, generally called positrons). The emission of charged particles from the nucleus may be accompanied by the emission of gamma rays. Gamma rays are also emitted in the process of isomeric transition. These emissions of gamma rays may be partly replaced by the ejection of electrons known as internal conversion electrons. This phenomenon, like the process of electron capture, causes a secondary emission of X-rays (due to the reorganisation of the electrons in the atom). This secondary emission may itself be partly replaced by the ejection of electrons known as Auger electrons. Radionuclides with a deficit of neutrons may decay by emitting positrons. These radionuclides are called positron emitters. Positrons are annihilated on contact with electrons, the process being accompanied by the emission of usually two gamma photons, each with an energy of 511 keV, generally emitted at 180° to each other, termed annihilation radiation.

The decay of a radionuclide is governed by the laws of probability with a characteristic decay constant and follows an exponential law. The time in which a given quantity of a radionuclide decays to half its initial value is termed the half-life ($T_{1/2}$).

The penetrating power of each radiation varies considerably according to its nature and its energy. Alpha particles are completely absorbed in a thickness of a few micrometers to some tens of micrometers of matter. Beta particles are completely absorbed in a thickness of several millimetres to several centimetres of matter. Gamma rays are not completely absorbed but only attenuated and a tenfold reduction may require, for example, several centimetres of lead. For most absorbents, the denser the absorbent, the shorter the range of alpha and beta particles and the greater the attenuation of gamma rays.

Each radionuclide is characterised by an invariable half-life, expressed in units of time and by the nature and energy of its radiation or radiations. The energy is expressed in electronvolts (eV), kilo-electronvolts (keV) or mega-electronvolts (MeV).

Generally the term "radioactivity" is used to describe the phenomenon of radioactive decay and to express the physical quantity (activity) of this phenomenon. The radioactivity of a preparation is the number of nuclear disintegrations or transformations per unit time.

In the International System (SI), radioactivity is expressed in becquerel (Bq) which is one nuclear transformation per second. Absolute radioactivity measurements require a specialised laboratory but identification and measurement of radiation can be carried out relatively by comparing with standardised preparations provided by laboratories recognised by the competent authority.

Radionuclidic purity: the ratio, expressed as a percentage, of the radioactivity of the radionuclide concerned to the total radioactivity of the radiopharmaceutical preparation. The relevant radionuclidic impurities are listed with their limits in the individual monographs.

Radiochemical purity: the ratio, expressed as a percentage, of the radioactivity of the radionuclide concerned which is present in the radiopharmaceutical preparation in the stated chemical form, to the total radioactivity of that radionuclide present in the radiopharmaceutical preparation. The relevant radiochemical impurities are listed with their limits in the individual monographs.

Chemical purity: in monographs on radiopharmaceutical preparations chemical purity is controlled by specifying limits on chemical impurities.

Isotopic carrier: a stable isotope of the element concerned either present or added to the radioactive preparation in the same chemical form as that in which the radionuclide is present.

Specific radioactivity: the radioactivity of a radionuclide per unit mass of the element or of the chemical form concerned.

Radioactive concentration: the radioactivity of a radionuclide per unit volume.

Total radioactivity: the radioactivity of the radionuclide, expressed per unit (vial, capsule, ampoule, generator, etc).

Starting materials: all the constituents which make up the radiopharmaceutical preparations.

General monographs

Period of validity: the time during which specifications described in the monograph must be fulfilled. Expiry date and, if necessary, time must be clearly stated.

PRODUCTION

A radiopharmaceutical preparation monograph describes as precisely as possible the method of production of the radionuclide. A radiopharmaceutical preparation contains its radionuclide:

- as an element in atomic or molecular form, e.g. [^{133}Xe], [^{15}O]O_2,
- as an ion, e.g. [^{131}I]iodide, [^{99m}Tc]pertechnetate,
- included in or attached to organic molecules by chelation, e.g. [^{111}In]oxine or by covalent bonding, e.g. 2-[^{18}F]fluoro-2-deoxy-D-glucose.

The practical ways of producing radionuclides for use in, or as radiopharmaceutical preparations are:

- neutron bombardment of target materials (generally in nuclear reactors),
- charged particles bombardment of target materials (in accelerators such as cyclotrons),
- nuclear fission of heavy nuclides of target materials (generally after neutron or particle bombardment),
- from a radionuclide generator.

NEUTRON OR CHARGED PARTICLE BOMBARDMENT

The nuclear reaction and the probability of its occurrence in unit time are dependent on the nature and physical properties of the target material and the nature, energy and quantity of the incident particles.

The nuclear transformation occurring through particle bombardment may be written in the form:

target nucleus (bombarding particle, emitted particle or radiation) produced nucleus.

Examples: ^{58}Fe(n,γ)^{59}Fe

^{18}O(p,n)^{18}F

In addition to the desired nuclear reaction adventitious transformations may occur. These will be influenced by the energy of the incident particle and the purity of the target material. Such adventitious transformations may give rise to radionuclidic impurities.

NUCLEAR FISSION

A small number of nuclides with a high atomic number are fissionable and the most frequently used reaction is the fission of uranium-235 by neutrons in a nuclear reactor. Iodine-131, molybdenum-99 and xenon-133 may be produced by nuclear fission of uranium-235. Their extraction from a mixture of more than 200 other radionuclides must be carefully controlled in order to minimise the radionuclidic impurities.

RADIONUCLIDE GENERATORS

Radionuclide generator systems use a relatively long-lived parent radionuclide which decays to a daughter radionuclide, usually with a shorter half-life.

By separating the daughter radionuclide from the parent radionuclide by a chemical or physical process, it is possible to use the daughter at a considerable distance from the production site of the generators despite its short half-life.

TARGET MATERIALS

The isotopic composition and purity of the target material will determine the relative percentages of the principal radionuclide and radionuclidic impurities. The use of isotopically enriched target material in which the abundance of the required target nuclide has been artificially increased, can improve the production yield and the purity of the desired radionuclide.

The chemical form, the purity, the physical state and the chemical additives, as well as the bombardment conditions and the direct physical and chemical environment will determine the chemical state and chemical purity of the radionuclides which are produced.

In the production of radionuclides and particularly of short-lived radionuclides it may not be possible to determine any of these quality criteria before further processing and manufacture of radiopharmaceutical preparations. Therefore each batch of target material must be tested in test production runs before its use in routine radionuclide production and manufacture of the radiopharmaceutical preparations, to ensure that under specified conditions, the target yields the radionuclide in the desired quantity and quality specified.

The target material is contained in a holder in gaseous, liquid or solid state, in order to be irradiated by a beam of particles. For neutron bombardment, the target material is commonly contained in quartz ampoules or high purity aluminium or titanium containers. It is necessary to ascertain that no interaction can occur between the container and its contents under the irradiation conditions (temperature, pressure, time).

For charged particle bombardment, the holder for target material is usually built of aluminium or another appropriate metal, with inlet and outlet ports, a surrounding cooling system and usually a thin metal foil target window. The nature and thickness of the target window have a particular influence on the yield of the nuclear reaction and may also affect the radionuclidic purity.

The production procedure clearly describes:

- target material,
- construction of the holder for target material,
- loading of target material into the irradiation system,
- method of irradiation (bombardment),
- separation of the desired radionuclide,

and evaluates all effects on the efficiency of the production in terms of quality and quantity of the produced radionuclide.

The chemical state of the isolated radionuclide may play a major role in all further processing.

PRECURSORS FOR SYNTHESIS

Generally, these precursors are not produced on a large scale. Some precursors are synthesised by the radiopharmaceutical production laboratory, others are supplied by specialised producers or laboratories.

Tests for identity, for chemical purity and the assay must be performed by validated procedures.

When batches of precursors are accepted using data from the certificates of analysis, suitable evidence has to be established to demonstrate the consistent reliability of the supplier's analyses and at least one identity test must be conducted. It is recommended to test precursor materials in production runs before their use for the manufacture of radiopharmaceutical preparations, to ensure that under specified production conditions, the precursor yields the radiopharmaceutical preparation in the desired quantity and quality specified.

PERFORMANCE OF THE PRODUCTION SYSTEM

All operations, from the preparation of the target to the dispensing of the final radiopharmaceutical preparation, must be clearly documented including their impact on the purity of the final product and the efficiency of the procedure.

Where possible, in-process controls are performed and the results recorded at each production step to identify at which level a possible discrepancy from the normal production pathway may have occurred.

a) The production of radiopharmaceutical preparations may make use of mechanical and automated processes that are used in the pharmaceutical industry, subject to adapting these to the specificity of the radioactive starting material and to the requirements of radioprotection.

b) For radiopharmaceutical preparations containing shortlived radionuclides, such as certain positron emitters, remotely controlled production and automated radiosynthesis are generally used. For radionuclides with a very short half-life (less than 20 min) the control of the performance of the production system is an important measure to assure the quality of the radiopharmaceutical preparation before its release.

c) Any production procedure must be validated in test production runs before its use in routine manufacture of radiopharmaceutical preparations, to ensure that under specified production conditions, the production system yields the radiopharmaceutical preparation in the desired quantity and specified quality.

d) The preparation of the dosage form of the final radiopharmaceutical preparation in the practice of nuclear medicine generally involves limited radioactivity starting from ready-to-use radiopharmaceutical preparations, generators, kits and radioactive precursors. All conditions which may affect the quality of the product (e.g. radiochemical purity and sterility) must be clearly defined and must include appropriate measures for radiation protection.

IDENTIFICATION

Radioactive decay: radioactivity decays at an exponential rate with a decay constant characteristic of each radionuclide.

The curve of exponential decay (decay curve) is described by the equation:

$$A_t = A_o e^{-\lambda t}$$

A_t = the radioactivity at time t,

A_o = the radioactivity at time $t = 0$,

λ = the decay constant characteristic of each radionuclide,

e = the base of Napierian logarithms.

The half-life ($T_{1/2}$) is related to the decay constant (λ) by the equation:

$$T_{1/2} = \frac{\ln 2}{\lambda} \qquad (\ln 2 \approx 0.693)$$

The radionuclide is generally identified by its half-life or by the nature and energy of its radiation or radiations or by both, as prescribed in the monograph.

Measurement of half-life. The half-life is measured with a suitable detection apparatus such as an ionisation chamber, a Geiger-Müller counter, a scintillation counter (solid crystal, liquid) or a semiconductor detector. The preparation to be tested is used as such or diluted or dried in a capsule after appropriate dilution. The radioactivity chosen, having regard to experimental conditions, must be of a sufficiently high level to allow detection during several estimated half-lives, but not too high to minimise count rate losses, for example due to dead time.

The radioactive source is prepared in a manner that will avoid loss of material during handling. If it is a liquid (solution), it is contained in bottles or sealed tubes. If it is a solid (residue from drying in a capsule), it is protected by a cover consisting of a sheet of adhesive cellulose acetate or of some other material.

The same source is measured in the same geometrical conditions and at intervals usually corresponding to half of the estimated half-life throughout a time equal to about three half-lives. The correct functioning of the apparatus is checked using a source of long half-life and, if necessary, corrections for any changes of the count rate have to be applied (see Measurement of Radioactivity).

A graph can be drawn with time as the abscissa and the logarithm of the relative instrument reading (e.g. count rate) as the ordinate. The calculated half-life differs by not more than 5 per cent from the half-life stated in the Pharmacopoeia, unless otherwise stated.

Determination of the nature and energy of the radiation. The nature and energy of the radiation emitted may be determined by several procedures including the construction of an attenuation curve and the use of spectrometry. The attenuation curve can be used for analysis of electron radiation; spectrometry is mostly used for identification of gamma rays and detectable X-rays.

The *attenuation curve* is drawn for pure electron emitters when no spectrometer for beta rays is available or for beta/gamma emitters when no spectrometer for gamma rays is available. This method of estimating the maximum energy of beta radiation gives only an approximate value. The source, suitably mounted to give constant geometrical conditions, is placed in front of the thin window of a Geiger-Müller counter or a proportional counter. The source is protected as described above. The count rate of the source is then measured. Between the source and the counter are placed, in succession, at least six aluminium screens of increasing mass per unit area within such limits that with a pure beta emitter this count rate is not affected by the addition of further screens. The screens are inserted in such a manner that constant geometrical conditions are maintained. A graph is drawn showing, as the abscissa, the mass per unit area of the screen expressed in milligrams per square centimetre and, as the ordinate, the logarithm of the count rate for each screen examined. A graph is drawn in the same manner for a standardised preparation. The mass attenuation coefficients are calculated from the median parts of the curves, which are practically rectilinear.

The *mass attenuation coefficient* μ_m, expressed in square centimetres per milligram, depends on the energy spectrum of the beta radiation and on the nature and the physical properties of the screen. It therefore allows beta emitters to be identified. It is calculated using the equation:

$$\mu_m = \frac{\ln A_1 - \ln A_2}{m_2 - m_1}$$

m_1 = mass per unit area of the lightest screen,

m_2 = mass per unit area of the heaviest screen, m_1 and m_2 being within the rectilinear part of the curve,

A_1 = count rate for mass per unit area m_1,

A_2 = count rate for mass per unit area m_2.

The mass attenuation coefficient μ_m thus calculated does not differ by more than 10 per cent from the coefficient obtained under identical conditions using a standardised preparation of the same radionuclide.

The range of beta particles is a further parameter which can be used for the determination of the beta energy. It is obtained from the graph described above as the mass per unit area corresponding to the intersection of the extrapolations of the descending rectilinear part of the attenuation curve and the horizontal line of background radioactivity.

Liquid scintillation counting may be used to obtain spectra of α and β^- emitters (see measurement of radioactivity).

Gamma spectrometry is used to identify radionuclides by the energy and intensity of their gamma rays and X-rays.

The preferred detector for gamma and X-ray spectrometry is a germanium semiconductor detector. A thallium-activated sodium iodide scintillation detector is also used but this has a much lower energy resolution.

The gamma detector has to be calibrated using standard sources because the detection efficiency is a function of the energy of the gamma and X-rays as well as the form of the source and the source-to-detector distance. The detection efficiency may be measured using a calibrated source of the radionuclide to be measured or, for more general work, a graph of efficiency against gamma and X-ray energy may be constructed from a series of calibrated sources of various radionuclides.

The gamma and X-ray spectrum of a radionuclide which emits gamma and X-rays is unique to that nuclide and is characterised by the energies and the number of photons of particular energies emitted per transformation from one energy level to another energy level. This property contributes to the identification of radionuclides present in a source and to their quantification. It allows the estimation of the degree of radionuclidic impurity by detecting peaks other than those expected.

It is possible to establish the rate of the decay of radioactivity using gamma spectrometry since the peaks diminish in amplitude as a function of the half-life. If, in such a source, a radioactive impurity with a different half-life is present, it is possible to detect the latter by identification of the characteristic peak or peaks whose amplitudes decrease at a different rate from that expected for the particular radionuclide. A determination of the half-life of the additional peaks by repeated measurements of the sample will help to identify the impurity.

The *Table of physical characteristics of radionuclides mentioned in the European Pharmacopoeia (5.7)* summarises the most commonly accepted physical characteristics of radionuclides used in preparations which are the subject of monographs in the European Pharmacopoeia. In addition, the Table states the physical characteristics of the main potential impurities of the radionuclides mentioned in the monographs.

By "transition probability" is meant the probability of the transformation of a nucleus in a given energy state, via the transition concerned. Instead of "probability" the terms "intensity" and "abundance" are frequently used.

By "emission probability" is meant the probability of an atom of a radionuclide giving rise to the emission of the particles or radiation concerned.

Irrespective of whether the one or the other meaning is intended, probability is usually measured in terms of 100 disintegrations.

MEASUREMENT OF RADIOACTIVITY

The radioactivity of a preparation is stated at a given date and, if necessary, time.

The absolute measurement of the radioactivity of a given sample may be carried out if the decay scheme of the radionuclide is known, but in practice many corrections are required to obtain accurate results. For this reason it is common to carry out the measurement with the aid of a primary standard source. Primary standards may not be available for short-lived radionuclides e.g. positron emitters. Measuring instruments are calibrated using suitable standards for the particular radionuclides. Standards are available from the laboratories recognised by the competent authority. Ionisation chambers and Geiger-Müller counters may be used to measure beta and beta/gamma emitters; scintillation or semiconductor counters or ionisation chambers may be used for measuring gamma emitters; low-energy beta emitters require a liquid-scintillation counter. For the detection and measurement of alpha emitters, specialised equipment and techniques are required. For an accurate comparison of radioactive sources, it is essential for samples and standards to be measured under similar conditions.

Low-energy beta emitters may be measured by liquid-scintillation counting. The sample is dissolved in a solution containing one or more often two organic fluorescent substances (primary and secondary scintillators), which convert part of the energy of disintegration into photons of light, which are detected by a photomultiplier and converted into electrical impulses. When using a liquid-scintillation counter, comparative measurements are corrected for light-quenching effects. Direct measurements are made, wherever possible, under similar conditions, (e.g. volumes and type of solutions) for the source to be examined and the standard source.

All measurements of radioactivity must be corrected by subtracting the background due to radioactivity in the environment and to spurious signals generated in the equipment itself.

With some equipment, when measurements are made at high levels of radioactivity, it may be necessary to correct for loss by coincidence due to the finite resolving time of the detector and its associated electronic equipment. For a counting system with a fixed dead time τ following each count, the correction is:

$$N = \frac{N_{obs}}{1 - N_{obs}\tau}$$

N = the true count rate per second,

N_{obs} = the observed count rate per second,

τ = the dead time, in seconds.

With some equipment this correction is made automatically. Corrections for loss by coincidence must be made before the correction for background radiation.

If the time of an individual measurement, t_m is not negligible short compared with the half-life, $T_{1/2}$, the decay during this measurement time must be taken into account. After having corrected the instrument reading (count rate, ionisation current, etc.) for background and, if necessary, for losses due to electronic effects, the decay correction during measurement time is:

$$R_{corr} = \frac{R\dfrac{t_m \ln 2}{T_{1/2}}}{1 - \exp\left(-\dfrac{t_m \ln 2}{T_{1/2}}\right)}$$

R_{corr} = instrument reading corrected to the beginning of the individual measurement,

R = instrument reading before decay correction, but already corrected for background, etc.

The results of determinations of radioactivity show variations which derive mainly from the random nature of nuclear transformation. A sufficient number of counts must be registered in order to compensate for variations in the number of transformations per unit of time. The standard deviation is the square root of the counts, so at least 10 000 counts are necessary to obtain a relative standard deviation of not more than 1 per cent (confidence interval: 1 sigma).

All statements of radioactive content are accompanied by a statement of the date and, if necessary, the time at which the measurement was made. This statement of the radioactive content must be made with reference to a time zone (GMT, CET). The radioactivity at other times may be calculated from the exponential equation or from tables.

The radioactivity of a solution is expressed per unit volume to give the radioactive concentration.

RADIONUCLIDIC PURITY

In most of the cases, to state the radionuclidic purity of a radiopharmaceutical preparation, the identity of every radionuclide present and their radioactivity must be known. The most generally useful method for examination of radionuclidic purity is that of gamma spectrometry. It is not a completely reliable method because alpha- and beta-emitting impurities are not usually easily detectable and, when sodium iodide detectors are employed, the peaks due to gamma emitting impurities are often obscured by the spectrum of the principal radionuclide.

The individual monographs prescribe the radionuclidic purity required (for example, the gamma-ray spectrum does not significantly differ from that of a standardised preparation) and may set limits for specific radionuclidic impurities (for example, cobalt-60 in cobalt-57). While these requirements are necessary, they are not in themselves sufficient to ensure that the radionuclidic purity of a preparation is sufficient for human use. The manufacturer must examine the product in detail and especially must examine preparations of radionuclides of short half-life for impurities of long half-life after a suitable period of decay. In this way, information on the suitability of the manufacturing processes and the adequacy of the testing procedures may be obtained. In cases where two or more positron emitting radionuclides need to be identified and/or differentiated, as e.g. 18F-impurities in 13N-preparations, half-life determinations need to be carried out in addition to gamma spectrometry.

Due to differences in the half-lives of the different radionuclides present in a radiopharmaceutical preparation, the radionuclidic purity changes with time. The requirement of the radionuclidic purity must be fulfilled throughout the period of validity. It is sometimes difficult to carry out these tests before authorising the release for use of the batch when the half-life of the radionuclide in the preparation is short. The test then constitutes a control of the quality of production.

RADIOCHEMICAL PURITY

The determination of radiochemical purity requires separation of the different chemical substances containing the radionuclide and estimating the percentage of radioactivity associated with the declared chemical substance. Radiochemical impurities may originate from:

- radionuclide production,
- subsequent chemical procedures,
- incomplete preparative separation,
- chemical changes during storage.

The requirement of the radiochemical purity must be fulfilled throughout the period of validity.

In principle, any method of analytical separation may be used in the determination of radiochemical purity. For example, the monographs for radiopharmaceutical products may include paper chromatography (*2.2.26*), thin-layer chromatography (*2.2.27*), electrophoresis (*2.2.31*), size-exclusion chromatography (*2.2.30*), gas chromatography (*2.2.28*) and liquid chromatography (*2.2.29*). The technical description of these analytical methods is set out in the monographs. Moreover certain precautions special to radioactivity must also be taken for radiation protection.

In a hospital environment thin-layer and paper chromatography are mostly used. In paper and thin-layer chromatography, a volume equal to that described in the monograph is deposited on the starting-line as prescribed in the general methods for chromatography. It is preferable not to dilute the preparation to be examined but it is important to avoid depositing such a quantity of radioactivity that counting losses by coincidence occur during measurement of the radioactivity. On account of the very small quantities of the radioactive material applied, a carrier may be added when specified in a particular monograph. After development, the support is dried and the positions of the radioactive areas are detected by autoradiography or by measurement of radioactivity over the length of the chromatogram, using suitable collimated counters or by cutting the strips and counting each portion. The positions of the spots or areas permit chemical identification by comparison with solutions of the same chemical substances (non-radioactive) using a suitable detection method.

Radioactivity may be measured by integration using an automatic-plotting instrument or a digital counter. The ratios of the areas under the peaks give the ratios of the radioactive concentration of the chemical substances. When the strips are cut into portions, the ratios of the quantities of radioactivity measured give the ratio of concentrations of the radioactive chemical species.

SPECIFIC RADIOACTIVITY

Specific radioactivity is usually calculated taking into account the radioactive concentration (radioactivity per unit volume) and the concentration of the chemical substance being studied, after verification that the radioactivity is attributable only to the radionuclide (radionuclidic purity) and the chemical species (radiochemical purity) concerned.

Specific radioactivity changes with time. The statement of the specific radioactivity therefore includes reference to a date and, if necessary, time. The requirement of the specific radioactivity must be fulfilled throughout the period of validity.

CHEMICAL PURITY

The determination of chemical purity requires quantification of the individual chemical impurities specified in the monograph.

ENANTIOMERIC PURITY

Where appropriate, the stereoisomeric purity has to be verified.

PHYSIOLOGICAL DISTRIBUTION

A physiological distribution test is prescribed, if necessary, for certain radiopharmaceutical preparations. The distribution pattern of radioactivity observed in specified organs, tissues or other body compartments of an appropriate animal species (usually rats or mice) can be a reliable indication of the expected distribution in humans and thus of the suitability for the intended purpose.

General monographs

The individual monograph prescribes the details concerning the performance of the test and the physiological distribution requirements which must be met for the radiopharmaceutical preparation. A physiological distribution conforming to the requirements will assure appropriate distribution of the radioactive compounds to the intended biological target in humans and limits its distribution to non-target areas.

In general, the test is performed as follows.

Each of three animals is injected intravenously with the preparation to be tested. If relevant, the species, sex, strain and weight and/or age of the animals is specified in the monograph. The test injection is the radiopharmaceutical preparation as it is intended for human use. Where applicable, products are reconstituted according to the manufacturer's instructions. In some cases, dilution immediately before injection may be necessary.

The administration will normally be made via the intravenous route for which purpose the caudal vein is used. Other veins such as the saphenous, femoral, jugular or penile veins may be used in special cases. Animals showing evidence of extravasation of the injection (observed at the time of injection or revealed by subsequent assay of tissue radioactivity) are rejected from the test.

Immediately after injection each animal is placed in a separate cage which will allow collection of excreta and prevent contamination of the body surface of the animal.

At the specified time after injection, the animals are killed by an appropriate method and dissected. Selected organs and tissues are assayed for their radioactivity using a suitable instrument as described elsewhere in this monograph. The physiological distribution is then calculated and expressed in terms of the percentage of the radioactivity which is found in each of the selected organs or tissues. For this purpose the radioactivity in an organ may be related to the injected radioactivity calculated from the radioactive content of the syringe measured before and after injection. For some radiopharmaceutical preparations it may be appropriate to determine the ratio of the radioactivity in weighed samples of selected tissues (radioactivity/mass).

For a preparation to meet the requirements of the test, the distribution of radioactivity in at least two of the three animals must comply with all the specified criteria.

STERILITY

Radiopharmaceutical preparations for parenteral administration must be prepared using precautions designed to exclude microbial contamination and to ensure sterility. The test for sterility is carried out as described in the general method for sterility (*2.6.1*). Special difficulties arise with radiopharmaceutical preparations because of the short half-life of some radionuclides small size of batches and the radiation hazards. It is not always possible to await the results of the test for sterility before authorisation of the release for use of the batch concerned. Parametric release (*5.1.1)* of the product manufactured by a fully validated process is the method of choice in such cases. When aseptic manufacturing is used, the test for sterility has to be executed as a control of the quality of production.

When the size of a batch of the radiopharmaceutical preparation is limited to one or a few samples (e.g. therapeutic or very short-lived radiopharmaceutical preparation), sampling the batch for sterility testing may not be applicable. If the radiopharmaceutical preparation is sterilised by filtration and/or aseptically processed (*5.1.1*) process validation is critical.

When the half-life of the radionuclide is very short (e.g. less than 20 min), the administration of the radiopharmaceutical preparation to the patient is generally on-line with a validated production system.

For safety reasons (high level of radioactivity) it is not possible to use the quantity of the radiopharmaceutical preparations as required in the test for sterility (*2.6.1*). The method by membrane filtration is to be preferred to limit irradiation of personnel.

Notwithstanding the requirements concerning the use of antimicrobial preservatives in *Parenteral preparations (0520)*, their addition to radiopharmaceutical preparations in multidose containers is not obligatory, unless prescribed in the monograph.

BACTERIAL ENDOTOXINS - PYROGENS

For certain radiopharmaceutical preparations a test for bacterial endotoxins is prescribed. The test is carried out as described in the general method (*2.6.14*), taking the necessary precautions to limit irradiation of the personnel carrying out the test.

The limit for bacterial endotoxins is indicated in the individual monograph.

When the nature of the radiopharmaceutical preparation results in an interference by inhibition or activation and it is not possible to eliminate the interfering factor(s), the test for pyrogens (*2.6.8*) may be specifically prescribed.

It is sometimes difficult to carry out these tests before releasing the batch for use when the half-life of the radionuclide in the preparation is short. The test then constitutes a control of the quality of production.

STORAGE

Store in an airtight container in a place that is sufficiently shielded to protect personnel from irradiation by primary or secondary emissions and that complies with national and international regulations concerning the storage of radioactive substances. During storage, containers may darken due to irradiation. Such darkening does not necessarily involve deterioration of the preparations.

Radiopharmaceutical preparations are intended for use within a short time and the end of the period of validity must be clearly stated.

LABELLING

The labelling of radiopharmaceutical preparations complies with the relevant national and European legislation.

The label on the direct container states:

- the name of the preparation and/or its reference,
- the name of the manufacturer,
- an identification number,
- for liquid and gaseous preparations: the total radioactivity in the container, or the radioactive concentration per millilitre at a stated date and, if necessary, time, and the volume of liquid in the container,
- for solid preparations (such as freeze-dried preparations): the total radioactivity at a stated date and, if necessary, time. After reconstitution with the appropriate solution, the preparation is considered as a liquid preparation,
- for capsules: the radioactivity per capsule at a stated date and, if necessary, time and the number of capsules in the container.

The labelling can be adapted in certain cases (e.g. radiopharmaceutical preparations containing short-lived radionuclides).

In addition, the label on the outer package states:
- the route of administration,
- the period of validity or the expiry date,
- the name and concentration of any added antimicrobial preservative,
- where applicable, any special storage conditions.

01/2005:0784

RECOMBINANT DNA TECHNOLOGY, PRODUCTS OF

Producta ab ADN recombinante

This monograph provides general requirements for the development and manufacture of products of recombinant DNA technology. These requirements are not necessarily comprehensive in a given case and requirements complementary or additional to those prescribed in this monograph may be imposed in an individual monograph or by the competent authority.

The monograph is not applicable to modified live organisms that are intended to be used directly in man and animals, for example as live vaccines.

DEFINITION

Products of rDNA technology are produced by genetic modification in which DNA coding for the required product is introduced, usually by means of a plasmid or a viral vector, into a suitable micro-organism or cell line, in which that DNA is expressed and translated into protein. The desired product is then recovered by extraction and purification. The cell or micro-organism before harbouring the vector is referred to as the host cell, and the stable association of the two used in the manufacturing process is referred to as the host-vector system.

PRODUCTION

Production is based on a validated seed-lot system using a host-vector combination that has been shown to be suitable to the satisfaction of the competent authority. The seed-lot system uses a master cell bank and a working cell bank derived from the master seed lot of the host-vector combination. A detailed description of cultivation, extraction and purification steps and a definition of the production batch shall be established.

The determination of the suitability of the host-vector combination and the validation of the seed-lot system include the following elements.

CLONING AND EXPRESSION

The suitability of the host-vector system, particularly as regards microbiological purity, is demonstrated by:

Characterisation of the host cell, including source, phenotype and genotype, and of the cell-culture media.

Documentation of the strategy for the cloning of the gene and characterisation of the recombinant vector including:

i. the origin and characterisation of the gene;

ii. nucleotide-sequence analysis of the cloned gene and the flanking control regions of the expression vector. The cloned sequences are kept to a minimum and all relevant expressed sequences are clearly identified and confirmed at the RNA level.

The DNA sequence of the cloned gene is normally confirmed at the seed-lot stage, up to and beyond the normal level of population doubling for full-scale fermentation. In certain systems, for example, where multiple copies of the gene are inserted into the genome of a continuous cell line, it may be inappropriate to sequence the cloned gene at the production level. Under these circumstances, Southern blot analysis of total cellular DNA or sequence analysis of the messenger RNA (m RNA) may be helpful, particular attention being paid to the characterisation of the expressed protein;

iii. the construction, genetics and structure of the complete expression vector.

Characterisation of the host-vector systemincluding:

i. mechanism of transfer of the vector into the host cells;

ii. copy number, physical state and stability of the vector inside the host cell;

iii. measures used to promote and control the expression.

CELL-BANK SYSTEM

The master cell bank is a homogeneous suspension of the original cells already transformed by the expression vector containing the desired gene, distributed in equal volumes into individual containers for storage (for example, in liquid nitrogen). In some cases it may be necessary to establish separate master cell banks for the expression vector and the host cells.

The working cell bank is a homogeneous suspension of the cell material derived from the master cell bank(s) at a finite passage level, distributed in equal volumes into individual containers for storage (for example, in liquid nitrogen).

In both cell banks, all containers are treated identically during storage and, once removed from storage, the containers are not returned to the cell stock.

The cell bank may be used for production at a finite passage level or for continuous-culture production.

Production at a finite passage level

This cultivation method is defined by a limited number of passages or population doublings which must not be exceeded during production. The maximum number of cell doublings, or passage levels, during which the manufacturing process routinely meets the criteria described below must be stated.

Continuous-culture production

By this cultivation method the number of passages or population doublings is not restricted from the beginning of production. Criteria for the harvesting as well as for the termination of production have to be defined by the manufacturer. Monitoring is necessary throughout the life of the culture; the required frequency and type of monitoring will depend on the nature of the production system and the product.

Information is required on the molecular integrity of the gene being expressed and on the phenotypic and genotypic characteristics of the host cell after long-term cultivation. The acceptance of harvests for further processing must be clearly linked to the schedule of monitoring applied and a clear definition of a "batch" of product for further processing is required.

VALIDATION OF THE CELL BANKS

Validation of the cell banks includes:

i. stability by measuring viability and the retention of the vector;

ii. identity of the cells by phenotypic features;

iii. where appropriate, evidence that the cell banks are free from potentially oncogenic or infective adventitious agents (viral, bacterial, fungal or mycoplasmal). Special attention has to be given to viruses that can commonly contaminate the species from which the cell line has been derived. Certain cell lines contain endogenous viruses, for example,

General monographs

retroviruses, which may not readily be eliminated. The expression of these organisms, under a variety of conditions known to cause their induction, shall be tested for;

iv. for mammalian cells, details of the tumorigenic potential of the cell bank shall be obtained.

CONTROL OF THE CELLS

The origin, form, storage, use and stability at the anticipated rate of use must be documented in full for all cell banks under conditions of storage and recovery. New cell banks must be fully validated.

VALIDATION OF THE PRODUCTION PROCESS

Extraction and purification

The capacity of each step of the extraction and purification procedure to remove and/or inactivate contaminating substances derived from the host cell or culture medium, including, in particular, virus particles, proteins, nucleic acids and added substances, must be validated.

Validation studies are carried out to demonstrate that the production process routinely meets the following criteria:

- exclusion of extraneous agents from the product. Studies including, for example, viruses with relevant physico-chemical features are undertaken, and a reduction capacity for such contaminants at each relevant stage of purification is established;
- adequate removal of vector, host-cell, culture medium and reagent-derived contaminants from the product. The reduction capacity for DNA is established by spiking. The reduction of proteins of animal origin can be determined by immunochemical methods;
- maintenance within stated limits of the yield of product from the culture;
- adequate stability of any intermediate of production and/or manufacturing when it is intended to use intermediate storage during the process.

Characterisation of the substance

The identity, purity, potency and stability of the final bulk product are established initially by carrying out a wide range of chemical, physical, immunochemical and biological tests. Prior to release, each batch of the product is tested by the manufacturer for identity and purity and an appropriate assay is carried out.

Production consistency

Suitable tests for demonstrating the consistency of the production and purification are performed. The tests include, especially characterisation tests, in-process controls and final-product tests, for example:

AMINO-ACID COMPOSITION

Partial amino-acid sequence analysis. The sequence data permit confirmation of the correct *N*-terminal processing and detection of loss of the *C*-terminal amino acids.

Peptide mapping. Peptide mapping using chemical and/or enzymatic cleavage of the protein product and analysis by a suitable method such as two-dimensional gel electrophoresis, capillary electrophoresis or liquid chromatography must show no significant difference between the test protein and the reference preparation. Peptide mapping can also be used to demonstrate correct disulphide bonding.

DETERMINATION OF MOLECULAR MASS

Cloned-gene retention. The minimum amount in percentage of the cells containing the vector or the cloned gene after cultivation is approved by the relevant authority.

Total protein. The yield of protein is determined.

Chemical purity. The purity of the protein product is analysed in comparison with a reference preparation by a suitable method such as liquid chromatography, capillary electrophoresis or sodium dodecyl sulphate polyacrylamide gel electrophoresis.

Host-cell-derived proteins. Host-cell-derived proteins are detected by immunochemical methods, using, for example, polyclonal antisera raised against protein components of the host-vector system used to manufacture the product, unless otherwise prescribed. The following types of procedure may be used: liquid-phase displacement assays (for example, radio-immunoassay), liquid-phase direct-binding assays and direct-binding assays using antigens immobilised on nitrocellulose (or similar) membranes (for example, dot-immunoblot assays, Western blots). General requirements for the validation of immunoassay procedures are given under *2.7.1. Immunochemical Methods.* In addition, immunoassay methods for host-cell contaminants meet the following criteria:

- *Antigen preparations.* Antisera are raised against a preparation of antigens derived from the host organism, into which has been inserted the vector used in the manufacturing process that lacks the specific gene coding for the product. This host cell is cultured, and proteins are extracted, using conditions identical to those used for culture and extraction in the manufacturing process. Partly purified preparations of antigens, using some of the purification steps in the manufacturing process, may also be used for the preparation of antisera.
- *Calibration and standardisation.* Quantitative data are obtained by comparison with dose-response curves obtained using standard preparations of host-derived protein antigens. Since these preparations are mixtures of poorly defined proteins, a standard preparation is prepared and calibrated by a suitable protein determination method. This preparation is stored in a stable state suitable for use over an extended period of time.
- *Antisera.* Antisera contain high-avidity antibodies recognising as many different proteins in the antigen mixture as possible, and do not cross-react with the product.

Host-cell- and vector-derived DNA. Residual DNA is detected by hybridisation analysis, using suitably sensitive, sequence-independent analytical techniques or other suitably sensitive analytical techniques.

Hybridisation analysis

DNA in the test sample is denatured to give single-stranded DNA, immobilised on a nitrocellulose or other suitable filter and hybridised with labelled DNA prepared from the host-vector manufacturing system (DNA probes). Although a wide variety of experimental approaches is available, hybridisation methods for measurement of host-vector DNA meet the following criteria:

- *DNA probes.* Purified DNA is obtained from the host-vector system grown under the same conditions as those used in the manufacturing process. Host chromosomal DNA and vector DNA may be separately prepared and used as probes.
- *Calibration and standardisation.* Quantitative data are obtained by comparison with responses obtained using standard preparations. Chromosomal DNA probes and vector DNA probes are used with chromosomal DNA and vector DNA standards, respectively. Standard preparations are calibrated by spectroscopic measurements and stored in a state suitable for use over an extended period of time.

– *Hybridisation conditions.* The stringency of hybridisation conditions is such as to ensure specific hybridisation between probes and standard DNA preparations and the drug substances must not interfere with hybridisation at the concentrations used.

Sequence-independent techniques

Suitable procedures include: detection of sulphonated cytosine residues in single-stranded DNA (where DNA is immobilised on a filter and cytosines are derivatised *in situ*, before detection and quantitation using an antibody directed against the sulphonated group); detection of single-stranded DNA using a fragment of single-stranded DNA bound to a protein and an antibody of this protein. Neither procedure requires the use of specific host or vector DNA as an assay standard. However, the method used must be validated to ensure parallelism with the DNA standard used, linearity of response and non-interference of either the drug substance or excipients of the formulation at the dilutions used in the assay.

IDENTIFICATION, TESTS AND ASSAY

The requirements with which the final product (bulk material or dose form) must comply throughout its period of validity, as well as specific test methods, are stated in the individual monograph.

STORAGE

See the individual monographs.

LABELLING

See the individual monographs.

01/2005:2034

SUBSTANCES FOR PHARMACEUTICAL USE

Corpora ad usum pharmaceuticum

The statements in this monograph are intended to be read in conjunction with individual monographs on substances in the Pharmacopoeia. Application of the monograph to other substances may be decided by the competent authority.

DEFINITION

Substances for pharmaceutical use are any organic or inorganic substances that are used as active substances or excipients for the production of medicinal products for human or veterinary use. They may be obtained from natural sources or produced by extraction from raw materials, fermentation or synthesis.

Substances for pharmaceutical use may be used as such or as starting materials for subsequent formulation to prepare medicinal products. Depending on the formulation, certain substances may be used either as active substances or excipients. Solid substances may be compacted, coated, granulated, powdered to a certain fineness or processed in other ways. Processing with addition of excipients is permitted only where this is specifically stated in the Definition of the individual monograph.

Substance for pharmaceutical use of special grade. Unless otherwise indicated or restricted in the individual monographs, a substance for pharmaceutical use is intended for human and veterinary use, and is of appropriate quality for manufacture of all dosage forms in which it can be used.

Polymorphism. Individual monographs do not usually specify crystalline or amorphous forms, unless bioavailability is affected. All forms of a substance for pharmaceutical use comply with the requirements of the monograph, unless otherwise indicated.

PRODUCTION

Substances for pharmaceutical use are manufactured by procedures that are designed to ensure a consistent quality and comply with the requirements of the individual monograph or approved specification.

The provisions of general chapter *5.10* apply to the control of impurities in substances for pharmaceutical use.

Whether or not it is specifically stated in the individual monograph that the substance for pharmaceutical use:

- is a recombinant protein or another substance obtained as a direct gene product based on genetic modification, where applicable, the substance also complies with the requirements of the general monograph on *Products of recombinant DNA technology (0784)*;
- is obtained from animals susceptible to transmissible spongiform encephalopathies other than by experimental challenge, where applicable, the substance also complies with the requirements of the general monograph on *Products with risk of transmitting agents of animal spongiform encephalopathies (1483)*;
- is a substance derived from a fermentation process whether or not the micro-organisms involved are modified by traditional procedures or recombinant DNA (rDNA) technology, where applicable, the substance complies with the requirements of the general monograph on *Products of fermentation (1468)*.

If solvents are used during production, they are of suitable quality. In addition, their toxicity and their residual level are taken into consideration (*5.4*). If water is used during production, it is of suitable quality.

If substances are produced or processed to yield a certain form or grade, that specific form or grade of the substance complies with the requirements of the monograph. Certain functionality-related tests may be described to control properties that may influence the suitability of the substance and subsequently the properties of dosage forms prepared from it.

Powdered substances may be processed to obtain a certain degree of fineness (*2.9.12*).

Compacted substances are processed to increase the particle size or to obtain particles of a specific form and/or to obtain a substance with a higher bulk density.

Coated active substances consist of particles of the active substance coated with one or more suitable excipients.

Granulated active substances are particles of a specified size and/or form produced from the active substance by granulation directly or with one or more suitable excipients.

If substances are processed with excipients, these excipients comply with the requirements of the relevant monograph or, where no such monograph exists, the approved specification.

CHARACTERS

The statements under the heading Characters (e.g. statements about the solubility or a decomposition point) are not to be interpreted in a strict sense and are not requirements. They are given for information.

Where a substance may show polymorphism, this may be stated under Characters in order to draw this to the attention of the user who may have to take this characteristic into consideration during formulation of a preparation.

IDENTIFICATION

Where under Identification an individual monograph contains subdivisions entitled *First identification* and *Second identification*, the test or tests that constitute the *First identification* may be used in all circumstances. The test or tests that constitute the *Second identification* may be used for identification, provided it can be demonstrated that the substance is fully traceable to a batch certified to comply with all the other requirements of the monograph.

TESTS

Polymorphism (*5.9*). If the nature of a crystalline or amorphous form imposes restrictions on its use in preparations, the nature of the specific crystalline or amorphous form is identified, its morphology is adequately controlled and its identity is stated on the label.

Related substances. Organic impurities in active substances are to be reported, identified wherever possible, and qualified as indicated in Table 2034.-1.

Specific thresholds may be applied for impurities known to be unusually potent or to produce toxic or unexpected pharmacological effects.

If the individual monograph does not provide suitable control for a new impurity, a suitable test for control must be developed and included in the specification for the substance.

The requirements above do not apply to biological and biotechnological products, peptides, oligonucleotides, radiopharmaceuticals, products of fermentation and semi-synthetic products derived therefrom, to crude products of animal or plant origin or herbal products.

Residual solvents are limited according to the principles defined in the chapter (*5.4*), using the general method (*2.4.24*) or other suitable methods. Where a quantitative determination of a residual solvent is carried out and a test for loss on drying is not carried out, the content of residual solvent is taken into account for calculation of the assay content of the substance.

Sterility (*2.6.1*). If intended for use in the manufacture of sterile dosage forms without a further appropriate sterilisation procedure, or if offered as sterile grade, the substance for pharmaceutical use complies with the test for sterility.

Bacterial endotoxins (*2.6.14*). If offered as bacterial endotoxin-free grade, the substance for pharmaceutical use complies with the test for bacterial endotoxins. The limit and test method (if not gelation method A) are stated in the individual monograph. The limit is calculated in accordance with *Test for bacterial endotoxins: guidelines* (*2.6.14*), unless a lower limit is justified from results from production batches or is required by the competent authority. Where a test for bacterial endotoxins is prescribed, a test for pyrogens is not required.

Pyrogens (*2.6.8*). If the test for pyrogens is justified rather than the test for bacterial endotoxins and if a pyrogen-free grade is offered, the substance for pharmaceutical use complies with the test for pyrogens. The limit and test method are stated in the individual monograph or approved by the competent authority. Based on appropriate test validation for bacterial endotoxins and pyrogens, the test for bacterial endotoxins may replace the test for pyrogens.

Additional properties. Control of additional properties (e.g. physical characteristics, functionality-related characteristics) may be necessary for individual manufacturing processes or formulations. Grades (such as sterile, endotoxin-free, pyrogen-free) may be produced with a view to manufacture of preparations for parenteral administration or other dosage forms and appropriate requirements may be specified in an individual monograph.

ASSAY

Unless justified and authorised, contents of substances for pharmaceutical use are determined. Suitable methods are used.

LABELLING

In general, labelling is subject to supranational and national regulation and to international agreements. The statements under the heading Labelling therefore are not comprehensive and, moreover, for the purposes of the Pharmacopoeia only those statements that are necessary to demonstrate compliance or non-compliance with the monograph are mandatory. Any other labelling statements are included as recommendations. When the term "label" is used in the Pharmacopoeia, the labelling statements may appear on the container, the package, a leaflet accompanying the package or a certificate of analysis accompanying the article, as decided by the competent authority.

Where appropriate, the label includes statements that the substance is:

- intended for a specific use,
- of a distinct crystalline form,
- of a specific degree of fineness,
- compacted,
- coated,
- granulated,
- sterile,
- free from bacterial endotoxins,
- free from pyrogens,
- containing gliding agents.

Where appropriate, the label indicates the degree of hydration, the nature of any added antimicrobial preservative, antioxidant or other excipient. When active substances are processed with addition of excipients, the label indicates the excipients used and the content of active substance and excipients.

Table 2034.-1. – *Reporting, identification and qualification of organic impurities in active substances*

Use	Maximum daily dose	Reporting threshold	Identification threshold	Qualification threshold
Human use or human and veterinary use	≤ 2 g/day	> 0.05 per cent	> 0.10 per cent or a daily intake of > 1.0 mg (whichever is the lower)	> 0.15 per cent or a daily intake of > 1.0 mg (whichever is the lower)
Human use or human and veterinary use	> 2 g/day	> 0.03 per cent	> 0.05 per cent	> 0.05 per cent
Veterinary use only	Not applicable	> 0.1 per cent	> 0.2 per cent	> 0.5 per cent

01/2005:0153

VACCINES FOR HUMAN USE

Vaccina ad usum humanum

For a combined vaccine, where there is no monograph to cover a particular combination, the vaccine complies with the monograph for each individual component, with any necessary modifications approved by the competent authority.

DEFINITION

Vaccines for human use are preparations containing antigenic substances capable of inducing a specific and active immunity in man against an infecting agent or the toxin or the antigen elaborated by it. They shall have been shown to have acceptable immunogenic activity in man with the intended vaccination schedule.

Vaccines for human use may contain: organisms inactivated by chemical or physical means that maintain adequate immunogenic properties; living organisms that are naturally avirulent or that have been treated to attenuate their virulence whilst retaining adequate immunogenic properties; antigens extracted from the organisms or secreted by them or produced by genetic engineering; the antigens may be used in their native state or may be detoxified by chemical or physical means and may be aggregated, polymerised or conjugated to a carrier to increase their immunogenicity.

Terminology used in monographs on vaccines for human use is defined in chapter *5.2.1*.

Bacterial vaccines are suspensions of various degrees of opacity in colourless or almost colourless liquids, or may be freeze-dried. The concentration of living or inactivated bacteria is expressed in terms of International Units of opacity or, where appropriate, is determined by direct cell count or, for living bacteria, by viable count.

Bacterial toxoids are prepared from toxins by diminishing their toxicity to a non-detectable level or by completely eliminating it by physical or chemical procedures whilst retaining adequate immunogenic properties. The toxins are obtained from selected strains of micro-organisms. The method of production is such that the toxoid does not revert to toxin. Toxoids may be liquid or freeze-dried. They may be purified and adsorbed. Adsorbed toxoids are suspensions of white or grey particles dispersed in colourless or pale yellow liquids and may form a sediment at the bottom of the container.

Viral vaccines are prepared from viruses grown in animals, in fertilised eggs, in suitable cell cultures or in suitable tissues or by culture of genetically engineered cells. They are liquids that vary in opacity according to the type of preparation or may be freeze-dried. Liquid preparations and freeze-dried preparations after reconstitution may be coloured if a pH indicator such as phenol red has been used in the culture medium.

PRODUCTION

General provisions. Requirements for production including in-process testing are included in individual monographs. Where justified and authorised, certain tests may be omitted where it can be demonstrated, for example by validation studies, that the production process consistently ensures compliance with the test.

Unless otherwise justified and authorised, vaccines are produced using a seed-lot system. The methods of preparation are designed to maintain adequate immunogenic properties, to render the preparation harmless and to prevent contamination with extraneous agents.

Unless otherwise justified and authorised, in the production of a final lot of vaccine, the number of passages of a virus, or the number of subcultures of a bacterium, from the master seed lot shall not exceed that used for production of the vaccine shown in clinical studies to be satisfactory with respect to safety and efficacy.

Vaccines are as far as possible free from ingredients known to cause toxic, allergic or other undesirable reactions in man. Suitable additives, including stabilisers and adjuvants may be incorporated. Penicillin and streptomycin are not used at any stage of production nor added to the final product; however, master seed lots prepared with media containing penicillin or streptomycin may, where justified and authorised, be used for production.

Substrates for propagation. Substrates for propagation comply with the relevant requirements of the Pharmacopoeia (*5.2.2, 5.2.3*) or in the absence of such requirements with those of the competent authority. Processing of cell banks and subsequent cell cultures is done under aseptic conditions in an area where no other cells are being handled. Serum and trypsin used in the preparation of cell suspensions shall be shown to be free from extraneous agents.

Seed lots. The strain of bacterium or virus used in a master seed lot is identified by historical records that include information on the origin of the strain and its subsequent manipulation. Suitable measures are taken to ensure that no micro-organism other than the seed strain is present in a seed lot.

Culture media. Culture media are as far as possible free from ingredients known to cause toxic, allergic or other undesirable reactions in man; if inclusion of such ingredients is necessary, it shall be demonstrated that the amount present in the final lot is reduced to such a level as to render the product safe. Approved animal (but not human) serum may be used in the growth medium for cell cultures but the medium used for maintaining cell growth during virus multiplication shall not contain serum, unless otherwise stated. Cell culture media may contain a pH indicator such as phenol red and approved antibiotics at the lowest effective concentration although it is preferable to have a medium free from antibiotics during production.

Propagation and harvest. The seed cultures are propagated and harvested under defined conditions. The purity of the harvest is verified by suitable tests as defined in the monograph.

Control cells. For vaccines produced in cell cultures, control cells are maintained and tested as prescribed. In order to provide a valid control, these cells must be maintained in conditions that are rigorously identical with those used for the production cell cultures, including use of the same batches of media and media changes.

Control eggs. For live vaccines produced in eggs, control eggs are incubated and tested as prescribed in the monograph.

Purification. Where applicable, validated purification procedures may be applied.

Inactivation. Inactivated vaccines are produced using a validated inactivation process whose effectiveness and consistency have been demonstrated. Where there are recognised potential contaminants of a harvest, for example in vaccines produced in eggs from healthy, non-SPF flocks, the inactivation process is also validated with respect to the

General monographs

potential contaminants. A test for inactivation is carried out as soon as possible after the inactivation process, unless otherwise justified and authorised.

Stability of intermediates. During production of vaccines, intermediates are obtained at various stages and are stored, sometimes for long periods. Such intermediates include:

- seed lots,
- live or inactivated harvests from bacterial or viral cultures,
- purified harvests that may consist of toxins or toxoids, polysaccharides, bacterial or viral suspensions,
- purified antigens,
- adsorbed antigens,
- conjugated polysaccharides,
- final bulk vaccine,
- vaccine in the final closed container stored at a temperature lower than that used for stability studies and intended for release without re-assay.

Except where they are used within a short period of time, stability studies are carried out on the intermediates in the intended storage conditions to establish the expected extent of degradation. For final bulk vaccine, stability studies may be carried out on representative samples in conditions equivalent to those intended to be used for storage. For each intermediate (except for seed lots), a period of validity applicable for the intended storage conditions is established, where appropriate in the light of stability studies.

Final bulk. The final bulk is prepared by aseptically blending the ingredients of the vaccine.

Adsorbents. Vaccines may be adsorbed on aluminium hydroxide, aluminium phosphate, calcium phosphate or other suitable adsorbent; the adsorbents are prepared in special conditions which confer the appropriate physical form and adsorptive properties.

Antimicrobial preservatives. Antimicrobial preservatives are used to prevent spoilage or adverse effects caused by microbial contamination occurring during the use of a vaccine. Antimicrobial preservatives are not included in freeze-dried products. For single-dose liquid preparations, inclusion of antimicrobial preservatives is not normally acceptable. For multidose liquid preparations, the need for effective antimicrobial preservation is evaluated taking into account likely contamination during use and the maximum recommended period of use after broaching of the container. If an antimicrobial preservative is used, it shall be shown that it does not impair the safety or efficacy of the vaccine. Addition of antibiotics as antimicrobial preservatives is not normally acceptable.

During development studies, the effectiveness of the antimicrobial preservative throughout the period of validity shall be demonstrated to the satisfaction of the competent authority.

The efficacy of the antimicrobial preservative is evaluated as described in chapter *5.1.3*. If neither the A criteria nor the B criteria can be met, then in justified cases the following criteria are applied to vaccines for human use: bacteria, no increase at 24 h and 7 days, 3 log reduction at 14 days, no increase at 28 days; fungi, no increase at 14 days and 28 days.

Final lot. For vaccines for parenteral administration, the final lot is prepared by aseptically distributing the final bulk into sterile tamper-proof containers which, after freeze-drying where applicable, are closed so as to exclude contamination. For vaccines for administration by a non-parenteral route, the final lot is prepared by distributing the final bulk under suitable conditions into sterile, tamper-proof containers.

Degree of adsorption. During development of an adsorbed vaccine, the degree of adsorption is evaluated as part of the consistency testing. A release specification for the degree of adsorption is established in the light of results found for batches used in clinical testing. From the stability data generated for the vaccine it must be shown that at the end of the period of validity the degree of adsorption will not be less than for batches used in clinical testing.

Stability. During development studies, maintenance of potency of the final lot throughout the period of validity shall be demonstrated; the loss of potency in the recommended storage conditions is assessed and excessive loss even within the limits of acceptable potency may indicate that the vaccine is unacceptable.

Expiry date. Unless otherwise stated, the expiry date is calculated from the beginning of the assay or from the beginning of the first assay for a combined vaccine. For vaccines stored at a temperature lower than that used for stability studies and intended for release without re-assay, the expiry date is calculated from the date of removal from cold storage. If, for a given vaccine, an assay is not carried out, the expiry date is calculated from the date of an approved stability-indicating test or failing this from the date of freeze-drying or the date of filling into the final containers. For a combined vaccine where components are presented in separate containers, the expiry date is that of the component which expires first.

The expiry date applies to vaccines stored in the prescribed conditions.

Animal tests. In accordance with the provisions of the European Convention for the Protection of Vertebrate Animals Used for Experimental and Other Scientific Purposes, tests must be carried out in such a way as to use the minimum number of animals and to cause the least pain, suffering, distress or lasting harm. The criteria for judging tests in monographs must be applied in the light of this. For example, if it is indicated that an animal is considered to show positive, infected etc. when typical clinical signs or death occur then as soon as sufficient indication of a positive result is obtained the animal in question shall be either humanely destroyed or given suitable treatment to prevent unnecessary suffering. In accordance with the General Notices, alternative test methods may be used to demonstrate compliance with the monograph and the use of such tests is particularly encouraged when this leads to replacement or reduction of animal use or reduction of suffering.

TESTS

Vaccines comply with the tests prescribed in individual monographs including, where applicable, the following:

Aluminium (*2.5.13*): maximum 1.25 mg of aluminium (Al) per single human dose where an aluminium adsorbent has been used in the vaccine, unless otherwise stated,

Calcium (*2.5.14*): maximum 1.3 mg of calcium (Ca) per single human dose where a calcium adsorbent has been used in the vaccine, unless otherwise stated,

Formaldehyde (*2.4.18*): maximum 0.2 g/l of free formaldehyde is present in the final product where formaldehyde has been used in the preparation of the vaccine, unless otherwise stated.

Phenol (*2.5.15*): maximum 2.5 g/l is present in the final product where phenol has been used in the preparation of the vaccine, unless otherwise stated.

Water (*2.5.12*): maximum 3.0 per cent *m/m* for freeze-dried vaccines, unless otherwise stated.

STORAGE

Store protected from light. Unless otherwise stated, the storage temperature is 5 ± 3 °C; liquid adsorbed vaccines must not be allowed to freeze.

LABELLING

The label states:

– the name of the preparation,
– a reference identifying the final lot,
– the recommended human dose and route of administration,
– the storage conditions,
– the expiry date,
– the name and amount of any antimicrobial preservative,
– the name of any antibiotic, adjuvant, flavour or stabiliser present in the vaccine,
– the name of any constituent that may cause adverse reactions and any contra-indications to the use of the vaccine,
– for freeze-dried vaccines:
  – the name or composition and the volume of the reconstituting liquid to be added,
  – the time within which the vaccine is to be used after reconstitution.

01/2005:0062
corrected

VACCINES FOR VETERINARY USE

Vaccina ad usum veterinarium

In the case of combined vaccines, for each component that is the subject of a monograph in the Pharmacopoeia, the provisions of that monograph apply to that component, modified where necessary as indicated (see Tests (Safety) below, Evaluation of safety of veterinary vaccines (5.2.6) and Evaluation of efficacy of veterinary vaccines (5.2.7)).

DEFINITION

Vaccines for veterinary use are preparations containing antigenic substances and are administered for the purpose of inducing a specific and active immunity against disease provoked by bacteria, toxins, viruses, fungi or parasites. The vaccines, live or inactivated, confer active immunity that may be transferred passively via maternal antibodies against the immunogens they contain and sometimes also against antigenically related organisms. Vaccines may contain bacteria, toxins, viruses or fungi, living or inactivated, parasites, or antigenic fractions or substances produced by these organisms and rendered harmless whilst retaining all or part of their antigenic properties; vaccines may also contain combinations of these constituents. The antigens may be produced by recombinant DNA technology. Suitable adjuvants may be included to enhance the immunising properties of the vaccines.

Terminology used in monographs on vaccines for veterinary use is defined in chapter *5.2.1*.

BACTERIAL VACCINES AND BACTERIAL TOXOIDS

Bacterial vaccines and bacterial toxoids are prepared from cultures grown on suitable solid or liquid media, or by other suitable means; the requirements of this section do not apply to bacterial vaccines prepared in cell cultures or in live animals. The strain of bacterium used may have been modified by genetic engineering. The identity, antigenic potency and purity of each bacterial culture used is carefully controlled.

Bacterial vaccines contain inactivated or live bacteria or their antigenic components; they are liquid preparations of various degrees of opacity or they may be freeze-dried.

Bacterial toxoids are prepared from toxins by diminishing their toxicity to a very low level or by completely eliminating it by physical or chemical means whilst retaining adequate immunising potency. The toxins are obtained from selected strains of specified micro-organisms grown in suitable media or are obtained by other suitable means, for example, chemical synthesis.

The toxoids may be:

– liquid,
– precipitated with alum or other suitable agent,
– purified and/or adsorbed on aluminium phosphate, aluminium hydroxide, calcium phosphate or other adsorbent prescribed in the monograph.

Bacterial toxoids are clear or slightly opalescent liquids. Adsorbed toxoids are suspensions or emulsions. Certain toxoids may be freeze-dried.

Unless otherwise indicated, statements and requirements given below for bacterial vaccines apply equally to bacterial vaccines, bacterial toxoids and products containing a combination of bacterial cells and toxoid.

VIRAL VACCINES

Viral vaccines are prepared by growth in suitable cell cultures (*5.2.4*), in tissues, in micro-organisms, in fertilised eggs or, where no other possibility is available, in live animals, or by other suitable means. The strain of virus used may have been modified by genetic engineering. They are liquid or freeze-dried preparations of one or more viruses or viral subunits or peptides.

Live viral vaccines are prepared from viruses of attenuated virulence or of natural low virulence for the target species.

Inactivated viral vaccines are treated by a validated procedure for inactivation of the virus and may be purified and concentrated.

VECTOR VACCINES

Vector vaccines are liquid or freeze-dried preparations of one or more types of live micro-organisms (bacteria or viruses) that are non-pathogenic or have low pathogenicity for the target species and in which have been inserted one or more genes encoding antigens that stimulate an immune response protective against other microorganisms.

PRODUCTION

The methods of preparation, which vary according to the type of vaccine, are such as to maintain the identity and immunogenicity of the antigen and to ensure freedom from contamination with extraneous agents.

Substances of animal origin used in the production of vaccines for veterinary use comply with the requirements of chapter *5.2.5*. Other substances used in the preparation of vaccines for veterinary use comply with requirements of the Pharmacopoeia (where a relevant monograph exists) and are prepared in a manner that avoids contamination of the vaccine.

SUBSTRATES FOR PRODUCTION

Cell cultures used in the production of vaccines for veterinary use comply with the requirements of chapter *5.2.4*.

Where a monograph refers to chicken flocks free from specified pathogens (SPF), these flocks comply with the requirements prescribed in chapter *5.2.2*.

General monographs

For production of inactivated vaccines, where vaccine organisms are grown in poultry embryos, such embryos are derived either from SPF flocks (*5.2.2*) or from healthy non-SPF flocks free from the presence of certain agents and their antibodies, as specified in the monograph. It may be necessary to demonstrate that the inactivation process is effective against specified potential contaminants. For the production of a master seed lot and for all passages of a micro-organism up to and including the working seed lot, eggs from SPF flocks (*5.2.2*) are used.

Where it is unavoidable to use animals or animal tissues in the production of veterinary vaccines, such animals shall be free from specified pathogens, as appropriate to the source species and the target animal for the vaccine.

MEDIA

At least the qualitative composition must be recorded of media used for seed culture preparation and for production. The grade of each named ingredient is specified. Where media or ingredients are claimed as proprietary, this is indicated and an appropriate description recorded. Ingredients that are derived from animals are specified as to the source species and country of origin, and must comply with the criteria described in chapter *5.2.5*. Preparation processes for media used, including sterilisation procedures, are documented.

The addition of antibiotics during the manufacturing process is normally restricted to cell culture fluids and other media, egg inocula and material harvested from skin or other tissues.

BACTERIAL SEED LOTS

General requirements. The genus and species (and varieties where appropriate) of the bacteria used in the vaccine are stated. Bacteria used in manufacture are handled in a seed-lot system wherever possible. Each master seed lot is tested as described below. A record of the origin, date of isolation, passage history (including purification and characterisation procedures) and storage conditions is maintained for each master seed lot. Each master seed lot is assigned a specific code for identification purposes.

Propagation. The minimum and maximum number of subcultures of each master seed lot prior to the production stage are specified. The methods used for the preparation of seed cultures, preparation of suspensions for seeding, techniques for inoculation of seeds, titre and concentration of inocula and the media used, are documented. It shall be demonstrated that the characteristics of the seed material (for example, dissociation or antigenicity) are not changed by these subcultures. The conditions under which each seed lot is stored are documented.

Identity and purity. Each master seed lot is shown to contain only the species and strain of bacterium stated. A brief description of the method of identifying each strain by biochemical, serological and morphological characteristics and distinguishing it as far as possible from related strains is recorded, as is also the method of determining the purity of the strain. If the master seed lot is shown to contain living organisms of any kind other than the species and strain stated, then it is unsuitable for vaccine production.

VIRUS SEED LOTS

General requirements. Viruses used in manufacture are handled in a seed-lot system. Each master seed lot is tested as described below. A record of the origin, date of isolation, passage history (including purification and characterisation procedures) and storage conditions is maintained for each seed lot. Each master seed lot is assigned a specific code for identification purposes. Production of vaccine is not normally undertaken using virus more than 5 passages from the master seed lot. In the tests on the master seed lot described below, the organisms used are not normally more than 5 passages from the master seed lot at the start of the tests, unless otherwise indicated.

Where the master seed lot is contained within a permanently infected master cell seed, the following tests are carried out on an appropriate volume of virus from disrupted master cell seed. Where relevant tests have been carried out on disrupted cells to validate the suitability of the master cell seed, these tests need not be repeated.

Propagation. The master seed lot and all subsequent passages are propagated on cells, on embryonated eggs or in animals that have been shown to be suitable for vaccine production (see above), and, where applicable, using substances of animal origin that meet the requirements prescribed in chapter *5.2.5*.

Identification. A suitable method to identify the vaccine strain and to distinguish it as far as possible from related strains must be used.

Bacterial and fungal contamination. The master seed lot complies with the test for sterility (*2.6.1*).

Mycoplasmas (*2.6.7*). The master seed lot complies with the test for mycoplasmas (culture method and indicator cell culture method).

Absence of extraneous viruses. Monographs may contain requirements for freedom from extraneous agents, otherwise the requirements stated below apply.

Preparations of monoclonal or polyclonal antibodies containing high levels of neutralising antibody to the virus of the seed lot are made on a batch basis, using antigen that is not derived from any passage level of the virus isolate giving rise to the master seed virus. Each batch of serum is maintained at 56 °C for 30 min to inactivate complement. Each batch is shown to be free of antibodies to potential contaminants of the seed virus and is shown to be free of any non-specific inhibiting effects on the ability of viruses to infect and propagate within cells (or eggs, where applicable). If such a serum cannot be obtained, other methods are used to remove or neutralise the seed virus specifically.

If the seed lot virus would interfere with the conduct and sensitivity of a test for extraneous viruses, a sample of the master seed lot is treated with a minimum amount of the monoclonal or polyclonal antibody so that the vaccine virus is neutralised as far as possible or removed. The final virus-serum mixture shall, if possible, contain at least the virus content of 10 doses of vaccine per 0.1 ml for avian vaccines and per millilitre for other vaccines. For avian vaccines, the testing to be carried out on seed lots is given in chapters *2.6.3*, *2.6.4*, *2.6.5* and *2.6.6*. For mammalian vaccines, the seed lot or the mixture of seed lot and antiserum is tested for freedom from extraneous agents as follows.

The mixture is inoculated onto cultures of at least 70 cm^2 of the required cell types. The cultures may be inoculated at any suitable stage of growth up to 70 per cent confluency. At least 1 monolayer of each type must be retained as a control. The cultures must be monitored daily for a week. At the end of this period the cultures are freeze thawed 3 times, centrifuged to remove cell debris and re-inoculated onto the same cell type as above. This is repeated twice. The final passage must produce sufficient cells in appropriate vessels to carry out the tests below.

Cytopathic and haemadsorbing agents are tested for using the methods described in the relevant sections on testing cell cultures (*5.2.4*) and techniques such as immuno-fluorescence are used for detection of specific contaminants for the tests in cell cultures. The master seed lot is inoculated onto:

- primary cells of the species of origin of the virus,
- cells sensitive to viruses pathogenic for the species for which the vaccine is intended,
- cells sensitive to pestiviruses.

If the master seed lot is shown to contain living organisms of any kind, other than the virus of the species and strain stated, or foreign viral antigens, then it is unsuitable for vaccine production.

INACTIVATION

Inactivated vaccines are subjected to a validated inactivation procedure. The testing of the inactivation kinetics described below is carried out once for a given production process. The rest of this section applies to each production run. When conducting tests for inactivation, it is essential to take account of the possibility that under the conditions of manufacture, organisms may be physically protected from inactivant.

Inactivation kinetics. The inactivating agent and the inactivation procedure shall be shown, under conditions of manufacture, to inactivate the vaccine micro-organism. Adequate data on inactivation kinetics shall be obtained. Normally, the time required for inactivation shall be not more than 67 per cent of the duration of the inactivation process.

Aziridine. If an aziridine compound is used as the inactivating agent then it shall be shown that no inactivating agent remains at the end of the inactivation procedure. This may be accomplished by neutralising the inactivating agent with thiosulphate and demonstrating residual thiosulphate in the inactivated harvest at the completion of the inactivation procedure.

Formaldehyde. If formaldehyde is used as the inactivating agent, then a test for free formaldehyde is carried out as prescribed under Tests.

Other inactivating agents. When other inactivation methods are used, appropriate tests are carried out to demonstrate that the inactivating agent has been removed or reduced to an acceptable residual level.

Inactivation and/or detoxification testing. A test for complete inactivation and/or detoxification is performed immediately after the inactivation and/or detoxification procedure and, if applicable, the neutralisation or removal of the inactivating or detoxifying agent.

Bacterial vaccines. The test selected shall be appropriate to the vaccine bacteria being used and shall consist of at least 2 passages in production medium or, if solid medium has been used for production, in a suitable liquid medium or in the medium prescribed in the monograph. The product complies with the test if no evidence of any live micro-organism is observed.

Bacterial toxoids. The test selected shall be appropriate to the toxin or toxins present and shall be the most sensitive available.

Viral vaccines. The test selected shall be appropriate to the vaccine virus being used and must consist of at least 2 passages in cells, embryonated eggs or, where no other suitably sensitive method is available, in animals. The quantity of cell samples, eggs or animals shall be sufficient to ensure appropriate sensitivity of the test. For tests in cell cultures, not less than 150 cm^2 of cell culture monolayer is inoculated with 1.0 ml of inactivated harvest. The product complies with the test if no evidence of the presence of any live virus or other micro-organism is observed.

CHOICE OF VACCINE COMPOSITION AND CHOICE OF VACCINE STRAIN

For the choice of vaccine composition and choice of vaccine strain, important aspects to be evaluated include safety, efficacy and stability. General requirements for evaluation of safety and efficacy are given in chapter *5.2.6* and chapter *5.2.7*. These requirements may be made more explicit or supplemented by the requirements of specific monographs.

For live vaccines, a maximum virus titre or bacterial count acceptable from the point of view of safety is established during development studies. This is then used as the maximum acceptable titre for each batch of vaccine at release.

Potency and immunogenicity. The tests given under the headings Potency and Immunogenicity in monographs serve 2 purposes:

- the Potency section establishes by a well-controlled test in experimental conditions, the minimum acceptable vaccinating capacity for all vaccines within the scope of the definition, which must be guaranteed throughout the period of validity;
- well-controlled experimental studies are normally a part of the overall demonstration of efficacy of a vaccine (see chapter *5.2.7*); the test referred to in the section 'Immunogenicity' (which is usually a cross-reference to the Potency section) is suitable as a part of this testing.

For most vaccines, the tests cited under Potency or Immunogenicity are not suitable for the routine testing of batches.

For live vaccines, the minimum acceptable virus titre or bacterial count that gives satisfactory results in the Potency test and other efficacy studies is established during development. For routine testing it must be demonstrated for each batch that the titre or count at release is such that at the end of the period of validity, in the light of stability studies, the vaccine, stored in the recommended conditions, will contain not less than the minimum acceptable virus titre or bacterial count determined during development studies.

For inactivated vaccines, if the test described under Potency is not used for routine testing, a batch potency test is established during development. The aim of the batch potency test is to ensure that each batch of vaccine would, if tested, comply with the test described under Potency or Immunogenicity. The acceptance criteria for the batch potency test are therefore established by correlation with the test described under Potency. Where a batch potency test is described in a monograph, this is given as an example of a test that is considered suitable, after establishment of correlation with the potency test; other test models can also be used.

Route of administration. During development of a vaccine, safety and immunogenicity are demonstrated for each route of administration to be recommended. The following is a non-exhaustive list of such routes of administration:

- intramuscular,
- subcutaneous,
- intravenous,
- ocular,
- oral,
- nasal,
- foot-stab,
- wing web,

General monographs

– intradermal,
– intraperitoneal,
– *in ovo*.

Methods of administration. During development of a vaccine, safety and immunogenicity are demonstrated for each method of administration to be recommended. The following is a non-exhaustive list of such methods of administration:

– injection,
– drinking water,
– spray,
– eye-drop,
– scarification,
– implantation,
– immersion.

Categories of animal. Monographs may indicate that a given test is to be carried out for each category of animal of the target species for which the product is recommended or is to be recommended. The following is a non-exhaustive list of categories that are to be taken into account.

– *Mammals*:
  – pregnant animals/non-pregnant animals,
  – animals raised primarily for breeding/animals raised primarily for food production,
  – animals of the minimum age or size recommended for vaccination.
– *Avian species*:
  – birds raised primarily for egg production/birds raised primarily for production of meat,
  – birds before point of lay/birds after onset of lay.
– *Fish*:
  – broodstock fish/fish raised primarily for food production.

Stability. Evidence of stability is obtained to justify the proposed period of validity. This evidence takes the form of the results of virus titrations, bacterial counts or potency tests carried out at regular intervals until 3 months beyond the end of the shelf life on not fewer than 3 representative consecutive batches of vaccine kept under recommended storage conditions together with results from studies of moisture content (for freeze-dried products), physical tests on the adjuvant, chemical tests on substances such as the adjuvant constituents and preservatives and pH, as appropriate.

Where applicable, studies on the stability of the reconstituted vaccine are carried out, using the product reconstituted in accordance with the proposed recommendations.

FINAL BULK VACCINE

The final bulk vaccine is prepared by combining one or more batches of antigen that comply with all the relevant requirements with any auxiliary substances, such as adjuvants, stabilisers, antimicrobial preservatives and diluents.

Antimicrobial preservatives. Antimicrobial preservatives are used to prevent spoilage or adverse effects caused by microbial contamination occurring during use of a vaccine which is expected to be no longer than 10 h after first broaching. Antimicrobial preservatives are not included in freeze-dried products but, if justified, taking into account the maximum recommended period of use after reconstitution, they may be included in the diluent for multi-dose freeze-dried products. For single-dose liquid preparations, inclusion of antimicrobial preservatives is not acceptable unless justified and authorised, but may be acceptable, for example where the same vaccine is filled in single-dose and multidose containers and is used in non-food-producing species. For multidose liquid preparations, the need for effective antimicrobial preservation is evaluated taking into account likely contamination during use and the maximum recommended period of use after broaching of the container.

During development studies the effectiveness of the antimicrobial preservative throughout the period of validity shall be demonstrated to the satisfaction of the competent authority.

The efficacy of the antimicrobial preservative is evaluated as described in chapter *5.1.3* and in addition samples are tested at suitable intervals over the proposed in use shelf-life. If neither the A criteria nor the B criteria can be met, then in justified cases the following criteria are applied to vaccines for veterinary use: bacteria, no increase from 24 h to 7 days, 3 log reduction at 14 days, no increase at 28 days; fungi, no increase at 14 days and 28 days.

Addition of antibiotics as antimicrobial preservative is generally not acceptable.

Test for inactivation and/or detoxification. For inactivated vaccines, where the auxiliary substances would interfere with a test for inactivation and/or detoxification, a test for inactivation or detoxification is carried out during preparation of the final bulk, after the different batches of antigen have been combined but before addition of auxiliary substances; the test for inactivation or detoxification may then be omitted on the final bulk and the batch.

Where there is a risk of reversion to toxicity, the test for detoxification performed at the latest stage of the production process at which the sensitivity of the test is not compromised (e.g. after the different batches of antigen have been combined but before the addition of auxiliary substances) is important to demonstrate a lack of reversion to toxicity.

In-process tests. Certain tests may be carried out on the final bulk vaccine rather than on the batch or batches prepared from it; such tests include those for antimicrobial preservatives, free formaldehyde and the potency determination for inactivated vaccines.

BATCH

Unless otherwise prescribed in the monograph, the final bulk vaccine is distributed aseptically into sterile, tamper-proof containers which are then closed so as to exclude contamination.

Only a batch that complies with each of the requirements given below under Identification, Tests and Potency or in the relevant individual monograph may be released for use. With the agreement of the competent authority, certain of the batch tests may be omitted where in-process tests give an equal or better guarantee that the batch would comply or where alternative tests validated with respect to the Pharmacopoeia method have been carried out.

The identification test can often be conveniently combined with the batch potency test to avoid unnecessary use of animals. For a given vaccine, a validated *in vitro* test can be used to avoid the unnecessary use of animals.

It is recognised that, in accordance with General Notices (*1.1. General statements*), for an established vaccine the routine application of the safety test will be waived by the competent authority in the interests of animal welfare when a sufficient number of consecutive production batches have been produced and found to comply with the test, thus demonstrating consistency of the manufacturing process. Significant changes to the manufacturing process may require resumption of routine testing to re-establish consistency. The number of consecutive batches to be tested

General monographs

depends on a number of factors such as the type of vaccine, the frequency of production of batches and experience with the vaccine during development safety testing and during application of the batch safety test. Without prejudice to the decision of the competent authority in the light of information available for a given vaccine, testing of 10 consecutive batches is likely to be sufficient for most products. For products with an inherent safety risk, it may be necessary to continue to conduct the safety test on each batch.

Animal tests. In accordance with the provisions of the European Convention for the Protection of Vertebrate Animals Used for Experimental and Other Scientific Purposes, tests must be carried out in such a way as to use the minimum number of animals and to cause the least pain, suffering, distress or lasting harm. The criteria for judging tests in monographs must be applied in the light of this. For example, if it is indicated that an animal is considered to be positive, infected etc. when typical clinical signs occur then as soon as it is clear that the result will not be affected the animal in question shall be either humanely killed or given suitable treatment to prevent unnecessary suffering. In accordance with the General Notices, alternative test methods may be used to demonstrate compliance with the monograph and the use of such tests is particularly encouraged when this leads to replacement or reduction of animal use or reduction of suffering.

Physical tests. A vaccine with an oily adjuvant is tested for viscosity by a suitable method and shown to be within the limits set for the product. The stability of the emulsion shall be demonstrated.

Chemical tests. Tests for the concentrations of appropriate substances such as aluminium and preservatives are carried out to show that these are within the limits set for the product.

pH. The pH of liquid products and diluents is measured and shown to be within the limits set for the product.

Water. Where applicable, the freeze-drying process is checked by a determination of water and shown to be within the limits set for the product.

IDENTIFICATION

For inactivated vaccines, the identification prescribed in monographs is usually an antibody induction test since this is applicable to all vaccines.

TESTS

The monographs also indicate tests to be carried out on each particular vaccine.

All hen eggs, chickens and chicken cell cultures for use in quality control tests shall be derived from an SPF flock (*5.2.2*).

Formaldehyde (*2.4.18*; use Method B if sodium metabisulphite has been used to neutralise excess formaldehyde). Where formaldehyde has been used in the preparation, the concentration of free formaldehyde is not greater than 0.5 g/l, unless a higher amount has been shown to be safe.

Phenol (*2.5.15*). When the vaccine contains phenol, the concentration is not greater than 5 g/l.

Sterility (*2.6.1*). Where prescribed in the monograph, vaccines comply with the test for sterility. Where the volume of liquid in a container is greater than 100 ml, the method of membrane filtration is used wherever possible. Where the method of membrane filtration cannot be used, the method of direct inoculation may be used. Where the volume of liquid in each container is at least 20 ml, the minimum volume to be used for each culture medium is 10 per cent of the contents or 5 ml, whichever is less. The appropriate number of items to be tested (*2.6.1*) is 1 per cent of the batch with a minimum of 4 and a maximum of 10.

For avian live viral vaccines, for non-parenteral use only, the requirement for sterility is usually replaced by requirements for absence of pathogenic micro-organisms and for a maximum of 1 non-pathogenic micro-organism per dose.

Extraneous agents. Monographs prescribe a set of measures that taken together give an acceptable degree of assurance that the final product does not contain infectious extraneous agents. These measures include:

1) Production within a seed-lot system and a cell-seed system, wherever possible;

2) Extensive testing of seed lots and cell seed for extraneous agents;

3) Requirements for SPF flocks used for providing substrates for vaccine production;

4) Testing of substances of animal origin, which must, wherever possible, undergo an inactivation procedure;

5) For live vaccines, testing of the final product for infectious extraneous agents; such tests are less extensive than those carried out at earlier stages because of the guarantees given by in-process testing.

In cases of doubt, the tests intended for the seed lot of a live vaccine may also be applied to the final product. If an extraneous agent is found in such a test, the vaccine does not comply the monograph.

Avian live viral vaccines comply with the tests for extraneous agents in batches of finished products (*2.6.4*).

Mycoplasmas (*2.6.7*). Where prescribed in a monograph, the vaccine complies with the test for mycoplasmas (culture method).

Safety. In general, 2 doses of an inactivated vaccine and/or 10 doses of a live vaccine are injected by a recommended route. It may be necessary to reduce the prescribed number of doses under certain circumstances or amend the method of re-constitution and injection, for example for a combined vaccine, where it is difficult to reconstitute 10 doses of the live component in 2 doses of the inactivated component. The animals are observed for the longest period stated in the monographs. No abnormal local or systemic reaction occurs. Where several batches are prepared from the same final bulk, the safety test is carried out on the first batch and then omitted for further batches prepared from the same final bulk.

During development studies, the type and degree of reactions expected with the vaccine are defined in the light of safety testing. This definition is then used as part of the operating procedure for the batch safety test to evaluate acceptable and unacceptable reactions.

The immune status of animals to be used for the safety test is specified in the individual monograph. For most monographs, one of the 3 following categories is specified:

1) the animals must be free from antibodies against the virus/bacterium/toxin etc. contained in the vaccine,

2) the animals are preferably free from antibodies but animals with a low level of antibody may be used as long as the animals have not been vaccinated and the administration of the vaccine does not cause an anamnestic response,

3) the animals must not have been vaccinated against the disease the vaccine is intended to prevent.

As a general rule, category 1 is specified for live vaccines. For other vaccines, category 2 is usually specified but where most animals available for use in tests would comply with category 1, this may be specified for inactivated vaccines also. Category 3 is specified for some inactivated vaccines where determination of antibodies prior to testing is unnecessary or impractical. For poultry vaccines, as a general rule the use of SPF birds is specified.

For avian vaccines, the safety test is generally carried out using 10 SPF chickens (*5.2.2*), except that for vaccines not recommended for use in chickens it is carried out using 10 birds of one of the species for which the vaccine is recommended, the birds being free from antibodies against the disease agent for which the vaccine is intended to provide protection.

POTENCY

See Choice of vaccine composition and choice of vaccine strain under Production.

STORAGE

Store protected from light at a temperature of 5 ± 3 °C, unless otherwise indicated. Liquid preparations are not to be allowed to freeze, unless otherwise indicated.

LABELLING

The label states:

- that the preparation is for veterinary use,
- the volume of the preparation and the number of doses in the container,
- the route of administration,
- the type or types of bacteria or viruses used and for live vaccines the minimum and the maximum number of live bacteria or the minimum and the maximum virus titre,
- where applicable, for inactivated vaccines, the minimum potency in International Units,
- where applicable, the name and amount of antimicrobial preservative or other substance added to the vaccine,
- the name of any substance that may cause an adverse reaction,
- for freeze-dried vaccines:
  - the name or composition and the volume of the reconstituting liquid to be added,
  - the period within which the vaccine is to be used after reconstitution,
- for vaccines with an oily adjuvant, that if the vaccine is accidentally injected into man, urgent medical attention is necessary,
- the animal species for which the vaccine is intended,
- the indications for the vaccine,
- the instructions for use,
- any contra-indications to the use of the product including any required warning on the dangers of administration of an overdose,
- the doses recommended for different species.

01/2005:1579

VEGETABLE FATTY OILS

Olea herbaria

DEFINITION

Vegetable fatty oils are mainly solid or liquid triglycerides of fatty acids. They may contain small amounts of other lipids such as waxes, free fatty acids, partial glycerides or unsaponifiable matters. Vegetable fatty oils are obtained from the seeds, the fruit or the pit/stone/kernel of various plants by expression and/or solvent extraction, then possibly refined and hydrogenated. A suitable antioxidant may be added if necessary.

Virgin oil: an oil obtained from raw materials of special quality by mechanical procedures (e.g. by cold expression or centrifugation).

Refined oil: an oil obtained by expression and/or solvent extraction, and subsequently, either alkali refining (followed by bleaching and deodorisation) or physical refining.

Hydrogenated oil: an oil obtained by expression and/or solvent extraction, and subsequently, either alkali refining or physical refining, then possible bleaching, followed by drying, hydrogenation and subsequent bleaching and deodorisation.

Only phosphoric acid and alkali refined oils are used in the preparation of parenteral dosage forms.

PRODUCTION

OBTAINING OF A CRUDE OIL

When the plant has a high oil content, the oil is generally obtained by expression under heating followed by an extraction; when the plant has a low oil content, the oil is generally obtained by direct extraction.

Mechanical procedures

A. Expression

High-pressure screw-pressing. It consists of some or all of the following steps: cleaning, drying, dehulling or decorticating, grinding, cooking and flaking.

During *cleaning* the foreign matter is eliminated. *Drying* may be necessary if the seed moisture content is higher than desirable for downstream processing. *Decorticating* is useful to obtain a high-protein meal by reduction of fibre and to reduce impurities in the oil. *Cooking* serves various purposes: completion of the breakdown of oil cells, lowering of the viscosity of the oil, coagulation of the protein in the meal, adjustment of the moisture level, sterilisation of the seed, detoxifying undesirable seed constituents (gossypol for cottonseed) and fixing certain phosphatides in the cake thus lowering subsequent refining losses. The efficacy of the expression process is such that only 3 per cent to 6 per cent of the oil is left in the cake.

Wet screw-pressing. The bunches are loaded into cages (for palm fruit) and moved into a horizontal steriliser with application of live steam and heating. The purposes of this steriliser are inactivation of enzymes, loosening of the fruit on the bunch, coagulation of proteins, etc. After heating in a digester, the pulp is fed to a screw-press. The oil is centrifugally clarified and vacuum-dried.

Pre-pressing followed by solvent extraction. The same sequence of steps is performed as above. The main function of pre-pressing is to obtain a cake of excellent permeability for the following solvent extraction stage. The extraction is performed either in a percolation type or in an immersion type apparatus. The efficacy of the solvent extraction process is such that residual oil levels in meal are generally below 1 per cent.

B. Centrifugation

Centrifugation separates the oily phase from the aqueous phase which contains water, water-soluble components and residual solid particles. This operation can be carried out using:

- self-cleaning bowl or disc centrifuges,

General monographs

- super-decanters, which are horizontal turbines equipped with a cylindrical bowl that tapers slightly at one end and which contains a continuously turning screw that scrapes the sides of the bowl. The screw and the bowl rotate at different speeds. The solid particles are discarded from the tapered end of the bowl and the oil flows out from the other end.

Solvent extraction. Prior to extraction, the following steps are carried out: the seeds are tempered for about a week at a temperature below 24 °C in order to loosen the hull from the seed and allow the seed moisture to attain equilibrium. Then the seeds are cleaned, ground, dehulled and flaked. The most widely used solvent is a mixture of mainly *n*-hexane and methylpentanes (bp: 65-70 °C) commonly referred to as "hexane". Due to the major fire and explosive risks of this mixture, liquified gases and supercritical gases may also be used.

REFINING

The objective of refining is to remove impurities and contaminants of the oil with the least possible damage to the triglycerides and with minimal loss of oil. The contents of the following substances are reduced:

- free fatty acids which may cause deterioration of the oil by oxidation, smoked taste when heated and sharp flavour (by alkali refining),
- water which favours the enzymatic hydrolysis reactions (by alkali refining, drying),
- partial glycerides which may cause foaming and bitter taste (by neutralisation, washing),
- phosphatides and phosphorous compounds which have emulsifying properties, may cause deposits, a darkening of the oil when heated, a cloudy appearance and bad organoleptic stability (by alkali refining),
- colouring matters such as chlorophyll (by alkali refining), carotenoids (by bleaching),
- glycolipids which may form colloidal solutions with water,
- free hydrocarbons, paraffin, waxes and resinous materials,
- metals (Fe, Cu, Pb, Sn, Pt, Pd, etc.) which are strong oxidation catalysts,
- pigments such as gossypol (in cottonseed oil) or mycotoxins such as aflatoxin (mainly in arachis oil),
- pesticides,
- oxidation products (aldehydes, peroxides),
- proteins having possible allergic reactions,
- unsaponifiable matters (e.g. lignins, sterols, tocopherols and other vitamins),
- polycyclic aromatic hydrocarbons.

Alkali refining. It involves the following steps: degumming, neutralisation using alkali, washing and drying.

Degumming. During this step of the refining, i.e. treatment with water and/or phosphoric acid, and/or sodium chloride, the phosphatides, phosphorous compounds and metals are eliminated. The use of this step depends on the nature of the oil.

Neutralisation with alkali. This step reduces the free fatty acid content below 0.1 per cent; the fatty acids are converted into oil-insoluble soaps, also called "soapstocks". Other substances may be removed by adsorption on these soaps: mucilaginous substances, phosphatides, oxidation products, colouring matters, etc. All substances that become insoluble in the oil on hydration are removed. Neutralisation with alkali has the disadvantage of saponifying a portion of neutral oil if the neutralisation is not well conducted.

Washing. This operation consists in removing the excess of soaps and alkali as well as the remaining traces of metals, phosphatides and other impurities, using hot water.

Drying. The remaining water is eliminated under vacuum before any further steps, such as bleaching.

Physical refining. It involves a steam treatment of the oil under high vacuum at a temperature greater than 235 °C. This technique must be applied to oils naturally low in phosphatides and metals (palm, coconut, olive) or from which phosphatides and metals have been removed by an acid treatment using concentrated phosphoric acid followed by an adsorptive treatment with activated bleaching earth (for sunflower, rapeseed, soya-bean). Moreover it cannot be used for heat sensitive oils (cottonseed oil) which darken.

Bleaching. The common method of bleaching is by adsorption treatment of the oil, which is generally heated at 90 °C for 30 min under vacuum, with bleaching earth (natural or activated) or carbon (activated or not); synthetic silica adsorbents may also be added. Substances which have not been totally removed during refining are eliminated, for example carotenoids and chlorophyll.

Deodorisation. Deodorisation eliminates odours, volatile substances and residual extraction solvents; it involves injecting dry vapour into the oil which is kept under vacuum at a high temperature. Different temperatures are used according to the oil: 200 °C to 235 °C for 1 h 30 min to 3 h or greater than 240 °C for 30 min.

One of the main side reactions is thermic decolourisation due to the destruction of carotenoids when the temperature is greater than 150 °C. This technique provokes a loss of substances which may be distilled (free fatty acids, sterols, tocopherols, part of the refined oil) and may cause *cis-trans* isomerisation of the unsaturated fatty-acid double bonds.

WINTERISATION

Elimination of solids and waxes by filtration at low temperature (also called dewaxing). These solids and waxes could affect the appearance of the oil and cause deposits.

HYDROGENATION

The hydrogenation of the dried and/or bleached oil is performed using a catalyst (e.g. Ni, Pt, Pd), at a temperature of about 100 °C to 200 °C under hydrogen pressure. The catalyst is then removed by filtration at 90 °C. The hydrogen must be pure: free of poisons for the catalyst, water-free, low in carbon dioxide, methane and nitrogen contents. Small amounts of *trans*-fatty acids or polymers may be obtained.

CHROMATOGRAPHIC PURIFICATION

In high purity applications, mainly for parenteral uses, the oil may be further purified by passing the oil through a column containing an activated earth. A solvent may sometimes be used to improve the efficiency. High polarity molecules such as oxidised materials, acids, alcohols, partial glycerides and free sterols are preferentially removed.

When the oil is used in the preparation of parenteral dosage forms, the limits set in the monograph for the acid value, the peroxide value and the water content may be different.

LABELLING

The label states:

- where applicable, that the oil was obtained by expression or extraction,
- where applicable, that the oil is suitable for use in the manufacture of parenteral dosage forms,
- the name and concentration of any added antioxidant.

DOSAGE FORMS

01/2005:1502

GLOSSARY

The following introductory text provides definitions and/or explanations of terms that may be found in, or used in association with, the general monographs on dosage forms, but that are not defined within them. Where relevant, reference is made to other equivalent terms that may be found in other publications or contexts.

This glossary is published for information.

Standard Term

Standard Terms for describing the pharmaceutical form of a medicinal product, the routes of administration and the containers used have been established by the European Pharmacopoeia Commission and are provided in a separate publication on Standard Terms.

Active substance

Equivalent terms: active ingredient, drug substance, medicinal substance, active pharmaceutical ingredient.

Vehicle

A vehicle is the carrier, composed of one or more excipients, for the active substance(s) in a liquid preparation.

Basis

A basis is the carrier, composed of one or more excipients, for the active substance(s) in semi-solid and solid preparations.

Conventional-release dosage forms

Conventional-release dosage forms are preparations showing a release of the active substance(s) which is not deliberately modified by a special formulation design and/or manufacturing method. In the case of a solid dosage form, the dissolution profile of the active substance depends essentially on its intrinsic properties. Equivalent term: immediate-release dosage form.

Modified-release dosage forms

Modified-release dosage forms are preparations where the rate and/or place of release of the active substance(s) is different from that of a conventional-release dosage form administered by the same route. This deliberate modification is achieved by a special formulation design and/or manufacturing method. Modified-release dosage forms include prolonged-release, delayed-release and pulsatile-release dosage forms.

Prolonged-release dosage forms

Prolonged-release dosage forms are modified-release dosage forms showing a slower release of the active substance(s) than that of a conventional-release dosage form administered by the same route. Prolonged-release is achieved by a special formulation design and/or manufacturing method. Equivalent term: extended-release dosage form.

Delayed-release dosage forms

Delayed-release dosage forms are modified-release dosage forms showing a release of the active substance(s) which is delayed. Delayed release is achieved by a special formulation design and/or manufacturing method. Delayed-release dosage forms include gastro-resistant preparations as defined in the general monographs on solid oral dosage forms.

Pulsatile-release dosage forms

Pulsatile-release dosage forms are modified-release dosage forms showing a sequential release of the active substance(s). Sequential release is achieved by a special formulation design and/or manufacturing method.

Large-volume parenterals

Infusions and injections supplied in containers with a nominal content of more than 100 ml.

Small-volume parenterals

Infusions and injections supplied in containers with a nominal content of 100 ml or less.

01/2005:0016

CAPSULES

Capsulae

The requirements of this monograph do not necessarily apply to preparations that are presented as capsules intended for use other than by oral administration. Requirements for such preparations may be found, where appropriate, in other general monographs, for example Rectal preparations (1145) and Vaginal preparations (1164).

DEFINITION

Capsules are solid preparations with hard or soft shells of various shapes and capacities, usually containing a single dose of active substance. They are intended for oral administration.

The capsule shells are made of gelatin or other substances, the consistency of which may be adjusted by the addition of substances such as glycerol or sorbitol. Excipients such as surface-active agents, opaque fillers, antimicrobial preservatives, sweeteners, colouring matter authorised by the competent authority and flavouring substances may be added. The capsules may bear surface markings.

The contents of capsules may be solid, liquid or of a paste-like consistency. They consist of one or more active substances with or without excipients such as solvents, diluents, lubricants and disintegrating agents. The contents do not cause deterioration of the shell. The shell, however, is attacked by the digestive fluids and the contents are released.

Where applicable, containers for capsules comply with the requirements of *Materials used for the manufacture of containers* (*3.1* and subsections) and *Containers* (*3.2* and subsections).

Several categories of capsules may be distinguished:

- hard capsules,
- soft capsules,
- gastro-resistant capsules,
- modified-release capsules,
- cachets.

PRODUCTION

In the manufacture, packaging, storage and distribution of capsules, suitable means are taken to ensure their microbial quality; recommendations on this aspect are provided in the text on *Microbiological quality of pharmaceutical preparations* (*5.1.4*).

TESTS

Uniformity of content (*2.9.6*). Unless otherwise prescribed or justified and authorised, capsules with a content of active substance less than 2 mg or less than 2 per cent of the total mass comply with test B for uniformity of content of single-dose preparations. If the preparation has more than one active substance, the requirement applies only to those ingredients which correspond to the above conditions.

Uniformity of mass (*2.9.5*). Capsules comply with the test for uniformity of mass of single-dose preparations. If the test for uniformity of content is prescribed for all the active substances, the test for uniformity of mass is not required.

Dissolution. A suitable test may be carried out to demonstrate the appropriate release of the active substance(s), for example one of the tests described in *Dissolution test for solid dosage forms* (*2.9.3*).

Where a dissolution test is prescribed, a disintegration test may not be required.

STORAGE

Store at a temperature not exceeding 30 °C.

LABELLING

The label states the name of any added antimicrobial preservative.

Hard capsules

DEFINITION

Hard capsules have shells consisting of two prefabricated cylindrical sections one end of which is rounded and closed, the other being open.

PRODUCTION

The active substance(s) usually in solid form (powder or granules) are filled into one of the sections which is then closed by slipping the other section over it. The security of the closure may be strengthened by suitable means.

TESTS

Disintegration. Hard capsules comply with the test for disintegration of tablets and capsules (*2.9.1*). Use *water R* as the liquid medium. When justified and authorised, *0.1 M hydrochloric acid* or *artificial gastric juice R* may be used as the liquid medium. If the capsules float on the surface of the water, a disc may be added. Operate the apparatus for 30 min, unless otherwise justified and authorised and examine the state of the capsules. The capsules comply with the test if all 6 have disintegrated.

Soft capsules

DEFINITION

Soft capsules have thicker shells than those of hard capsules. The shells consist of one part and are of various shapes.

PRODUCTION

Soft capsules are usually formed, filled and sealed in one operation but for extemporaneous use, the shell may be prefabricated. The shell material may contain an active substance.

Liquids may be enclosed directly; solids are usually dissolved or dispersed in a suitable vehicle to give a solution or dispersion of a paste-like consistency.

There may be partial migration of the constituents from the capsule contents into the shell and vice versa because of the nature of the materials and the surfaces in contact.

TESTS

Disintegration. Soft capsules comply with the test for disintegration of tablets and capsules (*2.9.1*). Use *water R* as the liquid medium. When justified and authorised, *0.1 M hydrochloric acid* or *artificial gastric juice R* may be used as the liquid medium. Add a disc to each tube. Liquid active substances dispensed in soft capsules may attack the disc; in such circumstances and where authorised, the disc may be omitted. Operate the apparatus for 30 min, unless otherwise justified and authorised and examine the state of the capsules. If the capsules fail to comply because of adherence to the discs, repeat the test on a further 6 capsules omitting the discs. The capsules comply with the test if all 6 have disintegrated.

Modified-release capsules

DEFINITION

Modified-release capsules are hard or soft capsules in which the contents or the shell or both contain special excipients or are prepared by a special process designed to modify the rate, the place or the time at which the active substance(s) are released.

Modified release capsules include prolonged-release capsules and delayed-release capsules.

PRODUCTION

A suitable test is carried out to demonstrate the appropriate release of the active substance(s).

Gastro-resistant capsules

DEFINITION

Gastro-resistant capsules are delayed-release capsules that are intended to resist the gastric fluid and to release their active substance or substances in the intestinal fluid. Usually they are prepared by filling capsules with granules or with particles covered with a gastro-resistant coating or in certain cases, by providing hard or soft capsules with a gastro-resistant shell (enteric capsules).

PRODUCTION

For capsules filled with granules or filled with particles covered with a gastro-resistant coating, a suitable test is carried out to demonstrate the appropriate release of the active substance(s).

TESTS

Disintegration. For capsules with a gastro-resistant shell carry out the test for disintegration (*2.9.1*) with the following modifications. Use *0.1 M hydrochloric acid* as the liquid medium and operate the apparatus for 2 h, or other such time as may be authorised, without the discs. Examine the state of the capsules. The time of resistance to the acid medium varies according to the formulation of the capsules to be examined. It is typically 2 h to 3 h but even with authorised deviations it must not be less than 1 h. No capsule shows signs of disintegration or rupture permitting the escape of the contents. Replace the acid by *phosphate buffer solution pH 6.8 R*. When justified and authorised, a buffer solution of pH 6.8 with added pancreas powder (for example, 0.35 g of *pancreas powder R* per 100 ml of buffer solution) may be used. Add a disc to each tube. Operate the apparatus for 60 min and examine the state of the capsules. If the capsules fail to comply because of adherence to the discs, repeat the test on a further 6 capsules omitting the discs. The capsules comply with the test if all 6 have disintegrated.

Dissolution. For capsules prepared from granules or particles already covered with a gastro-resistant coating, a suitable test is carried out to demonstrate the appropriate release of the active substance(s), for example the test described in *Dissolution test for solid dosage forms* (*2.9.3*).

Cachets

DEFINITION

Cachets are solid preparations consisting of a hard shell containing a single dose of one or more active substances. The cachet shell is made of unleavened bread usually from rice flour and consists of 2 prefabricated flat cylindrical sections. Before administration, the cachets are immersed in water for a few seconds, placed on the tongue and swallowed with a draught of water.

LABELLING

The label states the method of administration of the cachets.

01/2005:1239

CHEWING GUMS, MEDICATED

Masticabilia gummis medicata

DEFINITION

Medicated chewing gums are solid, single-dose preparations with a base consisting mainly of gum that are intended to be chewed but not swallowed.

They contain one or more active substances which are released by chewing. After dissolution or dispersion of the active substances in saliva, chewing gums are intended to be used for:

- local treatment of mouth diseases,
- systemic delivery after absorption through the buccal mucosa or from the gastrointestinal tract.

PRODUCTION

Medicated chewing gums are made with a tasteless masticatory gum base that consists of natural or synthetic elastomers. They may contain other excipients such as fillers, softeners, sweetening agents, flavouring substances, stabilisers and plasticisers and authorised colouring matter.

Medicated chewing gums are manufactured by compression or by softening or melting the gum bases and adding successively the other substances. In the latter case, chewing gums are then further processed to obtain the desired gum presentation. The medicated chewing gums may be coated, for example, if necessary to protect from humidity and light.

Unless otherwise justified and authorised, a suitable test is carried out to demonstrate the appropriate release of the active ingredient(s).

In the manufacture, packaging, storage and distribution of medicated chewing gums, suitable means must be taken to ensure their microbial quality; recommendations related to this aspect are provided in the general chapter on *Microbiological quality of pharmaceutical preparations* (*5.1.4*).

TESTS

Uniformity of content (*2.9.6*). Unless otherwise prescribed or justified and authorised, medicated chewing gums with a content of active ingredient less than 2 mg or less than 2 per cent of the total mass comply with test A for uniformity of content of single-dose preparations. If the preparation contains more than one active substance, the requirement applies only to those active substances which correspond to the above conditions.

Uniformity of mass (*2.9.5*). Uncoated medicated chewing gums and, unless otherwise justified and authorised, coated medicated chewing gums comply with the test for uniformity of mass of single-dose preparations. If the test for uniformity of content is prescribed for all the active substances, the test for uniformity of mass is not required.

STORAGE

Store uncoated medicated chewing gums protected from humidity and light.

01/2005:0652

EAR PREPARATIONS

Auricularia

DEFINITION

Ear preparations are liquid, semi-solid or solid preparations intended for instillation, for spraying, for insufflation, for application to the auditory meatus or as an ear wash.

Ear preparations usually contain one or more active substances in a suitable vehicle. They may contain excipients, for example, to adjust tonicity or viscosity, to adjust or stabilise the pH, to increase the solubility of the active substances, to stabilise the preparation or to provide adequate antimicrobial properties. The excipients do not adversely affect the intended medicinal action of the preparation or, at the concentrations used, cause toxicity or undue local irritation.

Preparations for application to the injured ear, particularly where the ear-drum is perforated, or prior to surgery are sterile, free from antimicrobial preservatives and supplied in single-dose containers.

Ear preparations are supplied in multi-dose or single-dose containers, provided, if necessary, with a suitable administration device which may be designed to avoid the introduction of contaminants.

Unless otherwise justified and authorised, aqueous ear preparations supplied in multidose containers contain a suitable antimicrobial preservative at a suitable concentration, except where the preparation itself has adequate antimicrobial properties.

Where applicable, containers for ear preparations comply with the requirements of *Materials used for the manufacture of containers* (*3.1* and subsections) and *Containers* (*3.2* and subsections).

Several categories of ear preparations may be distinguished:

- ear-drops and sprays,
- semi-solid ear preparations,
- ear powders,
- ear washes,
- ear tampons.

PRODUCTION

During the development of an ear preparation, the formulation for which contains an antimicrobial preservative, the effectiveness of the chosen preservative shall be demonstrated to the satisfaction of the competent authority. A suitable test method together with criteria for judging the preservative properties of the formulation are provided in the text on *Efficacy of antimicrobial preservation* (*5.1.3*).

In the manufacture, packaging, storage and distribution of ear preparations, suitable means are taken to ensure their microbial quality; recommendations on this aspect are provided in the text on *Microbiological quality of pharmaceutical preparations* (*5.1.4*).

Sterile ear preparations are prepared using materials and methods designed to ensure sterility and to avoid the introduction of contaminants and the growth of micro-organisms; recommendations on this aspect are provided in the text on *Methods of preparation of sterile products* (*5.1.1*).

In the manufacture of ear preparations containing dispersed particles, measures are taken to ensure a suitable and controlled particle size with regard to the intended use.

TESTS

Uniformity of content (*2.9.6*). Unless otherwise prescribed or justified and authorised, single-dose ear preparations with a content of active substance less than 2 mg or less than 2 per cent of the total mass comply with test B for uniformity of content of single-dose preparations. If the preparation has more than one active substance, the requirement applies only to those ingredients that correspond to the above conditions.

Uniformity of mass (*2.9.5*). Single-dose ear preparations comply with the test for uniformity of mass of single-dose preparations. If the test for uniformity of content is prescribed for all the active substances, the test for uniformity of mass is not required.

Sterility (*2.6.1*). Where the label indicates that the ear preparation is sterile, it complies with the test for sterility.

STORAGE

If the preparation is sterile, store in a sterile, airtight, tamper-proof container.

LABELLING

The label states:

- the name of any added antimicrobial preservative,
- where applicable, that the preparation is sterile,
- for multidose containers, the period after opening the container after which the contents must not be used. This period does not exceed 4 weeks, unless otherwise justified and authorised.

Ear-drops and sprays

DEFINITION

Ear-drops and sprays are solutions, emulsions or suspensions of one or more active substances in liquids suitable for application to the auditory meatus without exerting harmful pressure on the ear-drum (for example, water, glycols or fatty oils). They may also be placed in the auditory meatus by means of a tampon impregnated with the liquid.

Emulsions may show evidence of phase separation but are readily redispersed on shaking. Suspensions may show a sediment which is readily dispersed on shaking to give a suspension which remains sufficiently stable to enable the correct dose to be delivered.

Ear drops are usually supplied in multidose containers of glass or suitable plastic material that are fitted with an integral dropper or with a screw cap of suitable materials incorporating a dropper and rubber or plastic teat. Alternatively, such a cap assembly is supplied separately. Sprays are usually supplied in multi-dose containers fitted with an appropriate applicator. When sprays are supplied in pressurised containers, these comply with the requirements of the monograph on *Pressurised pharmaceutical preparations (0523)*.

Semi-solid ear preparations

DEFINITION

Semi-solid ear preparations are intended for application to the external auditory meatus, if necessary by means of a tampon impregnated with the preparation.

Semi-solid ear preparations comply with the requirements of the monograph on *Semi-solid preparations for cutaneous application (0132)*.

They are supplied in containers fitted with a suitable applicator.

Ear powders

DEFINITION

Ear powders comply with the requirements of the monograph on *Powders for cutaneous application (1166)*.

They are supplied in containers fitted with a suitable device for application or insufflation.

Ear washes

DEFINITION

Ear washes are preparations intended to cleanse the external auditory meatus. They are usually aqueous solutions with pH within physiological limits.

Ear washes intended for application to injured parts or prior to a surgical operation are sterile.

TESTS

Deliverable mass or volume (*2.9.28*). Ear washes supplied in single-dose containers comply with the test.

Ear tampons

DEFINITION

Ear tampons are intended to be inserted into the external auditory meatus. They comply with the requirements of the monograph on *Medicated tampons (1155)*.

01/2005:1163

EYE PREPARATIONS

Ophthalmica

DEFINITION

Eye preparations are sterile liquid, semi-solid or solid preparations intended for administration upon the eyeball and/or to the conjunctiva or for insertion in the conjunctival sac.

Where applicable, containers for eye preparations comply with the requirements of *Materials used for the manufacture of containers* (*3.1* and subsections) and *Containers* (*3.2* and subsections).

Several categories of eye preparations may be distinguished:

- eye drops,
- eye lotions,
- powders for eye drops and eye lotions,
- semi-solid eye preparations,
- ophthalmic inserts.

PRODUCTION

During the development of an eye preparation, the formulation for which contains an antimicrobial preservative, the effectiveness of the chosen preservative shall be demonstrated to the satisfaction of the competent authority. A suitable test method together with criteria for judging the preservative properties of the formulation are provided in the text on *Efficacy of antimicrobial preservation* (*5.1.3*).

Eye preparations are prepared using materials and methods designed to ensure sterility and to avoid the introduction of contaminants and the growth of micro-organisms; recommendations on this aspect are provided in the text on *Methods of preparation of sterile products (5.1.1)*.

In the manufacture of eye preparations containing dispersed particles, measures are taken to ensure a suitable and controlled particle size with regard to the intended use.

TESTS

Sterility (*2.6.1*). Eye preparations comply with the test for sterility. Applicators supplied separately also comply with the test for sterility. Remove the applicator with aseptic precautions from its package and transfer it to a tube of culture medium so that it is completely immersed. Incubate and interpret the results as described in the test for sterility.

Deliverable mass or volume (*2.9.28*). Liquid and semi-solid eye preparations supplied in single-dose containers comply with the test.

STORAGE

Unless otherwise prescribed, store in a sterile, airtight, tamper-proof container.

LABELLING

The label states the name of any added antimicrobial preservative.

Eye-drops

DEFINITION

Eye-drops are sterile aqueous or oily solutions or suspensions of one or more active substances intended for instillation into the eye.

Eye-drops may contain excipients, for example, to adjust the tonicity or the viscosity of the preparation, to adjust or stabilise the pH, to increase the solubility of the active substance, or to stabilise the preparation. These substances do not adversely affect the intended medicinal action or, at the concentrations used, cause undue local irritation.

Aqueous preparations supplied in multidose containers contain a suitable antimicrobial preservative in appropriate concentration except when the preparation itself has adequate antimicrobial properties. The antimicrobial preservative chosen must be compatible with the other ingredients of the preparation and must remain effective throughout the period of time during which eye-drops are in use.

If eye-drops are prescribed without antimicrobial preservatives they are supplied wherever possible in single-dose containers. Eye-drops intended for use in surgical procedures do not contain antimicrobial preservatives and are supplied in single-dose containers.

Eye-drops that are solutions, examined under suitable conditions of visibility, are practically clear and practically free from particles.

Eye-drops that are suspensions may show a sediment that is readily redispersed on shaking to give a suspension which remains sufficiently stable to enable the correct dose to be delivered.

Multidose preparations are supplied in containers that allow successive drops of the preparation to be administered. The containers contain at most 10 ml of the preparation, unless otherwise justified and authorised.

TESTS

Particle size. Unless otherwise justified and authorised, eye-drops in the form of a suspension comply with the following test: introduce a suitable quantity of the suspension into a counting cell or with a micropipette onto a slide, as appropriate, and scan under a microscope an area corresponding to 10 µg of the solid phase. For practical reasons, it is recommended that the whole sample is first scanned at low magnification (e.g. × 50) and particles greater than 25 µm are identified. These larger particles can then be measured at a larger magnification (e.g. × 200 to × 500). For each 10 µg of solid active substance, not more than 20 particles have a maximum dimension greater than 25 µm, and not more than 2 of these particles have a maximum dimension greater than 50 µm. None of the particles has a maximum dimension greater than 90 µm.

LABELLING

The label states for multidose containers, the period after opening the container after which the contents must not be used. This period does not exceed 4 weeks, unless otherwise justified and authorised.

Eye lotions

DEFINITION

Eye lotions are sterile aqueous solutions intended for use in washing or bathing the eye or for impregnating eye dressings.

Eye lotions may contain excipients, for example to adjust the tonicity or the viscosity of the preparation or to adjust or stabilise the pH. These substances do not adversely affect the intended action or, at the concentrations used, cause undue local irritation.

Eye lotions supplied in multidose containers contain a suitable antimicrobial preservative in appropriate concentration except when the preparation itself has adequate antimicrobial properties. The antimicrobial preservative chosen is compatible with the other ingredients of the preparation and remains effective throughout the period of time during which the eye lotions are in use.

If eye lotions are prescribed without an antimicrobial preservative, they are supplied in single-dose containers. Eye lotions intended for use in surgical procedures or in first-aid treatment do not contain an antimicrobial preservative and are supplied in single-dose containers.

Eye lotions examined under suitable conditions of visibility, are practically clear and practically free from particles.

The containers for multidose preparations do not contain more than 200 ml of eye lotion, unless otherwise justified and authorised.

LABELLING

The label states:

- where applicable, that the contents are to be used on one occasion only,
- for multidose preparations, the period after opening the container after which the contents must not be used. This period does not exceed 4 weeks, unless otherwise justified and authorised.

Powders for eye-drops and powders for eye lotions

DEFINITION

Powders for the preparation of eye-drops and eye lotions are supplied in a dry, sterile form to be dissolved or suspended in an appropriate liquid vehicle at the time of administration.

They may contain excipients to facilitate dissolution or dispersion, to prevent caking, to adjust the tonicity, to adjust or stabilise the pH or to stabilise the preparation.

After dissolution or suspension in the prescribed liquid, they comply with the requirements for eye-drops or eye lotions, as appropriate.

TESTS

Uniformity of content (*2.9.6*). Unless otherwise prescribed or justified and authorised, single-dose powders for eye-drops and eye lotions with a content of active substance less then 2 mg or less than 2 per cent of the total mass comply with test B for uniformity of content of single-dose preparations. If the preparation has more than one active substance, the requirement applies only to those substances which correspond to the above condition.

Uniformity of mass (*2.9.5*). Single-dose powders for eye-drops and eye lotions comply with the test for uniformity of mass of single-dose preparations. If the test for uniformity of content is prescribed for all the active substances, the test for uniformity of mass is not required.

Semi-solid eye preparations

DEFINITION

Semi-solid eye preparations are sterile ointments, creams or gels intended for application to the conjunctiva. They contain one or more active substances dissolved or dispersed in a suitable basis. They have a homogeneous appearance.

Semi-solid eye preparations comply with the requirements of the monograph on *Semi-solid preparations for cutaneous application (0132)*. The basis is non-irritant to the conjunctiva.

Semi-solid eye preparations are packed in small, sterilised collapsible tubes fitted or provided with a cannula and having a content of not more than 5 g of the preparation. The tubes must be well-closed to prevent microbial contamination. Semi-solid eye preparations may also be packed in suitably designed single-dose containers. The containers, or the nozzles of tubes, are of such a shape as to facilitate administration without contamination. Tubes are tamper-proof.

TESTS

Particle size. Semi-solid eye preparations containing dispersed solid particles comply with the following test: spread gently a quantity of the preparation corresponding to at least 10 μg of solid active substance as a thin layer. Scan under a microscope the whole area of the sample. For practical reasons, it is recommended that the whole sample is first scanned at a small magnification (e.g. × 50) and particles greater than 25 μm are identified. These larger particles can then be measured at a larger magnification (e.g. × 200 to × 500). For each 10 μg of solid active substance, not more than 20 particles have a maximum dimension greater than 25 μm, and not more than 2 of these particles have a maximum dimension greater than 50 μm. None of the particles has a maximum dimension greater than 90 μm.

Ophthalmic inserts

DEFINITION

Ophthalmic inserts are sterile, solid or semi-solid preparations of suitable size and shape, designed to be inserted in the conjunctival sac, to produce an ocular effect. They generally consist of a reservoir of active substance embedded in a matrix or bounded by a rate-controlling membrane. The active substance, which is more or less soluble in physiological fluids, is released over a determined period of time.

Ophthalmic inserts are individually distributed into sterile containers.

PRODUCTION

In the manufacture of ophthalmic inserts, means must be taken to ensure a suitable dissolution behaviour.

TESTS

Uniformity of content (*2.9.6*). Ophthalmic inserts comply, where applicable, with test A for uniformity of content.

LABELLING

The label states:

- where applicable, the total quantity of active substance per insert,
- where applicable, the dose released per unit time.

01/2005:1105

FOAMS, MEDICATED

Musci medicati

Additional requirements for medicated foams may be found, where appropriate, in other general monographs, for example on Rectal preparations (1145), Vaginal preparations (1164) and Liquid preparations for cutaneous application (0927).

DEFINITION

Medicated foams are preparations consisting of large volumes of gas dispersed in a liquid generally containing one or more active substances, a surfactant ensuring their formation and various other excipients. Medicated foams are usually intended for application to the skin or mucous membranes.

Medicated foams are usually formed at the time of administration from a liquid preparation in a pressurised container. The container is equipped with a device consisting of a valve and a push button suitable for the delivery of the foam.

Medicated foams intended for use on severely injured skin and on large open wounds are sterile.

Medicated foams supplied in pressurised containers comply with the requirements of the monograph on *Pressurised pharmaceutical preparations (0523)*.

PRODUCTION

Sterile medicated foams are prepared using materials and methods designed to ensure sterility and to avoid the introduction of contaminants and the growth of micro-organisms; recommendations on this aspect are provided in the text on *Methods of preparation of sterile products (5.1.1)*.

TESTS

Relative foam density. Maintain the container at about 25 °C for at least 24 h. Taking care not to warm the container, fit a rigid tube 70 mm to 100 mm long and about 1 mm in internal diameter onto the push button. Shake the container to homogenise the liquid phase of the contents and dispense 5 ml to 10 ml of foam to waste. Tare a flat-bottomed dish with a volume of about 60 ml and about 35 mm high. Place the end of the rigid tube attached to the push button in the corner of the dish, press the push button and fill the dish uniformly, using a circular motion. After the foam has

Dosage forms

completely expanded, level off by removing the excess foam with a slide. Weigh. Determine the mass of the same volume of *water R* by filling the same dish with *water R*.

The relative foam density is equivalent to the ratio:

$$\frac{m}{e}$$

m = mass of the test sample of foam, in grams,

e = mass of same volume of *water R*, in grams.

Carry out three measurements. None of the individual values deviate by more than 20 per cent from the mean value.

Duration of expansion. The apparatus (Figure 1105.-1) consists of a 50 ml burette, 15 mm in internal diameter, with 0.1 ml graduations and fitted with a 4 mm single bore stopcock. The graduation corresponding to 30 ml is at least 210 mm from the axis of the stopcock. The lower part of the burette is connected by means of a plastic tube not longer than 50 mm and 4 mm in internal diameter to the foam-generating container equipped with a push button fitted to this connection. Maintain the container at about 25 °C for at least 24 h. Shake the container, taking care not to warm it, to homogenise the liquid phase of the contents and dispense 5 ml to 10 ml of the foam to waste. Connect the push button to the outlet of the burette. Press the button and introduce about 30 ml of foam in a single delivery. Close the stopcock and at the same time start the chronometer and read the volume of foam in the burette. Every 10 s read the growing volume until the maximum volume is reached.

Carry out three measurements. None of the times needed to obtain the maximum volume is more than 5 min.

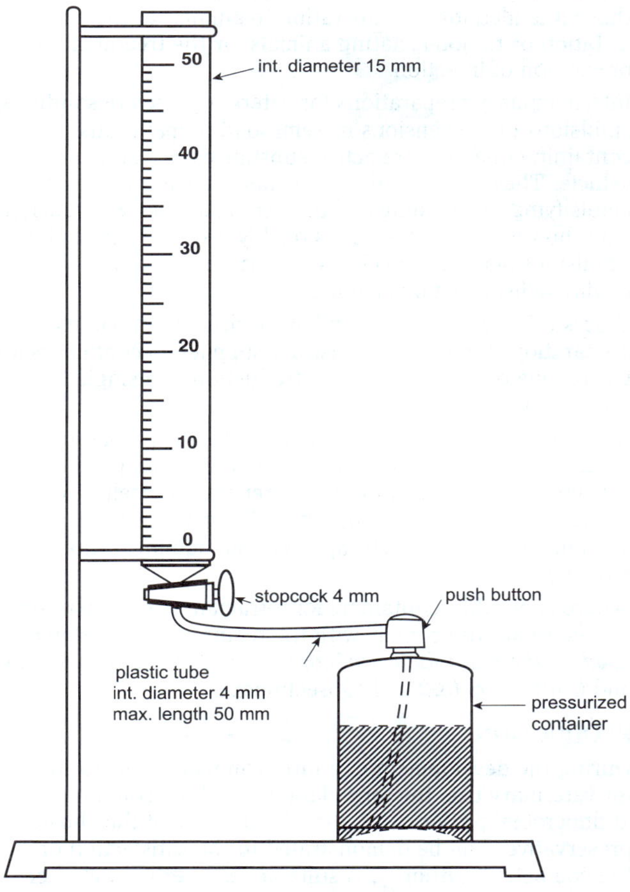

Figure 1105.-1. – *Apparatus for the determination of the duration of expansion*

Sterility (*2.6.1*). When the label indicates that the preparation is sterile, it complies with the test for sterility.

LABELLING

The label states, where applicable, that the preparation is sterile.

01/2005:0499

GRANULES

Granulata

Requirements for granules to be used for the preparation of oral solutions or suspensions are given in the monograph on Liquid preparations for oral use (0672). Where justified and authorised, the requirements of this monograph do not apply to granules for veterinary use.

DEFINITION

Granules are preparations consisting of solid, dry aggregates of powder particles sufficiently resistant to withstand handling. They are intended for oral administration. Some are swallowed as such, some are chewed and some are dissolved or dispersed in water or another suitable liquid before being administered.

Granules contain one or more active substances with or without excipients and, if necessary, colouring matter authorised by the competent authority and flavouring substances.

Granules are presented as single-dose or multidose preparations. Each dose of a multidose preparation is administered by means of a device suitable for measuring the quantity prescribed. For single-dose granules, each dose is enclosed in an individual container, for example a sachet or a vial.

Where applicable, containers for granules comply with the requirements of *Materials used for the manufacture of containers* (*3.1* and subsections) and *Containers* (*3.2* and subsections).

Several categories of granules may be distinguished:

– effervescent granules,
– coated granules,
– gastro-resistant granules,
– modified-release granules.

PRODUCTION

In the manufacture, packaging, storage and distribution of granules, suitable means are taken to ensure their microbial quality; recommendations on this aspect are provided in the text on *Microbiological quality of pharmaceutical preparations* (*5.1.4*).

TESTS

Uniformity of content (*2.9.6*). Unless otherwise prescribed or justified and authorised, single-dose granules with a content of active substance less than 2 mg or less than 2 per cent of the total mass comply with test B for uniformity of content of single-dose preparations. If the preparation has more than one active substance, the requirement applies only to those substances which correspond to the above conditions.

Uniformity of mass (*2.9.5*). Single-dose granules except for coated granules comply with the test for uniformity of mass of single-dose preparations. If the test for uniformity of content is prescribed for all the active substances, the test for uniformity of mass is not required.

Uniformity of mass of delivered doses from multidose containers (*2.9.27*). Granules supplied in multidose containers comply with the test.

STORAGE

If the preparation contains volatile ingredients or the contents have to be protected, store in an airtight container.

Effervescent granules

DEFINITION

Effervescent granules are uncoated granules generally containing acid substances and carbonates or hydrogen carbonates which react rapidly in the presence of water to release carbon dioxide. They are intended to be dissolved or dispersed in water before administration.

TESTS

Disintegration. Place one dose of the effervescent granules in a beaker containing 200 ml of *water R* at 15-25 °C; numerous bubbles of gas are evolved. When the evolution of gas around the individual grains ceases, the granules have disintegrated, being either dissolved or dispersed in the water. Repeat the operation on 5 other doses. The preparation complies with the test if each of the 6 doses used disintegrates within 5 min.

STORAGE

In an airtight container.

Coated granules

DEFINITION

Coated granules are usually multidose preparations and consist of granules coated with one or more layers of mixtures of various excipients.

PRODUCTION

The substances used as coatings are usually applied as a solution or suspension in conditions in which evaporation of the vehicle occurs.

TESTS

Dissolution. A suitable test may be carried out to demonstrate the appropriate release of the active substance(s), for example one of the tests described in *Dissolution test for solid dosage forms* (*2.9.3*).

Modified-release granules

DEFINITION

Modified-release granules are coated or uncoated granules which contain special excipients or which are prepared by special procedures, or both, designed to modify the rate, the place or the time at which the active substance or substances are released.

Modified-release granules include prolonged-release granules and delayed-release granules.

PRODUCTION

A suitable test is carried out to demonstrate the appropriate release of the active substance(s).

TESTS

Dissolution. Carry out a suitable test to demonstrate the appropriate release of the active substance(s), for example the test described in *Dissolution test for solid dosage forms* (*2.9.3*).

Gastro-resistant granules

DEFINITION

Gastro-resistant granules are delayed-release granules that are intended to resist the gastric fluid and to release the active substance(s) in the intestinal fluid. These properties are achieved by covering the granules with a gastro-resistant material (enteric-coated granules) or by other suitable means.

PRODUCTION

A suitable test is carried out to demonstrate the appropriate release of the active substance(s).

TESTS

Dissolution. Carry out a suitable test to demonstrate the appropriate release of the active substance(s), for example the test described in *Dissolution test for solid dosage forms* (*2.9.3*).

01/2005:0945

INTRAMAMMARY PREPARATIONS FOR VETERINARY USE

Praeparationes intramammariae ad usum veterinarium

DEFINITION

Intramammary preparations for veterinary use are sterile preparations intended for introduction into the mammary gland via the teat canal. There are two main categories: those intended for administration to lactating animals, and those intended for administration to animals at the end of lactation or to non-lactating animals for the treatment or prevention of infection.

Intramammary preparations for veterinary use are solutions, emulsions or suspensions or semi-solid preparations containing one or more active substances in a suitable vehicle. They may contain excipients such as stabilising, emulsifying, suspending and thickening agents. Suspensions may show a sediment which is readily dispersed on shaking. Emulsions may show evidence of phase separation but are readily redispersed on shaking.

Unless otherwise justified and authorised, intramammary preparations for veterinary use are supplied in containers for use on one occasion only for introduction in a single teat canal of an animal.

If supplied in multidose containers, aqueous preparations contain a suitable antimicrobial preservative at a suitable concentration, except where the preparation itself has adequate antimicrobial properties. Precautions for administration and for storage between administrations must be taken.

Where applicable, containers for intramammary preparations for veterinary use comply with the requirements of *Materials used for the manufacture of containers* (*3.1* and subsections) and *Containers* (*3.2* and subsections).

PRODUCTION

During the development of a intramammary preparation for veterinary use, the formulation for which contains an antimicrobial preservative, the effectiveness of the chosen preservative shall be demonstrated to the satisfaction of the competent authority. A suitable test method together with criteria for judging the preservative properties of the formulation are provided in the text on *Efficacy of antimicrobial preservation* (*5.1.3*).

Intramammary preparations for veterinary use are prepared using materials and methods designed to ensure sterility and to avoid the introduction of contaminants and the growth of micro-organisms; recommendations on this aspect are provided in the text on *Methods of preparation of sterile products* (*5.1.1*).

In the manufacture of intramammary preparations for veterinary use containing dispersed particles, measures are taken to ensure a suitable and controlled particle size with regard to the intended use.

TESTS

Deliverable mass or volume. Squeeze out as much as possible of the contents of ten containers according to the instructions on the label. The mean mass or volume does not differ by more than 10 per cent from the nominal mass or volume.

Sterility (*2.6.1*). Intramammary preparations for veterinary use comply with the test for sterility; use the technique of membrane filtration or, in justified cases, direct inoculation of the culture media. Squeeze out the contents of ten containers and mix thoroughly. For each medium, use 0.5 g to 1 g (or 0.5 ml to 1 ml as appropriate) taken from the mixed sample.

STORAGE

Store in a sterile, airtight, tamper-proof container.

LABELLING

The label states:

- the name of the active substance(s) and the mass or number of International Units of the active substance(s) that may be delivered from the container using normal technique,
- whether the preparation is intended for use in a lactating animal or a non-lactating animal,
- in the case of multidose containers, the name of any added antimicrobial preservative.

01/2005:1228

INTRARUMINAL DEVICES

Praeparationes intraruminales

The requirements of this monograph do not apply to preparations (sometimes known as boluses), such as large conventional tablets, capsules or moulded dosage forms which give immediate or prolonged release of the active substance(s). Such preparations comply with the relevant parts of the monographs on Capsules (0016) or Tablets (0478).

DEFINITION

Intraruminal devices are solid preparations each containing one or more active substances. They are intended for oral administration to ruminant animals and are designed to be retained in the rumen to deliver the active substance(s) in a continuous or pulsatile manner. The period of release of the active substance(s) may vary from days to weeks according to the nature of the formulation and/or the delivery device.

Intraruminal devices may be administered using a balling gun. Some intraruminal devices are intended to float on the surface of the ruminal fluid while others are intended to remain on the floor of the rumen or reticulum. Each device has a density appropriate for its intended purpose.

PRODUCTION

For continuous release, the intraruminal device is designed to release the active substance(s) at a defined rate over a defined period of time. This may be achieved by erosion, corrosion, diffusion, osmotic pressure or any other suitable chemical, physical or physico-chemical means.

For pulsatile-release, the intraruminal device is designed to release a specific quantity of active substance(s) at one or several defined intermediate times. This may be achieved by corrosion by ruminal fluids of the metallic elements of the intraruminal device which leads to sequential release of the constituent units which are usually in the form of tablets.

In the manufacture of intraruminal devices, means are taken to ensure an appropriate release of the active substance(s).

In the manufacture, packaging, storage and distribution of intraruminal devices, suitable means are taken to ensure their microbial quality; recommendations on this aspect are provided in the text on *Microbiological quality of pharmaceutical preparations* (*5.1.4*).

TESTS

Uniformity of content (*2.9.6*). Unless otherwise justified and authorised, constituent tablet units of intraruminal devices in which the active substances are present at levels less than 2 mg or less than 2 per cent of the total mass comply with test A for uniformity of content of single-dose preparations. If the preparation contains more than one active substance, the requirement applies only to those substances which correspond to the above conditions.

Uniformity of mass (*2.9.5*). Unless otherwise justified and authorised, the constituent tablet units of intraruminal devices comply with the test for uniformity of mass. If the test for uniformity of content is prescribed for all active substances, the test for uniformity of mass is not required.

LABELLING

The label states:

- for continuous-release devices, the dose released per unit time,
- for pulsatile-release devices, the dose released at specified times.

01/2005:0927

LIQUID PREPARATIONS FOR CUTANEOUS APPLICATION

Praeparationes liquidae ad usum dermicum

Where justified and authorised, the requirements of this monograph do not apply to preparations intended for systemic and veterinary use.

DEFINITION

Liquid preparations for cutaneous application are preparations of a variety of viscosities intended for local or transdermal delivery of active ingredients. They are solutions, emulsions or suspensions which may contain one or more active substances in a suitable vehicle. They may contain suitable antimicrobial preservatives, antioxidants and other excipients such as stabilisers, emulsifiers and thickeners.

Emulsions may show evidence of phase separation but are readily redispersed on shaking. Suspensions may show a sediment which is readily dispersed on shaking to give a suspension which is sufficiently stable to enable a homogeneous preparation to be delivered.

Where applicable, containers for liquid preparations for cutaneous application comply with the requirements of *Materials used for the manufacture of containers* (*3.1* and subsections) and *Containers* (*3.2* and subsections).

When liquid preparations for cutaneous application are dispensed in pressurised containers, the containers comply with the requirements of the monograph on *Pressurised pharmaceutical preparations (0523)*.

Preparations specifically intended for use on severely injured skin are sterile.

Several categories of liquid preparations for cutaneous application may be distinguished, for example:

- shampoos,
- cutaneous foams.

PRODUCTION

During the development of a liquid preparation for cutaneous application, the formulation for which contains an antimicrobial preservative, the effectiveness of the chosen preservative shall be demonstrated to the satisfaction of the competent authority. A suitable test method together with criteria for judging the preservative properties of the formulation are provided in the text on *Efficacy of antimicrobial preservation* (*5.1.3*).

In the manufacture, packaging, storage and distribution of liquid preparations for cutaneous application, suitable means are taken to ensure their microbial quality; recommendations on this aspect are provided in the text on *Microbiological quality of pharmaceutical preparations* (*5.1.4*).

Sterile liquid preparations for cutaneous application are prepared using materials and methods designed to ensure sterility and to avoid the introduction of contaminants and the growth of micro-organisms; recommendations on this aspect are provided in the text on *Methods of preparation of sterile products* (*5.1.1*).

In the manufacture of liquid preparations for cutaneous application containing dispersed particles, measures are taken to ensure a suitable and controlled particle size with regard to the intended use.

Dosage forms

TESTS

Deliverable mass or volume (*2.9.28*). Liquid preparations for cutaneous application supplied in single-dose containers comply with the test.

Sterility (*2.6.1*). Where the label indicates that the preparation is sterile, it complies with the test for sterility.

STORAGE

If the preparation is sterile, store in a sterile, airtight, tamper-proof container.

LABELLING

The label states:

- the name of any added antimicrobial preservative,
- where applicable, that the preparation is sterile.

Shampoos

DEFINITION

Shampoos are liquid or, occasionally semi-solid preparations intended for application to the scalp and subsequent washing away with water. Upon rubbing with water they usually form a foam.

They are emulsions, suspensions or solutions. Shampoos normally contain surface active agents.

Cutaneous foams

DEFINITION

Cutaneous foams comply with the requirements of the monograph on *Medicated foams (1105)*.

01/2005:0672

LIQUID PREPARATIONS FOR ORAL USE

Praeparationes liquidae peroraliae

Where justified and authorised, the requirements of this monograph do not apply to liquid preparations for oral use intended for veterinary use.

DEFINITION

Liquid preparations for oral use are usually solutions, emulsions or suspensions containing one or more active substances in a suitable vehicle; they may, however, consist of liquid active substances used as such (oral liquids).

Some preparations for oral use are prepared by dilution of concentrated liquid preparations, or from powders or granules for the preparation of oral solutions or suspensions, for oral drops or for syrups, using a suitable vehicle.

The vehicle for any preparations for oral use is chosen having regard to the nature of the active substance(s) and to provide organoleptic characteristics appropriate to the intended use of the preparation.

Liquid preparations for oral use may contain suitable antimicrobial preservatives, antioxidants and other excipients such as dispersing, suspending, thickening, emulsifying, buffering, wetting, solubilising, stabilising, flavouring and sweetening agents and colouring matter, authorised by the competent authority.

Emulsions may show evidence of phase separation but are readily redispersed on shaking. Suspensions may show a sediment which is readily dispersed on shaking to give a suspension which remains sufficiently stable to enable the correct dose to be delivered.

Where applicable, containers for liquid preparations for oral use comply with the requirements of *Materials used for the manufacture of containers* (*3.1* and subsections) and *Containers* (*3.2* and subsections).

Several categories of preparations may be distinguished:

- oral solutions, emulsions and suspensions,
- powders and granules for oral solutions and suspensions,
- oral drops,
- powders for oral drops,
- syrups,
- powders and granules for syrups.

PRODUCTION

During the development of a preparation for oral use, the formulation for which contains an antimicrobial preservative, the effectiveness of the chosen preservative shall be demonstrated to the satisfaction of the competent authority. A suitable test method together with criteria for judging the preservative properties of the formulation are provided in the text on *Efficacy of antimicrobial preservation* (*5.1.3*).

In the manufacturing, packaging, storage and distribution of liquid preparations for oral use, suitable means are taken to ensure their microbial quality; recommendations on this aspect are provided in the text on *Microbiological quality of pharmaceutical preparations* (*5.1.4*).

In the manufacture of liquid preparations for oral use containing dispersed particles, measures are taken to ensure a suitable and controlled particle size with regard to the intended use.

TESTS

Uniformity of content (*2.9.6*). Unless otherwise prescribed or justified and authorised, single-dose preparations that are suspensions comply with the following test. After shaking, empty each container as completely as possible and carry out the test on the individual contents. They comply with test B for uniformity of content of single-dose preparations.

Uniformity of mass. Single-dose preparations that are solutions or emulsions comply with the following test: weigh individually the contents of 20 containers, emptied as completely as possible, and determine the average mass. Not more than 2 of the individual masses deviate by more than 10 per cent from the average mass and none deviates by more than 20 per cent.

Dose and uniformity of dose of oral drops. Into a suitable, graduated cylinder, introduce by means of the dropping device the number of drops usually prescribed for one dose or introduce by means of the measuring device, the usually prescribed quantity. The dropping speed does not exceed 2 drops per second. Weigh the liquid, repeat the addition, weigh again and carry on repeating the addition and weighing until a total of 10 masses are obtained. No single mass deviates by more than 10 per cent from the average mass. The total of 10 masses does not differ by more than 15 per cent from the nominal mass of 10 doses. If necessary, measure the total volume of 10 doses. The volume does not differ by more than 15 per cent from the nominal volume of 10 doses.

Deliverable mass or volume (*2.9.28*). Liquid preparations for oral use supplied in single-dose containers comply with the test.

Uniformity of mass of delivered doses from multidose containers (*2.9.27*). Liquid preparations for oral use supplied in multidose containers comply with the test.

LABELLING

The label states the name of any added antimicrobial preservative.

Oral solutions, emulsions and suspensions

DEFINITION

Oral solutions, emulsions and suspensions are supplied in single-dose or multi-dose containers. Each dose from a multi-dose container is administered by means of a device suitable for measuring the prescribed volume. The device is usually a spoon or a cup for volumes of 5 ml or multiples thereof or an oral syringe for other volumes.

Powders and granules for oral solutions and suspensions

DEFINITION

Powders and granules for the preparation of oral solutions or suspensions generally conform to the definitions in the monographs on *Oral powders (1165)* or *Granules (0499)* as appropriate. They may contain excipients in particular to facilitate dispersion or dissolution and to prevent caking.

After dissolution or suspension, they comply with the requirements for oral solutions or oral suspensions, as appropriate.

TESTS

Uniformity of content (*2.9.6*). Unless otherwise prescribed or justified and authorised, single-dose powders and single-dose granules with a content of active substance less than 2 mg or less than 2 per cent of the total mass comply with test B for uniformity of content of single-dose preparations. If the preparation has more than one active substance, the requirement applies only to those substances that correspond to the above conditions.

Uniformity of mass (*2.9.5*). Single-dose powders and single-dose granules comply with the test for uniformity of mass of single-dose preparations. If the test for uniformity of content is prescribed for all the active substances, the test for uniformity of mass is not required.

LABELLING

The label states:

- the method of preparation of the solution or suspension,
- the conditions and the duration of storage after constitution.

Oral drops

DEFINITION

Oral drops are solutions, emulsions or suspensions which are administered in small volumes such as drops by the means of a suitable device.

LABELLING

The label states the number of drops per millilitre of preparation or per gram of preparation if the dose is measured in drops.

Powders for oral drops

DEFINITION

Powders for the preparation of oral drops generally conform to the definition of *Oral powders (1165)*. They may contain excipients to facilitate dissolution or suspension in the prescribed liquid or to prevent caking.

After dissolution or suspension, they comply with the requirements for oral drops.

TESTS

Uniformity of content (*2.9.6*). Unless otherwise prescribed or justified and authorised, single-dose powders for oral drops with a content of active substance less than 2 mg or less than 2 per cent of the total mass comply with test B for uniformity of content of single-dose preparations. If the preparation has more than one active substance, the requirement applies only to those substances that correspond to the above conditions.

Uniformity of mass (*2.9.5*). Single-dose powders for oral drops comply with the test for uniformity of mass of single-dose preparations. If the test for uniformity of content is prescribed for all the active substances, the test for uniformity of mass is not required.

Syrups

DEFINITION

Syrups are aqueous preparations characterised by sweet taste and a viscous consistency. They may contain sucrose at a concentration of at least 45 per cent *m/m*. The sweet taste can also be obtained by using other polyols or sweetening agents. Syrups usually contain aromatic or other flavouring agents. Each dose from a multi-dose container is administered by means of a device suitable for measuring the prescribed volume. The device is usually a spoon or a cup for volumes of 5 ml or multiples thereof.

LABELLING

The label states the name and concentration of the polyol or sweetening agent.

Powders and granules for syrups

DEFINITION

Powders and granules for syrups generally conform to the definitions in the monograph on *Oral powders (1165)* or *Granules (0499)*. They may contain excipients to facilitate dissolution.

After dissolution, they comply with the requirements for syrups.

TESTS

Uniformity of content (*2.9.6*). Unless otherwise prescribed or justified and authorised, single-dose powders and granules for syrups with a content of active substance less than 2 mg or less than 2 per cent of the total mass comply with test B for uniformity of content of single-dose preparations. If the preparation has more than one active substance, the requirement applies only to those substances that correspond to the above conditions.

Uniformity of mass (*2.9.5*). Single-dose powders and granules for syrups comply with the test for uniformity of mass of single-dose preparations. If the test for uniformity of content is prescribed for all the active substances, the test for uniformity of mass is not required.

01/2005:0676

NASAL PREPARATIONS

Nasalia

DEFINITION

Nasal preparations are liquid, semi-solid or solid preparations intended for administration to the nasal cavities to obtain a systemic or local effect. They contain one or more active substances. Nasal preparations are as far as possible non-irritating and do not adversely affect the functions of the nasal mucosa and its cilia. Aqueous nasal preparations are usually isotonic and may contain excipients, for example, to adjust the viscosity of the preparation, to adjust or stabilise the pH, to increase the solubility of the active substance, or to stabilise the preparation.

Nasal preparations are supplied in multidose or single-dose containers, provided, if necessary, with a suitable administration device which may be designed to avoid the introduction of contaminants.

Unless otherwise justified and authorised, aqueous nasal preparations supplied in multidose containers contain a suitable antimicrobial preservative in appropriate concentration, except where the preparation itself has adequate antimicrobial properties.

Where applicable, the containers comply with the requirements of *Materials used for the manufacture of containers* (*3.1* and subsections) and *Containers* (*3.2* and subsections).

Several categories of nasal preparations may be distinguished:

- nasal drops and liquid nasal sprays,
- nasal powders,
- semi-solid nasal preparations,
- nasal washes,
- nasal sticks.

PRODUCTION

During the development of a nasal preparation, the formulation for which contains an antimicrobial preservative, the effectiveness of the chosen preservative shall be demonstrated to the satisfaction of the competent authority. A suitable test method together with criteria for judging the preservative properties of the formulation are provided in the text on *Efficacy of antimicrobial preservation* (*5.1.3*).

In the manufacture, packaging, storage and distribution of nasal preparations, suitable means are taken to ensure their microbial quality; recommendations on this aspect are provided in the text on *Microbiological quality of pharmaceutical preparations* (*5.1.4*).

Sterile nasal preparations are prepared using materials and methods designed to ensure sterility and to avoid the introduction of contaminants and the growth of micro-organisms; recommendations on this aspect are provided in the text on *Methods of preparation of sterile products* (*5.1.1*).

In the manufacture of nasal preparations containing dispersed particles, measures are taken to ensure a suitable and controlled particle size with regard to the intended use.

TESTS

Sterility (*2.6.1*). Where the label states that the preparation is sterile, it complies with the test for sterility.

STORAGE

If the preparation is sterile, store in a sterile, airtight, tamper-proof container.

LABELLING

The label states:

- the name of any added antimicrobial preservative,
- where applicable, that the preparation is sterile.

Nasal drops and liquid nasal sprays

DEFINITION

Nasal drops and liquid nasal sprays are solutions, emulsions or suspensions intended for instillation or spraying into the nasal cavities.

Emulsions may show evidence of phase separation but are easily redispersed on shaking. Suspensions may show a sediment which is readily dispersed on shaking to give a suspension which remains sufficiently stable to enable the correct dose to be delivered.

Nasal drops are usually supplied in multidose containers provided with a suitable applicator.

Liquid nasal sprays are supplied in containers with atomising devices or in pressurised containers fitted with a suitable adapter and with or without a metering dose valve, which comply with the requirements of the monograph on *Pressurised pharmaceutical preparations (0523)*.

The size of droplets of the spray is such as to localise their deposition in the nasal cavity.

TESTS

Unless otherwise prescribed or justified and authorised, nasal drops supplied in single-dose containers and single doses of metered nasal sprays intended for systemic action, comply with the following tests.

Uniformity of mass. Nasal drops that are solutions comply with the following test: weigh individually the contents of ten containers emptied as completely as possible, and determine the average mass. Not more than two of the individual masses deviate by more than 10 per cent from the average mass and none deviates by more than 20 per cent.

Metered-dose nasal sprays that are solutions comply with the following test: discharge once to waste. Wait for not less than 5 s and discharge again to waste. Repeat this procedure for a further three actuations. Weigh the mass of the container, discharge once to waste and weigh the remaining mass of the container. Calculate the difference between the two masses. Repeat the procedure for a further nine containers. They comply with the test if not more than two of the individual values deviate by more than 25 per cent from the average value and none deviates by more than 35 per cent.

Uniformity of content (*2.9.6*). Nasal drops that are suspensions or emulsions comply with the following test: empty each container as completely as possible and carry out the test on the individual content. They comply with test B of uniformity of content.

Uniformity of delivered dose. Metered-dose nasal sprays that are suspensions or emulsions comply with the following test. Use an apparatus capable of quantitatively retaining the dose leaving the actuator of the atomising device.

Shake a container for 5 s and discharge once to waste. Wait for not less than 5 s, shake for 5 s and discharge again to waste. Repeat this procedure for a further three actuations. After 2 s, fire one dose of the metered-dose nasal spray into the collecting vessel by actuating the atomising device. Collect the contents of the collecting vessel by successive rinses. Determine the content of active substance in the combined rinses.

Repeat the procedure for a further nine containers.

Unless otherwise justified and authorised, the preparation complies with the test if not more than one of the individual contents is outside the limits of 75 per cent to 125 per cent and none is outside the limits of 65 per cent and 135 per cent of the average content.

If two or three individual contents are outside the limits of 75 per cent to 125 per cent but within the limits of 65 per cent to 135 per cent, repeat the test for twenty more containers. The preparation complies with the test if not more than three individual contents of the thirty individual contents are outside the limits of 75 per cent to 125 per cent and none is outside the limits of 65 per cent to 135 per cent of the average content.

Nasal powders

DEFINITION

Nasal powders are powders intended for insufflation into the nasal cavity by means of a suitable device.

They comply with the requirements of the monograph on *Powders for cutaneous application (1166)*.

The size of the particles is such as to localise their deposition in the nasal cavity and verified by adequate methods of particle-size determination.

Semi-solid nasal preparations

DEFINITION

Semi-solid nasal preparations comply with the requirements of the monograph on *Semi-solid preparations for cutaneous application (0132)*.

The containers are adapted to deliver the product to the site of application.

Nasal washes

DEFINITION

Nasal washes are generally aqueous isotonic solutions intended to cleanse the nasal cavities.

Nasal washes intended for application to injured parts or prior to a surgical operation are sterile.

TESTS

Deliverable mass or volume (*2.9.28*). Nasal washes supplied in single-dose containers comply with the test.

Nasal sticks

DEFINITION

Nasal sticks comply with the monograph on *Sticks (1154)*.

01/2005:1807

OROMUCOSAL PREPARATIONS

Praeparationes buccales

This monograph does not apply to dental preparations or to preparations such as chewable tablets (0478), medicated chewing gums (1239), oral lyophilisates and other solid or semi-solid preparations that are intended to be chewed or dispersed in the saliva before being swallowed. Where justified and authorised, this monograph does not apply to preparations for veterinary use.

DEFINITION

Oromucosal preparations are solid, semi-solid or liquid preparations, containing one or more active substances intended for administration to the oral cavity and/or the throat to obtain a local or systemic effect. Preparations intended for a local effect may be designed for application to a specific site within the oral cavity such as the gums (gingival preparations) or the throat (oropharyngeal preparations). Preparations intended for a systemic effect are designed to be absorbed primarily at one or more sites on the oral mucosa (e.g. sublingual preparations). Mucoadhesive preparations are intended to be retained in the oral cavity by adhesion to the mucosal epithelium and may modify systemic drug absorption at the site of application. For many oromucosal preparations, it is likely that some proportion of the active substance(s) will be swallowed and may be absorbed via the gastrointestinal tract.

Oromucosal preparations may contain suitable antimicrobial preservatives and other excipients such as dispersing, suspending, thickening, emulsifying, buffering, wetting, solubilising, stabilising, flavouring and sweetening agents. Solid preparations may in addition contain glidants, lubricants and excipients capable of modifying the release of the active substance(s).

Where applicable, containers for oromucosal preparations comply with the requirements for *Materials used for the manufacture of containers* (*3.1 and subsections*) and *Containers* (*3.2 and subsections*).

Several categories of preparations for oromucosal use may be distinguished:

– gargles,
– mouthwashes,
– gingival solutions,
– oromucosal solutions and oromucosal suspensions,

- semi-solid oromucosal preparations (including for example gingival gel, gingival paste, oromucosal gel, oromucosal paste),
- oromucosal drops, oromucosal sprays and sublingual sprays (including oropharyngeal sprays),
- lozenges and pastilles,
- compressed lozenges,
- sublingual tablets and buccal tablets,
- oromucosal capsules,
- mucoadhesive preparations.

PRODUCTION

During the development of an oromucosal preparation containing an antimicrobial preservative, the effectiveness of the chosen preservative shall be demonstrated to the satisfaction of the competent authority. A suitable test method together with the criteria for judging the preservative properties of the formulation are provided in *5.1.3 Efficacy of antimicrobial preservation*.

In the manufacture, packaging, storage and distribution of oromucosal preparations, suitable means are taken to ensure their microbiological quality; recommendations on this aspect are provided in the text on *Microbiological quality of pharmaceutical preparations* (*5.1.4*).

In the manufacture of semi-solid and liquid oromucosal preparations containing dispersed particles, measures are taken to ensure a suitable and controlled particle size with regard to the intended use.

TESTS

Uniformity of content (*2.9.6*). Unless otherwise prescribed or justified and authorised, single-dose preparations with a content of active substance less than 2 mg or less than 2 per cent of the total mass comply with test A (compressed and moulded dosage forms) or test B (capsules) for the uniformity of content of single-dose preparations. If the preparation contains more than one active substance, this requirement applies only to those substances that correspond to the above conditions.

Uniformity of mass (*2.9.5*). Solid single-dose preparations comply with the test for uniformity of mass. If the test for the uniformity of content is prescribed, or justified and authorised for all active substances, the test for uniformity of mass is not required.

LABELLING

The label states the name of any added antimicrobial preservative.

Gargles

DEFINITION

Gargles are aqueous solutions intended for gargling to obtain a local effect. They are not to be swallowed. They are supplied as ready-to-use solutions or concentrated solutions to be diluted. They may also be prepared from powders or tablets to be dissolved in water before use.

Gargles may contain excipients to adjust the pH which, as far as possible, is neutral.

Mouthwashes

DEFINITION

Mouthwashes are aqueous solutions intended for use in contact with the mucous membrane of the oral cavity, usually after dilution with water. They are not to be swallowed. They are supplied as ready-to-use solutions or concentrated solutions to be diluted. They may also be prepared from powders or tablets to be dissolved in water before use.

Mouthwashes may contain excipients to adjust the pH which, as far as possible, is neutral.

Gingival solutions

DEFINITION

Gingival solutions are intended for administration to the gingivae by means of a suitable applicator.

Oromucosal solutions and oromucosal suspensions

DEFINITION

Oromucosal solutions and oromucosal suspensions are liquid preparations intended for administration to the oral cavity by means of a suitable applicator.

Oromucosal suspensions may show a sediment which is readily dispersible on shaking to give a suspension which remains sufficiently stable to enable the correct dose to be delivered.

Semi-solid oromucosal preparations

DEFINITION

Semi-solid oromucosal preparations are hydrophilic gels or pastes intended for administration to the oral cavity or to a specific part of the oral cavity such as the gingivae (gingival gel, gingival paste). They may be provided as single-dose preparations.

Semi-solid oromucosal preparations comply with the requirements of the monograph on *Semi-solid preparations for cutaneous use (0132)*.

Oromucosal drops, oromucosal sprays and sublingual sprays

DEFINITION

Oromucosal drops, oromucosal sprays and sublingual sprays are solutions, emulsions or suspensions intended for local or systemic effect. They are applied by instillation or spraying into the oral cavity or onto a specific part of the oral cavity such as spraying under the tongue (sublingual spray) or into the throat (oropharyngeal spray).

Emulsions may show evidence of phase separation but are readily redispersed on shaking. Suspensions may show a sediment which is readily dispersed on shaking to give a suspension which remains sufficiently stable to enable the correct dose to be delivered.

Liquid oromucosal sprays are supplied in containers with atomising devices or in pressurised containers having a suitable adaptor, with or without a metering dose valve, which comply with the requirements of the monograph on *Pressurised pharmaceutical preparations (0523)*.

The size of the droplets of the spray is such as to localise their deposition in the oral cavity or the throat as intended.

TESTS

Unless otherwise prescribed or justified and authorised, oromucosal drops supplied in single-dose containers, single-doses of metered oromucosal sprays and sublingual sprays intended for systemic action comply with the following tests.

Dosage forms

Uniformity of mass. Oromucosal drops that are solutions comply with the following test: determine the individual masses of the contents of 10 containers emptied as completely as possible, and calculate the average mass. Not more than 2 of the individual masses deviate by more than 10 per cent from the average mass and none deviates by more than 20 per cent.

Metered-dose oromucosal sprays and sublingual sprays that are solutions comply with the following test: discharge once to waste. Wait for not less than 5 s and discharge again to waste. Repeat this procedure for a further 3 actuations. Weigh the mass of the container, discharge once to waste and weigh the remaining mass of the container. Calculate the difference between the 2 masses. Repeat the procedure for a further 9 containers. The preparation complies with the test if not more than 2 of the individual masses deviate by more than 25 per cent from the average value and none deviates by more than 35 per cent.

Uniformity of content (*2.9.6*). Oromucosal drops that are suspensions or emulsions comply with the following test: empty each container as completely as possible and carry out the test on the individual contents. They comply with test B of uniformity of content.

Uniformity of delivered dose. Metered-dose oromuscal sprays and sublingual sprays that are suspensions or emulsions comply with the following test: use an apparatus capable of quantitatively retaining the dose leaving the actuator of the atomising device.

Shake a container for 5 s and discharge once to waste. Wait for not less than 5 s, shake for 5 s and discharge again to waste. Repeat this procedure for a further 3 actuations. After 2 s, fire one dose of the metered-dose oromucosal spray into the collecting vessel by actuating the atomising device. Collect the contents of the collecting vessel by successive rinses. Determine the content of active substance in the combined rinses. Repeat the procedure for a further 9 containers. Unless otherwise justified and authorised, the preparation complies with the test if not more than one of the individual contents is outside the limits of 75 per cent to 125 per cent and none is outside the limits of 65 per cent to 135 per cent of the average content.

If 2 or 3 individual contents are outside the limits of 75 per cent to 125 per cent but within the limits of 65 per cent to 135 per cent, repeat the test for 20 more containers. The preparation complies with the test if not more than 3 individual contents of the 30 contents are outside the limits of 75 per cent to 125 per cent and none is outside the limits of 65 per cent to 135 per cent of the average content.

Lozenges and pastilles

DEFINITION

Lozenges and pastilles are solid, single-dose preparations intended to be sucked to obtain, usually, a local effect in the oral cavity and the throat. They contain one or more active substances, usually in a flavoured and sweetened base, and are intended to dissolve or disintegrate slowly in the mouth when sucked.

Lozenges are hard preparations prepared by moulding. Pastilles are soft, flexible preparations prepared by moulding of mixtures containing natural or synthetic polymers or gums and sweeteners.

Compressed lozenges

DEFINITION

Compressed lozenges are solid, single-dose preparations intended to be sucked to obtain a local or systemic effect. They are prepared by compression and are often rhomboid in shape.

Compressed lozenges conform with the general definition of tablets.

PRODUCTION

In the manufacture of compressed lozenges, means are taken to ensure that they possess a suitable mechanical strength to resist handling without crumbling or breaking. This may be demonstrated by examining the *Friability of uncoated tablets* (*2.9.7*) and the *Resistance to crushing of tablets* (*2.9.8*).

TESTS

Dissolution. For compressed lozenges intended for a systemic effect, a suitable test is carried out to demonstrate the appropriate release of the active substance(s).

Sublingual tablets and buccal tablets

DEFINITION

Sublingual tablets and buccal tablets are solid, single-dose preparations to be applied under the tongue or to the buccal cavity, respectively, to obtain a systemic effect. They are prepared by compression of mixtures of powders or granulations into tablets with a shape suited for the intended use.

Sublingual tablets and buccal tablets conform to the general definition of tablets.

PRODUCTION

In the manufacture of sublingual tablets and buccal tablets, means are taken to ensure that they possess suitable mechanical strength to resist handling without crumbling or breaking. This may be demonstrated by examining the *Friability of uncoated tablets* (*2.9.7*) and the *Resistance to crushing of tablets* (*2.9.8*).

TESTS

Dissolution. Unless otherwise justified and authorised, a suitable test is carried out to demonstrate the appropriate release of the active substance(s).

Oromucosal capsules

DEFINITION

Oromucosal capsules are soft capsules to be chewed or sucked.

Mucoadhesive preparations

DEFINITION

Mucoadhesive preparations contain one or more active substances intended for systemic absorption through the buccal mucosa over a prolonged period of time. They may be supplied as mucoadhesive buccal tablets or as other mucoadhesive solid or semi-solid preparations.

Mucoadhesive buccal tablets are prepared by compression of mono- or multi-layered tablets. They usually contain hydrophilic polymers, which on wetting with the saliva produce a flexible hydrogel that adheres to the buccal mucosa.

PRODUCTION

In the manufacture of mucoadhesive buccal tablets, means are taken to ensure that they possess suitable mechanical strength to resist handling without crumbling or breaking. This may be demonstrated by examining the *Friability of uncoated tablets* (*2.9.7*) and the *Resistance to crushing of tablets* (*2.9.8*).

TESTS

Dissolution. Unless otherwise justified and authorised, a suitable test is carried out to demonstrate the appropriate release of the active substance(s).

01/2005:0520

PARENTERAL PREPARATIONS

Parenteralia

The requirements of this monograph do not necessarily apply to products derived from human blood, to immunological preparations, or radiopharmaceutical preparations. Special requirements may apply to preparations for veterinary use depending on the species of animal for which the preparation is intended.

DEFINITION

Parenteral preparations are sterile preparations intended for administration by injection, infusion or implantation into the human or animal body.

Parenteral preparations may require the use of excipients, for example to make the preparation isotonic with blood, to adjust the pH, to increase solubility, to prevent deterioration of the active substances or to provide adequate antimicrobial properties but not to adversely affect the intended medicinal action of the preparation or, at the concentrations used, to cause toxicity or undue local irritation.

Containers for parenteral preparations are made as far as possible from materials that are sufficiently transparent to permit the visual inspection of the contents, except for implants and in other justified and authorised cases.

Where applicable, the containers for parenteral preparations comply with the requirements for *Materials used for the manufacture of containers* (*3.1* and subsections) and *Containers* (*3.2* and subsections).

Parenteral preparations are supplied in glass containers (*3.2.1*) or in other containers such as plastic containers (*3.2.2, 3.2.2.1* and *3.2.9*) and prefilled syringes. The tightness of the container is ensured by suitable means. Closures ensure a good seal, prevent the access of micro-organisms and other contaminants and usually permit the withdrawal of a part or the whole of the contents without removal of the closure. The plastic materials or elastomers (*3.2.9*) of which the closure is composed are sufficiently firm and elastic to allow the passage of a needle with the least possible shedding of particles. Closures for multidose containers are sufficiently elastic to ensure that the puncture is resealed when the needle is withdrawn.

Several categories of parenteral preparations may be distinguished:

- injections,
- infusions,
- concentrates for injections or infusions,
- powders for injections or infusions,
- implants.

PRODUCTION

During the development of a parenteral preparation, the formulation for which contains an antimicrobial preservative, the effectiveness of the chosen preservative shall be demonstrated to the satisfaction of the competent authority. A suitable test method together with criteria for judging the preservative properties of the formulation are provided under *Efficacy of antimicrobial preservation* (*5.1.3*).

Parenteral preparations are prepared using materials and methods designed to ensure sterility and to avoid the introduction of contaminants and the growth of micro-organisms; recommendations on this aspect are provided in the text on *Methods of preparation of sterile products* (*5.1.1*).

Water used in the manufacture of parenteral preparations complies with the requirements of water for injections in bulk stated in the monograph on *Water for injections (0169)*.

TESTS

Particulate contamination: sub-visible particles (*2.9.19*). For preparations for human use, solutions for infusion or solutions for injection supplied in containers with a nominal content of more than 100 ml comply with the test.

For preparations for veterinary use, when supplied in containers with a nominal content of more than 100 ml and when the content is equivalent to a dose of more than 1.4 ml per kilogram of body mass, solutions for infusion or solutions for injection comply with the test for particulate contamination: sub-visible particles.

Products for which the label states that the product is to be used with a final filter are exempt from these requirements.

Sterility (*2.6.1*). Parenteral preparations comply with the test for sterility.

STORAGE

Store in a sterile, airtight, tamper-proof container.

LABELLING

The label states:

- the name and concentration of any added antimicrobial preservative,
- where applicable, that the solution is to be used in conjunction with a final filter,
- where applicable, that the preparation is free from bacterial endotoxins or that it is apyrogenic.

Injections

DEFINITION

Injections are sterile solutions, emulsions or suspensions. They are prepared by dissolving, emulsifying or suspending the active substance(s) and any added excipients in *Water for injections (0169)*, in a suitable, sterile non-aqueous liquid or in a mixture of these vehicles.

Solutions for injection, examined under suitable conditions of visibility, are clear and practically free from particles.

Emulsions for injection do not show any evidence of phase separation. Suspensions for injection may show a sediment which is readily dispersed on shaking to give a suspension which remains sufficiently stable to enable the correct dose to be withdrawn.

Multidose preparations. Multidose aqueous injections contain a suitable antimicrobial preservative at an appropriate concentration except when the preparation itself has adequate antimicrobial properties. When it is necessary to present a preparation for parenteral use in a multidose

Dosage forms

container, the precautions to be taken for its administration and more particularly for its storage between successive withdrawals are given.

Antimicrobial preservatives. Aqueous preparations which are prepared using aseptic precautions and which cannot be terminally sterilised may contain a suitable antimicrobial preservative in an appropriate concentration.

No antimicrobial preservative is added when:

- the volume to be injected in a single dose exceeds 15 ml, unless otherwise justified,
- the preparation is intended for administration by routes where, for medical reasons, an antimicrobial preservative is not acceptable, such as intracisternally, epidurally, intrathecally or by any route giving access to the cerebrospinal fluid, or intra- or retro-ocularly.

Such preparations are presented in single-dose containers.

PRODUCTION

In the manufacture of injections containing dispersed particles, measures are taken to ensure a suitable and controlled particle size with regard to the intended use.

Single-dose preparations. The volume of the injection in a single-dose container is sufficient to permit the withdrawal and administration of the nominal dose using a normal technique.

TESTS

Uniformity of content (*2.9.6*). Unless otherwise prescribed or justified and authorised, single-dose suspensions for injection with a content of active substance less than 2 mg or less than 2 per cent of the total mass comply with test A for uniformity of content of single-dose preparations. If the preparation contains more than one active substance, the requirement applies only to those substances that correspond to the above conditions.

Bacterial endotoxins - pyrogens. A test for bacterial endotoxins (*2.6.14*) is carried out or, where justified and authorised, the test for pyrogens (*2.6.8*). Recommendations on the limits for bacterial endotoxins are given in chapter *2.6.14*.

Preparations for human use. The preparation complies with a test for bacterial endotoxins (*2.6.14*) or with the test for pyrogens (*2.6.8*).

Preparations for veterinary use. When the volume to be injected in a single dose is 15 ml or more and is equivalent to a dose of 0.2 ml or more per kilogram of body mass, the preparation complies with a test for bacterial endotoxins (*2.6.14*) or with the test for pyrogens (*2.6.8*).

Any preparation. Where the label states that the preparation is free from bacterial endotoxins or apyrogenic, respectively, the preparation complies with a test for bacterial endotoxins (*2.6.14*) or with the test for pyrogens (*2.6.8*), respectively.

Infusions

DEFINITION

Infusions are sterile, aqueous solutions or emulsions with water as the continuous phase; they are usually made isotonic with blood. They are principally intended for administration in large volume. Infusions do not contain any added antimicrobial preservative.

Solutions for infusion, examined under suitable conditions of visibility, are clear and practically free from particles.

Emulsions for infusion do not show any evidence of phase separation.

PRODUCTION

In the manufacture of infusions containing dispersed particles, measures are taken to ensure a suitable and controlled particle size with regard to the intended use.

The volume of the infusion in the container is sufficient to permit the withdrawal and administration of the nominal dose using a normal technique (*2.9.17*).

TESTS

Bacterial endotoxins - pyrogens. They comply with a test for bacterial endotoxins (*2.6.14*) or, where justified and authorised, with the test for pyrogens (*2.6.8*). For the latter test, inject 10 ml per kilogram of body mass into each rabbit, unless otherwise justified and authorised.

Concentrates for injections or infusions

DEFINITION

Concentrates for injections or infusions are sterile solutions intended for injection or infusion after dilution. They are diluted to a prescribed volume with a prescribed liquid before administration. After dilution, they comply with the requirements for injections or for infusions.

TESTS

Bacterial endotoxins - pyrogens. They comply with the requirements prescribed for injections or for infusions, after dilution to a suitable volume.

Powders for injections or infusions

DEFINITION

Powders for injections or infusions are solid, sterile substances distributed in their final containers and which, when shaken with the prescribed volume of a prescribed sterile liquid, rapidly form either clear and practically particle-free solutions or uniform suspensions. After dissolution or suspension, they comply with the requirements for injections or for infusions.

Freeze-dried products for parenteral use are considered as powders for injections or infusions.

PRODUCTION

The uniformity of content and uniformity of mass of freeze-dried products for parenteral use are ensured by the in-process control of the amount of the solution prior to freeze-drying.

TESTS

Uniformity of content (*2.9.6*). Unless otherwise prescribed or justified and authorised, powders for injections or infusions with a content of active substance less than 2 mg or less than 2 per cent of the total mass or with a unit mass equal to or less than 40 mg comply with test A for uniformity of content of single-dose preparations. If the preparation contains more than one active substance, the requirement applies only to those substances that correspond to the above conditions.

Uniformity of mass (*2.9.5*). Powders for injections or infusions comply with the test for uniformity of mass of single-dose preparations. If the test for uniformity of content is prescribed for all the active substances, the test for uniformity of mass is not required.

Bacterial endotoxins - pyrogens. They comply with the requirements prescribed for injections or for infusions, after dissolution or suspension in a suitable volume of liquid.

LABELLING

The label states the instructions for the preparation of injections and infusions.

Implants

DEFINITION

Implants are sterile, solid preparations of a size and shape suitable for parenteral implantation and release the active substance(s) over an extended period of time. Each dose is provided in a sterile container.

01/2005:1011

PATCHES, TRANSDERMAL

Emplastra transcutanea

DEFINITION

Transdermal patches are flexible pharmaceutical preparations of varying sizes, containing one or more active substances. They are intended to be applied to the unbroken skin in order to deliver the active substance(s) to the systemic circulation after passing through the skin barrier.

Transdermal patches normally consist of an outer covering which supports a preparation which contains the active substance(s). The transdermal patches are covered on the site of the release surface of the preparation by a protective liner, which is removed before applying the patch to the skin.

The outer covering is a backing sheet impermeable to the active substance(s) and normally impermeable to water, designed to support and protect the preparation. The outer covering may have the same dimensions as the preparation or it may be larger. In the latter case the overlapping border of the outer covering is covered by pressure-sensitive adhesive substances which assure the adhesion of the patch to the skin.

The preparation contains the active substance(s) together with excipients such as stabilisers, solubilisers or substances intended to modify the release rate or to enhance transdermal absorption. It may be a single layer or multi-layer solid or semi-solid matrix, and in this case it is the composition and structure of the matrix which determines the diffusion pattern of the active substance(s) to the skin. The matrix may contain pressure-sensitive adhesives which assure the adhesion of the preparation to the skin. The preparation may exist as a semi-solid reservoir one side of which is a membrane which may control the release and the diffusion of the active substance(s) from the preparation. The pressure-sensitive adhesive substances may, in this case, be applied to some or all parts of the membrane, or only around the border of the membrane of the outer covering.

When applied to the dried, clean and unbroken skin, the transdermal patch adheres firmly to the skin by gentle pressure of the hand or the fingers and can be peeled off without causing appreciable injury to the skin or detachment of the preparation from the outer covering. The patch must not be irritant or sensitising to the skin, even after repeated applications.

The protective liner generally consists of a sheet of plastic or metal material. When removed, the protective liner does not detach the preparation (matrix or reservoir) or the adhesive from the patch.

Transdermal patches are normally individually enclosed in sealed sachets.

PRODUCTION

In the manufacture, packaging, storage and distribution of transdermal patches suitable means are taken to ensure their microbial quality; recommendations on this aspect are provided in the text on *Microbiological quality of pharmaceutical preparations* (*5.1.4*).

TESTS

Uniformity of content (*2.9.6*). Unless otherwise prescribed or justified and authorised, transdermal patches comply with test C for uniformity of content of single-dose preparations.

Dissolution. A suitable test may be required to demonstrate the appropriate release of the active substance(s), for example one of the tests described in *Dissolution test for transdermal patches* (*2.9.4*). The disc assembly method, the cell method or the rotating cylinder method may be used, as suitable, according to the composition, dimensions and shape of the patch.

A membrane may be used. It can be of various materials, such as inert porous cellulose or silicones, and must not affect the release kinetics of the active substance(s) from the patch. Furthermore, it must be free of substances that may interfere with its performance (for example grease). The membrane may be suitably treated before the tests, for example, by maintaining it in the medium to be used in the test for 24 h. Apply the membrane above the releasing surface of the patch, avoiding the formation of air bubbles.

The test conditions and the requirements are to be authorised by the competent authority.

STORAGE

Store at room temperature, unless otherwise indicated.

LABELLING

The label states, where applicable, the total quantity of active substance(s) per patch, the dose released per unit time and the area of the releasing surface.

01/2005:1166

POWDERS FOR CUTANEOUS APPLICATION

Pulveres ad usum dermicum

Where justified and authorised, the requirements of this monograph do not apply to powders for cutaneous application intended for veterinary use.

DEFINITION

Powders for cutaneous application are preparations consisting of solid, loose, dry particles of varying degrees of fineness. They contain one or more active substances, with or without excipients and, if necessary, colouring matter authorised by the competent authority.

Powders for cutaneous application are presented as single-dose powders or multidose powders. They are free from grittiness. Powders specifically intended for use on large open wounds or on severely injured skin are sterile.

Multidose powders for cutaneous application may be dispensed in sifter-top containers, containers equipped with a mechanical spraying device or in pressurised containers.

Powders dispensed in pressurised containers comply with the requirements of *Pressurised pharmaceutical preparations (0523)*.

Where applicable, containers for powders comply with the requirements of *Materials used for the manufacture of containers* (*3.1* and subsections) and *Containers* (*3.2* and subsections).

PRODUCTION

In the manufacture of powders for cutaneous application, measures are taken to ensure a suitable particle size with regard to the intended use.

In the manufacture, packaging, storage and distribution of powders for cutaneous application, suitable means are taken to ensure their microbial quality; recommendations on this aspect are provided in the text on *Microbiological quality of pharmaceutical preparations* (*5.1.4*).

Sterile powders for cutaneous application are prepared using materials and methods designed to ensure sterility and to avoid the introduction of contaminants and the growth of micro-organisms; recommendations on this aspect are provided in the text on *Methods of preparation of sterile products* (*5.1.1*).

TESTS

Fineness. If prescribed, the fineness of a powder is determined by the sieve test (*2.9.12*) or another appropriate method.

Uniformity of content (*2.9.6*). Unless otherwise prescribed or justified and authorised, single-dose powders for cutaneous application with a content of active substance less than 2 mg or less than 2 per cent of the total mass comply with test B for uniformity of content of single-dose preparations. If the preparation has more than one active substance, the requirement applies only to those substances which correspond to the above conditions.

Uniformity of mass (*2.9.5*). Single-dose powders for cutaneous application comply with the test for uniformity of mass of single-dose preparations. If the test for uniformity of content is prescribed for all the active substances, the test for uniformity of mass is not required.

Sterility (*2.6.1*). Where the label indicates that the preparation is sterile, it complies with the test for sterility.

LABELLING

The label states:

– that the preparation is for external use,

– where applicable, that the preparation is sterile.

01/2005:1165

POWDERS, ORAL

Pulveres perorales

Requirements for powders to be used for the preparation of oral solutions or suspensions are given in the monograph for Liquid preparations for oral use (0672). Where justified and authorised, the requirements of this monograph do not apply to oral powders intended for veterinary use.

DEFINITION

Oral powders are preparations consisting of solid, loose, dry particles of varying degrees of fineness. They contain one or more active substances, with or without excipients and, if necessary, colouring matter authorised by the competent authority and flavouring substances. They are generally administered in or with water or another suitable liquid. They may also be swallowed directly. They are presented as single-dose or multidose preparations.

Where applicable, containers for oral powders comply with the requirements of *Materials used for the manufacture of containers* (*3.1* and subsections) and *Containers* (*3.2* and subsections).

Multidose oral powders require the provision of a measuring device capable of delivering the quantity prescribed.

Each dose of a single-dose powder is enclosed in an individual container, for example a sachet or a vial.

PRODUCTION

In the manufacture of oral powders, means are taken to ensure a suitable particle size with regard to the intended use.

In the manufacture, packaging, storage and distribution of oral powders, suitable means are taken to ensure their microbial quality; recommendations on this aspect are provided in the text on *Microbiological quality of pharmaceutical preparations* (*5.1.4*).

TESTS

Uniformity of content (*2.9.6*). Unless otherwise prescribed or justified and authorised, single-dose oral powders with a content of active substance less than 2 mg or less than 2 per cent of the total mass comply with test B for uniformity of content of single-dose preparations. If the preparation has more than one active substance, the requirement applies only to those substances which correspond to the above conditions.

Uniformity of mass (*2.9.5*). Single-dose oral powders comply with the test for uniformity of mass of single-dose preparations. If the test for uniformity of content is prescribed for all the active substances, the test for uniformity of mass is not required.

Uniformity of mass of delivered doses from multidose containers (*2.9.27*). Oral powders supplied in multidose containers comply with the test.

STORAGE

If the preparation contains volatile ingredients, or the contents have to be protected, store in an airtight container.

Effervescent powders

Effervescent powders are presented as single-dose or multidose preparations and generally contain acid substances and carbonates or hydrogen carbonates which react rapidly in the presence of water to release carbon dioxide. They are intended to be dissolved or dispersed in water before administration.

STORAGE

In an airtight container.

01/2005:1037

PREMIXES FOR MEDICATED FEEDING STUFFS FOR VETERINARY USE

Praeadmixta ad alimenta medicata ad usum veterinarium

DEFINITION

Mixtures of one or more active substances, usually in suitable bases, that are prepared to facilitate feeding the active substances to animals. They are used exclusively in the preparation of medicated feeding stuffs.

Premixes occur in granulated, powdered, semi-solid or liquid form. Used as powders or granules, they are free-flowing and homogeneous; any aggregates break apart during normal handling. Used in liquid form, they are homogeneous suspensions or solutions which may be obtained from thixotropic gels or structured liquids. The particle size and other properties are such as to ensure uniform distribution of the active substance(s) in the final feed. Unless otherwise justified and authorised, the instructions for use state that the concentration of a premix in granulated or powdered form is at least 0.5 per cent in the medicated feeding stuff.

PRODUCTION

Active substance. An active substance intended for incorporation into a medicated premix complies with the requirements of the relevant monograph of the European Pharmacopoeia, unless already otherwise justified and authorised for existing premixes.

TESTS

Loss on drying (*2.2.32*). Unless otherwise justified and authorised, for premixes occurring in granulated or powdered form, maximum 15.0 per cent, determined on 3.000 g by drying in an oven at 100-105 °C for 2 h.

LABELLING

The label states:

- the category of animal for which the premix is intended,
- the instructions for the preparation of the medicated feeding stuffs from the premix and the basic feed,
- where applicable, the time that must elapse between the cessation of feeding of the medicated feeding stuff and collection of the material intended for human consumption.

01/2005:0671

PREPARATIONS FOR INHALATION

Inhalanda

DEFINITION

Preparations for inhalation are liquid or solid preparations intended for administration as vapours or aerosols to the lung in order to obtain a local or systemic effect. They contain one or more active substances which may be dissolved or dispersed in a suitable vehicle.

Preparations for inhalation may, depending on the type of preparation, contain propellants, co-solvents, diluents, antimicrobial preservatives, solubilising and stabilising agents, etc. These excipients do not adversely affect the functions of the mucosa of the respiratory tract or its cilia.

Preparations for inhalation are supplied in multidose or single-dose containers. When supplied in pressurised containers, they comply with the requirements of the monograph on *Pressurised pharmaceutical preparations (0523)*.

Preparations intended to be administered as aerosols (dispersions of solid or liquid particles in a gas) are administered by one of the following devices:

- nebuliser,
- pressurised metered-dose inhaler,
- dry-powder inhaler.

PRODUCTION

During the development of a preparation for inhalation which contains an antimicrobial preservative, the effectiveness of the chosen preservative shall be demonstrated to the satisfaction of the competent authority. A suitable test method together with the criteria for judging the preservative properties of the formulation are described in the text on *Efficacy of antimicrobial preservation* (*5.1.3*).

The size of aerosol particles to be inhaled is controlled so that a significant fraction is deposited in the lung. The fine-particle characteristics of preparations for inhalation are determined by the method for *Aerodynamic assessment of fine particles* (*2.9.18*).

In assessing the uniformity of delivered dose of a multidose inhaler, it is not sufficient to test a single inhaler. Manufacturers must substitute procedures which take both inter- and intra-inhaler dose uniformity into account. A suitable procedure based on the intra-inhaler test would be to collect each of the specified doses at the beginning, middle and end of the number of doses stated on the label from separate inhalers.

Pressurised metered-dose inhalers are tested for leakage. All inhalers are tested for extraneous particulate contamination.

LABELLING

For metered-dose preparations the label states:

- the delivered dose, except for preparations for which the dose has been established as a metered-dose or as a predispensed-dose,
- where applicable, the number of deliveries from the inhaler to provide the minimum recommended dose,
- the number of deliveries per inhaler.

The label states, where applicable, the name of any added antimicrobial preservative.

Liquid preparations for inhalation

Three categories of liquid preparations for inhalation may be distinguished:

A. preparations intended to be converted into vapour,

B. liquid preparations for nebulisation,

C. pressurised metered-dose preparations for inhalation.

Liquid preparations for inhalation are solutions or dispersions.

Dispersions are readily dispersible on shaking and they remain sufficiently stable to enable the correct dose to be delivered. Suitable excipients may be used.

A. PREPARATIONS INTENDED TO BE CONVERTED INTO VAPOUR

DEFINITION

Preparations intended to be converted into vapour are solutions, dispersions or solid preparations. They are usually added to hot water and the vapour generated is inhaled.

B. LIQUID PREPARATIONS FOR NEBULISATION

DEFINITION

Liquid preparations for inhalation intended to be converted into aerosols by continuously operating nebulisers or metered-dose nebulisers are solutions, suspensions or emulsions. Suitable co-solvents or solubilisers may be used to increase the solubility of the active substances.

Liquid preparations for nebulisation in concentrated form for use in continuously operating nebulisers are diluted to the prescribed volume with the prescribed liquid before use. Liquids for nebulisation may also be prepared from powders.

The pH of the liquid preparations for use in continuously operating nebulisers is not lower than 3 and not higher than 8.5.

Suspensions and emulsions are readily dispersible on shaking and they remain sufficiently stable to enable the correct dose to be delivered.

Aqueous preparations for nebulisation supplied in multidose containers may contain a suitable antimicrobial preservative at a suitable concentration except where the preparation itself has adequate antimicrobial properties.

Continuously operating nebulisers are devices that convert liquids into aerosols by high-pressure gases, ultrasonic vibration or other methods. They allow the dose to be inhaled at an appropriate rate and particle size which ensures deposition of the preparation in the lungs.

Metered-dose nebulisers are devices that convert liquids into aerosols by high-pressure gases, ultrasonic vibration or other methods. The volume of liquid to be nebulised is metered so that the aerosol dose can be inhaled with one breath.

C. PRESSURISED METERED-DOSE PREPARATIONS FOR INHALATION

DEFINITION

Pressurised metered-dose preparations for inhalation are solutions, suspensions or emulsions supplied in special containers equipped with a metering valve and which are held under pressure with suitable propellants or suitable mixtures of liquefied propellants, which can act also as solvents. Suitable co-solvents, solubilisers and stabilisers may be added.

The delivered dose is the dose delivered from the inhaler to the patient. For some preparations, the dose has been established as a metered-dose. The metered-dose is determined by adding the amount deposited within the device to the delivered dose. It may also be determined directly.

TESTS

Uniformity of delivered dose. Containers usually operate in an inverted position. For containers that operate in an upright position, an equivalent test is applied using methods that ensure the complete collection of the delivered dose. In all cases, prepare the inhaler as directed in the instructions to the patient.

The dose collection apparatus must be capable of quantitatively capturing the delivered dose.

The following apparatus and procedure may be used.

The apparatus (Figure 0671.-1) consists of a filter-support base with an open-mesh filter-support, such as a stainless steel screen, a collection tube that is clamped or screwed to the filter-support base, and a mouthpiece adapter to ensure an airtight seal between the collection tube and the mouthpiece. Use a mouthpiece adapter which ensures that the front face of the inhaler mouthpiece is flush with the front face of the sample collection tube. The vacuum connector is connected to a system comprising a vacuum source and a flow regulator. The source should be adjusted to draw air through the complete assembly, including the filter and the inhaler to be tested, at 28.3 ± 1.5 litres/min. Air should be drawn continuously through the apparatus to avoid loss of the active substance into the atmosphere. The filter support base is designed to accommodate 25 mm diameter filter disks. The filter disk and other materials used in the construction of the apparatus must be compatible with the active substance and solvents that are used to extract the active substance from the filter. One end of the collection tube is designed to hold the filter disk tightly against the filter-support base. When assembled, the joints between the components of the apparatus are airtight so that when a vacuum is applied to the base of the filter, all of the air drawn through the collection tube passes through the inhaler.

Unless otherwise prescribed in the instructions to the patient, shake the inhaler for 5 s and discharge one delivery to waste. Fire the inverted inhaler into the apparatus, depressing the valve for a sufficient time to ensure complete discharge. Repeat the procedure until the number of deliveries that constitute the minimum recommended dose have been sampled. Quantitatively collect the contents of the apparatus and determine the amount of active substance.

Repeat the procedure for a further 2 doses.

Discharge the device to waste, waiting not less than 5 s between actuations until $(n/2)+1$ deliveries remain, where n is the number of deliveries stated on the label. Collect 4 doses using the procedure described above.

Discharge the device to waste, waiting not less than 5 s between actuations until 3 doses remain. Collect these 3 doses using the procedure described above.

For preparations containing more than one active substance, carry out the test for uniformity of delivered dose for each active substance.

Unless otherwise justified and authorised, the preparation complies with the test if 9 out of 10 results lie between 75 per cent and 125 per cent of the average value and all lie between 65 per cent and 135 per cent. If 2 or 3 values lie outside the range of 75 per cent to 125 per cent, repeat the test for 2 more inhalers. Not more than 3 of the 30 values lie outside the range 75 per cent to 125 per cent and no value lies outside the range 65 per cent to 135 per cent.

Fine particle dose. Using an apparatus and procedure described in *Aerodynamic assessment of fine particles (2.9.18 - apparatus C or D)*, calculate the fine particle dose.

Number of deliveries per inhaler. Take one inhaler and discharge the contents to waste, actuating the valve at intervals of not less than 5 s. The total number of deliveries so discharged from the inhaler is not less than the number stated on the label (this test may be combined with the test for uniformity of delivered dose).

Powders for inhalation

DEFINITION

Powders for inhalation are presented as single-dose powders or multidose powders. To facilitate their use, active substances may be combined with a suitable carrier. They are generally administered by dry-powder inhalers. In pre-metered systems, the inhaler is loaded with powders pre-dispensed in capsules or other suitable pharmaceutical forms. For devices using a powder reservoir, the dose is created by a metering mechanism within the inhaler.

The delivered dose is the dose delivered from the inhaler. For some preparations, the dose has been established as a metered dose or as a predispensed dose. The metered dose is determined by adding the amount deposited within the device to the delivered dose. It may also be determined directly.

TESTS

Uniformity of delivered dose. In all cases, prepare the inhaler as directed in the instructions to the patient. The dose collection apparatus must be capable of quantitatively capturing the delivered dose. A dose collection apparatus similar to that described for the evaluation of pressurised metered-dose inhalers may be used provided that the dimensions of the tube and the filter can accommodate

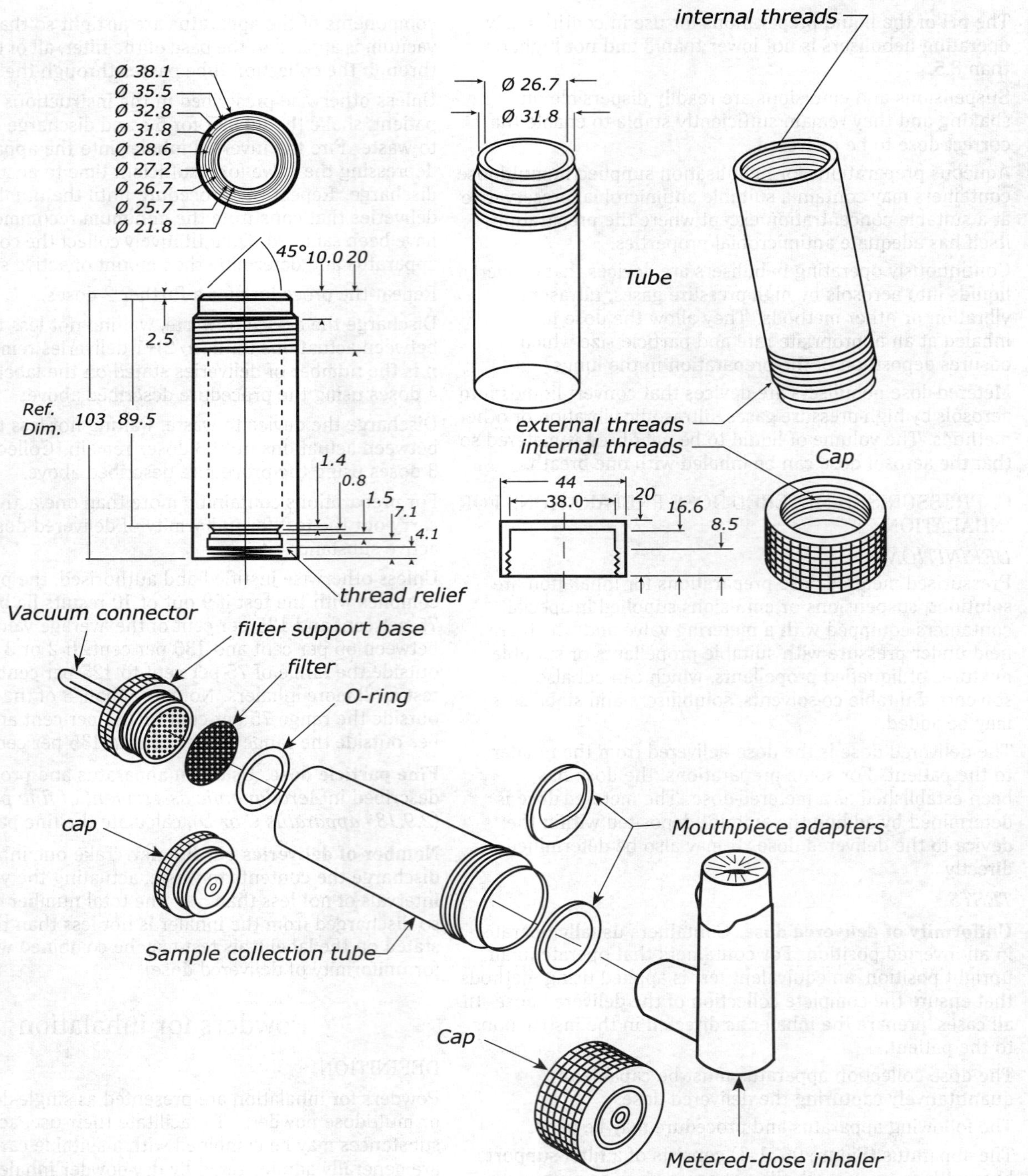

Figure 0671.-1. – *Dose collection apparatus for pressurised metered-dose preparations*
Dimensions in millimetres

the measured flow rate. A suitable tube is defined in Figure 0671.-1. Connect the tube to a flow system according to the scheme specified in Figure 0671.-2 and Table 0671.-1.

Unless otherwise stated, determine the test flow rate and duration using the dose collection tube, the associated flow system, a suitable differential pressure meter and a suitable volumetric flow meter, calibrated for the flow leaving the meter, according to the following procedure.

Prepare the inhaler for use and connect it to the inlet of the apparatus using a mouthpiece adapter to ensure an airtight seal. Use a mouthpiece adapter which ensures that the front face of the inhaler mouthpiece is flush with the front face of the sample collection tube. Connect one port of a differential pressure meter to the pressure reading point, P1, in Figure 0671.-2 and let the other be open to the atmosphere. Switch on the pump, open the two way valve and adjust the flow control valve until the pressure drop across the inhaler is 4.0 kPa (40.8 cm H_2O) as indicated by the differential pressure meter. Remove the inhaler from the mouthpiece adapter and without touching the flow control valve, connect a flow meter to the inlet of the sampling apparatus. If the flow rate is above 100 litres/min adjust the flow control valve to obtain a flow rate of 100 ± 5 litres/min. Note the volumetric airflow rate and define this as the test flow rate, Q, in litres per minute. Define the test flow duration, T, in seconds so that a volume of 4 litres of air is drawn through the inhaler.

Ensure that critical flow occurs in the flow control valve by the following procedure. With the inhaler in place and the test flow rate Q, measure the absolute pressure on both sides of the control valve (pressure reading points P2 and P3 in

Figure 0671.-2). A ratio P3/P2 ≤ 0.5 indicates critical flow. Switch to a more powerful pump and re-measure the test flow rate if critical flow is not indicated.

Predispensed systems. Prepare the inhaler as directed in the instructions to the patient and connect it to the apparatus using an adapter which ensures a good seal. Draw air through the inhaler using the predetermined conditions. Repeat the procedure until the number of deliveries which constitute the minimum recommended dose have been sampled. Quantitatively collect the contents of the apparatus and determine the amount of active substance.

Repeat the procedure for a further 9 doses.

Reservoir systems. Prepare the inhaler as directed in the instructions to the patient and connect it to the apparatus using an adapter which ensures a good seal. Draw air through the inhaler under the predetermined conditions. Repeat the procedure until the number of deliveries which constitute the minimum recommended dose have been sampled. Quantitatively collect the contents of the apparatus and determine the amount of active substance.

Repeat the procedure for a further 2 doses.

Discharge the device to waste until $(n/2)+1$ deliveries remain, where n is the number of deliveries stated on the label. If necessary, store the inhaler to discharge electrostatic charges. Collect 4 doses using the procedure described above.

Discharge the device to waste until 3 doses remain. If necessary, store the inhaler to discharge electrostatic charges. Collect 3 doses using the procedure described above.

For preparations containing more than 1 active substance, carry out the test for uniformity of delivered dose for each active substance.

The preparation complies with the test if 9 out of 10 results lie between 75 per cent and 125 per cent of the average value and all lie between 65 per cent and 135 per cent. If 2 or 3 values lie outside the range of 75 per cent to 125 per cent, repeat the test for 2 more inhalers. Not more than 3 of the 30 values lie outside the range 75 per cent to 125 per cent and no value lies outside the range 65 per cent to 135 per cent.

In justified and authorised cases, these ranges may be extended but no value should be greater than 150 per cent or less than 50 per cent of the average value.

Table 0671.-1. – *Specifications of the apparatus described in figure 0671.-2*

Code	Item	Description
A	Sample collection tube	Capable of quantitatively capturing the delivered dose, e.g. Dose collection tube similar to that described in Fig. 0671.-1 with dimensions of 34.85 mm ID × 12 cm length (e.g. product number XX40 047 00, Millipore Corporation, Bedford, MA 01732 with modified exit tube, ID ≥ 8 mm, fitted with Gelman product number 61631), or equivalent.
B	Filter	47 mm filter, e.g. A/E glass fibre filter (Gelman Sciences, Ann Arbor, MI 48106), or equivalent.
C	Connector	ID ≥ 8 mm, e.g., short metal coupling, with low-diameter branch to P3.
D	Vacuum tubing	8 ± 0.5 mm ID × 50 ± 10 cm length, e.g., silicone tubing with an OD of 14 mm and an ID of 8 mm.
E	Two-way solenoid valve	Minimum airflow resistance orifice having an ID of ≥ 8 mm and a maximum response time of 100 ms (e.g. type 256-A08, Bürkert GmbH, D-74653 Ingelfingen), or equivalent.
F	Vacuum pump	Pump must be capable of drawing the required flow rate through the assembled apparatus with the dry powder inhaler in the mouthpiece adapter (e.g. product type 1023, 1423 or 2565, Gast Manufacturing Inc., Benton Harbor, MI 49022), or equivalent. Connect the pump to the solenoid valve using short and/or wide (≥ 10 mm ID) vacuum tubing and connectors to minimise pump capacity requirements.
G	Timer	Timer capable of driving the solenoid valve for the required time period (e.g. type G814, RS Components International, Corby, NN17 9RS, UK), or equivalent.
P1	Pressure tap	2.2 mm ID, 3.1 mm OD, flush with internal surface of the sample collection tube, centred and burr-free, 59 mm from its inlet.
P1 P2 P3	Pressure measurements	Differential pressure to atmosphere (P1) or absolute pressure (P2 and P3).
H	Flow control valve	Adjustable regulating valve with maximum $Cv \geq 1$, (e.g. type 8FV12LNSS, Parker Hannifin plc., Barnstaple, EX31 1NP, UK), or equivalent.

Fine particle dose. Using the apparatus and procedure described in *Aerodynamic assessment of fine particles (2.9.18 - apparatus C or D)*, calculate the fine particle dose.

Number of deliveries per inhaler for multidose inhalers. Discharge doses from the inhaler until empty, at the predetermined flow rate. Record the deliveries discharged.

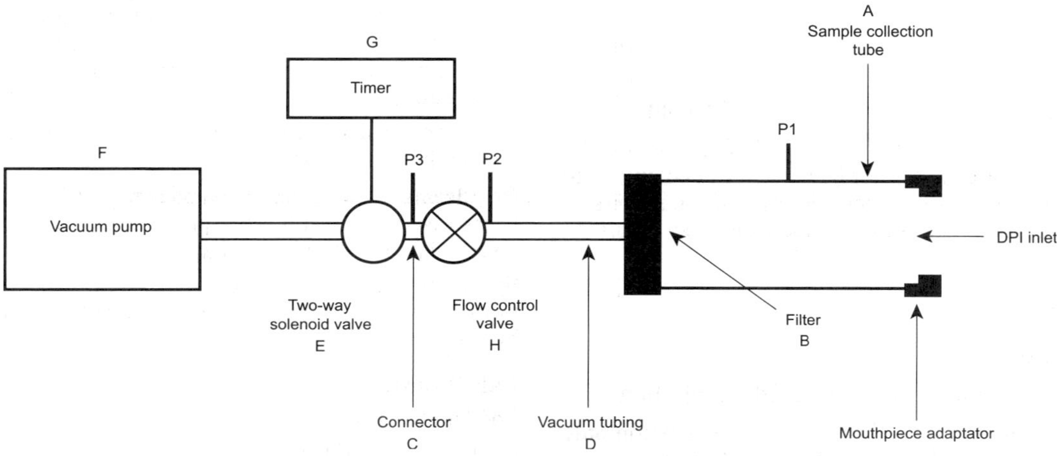

Figure 0671.-2. – *Apparatus suitable for measuring the uniformity of delivered dose for powder inhalers*

Dosage forms

The total number of doses delivered is not less than the number stated on the label (this test may be combined with the test for uniformity of delivered dose).

01/2005:1116

PREPARATIONS FOR IRRIGATION

Praeparationes ad irrigationem

DEFINITION

Preparations for irrigation are sterile, aqueous large volume preparations intended to be used for irrigation of body cavities, wounds and surfaces, for example during surgical procedures.

Preparations for irrigation are either solutions prepared by dissolving one or more active substances, electrolytes or osmotically active substances in water complying with the requirements for *Water for injections (0169)* or they consist of such water alone. In the latter case, the preparation may be labelled as water for irrigation. Irrigation solutions are usually adjusted to be isotonic with blood.

Examined in suitable conditions of visibility, preparations for irrigation are clear and practically free from particles.

Preparations for irrigation are supplied in single-dose containers. The containers and closures comply with the requirements for containers for preparations for parenteral use (*3.2.1* and *3.2.2*) but the administration port of the container is incompatible with intravenous administration equipment and does not allow the preparation for irrigation to be administered with such equipment.

PRODUCTION

Preparations for irrigation are prepared using materials and methods designed to ensure sterility and to avoid the introduction of contaminants and the growth of micro-organisms; recommendations on this aspect are provided in the text on *Methods of preparation of sterile products* (*5.1.1*).

TESTS

Deliverable mass or volume (*2.9.28*). Preparations for irrigation supplied in single-dose containers comply with the test.

Sterility (*2.6.1*). Preparations for irrigation comply with the test for sterility.

Bacterial endotoxins (*2.6.14*): less than 0.5 IU/ml.

Pyrogens (*2.6.8*). Preparations for which a validated test for bacterial endotoxins cannot be carried out comply with the test for pyrogens. Inject per kilogram of the rabbits mass, 10 ml of the preparation, unless otherwise justified and authorised.

LABELLING

The label states:

– that the preparation is not to be used for injection,

– that the preparation is to be used for one occasion only and that any unused portion of preparation is to be discarded.

Dosage forms

01/2005:0523

PRESSURISED PHARMACEUTICAL PREPARATIONS

Praeparationes pharmaceuticae in vasis cum pressu

Additional requirements for preparations presented in pressurised containers may be found, where appropriate, in other general monographs, for example Preparations for inhalation (0671), Liquid preparations for cutaneous application (0927), Powders for cutaneous application (1166), Nasal preparations (0676) and Ear preparations (0652).

DEFINITION

Pressurised pharmaceutical preparations are presented in special containers under pressure of a gas and contain one or more active substances. The preparations are released from the container, upon actuation of an appropriate valve, in the form of an aerosol (dispersion of solid or liquid particles in a gas, the size of the particles being adapted to the intended use) or of a liquid or semisolid jet such as a foam. The pressure for the release is generated by suitable propellants.

The preparations consist of a solution, an emulsion or a suspension and are intended for local application to the skin or to mucous membranes of various body orifices, or for inhalation. Suitable excipients may also be used, for example solvents, solubilisers, emulsifying agents, suspending agents and lubricants for the valve to prevent clogging.

Propellants. The propellants are either gases liquefied under pressure or compressed gases or low-boiling liquids. Liquefied gases are, for example, fluorinated hydrocarbons and low-molecular-mass hydrocarbons (such as propane and butane). Compressed gases are, for example, carbon dioxide, nitrogen and nitrous oxide.

Mixtures of these propellants may be used to obtain optimal solution properties and desirable pressure, delivery and spray characteristics.

Containers. The containers are tight and resistant to the internal pressure and may be made of metal, glass, plastic or combinations of these materials. They are compatible with their contents. Glass containers are protected with a plastic coating.

Spraying device. The valve keeps the container tightly closed when not in use and regulates the delivery of the contents during use. The spray characteristics are influenced by the type of spraying device, in particular by the dimensions, number and location of orifices. Some valves provide a continuous release, others ("metering dose valves") deliver a defined quantity of product upon each valve actuation.

The various valve materials in contact with the contents are compatible with them.

Requirements for pressurised pharmaceutical preparations. Pressurised preparations are provided with a delivery device appropriate for the intended application.

Special requirements may be necessary for the selection of propellants, for particle size and the single-dose delivered by the metering valves.

LABELLING

The label states:

– the method of use,

– any precautions to be taken,

– for a container with a metering dose valve, the amount of active substance in a unit-spray.

01/2005:1145

RECTAL PREPARATIONS

Rectalia

DEFINITION

Rectal preparations are intended for rectal use in order to obtain a systemic or local effect, or they may be intended for diagnostic purposes.

Where applicable, containers for rectal preparations comply with the requirements for *Materials used for the manufacture of containers* (*3.1* and subsections) and *Containers* (*3.2* and subsections).

Several categories of rectal preparations may be distinguished:

– suppositories,
– rectal capsules,
– rectal solutions, emulsions and suspensions,
– powders and tablets for rectal solutions and suspensions,
– semi-solid rectal preparations,
– rectal foams,
– rectal tampons.

PRODUCTION

During the development of a rectal preparation, the formulation for which contains an antimicrobial preservative, the effectiveness of the chosen preservative shall be demonstrated to the satisfaction of the competent authority. A suitable test method together with criteria for judging the preservative properties of the formulation are provided in the text on *Efficacy of antimicrobial preservation* (*5.1.3*).

In the manufacture, packaging, storage and distribution of rectal preparations, suitable means are taken to ensure their microbial quality; recommendations on this aspect are provided in the text on *Microbiological quality of pharmaceutical preparations* (*5.1.4*).

In the manufacture of semi-solid and liquid rectal preparations containing dispersed particles measures are taken to ensure a suitable and controlled particle size with regard to the intended use.

TESTS

Uniformity of content (*2.9.6*). Unless otherwise prescribed or justified and authorised, solid single-dose preparations with a content of active substance less than 2 mg or less than 2 per cent of the total mass comply with test A (tablets) or test B (suppositories, rectal capsules) for uniformity of content of single-dose preparations. If the preparation contains more than one active substance, this requirement applies only to those substances that correspond to the above conditions.

Uniformity of mass (*2.9.5*). Solid, single-dose preparations comply with the test for uniformity of mass. If the test for uniformity of content is prescribed for all active substances, the test for uniformity of mass is not required.

Deliverable mass or volume (*2.9.28*). Liquid and semi-solid rectal preparations supplied in single-dose containers comply with the test.

Dissolution. A suitable test may be required to demonstrate the appropriate release of the active substance(s) from solid, single-dose preparations, for example the dissolution test for suppositories and soft capsules (*2.9.3*).

Where a dissolution test is prescribed, a disintegration test may not be required.

LABELLING

The label states the name of any added antimicrobial preservative.

Suppositories

DEFINITION

Suppositories are solid, single-dose preparations. The shape, volume and consistency of suppositories are suitable for rectal administration.

They contain one or more active substances dispersed or dissolved in a suitable basis which may be soluble or dispersible in water or may melt at body temperature. Excipients such as diluents, adsorbents, surface-active agents, lubricants, antimicrobial preservatives and colouring matter, authorised by the competent authority, may be added if necessary.

PRODUCTION

Suppositories are prepared by compression or moulding. If necessary, the active substance(s) are previously ground and sieved through a suitable sieve. When prepared by moulding, the medicated mass, sufficiently liquified by heating, is poured into suitable moulds. The suppository solidifies on cooling. Various excipients are available for this process, such as hard fat, macrogols, cocoa butter, and various gelatinous mixtures consisting of, for example, gelatin, water and glycerol. Where applicable, the determination of the softening time of lipophilic suppositories (*2.9.22*) and/or the determination of the resistance to rupture of suppositories (*2.9.24*) are carried out.

A suitable test is carried out to demonstrate the appropriate release of the active substance(s) from suppositories intended for modified release or for prolonged local action.

In the manufacture of suppositories containing dispersed active substances, measures are taken to ensure a suitable and controlled particle size.

TESTS

Disintegration. Unless intended for modified release or for prolonged local action, they comply with the test for disintegration of suppositories and pessaries (*2.9.2*). For suppositories with a fatty base, examine after 30 min and for suppositories with a water-soluble base after 60 min, unless otherwise justified and authorised.

Rectal capsules

DEFINITION

Rectal capsules (shell suppositories) are solid, single-dose preparations generally similar to soft capsules as defined in the monograph on *Capsules (0016)* except that they may have lubricating coatings. They are of elongated shape, are smooth and have a uniform external appearance.

PRODUCTION

A suitable test is carried out to demonstrate the appropriate release of the active substance(s) from rectal capsules intended for modified release or for prolonged local action.

TESTS

Disintegration. Unless intended for modified release or for prolonged local action, they comply with the test for disintegration of suppositories and pessaries (*2.9.2*). Examine the state of the capsules after 30 min, unless otherwise justified and authorised.

Rectal solutions, emulsions and suspensions

DEFINITION

Rectal solutions, emulsions and suspensions are liquid preparations intended for rectal use in order to obtain a systemic or local effect, or they may be intended for diagnostic purposes.

Rectal solutions, emulsions and suspensions are supplied in single-dose containers and they contain one or more active substances dissolved or dispersed in water, glycerol or macrogols or other suitable solvents. Emulsions may show evidence of phase separation but are readily redispersed on shaking. Suspensions may show a sediment which is readily dispersible on shaking to give a suspension which remains sufficiently stable to enable the correct dose to be delivered.

Rectal solutions, emulsions and suspensions may contain excipients, for example to adjust the viscosity of the preparation, to adjust or stabilise the pH, to increase the solubility of the active substance(s) or to stabilise the preparation. These substances do not adversely affect the intended medical action or, at the concentrations used, cause undue local irritation.

Rectal solutions, emulsions and suspensions are supplied in containers containing a volume in the range of 2.5 ml to 2000 ml. The container is adapted to deliver the preparation to the rectum or it is accompanied by a suitable applicator.

Powders and tablets for rectal solutions and suspensions

DEFINITION

Powders and tablets intended for the preparation of rectal solutions or suspensions are single-dose preparations which are dissolved or dispersed in water at the time of administration. They may contain excipients to facilitate dissolution or dispersion or to prevent aggregation of the particles.

After dissolution or suspension, they comply with the requirements for rectal solutions or rectal suspensions, as appropriate.

TESTS

Disintegration. Tablets for rectal solutions or suspensions disintegrate within 3 min when tested according to the test for disintegration of tablets and capsules (*2.9.1*) but using *water R* at 15 °C to 25 °C.

LABELLING

The label states:

– the method of preparation of the rectal solution or suspension,
– the conditions and duration of storage of the solution or suspension after constitution.

Semi-solid rectal preparations

DEFINITION

Semi-solid rectal preparations are ointments, creams or gels.

They are often supplied as single-dose preparations in containers provided with a suitable applicator.

Semi-solid rectal preparations comply with the requirements of the monograph on *Semi-solid preparations for cutaneous application (0132)*.

Rectal foams

DEFINITION

Rectal foams comply with the requirements of the monograph on *Medicated foams (1105)*.

Rectal tampons

DEFINITION

Rectal tampons are solid, single-dose preparations intended to be inserted into the lower part of the rectum for a limited time.

They comply with the requirements of the monograph on *Medicated tampons (1155)*.

01/2005:0132

SEMI-SOLID PREPARATIONS FOR CUTANEOUS APPLICATION

Praeparationes molles ad usum dermicum

The requirements of this monograph apply to all semi-solid preparations for cutaneous application. Where appropriate, additional requirements specific to semi-solid preparations intended to be applied to particular surfaces or mucous membranes may be found in other general monographs, for example Ear preparations (0652), Nasal preparations (0676), Rectal preparations (1145), Eye preparations (1163) and Vaginal preparations (1164).

DEFINITION

Semi-solid preparations for cutaneous application are intended for local or transdermal delivery of active substances, or for their emollient or protective action. They are of homogeneous appearance.

Semi-solid preparations for cutaneous application consist of a simple or compound basis in which, usually, one or more active substances are dissolved or dispersed. According to its composition, the basis may influence the activity of the preparation.

The basis may consist of natural or synthetic substances and may be single phase or multiphase. According to the nature of the basis, the preparation may have hydrophilic or hydrophobic properties; it may contain suitable excipients such as antimicrobial preservatives, antioxidants, stabilisers, emulsifiers, thickeners and penetration enhancers.

Semi-solid preparations for cutaneous application intended for use on severely injured skin are sterile.

Where applicable, containers for semi-solid preparations for cutaneous application comply with the requirements for *Materials used for the manufacture of containers* (*3.1* and subsections) and *Containers* (*3.2* and subsections).

Several categories of semi-solid preparations for cutaneous application may be distinguished:

– ointments,
– creams,
– gels,
– pastes,

Dosage forms

– poultices,
– medicated plasters.

According to their structure, ointments, creams and gels generally show viscoelastic behaviour and are non-newtonian in character e.g. plastic, pseudoplastic or thixotropic type flow at high shear rates. Pastes frequently exhibit dilatancy.

PRODUCTION

During the development of semi-solid preparations for cutaneous application whose formulation contains an antimicrobial preservative, the necessity for and the effectiveness of the chosen preservative shall be demonstrated to the satisfaction of the competent authority. A suitable test method together with criteria for judging the preservative properties of the formulation are provided in *Efficacy of antimicrobial preservation* (*5.1.3*). In the manufacture, packaging, storage and distribution of semi-solid preparations for cutaneous application, suitable steps are taken to ensure their microbiological quality; recommendations on this are provided in *Microbiological Quality of Pharmaceutical Preparations* (*5.1.4*). Sterile semi-solid preparations for cutaneous application are prepared using materials and methods designed to ensure sterility and to avoid the introduction of contaminants and the growth of micro-organisms; recommendations on this are provided in *Methods of Preparation of Sterile Products* (*5.1.1*).

In the manufacture of semi-solid preparations for cutaneous application, suitable measures are taken to ensure that the defined rheological properties are fulfilled. Where appropriate, the following non-mandatory tests may be carried out: measurement of consistency by penetrometry (*2.9.9*), viscosity (apparent viscosity) (*2.2.10*) and a suitable test to demonstrate the appropriate release of the active substance(s).

In the manufacture of semi-solid preparations for cutaneous application containing (an) active substance(s) which is/are not dissolved in the basis (e.g. emulsions or suspensions), measures are taken to ensure appropriate homogeneity of the preparation to be delivered.

In the manufacture of semi-solid preparations for cutaneous application containing dispersed particles, measures are taken to ensure a suitable and controlled particle size with regard to the intended use.

TESTS

Deliverable mass or volume (*2.9.28*). Semi-solid preparations for cutaneous application supplied in single-dose containers comply with the test.

Sterility (*2.6.1*). Where the label indicates that the preparation is sterile, it complies with the test for sterility.

STORAGE

If the preparation contains water or other volatile ingredients, store in an airtight container. If the preparation is sterile, store in a sterile, airtight, tamper-proof container.

LABELLING

The label states:

– the name of any added antimicrobial preservative,
– where applicable, that the preparation is sterile.

Ointments

DEFINITION

An ointment consists of a single-phase basis in which solids or liquids may be dispersed.

Hydrophobic Ointments

Hydrophobic ointments can absorb only small amounts of water. Typical bases used for their formulation are hard, liquid and light liquid paraffins, vegetable oils, animal fats, synthetic glycerides, waxes and liquid polyalkylsiloxanes.

Water-emulsifying Ointments

Water-emulsifying ointments can absorb larger amounts of water and thereby produce water-in-oil or oil-in-water emulsions depending on the nature of the emulsifiers: water-in-oil emulsifying agents such as wool alcohols, sorbitan esters, monoglycerides and fatty alcohols, or oil-in-water emulsifying agents such as sulphated fatty alcohols, polysorbates, macrogol cetostearyl ether or esters of fatty acids with macrogols may be used for this purpose. Their bases are those of the hydrophobic ointments.

Hydrophilic Ointments

Hydrophilic ointments are preparations having bases that are miscible with water. The bases usually consist of mixtures of liquid and solid macrogols (polyethylene glycols). They may contain appropriate amounts of water.

Creams

DEFINITION

Creams are multiphase preparations consisting of a lipophilic phase and an aqueous phase.

Lipophilic Creams

Lipophilic creams have as the continuous phase the lipophilic phase. They contain water-in-oil emulsifying agents such as wool alcohols, sorbitan esters and monoglycerides.

Hydrophilic Creams

Hydrophilic creams have as the continuous phase the aqueous phase. They contain oil-in-water emulsifying agents such as sodium or trolamine soaps, sulphated fatty alcohols, polysorbates and polyoxyl fatty acid and fatty alcohol esters combined, if necessary, with water-in-oil emulsifying agents.

Gels

DEFINITION

Gels consist of liquids gelled by means of suitable gelling agents.

Lipophilic Gels

Lipophilic gels (oleogels) are preparations whose bases usually consist of liquid paraffin with polyethylene or fatty oils gelled with colloidal silica or aluminium or zinc soaps.

Hydrophilic Gels

Hydrophilic gels (hydrogels) are preparations whose bases usually consist of water, glycerol or propylene glycol gelled with suitable gelling agents such as starch, cellulose derivatives, carbomers and magnesium-aluminium silicates.

Pastes

DEFINITION

Pastes are semi-solid preparations for cutaneous application containing large proportions of solids finely dispersed in the basis.

Poultices

DEFINITION

Poultices consist of a hydrophilic heat-retentive basis in which solid or liquid active substances are dispersed. They are usually spread thickly on a suitable dressing and heated before application to the skin.

Medicated plasters

DEFINITION

Medicated plasters are flexible preparations containing one or more active substances. They are intended to be applied to the skin. They are designed to maintain the active substance(s) in close contact with the skin such that these may be absorbed slowly, or act as protective or keratolytic agents.

Medicated plasters consist of an adhesive basis, which may be coloured, containing one or more active substances, spread as a uniform layer on an appropriate support made of natural or synthetic material. It is not irritant or sensitising to the skin. The adhesive layer is covered by a suitable protective liner, which is removed before applying the plaster to the skin. When removed, the protective liner does not detach the preparation from the outer, supporting layer.

Medicated plasters are presented in a range of sizes directly adapted to their intended use or as larger sheets to be cut before use. Medicated plasters adhere firmly to the skin when gentle pressure is applied and can be peeled off without causing appreciable injury to the skin or detachment of the preparation from the outer, supporting layer.

TESTS

Dissolution. A suitable test may be required to demonstrate the appropriate release of the active substance(s), for example one of the tests described in *Dissolution test for transdermal patches* (*2.9.4*).

01/2005:1154

STICKS

Styli

Additional requirements for sticks may be found, where appropriate, in other general monographs, for example Nasal preparations (0676).

DEFINITION

Sticks are solid preparations intended for local application. They are rod-shaped or conical preparations consisting of one or more active substances alone or which are dissolved or dispersed in a suitable basis which may dissolve or melt at body temperature.

Urethral sticks and sticks for insertion into wounds are sterile.

PRODUCTION

In the manufacture, packaging, storage and distribution of sticks, suitable means are taken to ensure their microbial quality; recommendations on this aspect are provided in the text on *Microbiological quality of pharmaceutical preparations* (*5.1.4*).

Urethral sticks and other sterile sticks are prepared using materials and methods designed to ensure sterility and to avoid the introduction of contaminants and the growth of micro-organisms; recommendations on this aspect are provided in the text on *Methods of preparation of sterile products* (*5.1.1*).

In the manufacture of sticks means are taken to ensure that the preparation complies with a test for mass uniformity or, where appropriate, a test for uniformity of content.

TESTS

Sterility (*2.6.1*). Urethral sticks and sticks for insertion into wounds comply with the test for sterility.

LABELLING

The label states:

– the quantity of active substance(s) per stick,
– for urethral sticks and sticks to be inserted into wounds that they are sterile.

01/2005:0478

TABLETS

Compressi

The requirements of this monograph do not necessarily apply to preparations that are presented as tablets intended for use other than by oral administration. Requirements for such preparations may be found, where appropriate, in other general monographs; for example Rectal preparations (1145), Vaginal preparations (1164) and Oromucosal preparations (1807). This monograph does not apply to lozenges, oral lyophilisates, oral pastes and oral gums. Where justified and authorised, the requirements of this monograph do not apply to tablets for veterinary use.

DEFINITION

Tablets are solid preparations each containing a single dose of one or more active substances and usually obtained by compressing uniform volumes of particles. Tablets are intended for oral administration. Some are swallowed whole, some after being chewed, some are dissolved or dispersed in water before being administered and some are retained in the mouth where the active substance is liberated.

The particles consist of one or more active substances with or without excipients such as diluents, binders, disintegrating agents, glidants, lubricants, substances capable of modifying the behaviour of the preparation in the digestive tract, colouring matter authorised by the competent authority and flavouring substances.

Tablets are usually right, circular solid cylinders, the end surfaces of which are flat or convex and the edges of which may be bevelled. They may have lines or break-marks and may bear a symbol or other markings. Tablets may be coated.

Where applicable, containers for tablets comply with the requirements for *Materials used for the manufacture of containers* (*3.1* and subsections) and *Containers* (*3.2* and subsections).

Several categories of tablets for oral use may be distinguished:

– uncoated tablets,
– coated tablets,
– effervescent tablets,
– soluble tablets,
– dispersible tablets,
– orodispersible tablets,
– gastro-resistant tablets,
– modified-release tablets.

PRODUCTION

Tablets are usually prepared by compressing uniform volumes of particles or particle aggregates produced by granulation methods. In the manufacture of tablets, means are taken to ensure that they possess a suitable mechanical strength to avoid crumbling or breaking on handling or subsequent processing. This may be demonstrated by examining the *Friability of uncoated tablets* (*2.9.7*) and the *Resistance to crushing of tablets* (*2.9.8*). Chewable tablets are prepared to ensure that they are easily crushed by chewing.

Dosage forms

For tablets for which subdivision is authorised, it is demonstrated to the satisfaction of the competent authority that the subdivided parts comply either with test A for *Uniformity of content of single-dose preparations (2.9.6)* or with the test for *Uniformity of mass of single-dose preparations (2.9.5)*, as appropriate.

In the manufacture, packaging, storage and distribution of tablets, suitable means are taken to ensure their microbiological quality; recommendations on this aspect are provided in the text on *Microbiological quality of pharmaceutical preparations (5.1.4)*.

TESTS

Uniformity of content (*2.9.6*). Unless otherwise prescribed or justified and authorised, tablets with a content of active substance less than 2 mg or less than 2 per cent of the total mass comply with test A for uniformity of content of single-dose preparations. If the preparation has more than one active substance, the requirement applies only to those substances which correspond to the above conditions.

Unless otherwise justified and authorised, coated tablets other than film-coated tablets comply with test A for uniformity of content of single-dose preparations irrespective of their content of active substance(s).

Uniformity of mass (*2.9.5*). Uncoated tablets and, unless otherwise justified and authorised, film-coated tablets comply with the test for uniformity of mass of single-dose preparations. If the test for uniformity of content is prescribed or justified and authorised for all the active substances, the test for uniformity of mass is not required.

Dissolution. A suitable test may be carried out to demonstrate the appropriate release of the active substance(s), for example one of the tests described in *Dissolution test for solid dosage forms (2.9.3)*.

Where a dissolution test is prescribed, a disintegration test may not be required.

Uncoated tablets

DEFINITION

Uncoated tablets include single-layer tablets resulting from a single compression of particles and multi-layer tablets consisting of concentric or parallel layers obtained by successive compression of particles of different composition. The excipients used are not specifically intended to modify the release of the active substance in the digestive fluids.

Uncoated tablets conform to the general definition of tablets. A broken section, when examined under a lens, shows either a relatively uniform texture (single-layer tablets) or a stratified texture (multi-layer tablets) but no signs of coating.

TESTS

Disintegration. Uncoated tablets comply with the test for disintegration of tablets and capsules (*2.9.1*). Use *water R* as the liquid. Add a disc to each tube. Operate the apparatus for 15 min, unless otherwise justified and authorised, and examine the state of the tablets. If the tablets fail to comply because of adherence to the discs, repeat the test on a further 6 tablets omitting the discs. The tablets comply with the test if all 6 have disintegrated.

Chewable tablets are not required to comply with the test.

Coated tablets

DEFINITION

Coated tablets are tablets covered with one or more layers of mixtures of various substances such as natural or synthetic resins, gums, gelatin, inactive and insoluble fillers, sugars, plasticisers, polyols, waxes, colouring matter authorised by the competent authority and sometimes flavouring substances and active substances. The substances used as coatings are usually applied as a solution or suspension in conditions in which evaporation of the vehicle occurs. When the coating is a very thin polymeric coating, the tablets are known as film-coated tablets.

Coated tablets have a smooth surface which is often coloured and may be polished; a broken section, when examined under a lens, shows a core surrounded by one or more continuous layers with a different texture.

PRODUCTION

Where justified, uniformity of mass or uniformity of content of coated tablets other than film-coated tablets may be ensured by control of the cores.

TESTS

Disintegration. Coated tablets other than film-coated tablets comply with the test for disintegration of tablets and capsules (*2.9.1*). Use *water R* as the liquid. Add a disc to each tube. Operate the apparatus for 60 min, unless otherwise justified and authorised, and examine the state of the tablets. If any of the tablets has not disintegrated, repeat the test on a further 6 tablets, replacing *water R* with *0.1 M hydrochloric acid*. The tablets comply with the test if all 6 have disintegrated in the acid medium.

Film-coated tablets comply with the disintegration test prescribed above except that the apparatus is operated for 30 min, unless otherwise justified and authorised.

If coated tablets or film-coated tablets fail to comply because of adherence to the discs, repeat the test on a further 6 tablets omitting the discs. The tablets comply with the test if all 6 have disintegrated.

Chewable coated tablets are not required to comply with the test.

Effervescent tablets

DEFINITION

Effervescent tablets are uncoated tablets generally containing acid substances and carbonates or hydrogen carbonates which react rapidly in the presence of water to release carbon dioxide. They are intended to be dissolved or dispersed in water before administration.

TESTS

Disintegration. Place 1 tablet in a beaker containing 200 ml of *water R* at 15-25 °C; numerous bubbles of gas are evolved. When the evolution of gas around the tablet or its fragments ceases the tablet has disintegrated, being either dissolved or dispersed in the water so that no agglomerates of particles remain. Repeat the operation on 5 other tablets. The tablets comply with the test if each of the 6 tablets used disintegrates in the manner prescribed within 5 min, unless otherwise justified and authorised.

Soluble tablets

DEFINITION

Soluble tablets are uncoated or film-coated tablets. They are intended to be dissolved in water before administration. The solution produced may be slightly opalescent due to the added excipients used in the manufacture of the tablets.

TESTS

Disintegration. Soluble tablets disintegrate within 3 min when examined by the test for disintegration of tablets and capsules (*2.9.1*), but using *water R* at 15-25 °C.

Dispersible tablets

DEFINITION

Dispersible tablets are uncoated or film-coated tablets intended to be dispersed in water before administration giving a homogeneous dispersion.

TESTS

Disintegration. Dispersible tablets disintegrate within 3 min when examined by the test for disintegration of tablets and capsules (*2.9.1*), but using *water R* at 15-25 °C.

Fineness of dispersion. Place 2 tablets in 100 ml of *water R* and stir until completely dispersed. A smooth dispersion is produced, which passes through a sieve screen with a nominal mesh aperture of 710 μm.

Orodispersible tablets

DEFINITION

Orodispersible tablets are uncoated tablets intended to be placed in the mouth where they disperse rapidly before being swallowed.

TESTS

Disintegration. Orodispersible tablets disintegrate within 3 min when examined by the test for disintegration of tablets and capsules (*2.9.1*).

Modified-release tablets

DEFINITION

Modified-release tablets are coated or uncoated tablets which contain special excipients or which are prepared by special procedures, or both, designed to modify the rate, the place or the time at which the active substance(s) are released.

Modified-release tablets include prolonged-release tablets, delayed-release tablets and pulsatile-release tablets.

PRODUCTION

A suitable test is carried out to demonstrate the appropriate release of the active substance(s).

Gastro-resistant tablets

DEFINITION

Gastro-resistant tablets are delayed-release tablets that are intended to resist the gastric fluid and to release their active substance(s) in the intestinal fluid. Usually they are prepared from granules or particles already covered with a gastro-resistant coating or in certain cases by covering tablets with a gastro-resistant coating (enteric-coated tablets).

Tablets covered with a gastro-resistant coating conform to the definition of coated tablets.

PRODUCTION

For tablets prepared from granules or particles already covered with a gastro-resistant coating, a suitable test is carried out to demonstrate the appropriate release of the active substance(s).

TESTS

Disintegration. For tablets covered with a gastro-resistant coating carry out the test for disintegration (*2.9.1*) with the following modifications. Use *0.1 M hydrochloric acid* as the liquid. Operate the apparatus for 2 h, or other such time as may be justified and authorised, without the discs and examine the state of the tablets. The time of resistance to the acid medium varies according to the formulation of the tablets to be examined. It is typically 2 h to 3 h but even with authorised deviations is not less than 1 h. No tablet shows signs of either disintegration (apart from fragments of coating) or cracks that would allow the escape of the contents. Replace the acid by *phosphate buffer solution pH 6.8 R* and add a disc to each tube. Operate the apparatus for 60 min and examine the state of the tablets. If the tablets fail to comply because of adherence to the discs, repeat the test on a further 6 tablets omitting the discs. The tablets comply with the test if all 6 have disintegrated.

Dissolution. For tablets prepared from granules or particles already covered with a gastro-resistant coating, a suitable test is carried out to demonstrate the appropriate release of the active substance(s), for example the test described in *Dissolution test for solid dosage forms* (*2.9.3*).

Tablets for use in the mouth

DEFINITION

Tablets for use in the mouth are usually uncoated tablets. They are formulated to effect a slow release and local action of the active substance(s) or the release and absorption of the active substance or substances at a defined part of the mouth. They comply with the requirements of the monograph on *Oromucosal preparations (1807)*.

01/2005:1155

TAMPONS, MEDICATED

Tamponae medicatae

Additional requirements for medicated tampons may be found, where appropriate, in other general monographs, for example Rectal preparations (1145), Vaginal preparations (1164) and Ear preparations (0652).

DEFINITION

Medicated tampons are solid, single-dose preparations intended to be inserted into the body cavities for a limited period of time. They consist of a suitable material such as cellulose, collagen or silicone impregnated with one or more active substances.

PRODUCTION

In the manufacture, packaging, storage and distribution of medicated tampons, suitable means are taken to ensure their microbial quality; recommendations on this aspect are provided in the text on *Microbiological quality of pharmaceutical preparations* (*5.1.4*).

LABELLING

The label states the quantity of active substance(s) per tampon.

01/2005:1164

VAGINAL PREPARATIONS

Vaginalia

DEFINITION

Vaginal preparations are liquid, semi-solid or solid preparations intended for administration to the vagina usually in order to obtain a local effect. They contain one or more active substances in a suitable basis.

Where appropriate, containers for vaginal preparations comply with the requirements for *Materials used for the manufacture of containers* (*3.1* and subsections) and *Containers* (*3.2* and subsections).

Several categories of vaginal preparations may be distinguished:

- pessaries,
- vaginal tablets,
- vaginal capsules,
- vaginal solutions, emulsions and suspensions,
- tablets for vaginal solutions and suspensions,
- semi-solid vaginal preparations,
- vaginal foams,
- medicated vaginal tampons.

PRODUCTION

In the manufacturing, packaging, storage and distribution of vaginal preparations, suitable means are taken to ensure their microbial quality; recommendations on this aspect are provided in the text on *Microbiological quality of pharmaceutical preparations* (*5.1.4*).

TESTS

Uniformity of content (*2.9.6*). Unless otherwise prescribed or justified and authorised, solid single-dose preparations with a content of active substance less than 2 mg or less than 2 per cent of the total mass comply with test A (vaginal tablets) or test B (pessaries, vaginal capsules) for uniformity of content of single-dose preparations. If the preparation has more than one active substance, the requirement applies only to those substances which correspond to the above conditions.

Uniformity of mass (*2.9.5*). Solid single-dose vaginal preparations comply with the test for uniformity of mass of single-dose preparations. If the test for uniformity of content is prescribed for all the active substances, the test for uniformity of mass is not required.

Deliverable mass or volume (*2.9.28*). Liquid and semi-solid vaginal preparations supplied in single-dose containers comply with the test.

Dissolution. A suitable test may be carried out to demonstrate the appropriate release of the active substance(s) from solid single-dose preparations, for example one of the tests described in *Dissolution test for solid dosage forms* (*2.9.3*).

When a dissolution test is prescribed, a disintegration test may not be required.

Pessaries

DEFINITION

Pessaries are solid, single-dose preparations. They have various shapes, usually ovoid, with a volume and consistency suitable for insertion into the vagina. They contain one or more active substances dispersed or dissolved in a suitable basis that may be soluble or dispersible in water or may melt at body temperature. Excipients such as diluents, adsorbents, surface-active agents, lubricants, antimicrobial preservatives and colouring matter authorised by the competent authority may be added, if necessary.

PRODUCTION

Pessaries are usually prepared by moulding. Where appropriate in the manufacture of pessaries, measures are taken to ensure a suitable and controlled particle size of the active substance(s). If necessary, the active substance(s) are previously ground and sieved through a suitable sieve.

When prepared by moulding, the medicated mass, sufficiently liquified by heating, is poured into suitable moulds. The pessary solidifies on cooling. Various excipients are available for this process, such as hard fat, macrogols, cocoa butter, and various gelatinous mixtures consisting, for example, of gelatin, water and glycerol.

A suitable test is carried out to demonstrate the appropriate release of the active substance(s) from pessaries intended for prolonged local action.

Where appropriate, the determination of the resistance to rupture of pessaries (*2.9.24*) is carried out.

TESTS

Disintegration. Unless intended for prolonged local action, they comply with the test for disintegration of suppositories and pessaries (*2.9.2*). Examine the state of the pessaries after 60 min, unless otherwise justified and authorised.

Vaginal tablets

DEFINITION

Vaginal tablets are solid, single-dose preparations.
They generally conform to the definitions of uncoated or film-coated tablets given in the monograph on *Tablets (0478)*.

PRODUCTION

A suitable test is carried out to demonstrate the appropriate release of the active substance(s) from vaginal tablets intended for prolonged local action.

TESTS

Disintegration. Unless intended for prolonged local action, they comply with the test for disintegration of suppositories and pessaries (special method for vaginal tablets, *2.9.2*). Examine the state of the tablets after 30 min, unless otherwise justified and authorised.

Vaginal capsules

DEFINITION

Vaginal capsules (shell pessaries) are solid, single-dose preparations. They are generally similar to soft capsules, differing only in their shape and size. Vaginal capsules have various shapes, usually ovoid. They are smooth and have a uniform external appearance.

PRODUCTION

A suitable test is carried out to demonstrate the appropriate release of the active substance(s) from vaginal capsules intended for prolonged local action.

TESTS

Disintegration. Unless intended for prolonged local action, they comply with the test for disintegration of suppositories and pessaries (*2.9.2*). Examine the state of the capsules after 30 min, unless otherwise justified and authorised.

Vaginal solutions, emulsions and suspensions

DEFINITION

Vaginal solutions, emulsions and suspensions are liquid preparations intended for a local effect, for irrigation or for diagnostic purposes. They may contain excipients, for example to adjust the viscosity of the preparation, to adjust or stabilise the pH, to increase the solubility of the active substance(s) or to stabilise the preparation. The excipients do not adversely affect the intended medical action or, at the concentrations used, cause undue local irritation.

Vaginal emulsions may show evidence of phase separation but are readily redispersed on shaking. Vaginal suspensions may show a sediment that is readily dispersed on shaking to give a suspension which remains sufficiently stable to enable a homogeneous preparation to be delivered.

They are supplied in single-dose containers. The container is adapted to deliver the preparation to the vagina or it is accompanied by a suitable applicator.

PRODUCTION

In the manufacture of vaginal suspensions measures are taken to ensure a suitable and controlled particle size with regard to the intended use.

Tablets for vaginal solutions and suspensions

DEFINITION

Tablets intended for the preparation of vaginal solutions and suspensions are single-dose preparations which are dissolved or dispersed in water at the time of administration. They may contain excipients to facilitate dissolution or dispersion or to prevent caking.

Apart from the test for disintegration, tablets for vaginal solutions or suspensions conform with the definition for *Tablets (0478)*.

After dissolution or dispersion, they comply with the requirements for vaginal solutions or vaginal suspensions, as appropriate.

TESTS

Disintegration. Tablets for vaginal solutions or suspensions disintegrate within 3 min when tested according to the test for disintegration of tablets and capsules (*2.9.1*), but using *water R* at 15 °C to 25 °C.

LABELLING

The label states:

– the method of preparation of the vaginal solution or suspension,
– the conditions and duration of storage of the solution or suspension after constitution.

Semi-solid vaginal preparations

DEFINITION

Semi-solid vaginal preparations are ointments, creams or gels.

They are often supplied in single-dose containers. The container is provided with a suitable applicator.

Semi-solid vaginal preparations comply with the requirements of the monograph on *Semi-solid preparations for cutaneous application (0132)*.

Vaginal foams

DEFINITION

Vaginal foams comply with the requirements of the monograph on *Medicated foams (1105)*.

Medicated vaginal tampons

DEFINITION

Medicated vaginal tampons are solid, single-dose preparations intended to be inserted in the vagina for a limited time.

They comply with the requirements of the monograph on *Medicated tampons (1155)*.

01/2005:1808

VETERINARY LIQUID PREPARATIONS FOR CUTANEOUS APPLICATION

Praeparationes liquidae veterinariae ad usum dermicum

Unless otherwise justified and authorised, veterinary liquid preparations for cutaneous application comply with the requirements of the monograph on Liquid preparations for cutaneous application (0927). In addition to these requirements, the following statements apply to veterinary liquid preparations for cutaneous application.

DEFINITION

Veterinary liquid preparations for cutaneous application are liquid preparations intended to be applied to the skin to obtain a local and/or systemic effect. They are solutions, suspensions or emulsions which may contain one or more active substances in a suitable vehicle. They may be presented as concentrates in the form of wettable powders, pastes, solutions or suspensions, which are used to prepare diluted suspensions or emulsions of active substances. They may contain suitable antimicrobial preservatives, antioxidants and other excipients such as stabilisers, emulsifiers and thickeners.

Several categories of veterinary liquid preparations for cutaneous application may be distinguished:

– cutaneous foams (see *Liquid preparations for cutaneous application (0927)*),
– dip concentrates,
– pour-on preparations,
– shampoos (see *Liquid preparations for cutaneous application (0927)*),
– spot-on preparations,
– sprays,
– teat dips,
– teat sprays,
– udder-washes.

Dip concentrates

DEFINITION

Dip concentrates are preparations containing one or more active substances, usually in the form of wettable powders, pastes, solutions or suspensions, which are used to prepare diluted solutions, suspensions or emulsions of active substances. The diluted preparations are applied by complete immersion of the animal.

Dosage forms

Pour-on preparations

DEFINITION

Pour-on preparations contain one or more active substances for the prevention and treatment of ectoparasitic and/or endoparasitic infestations of animals. They are applied in volumes which are usually greater than 5 ml by pouring along the animal's dorsal midline.

Spot-on preparations

DEFINITION

Spot-on preparations contain one or more active substances for the prevention and treatment of ectoparasitic and/or endoparasitic infestations of animals. They are applied in volumes which are usually less than 10 ml, to a small area on the head or back, as appropriate, of the animal.

Sprays

DEFINITION

Sprays contain one or more active substances that are intended to be applied externally for therapeutic or prophylactic purposes. They are delivered in the form of an aerosol by the actuation of an appropriate valve or by means of a suitable atomising device that is either an integral part of the container or is supplied separately.

Sprays may be presented in pressurised containers (see *Pressurised pharmaceutical preparations (0523)*). When so presented, sprays usually consist of one or more active substances in a suitable vehicle held under pressure with suitable propellants or suitable mixtures of propellants. When otherwise presented, sprays are supplied in well-closed containers.

PRODUCTION

During the development and manufacture of a spray, measures are taken to ensure that the assembled product conforms to a defined spray rate and spray pattern.

Teat dips

DEFINITION

Teat dips contain one or more disinfectant active substances, usually in the form of solutions into which the teats of an animal are dipped pre- and, where necessary, post-milking to reduce the population of pathogenic micro-organisms on the surfaces. Teat dips may be supplied/presented as ready-to-use preparations or they may be prepared by dilution of teat dip concentrates. Pre- and post-milking teat dips often differ in formulation. Teat dips usually contain emollients to promote skin hydration, to soften the skin and allow healing of lesions that would otherwise harbour bacteria.

Teat sprays

DEFINITION

Teat sprays contain one or more disinfectant active substances, usually in the form of solutions which are sprayed onto the teats of an animal pre- and, where necessary, post-milking to reduce the population of pathogenic micro-organisms on the surfaces. Teat sprays may be supplied/presented as ready-to-use preparations or they may be prepared by dilution of teat spray concentrates. Pre- and post-milking sprays often differ in formulation. Teat sprays usually contain emollients to promote skin hydration, to soften the skin and allow healing of lesions that would otherwise harbour bacteria.

Udder-washes

DEFINITION

Udder-washes contain one or more disinfectant active substances, usually in the form of solutions which are sprayed onto the udder and teats of an animal to remove mud and faecal contamination before the application of teat dips or sprays. Udder-washes are usually prepared by the dilution either of concentrated preparations or of ready-to-use teat dips or teat sprays.

VACCINES FOR HUMAN USE

01/2005:1929

BCG FOR IMMUNOTHERAPY

BCG ad immunocurationem

DEFINITION

BCG for immunotherapy is a freeze-dried preparation of live bacteria derived from a culture of the bacillus of Calmette and Guérin (*Mycobacterium bovis* BCG) whose capacity for treatment has been established.

It complies with the monograph *Vaccines for human use (0153)*.

PRODUCTION

GENERAL PROVISIONS

BCG for immunotherapy shall be produced by a staff consisting of healthy persons who do not work with other infectious agents; in particular they shall not work with virulent strains of *Mycobacterium tuberculosis*, nor shall they be exposed to a known risk of tuberculosis infection. Staff are examined periodically for tuberculosis. BCG for immunotherapy is susceptible to sunlight: the procedures for production shall be so designed that all products are protected from direct sunlight and from ultraviolet light at all stages of manufacture, testing and storage.

Production is based on a seed-lot system. The production method shall have been shown to yield consistently BCG products that can be used for treatment of superficial bladder cancer and are safe. The product is prepared from cultures which are separated from the master seed lot by as few subcultures as possible and in any case not more than 8 subcultures. During the course of these subcultures the preparation is not freeze-dried more than once.

If a bioluminescence test or other biochemical method is used instead of viable count, the method is validated against the viable count for each stage of the process at which it is used.

SEED LOTS

The strain used to establish the master seed lot is chosen for and maintained to preserve its characteristics, its capacity to treat and prevent superficial bladder cancer, and its relative absence of pathogenicity for man and laboratory animals. The strain used shall be identified by historical records that include information on its origin and subsequent manipulation.

Before establishment of a working seed lot a batch is prepared and reserved for use as the comparison product. When a new working seed lot is established, a suitable test for delayed hypersensitivity in guinea-pigs is carried out on a batch of product prepared from the new working seed lot; the product is shown to be not significantly different in activity from the comparison product. Antimicrobial agent sensitivity testing is also carried out.

Only a working seed lot that complies with the following requirements may be used for propagation.

Identification. The bacteria in the working seed lot are identified as *Mycobacterium bovis* BCG using microbiological techniques, which may be supplemented by molecular biology techniques (for example, nucleic acid amplification and restriction-fragment-length polymorphism).

Bacterial and fungal contamination. Carry out the test for sterility (*2.6.1*), using 10 ml for each medium. The working seed lot complies with the test for sterility, except for the presence of mycobacteria.

Virulent mycobacteria. Examine the working seed lot as prescribed under Tests, using 10 guinea-pigs.

PROPAGATION AND HARVEST

The bacteria are grown in a suitable medium for not more than 21 days by surface or submerged culture. The culture medium does not contain substances known to cause toxic or allergic reactions in human beings or to cause the bacteria to become virulent for guinea-pigs. The culture is harvested and suspended in a sterile liquid medium that protects the viability of the culture as determined by a suitable method of viable count.

FINAL BULK

The final bulk is prepared from a single harvest or by pooling a number of single harvests. A stabiliser may be added; if the stabiliser interferes with the determination of bacterial concentration on the final bulk, the determination is carried out before addition of the stabiliser.

Only final bulk that complies with the following requirements may be used in the preparation of the final lot.

Bacterial and fungal contamination. Carry out the test for sterility (*2.6.1*), using 10 ml of final bulk for each medium. The final bulk complies with the test for sterility, except for the presence of mycobacteria.

Count of viable units. Determine the number of viable units per millilitre by viable count on solid medium using a method suitable for the product to be examined or by a suitable biochemical method. Carry out the test in parallel on a reference preparation of the same strain.

Bacterial concentration. Determine the total bacterial concentration by a suitable method, either directly by determining the mass of the micro-organisms, or indirectly by an opacity method that has been calibrated in relation to the mass of the micro-organisms; if the bacterial concentration is determined before addition of a stabiliser, the concentration in the final bulk is established by calculation. The total bacterial concentration is within the limits approved for the particular product.

The ratio of the count of viable units to the total bacterial concentration is not less than that approved for the particular product.

FINAL LOT

The final bulk is distributed into sterile containers and freeze-dried to a moisture content favourable to the stability of the product; the containers are closed either under vacuum or under an inert gas.

Except where the filled and closed containers are stored at a temperature of −20 °C or lower, the expiry date is not later than 4 years from the date of harvest.

Only a final lot that complies with the following requirement for count of viable units and with each of the requirements given below under Identification, Tests and Assay may be released for use. Provided the test for virulent mycobacteria has been carried out with satisfactory results on the final bulk, it may be omitted on the final lot.

Count of viable units. Determine the number of viable units per millilitre of the reconstituted product by viable count on solid medium using a method suitable for the product to be examined, or by a suitable biochemical method. The ratio of the count of viable units after freeze-drying to that before is not less than that approved for the particular product.

IDENTIFICATION

BCG for immunotherapy is identified by microscopic examination of the bacilli in stained smears demonstrating their acid-fast property and by the characteristic appearance of colonies grown on solid medium. Alternatively, molecular biology techniques (for example, nucleic acid amplification) may be used.

TESTS

Virulent mycobacteria. Inject subcutaneously or intramuscularly into each of 6 guinea-pigs, each weighing 250-400 g and having received no treatment likely to interfere with the test, a quantity of the product to be examined equivalent to at least 1/25 of 1 human dose. Observe the animals for at least 42 days. At the end of this period, kill the guinea-pigs and examine by autopsy for signs of infection with tuberculosis, ignoring any minor reactions at the site of injection. Animals that die during the observation period are also examined for signs of tuberculosis. The product complies with the test if none of the guinea-pigs shows signs of tuberculosis and if not more than 1 animal dies during the observation period. If 2 animals die during this period and autopsy does not reveal signs of tuberculosis, repeat the test on 6 other guinea-pigs. The product complies with the test if not more than 1 animal dies during the 42 days following the injection and autopsy does not reveal any sign of tuberculosis.

Bacterial and fungal contamination. The reconstituted product complies with the test for sterility (*2.6.1*) except for the presence of mycobacteria.

Temperature stability. Maintain samples of the freeze-dried product at 37 °C for 4 weeks. Determine the number of viable units in the heated product and in unheated product as described below. The number of viable units in the heated product is within the limits approved for the particular product but in any case not less than 20 per cent of that in unheated product.

Water. Not more than the limit approved for the particular product, determined by a suitable method.

ASSAY

Determine the number of viable units in the reconstituted product by viable count on solid medium using a method suitable for the product to be examined or by a suitable validated biochemical method. The number is within the range stated on the label. Determine the number of viable units in the comparison control in parallel.

LABELLING

The label states:

- the minimum and the maximum number of viable units per dose in the reconstituted product,
- that the product must be protected from direct sunlight.

01/2005:0163

BCG VACCINE, FREEZE-DRIED

Vaccinum tuberculosis (BCG) cryodesiccatum

DEFINITION

Freeze-dried BCG vaccine is a preparation of live bacteria derived from a culture of the bacillus of Calmette and Guérin (*Mycobacterium bovis* BCG) whose capacity to protect against tuberculosis has been established.

PRODUCTION

GENERAL PROVISIONS

BCG vaccine shall be produced by a staff consisting of healthy persons who do not work with other infectious agents; in particular they shall not work with virulent strains of *Mycobacterium tuberculosis*, nor shall they be exposed to a known risk of tuberculosis infection. Staff are examined periodically for tuberculosis. BCG vaccine is susceptible to sunlight: the procedures for the preparation of the vaccine shall be designed so that all cultures and vaccines are protected from direct sunlight and from ultraviolet light at all stages of manufacture, testing and storage.

Production of the vaccine is based on a seed-lot system. The production method shall have been shown to yield consistently BCG vaccines that induce adequate sensitivity to tuberculin in man, that have acceptable protective potency in animals and are safe. The vaccine is prepared from cultures which are derived from the master seed lot by as few subcultures as possible and in any case not more than 8 subcultures. During the course of these subcultures the preparation is not freeze-dried more than once.

If a bioluminescence test or other biochemical method is used instead of viable count, the method is validated against the viable count for each stage of the process at which it is used.

BACTERIAL SEED LOTS

The strain used to establish the master seed lot is chosen for and maintained to preserve its characteristics, its capacity to sensitise man to tuberculin and to protect animals against tuberculosis, and its relative absence of pathogenicity for man and laboratory animals. The strain used shall be identified by historical records that include information on its origin and subsequent manipulation.

A suitable batch of vaccine is prepared from the first working seed lot and is reserved for use as the comparison vaccine. When a new working seed lot is established, a suitable test for delayed hypersensitivity in guinea-pigs is carried out on a batch of vaccine prepared from the new working seed lot; the vaccine is shown to be not significantly different in activity from the comparison vaccine. Antimicrobial agent sensitivity testing is also carried out.

Only a working seed lot that complies with the following requirements may be used for propagation.

Identification. The bacteria in the working seed lot are identified as *Mycobacterium bovis* BCG using microbiological techniques, which may be supplemented by molecular biology techniques (for example, nucleic acid amplification and restriction-fragment-length polymorphism).

Bacterial and fungal contamination. Carry out the test for sterility (*2.6.1*), using 10 ml for each medium. The working seed lot complies with the test for sterility except for the presence of mycobacteria.

Virulent mycobacteria. Examine the working seed lot as prescribed under Tests, using 10 guinea-pigs.

PROPAGATION AND HARVEST

The bacteria are grown in a suitable medium for not more than 21 days by surface or submerged culture. The culture medium does not contain substances known to cause toxic or allergic reactions in humans or to cause the bacteria to become virulent for guinea-pigs. The culture is harvested and suspended in a sterile liquid medium that protects the viability of the vaccine as determined by a suitable method of viable count.

FINAL BULK VACCINE

The final bulk vaccine is prepared from a single harvest or by pooling a number of single harvests. A stabiliser may be added; if the stabiliser interferes with the determination of bacterial concentration in the final bulk vaccine, the determination is carried out before addition of the stabiliser.

Only final bulk vaccine that complies with the following requirements may be used in the preparation of the final lot.

Bacterial and fungal contamination. Carry out the test for sterility (*2.6.1*), using 10 ml for each medium. The final bulk vaccine complies with the test for sterility except for the presence of mycobacteria.

Count of viable units. Determine the number of viable units per millilitre by viable count on solid medium using a method suitable for the vaccine to be examined or by a suitable biochemical method. Carry out the test in parallel on a reference preparation of the same strain.

Bacterial concentration. Determine the total bacterial concentration by a suitable method, either directly by determining the mass of the micro-organisms, or indirectly by an opacity method that has been calibrated in relation to the mass of the organisms; if the bacterial concentration is determined before addition of a stabiliser, the concentration in the final bulk vaccine is established by calculation. The total bacterial concentration is within the limits approved for the particular product.

The ratio of the count of viable units to the total bacterial concentration is not less than that approved for the particular product.

FINAL LOT

The final bulk vaccine is distributed into sterile containers and freeze-dried to a moisture content favourable to the stability of the vaccine; the containers are closed either under vacuum or under an inert gas.

Except where the filled and closed containers are stored at a temperature of −20 °C or lower, the expiry date is not later than 4 years from the date of harvest.

Only a final lot that complies with the following requirement for count of viable units and with each of the requirements given below under Identification, Tests and Assay may be released for use. Provided the test for virulent mycobacteria has been carried out with satisfactory results on the final bulk vaccine, it may be omitted on the final lot. Provided the test for excessive dermal reactivity has been carried out with satisfactory results on the working seed lot and on 5 consecutive final lots produced from it, the test may be omitted on the final lot.

Count of viable units. Determine the number of viable units per millilitre of the reconstituted vaccine by viable count on solid medium using a method suitable for the vaccine to be examined or by a suitable biochemical method. The ratio of the count of viable units after freeze-drying to that before is not less than that approved for the particular product.

IDENTIFICATION

BCG vaccine is identified by microscopic examination of the bacilli in stained smears demonstrating their acid-fast property and by the characteristic appearance of colonies grown on solid medium. Alternatively, molecular biology techniques (for example nucleic acid amplification) may be used.

TESTS

Virulent mycobacteria. Inject subcutaneously or intramuscularly into each of 6 guinea-pigs, each weighing 250-400 g and having received no treatment likely to interfere with the test, a quantity of vaccine equivalent to at least 50 human doses. Observe the animals for at least 42 days. At the end of this period, kill the guinea-pigs and examine by autopsy for signs of infection with tuberculosis, ignoring any minor reactions at the site of injection. Animals that die during the observation period are also examined for signs of tuberculosis. The vaccine complies with the test if none of the guinea-pigs shows signs of tuberculosis and if not more than 1 animal dies during the observation period. If 2 animals die during this period and autopsy does not reveal signs of tuberculosis repeat the test on 6 other guinea-pigs. The vaccine complies with the test if not more than 1 animal dies during the 42 days following the injection and autopsy does not reveal any sign of tuberculosis.

Bacterial and fungal contamination. The reconstituted vaccine complies with the test for sterility (*2.6.1*) except for the presence of mycobacteria.

Excessive dermal reactivity. Use 6 healthy, white or pale-coloured guinea-pigs, each weighing not less than 250 g and having received no treatment likely to interfere with the test. Inject intradermally into each guinea-pig, according to a randomised plan, 0.1 ml of the reconstituted vaccine and of 2 tenfold serial dilutions of the vaccine and identical doses of the comparison vaccine. Observe the lesions formed at the site of the injection for 4 weeks. The vaccine complies with the test if the reaction it produces is not markedly different from that produced by the comparison vaccine.

Temperature stability. Maintain samples of the freeze-dried vaccine at 37 °C for 4 weeks. Determine the number of viable units in the heated vaccine and in unheated vaccine as described below. The number of viable units in the heated vaccine is not less than 20 per cent that in unheated vaccine.

Water. Not more than the limit approved for the particular product, determined by a suitable method.

ASSAY

Determine the number of viable units in the reconstituted vaccine by viable count on solid medium using a method suitable for the vaccine to be examined or by a suitable validated biochemical method. The number is within the range stated on the label. Determine the number of viable units in the comparison vaccine in parallel.

LABELLING

The label states:

- the minimum and maximum number of viable units per millilitre in the reconstituted vaccine,
- that the vaccine must be protected from direct sunlight.

01/2005:0154

CHOLERA VACCINE

Vaccinum cholerae

DEFINITION

Cholera vaccine is a homogeneous suspension of a suitable strain or strains of *Vibrio cholerae* containing not less than 8×10^9 bacteria in each human dose. The human dose does not exceed 1.0 ml.

PRODUCTION

The vaccine is prepared using a seed-lot system. The vaccine consists of a mixture of equal parts of vaccines prepared from smooth strains of the 2 main serological types, Inaba and Ogawa. These may be of the classical biotype with or without the El-Tor biotype. A single strain or several strains of each type may be included. All strains must contain, in addition to their type O antigens, the heat-stable O antigen common to Inaba and Ogawa. If more than one strain each of Inaba and Ogawa are used, these may be selected so as to contain other O antigens in addition. The World Health Organisation recommends new strains which may be used if necessary, in accordance with the regulations in force in the signatory States of the Convention on the Elaboration of a European Pharmacopoeia. In order to comply with the requirements for vaccination certificates required for international travel, the vaccine must contain not less than 8×10^9 organisms of the classical biotype. Each strain is grown separately. The bacteria are inactivated either by heating the suspensions (for example, at 56 °C for 1 h) or by treatment with formaldehyde or phenol or by a combination of the physical and chemical methods.

The production method is validated to demonstrate that the product, if tested, would comply with the test for abnormal toxicity for immunosera and vaccines for human use (*2.6.9*) modified as follows: inject 0.5 ml of the vaccine into each mouse and 1.0 ml into each guinea pig.

IDENTIFICATION

It is identified by specific agglutination tests.

TESTS

Phenol (*2.5.15*). If phenol has been used in the preparation, the concentration is not more than 5 g/l.

Antibody production. Test the ability of the vaccine to induce antibodies (such as agglutinating, vibriocidal or haemagglutinating antibodies) in the guinea-pig, the rabbit or the mouse. Administer the vaccine to a group of at least 6 animals. At the end of the interval of time necessary for maximum antibody formation, determined in preliminary tests, collect sera from the animals and titrate them individually for the appropriate antibody using a suitable method. The vaccine to be examined passes the test if each serotype has elicited a significant antibody response.

Sterility (*2.6.1*). It complies with the test for sterility.

LABELLING

The label states:

– the method used to inactivate the bacteria,

– the number of bacteria in each human dose.

01/2005:0155

CHOLERA VACCINE, FREEZE-DRIED

Vaccinum cholerae cryodesiccatum

DEFINITION

Freeze-dried cholera vaccine is a preparation of a suitable strain or strains of *Vibrio cholerae*. The vaccine is reconstituted as stated on the label to give a uniform suspension containing not less than 8×10^9 bacteria in each human dose. The human dose does not exceed 1.0 ml of the reconstituted vaccine.

PRODUCTION

The vaccine is prepared using a seed-lot system. The vaccine consists of a mixture of equal parts of vaccines prepared from smooth strains of the 2 main serological types, Inaba and Ogawa. These may be of the classical biotype with or without the El-Tor biotype. A single strain or several strains of each type may be included. All strains must contain, in addition to their type O antigens, the heat-stable O antigen common to Inaba and Ogawa. If more than one strain each of Inaba and Ogawa are used, these may be selected so as to contain other O antigens in addition. The World Health Organisation recommends new strains which may be used if necessary in accordance with the regulations in force in the signatory States of the Convention on the Elaboration of a European Pharmacopoeia. In order to comply with the requirements for vaccination certificates required for international travel, the vaccine must contain not less than 8×10^9 organisms of the classical biotype. Each strain is grown separately. The bacteria are inactivated either by heating the suspensions (for example, at 56 °C for 1 h) or by treatment with formaldehyde or by a combination of the physical and chemical methods. Phenol is not used in the preparation. The vaccine is distributed into sterile containers and freeze-dried to a moisture content favourable to the stability of the vaccine. The containers are then closed so as to exclude contamination.

The production method is validated to demonstrate that the product, if tested, would comply with the test for abnormal toxicity for immunosera and vaccines for human use (*2.6.9*) modified as follows: inject 0.5 ml of the vaccine into each mouse and 1.0 ml into each guinea pig.

IDENTIFICATION

The vaccine reconstituted as stated on the label is identified by specific agglutination tests.

TESTS

Phenol (*2.5.15*). If phenol has been used in the preparation, the concentration is not more than 5 g/l.

Antibody production. Test the ability of the vaccine to induce antibodies (such as agglutinating, vibriocidal or haemagglutinating antibodies) in the guinea-pig, the rabbit or the mouse. Administer the reconstituted vaccine to a group of at least 6 animals. At the end of the interval of time necessary for maximum antibody formation, determined in preliminary tests, collect sera from the animals and titrate them individually for the appropriate antibody using a suitable method. The vaccine to be examined passes the test if each serotype has elicited a significant antibody response.

Sterility (*2.6.1*). The reconstituted vaccine complies with the test for sterility.

LABELLING

The label states:

– the method used to inactivate the bacteria,

– the number of bacteria in each human dose.

01/2005:0444

DIPHTHERIA AND TETANUS VACCINE (ADSORBED)

Vaccinum diphtheriae et tetani adsorbatum

DEFINITION

Diphtheria and tetanus vaccine (adsorbed) is a preparation of diphtheria formol toxoid and tetanus formol toxoid with a mineral adsorbent. The formol toxoids are prepared from the toxins produced by the growth of *Corynebacterium diphtheriae* and *Clostridium tetani*, respectively.

PRODUCTION

GENERAL PROVISIONS

Specific toxicity of the diphtheria and tetanus components. The production method is validated to demonstrate that the product, if tested, would comply with the following test: inject subcutaneously 5 times the single human dose stated on the label into each of 5 healthy guinea-pigs, each weighing 250-350 g, that have not previously been treated with any material that will interfere with the test. If within 42 days of the injection any of the animals shows signs of or dies from diphtheria toxaemia or tetanus, the vaccine does not comply with the test. If more than 1 animal dies from non-specific causes, repeat the test once; if more than 1 animal dies in the second test, the vaccine does not comply with the test.

BULK PURIFIED DIPHTHERIA AND TETANUS TOXOIDS

The bulk purified diphtheria and tetanus toxoids are prepared as described in the monographs on *Diphtheria vaccine (adsorbed) (0443)* and *Tetanus vaccine (adsorbed) (0452)* and comply with the requirements prescribed therein.

FINAL BULK VACCINE

The final bulk vaccine is prepared by adsorption of suitable quantities of bulk purified diphtheria toxoid and tetanus toxoid onto a mineral carrier such as hydrated aluminium phosphate or aluminium hydroxide; the resulting mixture is approximately isotonic with blood. Suitable antimicrobial preservatives may be added. Certain antimicrobial preservatives, particularly those of the phenolic type, adversely affect the antigenic activity and must not be used. Only a final bulk vaccine that complies with the following requirements may be used in the preparation of the final lot.

Antimicrobial preservative. Where applicable, determine the amount of antimicrobial preservative by a suitable chemical method. The amount is not less than 85 per cent and not greater than 115 per cent of the intended amount.

Sterility (*2.6.1*). Carry out the test for sterility using 10 ml for each medium.

FINAL LOT

The final bulk vaccine is distributed aseptically into sterile, tamper-proof containers. The containers are closed so as to prevent contamination.

Only a final lot that is satisfactory with respect to each of the requirements given below under Identification, Tests and Assay may be released for use. Provided the test for antimicrobial preservative and the assay have been carried out with satisfactory results on the final bulk vaccine, they may be omitted on the final lot.

Provided the free formaldehyde content has been determined on the bulk purified antigens or on the final bulk and it has been shown that the content in the final lot will not exceed 0.2 g/l, the test for free formaldehyde may be omitted on the final lot.

IDENTIFICATION

A. Diphtheria toxoid is identified by a suitable immunochemical method (*2.7.1*). The following method, applicable to certain vaccines, is given as an example. Dissolve in the vaccine to be examined sufficient *sodium citrate R* to give a 100 g/l solution. Maintain at 37 °C for about 16 h and centrifuge until a clear supernatant liquid is obtained. The clear supernatant liquid reacts with a suitable diphtheria antitoxin, giving a precipitate.

B. Tetanus toxoid is identified by a suitable immunochemical method (*2.7.1*). The following method, applicable to certain vaccines, is given as an example. The clear supernatant liquid obtained as described in identification test A reacts with a suitable tetanus antitoxin, giving a precipitate.

TESTS

Aluminium (*2.5.13*): maximum 1.25 mg per single human dose, if aluminium hydroxide or hydrated aluminium phosphate is used as the adsorbent.

Free formaldehyde (*2.4.18*): maximum 0.2 g/l.

Antimicrobial preservative. Where applicable, determine the amount of antimicrobial preservative by a suitable chemical method. The content is not less than the minimum amount shown to be effective and is not greater than 115 per cent of the quantity stated on the label.

Sterility (*2.6.1*). The vaccine complies with the test for sterility.

ASSAY

Diphtheria component. Carry out one of the prescribed methods for the assay of diphtheria vaccine (adsorbed) (*2.7.6*).

The lower confidence limit (P = 0.95) of the estimated potency is not less than 30 IU per single human dose.

Tetanus component. Carry out one of the prescribed methods for the assay of tetanus vaccine (adsorbed) (*2.7.8*).

The lower confidence limit (P = 0.95) of the estimated potency is not less than 40 IU per single human dose.

LABELLING

The label states:

– the minimum number of International Units of each component per single human dose,
– where applicable, that the vaccine is intended for primary vaccination of children and is not necessarily suitable for reinforcing doses or for administration to adults,
– the name and the amount of the adsorbent,
– that the vaccine must be shaken before use,
– that the vaccine is not to be frozen.

01/2005:0647

DIPHTHERIA AND TETANUS VACCINE (ADSORBED) FOR ADULTS AND ADOLESCENTS

Vaccinum diphtheriae et tetani adulti et adulescentis adsorbatum

DEFINITION

Diphtheria and tetanus vaccine (adsorbed) for adults and adolescents is a preparation of diphtheria formol toxoid and tetanus formol toxoid with a mineral adsorbent. The formol toxoids are prepared from the toxins produced by the growth of *Corynebacterium diphtheriae* and *Clostridium tetani*, respectively. It shall have been demonstrated to the competent authority that the quantity of diphtheria toxoid used does not produce adverse reactions in subjects from the age groups for which the vaccine is intended.

PRODUCTION

GENERAL PROVISIONS

Specific toxicity of the diphtheria and tetanus components. The production method is validated to demonstrate that the product, if tested, would comply with the following test: inject subcutaneously 5 times the single human dose stated on the label into each of 5 healthy guinea-pigs, each weighing 250-350 g, that have not previously been treated with any material that will interfere with the test. If within 42 days of the injection any of the animals shows signs of or dies from diphtheria toxaemia or tetanus, the vaccine does not comply with the test. If more than 1 animal dies from non-specific causes, repeat the test once; if more than 1 animal dies in the second test, the vaccine does not comply with the test.

BULK PURIFIED DIPHTHERIA TOXOID AND TETANUS TOXOIDS

The bulk purified diphtheria and tetanus toxoids are prepared as described in the monographs on *Diphtheria vaccine (adsorbed) (0443)* and *Tetanus vaccine (adsorbed) (0452)* and comply with the requirements prescribed therein.

FINAL BULK VACCINE

The vaccine is prepared by adsorption of suitable quantities of bulk purified diphtheria toxoid and tetanus toxoid onto a mineral carrier such as hydrated aluminium phosphate or aluminium hydroxide; the resulting mixture is approximately isotonic with blood. Suitable antimicrobial preservatives may be added. Certain antimicrobial preservatives, particularly those of the phenolic type, adversely affect the antigenic activity and must not be used.

Only a final bulk vaccine that complies with the following requirements may be used in the preparation of the final lot.

Antimicrobial preservative. Where applicable, determine the amount of antimicrobial preservative by a suitable chemical method. The amount is not less than 85 per cent and not greater than 115 per cent of the intended amount.

Sterility (*2.6.1*). Carry out the test for sterility using 10 ml for each medium.

FINAL LOT

The final bulk vaccine is distributed aseptically into sterile, tamper-proof containers. The containers are closed so as to prevent contamination.

Only a final lot that is satisfactory with respect to each of the requirements given below under Identification, Tests and Assay may be released for use. Provided the test for antimicrobial preservative and the assay have been carried out with satisfactory results on the final bulk vaccine, they may be omitted on the final lot.

Provided the free formaldehyde content has been determined on the bulk purified toxoids or on the final bulk and it has been shown that the content in the final lot will not exceed 0.2 g/l, the test for free formaldehyde may be omitted on the final lot.

IDENTIFICATION

A. Diphtheria toxoid is identified by a suitable immunochemical method (*2.7.1*). The following method, applicable to certain vaccines, is given as an example. Dissolve in the vaccine to be examined sufficient *sodium citrate R* to give a 100 g/l solution. Maintain at 37 °C for about 16 h and centrifuge until a clear supernatant liquid is obtained. The clear supernatant liquid reacts with a suitable diphtheria antitoxin, giving a precipitate. If a satisfactory result is not obtained with a vaccine adsorbed on aluminium hydroxide, carry out the test as follows. Centrifuge 15 ml of the vaccine to be examined and suspend the residue in 5 ml of a freshly prepared mixture of 1 volume of a 56 g/l solution of *sodium edetate R* and 49 volumes of a 90 g/l solution of *disodium hydrogen phosphate R*. Maintain at 37 °C for not less than 6 h and centrifuge. The clear supernatant liquid reacts with a suitable diphtheria antitoxin, giving a precipitate.

B. Tetanus toxoid is identified by a suitable immunochemical method (*2.7.1*). The following method, applicable to certain vaccines, is given as an example. The clear supernatant liquid obtained during identification test A reacts with a suitable tetanus antitoxin, giving a precipitate.

TESTS

Aluminium (*2.5.13*): maximum 1.25 mg per single human dose, if aluminium hydroxide or hydrated aluminium phosphate is used as the adsorbent.

Free formaldehyde (*2.4.18*): maximum 0.2 g/l.

Antimicrobial preservative. Where applicable, determine the amount of antimicrobial preservative by a suitable chemical method. The content is not less than the minimum amount shown to be effective and is not greater than 115 per cent of the quantity stated on the label.

Sterility (*2.6.1*). The vaccine complies with the test for sterility.

ASSAY

Diphtheria component. Carry out one of the prescribed methods for the assay of diphtheria vaccine (adsorbed) (*2.7.6*).

The lower confidence limit (P = 0.95) of the estimated potency is not less than 2 IU per single human dose.

Tetanus component. Carry out one of the prescribed methods for the assay of tetanus vaccine (adsorbed) (*2.7.8*).

The lower confidence limit (P = 0.95) of the estimated potency is not less than 20 IU per single human dose.

LABELLING

The label states:

- the minimum number of International Units of each component per single human dose,
- the name and the amount of the adsorbent,
- that the vaccine must be shaken before use,
- that the vaccine is not to be frozen.

Vaccines

01/2005:2062

DIPHTHERIA, TETANUS AND HEPATITIS B (rDNA) VACCINE (ADSORBED)

Vaccinum diphtheriae, tetani et hepatitidis B (ADNr) adsorbatum

DEFINITION

Diphtheria, tetanus and hepatitis B (rDNA) vaccine (adsorbed) is a combined vaccine composed of: diphtheria formol toxoid; tetanus formol toxoid; hepatitis B surface antigen (HBsAg); a mineral adsorbent such as aluminium hydroxide or hydrated aluminium phosphate.

The formol toxoids are prepared from the toxins produced by the growth of *Corynebacterium diphtheriae* and *Clostridium tetani*, respectively.

HBsAg is a component protein of hepatitis B virus; the antigen is obtained by recombinant DNA technology.

PRODUCTION

GENERAL PROVISIONS

The production method shall have been shown to yield consistently vaccines comparable with the vaccine of proven clinical efficacy and safety in man.

The content of bacterial endotoxins (*2.6.14*) in the bulk purified diphtheria toxoid and tetanus toxoid is determined to monitor the purification procedure and to limit the amount in the final vaccine. For each component, the content of bacterial endotoxins is less than the limit approved for the particular vaccine and in any case the contents are such that the final vaccine contains less than 100 IU per single human dose.

Reference vaccine(s). Provided valid assays can be performed, monocomponent reference vaccines may be used for the assays on the combined vaccine. If this is not possible because of interaction between the components of the combined vaccine or because of the difference in composition between monocomponent reference vaccine and the test vaccine, a batch of combined vaccine shown to be effective in clinical trials or a batch representative thereof is used as a reference vaccine. For the preparation of a representative batch, strict adherence to the production process used for the batch tested in clinical trials is necessary. The reference vaccine may be stabilised by a method that has been shown to have no effect on the assay procedure.

Specific toxicity of the diphtheria and tetanus components. The production method is validated to demonstrate that the product, if tested, would comply with the following test: inject subcutaneously 5 times the single human dose stated on the label into each of 5 healthy guinea-pigs, each weighing 250-350 g, that have not previously been treated with any material that will interfere with the test. If within 42 days of the injection any of the animals shows signs of or dies from diphtheria toxaemia or tetanus, the vaccine does not comply with the test. If more than 1 animal dies from non-specific causes, repeat the test once; if more than 1 animal dies in the second test, the vaccine does not comply with the test.

PRODUCTION OF THE COMPONENTS

The production of the components complies with the requirements of the monographs on *Diphtheria vaccine (adsorbed) (0443)*, *Tetanus vaccine (adsorbed) (0452)* and *Hepatitis B vaccine (rDNA) (1056)*.

FINAL BULK VACCINE

The final bulk vaccine is prepared by adsorption, separately or together, of suitable quantities of bulk purified diphtheria toxoid, tetanus toxoid and HBsAg onto a mineral carrier such as aluminium hydroxide or hydrated aluminium phosphate. Suitable antimicrobial preservatives may be added.

Only a final bulk vaccine that complies with the following requirements may be used in the preparation of the final lot.

Antimicrobial preservative. Where applicable, determine the amount of antimicrobial preservative by a suitable chemical method. The amount is not less than 85 per cent and not greater than 115 per cent of the intended content.

Sterility (*2.6.1*). Carry out the test for sterility using 10 ml for each medium.

FINAL LOT

Only a final lot that is satisfactory with respect to the test for osmolality and with respect to each of the requirements given below under Identification, Tests and Assay may be released for use.

Provided the test for antimicrobial preservative and the assays for the diphtheria and tetanus components have been carried out with satisfactory results on the final bulk vaccine, they may be omitted on the final lot.

Provided the content of free formaldehyde has been determined on the bulk purified antigens or on the final bulk and it has been shown that the content in the final lot will not exceed 0.2 g/l, the test for free formaldehyde may be omitted on the final lot.

If an *in vivo* assay is used for the hepatitis B component, provided it has been carried out with satisfactory results on the final bulk vaccine, it may be omitted on the final lot.

Osmolality (*2.2.35*). The osmolality of the vaccine is within the limits approved for the particular preparation.

IDENTIFICATION

A. Diphtheria toxoid is identified by a suitable immunochemical method (*2.7.1*). The following method, applicable to certain vaccines, is given as an example. Dissolve in the vaccine to be examined sufficient *sodium citrate R* to give a 100 g/l solution. Maintain at 37 °C for about 16 h and centrifuge until a clear supernatant liquid is obtained. The clear supernatant liquid reacts with a suitable diphtheria antitoxin, giving a precipitate.

B. Tetanus toxoid is identified by a suitable immunochemical method (*2.7.1*). The following method, applicable to certain vaccines, is given as an example. The clear supernatant liquid obtained during identification test A reacts with a suitable tetanus antitoxin, giving a precipitate.

C. The assay or, where applicable, the electrophoretic profile, serves also to identify the hepatitis B component of the vaccine.

TESTS

Aluminium (*2.5.13*): maximum 1.25 mg per single human dose, if aluminium hydroxide or hydrated aluminium phosphate is used as the adsorbent.

Free formaldehyde (*2.4.18*): maximum 0.2 g/l.

Antimicrobial preservative. Where applicable, determine the amount of antimicrobial preservative by a suitable chemical method. The content is not less than the minimum amount shown to be effective and is not greater than 115 per cent of the quantity stated on the label.

Sterility (*2.6.1*). It complies with the test for sterility.

Vaccines

Pyrogens (*2.6.8*). It complies with the test for pyrogens. Inject the equivalent of 1 human dose into each rabbit.

ASSAY

Diphtheria component. Carry out one of the prescribed methods for the assay of diphtheria vaccine (adsorbed) (*2.7.6*).

The lower confidence limit (P = 0.95) of the estimated potency is not less than 30 IU per single human dose.

Tetanus component. Carry out one of the prescribed methods for the assay of tetanus vaccine (adsorbed) (*2.7.8*).

The lower confidence limit (P = 0.95) of the estimated potency is not less than 40 IU per single human dose.

Hepatitis B component. It complies with the assay of hepatitis B vaccine (*2.7.15*).

LABELLING

The label states:

- the minimum number of International Units of diphtheria and tetanus toxoid per single human dose,
- the amount of HBsAg per single human dose,
- the type of cells used for production of the HBsAg component,
- where applicable, that the vaccine is intended for primary vaccination of children and is not necessarily suitable for reinforcing doses or for administration to adults,
- the name and the amount of the adsorbent,
- that the vaccine must be shaken before use,
- that the vaccine is not to be frozen.

01/2005:1931

DIPHTHERIA, TETANUS AND PERTUSSIS (ACELLULAR, COMPONENT) VACCINE (ADSORBED)

Vaccinum diphtheriae, tetani et pertussis sine cellulis ex elementis praeparatum adsorbatum

DEFINITION

Diphtheria, tetanus and pertussis (acellular, component) vaccine (adsorbed) is a combined vaccine composed of: diphtheria formol toxoid; tetanus formol toxoid; individually purified antigenic components of *Bordetella pertussis*; a mineral adsorbent such as aluminium hydroxide or hydrated aluminium phosphate.

The formol toxoids are prepared from the toxins produced by the growth of *Corynebacterium diphtheriae* and *Clostridium tetani*, respectively.

The vaccine contains either pertussis toxoid or a pertussis-toxin-like protein free from toxic properties, produced by expression of a genetically modified form of the corresponding gene. Pertussis toxoid is prepared from pertussis toxin by a method that renders the latter harmless while maintaining adequate immunogenic properties and avoiding reversion to toxin. The vaccine may also contain filamentous haemagglutinin, pertactin (a 69 kDa outer-membrane protein) and other defined components of *B. pertussis* such as fimbrial-2 and fimbrial-3 antigens. The latter 2 antigens may be copurified. The antigenic composition and characteristics are based on evidence of protection and freedom from unexpected reactions in the target group for which the vaccine is intended.

PRODUCTION

GENERAL PROVISIONS

The production method shall have been shown to yield consistently vaccines comparable with the vaccine of proven clinical efficacy and safety in man.

The content of bacterial endotoxins (*2.6.14*) in the bulk purified diphtheria toxoid, tetanus toxoid and pertussis components is determined to monitor the purification procedure and to limit the amount in the final vaccine. For each component, the content of bacterial endotoxins is less than the limit approved for the particular vaccine and, in any case, the contents are such that the final vaccine contains less than 100 IU per single human dose.

Reference vaccine(s). Provided valid assays can be performed, monocomponent reference vaccines may be used for the assays on the combined vaccine. If this is not possible because of interaction between the components of the combined vaccine or because of the difference in composition between monocomponent reference vaccine and the test vaccine, a batch of combined vaccine shown to be effective in clinical trials or a batch representative thereof is used as a reference vaccine. For the preparation of a representative batch, strict adherence to the production process used for the batch tested in clinical trials is necessary. The reference vaccine may be stabilised by a method that has been shown to have no effect on the assay procedure.

PRODUCTION OF THE COMPONENTS

The production of the components complies with the requirements of the monographs on *Diphtheria vaccine (adsorbed) (0443)*, *Tetanus vaccine (adsorbed) (0452)* and *Pertussis vaccine (acellular, component, adsorbed) (1356)*.

FINAL BULK VACCINE

The final bulk vaccine is prepared by adsorption of suitable quantities of bulk purified diphtheria toxoid, tetanus toxoid and pertussis components separately or together onto a mineral carrier such as aluminium hydroxide or hydrated aluminium phosphate. Suitable antimicrobial preservatives may be added.

Only a final bulk vaccine that complies with the following requirements may be used in the preparation of the final lot.

Antimicrobial preservative. Where applicable, determine the amount of antimicrobial preservative by a suitable chemical method. The amount is not less than 85 per cent and not greater than 115 per cent of the intended content.

Sterility (*2.6.1*). Carry out the test for sterility using 10 ml for each medium.

FINAL LOT

Only a final lot that is satisfactory with respect to the test for osmolality and with respect to each of the requirements given below under Identification, Tests and Assay may be released for use.

Provided the tests for absence of residual pertussis toxin, irreversibility of pertussis toxoid, free formaldehyde and antimicrobial preservative and the assay have been carried out with satisfactory results on the final bulk vaccine, they may be omitted on the final lot.

Osmolality (*2.2.35*). The osmolality of the vaccine is within the limits approved for the particular preparation.

IDENTIFICATION

A. Diphtheria toxoid is identified by a suitable immunochemical method (*2.7.1*). The following method, applicable to certain vaccines, is given as an example. Dissolve in the vaccine to be examined sufficient *sodium citrate R* to give a 100 g/l solution. Maintain at 37 °C for about 16 h and centrifuge until a clear supernatant liquid is obtained. The clear supernatant liquid reacts with a suitable diphtheria antitoxin, giving a precipitate.

B. Tetanus toxoid is identified by a suitable immunochemical method (*2.7.1*). The following method, applicable to certain vaccines, is given as an example. The clear supernatant liquid obtained as described in identification test A reacts with a suitable tetanus antitoxin, giving a precipitate.

C. The pertussis components are identified by a suitable immunochemical method (*2.7.1*). The following method, applicable to certain vaccines, is given as an example. The clear supernatant liquid obtained as described in identification test A reacts with specific antisera to the pertussis components of the vaccine.

TESTS

Absence of residual pertussis toxin and irreversibility of pertussis toxoid. *This test is not necessary for the product obtained by genetic modification.* Use 3 groups each of not fewer than 5 histamine-sensitive mice. Inject intraperitoneally into the first group twice the single human dose of the vaccine stored at 2-8 °C. Inject intraperitoneally into the second group twice the single human dose of the vaccine incubated at 37 °C for 4 weeks. Inject diluent into the third group of mice. After 5 days, inject into each mouse 2 mg of histamine base intraperitoneally in a volume not exceeding 0.5 ml and observe for 24 h. The test is invalid if 1 or more control mice die following histamine challenge. The vaccine complies with the test if no animal in the first or second group dies following histamine challenge. If 1 mouse dies in either or both of the first and second groups, the test may be repeated with the same number of mice or with a greater number and the results of valid tests combined; the vaccine complies with the test if, in both of the groups given the vaccine, not more than 5 per cent of the total number of mice die following histamine challenge.

The histamine sensitivity of the strain of mice used is verified at suitable intervals as follows: inject intravenously threefold dilutions of a reference pertussis toxin preparation in phosphate-buffered saline solution containing 2 g/l of gelatin and challenge with histamine as above; the strain is suitable if more than 50 per cent of the animals are sensitised by 50 ng of pertussis toxin and none of the control animals injected with only diluent and challenged similarly with histamine show symptoms of sensitisation.

Aluminium (*2.5.13*): maximum 1.25 mg per single human dose, if aluminium hydroxide or hydrated aluminium phosphate is used as the adsorbent.

Free formaldehyde (*2.4.18*): maximum 0.2 g/l.

Antimicrobial preservative. Where applicable, determine the amount of antimicrobial preservative by a suitable chemical method. The content is not less than the minimum amount shown to be effective and is not greater than 115 per cent of the quantity stated on the label.

Sterility (*2.6.1*). The vaccine complies with the test for sterility.

ASSAY

Diphtheria component. Carry out one of the prescribed methods for the assay of diphtheria vaccine (adsorbed) (*2.7.6*).

The lower confidence limit (P = 0.95) of the estimated potency is not less than the minimum potency stated on the label.

Unless otherwise justified and authorised, the minimum potency stated on the label is 30 IU per single human dose.

Tetanus component. Carry out one of the prescribed methods for the assay of tetanus vaccine (adsorbed) (*2.7.8*).

The lower confidence limit (P = 0.95) of the estimated potency is not less than 40 IU per single human dose.

Pertussis component. The vaccine complies with the assay of pertussis vaccine (acellular) (*2.7.16*).

LABELLING

The label states:

- the minimum number of International Units of diphtheria and tetanus toxoid per single human dose,
- the names and amounts of the pertussis components per single human dose,
- where applicable, that the vaccine is intended for primary vaccination of children and is not necessarily suitable for reinforcing doses or for administration to adults,
- the name and the amount of the adsorbent,
- that the vaccine must be shaken before use,
- that the vaccine is not to be frozen,
- where applicable, that the vaccine contains a pertussis toxin-like protein produced by genetic modification.

01/2005:0445

DIPHTHERIA, TETANUS AND PERTUSSIS VACCINE (ADSORBED)

Vaccinum diphtheriae, tetani et pertussis adsorbatum

DEFINITION

Diphtheria, tetanus and pertussis vaccine (adsorbed) is a preparation of diphtheria formol toxoid and tetanus formol toxoid with a mineral adsorbent to which a suspension of inactivated *Bordetella pertussis* has been added. The formol toxoids are prepared from the toxins produced by the growth of *Corynebacterium diphtheriae* and *Clostridium tetani*, respectively.

PRODUCTION

GENERAL PROVISIONS

Specific toxicity of the diphtheria and tetanus components. The production method is validated to demonstrate that the product, if tested, would comply with the following test: inject subcutaneously 5 times the single human dose stated on the label into each of 5 healthy guinea-pigs, each weighing 250-350 g, that have not previously been treated with any material that will interfere with the test. If within 42 days of the injection any of the animals shows signs of or dies from diphtheria toxaemia or tetanus, the vaccine does not comply with the test. If more than 1 animal dies from non-specific causes, repeat the test once; if more than 1 animal dies in the second test, the vaccine does not comply with the test.

BULK PURIFIED DIPHTHERIA AND TETANUS TOXOIDS, BULK INACTIVATED B. PERTUSSIS SUSPENSION

The bulk purified diphtheria and tetanus toxoids and the inactivated *B. pertussis* suspension are prepared as described in the monographs on *Diphtheria vaccine (adsorbed) (0443)*, *Tetanus vaccine (adsorbed) (0452)* and *Pertussis vaccine (adsorbed) (0161)*, respectively, and comply with the requirements prescribed therein.

FINAL BULK VACCINE

The final bulk vaccine is prepared by adsorption of suitable quantities of bulk purified diphtheria toxoid and tetanus toxoid onto a mineral carrier such as hydrated aluminium phosphate or aluminium hydroxide and admixture of an appropriate quantity of a suspension of inactivated *B. pertussis*; the resulting mixture is approximately isotonic with blood. The *B. pertussis* concentration of the final bulk vaccine does not exceed that corresponding to an opacity of 20 IU per single human dose. If 2 or more strains of *B. pertussis* are used, the composition of consecutive lots of the final bulk vaccine shall be consistent with respect to the proportion of each strain as measured in opacity units. Suitable antimicrobial preservatives may be added to the bulk vaccine. Certain antimicrobial preservatives, particularly those of the phenolic type, adversely affect the antigenic activity and must not be used.

Only a final bulk vaccine that complies with the following requirements may be used in the preparation of the final lot.

Antimicrobial preservative. Where applicable, determine the amount of antimicrobial preservative by a suitable chemical method. The amount is not less than 85 per cent and not greater than 115 per cent of the intended amount.

Sterility (*2.6.1*). Carry out the test for sterility using 10 ml for each medium.

FINAL LOT

The final bulk vaccine is distributed aseptically into sterile, tamper-proof containers. The containers are closed so as to prevent contamination.

Only a final lot that is satisfactory with respect to each of the requirements given below under Identification, Tests and Assay may be released for use. Provided the tests for specific toxicity of the pertussis component, antimicrobial preservative and the assay have been carried out with satisfactory results on the final bulk vaccine, they may be omitted on the final lot.

Provided the free formaldehyde content has been determined on the bulk purified antigens or on the final bulk and it has been shown that the content in the final lot will not exceed 0.2 g/l, the test for free formaldehyde may be omitted on the final lot.

IDENTIFICATION

A. Diphtheria toxoid is identified by a suitable immunochemical method (*2.7.1*). The following method, applicable to certain vaccines, is given as an example. Dissolve in the vaccine to be examined sufficient *sodium citrate R* to give a 100 g/l solution. Maintain at 37 °C for about 16 h and centrifuge until a clear supernatant liquid is obtained; reserve the precipitate for identification test C. The clear supernatant liquid reacts with a suitable diphtheria antitoxin, giving a precipitate.

B. Tetanus toxoid is identified by a suitable immunochemical method (*2.7.1*). The following method, applicable to certain vaccines, is given as an example. The clear supernatant liquid obtained during identification test A reacts with a suitable tetanus antitoxin, giving a precipitate.

C. Dissolve in the vaccine to be examined sufficient *sodium citrate R* to give a 100 g/l solution. Maintain at 37 °C for about 16 h and centrifuge to obtain a bacterial precipitate. Other suitable methods for separating the bacteria from the adsorbent may also be used. Identify pertussis vaccine by agglutination of the bacteria from the resuspended precipitate by antisera specific to *B. pertussis* or by the assay.

TESTS

Specific toxicity of the pertussis component. Use not fewer than 5 mice each weighing 14 g to 16 g for the vaccine group and for the saline control. Use mice of the same sex or distribute males and females equally between the groups. Allow the animals access to food and water for at least 2 h before injection and during the test. Inject each mouse of the vaccine group intraperitoneally with 0.5 ml, containing a quantity of the vaccine equivalent to not less than half the single human dose. Inject each mouse of the control group with 0.5 ml of a 9 g/l sterile solution of *sodium chloride R*, preferably containing the same amount of antimicrobial preservative as that injected with the vaccine. Weigh the groups of mice immediately before the injection and 72 h and 7 days after the injection. The vaccine complies with the test if: (a) at the end of 72 h the total mass of the group of vaccinated mice is not less than that preceding the injection; (b) at the end of 7 days the average increase in mass per vaccinated mouse is not less than 60 per cent of that per control mouse; and (c) not more than 5 per cent of the vaccinated mice die during the test. The test may be repeated and the results of the tests combined.

Aluminium (*2.5.13*): maximum 1.25 mg per single human dose, if aluminium hydroxide or hydrated aluminium phosphate is used as the adsorbent.

Free formaldehyde (*2.4.18*): maximum 0.2 g/l.

Antimicrobial preservative. Where applicable, determine the amount of antimicrobial preservative by a suitable chemical method. The content is not less than the minimum amount shown to be effective and is not greater than 115 per cent of the quantity stated on the label.

Sterility (*2.6.1*). The vaccine complies with the test for sterility.

ASSAY

Diphtheria component. Carry out one of the prescribed methods for the assay of diphtheria vaccine (adsorbed) (*2.7.6*).

The lower confidence limit ($P = 0.95$) of the estimated potency is not less than 30 IU per single human dose.

Tetanus component. Carry out one of the prescribed methods for the assay of tetanus vaccine (adsorbed) (*2.7.8*).

If the test is carried out in guinea-pigs, the lower confidence limit ($P = 0.95$) of the estimated potency is not less than 40 IU per single human dose; if the test is carried out in mice, the lower confidence limit ($P = 0.95$) of the estimated potency is not less than 60 IU per single human dose.

Pertussis component. Carry out the assay of pertussis vaccine (*2.7.7*).

The estimated potency is not less than 4 IU per single human dose and the lower confidence limit ($P = 0.95$) of the estimated potency is not less than 2 IU per single human dose.

LABELLING

The label states:

- the minimum number of International Units of each component per single human dose,
- where applicable, that the vaccine is intended for primary vaccination of children and is not necessarily suitable for reinforcing doses or for administration to adults,
- the name and the amount of the adsorbent,
- that the vaccine must be shaken before use,
- that the vaccine is not to be frozen.

01/2005:1932

DIPHTHERIA, TETANUS, PERTUSSIS (ACELLULAR, COMPONENT) AND HAEMOPHILUS TYPE b CONJUGATE VACCINE (ADSORBED)

Vaccinum diphtheriae, tetani, pertussis sine cellulis ex elementis praeparatum et haemophili stirpe b coniugatum adsorbatum

DEFINITION

Diphtheria, tetanus, pertussis (acellular, component) and haemophilus type b conjugate vaccine (adsorbed) is a combined vaccine composed of: diphtheria formol toxoid; tetanus formol toxoid; individually purified antigenic components of *Bordetella pertussis*; polyribosylribitol phosphate (PRP) covalently bound to a carrier protein; a mineral absorbent such as aluminium hydroxide or hydrated aluminium phosphate. The product may be presented with the haemophilus type b component in a separate container, the contents of which are mixed with the other components immediately before use.

The formol toxoids are prepared from the toxins produced by the growth of *Corynebacterium diphtheriae* and *Clostridium tetani* respectively.

The vaccine contains either pertussis toxoid or a pertussis-toxin-like protein free from toxic properties produced by expression of a genetically modified form of the corresponding gene. Pertussis toxoid is prepared from pertussis toxin by a method that renders the toxin harmless while maintaining adequate immunogenic properties and avoiding reversion to toxin. The acellular pertussis component may also contain filamentous haemagglutinin, pertactin (a 69 kDa outer-membrane protein) and other defined components of *B. pertussis* such as fimbrial-2 and fimbrial-3 antigens. The latter 2 antigens may be copurified. The antigenic composition and characteristics are based on evidence of protection and freedom from unexpected reactions in the target group for which the vaccine is intended.

PRP is a linear copolymer composed of repeated units of 3-β-D-ribofuranosyl-(1→1)-ribitol-5-phosphate [$(C_{10}H_{19}O_{12}P)_n$], with a defined molecular size and derived from a suitable strain of *Haemophilus influenzae* type b. The carrier protein, when conjugated to PRP, is capable of inducing a T-cell-dependent B-cell immune response to the polysaccharide.

PRODUCTION

GENERAL PROVISIONS

The production method shall have been shown to yield consistently vaccines comparable with the vaccine of proven clinical efficacy and safety in man.

If the vaccine is presented with the haemophilus component in a separate vial, as part of consistency studies the assays of the diphtheria, tetanus and pertussis components are carried out on a suitable number of batches of vaccine reconstituted as for use. For subsequent routine control, the assays of these components may be carried out without mixing with the haemophilus component.

The content of bacterial endotoxins (*2.6.14*) in bulk purified diphtheria toxoid, tetanus toxoid, pertussis components and PRP conjugate is determined to monitor the purification procedure and to limit the amount in the final vaccine. For each component, the content of bacterial endotoxins is less than the limit approved for the particular vaccine; if the vaccine is presented with the haemophilus component in a separate container, the contents of the diphtheria, tetanus and pertussis antigens are in any case such that the final vial for these components contains less than 100 IU per single human dose.

The production method is validated to demonstrate that the product, if tested, would comply with the test for abnormal toxicity for immunosera and vaccines for human use (*2.6.9*).

During development studies and wherever revalidation is necessary, it shall be demonstrated by tests in animals that the vaccine induces a T-cell dependent B-cell immune response to PRP.

Reference vaccine(s). Provided valid assays can be performed, monocomponent reference vaccines may be used for the assays on the combined vaccine. If this is not possible because of interaction between the components of the combined vaccine or because of the difference in composition between monocomponent reference vaccine and the test vaccine, a batch of combined vaccine shown to be effective in clinical trials or a batch representative thereof is used as a reference vaccine. For the preparation of a representative batch, strict adherence to the production process used for the batch tested in clinical trials is necessary. The reference vaccine may be stabilised by a method that has been shown to have no effect on the assay procedure.

PRODUCTION OF THE COMPONENTS

The production of the components complies with the requirements of the monographs on *Diphtheria vaccine (adsorbed) (0443)*, *Tetanus vaccine (adsorbed) (0452)*, *Pertussis vaccine (acellular, component, adsorbed) (1356)* and *Haemophilus type b conjugate vaccine (1219)*.

FINAL BULK VACCINE

Different methods of preparation may be used: a final bulk vaccine may be prepared by adsorption, separately or together, of suitable quantities of bulk purified diphtheria toxoid, tetanus toxoid, acellular pertussis components and PRP conjugate onto a mineral carrier such as aluminium hydroxide or hydrated aluminium phosphate; or 2 final bulks may be prepared and filled separately, one containing the diphtheria, tetanus and pertussis components, the other the haemophilus component, which may be freeze-dried. Suitable antimicrobial preservatives may be added.

Only a final bulk vaccine that complies with the following requirements may be used in the preparation of the final lot.

Antimicrobial preservative. Where applicable, determine the amount of antimicrobial preservative by a suitable chemical method. The amount is not less than 85 per cent and not greater than 115 per cent of the intended content.

Sterility (*2.6.1*). Carry out the test for sterility using 10 ml for each medium.

FINAL LOT

Only a final lot that is satisfactory with respect to the test for osmolality shown below and with respect to each of the requirements given below under Identification, Tests and Assay may be released for use.

Provided the tests for absence of residual pertussis toxin, irreversibility of pertussis toxoid and antimicrobial preservative and the assay have been carried out with satisfactory results on the final bulk vaccine, they may be omitted on the final lot.

Vaccines

Provided the free formaldehyde content has been determined on the bulk purified antigens or the final bulk and it has been shown that the content in the final lot will not exceed 0.2 g/l, the test for free formaldehyde may be omitted on the final lot.

Osmolality. (*2.2.35*). The osmolality of the vaccine, reconstituted where applicable, is within the limits approved for the particular preparation.

pH (*2.2.3*). The pH of the vaccine, reconstituted if necessary, is within the range approved for the particular product.

Free PRP. Unbound PRP is determined after removal of the conjugate, for example by anion-exchange, size-exclusion or hydrophobic chromatography, ultrafiltration or other validated methods. The amount of free PRP is not greater than that approved for the particular product.

IDENTIFICATION

If the vaccine is presented with the haemophilus component in a separate vial: identification tests A, B and C are carried out using the vial containing the diphtheria, tetanus and pertussis components; identification test D is carried out on the vial containing the haemophilus components.

A. Diphtheria toxoid is identified by a suitable immunochemical method (*2.7.1*). The following method, applicable to certain vaccines, is given as an example. Dissolve in the vaccine to be examined sufficient *sodium citrate R* to give a 100 g/l solution. Maintain at 37 °C for about 16 h and centrifuge until a clear supernatant liquid is obtained. The clear supernatant liquid reacts with a suitable diphtheria antitoxin, giving a precipitate.

B. Tetanus toxoid is identified by a suitable immunochemical method (*2.7.1*). The following method, applicable to certain vaccines, is given as an example. The clear supernatant liquid obtained as described in identification test A reacts with a suitable tetanus antitoxin, giving a precipitate.

C. The pertussis components are identified by a suitable immunochemical method (*2.7.1*). The following method, applicable to certain vaccines, is given as an example. The clear supernatant liquid obtained as described in identification test A reacts with a specific antisera to the pertussis components of the vaccine.

D. The haemophilus component is identified by a suitable immunochemical method (*2.7.1*) for PRP.

TESTS

If the product is presented with the haemophilus component in a separate container: the tests for absence of residual pertussis toxin, irreversibility of pertussis toxoid, aluminium, free formaldehyde, antimicrobial preservative and sterility are carried out on the container with the diphtheria, tetanus and pertussis components; the tests for PRP content, water (where applicable), sterility and pyrogens are carried out on the container with the haemophilus component.

If the haemophilus component is freeze-dried, some tests may be carried out on the freeze-dried product rather than on the bulk conjugate where the freeze-drying process may affect the component to be tested.

Absence of residual pertussis toxin and irreversibility of pertussis toxoid. *This test is not necessary for the product obtained by genetic modification.* Use 3 groups each of not fewer than 5 histamine-sensitive mice. Inject intraperitoneally into the first group twice the single human dose of the vaccine stored at 2-8 °C. Inject intraperitoneally into the second group twice the single human dose of the vaccine incubated at 37 °C for 4 weeks. Inject diluent into the third group of mice. After 5 days, inject into each mouse 2 mg of histamine base intraperitoneally in a volume not exceeding 0.5 ml and observe for 24 h. The test is invalid if 1 or more control mice die following histamine challenge. The vaccine complies with the test if no animal in the first or second group dies following histamine challenge. If 1 mouse dies in either or both of the first and second groups, the test may be repeated with the same number of mice or with a greater number and the results of valid tests combined; the vaccine complies with the test if, in both of the groups given the vaccine, not more than 5 per cent of the total number of mice die following histamine challenge.

The histamine sensitivity of the strain of mice used is verified at suitable intervals as follows: inject intravenously threefold dilutions of a reference pertussis toxin preparation in phosphate-buffered saline solution containing 2 g/l of gelatin and challenge with histamine as above; the strain is suitable if more than 50 per cent of the animals are sensitised by 50 ng of pertussis toxin and none of the control animals injected with only diluent and challenged similarly with histamine show symptoms of sensitisation.

PRP: minimum 80 per cent of the amount of PRP stated on the label. PRP is determined either by assay of ribose (*2.5.31*) or phosphorus (*2.5.18*), by an immunochemical method (*2.7.1*) or by anion-exchange liquid chromatography (*2.2.29*) with pulsed-amperometric detection.

Aluminium (*2.5.13*): maximum 1.25 mg per single human dose, if aluminium hydroxide or hydrated aluminium phosphate is used as the adsorbent.

Free formaldehyde (*2.4.18*): maximum 0.2 g/l.

Antimicrobial preservative. Where applicable, determine the amount of antimicrobial preservative by a suitable chemical method. The content is not less than the minimum amount shown to be effective and is not greater than 115 per cent of the quantity stated on the label.

Water (*2.5.12*): maximum 3.0 per cent for the freeze-dried haemophilus component.

Sterility (*2.6.1*). It complies with the test for sterility.

Pyrogens (*2.6.8*). It complies with the test for pyrogens. Inject per kilogram of the rabbit's mass a quantity of the vaccine equivalent to: 1 μg of PRP for a vaccine with diphtheria toxoid or CRM 197 diphtheria protein as carrier; 0.1 μg of PRP for a vaccine with tetanus toxoid as carrier; 0.025 μg of PRP for a vaccine with OMP as carrier.

ASSAY

Diphtheria component. Carry out one of the prescribed methods for the assay of diphtheria vaccine (adsorbed) (*2.7.6*).

The lower confidence limit (P = 0.95) of the estimated potency is not less than the minimum potency stated on the label.

Unless otherwise justified and authorised, the minimum potency stated on the label is 30 IU per single human dose.

Tetanus component. Carry out one of the prescribed methods for the assay of tetanus vaccine (adsorbed) (*2.7.8*).

The lower confidence limit (P = 0.95) of the estimated potency is not less than 40 IU per single human dose.

Pertussis component. The vaccine complies with the assay of pertussis vaccine (acellular) (*2.7.16*).

LABELLING

The label states:

– the minimum number of International Units of diphtheria and tetanus toxoid per single human dose,

Vaccines

- the names and amounts of the pertussis components per single human dose,
- the number of micrograms of PRP per single human dose,
- the type and nominal amount of carrier protein per single human dose,
- where applicable, that the vaccine is intended for primary vaccination of children and is not necessarily suitable for reinforcing doses or for administration to adults,
- the name and the amount of the adsorbent,
- that the vaccine must be shaken before use,
- that the vaccine is not to be frozen,
- where applicable, that the vaccine contains a pertussis toxin-like protein produced by genetic modification.

01/2005:1933

DIPHTHERIA, TETANUS, PERTUSSIS (ACELLULAR, COMPONENT) AND HEPATITIS B (rDNA) VACCINE (ADSORBED)

Vaccinum diphtheriae, tetani, pertussis sine cellulis ex elementis praeparatum et hepatitidis B (ADNr) adsorbatum

DEFINITION

Diphtheria, tetanus, pertussis (acellular, component) and hepatitis B (rDNA) vaccine (adsorbed) is a combined vaccine composed of: diphtheria formol toxoid; tetanus formol toxoid; individually purified antigenic components of *Bordella pertussis*; hepatitis B surface antigen; a mineral adsorbent such as aluminium hydroxide or hydrated aluminium phosphate.

The formol toxoids are prepared from the toxins produced by the growth of *Corynebacterium diphtheriae* and *Clostridium tetani*, respectively.

The vaccine contains either pertussis toxoid or a pertussis-toxin-like protein free from toxic properties, produced by expression of a genetically modified form of the corresponding gene. Pertussis toxoid is prepared from pertussis toxin by a method that renders the latter harmless while maintaining adequate immunogenic properties and avoiding reversion to toxin. The vaccine may also contain filamentous haemagglutinin, pertactin (a 69 kDa outer-membrane protein) and other defined components of *B. pertussis* such as fimbrial-2 and fimbrial-3 antigens. The latter 2 antigens may be copurified. The antigenic composition and characteristics are based on evidence of protection and freedom from unexpected reactions in the target group for which the vaccine is intended.

Hepatitis B surface antigen is a component protein of hepatitis B virus; the antigen is obtained by recombinant DNA technology.

PRODUCTION

GENERAL PROVISIONS

The production method shall have been shown to yield consistently vaccines comparable with the vaccine of proven clinical efficacy and safety in man.

The content of bacterial endotoxins (*2.6.14*) in the bulk purified diphtheria toxoid, tetanus toxoid and pertussis components is determined to monitor the purification procedure and to limit the amount in the final vaccine. For each component, the content of bacterial endotoxins is less than the limit approved for the particular vaccine.

Reference vaccine(s). Provided valid assays can be performed, monocomponent reference vaccines may be used for the assays on the combined vaccine. If this is not possible because of interaction between the components of the combined vaccine or because of the difference in composition between monocomponent reference vaccine and the test vaccine, a batch of combined vaccine shown to be effective in clinical trials or a batch representative thereof is used as a reference vaccine. For the preparation of a representative batch, strict adherence to the production process used for the batch tested in clinical trials is necessary. The reference vaccine may be stabilised by a method that has been shown to have no effect on the assay procedure.

PRODUCTION OF THE COMPONENTS

The production of the components complies with the requirements of the monographs on *Diphtheria vaccine (adsorbed) (0443)*, *Tetanus vaccine (adsorbed) (0452)*, *Pertussis vaccine (acellular, component, adsorbed) (1356)* and *Hepatitis B vaccine (rDNA) (1056)*.

FINAL BULK VACCINE

The final bulk vaccine is prepared by adsorption, separately or together, of suitable quantities of bulk purified diphtheria toxoid, tetanus toxoid, acellular pertussis components and hepatitis B surface antigen onto a mineral carrier such as aluminium hydroxide or hydrated aluminium phosphate. Suitable antimicrobial preservatives may be added.

Only a final bulk vaccine that complies with the following requirements may be used in the preparation of the final lot.

Antimicrobial preservative. Where applicable, determine the amount of antimicrobial preservative by a suitable chemical method. The amount is not less than 85 per cent and not greater than 115 per cent of the intended content.

Sterility (*2.6.1*). Carry out the test for sterility using 10 ml for each medium.

FINAL LOT

Only a final lot that is satisfactory with respect to the test for osmolality and with respect to each of the requirements given below under Identification, Tests and Assay may be released for use.

Provided the tests for absence of residual pertussis toxin, irreversibility of pertussis toxoid and antimicrobial preservative and the assays for the diphtheria, tetanus and pertussis components have been carried out with satisfactory results on the final bulk vaccine, they may be omitted on the final lot.

Provided the content of free formaldehyde has been determined on the bulk purified antigens or on the final bulk and it has been shown that the content in the final lot will not exceed 0.2 g/l, the test for free formaldehyde may be omitted on the final lot.

If an *in vivo* assay is used for the hepatitis B component, provided it has been carried out with satisfactory results on the final bulk vaccine, it may be omitted on the final lot.

Osmolality (*2.2.35*). The osmolality of the vaccine is within the limits approved for the particular preparation.

IDENTIFICATION

A. Diphtheria toxoid is identified by a suitable immunochemical method (*2.7.1*). The following method, applicable to certain vaccines, is given as an example. Dissolve in the vaccine to be examined sufficient *sodium citrate R* to give a 100 g/l solution. Maintain at 37 °C for about 16 h and centrifuge until a clear supernatant liquid is obtained. The clear supernatant liquid reacts with a suitable diphtheria antitoxin, giving a precipitate.

Vaccines

B. Tetanus toxoid is identified by a suitable immunochemical method (*2.7.1*). The following method, applicable to certain vaccines, is given as an example. The clear supernatant liquid obtained as described in identification test A reacts with a suitable tetanus antitoxin, giving a precipitate.

C. The pertussis components are identified by a suitable immunochemical method (*2.7.1*). The following method, applicable to certain vaccines, is given as an example. The clear supernatant liquid obtained as described in identification test A reacts with a specific antisera to the pertussis components of the vaccine.

D. The assay or, where applicable, the electrophoretic profile, serves also to identify the hepatitis B component of the vaccine.

TESTS

Absence of residual pertussis toxin and irreversibility of pertussis toxoid. *This test is not necessary for the product obtained by genetic modification.* Use 3 groups each of not fewer than 5 histamine-sensitive mice. Inject intraperitoneally into the first group twice the single human dose of the vaccine stored at 2-8 °C. Inject intraperitoneally into the second group twice the single human dose of the vaccine incubated at 37 °C for 4 weeks. Inject diluent into the third group of mice. After 5 days, inject into each mouse 2 mg of histamine base intraperitoneally in a volume not exceeding 0.5 ml and observe for 24 h. The test is invalid if 1 or more control mice die following histamine challenge. The vaccine complies with the test if no animal in the first or second group dies following histamine challenge. If 1 mouse dies in either or both of the first and second groups, the test may be repeated with the same number of mice or with a greater number and the results of valid tests combined; the vaccine complies with the test if, in both of the groups given the vaccine, not more than 5 per cent of the total number of mice die following histamine challenge.

The histamine sensitivity of the strain of mice used is verified at suitable intervals as follows: inject intravenously threefold dilutions of a reference pertussis toxin preparation in phosphate-buffered saline solution containing 2 g/l of gelatin and challenge with histamine as above; the strain is suitable if more than 50 per cent of the animals are sensitised by 50 ng of pertussis toxin and none of the control animals injected with only diluent and challenged similarly with histamine show symptoms of sensitisation.

Aluminium (*2.5.13*): maximum 1.25 mg per single human dose, if aluminium hydroxide or hydrated aluminium phosphate is used as the adsorbent.

Free formaldehyde (*2.4.18*): maximum 0.2 g/l.

Antimicrobial preservative. Where applicable, determine the amount of antimicrobial preservative by a suitable chemical method. The content is not less than the minimum amount shown to be effective and is not greater than 115 per cent of the quantity stated on the label.

Sterility (*2.6.1*). The vaccine complies with the test for sterility.

Pyrogens (*2.6.8*). The vaccine complies with the test for pyrogens. Inject the equivalent of 1 human dose into each rabbit.

ASSAY

Diphtheria component. Carry out one of the prescribed methods for the assay of diphtheria vaccine (adsorbed) (*2.7.6*).

The lower confidence limit ($P = 0.95$) of the estimated potency is not less than the minimum potency stated on the label.

Unless otherwise justified and authorised, the minimum potency stated on the label is 30 IU per single human dose.

Tetanus component. Carry out one of the prescribed methods for the assay of tetanus vaccine (adsorbed) (*2.7.8*).

The lower confidence limit ($P = 0.95$) of the estimated potency is not less than 40 IU per single human dose.

Pertussis component. The vaccine complies with the assay of pertussis vaccine (acellular) (*2.7.16*).

Hepatitis B component. The vaccine complies with the assay of hepatitis B vaccine (*2.7.15*).

LABELLING

The label states:

– the minimum number of International Units of diphtheria and tetanus toxoid per single human dose,
– the names and amounts of the pertussis components per single human dose,
– the amount of HBsAg per single human dose,
– the type of cells used for production of the hepatitis B component,
– where applicable, that the vaccine is intended for primary vaccination of children and is not necessarily suitable for reinforcing doses or for administration to adults,
– the name and the amount of the adsorbent,
– that the vaccine must be shaken before use,
– that the vaccine is not to be frozen,
– where applicable, that the vaccine contains a pertussis toxin-like protein produced by genetic modification.

01/2005:1934

DIPHTHERIA, TETANUS, PERTUSSIS (ACELLULAR, COMPONENT) AND POLIOMYELITIS (INACTIVATED) VACCINE (ADSORBED)

Vaccinum diphtheriae, tetani, pertussis sine cellulis ex elementis praeparatum et poliomyelitidis inactivatum adsorbatum

DEFINITION

Diphtheria, tetanus, pertussis (acellular, component) and poliomyelitis (inactivated) vaccine (adsorbed) is a combined vaccine containing: diphtheria formol toxoid; tetanus formol toxoid; individually purified antigenic components of *Bordetella pertussis*; suitable strains of human polioviruses 1, 2 and 3 grown in suitable cell cultures and inactivated by a validated method; a mineral adsorbent such as aluminium hydroxide or hydrated aluminium phosphate.

The formol toxoids are prepared from the toxins produced by the growth of *Corynebacterium diphtheriae* and *Clostridium tetani* respectively.

The vaccine contains either pertussis toxoid or a pertussis-toxin-like protein free from toxic properties produced by expression of a genetically modified form of the corresponding gene. Pertussis toxoid is prepared from pertussis toxin by a method that renders the toxin harmless while maintaining adequate immunogenic properties and avoiding reversion to toxin. The vaccine may also contain filamentous haemagglutinin, pertactin (a 69 kDa outer-membrane protein) and other defined components of *B. pertussis* such as fimbrial-2 and fimbrial-3 antigens. The latter 2 antigens may be copurified. The antigenic composition and characteristics are based on evidence of protection and freedom from unexpected reactions in the target group for which the vaccine is intended.

PRODUCTION

GENERAL PROVISIONS

The production method shall have been shown to yield consistently vaccines comparable with the vaccine of proven clinical efficacy and safety in man.

The production method is validated to demonstrate that the product, if tested, would comply with the test for abnormal toxicity for immunosera and vaccines for human use (*2.6.9*).

The content of bacterial endotoxins (*2.6.14*) in bulk purified diphtheria toxoid, tetanus toxoid, pertussis components and purified, inactivated monovalent poliovirus harvests is determined to monitor the purification procedure and to limit the amount in the final vaccine. For each component, the content of bacterial endotoxins is less than the limit approved for the particular vaccine and, in any case, the contents are such that the final vaccine contains less than 100 IU per single human dose.

Reference vaccine(s). Provided valid assays can be performed, monocomponent reference vaccines may be used for the assays on the combined vaccine. If this is not possible because of interaction between the components of the combined vaccine or because of the difference in composition between monocomponent reference vaccine and the test vaccine, a batch of combined vaccine shown to be effective in clinical trials or a batch representative thereof is used as a reference vaccine. For the preparation of a representative batch, strict adherence to the production process used for the batch tested in clinical trials is necessary. The reference vaccine may be stabilised by a method that has been shown to have no effect on the assay procedure.

PRODUCTION OF THE COMPONENTS

The production of the components complies with the requirements of the monographs on *Diphtheria vaccine (adsorbed) (0443)*, *Tetanus vaccine (adsorbed) (0452)*, *Pertussis vaccine (acellular, component, adsorbed) (1356)* and *Poliomyelitis vaccine (inactivated) (0214)*.

FINAL BULK VACCINE

The final bulk vaccine is prepared by adsorption onto a mineral carrier such as aluminium hydroxide or hydrated aluminium phosphate, separately or together, of suitable quantities of bulk purified diphtheria toxoid, tetanus toxoid, acellular pertussis components and admixture of suitable quantities of purified monovalent harvests of human polioviruses 1, 2 and 3 or a suitable quantity of a trivalent pool of such purified monovalent harvests. Suitable antimicrobial preservatives may be added.

Only a final bulk vaccine that complies with the following requirements may be used in the preparation of the final lot.

Bovine serum albumin. Determined on the poliomyelitis components by a suitable immunochemical method (*2.7.1*) after virus harvest and before addition of the adsorbent in the preparation of the final bulk vaccine, the amount of bovine serum albumin is such that the content in the final vaccine will be not more than 50 ng per single human dose.

Antimicrobial preservative. Where applicable, determine the amount of antimicrobial preservative by a suitable chemical method. The amount is not less than 85 per cent and not greater than 115 per cent of the intended content.

Sterility (*2.6.1*). Carry out the test for sterility using 10 ml for each medium.

FINAL LOT

Only a final lot that is satisfactory with respect to the test for osmolality and with respect to each of the requirements given below under Identification, Tests and Assay may be released for use.

Provided the tests for absence of residual pertussis toxin, irreversibility of pertussis toxoid and antimicrobial preservative and the assays for the diphtheria, tetanus and pertussis components have been carried out with satisfactory results on the final bulk vaccine, they may be omitted on the final lot.

Provided the free formaldehyde content has been determined on the bulk purified antigens or on the final bulk and it has been shown that the content in the final lot will not exceed 0.2 g/l, the test for free formaldehyde may be omitted on the final lot.

Provided that the determination of D-antigen content has been carried out with satisfactory results during preparation of the final bulk before addition of the adsorbent, it may be omitted on the final lot.

Provided that the *in vivo* assay for the poliomyelitis component has been carried out with satisfactory results on the final bulk vaccine, it may be omitted on the final lot.

Osmolality (*2.2.35*). The osmolality of the vaccine is within the limits approved for the particular preparation.

IDENTIFICATION

A. Diphtheria toxoid is identified by a suitable immunochemical method (*2.7.1*). The following method, applicable to certain vaccines, is given as an example. Dissolve in the vaccine to be examined sufficient *sodium citrate R* to give a 100 g/l solution. Maintain at 37 °C for about 16 h and centrifuge until a clear supernatant liquid is obtained. The clear supernatant liquid reacts with a suitable diphtheria antitoxin, giving a precipitate.

B. Tetanus toxoid is identified by a suitable immunochemical method (*2.7.1*). The following method, applicable to certain vaccines, is given as an example. The clear supernatant liquid obtained as described in identification test A reacts with a suitable tetanus antitoxin, giving a precipitate.

C. The pertussis components are identified by a suitable immunochemical method (*2.7.1*). The following method, applicable to certain vaccines, is given as an example. The clear supernatant liquid obtained as described in identification test A reacts with a specific antisera to the pertussis components of the vaccine.

D. The vaccine is shown to contain human polioviruses 1, 2 and 3 by a suitable immunochemical method (*2.7.1*) such as the determination of D-antigen by enzyme-linked immunosorbent assay (ELISA).

TESTS

Absence of residual pertussis toxin and irreversibility of pertussis toxoid. *This test is not necessary for the product obtained by genetic modification.* Use 3 groups each of not fewer than 5 histamine-sensitive mice. Inject intraperitoneally into the first group twice the single human dose of the vaccine stored at 2-8 °C. Inject intraperitoneally into the second group twice the single human dose of the vaccine incubated at 37 °C for 4 weeks. Inject diluent into the third group of mice. After 5 days, inject into each mouse 2 mg of histamine base intraperitoneally in a volume not exceeding 0.5 ml and observe for 24 h. The test is invalid if 1 or more control mice die following histamine challenge. The vaccine complies with the test if no animal in the first or second group dies following histamine challenge. If 1 mouse dies in either or both of the first and second groups, the test may be repeated with the same number of mice or with a greater number and the results of valid tests combined; the vaccine complies with the test if, in both of the groups given the vaccine, not more than 5 per cent of the total number of mice die following histamine challenge.

The histamine sensitivity of the strain of mice used is verified at suitable intervals as follows: inject intravenously threefold dilutions of a reference pertussis toxin preparation in phosphate-buffered saline solution containing 2 g/l of gelatin and challenge with histamine as above; the strain is suitable if more than 50 per cent of the animals are sensitised by 50 ng of pertussis toxin and none of the control animals injected with only diluent and challenged similarly with histamine show symptoms of sensitisation.

Aluminium (*2.5.13*): maximum 1.25 mg per single human dose if aluminium hydroxide or hydrated aluminium phosphate is used as the adsorbent.

Free formaldehyde (*2.4.18*): maximum 0.2 g/l.

Antimicrobial preservative. Where applicable, determine the amount of antimicrobial preservative by a suitable chemical method. The content is not less than the minimum amount shown to be effective and is not greater than 115 per cent of the quantity stated on the label.

Sterility (*2.6.1*). It complies with the test for sterility.

ASSAY

Diphtheria component. Carry out one of the prescribed methods for the assay of diphtheria vaccine (adsorbed) (*2.7.6*).

The lower confidence limit ($P = 0.95$) of the estimated potency is not less than the minimum potency stated on the label.

Unless otherwise justified and authorised, the minimum potency stated on the label is 30 IU per single human dose.

Tetanus component. Carry out one of the prescribed methods for the assay of tetanus vaccine (adsorbed) (*2.7.8*).

The lower confidence limit ($P = 0.95$) of the estimated potency is not less than 40 IU per single human dose.

Pertussis component. The vaccine complies with the assay of pertussis vaccine (acellular) (*2.7.16*).

Poliomyelitis component

D-antigen content. As a measure of consistency of production, determine the D-antigen content for human polioviruses 1, 2 and 3 by a suitable immunochemical method (*2.7.1*) following desorption using a reference preparation calibrated in European Pharmacopoeia D-antigen units. For each type, the content, expressed with reference to the amount of D-antigen stated on the label, is within the limits approved for the particular product.

Poliomyelitis vaccine (inactivated) BRP is calibrated in European Pharmacopoeia units and intended for use in the assay of D-antigen. The European Pharmacopoeia unit and the International Unit are equivalent.

In vivo test. The vaccine complies with the *in vivo* assay of poliomyelitis vaccine (inactivated) (*2.7.20*).

LABELLING

The label states:

- the minimum number of International Units of diphtheria and tetanus toxoid per single human dose,
- the names and amounts of the pertussis components per single human dose,
- the types of poliovirus contained in the vaccine,
- the nominal amount of poliovirus of each type (1, 2 and 3), expressed in European Pharmacopoeia units of D-antigen, per single human dose,
- the type of cells used for production of the poliomyelitis component,
- where applicable, that the vaccine is intended for primary vaccination of children and is not necessarily suitable for reinforcing doses or for administration to adults,
- the name and the amount of the adsorbent,
- that the vaccine must be shaken before use,
- that the vaccine is not to be frozen,
- where applicable, that the vaccine contains a pertussis toxin-like protein produced by genetic modification.

01/2005:2067

DIPHTHERIA, TETANUS, PERTUSSIS (ACELLULAR, COMPONENT), HEPATITIS B (rDNA), POLIOMYELITIS (INACTIVATED) AND HAEMOPHILUS TYPE b CONJUGATE VACCINE (ADSORBED)

Vaccinum diphtheriae, tetani, pertussis sine cellulis ex elementis praeparatum, hepatitidis B (ADNr), poliomyelitidis inactivatum et haemophili stirpe b coniugatum adsorbatum

DEFINITION

Diphtheria, tetanus, pertussis (acellular, component), hepatitis B (rDNA), poliomyelitis (inactivated) and haemophilus type b conjugate vaccine (adsorbed) is a combined vaccine composed of: diphtheria formol toxoid; tetanus formol toxoid; individually purified antigenic components of *Bordetella pertussis*; hepatitis B surface antigen (HBsAg); human polioviruses 1, 2 and 3 grown in suitable cell cultures and inactivated by a suitable method; polyribosylribitol phosphate (PRP) covalently bound to a carrier protein. The antigens in the vaccine may be adsorbed on a mineral carrier such as aluminium hydroxide or hydrated aluminium phosphate. The product may be presented with the haemophilus component in a separate container, the contents of which are mixed with the other components immediately before or during use.

The formol toxoids are prepared from the toxins produced by the growth of *Corynebacterium diphtheriae* and *Clostridium tetani* respectively.

The vaccine contains either pertussis toxoid or a pertussis-toxin-like protein free from toxic properties produced by expression of a genetically modified form of the corresponding gene. Pertussis toxoid is prepared from pertussis toxin by a method that renders the toxin harmless while maintaining adequate immunogenic properties and avoiding reversion to toxin. The acellular pertussis component may also contain filamentous haemagglutinin, pertactin (a 69 kDa outer-membrane protein) and other defined components of *B. pertussis* such as fimbrial-2 and fimbrial-3 antigens. The latter 2 antigens may be copurified. The antigenic composition and characteristics are based on evidence of protection and freedom from unexpected reactions in the target group for which the vaccine is intended.

Hepatitis B surface antigen is a component protein of hepatitis B virus; the antigen is obtained by recombinant DNA technology.

PRP is a linear copolymer composed of repeated units of 3-β-D-ribofuranosyl-(1 → 1)-ribitol-5-phosphate [$(C_{10}H_{19}O_{12}P)_n$], with a defined molecular size and derived from a suitable strain of *Haemophilus influenzae* type b. The carrier protein, when conjugated to PRP, is capable of inducing a T-cell-dependent B-cell immune response to the polysaccharide.

PRODUCTION

GENERAL PROVISIONS

The production method shall have been shown to yield consistently vaccines comparable with the vaccine of proven clinical efficacy and safety in man.

If the vaccine is presented with the haemophilus component in a separate vial, as part of consistency studies the assays of the diphtheria, tetanus, pertussis, hepatitis B and poliomyelitis components are carried out on a suitable number of batches of vaccine reconstituted as for use. For subsequent routine control, the assays of these components may be carried out without mixing with the haemophilus component.

The content of bacterial endotoxins (*2.6.14*) in bulk purified diphtheria toxoid, bulk purified tetanus toxoid, bulk purified pertussis components, the hepatitis B surface antigen, the purified, inactivated monovalent poliovirus harvests and bulk PRP conjugate is determined to monitor the purification procedure and to limit the amount in the final vaccine. For each component, the content of bacterial endotoxins is not greater than the limit approved.

During development studies and wherever revalidation is necessary, a test for pyrogens in rabbits (*2.6.8*) is carried out by injection of a suitable dose of the final lot. The vaccine is shown to be acceptable with respect to absence of pyrogenic activity.

The production method is validated to demonstrate that the product, if tested, would comply with the following test for specific toxicity of the diphtheria and tetanus component: inject subcutaneously 5 times the single human dose stated on the label into each of 5 healthy guinea-pigs, each weighing 250-350 g, that have not previously been treated with any material that will interfere with the test. If within 42 days of the injection any of the animals shows signs of or dies from diphtheria, toxaemia or tetanus, the vaccine does not comply with the test. If more than 1 animal dies from non-specific causes, repeat the test once; if more than 1 animal dies in the second test, the vaccine does not comply with the test.

During development studies and wherever revalidation is necessary, it shall be demonstrated by tests in animals that the vaccine induces a T-cell-dependent B-cell immune response to PRP.

The stability of the final lot and relevant intermediates is evaluated using one or more indicator tests. For the haemophilus component, such tests may include determination of molecular size, determination of free PRP in the conjugate and kinetics of depolymerisation. Taking account of the results of the stability testing, release requirements are set for these indicator tests to ensure that the vaccine will be satisfactory at the end of the period of validity.

Reference vaccine(s). Provided valid assays can be performed, monocomponent reference vaccines may be used for the assays on the combined vaccine. If this is not possible because of interaction between the components of the combined vaccine or because of the difference in composition between monocomponent reference vaccine and the test vaccine, a batch of combined vaccine shown to be effective in clinical trials or a batch representative thereof is used as a reference vaccine. For the preparation of a representative batch, strict adherence to the production process used for the batch tested in clinical trials is necessary. The reference vaccine may be stabilised by a method that has been shown to have no effect on the assay procedure.

PRODUCTION OF THE COMPONENTS

The production of the components complies with the requirements of the monographs on *Diphtheria vaccine (adsorbed) (0443)*, *Tetanus vaccine (adsorbed) (0452)*, *Pertussis vaccine (acellular, component, adsorbed) (1356)*, *Hepatitis B vaccine (rDNA) (1056)*, *Poliomyelitis vaccine (inactivated) (0214)* and *Haemophilus type b conjugate vaccine (1219)*.

FINAL BULKS

Vaccine with all components in the same container. The final bulk is prepared by adsorption, separately or together, of suitable quantities of bulk purified diphtheria toxoid, bulk purified tetanus toxoid, bulk purified acellular pertussis components and bulk purified hepatitis B surface antigen onto a mineral carrier such as aluminium hydroxide or hydrated aluminium phosphate and admixture of a suitable quantity of PRP conjugate and suitable quantities of purified and inactivated, monovalent harvests of human polioviruses 1, 2 and 3 or a suitable quantity of a trivalent pool of such monovalent harvests. Suitable antimicrobial preservatives may be added.

Vaccine with the haemophilus component in a separate container. The final bulk of diphtheria, tetanus, pertussis, hepatitis B and poliovirus component is prepared by adsorption, separately or together, of suitable quantities of bulk purified diphtheria toxoid, bulk purified tetanus toxoid, bulk purified acellular pertussis components and bulk purified hepatitis B surface antigen onto a mineral carrier such as aluminium hydroxide or hydrated aluminium phosphate and admixture of suitable quantities of purified and inactivated, monovalent harvests of human polioviruses 1, 2 and 3 or a suitable pool of such monovalent harvests. This final bulk is filled separately. Suitable antimicrobial preservatives may be added. The final bulk of the haemophilus component is prepared by dilution of the bulk conjugate to the final concentration with a suitable diluent. A stabiliser may be added.

Only final bulks that comply with the following requirements may be used in the preparation of the final lot.

Bovine serum albumin. Determined on the poliomyelitis components by a suitable immunochemical method (*2.7.1*) after purification of the harvests and before preparation of the final bulk vaccine, before addition of the adsorbent, the amount of bovine serum albumin is such that the content in the final vaccine will be not more than 50 ng per single human dose.

Antimicrobial preservative. Where applicable, determine the amount of antimicrobial preservative by a suitable chemical method. The amount is not less than 85 per cent and not greater than 115 per cent of the intended content.

Sterility (*2.6.1*). Carry out the test for sterility using 10 ml for each medium.

FINAL LOT

Where the haemophilus component is in a separate container, the final bulk of the haemophilus component is freeze-dried. Only a final lot that is satisfactory with respect to the test for osmolality shown below and with respect to each of the requirements given below under Identification, Tests and Assay may be released for use.

Provided that the tests for osmolality, for absence of residual pertussis toxin and irreversibility of pertussis toxoid and for antimicrobial preservative and the diphtheria, tetanus and pertussis component assays have been carried out with satisfactory results on the final bulk vaccine, they may be omitted on the final lot.

Provided the free formaldehyde content has been determined on the bulk purified antigens and the purified monovalent harvests or the trivalent pool of polioviruses or the final bulk and it has been shown that the content in the final lot will not exceed 0.2 g/l, the test for free formaldehyde may be omitted on the final lot.

Provided that the test for bovine serum albumin has been carried out with satisfactory results on the trivalent pool of inactivated monovalent harvests of polioviruses or on the final bulk vaccine, it may be omitted on the final lot.

If an *in vivo* assay is used for the hepatitis B component, provided it has been carried out with satisfactory results on the final bulk vaccine, it may be omitted on the final lot.

Provided the *in vivo* assay for the poliomyelitis component has been carried out with satisfactory results on the final bulk vaccine, it may be omitted on the final lot.

Free PRP. For vaccines with all components in the same container, the free PRP content is determined on the non-absorbed fraction. Unbound PRP is determined on the haemophilus component after removal of the conjugate, for example by anion-exchange, size-exclusion or hydrophobic chromatography, ultrafiltration or other validated methods. The amount of free PRP is not greater than that approved for the particular product.

Bacterial endotoxins (*2.6.14*): less than the limit approved for the particular product.

Osmolality (*2.2.35*). The osmolality of the vaccine, reconstituted where applicable, is within the limits approved for the particular preparation.

IDENTIFICATION

If the vaccine is presented with the haemophilus component in a separate vial: identification tests A, B, C, D and E are carried out using the vial containing the diphtheria, tetanus, pertussis, hepatitis B and poliomyelitis components; identification test F is carried out on the vial containing the haemophilus components.

A. Diphtheria toxoid is identified by a suitable immunochemical method (*2.7.1*). The following method is given as an example. Dissolve in the vaccine to be examined sufficient *sodium citrate R* to give a 100 g/l solution. Maintain at 37 °C for about 16 h and centrifuge until a clear supernatant liquid is obtained. The clear supernatant liquid reacts with a suitable diphtheria antitoxin, giving a precipitate.

B. Tetanus toxoid is identified by a suitable immunochemical method (*2.7.1*). The following method is given as an example. The clear supernatant liquid obtained during identification test A reacts with a suitable tetanus antitoxin, giving a precipitate.

C. The clear supernatant liquid obtained during identification test A reacts with a specific antisera to the pertussis components of the vaccine when examined by suitable immunochemical methods (*2.7.1*).

D. The hepatitis B component is identified by a suitable immunochemical method (*2.7.1*), for example the *in vitro* assay or by a suitable electrophoretic method (*2.2.31*).

E. The vaccine is shown to contain human polioviruses 1, 2 and 3 by a suitable immunochemical method (*2.7.1*), such as determination of D-antigen by enzyme-linked immunosorbent assay (ELISA).

F. The PRP and the haemophilus carrier protein are identified by a suitable immunochemical method (*2.7.1*).

TESTS

If the product is presented with the haemophilus component in a separate container: the tests for absence of residual pertussis toxin and irreversibility of pertussis toxoid, free formaldehyde, aluminium, antimicrobial preservative and sterility are carried out on the container with the diphtheria, tetanus, pertussis, poliomyelitis and hepatitis B components; the tests for PRP content, water, antimicrobial preservative, aluminium (where applicable) and sterility are carried out on the container with the haemophilus component.

Some tests for the haemophilus component are carried out on the freeze-dried product rather than on the bulk conjugate where the freeze-drying process may affect the component to be tested.

Absence of residual pertussis toxin and irreversibility of pertussis toxoid. *This test is not necessary for the product obtained by genetic modification.* Use 3 groups each of not fewer than 5 histamine-sensitive mice. Inject intraperitoneally into the first group twice the single human dose of the vaccine stored at 2-8 °C. Inject intraperitoneally into the second group twice the single human dose of the vaccine incubated at 37 °C for 4 weeks. Inject diluent into the third group of mice. After 5 days, inject into each mouse 2 mg of histamine base intraperitoneally in a volume not exceeding 0.5 ml and observe for 24 h. The test is invalid if 1 or more control mice die following histamine challenge. The vaccine complies with the test if no animal in the first or second group dies following histamine challenge. If 1 mouse dies in either or both of the first and second groups, the test may be repeated with the same number of mice or with a greater number and the results of valid tests combined; the vaccine complies with the test if, in both of the groups given the vaccine, not more than 5 per cent of the total number of mice die following histamine challenge.

The histamine sensitivity of the strain of mice used is verified at suitable intervals as follows: inject intravenously threefold dilutions of a reference pertussis toxin preparation in phosphate-buffered saline solution containing 2 g/l of gelatin and challenge with histamine as above; the strain is suitable if more than 50 per cent of the animals are sensitised by 50 ng of pertussis toxin and none of the control animals injected with only diluent and challenged similarly with histamine show symptoms of sensitisation.

PRP: minimum 80 per cent of the amount of PRP stated on the label, for a vaccine with the haemophilus component in a separate container.

For a vaccine with all components in the same container: the PRP content determined on the non-absorbed fraction is not less than that approved for the product.

PRP is determined either by assay of ribose (*2.5.31*) or phosphorus (*2.5.18*), by an immunochemical method (*2.7.1*) or by anion-exchange liquid chromatography (*2.2.29*) with pulsed-amperometric detection.

Aluminium (*2.5.13*): maximum 1.25 mg of aluminium (Al) per single human dose, if aluminium hydroxide or hydrated aluminium phosphate is used as the adsorbent.

Free formaldehyde (*2.4.18*): maximum 0.2 g/l of free formaldehyde per single human dose.

Antimicrobial preservative. Where applicable, determine the amount of antimicrobial preservative by a suitable chemical method. The content is not less than the minimum amount shown to be effective and is not greater than 115 per cent of the quantity stated on the label.

Water (*2.5.12*): maximum 3.0 per cent for the freeze-dried haemophilus component.

Sterility (*2.6.1*). It complies with the test for sterility.

ASSAY

Diphtheria component. Carry out one of the prescribed methods for the assay of diphtheria vaccine (adsorbed) (*2.7.6*).

The lower confidence limit ($P = 0.95$) of the estimated potency is not less than the minimum potency stated on the label.

Unless otherwise justified and authorised, the minimum potency stated on the label is 30 IU per single human dose.

Tetanus component. Carry out one of the prescribed methods for the assay of tetanus vaccine (adsorbed) (*2.7.8*).

The lower confidence limit ($P = 0.95$) of the estimated potency is not less than 40 IU per single human dose.

Pertussis component. The vaccine complies with the assay of pertussis vaccine (acellular) (*2.7.16*).

Hepatitis B component. The vaccine complies with the assay of hepatitis B vaccine (*2.7.15*).

Poliomyelitis component

D-antigen content. As a measure of consistency of production, determine the D-antigen content for human polioviruses 1, 2 and 3 by a suitable immunochemical method (*2.7.1*) using a reference preparation calibrated in European Pharmacopoeia D-antigen units. For each type, the content, expressed with reference to the amount of D-antigen stated on the label, is within the limits approved for the particular product. *Poliomyelitis vaccine (inactivated) BRP* is calibrated in European Pharmacopoeia units and intended for use in the assay of D antigen. The European Pharmacopoeia unit and the International Unit are equivalent.

In vivo test. The vaccine complies with the *in vivo* assay of poliomyelitis vaccine (inactivated) (*2.7.20*).

LABELLING

The label states:

- the minimum number of International Units of diphtheria and tetanus toxoid per single human dose,
- the names and amounts of the pertussis components per single human dose,
- the amount of HBsAg per single human dose,
- the nominal amount of poliovirus of each type (1, 2 and 3), expressed in European Pharmacopoeia Units of D-antigen, per single human dose,
- the types of cells used for production of the poliomyelitis and the hepatitis B components,
- the number of micrograms of PRP per single human dose,
- the type and nominal amount of carrier protein per single human dose,
- where applicable, that the vaccine is intended for primary vaccination of children and is not necessarily suitable for reinforcing doses or for administration to adults,
- the name and the amount of the adsorbent,
- that the vaccine must be shaken before use,
- that the vaccine is not to be frozen,
- where applicable, that the vaccine contains a pertussis toxin-like protein produced by genetic modification.

01/2005:2065

DIPHTHERIA, TETANUS, PERTUSSIS (ACELLULAR, COMPONENT), POLIOMYELITIS (INACTIVATED) AND HAEMOPHILUS TYPE b CONJUGATE VACCINE (ADSORBED)

Vaccinum diphtheriae, tetani, pertussis sine cellulis ex elementis praeparatum poliomyelitidis inactivatum et haemophili stirpe b coniugatum adsorbatum

DEFINITION

Diphtheria, tetanus, pertussis (acellular, component), poliomyelitis (inactivated) and haemophilus type b conjugate vaccine (adsorbed) is a combined vaccine composed of: diphtheria formol toxoid; tetanus formol toxoid; individually purified antigenic components of *Bordetella pertussis*; suitable strains of human polioviruses 1, 2 and 3 grown in suitable cell cultures and inactivated by a suitable method; polyribosylribitol phosphate (PRP) covalently bound to a carrier protein; a mineral adsorbent such as aluminium hydroxide or hydrated aluminium phosphate. The product is presented with the haemophilus component in a separate container the contents of which are mixed with the other components immediately before use.

The formol toxoids are prepared from the toxins produced by the growth of *Corynebacterium diphtheriae* and *Clostridium tetani* respectively.

The vaccine contains either pertussis toxoid or a pertussis-toxin-like protein free from toxic properties produced by expression of a genetically modified form of the corresponding gene. Pertussis toxoid is prepared from pertussis toxin by a method that renders the toxin harmless while maintaining adequate immunogenic properties and avoiding reversion to toxin. The acellular pertussis component may also contain filamentous haemagglutinin, pertactin (a 69 kDa outer-membrane protein) and other defined components of *B. pertussis* such as fimbrial-2 and fimbrial-3 antigens. The latter 2 antigens may be co-purified. The antigenic composition and characteristics are based on evidence of protection and freedom from unexpected reactions in the target group for which the vaccine is intended.

PRP is a linear copolymer composed of repeated units of 3-β-D-ribofuranosyl-(1→1)-ribitol-5-phosphate [$(C_{10}H_{19}O_{12}P)_n$], with a defined molecular size and derived from a suitable strain of *Haemophilus influenzae* type b. The carrier protein, when conjugated to PRP, is capable of inducing a T-cell-dependent B-cell immune response to the polysaccharide.

Vaccines

PRODUCTION

GENERAL PROVISIONS

The production method shall have been shown to yield consistently vaccines comparable with the vaccine of proven clinical efficacy and safety in man.

The content of bacterial endotoxins (*2.6.14*) in bulk purified diphtheria toxoid, tetanus toxoid, pertussis components, purified, inactivated monovalent poliovirus harvests and bulk PRP conjugate is determined to monitor the purification procedure and to limit the amount in the final vaccine. For each component, the content of bacterial endotoxins is less than the limit approved for the particular vaccine and, in any case, the contents are such that the final vaccine contains less than 100 IU per single human dose.

The production method is validated to demonstrate that the product, if tested, would comply with the test for abnormal toxicity for immunosera and vaccines for human use (*2.6.9*), and with the following test for specific toxicity of the diphtheria and tetanus components: inject subcutaneously 5 times the single human dose stated on the label into each of 5 healthy guinea-pigs, each weighing 250-350 g, that have not previously been treated with any material that will interfere with the test. If within 42 days of the injection any of the animals shows signs of or dies from diphtheria, toxaemia or tetanus, the vaccine does not comply with the test. If more than 1 animal dies from non-specific causes, repeat the test once; if more than 1 animal dies in the second test, the vaccine does not comply with the test.

During development studies and wherever revalidation is necessary, it shall be demonstrated by tests in animals that the vaccine induces a T-cell dependent B-cell immune response to PRP.

As part of consistency studies the assays of the diphtheria, tetanus, pertussis and poliomyelitis components are carried out on a suitable number of batches of vaccine reconstituted as for use. For subsequent routine control, the assays of these components may be carried out without mixing with the haemophilus component.

Reference vaccine(s). Provided valid assays can be performed, monocomponent reference vaccines may be used for the assays on the combined vaccine. If this is not possible because of interaction between the components of the combined vaccine or because of the difference in composition between monocomponent reference vaccine and the test vaccine, a batch of combined vaccine shown to be effective in clinical trials or a batch representative thereof is used as a reference vaccine. For the preparation of a representative batch, strict adherence to the production process used for the batch tested in clinical trials is necessary. The reference vaccine may be stabilised by a method that has been shown to have no effect on the assay procedure.

PRODUCTION OF THE COMPONENTS

The production of the components complies with the requirements of the monographs on *Diphtheria vaccine (adsorbed) (0443)*, *Tetanus vaccine (adsorbed) (0452)*, *Pertussis vaccine (acellular, component, adsorbed) (1356)*, *Poliomyelitis vaccine (inactivated) (0214)* and *Haemophilus type b conjugate vaccine (1219)*.

FINAL BULKS

The final bulk of the diphtheria, tetanus, pertussis and poliomyelitis components is prepared by adsorption, separately or together, of suitable quantities of bulk purified diphtheria toxoid, bulk purified tetanus toxoid and bulk purified acellular pertussis components onto a mineral carrier such as aluminium hydroxide or hydrated aluminium phosphate and admixture of suitable quantities of purified, monovalent harvests of human polioviruses 1, 2 and 3 or a suitable quantity of a trivalent pool of such monovalent harvests. Suitable antimicrobial preservatives may be added.

The final bulk of the haemophilus component is prepared by dilution of the bulk conjugate to the final concentration with a suitable diluent. A stabiliser may be added.

Only final bulks that comply with the following requirements may be used in the preparation of the final lot.

Bovine serum albumin. Determined on the poliomyelitis components by a suitable immunochemical method (*2.7.1*) during preparation of the final bulk vaccine, before addition of the adsorbent, the amount of bovine serum albumin is such that the content in the final vaccine will be not more than 50 ng per single human dose.

Antimicrobial preservative. Where applicable, determine the amount of antimicrobial preservative by a suitable chemical method. The amount is not less than 85 per cent and not greater than 115 per cent of the intended content.

Sterility (*2.6.1*). Carry out the test for sterility using 10 ml for each medium.

FINAL LOT

The final bulk of the haemophilus component is freeze-dried.

Only a final lot that is satisfactory with respect to the test for osmolality shown below and with respect to each of the requirements given below under Identification, Tests and Assay may be released for use.

Provided that the test for absence of residual pertussis toxin and irreversibility of pertussis toxoid, the test for antimicrobial preservative and the assay have been carried out with satisfactory results on the final bulk vaccine, they may be omitted on the final lot.

Provided that the free formaldehyde content has been determined on the bulk purified antigens and the purified monovalent harvests or the trivalent pool of polioviruses or the final bulk and it has been shown that the content in the final lot will not exceed 0.2 g/l, the test for free formaldehyde may be omitted on the final lot.

Provided that the *in vivo* assay for the poliomyelitis component has been carried out with satisfactory results on the final bulk vaccine, it may be omitted on the final lot.

Osmolality (*2.2.35*). The osmolality of the vaccine, reconstituted where applicable, is within the limits approved for the particular preparation.

Free PRP. Unbound PRP is determined on the haemophilus component after removal of the conjugate, for example by anion-exchange, size-exclusion or hydrophobic chromatography, ultrafiltration or other validated methods. The amount of free PRP is not greater than that approved for the particular product.

IDENTIFICATION

Identification tests A, B, C and D are carried out using the vial containing the diphtheria, tetanus, pertussis and poliomyelitis components; identification test E is carried out on the vial containing the haemophilus component.

A. Diphtheria toxoid is identified by a suitable immunochemical method (*2.7.1*). The following method, applicable to certain vaccines, is given as an example. Dissolve in the vaccine to be examined sufficient *sodium citrate R* to give a 100 g/l solution. Maintain at 37 °C for about 16 h and centrifuge until a clear supernatant liquid is obtained. The clear supernatant liquid reacts with a suitable diphtheria antitoxin, giving a precipitate.

B. Tetanus toxoid is identified by a suitable immunochemical method (*2.7.1*). The following method, applicable to certain vaccines, is given as an example. The clear supernatant liquid obtained during identification test A reacts with a suitable tetanus antitoxin, giving a precipitate.

C. The pertussis components are identified by suitable immunochemical methods (*2.7.1*). The following method, applicable to certain vaccines, is given as an example. The clear supernatant liquid obtained during identification test A reacts with specific antisera to the pertussis components of the vaccine.

D. The vaccine is shown to contain human polioviruses 1, 2 and 3 by a suitable immunochemical method (*2.7.1*), such as determination of D-antigen by enzyme-linked immunosorbent assay (ELISA).

E. The haemophilus component is identified by a suitable immunochemical method (*2.7.1*) for PRP.

TESTS

The tests for absence of residual pertussis toxin, irreversibility of pertussis toxoid, aluminium, free formaldehyde, antimicrobial preservative and sterility are carried out on the container with the diphtheria, tetanus, pertussis and poliomyelitis components; the tests for PRP content, water, sterility and pyrogens are carried out on the container with the haemophilus component.

Some tests for the haemophilus component may be carried out on the freeze-dried product rather than on the bulk conjugate where the freeze-drying process may affect the component to be tested.

Absence of residual pertussis toxin and irreversibility of pertussis toxoid. *This test is not necessary for the product obtained by genetic modification.* Use 3 groups each of not fewer than 5 histamine-sensitive mice. Inject intraperitoneally into the first group twice the single human dose of the vaccine stored at 2-8 °C. Inject intraperitoneally into the second group twice the single human dose of the vaccine incubated at 37 °C for 4 weeks. Inject diluent into the third group of mice. After 5 days, inject into each mouse 2 mg of histamine base intraperitoneally in a volume not exceeding 0.5 ml and observe for 24 h. The test is invalid if 1 or more control mice die following histamine challenge. The vaccine complies with the test if no animal in the first or second group dies following histamine challenge. If 1 mouse dies in either or both of the first and second groups, the test may be repeated with the same number of mice or with a greater number and the results of valid tests combined; the vaccine complies with the test if, in both of the groups given the vaccine, not more than 5 per cent of the total number of mice die following histamine challenge.

The histamine sensitivity of the strain of mice used is verified at suitable intervals as follows: inject intravenously threefold dilutions of a reference pertussis toxin preparation in phosphate-buffered saline solution containing 2 g/l of gelatin and challenge with histamine as above; the strain is suitable if more than 50 per cent of the animals are sensitised by 50 ng of pertussis toxin and none of the control animals injected with only diluent and challenged similarly with histamine show symptoms of sensitisation.

PRP: minimum 80 per cent of the amount of PRP stated on the label. PRP is determined either by assay of ribose (*2.5.31*) or phosphorus (*2.5.18*), by an immunochemical method (*2.7.1*) or by anion-exchange liquid chromatography (*2.2.29*) with pulsed-amperometric detection.

Aluminium (*2.5.13*): maximum 1.25 mg per single human dose, if aluminium hydroxide or hydrated aluminium phosphate is used as the adsorbent.

Free formaldehyde (*2.4.18*): maximum 0.2 g/l.

Antimicrobial preservative. Where applicable, determine the amount of antimicrobial preservative by a suitable chemical method. The content is not less than the minimum amount shown to be effective and is not greater than 115 per cent of the quantity stated on the label.

Water (*2.5.12*): maximum 3.0 per cent for the haemophilus component.

Sterility (*2.6.1*). It complies with the test for sterility.

Pyrogens (*2.6.8*). It complies with the test for pyrogens. Inject per kilogram of the rabbit's mass a quantity of the vaccine equivalent to: 1 μg of PRP for a vaccine with diphtheria toxoid or CRM 197 diphtheria protein as carrier; 0.1 μg of PRP for a vaccine with tetanus toxoid as carrier; 0.025 μg of PRP for a vaccine with OMP as a carrier.

ASSAY

Diphtheria component. Carry out one of the prescribed methods for the assay of diphtheria vaccine (adsorbed) (*2.7.6*).

Unless otherwise justified and authorised, the lower confidence limit (*P* = 0.95) of the estimated potency is not less than 30 IU per single human dose.

Tetanus component. Carry out one of the prescribed methods for the assay of tetanus vaccine (adsorbed) (*2.7.8*). The lower confidence limit (P = 0.95) of the estimated potency is not less than 40 IU per single human dose.

Pertussis component. It complies with the assay of pertussis vaccine (acellular) (*2.7.16*).

Poliomyelitis component

D-antigen content. As a measure of consistency of production, determine the D-antigen content for human polioviruses 1, 2 and 3 by a suitable immunochemical method (*2.7.1*) using a reference preparation calibrated in Ph. Eur. Units of D-antigen. For each type, the content, expressed with reference to the amount of D-antigen stated on the label, is within the limits approved for the particular product. *Poliomyelitis vaccine (inactivated) BRP* is calibrated in Ph. Eur. Units and intended for use in the assay of D-antigen. The Ph. Eur. Unit and the IU are equivalent.

In vivo test. The vaccine complies with the *in vivo* assay of poliomyelitis vaccine (inactivated) (*2.7.20*).

LABELLING

The label states:

- the minimum number of International Units of diphtheria and tetanus toxoid per single human dose,
- the names and amounts of the pertussis components per single human dose,
- the nominal amount of poliovirus of each type (1, 2 and 3), expressed in European Pharmacopoeia Units of D-antigen, per single human dose,
- the type of cells used for production of the poliomyelitis component,
- the number of micrograms of PRP per single human dose,
- the type and nominal amount of carrier protein per single human dose,
- where applicable, that the vaccine is intended for primary vaccination of children and is not necessarily suitable for reinforcing doses or for administration to adults,
- the name and the amount of the adsorbent,
- that the vaccine must be shaken before use,
- that the vaccine is not to be frozen,
- where applicable, that the vaccine contains a pertussis toxin-like protein produced by genetic modification.

Vaccines

01/2005:2061

DIPHTHERIA, TETANUS, PERTUSSIS AND POLIOMYELITIS (INACTIVATED) VACCINE (ADSORBED)

Vaccinum diphtheriae, tetani, pertussis et poliomyelitidis inactivatum adsorbatum

DEFINITION

Diphtheria, tetanus, pertussis and poliomyelitis (inactivated) vaccine (adsorbed) is a combined vaccine containing: diphtheria formol toxoid; tetanus formol toxoid; an inactivated suspension of *Bordetella pertussis*; suitable strains of human polioviruses 1, 2 and 3 grown in suitable cell cultures and inactivated by a validated method; a mineral adsorbent such as aluminium hydroxide or hydrated aluminium phosphate.

The formol toxoids are prepared from the toxins produced by the growth of *Corynebacterium diphtheriae* and *Clostridium tetani* respectively.

PRODUCTION

GENERAL PROVISIONS

The production method shall have been shown to yield consistently vaccines comparable with the vaccine of proven clinical efficacy and safety in man.

Reference vaccine(s). Provided valid assays can be performed, monocomponent reference vaccines may be used for the assays on the combined vaccine. If this is not possible because of interaction between the components of the combined vaccine or because of the difference in composition between monocomponent reference vaccine and the test vaccine, a batch of combined vaccine shown to be effective in clinical trials or a batch representative thereof is used as a reference vaccine. For the preparation of a representative batch, strict adherence to the production process used for the batch tested in clinical trials is necessary. The reference vaccine may be stabilised by a method that has been shown to have no effect on the assay procedure.

Specific toxicity of the diphtheria and tetanus components. The production method is validated to demonstrate that the product, if tested, would comply with the following test: inject subcutaneously 5 times the single human dose stated on the label into each of 5 healthy guinea-pigs, each weighing 250-350 g, that have not previously been treated with any material that will interfere with the test. If within 42 days of the injection any of the animals shows signs of or dies from diphtheria toxaemia or tetanus, the vaccine does not comply with the test. If more than 1 animal dies from non-specific causes, repeat the test once; if more than 1 animal dies in the second test, the vaccine does not comply with the test.

PRODUCTION OF THE COMPONENTS

The production of the components complies with the requirements of the monographs on *Diphtheria vaccine (adsorbed) (0443)*, *Tetanus vaccine (adsorbed) (0452)*, *Pertussis vaccine (adsorbed) (0161)* and *Poliomyelitis vaccine (inactivated) (0214)*.

FINAL BULK VACCINE

The final bulk vaccine is prepared by adsorption onto a mineral carrier such as aluminium hydroxide or hydrated aluminium phosphate, separately or together, of suitable quantities of bulk purified diphtheria toxoid and bulk purified tetanus toxoid and admixture of suitable quantities of an inactivated suspension of *B. pertussis* and purified monovalent harvests of human polioviruses 1, 2 and 3 or a suitable quantity of a trivalent pool of such purified monovalent harvests. Suitable antimicrobial preservatives may be added.

Only a final bulk vaccine that complies with the following requirements may be used in the preparation of the final lot.

Bovine serum albumin. Determined on the poliomyelitis components by a suitable immunochemical method (*2.7.1*) during preparation of the final bulk vaccine, before addition of the adsorbent, the amount of bovine serum albumin is such that the content in the final vaccine will be not more than 50 ng per single human dose.

Antimicrobial preservative. Where applicable, determine the amount of antimicrobial preservative by a suitable chemical method. The amount is not less than 85 per cent and not greater than 115 per cent of the intended content.

Sterility (*2.6.1*). Carry out the test for sterility using 10 ml for each medium.

FINAL LOT

Only a final lot that is satisfactory with respect to the test for osmolality and with respect to each of the requirements given below under Identification, Tests and Assay may be released for use.

Provided that the tests for specific toxicity of the pertussis component and antimicrobial preservative, and the assays for the diphtheria, tetanus and pertussis components have been carried out with satisfactory results on the final bulk vaccine, they may be omitted on the final lot.

Provided that the free formaldehyde content has been determined on the bulk purified antigens, the inactivated *B. pertussis* suspension and the purified monovalent harvests or the trivalent pool of polioviruses or on the final bulk and it has been shown that the content in the final lot will not exceed 0.2 g/l, the test for free formaldehyde may be omitted on the final lot.

Provided that the *in vivo* assay for the poliomyelitis component has been carried out with satisfactory results on the final bulk vaccine, it may be omitted on the final lot.

Osmolality (*2.2.35*). The osmolality of the vaccine is within the limits approved for the particular preparation.

IDENTIFICATION

A. Diphtheria toxoid is identified by a suitable immunochemical method (*2.7.1*). The following method, applicable to certain vaccines, is given as an example. Dissolve in the vaccine to be examined sufficient *sodium citrate R* to give a 100 g/l solution. Maintain at 37 °C for about 16 h and centrifuge until a clear supernatant liquid is obtained. The clear supernatant liquid reacts with a suitable diphtheria antitoxin, giving a precipitate.

B. Tetanus toxoid is identified by a suitable immunochemical method (*2.7.1*). The following method, applicable to certain vaccines, is given as an example. The clear supernatant liquid obtained during identification test A reacts with a suitable tetanus antitoxin, giving a precipitate.

C. The centrifugation residue obtained in identification A may be used. Other suitable methods for separating the bacteria from the adsorbent may also be used. Identify pertussis vaccine by agglutination of the bacteria from the resuspended precipitate by antisera specific to *B. pertussis* or by the assay of the pertussis component prescribed under Assay.

D. The vaccine is shown to contain human polioviruses 1, 2 and 3 by a suitable immunochemical method (*2.7.1*) such as the determination of D-antigen by enzyme-linked immunosorbent assay (ELISA).

Vaccines

TESTS

Specific toxicity of the pertussis component. Use not fewer than 5 healthy mice each weighing 14-16 g for the vaccine group and for the saline control. Use mice of the same sex or distribute males and females equally between the groups. Allow the animals access to food and water for at least 2 h before injection and during the test. Inject each mouse of the vaccine group intraperitoneally with 0.5 ml, containing a quantity of the vaccine equivalent to not less than half the single human dose. Inject each mouse of the control group with 0.5 ml of a 9 g/l sterile solution of *sodium chloride R*, preferably containing the same amount of antimicrobial preservative as that injected with the vaccine. Weigh the groups of mice immediately before the injection and 72 h and 7 days after the injection. The vaccine complies with the test if: (a) at the end of 72 h the total mass of the group of vaccinated mice is not less than that preceding the injection; (b) at the end of 7 days the average increase in mass per vaccinated mouse is not less than 60 per cent of that per control mouse; and (c) not more than 5 per cent of the vaccinated mice die during the test. The test may be repeated and the results of the tests combined.

Aluminium (*2.5.13*): maximum 1.25 mg per single human dose, if aluminium hydroxide or hydrated aluminium phosphate is used as the adsorbent.

Free formaldehyde (*2.4.18*): maximum 0.2 g/l.

Antimicrobial preservative. Where applicable, determine the amount of antimicrobial preservative by a suitable chemical method. The content is not less than the minimum amount shown to be effective and is not greater than 115 per cent of the quantity stated on the label.

Sterility (*2.6.1*). It complies with the test for sterility.

ASSAY

Diphtheria component. Carry out one of the prescribed methods for the assay of diphtheria vaccine (adsorbed) (*2.7.6*).

The lower confidence limit (P = 0.95) of the estimated potency is not less than 30 IU per single human dose.

Tetanus component. Carry out one of the prescribed methods for the assay of tetanus vaccine (adsorbed) (*2.7.8*).

If the test is carried out in guinea pigs, the lower confidence limit (P = 0.95) of the estimated potency is not less than 40 IU per single human dose; if the test is carried out in mice, the lower confidence limit (P = 0.95) of the estimated potency is not less than 60 IU per single human dose.

Pertussis component. Carry out the assay of pertussis vaccine (*2.7.7*).

The estimated potency is not less than 4 IU per single human dose and the lower confidence limit (P = 0.95) of the estimated potency is not less than 2 IU per single human dose.

Poliomyelitis component

D-antigen content. As a measure of consistency of production, determine the D-antigen content for human polioviruses 1, 2 and 3 by a suitable immunochemical method (*2.7.1*) using a reference preparation calibrated in European Pharmacopoeia Units of D-antigen. For each type, the content, expressed with reference to the amount of D-antigen stated on the label, is within the limits approved for the particular product. *Poliomyelitis vaccine (inactivated) BRP* is calibrated in European Pharmacopoeia Units and intended for use in the assay of D-antigen. The European Pharmacopoeia Unit and the International Unit are equivalent.

In vivo test. The vaccine complies with the *in vivo* assay of poliomyelitis vaccine (inactivated) (*2.7.20*).

LABELLING

The label states:

- the minimum number of International Units of diphtheria and tetanus toxoid per single human dose,
- the minimum number of International Units of pertussis vaccine per single human dose,
- the nominal amount of poliovirus of each type (1, 2 and 3), expressed in European Pharmacopoeia Units of D-antigen, per single human dose,
- the type of cells used for production of the poliomyelitis component,
- where applicable, that the vaccine is intended for primary vaccination of children and is not necessarily suitable for reinforcing doses or for administration to adults,
- the name and the amount of the adsorbent,
- that the vaccine must be shaken before use,
- that the vaccine is not to be frozen.

01/2005:2066

DIPHTHERIA, TETANUS, PERTUSSIS, POLIOMYELITIS (INACTIVATED) AND HAEMOPHILUS TYPE b CONJUGATE VACCINE (ADSORBED)

Vaccinum diphtheriae, tetani, pertussis, poliomyelitidis inactivatum et haemophili stirpe b coniugatum adsorbatum

DEFINITION

Diphtheria, tetanus, pertussis, poliomyelitis (inactivated) and haemophilus type b conjugate vaccine (adsorbed) is a combined vaccine composed of: diphtheria formol toxoid; tetanus formol toxoid; an inactivated suspension of *Bordetella pertussis*; suitable strains of human polioviruses 1, 2 and 3 grown in suitable cell cultures and inactivated by a suitable method; polyribosylribitol phosphate (PRP) covalently bound to a carrier protein; a mineral adsorbent such as aluminium hydroxide or hydrated aluminium phosphate. The product is presented with the haemophilus component in a separate container, the contents of which are mixed with the other components immediately before use.

The formol toxoids are prepared from the toxins produced by the growth of *Corynebacterium diphtheriae* and *Clostridium tetani* respectively.

PRP is a linear copolymer composed of repeated units of 3-β-D-ribofuranosyl-(1→1)-ribitol-5-phosphate [$(C_{10}H_{19}O_{12}P)_n$], with a defined molecular size and derived from a suitable strain of *Haemophilus influenzae* type b. The carrier protein, when conjugated to PRP, is capable of inducing a T-cell-dependent B-cell immune response to the polysaccharide.

PRODUCTION

GENERAL PROVISIONS

The production method shall have been shown to yield consistently vaccines comparable with the vaccine of proven clinical efficacy and safety in man.

During development studies and wherever revalidation is necessary, it shall be demonstrated by tests in animals that the vaccine induces a T-cell dependent B-cell immune response to PRP.

As part of consistency studies the assays of the diphtheria, tetanus, pertussis and poliomyelitis components are carried out on a suitable number of batches of vaccine reconstituted as for use. For subsequent routine control, the assays of these components may be carried out without mixing with the haemophilus component.

Reference vaccine(s). Provided valid assays can be performed, monocomponent reference vaccines may be used for the assays on the combined vaccine. If this is not possible because of interaction between the components of the combined vaccine or because of the difference in composition between monocomponent reference vaccine and the test vaccine, a batch of combined vaccine shown to be effective in clinical trials or a batch representative thereof is used as a reference vaccine. For the preparation of a representative batch, strict adherence to the production process used for the batch tested in clinical trials is necessary. The reference vaccine may be stabilised by a method that has been shown to have no effect on the assay procedure.

Specific toxicity of the diphtheria and tetanus components. The production method is validated to demonstrate that the product, if tested, would comply with the following test: inject subcutaneously 5 times the single human dose stated on the label into each of 5 healthy guinea-pigs, each weighing 250-350 g, that have not previously been treated with any material that will interfere with the test. If within 42 days of the injection any of the animals shows signs of or dies from diphtheria toxaemia or tetanus, the vaccine does not comply with the test. If more than 1 animal dies from non-specific causes, repeat the test once; if more than 1 animal dies in the second test, the vaccine does not comply with the test.

PRODUCTION OF THE COMPONENTS

The production of the components complies with the requirements of the monographs on *Diphtheria vaccine (adsorbed) (0443)*, *Tetanus vaccine (adsorbed) (0452)*, *Pertussis vaccine (adsorbed) (0161)*, *Poliomyelitis vaccine (inactivated) (0214)* and *Haemophilus type b conjugate vaccine (1219)*.

FINAL BULKS

The final bulk of the diphtheria, tetanus, pertussis and poliomyelitis components is prepared by adsorption, separately or together, of suitable quantities of bulk purified diphtheria toxoid, and bulk purified tetanus toxoid onto a mineral carrier such as aluminium hydroxide or hydrated aluminium phosphate and admixture of suitable quantities of an inactivated suspension of *B. pertussis* and of purified, monovalent harvests of human polioviruses 1, 2 and 3 or a suitable quantity of a trivalent pool of such monovalent harvests. Suitable antimicrobial preservatives may be added.

The final bulk of the haemophilus component is prepared by dilution of the bulk conjugate to the final concentration with a suitable diluent. A stabiliser may be added.

Only final bulks that comply with the following requirements may be used in the preparation of the final lot.

Bovine serum albumin. Determined on the poliomyelitis components by a suitable immunochemical method (*2.7.1*) during preparation of the final bulk vaccine, before addition of the adsorbent, the amount of bovine serum albumin is such that the content in the final vaccine will be not more than 50 ng per single human dose.

Antimicrobial preservative. Where applicable, determine the amount of antimicrobial preservative by a suitable chemical method. The amount is not less than 85 per cent and not greater than 115 per cent of the intended content.

Sterility (*2.6.1*). Carry out the test for sterility using 10 ml for each medium.

FINAL LOT

The final bulk of the haemophilus component is freeze-dried.

Only a final lot that is satisfactory with respect to the test for osmolality shown below and with respect to each of the requirements given below under Identification, Tests and Assay may be released for use.

Provided that the tests for specific toxicity of the pertussis component and antimicrobial preservative, and the assays for the diphtheria, tetanus and pertussis components have been carried out with satisfactory results on the final bulk vaccine, they may be omitted on the final lot.

Provided that the free formaldehyde content has been determined on the bulk purified antigens, the inactivated *B. pertussis* suspension and the purified monovalent harvests or the trivalent pool of polioviruses or on the final bulk and it has been shown that the content in the final lot will not exceed 0.2 g/l, the test for free formaldehyde may be omitted on the final lot.

Provided that the *in vivo* assay for the poliomyelitis component has been carried out with satisfactory results on the final bulk vaccine, it may be omitted on the final lot.

Osmolality (*2.2.35*). The osmolality of the vaccine, reconstituted where applicable, is within the limits approved for the particular preparation.

Free PRP. Unbound PRP is determined on the haemophilus component after removal of the conjugate, for example by anion-exchange, size-exclusion or hydrophobic chromatography, ultrafiltration or other validated methods. The amount of free PRP is not greater than that approved for the particular product.

IDENTIFICATION

Identification tests A, B, C and D are carried out using the vial containing the diphtheria, tetanus, pertussis and poliomyelitis components; identification test E is carried out on the vial containing the haemophilus component.

A. Diphtheria toxoid is identified by a suitable immunochemical method (*2.7.1*). The following method, applicable to certain vaccines, is given as an example. Dissolve in the vaccine to be examined sufficient *sodium citrate R* to give a 100 g/l solution. Maintain at 37 °C for about 16 h and centrifuge until a clear supernatant liquid is obtained. The clear supernatant liquid reacts with a suitable diphtheria antitoxin, giving a precipitate.

B. Tetanus toxoid is identified by a suitable immunochemical method (*2.7.1*). The following method, applicable to certain vaccines, is given as an example. The clear supernatant liquid obtained during identification test A reacts with a suitable tetanus antitoxin, giving a precipitate.

C. The centrifugation residue obtained in identification A may be used. Other suitable methods for separating the bacteria from the adsorbent may also be used. Identify pertussis vaccine by agglutination of the bacteria from the resuspended precipitate by antisera specific to *B. pertussis* or by the assay of the pertussis component prescribed under Assay.

D. The vaccine is shown to contain human polioviruses 1, 2 and 3 by a suitable immunochemical method (*2.7.1*), such as determination of D-antigen by enzyme-linked immunosorbent assay (ELISA).

E. The haemophilus component is identified by a suitable immunochemical method (*2.7.1*) for PRP.

TESTS

The tests for specific toxicity of the pertussis component, aluminium, free formaldehyde, antimicrobial preservative and sterility are carried out on the container with diphtheria, tetanus, pertussis and poliomyelitis components; the tests for PRP, water, sterility and pyrogens are carried out on the container with the haemophilus component.

Some tests for the haemophilus component may be carried out on the freeze-dried product rather than on the bulk conjugate where the freeze-drying process may affect the component to be tested.

Specific toxicity of the pertussis component. Use not fewer than 5 healthy mice each weighing 14-16 g, for the vaccine group and for the saline control. Use mice of the same sex or distribute males and females equally between the groups. Allow the animals access to food and water for at least 2 h before injection and during the test. Inject each mouse of the vaccine group intraperitoneally with 0.5 ml, containing a quantity of the vaccine equivalent to not less than half the single human dose. Inject each mouse of the control group with 0.5 ml of a 9 g/l sterile solution of *sodium chloride R*, preferably containing the same amount of antimicrobial preservative as that injected with the vaccine. Weigh the groups of mice immediately before the injection and 72 h and 7 days after the injection. The vaccine complies with the test if: (a) at the end of 72 h the total mass of the group of vaccinated mice is not less than that preceding the injection; (b) at the end of 7 days the average increase in mass per vaccinated mouse is not less than 60 per cent of that per control mouse; and (c) not more than 5 per cent of the vaccinated mice die during the test. The test may be repeated and the results of the tests combined.

PRP: minimum 80 per cent of the amount of PRP stated on the label. PRP is determined either by assay of ribose (*2.5.31*) or phosphorus (*2.5.18*), by an immunochemical method (*2.7.1*) or by anion-exchange liquid chromatography (*2.2.29*) with pulsed-amperometric detection.

Aluminium (*2.5.13*): maximum 1.25 mg per single human dose, if aluminium hydroxide or hydrated aluminium phosphate is used as the adsorbent.

Free formaldehyde (*2.4.18*): maximum 0.2 g/l.

Antimicrobial preservative. Where applicable, determine the amount of antimicrobial preservative by a suitable chemical method. The content is not less than the minimum amount shown to be effective and is not greater than 115 per cent of the quantity stated on the label.

Water (*2.5.12*): maximum 3.0 per cent for the haemophilus component.

Sterility (*2.6.1*). It complies with the test for sterility.

Pyrogens (*2.6.8*). It complies with the test for pyrogens. Inject per kilogram of the rabbit's mass a quantity of the vaccine equivalent to: 1 µg of PRP for a vaccine with diphtheria toxoid or CRM 197 diphtheria protein as carrier; 0.1 µg of PRP for a vaccine with tetanus toxoid as carrier; 0.025 µg of PRP for a vaccine with OMP as carrier.

ASSAY

Diphtheria component. Carry out one of the prescribed methods for the assay of diphtheria vaccine (adsorbed) (*2.7.6*).

The lower confidence limit (P = 0.95) of the estimated potency is not less than 30 IU per single human dose.

Tetanus component. Carry out one of the prescribed methods for the assay of tetanus vaccine (adsorbed) (*2.7.8*).

If the test is carried out in guinea-pigs, the lower confidence limit (P = 0.95) of the estimated potency is not less than 40 IU per single human dose; if the test is carried out in mice, the lower confidence limit (P = 0.95) of the estimated potency is not less than 60 IU per single human dose.

Pertussis component. Carry out the assay of pertussis vaccine (*2.7.7*).

The estimated potency is not less than 4 IU per single human dose and the lower confidence limit (P = 0.95) of the estimated potency is not less than 2 IU per single human dose.

Poliomyelitis component

D-antigen content. As a measure of consistency of production, determine the D-antigen content for human polioviruses 1, 2 and 3 by a suitable immunochemical method (*2.7.1*) using a reference preparation calibrated in European Pharmacopoeia Units of D-antigen. For each type, the content, expressed with reference to the amount of D-antigen stated on the label, is within the limits approved for the particular product. *Poliomyelitis vaccine (inactivated) BRP* is calibrated in European Pharmacopoeia Units and intended for use in the assay of D-antigen. The European Pharmacopoeia Unit and the International Unit are equivalent.

In vivo test. The vaccine complies with the *in vivo* assay of poliomyelitis vaccine (inactivated) (*2.7.20*).

LABELLING

The label states:

- the minimum number of International Units of diphtheria and tetanus toxoid per single human dose,
- the minimum number of International Units of pertussis vaccine per single human dose,
- the nominal amount of poliovirus of each type (1, 2 and 3), expressed in European Pharmacopoeia Units of D-antigen, per single human dose,
- the type of cells used for production of the poliomyelitis component,
- the number of micrograms of PRP per single human dose,
- the type and nominal amount of carrier protein per single human dose,
- where applicable, that the vaccine is intended for primary vaccination of children and is not necessarily suitable for reinforcing doses or for administration to adults,
- the name and the amount of the adsorbent,
- that the vaccine must be shaken before use,
- that the vaccine is not to be frozen.

01/2005:0443

DIPHTHERIA VACCINE (ADSORBED)

Vaccinum diphtheriae adsorbatum

DEFINITION

Diphtheria vaccine (adsorbed) is a preparation of diphtheria formol toxoid with a mineral adsorbent. The formol toxoid is prepared from the toxin produced by the growth of *Corynebacterium diphtheriae*.

PRODUCTION

GENERAL PROVISIONS

Specific toxicity. The production method is validated to demonstrate that the product, if tested, would comply with the following test: inject subcutaneously 5 times the single human dose stated on the label into each of 5 healthy guinea-pigs, each weighing 250-350 g, that have not previously been treated with any material that will interfere with the test. If within 42 days of the injection any of the animals shows signs of or dies from diphtheria toxaemia, the vaccine does not comply with the test. If more than 1 animal dies from non-specific causes, repeat the test once; if more than 1 animal dies in the second test, the vaccine does not comply with the test.

BULK PURIFIED TOXOID

For the production of diphtheria toxin, from which toxoid is prepared, seed cultures are managed in a defined seed-lot system in which toxinogenicity is conserved and, where necessary, restored by deliberate reselection. A highly toxinogenic strain of *Corynebacterium diphtheriae* with known origin and history is grown in a suitable liquid medium. At the end of cultivation, the purity of each culture is tested and contaminated cultures are discarded. Toxin-containing culture medium is separated aseptically from the bacterial mass as soon as possible. The toxin content (Lf per millilitre) is checked to monitor consistency of production. Single harvests may be pooled to prepare the bulk purified toxoid. The toxin is purified to remove components likely to cause adverse reactions in humans. The purified toxin is detoxified with formaldehyde by a method that avoids destruction of the immunogenic potency of the toxoid and reversion of the toxoid to toxin, particularly on exposure to heat. Alternatively, purification may be carried out after detoxification.

Only bulk purified toxoid that complies with the following requirements may be used in the preparation of the final bulk vaccine.

Sterility (*2.6.1*). Carry out the test for sterility using 10 ml for each medium.

Absence of toxin and irreversibility of toxoid. Using the same buffer solution as for the final vaccine, without adsorbent, prepare a solution of bulk purified toxoid at 100 Lf/ml. Divide the solution into 2 equal parts. Maintain 1 part at 5 ± 3 °C and the other at 37 °C for 6 weeks. Carry out a test in Vero cells for active diphtheria toxin using 50 µl/well of both samples. The sample should not contain antimicrobial preservatives and detoxifying agents should be determined to be below the concentration toxic to Vero cells. Non-specific toxicity may be eliminated by dialysis.

Use freshly trypsinised Vero cells at a suitable concentration, for example 2.5×10^5 ml^{-1} and a reference diphtheria toxin diluted in 100 Lf/ml diphtheria toxoid. A suitable reference diphtheria toxin will contain either not less than 100 LD_{50}/ml or 67 to 133 lr/100 in 1 Lf and 25 000 to 50 000 minimal reacting doses for guinea-pig skin in 1 Lf (*diphtheria toxin BRP* is suitable for use as the reference toxin). Dilute the toxin in 100 Lf/ml diphtheria toxoid to a suitable concentration, for example 2×10^{-4} Lf/ml. Prepare serial twofold dilutions of the diluted diphtheria toxin and use undiluted test samples (50 µl/well). Distribute them in the wells of a sterile tissue culture plate containing a medium suitable for Vero cells. To ascertain that any cytotoxic effect noted is specific to diphtheria toxin, prepare in parallel dilutions where the toxin is neutralised by a suitable concentration of diphtheria antitoxin, for example 100 IU/ml. Include control wells without toxoid or toxin and with non-toxic toxoid at 100 Lf/ml on each plate to verify normal cell growth. Add cell suspension to each well, seal the plates and incubate at 37 °C for 5-6 days. Cytotoxic effect is judged to be present where there is complete metabolic inhibition of the Vero cells, indicated by the pH indicator of the medium. Confirm cytopathic effect by microscopic examination or suitable staining such as MTT dye. The test is invalid if 5×10^{-5} Lf/ml of reference diphtheria toxin in 100 Lf/ml toxoid has no cytotoxic effect on Vero cells or if the cytotoxic effect of this amount of toxin is not neutralised in the wells containing diphtheria antitoxin. The bulk purified toxoid complies with the test if no toxicity neutralisable by antitoxin is found in either sample.

Antigenic purity. Not less than 1500 Lf per milligram of protein nitrogen.

FINAL BULK VACCINE

The final bulk vaccine is prepared by adsorption of a suitable quantity of bulk purified toxoid onto a mineral carrier such as hydrated aluminium phosphate or aluminium hydroxide; the resulting mixture is approximately isotonic with blood. Suitable antimicrobial preservatives may be added. Certain antimicrobial preservatives, particularly those of the phenolic type, adversely affect the antigenic activity and must not be used.

Only a final bulk vaccine that complies with the following requirements may be used in the preparation of the final lot.

Antimicrobial preservative. Where applicable, determine the amount of antimicrobial preservative by a suitable chemical method. The amount is not less than 85 per cent and not greater than 115 per cent of the intended amount.

Sterility (*2.6.1*). Carry out the test for sterility using 10 ml for each medium.

FINAL LOT

The final bulk vaccine is distributed aseptically into sterile, tamper-proof containers. The containers are closed so as to prevent contamination.

Only a final lot that is satisfactory with respect to each of the requirements given below under Identification, Tests and Assay may be released for use. Provided the test for antimicrobial preservative and the assay have been carried out with satisfactory results on the final bulk vaccine, they may be omitted on the final lot.

Provided the free formaldehyde content has been determined on the bulk purified antigens or on the final bulk and it has been shown that the content in the final lot will not exceed 0.2 g/l, the test for free formaldehyde may be omitted on the final lot.

IDENTIFICATION

Diphtheria toxoid is identified by a suitable immunochemical method (*2.7.1*). The following method, applicable to certain vaccines, is given as an example. Dissolve in the vaccine to be examined sufficient *sodium citrate R* to give a 100 g/l solution. Maintain at 37 °C for about 16 h and centrifuge until a clear supernatant liquid is obtained. The clear supernatant liquid reacts with a suitable diphtheria antitoxin, giving a precipitate.

TESTS

Aluminium (*2.5.13*): maximum 1.25 mg per single human dose, if aluminium hydroxide or hydrated aluminium phosphate is used as the absorbent.

Free formaldehyde (*2.4.18*): maximum 0.2 g/l.

Antimicrobial preservative. Where applicable, determine the amount of antimicrobial preservative by a suitable chemical method. The content is not less than the minimum amount shown to be effective and is not greater than 115 per cent of the quantity stated on the label.

Sterility (*2.6.1*). The vaccine complies with the test for sterility.

ASSAY

Carry out one of the prescribed methods for the assay of diphtheria vaccine (adsorbed) (*2.7.6*).

The lower confidence limit ($P = 0.95$) of the estimated potency is not less than 30 IU per single human dose.

LABELLING

The label states:

- the minimum number of International Units per single human dose,
- where applicable, that the vaccine is intended for primary vaccination of children and is not necessarily suitable for reinforcing doses or for administration to adults,
- the name and the amount of the adsorbent,
- that the vaccine must be shaken before use,
- that the vaccine is not to be frozen.

01/2005:0646

DIPHTHERIA VACCINE (ADSORBED) FOR ADULTS AND ADOLESCENTS

Vaccinum diphtheriae adulti et adulescentis adsorbatum

DEFINITION

Diphtheria vaccine (adsorbed) for adults and adolescents is a preparation of diphtheria formol toxoid with a mineral adsorbent. The formol toxoid is prepared from the toxin produced by the growth of *Corynebacterium diphtheriae*. It shall have been demonstrated to the competent authority that the quantity of diphtheria toxoid used does not produce adverse reactions in subjects from the age groups for which the vaccine is intended.

PRODUCTION

GENERAL PROVISIONS

Specific toxicity. The production method is validated to demonstrate that the product, if tested, would comply with the following test: inject subcutaneously 5 times the single human dose stated on the label into each of 5 healthy guinea-pigs, each weighing 250-350 g, that have not previously been treated with any material that will interfere with the test. If within 42 days of the injection any of the animals shows signs of or dies from diphtheria toxaemia, the vaccine does not comply with the test. If more than 1 animal dies from non-specific causes, repeat the test once; if more than 1 animal dies in the second test, the vaccine does not comply with the test.

BULK PURIFIED TOXOID

The bulk purified toxoid is prepared as described in the monograph on *Diphtheria vaccine (adsorbed) (0443)* and complies with the requirements prescribed therein.

FINAL BULK VACCINE

The final bulk vaccine is prepared by adsorption of a suitable quantity of bulk purified toxoid onto a mineral carrier such as hydrated aluminium phosphate or aluminium hydroxide; the resulting mixture is approximately isotonic with blood. Suitable antimicrobial preservatives may be added. Certain antimicrobial preservatives, particularly those of the phenolic type, adversely affect the antigenic activity and must not be used.

Only a final bulk vaccine that complies with the following requirements may be used in the preparation of the final lot.

Antimicrobial preservative. Where applicable, determine the amount of antimicrobial preservative by a suitable chemical method. The amount is not less than 85 per cent and not greater than 115 per cent of the intended amount.

Sterility (*2.6.1*). Carry out the test for sterility using 10 ml for each medium.

FINAL LOT

The final bulk vaccine is distributed aseptically into sterile, tamper-proof containers. The containers are closed so as to prevent contamination.

Only a final lot that is satisfactory with respect to each of the requirements given below under Identification, Tests and Assay may be released for use. Provided the test for antimicrobial preservative and the assay have been carried out with satisfactory results on the final bulk vaccine, they may be omitted on the final lot.

Provided the free formaldehyde content has been determined on the bulk purified toxoid or on the final bulk and it has been shown that the content in the final lot will not exceed 0.2 g/l, the test for free formaldehyde may be omitted on the final lot.

IDENTIFICATION

Diphtheria toxoid is identified by a suitable immunochemical method (*2.7.1*). The following method, applicable to certain vaccines, is given as an example. Dissolve in the vaccine to be examined sufficient *sodium citrate R* to give a 100 g/l solution. Maintain at 37 °C for about 16 h and centrifuge until a clear supernatant liquid is obtained. The clear supernatant liquid reacts with a suitable diphtheria antitoxin, giving a precipitate. If a satisfactory result is not obtained with a vaccine adsorbed on aluminium hydroxide, carry out the test as follows. Centrifuge 15 ml of the vaccine to be examined and suspend the residue in 5 ml of a freshly prepared mixture of 1 volume of a 56 g/l solution of *sodium edetate R* and 49 volumes of a 90 g/l solution of *disodium hydrogen phosphate R*. Maintain at 37 °C for not less than 6 h and centrifuge. The clear supernatant liquid reacts with a suitable diphtheria antitoxin, giving a precipitate.

TESTS

Aluminium (*2.5.13*): maximum 1.25 mg per single human dose, if aluminium hydroxide or hydrated aluminium phosphate is used as the adsorbent.

Free formaldehyde (*2.4.18*): maximum 0.2 g/l.

Antimicrobial preservative. Where applicable, determine the amount of antimicrobial preservative by a suitable chemical method. The content is not less than the minimum amount shown to be effective and is not greater than 115 per cent of the quantity stated on the label.

Sterility (*2.6.1*). The vaccine complies with the test for sterility.

ASSAY

Carry out one of the prescribed methods for the assay of diphtheria vaccine (adsorbed) (*2.7.6*).

The lower confidence limit ($P = 0.95$) of the estimated potency is not less than 2 IU per single human dose.

LABELLING

The label states:

- the minimum number of International Units per single human dose,
- the name and the amount of the adsorbent,
- that the vaccine must be shaken before use,
- that the vaccine is not to be frozen.

01/2005:1219

HAEMOPHILUS TYPE b CONJUGATE VACCINE

Vaccinum haemophili stirpe b coniugatum

DEFINITION

Haemophilus type b conjugate vaccine is a liquid or freeze-dried preparation of a polysaccharide, derived from a suitable strain of *Haemophilus influenzae* type b, covalently bound to a carrier protein. The polysaccharide, polyribosylribitol phosphate, referred to as PRP, is a linear copolymer composed of repeated units of 3-β-D-ribofuranosyl-(1→1)-ribitol-5-phosphate [$(C_{10}H_{19}O_{12}P)_n$], with a defined molecular size. The carrier protein, when conjugated to PRP, is capable of inducing a T-cell-dependent B-cell immune response to the polysaccharide.

PRODUCTION

GENERAL PROVISIONS

The production method shall have been shown to yield consistently haemophilus type b conjugate vaccines of adequate safety and immunogenicity in man. The production of PRP and of the carrier are based on seed-lot systems.

The production method is validated to demonstrate that the product, if tested, would comply with the test for abnormal toxicity for immunosera and vaccines for human use (*2.6.9*).

During development studies and wherever revalidation of the manufacturing process is necessary, it shall be demonstrated by tests in animals that the vaccine consistently induces a T-cell-dependent B-cell immune response.

The stability of the final lot and relevant intermediates is evaluated using one or more indicator tests. Such tests may include determination of molecular size, determination of free PRP in the conjugate and the immunogenicity test in mice. Taking account of the results of the stability testing, release requirements are set for these indicator tests to ensure that the vaccine will be satisfactory at the end of the period of validity.

BACTERIAL SEED LOTS

The seed lots of *H. influenzae* type b are shown to be free from contamination by methods of suitable sensitivity. These may include inoculation into suitable media, examination of colony morphology, microscopic examination of Gram-stained smears and culture agglutination with suitable specific antisera.

No complex products of animal origin are included in the menstruum used for preservation of strain viability, either for freeze-drying or for frozen storage.

It is recommended that PRP produced by the seed lot be characterised using nuclear magnetic resonance spectrometry (*2.2.33*).

H. INFLUENZAE TYPE b POLYSACCHARIDE (PRP)

H. influenzae type b is grown in a liquid medium that does not contain high-molecular-mass polysaccharides; if any ingredient of the medium contains blood-group substances, the process shall be validated to demonstrate that after the purification step they are no longer detectable. The bacterial purity of the culture is verified by methods of suitable sensitivity. These may include inoculation into suitable media, examination of colony morphology, microscopic examination of Gram-stained smears and culture agglutination with suitable specific antisera. The culture may be inactivated. PRP is separated from the culture medium and purified by a suitable method. Volatile matter, including water, in the purified polysaccharide is determined by a suitable method such as thermogravimetry (*2.2.34*); the result is used to calculate the results of certain tests with reference to the dried substance, as prescribed below.

Only PRP that complies with the following requirements may be used in the preparation of the conjugate.

Identification. PRP is identified by an immunochemical method (*2.7.1*) or other suitable method, for example ^{1}H nuclear magnetic resonance spectrometry (*2.2.33*).

Molecular-size distribution. The percentage of PRP eluted before a given K_0 value or within a range of K_0 values is determined by size-exclusion chromatography (*2.2.30*); an acceptable value is established for the particular product and each batch of PRP must be shown to comply with this limit. Limits for currently approved products, using the indicated stationary phases, are shown for information in Table 1219.-1. Where applicable, the molecular-size distribution is also determined after chemical modification of the polysaccharide.

Liquid chromatography (*2.2.29*) with multiple-angle laser light-scattering detection may also be used for determination of molecular-size distribution.

A validated determination of the degree of polymerisation or of the weight-average molecular weight and the dispersion of molecular masses may be used instead of the determination of molecular size distribution.

Ribose (*2.5.31*). Not less than 32 per cent, calculated with reference to the dried substance.

Phosphorus (*2.5.18*): 6.8 per cent to 9.0 per cent, calculated with reference to the dried substance.

Protein (*2.5.16*). Not more than 1.0 per cent, calculated with reference to the dried substance. Use sufficient PRP to allow detection of proteins at concentrations of 1 per cent or greater.

Nucleic acid (*2.5.17*). Not more than 1.0 per cent, calculated with reference to the dried substance.

Bacterial endotoxins (*2.6.14*): less than 25 IU per microgram of PRP.

Residual reagents. Where applicable, tests are carried out to determine residues of reagents used during inactivation and purification. An acceptable value for each reagent is established for the particular product and each batch of PRP must be shown to comply with this limit. Where validation studies have demonstrated removal of a residual reagent, the test on PRP may be omitted.

Vaccines

Table 1219.-1. – *Product characteristics and specifications for PRP and carrier protein in currently approved products*

Carrier			**Haemophilus polysaccharide**		**Conjugation**	
Type	**Purity**	**Nominal amount per dose**	**Type of PRP**	**Nominal amount per dose**	**Coupling method**	**Procedure**
Diphtheria toxoid	> 1500 Lf per milligram of nitrogen	18 μg	Size-reduced PRP K_0: 0.6-0.7, using *cross-linked agarose for chromatography R*	25 μg	cyanogen bromide activation of PRP	activated diphtheria toxoid (D-AH$^+$), cyanogen bromide-activated PRP
Tetanus toxoid	> 1500 Lf per milligram of nitrogen	20 μg	PRP ≥ 50 % ≤ K_0: 0.30, using *cross-linked agarose for chromatography R*	10 μg	carbodi-imide mediated	ADH-activated PRP (PRP-cov.-AH) + tetanus toxoid + EDAC
CRM 197 diphtheria protein	> 90 % of diphtheria protein	25 μg	Size-reduced PRP Dp = 15-35 or 10-35	10 μg	reductive amination (1-step method) or *N*-hydroxysuccinimide activation	direct coupling of PRP to CRM 197 (cyanoborohydride activated)
Meningococcal group B outer membrane protein (OMP)	outer membrane protein vesicles: ≤ 8 % of lipopolysaccharide	125 μg or 250 μg	Size-reduced PRP K_0 < 0.6, using *cross-linked agarose for chromatography R* or M_w > 50 × 10^3	7.5 μg or 15 μg	thioether bond	PRP activation by CDI PRP-IM + BuA2 + BrAc = PRP-BuA2-BrAc + thioactivated OMP

ADH = adipic acid dihydrazide
BrAc = bromoacetyl chloride
BuA2 = butane-1,4-diamide
CDI = carbonyldiimidazole
Dp = degree of polymerisation
EDAC = 1-ethyl-3-(3-dimethylaminopropyl)carbodiimide
IM = imidazolium
M_w = weight-average molecular weight

CARRIER PROTEIN

The carrier protein is chosen so that when the PRP is conjugated it is able to induce a T-cell-dependent B-cell immune response. Currently approved carrier proteins and coupling methods are listed for information in Table 1219.-1. The carrier proteins are produced by culture of suitable micro-organisms; the bacterial purity of the culture is verified; the culture may be inactivated; the carrier protein is purified by a suitable method.

Only a carrier protein that complies with the following requirements may be used in the preparation of the conjugate.

Identification. The carrier protein is identified by a suitable immunochemical method (*2.7.1*).

Sterility (*2.6.1*). Carry out the test using for each medium 10 ml or the equivalent of one-hundred doses, whichever is less.

Diphtheria toxoid. Diphtheria toxoid is produced as described in *Diphtheria vaccine (adsorbed) (0443)* and complies with the requirements prescribed therein for bulk purified toxoid.

Tetanus toxoid. Tetanus toxoid is produced as described in *Tetanus vaccine (adsorbed) (0452)* and complies with the requirements prescribed therein for bulk purified toxoid, except that the antigenic purity is not less than 1500 Lf per milligram of protein nitrogen.

Diphtheria protein CRM 197. It contains not less than 90 per cent of diphtheria CRM 197 protein, determined by a suitable method. Suitable tests are carried out, for validation or routinely, to demonstrate that the product is nontoxic.

OMP (meningococcal group B Outer Membrane Protein complex). OMP complies with the following requirements for lipopolysaccharide and pyrogens.

Lipopolysaccharide. Not more than 8 per cent of lipopolysaccharide, determined by a suitable method.

Pyrogens (*2.6.8*). Inject into each rabbit 0.25 μg of OMP per kilogram of body mass.

BULK CONJUGATE

PRP is chemically modified to enable conjugation; it is usually partly depolymerised either before or during this procedure. Reactive functional groups or spacers may be introduced into the carrier protein or PRP prior to conjugation. As a measure of consistency, the extent of derivatisation is monitored. The conjugate is obtained by the covalent binding of PRP and carrier protein. Where applicable, unreacted but potentially reactogenic functional groups are made unreactive by means of capping agents; the conjugate is purified to remove reagents.

Only a bulk conjugate that complies with the following requirements may be used in the preparation of the final bulk vaccine. For each test and for each particular product, limits of acceptance are established and each batch of conjugate must be shown to comply with these limits. Limits applied to currently approved products for some of these tests are listed for information in Table 1219.-2. For a freeze-dried vaccine, some of the tests may be carried out on the final lot rather than on the bulk conjugate where the freeze-drying process may affect the component being tested.

PRP. The PRP content is determined by assay of phosphorus (*2.5.18*) or by assay of ribose (*2.5.31*) or by an immunochemical method (*2.7.1*).

Protein. The protein content is determined by a suitable chemical method (for example, *2.5.16*).

PRP to protein ratio. Determine the ratio by calculation.

Molecular-size distribution. Molecular-size distribution is determined by size-exclusion chromatography (*2.2.30*).

Free PRP. Unbound PRP is determined after removal of the conjugate, for example by anion-exchange, size-exclusion or hydrophobic chromatography, ultrafiltration or other validated methods.

Free carrier protein. Determine the content by a suitable method, either directly or by deriving the content by calculation from the results of other tests. The amount is within the limits approved for the particular product.

Table 1219.-2. – *Bulk conjugate requirements for currently approved products*

Test	Protein carrier			
	Diphtheria toxoid	Tetanus toxoid	CRM 197	OMP
Free PRP	< 37 %	< 20 %	< 25 %	< 15 %
Free protein	< 4 %	< 1 %, where applicable	< 1 % or < 2 %, depending on the coupling method	not applicable
PRP to protein ratio	1.25 - 1.8	0.30 - 0.55	0.3 - 0.7	0.05 - 0.1
Molecular size (K_o):				
cross-linked agarose for chromatography R	95 % < 0.75	60 % < 0.2	50 % 0.3 - 0.6	85 % < 0.3
cross-linked agarose for chromatography R1	0.6-0.7	85 % < 0.5		

Unreacted functional groups. No unreacted functional groups are detectable in the bulk conjugate unless process validation has shown that unreacted functional groups detectable at this stage are removed during the subsequent manufacturing process (for example, owing to short half-life).

Residual reagents. Removal of residual reagents such as cyanide, EDAC (ethyldimethylaminopropylcarbodi-imide) and phenol is confirmed by suitable tests or by validation of the process.

Sterility (*2.6.1*). Carry out the test using for each medium 10 ml or the equivalent of 100 doses, whichever is less.

FINAL BULK VACCINE

An adjuvant, an antimicrobial preservative and a stabiliser may be added to the bulk conjugate before dilution to the final concentration with a suitable diluent.

Only a final bulk vaccine that complies with the following requirements may be used in preparation of the final lot.

Antimicrobial preservative. Where applicable, determine the amount of antimicrobial preservative by a suitable chemical or physico-chemical method. The content is not less than 85 per cent and not greater than 115 per cent of the intended amount.

Sterility (*2.6.1*). It complies with the test for sterility, carried out using 10 ml for each medium.

FINAL LOT

Only a final lot that is satisfactory with respect to each of the requirements given below under Identification and Tests may be released for use. Provided the test for antimicrobial preservative has been carried out on the final bulk vaccine, it may be omitted on the final lot.

pH (*2.2.3*). The pH of the vaccine, reconstituted if necessary, is within the range approved for the particular product.

Free PRP. Unbound PRP is determined after removal of the conjugate, for example by anion-exchange, size-exclusion or hydrophobic chromatography, ultrafiltration or other validated methods. The amount of free PRP is not greater than that approved for the particular product.

IDENTIFICATION

The vaccine is identified by a suitable immunochemical method (*2.7.1*) for PRP.

TESTS

PRP. Not less than 80 per cent of the amount of PRP stated on the label. PRP is determined either by assay of ribose (*2.5.31*) or phosphorus (*2.5.18*), by an immunochemical method (*2.7.1*) or by anion-exchange liquid chromatography with pulsed amperometric detection (*2.2.29*).

Aluminium (*2.5.13*): maximum 1.25 mg per single human dose, if aluminium hydroxide or hydrated aluminium phosphate is used as the adsorbent.

Antimicrobial preservative. Where applicable, determine the amount of antimicrobial preservative by a suitable chemical or physico-chemical method. The content is not less than the minimum amount shown to be effective and not greater than 115 per cent of the quantity stated on the label.

Water (*2.5.12*): maximum 3.0 per cent for freeze-dried vaccines.

Sterility (*2.6.1*). It complies with the test for sterility.

Pyrogens (*2.6.8*). It complies with the test for pyrogens. Inject per kilogram of the rabbit's mass a quantity of the vaccine equivalent to: 1 μg of PRP for a vaccine with diphtheria toxoid or CRM 197 diphtheria protein as carrier; 0.1 μg of PRP for a vaccine with tetanus toxoid as carrier; 0.025 μg of PRP for a vaccine with OMP as carrier.

LABELLING

The label states:

– the number of micrograms of PRP per human dose,
– the type and nominal amount of carrier protein per single human dose.

01/2005:1526

HEPATITIS A (INACTIVATED) AND HEPATITIS B (rDNA) VACCINE (ADSORBED)

Vaccinum hepatitidis A inactivatum et hepatitidis B (ADNr) adsorbatum

DEFINITION

Hepatitis A (inactivated) and hepatitis B (rDNA) vaccine (adsorbed) is a suspension consisting of a suitable strain of hepatitis A virus, grown in cell cultures and inactivated by a validated method, and of hepatitis B surface antigen (HBsAg), a component protein of hepatitis B virus obtained by recombinant DNA technology; the antigens are adsorbed on a mineral carrier, such as aluminium hydroxide or hydrated aluminium phosphate.

PRODUCTION

GENERAL PROVISIONS

The two components are prepared as described in the monographs on *Hepatitis A vaccine (inactivated, adsorbed) (1107)* and *Hepatitis B vaccine (rDNA) (1056)* and comply with the requirements prescribed therein.

The production method is validated to demonstrate that the product, if tested, would comply with the test for abnormal toxicity for immunosera and vaccines for human use (*2.6.9*).

Reference preparation. The reference preparation is part of a representative batch shown to be at least as immunogenic in animals as a batch that, in clinical studies in young healthy adults, produced not less than 95 per cent seroconversion, corresponding to a level of neutralising antibody recognised to be protective, after a full-course primary immunisation. For hepatitis A, an antibody level not less than 20 mIU/ml determined by enzyme-linked immunosorbent assay is recognised as being protective. For hepatitis B, an antibody level not less than 10 mIU/ml against HBsAg is recognised as being protective.

FINAL BULK VACCINE

The final bulk vaccine is prepared from one or more inactivated harvests of hepatitis A virus and one or more batches of purified antigen.

Only a final bulk vaccine that complies with the following requirements may be used in the preparation of the final lot.

Antimicrobial preservative. Where applicable, determine the amount of antimicrobial preservative by a suitable chemical or physico-chemical method. The amount is not less than 85 per cent and not greater than 115 per cent of the intended amount.

Sterility (*2.6.1*). The final bulk vaccine complies with the test for sterility, carried out using 10 ml for each medium.

FINAL LOT

Only a final lot that complies with each of the requirements given below under Identification, Tests and Assay may be released for use. Provided that the tests for free formaldehyde (where applicable) and antimicrobial preservative content (where applicable) have been carried out on the final bulk vaccine with satisfactory results, they may be omitted on the final lot. If the assay of the hepatitis A and/or the hepatitis B component is carried out *in vivo*, then provided it has been carried out with satisfactory results on the final bulk vaccine, it may be omitted on the final lot.

IDENTIFICATION

The vaccine is shown to contain hepatitis A virus antigen and hepatitis B surface antigen by suitable immunochemical methods (*2.7.1*), using specific antibodies or by the mouse immunogenicity tests described under Assay.

TESTS

Aluminium (*2.5.13*): maximum 1.25 mg per single human dose, if aluminium hydroxide or hydrated aluminium phosphate is used as the adsorbent.

Free formaldehyde (*2.4.18*): maximum 0.2 g/l.

Antimicrobial preservative. Where applicable, determine the amount of antimicrobial preservative by a suitable chemical or physico-chemical method. The amount is not less than the minimum amount shown to be effective and is not greater than 115 per cent of that stated on the label.

Sterility (*2.6.1*). The vaccine complies with the test for sterility.

Bacterial endotoxins (*2.6.14*): less than 2 IU per human dose.

ASSAY

Hepatitis A component. The vaccine complies with the assay of hepatitis A vaccine (*2.7.14*).

Hepatitis B component. The vaccine complies with the assay of hepatitis B vaccine (rDNA) (*2.7.15*).

LABELLING

The label states:

- the amount of hepatitis A virus antigen and hepatitis B surface antigen per container,
- the type of cells used for production of the vaccine,
- the name and amount of the adsorbent used,
- that the vaccine must be shaken before use,
- that the vaccine must not be frozen.

01/2005:1107

HEPATITIS A VACCINE (INACTIVATED, ADSORBED)

Vaccinum hepatitidis A inactivatum adsorbatum

DEFINITION

Hepatitis A vaccine (inactivated, adsorbed) is a suspension consisting of a suitable strain of hepatitis A virus grown in cell cultures, inactivated by a validated method and adsorbed on a mineral carrier.

PRODUCTION

Production of the vaccine is based on a virus seed-lot system and a cell-bank system. The production method shall have been shown to yield consistently vaccines that comply with the requirements for immunogenicity, safety and stability.

The production method is validated to demonstrate that the product, if tested, would comply with the test for abnormal toxicity for immunosera and vaccines for human use (*2.6.9*).

Unless otherwise justified and authorised, the virus in the final vaccine shall not have undergone more passages from the master seed lot than were used to prepare the vaccine shown in clinical studies to be satisfactory with respect to safety and efficacy.

Reference preparation. A part of a batch shown to be at least as immunogenic in animals as a batch that, in clinical studies in young healthy adults, produced not less than 95 per cent seroconversion, corresponding to a level of neutralising antibody accepted to be protective, after a full-course primary immunisation is used as a reference preparation. An antibody level of 20 mIU/ml determined by enzyme-linked immunosorbent assay is recognised as being protective.

SUBSTRATE FOR VIRUS PROPAGATION

The virus is propagated in a human diploid cell line (*5.2.3*) or in a continuous cell line approved by the competent authority.

SEED LOTS

The strain of hepatitis A virus used to prepare the master seed lot shall be identified by historical records that include information on the origin of the strain and its subsequent manipulation.

Only a seed lot that complies with the following requirements may be used for virus propagation.

Identification. Each master and working seed lot is identified as hepatitis A virus using specific antibodies.

Virus concentration. The virus concentration of each master and working seed lot is determined to monitor consistency of production.

Extraneous agents. The master and working seed lots comply with the requirements for seed lots for virus vaccines (*2.6.16*). In addition, if primary monkey cells have been used for isolation of the strain, measures are taken to ensure that the strain is not contaminated with simian viruses such as simian immunodeficiency virus and filoviruses.

VIRUS PROPAGATION AND HARVEST

All processing of the cell bank and subsequent cell cultures is done under aseptic conditions in an area where no other cells are being handled. Animal serum (but not human

Vaccines

serum) may be used in the cell culture media. Serum and trypsin used in the preparation of cell suspensions and media are shown to be free from extraneous agents. The cell culture media may contain a pH indicator, such as phenol red, and antibiotics at the lowest effective concentration. Not less than 500 ml of the cell cultures employed for vaccine production is set aside as uninfected cell cultures (control cells). Multiple harvests from the same production cell culture may be pooled and considered as a single harvest.

Only a single harvest that complies with the following requirements may be used in the preparation of the vaccine. When the determination of the ratio of virus concentration to antigen content has been carried out on a suitable number of single harvests to demonstrate production consistency, it may subsequently be omitted as a routine test.

Identification. The test for antigen content also serves to identify the single harvest.

Bacterial and fungal contamination (*2.6.1*). The single harvest complies with the test for sterility, carried out using 10 ml for each medium.

Mycoplasmas (*2.6.7*). The single harvest complies with the test for mycoplasmas, carried out using 1 ml for each medium.

Control cells. The control cells of the production cell culture comply with a test for identification and the requirements for extraneous agents (*2.6.16*).

Antigen content. Determine the hepatitis A antigen content by a suitable immunochemical method (*2.7.1*) to monitor production consistency; the content is within the limits approved for the particular product.

Ratio of virus concentration to antigen content. The consistency of the ratio of the concentration of infectious virus, determined by a suitable cell culture method, to antigen content is established by validation on a suitable number of single harvests.

PURIFICATION AND PURIFIED HARVEST

The harvest, which may be a pool of several single harvests, is purified by validated methods. If continuous cell lines are used for production, the purification process shall have been shown to reduce consistently the level of host-cell DNA.

Only a purified harvest that complies with the following requirements may be used in the preparation of the inactivated harvest.

Virus concentration. The concentration of infectious virus in the purified harvest is determined by a suitable cell culture method to monitor production consistency and as a starting point for monitoring the inactivation curve.

Antigen:total protein ratio. Determine the hepatitis A virus antigen content by a suitable immunochemical method (*2.7.1*). Determine the total protein by a validated method. The ratio of hepatitis A virus antigen content to total protein content is within the limits approved for the particular product.

Bovine serum albumin. Not more than 50 ng in the equivalent of a single human dose, determined by a suitable immunochemical method (*2.7.1*). Where appropriate in view of the manufacturing process, other suitable protein markers may be used to demonstrate effective purification.

Residual host-cell DNA. If a continuous cell line is used for virus propagation, the content of residual host-cell DNA, determined using a suitable method, is not greater than 100 pg in the equivalent of a single human dose.

Residual chemicals. If chemical substances are used during the purification process, tests for these substances are carried out on the purified harvest (or on the inactivated harvest), unless validation of the process has demonstrated total clearance. The concentration must not exceed the limits approved for the particular product.

INACTIVATION AND INACTIVATED HARVEST

Several purified harvests may be pooled before inactivation. In order to avoid interference with the inactivation process, virus aggregation must be prevented or aggregates must be removed immediately before and/or during the inactivation process. The virus suspension is inactivated by a validated method; the method shall have been shown to be consistently capable of inactivating hepatitis A virus without destroying the antigenic and immunogenic activity; for each inactivation procedure, an inactivation curve is plotted representing residual live virus concentration measured at not fewer than three points in time (for example, on days 0, 1 and 2 of the inactivation process). If formaldehyde is used for inactivation, the presence of excess free formaldehyde is verified at the end of the inactivation process.

Only an inactivated harvest that complies with the following requirements may be used in the preparation of the final bulk vaccine.

Inactivation. Carry out an amplification test for residual infectious hepatitis A virus by inoculating a quantity of the inactivated harvest equivalent to 5 per cent of the batch or, if the harvest contains the equivalent of 30 000 doses or more, not less than 1500 doses of vaccine into cell cultures of the same type as those used for production of the vaccine; incubate for a total of not less than 70 days making not fewer than one passage of cells within that period. At the end of the incubation period, carry out a test of suitable sensitivity for residual infectious virus. No evidence of hepatitis A virus multiplication is found in the samples taken at the end of the inactivation process. Use infectious virus inocula concurrently as positive controls to demonstrate cellular susceptibility and absence of interference. Incubate for a total of not less than 70 days, making not fewer than one passage of cells within that period.

Sterility (*2.6.1*). The inactivated viral harvest complies with the test for sterility, carried out using 10 ml for each medium.

Bacterial endotoxins (*2.6.14*): less than 2 IU in the equivalent of a single human dose.

Antigen content. Determine the hepatitis A virus antigen content by a suitable immunochemical method (*2.7.1*).

Residual chemicals. See under Purification and purified harvest.

FINAL BULK VACCINE

The final bulk vaccine is prepared from one or more inactivated harvests. Approved adjuvants, stabilisers and antimicrobial preservatives may be added.

Only a final bulk vaccine that complies with the following requirements may be used in the preparation of the final lot.

Sterility (*2.6.1*). The final bulk vaccine complies with the test for sterility, carried out using 10 ml for each medium.

Antimicrobial preservative. Where applicable, determine the amount of antimicrobial preservative by a suitable chemical or physico-chemical method. The amount is not less than 85 per cent and not greater than 115 per cent of the intended amount.

FINAL LOT

The final bulk vaccine is distributed aseptically into sterile containers. The containers are then closed so as to avoid contamination.

Only a final lot that complies with each of the requirements given below under Identification, Tests and Assay may be released for use. Provided that the tests for free formaldehyde (where applicable) and antimicrobial preservative content (where applicable) have been carried out on the final bulk vaccine with satisfactory results, these tests may be omitted on the final lot. If the assay is carried out using mice or other animals, then provided it has been carried out with satisfactory results on the final bulk vaccine, it may be omitted on the final lot.

IDENTIFICATION

The vaccine is shown to contain hepatitis A virus antigen by a suitable immunochemical method (*2.7.1*) using specific antibodies or by the *in vivo* assay (*2.7.14*).

TESTS

Aluminium (*2.5.13*): maximum 1.25 mg per single human dose, if aluminium hydroxide or hydrated aluminium phosphate is used as the adsorbent.

Free formaldehyde (*2.4.18*): maximum 0.2 g/l.

Antimicrobial preservative. Where applicable, determine the amount of antimicrobial preservative by a suitable chemical or physico-chemical method. The amount is not less than the minimum amount shown to be effective and is not greater than 115 per cent of that stated on the label.

Sterility (*2.6.1*). The vaccine complies with the test for sterility.

ASSAY

The vaccine complies with the assay of hepatitis A vaccine (*2.7.14*).

LABELLING

The label states the biological origin of the cells used for the preparation of the vaccine.

01/2005:1935

HEPATITIS A VACCINE (INACTIVATED, VIROSOME)

Vaccinum hepatitidis A inactivatum virosomale

DEFINITION

Hepatitis A vaccine (inactivated, virosome) is a suspension of a suitable strain of hepatitis A virus grown in cell cultures and inactivated by a validated method. Virosomes composed of influenza proteins of a strain approved for the particular product and phospholipids are used as adjuvants.

PRODUCTION

GENERAL PROVISIONS

The production method shall have been shown to yield consistently vaccines comparable with the vaccine of proven clinical efficacy and safety in man.

The production method is validated to demonstrate that the product, if tested, would comply with the test for abnormal toxicity for immunosera and vaccines for human use (*2.6.9*).

Reference preparation. A reference preparation of inactivated hepatitis A antigen is calibrated against a batch of hepatitis A vaccine (inactivated, virosome) that, in clinical studies in young healthy adults, produced not less than 95 per cent seroconversion, corresponding to a level of neutralising antibody accepted to be protective, after a full-course primary immunisation. An antibody level not less than 20 mIU/ml determined by enzyme-linked immunosorbent assay is recognised as being protective.

PREPARATION OF HEPATITIS A ANTIGEN

Production of the hepatitis A antigen is based on a virus seed-lot system and a cell-bank system. The production method shall have been shown to yield consistently vaccines that comply with the requirements for immunogenicity, safety and stability.

Unless otherwise justified and authorised, the virus in the final vaccine shall not have undergone more passages from the master seed lot than were used to prepare the vaccine shown in clinical studies to be satisfactory with respect to safety and efficacy.

SUBSTRATE FOR PROPAGATION OF HEPATITIS A VIRUS

The virus is propagated in a human diploid cell line (*5.2.3*).

SEED LOTS OF HEPATITIS A VIRUS

The strain of hepatitis A virus used to prepare the master seed lot shall be identified by historical records that include information on the origin of the strain and its subsequent manipulation.

Only a seed lot that complies with the following requirements may be used for virus propagation.

Identification. Each master and working seed lot is identified as hepatitis A virus using specific antibodies.

Virus concentration. The virus concentration of each master and working seed lot is determined to monitor consistency of production.

Extraneous agents. The master and working seed lots comply with the requirements for seed lots for virus vaccines (*2.6.16*).

PROPAGATION AND HARVEST OF HEPATITIS A VIRUS

All processing of the cell bank and subsequent cell cultures is done under aseptic conditions in an area where no other cells are handled. Animal serum (but not human serum) may be used in the cell culture media. Serum and trypsin used in the preparation of cell suspensions and media are shown to be free from extraneous agents. The cell culture media may contain a pH indicator such as phenol red and antibiotics at the lowest effective concentration. Not less than 500 ml of the cell cultures employed for vaccine production is set aside as uninfected cell cultures (control cells). Multiple harvests from the same production cell culture may be pooled and considered as a single harvest.

Only a single harvest that complies with the following requirements may be used in the preparation of the vaccine. When the determination of the ratio of virus concentration to antigen content has been carried out on a suitable number of single harvests to demonstrate consistency, it may subsequently be omitted as a routine test.

Identification. The test for antigen content also serves to identify the single harvest.

Bacterial and fungal contamination (*2.6.1*). The single harvest complies with the test for sterility, carried out using 10 ml for each medium.

Mycoplasmas (*2.6.7*). The single harvest complies with the test for mycoplasmas.

Control cells. The control cells of the production cell culture comply with a test for identity and the requirements for extraneous agents (*2.6.16*).

Antigen content. Determine the hepatitis A antigen content by a suitable immunochemical method (*2.7.1*) to monitor production consistency; the content is within the limits approved for the particular product.

Ratio of virus concentration to antigen content. The consistency of the ratio of the concentration of infectious virus, as determined by a suitable cell culture method, to antigen content is established by validation on a suitable number of single harvests.

PURIFICATION AND PURIFIED HARVEST OF HEPATITIS A VIRUS

The harvest, which may be a pool of several single harvests, is purified by validated methods. If continuous cell lines are used for production, the purification process shall have been shown to reduce consistently the level of host-cell DNA.

Only a purified harvest that complies with the following requirements may be used in the preparation of the inactivated harvest.

Virus concentration. The concentration of infective virus in the purified harvest is determined by a suitable cell culture method to monitor production consistency and as a starting point for monitoring the inactivation curve.

Ratio of antigen to total protein. Determine the hepatitis A virus antigen content by a suitable immunochemical method (*2.7.1*). Determine the total protein by a validated method. The ratio of hepatitis A virus antigen content to total protein content is within the limits approved for the particular product.

Bovine serum albumin: maximum 50 ng per single human dose if foetal bovine serum is used, determined by a suitable immunochemical method (*2.7.1*). Where appropriate in view of the manufacturing process, other suitable protein markers may be used to demonstrate effective purification.

Residual chemicals. If chemical substances are used during the purification process, tests for these substances are carried out on the purified harvest (or on the inactivated harvest), unless validation of the process has demonstrated total clearance. The concentration must not exceed the limits approved for the particular product.

INACTIVATION AND INACTIVATED HARVEST OF HEPATITIS A VIRUS

Several purified harvests may be pooled before inactivation. In order to avoid interference with the inactivation process, virus aggregation must be prevented or aggregates must be removed immediately before and/or during the inactivation process. The virus suspension is inactivated by a validated method; the method shall have been shown to be consistently capable of inactivating hepatitis A virus without destroying the antigenic and immunogenic activity; for each inactivation procedure, an inactivation curve is plotted representing residual live virus concentration measured on at least 3 occasions (for example, on days 0, 1 and 2 of the inactivation process). If formaldehyde is used for inactivation, the presence of excess free formaldehyde is verified at the end of the inactivation process.

Only an inactivated harvest that complies with the following requirements may be used in the preparation of the final bulk vaccine.

Inactivation. Carry out an amplification test for residual infectious hepatitis A virus by inoculating a quantity of the inactivated harvest equivalent to 5 per cent of the batch or, if the harvest contains the equivalent of 30 000 doses or more, not less than 1500 doses of vaccine into cell cultures of the same type as those used for production of the vaccine; incubate for a total of not less than 70 days making not fewer than 1 passage of cells within that period. At the end of the incubation period, carry out a test of suitable sensitivity for residual infectious virus. No evidence of hepatitis A virus multiplication is found in the samples taken at the end of the inactivation process. Use infective virus inocula concurrently as positive controls to demonstrate cellular susceptibility and absence of interference.

Sterility (*2.6.1*). The inactivated viral harvest complies with the test for sterility, carried out using 10 ml for each medium.

Bacterial endotoxins (*2.6.14*): less than 2 IU of endotoxin in the equivalent of a single human dose.

Antigen content. Determine the hepatitis A virus antigen content by a suitable immunochemical method (*2.7.1*).

Residual chemicals. See under Purification and purified harvest.

PREPARATION OF INACTIVATED INFLUENZA VIRUS

The production of influenza viruses is based on a seed-lot system. Working seed lots represent not more than 15 passages from the approved reassorted virus or the approved virus isolate. The final production represents 1 passage from the working seed lot. The strain of influenza virus to be used is approved by the competent authority.

SUBSTRATE FOR PROPAGATION OF INFLUENZA VIRUS

Influenza virus seed to be used in the production of vaccine is propagated in fertilised eggs from chicken flocks free from specified pathogens (*5.2.2*) or in suitable cell cultures (*5.2.4*), such as chick-embryo fibroblasts or chick kidney cells obtained from chicken flocks free from specified pathogens (*5.2.2*). For production, the virus is grown in the allantoic cavity of fertilised hens' eggs from healthy flocks.

SEED LOTS OF INFLUENZA VIRUS

The haemagglutinin and neuraminidase antigens of each seed lot are identified as originating from the correct strain of influenza virus by suitable methods.

Only a working virus seed lot that complies with the following requirements may be used in the preparation of the monovalent pooled harvest.

Bacterial and fungal contamination. Carry out the test for sterility (*2.6.1*), using 10 ml for each medium.

Mycoplasmas (*2.6.7*). Carry out the test for mycoplasmas, using 10 ml.

PROPAGATION AND HARVEST OF INFLUENZA VIRUS

An antimicrobial agent may be added to the inoculum. After incubation at a controlled temperature, the allantoic fluids are harvested and combined to form the monovalent pooled harvest. An antimicrobial agent may be added at the time of harvest. At no stage in the production is penicillin or streptomycin used.

POOLED HARVEST OF INFLUENZA VIRUS

To limit the possibility of contamination, inactivation is initiated as soon as possible after preparation. The virus is inactivated by a method that has been demonstrated on 3 consecutive batches to be consistently effective for the manufacturer. The inactivation process shall have been shown to be capable of inactivating the influenza virus without destroying antigenicity of haemagglutinin. The inactivation process shall also have been shown to be capable of inactivating avian leucosis viruses and mycoplasmas. If the monovalent pooled harvest is stored after inactivation, it is held at a temperature of 5 ± 3 °C. If formaldehyde solution is used, the concentration does not exceed 0.2 g/l of CH_2O at any time during inactivation; if betapropiolactone is used, the concentration does not exceed 0.1 per cent *V/V* at any time during inactivation.

Only a pooled harvest that complies with the following requirements may be used in the preparation of the virosomes.

Haemagglutinin antigen. Determine the content of haemagglutinin antigen by an immunodiffusion test (*2.7.1*), by comparison with a haemagglutinin antigen reference preparation or with an antigen preparation calibrated against it. Carry out the test at 20-25 °C.

Sterility (*2.6.1*). Carry out the test for sterility, using 10 ml for each medium.

Viral inactivation. Inoculate 0.2 ml of the harvest into the allantoic cavity of each of 10 fertilised eggs and incubate at 33-37 °C for 3 days. The test is not valid unless at least 8 of the 10 embryos survive. Harvest 0.5 ml of the allantoic fluid from each surviving embryo and pool the fluids. Inoculate 0.2 ml of the pooled fluid into a further 10 fertilised eggs and incubate at 33-37 °C for 3 days. The test is not valid unless at least 8 of the 10 embryos survive. Harvest about 0.1 ml of the allantoic fluid from each surviving embryo and examine each individual harvest by a haemagglutination test. If haemagglutination is found for any of the fluids, carry out for that fluid a further passage in eggs and test for haemagglutination; no haemagglutination occurs.

Ovalbumin: maximum 1 µg of ovalbumin in the equivalent of 1 human dose, determined by a suitable technique using a suitable reference preparation of ovalbumin.

Antimicrobial preservative. Where applicable, determine the amount of antimicrobial preservative by a suitable chemical method. The content is not less than 85 per cent and not greater than 115 per cent of the intended amount.

Residual chemicals. Tests are carried out on the monovalent pooled harvest for the chemicals used for inactivation, the limits being approved by the competent authority.

PREPARATION OF VIROSOMES

Inactivated influenza virions are solubilised using a suitable detergent and are purified by high-speed centrifugation in order to obtain supernatants containing mainly influenza antigens. After the addition of suitable phospholipids, virosomes are formed by removal of the detergent either by adsorption chromatography or another suitable technique

Only virosomes that comply with the following requirements may be used in the preparation of the final bulk vaccine.

Haemagglutinin content. Determine the content of haemagglutinin antigen by an immunodiffusion test (*2.7.1*), by comparison with a haemagglutinin antigen reference preparation or with an antigen preparation calibrated against it.

Phospholipids. The content and identity of the phospholipids are determined by suitable immunochemical or physico-chemical methods.

Ratio of phospholipid to haemagglutinin. The ratio of phospholipid content to haemagglutinin content is within the limits approved for the particular product.

Residual chemicals. Tests are carried out for the chemicals used during the process. The concentration of each residual chemical is within the limits approved for the particular product.

FINAL BULK VACCINE

The bulk vaccine is prepared by adding virosomes to inactivated hepatitis A viruses to yield an approved hepatitis A antigen:haemagglutinin ratio. Several bulks may be pooled, and approved stabilisers and antimicrobial preservatives may be added.

Only a final bulk vaccine that complies with the following requirements may be used in the preparation of the final lot.

Protein content. The amount of protein is determined using a suitable technique, the limits being approved by the competent authorithy.

Phospholipids. The content and identity of the phospholipids are determined by suitable immunochemical or physico-chemical methods. The amount of phospholipids complies with the limits approved for the particular product.

Haemagglutinin content. Determine the content of haemagglutinin antigen by an immunodiffusion test (*2.7.1*). The amount of haemagglutinin must not exceed the limits approved for the particular product.

Hepatitis A antigen content. Determine the hepatitis A antigen content by a suitable immunochemical method. The amount of antigen must not exceed the limits approved for the particular product.

Ratio of hepatitis A antigen to haemagglutinin. The ratio of hepatitis A antigen content to haemagglutinin content is within the limits approved for the particular product.

Ovalbumin: maximum 1 µg of ovalbumin per human dose, determined by a suitable technique using a suitable reference preparation of ovalbumin.

Virosome size. The size distribution of the virosome-hepatitis A virus mixture is within the limits approved for the particular product.

Sterility (*2.6.1*). The final bulk vaccine complies with the test for sterility, carried out using 10 ml for each medium.

Antimicrobial preservative. Where applicable, determine the amount of antimicrobial preservative by a suitable chemical or physico-chemical method. The amount is not less than 85 per cent and not greater than 115 per cent of the intended amount.

Residual chemicals. If chemical substances are used during the formulation process, tests for these substances are carried out, the limits being approved by the competent authority.

FINAL LOT

The final bulk vaccine is distributed aseptically into sterile containers. The containers are then closed so as to avoid contamination.

Only a final lot that complies with each of the requirements given below under Identification, Tests and Assay may be released for use. Provided that the tests for free formaldehyde (where applicable) and antimicrobial preservative content (where applicable) have been carried out on the final bulk vaccine with satisfactory results, these tests may be omitted on the final lot. If the assay is carried out *in vivo*, provided it has been carried out with satisfactory results on the final bulk vaccine, it may be omitted on the final lot.

IDENTIFICATION

The vaccine is shown to contain hepatitis A virus antigen by a suitable immunochemical method (*2.7.1*) using specific antibodies.

TESTS

Free formaldehyde (*2.4.18*): maximum 0.2 g/l.

Antimicrobial preservative. Where applicable, determine the amount of antimicrobial preservative by a suitable chemical or physico-chemical method. The amount is not less than the minimum amount shown to be effective and is not greater than 115 per cent of that stated on the label.

Sterility (*2.6.1*). The vaccine complies with the test for sterility.

Bacterial endotoxins (*2.6.14*): less than 2 IU of endotoxin per human dose.

ASSAY

Determine the antigen content of the vaccine using a suitable immunochemical method (*2.7.1*) by comparison with the reference preparation. The acceptance criteria are approved for a given reference preparation by the competent authority.

LABELLING

The label states:

– the biological origin of the cells used for the preparation of the vaccine,
– that the carrier contains influenza proteins prepared in eggs,
– that the vaccine is not to be frozen,
– that the vaccine is to be shaken before use.

01/2005:1056

HEPATITIS B VACCINE (rDNA)

Vaccinum hepatitidis B (ADNr)

DEFINITION

Hepatitis B vaccine (rDNA) is a preparation of hepatitis B surface antigen (HBsAg), a component protein of hepatitis B virus; the antigen may be adsorbed on a mineral carrier such as aluminium hydroxide or hydrated aluminium phosphate. The antigen is obtained by recombinant DNA technology.

PRODUCTION

GENERAL PROVISIONS

The vaccine shall have been shown to induce specific, protective antibodies in man. The production method shall have been shown to yield consistently vaccines that comply with the requirements for immunogenicity and safety.

The production method is validated to demonstrate that the product, if tested, would comply with the test for abnormal toxicity for immunosera and vaccines for human use (*2.6.9*).

Hepatitis B vaccine (rDNA) is produced by the expression of the viral gene coding for HBsAg in yeast (*Saccharomyces cerevisiae*) or mammalian cells (Chinese hamster ovary (CHO) cells or other suitable cell lines), purification of the resulting HBsAg and the rendering of this antigen into an immunogenic preparation. The suitability and safety of the cells are approved by the competent authority.

The vaccine may contain the product of the S gene (major protein), a combination of the S gene and pre-S2 gene products (middle protein) or a combination of the S gene, the pre-S2 gene and pre-S1 gene products (large protein).

Reference preparation. The reference preparation is part of a representative batch shown to be at least as immunogenic in animals as a batch that, in clinical studies in young, healthy adults, produced not less than 95 per cent seroconversion, corresponding to a level of HBsAg neutralising antibody recognised to be protective, after a full-course primary immunisation. An antibody level not less than 10 mIU/ml is recognised as being protective.

CHARACTERISATION OF THE SUBSTANCE

Development studies are carried out to characterise the antigen. The complete protein, lipid and carbohydrate structure of the antigen is established. The morphological characteristics of the antigen particles are established by electron microscopy. The mean buoyant density of the antigen particles is determined by a physico-chemical method, such as gradient centrifugation. The antigenic epitopes are characterised. The protein fraction of the antigen is characterised in terms of the primary structure (for example, by determination of the amino-acid composition, by partial amino-acid sequence analysis and by peptide mapping).

CULTURE AND HARVEST

Identity, microbial purity, plasmid retention and consistency of yield are determined at suitable production stages. If mammalian cells are used, tests for extraneous agents and mycoplasmas are performed in accordance with *Tests for extraneous agents in viral vaccines for human use* (*2.6.16*), but using 200 ml of harvest in the test in cell culture for other extraneous agents.

PURIFIED ANTIGEN

Only a purified antigen that complies with the following requirements may be used in the preparation of the final bulk vaccine.

Total protein. The total protein is determined by a validated method. The content is within the limits approved for the specific product.

Antigen content and identification. The quantity and specificity of HBsAg is determined in comparison with the International Standard for HBsAg subtype *ad* or an in-house reference, by a suitable immunochemical method (*2.7.1*) such as radio-immunoassay (RIA), enzyme-linked immunosorbent assay (ELISA), immunoblot (preferably using a monoclonal antibody directed against a protective epitope) or single radial diffusion. The antigen/protein ratio is within the limits approved for the specific product.

The molecular weight of the major band revealed following sodium dodecyl sulphate polyacrylamide gel electrophoresis (SDS-PAGE) performed under reducing conditions corresponds to the value expected from the known nucleic acid and polypeptide sequences and possible glycosylation.

Antigenic purity. The purity of the antigen is determined by comparison with a reference preparation using liquid chromatography or other suitable methods such as SDS-PAGE with staining by acid blue 92 and silver. A suitable method is sensitive enough to detect a potential contaminant at a concentration of 1 per cent of total protein. Not less than 95 per cent of the total protein consists of hepatitis B surface antigen.

Composition. The content of proteins, lipids, nucleic acids and carbohydrates is determined.

Host-cell- and vector-derived DNA. If mammalian cells are used for production, not more than 10 pg of DNA in the quantity of purified antigen equivalent to a single human dose of vaccine.

Caesium. If a caesium salt is used during production, a test for residual caesium is carried out on the purified antigen. The content is within the limits approved for the specific product.

Sterility (*2.6.1*). The purified antigen complies with the test for sterility, carried out using 10 ml for each medium.

Additional tests on the purified antigen may be required depending on the production method used: for example, a test for residual animal serum where mammalian cells are used for production or tests for residual chemicals used during extraction and purification.

FINAL BULK VACCINE

An antimicrobial preservative and an adjuvant may be included in the vaccine.

Only a final bulk vaccine that complies with the following requirements may be used in the preparation of the final lot.

Antimicrobial preservative. Where applicable, determine the amount of antimicrobial preservative by a suitable chemical or physico-chemical method. The amount is not less than 85 per cent and not greater than 115 per cent of the intended amount.

Sterility (*2.6.1*). The final bulk vaccine complies with the test for sterility, carried out using 10 ml for each medium.

FINAL LOT

Only a final lot that complies with each of the requirements given below under Identification, Tests and Assay may be released for use. Provided that the tests for free formaldehyde (where applicable) and antimicrobial preservative content (where applicable) have been carried out on the final bulk vaccine with satisfactory results, they may be omitted on the final lot. If the assay is carried out *in vivo*, then provided it has been carried out with satisfactory results on the final bulk vaccine, it may be omitted on the final lot.

IDENTIFICATION

The assay or, where applicable, the electrophoretic profile, serves also to identify the vaccine.

TESTS

Aluminium (*2.5.13*): maximum 1.25 mg per single human dose, if aluminium hydroxide or hydrated aluminium phosphate is used as the adsorbent.

Free formaldehyde (*2.4.18*): maximum 0.2 g/l.

Antimicrobial preservative. Where applicable, determine the amount of antimicrobial preservative by a suitable chemical or physico-chemical method. The amount is not less than the minimum amount shown to be effective and is not greater than 115 per cent of that stated on the label.

Sterility (*2.6.1*). The vaccine complies with the test for sterility.

Pyrogens (*2.6.8*). The vaccine complies with the test for pyrogens. Inject the equivalent of one human dose into each rabbit.

ASSAY

The vaccine complies with the assay of hepatitis B vaccine (rDNA) (*2.7.15*).

LABELLING

The label states:

– the amount of HBsAg per container,
– the type of cells used for production of the vaccine,
– the name and amount of the adsorbent used,
– that the vaccine must be shaken before use,
– that the vaccine must not be frozen.

01/2005:0158

INFLUENZA VACCINE (SPLIT VIRION, INACTIVATED)

Vaccinum influenzae inactivatum ex virorum fragmentis praeparatum

DEFINITION

Influenza vaccine (split virion, inactivated) is a sterile, aqueous suspension of a strain or strains of influenza virus, type A or B, or a mixture of strains of the two types grown individually in fertilised hens' eggs, inactivated and treated so that the integrity of the virus particles has been disrupted without diminishing the antigenic properties of the haemagglutinin and neuraminidase antigens. The stated amount of haemagglutinin antigen for each strain present in the vaccine is 15 μg per dose, unless clinical evidence supports the use of a different amount.

The vaccine is a slightly opalescent liquid.

PRODUCTION

The production method is validated to demonstrate that the product, if tested, would comply with the test for abnormal toxicity for immunosera and vaccines for human use (*2.6.9*).

CHOICE OF VACCINE STRAIN

The World Health Organisation reviews the world epidemiological situation annually and if necessary recommends new strains corresponding to prevailing epidemiological evidence.

Such strains are used in accordance with the regulations in force in the signatory states of the Convention on the Elaboration of a European Pharmacopoeia. It is now common practice to use reassorted strains giving high yields of the appropriate surface antigens. The origin and passage history of virus strains shall be approved by the competent authority.

SUBSTRATE FOR VIRUS PROPAGATION

Influenza virus seed to be used in the production of vaccine is propagated in fertilised eggs from chicken flocks free from specified pathogens (*5.2.2*) or in suitable cell cultures (*5.2.4*), such as chick-embryo fibroblasts or chick kidney cells obtained from chicken flocks free from specified pathogens (*5.2.2*). For production, the virus of each strain is grown in the allantoic cavity of fertilised hens' eggs from healthy flocks.

VIRUS SEED LOT

The production of vaccine is based on a seed-lot system. Working seed lots represent not more than 15 passages from the approved reassorted virus or the approved virus isolate. The final vaccine represents 1 passage from the working seed lot. The haemagglutinin and neuraminidase antigens of each seed lot are identified as originating from the correct strain of influenza virus by suitable methods.

Only a working virus seed lot that complies with the following requirements may be used in the preparation of the monovalent pooled harvest.

Bacterial and fungal contamination. Carry out the test for sterility (*2.6.1*), using 10 ml for each medium.

Mycoplasmas (*2.6.7*). Carry out the test for mycoplasmas, using 10 ml.

VIRUS PROPAGATION AND HARVEST

An antimicrobial agent may be added to the inoculum. After incubation at a controlled temperature, the allantoic fluids are harvested and combined to form a monovalent pooled harvest. An antimicrobial agent may be added at the time of harvest. At no stage in the production is penicillin or streptomycin used.

MONOVALENT POOLED HARVEST

To limit the possibility of contamination, inactivation is initiated as soon as possible after preparation. The virus is inactivated by a method that has been demonstrated on three consecutive batches to be consistently effective for the manufacturer. The inactivation process shall have been shown to be capable of inactivating the influenza virus without destroying its antigenicity; the process should cause minimum alteration of the haemagglutinin and neuraminidase antigens. The inactivation process shall also have been shown to be capable of inactivating avian leucosis viruses and mycoplasmas. If the monovalent pooled harvest is stored after inactivation, it is held at a temperature of 5 ± 3 °C. If formaldehyde solution is used, the concentration does not exceed 0.2 g/l of CH_2O at any time during inactivation; if betapropiolactone is used, the concentration does not exceed 0.1 per cent *V/V* at any time during inactivation.

Before or after the inactivation procedure, the monovalent pooled harvest is concentrated and purified by high-speed centrifugation or other suitable method and the virus particles are disrupted into component subunits by the use of approved procedures. For each new strain, a validation test is carried out to show that the monovalent bulk consists predominantly of disrupted virus particles.

Only a monovalent pooled harvest that complies with the following requirements may be used in the preparation of the final bulk vaccine.

Haemagglutinin antigen. Determine the content of haemagglutinin antigen by an immunodiffusion test (*2.7.1*), by comparison with a haemagglutinin antigen reference preparation or with an antigen preparation calibrated against it[(1)]. Carry out the test at 20 °C to 25 °C.

For some vaccines, the physical form of the haemagglutinin particles prevents quantitative determination by immunodiffusion after inactivation of the virus. For these vaccines, a determination of haemagglutinin antigen is made on the monovalent pooled harvest before inactivation. The production process is validated to demonstrate suitable conservation of haemagglutinin antigen and a suitable tracer is used for formulation, for example, protein content.

Neuraminidase antigen. The presence and type of neuraminidase antigen are confirmed by suitable enzymatic or immunological methods on the first 3 monovalent pooled harvests from each working seed lot.

Sterility (*2.6.1*). Carry out the test for sterility, using 10 ml for each medium.

Viral inactivation. Carry out the test described below under Tests.

Chemicals used for disruption. Tests are carried out on the monovalent pooled harvest for the chemicals used for disruption, the limits being approved by the competent authority.

FINAL BULK VACCINE

Appropriate quantities of the monovalent pooled harvests are blended to make the final bulk vaccine.

Only a final bulk vaccine that complies with the following requirements may be used in the preparation of the final lot.

Antimicrobial preservative. Where applicable, determine the amount of antimicrobial preservative by a suitable chemical method. The content is not less than 85 per cent and not greater than 115 per cent of the intended amount.

Sterility (*2.6.1*). Carry out the test for sterility, using 10 ml for each medium.

FINAL LOT

The final bulk vaccine is distributed aseptically into sterile, tamper-proof containers. The containers are closed so as to prevent contamination.

Only a final lot that is satisfactory with respect to each of the requirements given below under Tests and Assay may be released for use. Provided that the test for viral inactivation has been performed with satisfactory results on each monovalent pooled harvest and that the tests for free formaldehyde, ovalbumin and total protein have been performed with satisfactory results on the final bulk vaccine, they may be omitted on the final lot.

IDENTIFICATION

The assay serves to confirm the antigenic specificity of the vaccine.

TESTS

Viral inactivation. Inoculate 0.2 ml of the vaccine into the allantoic cavity of each of 10 fertilised eggs and incubate at 33 °C to 37 °C for 3 days. The test is not valid unless at least 8 of the 10 embryos survive. Harvest 0.5 ml of the allantoic fluid from each surviving embryo and pool the fluids. Inoculate 0.2 ml of the pooled fluid into a further 10 fertilised eggs and incubate at 33 °C to 37 °C for 3 days. The test is not valid unless at least 8 of the 10 embryos survive. Harvest about 0.1 ml of the allantoic fluid from each surviving embryo and examine each individual harvest for live virus by a haemagglutination test. If haemagglutination is found for any of the fluids, carry out for that fluid a further passage in eggs and test for haemagglutination; no haemagglutination occurs.

Total protein. Not more than 6 times the total haemagglutinin content of the vaccine as determined in the assay, but in any case, not more than 100 µg of protein per virus strain per human dose and not more than a total of 300 µg of protein per human dose.

Ovalbumin. Not more than 1 µg of ovalbumin per human dose, determined by a suitable technique using a suitable reference preparation of ovalbumin.

Free formaldehyde (*2.4.18*): maximum 0.2 g/l.

Antimicrobial preservative. Where applicable, determine the amount of antimicrobial preservative by a suitable chemical method. The content is not less than the minimum amount shown to be effective and is not greater than 115 per cent of the quantity stated on the label.

Sterility (*2.6.1*). It complies with the test for sterility.

Bacterial endotoxins (*2.6.14*): less than 100 IU per human dose.

ASSAY

Determine the content of haemagglutinin antigen by an immunodiffusion test (*2.7.1*), by comparison with a haemagglutinin antigen reference preparation or with an antigen preparation calibrated against it[(1)]. Carry out the test at 20 °C to 25 °C. The confidence limits ($P = 0.95$) are not less than 80 per cent and not more than 125 per cent of the estimated haemagglutinin antigen content. The lower confidence limit ($P = 0.95$) is not less than 80 per cent of the amount stated on the label for each strain.

For some vaccines, quantitative determination of haemagglutinin antigen with respect to available reference preparations is not possible. An immunological identification of the haemagglutinin antigen and a semi-quantitative determination are carried out instead by suitable methods.

LABELLING

The label states:

- that the vaccine has been prepared on eggs,
- the strain or strains of influenza virus used to prepare the vaccine,
- the method of inactivation,

(1) Reference haemagglutinin antigens are available from the National Institute for Biological Standards and Control, Blanche Lane, South Mimms, Potters Bar, Hertfordshire EN6 3QG, Great Britain.

- the haemagglutinin content in micrograms per virus strain per dose,
- the season during which the vaccine is intended to protect.

01/2005:0869

INFLUENZA VACCINE (SURFACE ANTIGEN, INACTIVATED)

Vaccinum influenzae inactivatum ex corticis antigeniis praeparatum

DEFINITION

Influenza vaccine (surface antigen, inactivated) is a sterile suspension of a strain or strains of influenza virus, type A or B, or a mixture of strains of the 2 types grown individually in fertilised hens' eggs, inactivated and treated so that the preparation consists predominantly of haemagglutinin and neuraminidase antigens, without diminishing the antigenic properties of these antigens. The stated amount of haemagglutinin antigen for each strain present in the vaccine is 15 μg per dose, unless clinical evidence supports the use of a different amount. The vaccine may contain an adjuvant.

PRODUCTION

The production method is validated to demonstrate that the product, if tested, would comply with the test for abnormal toxicity for immunosera and vaccines for human use (*2.6.9*).

CHOICE OF VACCINE STRAIN

The World Health Organisation reviews the world epidemiological situation annually and if necessary recommends new strains corresponding to prevailing epidemiological evidence.

Such strains are used in accordance with the regulations in force in the signatory states of the Convention on the Elaboration of a European Pharmacopoeia. It is now common practice to use reassorted strains giving high yields of the appropriate surface antigens. The origin and passage history of virus strains shall be approved by the competent authority.

SUBSTRATE FOR VIRUS PROPAGATION

Influenza virus seed to be used in the production of vaccine is propagated in fertilised eggs from chicken flocks free from specified pathogens (SPF) (*5.2.2*) or in suitable cell cultures (*5.2.4*), such as chick-embryo fibroblasts or chick kidney cells obtained from SPF chicken flocks (*5.2.2*). For production, the virus of each strain is grown in the allantoic cavity of fertilised hens' eggs from healthy flocks.

VIRUS SEED LOT

The production of vaccine is based on a seed-lot system. Working seed lots represent not more than 15 passages from the approved reassorted virus or the approved virus isolate. The final vaccine represents one passage from the working seed lot. The haemagglutinin and neuraminidase antigens of each seed lot are identified as originating from the correct strain of influenza virus by suitable methods.

Only a working virus seed lot that complies with the following requirements may be used in the preparation of the monovalent pooled harvest.

Bacterial and fungal contamination. Carry out the test for sterility (*2.6.1*), using 10 ml for each medium.

Mycoplasmas (*2.6.7*). Carry out the test for mycoplasmas, using 10 ml.

VIRUS PROPAGATION AND HARVEST

An antimicrobial agent may be added to the inoculum. After incubation at a controlled temperature, the allantoic fluids are harvested and combined to form a monovalent pooled harvest. An antimicrobial agent may be added at the time of harvest. At no stage in the production is penicillin or streptomycin used.

MONOVALENT POOLED HARVEST

To limit the possibility of contamination, inactivation is initiated as soon as possible after preparation. The virus is inactivated by a method that has been demonstrated on 3 consecutive batches to be consistently effective for the manufacturer. The inactivation process shall have been shown to be capable of inactivating the influenza virus without destroying its antigenicity; the process should cause minimum alteration of the haemagglutinin and neuraminidase antigens. The inactivation process shall also have been shown to be capable of inactivating avian leucosis viruses and mycoplasmas. If the monovalent pooled harvest is stored after inactivation, it is held at 5 ± 3 °C. If formaldehyde solution is used, the concentration does not exceed 0.2 g/l of CH_2O at any time during inactivation; if betapropiolactone is used, the concentration does not exceed 0.1 per cent *V/V* at any time during inactivation.

Before or after the inactivation process, the monovalent pooled harvest is concentrated and purified by high-speed centrifugation or other suitable method. Virus particles are disrupted into component subunits by approved procedures and further purified so that the monovalent bulk consists mainly of haemagglutinin and neuraminidase antigens.

Only a monovalent pooled harvest that complies with the following requirements may be used in the preparation of the final bulk vaccine.

Haemagglutinin antigen. Determine the content of haemagglutinin antigen by an immunodiffusion test (*2.7.1*), by comparison with a haemagglutinin antigen reference preparation or with an antigen preparation calibrated against it[(2)]. Carry out the test at 20-25 °C.

Neuraminidase antigen. The presence and type of neuraminidase antigen are confirmed by suitable enzymatic or immunological methods on the first 3 monovalent pooled harvests from each working seed lot.

Sterility (*2.6.1*). Carry out the test for sterility, using 10 ml for each medium.

Viral inactivation. Carry out the test described below under Tests.

Purity. The purity of the monovalent pooled harvest is examined by polyacrylamide gel electrophoresis or by other approved techniques. Mainly haemagglutinin and neuraminidase antigens shall be present.

Chemicals used for disruption and purification. Tests are carried out on the monovalent pooled harvest for the chemicals used for disruption and purification, the limits being approved by the competent authority.

FINAL BULK VACCINE

Appropriate quantities of the monovalent pooled harvests are blended to make the final bulk vaccine. An adjuvant may be added.

Only a final bulk vaccine that complies with the following requirements may be used in the preparation of the final lot.

(2) Reference haemagglutinin antigens are available from the National Institute for Biological Standards and Control, Blanche Lane, South Mimms, Potters Bar, Hertfordshire EN6 3QG, Great Britain.

Vaccines

Antimicrobial preservative. Where applicable, determine the amount of antimicrobial preservative by a suitable chemical method. The content is not less than 85 per cent and not greater than 115 per cent of the intended amount.

Sterility (*2.6.1*). Carry out the test for sterility, using 10 ml for each medium.

FINAL LOT

The final bulk vaccine is distributed aseptically into sterile, tamper-proof containers. The containers are closed so as to prevent contamination.

Only a final lot that is satisfactory with respect to each of the requirements given below under Tests and Assay may be released for use.

Provided that the test for viral inactivation has been performed with satisfactory results on each monovalent pooled harvest and that the tests for free formaldehyde, ovalbumin and total protein have been performed with satisfactory results on the final bulk vaccine, they may be omitted on the final lot.

If the ovalbumin and formaldehyde content cannot be determined on the final lot, owing to interference from the adjuvant, they are determined on the monovalent pooled harvest, the acceptance limits being set to ensure that the limits for the final product will not be exceeded.

If the vaccine contains an adjuvant, suitable tests for identity and other relevant quality criteria are carried out on the final lot. These tests may include chemical and physical analysis, determination of particle size and determination of the number of particles per unit volume.

IDENTIFICATION

The assay serves to confirm the antigenic specificity of the vaccine.

TESTS

Viral inactivation. Inoculate 0.2 ml of the vaccine into the allantoic cavity of each of 10 fertilised eggs and incubate at 33-37 °C for 3 days. The test is not valid unless at least 8 of the 10 embryos survive. Harvest 0.5 ml of the allantoic fluid from each surviving embryo and pool the fluids. Inoculate 0.2 ml of the pooled fluid into a further 10 fertilised eggs and incubate at 33-37 °C for 3 days. The test is not valid unless at least 8 of the 10 embryos survive. Harvest about 0.1 ml of the allantoic fluid from each surviving embryo and examine each individual harvest for live virus by a haemagglutination test. If haemagglutination is found for any of the fluids, carry out for that fluid a further passage in eggs and test for haemagglutination; no haemagglutination occurs.

Total protein. Not more than 40 µg of protein other than haemagglutinin per virus strain per human dose and not more than a total of 120 µg of protein other than haemagglutinin per human dose.

Free formaldehyde (*2.4.18*): maximum 0.2 g/l.

Antimicrobial preservative. Where applicable, determine the amount of antimicrobial preservative by a suitable chemical method. The content is not less than the minimum amount shown to be effective and is not greater than 115 per cent of the quantity stated on the label.

Ovalbumin. Not more than 1 µg of ovalbumin per human dose, determined by a suitable immunochemical method (*2.7.1*) using a suitable reference preparation of ovalbumin.

Sterility. It complies with the test for sterility (*2.6.1*).

Bacterial endotoxins (*2.6.14*): less than 100 IU per human dose.

ASSAY

Determine the content of haemagglutinin antigen by an immunodiffusion test (*2.7.1*), by comparison with a haemagglutinin antigen reference preparation or with an antigen preparation calibrated against it[(2)]. Carry out the test at 20-25 °C. The confidence limits ($P = 0.95$) are not less than 80 per cent and not more than 125 per cent of the estimated haemagglutinin antigen content. The lower confidence limit ($P = 0.95$) is not less than 80 per cent of the amount stated on the label for each strain.

LABELLING

The label states:

- that the vaccine has been prepared on eggs,
- the strain or strains of influenza virus used to prepare the vaccine,
- the method of inactivation,
- the haemagglutinin content in micrograms per virus strain per dose,
- the season during which the vaccine is intended to protect,
- where applicable, the name and the quantity of adjuvant used.

01/2005:2053

INFLUENZA VACCINE (SURFACE ANTIGEN, INACTIVATED, VIROSOME)

Vaccinum influenzae inactivatum ex corticis antigeniis praeparatum virosomale

DEFINITION

Influenza vaccine (surface antigen, inactivated, virosome) is a sterile, aqueous suspension of a strain or strains of influenza virus, type A or B, or a mixture of strains of the 2 types grown individually in fertilised hens' eggs, inactivated and treated so that the preparation consists predominantly of haemagglutinin and neuraminidase antigens reconstituted to virosomes with phospholipids and without diminishing the antigenic properties of the antigens. The stated amount of haemagglutinin antigen for each strain present in the vaccine is 15 µg per dose, unless clinical evidence supports the use of a different amount.

CHARACTERS

The vaccine is a slightly opalescent liquid.

PRODUCTION

GENERAL PROVISIONS

The production method shall have been shown to yield consistently vaccines comparable with the vaccine of proven clinical efficacy and safety in man.

The production method is validated to demonstrate that the product, if tested, would comply with the test for abnormal toxicity for immunosera and vaccines for human use (*2.6.9*).

CHOICE OF VACCINE STRAIN

The World Health Organisation reviews the world epidemiological situation annually and if necessary recommends new strains corresponding to prevailing epidemiological evidence.

Such strains are used in accordance with the regulations in force in the signatory states of the Convention on the Elaboration of a European Pharmacopoeia. It is now common practice to use reassorted strains giving high yields of the appropriate surface antigens. The origin and passage history of virus strains shall be approved by the competent authority.

SUBSTRATE FOR VIRUS PROPAGATION

Influenza virus seed to be used in the production of vaccine is propagated in fertilised eggs from chicken flocks free from specified pathogens (*5.2.2*) or in suitable cell cultures (*5.2.4*), such as chick-embryo fibroblasts or chick kidney cells obtained from chicken flocks free from specified pathogens (*5.2.2*). For production, the virus of each strain is grown in the allantoic cavity of fertilised hens' eggs from healthy flocks.

VIRUS SEED LOT

The production of vaccine is based on a seed lot system. Working seed lots represent not more than 15 passages from the approved reassorted virus or the approved virus isolate. The final vaccine represents 1 passage from the working seed lot. The haemagglutinin and neuraminidase antigens of each seed lot are identified as originating from the correct strain of influenza virus by suitable methods.

Only a working virus seed lot that complies with the following requirements may be used in the preparation of the monovalent pooled harvest.

Bacterial and fungal contamination. Carry out the test for sterility (*2.6.1*), using 10 ml for each medium.

Mycoplasmas (*2.6.7*). Carry out the test for mycoplasmas, using 10 ml.

VIRUS PROPAGATION AND HARVEST

An antimicrobial agent may be added to the inoculum. After incubation at a controlled temperature, the allantoic fluids are harvested and combined to form a monovalent pooled harvest. An antimicrobial agent may be added at the time of harvest.

MONOVALENT POOLED HARVEST

To limit the possibility of contamination, inactivation is initiated as soon as possible after preparation. The virus is inactivated by a method that has been demonstrated on 3 consecutive batches to be consistently effective for the manufacturer. The inactivation process shall have been shown to be capable of inactivating the influenza virus without destroying its antigenicity; the process is designed so as to cause minimum alteration of the haemagglutinin and neuraminidase antigens. The inactivation process shall also have been shown to be capable of inactivating avian leucosis viruses and mycoplasmas. If the monovalent pooled harvest is stored after inactivation, it is held at a temperature of 5 ± 3 °C. If formaldehyde solution is used, the concentration does not exceed 0.2 g/l of CH_2O at any time during inactivation; if betapropiolactone is used, the concentration does not exceed 0.1 per cent *V/V* at any time during inactivation.

Before or after the inactivation process, the monovalent pooled harvest is concentrated and purified by high-speed centrifugation or other suitable method.

Only a monovalent pooled harvest that complies with the following requirements may be used for the preparation of virosomes.

Haemagglutinin antigen. Determine the content of haemagglutinin antigen by an immunodiffusion test (*2.7.1*), by comparison with a haemagglutinin antigen reference preparation or with an antigen preparation calibrated against it[(3)]. Carry out the test at 20-25 °C.

Neuraminidase antigen. The presence and type of neuraminidase antigen are confirmed by suitable enzymatic or immunological methods on the first 3 monovalent pooled harvests from each working seed lot.

Viral inactivation. Carry out the test described under Tests.

PREPARATION OF MONOVALENT VIROSOMES

Virus particles are disrupted into component subunits by a suitable detergent and further purified so that the monovalent bulk consists mainly of haemagglutinin and neuraminidase antigens. After addition of suitable phospholipids, solubilisation by ultrasonication and sterile filtration, virosomal preparations are formed by removal of the detergent either by adsorption chromatography or another suitable technique. Several monovalent virosomal preparations may be pooled.

Only a monovalent virosomal preparation that complies with the following requirements may be used in the preparation of the final bulk vaccine.

Haemagglutinin antigen. Determine the content of haemagglutinin antigen by an immunodiffusion test (*2.7.1*), by comparison with a haemagglutinin antigen reference preparation or with an antigen preparation calibrated against it[(3)]. Carry out the test at 20-25 °C.

Neuraminidase antigen. The presence and type of neuraminidase antigen are confirmed by suitable enzymatic or immunological methods on the first 3 virosomal preparations from each working seed lot.

Sterility (*2.6.1*). Carry out the test for sterility, using 10 ml for each medium.

Purity. The purity of the virosomal preparation is examined by polyacrylamide gel electrophoresis (*2.2.31*) or by other approved techniques. Mainly haemagglutinin and neuraminidase antigens are present.

Residual chemicals. Tests for the chemicals used for disruption and purification are carried out on the virosomal preparation, the limits being approved by the competent authority.

Phospholipid. The content and identity of the phospholipids is determined by suitable immunochemical or physico-chemical methods.

Ratio of haemagglutinin to phospholipid. The ratio of haemagglutinin content to phospholipid content is within the limits approved for the particular product.

Virosome size distribution. The size of the virosomes, determined by a suitable method such as laser light scattering, is not less than 100 nm and not greater than 500 nm.

FINAL BULK VACCINE

Appropriate quantities of the virosomal preparations are blended to make the final bulk vaccine.

Only a final bulk vaccine that complies with the following requirements may be used in the preparation of the final lot.

Antimicrobial preservative. Where applicable, determine the amount of antimicrobial preservative by a suitable chemical method. The content is not less than 85 per cent and not greater than 115 per cent of the intended amount.

Sterility (*2.6.1*). Carry out the test for sterility, using 10 ml for each medium.

FINAL LOT

The final bulk vaccine is distributed aseptically into sterile, tamper-proof containers. The containers are closed so as to prevent contamination.

Vaccines

(3) Reference haemagglutinin antigens are available from the National Institute for Biological Standards and Control (NIBSC), Blanche Lane, South Mimms, Potters Bar, Hertfordshire EN6 3QC, United Kingdom.

Only a final lot that is satisfactory with respect to each of the requirements given under Tests and Assay may be released for use. Provided that the test for viral inactivation has been performed with satisfactory results on each monovalent pooled harvest and that the tests for phospholipid, ratio of haemagglutinin to phospholipid, free formaldehyde, ovalbumin and total protein have been performed with satisfactory results on the final bulk vaccine, they may be omitted on the final lot.

IDENTIFICATION

The assay serves to confirm the antigenic specificity of the vaccine.

TESTS

Viral inactivation. Inoculate 0.2 ml of the vaccine into the allantoic cavity of each of 10 fertilised eggs and incubate at 33-37 °C for 3 days. The test is not valid unless at least 8 of the 10 embryos survive. Harvest 0.5 ml of the allantoic fluid from each surviving embryo and pool the fluids. Inoculate 0.2 ml of the pooled fluid into a further 10 fertilised eggs and incubate at 33-37 °C for 3 days. The test is not valid unless at least 8 of the 10 embryos survive. Harvest about 0.1 ml of the allantoic fluid from each surviving embryo and examine each individual harvest for live virus by a haemagglutination test. If haemagglutination is found for any of the fluids, carry out for that fluid a further passage in eggs and test for haemagglutination; no haemagglutination occurs.

pH (*2.2.3*): 6.5 to 7.8

Total protein: maximum 40 µg of protein other than haemagglutinin per virus strain per human dose and maximum 120 µg of protein other than hemagglutinin per human dose.

Phospholipid. The content and identity of the phospholipids is determined by a suitable immunochemical or physico-chemical method.

Ratio of haemagglutinin to phospholipid. The ratio of haemagglutinin content to phospholipid content is within the limits approved for the particular product.

Free formaldehyde (*2.4.18*): where applicable, maximum 0.2 g/l.

Antimicrobial preservative. Where applicable, determine the amount of antimicrobial preservative by a suitable chemical method. The content is not less than the minimum amount shown to be effective and is not greater than 115 per cent of the quantity stated on the label.

Ovalbumin: maximum 50 ng of ovalbumin per human dose, determined by a suitable technique using a suitable reference preparation of ovalbumin.

Sterility (*2.6.1*). It complies with the test for sterility.

Virosome size distribution. The size of the virosomes, determined by a suitable method such as laser light scattering, is not less than 100 nm and not greater than 500 nm.

Bacterial endotoxins (*2.6.14*): maximum 100 IU per human dose.

ASSAY

Determine the content of haemagglutinin antigen by an immunodiffusion test (*2.7.1*), by comparison with a haemagglutinin antigen reference preparation or with an antigen preparation calibrated against it[(3)]. Carry out the test at 20-25 °C. The confidence limits ($P = 0.95$) are not less than 80 per cent and not more than 125 per cent of the estimated haemaglutinin antigen content. The lower confidence limit ($P = 0.95$) is not less than 80 per cent of the amount stated on the label for each strain.

LABELLING

The label states:

– that the vaccine has been prepared on eggs,
– the strain or strains of influenza virus used to prepare the vaccine,
– the method of inactivation,
– the haemagglutinin content, in micrograms per virus strain per dose,
– the season during which the vaccine is intended to protect.

01/2005:0159

INFLUENZA VACCINE (WHOLE VIRION, INACTIVATED)

Vaccinum influenzae inactivatum ex viris integris praeparatum

DEFINITION

Influenza vaccine (whole virion, inactivated) is a sterile, aqueous suspension of a strain or strains of influenza virus, type A or B, or a mixture of strains of the two types grown individually in fertilised hens' eggs and inactivated in such a manner that their antigenic properties are retained. The stated amount of haemagglutinin antigen for each strain present in the vaccine is 15 µg per dose, unless clinical evidence supports the use of a different amount.

The vaccine is a slightly opalescent liquid.

PRODUCTION

The production method is validated to demonstrate that the product, if tested, would comply with the test for abnormal toxicity for immunosera and vaccines for human use (*2.6.9*).

CHOICE OF VACCINE STRAIN

The World Health Organisation reviews the world epidemiological situation annually and if necessary recommends new strains corresponding to prevailing epidemiological evidence.

Such strains are used in accordance with the regulations in force in the signatory states of the Convention on the Elaboration of a European Pharmacopoeia. It is now common practice to use reassorted strains giving high yields of the appropriate surface antigens. The origin and passage history of virus strains shall be approved by the competent authority.

SUBSTRATE FOR VIRUS PROPAGATION

Influenza virus seed to be used in the production of vaccine is propagated in fertilised eggs from chicken flocks free from specified pathogens (*5.2.2*) or in suitable cell cultures (*5.2.4*), such as chick-embryo fibroblasts or chick kidney cells obtained from chicken flocks free from specified pathogens (*5.2.2*). For production, the virus of each strain is grown in the allantoic cavity of fertilised hens' eggs from healthy flocks.

VIRUS SEED LOT

The production of vaccine is based on a seed-lot system. Working seed lots represent not more than 15 passages from the approved reassorted virus or the approved virus isolate. The final vaccine represents 1 passage from the working seed lot. The haemagglutinin and neuraminidase antigens of each seed lot are identified as originating from the correct strain of influenza virus by suitable methods.

Only a working virus seed lot that complies with the following requirements may be used in the preparation of the monovalent pooled harvest.

Bacterial and fungal contamination. Carry out the test for sterility (*2.6.1*), using 10 ml for each medium.

Mycoplasmas (*2.6.7*). Carry out the test for mycoplasmas, using 10 ml.

VIRUS PROPAGATION AND HARVEST

An antimicrobial agent may be added to the inoculum. After incubation at a controlled temperature, the allantoic fluids are harvested and combined to form a monovalent pooled harvest. An antimicrobial agent may be added at the time of harvest. At no stage in the production is penicillin or streptomycin used.

MONOVALENT POOLED HARVEST

To limit the possibility of contamination, inactivation is initiated as soon as possible after preparation. The virus is inactivated by a method that has been demonstrated on three consecutive batches to be consistently effective for the manufacturer. The inactivation process shall have been shown to be capable of inactivating the influenza virus without destroying its antigenicity; the process should cause minimum alteration of the haemagglutinin and neuraminidase antigens. The inactivation process shall also have been shown to be capable of inactivating avian leucosis viruses and mycoplasmas. If the monovalent pooled harvest is stored after inactivation, it is held at a temperature of 5 ± 3 °C. If formaldehyde solution is used, the concentration does not exceed 0.2 g/l of CH_2O at any time during inactivation; if betapropiolactone is used, the concentration does not exceed 0.1 per cent *V/V* at any time during inactivation.

Before or after the inactivation process, the monovalent pooled harvest is concentrated and purified by high-speed centrifugation or other suitable method.

Only a monovalent pooled harvest that complies with the following requirements may be used in the preparation of the final bulk vaccine.

Haemagglutinin antigen. Determine the content of haemagglutinin antigen by an immunodiffusion test (*2.7.1*), by comparison with a haemagglutinin antigen reference preparation or with an antigen preparation calibrated against it[(4)]. Carry out the test at 20 °C to 25 °C.

Neuraminidase antigen. The presence and type of neuraminidase antigen are confirmed by suitable enzymatic or immunological methods on the first 3 monovalent pooled harvests from each working seed lot.

Sterility (*2.6.1*). Carry out the test for sterility, using 10 ml for each medium.

Viral inactivation. Carry out the test described below under Tests.

FINAL BULK VACCINE

Appropriate quantities of the monovalent pooled harvests are blended to make the final bulk vaccine.

Only a final bulk vaccine that complies with the following requirements may be used in the preparation of the final lot.

Antimicrobial preservative. Where applicable, determine the amount of antimicrobial preservative by a suitable chemical method. The content is not less than 85 per cent and not greater than 115 per cent of the intended amount.

Sterility (*2.6.1*). Carry out the test for sterility using 10 ml for each medium.

FINAL LOT

The final bulk vaccine is distributed aseptically into sterile, tamper-proof containers. The containers are closed so as to prevent contamination.

Only a final lot that is satisfactory with respect to each of the requirements given below under Tests and Assay may be released for use. Provided that the test for viral inactivation has been performed with satisfactory results on each monovalent pooled harvest and that the tests for free formaldehyde, ovalbumin and total protein have been performed with satisfactory results on the final bulk vaccine, they may be omitted on the final lot.

IDENTIFICATION

The assay serves to confirm the antigenic specificity of the vaccine.

TESTS

Viral inactivation. Inoculate 0.2 ml of the vaccine into the allantoic cavity of each of 10 fertilised eggs and incubate at 33 °C to 37 °C for 3 days. The test is not valid unless at least 8 of the 10 embryos survive. Harvest 0.5 ml of the allantoic fluid from each surviving embryo and pool the fluids. Inoculate 0.2 ml of the pooled fluid into a further 10 fertilised eggs and incubate at 33 °C to 37 °C for 3 days. The test is not valid unless at least 8 of the 10 embryos survive. Harvest about 0.1 ml of the allantoic fluid from each surviving embryo and examine each individual harvest for live virus by a haemagglutination test. If haemagglutination is found for any of the fluids, carry out for that fluid a further passage in eggs and test for haemagglutination; no haemagglutination occurs.

Total protein. Not more than 6 times the total haemagglutinin content of the vaccine as determined in the assay, but in any case, not more than 100 µg of protein per virus strain per human dose and not more than a total of 300 µg of protein per human dose.

Ovalbumin. Not more than 1 µg of ovalbumin per human dose, determined by a suitable technique using a suitable reference preparation of ovalbumin.

Free formaldehyde (*2.4.18*): maximum 0.2 g/l.

Antimicrobial preservative. Where applicable, determine the amount of antimicrobial preservative by a suitable chemical method. The content is not less than the minimum amount shown to be effective and is not greater than 115 per cent of the quantity stated on the label.

Sterility (*2.6.1*). It complies with the test for sterility.

Bacterial endotoxins (*2.6.14*): less than 100 IU per human dose.

ASSAY

Determine the content of haemagglutinin antigen by an immunodiffusion test (*2.7.1*), by comparison with a haemagglutinin antigen reference preparation or with an antigen preparation calibrated against it[(1)]. Carry out the test at 20 °C to 25 °C. The confidence limits ($P = 0.95$) are not less than 80 per cent and not more than 125 per cent of

(4) Reference haemagglutinin antigens are available from the National Institute for Biological Standards and Control, Blanche Lane, South Mimms, Potters Bar, Hertfordshire EN6 3QG, Great Britain.

the estimated haemagglutinin antigen content. The lower confidence limit (P = 0.95) is not less than 80 per cent of the amount stated on the label for each strain.

LABELLING

The label states:

- that the vaccine has been prepared on eggs,
- the strain or strains of influenza virus used to prepare the vaccine,
- the method of inactivation,
- the haemagglutinin content in micrograms per virus strain per dose,
- the season during which the vaccine is intended to protect.

01/2005:1057
corrected

MEASLES, MUMPS AND RUBELLA VACCINE (LIVE)

Vaccinum morbillorum, parotitidis et rubellae vivum

DEFINITION

Measles, mumps and rubella vaccine (live) is a freeze-dried preparation of suitable attenuated strains of measles virus, mumps virus and rubella virus.

The vaccine is reconstituted immediately before use, as stated on the label, to give a clear liquid that may be coloured owing to the presence of a pH indicator.

PRODUCTION

The three components are prepared as described in the monographs on *Measles vaccine (live) (0213)*, *Mumps vaccine (live) (0538)* and *Rubella vaccine (live) (0162)* and comply with the requirements prescribed therein.

The production method is validated to demonstrate that the product, if tested, would comply with the test for abnormal toxicity for immunosera and vaccines for human use (*2.6.9*).

FINAL BULK VACCINE

Virus harvests for each component are pooled and clarified to remove cells. A suitable stabiliser may be added and the pooled harvests diluted as appropriate. Suitable quantities of the pooled harvest for each component are mixed.

Only a final bulk vaccine that complies with the following requirement may be used in the preparation of the final lot.

Bacterial and fungal contamination. Carry out the test for sterility (*2.6.1*), using 10 ml for each medium.

FINAL LOT

For each component, a minimum virus concentration for release of the product is established such as to ensure, in the light of stability data, that the minimum concentration stated on the label will be present at the end of the period of validity.

Only a final lot that complies with the requirements for minimum virus concentration of each component for release, with the following requirement for thermal stability and with each of the requirements given below under Identification and Tests may be released for use. Provided that the tests for bovine serum albumin and, where applicable, for ovalbumin have been carried out with satisfactory results on the final bulk vaccine, they may be omitted on the final lot.

Thermal stability. Maintain samples of the final lot of freeze-dried vaccine in the dry state at 37 °C for 7 days. Determine the virus concentration as described under Assay in parallel for the heated vaccine and for unheated vaccine stored at 5 ± 3 °C. For each component, the virus concentration of the heated vaccine is not more than 1.0 $\log_{10}$ lower than that of the unheated vaccine.

IDENTIFICATION

When the vaccine reconstituted as stated on the label is mixed with antibodies specific for measles virus, mumps virus and rubella virus, it is no longer able to infect cell cultures susceptible to these viruses. When the vaccine reconstituted as stated on the label is mixed with quantities of specific antibodies sufficient to neutralise any two viral components, the third viral component infects susceptible cell cultures.

TESTS

Bacterial and fungal contamination. The reconstituted vaccine complies with the test for sterility (*2.6.1*).

Bovine serum albumin. Not more than 50 ng per single human dose, determined by a suitable immunochemical method (*2.7.1*).

Ovalbumin. If the mumps component is produced in chick embryos, the vaccine contains not more than 1 µg of ovalbumin per single human dose, determined by a suitable immunochemical method (*2.7.1*).

Water (*2.5.12*). Not more than 3.0 per cent, determined by the semi-micro determination of water.

ASSAY

A. Mix the vaccine with a sufficient quantity of antibodies specific for mumps virus. Titrate the vaccine for infective measles virus at least in triplicate, using at least five cell cultures for each 0.5 $\log_{10}$ dilution step or by a method of equal precision. Use an appropriate virus reference preparation to validate each assay. The estimated measles virus concentration is not less than that stated on the label; the minimum measles virus concentration stated on the label is not less than 1×10^3 $CCID_{50}$ per single human dose. The assay is not valid if the confidence interval (P = 0.95) of the logarithm of the virus concentration is greater than ± 0.3.
Measles vaccine (live) BRP is suitable for use as a reference preparation.

B. Mix the vaccine with a sufficient quantity of antibodies specific for measles virus. Titrate the vaccine for infective mumps virus at least in triplicate, using at least five cell cultures for each 0.5 $\log_{10}$ dilution step or by a method of equal precision. Use an appropriate virus reference preparation to validate each assay. The estimated mumps virus concentration is not less than that stated on the label; the minimum mumps virus concentration stated on the label is not less than 5×10^3 $CCID_{50}$ per single human dose. The assay is not valid if the confidence interval (P = 0.95) of the logarithm of the virus concentration is greater than ± 0.3.
Mumps vaccine (live) BRP is suitable for use as a reference preparation.

C. Mix the vaccine with a sufficient quantity of antibodies specific for mumps virus. Titrate the vaccine for infective rubella virus at least in triplicate, using at least five cell cultures for each 0.5 $\log_{10}$ dilution step or by a method of equal precision. Use an appropriate virus reference preparation to validate each assay. The estimated rubella virus concentration is not less than that stated on the label; the minimum rubella virus concentration stated on the label is not less than 1×10^3 $CCID_{50}$

per single human dose. The assay is not valid if the confidence interval (P = 0.95) of the logarithm of the virus concentration is greater than ± 0.3.

Rubella vaccine (live) BRP is suitable for use as a reference preparation.

LABELLING

The label states:

- the strains of virus used in the preparation of the vaccine,
- where applicable, that chick embryos have been used for the preparation of the vaccine,
- the type and origin of the cells used for the preparation of the vaccine,
- the minimum virus concentration for each component of the vaccine,
- that contact with disinfectants is to be avoided,
- the time within which the vaccine must be used after reconstitution,
- that the vaccine must not be given to a pregnant woman and that a woman must not become pregnant within 2 months after having the vaccine.

01/2005:0213 corrected

MEASLES VACCINE (LIVE)

Vaccinum morbillorum vivum

DEFINITION

Measles vaccine (live) is a freeze-dried preparation of a suitable attenuated strain of measles virus. The vaccine is reconstituted immediately before use, as stated on the label, to give a clear liquid that may be coloured owing to the presence of a pH indicator.

PRODUCTION

The production of vaccine is based on a virus seed-lot system and, if the virus is propagated in human diploid cells, a cell-bank system. The production method shall have been shown to yield consistently live measles vaccines of adequate immunogenicity and safety in man. Unless otherwise justified and authorised, the virus in the final vaccine shall have undergone no more passages from the master seed lot than were used to prepare the vaccine shown in clinical studies to be satisfactory with respect to safety and efficacy; even with authorised exceptions, the number of passages beyond the level used for clinical studies shall not exceed five.

The production method is validated to demonstrate that the product, if tested, would comply with the test for abnormal toxicity for immunosera and vaccines for human use (*2.6.9*).

SUBSTRATE FOR VIRUS PROPAGATION

The virus is propagated in human diploid cells (*5.2.3*) or in cultures of chick-embryo cells derived from a chicken flock free from specified pathogens (*5.2.2*).

SEED LOT

The strain of measles virus used shall be identified by historical records that include information on the origin of the strain and its subsequent manipulation. To avoid the unnecessary use of monkeys in the test for neurovirulence, virus seed lots are prepared in large quantities and stored at temperatures below − 20 °C if freeze-dried, or below − 60 °C if not freeze-dried.

Only a seed lot that complies with the following requirements may be used for virus propagation.

Identification. The master and working seed lots are identified as measles virus by serum neutralisation in cell culture, using specific antibodies.

Virus concentration. The virus concentration of the master and working seed lots is determined to monitor consistency of production.

Extraneous agents (*2.6.16*). The working seed lot complies with the requirements for seed lots.

Neurovirulence (*2.6.18*). The working seed lot complies with the test for neurovirulence of live virus vaccines. *Macaca* and *Cercopithecus* monkeys susceptible to measles virus are suitable for the test.

PROPAGATION AND HARVEST

All processing of the cell bank and subsequent cell cultures is done under aseptic conditions in an area where no other cells are handled. Suitable animal (but not human) serum may be used in the growth medium, but the final medium for maintaining cell growth during virus multiplication does not contain animal serum. Serum and trypsin used in the preparation of cell suspensions and culture media are shown to be free from extraneous agents. The cell culture medium may contain a pH indicator such as phenol red and suitable antibiotics at the lowest effective concentration. It is preferable to have a substrate free from antibiotics during production. Not less than 500 ml of the production cell culture is set aside as uninfected cell cultures (control cells). The viral suspensions are harvested at a time appropriate to the strain of virus being used.

Only a single harvest that complies with the following requirements may be used in the preparation of the final bulk vaccine.

Identification. The single harvest contains virus that is identified as measles virus by serum neutralisation in cell culture, using specific antibodies.

Virus concentration. The virus concentration in the single harvest is determined as prescribed under Assay to monitor consistency of production and to determine the dilution to be used for the final bulk vaccine.

Extraneous agents (*2.6.16*). The single harvest complies with the tests for extraneous agents.

Control cells. If human diploid cells are used for production, the control cells comply with a test for identification. They comply with the tests for extraneous agents (*2.6.16*).

FINAL BULK VACCINE

Virus harvests that comply with the above tests are pooled and clarified to remove cells. A suitable stabiliser may be added and the pooled harvests diluted as appropriate.

Only a final bulk vaccine that complies with the following requirement may be used in the preparation of the final lot.

Bacterial and fungal contamination. The final bulk vaccine complies with the test for sterility (*2.6.1*), carried out using 10 ml for each medium.

FINAL LOT

A minimum virus concentration for release of the product is established such as to ensure, in the light of stability data, that the minimum concentration stated on the label will be present at the end of the period of validity.

Only a final lot that complies with the requirements for minimum virus concentration for release, with the following requirement for thermal stability and with each of the requirements given below under Identification and Tests may be released for use. Provided that the test for bovine serum albumin has been carried out with satisfactory results on the final bulk vaccine, it may be omitted on the final lot.

Thermal stability. Maintain samples of the final lot of freeze-dried vaccine in the dry state at 37 °C for 7 days. Determine the virus concentration as described under Assay in parallel for the heated vaccine and for unheated vaccine stored at 5 ± 3 °C. The virus concentration of the heated vaccine is not more than 1.0 $\log_{10}$ lower than that of the unheated vaccine.

IDENTIFICATION

When the vaccine reconstituted as stated on the label is mixed with specific measles antibodies, it is no longer able to infect susceptible cell cultures.

TESTS

Bacterial and fungal contamination. The reconstituted vaccine complies with the test for sterility (*2.6.1*).

Bovine serum albumin. Not more than 50 ng per single human dose, determined by a suitable immunochemical method (*2.7.1*).

Water (*2.5.12*). Not more than 3.0 per cent, determined by the semi-micro determination of water.

ASSAY

Titrate the vaccine for infective virus at least in triplicate, using at least five cell cultures for each 0.5 $\log_{10}$ dilution step or by a method of equal precision. Use an appropriate virus reference preparation to validate each assay. The estimated virus concentration is not less than that stated on the label; the minimum virus concentration stated on the label is not less than 1×10^3 $CCID_{50}$ per human dose. The assay is not valid if the confidence interval ($P = 0.95$) of the logarithm of the virus concentration is greater than ± 0.3.

Measles vaccine (live) BRP is suitable for use as a reference preparation.

LABELLING

The label states:

- the strain of virus used for the preparation of the vaccine,
- the type and origin of the cells used for the preparation of the vaccine,
- the minimum virus concentration,
- that contact with disinfectants is to be avoided,
- the time within which the vaccine must be used after reconstitution.

Vaccines

01/2005:2112

MENINGOCOCCAL GROUP C CONJUGATE VACCINE

Vaccinum meningococcale classis C coniugatum

DEFINITION

Meningococcal group C conjugate vaccine is a liquid or freeze-dried preparation of purified capsular polysaccharide derived from a suitable strain of *Neisseria meningitidis* group C covalently linked to a carrier protein. Meningococcal group C polysaccharide consists of partly *O*-acetylated or *O*-deacetylated repeating units of sialic acids, linked with 2α→ 9 glycosidic bonds. The carrier protein, when conjugated to group C polysaccharide, is capable of inducing a T-cell-dependent B-cell immune response to the polysaccharide. The vaccine may contain an adjuvant.

PRODUCTION

GENERAL PROVISIONS

The production method shall consistently have been shown to yield meningococcal group C conjugate vaccines of satisfactory immunogenicity and safety in man. The production of meningococcal group C polysaccharide and of the carrier protein are based on seed-lot systems.

During development studies and wherever revalidation is necessary, a test for pyrogens in rabbits (*2.6.8*) is carried out by injection of a suitable dose of the final lot. The vaccine is shown to be acceptable with respect to absence of pyrogenic activity.

The production method is validated to demonstrate that the vaccine, if tested, would comply with the test for abnormal toxicity for immunosera and vaccines for human use (*2.6.9*).

During development studies and wherever revalidation of the manufacturing process is necessary, it shall be demonstrated by tests in animals that the vaccine consistently induces a T-cell-dependent B-cell immune response.

The stability of the final lot and relevant intermediates is evaluated using 1 or more indicator tests. Such tests may include determination of molecular size, determination of free saccharide in the conjugate or an immunogenicity test in animals.

BACTERIAL SEED LOTS

The bacterial strains used for master seed lots shall be identified by historical records that include information on their origin and the tests used to characterise the strain. Cultures from the working seed lot shall have the same characteristics as the strain that was used to prepare the master seed lot.

Purity of bacterial cultures is verified by methods of suitable sensitivity. These may include inoculation into suitable media, examination of colony morphology, microscopic examination of Gram-stained smears and culture agglutination with suitable specific antisera.

MENINGOCOCCAL GROUP C POLYSACCHARIDE

N. meningitidis is grown in a liquid medium that does not contain high-molecular-mass polysaccharides and is free from ingredients that will form a precipitate upon addition of cetyltrimethylammonium bromide (CTAB). The culture may be inactivated by heat and filtered before the polysaccharide is precipitated by addition of CTAB. The precipitate is further purified using suitable methods to remove nucleic acids, proteins and lipopolysaccharides and the final purification step consists of ethanol precipitation. An *O*-deacetylation step may also be included. Volatile matter, including water, in the purified polysaccharide is determined by a suitable method such as thermogravimetry (*2.2.34*). The value is used to calculate the results of other tests with reference to the dried substance, as prescribed below.

Only meningococcal group C polysaccharide that complies with the following requirements may be used in the preparation of the conjugate.

Protein (*2.5.16*): maximum 1.0 per cent, calculated with reference to the dried substance.

Nucleic acid (*2.5.17*): maximum 1.0 per cent, calculated with reference to the dried substance.

***O*-acetyl groups**. Examine by a suitable method (for example *2.5.19*). An acceptable value is established for the particular product and each batch of meningococcal group C polysaccharide must be shown to comply with this limit.

Sialic acid (*2.5.23*): minimum 0.800 g of sialic acid per gram of meningococcal group C polysaccharide using *N-acetylneuraminic acid R* to prepare the reference solution.

Residual reagents. Where applicable, tests are carried out to determine residues of reagents used during inactivation and purification. An acceptable value for each reagent is established for the particular product and each batch of meningococcal group C polysaccharide must be shown to comply with this limit. Where validation studies have demonstrated removal of a residual reagent, the test on purified meningococcal group C polysaccharide may be omitted.

Molecular-size distribution. Examine by size-exclusion chromatography (*2.2.30*). An acceptable value is established for the particular product and each batch of meningococcal group C polysaccharide must be shown to comply with this limit. Where applicable, the molecular-size distribution is also determined after chemical modification of the meningococcal group C polysaccharide.

Identification and serological specificity. The identity and serological specificity are determined by a suitable immunochemical method (*2.7.1*) or other suitable method, for example ^{1}H nuclear magnetic resonance spectrometry (*2.2.33*).

Bacterial endotoxins (*2.6.14*): less than 100 IU per microgram of meningococcal group C polysaccharide.

CARRIER PROTEIN

The carrier protein is chosen so that when meningococcal group C polysaccharide is conjugated it is able to induce a T-cell-dependent immune response. Tetanus toxoid and the non-toxic mutant of diphtheria toxin-like protein, CRM197 are suitable. The carrier protein is produced by culture of a suitable microorganism, the bacterial purity of which is verified.

Only a carrier protein that complies with the following requirements may be used in preparation of the conjugate.

Identification. The carrier protein is identified by a suitable immunochemical method (*2.7.1*).

Diphtheria toxin-like protein. Where diphtheria toxin-like protein is used as the carrier, it contains not less than 90 per cent of CRM197, determined by a suitable method. Suitable tests are carried out, for validation or routinely, to demonstrate that the product is non-toxic.

Tetanus toxoid. Where tetanus toxoid is used as the carrier, it is produced as described in *Tetanus vaccine (adsorbed) (0452)* and complies with the requirements prescribed therein for bulk purified toxoid , except that the antigenic purity is not less than 1500 Lf per milligram of protein nitrogen.

BULK CONJUGATE

Meningococcal group C polysaccharide is chemically modified to enable conjugation; it is usually partly depolymerised either before or during this procedure. The conjugate is obtained by the covalent bonding of activated meningococcal group C oligosaccharide and carrier protein. The conjugate purification procedures are designed to remove residual reagents used for conjugation. The removal of residual reagents and reaction by-products is confirmed by suitable tests or by validation of the purification process.

Only a bulk conjugate that complies with the following requirements may be used in the preparation of the final bulk vaccine. For each test and for each particular product, limits of acceptance are established and each batch of conjugate must be shown to comply with these limits.

Molecular-size distribution. Examine by size-exclusion chromatography (*2.2.30*). An acceptable value is established for the particular product and each batch of bulk conjugate must be shown to comply with this limit.

Saccharide. The saccharide content is determined by a suitable validated assay, for example (*2.5.23*). Anion-exchange liquid chromatography with pulsed amperometric detection (*2.2.29*) may also be used for determination of saccharide content. An acceptable value is established for the particular product and each batch of bulk conjugate must be shown to comply with this limit.

Protein. The protein content is determined by a suitable chemical method, for example (*2.5.16*). An acceptable value is established for the particular product and each batch of bulk conjugate must be shown to comply with this limit.

Saccharide-to-protein ratio. Determine the ratio by calculation.

Free saccharide. Unbound saccharide is determined after removal of the conjugate, for example by anion-exchange liquid chromatography, size-exclusion or hydrophobic chromatography, ultrafiltration or other validated methods. An acceptable value is established for the particular product and each batch of bulk conjugate must be shown to comply with this limit.

Free carrier protein. Determine the content, either directly by a suitable method or by deriving the content by calculation from the results of other tests. An acceptable value is established for the particular product and each batch of bulk conjugate must be shown to comply with this limit.

Residual reagents. Removal of residual reagents such as cyanide is confirmed by suitable tests or by validation of the process.

Sterility (*2.6.1*). It complies with the test for sterility, carried out using 10 ml for each medium or the equivalent of 100 doses, whichever is less.

FINAL BULK VACCINE

An adjuvant and a stabiliser may be added to the bulk conjugate before dilution to the final concentration with a suitable diluent.

Only a final bulk vaccine that complies with the following requirement and is within the limits approved for the particular product may be used in preparation of the final lot.

Sterility (*2.6.1*). It complies with the test for sterility, carried out using 10 ml for each medium.

FINAL LOT

Only a final lot that is within the limits approved for the particular product and is satisfactory with respect to each of the requirement given below under Identification, Tests and Assay may be released for use.

IDENTIFICATION

The vaccine is identified by a suitable immunochemical method (*2.7.1*).

TESTS

pH (*2.2.3*). The pH of the vaccine, reconstituted if necessary, is within ± 0.5 pH units of the limit approved for the particular product.

Aluminium (*2.5.13*): maximum 1.25 mg per single human dose, if aluminium hydroxide or hydrated aluminium phosphate is used as the adsorbent.

Water (*2.5.12*): maximum 3.0 per cent for freeze-dried vaccines.

Free saccharide. Unbound saccharide is determined after removal of the conjugate, for example by anion-exchange liquid chromatography, size-exclusion or hydrophobic chromatography, ultrafiltration or other validated methods. An acceptable value consistent with adequate immunogenicity, as shown in clinical trials, is established for the particular product and each final lot must be shown to comply with this limit.

Sterility (*2.6.1*). It complies with the test for sterility.

Bacterial endotoxins (*2.6.14*): less than 25 IU per single human dose.

ASSAY

Saccharide: minimum 80 per cent of the amount of meningococcal group C polysaccharide stated on the label. The saccharide content is determined by a suitable validated assay, for example sialic acid assay (*2.5.23*) or anion-exchange liquid chromatography with pulsed amperometric detection (*2.2.29*).

LABELLING

The label states:

- the number of micrograms of meningococcal group C polysaccharide per human dose,
- the type and number of micrograms of carrier protein per human dose.

01/2005:0250

MENINGOCOCCAL POLYSACCHARIDE VACCINE

Vaccinum meningococcale polysaccharidicum

DEFINITION

Meningococcal polysaccharide vaccine is a freeze-dried preparation of one or more purified capsular polysaccharides obtained from one or more suitable strains of *Neisseria meningitidis* group A, group C, group Y and group W135 that are capable of consistently producing polysaccharides.

N. meningitidis group A polysaccharide consists of partly *O*-acetylated repeating units of *N*-acetylmannosamine, linked with 1α→6 phosphodiester bonds.

N. meningitidis group C polysaccharide consists of partly *O*-acetylated repeating units of sialic acid, linked with 2α→9 glycosidic bonds.

N. meningitidis group Y polysaccharide consists of partly *O*-acetylated alternating units of sialic acid and D-glucose, linked with 2α→6 and 1α→4 glycosidic bonds.

N. meningitidis group W135 polysaccharide consists of partly *O*-acetylated alternating units of sialic acid and D-galactose, linked with 2α→6 and 1α→4 glycosidic bonds.

The polysaccharide component or components stated on the label together with calcium ions and residual moisture account for over 90 per cent of the mass of the preparation.

PRODUCTION

Production of the meningococcal polysaccharides is based on a seed-lot system. The production method shall have been shown to yield consistently meningococcal polysaccharide vaccines of satisfactory immunogenicity and safety in man.

The production method is validated to demonstrate that the product, if tested, would comply with the test for abnormal toxicity for immunosera and vaccines for human use (*2.6.9*).

SEED LOTS

The strains of *N. meningitidis* used for the master seed lots shall be identified by historical records that include information on their origin and by their biochemical and serological characteristics.

Cultures from each working seed lot shall have the same characteristics as the strain that was used to prepare the master seed lot. The strains have the following characteristics:

- colonies obtained from a culture are rounded, uniform in shape and smooth with a mucous, opalescent, greyish appearance,
- Gram staining reveals characteristic Gram-negative diplococci in "coffee-bean" arrangement,
- the oxidase test is positive,
- the culture utilises glucose and maltose,
- suspensions of the culture agglutinate with suitable specific antisera.

Purity of bacterial strains used for the seed lots is verified by methods of suitable sensitivity. These may include inoculation into suitable media, examination of colony morphology, microscopic examination of Gram-stained smears and culture agglutination with suitable specific antisera.

PROPAGATION AND HARVEST

The working seed lots are cultured on solid media that do not contain blood-group substances or ingredients of mammalian origin. The inoculum may undergo 1 or more subcultures in liquid medium before being used for inoculating the final medium. The liquid media used and the final medium are semisynthetic and free from substances precipitated by cetrimonium bromide (hexadecyltrimethylammonium bromide) and do not contain blood-group substances or high-molecular-mass polysaccharides.

The bacterial purity of the culture is verified by methods of suitable sensitivity. These may include inoculation into suitable media, examination of colony morphology, microscopic examination of Gram-stained smears and culture agglutination with suitable specific antisera.

The cultures are centrifuged and the polysaccharides precipitated from the supernatant by addition of cetrimonium bromide. The precipitate obtained is harvested and may be stored at − 20 °C awaiting further purification.

PURIFIED POLYSACCHARIDES

The polysaccharides are purified, after dissociation of the complex of polysaccharide and cetrimonium bromide, using suitable procedures to remove successively nucleic acids, proteins and lipopolysaccharides.

The final purification step consists of ethanol precipitation of the polysaccharides which are then dried and stored at − 20 °C. The loss on drying is determined by thermogravimetry (*2.2.34*) and the value is used to calculate the results of the other chemical tests with reference to the dried substance.

Only purified polysaccharides that comply with the following requirements may be used in the preparation of the final bulk vaccine.

Protein (*2.5.16*). Not more than 10 mg of protein per gram of purified polysaccharide, calculated with reference to the dried substance.

Nucleic acids (*2.5.17*). Not more than 10 mg of nucleic acids per gram of purified polysaccharide, calculated with reference to the dried substance.

***O*-Acetyl groups** (*2.5.19*). Not less than 2 mmol of *O*-acetyl groups per gram of purified polysaccharide for group A, not less than 1.5 mmol per gram of polysaccharide for group C, not less than 0.3 mmol per gram of polysaccharide for groups Y and W135, all calculated with reference to the dried substance.

Phosphorus (*2.5.18*). Not less than 80 mg of phosphorus per gram of group A purified polysaccharide, calculated with reference to the dried substance.

Sialic acid (*2.5.23*). Not less than 800 mg of sialic acid per gram of group C polysaccharide and not less than 560 mg of sialic acid per gram of purified polysaccharide for groups Y and W135, all calculated with reference to the dried substance. Use the following reference solutions.

Group C polysaccharide: a 150 mg/l solution of *N-acetylneuraminic acid R*.

Group Y polysaccharide: a solution containing 95 mg/l of *N-acetylneuraminic acid R* and 55 mg/l of *glucose R*.

Group W135 polysaccharide: a solution containing 95 mg/l of *N-acetylneuraminic acid R* and 55 mg/l of *galactose R*.

Calcium. If a calcium salt is used during purification, a determination of calcium is carried out on the purified polysaccharide; the content is within the limits approved for the particular product.

Distribution of molecular size. Examine by size-exclusion chromatography (*2.2.30*) using *agarose for chromatography R* or *cross-linked agarose for chromatography R*. Use a column about 0.9 m long and 16 mm in internal diameter equilibrated with a solvent having an ionic strength of 0.2 mol/kg and a pH of 7.0-7.5. Apply to the column about 2.5 mg of polysaccharide in a volume of about 1.5 ml and elute at about 20 ml/h. Collect fractions of about 2.5 ml and determine the content of polysaccharide by a suitable method. At least 65 per cent of group A polysaccharide, 75 per cent of group C polysaccharide, 80 per cent of group Y polysaccharide and 80 per cent of group W135 polysaccharide is eluted before a distribution coefficient (K_0) of 0.50 is reached. In addition, the percentages eluted before this distribution coefficient are within the limits approved for the particular product.

Identification and serological specificity. The identity and serological specificity are determined by a suitable immunochemical method (*2.7.1*). Identity and purity of each polysaccharide shall be confirmed; it shall be shown that there is not more than 1 per cent *m/m* of group-heterologous *N. meningitidis* polysaccharide.

Pyrogens (*2.6.8*). The polysaccharide complies with the test for pyrogens. Inject into each rabbit per kilogram of body mass 1 ml of a solution containing 0.025 µg of purified polysaccharide per millilitre.

FINAL BULK VACCINE

One or more purified polysaccharides of 1 or more *N. meningitidis* groups are dissolved in a suitable solvent that may contain a stabiliser. When dissolution is complete, the solution is filtered through a bacteria-retentive filter.

Only a final bulk vaccine that complies with the following requirement may be used in the preparation of the final lot.

Sterility (*2.6.1*). The final bulk vaccine complies with the test for sterility, carried out using 10 ml for each medium.

FINAL LOT

The final bulk vaccine is distributed aseptically into sterile containers. The containers are then closed so as to avoid contamination.

Only a final lot that is satisfactory with respect to each of the requirements prescribed below under Identification, Tests and Assay may be released for use.

CHARACTERS

A white or cream-coloured powder or pellet, freely soluble in water.

IDENTIFICATION

Carry out an identification test for each polysaccharide present in the vaccine by a suitable immunochemical method (*2.7.1*).

TESTS

Distribution of molecular size. Examine by size-exclusion chromatography (*2.2.30*). Use a column about 0.9 m long and 16 mm in internal diameter equilibrated with a solvent having an ionic strength of 0.2 mol/kg and a pH of 7.0-7.5. Apply to the column about 2.5 mg of each polysaccharide in a volume of about 1.5 ml and elute at about 20 ml/h. Collect fractions of about 2.5 ml and determine the content of polysaccharide by a suitable method.

For a divalent vaccine (group A + group C), use *cross-linked agarose for chromatography R*. The vaccine complies with the test if:

- 65 per cent of group A polysaccharide is eluted before $K_0 = 0.50$,
- 75 per cent of group C polysaccharide is eluted before $K_0 = 0.50$.

For a tetravalent vaccine (group A + group C + group Y + group W135), use *cross-linked agarose for chromatography R1* and apply a suitable immunochemical method (*2.7.1*) to establish the elution pattern of the different polysaccharides. The vaccine complies with the test if K_0 for the principal peak is:

- not greater than 0.70 for group A and group C polysaccharide,
- not greater than 0.57 for group Y polysaccharide,
- not greater than 0.68 for group W135 polysaccharide.

Water (*2.5.12*). Not more than 3.0 per cent, determined by the semi-micro determination of water.

Sterility (*2.6.1*). It complies with the test for sterility.

Pyrogens (*2.6.8*). It complies with the test for pyrogens. Inject per kilogram of the rabbit's mass 1 ml of a solution containing:

- 0.025 µg of polysaccharide for a monovalent vaccine,
- 0.050 µg of polysaccharide for a divalent vaccine,
- 0.10 µg of polysaccharide for a tetravalent vaccine.

ASSAY

Carry out an assay of each polysaccharide present in the vaccine.

For a divalent vaccine (group A + group C), use measurement of phosphorus (*2.5.18*) to determine the content of polysaccharide A and measurement of sialic acid (*2.5.23*) to determine the content of polysaccharide C. To determine sialic acid, use as reference solution a 150 mg/l solution of *N-acetylneuraminic acid R*.

For a tetravalent vaccine (group A + group C + group Y + group W135) a suitable immunochemical method (*2.7.1*) is used with a reference preparation of purified polysaccharide for each group.

The vaccine contains not less than 70 per cent and not more than 130 per cent of the quantity of each polysaccharide stated on the label.

LABELLING

The label states:

- the group or groups of polysaccharides (A, C, Y or W135) present in the vaccine,
- the number of micrograms of polysaccharide per human dose.

01/2005:0538
corrected

MUMPS VACCINE (LIVE)

Vaccinum parotitidis vivum

DEFINITION

Mumps vaccine (live) is a freeze-dried preparation of a suitable attenuated strain of mumps virus. The vaccine is reconstituted immediately before use, as stated on the label, to give a clear liquid that may be coloured owing to the presence of a pH indicator.

PRODUCTION

The production of vaccine is based on a virus seed-lot system and, if the virus is propagated in human diploid cells, a cell-bank system. The production method shall have been shown to yield consistently live mumps vaccines of adequate immunogenicity and safety in man. Unless otherwise justified and authorised, the virus in the final vaccine shall have undergone no more passages from the master seed lot than were used to prepare the vaccine shown in clinical studies to be satisfactory with respect to safety and efficacy.

The production method is validated to demonstrate that the product, if tested, would comply with the test for abnormal toxicity for immunosera and vaccines for human use (*2.6.9*).

SUBSTRATE FOR VIRUS PROPAGATION

The virus is propagated in human diploid cells (*5.2.3*) or in chick-embryo cells or in the amniotic cavity of chick embryos derived from a chicken flock free from specified pathogens (*5.2.2*).

SEED LOT

The strain of mumps virus used shall be identified by historical records that include information on the origin of the strain and its subsequent manipulation. To avoid the unnecessary use of monkeys in the test for neurovirulence, virus seed lots are prepared in large quantities and stored at temperatures below −20 °C if freeze-dried, or below −60 °C if not freeze-dried.

Only a seed lot that complies with the following requirements may be used for virus propagation.

Identification. The master and working seed lots are identified as mumps virus by serum neutralisation in cell culture, using specific antibodies.

Virus concentration. The virus concentration of the master and working seed lots is determined to ensure consistency of production.

Extraneous agents (*2.6.16*). The working seed lot complies with the requirements for seed lots.

Neurovirulence (*2.6.18*). The working seed lot complies with the test for neurovirulence of live virus vaccines. *Macaca* and *Cercopithecus* monkeys are suitable for the test.

PROPAGATION AND HARVEST

All processing of the cell bank and subsequent cell cultures is done under aseptic conditions in an area where no other cells are handled. Suitable animal (but not human) serum may be used in the culture media. Serum and trypsin used in the preparation of cell suspensions and culture media are shown to be free from extraneous agents. The cell culture medium may contain a pH indicator such as phenol red and suitable antibiotics at the lowest effective concentration. It is preferable to have a substrate free from antibiotics during production. Not less than 500 ml of the production cell cultures is set aside as uninfected cell cultures (control cells). If the virus is propagated in chick embryos, 2 per cent but not less than twenty eggs are set aside as uninfected control eggs. The viral suspensions are harvested at a time appropriate to the strain of virus being used.

Only a single harvest that complies with the following requirements may be used in the preparation of the final bulk vaccine.

Identification. The single harvest contains virus that is identified as mumps virus by serum neutralisation in cell culture, using specific antibodies.

Virus concentration. The virus concentration in the single harvest is determined as prescribed under Assay to monitor consistency of production and to determine the dilution to be used for the final bulk vaccine.

Extraneous agents (*2.6.16*). The single harvest complies with the tests for extraneous agents.

Control cells or eggs. If human diploid cells are used for production, the control cells comply with a test for identification; the control cells and the control eggs comply with the tests for extraneous agents (*2.6.16*).

FINAL BULK VACCINE

Single harvests that comply with the above tests are pooled and clarified to remove cells. A suitable stabiliser may be added and the pooled harvests diluted as appropriate.

Only a final bulk vaccine that complies with the following requirement may be used in the preparation of the final lot.

Bacterial and fungal contamination. The final bulk vaccine complies with the test for sterility (*2.6.1*), carried out using 10 ml for each medium.

FINAL LOT

A minimum virus concentration for release of the product is established such as to ensure, in the light of stability data, that the minimum concentration stated on the label will be present at the end of the period of validity.

Only a final lot that complies with the requirements for minimum virus concentration for release, with the following requirement for thermal stability and with each of the requirements given below under Identification and Tests may be released for use. Provided that the tests for bovine serum albumin and, where applicable, for ovalbumin have been carried out with satisfactory results on the final bulk vaccine, they may be omitted on the final lot.

Thermal stability. Maintain samples of the final lot of freeze-dried vaccine in the dry state at 37 °C for 7 days. Determine the virus concentration as described under Assay in parallel for the heated vaccine and for unheated vaccine stored at 5 ± 3 °C. The virus concentration of the heated vaccine is not more than 1.0 $\log_{10}$ lower than that of the unheated vaccine.

IDENTIFICATION

When the vaccine reconstituted as stated on the label is mixed with specific mumps antibodies, it is no longer able to infect susceptible cell cultures.

TESTS

Bacterial and fungal contamination. The reconstituted vaccine complies with the test for sterility (*2.6.1*).

Bovine serum albumin. Not more than 50 ng per single human dose, determined by a suitable immunochemical method (*2.7.1*).

Ovalbumin. If the vaccine is produced in chick embryos, it contains not more than 1 µg of ovalbumin per single human dose, determined by a suitable immunochemical method (*2.7.1*).

Water (*2.5.12*). Not more than 3.0 per cent, determined by the semi-micro determination of water.

ASSAY

Titrate the vaccine for infective virus at least in triplicate, using at least five cell cultures for each 0.5 $\log_{10}$ dilution step or by a method of equal precision. Use an appropriate virus reference preparation to validate each assay. The estimated virus concentration is not less than that stated on the label; the minimum virus concentration stated on the label is not less than 5×10^3 $CCID_{50}$ per human dose. The assay is not valid if the confidence interval ($P = 0.95$) of the logarithm of the virus concentration is greater than ± 0.3.

Mumps vaccine (live) BRP is suitable for use as a reference preparation.

LABELLING

The label states:

- the strain of virus used for the preparation of the vaccine,
- that the vaccine has been prepared in chick embryos or the type and origin of cells used for the preparation of the vaccine,
- the minimum virus concentration,
- that contact with disinfectants is to be avoided,
- the time within which the vaccine must be used after reconstitution.

01/2005:0160

PERTUSSIS VACCINE

Vaccinum pertussis

DEFINITION

Pertussis vaccine is a sterile saline suspension of inactivated whole cells of one or more strains of *Bordetella pertussis*.

PRODUCTION

INACTIVATED B. PERTUSSIS SUSPENSION

The inactivated *B. pertussis* suspension is prepared as described in the monograph on *Pertussis vaccine (adsorbed) (0161)* and complies with the requirements prescribed therein.

FINAL BULK VACCINE

Suitable quantities of the inactivated single harvests are pooled to prepare the final bulk vaccine. Suitable antimicrobial preservatives may be added. The bacterial concentration of the final bulk vaccine does not exceed that corresponding to an opacity of 20 IU per single human dose. If 2 or more strains of *B. pertussis* are used, the composition of consecutive lots of the final bulk vaccine shall be consistent with respect to the proportion of each strain as measured in opacity units.

Only a final bulk vaccine that complies with the following requirements may be used in the preparation of the final lot.

Antimicrobial preservative. Where applicable, determine the amount of antimicrobial preservative by a suitable chemical method. The amount is not less than 85 per cent and not greater than 115 per cent of the intended amount.

Sterility (*2.6.1*). Carry out the test for sterility using 10 ml for each medium.

FINAL LOT

The final bulk vaccine is distributed aseptically into sterile, tamper-proof containers. The containers are closed so as to prevent contamination.

Only a final lot that is satisfactory with respect to each of the requirements given below under Identification, Tests and Assay may be released for use. Provided the tests for specific toxicity, free formaldehyde and antimicrobial preservative and the assay have been carried out with satisfactory results on the final bulk vaccine, they may be omitted on the final lot.

IDENTIFICATION

Identify pertussis vaccine by agglutination of the bacteria in the vaccine by antisera specific to *B. pertussis*.

TESTS

Specific toxicity. Use not fewer than 5 healthy mice each weighing 14 g to 16 g for the vaccine group and for the saline control. Use mice of the same sex or distribute males and females equally between the groups. Allow the animals access to food and water for at least 2 h before injection and during the test. Inject each mouse of the vaccine group intraperitoneally with 0.5 ml, containing a quantity of the vaccine equivalent to not less than half the single human dose. Inject each mouse of the control group with 0.5 ml of a 9 g/l sterile solution of *sodium chloride R*, preferably containing the same amount of antimicrobial preservative as that injected with the vaccine. Weigh the groups of mice immediately before the injection and 72 h and 7 days after the injection. The vaccine complies with the test if: (a) at the end of 72 h the total mass of the group of vaccinated mice is not less than that preceding the injection; (b) at the end of 7 days the average increase in mass per vaccinated mouse is not less than 60 per cent of that per control mouse; and (c) not more than 5 per cent of the vaccinated mice die during the test. The test may be repeated and the results of the tests combined.

Free formaldehyde (*2.4.18*): maximum 0.2 g/l.

Antimicrobial preservative. Where applicable, determine the amount of antimicrobial preservative by a suitable chemical method. The content is not less than the minimum amount shown to be effective and is not greater than 115 per cent of the quantity stated on the label.

Sterility (*2.6.1*). The vaccine complies with the test for sterility.

ASSAY

Carry out the assay of pertussis vaccine (*2.7.7*).

The estimated potency is not less than 4 IU per single human dose and the lower confidence limit ($P = 0.95$) of the estimated potency is not less than 2 IU per single human dose.

LABELLING

The label states:

- the minimum number of International Units per single human dose,
- that the vaccine must be shaken before use,
- that the vaccine is not to be frozen.

01/2005:1356

PERTUSSIS VACCINE (ACELLULAR, COMPONENT, ADSORBED)

Vaccinum pertussis sine cellulis ex elementis praeparatum adsorbatum

DEFINITION

Pertussis vaccine (acellular, component, adsorbed) is a preparation of individually prepared and purified antigenic components of *Bordetella pertussis* adsorbed on a mineral carrier such as aluminium hydroxide or hydrated aluminium phosphate.

The vaccine contains either pertussis toxoid or a pertussis-toxin-like protein free from toxic properties, produced by expression of a genetically modified form of the corresponding gene. Pertussis toxoid is prepared from pertussis toxin by a method that renders the latter harmless while maintaining adequate immunogenic properties and avoiding reversion to toxin. The vaccine may also contain filamentous haemagglutinin, pertactin (a 69 kDa outer-membrane protein) and other defined components of *B. pertussis* such as fimbrial-2 and fimbrial-3 antigens. The latter 2 antigens may be copurified. The antigenic composition and characteristics are based on evidence of protection and freedom from unexpected reactions in the target group for which the vaccine is intended.

PRODUCTION

The production method shall have been shown to yield consistently vaccines comparable with the vaccine of proven clinical efficacy and safety in man.

Where a genetically modified form of *B. pertussis* is used for production consistency and genetic stability shall be established in conformity with the requirements of the monograph *Products of recombinant DNA technology (0784)*.

Reference vaccine. A batch of vaccine shown to be effective in clinical trials or a batch representative thereof is used as a reference vaccine. For the preparation of a representative batch, strict adherence to the production process used for the batch tested in clinical trials is necessary. The reference vaccine is preferably stabilised by a method that has been shown to have no significant effect on the assay procedure when the stabilised and non-stabilised batches are compared.

CHARACTERISATION OF COMPONENTS

During development of the vaccine, the production process shall be validated to demonstrate that it yields consistently individual components that comply with the following requirements; after demonstration of consistency, the tests need not be applied routinely to each batch.

Adenylate cyclase. Not more than 500 ng in the equivalent of 1 dose of the final vaccine, determined by immunoblot analysis or another suitable method.

Tracheal cytotoxin. Not more than 2 pmol in the equivalent of 1 dose of the final vaccine, determined by a suitable method such as a biological assay or liquid chromatography (*2.2.29*).

Absence of residual dermonecrotic toxin. Inject intradermally into each of 3 unweaned mice, in a volume of 0.1 ml, the amount of component or antigenic fraction equivalent to 1 dose of the final vaccine. Observe for 48 h. No dermonecrotic reaction is demonstrable.

Specific properties. The components of the vaccine are analysed by one or more of the methods shown below in order to determine their identity and specific properties (activity per unit amount of protein) in comparison with reference preparations.

Pertussis toxin. Chinese hamster ovary (CHO) cell-clustering effect and haemagglutination as *in vitro* methods; lymphocytosis-promoting activity, histamine-sensitising activity and insulin secretory activity as *in vivo* methods. The toxin shows ADP-ribosyl transferase activity using transducin as the acceptor.

Filamentous haemagglutinin. Haemagglutination and inhibition by specific antibody.

Pertactin, fimbrial-2 and fimbrial-3 antigens. Reactivity with specific antibody.

Pertussis toxoid. The toxoid induces in animals production of antibodies capable of inhibiting all the properties of pertussis toxin.

PURIFIED COMPONENTS

Production of each component is based on a seed-lot system. The seed cultures from which toxin is prepared are managed to conserve or where necessary restore toxinogenicity by deliberate selection.

None of the media used at any stage contains blood or blood products of human origin. Media used for the preparation of seed lots and inocula may contain blood or blood products of animal origin.

Pertussis toxin and, where applicable, filamentous haemagglutinin and pertactin are purified and, after appropriate characterisation, detoxified using suitable chemical reagents, by a method that avoids reversion of the toxoid to toxin, particularly on storage or exposure to heat. Other components such as fimbrial-2 and fimbrial-3 antigens are purified either separately or together, characterised and shown to be free from toxic substances. The purification procedure is validated to demonstrate appropriate clearance of substances used during culture or purification.

The content of bacterial endotoxins (*2.6.14*) is determined to monitor the purification procedure and to limit the amount in the final vaccine. The limits applied for the individual components are such that the final vaccine contains less than 100 IU per single human dose.

Before detoxification, the purity of the components is determined by a suitable method such as polyacrylamide gel electrophoresis (PAGE) or liquid chromatography. SDS-PAGE or immunoblot analysis with specific monoclonal or polyclonal antibodies may be used to characterise subunits. Requirements are established for each individual product.

Only purified components that comply with the following requirements may be used in the preparation of the final bulk vaccine.

Sterility (*2.6.1*). Carry out the test for sterility using for each medium a quantity of purified component equivalent to not less than 100 doses.

Absence of residual pertussis toxin. *This test is not necessary for the product obtained by genetic modification.* Use a group of not fewer than 5 histamine-sensitive mice each weighing 18-26 g. Inject into each mouse the equivalent of 1 human dose intravenously or twice the human dose intraperitoneally, diluted to not more than 0.5 ml with phosphate-buffered saline solution containing 2 g/l of gelatin. Inject diluent into a second group of control mice.

After 5 days, inject 2 mg of histamine base intraperitoneally in a volume not exceeding 0.5 ml and observe for 24 h. If no animal dies, the preparation complies with the test.

The histamine sensitivity of the strain of mice used is verified at suitable intervals as follows: inject threefold dilutions of a reference pertussis toxin preparation in phosphate-buffered saline solution containing 2 g/l of gelatin and challenge with histamine as above; the strain is suitable if more than 50 per cent of the animals are sensitised by 50 ng of pertussis toxin and none of the control animals injected with only diluent and challenged similarly with histamine show symptoms of sensitisation.

A validated test based on the clustering effect of the toxin for Chinese hamster ovary (CHO) cells may be used instead of the test in mice.

Residual detoxifying agents and other reagents. The content of residual detoxifying agents and other reagents is determined and shown to be below approved limits unless validation of the process has demonstrated acceptable clearance.

Antigen content. Determine the antigen content by a suitable immunochemical method (*2.7.1*) and protein nitrogen by sulphuric acid digestion (*2.5.9*) or another suitable method. The ratio of antigen content to protein nitrogen is within the limits established for the product.

FINAL BULK VACCINE

The vaccine is prepared by adsorption of suitable quantities of purified components, separately or together, onto aluminium hydroxide or hydrated aluminium phosphate. A suitable antimicrobial preservative may be added.

Only a final bulk vaccine that complies with the following requirements may be used in the preparation of the final lot.

Antimicrobial preservative. Where applicable, determine the amount of antimicrobial preservative by a suitable chemical or physico-chemical method. The amount is not less than 85 per cent and not greater than 115 per cent of the intended content.

Sterility (*2.6.1*). Carry out the test for sterility using 10 ml for each medium.

FINAL LOT

Only a final lot that is satisfactory with respect to each of the requirements given below under Identification, Tests and Assay may be released for use. Provided that the tests for absence of residual pertussis toxin and irreversibility of pertussis toxoid, antimicrobial preservative, free formaldehyde and the assay have been carried out with satisfactory results on the final bulk vaccine, these tests may be omitted on the final lot.

IDENTIFICATION

Subject the vaccine to a suitable desorption procedure such as the following: dissolve in the vaccine to be examined sufficient *sodium citrate R* to give a 10 g/l solution; maintain at 37 °C for about 16 h and centrifuge until a clear supernatant liquid is obtained. Examined by a suitable immunochemical method (*2.7.1*), the clear supernatant liquid reacts with specific antisera to the components stated on the label.

TESTS

Absence of residual pertussis toxin and irreversibility of pertussis toxoid. *This test is not necessary for the product obtained by genetic modification.* Use 3 groups each of not fewer than 5 histamine-sensitive mice. Inject intraperitoneally into the first group twice the single human dose of the vaccine stored at 2-8 °C. Inject intraperitoneally into the second group twice the single human dose of the vaccine incubated at 37 °C for 4 weeks. Inject diluent into the third group of mice. After 5 days, inject into each mouse 2 mg of histamine base intraperitoneally in a volume not exceeding 0.5 ml and observe for 24 h. The test is invalid if 1 or more control mice die following histamine challenge. The vaccine complies with the test if no animal in the first or second group dies following histamine challenge. If 1 mouse dies in either or both of the first and second groups, the test may be repeated with the same number of mice or with a greater number and the results of valid tests combined; the vaccine complies with the test if, in both of the groups given the vaccine, not more than 5 per cent of the total number of mice die following histamine challenge.

The histamine sensitivity of the strain of mice used is verified at suitable intervals as follows: inject intravenously threefold dilutions of a reference pertussis toxin preparation in phosphate-buffered saline solution containing 2 g/l of gelatin and challenge with histamine as above; the strain is suitable if more than 50 per cent of the animals are sensitised by 50 ng of pertussis toxin and none of the control animals injected with only diluent and challenged similarly with histamine show symptoms of sensitisation.

Aluminium (*2.5.13*): maximum 1.25 mg per single human dose, if aluminium hydroxide or hydrated aluminium phosphate is used as the adsorbent.

Free formaldehyde (*2.4.18*): maximum 0.2 g/l.

Antimicrobial preservative. Where applicable, determine the amount of antimicrobial preservative by a suitable chemical or physico-chemical method. The amount is not less than the minimum amount shown to be effective and is not greater than 115 per cent of the quantity stated on the label.

Sterility (*2.6.1*). It complies with the test for sterility.

ASSAY

The capacity of the vaccine to induce the formation of specific antibodies is compared with the same capacity of a reference preparation examined in parallel; antibodies are determined using suitable immunochemical methods (*2.7.1*) such as enzyme-linked immunosorbent assay (ELISA). The test in mice shown below uses a three-point model but, after validation, for routine testing a single-dilution method may be used.

Requirement. The capacity to induce antibodies is not significantly ($P = 0.95$) less than that of the reference vaccine.

The following test model is given as an example of a method that has been found to be satisfactory.

Selection and distribution of test animals. Use in the test healthy mice (for example, CD1 strain) of the same stock 4 to 8 weeks old. Distribute the animals in 6 groups of a number appropriate to the requirements of the assay. Use 3 dilutions of the vaccine to be examined and 3 dilutions of a reference preparation and attribute each dilution to a group of mice. Inject intraperitoneally or subcutaneously into each mouse 0.5 ml of the dilution attributed to its group.

Collection of serum samples. 4 to 5 weeks after vaccination, bleed the mice individually under anaesthesia. Store the sera at − 20 °C until tested for antibody content.

Antibody determination. Assay the individual sera for content of specific antibodies to each component using a validated method such as the ELISA test shown below.

ELISA test. Microtitre plates (poly(vinyl chloride) or polystyrene as appropriate for the specific antigen) are coated with the purified antigen at a concentration of 100 ng per well. After washing, unreacted sites are blocked by incubating with a solution of bovine serum albumin and then

Vaccines

washed. Two-fold dilutions of sera from mice immunised with test or reference vaccines are made on the plates. After incubation at 22-25 °C for 1 h, the plates are washed. A suitable solution of anti-mouse IgG enzyme conjugate is added to each well and incubated at 22-25 °C for 1 h. After washing, a substrate is added from which the bound enzyme conjugate liberates a chromophore which can be quantified by measurement of absorbance (*2.2.25*). The test conditions are designed to obtain a linear response for absorbance with respect to antibody content over the range of measurement used and absorbance values within the range 0.1 to 2.0.

A reference antiserum of assigned potency is used in the test and serves as the basis for calculation of the antibody levels in test sera. A standardised control serum is also included in the test.

The test is not valid if:

– the value found for the control serum differs by more than 2 standard deviations from the assigned value,
– the confidence limits ($P = 0.95$) are less than 50 per cent or more than 200 per cent of the estimated potency.

Calculation. The antibody titres in the sera of mice immunised with reference and test vaccines are calculated and from the values obtained the potency of the test vaccine in relation to the reference vaccine is calculated by the usual statistical methods.

LABELLING

The label states:

– the names and amounts of the components present in the vaccine,
– where applicable, that the vaccine contains a pertussis toxin-like protein produced by genetic modification,
– the name and amount of the adsorbent,
– that the vaccine must be shaken before use,
– that the vaccine is not to be frozen.

01/2005:1595 corrected

PERTUSSIS VACCINE (ACELLULAR, CO-PURIFIED, ADSORBED)

Vaccinum pertussis sine cellulis copurificatum adsorbatum

DEFINITION

Pertussis vaccine (acellular, co-purified, adsorbed) is a preparation of antigenic components of *Bordetella pertussis* adsorbed on a mineral carrier such as aluminium hydroxide or hydrated aluminium phosphate.

The vaccine contains an antigenic fraction purified without separation of the individual components. The antigenic fraction is treated by a method that transforms pertussis toxin to toxoid, rendering it harmless while maintaining adequate immunogenic properties of all the components and avoiding reversion to toxin. The antigenic fraction is composed of pertussis toxoid, filamentous haemagglutinin, pertactin (a 69 kDa outer-membrane protein) and other defined components of *B. pertussis* such as fimbrial-2 and fimbrial-3 antigens. It may contain residual pertussis toxin up to a maximum level approved by the competent authority. The antigenic composition and characteristics are based on evidence of protection and freedom from unexpected reactions in the target group for which the vaccine is intended.

PRODUCTION

GENERAL PROVISIONS

The production method shall have been shown to yield consistently vaccines comparable with the vaccine of proven clinical efficacy and safety in man.

Reference vaccine. A batch of vaccine shown to be effective in clinical trials or a batch representative thereof is used as a reference vaccine. For the preparation of a representative batch, strict adherence to the production process used for the batch tested in clinical trials is necessary. The reference vaccine is preferably stabilised, by a method that has been shown to have no significant effect on the assay procedure when the stabilised and non-stabilised batches are compared.

CHARACTERISATION OF COMPONENTS

During development of the vaccine, the production process shall be validated to demonstrate that it yields consistently an antigenic fraction that complies with the following requirements; after demonstration of consistency, the tests need not be applied routinely to each batch.

Adenylate cyclase. Not more than 500 ng in the equivalent of 1 dose of the final vaccine, determined by immunoblot analysis or another suitable method.

Tracheal cytotoxin. Not more than 2 pmol in the equivalent of 1 dose of the final vaccine, determined by a suitable method such as a biological assay or liquid chromatography (*2.2.29*).

Absence of residual dermonecrotic toxin. Inject intradermally into each of 3 unweaned mice, in a volume of 0.1 ml, the amount of antigenic fraction equivalent to 1 dose of the final vaccine. Observe for 48 h. No dermonecrotic reaction is demonstrable.

Specific properties. The antigenic fraction is analysed by one or more of the methods shown below in order to determine the identity and specific properties (activity per unit amount of protein) of its components in comparison with reference preparations.

Pertussis toxin. Chinese hamster ovary (CHO) cell-clustering effect and haemagglutination as *in vitro* methods; lymphocytosis-promoting activity, histamine-sensitising activity and insulin secretory activity as *in vivo* methods. The toxin shows ADP-ribosyl transferase activity using transducin as the acceptor.

Filamentous haemagglutinin. Haemagglutination and inhibition by specific antibody.

Pertactin, fimbrial-2 and fimbrial-3 antigens. Reactivity with specific antibody.

Pertussis toxoid. The toxoid induces in animals the production of antibodies capable of inhibiting all the properties of pertussis toxin.

PURIFIED ANTIGENIC FRACTION

Production of the antigenic fraction is based on a seed-lot system. The seed cultures are managed to conserve or, where necessary, restore toxinogenicity by deliberate selection. None of the media used at any stage contains blood or blood products of human origin. Media used for the preparation of seed batches and inocula may contain blood or blood products of animal origin.

The antigenic fraction is purified and, after appropriate characterisation, detoxified using suitable reagents by a method that ensures minimal reversion of toxoid to toxin, particularly on storage or exposure to heat. The purification procedure is validated to demonstrate appropriate clearance of substances used during culture or purification.

The content of bacterial endotoxins (*2.6.14*) is determined to monitor the purification procedure and to limit the amount in the final vaccine. The limits applied are such that the final vaccine contains not more than 100 IU per single human dose.

Before detoxification, the purity of the antigenic fraction is determined by a suitable method such as polyacrylamide gel electrophoresis (PAGE) or liquid chromatography. SDS-PAGE or immunoblot analysis with specific monoclonal or polyclonal antibodies may be used to characterise subunits. Requirements are established for each individual product.

Only a purified antigenic fraction that complies with the following requirements may be used in the preparation of the final bulk vaccine.

Sterility (*2.6.1*). Carry out the test for sterility using for each medium a quantity of purified antigenic fraction equivalent to not less than 100 doses of the final vaccine.

Test for residual pertussis toxin. Use 3 groups of not fewer than 5 histamine-sensitive mice each weighing 18 g to 26 g. Using phosphate-buffered saline containing 2 g/l of gelatin, prepare a series of dilutions of the purified antigenic fraction that have been shown to yield a graded response and attribute each dilution to a separate group of mice. Inject intraperitoneally into each mouse the dilution attributed to its group. Inject diluent into a fourth group of control mice. After 5 days, inject intraperitoneally into each mouse 1 mg of histamine base in a volume not exceeding 0.5 ml. Record the number of animals that die within 24 h of histamine challenge. Calculate the weight or volume of a preparation that sensitises 50 per cent of the mice injected using a suitable statistical method such as probit analysis (see *5.3*). The residual activity of pertussis toxin does not exceed that of batches shown to be safe in clinical studies.

The histamine sensitivity of the strain of mice used is verified at suitable intervals as follows: inject threefold dilutions of a reference pertussis toxin preparation in phosphate-buffered saline solution containing 2 g/l of gelatin and challenge with histamine as described above; the strain is suitable if more than 50 per cent of the animals are sensitised by 50 ng of pertussis toxin and none of the control animals injected with only diluent and challenged similarly with histamine show symptoms of sensitisation.

Pertussis toxin BRP is suitable for use as a reference pertussis toxin.

A validated test based on the clustering effect of the toxin for Chinese hamster ovary (CHO) cells may be used instead of the test in mice.

Residual detoxifying agents and other reagents. The content of residual detoxifying agents and other reagents is determined and shown to be below approved limits unless validation of the process has demonstrated acceptable clearance.

Antigen content. Determine the complete quantitative antigen composition of the antigenic fraction by suitable immunochemical methods (*2.7.1*) and protein nitrogen by sulphuric acid digestion (*2.5.9*) or another suitable method. The ratio of total antigen content to protein nitrogen is within the limits established for the product.

FINAL BULK VACCINE

The vaccine is prepared by adsorption of a suitable quantity of the antigenic fraction onto aluminium hydroxide or hydrated aluminium phosphate. A suitable antimicrobial preservative may be added.

Only a final bulk vaccine that complies with the following requirements may be used in the preparation of the final lot.

Antimicrobial preservative. Where applicable, determine the amount of antimicrobial preservative by a suitable chemical or physico-chemical method. The amount is not less than 85 per cent and not greater than 115 per cent of the intended content.

Sterility (*2.6.1*). The final bulk vaccine complies with the test for sterility, carried out using 10 ml for each medium.

FINAL LOT

Only a final lot that is satisfactory with respect to each of the requirements given below under Identification, Tests and Assay may be released for use.

Provided that the tests for residual pertussis toxin, reversibility of toxoid, antimicrobial preservative, free formaldehyde and the assay have been carried out with satisfactory results on the final bulk vaccine, these tests may be omitted on the final lot.

IDENTIFICATION

Subject the vaccine to a suitable desorption procedure such as the following: dissolve in the vaccine to be examined sufficient *sodium citrate R* to give a 10 g/l solution; maintain at 37 °C for about 16 h and centrifuge until a clear supernatant liquid is obtained. Examined by a suitable immunochemical method (*2.7.1*), the clear supernatant liquid reacts with specific antisera to the components in the vaccine.

TESTS

Test for residual pertussis toxin. Use 3 groups of not fewer than 5 histamine-sensitive mice (see under Production) each weighing 18 g to 26 g. Using phosphate-buffered saline containing 2 g/l of gelatin, prepare a series of dilutions of the vaccine to be examined that have been shown to yield a graded response and attribute each dilution to a separate group of mice. Inject intraperitoneally into each mouse the dilution attributed to its group. Inject diluent into a fourth group of control mice. After 5 days, inject intraperitoneally into each mouse 1 mg of histamine base in a volume not exceeding 0.5 ml. Note the number of animals that die within 24 h of histamine challenge. Calculate the weight or volume of a preparation that sensitises 50 per cent of the mice injected using a suitable statistical method such as probit analysis (see *5.3*). The residual activity of pertussis toxin does not exceed that of batches shown to be safe in clinical studies.

Reversibility of toxoid. Carry out the test for residual pertussis toxin described above using the vaccine incubated at 37 °C for 4 weeks in parallel with a sample stored at 2 °C to 8 °C. The degree of reversibility does not exceed that of batches shown to be safe in clinical studies.

Antimicrobial preservative. Where applicable, determine the amount of antimicrobial preservative by a suitable chemical or physico-chemical method. The amount is not less than the minimum amount shown to be effective and is not greater than 115 per cent of the quantity stated on the label.

Aluminium (*2.5.13*): maximum 1.25 mg per single human dose, if aluminium hydroxide or hydrated aluminium phosphate is used as the adsorbent.

Free formaldehyde (*2.4.18*): maximum 0.2 g/l.

Sterility (*2.6.1*). It complies with the test for sterility.

ASSAY

The vaccine complies with the assay of pertussis vaccine (acellular) (*2.7.16*).

LABELLING

The label states:

- the names and amounts of the antigenic components present in the vaccine,
- the maximum amount of residual pertussis toxin present in the vaccine,
- the maximum degree of reversion of toxoid to toxin during the period of validity,
- the name and amount of the adsorbent,
- that the vaccine must be shaken before use,
- that the vaccine is not to be frozen.

01/2005:0161

PERTUSSIS VACCINE (ADSORBED)

Vaccinum pertussis adsorbatum

DEFINITION

Pertussis vaccine (adsorbed) is a sterile saline suspension of inactivated whole cells of one or more strains of *Bordetella pertussis* with a mineral adsorbent such as hydrated aluminium phosphate or aluminium hydroxide.

PRODUCTION

INACTIVATED B. PERTUSSIS SUSPENSION

Production is based on a seed-lot system. One or more strains of *B. pertussis* with known origin and history are used. Strains, culture medium and cultivation method are chosen in such a way that agglutinogens 1, 2 and 3 are present in the final vaccine. Each strain is grown for 24 h to 72 h in a liquid medium or on a solid medium; the medium used in the final cultivation stage does not contain blood or blood products. Human blood or blood products are not used in any culture media. The bacteria are harvested, washed to remove substances derived from the medium and suspended in a 9 g/l solution of sodium chloride or other suitable isotonic solution. The opacity of the suspension is determined not later than 2 weeks after harvest by comparison with the International Reference Preparation of Opacity and used as the basis of calculation for subsequent stages in vaccine preparation. The equivalence in International Units of the International Reference Preparation is stated by the World Health Organisation.

Single harvests are not used for the final bulk vaccine unless they have been shown to contain *B. pertussis* cells with the same characteristics, with regard to growth and agglutinogens, as the parent strain and to be free from contaminating bacteria and fungi. The bacteria are killed and detoxified in controlled conditions by means of a suitable chemical agent or by heating or by a combination of these methods. Freedom from live *B. pertussis* is tested using a suitable culture medium. The suspension is maintained at 5 ± 3 °C for a suitable period to diminish its toxicity.

FINAL BULK VACCINE

Suitable quantities of the inactivated single harvests are pooled to prepare the final bulk vaccine. A mineral adsorbent such as hydrated aluminium phosphate or aluminium hydroxide is added to the cell suspension. Suitable antimicrobial preservatives may be added. The bacterial concentration of the final bulk vaccine does not exceed that corresponding to an opacity of 20 IU per single human dose. If 2 or more strains of *B. pertussis* are used, the composition of consecutive lots of the final bulk vaccine shall be consistent with respect to the proportion of each strain as measured in opacity units.

Only a final bulk vaccine that complies with the following requirements may be used in the preparation of the final lot.

Antimicrobial preservative. Where applicable, determine the amount of antimicrobial preservative by a suitable chemical method. The amount is not less than 85 per cent and not greater than 115 per cent of the intended amount.

Sterility (*2.6.1*). Carry out the test for sterility using 10 ml for each medium.

FINAL LOT

The final bulk vaccine is distributed aseptically into sterile, tamper-proof containers. The containers are closed so as to prevent contamination.

Only a final lot that is satisfactory with respect to each of the requirements given below under Identification, Tests and Assay may be released for use. Provided the tests for specific toxicity, free formaldehyde and antimicrobial preservative and the assay have been carried out with satisfactory results on the final bulk vaccine, they may be omitted on the final lot.

IDENTIFICATION

Dissolve in the vaccine to be examined sufficient *sodium citrate R* to give a 100 g/l solution. Maintain at 37 °C for about 16 h and centrifuge to obtain a bacterial precipitate. Other suitable methods for separating the bacteria from the adsorbent may also be used. Identify pertussis vaccine by agglutination of the bacteria from the resuspended precipitate by antisera specific to *B. pertussis* or by the assay.

TESTS

Specific toxicity. Use not fewer than 5 healthy mice each weighing 14 g to 16 g for the vaccine group and for the saline control. Use mice of the same sex or distribute males and females equally between the groups. Allow the animals access to food and water for at least 2 h before injection and during the test. Inject each mouse of the vaccine group intraperitoneally with 0.5 ml, containing a quantity of the vaccine equivalent to not less than half the single human dose. Inject each mouse of the control group with 0.5 ml of a 9 g/l sterile solution of *sodium chloride R*, preferably containing the same amount of antimicrobial preservative as that injected with the vaccine. Weigh the groups of mice immediately before the injection and 72 h and 7 days after the injection. The vaccine complies with the test if: (a) at the end of 72 h the total mass of the group of vaccinated mice is not less than that preceding the injection; (b) at the end of 7 days the average increase in mass per vaccinated mouse is not less than 60 per cent of that per control mouse; and (c) not more than 5 per cent of the vaccinated mice die during the test. The test may be repeated and the results of the tests combined.

Aluminium (*2.5.13*): maximum 1.25 mg per single human dose, if aluminium hydroxide or hydrated aluminium phosphate is used as the adsorbent.

Free formaldehyde (*2.4.18*): maximum 0.2 g/l.

Antimicrobial preservative. Where applicable, determine the amount of antimicrobial preservative by a suitable chemical method. The content is not less than the minimum amount shown to be effective and is not greater than 115 per cent of the quantity stated on the label.

Sterility (*2.6.1*). The vaccine complies with the test for sterility.

ASSAY

Carry out the assay of pertussis vaccine (*2.7.7*).

Vaccines

The estimated potency is not less than 4 IU per single human dose and the lower confidence limit ($P = 0.95$) of the estimated potency is not less than 2 IU per single human dose.

LABELLING

The label states:

– the minimum number of International Units per single human dose,
– the name and the amount of the adsorbent,
– that the vaccine must be shaken before use,
– that the vaccine is not to be frozen.

01/2005:0966

PNEUMOCOCCAL POLYSACCHARIDE VACCINE

Vaccinum pneumococcale polysaccharidicum

DEFINITION

Pneumococcal polysaccharide vaccine consists of a mixture of equal parts of purified capsular polysaccharide antigens prepared from suitable pathogenic strains of *Streptococcus pneumoniae* whose capsules have been shown to be made up of polysaccharides that are capable of inducing satisfactory levels of specific antibodies in man. It contains the 23 immunochemically different capsular polysaccharides listed in Table 0966-1.

The vaccine is a clear, colourless liquid.

PRODUCTION

Production of the vaccine is based on a seed-lot system for each type. The production method shall have been shown to yield consistently pneumococcal polysaccharide vaccines of adequate safety and immunogenicity in man.

The production method is validated to demonstrate that the product, if tested, would comply with the test for abnormal toxicity for immunosera and vaccines for human use (*2.6.9*) modified as follows for the test in guinea-pigs: inject 10 human doses into each guinea-pig and observe for 12 days.

MONOVALENT BULK POLYSACCHARIDES

The bacteria are grown in a suitable liquid medium that does not contain blood-group substances or high-molecular-mass polysaccharides. The bacterial purity of the culture is verified and the culture is inactivated with phenol. Impurities are removed by such techniques as fractional precipitation, enzymatic digestion and ultrafiltration. The polysaccharide is obtained by fractional precipitation, washed, and dried in a vacuum to a residual moisture content shown to be favourable to the stability of the polysaccharide. The residual moisture content is determined by drying under reduced pressure over diphosphorus pentoxide or by thermogravimetric analysis and the value obtained is used to calculate the results of the tests shown below with reference to the dried substance. The monovalent bulk polysaccharide is stored at a suitable temperature in conditions that avoid the uptake of moisture.

Only a monovalent bulk polysaccharide that complies with the following requirements may be used in the preparation of the final bulk vaccine. Percentage contents of components, determined by the methods prescribed below, are shown in Table 0966-1.

Protein (*2.5.16*).

Nucleic acids (*2.5.17*).

Total nitrogen (*2.5.9*).

Phosphorus (*2.5.18*).

Molecular size. Determine by size-exclusion chromatography (*2.2.30*) using *cross-linked agarose for chromatography R* or *cross-linked agarose for chromatography R1*.

Uronic acids (*2.5.22*).

Hexosamines (*2.5.20*).

Methylpentoses (*2.5.21*).

***O*-Acetyl groups** (*2.5.19*).

Identification (*2.7.1*). Confirm the identity of the monovalent bulk polysaccharide by double immunodiffusion or electroimmunodiffusion (except for polysaccharides 7F, 14 and 33F), using specific antisera.

Specificity. No reaction occurs when the antigens are tested against all the antisera specific for the other polysaccharides of the vaccine, including factor sera for distinguishing types within groups. The polysaccharides are tested at a concentration of 50 µg/ml using a method capable of detecting 0.5 µg/ml.

FINAL BULK VACCINE

The final bulk vaccine is obtained by aseptically mixing the different polysaccharide powders. The uniform mixture is aseptically dissolved in a suitable isotonic solution so that one human dose of 0.50 ml contains 25 µg of each polysaccharide. An antimicrobial preservative may be added. The solution is sterilised by filtration through a bacteria-retentive filter.

Only a final bulk vaccine that complies with the following requirements may be used in the preparation of the final lot.

Antimicrobial preservative. Where applicable, determine the amount of antimicrobial preservative by a suitable chemical method. The content is not less than 85 per cent and not greater than 115 per cent of the intended amount.

Sterility (*2.6.1*). The final bulk vaccine complies with the test for sterility, using 10 ml for each medium.

FINAL LOT

The final bulk vaccine is distributed aseptically into sterile, tamper-proof containers.

Only a final lot that is satisfactory with respect to each of the requirements given below under identification, tests and assay may be released for use. Provided that the tests for phenol and for antimicrobial preservative have been carried out with satisfactory results on the final bulk vaccine, they may be omitted on the final lot. When consistency of production has been established on a suitable number of consecutive batches, the assay may be replaced by a qualitative test that identifies each polysaccharide, provided that an assay has been performed on each monovalent bulk polysaccharide used in the preparation of the final lot.

IDENTIFICATION

The assay serves also to identify the vaccine.

TESTS

pH (*2.2.3*). The pH of the vaccine is 4.5 to 7.4.

Antimicrobial preservative. Where applicable, determine the amount of antimicrobial preservative by a suitable chemical method. The content is not less than the minimum amount shown to be effective and is not greater than 115 per cent of the quantity stated on the label.

Phenol (*2.5.15*). Not more than 2.5 g/l.

Sterility (*2.6.1*). It complies with the test for sterility.

Table 0966.-1 – *Percentage contents of components of monovalent bulk polysaccharides*

Molecular type*	Protein	Nucleic acids	Total nitrogen	Phosphorus	Molecular size (K_o)		Uronic acids	Hexos-amines	Methyl-pentoses	O-acetyl Groups
					**	***				
1	≤ 2	≤ 2	3.5-6	0-1.5	≤ 0.15		≥ 45			≥ 1.8
2	≤ 2	≤ 2	0-1	0-1.0	≤ 0.15		≥ 15		≥ 38	
3	≤ 5	≤ 2	0-1	0-1.0	≤ 0.15		≥ 40			
4	≤ 3	≤ 2	4-6	0-1.5	≤ 0.15			≥ 40		
5	≤ 7.5	≤ 2	2.5-6.0	≤ 2		≤ 0.60	≥ 12	≥ 20		
6B	≤ 2	≤ 2	0-2	2.5-5.0		≤ 0.50			≥ 15	
7F	≤ 5	≤ 2	1.5-4.0	0-1.0	≤ 0.20				≥13	
8	≤ 2	≤ 2	0-1	0-1.0	≤ 0.15		≥ 25			
9N	≤ 2	≤ 1	2.2-4	0-1.0	≤ 0.20		≥ 20	≥ 28		
9V	≤ 2	≤ 2	0.5-3	0-1.0		≤ 0.45	≥ 15	≥ 13		
10A	≤ 7	≤ 2	0.5-3.5	1.5-3.5		≤ 0.65		≥ 12		
11A	≤ 3	≤ 2	0-2.5	2.0-5.0		≤ 0.40				≥ 9
12F	≤ 3	≤ 2	3-5	0-1.0	≤ 0.25			≥ 25		
14	≤ 5	≤ 2	1.5-4	0-1.0	≤ 0.30			≥ 20		
15B	≤ 3	≤ 2	1-3	2.0-4.5		≤0.55		≥ 15		
17A or17F	≤ 2	≤ 2	0-1.5	0-3.5		≤ 0.45			≥ 20	
18C	≤ 3	≤ 2	0-1	2.4-4.9	≤ 0.15				≥ 14	
19A	≤ 2	≤ 2	0.6-3.5	3.0-7.0	≤ 0.45			≥ 12	≥ 20	
19F	≤ 3	≤ 2	1.4-3.5	3.0-5.5	≤ 0.20			≥ 12.5	≥ 20	
20	≤ 2	≤ 2	0.5-2.5	1.5-4.0		≤ 0.60		≥ 12		
22F	≤ 2	≤ 2	0-2	0-1.0		≤ 0.55	≥ 15		≥ 25	
23F	≤ 2	≤ 2	0-1	3.0-4.5	≤ 0.15				≥ 37	
33F	≤ 2.5	≤ 2	0-2	0-1.0		≤ 0.50				

* The different types are indicated using the Danish nomenclature.

** *Cross-linked agarose for chromatography R.*

*** *Cross-linked agarose for chromatography R1.*

Pyrogens (*2.6.8*). It complies with the test for pyrogens. Inject per kilogram of the rabbit's mass 1 ml of a dilution of the vaccine containing 2.5 μg/ml of each polysaccharide.

ASSAY

Determine the content of each polysaccharide by a suitable immunochemical method (*2.7.1*), using antisera specific for each polysaccharide contained in the vaccine, including factor sera for types within groups, and purified polysaccharides of each type as standards.

The vaccine contains not less than 70 per cent and not more than 130 per cent of the quantity stated on the label for each polysaccharide. The confidence limits ($P = 0.95$) are not less than 80 per cent and not more than 120 per cent of the estimated content.

LABELLING

The label states:

– the number of micrograms of each polysaccharide per human dose,

– the total amount of polysaccharide in the container.

01/2005:0214

POLIOMYELITIS VACCINE (INACTIVATED)

Vaccinum poliomyelitidis inactivatum

DEFINITION

Poliomyelitis vaccine (inactivated) is a liquid preparation of suitable strains of human polioviruses 1, 2 and 3 grown in suitable cell cultures and inactivated by a validated method. It is a clear liquid that may be coloured owing to the presence of a pH indicator.

PRODUCTION

The production method shall have been shown to yield consistently vaccines of acceptable safety and immunogenicity in man.

Production of the vaccine is based on a virus seed-lot system. Cell lines are used according to a cell-bank system. If primary, secondary or tertiary monkey kidney cells are used, production complies with the requirements indicated below.

Unless otherwise justified and authorised, the virus in the final vaccine shall not have undergone more passages from the master seed lot than was used to prepare the vaccine shown in clinical studies to be satisfactory with respect to safety and efficacy.

The production method is validated to demonstrate that the product, if tested, would comply with the test for abnormal toxicity for immunosera and vaccines for human use (*2.6.9*).

SUBSTRATE FOR VIRUS PROPAGATION

The virus is propagated in a human diploid cell line (*5.2.3*), in a continuous cell line (*5.2.3*) or in primary, secondary or tertiary monkey kidney cells.

Primary, secondary or tertiary monkey kidney cells. The following special requirements for the substrate for virus propagation apply to primary, secondary or tertiary monkey kidney cells.

Monkeys used in the preparation of kidney cell cultures for production and control of the vaccine. The animals used are of a species approved by the competent authority, in good health and, unless otherwise justified and authorised, have not been previously employed for experimental purposes. Kidney cells used for vaccine production and control are derived from monitored, closed colonies of monkeys bred in captivity, not from animals caught in the wild; a previously approved seed lot prepared using virus passaged in cells from wild monkeys may, subject to approval by the competent authority, be used for vaccine production if historical data on safety justify this.

Monitored, closed colonies of monkeys. The monkeys are kept in groups in cages. Freedom from extraneous agents is achieved by the use of animals maintained in closed colonies that are subject to continuous and systematic veterinary and laboratory monitoring for the presence of infectious agents. The supplier of animals is certified by the competent authority. Each monkey is tested serologically at regular intervals during a quarantine period of not less than 6 weeks imposed before entering the colony and then during its stay in the colony.

The monkeys used are shown to be tuberculin-negative and free from antibodies to simian virus 40 (SV40) and simian immunodeficiency virus. The blood sample used in testing for SV40 antibodies must be taken as close as possible to the time of removal of the kidneys. If *Macaca* sp. monkeys are used for production, the monkeys are also shown to be free from antibodies to herpesvirus B (cercopithecine herpesvirus 1) infection. Human herpesvirus 1 has been used as an indicator for freedom from herpesvirus B antibodies on account of the danger of handling herpesvirus B (cercopithecine herpesvirus 1).

Monkeys from which kidneys are to be removed are thoroughly examined, particularly for evidence of tuberculosis and herpesvirus B (cercopithecine herpesvirus 1) infection. If a monkey shows any pathological lesion relevant to the use of its kidneys in the preparation of a seed lot or vaccine, it is not to be used nor are any of the remaining monkeys of the group concerned unless it is evident that their use will not impair the safety of the product.

All the operations described in this section are conducted outside the area where the vaccine is produced.

Monkey cell cultures for vaccine production. Kidneys that show no pathological signs are used for preparing cell cultures. Each group of cell cultures derived from a single monkey forms a separate production cell culture giving rise to a separate single harvest.

The primary monkey kidney cell suspension complies with the test for mycobacteria (*2.6.2*); disrupt the cells before carrying out the test.

If secondary or tertiary cells are used, it shall be demonstrated by suitable validation tests that cell cultures beyond the passage level used for production are free from tumorigenicity.

SEED LOTS

Each of the 3 strains of poliovirus used shall be identified by historical records that include information on the origin of the strain and its subsequent manipulation.

Only a working seed lot that complies with the following requirements may be used for virus propagation.

Identification. Each working seed lot is identified as human poliovirus 1, 2 or 3 by virus neutralisation in cell culture using specific antibodies.

Virus concentration. The virus concentration of each working seed lot is determined to define the quantity of virus to be used for inoculation of production cell cultures.

Extraneous agents. The working seed lot complies with the requirements for seed lots for virus vaccines (*2.6.16*). In addition, if primary, secondary or tertiary monkey kidney cells have been used for isolation of the strain, measures are taken to ensure that the strain is not contaminated with simian viruses such as simian immunodeficiency virus, simian virus 40, filoviruses and herpesvirus B (cercopithecine herpesvirus 1). A working seed lot produced in primary, secondary or tertiary monkey kidney cells complies with the requirements given below under Virus propagation and harvest for single harvests produced in such cells.

PROPAGATION AND HARVEST

All processing of the cell bank and cell cultures is done under aseptic conditions in an area where no other cells or viruses are being handled. Approved animal serum (but not human serum) may be used in the cell culture media. Serum and trypsin used in the preparation of cell suspensions and media are shown to be free from extraneous agents. The cell culture media may contain a pH indicator such as phenol red and approved antibiotics at the lowest effective concentration. Not less than 500 ml of the cell cultures employed for vaccine production is set aside as uninfected cell cultures (control cells); where continuous cell lines in a fermenter are used for production, 200×10^6 cells are set aside to prepare control cells; where primary, secondary or tertiary monkey kidney cells are used for production, a cell sample equivalent to at least 500 ml of the cell suspension, at the concentration employed for vaccine production, is taken to prepare control cells.

Only a single harvest that complies with the following requirements may be used in the preparation of the vaccine. The tests for identification and bacterial and fungal contamination may be carried out instead on the purified, pooled monovalent harvest. After demonstration of consistency of production at the stage of the single harvest, the test for virus concentration may be carried out instead on the purified, pooled monovalent harvest.

Control cells. The control cells of the production cell culture comply with a test for identification (if a cell-bank system is used for production) and with the requirements for extraneous agents (*2.6.16*; where primary, secondary or tertiary monkey kidney cells are used, the tests in cell cultures are carried out as shown below under Test in rabbit kidney cell cultures and Test in cercopithecus kidney cell cultures).

– *Test in rabbit kidney cell cultures.* Test a sample of at least 10 ml of the pooled supernatant fluid from the control cultures for the absence of herpesvirus B (cercopithecine herpesvirus 1) and other viruses by inoculation onto rabbit kidney cell cultures. The dilution of supernatant in the nutrient medium is not

Vaccines

greater than 1/4 and the area of the cell layer is at least 3 cm² per millilitre of inoculum. Set aside one or more containers of each batch of cells with the same medium as non-inoculated control cells. Incubate the cultures at 37 °C and observe for at least 2 weeks. The test is not valid if more than 20 per cent of the control cells are discarded for non-specific, accidental reasons.

– *Test in cercopithecus kidney cell cultures*. Test a sample of at least 10 ml of the pooled supernatant fluid from the control cultures for the absence of SV40 virus and other extraneous agents by inoculation onto cell cultures prepared from the kidneys of cercopithecus monkeys, or other cells shown to be at least as sensitive for SV40, by the method described under Test in rabbit kidney cell cultures. The test is not valid if more than 20 per cent of the control cell cultures are discarded for non-specific, accidental reasons.

Identification. The single harvest is identified as containing human poliovirus 1, 2 or 3 by virus neutralisation in cell cultures using specific antibodies.

Virus concentration. The virus concentration of each single harvest is determined by titration of infectious virus in cell cultures.

Bacterial and fungal contamination. The single harvest complies with the test for sterility (*2.6.1*), carried out using 10 ml for each medium.

Mycoplasmas (*2.6.7*). The single harvest complies with the test for mycoplasmas, carried out using 10 ml.

Test in rabbit kidney cell cultures. Where primary, secondary or tertiary monkey kidney cells are used for production, test a sample of at least 10 ml of the single harvest for the absence of herpesvirus B (cercopithecine herpesvirus 1) and other viruses by inoculation onto rabbit kidney cell cultures as described above for the control cells.

Test in cercopithecus kidney cell cultures. Where primary, secondary or tertiary monkey kidney cells are used for production, test a sample of at least 10 ml of the single harvest for the absence of SV40 virus and other extraneous agents. Neutralise the sample by a high-titre antiserum against the specific type of poliovirus. Test the sample in primary cercopithecus kidney cell cultures or cells that have been demonstrated to be at least as susceptible for SV40. Incubate the cultures at 37 °C and observe for 14 days. At the end of this period, make at least one subculture of fluid in the same cell culture system and observe both primary cultures and subcultures for an additional 14 days.

PURIFICATION AND PURIFIED MONOVALENT HARVEST

Several single harvests of the same type may be pooled and may be concentrated. The monovalent harvest or pooled monovalent harvest is purified by validated methods. If continuous cell lines are used for production, the purification process shall have been shown to reduce consistently the content of substrate-cell DNA to not more than 100 pg per single human dose.

Only a purified monovalent harvest that complies with the following requirements may be used for the preparation of the inactivated monovalent harvest.

Identification. The virus is identified by virus neutralisation in cell cultures using specific antibodies or by determination of D-antigen.

Virus concentration. The virus concentration is determined by titration of infectious virus.

Specific activity. The ratio of the virus concentration or the D-antigen content, determined by a suitable immunochemical method (*2.7.1*), to the total protein content (specific activity) of the purified monovalent harvest is within the limits approved for the particular product.

INACTIVATION AND INACTIVATED MONOVALENT HARVEST

Several purified monovalent harvests of the same type may be mixed before inactivation. To avoid failures in inactivation caused by the presence of virus aggregates, filtration is carried out before and during inactivation; inactivation is started within a suitable period, preferably not more than 24 h and in any case not more than 72 h, of the prior filtration. The virus suspension is inactivated by a validated method that has been shown to inactivate poliovirus without destruction of immunogenicity; during validation studies, an inactivation curve with at least 4 points (for example, time 0 h, 24 h, 48 h and 96 h) is established showing the decrease in concentration of live virus with time. If formaldehyde is used for inactivation, the presence of an excess of formaldehyde at the end of the inactivation period is verified.

Only an inactivated monovalent harvest that complies with the following requirements may be used in the preparation of a trivalent pool of inactivated monovalent harvests or a final bulk vaccine.

Test for effective inactivation. After neutralisation of the formaldehyde with sodium bisulphite (where applicable), verify the absence of residual live poliovirus by inoculation on suitable cell cultures of 2 samples of each inactivated monovalent harvest, corresponding to at least 1500 human doses. Take one sample not later than three-quarters of the way through the inactivation period and the other at the end. Inoculate the samples in cell cultures such that the dilution of vaccine in the nutrient medium is not greater than 1/4 and the area of the cell layer is at least 3 cm² per millilitre of inoculum. Set aside one or more containers with the same medium as non-inoculated control cells. Observe the cell cultures for at least 3 weeks. Make not fewer than 2 passages from each container, one at the end of the observation period and the other 1 week before; for the passages, use cell culture supernatant and inoculate as for the initial sample. Observe the subcultures for at least 2 weeks. No sign of poliovirus multiplication is present in the cell cultures. At the end of the observation period, test the susceptibility of the cell culture used by inoculation of live poliovirus of the same type as that present in the inactivated monovalent harvest.

Sterility (*2.6.1*). The inactivated monovalent harvest complies with the test for sterility, carried out using 10 ml for each medium.

D-antigen content. The content of D-antigen determined by a suitable immunochemical method (*2.7.1*) is within the limits approved for the particular preparation.

FINAL BULK VACCINE

The final bulk vaccine is prepared directly from the inactivated monovalent harvests of human polioviruses 1, 2 and 3 or from a trivalent pool of inactivated monovalent harvests. If a trivalent pool of inactivated monovalent harvests is used, a test for effective inactivation is carried out on this pool instead of on the final bulk vaccine. A stabiliser and an antimicrobial preservative may be added.

Only a final bulk vaccine that complies with the following requirements may be used in the preparation of the final lot.

Sterility (*2.6.1*). The final bulk vaccine complies with the test for sterility, carried out using 10 ml for each medium.

Antimicrobial preservative. Where applicable, determine the amount of antimicrobial preservative by a suitable chemical or physicochemical method. The amount is not less than 85 per cent and not greater than 115 per cent of the intended amount.

Inactivation. Before addition of any antimicrobial preservative, a sample of at least 1500 ml or, for a purified and concentrated vaccine, the equivalent of 1500 doses is tested for residual live poliovirus in cell cultures, as described for the inactivated monovalent harvest. If the final bulk vaccine is prepared from a trivalent pool of inactivated monovalent harvests, the test for inactivation is carried out on that pool rather than on the final bulk vaccine.

FINAL LOT

Only a final lot that complies with each of the requirements given below under Identification, Tests and Assay may be released for use. Provided that the tests for free formaldehyde and antimicrobial preservative and the *in vivo* assay have been performed with satisfactory results on the final bulk vaccine, they may be omitted on the final lot. Provided that the test for bovine serum albumin has been performed with satisfactory results on the trivalent pool of inactivated monovalent harvests or on the final bulk vaccine, it may be omitted on the final lot.

IDENTIFICATION

The vaccine is shown to contain human polioviruses 1, 2 and 3 by a suitable immunochemical method (*2.7.1*) such as the determination of D-antigen by enzyme-linked immunosorbent assay (ELISA).

TESTS

Free formaldehyde (*2.4.18*): maximum 0.2 g/l.

Antimicrobial preservative. Where applicable, determine the amount of antimicrobial preservative by a suitable chemical or physicochemical method. The amount is not less than the minimum amount shown to be effective and is not greater than 115 per cent of that stated on the label.

Protein nitrogen content (*Lowry method*). Not more than 10 μg of protein nitrogen per single human dose.

Bovine serum albumin. Not more than 50 ng per single human dose, determined by a suitable immunochemical method (*2.7.1*).

Sterility (*2.6.1*). The vaccine complies with the test for sterility.

Bacterial endotoxins (*2.6.14*): less than 5 IU per single human dose.

ASSAY

D-antigen content. As a measure of consistency of production, determine the D-antigen content for human polioviruses 1, 2 and 3 by a suitable immunochemical method (*2.7.1*) using a reference preparation calibrated in European Pharmacopoeia D-antigen units. For each type, the content, expressed with reference to the amount of D-antigen stated on the label, is within the limits approved for the particular product.

Poliomyelitis vaccine (inactivated) BRP is calibrated in European Pharmacopoeia units and intended for use in the assay of D-antigen. The European Pharmacopoeia unit and the International Unit are equivalent.

***In vivo* test**. The vaccine complies with the *in vivo* assay of poliomyelitis vaccine (inactivated) (*2.7.20*).

LABELLING

The label states:

– the types of poliovirus contained in the vaccine,
– the nominal amount of virus of each type (1, 2 and 3), expressed in Ph. Eur. units of D-antigen, per single human dose,
– the cell substrate used to prepare the vaccine.

01/2005:0215

POLIOMYELITIS VACCINE (ORAL)

Vaccinum poliomyelitidis perorale

DEFINITION

Oral poliomyelitis vaccine is a preparation of approved strains of live attenuated poliovirus type 1, 2 or 3 grown in *in vitro* cultures of approved cells, containing any one type or any combination of the 3 types of Sabin strains, presented in a form suitable for oral administration.

The vaccine is a clear liquid that may be coloured owing to the presence of a pH indicator.

PRODUCTION

The vaccine strains and the production method shall have been shown to yield consistently vaccines that are both immunogenic and safe in man.

The production of vaccine is based on a virus seed-lot system. Cell lines are used according to a cell-bank system. If primary monkey kidney cell cultures are used, production complies with the requirements indicated below. Unless otherwise justified and authorised, the virus in the final vaccine shall not have undergone more than 2 passages from the master seed lot.

SUBSTRATE FOR VIRUS PROPAGATION

The virus is propagated in human diploid cells (*5.2.3*), in continuous cell lines (*5.2.3*) or in primary monkey kidney cell cultures (including serially passaged cells from primary monkey kidney cells).

Primary monkey kidney cell cultures. *The following special requirements for the substrate for virus propagation apply to primary monkey kidney cell cultures.*

Monkeys used for preparation of primary monkey kidney cell cultures and for testing of virus. If the vaccine is prepared in primary monkey kidney cell cultures, animals of a species approved by the competent authority, in good health, kept in closed or intensively monitored colonies and not previously employed for experimental purposes shall be used.

The monkeys shall be kept in well-constructed and adequately ventilated animal rooms in cages spaced as far apart as possible. Adequate precautions shall be taken to prevent cross-infection between cages. Not more than 2 monkeys shall be housed per cage and cage-mates shall not be interchanged. The monkeys shall be kept in the country of manufacture of the vaccine in quarantine groups for a period of not less than 6 weeks before use. A quarantine group is a colony of selected, healthy monkeys kept in one room, with separate feeding and cleaning facilities, and having no contact with other monkeys during the quarantine period. If at any time during the quarantine period the overall death rate of a shipment consisting of one or more groups reaches 5 per cent (excluding deaths from accidents or where the cause was specifically determined not to be an infectious disease), monkeys from that entire shipment shall continue in quarantine from that time for a minimum of 6 weeks. The groups shall be kept continuously in isolation, as in

Vaccines

quarantine, even after completion of the quarantine period, until the monkeys are used. After the last monkey of a group has been taken, the room that housed the group shall be thoroughly cleaned and decontaminated before being used for a fresh group. If kidneys from near-term monkeys are used, the mother is quarantined for the term of pregnancy.

Monkeys from which kidneys are to be removed shall be anaesthetised and thoroughly examined, particularly for evidence of tuberculosis and cercopithecid herpesvirus 1 (B virus) infection.

If a monkey shows any pathological lesion relevant to the use of its kidneys in the preparation of a seed lot or vaccine, it shall not be used, nor shall any of the remaining monkeys of the quarantine group concerned be used unless it is evident that their use will not impair the safety of the product.

All the operations described in this section shall be conducted outside the areas where the vaccine is produced.

The monkeys used shall be shown to be free from antibodies to simian virus 40 (SV40), simian immunodeficiency virus and spumaviruses. The blood sample used in testing for SV40 antibodies must be taken as close as possible to the time of removal of the kidneys. If *Macaca* spp. are used for production, the monkeys shall also be shown to be free from antibodies to cercopithecid herpesvirus 1 (B virus). Human herpesvirus has been used as an indicator for freedom from B virus antibodies on account of the danger of handling cercopithecid herpesvirus 1 (B virus).

Primary monkey kidney cell cultures for vaccine production. Kidneys that show no pathological signs are used for preparing cell cultures. If the monkeys are from a colony maintained for vaccine production, serially passaged monkey kidney cell cultures from primary monkey kidney cells may be used for virus propagation, otherwise the monkey kidney cells are not propagated in series. Virus for the preparation of vaccine is grown by aseptic methods in such cultures. If animal serum is used in the propagation of the cells, the maintenance medium after virus inoculation shall contain no added serum.

Each group of cell cultures derived from a single monkey or from foetuses from no more than 10 near-term monkeys is prepared and tested as an individual group.

VIRUS SEED LOTS

The strains of poliovirus used shall be identified by historical records that include information on the origin and subsequent manipulation of the strains.

Working seed lots are prepared by a single passage from a master seed lot and at an approved passage level from the original Sabin virus. Virus seed lots are prepared in large quantities and stored at a temperature below − 60 °C.

Only a virus seed lot that complies with the following requirements may be used for virus propagation.

Identification. Each working seed lot is identified as poliovirus of the given type, using specific antibodies.

Virus concentration. Determined by the method described below, the virus concentration is the basis for the quantity of virus used in the neurovirulence test.

Extraneous agents (*2.6.16*). If the working seed lot is produced in human diploid cells or in a continuous cell line, it complies with the requirements for seed lots for virus vaccines. If the working seed lot is produced in primary monkey kidney cell cultures, it complies with the requirements given below under Virus Propagation and Harvest and Monovalent Pooled Harvest and with the tests in adult mice, suckling mice and guinea-pigs given under *2.6.16. Tests for extraneous agents in viral vaccines for human use.*

Working seed lots shall be free from detectable DNA sequences from simian virus 40 (SV40).

Neurovirulence (*2.6.19*). Each master and working seed lot complies with the test for neurovirulence of poliomyelitis vaccine (oral). Furthermore, the seed lot shall cease to be used in vaccine production if the frequency of failure of the monovalent pooled harvests produced from it is greater than predicted statistically. This statistical prediction is calculated after each test on the basis of all the monovalent pooled harvests tested; it is equal to the probability of false rejection on the occasion of a first test (i.e. 1 per cent), the probability of false rejection on retest being negligible. If the test is carried out only by the manufacturer, the test slides are provided to the control authority for assessment. Reference preparations of the 3 types of poliovirus at the Sabin Original + 2 passage levels are available on application to Biologicals, WHO, Geneva, Switzerland.

Genetic markers. Each working seed lot is tested for its replicating properties at temperatures ranging from 36 °C to 40 °C as described under Monovalent Pooled Harvest.

VIRUS PROPAGATION AND HARVEST

All processing of the cell banks and subsequent cell cultures is done under aseptic conditions in an area where no other cells are handled. Approved animal (but not human) serum may be used in the media, but the final medium for maintaining cell growth during virus multiplication does not contain animal serum. Serum and trypsin used in the preparation of cell suspensions and media are shown to be free from live extraneous agents. The cell-culture medium may contain a pH indicator such as phenol red and approved antibiotics at the lowest effective concentration. It is preferable to have a substrate free from antibiotics during production. On the day of inoculation with the virus working seed lot, not less than 5 per cent or 1000 ml, whichever is less, of the cell cultures employed for vaccine production are set aside as uninfected cell cultures (control cells); special requirements, given below, apply to control cells when the vaccine is produced in primary monkey kidney cell cultures. The virus suspension is harvested not later than 4 days after virus inoculation. After inoculation of the production cell culture with the virus working seed lot, inoculated cells are maintained at a fixed temperature, shown to be suitable, within the range 33 °C to 35 °C; the temperature is maintained constant to ± 0.5 °C; control cell cultures are maintained at 33-35 °C for the relevant incubation periods.

Only a single virus harvest that complies with the following requirements may be used in the preparation of the monovalent pooled harvest.

Virus concentration. The virus concentration of virus harvests is determined as prescribed under Assay to monitor consistency of production and to determine the dilution to be used for the final bulk vaccine.

Extraneous agents (*2.6.16*).

Control cells. The control cells of the production cell culture from which the virus harvest is derived comply with a test for identity and with the requirements for extraneous agents (*2.6.16*) or, where primary monkey kidney cell cultures are used, as shown below.

Primary monkey kidney cell cultures. *The following special requirements apply to virus propagation and harvest in primary monkey kidney cell cultures.*

Cell cultures. On the day of inoculation with virus working seed lot, each cell culture is examined for degeneration caused by an infective agent. If, in this examination, evidence is found of the presence in a cell culture of any extraneous agent, the entire group of cultures concerned shall be rejected.

On the day of inoculation with the virus working seed lot, a sample of at least 30 ml of the pooled fluid removed from the cell cultures of the kidneys of each single monkey or from foetuses from not more than 10 near-term monkeys is divided into 2 equal portions. 1 portion of the pooled fluid is tested in monkey kidney cell cultures prepared from the same species, but not the same animal, as that used for vaccine production. The other portion of the pooled fluid is, where necessary, tested in monkey kidney cell cultures from another species so that tests on the pooled fluids are done in cell cultures from at least 1 species known to be sensitive to SV40. The pooled fluid is inoculated into bottles of these cell cultures in such a way that the dilution of the pooled fluid in the nutrient medium does not exceed 1 in 4. The area of the cell sheet is at least 3 cm^2/ml of pooled fluid. At least 1 bottle of each kind of cell culture remains uninoculated to serve as a control. If the monkey species used for vaccine production is known to be sensitive to SV40, a test in a second species is not required. Animal serum may be used in the propagation of the cells, provided that it does not contain SV40 antibody, but the maintenance medium after inoculation of test material contains no added serum except as described below.

The cultures are incubated at a temperature of 35-37 °C and are observed for a total period of at least 4 weeks. During this observation period and after not less than 2 weeks' incubation, at least 1 subculture of fluid is made from each of these cultures in the same cell culture system. The subcultures are also observed for at least 2 weeks.

Serum may be added to the original culture at the time of subculturing, provided that the serum does not contain SV40 antibody.

Fluorescent-antibody techniques may be useful for detecting SV40 virus and other viruses in the cells.

A further sample of at least 10 ml of the pooled fluid is tested for cercopithecid herpesvirus 1 (B virus) and other viruses in rabbit kidney cell cultures. Serum used in the nutrient medium of these cultures shall have been shown to be free from inhibitors of B virus. Human herpesvirus has been used as an indicator for freedom from B virus inhibitors on account of the danger of handling cercopithecid herpesvirus 1 (B virus). The sample is inoculated into bottles of these cell cultures in such a way that the dilution of the pooled fluid in the nutrient medium does not exceed 1 in 4. The area of the cell sheet is at least 3 cm^2/ml of pooled fluid. At least 1 bottle of the cell cultures remains uninoculated to serve as a control.

The cultures are incubated at a temperature of 35-37 °C and observed for at least 2 weeks.

A further sample of 10 ml of the pooled fluid removed from the cell cultures on the day of inoculation with the seed lot virus is tested for the presence of extraneous agents by inoculation into human cell cultures sensitive to measles virus.

The tests are not valid if more than 20 per cent of the culture vessels have been discarded for non-specific accidental reasons by the end of the respective test periods.

If, in these tests, evidence is found of the presence of an extraneous agent, the single harvest from the whole group of cell cultures concerned is rejected.

If the presence of cercopithecid herpesvirus 1 (B virus) is demonstrated, the manufacture of oral poliomyelitis vaccine shall be discontinued and the competent authority shall be informed. Manufacturing shall not be resumed until a thorough investigation has been completed and precautions have been taken against any reappearance of the infection, and then only with the approval of the competent authority.

If these tests are not done immediately, the samples of pooled cell-culture fluid shall be kept at a temperature of − 60 °C or below, with the exception of the sample for the test for B virus, which may be held at 4 °C, provided that the test is done not more than 7 days after it has been taken.

Control cell cultures. On the day of inoculation with the virus working seed lot, 25 per cent (but not more than 2.5 litres) of the cell suspension obtained from the kidneys of each single monkey or from not more than 10 near-term monkeys is taken to prepare uninoculated control cell cultures. These control cell cultures are incubated in the same conditions as the inoculated cultures for at least 2 weeks and are examined during this period for evidence of cytopathic changes. The tests are not valid if more than 20 per cent of the control cell cultures have been discarded for non-specific, accidental reasons. At the end of the observation period, the control cell cultures are examined for degeneration caused by an infectious agent. If this examination or any of the tests required in this section shows evidence of the presence in a control culture of any extraneous agent, the poliovirus grown in the corresponding inoculated cultures from the same group shall be rejected.

Tests for haemadsorbing viruses. At the time of harvest or within 4 days of inoculation of the production cultures with the virus working seed lot, a sample of 4 per cent of the control cell cultures is taken and tested for haemadsorbing viruses. At the end of the observation period, the remaining control cell cultures are similarly tested. The tests are made as described in *2.6.16. Tests for extraneous agents in viral vaccines for human use*.

Tests for other extraneous agents. At the time of harvest, or within 7 days of the day of inoculation of the production cultures with the working seed lot, a sample of at least 20 ml of the pooled fluid from each group of control cultures is taken and tested in 2 kinds of monkey kidney cell culture, as described above.

At the end of the observation period for the original control cell cultures, similar samples of the pooled fluid are taken and the tests referred to in this section in the 2 kinds of monkey kidney cell culture and in the rabbit cell cultures are repeated, as described above under Cell cultures.

If the presence of cercopithecid herpesvirus 1 (B virus) is demonstrated, the production cell cultures shall not be used and the measures concerning vaccine production described above must be undertaken.

The fluids collected from the control cell cultures at the time of virus harvest and at the end of the observation period may be pooled before testing for extraneous agents. A sample of 2 per cent of the pooled fluid is tested in each of the cell culture systems specified.

Single harvests.

Tests for neutralised single harvests in primary monkey kidney cell cultures. A sample of at least 10 ml of each single harvest is neutralised by a type-specific poliomyelitis antiserum prepared in animals other than monkeys. In preparing antisera for this purpose, the immunising antigens used shall be prepared in non-simian cells.

Half of the neutralised suspension (corresponding to at least 5 ml of single harvest) is tested in monkey kidney cell cultures prepared from the same species, but not the same animal, as that used for vaccine production. The other half of the neutralised suspension is tested, if necessary, in monkey kidney cell cultures from another species so that the tests on the neutralised suspension are done in cell cultures from at least 1 species known to be sensitive to SV40.

The neutralised suspensions are inoculated into bottles of these cell cultures in such a way that the dilution of the suspension in the nutrient medium does not exceed 1 in 4. The area of the cell sheet is at least 3 cm^2/ml of neutralised suspension. At least 1 bottle of each type of cell culture remains uninoculated to serve as a control and is maintained by nutrient medium containing the same concentration of the specific antiserum used for neutralisation.

Animal serum may be used in the propagation of the cells, provided that it does not contain SV40 antibody, but the maintenance medium, after the inoculation of the test material, contains no added serum other than the poliovirus neutralising antiserum, except as described below.

The cultures are incubated at a temperature of 35-37 °C and observed for a total period of at least 4 weeks. During this observation period and after not less than 2 weeks' incubation, at least 1 subculture of fluid is made from each of these cultures in the same cell-culture system. The subcultures are also observed for at least 2 weeks.

Serum may be added to the original cultures at the time of subculturing, provided that the serum does not contain SV40 antibody.

Additional tests are made for extraneous agents on a further sample of the neutralised single harvests by inoculation of 10 ml into human cell cultures sensitive to measles virus.

Fluorescent-antibody techniques may be useful for detecting SV40 virus and other viruses in the cells.

The tests are not valid if more than 20 per cent of the culture vessels have been discarded for non-specific accidental reasons by the end of the respective test periods.

If any cytopathic changes occur in any of the cultures, the causes of these changes are investigated. If the cytopathic changes are shown to be due to unneutralised poliovirus, the test is repeated. If there is evidence of the presence of SV40 or other extraneous agents attributable to the single harvest, that single harvest is rejected.

MONOVALENT POOLED HARVEST

Monovalent pooled harvests are prepared by pooling a number of satisfactory single harvests of the same virus type. Monovalent pooled harvests from continuous cell lines may be purified. Each monovalent pooled harvest is filtered through a bacteria-retentive filter.

Only a monovalent pooled harvest that complies with the following requirements may be used in the preparation of the final bulk vaccine.

Identification. Each monovalent pooled harvest is identified as poliovirus of the given type, using specific antibodies.

Virus concentration. The virus concentration is determined by the method described below and serves as the basis for calculating the dilutions for preparation of the final bulk, for the quantity of virus used in the neurovirulence test and to establish and monitor production consistency.

Genetic markers. A ratio of the replication capacities of the virus in the monovalent pooled harvest is obtained over a temperature range between 36 °C and 40 °C in comparison with the seed lot or a reference preparation for the marker tests and with appropriate rct/40− and rct/40+ strains of poliovirus of the same type. The incubation temperatures used in this test are controlled to within ± 0.1 °C. The monovalent pooled harvest passes the test if, for both the virus in the harvest and the appropriate reference material, the titre determined at 36 °C is at least 5.0 log greater than that determined at 40 °C. If growth at 40 °C is so low that a valid comparison cannot be established, a temperature in the region of 39.0 °C to 39.5 °C is used, at which temperature the reduction in titre of the reference material must be in the range 3.0 to 5.0 log of its value at 36 °C; the acceptable minimum reduction is determined for each virus strain at a given temperature. If the titres obtained for 1 or more of the reference viruses are not concordant with the expected values, the test must be repeated.

Neurovirulence (*2.6.19*). Each monovalent pooled harvest complies with the test for neurovirulence of poliomyelitis vaccine (oral). If the test is carried out only by the manufacturer, the test slides are provided to the competent authority for assessment.

Primary monkey kidney cell cultures. *The following special requirements apply to monovalent pooled harvests derived from primary monkey kidney cell cultures.*

Retroviruses. The monovalent pooled harvest is examined using a reverse transcriptase assay. No indication of the presence of retroviruses is found.

Test in rabbits. A sample of the monovalent pooled harvest is tested for cercopithecid herpesvirus 1 (B virus) and other viruses by injection of not less than 100 ml into not fewer than 10 healthy rabbits each weighing 1.5-2.5 kg. Each rabbit receives not less than 10 ml and not more than 20 ml, of which 1 ml is given intradermally at multiple sites, and the remainder subcutaneously. The rabbits are observed for at least 3 weeks for death or signs of illness.

All rabbits that die after the first 24 h of the test and those showing signs of illness are examined by autopsy, and the brain and organs removed for detailed examination to establish the cause of death.

The test is not valid if more than 20 per cent of the inoculated rabbits show signs of intercurrent infection during the observation period. The monovalent pooled harvest passes the test if none of the rabbits shows evidence of infection with B virus or with other extraneous agents or lesions of any kind attributable to the bulk suspension.

If the presence of B virus is demonstrated, the measures concerning vaccine production described above under Cell cultures are taken.

Test in guinea-pigs. If the primary monkey kidney cell cultures are not derived from monkeys kept in a closed colony, the monovalent pooled harvest shall be shown to comply with the following test. Administer to not fewer than 5 guinea-pigs, each weighing 350-450 g, 0.1 ml of the monovalent pooled harvest by intracerebral injection and 0.5 ml by intraperitoneal injection. Measure the rectal temperature of each animal on each working day for 6 weeks. At the end of the observation period carry out autopsy on each animal.

In addition, administer to not fewer than 5 guinea-pigs 0.5 ml by intraperitoneal injection and observe as described above for 2-3 weeks. At the end of the observation period, carry out a passage from these animals to not fewer than 5 guinea-pigs using blood and a suspension of liver or spleen tissue. Measure the rectal temperature of the latter guinea-pigs for 2-3 weeks. Examine by autopsy all animals that, after the first day of the test, die or are killed because they show disease or show on 3 consecutive days a body temperature higher than 40.1 °C; carry out histological examination to detect infection with filoviruses; in addition, inject a suspension of liver or spleen tissue or of blood intraperitoneally into not fewer than 3 guinea-pigs. If any signs of infection with filoviruses are noted, confirmatory serological tests are carried out on the blood of the affected animals. The monovalent pooled harvest complies with the

Vaccines

test if not fewer than 80 per cent of the guinea-pigs survive to the end of the observation period and remain in good health and no animal shows signs of infection with filoviruses.

FINAL BULK VACCINE

The final bulk vaccine is prepared from one or more satisfactory monovalent pooled harvests and may contain more than one virus type. Suitable flavouring substances and stabilisers may be added.

Only a final bulk vaccine that complies with the following requirement may be used in the preparation of the final lot.

Bacterial and fungal contamination. Carry out the test for sterility (*2.6.1*), using 10 ml for each medium.

FINAL LOT

Only a final lot that complies with the following requirement for thermal stability and is satisfactory with respect to each of the requirements given below under Identification, Tests and Assay may be released for use.

Thermal stability. Maintain samples of the final lot at 37 °C for 48 h. Determine the total virus concentration as described under Assay in parallel for the heated vaccine and for unheated vaccine. The estimated difference between the total virus concentration of the unheated and heated vaccines is not greater than 0.5 $\log_{10}$ infectious virus units ($CCID_{50}$) per single human dose.

IDENTIFICATION

The vaccine is shown to contain poliovirus of each type stated on the label, using specific antibodies.

TESTS

Bacterial and fungal contamination. The vaccine complies with the test for sterility (*2.6.1*).

ASSAY

Titrate for infectious virus at least in triplicate using the method described below. Use an appropriate virus reference preparation to validate each assay. If the vaccine contains more than one poliovirus type, titrate each type separately, using appropriate type-specific antiserum (or preferably a monoclonal antibody) to neutralise each of the other types present.

For a trivalent vaccine, the estimated mean virus titres must be: not less than $1 \times 10^{6.0}$ infectious virus units ($CCID_{50}$) per single human dose for type 1; not less than $1 \times 10^{5.0}$ infectious virus units ($CCID_{50}$) for type 2; and not less than $1 \times 10^{5.5}$ infectious virus units ($CCID_{50}$) for type 3.

For monovalent or divalent vaccine, the minimum virus titres are decided by the competent authority.

Method. Inoculate groups of 8 to 12 flat-bottomed wells in a microtitre plate with 0.1 ml of each of the selected dilutions of virus followed by a suitable cell suspension of the Hep-2 (Cincinnati) line. Incubate the plates at a suitable temperature. Examine the cultures on days 7-9. The assay is not valid if the confidence interval ($P = 0.95$) of the logarithm of the virus concentration is greater than ± 0.3.

LABELLING

The label states:

– the types of poliovirus contained in the vaccine,

– the minimum amount of virus of each type contained in 1 single human dose,

– the cell substrate used for the preparation of the vaccine,

– that the vaccine is not to be injected.

01/2005:0216

RABIES VACCINE FOR HUMAN USE PREPARED IN CELL CULTURES

Vaccinum rabiei ex cellulis ad usum humanum

DEFINITION

Rabies vaccine for human use prepared in cell cultures is a freeze-dried preparation of a suitable strain of fixed rabies virus grown in cell cultures and inactivated by a validated method.

The vaccine is reconstituted immediately before use as stated on the label to give a clear liquid that may be coloured owing to the presence of a pH indicator.

PRODUCTION

The production of the vaccine is based on a virus seed-lot system and, if a cell line is used for virus propagation, a cell-bank system. The production method shall have been shown to yield consistently vaccines that comply with the requirements for immunogenicity, safety and stability. Unless otherwise justified and authorised, the virus in the final vaccine shall not have undergone more passages from the master seed lot than was used to prepare the vaccine shown in clinical studies to be satisfactory with respect to safety and efficacy; even with authorised exceptions, the number of passages beyond the level used for clinical studies shall not exceed five.

The production method is validated to demonstrate that the product, if tested, would comply with the test for abnormal toxicity for immunosera and vaccines for human use (*2.6.9*).

SUBSTRATE FOR VIRUS PROPAGATION

The virus is propagated in a human diploid cell line (*5.2.3*), in a continuous cell line approved by the competent authority or in cultures of chick-embryo cells derived from a flock free from specified pathogens (*5.2.2*).

SEED LOTS

The strain of rabies virus used shall be identified by historical records that include information on the origin of the strain and its subsequent manipulation.

Working seed lots are prepared by not more than five passages from the master seed lot.

Only a working seed lot that complies with the following tests may be used for virus propagation.

Identification. Each working seed lot is identified as rabies virus using specific antibodies.

Virus concentration. The virus concentration of each working seed lot is determined by a cell culture method using immunofluorescence, to ensure consistency of production.

Extraneous agents (*2.6.16*). The working seed lot complies with the requirements for virus seed lots. If the virus has been passaged in mouse brain, specific tests for murine viruses are carried out.

VIRUS PROPAGATION AND HARVEST

All processing of the cell bank and subsequent cell cultures are done under aseptic conditions in an area where no other cells are handled. Approved animal (but not human) serum may be used in the media, but the final medium for maintaining cell growth during virus multiplication does not contain animal serum; the media may contain human albumin complying with the monograph on *Human albumin solution (0255)*. Serum and trypsin used in the preparation of cell suspensions and media are shown to be free from infectious extraneous agents; trypsin complies with the monograph on *Trypsin (0694)*. The cell culture media may contain a pH indicator such as phenol red and approved antibiotics at the lowest effective concentration. Not less than 500 ml of the cell cultures employed for vaccine production are set aside as uninfected cell cultures (control cells). The virus suspension is harvested on one or more occasions during incubation. Multiple harvests from the same production cell culture may be pooled and considered as a single harvest.

Only a single harvest that complies with the following requirements may be used in the preparation of the inactivated viral harvest.

Identification. The single harvest contains virus that is identified as rabies virus using specific antibodies.

Virus concentration. Titrate for infective virus in cell cultures; the titre is used to monitor consistency of production.

Control cells. The control cells of the production cell culture from which the single harvest is derived comply with a test for identification and with the requirements for extraneous agents (*2.6.16*).

PURIFICATION AND INACTIVATION

The virus harvest may be concentrated and/or purified by suitable methods; the virus harvest is inactivated by a validated method at a fixed, well defined stage of the process which may be before, during or after any concentration or purification. The method shall have been shown to be capable of inactivating rabies virus without destruction of the immunogenic activity. If betapropiolactone is used, the concentration shall at no time exceed 1:3500.

Only an inactivated viral suspension that complies with the following requirements may be used in the preparation of the final bulk vaccine.

Inactivation. Carry out an amplification test for residual infectious rabies virus immediately after inactivation or using a sample frozen immediately after inactivation and stored at −70 °C. Inoculate a quantity of inactivated viral suspension equivalent to not less than 25 doses of vaccine into cell cultures of the same type as those used for production of the vaccine. Make a passage after 7 days. Maintain the cultures for a further 14 days and then examine the cell cultures for rabies virus using an immunofluorescence test. No rabies virus is detected.

Residual host-cell DNA. If a continuous cell line is used for virus propagation, the content of residual host-cell DNA, determined using a suitable method as described in *Products of recombinant DNA technology (0784)*, is not greater than 100 pg per single human dose.

FINAL BULK VACCINE

The final bulk vaccine is prepared from one or more inactivated viral suspensions. An approved stabiliser may be added to maintain the activity of the product during and after freeze-drying.

Only a final bulk vaccine that complies with the following requirements may be used in the preparation of the final lot.

Glycoprotein content. Determine the glycoprotein content by a suitable immunochemical method (*2.7.1*), for example, single-radial immunodiffusion, enzyme-linked immunosorbent assay or an antibody-binding test. The content is within the limits approved for the particular product.

Sterility (*2.6.1*). The final bulk vaccine complies with the test for sterility, carried out using 10 ml for each medium.

FINAL LOT

The final bulk vaccine is distributed aseptically into sterile containers and freeze-dried to a moisture content shown to be favourable to the stability of the vaccine. The containers are then closed so as to avoid contamination and the introduction of moisture.

Only a final lot that complies with each of the requirements given below under Identification, Tests and Assay may be released for use. Provided that the test for inactivation has been carried out with satisfactory results on the inactivated viral suspension and the test for bovine serum albumin has been carried out with satisfactory results on the final bulk vaccine, these tests may be omitted on the final lot.

IDENTIFICATION

The vaccine is shown to contain rabies virus antigen by a suitable immunochemical method (*2.7.1*) using specific antibodies, preferably monoclonal; alternatively, the assay serves also to identify the vaccine.

TESTS

Inactivation. Inoculate a quantity equivalent to not less than 25 human doses of vaccine into cell cultures of the same type as those used for production of the vaccine. Make a passage after 7 days. Maintain the cultures for a further 14 days and then examine the cell cultures for rabies virus using an immunofluorescence test. No rabies virus is detected.

Bovine serum albumin. Not more than 50 ng per single human dose, determined by a suitable immunochemical method (*2.7.1*).

Sterility (*2.6.1*). The vaccine complies with the test for sterility.

Bacterial endotoxins (*2.6.14*): less than 25 IU per single human dose.

Pyrogens (*2.6.8*). The vaccine complies with the test for pyrogens. Unless otherwise justified and authorised, inject into each rabbit a single human dose of the vaccine diluted to ten times its volume.

Water (*2.5.12*). Not more than 3.0 per cent, determined by the semi-micro determination of water.

ASSAY

The potency of rabies vaccine is determined by comparing the dose necessary to protect mice against the effects of a lethal dose of rabies virus, administered intracerebrally, with the quantity of a reference preparation of rabies vaccine necessary to provide the same protection. For this comparison a reference preparation of rabies vaccine, calibrated in International Units, and a suitable preparation of rabies virus for use as the challenge preparation are necessary.

The International Unit is the activity contained in a stated quantity of the International Standard. The equivalence in International Units of the International Standard is stated by the World Health Organisation.

The test described below uses a parallel-line model with at least three points for the vaccine to be examined and the reference preparation. Once the analyst has experience with the method for a given vaccine, it is possible to carry out a simplified test using a single dilution of the vaccine to be examined. Such a test enables the analyst to determine that the vaccine has a potency significantly higher than the required minimum but will not give full information on the validity of each individual potency determination. The use of a single dilution allows a considerable reduction in the number of animals required for the test and must be considered by each laboratory in accordance with the

Vaccines

provisions of the European Convention for the Protection of Vertebrate Animals used for Experimental and other Scientific Purposes.

Selection and distribution of the test animals. Use in the test healthy female mice about 4 weeks old, each weighing 11 g to 15 g, and from the same stock. Distribute the mice into six groups of a size suitable to meet the requirements for validity of the test and, for titration of the challenge suspension, four groups of five.

Preparation of the challenge suspension. Inoculate mice intracerebrally with the CVS strain of rabies virus and when the mice show signs of rabies, but before they die, sacrifice them, remove the brains and prepare a homogenate of the brain tissue in a suitable diluent. Separate gross particulate matter by centrifugation and use the supernatant liquid as the challenge suspension. Distribute the suspension in small volumes in ampoules, seal and store at a temperature below − 60 °C. Thaw one ampoule of the suspension and make serial dilutions in a suitable diluent. Allocate each dilution to a group of five mice and inject intracerebrally into each mouse 0.03 ml of the dilution allocated to its group. Observe the mice for 14 days. Calculate the LD_{50} of the undiluted suspension using the number in each group that, between the fifth and fourteenth days, die or develop signs of rabies.

Determination of potency of the vaccine to be examined. Prepare three fivefold serial dilutions of the vaccine to be examined and three fivefold serial dilutions of the reference preparation. Prepare the dilutions such that the most concentrated suspensions may be expected to protect more than 50 per cent of the animals to which they are administered and the least concentrated suspensions may be expected to protect less than 50 per cent of the animals to which they are administered. Allocate the six dilutions one to each of the six groups of mice and inject intraperitoneally into each mouse 0.5 ml of the dilution allocated to its group. After 7 days, prepare three identical dilutions of the vaccine to be examined and of the reference preparation and repeat the injections. Seven days after the second injection, prepare a suspension of the challenge virus such that, on the basis of the preliminary titration, 0.03 ml contains about 50 LD_{50}. Inject intracerebrally into each vaccinated mouse 0.03 ml of this suspension. Prepare three suitable serial dilutions of the challenge suspension. Allocate the challenge suspension and the three dilutions one to each of the four groups of five control mice and inject intracerebrally into each mouse 0.03 ml of the suspension or one of the dilutions allocated to its group. Observe the animals in each group for 14 days and record the number in each group that die or show signs of rabies in the period 5 days to 14 days after challenge.

The test is not valid unless: for both the vaccine to be examined and the reference preparation the 50 per cent protective dose lies between the largest and smallest doses given to the mice; the titration of the challenge suspension shows that 0.03 ml of the suspension contained not less than 10 LD_{50}; the statistical analysis shows a significant slope and no significant deviations from linearity or parallelism of the dose-response lines; the confidence limits ($P = 0.95$) are not less than 25 per cent and not more than 400 per cent of the estimated potency.

The vaccine complies with the test if the estimated potency is not less than 2.5 IU per human dose.

LABELLING

The label states the biological origin of the cells used for the preparation of the vaccine.

01/2005:0162
corrected

RUBELLA VACCINE (LIVE)

Vaccinum rubellae vivum

DEFINITION

Rubella vaccine (live) is a freeze-dried preparation of a suitable attenuated strain of rubella virus. The vaccine is reconstituted immediately before use, as stated on the label, to give a clear liquid that may be coloured owing to the presence of a pH indicator.

PRODUCTION

The production of vaccine is based on a virus seed-lot system and a cell-bank system. The production method shall have been shown to yield consistently live rubella vaccines of adequate immunogenicity and safety in man. Unless otherwise justified and authorised, the virus in the final vaccine shall have undergone no more passages from the master seed lot than were used to prepare the vaccine shown in clinical studies to be satisfactory with respect to safety and efficacy.

The production method is validated to demonstrate that the product, if tested, would comply with the test for abnormal toxicity for immunosera and vaccines for human use (*2.6.9*).

SUBSTRATE FOR VIRUS PROPAGATION

The virus is propagated in human diploid cells (*5.2.3*).

SEED LOT

The strain of rubella virus used shall be identified by historical records that include information on the origin of the strain and its subsequent manipulation. To avoid the unnecessary use of monkeys in the test for neurovirulence, virus seed lots are prepared in large quantities and stored at temperatures below − 20 °C if freeze-dried, or below − 60 °C if not freeze-dried.

Only a seed lot that complies with the following requirements may be used for virus propagation.

Identification. The master and working seed lots are identified as rubella virus by serum neutralisation in cell culture, using specific antibodies.

Virus concentration. The virus concentration of the master and working seed lots is determined to ensure consistency of production.

Extraneous agents (*2.6.16*). The working seed lot complies with the requirements for seed lots.

Neurovirulence (*2.6.18*). The working seed lot complies with the test for neurovirulence of live virus vaccines. *Macaca* and *Cercopithecus* monkeys are suitable for the test.

PROPAGATION AND HARVEST

All processing of the cell bank and subsequent cell cultures is done under aseptic conditions in an area where no other cells are handled. Suitable animal (but not human) serum may be used in the growth medium, but the final medium for maintaining cell growth during virus multiplication does not contain animal serum. Serum and trypsin used in the preparation of cell suspensions and culture media are shown to be free from extraneous agents. The cell culture medium may contain a pH indicator such as phenol red and suitable antibiotics at the lowest effective concentration. It is preferable to have a substrate free from antibiotics during production. Not less than 500 ml of the production cell cultures is set aside as uninfected cell cultures (control cells). The temperature of incubation is controlled during the growth of the virus. The virus suspension is harvested,

Vaccines

on one or more occasions, within 28 days of inoculation. Multiple harvests from the same production cell culture may be pooled and considered as a single harvest.

Only a single harvest that complies with the following requirements may be used in the preparation of the final bulk vaccine.

Identification. The single harvest contains virus that is identified as rubella virus by serum neutralisation in cell culture, using specific antibodies.

Virus concentration. The virus concentration in the single harvest is determined as prescribed under Assay to monitor consistency of production and to determine the dilution to be used for the final bulk vaccine.

Extraneous agents (*2.6.16*). The single harvest complies with the tests for extraneous agents.

Control cells. The control cells comply with a test for identification and with the tests for extraneous agents (*2.6.16*).

FINAL BULK VACCINE

Single harvests that comply with the above tests are pooled and clarified to remove cells. A suitable stabiliser may be added and the pooled harvests diluted as appropriate.

Only a final bulk vaccine that complies with the following requirement may be used in the preparation of the final lot.

Bacterial and fungal contamination. The final bulk vaccine complies with the test for sterility (*2.6.1*), carried out using 10 ml for each medium.

FINAL LOT

A minimum virus concentration for release of the product is established such as to ensure, in the light of stability data, that the minimum concentration stated on the label will be present at the end of the period of validity.

Only a final lot that complies with the requirements for minimum virus concentration for release, with the following requirement for thermal stability and with each of the requirements given below under Identification and Tests may be released for use. Provided that the test for bovine serum albumin has been carried out with satisfactory results on the final bulk vaccine, it may be omitted on the final lot.

Thermal stability. Maintain samples of the final lot of freeze-dried vaccine in the dry state at 37 °C for 7 days. Determine the virus concentration as described under Assay in parallel for the heated vaccine and for unheated vaccine stored at 5 ± 3 °C. The virus concentration of the heated vaccine is not more than 1.0 $\log_{10}$ lower than that of the unheated vaccine.

IDENTIFICATION

When the vaccine reconstituted as stated on the label is mixed with specific rubella antibodies, it is no longer able to infect susceptible cell cultures.

TESTS

Bacterial and fungal contamination. The reconstituted vaccine complies with the test for sterility (*2.6.1*).

Bovine serum albumin. Not more than 50 ng per single human dose, determined by a suitable immunochemical method (*2.7.1*).

Water (*2.5.12*). Not more than 3.0 per cent, determined by the semi-micro determination of water.

ASSAY

Titrate the vaccine for infective virus at least in triplicate, using at least 5 cell cultures for each 0.5 $\log_{10}$ dilution step or by a method of equal precision. Use an appropriate virus reference preparation to validate each assay. The estimated virus concentration is not less than that stated on the label; the minimum virus concentration stated on the label is not less than 1×10^3 $CCID_{50}$ per human dose. The assay is not valid if the confidence interval ($P = 0.95$) of the logarithm of the virus concentration is greater than ± 0.3.

Rubella vaccine (live) BRP is suitable for use as a reference preparation.

LABELLING

The label states:

- the strain of virus used for the preparation of the vaccine,
- the type and origin of the cells used for the preparation of the vaccine,
- the minimum virus concentration,
- that contact with disinfectants is to be avoided,
- the time within which the vaccine must be used after reconstitution,
- that the vaccine must not be given to a pregnant woman and that a woman must not become pregnant within 2 months after having the vaccine.

01/2005:0452

TETANUS VACCINE (ADSORBED)

Vaccinum tetani adsorbatum

DEFINITION

Tetanus vaccine (adsorbed) is a preparation of tetanus formol toxoid with a mineral adsorbent. The formol toxoid is prepared from the toxin produced by the growth of *Clostridium tetani*.

PRODUCTION

GENERAL PROVISIONS

Specific toxicity. The production method is validated to demonstrate that the product, if tested, would comply with the following test: inject subcutaneously 5 times the single human dose stated on the label into each of 5 healthy guinea-pigs, each weighing 250-350 g, that have not previously been treated with any material that will interfere with the test. If within 21 days of the injection any of the animals shows signs of or dies from tetanus, the vaccine does not comply with the test. If more than 1 animal dies from non-specific causes, repeat the test once; if more than 1 animal dies in the second test, the vaccine does not comply with the test.

BULK PURIFIED TOXOID

For the production of tetanus toxin, from which toxoid is prepared, seed cultures are managed in a defined seed-lot system in which toxinogenicity is conserved and, where necessary, restored by deliberate reselection. A highly toxinogenic strain of *Clostridium tetani* with known origin and history is grown in a suitable liquid medium. At the end of cultivation, the purity of each culture is tested and contaminated cultures are discarded. Toxin-containing culture medium is collected aseptically. The toxin content (Lf per millilitre) is checked to monitor consistency of production. Single harvests may be pooled to prepare the bulk purified toxoid. The toxin is purified to remove components likely to cause adverse reactions in humans. The purified toxin is detoxified with formaldehyde by a method that avoids destruction of the immunogenic potency of the toxoid and reversion of toxoid to toxin, particularly on exposure to heat. Alternatively, purification may be carried out after detoxification.

Only bulk purified toxoid that complies with the following requirements may be used in the preparation of the final bulk vaccine.

Sterility (*2.6.1*). Carry out the test for sterility using 10 ml for each medium.

Absence of toxin and irreversibility of toxoid. Using the same buffer solution as for the final vaccine, without adsorbent, prepare a solution of bulk purified toxoid at the same concentration as in the final vaccine. Divide the dilution into 2 equal parts. Keep one of them at 5 ± 3 °C and the other at 37 °C for 6 weeks. Test both dilutions as described below. Use 15 guinea-pigs, each weighing 250-350 g and that have not previously been treated with any material that will interfere with the test. Inject subcutaneously into each of 5 guinea-pigs 5 ml of the dilution incubated at 5 ± 3 °C. Inject subcutaneously into each of 5 other guinea-pigs 5 ml of the dilution incubated at 37 °C. Inject subcutaneously into each of 5 guinea-pigs at least 500 Lf of the non-incubated bulk purified toxoid in a volume of 1 ml. The bulk purified toxoid complies with the test if during the 21 days following the injection no animal shows signs of or dies from tetanus. If more than 1 animal dies from non-specific causes, repeat the test; if more than 1 animal dies in the second test, the toxoid does not comply with the test.

Antigenic purity. Not less than 1000 Lf per milligram of protein nitrogen.

FINAL BULK VACCINE

The final bulk vaccine is prepared by adsorption of a suitable quantity of bulk purified toxoid onto a mineral carrier such as hydrated aluminium phosphate or aluminium hydroxide; the resulting mixture is approximately isotonic with blood. Suitable antimicrobial preservatives may be added. Certain antimicrobial preservatives, particularly those of the phenolic type, adversely affect the antigenic activity and must not be used.

Only final bulk vaccine that complies with the following requirements may be used in the preparation of the final lot.

Antimicrobial preservative. Where applicable, determine the amount of antimicrobial preservative by a suitable chemical method. The amount is not less than 85 per cent and not greater than 115 per cent of the intended amount.

Sterility (*2.6.1*). Carry out the test for sterility using 10 ml for each medium.

FINAL LOT

The final bulk vaccine is distributed aseptically into sterile, tamper-proof containers. The containers are closed so as to prevent contamination.

Only a final lot that is satisfactory with respect to each of the requirements given below under Identification, Tests and Assay may be released for use. Provided the test for antimicrobial preservative and the assay have been carried out with satisfactory results on the final bulk vaccine, they may be omitted on the final lot.

Provided the free formaldehyde content has been determined on the bulk purified toxoid or on the final bulk and it has been shown that the content in the final lot will not exceed 0.2 g/l, the test for free formaldehyde may be omitted on the final lot.

IDENTIFICATION

Tetanus toxoid is identified by a suitable immunochemical method (*2.7.1*). The following method, applicable to certain vaccines, is given as an example. Dissolve in the vaccine to be examined sufficient *sodium citrate R* to give a 100 g/l solution. Maintain at 37 °C for about 16 h and centrifuge until a clear supernatant liquid is obtained. The clear supernatant liquid reacts with a suitable tetanus antitoxin, giving a precipitate.

TESTS

Aluminium (*2.5.13*): maximum 1.25 mg per single human dose, if aluminium hydroxide or hydrated aluminium phosphate is used as the adsorbent.

Free formaldehyde (*2.4.18*): maximum 0.2 g/l.

Antimicrobial preservative. Where applicable, determine the amount of antimicrobial preservative by a suitable chemical method. The content is not less than the minimum amount shown to be effective and is not greater than 115 per cent of the quantity stated on the label.

Sterility (*2.6.1*). The vaccine complies with the test for sterility.

ASSAY

Carry out one of the prescribed methods for the assay of tetanus vaccine (adsorbed) (*2.7.8*).

The lower confidence limit (P = 0.95) of the estimated potency is not less than 40 IU per single human dose.

LABELLING

The label states:

- the minimum number of International Units per single human dose,
- the name and the amount of the adsorbent,
- that the vaccine must be shaken before use,
- that the vaccine is not to be frozen.

01/2005:1375

TICK-BORNE ENCEPHALITIS VACCINE (INACTIVATED)

Vaccinum encephalitidis ixodibus advectae inactivatum

DEFINITION

Tick-borne encephalitis vaccine (inactivated) is a liquid preparation of a suitable strain of tick-borne encephalitis virus grown in cultures of chick-embryo cells or other suitable cell cultures and inactivated by a suitable, validated method.

PRODUCTION

Production of the vaccine is based on a virus seed-lot system. The production method shall have been shown to yield consistently vaccines comparable with the vaccine of proven clinical efficacy and safety in man. Unless otherwise justified and authorised, the virus in the final vaccine shall not have undergone more passages from the master seed lot than the virus in the vaccine used in clinical trials.

The production method is validated to demonstrate that the product, if tested, would comply with the test for abnormal toxicity for immunosera and vaccines for human use (*2.6.9*).

SUBSTRATE FOR VIRUS PROPAGATION

The virus is propagated in chick embryo cells prepared from eggs derived from a chicken flock free from specified pathogens (*5.2.2*) or in other suitable cell cultures (*5.2.3*).

SEED LOTS

The strain of virus used is identified by historical records that include information on the origin of the strain and its subsequent manipulation. Virus seed lots are stored at or below −60 °C.

Only a seed lot that complies with the following requirements may be used for virus propagation.

Identification. Each seed lot is identified as containing the vaccine strain of tick-borne encephalitis virus by a suitable immunochemical method (*2.7.1*), preferably using monoclonal antibodies.

Virus concentration. The virus concentration of each seed lot is determined by titration in suitable cell cultures to monitor consistency of production.

Extraneous agents (*2.6.16*). Each seed lot complies with the requirements for extraneous agents in viral vaccines for human use; the tests in cell cultures are carried out in human and simian cells only. For neutralisation of the vaccine virus, the use of monoclonal antibodies is preferable.

VIRUS PROPAGATION AND HARVEST

All processing of the cell cultures is performed under aseptic conditions in an area where no other cells are being handled. Serum and trypsin used in the preparation of cell suspensions and media used must be shown to be free from extraneous agents. The cell culture media may contain a pH indicator such as phenol red and approved antibiotics at the lowest effective concentration. At least 500 ml of the cell cultures employed for vaccine production is set aside as uninfected cell cultures (control cells).

Only a single harvest that complies with the following requirements may be used in the preparation of the inactivated harvest.

Identification. The single harvest is shown to contain tick-borne encephalitis virus by a suitable immunochemical method (*2.7.1*), preferably using monoclonal antibodies, or by virus neutralisation in cell cultures.

Bacterial and fungal contamination (*2.6.1*). The single harvest complies with the test for sterility, carried out using 10 ml for each medium.

Mycoplasmas (*2.6.7*). The single harvest complies with the test for mycoplasmas carried out using 1 ml for each medium.

Control cells. The control cells comply with the tests for extraneous agents (*2.6.16*). If the vaccine is produced using a cell-bank system, the control cells comply with a test for identification.

Virus concentration. Determine the virus concentration by titration in suitable cell cultures to monitor consistency of production.

INACTIVATION

To avoid interference, viral aggregates are removed by filtration immediately before the inactivation process. The virus suspension is inactivated by a validated method; the method shall have been shown to be consistently capable of inactivating tick-borne encephalitis virus without destroying the antigenic and immunogenic activity; as part of the validation studies, an inactivation curve is plotted representing residual live virus concentration measured on not fewer than three occasions. If formaldehyde is used for inactivation, the presence of an excess of free formaldehyde is verified at the end of the inactivation process.

Only an inactivated harvest that complies with the following requirements may be used in the preparation of the final bulk vaccine.

Residual infective virus. Inoculate a quantity of the inactivated harvest equivalent to not less than ten human doses of vaccine in the final lot into primary chicken fibroblast cell cultures, or other cells shown to be at least as sensitive to tick-borne encephalitis virus, with not less than 3 cm^2 of cell sheet per millilitre of inoculum. Incubate at 37 ± 1 °C for 14 days. No cytopathic effect is detected at the end of the incubation period. Collect the culture fluid and inoculate 0.03 ml intracerebrally into each of not fewer than ten mice about 4 weeks old. Observe the mice for 14 days. They show no evidence of tick-borne encephalitis virus infection.

PURIFICATION

Several inactivated single harvests may be pooled before concentration and purification by suitable methods, preferably by continuous-flow, sucrose density-gradient centrifugation.

Only a purified, inactivated harvest that complies with the following requirements may be used in the preparation of the final bulk vaccine.

Sterility (*2.6.1*). The purified, inactivated harvest complies with the test for sterility carried out using 10 ml for each medium.

Specific activity. Determine the antigen content of the purified, inactivated harvest by a suitable immunochemical method (*2.7.1*). Determine the total protein content by a suitable method. The specific activity, calculated as the antigen content per unit mass of protein, is within the limits approved for the specific product.

FINAL BULK VACCINE

The final bulk vaccine is prepared from one or more purified, inactivated harvests.

Only a final bulk vaccine that complies with the following requirement may be used in the preparation of the final lot.

Sterility (*2.6.1*). The final bulk vaccine complies with the test for sterility, carried out using 10 ml for each medium.

FINAL LOT

Only a final lot that is satisfactory with respect to each of the requirements given below under Identification, Tests and Assay may be released for use. Provided that the tests for free formaldehyde, bovine serum albumin (where applicable) and pyrogens and the assay have been carried out with satisfactory results on the final bulk vaccine, they may be omitted on the final lot.

IDENTIFICATION

The vaccine is shown to contain tick-borne encephalitis virus antigen by a suitable immunochemical method (*2.7.1*) using specific antibodies or by the mouse immunogenicity test described under Assay.

TESTS

Aluminium (*2.5.13*): maximum 1.25 mg per single human dose, if aluminium hydroxide or hydrated aluminium phosphate is used as the adsorbent.

Free formaldehyde (*2.4.18*): maximum of 0.1 g/l.

Bovine serum albumin. If bovine serum albumin has been used during production, the vaccine contains not more than 50 ng per single human dose, determined by a suitable immunochemical method (*2.7.1*).

Sterility (*2.6.1*). The vaccine complies with the test for sterility.

Pyrogens (*2.6.8*). The vaccine complies with the test for pyrogens. Inject into each rabbit, per kilogram of body mass, one dose of vaccine.

ASSAY

The potency is determined by comparing the dose necessary to protect a given proportion of mice against the effects of a lethal dose of tick-borne encephalitis virus, administered intraperitoneally, with the quantity of a reference preparation of tick-borne encephalitis vaccine necessary to provide the same protection. For this comparison an approved reference preparation and a suitable preparation of tick-borne encephalitis virus from an approved strain for use as the challenge preparation are necessary.

The following is cited as an example of a method that has been found suitable for a given vaccine.

Selection and distribution of test animals. Use healthy mice weighing 11 g to 17 g and derived from the same stock. Distribute the mice into not fewer than six groups of a suitable size to meet the requirements for validity of the test; for titration of the challenge suspension, use not fewer than four groups of ten mice. Use mice of the same sex or distribute males and females equally between groups.

Determination of potency of the vaccine. Prepare not fewer than three suitable dilutions of the vaccine to be examined and of the reference preparation; in order to comply with validity criteria four to five dilutions will usually be necessary. Prepare dilutions such that the most concentrated suspension is expected to protect more than 50 per cent of the animals and the least concentrated suspension less than 50 per cent. Allocate each dilution to a different group of mice and inject subcutaneously into each mouse 0.2 ml of the dilution allocated to its group. 7 days later make a second injection using the same dilution scale. 14 days after the second injection prepare a suspension of the challenge virus containing not less than 100 LD_{50} in 0.2 ml. Inject 0.2 ml of this virus suspension intraperitoneally into each vaccinated mouse. To verify the challenge dose, prepare a series of not fewer than three dilutions of the challenge virus suspension at not greater than one-hundredfold intervals. Allocate the challenge suspension and the four dilutions, one to each of the five groups of ten mice, and inject intraperitoneally into each mouse 0.2 ml of the challenge suspension or the dilution allocated to its group. Observe the animals for 21 days after the challenge and record the number of mice that die in the period between 7 days and 21 days after the challenge.

Calculations. Calculate the results by the usual statistical methods for an assay with quantal responses (for example, *5.3.*).

Validity criteria. The test is not valid unless:

- the concentration of the challenge virus is not less than 100 LD_{50},
- for both the vaccine to be examined and the reference preparation the 50 per cent protective dose (PD_{50}) lies between the largest and smallest doses given to the mice,
- the statistical analysis shows a significant slope and no significant deviation from linearity and parallelism of the dose-response lines,
- the confidence limits (P = 0.95) are not less than 33 per cent and not more than 300 per cent of the estimated potency.

Potency requirement. Include all valid tests to estimate the mean potency and the confidence limits (P = 0.95) for the mean potency; compute weighted means with the inverse of the squared standard error as weights. The vaccine complies with the test if the estimated potency is not less than that approved by the competent authority, based on data from clinical efficacy trials.

LABELLING

The label states:

- the strain of virus used in preparation,
- the type of cells used for production of the vaccine.

01/2005:1160

TYPHOID POLYSACCHARIDE VACCINE

Vaccinum febris typhoidis polysaccharidicum

DEFINITION

Typhoid polysaccharide vaccine is a preparation of purified Vi capsular polysaccharide obtained from *Salmonella typhi* Ty 2 strain or some other suitable strain that has the capacity to produce Vi polysaccharide.

Capsular Vi polysaccharide consists of partly 3-*O*-acetylated repeated units of 2-acetylamino-2-deoxy-D-galactopyranuronic acid with α-(1$\rightarrow$4) linkages.

PRODUCTION

The production of Vi polysaccharide is based on a seed-lot system. The method of production shall have been shown to yield consistently typhoid polysaccharide vaccines of adequate immunogenicity and safety in man.

The production method is validated to demonstrate that the product, if tested, would comply with the test for abnormal toxicity for immunosera and vaccines for human use (*2.6.9*).

BACTERIAL SEED LOTS

The strain of *S. typhi* used for the master seed lot shall be identified by historical records that include information on its origin and by its biochemical and serological characteristics. Cultures from the working seed lot shall have the same characteristics as the strain that was used to prepare the master seed lot.

Only a strain that has the following characteristics may be used in the preparation of the vaccine: (a) stained smears from a culture are typical of enterobacteria; (b) the culture utilises glucose without production of gas; (c) colonies on agar are oxidase-negative; (d) a suspension of the culture agglutinates specifically with a suitable Vi antiserum or colonies form haloes on an agar plate containing a suitable Vi antiserum.

Purity of bacterial strain used for the seed lot is verified by methods of suitable sensitivity. These may include inoculation into suitable media, examination of colony morphology, microscopic examination of Gram-stained smears and culture agglutination with suitable specific antisera.

CULTURE AND HARVEST

The working seed lot is cultured on a solid medium, which may contain blood-group substances, or a liquid medium; the inoculum obtained is transferred to a liquid medium which is used to inoculate the final medium. The liquid medium used and the final medium are semi-synthetic, free from substances that are precipitated by cetrimonium bromide and do not contain blood-group substances or high-molecular-mass polysaccharides, unless it has been demonstrated that they are removed by the purification process.

The bacterial purity of the culture is verified by methods of suitable sensitivity. These may include inoculation into suitable media, examination of colony morphology, microscopic examination of Gram-stained smears and culture agglutination with suitable specific antisera.

The culture is then inactivated at the beginning of the stationary phase by the addition of formaldehyde. Bacterial cells are eliminated by centrifugation; the polysaccharide is precipitated from the culture medium by addition of hexadecyltrimethylammonium bromide (cetrimonium bromide). The precipitate is harvested and may be stored at − 20 °C before purification.

PURIFIED VI POLYSACCHARIDE

The polysaccharide is purified, after dissociation of the polysaccharide/cetrimonium bromide complex, using suitable procedures to eliminate successively nucleic acids, proteins and lipopolysaccharides. The polysaccharide is precipitated as the calcium salt in the presence of ethanol and dried at 2-8 °C; the powder obtained constitutes the purified Vi polysaccharide. The loss on drying is determined by thermogravimetry (*2.2.34*) and is used to calculate the results of the chemical tests shown below with reference to the dried substance.

Only a purified Vi polysaccharide that complies with the following requirements may be used in the preparation of the final bulk.

Protein (*2.5.16*): maximum 10 mg per gram of polysaccharide, calculated with reference to the dried substance.

Nucleic acids (*2.5.17*): maximum 20 mg per gram of polysaccharide, calculated with reference to the dried substance.

***O*-Acetyl groups** (*2.5.19*): minimum 2 mmol per gram of polysaccharide, calculated with reference to the dried substance.

Molecular size. Examine by size-exclusion chromatography (*2.2.30*) using *cross-linked agarose for chromatography R*. Use a column 0.9 m long and 16 mm in internal diameter equilibrated with a solvent having an ionic strength of 0.2 mol/kg and a pH of 7.0-7.5. Apply about 5 mg of polysaccharide in a volume of 1 ml to the column and elute at about 20 ml/h. Collect fractions of about 2.5 ml. Determine the point corresponding to K_0 = 0.25 and make 2 pools consisting of fractions eluted before and after this point. Determine *O*-acetyl groups on the 2 pools (*2.5.19*). Not less than 50 per cent of the polysaccharide is found in the pool containing fractions eluted before K_0 = 0.25.

Identification. Carry out an identification test using a suitable immunochemical method (*2.7.1*).

Bacterial endotoxins. The content of bacterial endotoxins determined by a suitable method (*2.6.14*) is within the limits approved for the specific product.

FINAL BULK VACCINE

One or more batches of purified Vi polysaccharide are dissolved in a suitable solvent, which may contain an antimicrobial preservative, so that the volume corresponding to 1 dose contains 25 μg of polysaccharide and the solution is isotonic with blood (250 mosmol/kg to 350 mosmol/kg).

Only a final bulk vaccine that complies with the following tests may be used in the preparation of the final lot.

Sterility (*2.6.1*). The final bulk vaccine complies with the test for sterility, carried out using 10 ml for each medium.

Antimicrobial preservative. Where applicable, determine the amount of antimicrobial preservative by a suitable physicochemical method. The amount is not less than 85 per cent and not greater than 115 per cent of the intended amount.

FINAL LOT

The final bulk vaccine is distributed aseptically into sterile tamper-proof containers that are then closed so as to prevent contamination.

Only a final lot that is satisfactory with respect to each of the requirements prescribed below under Identification, Tests and Assay and with the requirement for bacterial endotoxins may be released for use. Provided the tests for free formaldehyde and antimicrobial preservative have been carried out on the final bulk vaccine, they may be omitted on the final lot.

Bacterial endotoxins. The content of bacterial endotoxins determined by a suitable method (*2.6.14*) is within the limit approved for the specific product.

CHARACTERS

Clear colourless liquid, free from visible particles.

IDENTIFICATION

Carry out an identification test using a suitable immunochemical method (*2.7.1*).

TESTS

pH (*2.2.3*): 6.5 to 7.5.

***O*-Acetyl groups**: 0.085 (± 25 per cent) μmol per dose (25 μg of polysaccharide).

Test solution. Place 3 ml of the vaccine in each of 3 tubes (2 reaction solutions and 1 correction solution).

Reference solutions. Dissolve 0.150 g of *acetylcholine chloride R* in 10 ml of *water R* (stock solution containing 15 g/l of acetylcholine chloride). Immediately before use, dilute 0.5 ml of the stock solution to 50 ml with *water R* (working dilution containing 150 μg/ml of acetylcholine chloride). In 10 tubes, place in duplicate (reaction and correction solutions) 0.1 ml, 0.2 ml, 0.5 ml, 1.0 ml and 1.5 ml of the working dilution.

Prepare a blank using 3 ml of *water R*.

Make up the volume in each tube to 3 ml with *water R*. Add 0.5 ml of a mixture of 1 volume of *water R* and 2 volumes of *dilute hydrochloric acid R* to each of the correction tubes and to the blank. Add 1.0 ml of *alkaline hydroxylamine solution R* to each tube. Allow the reaction to proceed for exactly 2 min and add 0.5 ml of a mixture of 1 volume of *water R* and 2 volumes of *dilute hydrochloric acid R* to each of the reaction tubes. Add 0.5 ml of a 200 g/l solution of *ferric chloride R* in *0.2 M hydrochloric acid* to each tube, stopper the tubes and shake vigorously to remove bubbles.

Measure the absorbance (*2.2.25*) of each solution at 540 nm using the blank as the compensation liquid. For each reaction solution, subtract the absorbance of the corresponding correction solution. Draw a calibration curve from the corrected absorbances for the 5 reference solutions and the corresponding content of acetylcholine chloride and read from the curve the content of acetylcholine chloride in the test solution for each volume tested. Calculate the mean of the 2 values.

1 mole of acetylcholine chloride (181.7 g) is equivalent to 1 mole of *O*-acetyl (43.05 g).

Free formaldehyde (*2.4.18*): maximum 0.2 g/l.

Vaccines

Antimicrobial preservative. Where applicable, determine the amount of antimicrobial preservative by a suitable physicochemical method. The content is not less than the minimum amount shown to be effective and not more than 115 per cent of the content stated on the label. If phenol has been used in the preparation, the content is not more than 2.5 g/l (*2.5.15*).

Sterility (*2.6.1*). The vaccine complies with the test for sterility.

ASSAY

Determine Vi polysaccharide by a suitable immunochemical method (*2.7.1*), using a reference purified polysaccharide. The estimated amount of polysaccharide per dose is 80 per cent to 120 per cent of the content stated on the label. The confidence limits ($P = 0.95$) of the estimated amount of polysaccharide are not less than 80 per cent and not more than 120 per cent.

LABELLING

The label states:

- the number of micrograms of polysaccharide per human dose (25 µg),
- the total quantity of polysaccharide in the container.

01/2005:0156

TYPHOID VACCINE

Vaccinum febris typhoidi

DEFINITION

Typhoid vaccine is a sterile suspension of inactivated *Salmonella typhi* containing not less than 5×10^8 and not more than 1×10^9 bacteria (*S. typhi*) per human dose. The human dose does not exceed 1.0 ml.

PRODUCTION

The vaccine is prepared using a seed-lot system from a suitable strain, such as Ty 2[(5)], of *S. typhi*. The final vaccine represents not more than 3 subcultures from the strain on which were made the laboratory and clinical tests that showed it to be suitable. The bacteria are inactivated by acetone, by formaldehyde, by phenol or by heating or by a combination of the last 2 methods.

The production method is validated to demonstrate that the product, if tested, would comply with the test for abnormal toxicity for immunosera and vaccines for human use (*2.6.9*) modified as follows: inject 0.5 ml of the vaccine into each mouse and 1.0 ml into each guinea pig.

IDENTIFICATION

It is identified by specific agglutination.

TESTS

Phenol (*2.5.15*). If phenol has been used in the preparation, the concentration is not more than 5 g/l.

Antigenic power. When injected into susceptible laboratory animals, it elicits anti-O, anti-H and, to a lesser extent, anti-Vi agglutinins.

Sterility (*2.6.1*). It complies with the test for sterility.

LABELLING

The label states:

- the method used to inactivate the bacteria,
- the number of bacteria per human dose.

01/2005:0157

TYPHOID VACCINE, FREEZE-DRIED

Vaccinum febris typhoidi cryodesiccatum

DEFINITION

Freeze-dried typhoid vaccine is a freeze-dried preparation of inactivated *Salmonella typhi*. The vaccine is reconstituted as stated on the label to give a uniform suspension containing not less than 5×10^8 and not more than 1×10^9 bacteria (*S. typhi*) per human dose. The human dose does not exceed 1.0 ml of the reconstituted vaccine.

PRODUCTION

The vaccine is prepared using a seed-lot system from a suitable strain, such as Ty 2[(6)], of *S. typhi*. The final vaccine represents not more than 3 subcultures from the strain on which were made the laboratory and clinical tests that showed it to be suitable. The bacteria are inactivated either by acetone or by formaldehyde or by heat. Phenol is not used in the preparation. The vaccine is distributed into sterile containers and freeze-dried to a moisture content favourable to the stability of the vaccine. The containers are then closed so as to exclude contamination.

The production method is validated to demonstrate that the product, if tested, would comply with the test for abnormal toxicity for immunosera and vaccines for human use (*2.6.9*) modified as follows: inject 0.5 ml of the vaccine into each mouse and 1.0 ml into each guinea pig.

IDENTIFICATION

The vaccine reconstituted as stated on the label is identified by specific agglutination.

TESTS

Phenol (*2.5.15*). If phenol has been used in the preparation, the concentration is not more than 5 g/l.

Antigenic power. When injected into susceptible laboratory animals, the reconstituted vaccine elicits anti-O, anti-H and, to a lesser extent, anti-Vi agglutinins.

Sterility (*2.6.1*). The reconstituted vaccine complies with the test for sterility.

LABELLING

The label states:

- the method used to inactivate the bacteria,
- the number of bacteria per human dose,
- that the vaccine should be used within 8 h of reconstitution.

(5) This strain is issued by the World Health Organisation Collaborating Centre for Reference and Research on Bacterial Vaccines, Human Serum and Vaccine Institute, Szallas Utea 5, H-1107, Budapest, Hungary.
(6) This strain is issued by the World Health Organisation Collaborating Centre for Reference and Research on Bacterial Vaccines, Human Serum and Vaccine Institute, Szallas Utea 5, H-1107, Budapest, Hungary.

01/2005:1055

TYPHOID VACCINE (LIVE, ORAL, STRAIN Ty 21a)

Vaccinum febris typhoidis vivum perorale (stirpe Ty 21a)

DEFINITION

Typhoid vaccine (live, oral, strain Ty 21a) is a freeze-dried preparation of live *Salmonella typhi* strain Ty 21a grown in a suitable medium. When presented in capsules, the vaccine complies with the monograph on *Capsules (0016)*.

PRODUCTION

CHOICE OF VACCINE STRAIN

The main characteristic of the strain is the defect of the enzyme uridine diphosphate-galactose-4-epimerase. The activities of galactopermease, galactokinase and galactose-1-phosphate uridyl-transferase are reduced by 50 per cent to 90 per cent. Whatever the growth conditions, the strain does not contain Vi antigen. The strain agglutinates to anti-O:9 antiserum only if grown in medium containing galactose. It contains the flagellar H:d antigen and does not produce hydrogen sulphide on Kligler iron agar. The strain is nonvirulent for mice. Cells of strain Ty 21a lyse if grown in the presence of 1 per cent of galactose.

BACTERIAL SEED LOTS

The vaccine is prepared using a seed-lot system. The working seed lots represent not more than one subculture from the master seed lot. The final vaccine represents not more than four subcultures from the original vaccine on which were made the laboratory and clinical tests showing the strain to be suitable.

Only a master seed lot that complies with the following requirements may be used in the preparation of working seed lots.

Galactose metabolism. In a spectrophotometric assay, no activity of the enzyme uridine diphosphate-galactose-4-epimerase is found in the cytoplasm of strain Ty 21a compared to strain Ty 2.

Biosynthesis of lipopolysaccharide. Lipopolysaccharides are extracted by the hot-phenol method and examined by size-exclusion chromatography. Strain Ty 21a grown in medium free of galactose shows only the rough (R) type of lipopolysaccharide.

Serological characteristics. Strain Ty 21a grown in a synthetic medium without galactose does not agglutinate to specific anti-O:9 antiserum. Whatever the growth conditions, strain Ty 21a does not agglutinate to Vi antiserum. Strain Ty 21a agglutinates to H:d flagellar antiserum.

Biochemical markers. Strain Ty 21a does not produce hydrogen sulphide on Kligler iron agar. This property serves to distinguish Ty 21a from other galactose-epimerase-negative *S. typhi* strains.

Cell growth. Strain Ty 21a cells lyse when grown in the presence of 1 per cent of galactose.

BACTERIAL PROPAGATION AND HARVEST

The bacteria from the working seed lot are multiplied in a preculture, subcultured once and are then grown in a suitable medium containing 0.001 per cent of galactose at 30 °C for 13 h to 15 h. The bacteria are harvested. The harvest must be free from contaminating micro-organisms.

Only a single harvest that complies with the following requirements may be used for the preparation of the freeze-dried harvest.

pH. The pH of the culture is 6.8 to 7.5.

Optical density. The optical density of the culture, measured at 546 nm, is 6.5 to 11.0. Before carrying out the measurement, dilute the culture so that a reading in the range 0.1 to 0.5 is obtained and correct the reading to take account of the dilution.

Identification. Culture bacteria on an agar medium containing 1 per cent of galactose and bromothymol blue. Light blue, concave colonies, transparent due to lysis of cells, are formed. No yellow colonies (galactose-fermenting) are found.

FREEZE-DRIED HARVEST

The harvest is mixed with a suitable stabiliser and freeze-dried by a process that ensures the survival of at least 10 per cent of the bacteria and to a water content shown to be favourable to the stability of the vaccine. No antimicrobial preservative is added to the vaccine.

Only a freeze-dried harvest that complies with the following tests may be used for the preparation of the final bulk.

Identification. Culture bacteria are examined on an agar medium containing 1 per cent of galactose and bromothymol blue. Light blue, concave colonies, transparent due to lysis of cells, are formed. No yellow colonies (galactose-fermenting) are found.

Number of live bacteria. Not fewer than 1×10^{11} live *S. typhi* strain Ty 21a per gram.

Water (*2.5.12*): 1.5 per cent to 4.0 per cent, determined by the semi-micro determination of water.

FINAL BULK VACCINE

The final bulk vaccine is prepared by aseptically mixing one or more freeze-dried harvests with a suitable sterile excipient.

Only a final bulk that complies with the following requirement may be used in the preparation of the final lot.

Number of live bacteria. Not fewer than 40×10^9 live *S. typhi* strain Ty 21a per gram.

FINAL LOT

The final bulk vaccine is distributed under aseptic conditions into capsules with a gastro-resistant shell or into suitable containers.

Only a final lot that is satisfactory with respect to each of the requirements given below under Identification, Tests and Number of live bacteria may be released for use, except that in the determination of the number of live bacteria each dosage unit must contain not fewer than 4×10^9 live bacteria.

IDENTIFICATION

Culture bacteria from the vaccine to be examined on an agar medium containing 1 per cent of galactose and bromothymol blue. Light blue, concave colonies, transparent due to lysis of cells, are formed. No yellow colonies (galactose-fermenting) are found.

TESTS

Contaminating micro-organisms (*2.6.12, 2.6.13*). Carry out the test using suitable selective media. Determine the total viable count using the plate-count method. The number of contaminating micro-organisms per dosage unit is not greater than 10^2 bacteria and 20 fungi. No pathogenic bacterium, particularly *Escherichia coli, Staphylococcus aureus, Pseudomonas aeruginosa,* and no salmonella other than strain Ty 21a are found.

Water (*2.5.12*): 1.5 per cent to 4.0 per cent, determined on the contents of the capsule or of the container by the semi-micro determination of water.

NUMBER OF LIVE BACTERIA

Carry out the test using not fewer than five dosage units. Homogenise the contents of the dosage units in a 9 g/l solution of *sodium chloride R* at 4 °C using a mixer in a cold room with sufficient glass beads to emerge from the liquid. Immediately after homogenisation prepare a suitable dilution of the suspension using cooled diluent and inoculate brain heart infusion agar; incubate at 36 ± 1 °C for 20 h to 36 h. The vaccine contains not fewer than 2×10^9 live *S. typhi* Ty 21a bacteria per dosage unit.

LABELLING

The label states:
- the minimum number of live bacteria per dosage unit,
- that the vaccine is for oral use only.

01/2005:0648

VARICELLA VACCINE (LIVE)

Vaccinum varicellae vivum

DEFINITION

Varicella vaccine (live) is a freeze-dried preparation of a suitable attenuated strain of *Herpesvirus varicellae*. The vaccine is reconstituted immediately before use, as stated on the label, to give a clear liquid that may be coloured owing to the presence of a pH indicator.

PRODUCTION

The production of vaccine is based on a virus seed-lot system and a cell-bank system. The production method shall have been shown to yield consistently live varicella vaccines of adequate immunogenicity and safety in man. The virus in the final vaccine shall not have been passaged in cell cultures beyond the 38th passage from the original isolated virus.

The production method is validated to demonstrate that the product, if tested, would comply with the test for abnormal toxicity for immunosera and vaccines for human use (*2.6.9*).

SUBSTRATE FOR VIRUS PROPAGATION

The virus is propagated in human diploid cells (*5.2.3*).

VIRUS SEED LOT

The strain of varicella virus shall be identified as being suitable by historical records which shall include information on the origin of the strain and its subsequent manipulation. The virus shall at no time have been passaged in continuous cell lines. Seed lots are prepared in the same kind of cells as those used for the production of the final vaccine. To avoid the unnecessary use of monkeys in the test for neurovirulence, virus seed lots are prepared in large quantities and stored at temperatures below − 20 °C, if freeze-dried, or below − 60 °C, if not freeze-dried.

Only a virus seed lot that complies with the following requirements may be used for virus propagation.

Identification. The master and working seed lots are identified as varicella virus by serum neutralisation in cell culture, using specific antibodies.

Virus concentration. The virus concentration of the master and working seed lots is determined as prescribed under Assay to monitor consistency of production.

Extraneous agents (*2.6.16*). The working seed lot complies with the requirements for seed lots for live virus vaccines; a sample of 50 ml is taken for the test in cell cultures.

Neurovirulence (*2.6.18*). The working seed lot complies with the test for neurovirulence of live virus vaccines.

VIRUS PROPAGATION AND HARVEST

All processing of the cell bank and subsequent cell cultures is done under aseptic conditions in an area where no other cells are handled. Approved animal (but not human) serum may be used in the media. Serum and trypsin used in the preparation of cell suspensions and media are shown to be free from extraneous agents. The cell culture medium may contain a pH indicator such as phenol red and approved antibiotics at the lowest effective concentration. It is preferable to have a substrate free from antibiotics during production. 5 per cent, but not less than 50 ml, of the cell cultures employed for vaccine production is set aside as uninfected cell cultures (control cells). The infected cells constituting a single harvest are washed, released from the support surface and pooled. The cell suspension is disrupted by sonication.

Only a virus harvest that complies with the following requirements may be used in the preparation of the final bulk vaccine.

Identification. The virus harvest contains virus that is identified as varicella virus by serum neutralisation in cell culture, using specific antibodies.

Virus concentration. The concentration of infective virus in virus harvests is determined as prescribed under Assay to monitor consistency of production and to determine the dilution to be used for the final bulk vaccine.

Extraneous agents (*2.6.16*). Use 50 ml for the test in cell cultures.

Control cells. The control cells of the production cell culture from which the single harvest is derived comply with a test for identity and with the requirements for extraneous agents (*2.6.16*).

FINAL BULK VACCINE

Virus harvests that comply with the above tests are pooled and clarified to remove cells. A suitable stabiliser may be added and the pooled harvests diluted as appropriate.

Only a final bulk vaccine that complies with the following requirements may be used in the preparation of the final lot.

Bacterial and fungal contamination. Carry out the test for sterility (*2.6.1*) using 10 ml for each medium.

FINAL LOT

The final bulk vaccine is distributed aseptically into sterile, tamper-proof containers and freeze-dried to a moisture content shown to be favourable to the stability of the vaccine. The containers are then closed so as to prevent contamination and the introduction of moisture.

Only a final lot that is satisfactory with respect to each of the requirements given below under Identification, Tests and Assay may be released for use. Provided that the test for bovine serum albumin has been carried out with satisfactory results on the final bulk vaccine, it may be omitted on the final lot.

IDENTIFICATION

When the vaccine reconstituted as stated on the label is mixed with specific *Herpesvirus varicellae* antibodies, it is no longer able to infect susceptible cell cultures.

TESTS

Bacterial and fungal contamination. The reconstituted vaccine complies with the test for sterility (*2.6.1*).

Bovine serum albumin. Not more than 0.5 µg per human dose, determined by a suitable immunochemical method (*2.7.1*).

Water (*2.5.12*). Not more than 3.0 per cent, determined by the semi-micro determination of water.

ASSAY

Titrate for infective virus, using at least 10 cell cultures for each fourfold dilution or by a technique of equal precision. Use a suitable virus reference preparation to validate each assay. The virus concentration is not less than the minimum stated on the label.

LABELLING

The label states:

- the strain of virus used for the preparation of the vaccine,
- the type and origin of the cells used for the preparation of the vaccine,
- that contact with disinfectants is to be avoided,
- the minimum virus concentration,
- that the vaccine is not to be administered to pregnant women,
- the time within which the vaccine must be used after reconstitution.

01/2005:0537

YELLOW FEVER VACCINE (LIVE)

Vaccinum febris flavae vivum

DEFINITION

Yellow fever vaccine (live) is a freeze-dried preparation of the 17D strain of yellow fever virus grown in fertilised hen eggs. The vaccine is reconstituted immediately before use, as stated on the label, to give a clear liquid.

PRODUCTION

The production of vaccine is based on a virus seed-lot system. The production method shall have been shown to yield consistently yellow fever vaccine (live) of acceptable immunogenicity and safety for man.

The production method is validated to demonstrate that the product, if tested, would comply with the test for abnormal toxicity for immunosera and vaccines for human use (*2.6.9*) modified as follows for the test in guinea-pigs: inject ten human doses into each guinea-pig and observe for 21 days.

Reference preparation. In the test for neurotropism, a suitable batch of vaccine known to have satisfactory properties in man is used as the reference preparation.

SUBSTRATE FOR VIRUS PROPAGATION

Virus for the preparation of master and working seed lots and of all vaccine batches is grown in the tissues of chick embryos from a flock free from specified pathogens (*5.2.2*).

SEED LOTS

The 17D strain shall be identified by historical records that include information on the origin of the strain and its subsequent manipulation. Virus seed lots are prepared in large quantities and stored at a temperature below −60 °C. Master and working seed lots shall not contain any human protein or added serum.

Unless otherwise justified and authorised, the virus in the final vaccine shall be between passage levels 204 and 239 from the original isolate of strain 17D. A working seed lot shall be only one passage from a master seed lot. A working seed lot shall be used without intervening passage as the inoculum for infecting the tissues used in the production of a vaccine lot, so that no vaccine virus is more than one passage from a seed lot that has passed all the safety tests.

Only a virus seed lot that complies with the following requirements may be used for virus propagation.

Identification. The master and working seed lots are identified as containing yellow fever virus by serum neutralisation in cell culture, using specific antibodies.

Extraneous agents (*2.6.16*). Each working seed lot complies with the following tests:

Bacterial and fungal sterility

Mycoplasmas

Mycobacteria

Avian viruses

Test in adult mice (intraperitoneal inoculation only)

Test in guinea-pigs

Tests in monkeys. Each master and working seed lot complies with the following tests in monkeys for viraemia (viscerotropism), immunogenicity and neurotropism.

The monkeys shall be *Macaca* sp. susceptible to yellow fever virus and shall have been shown to be non-immune to yellow fever at the time of injecting the seed virus. They shall be healthy and shall not have received previously intracerebral or intraspinal inoculation. Furthermore, they shall not have been inoculated by other routes with neurotropic viruses or with antigens related to yellow fever virus. Not fewer than ten monkeys are used for each test.

Use a test dose of 0.25 ml containing the equivalent of not less than 5000 mouse LD_{50} and not more than 50 000 mouse LD_{50}, determined by a titration for infectious virus and using the established equivalence between virus concentration and mouse LD_{50} (see under Assay). Inject the test dose into one frontal lobe of each monkey under anaesthesia and observe the monkeys for not less than 30 days.

Viraemia (Viscerotropism). Viscerotropism is indicated by the amount of virus present in serum. Take blood from each of the test monkeys on the second, fourth and sixth days after inoculation and prepare serum from each sample. Prepare 1:10, 1:100 and 1:1000 dilutions from each serum and inoculate each dilution into a group of at least six cell culture vessels used for the determination of the virus concentration. The seed lot complies with the test if none of the sera contains more than the equivalent of 500 mouse LD_{50} in 0.03 ml and at most one serum contains more than the equivalent of 100 mouse LD_{50} in 0.03 ml.

Immunogenicity. Take blood from each monkey 30 days after the injection of the test dose and prepare serum from each sample. The seed lot complies with the test if at least 90 per cent of the test monkeys are shown to be immune, as determined by examining their sera in the test for neutralisation of yellow fever virus described below.

It has been shown that a low dilution of serum (for example, 1:10) may contain non-specific inhibitors that influence this test; such serum shall be treated to remove inhibitors. Mix dilutions of at least 1:10, 1:40 and 1:160 of serum from each monkey with an equal volume of 17D vaccine virus at a dilution that will yield an optimum number of plaques with the titration method used. Incubate the serum-virus mixtures in a water-bath at 37 °C for 1 h and then cool in iced water; add 0.2 ml of each serum-virus mixture to each of four cell-culture plates and proceed as for the determination of virus concentration. Inoculate similarly ten plates with the same amount of virus plus an equal volume of a 1:10 dilution of monkey serum known to contain no neutralising antibodies to yellow fever virus. At the end of the observation period, compare the mean number of plaques in the plates

Vaccines

receiving virus plus non-immune serum with the mean number of plaques in the plates receiving virus plus dilutions of each monkey serum. Not more than 10 per cent of the test monkeys have serum that fails to reduce the number of plaques by 50 per cent at the 1:10 dilution.

Neurotropism. Neurotropism is assessed from clinical evidence of encephalitis, from incidence of clinical manifestations and by evaluation of histological lesions, in comparison with ten monkeys injected with the reference preparation. The seed lot is not acceptable if either the onset and duration of the febrile reaction or the clinical signs of encephalitis and pathological findings are such as to indicate a change in the properties of the virus.

Clinical evaluation. - The monkeys are examined daily for 30 days by personnel familiar with clinical signs of encephalitis in primates (if necessary, the monkeys are removed from their cage and examined for signs of motor weakness or spasticity). The seed lot is not acceptable if in the monkeys injected with it the incidence of severe signs of encephalitis, such as paralysis or inability to stand when stimulated, or mortality is greater than for the reference vaccine. These and other signs of encephalitis, such as paresis, inco-ordination, lethargy, tremors or spasticity are assigned numerical values for the severity of symptoms by a grading method. Each day each monkey in the test is given a score based on the scale:

Grade 1 - rough coat, not eating,

Grade 2 - high-pitched voice, inactive, slow moving,

Grade 3 - shaky, tremors, unco-ordinated, limb weakness,

Grade 4 - inability to stand, limb paralysis or death (a dead monkey receives a daily score of 4 from the day of death until day 30).

A clinical score for a particular monkey is the average of its daily scores; the clinical score for the seed lot is the mean of the individual monkey scores. The seed lot is not acceptable if the mean of the clinical severity scores for the group of monkeys inoculated with it is significantly greater ($P = 0.95$) than the mean for the group of monkeys injected with the reference preparation. In addition, special consideration is given to any animal showing unusually severe signs when deciding on the acceptability of the seed lot.

Histological evaluation. - Five levels of the brain are examined including:

Block I - the corpus striatum at the level of the optic chiasma,

Block II - the thalamus at the level of the mamillary bodies,

Block III - the mesencephalon at the level of the superior colliculi,

Block IV - the pons and cerebellum at the level of the superior olives,

Block V - the medulla oblongata and cerebellum at the level of the mid-inferior olivary nuclei.

Cervical and lumbar enlargements of the spinal cord are each divided equally into six blocks; 15 μm sections are cut from the tissue blocks embedded in paraffin wax and stained with gallocyanin. Numerical scores are given to each hemisection of the cord and to structures in each hemisection of the brain as listed below. Lesions are scored as follows:

Grade 1. Minimal: 1 to 3 small focal inflammatory infiltrates. Degeneration or loss of a few neurons.

Grade 2. Moderate: 4 or more focal inflammatory infiltrates. Degeneration or loss of neurons affecting not more than one third of cells.

Grade 3. Severe: moderate focal or diffuse inflammatory infiltration. Degeneration or loss of up to two thirds of the neurons.

Grade 4. Overwhelming: variable but often severe inflammatory reaction. Degeneration or loss of more than 90 per cent of neurons.

It has been found that inoculation of yellow fever vaccine into the monkey brain causes histological lesions in different anatomical formations of the central nervous system with varying frequency and severity (I. S. Levenbook *et al.*, *Journal of Biological Standardization*, 1987, 15, 305-313). Based on these two indicators, the anatomical structures can be divided into target, spared and discriminator areas. Target areas are those which show more severe specific lesions in a majority of monkeys irrespective of the degree of neurovirulence of the seed lot. Spared areas are those which show only minimal specific lesions and in a minority of monkeys. Discriminator areas are those where there is a significant increase in the frequency of more severe specific lesions with seed lots having a higher degree of neurovirulence. Discriminator and target areas for *Macaca cynomolgus* and *Macaca rhesus* monkeys are shown in Table 0537.-1.

Table 0537.-1

Type of monkey	Discriminator areas	Target areas
Macaca cynomolgus	globus pallidus	substantia nigra
	putamen	
	anterior/median thalamic nucleus	
	lateral thalamic nucleus	
Macaca rhesus	caudate nucleus	substantia nigra
	globus pallidus	cervical enlargement
	putamen	lumbar enlargement
	anterior/median thalamic nucleus	
	lateral thalamic nucleus	
	cervical enlargement	
	lumbar enlargement	

Scores for discriminator and target areas are used for the final evaluation of the seed lot. The individual monkey score is calculated from the sum of individual target area scores in each hemisection divided by the number of areas examined. A separate score is calculated similarly for the discriminator areas.

Mean scores for the test group are calculated in two ways: (1) by dividing the sum of the individual monkey discriminator scores by the number of monkeys and (2) by dividing the sum of the individual monkey target and discriminator scores by the number of monkeys. These two mean scores are taken into account when deciding on the acceptability of the seed lot. The seed lot is not acceptable if either of the mean lesion scores is significantly greater ($P = 0.95$) than for the reference preparation.

PROPAGATION AND HARVEST

All processing of the fertilised eggs is done under aseptic conditions in an area where no other infectious agents or cells are handled at the same time. 2 per cent but not less than twenty and not more than fifty eggs are set aside as uninfected control eggs. After inoculation and incubation at a controlled temperature, only living and typical chick embryos are harvested. The age of the embryo at the time of virus harvest is reckoned from the initial introduction of the egg into the incubator and shall be not more than 12 days. After homogenisation and clarification by centrifugation, the extract of embryonic pulp is tested as described below

Vaccines

and kept at − 70 °C or colder until further processing. Virus harvests that comply with the prescribed tests may be pooled. No human protein is added to the virus suspension at any stage during production. If stabilisers are added, they shall have been shown to have no antigenic or sensitising properties for man.

Only a single harvest that complies with the following requirements may be used in the preparation of the final bulk vaccine.

Identification. The single harvest contains virus that is identified as yellow fever virus by serum neutralisation in cell culture, using specific antibodies.

Extraneous agents (*2.6.16*). The single harvest complies with the tests for extraneous agents.

Control eggs (*2.6.16*). The control eggs comply with the tests for extraneous agents.

Virus concentration. In order to calculate the dilution for formulation of the final bulk, each single harvest is titrated as described under Assay.

FINAL BULK VACCINE

Single harvests that comply with the tests prescribed above are pooled and clarified again. A test for protein nitrogen content is carried out. A suitable stabiliser may be added and the pooled harvests diluted as appropriate.

Only a final bulk vaccine that complies with the following requirements may be used in the preparation of the final lot.

Bacterial and fungal contamination. Carry out the test for sterility (*2.6.1*), using 10 ml for each medium.

Protein nitrogen content. The protein nitrogen content, before the addition of any stabiliser, is not more than 0.25 mg per human dose.

FINAL LOT

The final bulk vaccine is distributed aseptically into sterile, tamper-proof containers and freeze-dried to a moisture content shown to be favourable to the stability of the vaccine. The containers are then closed so as to prevent contamination and the introduction of moisture.

Only a final lot that is satisfactory with respect to thermal stability and each of the requirements given below under Identification, Tests and Assay may be released for use. Provided that the test for ovalbumin has been performed with satisfactory results on the final bulk vaccine, it may be omitted on the final lot.

Thermal stability. Maintain samples of the final lot of freeze-dried vaccine in the dry state at 37 °C for 14 days. Determine the virus concentration as described under Assay in parallel for the heated vaccine and for unheated vaccine. The difference in the virus concentration between unheated and heated vaccine does not exceed 1.0 $\log_{10}$ and the virus concentration of the heated vaccine is not less than the number of plaque-forming units (PFU) equivalent to 1×10^3 mouse LD_{50} per human dose.

IDENTIFICATION

When the vaccine reconstituted as stated on the label is mixed with specific yellow fever virus antibodies, there is a significant reduction in its ability to infect susceptible cell cultures.

TESTS

Bacterial and fungal contamination. The reconstituted vaccine complies with the test for sterility (*2.6.1*).

Ovalbumin. Not more than 5 µg of ovalbumin per human dose, determined by a suitable immunochemical method (*2.7.1*).

Bacterial endotoxins (*2.6.14*): less than 5 IU per human dose.

Water (*2.5.12*). Not more than 3.0 per cent, determined by the semi-micro determination of water.

ASSAY

Titrate for infective virus in cell cultures. Use an appropriate virus reference preparation to validate each assay.

The virus concentration is not less than the equivalent in PFU of 1×10^3 mouse LD_{50} per human dose. The relationship between mouse LD_{50} and PFU is established by each laboratory and approved by the competent authority.

The method shown below, or another suitable technique, may be used to determine the mouse LD_{50}.

Suggested method for determination of the mouse LD_{50}

Mouse LD_{50}. The statistically calculated quantity of virus suspension that is expected to produce fatal specific encephalitis in 50 per cent of mice of a highly susceptible strain, 4 to 6 weeks of age, after intracerebral inoculation.

Appropriate serial dilutions of the reconstituted vaccine are made in diluent for yellow fever virus (a 7.5 g/l solution of *bovine albumin R* in *phosphate-buffered saline pH 7.4 R*, or any other diluent that has been shown to be equivalent for maintaining the infectivity of the virus).

Mice of a highly susceptible strain, 4 to 6 weeks of age, are injected intracerebrally under anaesthesia with 0.03 ml of the vaccine dilution. Groups of not fewer than six mice are used for each dilution; the series of dilutions is chosen so as to cover the range 0 to 100 per cent mortality of the mice. Injection of the mice is performed immediately after the dilutions have been made. The mice are observed for 21 days and all deaths are recorded. Only survivors and deaths caused by typical yellow fever infections are counted in the computations. Mice paralysed on the twenty-first day of observation are counted as survivors.

LABELLING

The label states:

- the strain of virus used in preparation,
- that the vaccine has been prepared in chick embryos,
- the minimum virus concentration,
- that contact with disinfectants is to be avoided,
- the period of time within which the vaccine is to be used after reconstitution.

VACCINES FOR VETERINARY USE

01/2005:0441

ANTHRAX SPORE VACCINE (LIVE) FOR VETERINARY USE

Vaccinum anthracis vivum ad usum veterinarium

DEFINITION

Anthrax spore live vaccine for veterinary use consists of a suspension of live spores of an attenuated, non-capsulated strain of *Bacillus anthracis*.

PRODUCTION

The strain used is either: not lethal to the guinea-pig or the mouse; or lethal to the guinea-pig but not to the rabbit; or lethal to some rabbits. *B. anthracis* is grown in an appropriate medium. At the end of growth the spores are suspended in a stabilising solution and counted. The vaccine may contain an adjuvant.

IDENTIFICATION

B. anthracis present in the vaccine is identified by means of morphological and serological tests, culture and biochemical tests.

TESTS

Safety. Carry out the test on one of the species of animals for which the vaccine is intended. If the vaccine is intended for several species, including the goat, carry out the test on goats. Administer subcutaneously or intradermally to each of 2 animals, of the minimum age recommended for vaccination and having no antibodies against *B. anthracis*, twice the dose stated on the label for the species used and observe the animals for 14 days. No abnormal systemic reaction is produced but a local reaction may occur at the site of injection. The severity of the local reaction may vary according to the strain of the spores and the adjuvants used in the preparation, but necrosis does not occur.

Spore count. The number of live spores determined by plate count is not less than 80 per cent of that stated on the label.

Bacterial and fungal contamination. Carry out the test by microscopic examination and by inoculation of suitable media. The vaccine does not contain contaminating bacteria or fungi.

POTENCY

For a strain of *B. anthracis* which is not lethal to the guinea-pig or the mouse, the test may be carried out in guinea-pigs. For a strain which is lethal to the guinea-pig but not to the rabbit, the test may be carried out in rabbits. For a strain which is lethal to some rabbits, carry out the test in sheep.

If the test is carried out in guinea-pigs or in rabbits, use 10 healthy animals (group a). Inject subcutaneously or intradermally into each animal 1/10 of the smallest dose of the vaccine stated on the label for sheep. Observe the animals for 21 days. If more than 2 animals die from non-specific causes, repeat the test. Use as controls 3 animals of the same species and of the same origin.

If the test is carried out in sheep, use 5 healthy animals (group b). Inject subcutaneously or intradermally into each animal 1/10 of the smallest dose of the vaccine stated on the label for sheep. Observe the animals for 21 days. Use as controls 3 sheep of the same origin. Inject subcutaneously into each vaccinated animal of group (a) or group (b) at least 100 MLD and into each control animal 10 MLD of a strain of *B. anthracis* pathogenic for the species of animal used in the test. Observe all the animals for 10 days. All the vaccinated animals survive and all the controls die from anthrax during the observation period. If a vaccinated animal dies after the challenge, repeat the test. If in the second test a vaccinated animal dies, the vaccine fails the test.

LABELLING

The label states:

– the strain used for preparation of the vaccine,
– the number of viable spores per millilitre.

01/2005:0744

AUJESZKY'S DISEASE VACCINE (INACTIVATED) FOR PIGS

Vaccinum morbi Aujeszkyi ad suem inactivatum

DEFINITION

Aujeszky's disease vaccine (inactivated) for pigs consists of a suspension of an appropriate strain of Aujeszky's disease virus inactivated without affecting its immunogenic properties or a suspension of an inactivated fraction of the virus having adequate immunogenic properties.

PRODUCTION

The virus strain is grown in suitable cell cultures (*5.2.4*). The viral suspension is harvested and inactivated; it may be treated to fragment the virus and the viral fragments may be purified and concentrated.

The test for inactivation is carried out using two passages in the same type of cell culture as that used in the production of the vaccine or cells shown to be at least as sensitive. The quantity of inactivated virus used in the test is equivalent to not less than twenty-five doses of the vaccine. No live virus is detected.

Suitable adjuvants and antimicrobial preservatives may be added. The vaccine may be freeze-dried.

CHOICE OF VACCINE COMPOSITION

The vaccine is shown to be satisfactory with respect to safety and immunogenicity. The following tests may be used during demonstration of safety (*5.2.6*) and efficacy (*5.2.7*).

Safety

A. A test is carried out in each category of animals for which the vaccine is intended (sows, fattening pigs). The animals used do not have antibodies against Aujeszky's disease virus or against a fraction of the virus. Two doses of vaccine are injected by a recommended route into each of not fewer than ten animals. After 14 days, one dose of vaccine is injected into each of the animals. The animals are observed for a further 14 days. No abnormal local or systemic reaction is produced during the 28 days of the test. If the vaccine is intended for use in pregnant sows, for the test in this category of animal the observation period is prolonged up to farrowing and any effects on gestation or the offspring are noted.

B. The animals used in the test for immunogenicity are also used to evaluate safety. The rectal temperature of each vaccinated animal is measured at the time of vaccination and 6 h, 24 h and 48 h later. No animal shows a temperature rise greater than 1.5 °C and the number of animals showing a temperature greater than 41 °C does not exceed 10 per cent of the group. No other systemic reactions (for example, anorexia) are noted. At slaughter,

Vaccines

the injection site is examined for local reactions. No abnormal local reactions attributable to the vaccine are produced.

C. The animals used for field trials are also used to evaluate safety. A test is carried out in each category of animals for which the vaccine is intended (sows, fattening pigs). Not fewer than three groups each of not fewer than twenty animals are used with corresponding groups of not fewer than ten controls. The rectal temperature of each vaccinated animal is measured at the time of vaccination and 6 h, 24 h and 48 h later. No animal shows a temperature rise greater than 1.5 °C and the number of animals showing a temperature greater than 41 °C does not exceed 25 per cent of the group. At slaughter, the injection site is examined for local reactions. No abnormal local reactions attributable to the vaccine are produced.

Immunogenicity. Not fewer than ten fattening pigs of the age recommended for vaccination and which do not have antibodies against Aujeszky's disease virus or against a fraction of the virus are used. The body mass of none of the pigs differs from the average body mass of the group by more than 20 per cent. Each pig is vaccinated according to the recommended schedule and by a recommended route. Five similar pigs are used as controls. At the end of the fattening period (80 kg to 90 kg), each pig is weighed and then challenged by the intranasal route with a suitable quantity of a virulent strain of Aujeszky's disease virus (challenge with at least 10^6 $CCID_{50}$ of a virulent strain having undergone not more than three passages and administered in not less than 4 ml of diluent has been found to be satisfactory). The titre of challenge virus is determined in swabs taken from the nasal cavity of each animal daily from the day before challenge until virus is no longer detected. Each animal is weighed 7 days after challenge or at the time of death if this occurs earlier and the average daily gain is calculated as a percentage. For each group (vaccinated and controls), the average of the average daily gains is calculated. The vaccine complies with the test if:

- all the vaccinated pigs survive and the difference between the averages of the daily gains for the two groups is not less than 1.5,
- the geometrical mean titres and the duration of excretion of the challenge virus are significantly lower in vaccinates than in controls.

The test is not valid unless all the control pigs display signs of Aujeszky's disease and the average of their daily gains is less than − 0.5.

If the vaccine is intended for use in sows for the passive protection of piglets, the suitability of the strain for this purpose may be demonstrated by the following method. Eight sows which do not have antibodies against Aujeszky's disease virus or against a fraction of the virus are vaccinated according to the recommended schedule and by a recommended route; four sows are kept as controls. The piglets from the sows are challenged with a suitable quantity of a virulent strain of Aujeszky's disease virus at 6 to 10 days of age. The piglets are observed for 21 days. The vaccine is satisfactory if not less than 80 per cent protection against mortality is found in the piglets from the vaccinated sows compared to those from the control sows. The test is not valid if the average number of piglets per litter for each group is less than six.

BATCH TESTING

The test described under Potency is not necessarily carried out for routine testing of batches of vaccine. It is carried out for a given vaccine, on one or more occasions, as decided by or with the agreement of the competent authority; where the test is not carried out a suitable, validated, alternative test is carried out, the criteria for acceptance being set with reference to a batch of vaccine that has given satisfactory results in the test described under Potency.

IDENTIFICATION

In animals having no antibodies against Aujeszky's disease virus or against a fraction of the virus, the vaccine stimulates the production of specific antibodies against Aujeszky's disease virus or the fraction of the virus used in the production of the vaccine.

TESTS

Safety. Inject two doses of the vaccine by a recommended route into each of not fewer than two pigs of the minimum age recommended for vaccination and having no antibodies against Aujeszky's disease virus or against a fraction of the virus. Observe the animals for 14 days and then inject one dose of the vaccine into each piglet. Observe the animals for a further 14 days. No abnormal local or systemic reaction occurs during the 28 days of the test.

Inactivation. Wherever possible, carry out a suitable test for residual infectious Aujeszky's disease virus using two passages in the same type of cell culture as used in the production of the vaccine or cells shown to be at least as sensitive. Otherwise, inject one dose of the vaccine subcutaneously into each of five healthy non-immunised rabbits. Observe the animals for 14 days after the injection. No abnormal reaction (in particular a local rash) occurs. If the vaccine strain is not pathogenic for the rabbit, carry out the test in two sheep.

Extraneous viruses. On the pigs used for the safety test carry out tests for antibodies. The vaccine does not stimulate the formation of antibodies, other than those against Aujeszky's disease virus, against viruses pathogenic for pigs or against viruses that could interfere with the diagnosis of infectious diseases of pigs (including the viruses of the pestivirus group).

Sterility. The vaccine complies with the test for sterility prescribed in the monograph on *Vaccines for veterinary use (0062)*.

POTENCY

Use not fewer than five pigs each weighing 15 kg to 35 kg and which do not have antibodies against Aujeszky's disease virus or against a fraction of the virus. The body mass of none of the pigs differs from the average body mass of the group by more than 25 per cent. Administer to each pig by a recommended route one dose of the vaccine. Use five similar pigs as controls. Three weeks later weigh each pig and then challenge by the intranasal route with a suitable quantity of a virulent strain of Aujeszky's disease virus. Weigh each animal 7 days after challenge or at the time of death if this occurs earlier and calculate the average daily gain as a percentage. For each group (vaccinated and controls), calculate the average of the average daily gains. The vaccine passes the test if the vaccinated pigs survive and the difference between the averages of the daily gains for the two groups is not less than 1.1. The test is not valid unless all the control pigs display signs of Aujeszky's disease and the average of their daily gains is less than − 0.5.

LABELLING

The label states:

- whether the vaccine strain is pathogenic for the rabbit,
- whether the vaccine is a whole-virus vaccine or a subunit vaccine.

01/2005:0745

AUJESZKY'S DISEASE VACCINE (LIVE) FOR PIGS FOR PARENTERAL ADMINISTRATION, FREEZE-DRIED

Vaccinum morbi Aujeszkyi ad suem vivum cryodesiccatum ad usum parenterale

DEFINITION

Freeze-dried Aujeszky's disease vaccine (live) for pigs for parenteral administration is a preparation of an attenuated strain of Aujeszky's disease virus. It may be administered after mixing with an adjuvant.

PRODUCTION

The virus strain is grown in suitable cell cultures (*5.2.4*) or in fertilised hen eggs from flocks free from specified pathogens (*5.2.2*). The viral suspension is harvested, mixed with a suitable stabilising liquid and freeze-dried.

CHOICE OF VACCINE STRAIN

Only a virus strain shown to be satisfactory with respect to the following characteristics may be used in the preparation of the vaccine: safety; transmissibility, including transmission across the placenta and by semen; irreversibility of attenuation; immunogenicity. The strain may have a genetic marker. The following tests may be used during demonstration of safety (*5.2.6*) and efficacy (*5.2.7*).

Safety.

A. 10 piglets, 3 to 4 weeks old and which do not have antibodies against Aujeszky's disease virus or against a fraction of the virus, each receive by a recommended route a quantity of virus corresponding to 10 doses of vaccine. 10 piglets of the same origin and age and which do not have antibodies against Aujeszky's disease virus or against a fraction of the virus are kept as controls. The animals are observed for 21 days. The piglets remain in good health. The weight curve of the vaccinated piglets does not differ significantly from that of the controls.

B. The animals used in the test for immunogenicity are also used to evaluate safety. The rectal temperature of each vaccinated animal is measured at the time of vaccination and 6 h, 24 h and 48 h later. No animal shows a temperature rise greater than 1.5 °C and the number of animals showing a temperature greater than 41 °C does not exceed 10 per cent of the group. No other systemic reactions (for example, anorexia) are noted. At slaughter, the injection site is examined for local reactions. No abnormal local reactions attributable to the vaccine are produced.

C. The animals used for field trials are also used to evaluate safety. A test is carried out in each category of animals for which the vaccine is intended (sows, fattening pigs). Not fewer than 3 groups each of not fewer than 20 animals are used with corresponding groups of not fewer than 10 controls. The rectal temperature of each animal is measured at the time of vaccination and 6 h, 24 h and 48 h later. No animal shows a temperature rise greater than 1.5 °C and the number of animals showing a temperature greater than 41 °C does not exceed 25 per cent of the group. At slaughter, the injection site is examined for local reactions. No abnormal local reactions attributable to the vaccine are produced.

D. 10 piglets, 3 to 5 days old and which do not have antibodies against Aujeszky's disease virus or against a fraction of the virus, each receive by the intranasal route a quantity of virus corresponding to 10 doses of vaccine. The animals are observed for 21 days. None of the piglets dies or shows signs of neurological disorder attributable to the vaccine virus.

E. This test is not necessary for gE-negative strains. 5 piglets, 3 to 5 days old, each receive $10^{4.5}$ $CCID_{50}$ of vaccine virus intracerebrally. None of the piglets dies or shows signs of neurological disorder.

F. 10 piglets, 3 to 4 weeks old and which do not have antibodies against Aujeszky's disease virus or against a fraction of the virus, each receive a daily injection of 2 mg of prednisolone per kilogram of body mass for 5 consecutive days. On the third day each piglet receives a quantity of virus corresponding to 1 dose of vaccine by a recommended route. Antimicrobial agents may be administered to prevent aspecific signs. Observe the animals for 21 days following administration of the virus. The piglets remain in good health.

G. 15 pregnant sows which do not have antibodies against Aujeszky's disease virus or against a fraction of the virus are used. Each of 5 sows receive by a recommended route a quantity of virus corresponding to 10 doses of vaccine during the fourth or fifth week of gestation. 5 other sows each receive the same dose of virus by the same route during the tenth or eleventh week of gestation. The other 5 pregnant sows are kept as controls. The number of piglets born to the vaccinated sows, any abnormalities in the piglets and the duration of gestation do not differ significantly from those of the controls. For the piglets from vaccinated sows: carry out tests for serum antibodies against Aujeszky's disease virus; carry out tests for Aujeszky's disease virus antigen in the liver and lungs of those piglets showing abnormalities and in a quarter of the remaining healthy piglets. No Aujeszky's disease virus antigen is found in piglets born to the vaccinated sows and no antibodies against Aujeszky's disease virus are found in the serum taken before ingestion of colostrum.

Virus excretion. 18 pigs, 3 to 4 weeks old and which do not have antibodies against Aujeszky's disease virus or against a fraction of the virus are used. 14 of the pigs each receive 1 dose of vaccine by the recommended route and at the recommended site and the remaining 4 pigs are kept as contact controls. Suitably sensitive tests for the virus are carried out individually on the nasal and oral secretions as follows: nasal and oral swabs are collected daily from the day before vaccination until 10 days after vaccination. The vaccine is acceptable if the virus is not isolated from the secretions collected.

Transmissibility. The test is carried out on 4 separate occasions. Each time 4 piglets, 3 to 4 weeks old and which do not have antibodies against Aujeszky's disease virus or against a fraction of the virus, each receive by a recommended route a quantity of virus corresponding to 1 dose of vaccine. 1 day after the administration, 2 other piglets of the same age which do not have antibodies against Aujeszky's disease virus or against a fraction of the virus are kept close together with them. After 5 weeks all the animals are tested for the presence of antibodies against Aujeszky's disease virus. Antibodies against Aujeszky's disease virus are not detected in any group of contact controls. All the treated piglets show an antibody response.

Reversion to virulence. 2 piglets, 3 to 5 days old and which do not have antibodies against Aujeszky's disease virus or against a fraction of the virus, each receive by the intranasal route a quantity of virus corresponding to 1 dose of vaccine. 3 to 5 days later brain, lung, tonsils and local lymph glands are taken from each piglet and the samples are pooled. 1 ml of the pooled organ suspension is administered intranasally into each of 2 other piglets of the same age and susceptibility. This operation is then repeated not fewer than 4 times, the last time in not fewer than 5 piglets. The presence of the virus is verified at each passage by direct or indirect means. If the virus has disappeared, a second series of passages is carried out. The piglets do not die or show neurological disorders from causes attributable to the vaccine virus. There is no indication of an increase of virulence as compared with the non-passaged virus.

Immunogenicity. Not fewer than 10 fattening pigs of the age recommended for vaccination and which do not have antibodies against Aujeszky's disease virus or against a fraction of the virus are used. The body mass of none of the pigs differs from the average body mass of the group by more than 20 per cent. Each pig is vaccinated according to the recommended schedule and by a recommended route. 5 similar pigs are used as controls. At the end of the fattening period (80 kg to 90 kg), each pig is weighed and then challenged by the intranasal route with a suitable quantity of a virulent strain of Aujeszky's disease virus (challenge with at least 10^6 $CCID_{50}$ of a virulent strain having undergone not more than 3 passages and administered in not less than 4 ml of diluent has been found to be satisfactory). The titre of virus is determined in swabs taken from the nasal cavity of each pig daily from the day before challenge until virus is no longer detected. Each pig is weighed 7 days after challenge or at the time of death if this occurs earlier and the average daily gain is calculated as a percentage. For each group (vaccinated and controls), the average of the average daily gains is calculated. The vaccine complies with the test if:

- all the vaccinated pigs survive and the difference between the averages of the average daily gains for the 2 groups is not less than 1.5,
- the geometrical mean titres and the duration of excretion of the challenge virus are significantly lower in vaccinates than in controls.

The test is not valid unless all the control pigs display signs of Aujeszky's disease and the average of their average daily gains is less than − 0.5.

If the vaccine is intended for use in sows for the passive protection of piglets, the suitability of the strain for this purpose may be demonstrated by the following method. 8 sows which do not have antibodies against Aujeszky's disease virus or against a fraction of the virus are vaccinated according to the recommended schedule and by the recommended route; 4 sows are kept as controls. The piglets from the sows are challenged with a suitable quantity of a virulent strain of Aujeszky's disease virus at 6 to 10 days of age. The piglets are observed for 21 days. The vaccine is satisfactory if not less than 80 per cent protection against mortality is found in the piglets from the vaccinated sows compared to those from the control sows. The test is not valid if the average number of piglets per litter for each group is less than 6.

BATCH TESTING

The test described under Potency is not necessarily carried out for routine testing of batches of vaccine. It is carried out for a given vaccine, on one or more occasions, as decided by or with the agreement of the competent authority; where the test is not carried out a suitable, validated alternative test is carried out, the criteria for acceptance being set with reference to a batch of vaccine that has given satisfactory results in the test described under Potency.

IDENTIFICATION

In animals having no antibodies against Aujeszky's disease virus or against a fraction of the virus, the vaccine stimulates the production of specific neutralising antibodies.

TESTS

Safety. Administer 10 doses of the vaccine in a suitable volume by a recommended route to each of not fewer than 2 pigs of the minimum age recommended for vaccination and which do not have antibodies against Aujeszky's disease virus or against a fraction of the virus. Observe the animals for 14 days. No abnormal local or systemic reaction occurs.

Extraneous viruses. Neutralise the vaccine using a monospecific antiserum or monoclonal antibodies and inoculate into cell cultures known to be sensitive to viruses pathogenic for pigs and to pestiviruses. Maintain these cultures for 14 days and make at least 1 passage during this period. No cytopathic effect develops; the cells show no evidence of the presence of haemadsorbing agents. Carry out a specific test for pestiviruses.

Sterility. The vaccine complies with the test for sterility prescribed in the monograph on *Vaccines for veterinary use (0062)*.

Mycoplasmas (*2.6.7*). The vaccine complies with the test for mycoplasmas.

Virus titre. Titrate the reconstituted vaccine on the same substrate as used for production (cell cultures or inoculation into the allantoic cavity of fertilised hen eggs). 1 dose of the vaccine contains not less than the quantity of virus equivalent to the minimum virus titre stated on the label.

POTENCY

Use not fewer than 5 pigs weighing 15 kg to 35 kg and which do not have antibodies against Aujeszky's disease virus or against a fraction of the virus. The body mass of none of the pigs differs from the average body mass of the group by more than 25 per cent. Administer to each pig by a recommended route 1 dose of the vaccine. Use 5 similar pigs as controls. 3 weeks later weigh each pig and then challenge by the intranasal route with a suitable quantity of a virulent strain of Aujeszky's disease virus. Weigh each animal 7 days after challenge or at the time of death if this occurs earlier and calculate the average daily gain as a percentage. For each group (vaccinated and controls), calculate the average of the average daily gains. The vaccine complies with the test if all the vaccinated pigs survive and the difference between the averages of the average daily gains for the 2 groups is not less than 1.6. The test is not valid unless all the control pigs display signs of Aujeszky's disease and the average of their average daily gains is less than − 0.5.

LABELLING

The label states:

- the substrate used for production of the vaccine (cell cultures or eggs),
- the minimum virus titre.

01/2005:0959

AVIAN INFECTIOUS BRONCHITIS VACCINE (INACTIVATED)

Vaccinum bronchitidis infectivae aviariae inactivatum

DEFINITION

Avian infectious bronchitis vaccine (inactivated) consists of an emulsion or a suspension of one or more serotypes of avian infectious bronchitis virus which have been inactivated in such a manner that the immunogenic activity is retained. This monograph describes vaccines intended to protect

Vaccines

against drop of egg production or quality; for vaccines also intended to protect against respiratory symptoms, a demonstration of efficacy additional to that described under Potency is required.

PRODUCTION

The virus is propagated in fertilised hen eggs from healthy flocks (*5.2.2*) or in suitable cell cultures (*5.2.4*).

An amplification test for residual live avian infectious bronchitis virus is carried out on each batch of antigen immediately after inactivation and on the final bulk vaccine or, if the vaccine contains an adjuvant, on the bulk antigen or the mixture of bulk antigens immediately before the addition of adjuvant; the test is carried out in fertilised hen eggs from flocks free from specified pathogens (*5.2.2*) or in suitable cell cultures (*5.2.4*) and the quantity of inactivated virus used is equivalent to not less than 10 doses of vaccine. No live virus is detected.

The vaccine may contain one or more suitable adjuvants.

CHOICE OF VACCINE COMPOSITION

The vaccine is shown to be satisfactory with respect to safety and immunogenicity for each category of chickens for which it is intended. The following test may be used during demonstration of efficacy (*5.2.7*).

Immunogenicity. The test described under Potency is suitable to demonstrate immunogenicity.

BATCH POTENCY TEST

The test described under Potency is not carried out for routine testing of batches of vaccine. It is carried out, for a given vaccine, on one or more occasions, as decided by or with the agreement of the competent authority; where the test is not carried out, a suitable validated test is carried out, the criteria for acceptance being set with reference to a batch of vaccine that has given satisfactory results in the test described under Potency. The following test may be used after a satisfactory correlation with the test described under Potency has been established by a statistical evaluation.

Administer 1 dose of vaccine intramuscularly to each of ten chickens, between 2 weeks of age and the minimum age stated for vaccination and from a flock free from specified pathogens and keep five hatch mates as unvaccinated controls. Collect serum samples from each chicken just before administration of the vaccine and after the period defined when testing the reference vaccine; determine the antibody titre of each serum, for each serotype in the vaccine, by a suitable serological method, for example, serum neutralisation. The antibody levels are not significantly less than those obtained with a batch that has given satisfactory results in the test described under Potency (reference vaccine). The test is not valid unless the sera collected from the unvaccinated controls and from the chickens just before the administration of the vaccine are free from detectable specific antibody.

IDENTIFICATION

In susceptible animals, the vaccine stimulates the production of specific antibodies against each of the virus serotypes in the vaccine, detectable by virus neutralisation.

TESTS

Safety. Inject a double dose of vaccine by a recommended route into each of ten 14- to 28-day-old chickens from a flock free from specified pathogens (*5.2.2*). Observe the chickens for 21 days. No abnormal local or systemic reaction occurs.

Inactivation.

A. For vaccine prepared with embryo-adapted strains of virus, inject two-fifths of a dose into the allantoic cavity of ten 9- to 11-day-old fertilised hen eggs from a flock free from specified pathogens (SPF hen eggs) (*5.2.2*) and incubate. Observe for 5 to 6 days and pool separately the allantoic liquid from eggs containing live embryos and that from eggs containing dead embryos, excluding those that die within the first 24 h after injection. Examine for abnormalities all embryos which die after 24 h of injection or which survive 5 to 6 days. No death or abnormality attributable to the vaccine virus occurs.

   Inject into the allantoic cavity of each of ten 9- to 11-day-old fertilised SPF hen eggs 0.2 ml of the pooled allantoic liquid from the live embryos and into each of ten similar eggs 0.2 ml of the pooled liquid from the dead embryos and incubate for 5 to 6 days. Examine for abnormalities all embryos which die after 24 h of injection or which survive 5 to 6 days. No death or abnormality attributable to the vaccine virus occurs.

   If more than 20 per cent of the embryos die at either stage repeat the test from that stage. The vaccine complies with the test if there is no death or abnormality attributable to the vaccine virus.

B. For vaccine prepared with cell-culture-adapted strains of virus, inoculate ten doses of the vaccine into suitable cell cultures. If the vaccine contains an oil adjuvant, eliminate it by suitable means. Incubate at 38 ± 1 °C for 7 days. Make a passage on another set of cell cultures and incubate at 38 ± 1 °C for 7 days. None of the cultures shows signs of infection.

Extraneous agents. Use the chickens from the test for safety. 21 days after injection of the double dose of vaccine, inject one dose by the same route into each chicken. Collect serum samples from each chicken 2 weeks later and carry out tests for antibodies to the following agents by the methods prescribed for *chicken flocks free from specified pathogens for the production and quality control of vaccines* (*5.2.2*): avian encephalomyelitis virus, avian leucosis viruses, haemagglutinating avian adenovirus, infectious bursal disease virus, infectious laryngotracheitis virus, influenza A virus, Marek's disease virus, Newcastle disease virus. The vaccine does not stimulate the formation of antibodies against these agents.

Sterility. The vaccine complies with the test for sterility prescribed in the monograph on *Vaccines for veterinary use (0062)*.

POTENCY

Carry out a potency test for each serotype in the vaccine. Use four groups of not fewer than thirty chickens from a flock free from specified pathogens (*5.2.2.*), treated as follows:

Group A: unvaccinated controls.

Group B: vaccinated with inactivated avian infectious bronchitis vaccine.

Group C: vaccinated with live avian infectious bronchitis vaccine and inactivated avian infectious bronchitis vaccine according to the recommended schedule.

Group D: vaccinated with live avian infectious bronchitis vaccine.

Monitor egg production and quality in all birds from point of lay until at least 4 weeks after challenge. At the peak of lay, challenge all groups with a quantity of virulent avian infectious bronchitis virus sufficient to cause a drop in egg production or quality over three consecutive weeks during the 4 weeks following challenge. The vaccine complies with the test if egg production or quality is significantly better in group C than in group D and significantly better in group B than in group A. The test is not valid unless there is a drop in egg production in group A compared to the normal level noted before challenge of at least 35 per cent where challenge has been made with a Massachusetts-type strain; where it is necessary to carry out a challenge with a strain of another serotype for which there is documented evidence that the strain will not cause a 35 per cent drop in egg production, the challenge must produce a drop in egg production commensurate with the documented evidence and in any case not less than 15 per cent.

LABELLING

The label states:

- the category and age of the chickens for which the vaccine is intended,
- the strains and serotypes of virus used in the production of the vaccine and the serotypes against which the vaccine is intended to protect,
- whether the strain in the vaccine is embryo-adapted or cell-culture-adapted.

01/2005:0442

AVIAN INFECTIOUS BRONCHITIS VACCINE (LIVE)

Vaccinum bronchitidis infectivae aviariae vivum

1. DEFINITION

Avian infectious bronchitis vaccine (live) is a preparation of one or more suitable strains of different types of avian infectious bronchitis virus. This monograph applies to vaccines intended for administration to chickens for active immunisation against respiratory disease caused by avian infectious bronchitis virus.

2. PRODUCTION

2-1. *PREPARATION OF THE VACCINE*

The vaccine virus is grown in embryonated hens' eggs or in cell cultures.

2-2. *SUBSTRATE FOR VIRUS PROPAGATION*

2-2-1. **Embryonated hens' eggs**. If the vaccine virus is grown in embryonated hens' eggs, they are obtained from flocks free from specified pathogens (SPF) (*5.2.2*).

2-2-2. **Cell cultures**. If the vaccine virus is grown in cell cultures, they comply with the requirements for cell cultures for production of veterinary vaccines (*5.2.4*).

2-3. *SEED LOTS*

2-3-1. **Extraneous agents**. The master seed lot complies with the tests for extraneous agents in seed lots (*2.6.24*). In these tests on the master seed lot, the organisms used are not more that 5 passages from the master seed lot at the start of the test.

2-4. *CHOICE OF VACCINE VIRUS*

The vaccine virus shall be shown to be satisfactory with respect to safety (*5.2.6*) and efficacy (*5.2.7*) for the chickens for which it is intended.

The following tests for safety (section 2-4-1), increase in virulence (section 2-4-2) and immunogenicity (section 2-4-3) may be used during the demonstration of safety and immunogenicity.

2-4-1. **Safety**

2-4-1-1. *Safety for the respiratory tract and kidneys.* Carry out the test in chickens not older than the youngest age to be recommended for vaccination. Use vaccine virus at the least attenuated passage level that will be present between the master seed lot and a batch of the vaccine. Use not fewer than 15 chickens from an SPF flock (*5.2.2*) and from the same origin. Administer to each chicken by the oculonasal route a quantity of the vaccine virus equivalent to not less than 10 times the maximum virus titre likely to be contained in 1 dose of the vaccine. On each of days 5, 7 and 10 after administration of the virus, kill not fewer than 5 of the chickens, take samples of trachea and kidney. Fix kidney samples for histological examination. Remove the tracheas and cut 10 rings from each trachea (3 from the top, 4 from the mid-part and 3 from the bottom); examine each ring under low magnification and score for ciliostasis on a scale from 0 (100 per cent ciliary activity) to 4 (no activity, complete ciliostasis); calculate the mean ciliostasis score (the maximum for each trachea being 40) for the 5 chickens killed on each of days 5, 7 and 10. The test is not valid if more than 10 per cent of the chickens die from causes not attributable to the vaccine virus. The vaccine virus complies with the test if:

- no chicken shows notable clinical signs of avian infectious bronchitis or dies from causes attributable to the vaccine virus,
- the average ciliostasis score is not more than 25,
- at most moderate inflammatory lesions are seen during kidney histological examination.

2-4-1-2. *Safety for the reproductive tract.* If the recommendations for use state or imply that the vaccine may be used in females of less than 3 weeks old that are subsequently kept to sexual maturity, it shall be demonstrated that there is no damage to development of the reproductive tract when the vaccine is given to chickens of the minimum age to be recommended for vaccination. The following test may be carried out: use not fewer than 40 female chickens not older than the minimum age recommended for vaccination and from an SPF flock (*5.2.2*); use the vaccine virus at the least attenuated passage level that will be present in a batch of vaccine; administer to each chicken by a recommended route a quantity of virus equivalent to not less than the maximum titre likely to be present in 1 dose of vaccine; at least 10 weeks after administration of the vaccine virus, kill the chickens and carry out macroscopic examination of the oviducts. The vaccine virus complies with the test if abnormalities are present in not more than 5 per cent of the oviducts.

2-4-2. **Increase in virulence**. The test for increase in virulence consists of the administration of the vaccine virus, at the least attenuated virus passage level that will be present between the master seed lot and a batch of the vaccine, to a group of five 2-week-old chickens from an SPF flock (*5.2.2*), sequential passages, 5 times where possible, to further similar groups and testing of the final recovered virus for increase in virulence. If the properties of the vaccine virus allow sequential passage to 5 groups via natural spreading, this method may be used, otherwise passage as described below is carried out and the maximally passaged virus that has been recovered is tested for increase in virulence. Care must be taken to avoid contamination by virus from previous passages. Administer by eye-drop a quantity of the vaccine virus that will allow recovery of virus for the passages described below. 2 to 4 days after administration of the vaccine virus, prepare a suspension from the mucosa of the trachea of each chicken and pool these samples. Administer 0.05 ml of the pooled samples by eye-drop to each of 5

Vaccines

other 2-week-old chickens from an SPF flock (*5.2.2*). Carry out this passage operation not fewer than 5 times; verify the presence of the virus at each passage. If the virus is not found at a passage level, carry out a second series of passages. Carry out the test for safety for the respiratory tract and kidney (section 2-4-1-1) and, where applicable, the test for safety for the reproductive tract (section 2-4-1-2) using the unpassaged vaccine virus and the maximally passaged virus that has been recovered. Administer the virus by the route to be recommended for vaccination likely to be the least safe. The vaccine virus complies with the test if no indication of increase in virulence of the maximally passaged virus compared with the unpassaged virus is observed. If virus is not recovered at any passage level in the first and second series of passages, the vaccine virus also complies with the test.

2-4-3. **Immunogenicity**. Immunogenicity is demonstrated for each strain of virus to be included in the vaccine. A test is carried out for each route and method of administration to be recommended using in each case chickens from an SPF flock (*5.2.2*) not older than the youngest age to be recommended for vaccination. The quantity of the vaccine virus administered to each chicken is not greater than the minimum virus titre to be stated on the label and the virus is at the most attenuated passage level that will be present in a batch of the vaccine. 1 or both of the tests below may be used during the demonstration of immunogenicity.

2-4-3-1. *Ciliary activity of tracheal explants.* Use not fewer than 25 chickens of the same origin and from an SPF flock (*5.2.2*). Vaccinate by a recommended route not fewer than 20 chickens. Maintain not fewer than 5 chickens as controls. Challenge each chicken after 21 days by eye-drop with a sufficient quantity of virulent avian infectious bronchitis virus of the same type as the vaccine virus to be tested. Kill the chickens 4 to 7 days after challenge and prepare transverse sections from the upper part (3), the middle part (4) and the lower part (3) of the trachea of each chicken. Examine all explants as soon as possible and at the latest 2 h after sampling by low-magnification microscopy for ciliary activity. For a given tracheal section, ciliary activity is considered as normal when at least 50 per cent of the internal ring shows vigorous ciliary movement. A chicken is considered not affected if not fewer than 9 out of 10 rings show normal ciliary activity.

The test is not valid if:

- fewer than 80 per cent of the control chickens show cessation or extreme loss of vigour of ciliary activity,
- and/or during the period between the vaccination and challenge more than 10 per cent of vaccinated or control chickens show abnormal clinical signs or die from causes not attributable to the vaccine.

The vaccine virus complies with the test if not fewer than 80 per cent of the vaccinated chickens show normal ciliary activity.

2-4-3-2. *Virus recovery from tracheal swabs.*Use not fewer than 30 chickens of the same origin and from an SPF flock (*5.2.2*). Vaccinate by a recommended route not fewer than 20 chickens. Maintain not fewer than 10 chickens as controls. Challenge each chicken after 21 days by eye-drop with a sufficient quantity of virulent avian infectious bronchitis virus of the same type as the vaccine virus to be tested. Kill the chickens 4 to 7 days after challenge and prepare a suspension from swabs of the tracheal mucosa of each chicken. Inoculate 0.2 ml of the suspension into the allantoic cavity of each of 5 embryonated hens' eggs, 9 to 11 days old, from an SPF flock (*5.2.2*). Incubate the eggs for 6-8 days after inoculation. Eggs that after 1 day of incubation do not contain a live embryo are eliminated and considered as non-specific deaths. Record the other eggs containing a dead embryo and after 6-8 days' incubation examine each egg containing a live embryo for lesions characteristic of avian infectious bronchitis. Make successively 3 such passages. If 1 embryo of a series of eggs dies or shows characteristic lesions, the inoculum is considered to be a carrier of avian infectious bronchitis virus. The examination of a series of eggs is considered to be definitely negative if no inoculum concerned is a carrier. The test is not valid if:

- the challenge virus is re-isolated from fewer than 80 per cent of the control chickens,
- and/or during the period between vaccination and challenge more than 10 per cent of the vaccinated or control chickens show abnormal clinical signs or die from causes not attributable to the vaccine,
- and/or more than 1 egg in any group is eliminated because of non-specific embryo death.

The vaccine virus complies with the test if the challenge virus is re-isolated from not more than 20 per cent of the vaccinated chickens.

3. BATCH TESTS

3-1. **Identification**

3-1-1. *Vaccines containing one type of virus.* The vaccine, diluted if necessary and mixed with avian infectious bronchitis virus antiserum specific for the virus type, no longer infects embryonated hens' eggs from an SPF flock (*5.2.2*) or susceptible cell cultures (*5.2.4*) into which it is inoculated.

3-1-2. *Vaccines containing more than one type of virus.* The vaccine, diluted if necessary and mixed with type-specific antisera against each strain present in the vaccine except that to be identified, infects embryonated hens' eggs from an SPF flock (*5.2.2*) or susceptible cell cultures (*5.2.4*) into which it is inoculated whereas after further admixture with type-specific antiserum against the strain to be identified it no longer produces such infection.

3-2. **Bacteria and fungi**

Vaccines intended for administration by injection comply with the test for sterility prescribed in the monograph *Vaccines for veterinary use (0062).*

Vaccines not intended for administration by injection either comply with the test for sterility prescribed in the monograph *Vaccines for veterinary use (0062)* or with the following test: carry out a quantitative test for bacterial and fungal contamination; carry out identification tests for microorganisms detected in the vaccine; the vaccine does not contain pathogenic microorganisms and contains not more than 1 non-pathogenic microorganism per dose.

Any liquid supplied with the vaccine complies with the test for sterility prescribed in the monograph *Vaccines for veterinary use (0062).*

3-3. **Mycoplasmas**. The vaccine complies with the test for mycoplasmas (*2.6.7*).

3-4. **Extraneous agents**. The vaccine complies with the tests for extraneous agents in batches of finished product (*2.6.25*).

3-5. **Safety**. Use not fewer than 10 chickens from an SPF flock (*5.2.2*) and of the youngest age recommended for vaccination. Administer by a recommended route to each chicken, 10 doses of the vaccine. Observe the chickens at least daily for 21 days. The test is not valid if more than 20 per cent of the chickens show abnormal clinical signs or die from causes not attributable to the vaccine. The vaccine complies with the test if no chicken shows notable clinical signs of disease or dies from causes attributable to the vaccine.

3-6. **Virus titre**. Titrate the vaccine virus by inoculation into embryonated hens' eggs from an SPF flock (*5.2.2*) or into suitable cell cultures (*5.2.4*). If the vaccine contains more than 1 strain of virus, titrate each strain after having neutralised the others with type-specific avian infectious bronchitis antisera. The vaccine complies with the test if 1 dose contains for each vaccine virus not less than the minimum titre stated on the label.

3-7. **Potency**. The vaccine complies with the requirements of 1 of the tests prescribed under Immunogenicity (section 2-4-3) when administered according to the recommended schedule by a recommended route and method. It is not necessary to carry out the potency test for each batch of the vaccine if it has been carried out on a representative batch using a vaccinating dose containing not more than the minimum virus titre stated on the label.

01/2005:0960

AVIAN INFECTIOUS BURSAL DISEASE VACCINE (INACTIVATED)

Vaccinum bursitidis infectivae aviariae inactivatum

DEFINITION

Inactivated infectious avian bursal disease vaccine consists of an emulsion or a suspension of a suitable strain of infectious avian bursal disease virus type 1 which has been inactivated in such a manner that immunogenic activity is retained. The vaccine is for use in breeding domestic fowl to protect their progeny from infectious avian bursal disease.

PRODUCTION

The virus is propagated in fertilised eggs from healthy flocks, in suitable cell cultures (*5.2.4*) or in chickens from a flock free from specified pathogens (*5.2.2*).

An amplification test for residual live infectious avian bursal disease virus is carried out on each batch of antigen immediately after inactivation and on the final bulk vaccine or, if the vaccine contains an adjuvant, on the bulk antigen or the mixture of bulk antigens immediately before the addition of any adjuvant, to confirm inactivation; the test is carried out in fertilised hen eggs or in suitable cell cultures or, where chickens have been used for production of the vaccine, in chickens from a flock free from specified pathogens (*5.2.2*); the quantity of inactivated virus used in the test is equivalent to not less than ten doses of the vaccine. No live virus is detected.

The vaccine may contain one or more suitable adjuvants.

CHOICE OF VACCINE COMPOSITION

The vaccine is shown to be satisfactory with respect to safety (*5.2.6*) and immunogenicity (*5.2.7*). The following test may be used during demonstration of efficacy.

Immunogenicity. Each of at least twenty chickens from a flock free from specified pathogens (*5.2.2*), and of the recommended age for vaccination (close to the point of lay), is injected with the minimum recommended dose of vaccine by one of the recommended routes. 4 to 6 weeks later serum samples are collected from each bird and the antibody response is measured in a serum-neutralisation (SN) test. A suitable standard, calibrated in Ph. Eur. Units against *infectious avian bursal disease serum BRP*, is included in the test. The vaccine complies with the test if the mean antibody level in the sera from the vaccinated birds is at least 10 000 Ph. Eur. Units per millilitre.

Eggs are collected for hatching 5 to 7 weeks after vaccination and the test described below is carried out with 3-week-old chickens from that egg collection. Eggs are collected again towards the end of the period of lay and the test is repeated with chickens from that egg collection which are at least 15 days old.

Twenty-five chickens from vaccinated hens and ten control chickens of the same breed and age from unvaccinated hens are challenged with an eye-drop application of a quantity of a virulent strain of infectious avian bursal disease virus sufficient to produce severe signs of disease, including lesions of the bursa of Fabricius, in all unvaccinated chickens. 3 to 4 days after challenge, the bursa of Fabricius is removed from each chicken. The bursae are examined for evidence of infection by histological examination or by testing for the presence of infectious avian bursal disease antigen in an agar-gel precipitation test. The vaccine complies with the test if three or fewer of the chickens from vaccinated hens show evidence of infectious avian bursal disease infection. The test is not valid unless all the chickens from unvaccinated hens are affected.

Where there is more than one recommended route of administration, the test described under Potency is carried out in parallel with the above immunogenicity test, using different groups of birds for each recommended route. The serological response of the birds inoculated by routes other than that used in the immunogenicity test is not significantly less than that of the group vaccinated by that route.

IDENTIFICATION

In chickens with no antibodies to infectious avian bursal disease virus type 1, the vaccine stimulates the production of specific antibodies.

TESTS

Safety. Inject twice the vaccinating dose by one of the recommended routes into each of ten chickens, 14 to 28 days old, from flocks free from specified pathogens (*5.2.2*). Observe the birds for 21 days. No abnormal local or systemic reaction occurs. *Note: this test may be omitted if inactivation test C is carried out.*

Inactivation

A. For vaccine prepared with embryo-adapted strains of virus, inject two-fifths of a dose into the allantoic cavity or onto the chorio-allantoic membrane of ten 9- to 11-day-old fertilised hen eggs from a flock free from specified pathogens (SPF eggs) (*5.2.2*). Incubate the eggs and observe for 6 days. Pool separately the allantoic liquid or membranes from eggs containing live embryos, and that from eggs containing dead embryos, excluding those that die from non-specific causes within 24 h of the injection.

Inject into the allantoic cavity or onto the chorio-allantoic membrane of each of ten 9- to 11-day-old SPF eggs 0.2 ml of the pooled allantoic liquid or crushed chorio-allantoic membranes from the live embryos and, into each of ten similar eggs, 0.2 ml of the pooled liquid or membranes from the dead embryos and incubate for 6 days. Examine each embryo for lesions of infectious avian bursal disease.

If more than 20 per cent of the embryos die at either stage repeat that stage. The vaccine complies with the test if there is no evidence of lesions of infectious avian bursal disease and if, in any repeat test, not more than 20 per cent of the embryos die from non-specific causes.

Antibiotics may be used in the test to control extraneous bacterial infection.

Vaccines

B. For vaccine prepared with cell-culture-adapted strains of virus, inoculate ten doses of the vaccine into suitable cell cultures. If the vaccine contains an oil adjuvant, eliminate it by suitable means. Incubate at 38 ± 1 °C for 7 days. Make a passage on another set of cell cultures and incubate at 38 ± 1 °C for 7 days. The cultures show no signs of infection.

C. For vaccine prepared with strains of virus not adapted to embryos or cell cultures, inject two doses intramuscularly into each of twenty 14- to 28-day-old chickens from flocks free from specified pathogens (*5.2.2*). 4 days later, kill ten of the chickens and remove the bursa of Fabricius from each chicken. Pool the bursae and homogenise in an equal volume of a suitable liquid. Inject 1 ml of the bursal homogenate into each of a further ten chickens of the same age and from the same source. Examine microscopically the bursa of Fabricius of each remaining chicken from the first group and of each chicken from the second group 21 days after the injection; there is no evidence of infectious avian bursal disease infection. In addition there are no signs of any disease attributable to the vaccine and no abnormal local reaction develops. The chickens of the second group do not have antibodies against infectious avian bursal disease virus when examined 21 days after the injection.

Extraneous agents. Collect serum samples from each of the birds used in the safety test or inactivation test C, three weeks after vaccination. Carry out tests for antibodies to the following agents by the methods prescribed for *chicken flocks free from specified pathogens for the production and quality control of vaccines* (*5.2.2*): avian encephalomyelitis virus, avian leucosis viruses, haemagglutinating avian adenovirus, infectious bronchitis virus, infectious laryngotracheitis virus, influenza A virus, Marek's disease virus, Newcastle disease virus. The vaccine does not stimulate the formation of antibodies against these agents.

Sterility. The vaccine complies with the test for sterility prescribed in the monograph on *Vaccines for veterinary use (0062)*.

POTENCY

Vaccinate each of not fewer than ten chickens, 4 weeks of age and from a flock free from specified pathogens (*5.2.2*), with one dose of vaccine by one of the recommended routes. 4 to 6 weeks later, collect serum samples from each bird and ten unvaccinated control birds of the same age and from the same source. Measure the antibody response in a serum-neutralisation test. Include in the test a suitable standard, calibrated in Ph.Eur. Units against *infectious avian bursal disease serum BRP*. The mean antibody level in the sera from the vaccinated birds is not less than 10 000 Ph. Eur. Units per millilitre. There are no antibodies in the sera of the unvaccinated birds.

LABELLING

The label states whether the strain in the vaccine is embryo-adapted or cell-culture-adapted.

01/2005:0587

AVIAN INFECTIOUS BURSAL DISEASE VACCINE (LIVE)

Vaccinum bursitidis infectivae aviariae vivum

1. DEFINITION

Avian infectious bursal disease vaccine (live) [Gumboro disease vaccine (live)] is a preparation of a suitable strain of infectious bursal disease virus type 1. This monograph applies to vaccines intended for administration to chickens for active immunisation; it applies to vaccines containing strains of low virulence but not to those containing strains of higher virulence that may be needed for disease control in certain epidemiological situations.

2. PRODUCTION

2-1. *PREPARATION OF THE VACCINE*

The vaccine virus is grown in embryonated hens' eggs or in cell cultures.

2-2. *SUBSTRATE FOR VIRUS PROPAGATION*

2-2-1. **Embryonated hens' eggs**. If the vaccine virus is grown in embryonated hens' eggs, they are obtained from flocks free from specified pathogens (SPF) (*5.2.2*).

2-2-2. **Cell cultures**. If the vaccine virus is grown in cell cultures, they comply with the requirements for cell cultures for production of veterinary vaccines (*5.2.4*).

2-3. *SEED LOTS*

2-3-1. **Extraneous agents**. The master seed lot complies with the tests for extraneous agents in seed lots (*2.6.24*). In these tests on the master seed lot, the organisms used are not more than 5 passages from the master seed lot at the start of the tests.

2-4. *CHOICE OF VACCINE VIRUS*

The vaccine virus shall be shown to be satisfactory with respect to safety (*5.2.6*) and efficacy (*5.2.7*) for the chickens for which it is intended.

The following tests for safety (section 2-4-1), damage to the bursa of Fabricius (section 2-4-2), immunosuppression (section 2-4-3), increase in virulence (section 2-4-4) and immunogenicity (section 2-4-5) may be used during the demonstration of safety and immunogenicity.

2-4-1. **Safety**. Carry out the test for each route and method of administration to be recommended for vaccination using in each case chickens not older than the youngest age to be recommended for vaccination. Use vaccine virus at the least attenuated passage level that will be present between the master seed lot and a batch of the vaccine. For each test, use not fewer than 20 chickens from an SPF flock (*5.2.2*). Administer to each chicken a quantity of the vaccine virus equivalent to not less than 10 times the maximum virus titre likely to be contained in 1 dose of the vaccine. Observe the chickens at least daily for 21 days. The test is not valid if more than 10 per cent of the chickens die from causes not attributable to the vaccine virus. The vaccine virus complies with the test if no chicken shows notable clinical signs of avian infectious bursal disease or dies from causes attributable to the vaccine virus.

2-4-2. **Damage to the bursa of Fabricius**. Carry out the test for the route to be recommended for vaccination likely to be the least safe using chickens not older than the youngest age to be recommended for vaccination. Use virus at the least attenuated passage level that will be present between

Vaccines

the master seed lot and a batch of the vaccine. Use not fewer than 20 chickens from an SPF flock (*5.2.2*). Administer to each chicken a quantity of the vaccine virus equivalent to 10 times the maximum titre likely to be contained in a dose of the vaccine. On each of days 7, 14, 21 and 28 after administration of the vaccine virus, kill not fewer than 5 chickens and prepare a section from the site with the greatest diameters of the bursa of Fabricius of each chicken. Carry out histological examination of the section and score the degree of bursal damage using the following scale.

0	No lesion, normal bursa.
1	1 per cent to 25 per cent of the follicles show lymphoid depletion (i.e. less than 50 per cent depletion in 1 affected follicle) influx of heterophils in lesions.
2	26 per cent to 50 per cent of the follicles show nearly complete lymphoid depletion (i.e. more than 75 per cent depletion in 1 affected follicle), affected follicles show necrosis and severe influx of heterophils may be detected.
3	51 per cent to 75 per cent of the follicles show lymphoid depletion; affected follicles show necrosis and severe influx of heterophils is detected.
4	76 per cent to100 per cent of the follicles show nearly complete lymphoid depletion, hyperplasia and cyst structures are detected; affected follicles show necrosis and severe influx of heterophils is detected.
5	100 per cent of the follicles show nearly complete lymphoid depletion; complete loss of follicular structure, thickened and folded epithelium, fibrosis of bursal tissue.

Calculate the average score for each group of chickens. The vaccine virus complies with the test if:

– no chicken shows notable clinical signs of disease or dies from causes attributable to the vaccine virus,

– the average score for bursal damage 21 days after administration of the vaccine virus is less than or equal to 2.0 and 28 days after administration is less than or equal to 0.6,

– during the 21 days after administration a notable repopulation of the bursae by lymphocytes has taken place.

2-4-3. **Immunosuppression**. Carry out the tests for the route recommended for vaccination likely to be the least safe using chickens not older than the youngest age recommended for vaccination. Use vaccine virus at the least attenuated passage level that will be present between the master seed lot and a batch of the vaccine. Use not fewer than 30 chickens from an SPF flock (*5.2.2*). Divide them randomly into 3 groups each of not fewer than 10 and maintain the groups separately. Administer by eye-drop to each chicken of 1 group a quantity of the vaccine virus equivalent to not less than the maximum titre likely to be contained in 1 dose of the vaccine. At the time after administration when maximal bursal damage is likely to be present, as judged from the results obtained in the test for damage to the bursa of Fabricius (section 2-4-2), administer to each vaccinated chicken and to each chicken of another group 1 dose of Hitchner B1 strain Newcastle disease vaccine (live). Determine the seroresponse of each chicken of the 2 groups to the Newcastle disease virus 14 days after administration. Challenge each chicken of the 3 groups by the intramuscular route with not less than 10^5 EID_{50} of virulent Newcastle disease virus and note the degree of protection in the 2 groups vaccinated with Hitchner B1 strain Newcastle vaccine compared with the non-vaccinated group. The test is not valid if 1 or more of the non-vaccinated chickens does not die within 7 days of challenge. The degree of immunosuppression is estimated from the comparative seroresponses and protection rates of the 2 Hitchner B1 vaccinated groups. The vaccine complies with the test if there is no significant difference between the 2 groups.

2-4-4. **Increase in virulence**. The test for increase in virulence consists of the administration of the vaccine virus at the least attenuated passage level that will be present between the master seed lot and a batch of the vaccine to a group of 5 chickens from an SPF flock (*5.2.2*) and not older than the youngest age to be recommended for vaccination, sequential passages, 5 times where possible, to further similar groups and testing of the final recovered virus for increase in virulence. If the properties of the vaccine virus allow sequential passage to 5 groups via natural spreading, this method may be used, otherwise passage as described below is carried out and the maximally passaged virus that has been recovered is tested for increase in virulence. Care must be taken to avoid contamination by virus from previous passages. Administer by eye-drop a quantity of the vaccine virus that will allow recovery of virus for the passages described below. Prepare 3 to 4 days after administration a suspension from the bursa of Fabricius of each chicken and pool these samples. Administer 0.05 ml of the pooled samples by eye-drop to each of 5 other chickens of the same age and origin. Carry out this passage operation not fewer than 5 times; verify the presence of the virus at each passage. If the virus is not found at a passage level, carry out a second series of passages. Carry out the test for damage to the bursa of Fabricius (section 2-4-2) using the unpassaged vaccine virus and the maximally passaged virus that has been recovered. Administer the virus by the route recommended for vaccination likely to be the least safe. The vaccine virus complies with the test if no indication of increasing virulence of the maximally passaged virus compared with the unpassaged virus is observed. If virus is not recovered at any passage level in the first and second series of passages, the vaccine virus also complies with the test.

2-4-5. **Immunogenicity**. A test is carried out for each route and method of administration to be recommended using in each case chickens not older than the youngest age to be recommended for vaccination. The quantity of vaccine virus administered to each chicken is not greater than the minimum virus titre to be stated on the label and the virus is at the most attenuated passage level that will be present in a batch of the vaccine. Use not fewer than 30 chickens of the same origin and from an SPF flock (*5.2.2*). Vaccinate by a recommended route not fewer than 20 chickens. Maintain not fewer than 10 chickens as controls. Challenge each chicken after 14 days by eye-drop with a sufficient quantity of virulent avian infectious bursal disease virus. Observe the chickens at least daily for 10 days after challenge. Record the deaths due to infectious bursal disease and the surviving chickens that show clinical signs of disease. At the end of the observation period, kill all the surviving chickens and carry out histological examination for lesions of the bursa of Fabricius. The test is not valid if one or more of the following applies:

– during the observation period following challenge, fewer than 50 per cent of the control chickens show characteristic signs of avian infectious bursal disease,

– 1 or more of the surviving control chickens does not show degree 3 lesions of the bursa of Fabricius,

– during the period between the vaccination and challenge more than 10 per cent of the vaccinated or control chickens show abnormal clinical signs or die from causes not attributable to the vaccine.

The vaccine virus complies with the test if during the observation period after challenge not fewer than 90 per cent of the vaccinated chickens survive and show no notable clinical signs of disease nor degree 3 lesions of the bursa of Fabricius.

3. BATCH TESTS

3-1. **Identification**. The vaccine, diluted if necessary and mixed with a monospecific infectious bursal disease virus type 1 antiserum, no longer infects embryonated hens' eggs from an SPF flock (*5.2.2*) or susceptible cell cultures (*5.2.4*) into which it is inoculated.

3-2. **Bacteria and fungi**

Vaccines intended for administration by injection comply with the test for sterility prescribed in the monograph *Vaccines for veterinary use (0062)*.

Vaccines not intended for administration by injection either comply with the test for sterility prescribed in the monograph *Vaccines for veterinary use (0062)* or with the following test: carry out a quantitative test for bacterial and fungal contamination; carry out identification tests for microorganisms detected in the vaccine; the vaccine does not contain pathogenic microorganisms and contains not more than 1 non-pathogenic microorganism per dose.

Any liquid supplied with the vaccine complies with the test for sterility prescribed in the monograph *Vaccines for veterinary use (0062)*.

3-3. **Mycoplasmas**. The vaccine complies with the test for mycoplasmas (*2.6.7*).

3-4. **Extraneous agents**. The vaccine complies with the tests for extraneous agents in batches of finished product (*2.6.25*).

3-5. **Safety**. Use not fewer than 10 chickens from an SPF flock (*5.2.2*) and of the youngest age recommended for vaccination. Administer by a recommended route and method to each chicken 10 doses of the vaccine. Observe the chickens at least daily for 21 days. The test is not valid if more than 20 per cent of the chickens show abnormal clinical signs or die from causes not attributable to the vaccine. The vaccine complies with the test if no chicken shows notable clinical signs of disease or dies from causes attributable to the vaccine.

3-6. **Virus titre**. Titrate the vaccine virus by inoculation into embryonated hens' eggs from an SPF flock (*5.2.2*) or into suitable cell cultures (*5.2.4*). The vaccine complies with the test if 1 dose contains not less than the minimum virus titre stated on the label.

3-7. **Potency**. The vaccine complies with the requirements of the test prescribed under Immunogenicity (section 2-4-5) when administered by a recommended route and method. It is not necessary to carry out the potency test for each batch of the vaccine if it has been carried out on a representative batch using a vaccinating dose containing not more than the minimum virus titre stated on the label.

01/2005:0588

AVIAN INFECTIOUS ENCEPHALOMYELITIS VACCINE (LIVE)

Vaccinum encephalomyelitidis infectivae aviariae vivum

1. DEFINITION

Avian infectious encephalomyelitis vaccine (live) is a preparation of a suitable strain of avian encephalomyelitis virus. This monograph applies to vaccines intended for administration to non-laying breeder chickens to protect passively their future progeny and/or to prevent vertical transmission of virus via the egg.

2. PRODUCTION

2-1. *PREPARATION OF THE VACCINE*

The vaccine virus is grown in embryonated hens' eggs or in cell cultures.

2-2. *SUBSTRATE FOR VIRUS PROPAGATION*

2-2-1. **Embryonated hens' eggs**. If the vaccine virus is grown in embryonated hens' eggs, they are obtained from flocks free from specified pathogens (SPF) (*5.2.2*).

2-2-2. **Cell cultures**. If the vaccine virus is grown in cell cultures, they comply with the requirements for cell cultures for production of veterinary vaccines (*5.2.4*).

2-3. *SEED LOTS*

2-3-1. **Extraneous agents**. The master seed lot complies with the tests for extraneous agents in seed lots (*2.6.24*). In these tests on the master seed lot, the organisms used are not more than 5 passages from the master seed lot at the start of the tests.

2-4. *CHOICE OF VACCINE VIRUS*

The vaccine virus shall be shown to be satisfactory with respect to safety (*5.2.6*) and efficacy (*5.2.7*) for the chickens for which it is intended.

The following tests for safety (section 2-4-1), increase in virulence (section 2-4-2) and immunogenicity (section 2-4-3) may be used during the demonstration of safety and immunogenicity.

2-4-1. **Safety**. Carry out the test for each route and method of administration to be recommended for vaccination using in each case non-laying breeder chickens not older than the youngest age to be recommended for vaccination. Use vaccine virus at the least attenuated passage level that will be present between the master seed lot and a batch of the vaccine. For each test, use not fewer than 20 chickens from an SPF flock (*5.2.2*). Administer to each chicken a quantity of the vaccine virus equivalent to not less than 10 times the maximum virus titre likely to be contained in 1 dose of the vaccine. Observe the chickens at least daily for 21 days. The test is not valid if more than 10 per cent of the chickens show abnormal clinical signs or die from causes not attributable to the vaccine virus. The vaccine virus complies with the test if no chicken shows notable clinical signs of avian infectious encephalomyelitis or dies from causes attributable to the vaccine virus.

2-4-2. **Increase in virulence**. The test for increase in virulence consists of the administration of the vaccine virus at the least attenuated passage level that will be present between the master seed lot and a batch of vaccine to a group of five 1-day-old chickens from an SPF flock (*5.2.2*), sequential passages, 5 times where possible, to further

Vaccines

similar groups of 1-day-old chickens, and testing of the final recovered virus for increase in virulence. If the properties of the vaccine virus allow sequential passage to 5 groups via natural spreading, this method may be used, otherwise passage as described below is carried out and the maximally passaged virus that has been recovered is tested for increase in virulence. Care must be taken to avoid contamination by virus from previous passages. Administer by a recommended route and method, a quantity of the vaccine virus that will allow recovery of virus for the passages described below. 5 to 7 days later, prepare a suspension from the brain of each chick and pool these samples. Administer a suitable volume of the pooled samples by the oral route to each of 5 other chickens of the same age and origin. Carry out this passage operation not fewer than 5 times; verify the presence of the virus at each passage. If the virus is not found at a passage level, carry out a second series of passages. Carry out the test for safety (section 2-4-1) using the unpassaged vaccine virus and the maximally passaged vaccine virus that has been recovered. The vaccine virus complies with the test if no indication of increase in virulence of the maximally passaged virus compared with the unpassaged virus is observed. If virus is not recovered at any passage level in the first and second series of passages, the vaccine virus also complies with the test.

2-4-3. **Immunogenicity**. If the vaccine is recommended for passive protection of future progeny carry out test 2-4-3-1. If the vaccine is recommended for prevention of vertical transmission of virus via the egg, carry out test 2-4-3-2. A test is carried out for each route and method of administration to be recommended, using in each case chickens from an SPF flock (*5.2.2*) not older than the youngest age to be recommended for vaccination. The quantity of the vaccine virus administered to each chicken is not greater than the minimum titre to be stated on the label and the virus is at the most attenuated passage level that will be present in a batch of the vaccine.

2-4-3-1. *Passive immunity in chickens*. Vaccinate not fewer than 20 breeder chickens from an SPF flock (*5.2.2*). Maintain separately not fewer than 10 breeder chickens of the same age and origin as controls. At the peak of lay, hatch not fewer than 25 chickens from eggs from vaccinated breeder chickens and 10 chickens from non-vaccinated breeder chickens. At 2 weeks of age, challenge each chicken by the intracerebral route with a sufficient quantity of virulent avian encephalomyelitis virus. Observe the chickens at least daily for 21 days after challenge. Record the deaths and the number of surviving chickens that show clinical signs of disease. The test is not valid if:

- during the observation period after challenge fewer than 80 per cent of the control chickens die or show severe clinical signs of avian infectious encephalomyelitis,
- and/or during the period between the vaccination and challenge more than 15 per cent of control or vaccinated chickens show abnormal clinical signs or die from causes not attributable to the vaccine.

The vaccine virus complies with the test if during the observation period after challenge not fewer than 80 per cent of the progeny of vaccinated chickens survive and show no notable clinical signs of disease.

2-4-3-2. *Passive immunity in embryos*. Vaccinate not fewer than 20 breeder chickens from an SPF flock (*5.2.2*). Maintain separately not fewer than 10 breeder chickens of the same age and origin as controls. At the peak of lay, incubate not fewer than 36 eggs from the 2 groups, vaccinated and controls, and carry out an embryo sensitivity test. On the sixth day of incubation inoculate 100 EID_{50} of the Van Roekel strain of avian encephalomyelitis virus into the yolk sacs of the eggs. 12 days after inoculation examine the embryos for specific lesions of avian encephalomyelitis (muscular atrophy). Deaths during the first 24 h are considered to be non-specific. The test is not valid if fewer than 80 per cent of the control embryos show lesions of avian encephalomyelitis. The test is not valid if fewer than 80 per cent of the embryos can be given an assessment. The vaccine virus complies with the test if not fewer than 80 per cent of the embryos in the vaccinated group show no lesions of avian encephalomyelitis.

3. BATCH TESTS

3-1. **Identification**. The vaccine, diluted if necessary and mixed with a monospecific avian encephalomyelitis virus antiserum, no longer infects embryonated hens' eggs from an SPF flock (*5.2.2*) or susceptible cell cultures (*5.2.4*) into which it is inoculated.

3-2. **Bacteria and fungi**

Vaccines intended for administration by injection comply with the test for sterility prescribed in the monograph *Vaccines for veterinary use (0062)*.

Vaccines not intended for administration by injection either comply with the test for sterility prescribed in the monograph *Vaccines for veterinary use (0062)* or with the following test: carry out a quantitative test for bacterial and fungal contamination; carry out identification tests for microorganisms detected in the vaccine; the vaccine does not contain pathogenic microorganisms and contains not more than 1 non-pathogenic microorganism per dose.

Any liquid supplied with the vaccine complies with the test for sterility prescribed in the monograph *Vaccines for veterinary use (0062)*.

3-3. **Mycoplasmas**. The vaccine complies with the test for mycoplasmas (*2.6.7*).

3-4. **Extraneous agents**. The vaccine complies with the tests for extraneous agents in batches of finished product (*2.6.25*).

3-5. **Safety**. Use not fewer than 10 chickens not older than the minimum age recommended for vaccination and from an SPF flock (*5.2.2*). Administer by a recommended route and method to each chicken 10 doses of the vaccine. Observe the chickens at least daily for 21 days. The test is not valid if more than 20 per cent of the chickens show abnormal clinical signs or die from causes not attributable to the vaccine. The vaccine complies with the test if no chicken shows notable clinical signs of disease or dies from causes attributable to the vaccine.

3-6. **Virus titre**. Titrate the vaccine virus by inoculation into embryonated hens' eggs from an SPF flock (*5.2.2*) or into suitable cell cultures (*5.2.4*). The vaccine complies with the test if 1 dose contains not less than the minimum virus titre stated on the label.

3-7. **Potency**. Depending on the indications, the vaccine complies with the requirements of 1 or both of the tests prescribed under Immunogenicity (section 2-4-3-1, 2-4-3-2), when administered by a recommended route and method. It is not necessary to carry out the potency test for each batch of the vaccine if it has been carried out on a representative batch using a vaccinating dose containing not more than the minimum virus titre stated on the label.

Vaccines

01/2005:1068

AVIAN INFECTIOUS LARYNGOTRACHEITIS VACCINE (LIVE)

Vaccinum laryngotracheitidis infectivae aviariae vivum

1. DEFINITION

Avian infectious laryngotracheitis vaccine (live) is a preparation of a suitable strain of avian infectious laryngotracheitis virus (gallid herpesvirus 1). This monograph applies to vaccines intended for administration to chickens for active immunisation.

2. PRODUCTION

2-1. *PREPARATION OF THE VACCINE*

The vaccine virus is grown in embryonated hens' eggs or in cell cultures.

2-2. *SUBSTRATE FOR VIRUS PROPAGATION*

2-2-1. **Embryonated hens' eggs**. If the vaccine virus is grown in embryonated hens' eggs, they are obtained from flocks free from specified pathogens (SPF) (*5.2.2*).

2-2-2. **Cell cultures**. If the vaccine virus is grown in cell cultures, they comply with the requirements for cell cultures for production of veterinary vaccines (*5.2.4*).

2-3. *SEED LOTS*

2-3-1. **Extraneous agents**. The master seed lot complies with the tests for extraneous agents in seed lots (*2.6.24*). In these tests on the master seed lot, the organisms used are not more than 5 passages from the master seed lot at the start of the tests.

2-4. *CHOICE OF VACCINE VIRUS*

The vaccine virus shall be shown to be satisfactory with respect to safety (*5.2.6*) and efficacy (*5.2.7*) for the chickens for which it is intended.
The following tests for index of respiratory virulence (section 2-4-1), safety (section 2-4-2), increase in virulence (section 2-4-3) and immunogenicity (section 2-4-4) may be used during the demonstration of safety and immunogenicity.

2-4-1. **Index of respiratory virulence**. Use for the test not fewer than sixty 10-day-old chickens from an SPF flock (*5.2.2*). Divide them randomly into 3 groups, maintained separately. Prepare 2 tenfold serial dilutions starting from a suspension of the vaccine virus having a titre of 10^5 EID_{50} or 10^5 $CCID_{50}$ per 0.2 ml or, if not possible, having the maximum attainable titre. Use vaccine virus at the least attenuated passage level that will be present in a batch of the vaccine. Allocate the undiluted virus suspension and the 2 virus dilutions each to a different group of chickens. Administer by the intratracheal route to each chicken 0.2 ml of the virus suspension attributed to its group. Observe the chickens for 10 days after administration and record the number of deaths. The index of respiratory virulence is the total number of deaths in the 3 groups divided by the total number of chickens. The vaccine virus complies with the test if its index of respiratory virulence is not greater than 0.33.

2-4-2. **Safety**. Carry out the test for each route and method of administration to be recommended for vaccination, using in each case chickens not older than the youngest age to be recommended for vaccination. Use vaccine virus at the least attenuated passage level that will be present between the master seed lot and a batch of the vaccine. For each test use not fewer than 20 chickens, from an SPF flock (*5.2.2*). Administer to each chicken a quantity of the vaccine virus equivalent to not less than 10 times the maximum virus titre likely to be contained in 1 dose of the vaccine. Observe the chickens at least daily for 21 days. The test is not valid if more than 10 per cent of the chickens die from causes not attributable to the vaccine virus. The vaccine virus complies with the test if no chicken shows notable clinical signs of avian infectious laryngotracheitis or dies from causes attributable to the vaccine virus.

2-4-3. **Increase in virulence**. The test for increase in virulence consists of the administration of the vaccine virus at the least attenuated passage level that will be present between the master seed lot and a batch of the vaccine to a group of 5 chickens not more than 2 weeks old, from an SPF flock (*5.2.2*), sequential passages, 5 times where possible, to further similar groups and testing of the final recovered virus for increase in virulence. If the properties of the vaccine virus allow sequential passage to 5 groups via natural spreading, this method may be used, otherwise passage as described below is carried out and the maximally passaged virus that has been recovered is tested for increase in virulence. Care must be taken to avoid contamination by virus from previous passages. Administer by eye-drop a quantity of the vaccine virus that will allow recovery of virus for the passages described below. After the period shown to correspond to maximum replication of the virus, prepare a suspension from the mucosae of suitable parts of the respiratory tract of each chicken and pool these samples. Administer 0.05 ml of the pooled samples by eye-drop to each of 5 other chickens that are 2 weeks old and from an SPF flock (*5.2.2*). Carry out this passage operation not fewer than 5 times; verify the presence of the virus at each passage. If the virus is not found at a passage level, carry out a second series of passages. Determine the index of respiratory virulence (section 2-4-1) using the unpassaged vaccine virus and the maximally passaged virus that has been recovered; if the titre of the maximally passaged virus is less than 10^5 EID_{50} or 10^5 $CCID_{50}$, prepare the tenfold, serial dilutions using the highest titre available. The vaccine virus complies with the test if no indication of increase in virulence of the maximally passaged virus compared with the unpassaged virus is observed. If virus is not recovered at any passage level in the first and second series of passages, the vaccine virus also complies with the test.

2-4-4. **Immunogenicity**. A test is carried out for each route and method of administration to be recommended using in each case chickens not older than the youngest age to be recommended for vaccination. The quantity of the vaccine virus administered to each chicken is not greater than the minimum virus titre to be stated on the label and the virus is at the most attenuated passage level that will be present in a batch of the vaccine. Use for the test not fewer than 30 chickens of the same origin and from an SPF flock (*5.2.2*). Vaccinate by a recommended route not fewer than 20 chickens. Maintain not fewer than 10 chickens as controls. Challenge each chicken after 21 days by the intratracheal route with a sufficient quantity of virulent infectious laryngotracheitis virus. Observe the chickens at least daily for 7 days after challenge. Record the deaths and the number of surviving chickens that show clinical signs of disease. At the end of the observation period kill all the surviving chickens and carry out examination for macroscopic lesions: mucoid, haemorrhagic and pseudomembraneous inflammation of the trachea and orbital sinuses. The test is not valid if:

Vaccines

– during the observation period after challenge fewer than 90 per cent of the control chickens die or show severe clinical signs of avian infectious laryngotracheitis or notable macroscopic lesions of the trachea and orbital sinuses,
– or if during the period between the vaccination and challenge more than 10 per cent of the vaccinated or control chickens show notable clinical signs of disease or die from causes not attributable to the vaccine.

The vaccine virus complies with the test if during the observation period after challenge not fewer than 90 per cent of the vaccinated chickens survive and show no notable clinical signs of disease and/or macroscopical lesions of the trachea and orbital sinuses.

3. BATCH TESTS

3-1. **Identification**. The vaccine, diluted if necessary and mixed with a monospecific infectious laryngotracheitis virus antiserum, no longer infects embryonated hens' eggs from an SPF flock (*5.2.2*) or susceptible cell cultures (*5.2.4*) into which it is inoculated.

3-2. **Bacteria and fungi**

Vaccines intended for administration by injection comply with the test for sterility prescribed in the monograph *Vaccines for veterinary use (0062)*.

Vaccines not intended for administration by injection either comply with the test for sterility prescribed in the monograph *Vaccines for veterinary use (0062)* or with the following test: carry out a quantitative test for bacterial and fungal contamination; carry out identification tests for micro-organisms detected in the vaccine; the vaccine does not contain pathogenic micro-organisms and contains not more than 1 non-pathogenic micro-organism per dose.

Any liquid supplied with the vaccine complies with test for sterility in the monograph *Vaccines for veterinary use (0062)*.

3-3. **Mycoplasmas**. The vaccine complies with the test for mycoplasmas (*2.6.7*).

3-4. **Extraneous agents**. The vaccine complies with the tests for extraneous agents in batches of finished product (*2.6.25*).

3-5. **Safety**. Use not fewer than 10 chickens from an SPF flock (*5.2.2*) and of the youngest age recommended for vaccination. Administer by eye-drop to each chicken 10 doses of the vaccine. Observe the chickens at least daily for 21 days. The test is not valid if more than 20 per cent of the chickens show abnormal clinical signs or die from causes not attributable to the vaccine. The vaccine complies with the test if no chicken shows notable clinical signs of disease or dies from causes attributable to the vaccine.

3-6. **Virus titre**. Titrate the vaccine virus by inoculation into embryonated hens' eggs from an SPF flock (*5.2.2*) or into suitable cell cultures (*5.2.4*). The vaccine complies with the test if 1 dose contains not less than the minimum titre stated on the label.

3-7. **Potency**. The vaccine complies with the requirements of the test prescribed under Immunogenicity (section 2-4-4) when administered according to the recommended schedule by a recommended route and method. It is not necessary to carry out the potency test for each batch of the vaccine if it has been carried out on a representative batch using a vaccinating dose containing not more than the minimum virus titre stated on the label.

Vaccines

01/2005:1392

AVIAN PARAMYXOVIRUS 3 VACCINE (INACTIVATED)

Vaccinum paramyxoviris 3 aviarii inactivatum

DEFINITION

Avian paramyxovirus 3 vaccine (inactivated) consists of an emulsion or a suspension of a suitable strain of avian paramyxovirus 3 that has been inactivated in such a manner that immunogenic activity is retained. The vaccine is used for protection against loss in egg production and egg quality in turkeys.

PRODUCTION

The virus is propagated in embryonated eggs from healthy flocks or in suitable cell cultures (*5.2.4*).

The test for inactivation is carried out in embryonated eggs or suitable cell cultures and the quantity of inactivated virus used is equivalent to not less than ten doses of vaccine. No live virus is detected.

The vaccine may contain an adjuvant.

CHOICE OF VACCINE COMPOSITION

The vaccine is shown to be satisfactory with respect to safety (*5.2.6*) and immunogenicity (*5.2.7*) for each category of turkeys for which it is intended. The following test may be used during demonstration of immunogenicity.

Immunogenicity. The test described under Potency is suitable for demonstrating immunogenicity.

BATCH TESTING

Batch potency test. Carry out a suitable validated test for which satisfactory correlation with the test described under Potency has been established, the criteria for acceptance being set with reference to a batch that has given satisfactory results in the latter test.

IDENTIFICATION

When injected into animals free from antibodies against avian paramyxovirus 3, the vaccine stimulates the production of such antibodies.

TESTS

Safety. Inject twice the vaccinating dose by a recommended route into each of ten turkeys, 14 to 28 days old and free from antibodies against avian paramyxovirus 3. Observe the birds for 21 days. No abnormal local or systemic reaction occurs.

Inactivation. Inject two-fifths of a dose into the allantoic cavity of each of ten embryonated hen eggs, 9 to 11 days old, from flocks free from specified pathogens (*5.2.2*) (SPF eggs) and incubate. Observe for 6 days and pool separately the allantoic fluid from eggs containing live embryos, and that from eggs containing dead embryos, excluding those dying within 24 h of the injection. Examine embryos that die within 24 h of injection for the presence of avian paramyxovirus 3: the vaccine does not comply with the test if avian paramyxovirus 3 is found.

Inject into the allantoic cavity of each of ten SPF eggs, 9 to 11 days old, 0.2 ml of the pooled allantoic fluid from the live embryos and, into each of ten similar eggs, 0.2 ml of the pooled fluid from the dead embryos and incubate for 5 to 6 days. Test the allantoic fluid from each egg for the presence of haemagglutinins using chicken erythrocytes.

The vaccine complies with the test if there is no evidence of haemagglutinating activity and if not more than 20 per cent of the embryos die at either stage. If more than 20 per cent of the embryos die at one of the stages, repeat that stage; the vaccine complies with the test if there is no evidence of haemagglutinating activity and not more than 20 per cent of the embryos die at that stage.

Antibiotics may be used in the test to control extraneous bacterial infection.

Extraneous agents. Inject a double dose by a recommended route into each of ten chickens, 14 to 28 days old and from a flock free from specified pathogens (*5.2.2*). After 3 weeks, inject one dose by the same route. Collect serum samples from each chicken 2 weeks later and carry out tests for antibodies against the following agents by the methods prescribed for chicken flocks free from specified pathogens (*5.2.2*): avian encephalomyelitis virus, avian infectious bronchitis virus, avian leucosis viruses, egg-drop syndrome virus, avian bursal disease virus, avian infectious laryngotracheitis virus, influenza A virus, Marek's disease virus. The vaccine does not stimulate the formation of antibodies against these agents.

Sterility. The vaccine complies with the test for sterility prescribed in the monograph on *Vaccines for veterinary use (0062)*.

POTENCY

Use two groups each of not fewer than twenty turkeys free from antibodies against avian paramyxovirus 3. Vaccinate one group in accordance with the recommendations for use. Keep the other group as controls. The test is invalid if serological tests carried out on serum samples obtained at the time of first vaccination show the presence of antibodies against avian paramyxovirus 3 in either vaccinates or controls or if tests carried out at the time of challenge show such antibodies in controls. At the egg-production peak, challenge the two groups by the oculo-nasal route with a sufficient quantity of a virulent strain of avian paramyxovirus 3. For not less than 6 weeks after challenge, record the number of eggs laid weekly for each group, distinguishing between normal and abnormal eggs. The vaccine complies with the test if egg production and quality are significantly better in the vaccinated group than in the control group.

01/2005:1956

AVIAN VIRAL TENOSYNOVITIS VACCINE (LIVE)

Vaccinum tenosynovitidis viralis aviariae vivum

1. DEFINITION

Avian viral tenosynovitis vaccine (live) is a preparation of a suitable strain of avian tenosynovitis virus (avian orthoreovirus). This monograph applies to vaccines intended for administration to chickens for active immunisation.

2. PRODUCTION

2-1. *PREPARATION OF THE VACCINE*

The vaccine virus is grown in cell cultures.

2-2. *SUBSTRATE FOR VIRUS PROPAGATION*

2-2-1. **Cell cultures**. Cell cultures comply with the requirements for cell cultures for production of veterinary vaccines (*5.2.4*).

2-3. *SEED LOTS*

2-3-1. **Extraneous agents**. The master seed lot complies with the tests for extraneous agents in seed lots (*2.6.24*). In these tests on the master seed lot, the organisms used are not more than 5 passages from the master seed lot at the start of the tests.

2-4. *CHOICE OF VACCINE VIRUS*

The vaccine virus shall be shown to be satisfactory with respect to safety (*5.2.6*) and efficacy (*5.2.7*) for the chickens for which it is intended.

The following tests for safety (section 2-4-1), increase in virulence (section 2-4-2) and immunogenicity (section 2-4-3) may be used during the demonstration of safety and immunogenicity.

2-4-1. **Safety**. Carry out the test for each route and method of administration to be recommended for vaccination using in each case chickens not older than the youngest age to be recommended for vaccination. Use vaccine virus at the least attenuated passage level that will be present between the master seed lot and a batch of the vaccine. For each test use not fewer than 20 chickens, from an SPF flock (*5.2.2*). Administer to each chicken a quantity of the vaccine virus not less than 10 times the maximum virus titre likely to be contained in 1 dose of the vaccine. Observe the chickens at least daily for 21 days. Carry out histological examination of the joints and tendon sheaths of the legs and feet at the end of the observation period (as a basis for comparison in the test for increase in virulence). The test is not valid if more than 10 per cent of the chickens die from causes not attributable to the vaccine virus. The vaccine virus complies with the test if no chicken shows notable clinical signs of avian viral tenosynovitis or dies from causes attributable to the vaccine virus.

2-4-2. **Increase in virulence**. The test for increase in virulence consists of the administration of the vaccine virus at the least attenuated passage level that will be present between the master seed lot and a batch of the vaccine to a group of five 1-day-old chicks from an SPF flock (*5.2.2*), sequential passages, 5 times where possible, to further groups of 1-day-old chicks and testing of the final recovered virus for increase in virulence. If the properties of the vaccine virus allow sequential passage to 5 groups via natural spreading, this method may be used, otherwise passage as described below is carried out and the maximally passaged virus that has been recovered is tested for increase in virulence. Care must be taken to avoid contamination by virus from previous passages. Administer by a suitable route a quantity of the vaccine virus that will allow recovery of virus for the passages described below. Kill the chickens at the moment when the virus concentration in the most suitable material (for example, tendons, tendon sheaths and liquid exudates from the hock joints, spleen) is sufficient. Prepare a suspension from this material from each chicken and pool these samples. Administer 0.1 ml of the pooled samples by the route of administration most likely to lead to increase in virulence to each of 5 other chickens of the same age and origin. Carry out this passage operation not fewer than 5 times; verify the presence of the virus at each passage. If the virus is not found at a passage level, carry out a second series of passages. Carry out the test for safety (section 2-4-1) using the unpassaged vaccine virus and the maximally passaged vaccine virus that has been recovered. The vaccine virus complies with the test if no indication of increase in virulence of the maximally passaged virus compared with the unpassaged virus is observed. If the virus is not recovered at any passage level in the first and second series of passages, the vaccine virus also complies with the test.

2-4-3. **Immunogenicity**. A test is carried out for each route and method of administration to be recommended using in each case chickens not older than the youngest age to be recommended for vaccination. The quantity of the vaccine virus administered to each chicken is not greater than the minimum virus titre to be stated on the label and the virus is at the most attenuated passage level that will be present in a batch of the vaccine. Use not fewer than 30 chickens of the same origin and from an SPF flock (*5.2.2*). Administer the vaccine by a recommended route to not fewer than 20 chickens. Maintain not fewer than 10 chickens as controls. Challenge each chicken after 21 days by a suitable route with a sufficient quantity of virulent avian tenosynovitis virus. Observe the chickens at least daily for 21 days after challenge. Record the deaths and the surviving chickens that show clinical signs of disease. If the challenge is administered by the foot pad, any transient swelling of the foot pad during the first 5 days after challenge may be considered non-specific. At the end of the observation period, kill all the surviving chickens and carry out macroscopic and/or microscopic examination for lesions of the joints and tendon sheaths of the legs and feet, e.g. exudate and swelling. The test is not valid if:

- during the observation period after challenge fewer than 80 per cent of the control chickens die or show severe clinical signs of avian viral tenosynovitis or show macroscopical and/or microscopical lesions in the joints and tendon sheaths of the legs and feet,
- or if during the period between vaccination and challenge more than 10 per cent of the control or vaccinated chickens show abnormal clinical signs or die from causes not attributable to the vaccine.

The vaccine virus complies with the test if during the observation period after challenge not fewer than 90 per cent of the vaccinated chickens survive and show no notable clinical signs of disease or show macroscopical and/or microscopical lesions in the joints and tendon sheaths of the legs and feet.

3. BATCH TESTS

3-1. **Identification**. Carry out an immunostaining test in cell cultures to identify the vaccine virus.

3-2. **Bacteria and fungi**

Vaccines intended for administration by injection comply with the test for sterility prescribed in the monograph *Vaccines for veterinary use (0062)*.

Vaccines not intended for administration by injection either comply with the test for sterility prescribed in the monograph *Vaccines for veterinary use (0062)* or with the following test: carry out a quantitative test for bacterial and fungal contamination; carry out identification tests for microorganisms detected in the vaccine; the vaccine does not contain pathogenic microorganisms and contains not more than 1 non-pathogenic microorganism per dose.

Any liquid supplied with the vaccine complies with the test for sterility prescribed in the monograph *Vaccines for veterinary use (0062)*.

3-3. **Mycoplasmas**. The vaccine complies with the test for mycoplasmas (*2.6.7*).

3-4. **Extraneous agents**. The vaccine complies with the tests for extraneous agents in batches of finished product (*2.6.25*).

3-5. **Safety**. Use not fewer than 10 chickens from an SPF flock (*5.2.2*) and of the youngest age recommended for vaccination. Administer by a recommended route and method to each chicken 10 doses of the vaccine. Observe the chickens at least daily for 21 days. The test is not valid if more than 20 per cent of the chickens show abnormal clinical signs or die from causes not attributable to the vaccine. The vaccine complies with the test if no chicken shows notable clinical signs of disease or dies from causes attributable to the vaccine.

3-6. **Virus titre**. Titrate the vaccine virus by inoculation into suitable cell cultures (*5.2.4*). The vaccine complies with the test if 1 dose contains not less than the minimum virus titre stated on the label.

3-7. **Potency**. The vaccine complies with the requirements of the test prescribed under Immunogenicity (section 2-4-3) when administered by a recommended route and method. It is not necessary to carry out the potency test for each batch of the vaccine if it has been carried out on a representative batch using a vaccinating dose containing not more than the minimum virus titre stated on the label.

01/2005:1939

BOVINE LEPTOSPIROSIS VACCINE (INACTIVATED)

Vaccinum leptospirosis bovinae inactivatum

DEFINITION

Bovine leptospirosis vaccine (inactivated) is a suspension of inactivated whole organisms and/or antigenic extract(s) of one or more suitable strains of one or more of *Leptospira borgpetersenii* serovar hardjo, *Leptospira interrogans* serovar hardjo or other *L. interrogans* serovars, inactivated and prepared in such a way that adequate immunogenicity is maintained. This monograph applies to vaccines intended for active immunisation of cattle against leptospirosis.

PRODUCTION

The seed material is cultured in a suitable medium; each strain is cultivated separately. During production, various parameters such as growth rate are monitored by suitable methods; the values are within the limits approved for the particular product. Purity and identity are verified on the harvest using suitable methods. After cultivation, the bacterial harvest is inactivated by a suitable method. The antigen may be concentrated. The vaccine may contain an adjuvant.

CHOICE OF VACCINE COMPOSITION

The vaccine is shown to be satisfactory with respect to safety (*5.2.6*) and efficacy (*5.2.7*) in cattle. As part of the studies to demonstrate the suitability of the vaccine with respect to these characteristics the following tests may be carried out.

Safety

A. The test is carried out for each route of administration to be stated on the label and in animals of each category (for example, young calves, pregnant cattle) for which the vaccine is intended. For each test, use not fewer than 10 animals that do not have antibodies against *L. borgpetersenii* serovar hardjo and the principal serovars of *L. interrogans* (icterohaemorrhagiae, canicola, grippotyphosa, sejroe, hardjo, hebdomonadis, pomona, australis and autumnalis). Use a batch of vaccine containing not less than the maximum potency that may be expected in a batch of vaccine. Administer to each animal a double dose of vaccine. If the recommended schedule requires a second dose, administer 1 dose after the recommended interval. Observe the animals for at least 14 days after the last administration. Record body temperatures the day before each vaccination, at vaccination, 4 h later and daily for 4 days. If the vaccine is intended for use or may be used in pregnant cattle, vaccinate the animals at the relevant stages of pregnancy and prolong the observation period until 1 day after calving. The vaccine complies with the test if no animal shows an abnormal local or systemic reaction or clinical signs of disease or dies from a cause attributable to the vaccine. In addition, if the vaccine is for use in pregnant animals, no adverse effects on the pregnancy and offspring are noted.

B. The animals used for the field trials are also used to evaluate safety. Use not fewer than 3 groups of 20 animals with corresponding groups of not fewer than 10 controls in 3 different locations. Examine the injection sites for local reactions after vaccination. Record body temperatures the day before vaccination, at vaccination and on the 2 days following vaccination. The vaccine complies with the test if no animal shows an abnormal local or systemic reaction or clinical signs of disease or dies from a cause attributable to the vaccine. In addition, if the vaccine is for use in pregnant animals, no adverse effects on the pregnancy and offspring are noted.

Immunogenicity. As part of the studies to demonstrate the suitability of the vaccine with respect to immunogenicity and in support of the claims for a beneficial effect on the rates of infection and urinary excretion, the test described under Potency may be carried out for each proposed route of administration, using vaccine of minimum potency. Urine samples are collected from each animal on days 0, 14, 21, 28 and 35 post-challenge. For leptospiral species other than *L. borgpetersenii* serovar hardjo, appropriate days are determined by the characteristics of the challenge model. In the case of other serovars for which there is published evidence that the serovar has a lower tropism for the urinary tract, a lower rate of infection may be justified. Depending on their tissue tropism, for some leptospira serovars, samples from other tissues/body fluids can be used to establish whether the animals are infected or not by the challenge organism. If claims are to be made for protection against reproductive or production losses, further specific studies will be required.

BATCH POTENCY TEST

The test described under Potency is not carried out for routine testing of batches of vaccine. It is carried out, for a given vaccine, on one or more occasions, as decided by or with the agreement of the competent authority; where the test is not carried out, a suitable validated test is carried out, the criteria for acceptance being set with reference to a batch of vaccine that has given satisfactory results in the test described under Potency. The following test may be used after a suitable correlation with the test described under Potency has been established.

For each of the serovars for which protection is claimed, the antibody response from vaccinated animals is measured. Use guinea pigs weighing 250-350 g which do not have antibodies to *L. borgpetersenii* serovar hardjo and the principal serovars of *L. interrogans* (icterohaemorrhagiae, canicola, grippotyphosa, sejroe, hardjo, hebdomonadis, pomona, australis and autumnalis) and which have been obtained from a regularly tested and certified leptospira-free source. The dose to be administered to the animals is that fraction of a cattle dose which has been shown in the validation studies to provide a suitably sensitive test. Vaccinate each of 10 animals with the suitable dose. Maintain not fewer than 2 guinea-pigs as unvaccinated controls. At a given interval within the range of 19 to 23 days after the injection, collect blood from each animal and prepare serum samples. Use a suitable validated method such as a micro-agglutination test to measure the antibody responses in each sample. The antibody levels are equal to or greater than those obtained with a batch that has given satisfactory results in the test described under Potency and there is no significant increase in antibody titre in the controls.

IDENTIFICATION

When injected into healthy seronegative animals, the vaccine stimulates the production of specific antibodies to the leptospira serovar(s) present in the vaccine.

TESTS

Safety. For vaccines recommended for use in cattle older than 6 months of age, use cattle not older than the minimum age recommended for vaccination and not younger than 6 months of age. For vaccines recommended for use in cattle less than 6 months of age, use cattle of the minimum age recommended for vaccination. Inject 2 doses of the vaccine into each of 2 cattle, free from specific antibodies to the leptospira serovar(s) present in the vaccine, by a recommended route. Observe the animals for 14 days. The animals remain in good health and no abnormal local or systemic reaction occurs.

Inactivation. Carry out a test for live leptospirae by inoculation of a specific medium. Inoculate 1 ml of the vaccine into 100 ml of the medium. Incubate at 30 °C for 14 days, subculture into a further quantity of the medium and incubate both media at 30 °C for 14 days: no growth occurs in either medium. At the same time, carry out a control test by inoculating a further quantity of the medium with the vaccine together with a quantity of a culture containing approximately 100 leptospirae and incubating at 30 °C: growth of leptospirae occurs within 14 days.

Sterility. The vaccine complies with the test for sterility prescribed in the monograph *Vaccines for veterinary use (0062)*.

POTENCY

Carry out a separate test for each of the serovars for which a claim is made for a beneficial effect on the rates of infection and urinary excretion.

Use not fewer than 15 cattle of the minimum age recommended for vaccination and free from specific antibodies against *L. borgpetersenii* serovar hardjo and the principal serovars of *L. interrogans* (icterohaemorrhagiae, canicola, grippotyphosa, sejroe, hardjo, hebdomonadis, pomona, australis and autumnalis). Vaccinate not fewer than 10 animals by a recommended route and according to the recommended schedule. Keep not fewer than 5 animals as controls. 21 days after the last vaccination, infect all the animals by a suitable mucosal route with a suitable quantity of a virulent strain of the relevant serovar. Observe the animals for a further 35 days. Collect urine samples from each animal on days 0, 14, 21, 28 and 35 post-challenge. Kill surviving animals at the end of the observation period. Carry out post-mortem examination on any animal that dies and on those killed at the end of the observation period. In particular, examine the kidneys for macroscopic and microscopic signs of leptospira infection. A sample of each kidney is collected and each urine and kidney sample is tested for the presence of the challenge organisms by re-isolation or by another suitable method.

For the test conducted with *L. borgpetersenii* serovar hardjo, control animals are regarded as infected if the challenge organisms are re-isolated from at least 2 samples. The test is invalid if infection has been established in fewer than 80 per cent of the control animals.

The vaccine complies with the requirements of the test if the challenge organisms are re-isolated from any urine or kidney sample from not more than 20 per cent of the vaccinated animals.

LABELLING

The label states:
– the serovar(s) used to prepare the vaccine,
– the serovar(s) against which protection is claimed.

01/2005:1176

BOVINE PARAINFLUENZA VIRUS VACCINE (LIVE), FREEZE-DRIED

Vaccinum parainfluenzae viri bovini vivum cryodesiccatum

DEFINITION

Freeze-dried bovine parainfluenza virus vaccine (live) is a preparation of a suitable strain of bovine parainfluenza 3 virus.

PRODUCTION

The vaccine strain is grown in suitable cell cultures (*5.2.4*). The viral suspension is harvested, mixed with a suitable stabilising liquid and freeze-dried.

CHOICE OF VACCINE STRAIN

Only a virus strain shown to be satisfactory with respect to reversion to virulence, safety and immunogenicity may be used in the preparation of the vaccine. The following tests may be used during demonstration of safety (*5.2.6*) and efficacy (*5.2.7*).

Reversion to virulence. Administer by the intranasal route to 2 susceptible calves that do not have antibodies against bovine parainfluenza virus 3 a quantity of virus that will allow optimal re-isolation of the virus for subsequent passages. On each of days 3 to 7 after administration of the virus, take nasal swabs from each calf and collect in not more than 5 ml of a suitable medium which is then used to inoculate cell cultures to verify the presence of virus; use about 1 ml of the suspensions from swabs that contain the maximum amount of virus, as indicated by the titration in cell cultures, to inoculate 2 other calves of the same age and sensitivity; repeat these operations until 5 passages on calves have been carried out. No calf shows clinical signs attributable to the vaccinal virus. No indication of increase of virulence, compared to the original vaccinal virus is observed; account is taken of the titre of excreted virus in the nasal swabs.

Safety. The test is carried out for each recommended route of administration. Use calves of the minimum age recommended for vaccination and preferably having no antibodies against bovine parainfluenza 3 virus or, where justified, use calves with a very low level of such antibodies as long as they have not been vaccinated against bovine parainfluenza virus and administration of the vaccine does not cause an anamnestic response. Administer to 5 calves a quantity of virus corresponding to not less than 10 times the maximum virus titre that may be expected in a batch of vaccine. Observe the animals for 21 days. Measure the body temperature of each animal on the day before vaccination, at the time of vaccination and for the 4 subsequent days. No abnormal effect on body temperature and no abnormal local or systemic reactions occur.

Immunogenicity. The test described under Potency is suitable to demonstrate immunogenicity of the vaccine strain.

BATCH TESTING

If the test for potency has been carried out with satisfactory results on a representative batch of vaccine, this test may be omitted as a routine control on other batches of vaccine prepared from the same seed lot, subject to agreement by the competent authority.

IDENTIFICATION

Carry out an immunofluorescence test in suitable cell cultures, using a monospecific antiserum.

TESTS

Safety. Use calves of the minimum age recommended for vaccination and preferably having no antibodies against bovine parainfluenza 3 virus or, where justified, use calves with a very low level of such antibodies as long as they have not been vaccinated against bovine parainfluenza virus and administration of the vaccine does not cause an anamnestic response. Administer 10 doses of the vaccine by a recommended route to each of 2 calves. Observe the animals for 21 days. No abnormal local or systemic reaction occurs.

Extraneous viruses. Neutralise the vaccine using a monospecific antiserum against bovine parainfluenza 3 virus and inoculate into cell cultures known to be sensitive to viruses pathogenic for cattle. Maintain these cultures for 14 days and make at least one passage during this period. No cytopathic effect develops; the cells show no evidence of the presence of haemadsorbing agents. Carry out a specific test for pestiviruses.

Bacterial and fungal contamination. The vaccine complies with the test for sterility prescribed under *Vaccines for veterinary use (0062)*.

Mycoplasmas (*2.6.7*). The vaccine complies with the test for mycoplasmas.

Virus titre. Titrate the vaccine in suitable cell cultures. One dose of the vaccine contains not less than the quantity of virus equivalent to the minimum virus titre stated on the label.

POTENCY

Use not fewer than 10 calves of the minimum age recommended for vaccination and that do not have antibodies against bovine parainfluenza 3 virus; calves having low levels of such antibodies may be used if it has been demonstrated that valid results are obtained in these conditions. Collect sera from the animals before vaccination, 7 days and 14 days after the time of vaccination and just before challenge. Vaccinate not fewer than 5 of the calves according to the instructions for use. Keep 5 calves as controls. Observe the animals for 21 days and then administer to each of them by a respiratory tract route a suitable quantity of a low-passage virulent strain of bovine parainfluenza 3 virus. Monitor each animal for clinical signs, in particular respiratory symptoms, and virus shedding (by nasal swabs or tracheobronchial washing) for 14 days after challenge. The vaccine complies with the test if in vaccinated animals compared to controls there is (a) a significant reduction in mean titre and in mean duration of virus excretion and (b) a notable reduction in general and local signs (if the challenge virus used produces such signs). The test is not valid if tests for antibodies against bovine parainfluenza 3 virus on the sera indicate that there was intercurrent infection with the virus during the test or if more than 2 of the 5 control animals show no excretion of the challenge virus, as shown by nasal swabs or samples harvested by tracheobronchial washing.

01/2005:1177

BOVINE RESPIRATORY SYNCYTIAL VIRUS VACCINE (LIVE), FREEZE-DRIED

Vaccinum viri syncytialis meatus spiritus bovini vivum cryodesiccatum

DEFINITION

Freeze-dried bovine respiratory syncytial virus vaccine (live) is a preparation of a suitable strain of bovine respiratory syncytial virus.

PRODUCTION

The vaccine strain is grown in suitable cell cultures (*5.2.4*). The viral suspension is harvested, mixed with a suitable stabilising solution and freeze-dried.

CHOICE OF VACCINE STRAIN

Only a virus strain shown to be satisfactory with respect to reversion to virulence, safety and immunogenicity may be used in the preparation of the vaccine. The following tests may be used during demonstration of safety (*5.2.6*) and efficacy (*5.2.7*).

Reversion to virulence. Administer by the intranasal route to two susceptible calves that do not have antibodies against bovine respiratory syncytial virus a quantity of virus that will allow optimal re-isolation of the virus for subsequent passages. On each of days 3 to 7 after administration of the virus, take nasal swabs from each calf and collect in not more than 5 ml of a suitable medium which is then used to inoculate cell cultures to verify the presence of virus; use about 1 ml of the suspensions from swabs that contain the maximum amount of virus, as indicated by the titration in cell cultures, to inoculate two other calves of the same age and sensitivity; repeat these operations until five passages on calves have been carried out. No calf shows clinical signs attributable to the vaccinal virus. No indication of increase of virulence compared to the original vaccinal virus is observed; account is taken of the titre of excreted virus in the nasal swabs.

Safety. Safety studies are conducted in calves of the minimum age for which the vaccine is recommended and for each recommended route of administration.

A. Administer by a recommended route to five calves, without antibodies against bovine respiratory syncytial virus, a quantity of virus corresponding to not less than ten times the maximum virus titre that may be expected in a batch of vaccine. Observe the animals for 21 days. Measure the rectal temperature of each animal on the day before vaccination, at the time of vaccination and daily for the following 7 days. No abnormal effect on body temperature and no abnormal local or systemic reaction are noted.

B. The animals used for the field trials are also used to evaluate the incidence of hypersensitivity reactions in vaccinated animals following subsequent exposure to the vaccine or to wild virus. The vaccine is satisfactory if it is not associated with an abnormal incidence of immediate hypersensitivity reactions.

Immunogenicity. The test described under Potency is suitable to demonstrate immunogenicity of the vaccine strain.

BATCH TESTING

If the test for potency has been carried out with satisfactory results on a representative batch of vaccine, this test may be omitted as a routine control on other batches of vaccine prepared from the same seed lot, subject to agreement by the competent authority.

IDENTIFICATION

Identify the vaccine by an immunofluorescence test in suitable cell cultures using a monospecific antiserum.

TESTS

Safety. Administer ten doses of the vaccine by a recommended route to each of two calves of the minimum age recommended for vaccination and that do not have antibodies against bovine respiratory syncytial virus. Observe the animals for 21 days. No abnormal local or systemic reaction occurs.

Extraneous viruses. Neutralise the vaccine using a monospecific antiserum against bovine respiratory syncytial virus and inoculate into cell cultures known to be sensitive to viruses pathogenic for cattle. Maintain the cultures for 14 days and make at least one passage during this period. No cytopathic effect develops; the cells show no evidence of the presence of haemadsorbing agents. Carry out a specific test for pestiviruses.

Bacterial and fungal contamination. The vaccine complies with the test for sterility prescribed under *Vaccines for veterinary use (0062)*.

Mycoplasmas (*2.6.7*). The vaccine complies with the test for mycoplasmas.

Virus titre. Titrate the vaccine in suitable cell cultures. One dose of the vaccine contains not less than the quantity of virus equivalent to the minimum titre stated on the label.

POTENCY

Use not fewer than ten calves of the minimum age recommended for vaccination and that do not have antibodies against bovine respiratory syncytial virus. Collect sera from the animals before the time of vaccination, 7 and 14 days after the time of vaccination and just before challenge. Vaccinate not fewer than five of the calves according to the instructions for use. Keep five calves as controls. Observe the animals for 21 days and then administer to each of them by a respiratory tract route a suitable quantity of a low-passage virulent strain of bovine respiratory syncytial virus. Monitor each animal for clinical signs, in particular respiratory symptoms, and virus shedding (by nasal swabs or tracheobronchial washing) for 14 days after challenge. The vaccine complies with the test if there is: (a) a significant reduction in mean titre and in mean duration of virus excretion in vaccinates compared to controls and (b) a notable reduction in general and local clinical signs in vaccinated animals (if the challenge virus used produces such signs). The test is not valid if antibodies to bovine respiratory syncytial virus are detected in any sample from control animals before challenge or if more than two of the five control animals show no excretion of the challenge virus, as shown by nasal swabs or samples harvested by tracheobronchial washing.

Vaccines

01/2005:1952

BOVINE VIRAL DIARRHOEA VACCINE (INACTIVATED)

Vaccinum diarrhoeae viralis bovinae inactivatum

DEFINITION

Bovine viral diarrhoea vaccine (inactivated) is a preparation of one or more suitable strains of bovine diarrhoea virus inactivated by a suitable method. This monograph applies to vaccines intended for vaccination of heifers and cows to protect the foetus against transplacental infection.

PRODUCTION

The vaccine virus strain or strains are grown in suitable cell cultures (*5.2.4*).

The test for inactivation is carried out using a quantity of virus equivalent to not less than 25 doses of vaccine in cells of the same type as those used for production of the vaccine or cells shown to be at least as sensitive; the cells are passaged after 7 days and observed for a total of not less than 14 days. No infectious virus is detected.

CHOICE OF VACCINE COMPOSITION

The vaccine shall be shown to be satisfactory with respect to safety (*5.2.6*) and immunogenicity (*5.2.7*) in cattle.

The following tests may be used during the demonstration of safety and immunogenicity.

Safety. Carry out a safety test for each recommended route and for each category of cattle for which the vaccine is intended. Use cattle of the minimum age recommended for vaccination and that are free from bovine diarrhoea virus and from antibodies against the virus. Inject a double dose of vaccine into each of not fewer than 10 animals. Observe the animals for 14 days. No abnormal local or systemic reaction occurs. If the vaccine is intended for administration to pregnant cattle, carry out the test in these animals at the beginning of each trimester for which use is not contra-indicated and extend the observation period to calving. No undesirable effect on gestation or the offspring occurs. If the vaccine is intended for administration shortly before or at insemination, absence of undesirable effects on conception rate must be demonstrated.

Immunogenicity. The test for potency is suitable to demonstrate the immunogenicity of the vaccine with respect to bovine diarrhoea virus of genotype 1; if protection against bovine diarrhoea virus of genotype 2 is claimed, an additional test, similar to that described under Potency, but using bovine diarrhoea virus of genotype 2 for challenge, is carried out.

BATCH POTENCY TEST

The test described under Potency is not carried out for routine testing of batches of vaccine. It is carried out for a given vaccine on one or more occasions as decided by or with the agreement of the competent authority. Where the test is not carried out, a suitable validated test is carried out, the criteria for acceptance being set with reference to a batch of vaccine that has given satisfactory results in the test described under Potency. The following test may be used after a satisfactory correlation with the test described under Potency has been established.

Inject subcutaneously a suitable dose of the vaccine into each of 5 suitable seronegative laboratory animals or calves. Keep 2 animals as controls. A second dose of vaccine may be administered after a suitable interval if this has been shown to provide a suitably discriminating test system. Collect blood samples before the first vaccination and at a given interval between 14 and 21 days after the last vaccination. Determine the antibody titres against bovine diarrhoea virus by seroneutralisation on suitable cell cultures. The test is invalid if the control animals show antibodies against bovine diarrhoea virus. The vaccine complies with the test if the level of antibodies is not lower than that found for a batch of vaccine that has given satisfactory results in the test described under Potency.

IDENTIFICATION

When administered to animals free from specific neutralising antibodies against bovine diarrhoea virus, the vaccine stimulates the production of such antibodies.

TESTS

Safety. Inject a double dose of the vaccine by a recommended route into each of 2 cattle not older than the minimum age recommended for vaccination and that are free from bovine diarrhoea virus and antibodies against the virus. Observe the animals for 14 days. No abnormal local or systemic reaction occurs.

Inactivation. Carry out a test for residual infectious bovine diarrhoea virus by inoculating not less than 10 doses onto cells known to be sensitive to bovine diarrhoea virus; passage the cells after 7 days and observe the second culture for not less than 7 days. No live virus is detected. If the vaccine contains an adjuvant, separate the adjuvant if possible from the liquid phase by a method that does not interfere with the detection of possible live virus.

Bacteria and fungi. The vaccine complies with the requirement for sterility prescribed in the monograph on *Vaccines for veterinary use (0062)*.

POTENCY

Use heifers free from bovine diarrhoea virus that do not have neutralising antibodies against bovine diarrhoea virus. Vaccinate not fewer than 13 animals using the recommended schedule. Keep not fewer than 7 heifers as non-vaccinated controls. Keep all the animals as one group. Inseminate the heifers. Take a blood sample from non-vaccinated heifers shortly before challenge. The test is discontinued if fewer than 10 vaccinated heifers or 5 non-vaccinated heifers are pregnant at the time of challenge. Between the 60th and 90th days of gestation, challenge the animals. For both test models described (observation until calving and harvest of foetuses at 28 days), challenge may be made by the intranasal inoculation of a suitable quantity of a non-cytopathic strain of bovine diarrhoea virus or alternatively, where the animals are observed until calving, challenge may be made by contact with a persistently viraemic animal. Observe the animals clinically from challenge either until the end of gestation or until harvest of foetuses after 28 days. If abortion occurs, examine the aborted foetus for bovine diarrhoea virus by suitable methods. If animals are observed until calving, immediately after birth and prior to ingestion of colostrum, examine all calves for viraemia and antibodies against bovine diarrhoea virus. If foetuses are harvested 28 days after challenge, examine the foetuses for bovine diarrhoea virus by suitable methods. Transplacental infection is considered to have occurred if virus is detected in foetal organs or in the blood of newborn calves or if antibodies are detected in precolostral sera of calves. The test is invalid if any of the non-vaccinated heifers have neutralising antibody before challenge or if transplacental infection fails to occur in more than 10 per cent of non-vaccinated heifers. The vaccine complies with the test if 90 per cent or more of the vaccinated animals are protected from transplacental infection.

01/2005 :0793

BRUCELLOSIS VACCINE (LIVE) (BRUCELLA MELITENSIS REV. 1 STRAIN), FREEZE-DRIED, FOR VETERINARY USE

Vaccinum brucellosis (Brucella melitensis stirpe Rev. 1) vivum cryodesiccatum ad usum veterinarium

DEFINITION

Brucellosis vaccine (live) (Brucella melitensis Rev. 1 strain), freeze-dried, for veterinary use is a freeze-dried suspension of live *Brucella melitensis* Rev. 1 strain. The vaccine contains not fewer than 0.5×10^9 and not more than 4×10^9 live bacteria per dose.

PRODUCTION

Brucella melitensis Rev. 1 strain is cultured in a suitable medium. The method of culture is such as to avoid bacterial dissociation and thus maintain the smooth characteristic of the culture. The bacteria are suspended in a buffer solution which may contain a suitable stabiliser. The suspension is distributed into containers and freeze-dried.

CHOICE OF VACCINE STRAIN

Only a vaccine strain shown to be satisfactory with respect to safety and immunogenicity may be used in the production of the vaccine. The following test may be used during demonstration of efficacy (*5.2.7*).

Immunogenicity. 40 ewe lambs, 4 to 5 months old, from a non-vaccinated flock free from brucellosis are used. For the challenge strain, a 24-hour culture of *Brucella melitensis* strain H38 in trypticase agar is used. A preliminary test using animals of the same breed and age as for the main test is carried out to determine the challenge dose, which is between 10^7 and 10^8 colony-forming units and is chosen so as to produce abortion in all non-vaccinated animals. Half the animals are vaccinated at 4 to 6 months of age, according to the recommended schedule and using the minimum recommended dose. Oestrus is synchronised in the 40 animals which are then inseminated at 10 to 12 months of age. A diagnosis of pregnancy is made on all animals 2 to 3 months after insemination and all non-gravid animals are excluded from the test. All gravid animals are challenged by conjunctival instillation of the challenge dose of *Brucella melitensis* strain H38. The occurrence of abortion is noted and aetiology confirmed by testing for the presence of the challenge strain in the aborted foetus and in the ewe (using selective media of Kuzdas and Morse or of Farrell). Tests for the presence of the challenge strain are carried out on each animal at lambing. Tests for the presence of the challenge strain in the prescapular and retromammary lymph nodes are carried out at slaughter of the animals 4 to 6 weeks after lambing. The test is not valid unless at least 70 per cent of non-vaccinated animals: show abortion caused by the challenge strain; show infection with the challenge strain at lambing; show infection of the prescapular and retromammary lymph nodes at slaughter. The vaccine complies with the test if: not more than 30 per cent of vaccinated animals show abortion caused by the challenge strain; the challenge strain is found in not more than 50 per cent of vaccinated animals at lambing; the challenge strain is found in not more than 40 per cent of vaccinated animals at slaughter.

IDENTIFICATION

Brucella melitensis present in the vaccine is identified by suitable morphological, serological and biochemical tests and by culture: Rev. 1 strain is inhibited by addition to the suitable culture medium of 3 µg of benzylpenicillin sodium per millilitre; the strain grows on agar containing 2.5 µg of streptomycin per millilitre.

TESTS

Safety. Use 2 sheep, 4 to 6 months old and having no antibodies against *B. melitensis*. Administer 1 dose of vaccine by a recommended route to each sheep. Observe the animals for 21 days. No abnormal local or systemic reaction occurs.

Determination of dissociation phase. Examine not fewer than 200 colonies by a suitable technique. The culture of the vaccine strain is seen to be in the smooth (S) phase. Not fewer than 95 per cent of the colonies are of the smooth type.

Extraneous micro-organisms. The reconstituted vaccine does not contain extraneous micro-organisms. Verify the absence of micro-organisms other than *Brucella melitensis* Rev. 1 strain as described in the test for sterility prescribed in the monograph on *Vaccines for veterinary use (0062)*.

Live bacteria. Make a count of live bacteria on a solid medium suitable for the culture of *Brucella melitensis* Rev. 1 strain. The vaccine contains not fewer than 0.5×10^9 and not more than 4×10^9 live bacteria per dose.

Fifty per cent persistence time. Inject subcutaneously a suspension containing 10^8 live bacteria of the vaccine to be examined into each of 32 female CD1 mice, aged 5 to 6 weeks. Kill the mice in groups of eight, selected at random, 3, 6, 9 and 12 weeks later. Remove the spleens and homogenise individually and aseptically in 10 volumes of *phosphate buffered saline pH 6.8 R*. Spread the suspension on plates containing a suitable culture medium, using 0.4 ml per plate and not fewer than 3 plates per spleen (lower limit of detection: 5 bacteria per spleen). Carry out in parallel a similar test using *Brucella melitensis Rev. 1 strain BRP* (reference strain). Calculate the 50 per cent persistence time by the usual statistical methods (*5.3*) for probit analysis. The 50 per cent persistence time for the vaccine strain does not differ significantly from that of the reference strain. For Rev. 1 strain, the 50 per cent persistence time and confidence limits ($P = 0.05$) are usually 7.9 ± 1.2 weeks.

STORAGE

Store at a temperature of 2 °C to 8 °C.

LABELLING

The label states:

- the number of *Brucella melitensis* Rev. 1 strain per dose,
- that the vaccine is intended for sheep and goats 4 to 6 months old,
- that the vaccine may be dangerous for man,
- that the vaccine is not to be used in pregnant or lactating animals,
- that the vaccine may be dangerous for cattle and that they are not to be kept in contact with vaccinated animals.

01/2005:1953

CALF CORONAVIRUS DIARRHOEA VACCINE (INACTIVATED)

Vaccinum inactivatum diarrhoeae vituli coronaviro illatae

DEFINITION

Calf coronavirus diarrhoea vaccine (inactivated) is a preparation of one or more suitable strains of bovine coronavirus, inactivated in such a manner that immunogenic properties are maintained. The vaccine is administered to the dam to aid in the control of coronavirus diarrhoea in offspring during the first few weeks of life.

PRODUCTION

Each virus strain is grown separately in suitable cell cultures (*5.2.4*). The viral suspensions of each strain are harvested separately and inactivated by a method that maintains immunogenicity. The viral suspensions may be purified and concentrated.

The test for inactivation is carried out using 2 passages in cell cultures of the same type as those used for production or in cells shown to be at least as sensitive. The quantity of virus used in the test is equivalent to not less than 10 doses of vaccine. No live virus is detected.

The vaccine may contain an adjuvant.

CHOICE OF VACCINE COMPOSITION

The vaccine is shown to be satisfactory with respect to safety (*5.2.6*) and efficacy (*5.2.7*) in the pregnant cow. The following tests may be used during demonstration of safety and immunogenicity.

Safety. Carry out the test for each proposed route of administration. Administer by a proposed route and at the proposed stage or stages of pregnancy, a double dose of vaccine to each of not fewer than 10 pregnant cows that have not been vaccinated against bovine coronavirus. After the proposed interval, inject 1 dose into each cow. After each injection, measure the body temperature on the day of the injection and on the 4 following days. Observe the cows until calving. No abnormal local or systemic reaction occurs; any effects on gestation and the offspring are noted.

Immunogenicity. The test described under Potency is suitable to demonstrate immunogenicity of the strain.

BATCH TESTING

Batch potency test. The test described under Potency is not carried out for routine testing of batches of vaccine. It is carried out, for a given vaccine, on one or more occasions, as decided by or with the agreement of the competent authority; where the test is not carried out, a suitable validated test is carried out, the criteria for acceptance being set with reference to a batch of vaccine that has given satisfactory results in the test described under Potency. The following test may be used after a suitable correlation with the test described under Potency has been established.

To obtain a valid assay, it may be necessary to carry out a test using several groups of animals, each receiving a different dose. For each dose required, carry out the test as follows. Vaccinate not fewer than 5 animals of a suitable species, free from specific antibodies against bovine coronavirus, using 1 injection of a suitable dose. Maintain not fewer than 2 animals as unvaccinated controls. Where the recommended schedule requires a booster injection to be given, a booster vaccination may also be given in this test provided it has been demonstrated that this will still provide a suitably sensitive test system. At a given interval not less than 14 days after the last injection, collect blood from each animal and prepare serum samples. Use a suitable validated test to measure the antibody response. The antibody level is not significantly less than that obtained with a batch that has given satisfactory results in the test described under Potency and there is no significant increase in antibody titre in the controls.

IDENTIFICATION

Injected into animals free from specific antibodies against bovine coronavirus, the vaccine stimulates the formation of such antibodies.

TESTS

Safety. Use cattle not less than 6 months old and preferably having no antibodies against bovine coronavirus or, where justified, use cattle with a low level of such antibodies as long as they have not been vaccinated against bovine coronavirus and administration of the vaccine does not cause an anamnestic response. Administer to each of 2 animals a double dose of vaccine by a recommended route. After 14 days, administer 1 dose to each animal. Observe the animals for 14 days. No abnormal local or systemic reaction occurs.

Inactivation. Carry out a test for residual infectious virus using 10 doses of vaccine and 2 passages in cell cultures of the same type as those used for production of the vaccine or other cell cultures of suitable sensitivity. No live virus is detected. If the vaccine contains an adjuvant which interferes with the test, separate it if possible from the liquid phase of the vaccine by a method that does not inactivate virus nor interfere in any other way with detection of live viruses.

Extraneous viruses. Carry out tests for antibodies on the cattle used for the safety test. Take a blood sample at the end of the second observation period. The vaccine does not stimulate the formation of antibodies against bovine herpes virus 1 (BHV1), bovine leukaemia virus (BLV) and bovine viral diarrhoea virus (BVDV).

Sterility. The vaccine complies with the test for sterility prescribed in the monograph on *Vaccines for veterinary use (0062)*.

POTENCY

Use not fewer than 15 pregnant cows, where possible having no antibodies against bovine coronavirus. Where such cows are not available, use cows that: have not been vaccinated against bovine coronavirus; come from a farm where there is no recent history of infection with bovine coronavirus; and have a low level of antibodies against bovine coronavirus, the levels being comparable in all animals. Vaccinate not fewer than 10 pregnant cows according to the recommended schedule. Keep not fewer than 5 pregnant cows as unvaccinated controls. Starting at calving, take the colostrum and then milk from each cow and keep it in suitable conditions. Determine individually the protective activity of the colostrum and milk from each cow using calves born from healthy cows, and which may be born by Caesarean section, and maintained in an environment where they are not exposed to infection by bovine coronavirus. Feed colostrum and then milk to each calf every 6 h or according to the recommended schedule. At 5-7 days after birth, challenge each calf by the oral administration of a suitable quantity of a virulent strain of bovine coronavirus. Observe the calves for 7 days. Note the incidence, severity and duration of diarrhoea and the duration and quantity of virus excretion. The vaccine complies with the test if there

Vaccines

is a significant reduction in diarrhoea and virus excretion in calves given colostrum and milk from vaccinated cows compared to those given colostrum and milk from controls.

LABELLING

The label states the recommended schedule for administering colostrum and milk, *post-partum*.

01/2005:1954

CALF ROTAVIRUS DIARRHOEA VACCINE (INACTIVATED)

Vaccinum inactivatum diarrhoeae vituli rotaviro illatae

DEFINITION

Calf rotavirus diarrhoea vaccine (inactivated) is a preparation of one or more suitable strains of bovine rotavirus, inactivated in such a manner that immunogenic properties are maintained. The vaccine is administered to the dam to aid in the control of rotavirus diarrhoea in offspring during the first few weeks of life.

PRODUCTION

Each virus strain is grown separately in suitable cell cultures (*5.2.4*). The viral suspensions of each strain are harvested separately and inactivated by a method that maintains immunogenicity. The viral suspensions may be purified and concentrated.

The test for inactivation is carried out using 2 passages in cell cultures of the same type as those used for production or in cells shown to be at least as sensitive. The quantity of virus used in the test is equivalent to not less than 100 doses of vaccine. No live virus is detected.

The vaccine may contain an adjuvant.

CHOICE OF VACCINE COMPOSITION

The vaccine is shown to be satisfactory with respect to safety (*5.2.6*) and efficacy (*5.2.7*) in the pregnant cow. The following tests may be used during demonstration of safety and immunogenicity.

Safety. Carry out the test for each proposed route of administration. Administer by a proposed route and at the proposed stage or stages of pregnancy, a double dose of vaccine to each of not fewer than 10 pregnant cows that have not been vaccinated against bovine rotavirus. After the proposed interval, inject 1 dose into each cow. After each injection, measure the body temperature on the day of the injection and on the 4 following days. Observe the cows until calving. No abnormal local or systemic reaction occurs; any effects on gestation and the offspring are noted.

Immunogenicity. The test described under Potency is suitable to demonstrate immunogenicity of the strain.

BATCH TESTING

Batch potency test. The test described under Potency is not carried out for routine testing of batches of vaccine. It is carried out, for a given vaccine, on one or more occasions, as decided by or with the agreement of the competent authority; where the test is not carried out, a suitable validated test is carried out, the criteria for acceptance being set with reference to a batch of vaccine that has given satisfactory results in the test described under Potency. The following test may be used after a suitable correlation with the test described under Potency has been established.

To obtain a valid assay, it may be necessary to carry out a test using several groups of animals, each receiving a different dose. For each dose required, carry out the test as follows. Vaccinate not fewer than 5 animals of a suitable species, free from specific antibodies against bovine rotavirus, using 1 injection of a suitable dose. Maintain not fewer than 2 animals as unvaccinated controls. Where the recommended schedule requires a booster injection to be given, a booster vaccination may also be given in this test provided it has been demonstrated that this will still provide a suitably sensitive test system. At a given interval not less than 14 days after the last injection, collect blood from each animal and prepare serum samples. Use a suitable validated test to measure the antibody response. The antibody level is not significantly less than that obtained with a batch that has given satisfactory results in the test described under Potency and there is no significant increase in antibody titre in the controls.

IDENTIFICATION

Injected into animals free from specific antibodies against bovine rotavirus, the vaccine stimulates the formation of such antibodies.

TESTS

Safety. Use cattle not less than 6 months old and preferably having no antibodies against bovine rotavirus or, where justified, use cattle with a low level of such antibodies as long as they have not been vaccinated against bovine rotavirus and administration of the vaccine does not cause an anamnestic response. Administer to each of 2 animals a double dose of vaccine by a recommended route. After 14 days, administer 1 dose to each animal. Observe the animals for 14 days. No abnormal local or systemic reaction occurs.

Inactivation. Carry out a test for residual infectious virus using 10 doses of vaccine and 2 passages in cell cultures of the same type as those used for production of the vaccine or other cell cultures of suitable sensitivity. No live virus is detected. If the vaccine contains an adjuvant which interferes with the test, separate it if possible from the liquid phase of the vaccine by a method that does not inactivate virus nor interfere in any other way with detection of live viruses.

Extraneous viruses. Carry out tests for antibodies on the cattle used for the safety test. Take a blood sample at the end of the second observation period. The vaccine does not stimulate the formation of antibodies against bovine herpes virus 1 (BHV 1), bovine leukaemia virus (BLV) and bovine viral diarrhoea virus (BVDV).

Sterility. The vaccine complies with the test for sterility prescribed in the monograph on *Vaccines for veterinary use (0062)*.

POTENCY

Use not fewer than 15 pregnant cows, where possible having no antibodies against bovine rotavirus. Where such cows are not available, use cows that: have not been vaccinated against bovine rotavirus; come from a farm where there is no recent history of infection with bovine rotavirus; and have a low level of antibodies against bovine rotavirus, the levels being comparable in all animals. Vaccinate not fewer than 10 pregnant cows according to the recommended schedule. Keep not fewer than 5 pregnant cows as unvaccinated controls. Starting at calving, take the colostrum and then milk from each cow and keep it in suitable conditions. Determine individually the protective activity of the colostrum and milk from each cow using calves born from healthy cows, and which may be born by Caesarean section, and maintained in an environment where they are not exposed to infection by bovine rotavirus. Feed colostrum and then milk to each calf every 6 h or according to the recommended schedule. At 5-7 days after birth, challenge each calf by the oral administration of a suitable quantity of a virulent strain of bovine rotavirus. Observe the calves for 7 days. Note the incidence, severity and duration of diarrhoea and the duration and quantity of virus excretion. The vaccine complies with the test if there is a significant reduction in diarrhoea and virus excretion in calves given colostrum and milk from vaccinated cows compared to those given colostrum and milk from controls.

LABELLING

The label states the recommended schedule for administering colostrum and milk, *post-partum*.

01/2005:1298

CANINE ADENOVIRUS VACCINE (INACTIVATED)

Vaccinum adenovirosis caninae inactivatum

DEFINITION

Canine adenovirus vaccine (inactivated) is a suspension of one or more suitable strains of canine adenovirus 1 (canine contagious hepatitis virus) and/or canine adenovirus 2, inactivated in such a way that adequate immunogenicity is maintained.

PRODUCTION

The test for inactivation is carried out using a quantity of virus equivalent to at least 10 doses of vaccine with 2 passages in cell cultures of the same type as those used for production or in cell cultures shown to be at least as sensitive. No live virus is detected.

The vaccine may contain an adjuvant.

CHOICE OF VACCINE COMPOSITION

The vaccine is shown to be satisfactory with respect to safety (*5.2.6*) and efficacy (*5.2.7*). The following tests may be used during demonstration of safety and immunogenicity.

Safety. Carry out the test for each recommended route of administration in animals of the minimum age recommended for vaccination. Use a batch of vaccine of the maximum potency likely to be attained.

Use for each test not fewer than 10 dogs that do not have antibodies against canine adenovirus 1 or 2. Administer to each dog a double dose of vaccine. If the recommended schedule requires a second dose, administer one dose after the recommended interval. Observe the dogs for 14 days after the last administration. No abnormal local or systemic reaction occurs.

If the vaccine is intended for use in pregnant bitches, vaccinate bitches at the stage of pregnancy or at different stages of pregnancy according to the recommended schedule. Prolong observation until 1 day after parturition. No abnormal local or systemic reaction occurs. No adverse effects on the pregnancy and offspring are noted.

Immunogenicity. For vaccines intended to protect against hepatitis, the test described under Potency is suitable for demonstration of immunogenicity. If the vaccine is indicated for protection against respiratory signs, a further test to demonstrate immunogenicity for this indication is also necessary.

BATCH TESTING

Batch potency test. The test described under Potency is not carried out for routine testing of batches of vaccine. It is carried out for a given vaccine on one or more occasions as decided by or with the agreement of the competent authority. Where the test is not carried out, a suitable validated alternative test is carried out, the criteria for acceptance being set with reference to a batch of vaccine that has given satisfactory results in the test described under Potency.

IDENTIFICATION

When injected into susceptible animals, the vaccine stimulates the formation of specific antibodies against the type or types of canine adenovirus stated on the label.

TESTS

Safety. Use dogs of the minimum age recommended for vaccination and preferably having no canine adenovirus-neutralising antibodies or, where justified, use dogs with a low level of such antibodies as long as they have not been vaccinated against canine adenovirus and administration of the vaccine does not cause an anamnestic response. Administer a double dose of vaccine by a recommended route to each of 2 dogs. Observe the dogs for 14 days. No abnormal local or systemic reaction occurs.

Inactivation. Carry out a test for residual infectious canine adenovirus using 10 doses of vaccine by inoculation into sensitive cell cultures; make a passage after 6-8 days and maintain the cultures for 14 days. No live virus is detected. If the vaccine contains an adjuvant, separate the adjuvant from the liquid phase by a method that does not inactivate or otherwise interfere with the detection of live virus.

Sterility. The vaccine complies with the test for sterility prescribed in the monograph on *Vaccines for veterinary use (0062)*.

POTENCY

Use 7 dogs of the minimum age recommended for vaccination and that do not have antibodies against canine adenovirus. Vaccinate 5 of the animals by a recommended route and according to the recommended schedule. Keep the other 2 dogs as controls. 21 days later inject intravenously into each of the 7 animals a quantity of a virulent strain of canine adenovirus sufficient to cause death or typical signs of the disease in a susceptible dog. Observe the animals for a further 21 days. Dogs displaying typical signs of serious infection with canine adenovirus are killed humanely to avoid unnecessary suffering. The test is invalid and must be repeated if one or both of the controls do not die from or display typical signs of serious infection with canine adenovirus. The vaccine complies with the test if the vaccinated animals remain in good health.

LABELLING

The label states the type or types of canine adenovirus present in the vaccine.

01/2005:1951

CANINE ADENOVIRUS VACCINE (LIVE)

Vaccinum adenovirosidis caninae vivum

DEFINITION

Canine adenovirus vaccine (live) is a preparation of 1 or more suitable strains of canine adenovirus 2. This monograph applies to vaccines intended for active immunisation of dogs against canine contagious hepatitis and/or respiratory disease caused by canine adenovirus.

Vaccines

PRODUCTION

The virus strain is propagated in suitable cell cultures (*5.2.4*). The viral suspension is harvested, titrated and may be mixed with a suitable stabilising solution. The vaccine may be freeze-dried.

CHOICE OF VACCINE STRAIN

The vaccine is shown to be satisfactory with respect to safety (*5.2.6*), absence of increase in virulence and immunogenicity (*5.2.7*). The following tests may be used during demonstration of safety, absence of increase in virulence and immunogenicity.

Safety. The test is carried out for each route of administration to be stated on the label. Use not fewer than 5 puppies of the minimum age recommended for vaccination and that do not have antibodies to canine adenovirus. Administer to each puppy by a recommended route a quantity of virus corresponding to not less than 10 times the maximum titre that may be expected in a dose of vaccine. Observe the dogs for 14 days. The puppies remain in good health and no abnormal local or systemic reaction occurs.

If the vaccine is intended for use or may be used in pregnant bitches, administer the virus to 5 bitches at the recommended stage or at a range of stages of pregnancy according to the recommended schedule. Prolong the observation period until 1 day after parturition. The bitches remain in good health and there is no abnormal local or systemic reaction. No adverse effects on the pregnancy or the offspring are noted.

Increase in virulence. Administer by a recommended route to each of 2 puppies, 5-7 weeks old and which do not have antibodies against canine adenovirus, a quantity of virus that will allow recovery of virus for the passages described below. Kill the puppies 4-6 days later. Remove from each puppy nasal and pharyngeal mucosa, tonsils, lung, spleen and, if they are likely to contain virus, liver and kidney. Pool the samples; administer by a suitable route, for example intranasally, 1 ml of the pooled organ suspension to each of 2 other puppies of the same age and susceptibility; carry out these operations at least 5 times; verify the presence of the virus at each passage by direct or indirect means. If the virus has disappeared, carry out a second series of passages. Inoculate virus from the highest recovered passage level to 5 puppies of the minimum age recommended for vaccination, observe for 14 days and compare the reactions that occur with those seen in the test for safety described above. There is no indication of an increase of virulence as compared with the non-passaged virus.

Immunogenicity. For vaccines intended to protect against hepatitis, test A described under Potency is suitable for demonstration of Immunogenicity. For vaccines intended to protect against respiratory signs, test B described under Potency is suitable for demonstration of immunogenicity.

BATCH TESTING

If the test for Potency has been carried out with satisfactory results on a representative batch of vaccine, this test may be omitted as a routine control on other batches of vaccine prepared from the same seed lot.

IDENTIFICATION

The vaccine mixed with monospecific antiserum against canine adenovirus 2 no longer infects susceptible cell cultures.

TESTS

Safety. Use 2 puppies not older than the minimum age recommended for vaccination and which do not have antibodies against canine adenovirus. Administer 10 doses of the vaccine to each dog by a recommended route. Observe for 14 days. The dogs remain in good health and no abnormal local or systemic reaction occurs.

Extraneous viruses. Mix the vaccine with a suitable monospecific antiserum against canine adenovirus 2 and inoculate into cell cultures known for their susceptibility to viruses pathogenic for the dog. Carry out a passage after 6-8 days and maintain the cultures for a total of 14 days. No cytopathic effect develops and the cells show no evidence of the presence of haemadsorbing agents.

Bacterial and fungal contamination. The vaccine, reconstituted if necessary, complies with the test for sterility prescribed in the monograph on *Vaccines fo veterinary use (0062)*.

Mycoplasmas (*2.6.7*). The vaccine, reconstituted if necessary, complies with the test for mycoplasmas.

Virus titre. Reconstitute the vaccine, if necessary, and titrate in suitable cell cultures. 1 dose of the vaccine contains not less than the quantity of virus equivalent to the minimum virus titre stated on the label.

POTENCY

Depending on the indications for the vaccine, it complies with test A and/or B for potency.

A. Use 7 puppies of the minimum age recommended for vaccination and that do not have antibodies against canine adenovirus. Vaccinate 5 of the animals by a recommended route and according to the recommended schedule. Keep the other 2 dogs as controls. 21 days later, inject intravenously into each of the 7 animals a quantity of a virulent strain of canine adenovirus 1 (canine contagious hepatitis virus) sufficient to cause death or typical signs of the disease in a susceptible dog. Observe the animals for a further 21 days. Dogs displaying typical signs of serious infection with canine adenovirus are killed humanely to avoid unnecessary suffering. The test is invalid and must be repeated if 1 or both of the controls do not die from or display typical signs of serious infection with canine adenovirus. The vaccine complies with the test if the vaccinated animals remain in good health showing no clinical signs except for a possible transient elevated rectal temperature.

B. Use 20 dogs of the minimum age recommended for vaccination and that do not have antibodies against canine adenovirus. Vaccinate 10 of the dogs by a recommended route and according to the recommended schedule. Keep the other 10 dogs as controls. 21 days later, administer intranasally to each of the 20 animals a quantity of a virulent strain of canine adenovirus 2 sufficient to cause typical signs of respiratory disease in a susceptible dog. Observe the animals daily for a further 10 days. Record the incidence of signs of respiratory and general disease in each dog (for example, sneezing, coughing, nasal and lachrymal discharge, loss of appetite). Collect nasal swabs or washings from each dog daily from days 2 to 10 after challenge and test these samples to determine the presence and titre of excreted virus. The vaccine complies with the test if there is a notable decrease in the incidence and severity of clinical signs and in virus excretion in vaccinates compared to controls.

01/2005:0448

CANINE DISTEMPER VACCINE (LIVE), FREEZE-DRIED

Vaccinum morbi Carrei vivum cryodesiccatum ad canem

DEFINITION

Freeze-dried canine distemper vaccine (live) is a preparation of a strain of distemper virus that is attenuated for dogs.

PRODUCTION

The virus is propagated in suitable cell cultures (*5.2.4*) or in fertilised hen eggs from flocks free from specified pathogens (*5.2.2*). The viral suspension is harvested, titrated and may be mixed with a suitable stabilising solution. The vaccine is then freeze-dried.

CHOICE OF VACCINE STRAIN

The vaccine strain is shown to be satisfactory with respect to safety (*5.2.6*), absence of increase in virulence and immunogenicity (*5.2.7*). The following tests may be used during demonstration of safety, absence of increase in virulence and immunogenicity.

Safety. The test is carried out for each recommended route of administration. Use five susceptible puppies of the minimum age recommended for vaccination and that do not have antibodies against canine distemper virus. Administer to each puppy by a recommended route a quantity of virus corresponding to not less than ten times the maximum titre that may be expected in a dose of vaccine. Observe the puppies for 42 days. The puppies remain in good health and there is no abnormal local or systemic reaction.

If the vaccine is intended for use in pregnant bitches, administer the virus to five bitches at the recommended stage of pregnancy or at a range of stages of pregnancy according to the recommended schedule. Prolong observation until 1 day after parturition. The dogs remain in good health and there is no abnormal local or systemic reaction. No adverse effects on the pregnancy or the offspring are noted.

Increase in virulence. Administer by a recommended route to each of two puppies, 5 to 7 weeks old and which do not have antibodies against canine distemper virus a quantity of virus corresponding to one dose of vaccine. Kill the puppies 5 to 10 days later, remove nasal mucosa, tonsils, thymus, spleen and the lungs and their local lymph nodes from each puppy and pool the samples; administer intranasally 1 ml of the pooled organ suspension to each of two other puppies of the same age and susceptibility; carry out these operations at least five times; verify the presence of the virus at each passage by direct or indirect means. If the virus has disappeared, carry out a second series of passages. Inoculate virus from the highest recovered passage level to puppies, observe for 42 days and compare any reactions that occur with those seen in the test for safety described above. There is no indication of an increase of virulence as compared with the non-passaged virus.

Immunogenicity. The test described under Potency may be used to demonstrate the immunogenicity of the strain.

BATCH TESTING

If the test for potency has been carried out with satisfactory results on a representative batch of vaccine, this test may be omitted as a routine control on other batches of vaccine prepared from the same seed lot.

IDENTIFICATION

The vaccine reconstituted as stated on the label and mixed with a monospecific distemper antiserum against canine distemper virus no longer provokes cytopathic effects in susceptible cell cultures.

TESTS

Safety. Use two puppies of the minimum age recommended for vaccination and which do not have antibodies against canine distemper virus. Administer ten doses of the vaccine to each dog by a recommended route. Observe for 14 days. The dogs remain in good health and no abnormal local or systemic reaction occurs.

Extraneous viruses. Mix the vaccine with a suitable monospecific antiserum against canine distemper virus and inoculate into cell cultures known for their susceptibility to viruses pathogenic for the dog. Carry out a passage after 6 to 8 days and maintain the cultures for 14 days. No cytopathic effect develops and the cells show no evidence of the presence of haemadsorbing agents.

Bacterial and fungal contamination. The reconstituted vaccine complies with the test for sterility prescribed under *Vaccines for veterinary use (0062)*.

Mycoplasmas (*2.6.7*). The reconstituted vaccine complies with the test for mycoplasmas.

Virus titre. Titrate the reconstituted vaccine in suitable cell cultures. One dose of the vaccine contains not less than the quantity of virus equivalent to the minimum virus titre stated on the label.

POTENCY

Use seven susceptible puppies, 8 to 16 weeks old and free from antibodies against canine distemper virus. Vaccinate five puppies according to the instructions for use. Keep the two other animals as controls. Observe all the animals for 21 days. Inject intravenously into each animal a quantity of canine distemper virus sufficient to cause in a susceptible dog death or typical signs of the disease. Observe the animals for a further 21 days. Dogs displaying typical signs of serious infection with canine distemper virus are killed humanely to avoid unnecessary suffering. The test is not valid and must be repeated if one or more of the control animals do not either die of distemper or display typical signs of serious infection. The vaccine complies with the test if the vaccinated animals remain in good health.

01/2005:0447

CANINE LEPTOSPIROSIS VACCINE (INACTIVATED)

Vaccinum leptospirosis caninae inactivatum

DEFINITION

Canine leptospirosis vaccine (inactivated) is a suspension of inactivated whole organisms and/or antigenic extract(s) of one or more suitable strains of one or more of *Leptospira interrogans* serovar canicola, serovar icterohaemorrhagiae or any other epidemiologically appropriate serovar, inactivated and prepared in such a way that adequate immunogenicity is maintained. This monograph applies to vaccines intended for active immunisation of dogs against leptospirosis.

PRODUCTION

The seed material is cultured in a suitable medium; each strain is cultivated separately. During production, various parameters such as growth rate are monitored by suitable methods; the values are within the limits approved for the particular product. Purity and identity are verified on the harvest using suitable methods. After cultivation, the bacterial harvests are collected separately and inactivated by a suitable method. The antigen may be concentrated. The vaccine may contain an adjuvant.

CHOICE OF VACCINE COMPOSITION

The vaccine is shown to be satisfactory with respect to safety (*5.2.6*) and efficacy (*5.2.7*) in dogs. As part of the studies to demonstrate the suitability of the vaccine with respect to these characteristics the following tests may be carried out.

Safety. The test is carried out for each route of administration to be stated on the label and in animals of each category for which the vaccine is intended. For each test, use not fewer than 10 dogs that do not have antibodies against the principal *L. interrogans* serovars (icterohaemorrhagiae, canicola, grippotyphosa, sejroe, hardjo, hebdomonadis, pomona, australis and autumnalis). Use a batch of vaccine containing not less than the maximum antigen content and/or potency that may be expected in a batch of vaccine. Administer to each animal a double dose of vaccine. If the recommended schedule requires a second dose, administer 1 dose after the recommended interval. Observe the animals for at least 14 days after the last administration. Record body temperatures the day before each vaccination, at vaccination, 4 h later and daily for 4 days. If the vaccine is intended for use or may be used in pregnant bitches, vaccinate the animals at the recommended stage of pregnancy or at a range of stages of pregnancy and prolong the observation period until 1 day after whelping. The vaccine complies with the test if no animal shows an abnormal local or systemic reaction or clinical signs of disease or dies from a cause attributable to the vaccine. In addition, if the vaccine is for use in pregnant animals, no adverse effects on the pregnancy and offspring are noted.

Immunogenicity. As part of the studies to demonstrate the suitability of the vaccine with respect to immunogenicity and compliance with the claims to be stated on the label, the test described under Potency may be carried out for each proposed route of administration and using vaccine of minimum antigen content and/or potency.

BATCH POTENCY TEST

The test described under Potency is not carried out for routine testing of batches of vaccine. It is carried out, for a given vaccine, on one or more occasions, as decided by or with the agreement of the competent authority. Where the test is not carried out, one of the following tests may be used.

A. For vaccines with or without adjuvants

If leptospira from more than 1 serovar (for example *L. interrogans* serovar canicola and serovar icterohaemorrhagiae) has been used to prepare the vaccine, carry out a batch potency test for each serovar against which protective immunity is claimed on the label. Inject 1/40 of the dose for dogs stated on the label subcutaneously into each of 5 healthy hamsters not more than 3 months old, which do not have antibodies to the principal serovars of *L. interrogans* (icterohaemorrhagiae, canicola, grippotyphosa, sejroe, hardjo, hebdomonadis, pomona, australis and autumnalis) and which have been obtained from a regularly tested and certified leptospira-free source. After 15-20 days, inoculate intraperitoneally into each of the vaccinated animals and into an equal number of non-vaccinated controls derived from the same certified leptospira-free source, a suitable quantity of a virulent culture of leptospirae of the serovar against which protective immunity is claimed on the label. The vaccine complies with the test if not fewer than 4 of the 5 control animals die showing typical signs of leptospira infection within 14 days of receiving the challenge suspension and if not fewer than 4 of the 5 vaccinated animals remain in good health for 14 days after the death of 4 control animals.

B. For vaccines with or without adjuvants

A suitable validated sero-response test may be carried out. Vaccinate each animal in a group of experimental animals with a suitable dose. Collect blood samples after a suitable, fixed time after vaccination. For each of the serovars present in the vaccine, an *in vitro* test is carried out on individual blood samples to determine the antibody response to one or more antigenic components which are indicators of protection and which are specific for that serovar. The criteria for acceptance are set with reference to a batch of vaccine that has given satisfactory results in the test described under Potency.

C. For vaccines without adjuvants

For each of the serovars present in the vaccine, a suitable validated *in vitro* test may be carried out to determine the content of one or more antigenic components which are indicators of protection and which are specific for that serovar. The criteria for acceptance are set with reference to a batch of vaccine that has given satisfactory results in the test described under Potency.

IDENTIFICATION

When injected into healthy seronegative animals, the vaccine stimulates the production of specific antibodies to the leptospira serovar(s) present in the vaccine. If test C is used for batch potency test, it also serves to identify the vaccine.

TESTS

Safety. Use 2 dogs of the minimum age recommended for vaccination and which do not have antibodies to the leptospira serovar(s) present in the vaccine. Administer 2 doses of the vaccine to each dog by a recommended route. Observe the animals for 14 days. The animals remain in good health and no abnormal local or systemic reaction occurs.

Inactivation. Carry out a test for live leptospirae by inoculation of a specific medium. Inoculate 1 ml of the vaccine into 100 ml of the medium. Incubate at 30 °C for 14 days, subculture into a further quantity of the medium and incubate both media at 30 °C for 14 days: no growth occurs in either medium. At the same time, carry out a control test by inoculating a further quantity of the medium with the vaccine together with a quantity of a culture containing approximately 100 leptospirae and incubating at 30 °C: growth of leptospirae occurs within 14 days.

Sterility. The vaccine complies with the test for sterility prescribed in the monograph *Vaccines for veterinary use (0062)*.

POTENCY

For each type of the serovars against which protective immunity is claimed on the label, carry out a separate test with a challenge strain representative of that serovar.

Use not fewer than 12 dogs of the minimum age recommended for vaccination and free from specific antibodies against the principal serovars of *L. interrogans* (icterohaemorrhagiae, canicola, grippotyphosa, sejroe, hardjo, hebdomonadis, pomona, australis and autumnalis). Vaccinate half of the animals by a recommended route and according to the recommended schedule. Keep the remaining animals as controls. 25-28 days after the last vaccination, infect all the animals by the conjunctival and/or intraperitoneal route with a suitable quantity of a virulent strain of the relevant *L. interrogans* serovar. Observe the animals for a further 28 days. Examine the dogs daily and record and score clinical signs observed post-challenge and any deaths that occur. If an animal shows marked signs of disease, it is killed. Monitor body temperatures each day for the first week after challenge. Collect blood samples from each animal on days 0, 2, 3, 4, 5, 8 and 11 post challenge. Collect urine samples from each animal on days 0, 3, 5, 8, 11, 14, 21 and 28 post challenge. Kill surviving animals at the end of the observation period. Carry out post-mortem examination on any animal that dies during the observation period and on the remainder when killed at the end of the observation period. In particular, examine the liver and kidneys for macroscopic and microscopic signs of leptospira infection. A sample of each kidney is collected and each blood, urine and kidney sample is tested for the presence of challenge organisms by re-isolation or by another suitable method. The blood samples are also analysed to detect biochemical and haematological changes indicative of infection and these are also scored.

The test is invalid if: samples give positive results on day 0; *L. interrogans* serovar challenge strain is re-isolated from or demonstrated by another suitable method to be present in fewer than 2 samples on fewer than 2 different days, to show infection has been established in fewer than 80 per cent of the control animals.

The vaccine complies with the test if: at least 80 per cent of the vaccinates show no more than mild signs of disease (for example, transient hyperthermia) and, depending on the *L. interrogans* serovar used for the challenge, one or more of the following is also shown:

- where the vaccine is intended to have a beneficial effect against clinical signs, the clinical scores and haematological and biochemical scores are statistically lower for the vaccinates than for the controls,
- where the vaccine is intended to have a beneficial effect against infection, the number of days that the organisms are detected in the blood is statistically lower for the vaccinates than for the controls,
- where the vaccine is intended to have a beneficial effect against urinary tract infection and excretion, the number of days that the organisms are detected in the urine and the number of kidney samples in which the organisms are detected is statistically lower for the vaccinates than for the controls.

LABELLING

The label states:

- the serovar(s) used to prepare the vaccine,
- the serovar(s) against which the protection is claimed.

01/2005:1955

CANINE PARAINFLUENZA VIRUS VACCINE (LIVE)

Vaccinum parainfluenzae viri canini vivum

DEFINITION

Canine parainfluenza virus vaccine (live) is a preparation of a suitable attenuated strain of canine parainfluenza virus for dogs. The vaccine is intended for the protection of dogs against respiratory signs of infection with parainfluenza virus of canine origin.

PRODUCTION

The virus is propagated in suitable cell cultures (*5.2.4*). The viral suspension is harvested, titrated and may be mixed with a suitable stabilising solution. The vaccine may be freeze-dried.

CHOICE OF VACCINE STRAIN

The vaccine is shown to be satisfactory with respect to safety, absence of increase in virulence and immunogenicity. The following tests may be used during demonstration of safety (*5.2.6*), absence of increase in virulence and immunogenicity (*5.2.7*).

Safety. The test is carried out for each route of administration stated on the label. Use not fewer than 5 susceptible puppies of the recommended minimum age for vaccination and that do not have antibodies against parainfluenza virus of canine origin. Administer to each puppy by a recommended route a quantity of virus corresponding to not less than 10 times the maximum titre that may be expected in a dose of vaccine. Observe the puppies for 21 days. The puppies remain in good health and there is no abnormal local or systemic reaction.

If the vaccine is intended for use in pregnant bitches, administer the virus to not fewer than 5 bitches at the recommended stage or stages of pregnancy and according to the recommended schedule. Prolong the observation period until 1 day after whelping. The dogs remain in good health and there is no abnormal local or systemic reaction. No adverse effects on the pregnancy or the offspring are noted.

Increase in virulence. Administer intranasally and by a recommended route to each of 2 puppies, 5 to 7 weeks old and which do not have antibodies against parainfluenza virus of canine origin, a quantity of virus that will allow recovery of virus for the passages described below. Use vaccine virus at the least attenuated passage level that will be present in a batch of the vaccine. Collect nasal swabs from each dog daily from 3 to 10 days after inoculation. Inoculate the suspension from the swabs into suitable cell cultures to verify the presence of virus. Use the suspension from the swabs that contain the maximum amount of virus and administer intranasally 1 ml of the suspension into each of 2 other puppies of the same age and susceptibility. This operation is then repeated at least 5 times. If the virus is not recovered at a given passage level, a second series of passages is carried out. Inoculate virus from the highest recovered passage level to not fewer than 5 puppies, observe for 21 days and compare any reactions that occur with those seen in the test for safety described above. There is no indication of an increase in virulence as compared with the non-passaged virus.

Immunogenicity. The test described under Potency is suitable to demonstrate the immunogenicity of the strain.

BATCH TESTING

If the test for potency has been carried out with satisfactory results on a representative batch of vaccine, this test may be omitted as a routine control on other batches of vaccine prepared from the same seed lot.

IDENTIFICATION

Carry out an immunofluorescence test in suitable cell cultures, using a monospecific antiserum.

TESTS

Safety. Use 2 puppies not older than the minimum age recommended for vaccination and which do not have antibodies against parainfluenza virus of canine origin. Administer a volume containing 10 doses of the vaccine into each puppy by a recommended route. Observe for 14 days. The puppies remain in good health and no abnormal local or systemic reaction occurs.

Extraneous viruses. Neutralise the vaccine virus using a monospecific antiserum and inoculate into cell cultures known for their susceptibility to viruses pathogenic for the dog. Carry out a passage after 6 to 8 days and maintain the cultures for a total of 14 days. No cytopathic effect develops and the cells show no evidence of the presence of haemadsorbing agents.

Bacterial and fungal contamination. The vaccine, reconstituted if necessary, complies with the test for sterility prescribed in the monograph on *Vaccines for veterinary use (0062)*.

Mycoplasmas (*2.6.7*). The vaccine, reconstituted if necessary, complies with the test for mycoplasmas.

Virus titre. Reconstitute the vaccine, if necessary, and titrate in suitable cell cultures. 1 dose of the vaccine contains not less than the quantity of virus equivalent to the minimum virus titre stated on the label.

POTENCY

Use not fewer than 15 susceptible puppies of the minimum age recommended for vaccination and which do not have antibodies against parainfluenza virus of canine origin. Vaccinate not fewer than 10 of the puppies according to the instructions for use. Keep not fewer than 5 other puppies as controls. Observe all the animals for not less than 21 days after the last vaccination. Administer by the intratracheal or intranasal route to each animal a quantity of a virulent strain of parainfluenza virus of canine origin sufficient to establish infection with the virus in a susceptible dog. Observe the animals for a further 14 days. Collect nasal swabs or washings from each dog daily from day 2 to 10 after challenge and test these samples for the presence of excreted virus. Use a scoring system to record the incidence of coughing in each dog. The test is not valid if more than 1 of the control animals shows neither coughing nor the excretion of the challenge virus. The vaccine complies with the test if the scores for coughing or virus excretion for the vaccinated animals are significantly lower than in the controls.

01/2005:0795

CANINE PARVOVIROSIS VACCINE (INACTIVATED)

Vaccinum parvovirosis caninae inactivatum

DEFINITION

Inactivated canine parvovirosis vaccine is a liquid or freeze-dried preparation of canine parvovirus inactivated by a suitable method.

PRODUCTION

The virus is propagated in suitable cell cultures (*5.2.4*). The virus may be purified and concentrated.

A test for residual live virus is carried out on the bulk harvest of each batch to confirm inactivation of the canine parvovirus. The quantity of inactivated virus used in the test is equivalent to not less than 100 doses of the vaccine. The vaccine is inoculated into suitable non-confluent cells; after incubation for 8 days, a subculture is made using trypsinised cells. After incubation for a further 8 days, the cultures are examined for residual live parvovirus by an immunofluorescence test. The immunofluorescence test may be supplemented by a haemagglutination test or other suitable tests on the supernatant of the cell cultures. No live virus is detected.

The vaccine may contain an adjuvant or adjuvants.

CHOICE OF VACCINE COMPOSITION

The vaccine is shown to be satisfactory with respect to safety and immunogenicity in dogs. The following test may be used in the demonstration of efficacy (*5.2.7*).

Immunogenicity. 7 susceptible dogs of the minimum age recommended for vaccination are used. A blood sample is drawn from each dog and tested individually for antibodies against canine parvovirus to determine susceptibility. 5 dogs are vaccinated according to the recommended schedule. 2 dogs are kept as controls. 20 to 22 days after the last vaccination each of the dogs receives by the oronasal route a suspension of pathogenic canine parvovirus. The dogs are observed for 14 days. Haemagglutination tests are carried out to detect virus in the faeces. The test is not valid unless the 2 control dogs show typical signs of the disease or leucopenia and excretion of the virus. The vaccine complies with the test if the 5 vaccinated dogs remain in excellent health and show no sign of the disease nor leucopenia and if the maximum titre of virus excreted in the faeces is less than 1/100 of the geometric mean of the maximum titres found in the controls.

IDENTIFICATION

When injected into dogs, the vaccine stimulates the production of antibodies against canine parvovirus.

TESTS

Safety. Use dogs of the minimum age recommended for vaccination and preferably having no canine parvovirus antibodies or, where justified, use dogs with a low level of such antibodies as long as they have not been vaccinated against canine parvovirus and administration of the vaccine does not cause an anamnestic response. Administer a double dose of vaccine by a recommended route to each of 2 dogs. Observe the animals for 14 days. No abnormal local or systemic reaction occurs.

Sterility. The vaccine complies with the test for sterility prescribed in the monograph on *Vaccines for veterinary use (0062)*.

POTENCY

Carry out test A or test B.

A. Inject subcutaneously into each of 5 guinea-pigs, free from specific antibodies, half of the dose stated on the label. After 14 days, inject again half of the dose stated on the label. 14 days later, collect blood samples and separate the serum. Inactivate each serum by heating at 56 °C for 30 min. To 1 volume of each serum add 9 volumes of a 200 g/l suspension of *light kaolin R* in *phosphate buffered saline pH 7.4 R*. Shake each mixture for 20 min. Centrifuge, collect the supernatant liquid and mix with 1 volume of a concentrated suspension of pig erythrocytes. Allow to stand at 4 °C for 60 min and centrifuge. The dilution of the serum obtained is 1:10. Using each serum, prepare a series of twofold dilutions. To 0.025 ml of each of the latter dilutions add 0.025 ml of a suspension of canine parvovirus antigen containing 4 haemagglutinating units. Allow to stand at 37 °C for 30 min and add 0.05 ml of a suspension of pig erythrocytes containing 30×10^6 cells per millilitre. Allow to stand at 4 °C for 90 min and note the last dilution of serum that still completely inhibits haemagglutination.

Vaccines

The vaccine complies with the test if the median antibody titre of the sera collected after the second vaccination is not less than 1/80.

B. Vaccinate, according to the schedule stated on the label, 2 healthy susceptible dogs, 8 to 12 weeks old and having antibody titres less than 4 ND_{50} (50 per cent neutralising dose) per 0.1 ml of serum measured by the method described below. 14 days after vaccination, examine the serum of each animal as follows. Heat the serum at 56 °C for 30 min and prepare serial dilutions using a medium suitable for canine cells. Add to each dilution an equal volume of a virus suspension containing an amount of virus such that when the volume of serum-virus mixture appropriate for the assay system is inoculated into cell cultures, each culture receives approximately 10^4 $CCID_{50}$. Incubate the mixtures at 37 °C for 1 h and inoculate 4 canine cell cultures with a suitable volume of each mixture. Incubate the cell cultures at 37 °C for 7 days, passage and incubate for a further 7 days. Examine the cultures for evidence of specific cytopathic effects and calculate the antibody titre. The vaccine complies with the test if the mean titre is not less than 32 ND_{50} per 0.1 ml of serum. If one dog fails to respond, repeat the test using 2 more dogs and calculate the result as the mean of the titres obtained from all of the 3 dogs that have responded.

01/2005:0964

CANINE PARVOVIROSIS VACCINE (LIVE)

Vaccinum parvovirosis caninae vivum

DEFINITION

Canine parvovirosis vaccine (live) is a preparation of a strain of canine parvovirus that is attenuated for the dog.

PRODUCTION

The attenuated virus is grown in suitable cell cultures (*5.2.4*). The viral suspension is harvested, titrated and mixed with a suitable stabilising solution. The vaccine may be freeze-dried.

CHOICE OF VACCINE STRAIN

Only a virus strain shown to be satisfactory with respect to safety, irreversibility of attenuation, and immunogenicity may be used in the preparation of the vaccine. The following tests are used in the demonstration of safety (*5.2.6*) and efficacy (*5.2.7*).

Safety. Each test is carried out for each recommended route of administration.

5 susceptible puppies of the minimum age recommended for vaccination and having no haemagglutination-inhibiting antibodies against canine parvovirus are used for the test. A count of white blood cells in circulating blood is made on days 4, 2 and 0 before injection of the vaccine strain. Each puppy receives by a recommended route a quantity of virus corresponding to not less than 10 times the maximum virus titre that may be expected in a batch of vaccine and at the lowest passage level. The puppies are observed for 21 days. A count of white blood cells in circulating blood is made on days 3, 5, 7 and 10 after the injection. The puppies remain in good health and there is no abnormal local or systemic reaction. Any diminution in the number of circulating white blood cells is not greater than 50 per cent of the initial number determined as the average of the 3 values found before injection of the vaccine strain.

A quantity of virus corresponding to not less than 10 times the maximum titre that may be expected in a batch of vaccine and at the lowest passage level is administered by one of the recommended routes to each of 5 susceptible puppies. Five puppies are kept as controls. 2 puppies from each group are killed at 14 days and the 3 remaining puppies from each group at 21 days and histological examination of the thymus of each animal is carried out. Slight hypoplasia of the thymus may be evident after 14 days. The strain is not acceptable if damage is evident after 21 days.

Irreversibility of attenuation. Use 2 susceptible puppies of the minimum age recommended for vaccination and which do not have haemagglutination-inhibiting antibodies against canine parvovirus. Administer to each puppy, by a recommended route, a quantity of virus corresponding to 10 times the maximum titre that may be expected in a batch of vaccine. From the second to the tenth day after administration of the virus, the faeces are collected from each puppy and checked for the presence of the virus; faeces containing virus are pooled. 1 ml of the suspension of pooled faeces is administered by the oronasal route to each of 2 other puppies of the same age and susceptibility; this operation is carried out 4 times. The presence of virus is verified at each passage. If the virus is not found, a second identification of passages is carried out; if the virus is not found in one of the second identification of passages, the vaccine strain complies with the test. No puppy dies or shows signs attributable to the vaccine. No indication of increase of virulence compared to the original vaccinal virus is observed; account is taken, notably, of the count of white blood cells, of results of histological examination of the thymus and of the titre of excreted virus.

Immunogenicity. The test described under Potency is suitable to demonstrate immunogenicity of the strain.

BATCH TESTING

If the test for potency has been carried out with satisfactory results on a representative batch of vaccine, this test may be omitted as a routine control on other batches of vaccine prepared from the same seed lot, subject to agreement by the competent authority.

IDENTIFICATION

The vaccine is grown in a susceptible cell line in a substrate suitable for presenting for fluorescent antibody or immunoperoxidase tests. Suitable controls are included. A proportion of the cells is tested with a monoclonal antibody specific for canine parvovirus and a proportion of the cells tested with a monoclonal antibody specific for feline parvovirus. Canine parvovirus antigen is detected but no feline parvovirus is detected in the cells inoculated with the vaccine.

TESTS

Safety. Use 2 dogs of the minimum age recommended for vaccination and having no haemagglutination-inhibiting antibodies against canine parvovirus. Administer 10 doses of the vaccine to each dog by a recommended route. Observe for 14 days. No abnormal local or systemic reaction occurs.

Extraneous viruses. Mix the vaccine with a suitable antiserum against canine parvovirus and inoculate into cell cultures known for their susceptibility to viruses pathogenic for the dog. No cytopathic effect develops. There is no sign of haemagglutinating or haemadsorbing agents and no other sign of the presence of extraneous viruses.

Bacterial and fungal contamination. The vaccine, reconstituted if necessary, complies with the test for sterility prescribed in the monograph on *Vaccines for veterinary use (0062)*.

Mycoplasmas (*2.6.7*). The vaccine, reconstituted if necessary, complies with the test for mycoplasmas.

Virus titre. Reconstitute the vaccine, if necessary, as stated on the label and titrate in suitable cell cultures. One dose of the vaccine contains not less than the quantity of virus equivalent to the minimum virus titre stated on the label.

POTENCY

Use 7 susceptible puppies of the minimum age recommended for vaccination and which do not have haemagglutination-inhibiting antibodies against canine parvovirus. Keep 2 of the puppies as controls and to each of the others inject by a recommended route the quantity of virus equivalent to the minimum titre stated on the label. Observe all the puppies for 20 to 22 days and then inoculate to each of them by the oronasal route a suspension of virulent canine parvovirus. Observe all the animals for 14 days. Carry out a haemagglutination test for the virus in the faeces. The test is not valid unless the 2 control puppies show typical signs of the disease and/or leucopenia and excretion of the virus. The vaccine complies with the test if the 5 vaccinated puppies remain in excellent health and show no sign of the disease nor leucopenia and if the maximum titre of virus excreted in the faeces is less than 1/100 of the geometric mean of the maximum titres found in the controls.

01/2005:0360

CLOSTRIDIUM BOTULINUM VACCINE FOR VETERINARY USE

Vaccinum clostridii botulini ad usum veterinarium

DEFINITION

Clostridium botulinum vaccine for veterinary use is prepared from a culture in liquid medium of *Clostridium botulinum* type C or type D or a mixture of these types. The whole culture or its filtrate or a mixture of the two is inactivated in such a manner that toxicity is eliminated and immunogenic activity is retained.

The preparation may be adsorbed, precipitated or concentrated. It may be treated with a suitable adjuvant and may be freeze-dried.

The identification, the tests and the determination of potency apply to the liquid preparation and to the freeze-dried preparation reconstituted as stated on the label.

IDENTIFICATION

When injected into a healthy susceptible animal, the vaccine provokes the formation of specific antibodies against the type or types of *C. botulinum* from which the vaccine was prepared.

TESTS

Safety. Use 2 animals of one of the species for which the vaccine is intended and that have not been vaccinated against *C. botulinum*. Administer to each animal, by a recommended route, twice the maximum dose stated on the label. Observe the animals for 7 days. No abnormal local or systemic reaction occurs.

Residual toxicity. Inject 0.5 ml of the vaccine subcutaneously into each of 5 mice, each weighing 17 g to 22 g. Observe the animals for 7 days. No abnormal local or systemic reaction occurs.

Sterility. It complies with the test for sterility prescribed in the monograph on *Vaccines for veterinary use (0062)*.

POTENCY

Use healthy white mice from a uniform stock, each weighing 18 g to 20 g. Use as challenge dose a quantity of a toxin of *C. botulinum* of the same type as that used in the preparation of the vaccine corresponding to 25 times the paralytic dose 50 per cent, a paralytic dose 50 per cent being the quantity of toxin which, when injected intraperitoneally into mice, causes paralysis in 50 per cent of the animals within an observation period of 7 days. If 2 types of *C. botulinum* have been used in the preparation of the vaccine, carry out the potency determination for each. Dilute the vaccine to be examined 1 in 8 using a 9 g/l solution of *sodium chloride R*. Inject 0.2 ml of the dilution subcutaneously into each of 20 mice. After 21 days, inject the challenge dose intraperitoneally into each of the vaccinated mice and into each of 10 control mice. Observe the mice for 7 days and record the number of animals which show signs of botulism. All the control mice show signs of botulism during the observation period. The vaccine passes the test if not fewer than 80 per cent of the vaccinated mice are protected.

LABELLING

The label states:

- the type or types of *C. botulinum* from which the vaccine has been prepared,
- whether the preparation is a toxoid or a vaccine prepared from a whole inactivated culture or a mixture of the two,
- that the preparation be shaken before use.

01/2005:0361

CLOSTRIDIUM CHAUVOEI VACCINE FOR VETERINARY USE

Vaccinum clostridii chauvoei ad usum veterinarium

DEFINITION

Clostridium chauvoei vaccine for veterinary use is prepared from a culture in liquid medium of one or more suitable strains of *Clostridium chauvoei*. The whole culture is inactivated in such a manner that toxicity is eliminated and immunogenic activity is retained. Inactivated cultures may be treated with a suitable adjuvant.

IDENTIFICATION

The vaccine protects susceptible animals against infection with *C. chauvoei*.

TESTS

Safety. Use 2 animals of one of the species for which the vaccine is intended and that have not been vaccinated against *C. chauvoei*. Administer to each animal at a single site, by a recommended route, twice the maximum dose stated on the label. Observe the animals for 7 days. No abnormal local or systemic reaction occurs.

Sterility. It complies with the test for sterility prescribed in the monograph on *Vaccines for veterinary use (0062)*.

POTENCY

Inject subcutaneously into not fewer than 10 healthy guinea-pigs, each weighing 350 g to 450 g, a quantity of the vaccine not exceeding the minimum dose stated on the label as the first dose. After 28 days, inject into the same animals a quantity of the vaccine not exceeding the minimum dose stated on the label as the second dose. 14 days after the second vaccination, inoculate intramuscularly into each

Vaccines

of the vaccinated guinea-pigs and into each of 5 control animals a suitable quantity of a virulent culture, or of a spore suspension, of *C. chauvoei*, activated if necessary with an activating agent such as calcium chloride. The vaccine complies with the test if not more than 10 per cent of the vaccinated guinea-pigs die from *C. chauvoei* infection within 5 days and all the control animals die from *C. chauvoei* infection within 48 h of challenge or within 72 h if a spore suspension was used for the challenge. If more than 10 per cent but not more than 20 per cent of the vaccinated animals die, repeat the test. The vaccine complies with the test if not more than 10 per cent of the second group of vaccinated animals die within 5 days and all of the second group of control animals die within 48 h of challenge or within 72 h if a spore suspension was used for the challenge. To avoid unnecessary suffering following virulent challenge, moribund animals are killed and are then considered to have died from *C. chauvoei* infection.

LABELLING

The label states that the preparation is to be shaken before use.

01/2005:0362
corrected

CLOSTRIDIUM NOVYI (TYPE B) VACCINE FOR VETERINARY USE

Vaccinum clostridii novyi B ad usum veterinarium

DEFINITION

Clostridium novyi (type B) vaccine for veterinary use is prepared from a liquid culture of a suitable strain of *Clostridium novyi* (type B).

PRODUCTION

The whole culture or its filtrate or a mixture of the two is inactivated in such a manner that toxicity is eliminated and immunogenic activity is retained. Toxoids and/or inactivated cultures may be treated with a suitable adjuvant, after concentration if necessary.

CHOICE OF VACCINE COMPOSITION

The vaccine is shown to be satisfactory with respect to safety (*5.2.6*) and efficacy (*5.2.7*). For the latter, it shall be demonstrated that for each target species the vaccine, when administered according to the recommended schedule, stimulates an immune response (for example, induction of antibodies) consistent with the claims made for the product.

BATCH TESTING

Residual toxicity. The test for residual toxicity may be omitted by the manufacturer, since a test for detoxification is carried out immediately after the detoxification process and, when there is risk of reversion, a second test is carried out at as late a stage as possible during the production process.

Batch potency test. The test described under Potency is not necessarily carried out for routine testing of batches of vaccine. It is carried out for a given vaccine on one or more occasions as decided by or with the agreement of the competent authority. Where the test is not carried out, a suitable validated alternative test is carried out, the criteria for acceptance being set with reference to a batch of vaccine that has given satisfactory results in the test described under Potency and that has been shown to be satisfactory with respect to immunogenicity in the target species. The following test may be used after a satisfactory correlation with the test described under Potency has been established.

Vaccinate rabbits as described under Potency and prepare sera. Determine the level of antibodies against the alpha toxin of *C. novyi* in the individual sera by a suitable method such as an immunochemical method (*2.7.1*) or neutralisation in cell cultures. Use a homologous reference serum calibrated in International Units of *C. novyi* alpha antitoxin. *Clostridia (multicomponent) rabbit antiserum BRP* is suitable for use as a reference serum. The vaccine complies with the test if the level of antibodies is not less than that found for a batch of vaccine that has given satisfactory results in the test described under Potency and that has been shown to be satisfactory with respect to immunogenicity in the target species.

IDENTIFICATION

The vaccine stimulates the formation of novyi alpha antitoxin when injected into animals that do not have this antitoxin.

TESTS

Safety. Administer by a recommended route, to each of 2 sheep that have not been vaccinated against *C. novyi* (type B) twice the maximum dose of the vaccine stated on the label. Observe the animals for not less than 14 days. No abnormal local or systemic reaction occurs.

Residual toxicity. Inject 0.5 ml of the vaccine subcutaneously into each of 5 mice, each weighing 17 g to 22 g. Observe the animals for 7 days. No abnormal local or systemic reaction occurs.

Sterility. It complies with the test for sterility prescribed in the monograph on *Vaccines for veterinary use (0062)*.

POTENCY

Inject subcutaneously into each of not fewer than 10 healthy rabbits, 3 to 6 months old, a quantity of vaccine not exceeding the minimum dose stated on the label as the first dose. After 21 to 28 days, inject into the same animals a quantity of the vaccine not exceeding the minimum dose stated on the label as the second dose. 10 to 14 days after the second injection, bleed the rabbits and pool the sera. The potency of the pooled sera is not less than 3.5 IU/ml.

The International Unit is the specific neutralising activity for *C. novyi* alpha toxin contained in a stated amount of the International Standard, which consists of a quantity of dried immune horse serum. The equivalence in International Units of the International Standard is stated by the World Health Organisation.

The potency of the pooled sera obtained from the rabbits is determined by comparing the quantity necessary to protect mice or other suitable animals against the toxic effects of a fixed dose of *C. novyi* alpha toxin with the quantity of a reference preparation of Clostridium novyi alpha antitoxin, calibrated in International Units, necessary to give the same protection. For this comparison, a suitable preparation of *C. novyi* alpha toxin for use as a test toxin is required. The dose of the test toxin is determined in relation to the reference preparation; the potency of the serum to be examined is determined in relation to the reference preparation using the test toxin.
Clostridia (multicomponent) rabbit antiserum BRP is suitable for use as a reference serum.

Preparation of test toxin. Prepare the test toxin from a sterile filtrate of an approximately 5-day culture in liquid medium of *C. novyi* type B and dry by a suitable method. Select the test toxin by determining for mice the L+/10 dose and the LD_{50}, the observation period being 72 h.

A suitable alpha toxin contains not less than one L+/10 dose in 0.05 mg and not less than 10 LD_{50} in each L+/10 dose.

Determination of test dose of toxin. Prepare a solution of the reference preparation in a suitable liquid so that it contains 1 IU/ml. Prepare a solution of the test toxin in a suitable liquid so that 1 ml contains a precisely known amount such as 1 mg. Prepare mixtures of the solution of the reference preparation and the solution of the test toxin such that each mixture contains 1.0 ml of the solution of the reference preparation (1 IU), one of a series of graded volumes of the solution of the test toxin and sufficient of a suitable liquid to bring the total volume to 2.0 ml. Allow the mixtures to stand at room temperature for 60 min. Using not fewer than 2 mice, each weighing 17 g to 22 g, for each mixture, inject a dose of 0.2 ml intramuscularly or subcutaneously into each mouse. Observe the mice for 72 h. If all the mice die, the amount of toxin present in 0.2 ml of the mixture is in excess of the test dose. If none of the mice die, the amount of toxin present in 0.2 ml of the mixture is less than the test dose. Prepare fresh mixtures such that 2.0 ml of each mixture contains 1.0 ml of the solution of the reference preparation (1 IU) and one of a series of graded volumes of the solution of the test toxin separated from each other by steps of not more than 20 per cent and covering the expected end-point. Allow the mixtures to stand at room temperature for 60 min. Using not fewer than two mice for each mixture, inject a dose of 0.2 ml intramuscularly or subcutaneously into each mouse. Observe the mice for 72 h. Repeat the determination at least once and combine the results of the separate tests that have been made with mixtures of the same composition so that a series of totals is obtained, each total representing the mortality due to a mixture of a given composition.

The test dose of toxin is the amount present in 0.2 ml of that mixture which causes the death of one half of the total number of mice injected with it.

Determination of the potency of the serum obtained from rabbits

Preliminary test. Dissolve a quantity of the test toxin in a suitable liquid so that 1 ml contains 10 times the test dose (solution of the test toxin). Prepare a series of mixtures of the solution of the test toxin and of the serum to be examined such that each mixture contains 1.0 ml of the solution of the test toxin, one of a series of graded volumes of the serum to be examined and sufficient of a suitable liquid to bring the final volume to 2.0 ml. Allow the mixtures to stand at room temperature for 60 min. Using not fewer than 2 mice for each mixture, inject a dose of 0.2 ml intramuscularly or subcutaneously into each mouse. Observe the mice for 72 h. If none of the mice dies, 0.2 ml of the mixture contains more than 0.1 IU. If all the mice die, 0.2 ml of the mixture contains less than 0.1 IU.

Final test. Prepare a series of mixtures of the solution of the test toxin and of the serum to be examined such that 2.0 ml of each mixture contains 1.0 ml of the solution of the test toxin and one of a series of graded volumes of the serum to be examined, separated from each other by steps of not more than 20 per cent and covering the expected end-point as determined by the preliminary test. Prepare further mixtures of the solution of the test toxin and of the solution of the reference preparation such that 2.0 ml of each mixture contains 1.0 ml of the solution of the test toxin and one of a series of graded volumes of the solution of the reference preparation, in order to confirm the test dose of the toxin. Allow the mixtures to stand at room temperature for 60 min. Using not fewer than 2 mice for each mixture, proceed as described in the preliminary test. The test mixture which contains 0.1 IU in 0.2 ml is that mixture which kills the same or almost the same number of mice as the reference mixture containing 0.1 IU in 0.2 ml. Repeat the determination at least once and calculate the average of all valid estimates. The test is valid only if the reference preparation gives a result within 20 per cent of the expected value.

The confidence limits ($P = 0.95$) have been estimated to be:

- 85 per cent and 114 per cent when 2 animals per dose are used,
- 91.5 per cent and 109 per cent when 4 animals per dose are used,
- 93 per cent and 108 per cent when 6 animals per dose are used.

LABELLING

The label states:

- whether the product is a toxoid, a vaccine prepared from a whole inactivated culture or a mixture of the two,
- that the preparation is to be shaken before use,
- for each target species, the immunising effect produced (for example, antibody production, protection against signs of disease or infection).

01/2005:0363
corrected

CLOSTRIDIUM PERFRINGENS VACCINE FOR VETERINARY USE

Vaccinum clostridii perfringentis ad usum veterinarium

DEFINITION

Clostridium perfringens vaccine for veterinary use is prepared from liquid cultures of suitable strains of *Clostridium perfringens* type B, *C. perfringens* type C or *C. perfringens* type D or a mixture of these types.

PRODUCTION

The whole cultures or their filtrates or a mixture of the two are inactivated in such a manner that toxicity is eliminated and immunogenic activity is retained. Toxoids and/or inactivated cultures may be treated with a suitable adjuvant.

CHOICE OF VACCINE COMPOSITION

The vaccine is shown to be satisfactory with respect to safety (*5.2.6*) and efficacy (*5.2.7*). For the latter, it shall be demonstrated that for each target species the vaccine, when administered according to the recommended schedule, stimulates an immune response (for example, induction of antibodies) consistent with the claims made for the product.

BATCH TESTING

Residual toxicity. The test for residual toxicity may be omitted by the manufacturer, since a test for detoxification is carried out immediately after the detoxification process and, when there is risk of reversion, a second test is carried out at as late a stage as possible during the production process.

Batch potency test. The test described under Potency is not necessarily carried out for routine testing of batches of vaccine. It is carried out for a given vaccine on one or more occasions as decided by or with the agreement of the competent authority. Where the test is not carried out, a suitable validated alternative test is carried out, the criteria for acceptance being set with reference to a batch of vaccine that has given satisfactory results in the test described under Potency and that has been shown to be satisfactory with respect to immunogenicity in the target species. The following test may be used after a satisfactory correlation with the test described under Potency has been established.

Vaccinate rabbits as described under Potency and prepare sera. Determine the level of antibodies against the beta and/or epsilon toxins of *C. perfringens* in the individual sera by a suitable method such as an immunochemical method (*2.7.1*) or neutralisation in cell cultures. Use a homologous reference serum calibrated in International Units of *C. perfringens* beta and/or epsilon antitoxin. *Clostridia (multicomponent) rabbit antiserum BRP* is suitable for use as a reference serum. The vaccine complies with the test if the level or levels of antibodies are not less than that found for a batch of vaccine that has given satisfactory results in the test described under Potency and that has been shown to be satisfactory with respect to immunogenicity in the target species.

IDENTIFICATION

Type B. The vaccine stimulates the formation of beta and epsilon antitoxins when injected into animals that do not have these antitoxins.

Type C. The vaccine stimulates the formation of beta antitoxin when injected into animals that do not have this antitoxin.

Type D. The vaccine stimulates the formation of epsilon antitoxin when injected into animals that do not have this antitoxin.

TESTS

Safety. Use 2 animals of one of the species for which the vaccine is intended and that have not been vaccinated against *C. perfringens*. Administer by a recommended route to each animal, twice the maximum dose stated on the label. Observe the animals for 14 days. No abnormal local or systemic reaction occurs.

Residual toxicity. Inject 0.5 ml of the vaccine subcutaneously into each of 5 mice, each weighing 17 g to 22 g. Observe the animals for 7 days. No abnormal local or systemic reaction occurs.

Sterility. It complies with the test for sterility prescribed in the monograph on *Vaccines for veterinary use (0062)*.

POTENCY

Inject subcutaneously into each of not fewer than 10 healthy rabbits, 3 to 6 months old, a quantity of vaccine not exceeding the minimum dose stated on the label as the first dose. After 21 to 28 days inject into the same animals a quantity of the vaccine not exceeding the minimum dose stated on the label as the second dose. 10 to 14 days after the second injection, bleed the rabbits and pool the sera.

Type B. The potency of the pooled sera is not less than 10 IU of beta antitoxin and not less than 5 IU of epsilon antitoxin per millilitre.

Type C. The potency of the pooled sera is not less than 10 IU of beta antitoxin per millilitre.

Type D. The potency of the pooled sera is not less than 5 IU of epsilon antitoxin per millilitre.

International standard for clostridium perfringens beta antitoxin

The International Unit is the specific neutralising activity for *C. perfringens* beta toxin contained in a stated amount of the International Standard which consists of a quantity of dried immune horse serum. The equivalence in International Units of the International Standard is stated by the World Health Organisation.

International standard for clostridium perfringens epsilon antitoxin

The International Unit is the specific neutralising activity for *C. perfringens* epsilon toxin contained in a stated amount of the International Standard which consists of a quantity of dried immune horse serum. The equivalence in International Units of the International Standard is stated by the World Health Organisation.

The potency of the pooled sera obtained from the rabbits is determined by comparing the quantity necessary to protect mice or other suitable animals against the toxic effects of a fixed dose of *C. perfringens* beta toxin or *C. perfringens* epsilon toxin with the quantity of a reference preparation of clostridium perfringens beta antitoxin or clostridium perfringens epsilon antitoxin, as appropriate, calibrated in International Units, necessary to give the same protection. For this comparison, a suitable preparation of *C. perfringens* beta or epsilon toxin for use as a test toxin is required. The dose of the test toxin is determined in relation to the appropriate reference preparation; the potency of the serum to be examined is determined in relation to the appropriate reference preparation using the appropriate test toxin.

Clostridia (multicomponent) rabbit antiserum BRP is suitable for use as a reference serum.

Preparation of test toxin. Prepare the test toxin from a sterile filtrate of an early culture in liquid medium of *C. perfringens* type B, type C or type D as appropriate and dry by a suitable method. Use a beta or epsilon toxin as appropriate. Select the test toxin by determining for mice the L+ and the LD_{50} for the beta toxin and the L+/10 dose and the LD_{50} for the epsilon toxin, the observation period being 72 h.

A suitable beta toxin contains not less than one L+ in 0.2 mg and not less than 25 LD_{50} in one L+ dose. A suitable epsilon toxin contains not less than one L+/10 dose in 0.005 mg and not less than 20 LD_{50} in one L+/10 dose.

Determination of test dose of toxin. Prepare a solution of the reference preparation in a suitable liquid so that it contains 5 IU/ml for clostridium perfringens beta antitoxin and 0.5 IU/ml for clostridium perfringens epsilon antitoxin. Prepare a solution of the test toxin in a suitable liquid so that 1 ml contains a precisely known amount such as 10 mg for beta toxin and 1 mg for epsilon toxin. Prepare mixtures of the solution of the reference preparation and the solution of the test toxin such that each contains 2.0 ml of the solution of the reference preparation, one of a series of graded volumes of the solution of the test toxin and sufficient of a suitable liquid to bring the total volume to 5.0 ml. Allow the mixtures to stand at room temperature for 30 min. Using not fewer than 2 mice, each weighing 17 g to 22 g, for each mixture, inject a dose of 0.5 ml intravenously or intraperitoneally into each mouse. Observe the mice for 72 h. If all the mice die, the amount of toxin present in 0.5 ml of the mixture is in excess of the test dose. If none of the mice dies the amount of toxin present in 0.5 ml of the mixture is less than the test dose. Prepare fresh mixtures such that 5.0 ml of each mixture contains 2.0 ml of the solution of the reference preparation and one of a series of graded volumes of the solution of the test toxin separated from each other by steps of not more than 20 per cent and covering the expected end-point. Allow the mixtures to stand at room temperature for 30 min. Using not fewer than two mice for each mixture, inject a dose of 0.5 ml intravenously or intraperitoneally into each mouse. Observe the mice for 72 h. Repeat the determination at least once and add together the results of the separate tests that have been made with mixtures of the same composition so that a series of totals is obtained, each total representing the mortality due to a mixture of given composition.

The test dose of toxin is the amount present in 0.5 ml of that mixture which causes the death of one half of the total number of mice injected with it.

Determination of the potency of the serum obtained from rabbits

Preliminary test. Dissolve a quantity of the test toxin in a suitable liquid so that 2.0 ml contains 10 times the test dose (solution of the test toxin). Prepare a series of mixtures of the solution of the test toxin and of the serum to be examined such that each contains 2.0 ml of the solution of the test toxin, one of a series of graded volumes of the serum to be examined and sufficient of a suitable liquid to bring the final volume to 5.0 ml. Allow the mixtures to stand at room temperature for 30 min. Using not fewer than 2 mice for each mixture, inject a dose of 0.5 ml intravenously or intraperitoneally into each mouse. Observe the mice for 72 h. If none of the mice die, 0.5 ml of the mixture contains more than 1 IU of beta antitoxin or 0.1 IU of epsilon antitoxin. If all the mice die, 0.5 ml of the mixture contains less than 1 IU of beta antitoxin or 0.1 IU of epsilon antitoxin.

Final test. Prepare a series of mixtures of the solution of the test toxin and the serum to be examined such that 5.0 ml of each mixture contains 2.0 ml of the solution of the test toxin and one of a series of graded volumes of the serum to be examined separated from each other by steps of not more than 20 per cent and covering the expected end-point as determined by the preliminary test. Prepare further mixtures of the solution of the test toxin and of the solution of the reference preparation such that 5.0 ml of each mixture contains 2.0 ml of the solution of the test toxin and one of a series of graded volumes of the solution of the reference preparation, in order to confirm the test dose of the toxin. Allow the mixtures to stand at room temperature for 30 min. Using not fewer than 2 mice for each mixture proceed as described in the preliminary test.

Beta antitoxin. The test mixture which contains 1 IU in 0.5 ml is that mixture which kills the same or almost the same number of mice as the reference mixture containing 1 IU in 0.5 ml.

Epsilon antitoxin. The test mixture which contains 0.1 IU in 0.5 ml is that mixture which kills the same or almost the same number of mice as the reference mixture containing 0.1 IU in 0.5 ml. Repeat the determination at least once and calculate the average of all valid estimates. The test is valid only if the reference preparation gives a result within 20 per cent of the expected value.

The confidence limits ($P = 0.95$) have been estimated to be:

- 85 per cent and 114 per cent when 2 animals per dose are used,
- 91.5 per cent and 109 per cent when 4 animals per dose are used,
- 93 per cent and 108 per cent when 6 animals per dose are used.

LABELLING

The label states:

- the type or types of *C. perfringens* from which the vaccine has been prepared,
- whether the preparation is a toxoid or a vaccine prepared from a whole inactivated culture or a mixture of the two,
- that the preparation is to be shaken before use,
- for each target species, the immunising effect produced (for example, antibody production, protection against signs of disease or infection).

01/2005:0364
corrected

CLOSTRIDIUM SEPTICUM VACCINE FOR VETERINARY USE

Vaccinum clostridii septici ad usum veterinarium

DEFINITION

Clostridium septicum vaccine for veterinary use is prepared from a liquid culture of a suitable strain of *Clostridium septicum*.

PRODUCTION

The whole culture or its filtrate or a mixture of the two is inactivated in such a manner that toxicity is eliminated and immunogenic activity is retained. Toxoid and/or inactivated cultures may be treated with a suitable adjuvant.

CHOICE OF VACCINE COMPOSITION

The vaccine is shown to be satisfactory with respect to safety (*5.2.6*) and efficacy (*5.2.7*). For the latter, it shall be demonstrated that for each target species the vaccine, when administered according to the recommended schedule, stimulates an immune response (for example, induction of antibodies) consistent with the claims made for the product.

BATCH TESTING

Residual toxicity. The test for residual toxicity may be omitted by the manufacturer, since a test for detoxification is carried out immediately after the detoxification process and, when there is risk of reversion, a second test is carried out at as late a stage as possible during the production process.

Batch potency test. The test described under Potency is not necessarily carried out for routine testing of batches of vaccine. It is carried out for a given vaccine on one or more occasions as decided by or with the agreement of the competent authority. Where the test is not carried out, a suitable validated alternative test is carried out, the criteria for acceptance being set with reference to a batch of vaccine that has given satisfactory results in the test described under Potency and that has been shown to be satisfactory with respect to immunogenicity in the target species. The following test may be used after a satisfactory correlation with the test described under Potency has been established.

Vaccinate rabbits as described under Potency and prepare sera. Determine the level of antibodies against the toxin of *C. septicum* in the individual sera by a suitable method such as an immunochemical method (*2.7.1*) or neutralisation in cell cultures. Use a homologous reference serum calibrated in International Units of *C. septicum* antitoxin. *Clostridia (multicomponent) rabbit antiserum BRP* is suitable for use as a reference serum. The vaccine complies with the test if the level of antibodies is not less than that found for a batch of vaccine that has given satisfactory results in the test described under Potency and that has been shown to be satisfactory with respect to immunogenicity in the target species.

IDENTIFICATION

The vaccine stimulates the formation of *C. septicum* antitoxin when injected into animals that do not have this antitoxin.

Vaccines

TESTS

Safety. Use 2 animals of one of the species for which the vaccine is intended and that have not been vaccinated against *C. septicum*. Administer to each animal, by a recommended route, twice the maximum dose stated on the label. Observe the animals for 14 days. No abnormal local or systemic reaction occurs.

Residual toxicity. Inject 0.5 ml of the vaccine subcutaneously into each of 5 mice, each weighing 17 g to 22 g. Observe the animals for 7 days. No abnormal local or systemic reaction occurs.

Sterility. It complies with the test for sterility prescribed in the monograph on *Vaccines for veterinary use (0062)*.

POTENCY

Inject subcutaneously into each of not fewer than 10 healthy rabbits, 3 to 6 months old, a quantity of vaccine not exceeding the minimum dose stated on the label as the first dose. After 21 to 28 days, inject into the same animals a quantity of the vaccine not exceeding the minimum dose stated on the label as the second dose. 10 to 14 days after the second injection, bleed the rabbits and pool the sera.

The potency of the pooled sera is not less than 2.5 IU/ml.

The International Unit is the specific neutralising activity for *C. septicum* toxin contained in a stated amount of the International Standard which consists of a quantity of dried immune horse serum. The equivalence in International Units of the International Standard is stated by the World Health Organisation.

The potency of the pooled sera obtained from the rabbits is determined by comparing the quantity necessary to protect mice or other suitable animals against the toxic effects of a dose of *C. septicum* toxin with the quantity of a reference preparation of clostridium septicum antitoxin, calibrated in International Units, necessary to give the same protection. For this comparison, a suitable preparation of *C. septicum* toxin for use as a test toxin is required. The dose of the test toxin is determined in relation to the reference preparation; the potency of the serum to be examined is determined in relation to the reference preparation using the test toxin. *Clostridia (multicomponent) rabbit antiserum BRP* is suitable for use as a reference serum.

Preparation of test toxin. Prepare the test toxin from a sterile filtrate of a 1- to 3-day culture of *C. septicum* in liquid medium and dry by a suitable method. Select the test toxin by determining for mice the L+/5 dose and the LD_{50} the observation period being 72 h.

A suitable toxin contains not less than one L+/5 dose in 1.0 mg and not less than 10 LD_{50} in each L+/5 dose.

Determination of test dose of toxin. Prepare a solution of the reference preparation in a suitable liquid so that it contains 1.0 IU/ml. Prepare a solution of the test toxin in a suitable liquid so that 1 ml contains a precisely known amount, such as 4 mg. Prepare mixtures of the solution of the reference preparation and the solution of the test toxin such that each mixture contains 2.0 ml of the solution of the reference preparation (2 IU), one of a series of graded volumes of the solution of the test toxin and sufficient of a suitable liquid to bring the total volume to 5.0 ml. Allow the mixtures to stand at room temperature for 60 min. Using not fewer than 2 mice, each weighing 17 g to 22 g, for each mixture, inject a dose of 0.5 ml intravenously or intraperitoneally into each mouse. Observe the mice for 72 h. If all the mice die, the amount of toxin present in 0.5 ml of the mixture is in excess of the test dose. If none of the mice die, the amount of toxin present in 0.5 ml of the mixture is less than the test dose. Prepare fresh mixtures such that 5.0 ml of each mixture contains 2.0 ml of the reference preparation (2 IU) and one of a series of graded volumes of the solution of the test toxin separated from each other by steps of not more than 20 per cent and covering the expected end-point. Allow the mixtures to stand at room temperature for 60 min. Using not fewer than 2 mice for each mixture, inject a dose of 0.5 ml intravenously or intraperitoneally into each mouse. Observe the mice for 72 h. Repeat the determination at least once and add together the results of the separate tests that have been made with mixtures of the same composition so that a series of totals is obtained, each total representing the mortality due to a mixture of a given composition.

The test dose of toxin is the amount present in 0.5 ml of that mixture which causes the death of one half of the total number of mice injected with it.

Determination of the potency of the serum obtained from rabbits

Preliminary test. Dissolve a quantity of the test toxin in a suitable liquid so that 2.0 ml contains ten times the test dose (solution of the test toxin). Prepare a series of mixtures of the solution of the test toxin and of the serum to be examined such that each contains 2.0 ml of the solution of the test toxin, one of a series of graded volumes of the serum to be examined and sufficient of a suitable liquid to bring the final volume to 5.0 ml. Allow the mixtures to stand at room temperature for 60 min. Using not fewer than 2 mice for each mixture, inject a dose of 0.5 ml intravenously or intraperitoneally into each mouse. Observe the mice for 72 h. If none of the mice dies, 0.5 ml of the mixture contains more than 0.2 IU. If all the mice die, 0.5 ml of the mixture contains less than 0.2 IU.

Final test. Prepare a series of mixtures of the solution of the test toxin and of the serum to be examined such that 5.0 ml of each mixture contains 2.0 ml of the solution of the test toxin and one of a series of graded volumes of the serum to be examined, separated from each other by steps of not more than 20 per cent and covering the expected end-point as determined by the preliminary test. Prepare further mixtures of the solution of the test toxin and of the solution of the reference preparation such that 5.0 ml of each mixture contains 2.0 ml of the solution of the test toxin and one of a series of graded volumes of the solution of the reference preparation to confirm the test dose of the toxin. Allow the mixtures to stand at room temperature for 60 min. Using not fewer than 2 mice for each mixture proceed as described in the preliminary test. The test mixture which contains 0.2 IU in 0.5 ml is that mixture which kills the same or almost the same number of mice as the reference mixture containing 0.2 IU in 0.5 ml. Repeat the determination at least once and calculate the average of all valid estimates. The test is valid only if the reference preparation gives a result within 20 per cent of the expected value.

The confidence limits ($P = 0.95$) have been estimated to be:

- 85 per cent and 114 per cent when 2 animals per dose are used,
- 91.5 per cent and 109 per cent when 4 animals per dose are used,
- 93 per cent and 108 per cent when 6 animals per dose are used.

LABELLING

The label states:

- whether the preparation is a toxoid or a vaccine prepared from a whole inactivated culture, or a mixture of the two,
- that the preparation is to be shaken before use,

– for each target species, the immunising effect produced (for example, antibody production, protection against signs of disease or infection).

01/2005:0449

DISTEMPER VACCINE (LIVE) FOR MUSTELIDS, FREEZE-DRIED

Vaccinum morbi Carrei vivum cryodesiccatum ad mustelidas

DEFINITION

Freeze-dried distemper vaccine (live) for mustelids is a preparation of a strain of distemper virus that is attenuated for ferrets.

PRODUCTION

The attenuated strain is grown in suitable cell cultures (*5.2.4*) or in fertilised hen eggs, obtained from healthy flocks.

CHOICE OF VACCINE STRAIN

Only a virus strain shown to be satisfactory with respect to attenuation and immunogenicity may be used in the preparation of the vaccine. The following tests may be used during demonstration of safety (*5.2.6*) and immunogenicity (*5.2.7*).

Attenuation. When a volume of a viral suspension equivalent to five doses of the vaccine is injected intramuscularly into each of two susceptible ferrets, it does not provoke pathogenic effects within 21 days.

Immunogenicity. The test described under Potency is suitable to demonstrate the immunogenicity of the strain.

BATCH TESTING

If the test for potency has been carried out with satisfactory results on a representative batch of vaccine, this test may be omitted as a routine control on other batches of vaccine prepared from the same seed lot, subject to agreement by the competent authority.

IDENTIFICATION

The vaccine reconstituted as stated on the label and mixed with a specific distemper antiserum no longer provokes cytopathic effects in susceptible cell cultures or lesions on the chorio-allantoic membranes of fertilised hen eggs 9 to 11 days old.

TESTS

Safety. Inject by the route stated on the label twice the dose of the reconstituted vaccine into each of two susceptible ferrets free from distemper-virus-neutralising antibodies. Observe the animals for 21 days. They remain in normal health and no abnormal local or systemic reaction occurs.

Extraneous viruses. Mix the reconstituted vaccine with a monospecific antiserum. It no longer provokes cytopathic effects in susceptible cell cultures. It shows no evidence of haemagglutinating or haemadsorbing agents.

Bacterial and fungal contamination. The reconstituted vaccine complies with the test for sterility prescribed in the monograph on *Vaccines for veterinary use (0062)*.

Mycoplasmas (*2.6.7*). The reconstituted vaccine complies with the test for mycoplasmas.

Virus titre. Titrate the reconstituted vaccine in suitable cell cultures or fertilised hen eggs 9 to 11 days old. One dose of the vaccine contains not less than the quantity of virus equivalent to the minimum titre stated on the label.

POTENCY

Use seven susceptible ferrets free from distemper-virus-neutralising antibodies. Vaccinate five of the ferrets according to the instructions for use. Keep the two other animals as controls. Observe all the animals for 21 days. Inject intramuscularly into each animal a quantity of distemper virus sufficient to cause the death of a susceptible ferret. Observe the animals for a further 21 days. The test is invalid if one or both of the control ferrets do not die of distemper. The vaccine complies with the test if the vaccinated ferrets remain in normal health.

01/2005:1315

DUCK VIRAL HEPATITIS TYPE I VACCINE (LIVE)

Vaccinum hepatitidis viralis anatis stirpe I vivum

1. DEFINITION

Duck viral hepatitis type I vaccine (live) is a preparation of a suitable strain of duck hepatitis virus type I. This monograph applies to vaccines intended for the active immunisation of breeder ducks in order to protect passively their progeny and/or for the active immunisation of ducklings.

2. PRODUCTION

2-1. *PREPARATION OF THE VACCINE*

The vaccine virus is grown in embryonated hens' eggs or in cell cultures.

2-2. *SUBSTRATE FOR VIRUS PROPAGATION*

2-2-1. **Embryonated hens' eggs**. If the vaccine virus is grown in embryonated hens' eggs, they are obtained from flocks free from specified pathogens (SPF) (*5.2.2*).

2-2-2. **Cell cultures**. If the vaccine virus is grown in cell cultures, they comply with the requirements for cell cultures for production of veterinary vaccines (*5.2.4*).

2-3. *SEED LOTS*

2-3-1. **Extraneous agents**. The master seed lot complies with the tests for extraneous agents in seed lots (*2.6.24*). In these tests on the master seed lot, the organisms used are not more than 5 passages from the master seed lot at the start of the tests.

2-4. *CHOICE OF VACCINE VIRUS*

The vaccine virus shall be shown to be satisfactory with respect to safety (*5.2.6*) and efficacy (*5.2.7*) for the ducks for which it is intended.

The following tests for safety (section 2-4-1), increase in virulence (section 2-4-2) and immunogenicity (section 2-4-3) may be used during demonstration of safety and immunogenicity.

2-4-1. **Safety**. Carry out the test for each route and method of administration to be recommended for vaccination using in each case ducks not older than the youngest age to be recommended for vaccination. Use vaccine virus at the least attenuated passage level that will be present between the master seed lot and a batch of the vaccine. For each test, use not fewer than 20 susceptible domestic ducklings (*Anas platyrhynchos*) that do not have antibodies against duck hepatitis virus type I. Administer to each duckling a quantity of vaccine virus equivalent to not less than 10 times the maximum virus titre likely to be contained in 1 dose of vaccine. Observe the ducklings at least daily for 21 days. The test is not valid if more than 10 per cent of the ducklings

Vaccines

die from causes not attributable to the vaccine virus. The vaccine virus complies with the test if no duckling shows notable signs of duck viral hepatitis or dies from causes attributable to the vaccine virus.

2-4-2. **Increase in virulence**. The test for increase in virulence consists of the administration of the vaccine virus at the least attenuated passage level that will be present between the master seed lot and a batch of vaccine to a group of five 1-day-old domestic ducklings that do not have antibodies against duck hepatitis virus type I, sequential passages, 5 times where possible, to further similar groups of 1-day-old ducklings and testing of the final recovered virus for increase in virulence. If the properties of the vaccine virus allow sequential passage to 5 groups via natural spreading, this method may be used, otherwise passage as described below is carried out and the maximally passaged virus that has been recovered is tested for increase in virulence. Care must be taken to avoid contamination by virus from previous passages. Administer by the oro-nasal route a quantity of vaccine virus that will allow recovery of virus for the passages described below. 2 to 4 days later, take samples of liver from each duckling and pool the samples. Administer 1 ml of the pooled liver suspension by the oro-nasal route to each of five 1-day-old seronegative domestic ducklings. Carry out this operation 5 times. Verify the presence of the virus at each passage. If the virus is not found at a passage level, carry out a second series of passages. Observe the ducklings given the last passage at least daily for 21 days. Compare the results obtained with unpassaged virus in the safety studies and those obtained with maximally passaged virus to assess the degree of increase in virulence. If the virus is not recovered at any passage level in the first and second series of passages, it is considered not to show increase in virulence.

2-4-3. **Immunogenicity**. A test is carried out for each route and method of administration to be recommended, using in each case domestic ducks not older than the youngest age to be recommended for vaccination. The quantity of the vaccine virus administered to each bird is not greater than the minimum virus titre to be stated on the label and the virus is at the most attenuated passage level that will be present in a batch of the vaccine.

2-4-3-1. *Vaccines for passive immunisation of ducklings*. Use for the test not fewer than 15 laying ducks or ducks intended for laying, as appropriate, of the same origin and that do not have antibodies against duck hepatitis virus type I. Vaccinate by a recommended route not fewer than 10 ducks using the schedule to be recommended. Maintain not fewer than 5 ducks as controls. Starting from 4 weeks after onset of lay, collect embryonated eggs from vaccinated and control ducks and incubate them. Challenge not fewer than twenty 1-week-old ducklings representative of the vaccinated group and not fewer than 10 from the control group by the oro-nasal route with a sufficient quantity of virulent duck hepatitis virus type I. Observe the ducklings at least daily for 14 days after challenge. Record the deaths and the number of surviving ducklings that show clinical signs of disease.

The test is not valid if:

- during the observation period after challenge fewer than 70 per cent of the challenged ducklings from the control ducks die or show typical signs of the disease,
- and/or during the period between vaccination and collection of the eggs more than 10 per cent of the control or vaccinated ducks show abnormal clinical signs or die from causes not attributable to the vaccine.

The vaccine virus complies with the test if during the observation period after challenge the percentage relative protection calculated using the following expression is not less than 80 per cent:

$$\frac{V - C}{100 - C} \times 100$$

V = percentage of challenged ducklings from vaccinated ducks that survive to the end of the observation period without clinical signs of the disease.

C = percentage of challenged ducklings from unvaccinated control ducks that survive to the end of the observation period without clinical signs of the disease.

2-4-3-2. *Vaccines for active immunisation of ducklings*. Use for the test not fewer than 30 ducklings of the same origin and that do not have antibodies against duck hepatitis virus type I. Vaccinate by a recommended route not fewer than 20 ducklings. Maintain not fewer than 10 ducklings as controls. Challenge each duckling after at least 5 days by the oro-nasal route with a sufficient quantity of virulent duck hepatitis virus type I. Observe the ducklings at least daily for 14 days after challenge. Record the deaths and the number of surviving ducklings that show clinical signs of disease.

The test is not valid if:

- during the observation period after challenge fewer than 70 per cent of the control ducklings die or show typical signs of the disease,
- and/or during the period between vaccination and challenge more than 10 per cent of the control or vaccinated ducklings show abnormal clinical signs or die from causes not attributable to the vaccine.

The vaccine virus complies with the test if during the observation period after challenge the percentage relative protection calculated using the following expression is not less than 80 per cent:

$$\frac{V - C}{100 - C} \times 100$$

V = percentage of challenged vaccinated ducklings that survive to the end of the observation period without clinical signs of the disease.

C = percentage of challenged unvaccinated control ducklings that survive to the end of the observation period without clinical signs of the disease.

3. BATCH TESTS

3-1. **Identification**. The vaccine, diluted if necessary and mixed with a monospecific duck hepatitis virus type I antiserum, no longer infects embryonated hens' eggs from an SPF flock (*5.2.2*) or susceptible cell cultures (*5.2.4*) into which it is inoculated.

3-2. **Bacteria and fungi**

Vaccines intended for administration by injection comply with the test for sterility prescribed in the monograph *Vaccines for veterinary use (0062)*.

Vaccines not intended for administration by injection either comply with the test for sterility prescribed in the monograph *Vaccines for veterinary use (0062)* or with the following test: carry out a quantitative test for bacterial and fungal contamination; carry out identification tests for micro-organisms detected in the vaccine; the vaccine does not contain pathogenic micro-organisms and contains not more than 1 non-pathogenic micro-organism per dose.

Any liquid supplied with the vaccine complies with the test for sterility prescribed in the monograph *Vaccines for veterinary use (0062)*.

3-3. **Mycoplasmas**. The vaccine complies with the test for mycoplasmas (*2.6.7*).

3-4. **Extraneous agents**. The vaccine complies with the tests for extraneous agents in batches of finished product (*2.6.25*).

3-5. **Safety**. Use not fewer than 10 domestic ducks that do not have antibodies against duck hepatitis virus type I and of the youngest age recommended for vaccination. For vaccines recommended for use in ducks older than 2 weeks, ducks 2 weeks old may be used. Administer by a recommended route and method to each duck 10 doses of the vaccine. Observe the ducks at least daily for 21 days. The test is not valid if more than 20 per cent of ducks show abnormal clinical signs or die from causes not attributable to the vaccine. The vaccine complies with the test if no duck shows notable clinical signs of disease or dies from causes attributable to the vaccine.

3-6. **Virus titre**. Titrate the vaccine virus by inoculation into embryonated hens' eggs from an SPF flock (*5.2.2*) or into suitable cell cultures (*5.2.4*). The vaccine complies with the test if 1 dose contains not less than the minimum virus titre stated on the label.

3-7. **Potency**. Depending on the indications, the vaccine complies with 1 or both of the tests prescribed under Immunogenicity (section 2-4-3), when administered by a recommended route and method. It is not necessary to carry out the potency test for each batch of the vaccine if it has been carried out on a representative batch using a vaccinating dose containing not more than the minimum virus titre stated on the label.

4. LABELLING

If it has been found that the vaccine may show reversion to virulence, the label indicates the precautions necessary to avoid transmission of virulent virus to unvaccinated ducklings.

01/2005:1202

EGG DROP SYNDROME '76 VACCINE (INACTIVATED)

Vaccinum morbi partus diminutionis MCMLXXVI inactivatum ad pullum

DEFINITION

Egg drop syndrome '76 vaccine (inactivated) consists of an emulsion or a suspension of a suitable strain of egg drop syndrome '76 virus (haemagglutinating avian adenovirus) which has been inactivated in such a manner that immunogenic activity is retained.

PRODUCTION

The vaccine strain is propagated in fertilised hen or duck eggs from healthy flocks or in suitable cell cultures (*5.2.4*).

The test for inactivation is carried out in fertilised duck eggs from a flock free from egg drop syndrome '76 virus infection or hen eggs from a flock free from specified pathogens (*5.2.2*), or in suitable cell cultures, whichever is the most sensitive for the vaccine strain; the quantity of virus used in the test is equivalent to not less than ten doses of the vaccine. No live virus is detected.

The vaccine may contain adjuvants.

CHOICE OF VACCINE COMPOSITION

The vaccine is shown to be satisfactory with respect to safety and immunogenicity. The following test may be used during demonstration of efficacy (*5.2.7*).

Immunogenicity. The test described under Potency is suitable to demonstrate immunogenicity.

BATCH TESTING

The test described under Potency is not necessarily carried out for routine testing of batches of vaccine. It is carried out, for a given vaccine, on one or more occasions, as decided by or with the agreement of the competent authority; where the test is not carried out, an alternative validated method is used, the criteria for acceptance being set with reference to a batch of vaccine that has given satisfactory results in the test described under Potency. The following test may be used after a satisfactory correlation with the test described under Potency has been established.

Batch potency test. Vaccinate not fewer than ten 14- to 28-day-old chickens from a flock free from specified pathogens (*5.2.2*) with one dose of vaccine by one of the recommended routes. Four weeks later, collect serum samples from each bird and from five unvaccinated control birds of the same age and from the same source. Measure the antibody response in a haemagglutination (HA) inhibition test on each serum using four HA units of antigen and chicken erythrocytes. The test is not valid if there are specific antibodies in the sera of the unvaccinated birds. The vaccine complies with the test if the mean titre of the vaccinated group is not less than that found previously for a batch of vaccine that has given satisfactory results in the test described under Potency.

IDENTIFICATION

In chickens with no antibodies to egg drop syndrome '76 virus, the vaccine stimulates the production of specific antibodies.

TESTS

Safety. Inject a double dose by a recommended route into each of 10 chickens, 14 to 28 days old, from a flock free from specified pathogens (*5.2.2*). Observe the birds for 21 days. No abnormal local or systemic reaction occurs.

Inactivation

A. For a vaccine prepared in eggs, carry out the test in fertilised duck eggs from a flock free from egg drop syndrome '76 virus infection or, if it is known to provide a more sensitive test system, in hen eggs from a flock free from specified pathogens (*5.2.2*).

Inject two-fifths of a dose into the allantoic cavity of each of ten 10- to 14-day-old fertilised eggs that are free from parental antibodies to egg drop syndrome '76 virus. Incubate the eggs and observe for 8 days. Pool separately the allantoic fluid from eggs containing live embryos, and that from eggs containing dead embryos, excluding those that die from non-specific causes within 24 h of the injection.

Inject into the allantoic cavity of each of ten 10- to 14-day-old fertilised eggs that are free from parental antibodies to egg drop syndrome '76 virus, 0.2 ml of the pooled allantoic fluid from the live embryos and into each of ten similar eggs, 0.2 ml of the pooled allantoic fluid from the dead embryos and incubate for 8 days. Examine the allantoic fluid from each egg for the presence of haemagglutinating activity using chicken erythrocytes.

If more than 20 per cent of the embryos die at either stage, repeat that stage. The vaccine complies with the test if there is no evidence of haemagglutinating activity and if, in any repeat test, not more than 20 per cent of the embryos die from non-specific causes.

Antibiotics may be used in the test to control extraneous bacterial infection.

B. For a vaccine adapted to growth in cell cultures, inoculate ten doses into suitable cell cultures. If the vaccine contains an oily adjuvant, eliminate it by suitable means. Incubate the cultures at 38 ± 1 °C for 7 days. Make a passage on another set of cell cultures and incubate at 38 ± 1 °C for 7 days. Examine the cultures regularly and at the end of the incubation period examine the supernatant liquid for the presence of haemagglutinating activity. The vaccine complies with the test if the cell cultures show no sign of infection and if the there is no haemagglutinating activity in the supernatant liquid.

Extraneous agents. Use the chickens from the test for safety. 21 days after injection of the double dose of vaccine, inject one dose by the same route into each chicken. Collect serum samples from each chicken 2 weeks later and carry out tests for antibodies to the following agents by the methods prescribed for chicken flocks free from specified pathogens (*5.2.2*): avian encephalomyelitis virus, avian leucosis viruses, infectious bronchitis virus, infectious bursal disease virus, infectious laryngotracheitis virus, influenza A virus, Marek's disease virus, Newcastle disease virus and, for vaccine produced in duck eggs, *Chlamydia* (by a complement-fixation test or agar gel precipitation test), duck hepatitis virus type I (by a fluorescent-antibody test or serum-neutralisation test) and Derzsy's disease virus (by a serum-neutralisation test). The vaccine does not stimulate the formation of antibodies against these agents.

Sterility. The vaccine complies with the test for sterility prescribed in the monograph on *Vaccines for veterinary use (0062)*.

POTENCY

Vaccinate each of 2 groups of 30 hens from a flock free from specified pathogens (*5.2.2*) and of the age at which vaccination is recommended. Maintain two control groups one of 10 hens and the other of 30 hens, of the same age and from the same source as the vaccinates. Keep individual egg production records from point of lay until 4 weeks after challenge.

At 30 weeks of age, 1 group of 30 vaccinates and the group of 10 control birds are challenged with a dose of egg drop syndrome ′76 virus sufficient to cause a well marked drop in egg production and/or quality. The vaccine complies with the test if the vaccinated birds show no marked drop in egg production and/or quality. The test is not valid unless there is a well marked drop in egg production and/or quality in the control birds.

When the second group of vaccinated birds and the group of 30 control birds are nearing the end of lay, challenge these birds, as before. The vaccine complies with the test if the vaccinated birds show no marked drop in egg production and/or quality. The test is not valid unless there is a well marked drop in egg production and/or quality in the control birds.

Carry out serological tests on serum samples obtained at the time of vaccination, 4 weeks later and just prior to challenge. The test is not valid if antibodies to egg drop syndrome ′76 virus are detected in any sample from control birds.

LABELLING

The label states whether the strain in the vaccine is duck- or hen-embryo-adapted or cell-culture-adapted.

01/2005:1613

EQUINE HERPESVIRUS VACCINE (INACTIVATED)

Vaccinum herpesviris equini inactivatum

DEFINITION

Equine herpesvirus vaccine (inactivated) is a preparation of one or more suitable strains of equid herpesvirus 1 and/or equid herpesvirus 4 inactivated without impairing their immunogenic activity or a suspension of an inactivated fraction of the virus.

PRODUCTION

Each strain of virus is propagated separately in suitable cell cultures (*5.2.4*). The viral suspensions may be purified and concentrated and are inactivated; they may be treated to fragment the virus and the viral fragments may be purified and concentrated.

The test for residual infectious equid herpesvirus is carried out using 2 passages in the same type of cell culture as that used in the production or in cell cultures shown to be at least as sensitive. The quantity of inactivated virus used in the test is equivalent to not less than 25 doses of the vaccine. No live virus is detected.

The vaccine may contain a suitable adjuvant.

CHOICE OF VACCINE COMPOSITION

The vaccine is shown to be satisfactory with respect to safety (*5.2.6*) and immunogenicity (*5.2.7*) in horses. Where a particular breed of horse is known to be especially sensitive to the vaccine, horses from that breed are included in the test for safety. The following tests may be used during demonstration of safety and immunogenicity.

Safety. A test is carried out in each category of animals for which the vaccine is intended and by each recommended route. 2 doses of vaccine are administered to each of not fewer than 10 animals which have not been previously vaccinated with an equine herpesvirus vaccine, which have at most a low antibody titre not indicative of recent infection and which do not excrete equid herpesvirus. After 14 days, 1 dose of vaccine is injected into each of the animals. The animals are observed for a further 14 days. During the 28 days of the test, no abnormal or systemic reaction occurs. If the vaccine is intended for use in pregnant horses, for the test in this category of animal, mares are vaccinated during the relevant trimester or trimesters of pregnancy and the observation period is prolonged up to foaling; any effects on gestation or the offspring are noted.

Immunogenicity. The claims of the product reflect the type of immunogenicity demonstrated (protection against the disease of the respiratory tract and/or protection against abortion). The tests described under Potency are suitable to demonstrate the immunogenicity of the strains present in the vaccine.

BATCH TESTING

The test described under Potency is not carried out for routine testing of batches of vaccine. It is carried out, for a given vaccine on one or more occasions; where the test is not carried out, an alternative validated method is used, the criteria for acceptance being set with reference to a batch of vaccine that has given satisfactory results in the tests described under Potency. The following test may be used.

Batch potency test. Vaccinate not fewer than 5 rabbits, guinea-pigs or mice with a single injection of a suitable dose. Where the schedule stated on the label requires a second injection to be given, the recommended schedule may be used in laboratory animals provided it has been demonstrated that this will still provide a suitably sensitive test system. At a given interval within the range of 14 to 21 days after the last injection, collect blood from each animal and prepare serum samples. Use a suitable validated test such as an enzyme-linked immunosorbent assay to measure the response to each of the antigens stated on the label. The antibody levels are not significantly less than those obtained with a batch that has given satisfactory results in the test described under Potency.

IDENTIFICATION

In animals having no antibodies against equid herpesvirus 1 and equid herpesvirus 4 or a fraction of the viruses, the vaccine stimulates the production of specific antibodies against the virus type or types included in the product. The method used must distinguish between antibodies against equid herpesviruses 1 and 4.

TESTS

Safety. Use for the test horses that have not been vaccinated against equid herpesviruses 1 and 4. Administer by a recommended route twice the vaccinating dose into each of not fewer than 2 horses. After 2 weeks, administer a single dose to each of the animals. Observe the animals for a further 10 days. The animals remain in good health and no abnormal local or systemic reaction occurs.

Inactivation. Carry out a test for residual infectious equid herpesvirus using not less than 25 doses of vaccine by inoculating cell cultures sensitive to equid herpesviruses 1 and 4; make a passage after 5 to 7 days and maintain the cultures for 14 days. No live virus is detected. If the vaccine contains an adjuvant, separate the adjuvant from the liquid phase, by a method that does not inactivate or otherwise interfere with the detection of live virus, or carry out a test for inactivation on the mixture of bulk antigens before addition of the adjuvant.

Sterility. The vaccine complies with the test for sterility prescribed in the monograph on *Vaccines for veterinary use (0062)*.

POTENCY

The type of potency test depends on the claims for the product. For vaccines intended to protect against the disease of the respiratory tract carry out test A, using equid herpesvirus 1 and/or equid herpesvirus 4 depending on the claims for protection. For vaccines intended to protect against abortion carry out test B.

Use horses which have not been vaccinated with an equine herpesvirus vaccine, which have at most a low antibody titre not indicative of recent infection, and which do not excrete equid herpesvirus. To demonstrate that no recent infection occurs, immediately before vaccination: draw a blood sample from each animal and test individually for antibodies against equid herpesviruses 1 and 4; collect 10 ml of heparinised blood and test the washed leucocytes for equid herpesviruses 1 and 4; collect a nasopharyngeal swab and test for equid herpesviruses 1 and 4. There is no indication of an active infection. Immediately before challenge collect a nasopharyngeal swab and test for equid herpesviruses 1 and 4. If there is an indication of virus excretion remove the animal from the test. Keep the horses in strict isolation.

A. Use not fewer than 10 horses, not less than 6 months old. Vaccinate not fewer than 6 horses using the recommended schedule. Keep not fewer than 4 unvaccinated horses as controls. At least 2 weeks after the last vaccination, administer by nasal instillation to all horses a quantity of equid herpesvirus 1 or 4, sufficient to produce in a susceptible horse characteristic signs of the disease such as pyrexia and virus excretion (and possibly nasal discharge and coughing). Observe the horses for 14 days. Collect nasopharyngeal swabs daily from each individual animal to isolate the virus. The vaccinated horses show no more than slight signs; the signs in vaccinates are less severe than in controls. The average number of days on which virus is excreted, and the respective virus titres are significantly lower in vaccinated horses than in controls.

B. Use not fewer than 10 pregnant mares. In addition to the testing described above, 6, 4, 3, 2 and 1 month before the first vaccination draw a blood sample from each horse and test individually for antibodies against equid herpesvirus 1 and equid herpesvirus 4. There is no evidence of recent infection or virus excretion. Vaccinate not fewer than 6 mares using the recommended schedule. Keep not fewer than 4 horses as unvaccinated controls. Between day 260 and 290 of pregnancy but not earlier than 3 weeks after the last vaccination administer by nasal instillation to all horses a quantity of equid herpesvirus 1 sufficient to produce abortion in susceptible mares. Observe the mares up to foaling or abortion. Collect samples of fetal lung and liver tissues from aborted fetuses and carry out tests for virus in cell cultures. The test is invalid if more than one control horse gives birth to a healthy foal and if the challenge virus is not isolated from the aborted fetuses. The vaccine complies with the test if not more than one vaccinated mare aborts.

LABELLING

The label states:

- the strains of virus included in the vaccine,
- the claims of protection.

01/2005:0249
corrected

EQUINE INFLUENZA VACCINE (INACTIVATED)

Vaccinum influenzae equi inactivatum

DEFINITION

Equine influenza vaccine (inactivated) is a preparation of one or more suitable strains of equine influenza virus, inactivated in such a manner that immunogenic activity is maintained. Suitable strains contain both haemagglutinin and neuraminidase.

PRODUCTION

Each strain of virus is propagated separately in fertilised hen eggs from healthy flocks or in suitable cell cultures (*5.2.4*). The viral suspensions may be purified and concentrated. The antigen content of the vaccine is based on the haemagglutinin content of the viral suspensions determined as described under In-process Tests; the amount of haemagglutinin for each strain is not less than that in the vaccine shown to be satisfactory in the test for potency.

The test for residual infectious influenza virus is carried out using method A or method B whichever is the more sensitive. The quantity of inactivated virus used is equivalent to not less than 10 doses of vaccine.

A. The vaccine is inoculated into suitable cells; after incubation for 8 days, a subculture is made. It is incubated for a further 6 to 8 days. Harvest about 0.1 ml of the supernatant and examine for live virus by a haemagglutination test. If haemagglutination is found, carry out a further passage in cell culture and test for haemagglutination; no haemagglutination occurs.

B. Inoculate 0.2 ml into the allantoic cavity of each of 10 fertilised eggs and incubate at 33 °C to 37 °C for 3 to 4 days. The test is not valid unless not fewer than 8 of the 10 embryos survive. Harvest 0.5 ml of the allantoic fluid from each surviving embryo and pool the fluids. Inoculate 0.2 ml of the pooled fluid into a further 10 fertilised eggs and incubate at 33 °C to 37 °C for 3 to 4 days. The test is not valid unless at least 8 of the 10 embryos survive. Harvest about 0.1 ml of the allantoic fluid from each surviving embryo and examine each individual harvest for live virus by a haemagglutination test. If haemagglutination is found for any of the fluids, carry out a further passage of that fluid in eggs and test for haemagglutination; no haemagglutination occurs.

The vaccine may contain suitable adjuvants.

CHOICE OF VACCINE COMPOSITION

The choice of strains used in the vaccine is based on epidemiological data. The Office international des épizooties reviews the epidemiological data periodically and if necessary recommends new strains corresponding to prevailing epidemiological evidence. Such strains are used in accordance with the regulations in force in the signatory States of the Convention on the Elaboration of a European Pharmacopoeia.

The vaccine is shown to be satisfactory with respect to safety and immunogenicity in horses. Where a particular breed of horse is known to be especially sensitive to the vaccine, horses from that breed are included in the tests for safety. The following tests may be used during demonstration of safety (*5.2.6*) and efficacy (*5.2.7*).

Safety. A test is carried out in each category of animals for which the vaccine is intended and by each recommended route. Use animals that preferably have no equine influenza antibodies or, where justified, use animals with a low level of such antibodies as long as they have not been vaccinated against equine influenza and administration of the vaccine does not cause an anamnestic response. 2 doses of vaccine are injected by the intended route into each of not fewer than 10 animals. After 14 days, 1 dose of vaccine is injected into each of the animals. The animals are observed for a further 14 days. During the 28 days of the test, no abnormal local or systemic reaction occurs. If the vaccine is intended for use in pregnant horses, for the test in this category of animal, horses are vaccinated during the relevant trimester or trimesters of pregnancy and the observation period is prolonged up to foaling; any effects on gestation or the offspring are noted.

Immunogenicity. The test described under Potency is suitable to demonstrate the immunogenicity of the strains present in the vaccine.

A test with virulent challenge is carried out for at least one vaccine strain. For other strains in the vaccine, demonstration of immunogenicity may, where justified, be based on the serological response induced in horses by the vaccine; justification for protection against these strains may be based on published data on the correlation of the antibody titre with protection against antigenically related strains.

Where serology is used, the test is carried out as described under Potency but instead of virulent challenge, a blood sample is drawn 2 weeks after the last vaccination and the antibody titre of each serum is determined by a suitable immunochemical method (*2.7.1*), such as the single radial haemolysis test or the haemagglutination-inhibition test shown below; a reference serum is used to validate the test. The acceptance criteria depend on the strain and are based on available data; for A/equine-2 virus, vaccines have usually been found satisfactory if the antibody titre of each serum is not less than 85 mm^2 where the single radial haemolysistest is used, or not less than 1:64 (before mixture with the suspension of antigen and erythrocytes) where the haemagglutination-inhibition test is used.

Equine influenza subtype I horse antiserum BRP, *equine influenza subtype 2 American-like horse antiserum BRP* and *equine influenza subtype 2 European-like horse antiserum BRP* are suitable for use as reference sera for the single radial haemolysis test.

The claims for the product reflect the type of immunogenicity demonstrated (protection against challenge or antibody production).

Single radial haemolysis. Heat each serum at 56 °C for 30 min. Perform tests on each serum using respectively the antigen or antigens prepared from the strain(s) used in the production of the vaccine. Mix 1 ml of sheep erythrocyte suspension in barbital buffer solution (1 volume of erythrocytes in 10 volumes of final suspension) with 1 ml of a suitable dilution of the influenza virus strain in barbital buffer solution and incubate the mixture at 4 °C for 30 min. To 2 ml of the virus/erythrocyte mixture, add 1 ml of a 3 g/l solution of *chromium(III) chloride hexahydrate R*, mix and allow to stand for 10 min. Heat the sensitised erythrocytes to 47 °C in a water-bath. Mix 15 ml of a 10 g/l solution of *agarose for electrophoresis R* in barbital buffer solution, 0.7 ml of sensitised erythrocyte suspension and the appropriate amount of diluted guinea-pig complement in barbital buffer solution at 47 °C. Pour the mixture into Petri dishes and allow the agar to set. Punch holes in the agar layer and place in each hole, 5 µl of the undiluted serum to be tested or control serum. Incubate the Petri dishes at 37 °C for 18 h. Measure the diameter of the haemolysis zone and calculate its area, which expresses the antibody titre, in square millimetres.

Equine influenza subtype I horse antiserum BRP, *equine influenza subtype 2 American-like horse antiserum BRP* and *equine influenza subtype 2 European-like horse antiserum BRP* are suitable for use as reference sera for the single radial haemolysis test.

Haemagglutination-inhibition test. Inactivate each serum by heating at 56 °C for 30 min. To one volume of each serum add three volumes of *phosphate-buffered saline pH 7.4 R* and four volumes of a 250 g/l suspension of *light kaolin R* in the same buffer solution. Shake each mixture for 10 min. Centrifuge, collect the supernatant liquid and mix with a concentrated suspension of chicken erythrocytes. Allow to stand at 37 °C for 60 min and centrifuge. The dilution of the serum obtained is 1:8. Perform tests on each serum using each antigen prepared from the strains used in the production of the vaccine. Using each diluted serum, prepare a series of twofold dilutions. To 0.025 ml of each of the latter dilutions add 0.025 ml of a suspension of antigen treated with *ether R* and containing four haemagglutinating units. Allow the mixture to stand for 30 min and add 0.05 ml of a suspension

Vaccines

of chicken erythrocytes containing 2×10^7 erythrocytes/ml. Allow to stand for 1 h and note the last dilution of serum that still completely inhibits haemagglutination.

IN-PROCESS TESTS

The content of haemagglutinin in the inactivated virus suspension, after purification and concentration where applicable, is determined by a suitable immunochemical method (*2.7.1*), such as single radial immunodiffusion, using a suitable haemagglutinin reference preparation; the content is shown to be within the limits shown to allow preparation of a satisfactory vaccine. For vaccines produced in eggs, the content of bacterial endotoxins is determined on the virus harvest to monitor production.

BATCH TESTING

The test described under Potency is not carried out for routine testing of batches of vaccine. It is carried out, for a given vaccine, on one or more occasions, as decided by or with the agreement of the competent authority; where the test is not carried out, an alternative validated method is used, the criteria for acceptance being set with reference to a batch of vaccine that has given satisfactory results in the test described under Potency. The following test may be used.

Batch potency test. Inject one dose of vaccine subcutaneously into each of 5 guinea-pigs free from specified antibodies. 21 days later, collect blood samples and separate the serum. Carry out tests on the serum for specific antibodies by a suitable immunochemical method (*2.7.1*) such as single radial haemolysis or haemagglutinin inhibition, using reference sera to validate the test. The antibody titres are not significantly lower than those obtained in guinea-pigs with a reference batch of vaccine shown to have satisfactory potency in horses.

IDENTIFICATION

In susceptible animals, the vaccine stimulates the production of specific antibodies.

TESTS

Safety. Use horses that preferably have no equine influenza virus antibodies or, where justified, use horses with a low level of such antibodies as long as they have not been vaccinated against equine influenza and administration of the vaccine does not cause an anamnestic response. Administer by a recommended route a double dose of vaccine to each of not fewer than 2 horses. After 2 weeks, administer a single dose to each horse. Observe the animals for a further 10 days. No abnormal local or systemic reaction occurs.

Inactivation. Inoculate 0.2 ml of the vaccine into the allantoic cavity of each of 10 fertilised eggs and incubate at 33 °C to 37 °C for 3 to 4 days. The test is not valid unless at least 8 of the 10 embryos survive. Harvest 0.5 ml of the allantoic fluid from each surviving embryo and pool the fluids. Inoculate 0.2 ml of the pooled fluid into a further 10 fertilised eggs and incubate at 33 °C to 37 °C for 3 to 4 days. The test is not valid unless not fewer than 8 of the 10 embryos survive. Harvest about 0.1 ml of the allantoic fluid from each surviving embryo and examine each individual harvest for live virus by a haemagglutination test. If haemagglutination is found for any of the fluids, carry out for that fluid a further passage in eggs and test for haemagglutination; no haemagglutination occurs.

Sterility. The vaccine complies with the test for sterility prescribed in the monograph on *Vaccines for veterinary use (0062)*.

POTENCY

Carry out the potency test using a challenge strain against which the vaccine is stated to provide protection. Use where possible a recent isolate.

Use 10 horses, at least 6 months old, that do not have specific antibodies against equine influenza virus. Draw a blood sample from each animal and test individually for antibodies against equine influenza virus to determine seronegativity. Vaccinate 6 animals using the recommended schedule. Draw a second blood sample from each animal 7 days after the first vaccination and test individually for antibodies against equine influenza virus, to detect an anamnestic sero-response. Animals showing sero-conversion at this stage are excluded from the test. At least 2 weeks after the last vaccination, administer by aerosol to the 10 animals a quantity of equine influenza virus sufficient to produce characteristic signs of disease such as fever, nasal discharge and coughing in a susceptible animal. Observe the animals for 14 days. Collect nasal swabs daily from each individual animal to isolate the virus. The vaccinated animals show no more than slight signs; the controls show characteristic signs. The average number of days on which virus is excreted, and the respective virus titres are significantly lower in vaccinated animals than in control animals.

LABELLING

The label states:

- the age at which animals should be vaccinated,
- the period of time that should elapse between the first and second injections,
- any booster injections required,
- the strains of virus included in the vaccine.

01/2005:1101

FELINE CALICIVIROSIS VACCINE (INACTIVATED)

Vaccinum calicivirosis felinae inactivatum

DEFINITION

Inactivated feline calicivirosis vaccine is a suspension of one or more suitable strains of feline calicivirus which have been inactivated while maintaining adequate immunogenic properties or of fractions of one or more strains of feline calicivirus with adequate immunogenic properties.

PRODUCTION

The virus is grown in suitable cell lines (*5.2.4*). The viral suspension is harvested and inactivated.

The test for residual infectious calicivirus is carried out using 2 passages in cell cultures of the same type as those used for preparation of the vaccine or in cell cultures shown to be at least as sensitive; the quantity of inactivated virus used in the test is equivalent to not less than 25 doses of vaccine. No live virus is detected.

The vaccine may contain one or more suitable adjuvants.

CHOICE OF VACCINE COMPOSITION

The vaccine is shown to be satisfactory with respect to safety and immunogenicity in cats. The following test may be used during demonstration of efficacy (*5.2.7*).

Immunogenicity. The test described under Potency is suitable to demonstrate immunogenicity of the vaccine.

BATCH TESTING

Batch potency test. *The test described under Potency is not carried out for routine testing of batches of vaccine. It is carried out, for a given vaccine, on one or more occasions, as decided by or with the agreement of the competent authority; where the test is not carried out, a suitable validated alternative test is carried out, the criteria for acceptance being set with reference to a batch of vaccine that has given satisfactory results in the test described under Potency. The following test may be used after a satisfactory correlation with the test described under Potency has been established.*

Use groups of 15 seronegative mice. Administer half a dose of the vaccine to each mouse and 7 days later repeat the administration. 21 days after the first injection, take blood samples and determine the level of antibodies against feline calicivirus by an immunofluorescence technique using pools of serum from groups of 3 mice. The antibody levels are not significantly lower than those obtained with a batch of vaccine that has given satisfactory results in the test described under Potency.

IDENTIFICATION

When injected into susceptible animals, the vaccine stimulates the formation of specific antibodies against feline calicivirus.

TESTS

Safety. Use cats 8 to 12 weeks old and preferably having no feline calicivirus antibodies or, where justified, use cats with a low level of such antibodies as long as they have not been vaccinated against feline calicivirosis and administration of the vaccine does not cause an anamnestic response. Administer a double dose of vaccine by a recommended route to each of 2 cats. Observe the cats for 14 days. No abnormal local or systemic reaction occurs.

Inactivation. Carry out a test for residual infectious calicivirus using 10 doses of vaccine and 2 passages in cell cultures of the same type as those used for preparation of the vaccine or in cell cultures shown to be at least as sensitive. No live virus is detected. If the vaccine contains an adjuvant that would interfere with the test, where possible separate the adjuvant from the liquid phase by a method that does not inactivate or otherwise interfere with detection of live virus.

Sterility. The reconstituted vaccine complies with the test for sterility prescribed in *Vaccines for veterinary use (0062)*.

POTENCY

Carry out a potency test for each strain of feline calicivirus in the vaccine.

Use cats 8 to 12 weeks old and that do not have antibodies against feline calicivirus. Vaccinate 10 cats by a recommended route and according to the recommended schedule. Keep 10 cats as controls. 4 weeks after the last injection, administer intranasally to each vaccinated and control cat a quantity of a virulent strain of calicivirus of the same type as the vaccine strain sufficient to produce typical signs of the disease (hyperthermia, buccal ulcers, respiratory signs) in at least 8 of the control cats. Observe the cats for 14 days after challenge; collect nasal washings daily on days 2 to 14 to test for virus excretion. Note daily the body temperature and signs of disease using the scoring system shown below. The vaccine complies with the test if the score for the vaccinated cats is significantly lower than that for the controls.

Observed signs	Score
Death	10
Depressed state	2
Temperature ≥ 39.5 °C	1
Temperature ≤ 37 °C	2
Ulcer (nasal or oral)	
– small and few in number	1
– large and numerous	3
Nasal discharge	
– slight	1
– copious	2
Ocular discharge	1
Weight loss	2
Virus excretion (total number of days):	
≤ 4 days	1
5-7 days	2
>7 days	3

01/2005:1102

FELINE CALICIVIROSIS VACCINE (LIVE), FREEZE-DRIED

Vaccinum calicivirosis felinae vivum cryodesiccatum

DEFINITION

Freeze-dried feline calicivirosis vaccine (live) is a preparation of one or more suitable strains of feline calicivirus.

PRODUCTION

The virus is grown in suitable cell lines (*5.2.4*). The viral suspension is harvested and mixed with a suitable stabilising solution. The mixture is subsequently freeze-dried.

CHOICE OF VACCINE STRAIN

The vaccine strain shall have been shown to be satisfactory with respect to safety (including safety for pregnant queens if such use is not contra-indicated), absence of reversion to virulence, and immunogenicity. The following tests may be used during demonstration of safety (*5.2.6*) and efficacy (*5.2.7*).

Safety. To 10 cats of the minimum age stated for vaccination and which do not have antibodies against feline calicivirus, administer by a recommended route, a quantity of virus equivalent to 10 times the maximum titre that may be expected in a batch of vaccine. Observe the cats for 21 days. No abnormal local or systemic reaction occurs.

Reversion to virulence. To 2 cats which do not have antibodies against feline calicivirus administer by a recommended route a quantity of virus (for example, approximately 10 doses) that will allow maximum recovery of virus for the passages described below. 5 days later, kill the cats, remove the nasal mucus, tonsils and the trachea, mix, homogenise in 10 ml of buffered saline and decant; inoculate the supernatant intranasally into 2 other cats; carry out this operation five times. Verify the presence of virus at each passage. If the virus is not recovered, carry out a second series of passages. Observe the cats given the last passage for 21 days and compare the reactions observed with those seen in the cats in the safety test described above. The strain complies with the test if no evidence of an increase in virulence is seen compared to the original virus.

Immunogenicity. The test described under Potency is suitable to demonstrate immunogenicity.

BATCH TESTING

If the test for potency has been carried out with satisfactory results on a representative batch of vaccine, this test may be omitted as a routine control on other batches of vaccine prepared from the same seed lot, subject to agreement by the competent authority.

IDENTIFICATION

When neutralised by one or more monospecific antisera, the reconstituted vaccine no longer infects susceptible cell cultures into which it is inoculated.

TESTS

Safety. Administer 10 doses of vaccine , by a recommended route to 2 cats, 8 to 12 weeks old and having no antibodies against feline calicivirus. Observe the cats for 14 days. No abnormal local or systemic reaction occurs.

Bacterial and fungal contamination. The reconstituted vaccine complies with the test for sterility prescribed in *Vaccines for veterinary use (0062)*.

Mycoplasmas (*2.6.7*). The reconstituted vaccine complies wtith the test for mycoplasmas.

Extraneous viruses. Neutralise the vaccine using one or more monospecific antisera and inoculate into suitable cell cultures; make at least one passage and maintain the cultures for 14 days. Examine the cultures for cytopathic effects and carry out tests for haemadsorbing agents. No signs of viral contamination occur in the cell cultures.

Virus titre. Titrate the reconstituted vaccine in susceptible cell cultures at a temperature favourable to replication of the virus. One dose of the vaccine contains not less than the quantity of virus equivalent to the minimum titre stated on the label.

POTENCY

Carry out a potency test for each strain of feline calicivirus in the vaccine.

Use cats 8 to 12 weeks old that do not have antibodies against feline calicivirus. Vaccinate 10 cats by one of the recommended routes and according to the recommended schedule. Keep 10 cats as controls. 4 weeks after the last injection, administer intranasally to each vaccinated and control cat a quantity of a virulent strain of calicivirus of the same type as the vaccine strain sufficient to produce typical signs of the disease (hyperthermia, buccal ulcers, respiratory signs) in not fewer than 8 of the control cats. Observe the cats for 14 days after challenge; collect nasal washings daily on days 2 to 14 to test for virus excretion. Note daily the body temperature and signs of disease using the scoring system shown below. The vaccine complies with the test if the score for the vaccinated cats is significantly lower than that for the controls.

Observed signs	**Score**
Death	10
Depressed state	2
Temperature ≥ 39.5 °C	1
Temperature ≤ 37 °C	2
Ulcer (nasal or oral)	
– small and few in number	1
– large and numerous	3
Nasal discharge	
– slight	1
– copious	2
Ocular discharge	1
Weight loss	2
Virus excretion (total number of days):	
≤ 4 days	1
5-7 days	2
>7 days	3

01/2005:0794

FELINE INFECTIOUS ENTERITIS (FELINE PANLEUCOPENIA) VACCINE (INACTIVATED)

Vaccinum panleucopeniae felinae infectivae inactivatum

DEFINITION

Feline infectious enteritis (feline panleucopenia) vaccine (inactivated) is a liquid or freeze-dried preparation of feline panleucopenia virus or canine parvovirus inactivated by a suitable method.

PRODUCTION

The virus is propagated in suitable cell cultures (*5.2.4*). The virus is harvested and may be purified and concentrated.

The test for inactivation is carried out using a quantity of inactivated virus equivalent to not less than 100 doses of the vaccine by a validated method such as the following: inoculate into suitable non-confluent cells and after incubation for 8 days, make a subculture using trypsinised cells. After incubation for a further 8 days, examine the cultures for residual live parvovirus by an immunofluorescence test. The immunofluorescence test may be supplemented by a haemagglutination test or other suitable tests on the supernatant of the cell cultures. No live virus is detected.

The vaccine may contain an adjuvant and may be freeze-dried.

CHOICE OF VACCINE COMPOSITION

The vaccine is shown to be satisfactory with respect to safety (*5.2.6*) and efficacy (*5.2.7*) in cats. The following test may be used during demonstration of immunogenicity.

Immunogenicity. Use 10 susceptible cats, 8 to 12 weeks old. Draw a blood sample from each cat and test individually for antibodies against feline panleucopenia virus and canine parvovirus to determine susceptibility. Vaccinate 5 cats by the recommended schedule. Carry out leucocyte counts 8 days and 4 days before challenge and calculate the mean of the 2 counts to serve as the initial value. 20 to 22 days after the last vaccination, challenge each cat by the intraperitoneal injection of a suspension of pathogenic feline panleucopenia virus. Observe the cats for 14 days. Carry out leucocyte counts on the fourth, sixth, eighth and tenth days after challenge. The test is not valid unless the 5 control cats all show on not fewer than one occasion a diminution in the number of leucocytes of at least 75 per cent of the initial value; these animals may die from panleucopenia. The vaccine complies with the test if the 5 vaccinated cats remain in excellent health and show no sign of leucopenia; that is to say, the diminution in the number of leucocytes does not exceed, in any of the four counts, 50 per cent of the initial value.

BATCH TESTING

Batch potency test. For routine testing of batches of vaccine a test based on production of haemagglutination-inhibiting antibodies in guinea-pigs may be used instead of test A or B described under Potency if a satisfactory correlation with the test for immunogenicity has been established.

IDENTIFICATION

When injected into animals, the vaccine stimulates the production of antibodies against the parvovirus present in the vaccine.

TESTS

Safety. Use cats of the minimum age recommended for vaccination and preferably having no antibodies against feline panleucopenia virus or against canine parvovirus or, where justified, use cats with a low level of such antibodies as long as they have not been vaccinated against feline panleucopenia virus or against canine parvovirus, and administration of the vaccine does not cause an anamnestic response. Administer by a recommended route a double dose of vaccine to each of 2 cats. Observe the animals for 14 days. No abnormal local or systemic reaction occurs.

Sterility. The vaccine complies with the test for sterility prescribed in the monograph on *Vaccines for veterinary use (0062)*.

POTENCY

Carry out test A or test B.

A. Use 4 cats, 8 to 12 weeks old. Draw a blood sample from each cat and test individually for antibodies against feline panleucopenia virus and canine parvovirus to determine susceptibility. Inject by a recommended route one dose of vaccine into each of 2 cats. After 21 days, draw a blood sample from each cat and separate the serum from each sample. Inactivate each serum by heating at 56 °C for 30 min. To 1 volume of each serum add 9 volumes of a 200 g/l suspension of *light kaolin R* in *phosphate buffered saline pH 7.4 R*. Shake each mixture for 20 min. Centrifuge, collect the supernatant liquid and mix with 1 volume of a concentrated suspension of pig erythrocytes. Allow to stand at 4 °C for 60 min and centrifuge. The dilution of the serum obtained is 1:10. Using each serum, prepare a series of twofold dilutions. To 0.025 ml of each of the latter dilutions add 0.025 ml of a suspension of canine parvovirus or feline panleucopenia virus antigen containing 4 haemagglutinating units. Allow to stand at 37 °C for 30 min and add 0.05 ml of a suspension of pig erythrocytes containing 30×10^6 cells per millilitre. Allow to stand at 4 °C for 90 min and note the last dilution of serum that still completely inhibits haemagglutination. The vaccine complies with the test if both vaccinated cats have developed titres of at least 1:20. The test is not valid if either control cat develops antibodies against canine parvovirus or feline panleucopenia virus.

B. Vaccinate according to the recommended schedule, 2 cats, 8 to 12 weeks old and having antibody titres less than 4 ND_{50} (neutralising dose 50 per cent) per 0.1 ml of serum measured by the method described below. 14 days after vaccination, examine the serum of each animal as follows. Heat the serum at 56 °C for 30 min and prepare serial dilutions using a medium suitable for feline cells. Add to each dilution an equal volume of a virus suspension containing an amount of virus such that when the volume of serum-virus mixture appropriate for the assay system is inoculated into cell cultures, each culture receives approximately 10^4 $CCID_{50}$. Incubate the mixtures at 37 °C for 1 h and inoculate four feline cell cultures with a suitable volume of each mixture. Incubate the cell cultures at 37 °C for 7 days, passage and incubate for a further 7 days. Examine the cultures for evidence of specific cytopathic effects and calculate the antibody titre. The vaccine complies with the test if the mean titre is not less than 32 ND_{50} per 0.1 ml of serum. If one cat fails to respond, repeat the test using 2 more cats and calculate the result as the mean of the titres obtained from all of the 3 cats that have responded.

01/2005:0251

FELINE INFECTIOUS ENTERITIS (FELINE PANLEUCOPENIA) VACCINE (LIVE)

Vaccinum panleucopeniae felinae infectivae vivum

DEFINITION

Feline infectious enteritis (feline panleucopenia) vaccine (live) is a preparation of a suitable strain of feline panleucopenia virus.

PRODUCTION

The virus is propagated in suitable cell cultures (*5.2.4*). The virus suspension is harvested and may be purified and concentrated. It is mixed with a suitable stabilising solution. The vaccine may be freeze-dried.

CHOICE OF VACCINE STRAIN

The vaccine strain shall have been shown to be satisfactory with respect to safety (including safety for pregnant queens if such use is not contra-indicated or if the virus is excreted in the faeces), absence of increase in virulence and immunogenicity.

The following tests may be used during demonstration of safety (*5.2.6*) and efficacy (*5.2.7*).

Safety. Each test is carried out for each recommended route of administration. Use 5 cats, of the minimum age recommended for vaccination and free from specific haemagglutination-inhibiting antibodies against feline panleucopenia virus and canine parvovirus. Make counts of leucocytes in circulating blood on days 8 and 4 before injection of the vaccine strain and calculate the mean of the 2 counts to serve as the initial value. Administer to each cat by a recommended route a quantity of virus corresponding to at least 10 times the maximum virus titre that may be expected in a batch of vaccine and at the lowest level of attenuation. Observe the animals for 21 days. Make leucocyte counts on the fourth, sixth, eighth and tenth days after inoculation. The strain complies with the test if: the

Vaccines

cats remain in good health and there is no abnormal local or systemic reaction; for each animal and for each blood count, the number of leucocytes is not less than 50 per cent of the initial value.

Increase in virulence. Use 2 cats of the minimum age recommended for vaccination and which do not have haemagglutination-inhibiting antibodies against feline panleucopenia virus and canine parvovirus. Administer to each cat, by a recommended route, a quantity of virus suitable to allow maximum recovery of the virus for subsequent passages. From the second to the tenth day after administration of the virus, collect the faeces from each cat and check for the presence of the virus; pool faeces containing virus. Administer 1 ml of the suspension of pooled faeces by the oronasal route to each of 2 other cats of the same age and susceptibility; repeat this operation a further 4 times. Verify the presence of virus at each passage. If the virus is not found, carry out a second series of passages; if the virus is not found in one of the second series of passages, the vaccine strain complies with the test. The vaccine strain complies with the test if: no cat dies or shows signs attributable to the vaccine; no indication of increase of virulence compared to the original vaccinal virus is observed; account is taken, notably, of the count of white blood cells, of results of histological examination of the thymus and of the titre of excreted virus.

Immunogenicity. The test described under Potency is suitable to demonstrate immunogenicity of the strain.

BATCH TESTING

If the test for potency has been carried out with satisfactory results on a representative batch of vaccine, this test may be omitted as a routine control on other batches of vaccine prepared from the same seed lot, subject to agreement by the competent authority.

IDENTIFICATION

Carry out replication of the vaccine virus in a susceptible cell line in a substrate suitable for a fluorescent antibody test or peroxidase test. Prepare suitable controls. Test a proportion of the cells with monoclonal antibodies specific for feline panleucopenia virus and a proportion with monoclonal antibodies specific for canine parvovirus. Feline panleucopenia virus is detected but no canine parvovirus is detected in the cells inoculated with the vaccine.

TESTS

Safety. Use 2 cats of the minimum age recommended for vaccination and having no antibodies against feline panleucopenia virus or against canine parvovirus. Administer 10 doses of the vaccine to each cat, by a recommended route. Observe the animals for 14 days. No abnormal local or systemic reaction occurs.

Extraneous viruses. Neutralise the vaccine using a suitable monospecific antiserum against feline panleucopenia virus and inoculate into suitable cell cultures; make at least one passage and maintain the cultures for 14 days. Examine the cultures for cytopathic effects and carry out tests for haemadsorbing agents. No signs of viral contamination occur in the cell cultures.

Bacterial and fungal contamination. The vaccine, reconstituted if necessary, complies with the test for sterility prescribed in the monograph on *Vaccines for veterinary use (0062)*.

Mycoplasmas (*2.6.7*). The vaccine complies with the test for mycoplasmas.

Virus titre. Reconstitute the vaccine, if necessary, and titrate in suitable cell cultures. One dose of vaccine contains not less than the quantity of virus equivalent to the minimum titre stated on the label.

POTENCY

Use 10 susceptible cats, 8 to 12 weeks old. Draw a blood sample from each cat and test individually for antibodies against feline panleucopenia virus and canine parvovirus to determine susceptibility. Vaccinate 5 cats by the recommended schedule. Carry out leucocyte counts 8 days and 4 days before challenge and calculate the mean of the 2 counts to serve as the initial value. 20 to 22 days after the last vaccination, challenge each cat by the intraperitoneal injection of a suspension of pathogenic feline panleucopenia virus. Observe the cats for 14 days. Carry out leucocyte counts on the fourth, sixth, eighth and tenth days after challenge. The test is not valid unless the 5 control cats all show on not fewer than one occasion a diminution in the number of leucocytes of at least 75 per cent of the initial value; these animals may die from panleucopenia. The vaccine complies with the test if the 5 vaccinated cats remain in excellent health and show no sign of leucopenia; that is to say, the diminution in the number of leucocytes does not exceed, in any of the four counts, 50 per cent of the initial value.

LABELLING

The label states that the vaccine should not be used in pregnant queens (unless it has been shown to be safe in such conditions).

01/2005:1321

FELINE LEUKAEMIA VACCINE (INACTIVATED)

Vaccinum leucosis felinae inactivatum

DEFINITION

Feline leukaemia vaccine (inactivated) is a preparation of immunogens from a suitable strain of feline leukaemia virus.

PRODUCTION

The immunogens consist either of a suitable strain of feline leukaemia virus inactivated in such a manner that adequate immunogenicity is maintained or of a fraction of the virus with adequate immunogenic properties; the immunogenic fraction may be produced by recombinant DNA technology.

Where applicable, the test for inactivation is carried out using a quantity of inactivated virus equivalent to not less than 25 doses of vaccine and two passages in the same type of cell cultures as used for the production of the vaccine or in cell cultures shown to be at least as sensitive; no live virus is detected.

The vaccine may contain an adjuvant.

CHOICE OF VACCINE COMPOSITION

The choice of the feline leukaemia virus strains and/or of the antigens included in the vaccine composition is made in such a manner as to ensure the safety (*5.2.6*) (including safety for pregnant queens if the vaccine may be used in such animals) and immunogenicity (*5.2.7*) of the vaccine. The following tests may be used during demonstration of safety and immunogenicity.

Safety. Carry out the test for each intended route of administration. Use animals that do not have antibodies against gp 70 antigen of feline leukaemia virus nor display

Vaccines

viraemia or antigenaemia at the time of the test; absence of antibodies and antigen is demonstrated by enzyme-linked immunosorbent assay (*2.7.1*).

A. Vaccinate, according to the intended schedule, not fewer than ten cats of the minimum age recommended for vaccination. Keep five cats as controls. Record the rectal temperature of each cat on the day before each vaccination, at the time of vaccination, 4 h and 8 h later, and once per day during the four following days. Observe the animals for at least 4 weeks after the last vaccination. No abnormal local or systemic reaction occurs during the test. 1, 2 and 4 weeks after the last vaccination, submit the animals to suitable tests for evidence of an immunosuppressive effect. The vaccine complies with the test if no significant difference is observed in vaccinated animals compared with controls.

B. Inject two doses of vaccine by one of the intended routes to not fewer than ten cats of the minimum age recommended for vaccination. At the end of the period of time stated in the instructions for use, inject one dose of vaccine to each animal. Where the instructions for use recommend it, administer a third injection after the period indicated. Observe the animals for 14 days after the last administration. The vaccine complies with the test if no abnormal local or systemic reaction occurs during the test.

C. If the vaccine is not contra-indicated for use in pregnant queens, inject two doses of vaccine into each of not fewer than ten cats at different stages of pregnancy. Observe the cats until parturition and note any effects on gestation and the offspring. The vaccine complies with the test if no abnormal local or systemic reaction occurs during the test.

Immunogenicity. The test described under Potency is suitable to demonstrate immunogenicity of the vaccine.

IN-PROCESS CONTROL TESTS

During production, suitable immunochemical tests are carried out for the evaluation of the quality and purity of the viral antigens included in the vaccine composition. The values found are within the limits approved for the particular vaccine.

BATCH TESTING

Potency. The test described under Potency is not carried out for routine testing of batches of vaccine. It is carried out, for a given vaccine, on one or more occasions, as decided by or with the agreement of the competent authority; where the test is not carried out, a suitable validated alternative method is used, the criteria for acceptance being set with reference to a batch of vaccine that has given satisfactory results in the test described under Potency.

Bacterial endotoxins. For vaccines produced by recombinant DNA technology with a bacterial host cell such as *Escherichia coli*, a test for bacterial endotoxins (*2.6.14*) is carried out on each final lot or, where the nature of the adjuvant prevents performance of a satisfactory test, on the antigen immediately before addition of the adjuvant. The value found is within the limit approved for the particular vaccine and which has been shown to be safe for cats.

IDENTIFICATION

When injected into healthy, seronegative cats, the vaccine stimulates the production of specific antibodies against the antigen or antigens stated on the label.

TESTS

Safety. Use two cats of the minimum age recommended for vaccination and that do not have antibodies against feline leukaemia virus. Inject by a recommended route a double dose of vaccine into each animal. Observe the animals for 14 days. The vaccine complies with the test if no abnormal local or systemic reaction is produced.

Inactivation. If the vaccine contains inactivated virus, carry out a test for residual live feline leukaemia virus by making two passages on susceptible cell cultures. No virus is detected. If the vaccine contains an adjuvant, if possible separate the adjuvant from the liquid phase by a method that does not inactivate the virus nor interfere in any other way with the detection of virus.

Sterility. The vaccine complies with the test for sterility prescribed in *Vaccines for veterinary use (0062)*.

POTENCY

Use not fewer than twenty-five susceptible cats of the minimum age recommended for vaccination, free from antibodies against the antigens of feline leukaemia virus and against the feline oncogene membrane antigen (anti-FOCMA antibodies), and showing no viraemia or antigenaemia at the time of the test. Vaccinate not fewer than fifteen cats by a recommended route in accordance with the instructions for use. Keep not fewer than ten cats as controls. Observe the animals for at least 14 days after the last administration of vaccine. Inject by the peritoneal or oronasal route, on one or several occasions, a quantity of a virulent strain of feline leukaemia virus sufficient to induce persistent viraemia or antigenaemia in not fewer than 80 per cent of susceptible animals; use for the challenge an epidemiologically relevant strain consisting predominantly of type A virus. Observe the animals for 15 weeks and, from the third week onwards, test each week for viraemia or antigenaemia (p27 protein) by suitable methods such as immunofluorescence on circulating leucocytes or enzyme-linked immunosorbent assay. A cat is considered persistently infected if it shows positive viraemia or antigenaemia for three consecutive weeks or on five occasions, consecutively or not, between the third and the fifteenth week. The test is not valid if fewer than 80 per cent of the control cats are persistently infected. The vaccine complies with the test if not fewer than 80 per cent of the vaccinated cats show no persistent infection.

LABELLING

The label states the antigen or antigens contained in the vaccine.

01/2005:1207

FELINE VIRAL RHINOTRACHEITIS VACCINE (INACTIVATED)

Vaccinum rhinotracheitidis viralis felinae inactivatum

DEFINITION

Feline viral rhinotracheitis vaccine (inactivated) is a preparation of a suitable strain of feline rhinotracheitis virus (feline herpesvirus 1) that has been inactivated while maintaining adequate immunogenic properties or of an inactivated fraction of the virus having adequate immunogenic properties.

PRODUCTION

The vaccine strain is grown in suitable cell cultures (*5.2.4*). The viral suspension is harvested and inactivated.

The test for inactivation is carried out using 2 passages in cell cultures of the same type as those used for preparation of the vaccine or in cell cultures shown to be at least as sensitive; the quantity of virus used in the test is equivalent to not less than 25 doses of vaccine. No live virus is detected.

The virus may be fragmented and the fragments may be purified and concentrated. The vaccine may be adjuvanted; it may be freeze-dried.

CHOICE OF VACCINE COMPOSITION

The vaccine is shown to be satisfactory with respect to safety and immunogenicity in cats. The following test may be used during demonstration of efficacy (*5.2.7*).

Immunogenicity. The test described under Potency, carried out using vaccine prepared from the most attenuated virus that will be attained during production, is suitable to demonstrate immunogenicity of the strain.

BATCH TESTING

The test described under Potency is not necessarily carried out for routine testing of batches of vaccine. It is carried out, for a given vaccine, on one or more occasions, as decided by or with the agreement of the competent authority. Where the test is not carried out, a suitable alternative validated test is carried out, the criteria for acceptance being set with reference to a batch of vaccine that has given satisfactory results in the test described under Potency. The following test may be used after a satisfactory correlation with the test described under Potency has been established.

Batch potency test. Use a group of 15 seronegative mice. Administer half a dose of the vaccine to each mouse and 7 days later repeat the administration. 21 days after the first injection, take blood samples and determine the level of antibodies against feline rhinotracheitis virus by a suitable immunochemical method (*2.7.1*), such as an immunofluorescence technique using pools of serum from groups of 3 mice. The antibody levels are not significantly lower than those obtained with a batch of vaccine that has given satisfactory results in the test described under Potency.

IDENTIFICATION

When administered to susceptible animals, the vaccine stimulates the production of specific serum antibodies against feline rhinotracheitis virus or against the fraction of the virus used to produce the vaccine.

TESTS

Safety. Use cats 8 to 12 weeks old and preferably having no feline rhinotracheitis virus antibodies or antibodies to a fraction of the virus, or, where justified, use cats with a low level of such antibodies as long as they have not been vaccinated against viral rhinotracheitis and administration of the vaccine does not cause an anamnestic response. Administer a double dose of vaccine by a recommended route to each of 2 cats. Observe the cats for 14 days. No abnormal local or systemic reaction occurs.

Inactivation. Carry out a test for residual infectious feline rhinotracheitis virus using 10 doses of vaccine and 2 passages in cell cultures of the same type as those used for preparation of the vaccine or in other suitably sensitive cell cultures. No live virus is detected. If the vaccine contains an adjuvant that interferes with the test, where possible separate the adjuvant from the liquid phase by a method that does not inactivate or otherwise interfere with detection of live virus.

Sterility. The reconstituted vaccine complies with the test for sterility prescribed under *Vaccines for veterinary use (0062)*.

POTENCY

Use cats 8 to 12 weeks old and which do not have antibodies against feline rhinotracheitis virus or against a fraction of the virus. Vaccinate 10 cats according to the instructions for use and keep 10 cats as controls. 4 weeks after the last administration of vaccine, administer intranasally to each of the 20 cats, a quantity of virulent feline rhinotracheitis virus sufficient to produce in susceptible cats typical signs of disease such as fever, nasal discharge and cough. Observe the cats for 14 days; collect nasal washings daily on days 2 to 14 after challenge to test for virus excretion. Note daily the body temperature and signs of disease using the scoring system shown below. If any sign of disease is observed on more than one day, record the score once only. The vaccine complies with the test if the score for the vaccinated cats is significantly lower than that for the controls.

Sign	**Score**
Death	10
Depressed state	2
Temperature:	
39.5 °C - 40.0 °C	1
≥ 40.0 °C	2
≤ 37.0 °C	3
Glossitis	3
Nasal discharge, slight	1
Nasal discharge, copious	2
Cough	2
Sneezing	1
Sneezing, paroxysmal	2
Ocular discharge, slight	1
Ocular discharge, serious	2
Conjunctivitis	2
Weight loss ≥ 5.0 per cent	5
Virus excretion (total number of days):	
≤ 4 days	1
5-7 days	2
> 7 days	3

01/2005:1206

FELINE VIRAL RHINOTRACHEITIS VACCINE (LIVE), FREEZE-DRIED

Vaccinum rhinotracheitidis viralis felinae vivum cryodesiccatum

DEFINITION

Freeze-dried feline viral rhinotracheitis vaccine (live) is a preparation of a suitable strain of feline rhinotracheitis virus (feline herpesvirus 1).

PRODUCTION

The vaccine strain is grown in suitable cell cultures (*5.2.4*). The viral suspension is harvested and mixed with a suitable stabilising solution. The mixture is subsequently freeze-dried.

CHOICE OF VACCINE STRAIN

Only a virus strain shown to be satisfactory with respect to safety, reversion to virulence and immunogenicity may be used in the preparation of the vaccine; if the vaccine is not contra-indicated in pregnant queens, the safety for such use is demonstrated. The following tests may be used during demonstration of safety (*5.2.6*) and efficacy (*5.2.7*).

Safety. Administer by a recommended route to each of ten cats, of the minimum age stated for vaccination and which do not have antibodies against feline rhinotracheitis virus, a quantity of virus equivalent to ten times the maximum titre that may be expected in a batch of vaccine. Observe the cats for 21 days. They remain in good health and show no abnormal local or systemic reaction.

Reversion to virulence. Administer by a recommended route to each of two cats that do not have antibodies against feline rhinotracheitis virus, a quantity of virus that will allow optimal re-isolation of the virus for subsequent passages (for example ten times the minimum titre to be stated on the label). Kill the cats 2 to 4 days after the inoculation and remove the nasal mucus, tonsils and local lymphatic ganglia and the trachea; mix the samples, homogenise in 10 ml of buffered saline and allow to settle; inoculate 1 ml of supernatant intranasally into two cats; repeat this operation not fewer than five times; verify the presence of virus at each passage; if the virus is not recovered, carry out a second series of passages. Observe the cats given the last passage for 21 days and compare any reactions with those seen in the safety test described above. No evidence of an increase in virulence is seen compared to the original virus.

Immunogenicity. The test described under Potency is suitable to demonstrate immunogenicity of the strain.

BATCH TESTING

If the test for potency has been carried out with satisfactory results on a representative batch of vaccine, this test may be omitted as a routine control on other batches of vaccine prepared from the same seed lot, subject to agreement by the competent authority.

IDENTIFICATION

When mixed with a monospecific antiserum, the reconstituted vaccine no longer infects susceptible cell cultures into which it is inoculated.

TESTS

Safety. Administer ten doses of the vaccine in a suitable volume by a recommended route to two cats, 8 to 12 weeks old, that do not have antibodies against feline rhinotracheitis virus. Observe the cats for 14 days. They remain in good health and show no abnormal local or systemic reaction.

Bacterial and fungal contamination. The reconstituted vaccine complies with the test for sterility prescribed in the monograph on *Vaccines for veterinary use (0062)*.

Mycoplasmas (*2.6.7*). The reconstituted vaccine complies with the test for mycoplasmas.

Extraneous viruses. Neutralise the vaccinal virus using a monospecfic antiserum and inoculate into suitable cell cultures; make at least one passage and maintain the cultures for 14 days. No cytopathic effect develops; the cells show no evidence of the presence of haemadsorbing agents or other signs of viral contamination.

Virus titre. Titrate the reconstituted vaccine in susceptible cell cultures at a temperature favourable to replication of the virus. One dose of vaccine contains not less than the quantity of virus corresponding to the minimum virus titre stated on the label.

POTENCY

Use cats 8 to 12 weeks old and which do not have antibodies against feline viral rhinotracheitis virus. Vaccinate ten cats according to the instructions for use and keep ten cats as controls. Four weeks after the last administration of vaccine, administer intranasally to each cat a quantity of virulent feline rhinotracheitis virus sufficient to produce in susceptible cats typical signs of disease such as fever, nasal discharge and cough. Observe the cats for 14 days; collect nasal washings daily on days 2 to 14 after challenge to test for virus excretion. Note daily the body temperature and signs of disease using the scoring system shown below. If any sign of disease is observed on more than one day, record the score once only. The vaccine complies with the test if the score for the vaccinated cats is significantly lower than that for the controls.

Sign	**Score**
Death	10
Depressed state	2
Temperature:	
39.5 °C - 40.0 °C	1
≥ 40.0 °C	2
≤ 37.0 °C	3
Glossitis	3
Nasal discharge, slight	1
Nasal discharge, copious	2
Cough	2
Sneezing	1
Sneezing, paroxysmal	2
Ocular discharge, slight	1
Ocular discharge, serious	2
Conjunctivitis	2
Weight loss ≥ 5.0 per cent	5
Virus excretion (total number of days):	
≤ 4 days	1
5-7 days	2
> 7 days	3

01/2005:0063
corrected

FOOT-AND-MOUTH DISEASE (RUMINANTS) VACCINE (INACTIVATED)

Vaccinum aphtharum epizooticarum inactivatum ad ruminantes

DEFINITION

Foot-and-mouth disease (ruminants) vaccine (inactivated) is a liquid preparation containing one or more types or sub-types of foot-and-mouth disease virus inactivated without impairing their immunogenic activity.

PRODUCTION

The virus is grown either in suspensions of cattle-tongue epithelium obtained immediately after slaughter of healthy animals, or, preferably, in suitable cell cultures (*5.2.4*). The

Vaccines

virus is separated from cellular material by filtration or other suitable procedures and the virus is inactivated in suitable conditions.

The vaccine is prepared from inactivated antigen by blending with one or more adjuvants. The antigen may be concentrated and purified by a number of procedures. The concentrated antigen is used for the preparation of vaccine immediately or after storage at a temperature not exceeding − 90 °C, unless stability of the antigen at a higher temperature has been demonstrated.

Validation of the inactivation procedure. During inactivation, the virus titre is monitored by a sensitive and reproducible technique. The inactivation procedure is not satisfactory unless the decrease in virus titre, plotted logarithmically, is linear and extrapolation indicates that there is less than 1 infectious virus unit per 10^4 litres of liquid preparation at the end of inactivation.

BULK INACTIVATED ANTIGEN

Inactivation. A proportion of each batch of bulk inactivated antigen representing at least 200 doses is tested for freedom from infectious virus by inoculation into sensitive cell cultures. For this purpose, the sample of the inactivated antigen is concentrated to allow testing of such large samples in cell cultures. It must be shown that the selected concentration and assay systems are not detrimental to detection of infectious virus within the test sample and that the concentrated inactivated antigen does not interfere with virus replication or cause toxic changes.

Antigenicity. The antigen content of each batch of bulk inactivated antigen is determined by an *in vitro* method (for example, 146S-particle measurement by sucrose density gradient centrifugation and ultraviolet spectophotometry at 259 nm).

Safety. A representative sample of the bulk inactivated antigen may be diluted and blended with the adjuvants for safety testing in cattle, as described below.

Sterility. The bulk inactivated antigen, the adjuvants and all dilution buffers comply with the test for sterility prescribed in the monograph on *Vaccines for veterinary use (0062)*.

Potency. A representative sample of the bulk inactivated antigen may be diluted and blended with the adjuvants for potency testing in cattle, as described below.

In situations of extreme urgency and subject to agreement by the competent authority, a batch of vaccine may be released before completion of the tests and the determination of potency if a test for sterility has been carried out on the bulk inactivated antigen and all other components of the vaccine and if the test for safety and the determination of potency have been carried out on a representative batch of vaccine prepared from the same bulk inactivated antigen. In this context, a batch is not considered to be representative unless it has been prepared using the same amount of antigen and with the same formulation as the batch to be released.

IDENTIFICATION

The serum of a susceptible animal that has been immunised with the vaccine neutralises the types or sub-types of the virus used to prepare the vaccine, when tested by a suitably sensitive method.

TESTS

Safety. Use three non-vaccinated cattle not less than 6 months old having serum free from foot-and-mouth disease antibodies and coming from regions free from foot-and-mouth disease. Inoculate each animal intradermally into the tongue at not fewer than twenty points, using 0.1 ml of the vaccine at each point. Observe the animals for not less than 4 days. No lesions or signs of foot-and-mouth disease occur. At the end of the observation period, inject into the same animals by the prescribed route three times the dose stated on the label. Observe the animals for 6 days after this inoculation. No lesions or clinical signs of foot-and-mouth disease occur on the feet or tongue and any reaction at the site of injection remains insignificant.

Sterility. It complies with the test for sterility prescribed in the monograph on *Vaccines for veterinary use (0062)*.

POTENCY

The potency of the vaccine is expressed as the number of 50 per cent cattle protective doses (PD_{50}) contained in the dose stated on the label. The PD_{50} is determined in animals given primary vaccination and challenged by the inoculation of 10 000 ID_{50} of virulent bovine virus of the same type or sub-type as that used in the preparation of the vaccine in the conditions described below.

The vaccine contains at least 3 PD_{50} per dose for cattle.

Carry out a potency test for each type and sub-type of foot-and-mouth disease virus present in the vaccine.

Use cattle not less than 6 months old, obtained from areas free from foot-and-mouth disease, which have never been vaccinated against foot-and-mouth disease and are free from antibodies neutralising the different types of foot-and-mouth disease virus. Vaccinate not fewer than three groups of not fewer than five cattle per group by the route stated on the label. Use a different dose of the vaccine for each group. Administer the different doses by injecting different volumes of the vaccine rather than by dilution of the vaccine. For example, if the label states that the injection of 2 ml corresponds to the administration of 1 dose of vaccine, a 1/4 dose of vaccine would be obtained by injecting 0.5 ml, and a 1/10 dose would be would be obtained by injecting 0.2 ml. Three weeks after the vaccination, challenge the vaccinated animals and a control group of two animals with a suspension of virus that has been obtained from cattle and that is fully virulent and of the same type or sub-type as that used in the preparation of the vaccine, by inoculating a total of 10 000 ID_{50} intradermally into two sites on the upper surface of the tongue (0.1 ml per site). Observe the animals for 8 days and then slaughter. Unprotected animals show lesions at sites other than the tongue. Protected animals may display lingual lesions. The test is not valid unless each control animal shows lesions on at least three feet. From the number of protected animals in each group, calculate the PD_{50} content of the vaccine.

STORAGE

The vaccine must not be frozen.

LABELLING

The label states:

- the method of preparation,
- the types and sub-types of virus used to prepare the vaccine.

01/2005:0649

FOWL-POX VACCINE (LIVE)

Vaccinum variolae gallinaceae vivum

1. DEFINITION

Fowl-pox vaccine (live) is a preparation of a suitable strain of avian pox virus. This monograph applies to vaccines intended for administration to chickens for active immunisation.

2. PRODUCTION

2-1. *PREPARATION OF THE VACCINE*

The vaccine virus is grown in embryonated hens' eggs or in cell cultures.

2-2. *SUBSTRATE FOR VIRUS PROPAGATION*

2-2-1. **Embryonated hens' eggs**. If the vaccine virus is grown in embryonated hens' eggs, they are obtained from flocks free from specified pathogens (SPF) (*5.2.2*).

2-2-2. **Cell cultures**. If the vaccine virus is grown in cell cultures, they comply with the requirements for cell cultures for production of veterinary vaccines (*5.2.4*).

2-3. *SEED LOTS*

2-3-1. **Extraneous agents**. The master seed lot complies with the tests for extraneous agents in seed lots (*2.6.24*). In these tests on the master seed lot, the organisms used are not more than 5 passages from the master seed lot at the start of the tests.

2-4. *CHOICE OF VACCINE VIRUS*

The vaccine virus shall be shown to be satisfactory with respect to safety (*5.2.6*) and efficacy (*5.2.7*) for the chickens for which it is intended.
The following tests for safety (section 2-4-1), increase in virulence (section 2-4-2) and immunogenicity (section 2-4-3) may be used during demonstration of safety and immunogenicity.

2-4-1. **Safety**. Carry out the test for each route and method of administration to be recommended for vaccination using in each case chickens not older than the youngest age to be recommended for vaccination. Use vaccine virus at the least attenuated passage level that will be present between the master seed lot and a batch of the vaccine. For each test use not fewer than 20 chickens, from an SPF flock (*5.2.2*). Administer to each chicken a quantity of the vaccine virus equivalent to not less than 10 times the maximum virus titre likely to be contained in a dose of the vaccine. Observe the chickens at least daily for 21 days. The test is not valid if more than 10 per cent of the chickens die from causes not attributable to the vaccine virus. The vaccine virus complies with the test if no chicken shows notable clinical signs of fowl pox or dies from causes attributable to the vaccine virus.

2-4-2. **Increase in virulence**. Administer by a suitable route a quantity of the vaccine virus that will allow recovery of virus for the passages described below to each of 5 chickens not older than the minimum age to be recommended for vaccination and from an SPF flock (*5.2.2*). Use the vaccine virus at the least attenuated passage level that will be present between the master seed lot and a batch of the vaccine. Prepare 4 to 7 days after administration a suspension from the induced skin lesions of each chicken and pool these samples. Administer 0.2 ml of the pooled samples by cutaneous scarification of the comb or other unfeathered part of the body, or by another suitable method to each of 5 other chickens not older than the minimum age to be recommended for vaccination and from an SPF flock (*5.2.2*). Carry out this passage operation not fewer than 5 times; verify the presence of the virus at each passage. Care must be taken to avoid contamination by virus from previous passages. If the virus is not found at a passage level, carry out a second series of passages. Carry out the test for safety (section 2-4-1) using the unpassaged vaccine virus and the maximally passaged virus that has been recovered. Administer the virus by the route recommended for vaccination likely to be the least safe. The vaccine virus complies with the test if no indication of increase in virulence of the maximally passaged virus compared with the unpassaged virus is observed. If virus is not recovered at any passage level in the first and second series of passages, the vaccine virus also complies with the test.

2-4-3. **Immunogenicity**. A test is carried out for each route and method of administration to be recommended using in each case chickens not older than the youngest age to be recommended for vaccination. The quantity of the vaccine virus administered to each chicken is not greater than the minimum virus titre to be stated on the label and the virus is at the most attenuated passage level that will be present in a batch of the vaccine. Use for the test not fewer than 30 chickens of the same origin and from an SPF flock (*5.2.2*). Vaccinate by a recommended route not fewer than 20 chickens. Maintain not fewer than 10 chickens as controls. Challenge each chicken after 21 days by the feather-follicle route with a sufficient quantity of virulent fowl-pox virus. Observe the chickens at least daily for 21 days after challenge. Record the deaths and the number of surviving chickens that show clinical signs of disease. Examine each surviving chicken for macroscopic lesions: cutaneous lesions of the comb, wattle and other unfeathered areas of the skin and diphtherical lesions of the mucous membranes of the oro-pharyngeal area.

The test is not valid if:

– during the observation period after challenge fewer than 90 per cent of the control chickens die or show severe clinical signs of fowl pox, including notable macroscopical lesions of the skin or mucous membranes of the oro-pharyngeal area,

– and/or during the period between vaccination and challenge, more than 10 per cent of the control or vaccinated chickens show abnormal clinical signs or die from causes not attributable to the vaccine.

The vaccine virus complies with the test if during the observation period after challenge not less than 90 per cent of the vaccinated chickens survive and show no notable clinical signs of disease, including macroscopical lesions of the skin and mucous membranes of the oro-pharyngeal area.

3. BATCH TESTS

3-1. **Identification**. Carry out an immunostaining test in cell cultures to demonstrate the presence of the vaccine virus. For egg adapted strains, inoculate the vaccine into eggs and notice the characteristic lesions.

3-2. **Bacteria and fungi**

Vaccines intended for administration by injection, scarification or piercing of the wing web comply with the test for sterility prescribed in the monograph *Vaccines for veterinary use (0062)*.

Vaccines not intended for administration by injection, scarification or piercing of the wing web either comply with the test for sterility prescribed in the monograph *Vaccines for veterinary use (0062)* or with the following test: carry out a quantitative test for bacterial and fungal contamination; carry out identification tests for

Vaccines

microorganisms detected in the vaccine; the vaccine does not contain pathogenic microorganisms and contains not more than 1 non-pathogenic microorganism per dose.

Any liquid supplied with the vaccine complies with the test for sterility prescribed in the monograph *Vaccines for veterinary use (0062)*.

3-3. **Mycoplasmas**. The vaccine complies with the test for mycoplasmas (*2.6.7*).

3-4. **Extraneous agents**. The vaccine complies with the tests for extraneous agents in batches of finished product (*2.6.25*).

3-5. **Safety**. Use not fewer than 10 chickens from an SPF flock (*5.2.2*) of the youngest age recommended for vaccination. For vaccines recommended for use in chickens older than 6 weeks, chickens 6 weeks old may be used. Administer 10 doses of the vaccine to each chicken by a recommended route. Observe the chickens at least daily for 21 days. The test is not valid if more than 20 per cent of the chickens show abnormal clinical signs or die from causes not attributable to the vaccine.

The vaccine complies with the test if no chicken shows notable clinical signs of disease or dies from causes attributable to the vaccine.

3-6. **Virus titre**. Titrate the vaccine virus by inoculation into embryonated hens' eggs from an SPF flock (*5.2.2*) or into suitable cell cultures (*5.2.4*). The vaccine complies with the test if 1 dose contains not less than the minimum virus titre stated on the label.

3-7. **Potency**. The vaccine complies with the requirements of the test prescribed under Immunogenicity (section 2-4-3) when administered according to the recommended schedule by a recommended route and method. It is not necessary to carry out the potency test for each batch of the vaccine if it has been carried out on a representative batch using a vaccinating dose containing not more than the minimum virus titre stated on the label.

01/2005:1521

FURUNCULOSIS VACCINE (INACTIVATED, OIL-ADJUVANTED, INJECTABLE) FOR SALMONIDS

Vaccinum furunculosidis ad salmonidas inactivatum cum adiuvatione oleosa ad iniectionem

DEFINITION

Furunculosis vaccine (inactivated, oil-adjuvanted, injectable) for salmonids is prepared from cultures of one or more suitable strains of *Aeromonas salmonicida* subsp. *salmonicida*.

PRODUCTION

The strains of *A. salmonicida* are cultured and harvested separately. The harvests are inactivated by a suitable method. They may be purified and concentrated. Whole or disrupted cells may be used and the vaccine may contain extracellular products of the bacterium released into the growth medium. The vaccine contains an oily adjuvant.

CHOICE OF VACCINE COMPOSITION

The strains included in the vaccine are shown to be suitable with respect to production of antigens of assumed immunological importance. The vaccine is shown to be satisfactory with respect to safety (*5.2.6*) and efficacy (*5.2.7*) in the species of fish for which it is intended. The following tests may be used during demonstration of safety and immunogenicity.

Safety

A. During development of the vaccine, safety is tested on 3 different batches. A test is carried out in each species of fish for which the vaccine is intended. The fish used are from a population that does not have specific antibodies against *A. salmonicida* subsp. *salmonicida* and has not been vaccinated against or exposed to furunculosis. The test is carried out in the conditions recommended for the use of the vaccine with a water temperature not less than 10 °C. An amount of vaccine corresponding to twice the recommended dose per mass unit is administered intraperitoneally into each of not fewer than 50 fish of the minimum body mass recommended for vaccination. The fish are observed for 21 days. No abnormal local or systemic reaction occurs. The test is invalid if more than 6 per cent of the fish die from causes not attributable to the vaccine.

B. Safety is also demonstrated in field trials by administering the intended dose to a sufficient number of fish in not fewer than 2 sets of premises. Samples of 30 fish are taken on 3 occasions (after vaccination, at the middle of the rearing period and at slaughter) and examined for local reactions in the body cavity. Moderate lesions involving localised adhesions between viscera or between viscera and the abdominal wall and slight opaqueness and/or sparse pigmentation of the peritoneum are acceptable. Extensive lesions including adhesions between greater parts of the abdominal organs, massive pigmentation and/or obvious thickening and opaqueness of greater areas of the peritoneum are unacceptable if they occur in more than 10 per cent of the fish in any sample. Such lesions include adhesions that give the viscera a "one-unit" appearance and/or lead to manifest laceration of the peritoneum following evisceration.

Immunogenicity. The test described under Potency is suitable to demonstrate the immunogenicity of the vaccine.

BATCH TESTING

Batch potency test. For routine testing of batches of vaccine, the test described under Potency may be carried out using not fewer than 30 fish per group; alternatively, a suitable validated test based on antibody response may be carried out, the criteria being set with reference to a batch of vaccine that has given satisfactory results in the test described under Potency. The following test may be used after a satisfactory correlation with the test described under Potency has been established.

Use fish from a population that does not have specific antibodies against *A. salmonicida* subsp. *salmonicida* and that are within defined limits for body mass. Carry out the test at a defined temperature. Inject intraperitoneally into each of not fewer than 25 fish one dose of vaccine, according to the instructions for use. Perform mock vaccination on a control group of not fewer than 10 fish. Collect blood samples at a defined time after vaccination. Determine for each sample the level of specific antibodies against *A. salmonicida* subsp. *salmonicida* by a suitable immunochemical method (*2.7.1*). The vaccine complies with the test if the mean level of antibodies is not significantly lower than that found for a batch that gave satisfactory results in the test described under Potency. The test is not valid if the control group shows antibodies against *A. salmonicida* subsp. *salmonicida*.

Vaccines

IDENTIFICATION

When injected into fish that do not have specific antibodies against *A. salmonicida,* the vaccine stimulates the production of such antibodies.

TESTS

Safety. Use not fewer than 10 fish of one of the species for which the vaccine is intended, having, where possible, the minimum body mass recommended for vaccination; if fish of the minimum body mass are not available, use fish not greater than twice this mass. Use fish from a population that preferably does not have specific antibodies against *A. salmonicida* subsp. *salmonicida* or, where justified, use fish from a population with a low level of such antibodies as long as they have not been vaccinated against or exposed to furunculosis and administration of the vaccine does not cause an anamnestic response. Carry out the test in the conditions recommended for use of the vaccine with a water temperature not less than 10 °C. Administer intraperitoneally to each fish an amount of vaccine corresponding to twice the recommended dose per mass unit. Observe the animals for 21 days. No abnormal local or systemic reaction attributable to the vaccine occurs. The test is invalid if more than 10 per cent of the fish die from causes not attributable to the vaccine.

Sterility. The vaccine complies with the test for sterility prescribed in the monograph on *Vaccines for veterinary use (0062)*.

POTENCY

Carry out the test according to a protocol defining limits of body mass for the fish, water source, water flow and temperature limits, and preparation of a standardised challenge. Vaccinate not fewer than 100 fish by a recommended route, according to the instructions for use. Perform mock vaccination on a control group of not fewer than 100 fish; mark vaccinated and control fish for identification. Keep all the fish in the same tank or mix equal numbers of controls and vaccinates in each tank if more than one tank is used. Carry out challenge by injection at a fixed time interval after vaccination, defined according to the statement regarding development of immunity. Use for challenge a culture of *A. salmonicida* subsp. *salmonicida* whose virulence has been verified. Observe the fish daily until at least 60 per cent specific mortality is reached in the control group. Plot for both vaccinates and controls a curve of specific mortality against time from challenge and determine by interpolation the time corresponding to 60 per cent specific mortality in controls. The test is invalid if the specific mortality is less than 60 per cent in the control group 21 days after the first death in the fish. Read from the curve for vaccinates the mortality (M) at the time corresponding to 60 per cent mortality in controls. Calculate the relative percentage survival (RPS) from the expression:

$$\left(1 - \frac{M}{60}\right) \times 100$$

The vaccine complies with the test if the RPS is not less than 80 per cent.

LABELLING

The label states information on the time needed for development of immunity after vaccination under the range of conditions corresponding to the recommended use.

01/2005:0696

INFECTIOUS BOVINE RHINOTRACHEITIS VACCINE (LIVE), FREEZE-DRIED

Vaccinum rhinotracheitidis infectivae bovinae vivum cryodesiccatum

DEFINITION

Freeze-dried infectious bovine rhinotracheitis vaccine (live) is a preparation of one or more attenuated strains of infectious bovine rhinotracheitis virus (bovine herpesvirus 1).

PRODUCTION

The virus is grown in suitable cell cultures (*5.2.4*). The viral suspension is collected and mixed with a suitable stabilising solution. The mixture is subsequently freeze-dried.

CHOICE OF VACCINE STRAIN

Only a virus strain shown to be satisfactory with respect to the following characteristics may be used in the preparation of the vaccine: safety (including absence of abortigenicity and passage through the placenta); reversion to virulence and immunogenicity. The strain may have markers. The following tests may be used during demonstration of safety (*5.2.6*) and efficacy (*5.2.7*).

Safety. Use 5 calves 3 months old, or of the minimum age to be recommended for vaccination if this is less than 3 months, and that do not have antibodies against infectious bovine rhinotracheitis virus. Administer to each calf, by the intended route, a quantity of virus corresponding to 10 doses of vaccine. The calves are observed for 21 days. No abnormal local or systemic reaction occurs.

Abortigenicity and passage through the placenta. 24 pregnant cows that do not have antibodies against infectious bovine rhinotracheitis virus are used for the test: 8 of the cows are in the fourth month of pregnancy, 8 in the fifth month and 8 in the sixth or seventh month. A quantity of virus equivalent to ten doses of vaccine is administered by the intended route to each cow. The cows are observed until the end of pregnancy. If abortion occurs, tests for infectious bovine rhinotracheitis virus are carried out; neither the virus nor viral antigens are present in the foetus or placenta. A test for antibodies against infectious bovine rhinotracheitis virus is carried out on calves born at term before ingestion of colostrum; no such antibodies are found.

Reversion to virulence. Suitable samples are taken from the 5 calves used for the test for safety at a time when the vaccinal virus can be easily detected. The presence and titre of virus in the samples are verified. The samples are then mixed and administered intranasally to 2 other calves of the same age having no antibodies against bovine rhinotracheitis virus. 5 further serial passages are carried out. The presence of the virus is verified at each passage. No abnormal local or systemic reaction occurs.

Immunogenicity. The test described under Potency is suitable to demonstrate immunogenicity.

BATCH TESTING

If the test for potency has been carried out with satisfactory results on a representative batch of vaccine, this test may be omitted as a routine control on other batches of vaccine prepared from the same seed lot, subject to agreement by the competent authority.

IDENTIFICATION

A. Reconstitute the vaccine as stated on the label. When mixed with a suitable quantity of a monospecific antiserum, the reconstituted vaccine is no longer able to infect susceptible cell cultures into which it is inoculated.

B. Any markers of the strain are verified.

TESTS

Safety. Use 2 calves 3 months old or of the minimum age recommended for vaccination if this is less than 3 months, having no antibodies against bovine rhinotracheitis virus. Administer 10 doses of the reconstituted vaccine to each calf by a recommended route. Observe the calves for 21 days. No abnormal local or systemic reaction occurs.

Bacterial and fungal contamination. The reconstituted vaccine complies with the test for sterility prescribed in the monograph on *Vaccines for veterinary use (0062)*.

Mycoplasmas (*2.6.7*). The reconstituted vaccine complies with the test for mycoplasmas.

Extraneous viruses. Neutralise the vaccine using a monospecific antiserum and inoculate into suitable cell cultures. Maintain the cultures for 14 days and make a passage at 7 days. The cell cultures show no signs of viral contamination.

Virus titre. Titrate the reconstituted vaccine in susceptible cell cultures at a temperature favourable to replication of the virus. One dose of the vaccine contains not less than the quantity of virus equivalent to the minimum virus titre stated on the label.

POTENCY

Use susceptible calves, 2 to 3 months old and free from antibodies neutralising infectious bovine rhinotracheitis virus. Administer to five calves, by the route stated on the label a volume of the reconstituted vaccine containing a quantity of virus equivalent to the minimum virus titre stated on the label. Keep 2 calves as controls. After 21 days, administer intranasally to the seven calves a quantity of infectious bovine rhinotracheitis virus sufficient to produce typical signs of disease such as fever, ocular and nasal discharge and ulceration of the nasal mucosa in a susceptible calf. Observe the animals for 21 days. The vaccinated calves show no more than mild signs; the controls show typical signs. In not fewer than 4 of the 5 vaccinated calves, the maximum virus titre found in the nasal mucus is at least 100 times lower than the average of the maximum titres found in the control calves; the average number of days on which virus is excreted is at least 3 days less in vaccinated calves than in the control calves.

01/2005:2038

INFECTIOUS CHICKEN ANAEMIA VACCINE (LIVE)

Vaccinum anaemiae infectivae pulli vivum

1. DEFINITION

Infectious chicken anaemia vaccine (live) is a preparation of a suitable strain of chicken anaemia virus. This monograph applies to vaccines intended for administration to breeder chickens for active immunisation, to prevent excretion of the virus, to prevent or reduce egg transmission and to protect passively their future progeny.

2. PRODUCTION

2-1. *PREPARATION OF THE VACCINE*

The vaccine virus is grown in embryonated hens' eggs or in cell cultures.

2-2. *SUBSTRATE FOR VIRUS PROPAGATION*

2-2-1. **Embryonated hens' eggs**. If the vaccine virus is grown in embryonated hens' eggs, they are obtained from flocks free from specified pathogens (SPF) (*5.2.2*).

2-2-2. **Cell cultures**. If the vaccine virus is grown in cell cultures, they comply with the requirements for cell cultures for production of veterinary vaccines (*5.2.4*).

2-3. *SEED LOTS*

2-3-1. **Extraneous agents**. The master seed lot complies with the tests for extraneous agents in seed lots (*2.6.24*). In these tests on the master seed lot, the organisms used are not more than 5 passages from the master seed lot at the start of the tests.

2-4. *CHOICE OF VACCINE VIRUS*

The vaccine virus shall be shown to be satisfactory with respect to safety (*5.2.6*) and efficacy (*5.2.7*) for the chickens for which it is intended.

The following tests for safety (section 2-4-1), increase in virulence (section 2-4-2) and immunogenicity (section 2-4-3) may be used during the demonstration of safety and immunogenicity.

2-4-1. **Safety**

2-4-1-1. *General test*. Carry out the test for each route and method of administration to be recommended for vaccination in chickens not older than the youngest age to be recommended for vaccination and from an SPF flock (*5.2.2*). Use vaccine virus at the least attenuated passage level that will be present between the master seed lot and a batch of the vaccine. For each test use not fewer than 20 chickens. Administer to each chicken a quantity of the vaccine virus not less than 10 times the maximum virus titre likely to be contained in 1 dose of the vaccine. 14 days after vaccination, collect blood samples from half of the chickens and determine the haematocrit value. Kill these chickens and carry out post-mortem examination. Note any pathological changes attributable to chicken anaemia virus, such as thymic atrophy and specific bone-marrow lesions. Observe the remaining chickens at least daily for 21 days. The vaccine virus complies with the test if during the observation period no chicken shows notable clinical signs of chicken anaemia or dies from causes attributable to the vaccine virus.

2-4-1-2. *Safety for young chicks*. Use not fewer than twenty 1-day-old chicks from an SPF flock (*5.2.2*). Administer to each chick by the oculonasal route a quantity of the vaccine virus equivalent to not less than the maximum titre likely to be contained in 1 dose of the vaccine. Observe the chicks at least daily. Record the incidence of any clinical signs attributable to the vaccine virus, such as depression, and any deaths. 14 days after vaccination, collect blood samples from half of the chicks and determine the haematocrit value. Kill these chicks and carry out post-mortem examination. Note any pathological changes attributable to chicken anaemia virus, such as thymic atrophy and specific bone marrow lesions. Observe the remaining chicks at least daily for 21 days. Assess the extent to which the vaccine strain is pathogenic for 1-day-old susceptible chicks from the results of the clinical observations and mortality rates and the proportion of chicks examined at 14 days that show anaemia (haematocrit value less than 27 per cent) and signs of infectious chicken anaemia on post-mortem examination. The results are used to formulate the label statement on safety for young chicks.

2-4-2. **Increase in virulence**. The test for increase in virulence consists of the administration of the vaccine virus at the least attenuated passage level that will be present between the master seed lot and a batch of the vaccine to a group of five 1-day-old chicks from an SPF flock (*5.2.2*), sequential passages, 5 times where possible, to further similar groups of 1-day-old chicks and testing of the final recovered virus for increase in virulence. If the properties of the vaccine virus allow sequential passage to 5 groups via natural spreading, this method may be used, otherwise passage as described below is carried out and the maximally passaged virus that has been recovered is tested for increase in virulence. Care must be taken to avoid contamination by virus from previous passages. Administer by the intramuscular route a quantity of the vaccine virus that will allow recovery of virus for the passages described below. Prepare 7 to 9 days after administration a suspension from the liver of each chick and pool these samples. Depending on the tropism of the virus, other tissues such as spleen or bone marrow may be used. Administer 0.1 ml of the pooled samples by the intramuscular route to each of 5 other chicks of the same age and origin. Carry out this passage operation at least 5 times; verify the presence of the virus at each passage. If the virus is not found at a passage level, carry out a second series of passages. Carry out the tests for safety (section 2-4-1) using the unpassaged vaccine virus and the maximally passaged vaccine virus that has been recovered. The vaccine virus complies with the test if no indication of increase in virulence of the maximally passaged virus compared with the unpassaged virus is observed. If virus is not recovered at any passage level in the first and second series of passages, the vaccine virus also complies with the test.

2-4-3. **Immunogenicity**. A test is carried out for each route and method of administration to be recommended using chickens from an SPF flock (*5.2.2*) not older than the youngest age to be recommended for vaccination. The test for prevention of virus excretion is intended to demonstrate absence of egg transmission. The quantity of the vaccine virus administered to each chicken is not greater than the minimum titre to be stated on the label and the virus is at the most attenuated passage level that will be present in a batch of the vaccine.

2-4-3-1 *Passive immunisation of chickens*. Vaccinate according to the recommended schedule not fewer than 10 breeder chickens not older than the minimum age recommended for vaccination and from an SPF flock (*5.2.2*); keep not fewer than 10 unvaccinated breeder chickens of the same origin and from an SPF flock (*5.2.2*). At a suitable time after excretion of vaccine virus has ceased, collect fertilised eggs from each vaccinated and control breeder chicken and incubate them. Challenge at least 3 randomly chosen 1-day-old chickens from each vaccinated and control breeder chicken by intramuscular administration of a sufficient quantity of virulent chicken anaemia virus. Observe the chickens at least daily for 14 days after challenge. Record the deaths and the surviving chickens that show clinical signs of disease. At the end of the observation period determine the haematocrit value of each surviving chicken. Kill these chickens and carry out post-mortem examination. Note any pathological signs attributable to chicken anaemia virus, such as thymic atrophy and specific bone-marrow lesions. The test is not valid if:

- during the observation period after challenge fewer than 90 per cent of the chickens of the control breeder chickens die or show severe clinical signs of infectious chicken anaemia, including haematocrit value under 27 per cent, and/or notable macroscopic lesions of the bone marrow and thymus,
- and/or during the period between vaccination and egg collection more than 10 per cent of vaccinated or control breeder chickens show notable clinical signs of disease or die from causes not attributable to the vaccine.

The vaccine complies with the test if during the observation period after challenge not fewer than 90 per cent of the chickens of the vaccinated breeder chickens survive and show no notable clinical signs of disease and/or macroscopic lesions of the bone marrow and thymus.

2-4-3-2. *Prevention of virus excretion*. Vaccinate according to the recommended schedule not fewer than 10 chickens not older than the minimum age recommended for vaccination and from an SPF flock (*5.2.2*). Maintain separately not fewer than 10 chickens of the same age and origin as controls. At a suitable time after excretion of vaccine virus has ceased, challenge all the chickens by intramuscular administration of a sufficient quantity of virulent chicken anaemia virus. Collect blood and faecal samples from the chickens on days 3, 5 and 7 after challenge and carry out a test for virus isolation to determine whether or not the chickens are viraemic and are excreting the virus. The test is not valid if:

- fewer than 70 per cent of the control chickens are viraemic and excrete the virus at one or more times of sampling,
- and/or during the period between vaccination and challenge more than 10 per cent of control or vaccinated chickens show abnormal clinical signs or die from causes not attributable to the vaccine.

The vaccine complies with the test if not fewer than 90 per cent of the vaccinated chickens do not develop viraemia or excrete the virus.

3 BATCH TESTING

3-1. **Identification**. The vaccine, diluted if necessary and mixed with a monospecific chicken anaemia virus antiserum, no longer infects susceptible cell cultures or eggs from an SPF flock (*5.2.2*) into which it is inoculated.

3-2. **Bacteria and fungi**. Vaccines intended for administration by injection comply with the test for sterility prescribed in the monograph *Vaccines for veterinary use (0062)*.

Vaccines not intended for administration by injection either comply with the test for sterility prescribed in the monograph *Vaccines for veterinary use (0062)* or with the following test: carry out a quantitative test for bacterial and fungal contamination; carry out identification tests for microorganisms detected in the vaccine; the vaccine does not contain pathogenic microorganisms and contains not more than 1 non-pathogenic microorganism per dose.

Any liquid supplied with the vaccine complies with the test for sterility prescribed in the monograph *Vaccines for veterinary use (0062)*.

3-3. **Mycoplasmas**. The vaccine complies with the test for mycoplasmas (*2.6.7*).

3-4. **Extraneous agents**. The vaccine complies with the tests for extraneous agents in batches of finished product (*2.6.25*).

3-5. **Safety**. Use not fewer than 10 chickens not older than the minimum age recommended for vaccination and from an SPF flock (*5.2.2*). Administer by a recommended route to each chicken 10 doses of the vaccine. Observe the chickens at least daily for 21 days. The test is not valid if more than 20 per cent of the chickens show abnormal clinical signs or die from causes not attributable to the vaccine. The vaccine complies with the test if no chicken shows notable clinical signs of disease or dies from causes attributable to the vaccine.

3-6. **Virus titre**. Titrate the vaccine virus by inoculation into suitable cell cultures (*5.2.4*) or eggs from an SPF flock (*5.2.2*). The vaccine complies with the test if 1 dose contains not less than the minimum virus titre stated on the label.

3-7. **Potency**. The vaccine complies with the requirements of the tests prescribed under Immunogenicity (sections 2-4-3-1 and 2-4-3-2) when administered by a recommended route and method. It is not necessary to carry out the potency test for each batch of the vaccine if it has been carried out on a representative batch using a vaccinating dose containing not more than the minimum virus titre stated on the label.

4. LABELLING

The label states to which extent the vaccine virus causes disease if it spreads to susceptible young chicks.

01/2005:1944

MANNHEIMIA VACCINE (INACTIVATED) FOR CATTLE

Vaccinum mannheimiae inactivatum ad bovidas

DEFINITION

Mannheimia vaccine (inactivated) for cattle is a preparation from cultures of one or more suitable strains of *Mannheimia haemolytica* (formerly *Pasteurella haemolytica*). This monograph applies to vaccines intended for administration to cattle of different ages for protection against respiratory diseases caused by *M. haemolytica*.

PRODUCTION

Production of the vaccine is based on a seed-lot system. The seed material is cultured in a suitable medium; each strain is cultivated separately and identity is verified using a suitable method. During production, various parameters such as growth rate are monitored by suitable methods; the values are within the limits approved for the particular product. Purity and identity of the harvest are verified using suitable methods. After cultivation, the bacterial suspensions are collected separately and inactivated by a suitable method. The vaccine may contain an adjuvant and may be freeze-dried.

CHOICE OF VACCINE COMPOSITION

The choice of composition and the strains to be included in the vaccine is based on epidemiological data on the prevalence of the different serovars of *M. haemolytica* and on the claims being made. The vaccine is shown to be satisfactory with respect to safety (*5.2.6*) and efficacy (*5.2.7*) in cattle. As part of the studies to demonstrate the suitability of the vaccine with respect to these characteristics the following tests may be carried out.

Safety

A. The test is carried out for each route of administration to be stated on the label and in animals of each category for which the vaccine is intended.

   For each test, use not fewer than 10 animals that preferably do not have antibodies against the serovars of *M. haemolytica* or against the leucotoxin present in the vaccine. Where justified, animals with a known history of no previous mannheimia vaccination and with low antibody titres (measured in a sensitive test system such as an ELISA) may be used.

   Administer to each animal a double dose of vaccine containing not less than the maximum potency that may be expected in a batch of vaccine. Administer a single dose of vaccine to each animal after the recommended interval. Observe the animals for at least 14 days after the last administration. Record body temperature the day before vaccination, at vaccination, 2 h, 4 h and 6 h later and then daily for 4 days; note the maximum temperature increase for each animal. No abnormal local or systemic reaction occurs; the average body temperature increase for all animals does not exceed 1.5 °C and no animal shows a rise greater than 2 °C. If the vaccine is intended for use or may be used in pregnant cows, vaccinate the cows at the relevant stages of pregnancy and prolong the observation period until 1 day after parturition.

   The vaccine complies with the test if no animal shows abnormal local or systemic reactions or clinical signs of disease or dies from causes attributable to the vaccine. In addition, if the vaccine is intended for use in pregnant cows, no significant effects on the pregnancy and offspring are demonstrated.

B. The animals used for the field trials are also used to evaluate safety. Carry out a test in each category of animals for which the vaccine is intended. Use not fewer than 3 groups of 20 animals with corresponding groups of not fewer than 10 controls in 3 different locations. Examine the injection sites for local reactions after vaccination. Record body temperatures the day before vaccination, at vaccination and on the 2 days following vaccination. The vaccine complies with the test if no animal shows abnormal local or systemic reactions or clinical signs of disease or dies from causes attributable to the vaccine. The average body temperature increase for all animals does not exceed 1.5 °C and no animal shows a rise greater than 2 °C. In addition, if the vaccine is intended for use in pregnant cows, no significant effects on the pregnancy and offspring are demonstrated.

Immunogenicity. As part of the studies to demonstrate the suitability of the vaccine with respect to immunogenicity, the test described under Potency may be carried out for each proposed route of administration and using vaccine of minimum potency.

BATCH TESTING

Batch potency test. The test described under Potency is not carried out for routine testing of batches of vaccine. It is carried out, for a given vaccine, on one or more occasions, as decided by or with the agreement of the competent authority. Where the test is not carried out, a suitable validated test is carried out, the criteria for acceptance being set with reference to the results obtained with a batch of vaccine that has given satisfactory results in the test described under Potency.

Bacterial endotoxins. A test for bacterial endotoxins (*2.6.14*) is carried out on the final lot or, where the nature of the adjuvant prevents performance of a satisfactory test, on the bulk antigen or the mixture of bulk antigens immediately before addition of the adjuvant. The maximum acceptable amount of bacterial endotoxins is that found for a batch of vaccine that has been shown satisfactory in safety test A given under Choice of vaccine composition or in the safety test described under Tests, carried out using 10 animals. Where the latter test is used, note the maximum temperature increase for each animal; the average body temperature increase for all animals does not exceed 1.5 °C. The method chosen for determining the amount of bacterial endotoxin present in the vaccine batch used in the safety test for determining the maximum acceptable level of endotoxin is used subsequently for testing of each batch.

IDENTIFICATION

When injected into healthy seronegative animals, the vaccine stimulates the production of specific antibodies against the serovars of *M. haemolytica* and/or against the leucotoxin present in the vaccine.

TESTS

Safety. Use 2 cattle of the minimum age recommended for vaccination that have not been vaccinated against mannheimiosis. Administer a double dose of vaccine to each animal by a recommended route. Observe the animals for 14 days. Record body temperature the day before vaccination, at vaccination, 2 h, 4 h and 6 h later and then daily for 2 days. The animals remain in good health and no abnormal local or systemic reaction occurs; a transient temperature increase not exceeding 2 °C may occur.

Sterility. It complies with the test for sterility prescribed in the monograph on *Vaccines for veterinary use (0062)*.

POTENCY

Carry out a test for each serovar for which protection is claimed on the label.

Use not fewer than 16 animals of the minimum age recommended for vaccination, free from antibodies against *M. haemolytica* and against the leucotoxin of *M. haemolytica*. Vaccinate not fewer than 8 of the animals by a recommended route and according to the recommended schedule. Keep 8 animals as controls. 21 days after the last vaccination, challenge all the animals by the intratracheal route or by another appropriate route, with a suitable quantity of a low-passage, virulent strain of a serovar of *M. haemolytica*. Observe the animals for a further 7 days; to avoid unnecessary suffering, severely ill animals are killed and are then considered to have died from the disease. During the observation period, the animals are examined for signs of disease for example, increased body temperature, dullness, abnormal breathing and the mortality is recorded. Kill surviving animals at the end of the observation period. Post-mortem examination is carried out on any animal that dies and those killed at the end of the observation period. The lungs are examined and the extent of lung lesions due to mannheimiosis is evaluated. Samples of lung tissue are collected for re-isolation of the challenge organisms. The clinical observations and lung lesions are scored and the results obtained for these parameters and the bacterial re-isolation results compared for the 2 groups.

The test is invalid if signs of *M. haemolytica* infection occur in less than 70 per cent of the control animals.

The vaccine complies with the requirements of the test if there is a significant difference between the scores obtained for the clinical and post-mortem observations in the vaccinates compared to the controls. For vaccines with a claim for a beneficial effect on the extent of infection against the serovar, the results for the infection rates are also significantly better for the vaccinates compared to the controls.

LABELLING

The label states:

– the serovar(s) of *M. haemolytica* against which protection is claimed,
– the serovar(s) of *M. haemolytica* and/or the leucotoxin present in the vaccine.

Vaccines

01/2005:1946

MANNHEIMIA VACCINE (INACTIVATED) FOR SHEEP

Vaccinum mannheimiae inactivatum ad ovem

DEFINITION

Mannheimia vaccine (inactivated) for sheep is a preparation of one or more suitable strains of *Mannheimia haemolytica* (formerly *Pasteurella haemolytica*). This monograph applies to vaccines intended for administration to sheep for active immunisation and to protect passively their future progeny against disease caused by *M. haemolytica*.

PRODUCTION

Production of the vaccine is based on a seed lot system. The seed material is cultured in a suitable medium; each strain is cultivated separately and identity is verified using a suitable method. During production, various parameters such as growth rate are monitored by suitable methods; the values are within the limits approved for the particular product. Purity and identity of the harvest are verified using suitable methods. After cultivation, the bacterial suspensions are collected separately and inactivated by a suitable method. The vaccine may contain an adjuvant and may be freeze-dried.

CHOICE OF VACCINE COMPOSITION

The choice of composition and the strains to be included in the vaccine is based on epidemiological data on the prevalence of the different serovars of *M. haemolytica* and on the claims being made for the product, for example active and/or passive protection. The vaccine is shown to be satisfactory with respect to safety (*5.2.6*) and efficacy (*5.2.7*) in sheep. As part of the studies to demonstrate the suitability of the vaccine with respect to these characteristics the following tests may be carried out.

Safety

A. The test is carried out for each of the routes of administration to be stated on the label and in animals of each category (for example, young sheep, pregnant ewes) for which the vaccine is intended.

For each test, use not fewer than 10 animals that preferably do not have antibodies against the serovars of *M. haemolytica* or against the leucotoxin present in the vaccine. Where justified, animals with a known history of no previous mannheimia vaccination and with low antibody titres (measured in a sensitive test system such as an ELISA) may be used.

Administer to each animal a double dose of vaccine containing not less than the maximum potency that may be expected in a batch of vaccine. Administer a single dose of vaccine to each animal after the recommended interval. Observe the animals for at least 14 days after the last administration. Record body temperature the day before vaccination, at vaccination, 2 h, 4 h and 6 h later and then daily for 4 days; note the maximum temperature increase for each animal. No abnormal local or systemic reaction occurs; the average body temperature increase for all animals does not exceed 1.5 °C and no animal shows a rise greater than 2 °C. If the vaccine is intended for use or may be used in pregnant ewes, vaccinate the ewes at the relevant stages of pregnancy and prolong the observation period until 1 day after lambing.

The vaccine complies with the test if no animal shows abnormal local reactions or clinical signs of disease or dies from causes attributable to the vaccine. In addition, if the vaccine is intended for use in pregnant ewes, no significant effects on the pregnancy and offspring are demonstrated.

B. The animals used for the field trials are also used to evaluate safety. Carry out a test in each category of animals for which the vaccine is intended. Use not fewer than 3 groups of 20 animals with corresponding groups of not fewer than 10 controls in 3 different locations. Examine the injection sites for local reactions after vaccination. Record body temperatures the day before vaccination, at vaccination and on the 2 days following vaccination. The vaccine complies with the test if no animal shows abnormal local or systemic reactions or clinical signs of disease or dies from causes attributable to the vaccine. The average body temperature increase for all animals does not exceed 1.5 °C and no animal shows a rise greater than 2 °C. In addition, if the vaccine is intended for use in pregnant ewes, no significant effects on the pregnancy and offspring are demonstrated.

Immunogenicity. As part of the studies to demonstrate the suitability of the vaccine with respect to immunogenicity, the tests described under Potency may be carried out for each proposed route of administration and using vaccine of minimum potency.

BATCH TESTING

Batch potency test. The relevant test or tests described under Potency are not carried out for routine testing of batches of vaccine. They are carried out, for a given vaccine, on one or more occasions, as decided by or with the agreement of the competent authority. Where the relevant test or tests are not carried out, a suitable validated batch potency test is carried out, the criteria for acceptance being set with reference to the results obtained with a batch of vaccine that has given satisfactory results in the test(s) described under Potency.

Bacterial endotoxins. A test for bacterial endotoxins (*2.6.14*) is carried out on the final lot or, where the nature of the adjuvant prevents performance of a satisfactory test, on the bulk antigen or the mixture of bulk antigens immediately before addition of the adjuvant. The maximum acceptable amount of bacterial endotoxins is that found for a batch of vaccine that has been shown satisfactory in safety test A given under Choice of vaccine composition or in the safety test described under Tests, carried out using 10 animals. Where the latter test is used, note the maximum temperature increase for each animal; the average body temperature increase for all animals does not exceed 1.5 °C. The method chosen for determining the amount of bacterial endotoxin present in the vaccine batch used in the safety test for determining the maximum acceptable level of endotoxin is used subsequently for testing of each batch.

IDENTIFICATION

When injected into healthy seronegative animals, the vaccine stimulates the production of specific antibodies against the serovars of *M. haemolytica* and/or against the leucotoxin present in the vaccine.

TESTS

Safety. Use 2 sheep of the minimum age recommended for vaccination or, if not available, of an age as close as possible to the minimum recommended age, and that have not been vaccinated against mannheimiosis. Administer a double dose of vaccine to each animal by a recommended route. Observe the animals for 14 days. Record body temperature the day before vaccination, at vaccination, 2 h, 4 h and 6 h later and then daily for 2 days. The animals remain in good health and no abnormal local or systemic reaction occurs; a transient temperature increase not exceeding 2 °C may occur.

Sterility. It complies with the test for sterility prescribed in the monograph on *Vaccines for veterinary use (0062)*.

POTENCY

Active immunisation. For vaccines with claims for active immunisation due to *M. haemolytica*, carry out a test for each serovar of *M. haemolytica* for which protection is claimed on the label.

Use not fewer than 20 lambs of the minimum age recommended for vaccination, free from antibodies against *M. haemolytica* and against the leucotoxin of *M. haemolytica*. Vaccinate not fewer than 10 of the animals by a recommended route and according to the recommended schedule. Keep 10 animals as controls. 21 days after the last vaccination, challenge all the lambs by the intratracheal route or by another appropriate route, with a suitable quantity of a low-passage, virulent strain of a serovar of *M. haemolytica*. Where necessary for a given serovar, prechallenge with parainfluenza type 3 (PI3) virus or another appropriate respiratory pathogen may be used. Observe the animals for a further 7 days; to avoid unnecessary suffering, severely ill animals are killed and are then considered to have died from the disease. During the observation period, the animals are examined for signs of disease (for example, increased body temperature, dullness, abnormal respiration) and the mortality is recorded. Kill surviving animals at the end of the observation period. Post-mortem examination is carried out on any animal that dies and those killed at the end of the observation period. The lungs are examined and the extent of lung lesions due to mannheimiosis is evaluated. Samples of lung tissue are collected for re-isolation of the challenge organisms. The clinical observations and lung lesions are scored and the results obtained for these parameters and the bacterial re-isolation results compared for the 2 groups.

The test is invalid if signs of *M. haemolytica* infection occur in less than 70 per cent of the control lambs.

The vaccine complies with the requirements of the test if there is a significant difference between the scores obtained for the clinical and post-mortem observations in the vaccinates compared to the controls. For vaccines with a claim for a beneficial effect on the extent of infection against the serovar, the results for the infection rates are also significantly better for the vaccinates compared to the controls.

Passive protection. For vaccines with claims for passive protection against mannheimiosis carry out a test for each serovar of *M. haemolytica* for which protection is claimed on the label.

Use at least 6 ewes that preferably do not have antibodies against the serovars of *M. haemolytica* or against the leucotoxin present in the vaccine. Where justified, animals with a known history of no previous mannheimia vaccination, from a source with a low incidence of respiratory disease and with low antibody titres (measured in a sensitive test system such as an ELISA) may be used. Vaccinate the animals by 1 of the recommended routes, at the recommended stages of pregnancy and according to the recommended schedule. A challenge study is conducted with 20 newborn, colostrum-deprived lambs. 10 of these lambs are given colostrum from the vaccinated ewes and 10 control lambs are given colostrum or colostrum substitute without detectable antibodies to *M. haemolytica*. When the lambs are at the age claimed for the duration of the passive protection, challenge by the intratracheal route with a suitable quantity of a low-passage, virulent strain of a serovar of *M. haemolytica*. Observe the animals for a further 7 days; to avoid unnecessary suffering, severely ill animals are killed and are then considered to have died from the disease. Observe the animals and assess the effect of the challenge on the offspring of the vaccinates and the controls as described in the test for active immunisation.

The test is invalid if clinical signs or lesions of *M. haemolytica* infection occur in less than 70 per cent of the control lambs.

The vaccine complies with the requirements of the test if there is a significant difference between the scores obtained for the clinical and post-mortem observations in the lambs from the vaccinates compared to those from the controls. For vaccines with a claim for a beneficial effect on the extent of infection against the serovar, the results for the infection rates are also significantly better for the lambs from the vaccinates compared to those from the controls.

LABELLING

The label states:

– the serovar(s) of *M. haemolytica* against which protection is claimed,
– the serovar(s) of *M. haemolytica* and/or the leucotoxin present in the vaccine,
– for vaccines for passive protection, the length of time for which the passive protection is claimed.

01/2005:0589

MAREK'S DISEASE VACCINE (LIVE)

Vaccinum morbi Marek vivum

1. DEFINITION

Marek's disease vaccine (live) is a preparation of a suitable strain or strains of Marek's disease virus (gallid herpesvirus 2 or 3) and/or turkey herpesvirus (meleagrid herpesvirus 1). This monograph applies to vaccines intended for administration to chickens for active immunisation.

2. PRODUCTION

2-1. *PREPARATION OF THE VACCINE*

The vaccine virus is grown in cell cultures. If the vaccine contains more than 1 type of virus, the different types are grown separately. The vaccine may be freeze-dried or stored in liquid nitrogen.

2-2. *SUBSTRATE FOR VIRUS PROPAGATION*

2-2-1. **Cell cultures**. The cell cultures comply with the requirements for cell cultures for production of veterinary vaccines (*5.2.4*).

2-3. *SEED LOTS*

2-3-1. **Extraneous agents**. The master seed lot complies with the tests for extraneous agents in seed lots (*2.6.24*). In these tests on the master seed lot, the organisms used are not more than 5 passages from the master seed lot at the start of the tests.

2-4. *CHOICE OF VACCINE VIRUS*

The vaccine virus shall be shown to be satisfactory with respect to safety (*5.2.6*) and efficacy (*5.2.7*) for the chickens for which it is intended.

The tests shown below for safety of the strain (section 2-4-1), increase in virulence (section 2-4-2) and immunogenicity (section 2-4-3) may be used during the demonstration of safety and immunogenicity. Additional testing may be needed to demonstrate safety in breeds of chickens known to be particularly susceptible to Marek's disease virus, unless the vaccine is to be contra-indicated.

2-4-1. **Safety**. Carry out the test for the route to be recommended for vaccination likely to be the least safe and in the category of chickens for which the vaccine is intended likely to be the most susceptible for Marek's disease. Use vaccine virus at the least attenuated passage level that will be present between the master seed lot and a batch of the vaccine. Use not fewer than eighty 1-day-old chickens from a flock free from specified pathogens (SPF) (*5.2.2*). Divide them randomly into 2 groups of not fewer than 40 chickens and maintain the groups separately. Carry out examination for macroscopic lesions of each chicken that dies and of the surviving chickens at the end of the observation periods. Administer to each chicken of one group (I) a quantity of the vaccine virus equivalent to not less than 10 times the maximum virus titre likely to be contained in 1 dose of the vaccine. Administer by a suitable route to each chicken of the other group (II) a quantity of virulent Marek's disease virus that will cause mortality and/or severe macroscopic lesions of Marek's disease in not fewer than 70 per cent of the effective number of chickens within 70 days (initial number reduced by the number that die within the first 7 days of the test). Observe the chickens of group II at least daily for 70 days and those of group I at least daily for 120 days. The test is not valid if 1 or more of the following apply: more than 10 per cent of the chickens in any group die within the first 7 days of the test; fewer than 70 per cent of the effective number of chickens in group II show macroscopic lesions of Marek's disease. The vaccine virus complies with the test if:

– no chicken of group I shows notable clinical signs or macroscopic lesions of Marek's disease or dies from causes attributable to the vaccine virus,
– at 120 days the number of surviving chickens of group I is not fewer than 80 per cent of the effective number.

2-4-2. **Increase in virulence**. The test for increase in virulence is required for Marek's disease virus vaccine strains but not for turkey herpesvirus vaccine strains, which are naturally apathogenic. Administer by the intramuscular route a quantity of the vaccine virus that will allow recovery of virus for the passages described below to each of five 1-day-old chickens from an SPF flock (*5.2.2*). Use vaccine virus at the least attenuated passage level that will be present between the master seed lot and a batch of the vaccine. Prepare 5 to 7 days later a suspension of white blood cells of each chicken and pool these samples. Administer a suitable volume of the pooled samples by the intraperitoneal route to each of 5 other chickens that are 1-day-old and from an SPF flock (*5.2.2*). Carry out this passage operation not fewer than 5 times; verify the presence of the virus at each passage. Care must be taken to avoid contamination by virus from previous passages. If the virus is not found at a passage level, carry out a second series of passages. Carry out the safety test (section 2-4-1) using the unpassaged vaccine virus and the maximally passaged virus that has been recovered. Administer the virus by the route to be recommended for vaccination likely to be the least safe for use in these birds. The vaccine virus complies with the test if no indication of increase in virulence of the maximally passaged virus compared with the unpassaged virus is observed. If virus is not recovered at any passage level in the first and second series of passages, the vaccine virus also complies with the test.

2-4-3. **Immunogenicity**. A test is carried out for each route and method of administration to be recommended using in each case chickens of the youngest age to be recommended for vaccination. The quantity of the vaccine virus administered to each chicken is not greater than the minimum virus titre to be stated on the label and the virus is at the most attenuated passage level that will be present in a batch of the vaccine. Use for the test not fewer than 60 chickens of the same origin and from an SPF flock (*5.2.2*). Vaccinate by a recommended route not fewer than 30 chickens. Maintain not fewer than 30 chickens as controls. Challenge each chicken after 9 days by a suitable route with a sufficient quantity of virulent Marek's disease virus. Observe the chickens at least daily for 70 days after challenge. Record the deaths and the number of surviving chickens that show clinical signs of disease. At the end of the observation period kill all the surviving chickens and carry out examination for macroscopic lesions of Marek's disease. The test is not valid if:

– during the observation period after challenge fewer than 70 per cent of the control chickens die or show severe clinical signs or macroscopic lesions of Marek's disease,
– and/or during the period between the vaccination and challenge more than 10 per cent of the control or vaccinated chickens show abnormal clinical signs or die from causes not attributable to the vaccine.

The vaccine virus complies with the test if the percentage relative protection, calculated using the following expression, is not less than 80 per cent:

$$\frac{V - C}{100 - C} \times 100$$

V = percentage of challenged vaccinated chickens that survive to the end of the observation period without notable clinical signs or macroscopic lesions of Marek's disease,

C = percentage of challenged control chickens that survive to the end of the observation period without notable clinical signs or macroscopic lesions of Marek's disease.

3. BATCH TESTS

3-1. **Identification**. Carry out an immunostaining test in cell cultures using monoclonal antibodies to demonstrate the presence of each type of virus stated on the label.

3-2. **Bacteria and fungi**. The vaccine and, where applicable, the liquid supplied with it comply with the requirement for sterility prescribed in the monograph *Vaccines for veterinary use (0062)*.

3-3. **Mycoplasmas**. The vaccine complies with the test for mycoplasmas (*2.6.7*).

3-4. **Extraneous agents**. The vaccine complies with the tests for extraneous agents in batches of finished product (*2.6.25*).

3-5. **Safety**. Use not fewer than 10 chickens from an SPF flock (*5.2.2*) and not older than the youngest age recommended for vaccination. Administer by a recommended route and method to each chicken 10 doses of the vaccine. Observe the chickens at least daily for 21 days. The test is not valid if more than 20 per cent of the chickens show abnormal clinical signs or die from causes not attributable to the vaccine. The vaccine complies with the test if no chicken shows notable clinical signs of disease or dies from causes attributable to the vaccine.

3-6. **Virus titre**

3-6-1 *Vaccines containing one type of virus*. Titrate the vaccine virus by inoculation into suitable cell cultures (*5.2.4*). If the virus titre is determined in plaque-forming units (PFU), only primary plaques are taken into consideration. The vaccine complies with the test if 1 dose contains not less than the minimum virus titre stated on the label.

3-6-2. *Vaccines containing more than one type of virus*. For vaccines containing more than 1 type of virus, titrate each virus by inoculation into suitable cell cultures (*5.2.4*), reading the results by immunostaining using antibodies. The vaccine complies with the test if 1 dose contains for each vaccine virus not less than the minimum virus titre stated on the label.

3-7. **Potency**. The vaccine complies with the requirements of the test prescribed under Immunogenicity (section 2-4-3) when administered according to the recommended schedule by a recommended route and method. It is not necessary to carry out the potency test for each batch of the vaccine if it has been carried out on a representative batch using a vaccinating dose containing not more than the minimum virus titre stated on the label.

01/2005:1943

MYXOMATOSIS VACCINE (LIVE) FOR RABBITS

Vaccinum myxomatosidis vivum ad cuniculum

DEFINITION

Myxomatosis vaccine (live) for rabbits is a preparation of a suitable strain of either myxoma virus that is attenuated for rabbits or Shope fibroma virus. The vaccine is intended for the active immunisation of rabbits against myxomatosis.

PRODUCTION

The virus is propagated in suitable cell cultures (*5.2.4*). The viral suspension is harvested, titrated and may be mixed with a suitable stabilising solution. The vaccine may be freeze-dried.

CHOICE OF VACCINE STRAIN

The vaccine is shown to be satisfactory with respect to safety, absence of increase in virulence and immunogenicity. The following tests may be used during demonstration of safety, absence of increase in virulence (*5.2.6*) and efficacy (*5.2.7*).

Safety. The test is carried out for each route of administration to be stated on the label. Use at least 10 rabbits of the minimum age to be recommended for vaccination and that do not have antibodies against myxoma virus. Administer to each rabbit by a recommended route a quantity of virus corresponding to not less than 10 times the maximum titre that may be expected in a dose of vaccine. Observe the rabbits for 28 days. Record the body temperature the day before vaccination, at vaccination, 4 h after vaccination and then daily for 4 days; note the maximum temperature increase for each animal. No abnormal local or systemic reaction occurs; the average temperature increase does not exceed 1 °C and no animal shows a rise greater than 2 °C. A local reaction lasting less than 28 days may occur.

If the vaccine is intended for use in pregnant rabbits, administer the virus to not less than 10 pregnant rabbits according to the schedule to be recommended on the label. Prolong the observation period until 1 day after parturition. The rabbits remain in good health and there is no abnormal local or systemic reaction. No adverse effects on the pregnancy or the offspring are noted.

Increase in virulence. (This test is performed only for vaccines based on attenuated strains of myxoma virus). Administer by a recommended route to each of 2 rabbits, 5 to 7 weeks old and which do not have antibodies against

Vaccines

myxoma virus, a quantity of virus that will allow recovery of virus for the passages described below. Use vaccine virus at the least attenuated passage level that will be present between the master seed lot and a batch of the vaccine. Kill the rabbits 5 to 10 days after inoculation and remove from each rabbit organs, or tissues with sufficient virus to allow passage; homogenise the organs and tissues in a suitable buffer solution, centrifuge the suspension and use the supernatant for further passages. Inoculate the supernatant into suitable cell cultures to verify the presence of virus. Administer by an appropriate route, at a suitable rate, a suitable volume of the supernatant to each of 2 other rabbits of the same age and the same susceptibility. This operation is then repeated at least 5 times. If the virus has disappeared, a second series of passages is carried out. Inoculate virus from the highest recovered passage level to rabbits, observe for 28 days and compare any reactions that occur with those seen in the test for safety described above. There is no indication of an increase in virulence as compared with the non-passaged virus. If virus is not recovered in either of 2 series of passages, the vaccine virus also complies with the test.

Immunogenicity. The test described under Potency may be used to demonstrate the immunogenicity of the strain.

BATCH POTENCY TEST

If the test for potency has been carried out with satisfactory results on a representative batch of vaccine, using a vaccinating dose containing not more than the minimum virus titre stated on the label, this test may be omitted as a routine control on other batches of vaccine prepared from the same seed lot.

IDENTIFICATION

Carry out an immunofluorescence test in suitable cell cultures, using a monospecific antiserum.

TESTS

Safety. Use not fewer than 2 rabbits, not older than the minimum age recommended for vaccination, that do not have antibodies against myxoma virus and rabbit haemorrhagic disease virus and that have been reared in suitable isolation conditions to avoid contact with myxoma virus. Administer by a recommended route to each rabbit 10 doses of vaccine. Observe the rabbits at least daily for 14 days. No abnormal local or systemic reaction occurs.

Extraneous agents. At the end of the 14 day observation period of the safety test, administer by a recommended route to each rabbit, a further 10 doses of vaccine. After 14 days take a blood sample from each rabbit and carry out a test for antibodies against rabbit haemorrhagic disease virus. No antibodies are found.

Bacterial and fungal contamination. The vaccine, reconstituted if necessary, complies with the test for sterility prescribed in the monograph on *Vaccines for Veterinary Use (0062)*.

Mycoplasmas (*2.6.7*). The vaccine, reconstituted if necessary, complies with the test for mycoplasmas.

Virus titre. Reconstitute the vaccine, if necessary, and titrate in suitable cell cultures. 1 dose of the vaccine contains not less than the quantity of virus equivalent to the minimum virus titre stated on the label.

POTENCY

Use not fewer than 15 susceptible rabbits of the minimum age to be recommended for vaccination, free from antibodies against myxoma virus and reared in suitable isolation conditions to ensure absence of contact with myxoma virus. Administer 1 dose of vaccine to each of not fewer than 10 of the rabbits according to the instructions for use. Keep not less than 5 other rabbits as controls. Not less than 21 days after the last vaccination, administer by a suitable route to each rabbit a quantity of a virulent strain of myxoma virus sufficient to cause typical signs of myxomatosis in a susceptible rabbit. Observe the rabbits for a further 21 days. The test is not valid if fewer than 90 per cent of the control rabbits display typical signs of myxomatosis. A vaccine containing myxoma virus complies with the test if not fewer than 90 per cent of vaccinated rabbits show no signs of myxomatosis. A vaccine containing Shope fibroma virus complies with the test if not fewer than 75 per cent of vaccinated rabbits show no signs of myxomatosis.

LABELLING

The label states, where applicable, that a local reaction may occur.

01/2005:0962

NEONATAL PIGLET COLIBACILLOSIS VACCINE (INACTIVATED)

Vaccinum colibacillosis fetus a partu recentis inactivatum ad suem

DEFINITION

Neonatal piglet colibacillosis vaccine (inactivated) is prepared from cultures of one or more suitable strains of *Escherichia coli*, carrying one or more adhesins or enterotoxins. This monograph applies to vaccines administered by injection to sows and gilts for protection of newborn piglets against enteric forms of colibacillosis.

PRODUCTION

The *E. coli* strains used for production are cultured separately in a suitable medium. The cells or toxins are processed to render them safe and are blended.

The vaccine may contain one or more suitable adjuvants.

CHOICE OF VACCINE COMPOSITION

The *E. coli* strains used in the production of the vaccine are shown to be satisfactory with respect to expression of antigens and the vaccine is shown to be satisfactory with respect to safety and immunogenicity. The following tests may be used during demonstration of safety (*5.2.6*) and efficacy (*5.2.7*).

Expression of antigens. The expression of antigens that stimulate a protective immune response is verified by a suitable immunochemical method (*2.7.1*) carried out on the antigen obtained from each of the vaccine strains under the conditions used for the production of the vaccine.

Safety

A. Administer a double dose of vaccine by a recommended route to each of not fewer than 10 pregnant sows that have not been vaccinated against colibacillosis. Administer 1 dose of vaccine to each of the animals after the recommended interval. Observe the animals until farrowing. Record body temperature the day before vaccination, at vaccination, 2 h, 4 h and 6 h later and then daily for 4 days; note the maximum temperature increase for each animal. Note any effects on gestation or the offspring. No abnormal local or systemic reaction occurs: the average temperature increase for all animals does not exceed 1.5 °C and no animal shows a rise greater than 2 °C.

B. The animals used for field trials are also used to evaluate safety. Use not fewer than 3 groups each of not fewer than 20 animals with corresponding groups of not fewer than 10 controls. Examine the injection site for local reactions after vaccination. Record body temperature the day before vaccination, at vaccination, at the time interval after which a rise in temperature, if any, was seen in test A, and daily during the 2 days following vaccination; note the maximum temperature increase for each animal. No abnormal local or systemic reaction occurs: the average temperature increase for all animals does not exceed 1.5 °C and no animal shows a rise greater than 2 °C.

Immunogenicity. The suitability of the vaccine with respect to immunogenicity may be demonstrated by the test described under Potency.

BATCH TESTING

Batch potency test. *The test described under Potency is not carried out for routine testing of batches of vaccine. It is carried out, for a given vaccine, on one or more occasions, as decided by or with the agreement of the competent authority; where the test is not carried out, a suitable validated test is carried out, the criteria for acceptance being set with reference to a batch of vaccine that has given satisfactory results in the test described under Potency. The following test may be used after a suitable correlation with the test described under Potency has been established by a statistical evaluation.*

Use pigs not less than 3 weeks old and free from specific antibodies against the antigens stated on the label: vaccinate each of 5 pigs by the route and according to the schedule stated on the label. Maintain 2 pigs as unvaccinated controls. Alternatively, if the nature of the antigens allows reproducible results to be obtained, a test in laboratory animals (for example, guinea-pigs, mice, rabbits or rats) may be carried out. To obtain a valid assay, it may be necessary to carry out a test using several groups of animals, each receiving a different dose. For each dose, carry out the test as follows. Vaccinate not fewer than 5 animals with a single injection of a suitable dose. Maintain not fewer than 2 animals as unvaccinated controls. Where the schedule stated on the label requires a booster injection to be given, a booster vaccination may also be given in this test provided it has been demonstrated that this will still provide a suitably sensitive test system. At a given interval within the range of 14 to 21 days after the last injection, collect blood from each animal and prepare serum samples. Use a suitable validated test such as an enzyme-linked immunosorbent assay (*2.7.1*) to measure the antibody response to each of the antigens stated on the label. The antibody levels are not significantly less than those obtained with a batch that has given satisfactory results in the test described under Potency and there is no significant increase in antibody titre in the controls.

Where seronegative animals are not available, seropositive animals may be used in the above test. During the development of a test with seropositive animals, particular care will be required during the validation of the test system to establish that the test is suitably sensitive and to specify acceptable pass, fail and retest criteria. It will be necessary to take into account the range of possible prevaccination titres and establish the acceptable minimum titre rise after vaccination in relation to these.

Bacterial endotoxins. A test for bacterial endotoxins (*2.6.14*) is carried out on the final lot or, where the nature of the adjuvant prevents performance of a satisfactory test, on the bulk antigen or the mixture of bulk antigens immediately before addition of the adjuvant. The maximum acceptable amount of bacterial endotoxins is that found for a batch of vaccine that has been shown satisfactory in safety test A given under Choice of vaccine composition or in the safety test described under Tests, carried out using 10 piglets. Where the latter test is used, note the maximum temperature increase for each animal; the average temperature increase for all animals does not exceed 1.5 °C. The method chosen for determining the amount of bacterial endotoxin present in the vaccine batch used in the safety test for determining the maximum acceptable level of endotoxin is used subsequently for testing of each batch.

IDENTIFICATION

In animals free from specific antibodies against the antigens stated on the label, the vaccine stimulates the production of antibodies against these antigens.

TESTS

Safety. Use pigs preferably having no specific antibodies against the antigens stated on the label or, where justified, pigs with a low level of such antibodies as long as they have not been vaccinated against colibacillosis and administration of the vaccine does not cause an anamnestic response. Administer to each of 2 pigs a double dose of vaccine by a recommended route. Observe the animals for 14 days. Record body temperature before vaccination, at vaccination, 2 h, 4 h and 6 h later and then daily for 2 days. No abnormal local or systemic reaction occurs; a transient temperature increase not exceeding 2 °C may occur.

Sterility. The vaccine complies with the test for sterility prescribed in the monograph on *Vaccines for veterinary use (0062)*.

POTENCY

Carry out the test with a challenge strain representing each type of antigen against which the vaccine is intended to protect: if a single strain with all the necessary antigens is not available, repeat the test using different challenge strains.

Use not fewer than 8 susceptible gilts free from specific antibodies against the antigens stated on the label. Take not fewer than 4 at random and vaccinate these at the stage of pregnancy and according to the recommended vaccination scheme. Within 12 h of their giving birth, take not fewer than 15 healthy piglets from the vaccinated animals and 15 healthy piglets from the unvaccinated controls, taking at least 3 from each litter. Challenge all the piglets orally with a pathogenic strain of *E. coli* before or after colostrum feeding and using the same conditions for vaccinated animals and controls. The strain used must not be one used in the manufacture of the vaccine. Return the piglets to their dam and observe for 8 days.

On each day, note clinical signs in each piglet and score using the following scale:

0	no signs
1	slight diarrhoea
2	marked diarrhoea (watery faeces)
3	dead

Total scores for each piglet over 8 days are calculated. The test is not valid unless at least 40 per cent of the piglets from the control animals die and not more than 15 per cent of the piglets from the control animals show no signs of illness. The vaccine complies with the test if there is a significant reduction in score in the group of piglets from the vaccinated gilts compared with the group from the unvaccinated controls.

For some adhesins (for example, F5 and F41), there is published evidence that high mortality cannot be achieved under experimental conditions. If challenge has to be carried out with a strain having such adhesins: the test is not valid if fewer than 70 per cent of the control piglets show clinical signs expected with the challenge strain; the vaccine complies with the test if there is a significant reduction in score in the group of piglets from the vaccinated gilts compared with the group from the unvaccinated controls.

LABELLING

The label states the antigen or antigens contained in the vaccine that stimulate a protective immune response.

01/2005:0961

NEONATAL RUMINANT COLIBACILLOSIS VACCINE (INACTIVATED)

Vaccinum colibacillosis fetus a partu recentis inactivatum ad ruminantes

DEFINITION

Neonatal ruminant colibacillosis vaccine (inactivated) is prepared from cultures of one or more suitable strains of *Escherichia coli*, carrying one or more adhesin factors or enterotoxins. This monograph applies to vaccines administered by injection to dams for protection of newborn offspring against enteric forms of colibacillosis.

PRODUCTION

The *E. coli* strains used for production are cultured separately in a suitable medium. The cells or toxins are processed to render them safe and are blended.

The vaccine may contain one or more suitable adjuvants.

CHOICE OF VACCINE COMPOSITION

The *E. coli* strains used in the production of the vaccine are shown to be satisfactory with respect to expression of antigens and the vaccine is shown to be satisfactory with respect to safety and immunogenicity. The following tests may be used during demonstration of safety (*5.2.6*) and efficacy (*5.2.7*).

Expression of antigens. The expression of antigens that stimulate a protective immune response is verified by a suitable immunochemical method (*2.7.1*) carried out on the antigen obtained from each of the vaccine strains under the conditions used for the production of the vaccine.

Safety

A. A double dose of vaccine is administered to each of 10 pregnant animals of each of the species for which the vaccine is intended and that have not been vaccinated against colibacillosis. 1 dose is administered to each animal after the interval stated on the label. The animals are observed until parturition has occurred. Record body temperature the day before vaccination, at vaccination, 2 h, 4 h and 6 h later and then daily for 4 days; note the maximum temperature increase for each animal. No abnormal local or systemic reaction occurs; the average temperature increase for all animals does not exceed 1.5 °C and no animal shows a rise greater than 2 °C. Any effects on gestation or the offspring are noted.

B. Safety is demonstrated in field trials for each species for which the vaccine is intended by administering the intended dose to at least 60 animals from 3 different stocks, by the route and according to the schedule stated on the label. At least 30 animals from the same stocks are assigned to control groups. The animals are observed for 14 days after the last dose. No abnormal local or systemic reaction is noted and, in particular, no rise in temperature of more than 1.5 °C occurs within 2 days of administration of each dose of vaccine.

Immunogenicity. The suitability of the vaccine with respect to immunogenicity must be demonstrated for each species for which it is intended. This may be demonstrated by the test described under Potency.

BATCH TESTING

Batch potency test. *The test described under Potency is not carried out for routine testing of batches of vaccine. It is carried out, for a given vaccine, on one or more occasions, as decided by or with the agreement of the competent authority; where the test is not carried out, a suitable validated test is carried out, the criteria for acceptance being set with reference to a batch of vaccine that has given satisfactory results in the test described under Potency. The following test may be used after a suitable correlation with the test described under Potency has been established by a statistical evaluation.*

To obtain a valid assay, it may be necessary to carry out a test using several groups of animals, each receiving a different dose. For each dose required, carry out the test as follows. Vaccinate not fewer than 5 animals (for example rabbits, guinea-pigs, rats or mice), free from specific antibodies against the antigens stated on the label, using one injection of a suitable dose. Maintain 2 animals as unvaccinated controls. Where the schedule stated on the label requires a booster injection to be given, a booster vaccination may also be given in this test provided it has been demonstrated that this will still provide a suitably sensitive test system. At a given interval within the range of 14 to 21 days after the last injection, collect blood from each animal and prepare serum samples. Use a suitable validated test such as an enzyme-linked immunosorbent assay (*2.7.1*) to measure the antibody response to each of the protective antigens stated on the label. The antibody levels are not significantly less than those obtained with a batch that has given satisfactory results in the test described under Potency and there is no significant increase in antibody titre in the controls.

Where seronegative animals are not available, seropositive animals may be used in the above test. During the development of a test with seropositive animals, particular care will be required during the validation of the test system to establish that the test is suitably sensitive and to specify acceptable pass, fail and retest criteria. It will be necessary to take into account the range of possible prevaccination titres and establish the acceptable minimum titre rise after vaccination in relation to these.

Bacterial endotoxins. A test for bacterial endotoxins (*2.6.14*) is carried out on the final lot or, where the nature of the adjuvant prevents performance of a satisfactory test, on the bulk antigen or the mixture of bulk antigens immediately before addition of the adjuvant. The maximum acceptable amount of bacterial endotoxins is that found for a batch of vaccine that has been shown satisfactory in safety test A given under Choice of vaccine composition or in the safety test described under Tests, carried out using 10 animals. Where the latter test is used, note the maximum temperature increase for each animal; the average temperature increase for all animals does not exceed 1.5 °C. The method chosen for determining the amount of bacterial endotoxin present

Vaccines

in the vaccine batch used in the safety test for determining the maximum acceptable level of endotoxins is used subsequently for testing of each batch.

IDENTIFICATION

In animals free from specific antibodies against the antigens stated on the label, the vaccine stimulates the production of antibodies against these antigens.

TESTS

Safety. Use animals of one of the species for which the vaccine is recommended and preferably having no specific antibodies against the antigens stated on the label or, where justified, use animals with a low level of such antibodies as long as they have not been vaccinated against colibacillosis and administration of the vaccine does not cause an anamnestic response. Administer by a recommended route a double dose of vaccine to each of 2 animals. Observe the animals for 14 days. Record body temperature before vaccination, at vaccination, 2 h, 4 h and 6 h later and then daily for 2 days. No abnormal local or systemic reaction occurs; a transient temperature increase not exceeding 2 °C may occur.

Sterility. The vaccine complies with the test for sterility prescribed in the monograph on *Vaccines for veterinary use (0062)*.

POTENCY

Carry out the test with a challenge strain representing each type of antigen against which the vaccine is intended to protect: if a single strain with all the necessary antigens is not available, repeat the test using different challenge strains.

Use not fewer than 15 susceptible animals of one of the species for which the vaccine is recommended and which are free from specific antibodies against the antigens stated on the label. Take not fewer than 10 at random and vaccinate these at the recommended stage of pregnancy and according to the recommended schedule. Collect colostrum from all animals after parturition and store the samples individually in conditions that maintain antibody levels. Take not fewer than 15 newborn unsuckled animals and house them in an environment ensuring absence of enteric pathogens. Allocate a colostrum sample from not fewer than 10 vaccinated dams and not fewer than 5 controls to the offspring. After birth, feed the animals with the colostrum sample allocated to it. After feeding the colostrum and within 12 h of birth, challenge the animals orally with a pathogenic strain of *E. coli* and observe for 10 days. The strain must not be one used in the manufacture of the vaccine.

On each day, note clinical signs in each animal and score using the following scale:

0 no signs

1 slight diarrhoea

2 marked diarrhoea (watery faeces)

3 dead

Total scores for each animal over 10 days are calculated. The test is not valid unless 80 per cent of the offspring from the control animals die or show severe signs of disease. The vaccine complies with the test if there is a significant reduction in score in the group of animals from vaccinated dams compared with the group from the unvaccinated controls.

LABELLING

The label states the antigen or antigens contained in the vaccine that stimulate a protective immune response.

01/2005:0870

NEWCASTLE DISEASE VACCINE (INACTIVATED)

Vaccinum pseudopestis aviariae inactivatum

DEFINITION

Newcastle disease vaccine (inactivated) [also known as avian paramyxovirus 1 vaccine (inactivated) for vaccines intended for some species] consists of an emulsion or a suspension of a suitable strain of Newcastle disease virus (avian paramyxovirus 1) that has been inactivated in such a manner that immunogenic activity is retained.

PRODUCTION

The virus is propagated in embryonated eggs from healthy flocks or in suitable cell cultures (*5.2.4*).

The test for inactivation is carried out in embryonated eggs or suitable cell cultures and the quantity of inactivated virus used is equivalent to not less than ten doses of vaccine. No live virus is detected.

The vaccine may contain an adjuvant.

CHOICE OF VACCINE COMPOSITION

The vaccine is shown to be satisfactory with respect to safety (*5.2.6*) and immunogenicity (*5.2.7*) for each species and category of birds for which it is intended. The following tests may be used during demonstration of immunogenicity.

Immunogenicity. For domestic fowl, the test with virulent challenge (test B) described under Potency is suitable for demonstrating immunogenicity. For other species of birds (for example, pigeons or turkeys), test C described under Potency is suitable for demonstrating immunogenicity.

BATCH TESTING

Batch potency test

For vaccines used in domestic fowl, carry out test A described under Potency but, if the nature of the product does not allow valid results to be obtained with test A or if the batch does not comply with test A, carry out test B. A test using fewer than twenty birds per group and a shorter observation period after challenge may be used if this has been shown to give a valid potency test.

For vaccines used in species other than domestic fowl, carry out a suitable validated test for which a satisfactory correlation has been established with test C described under Potency, the criteria for acceptance being set with reference to a batch that has given satisfactory results in the latter test. A test in chickens from a flock free from specified pathogens (*5.2.2*) and consisting of a measure of the serological response to graded amounts of vaccine (for example, 1/25, 1/50 and 1/100 dose with serum sampling 17 to 21 days later) may be used.

IDENTIFICATION

When injected into animals free from antibodies against Newcastle disease virus, the vaccine stimulates the production of such antibodies.

TESTS

Safety. If the vaccine is intended for use in domestic fowl, vaccinate ten chickens from a flock free from specified pathogens (*5.2.2*). If the vaccine is not for use in domestic fowl, use ten birds of one of the species for which the vaccine is intended, free from antibodies against Newcastle disease virus. Inject twice the vaccinating dose by a recommended route into each of ten birds, 14 to 28 days old. Observe the birds for 21 days. No abnormal local or systemic reaction occurs.

Inactivation. Inject two-fifths of a dose into the allantoic cavity of each of ten embryonated hen eggs, 9 to 11 days old, from flocks free from specified pathogens (*5.2.2*) (SPF eggs) and incubate. Observe for 6 days and pool separately the allantoic fluid from eggs containing live embryos, and that from eggs containing dead embryos, excluding those dying within 24 h of the injection. Examine embryos that die within 24 h of injection for the presence of Newcastle disease virus: the vaccine does not comply with the test if Newcastle disease virus is found.

Inject into the allantoic cavity of each of ten SPF eggs, 9 to 11 days old, 0.2 ml of the pooled allantoic fluid from the live embryos and, into each of ten similar eggs, 0.2 ml of the pooled fluid from the dead embryos and incubate for 5 to 6 days. Test the allantoic fluid from each egg for the presence of haemagglutinins using chicken erythrocytes.

The vaccine complies with the test if there is no evidence of haemagglutinating activity and if not more than 20 per cent of the embryos die at either stage. If more than 20 per cent of the embryos die at one of the stages, repeat that stage; the vaccine complies with the test if there is no evidence of haemagglutinating activity and not more than 20 per cent of the embryos die at that stage.

Antibiotics may be used in the test to control extraneous bacterial infection.

Extraneous agents. Inject a double dose by a recommended route into each of ten chickens, 14 to 28 days old and from a flock free from specified pathogens (*5.2.2*). After 3 weeks, inject one dose by the same route. Collect serum samples from each chicken 2 weeks later and carry out tests for antibodies to the following agents by the methods prescribed for chicken flocks free from specified pathogens (*5.2.2*): avian encephalomyelitis virus, avian infectious bronchitis virus, avian leucosis viruses, egg-drop syndrome virus, avian bursal disease virus, avian infectious laryngotracheitis virus, influenza A virus, Marek's disease virus. The vaccine does not stimulate the formation of antibodies against these agents.

Sterility. The vaccine complies with the test for sterility prescribed in the monograph on *Vaccines for veterinary use (0062)*.

POTENCY

For vaccines for use in domestic fowl carry out test A. If an unsatisfactory result is obtained with test A but a satisfactory result is obtained with test B, the vaccine complies with the requirements. For vaccines for use only in other species, such as pigeons, carry out test C.

A. Inject intramuscularly into each of not fewer than ten chickens, 21 to 28 days old and from a flock free from specified pathogens (*5.2.2*), a volume of the vaccine equivalent to 1/50 of a dose. 17 to 21 days later, collect serum samples from each vaccinated chicken and from each of not fewer than five control chickens of the same age and from the same source. Measure the antibody levels in the sera by the haemagglutination-inhibition (HI) test using the technique described below or an equivalent technique with the same numbers of haemagglutinating units and red blood cells. The test system used must include negative and positive control sera, the latter having an HI titre of 5.0 $\log_2$ to 6.0 $\log_2$. The vaccine complies with the test if the mean HI titre of the vaccinated group is equal to or greater than 4.0 $\log_2$ and that of the unvaccinated group is 2.0 $\log_2$ or less. If the HI titres are not satisfactory, carry out test B.

   Haemagglutination-inhibition test. Inactivate the test sera by heating at 56 °C for 30 min. Add 0.025 ml to the first row of wells in a microtitre plate. Add 0.025 ml of a buffered 9 g/l solution of *sodium chloride R* at pH 7.2 to pH 7.4 to the rest of the wells. Prepare twofold dilutions of the sera across the plate. To each well add 0.025 ml of a suspension containing 4 haemagglutinating units of inactivated Newcastle disease virus. Incubate the plate at 4 °C for 1 h. Add 0.025 ml of a 1 per cent *V/V* suspension of red blood cells collected from chickens, 3 to 4 weeks old and free from antibodies against Newcastle disease virus. Incubate the plate at 4 °C for 1 h. The HI titre is equal to the highest dilution that produces complete inhibition.

B. Use chickens 21 to 28 days old and from a flock free from specified pathogens (*5.2.2*). For vaccination, use not fewer than three groups, each of not fewer than twenty chickens; keep a group of ten chickens as controls. Choose a number of different volumes of the vaccine corresponding to the number of groups: for example, volumes equivalent to 1/25, 1/50 and 1/100 of a dose. Allocate a different volume to each vaccination group. Inject intramuscularly into each chicken the volume of vaccine allocated to its group. 17 to 21 days later, challenge all the chickens by intramuscular injection of 6 $\log_{10}$ embryo LD_{50} of the Herts (Weybridge 33/56) strain of Newcastle disease virus. Observe the chickens for 21 days. Calculate the PD_{50} by standard statistical methods from the number of chickens that survive in each vaccinated group without showing any clinical evidence of Newcastle disease during the 21 days. The vaccine complies with the test if the smallest dose stated on the label corresponds to not less than 50 PD_{50} and the lower confidence limit is not less than 35 PD_{50} per dose. If the lower confidence limit is less than 35 PD_{50} per dose, repeat the test; the vaccine must be shown to contain not less than 50 PD_{50} in the repeat test. The test is not valid unless all the control birds die within 6 days of challenge.

C. Vaccinate not fewer than twenty birds of the target species, free from antibodies against avian paramyxovirus 1, in accordance with the recommendations for use. Maintain as unvaccinated controls a group of not fewer than ten birds of the same age, from the same source and free from antibodies against avian paramyxovirus 1. The test is invalid if serum samples obtained at the time of the first vaccination show the presence of antibodies against avian paramyxovirus 1 in either vaccinates or controls or if tests carried out at the time of challenge show such antibodies in controls. 4 weeks after the last vaccination, challenge each bird intramuscularly with a sufficient quantity of virulent avian paramyxovirus 1. The test is not valid if fewer than 90 per cent of the control birds die or show serious signs of Newcastle disease virus infection. The vaccine complies with the test if not fewer than 90 per cent of the vaccinated birds survive and show no serious signs of avian paramyxovirus 1 infection.

Vaccines

01/2005:0450

NEWCASTLE DISEASE VACCINE (LIVE)

Vaccinum pseudopestis aviariae vivum

1. DEFINITION

Newcastle disease vaccine (live) is a preparation of a suitable strain of Newcastle disease virus (avian paramyxovirus 1). This monograph applies to vaccines intended for administration to chickens and/or other avian species for active immunisation.

2. PRODUCTION

2-1. *PREPARATION OF THE VACCINE*

The vaccine virus is grown in embryonated hens' eggs or in cell cultures.

2-2. *SUBSTRATE FOR VIRUS PROPAGATION*

2-2-1. **Embryonated hens' eggs**. If the vaccine virus is grown in embryonated hens' eggs, they are obtained from flocks free from specified pathogens (SPF) (*5.2.2*).

2-2-2. **Cell cultures**. If the vaccine virus is grown in cell cultures, they comply with the requirements for cell cultures for production of veterinary vaccines (*5.2.4*).

2-3. *SEED LOTS*

2-3-1. **Extraneous agents**. The master seed lot complies with the tests for extraneous agents in seed lots (*2.6.24*). In these tests on the master seed lot, the organisms used are not more than 5 passages from the master seed lot at the start of the tests.

2-4. *CHOICE OF VACCINE VIRUS*

The vaccine virus shall be shown to be satisfactory with respect to safety (*5.2.6*) and efficacy (*5.2.7*) for the birds for which it is intended.

The following tests for intracerebral pathogenicity index (section 2-4-1), amino-acid sequence (section 2-4-2), safety (section 2-4-3), increase in virulence (section 2-4-4) and immunogenicity (section 2-4-5) may be used during the demonstration of safety and immunogenicity.

2-4-1. **Intracerebral pathogenicity index**. Use vaccine virus at the least attenuated passage level that will be present in a batch of the vaccine. Inoculate the vaccine virus into the allantoic cavity of embryonated hens' eggs, 9- to 11- days-old, from an SPF flock (*5.2.2*). Incubate the inoculated eggs for a suitable period and harvest and pool the allantoic fluids. Use not fewer than ten 1-day-old chickens (i.e. more than 24 h but less than 40 h after hatching), from an SPF flock (*5.2.2*). Administer by the intracerebral route to each chick 0.05 ml of the pooled allantoic fluids containing not less than $10^{8.0}$ EID_{50} or, if this virus quantity cannot be achieved, not less than $10^{7.0}$ EID_{50}. Observe the chickens at least daily for 8 days after administration and score them once every 24 h. A score of 0 is attributed to a chicken if it is clinically normal, 1 if it shows clinical signs of disease and 2 if it is dead. The intracerebral pathogenicity index is the mean of the scores per chicken per observation over the 8 day period.

If an inoculum of not less than $10^{8.0}$ EID_{50} is used, the vaccine virus complies with the test if its intracerebral pathogenicity index is not greater than 0.5; if an inoculum of not less than $10^{7.0}$ EID_{50} but less than $10^{8.0}$ EID_{50} is used, the vaccine virus complies with the test if its intracerebral pathogenicity index is not greater than 0.4.

2-4-2. **Amino-acid sequence**. Determine the sequence of a fragment of RNA from the vaccine virus containing the region encoding for the F0 cleavage site by a suitable method. The encoded amino-acid sequence is shown to be one of the following:

			F2				Cleavage site		F1	
Site	111	112	113	114	115	116	˅	117	118	119
	Gly	Gly	Lys	Gln	Gly	Arg		Leu	Ile	Gly
or	Gly	Gly	Arg	Gln	Gly	Arg		Leu	Ile	Gly
or	Gly	Glu	Arg	Gln	Glu	Arg		Leu	Val	Gly

or equivalent with leucine at 117 and no basic amino acids at sites 111, 112, 114 and 115.

2-4-3. **Safety**. Carry out the test for each route and method of administration to be recommended for vaccination and in each avian species for which the vaccine is intended, using in each case birds not older than the youngest age to be recommended for vaccination. Use vaccine virus at the least attenuated passage level that will be present between the master seed lot and a batch of the vaccine. For tests in chickens, use not fewer than 20 chickens, from an SPF flock (*5.2.2*). For species other than the chicken, use not fewer than 20 birds that do not have antibodies against Newcastle disease virus. Administer to each bird a quantity of the vaccine virus equivalent to not less than 10 times the maximum virus titre likely to be contained in 1 dose of the vaccine. Observe the birds at least daily for 21 days. The test is not valid if more than 10 per cent of the birds show abnormal clinical signs or die from causes not attributable to the vaccine virus. The vaccine virus complies with the test if no bird shows notable clinical signs of Newcastle disease or dies from causes attributable to the vaccine virus.

2-4-4. **Increase in virulence**. The test for increase in virulence consists of the administration of the vaccine virus at the least attenuated passage level that will be present between the master seed lot and a batch of the vaccine to a group of 5 birds not more than 2 weeks old, sequential passages, 5 times where possible, to further similar groups and testing of the final recovered virus for increase in virulence. If the properties of the vaccine virus allow sequential passage to 5 groups via natural spreading, this method may be used, otherwise passage as described below is carried out and the maximally passaged virus that has been recovered is tested for increase in virulence. Care must be taken to avoid contamination by virus from previous passages. Carry out the test in a target species, using the chicken if it is one of the target species. For the test in chickens, use chickens from an SPF flock (*5.2.2*). For other species, carry out the test in birds that do not have antibodies against Newcastle disease virus. Administer by eye-drop a quantity of the vaccine virus that will allow recovery of virus for the passages described below. Observe the birds for the period shown to correspond to maximum replication of the vaccine virus, kill them and prepare a suspension from the brain of each bird and from a suitable organ depending on the tropism of the strain (for example, mucosa of the entire trachea, intestine, pancreas); pool the samples. Administer 0.05 ml of the pooled samples by eye-drop to each of 5 other birds of the same species, age and origin. Carry out this passage operation not fewer than 5 times; verify the presence of the virus at each passage. If the virus is not found at a passage level, carry out a second series of passages.

A. Carry out the test for intracerebral pathogenicity index (section 2-4-1) using unpassaged vaccine virus and the maximally passaged virus that has been recovered.

B. Carry out the test for amino-acid sequence (section 2-4-2) using unpassaged vaccine virus and the maximally passaged virus that has been recovered.

C. Carry out the test for safety (section 2-4-3) using unpassaged vaccine virus and the maximally passaged virus that has been recovered. Administer the virus by the route to be recommended for vaccination likely to be the least safe and to the avian species for which the vaccine is intended that is likely to be the most susceptible to Newcastle disease.

The vaccine virus complies with the test if, in the tests 2-4-4A, 2-4-4B and 2-4-4C, no indication of increase in virulence of the maximally passaged virus compared with the unpassaged virus is observed. If virus is not recovered at any passage level in the first and second series of passages, the vaccine virus also complies with the test.

2-4-5. **Immunogenicity**. For each avian species for which the vaccine is intended, a test is carried out for each route and method of administration to be recommended using in each case birds not older than the youngest age to be recommended for vaccination. The quantity of the vaccine virus administered to each bird is not greater than the minimum titre to be stated on the label and the virus is at the most attenuated passage level that will be present in a batch of the vaccine.

2-4-5-1. *Vaccines for use in chickens*. Use not fewer than 30 chickens of the same origin and from an SPF flock (*5.2.2*). Vaccinate by a recommended route not fewer than 20 chickens. Maintain not fewer than 10 chickens as controls. Challenge each chicken after 21 days by the intramuscular route with not less than $10^{5.0}$ embryo LD_{50} of the Herts (Weybridge 33/56) strain of Newcastle disease virus. Observe the chickens at least daily for 14 days after challenge. Record the deaths and the number of surviving chickens that show clinical signs of disease. The test is not valid if 6 days after challenge fewer than 100 per cent of the control chickens have died or if during the period between vaccination and challenge more than 10 per cent of the vaccinated or control chickens show abnormal clinical signs or die from causes not attributable to the vaccine. The vaccine virus complies with the test if during the observation period after challenge not fewer than 90 per cent of the vaccinated chickens survive and show no notable clinical signs of Newcastle disease.

2-4-5-2. *Vaccines for use in avian species other than the chicken*. Use not fewer than 30 birds of the species for which the vaccine is intended for Newcastle disease, of the same origin and that do not have antibodies against avian paramyxovirus 1. Vaccinate by a recommended route not fewer than 20 birds. Maintain not fewer than 10 birds as controls. Challenge each bird after 21 days by the intramuscular route with a sufficient quantity of virulent avian paramyxovirus 1. Observe the birds at least daily for 21 days after challenge. Record the deaths and the surviving birds that show clinical signs of disease. The test is not valid if:

- during the observation period after challenge fewer than 90 per cent of the control birds die or show severe clinical signs of Newcastle disease,
- or if during the period between the vaccination and challenge more than 10 per cent of the vaccinated or control birds show abnormal clinical signs or die from causes not attributable to the vaccine.

The vaccine virus complies with the test if during the observation period after challenge not fewer than 90 per cent of the vaccinated birds survive and show no notable clinical signs of Newcastle disease. For species where there is published evidence that it is not possible to achieve this level of protection, the vaccine complies with the test if there is a significant reduction in morbidity and mortality of the vaccinated birds compared with the control birds.

3. BATCH TESTS

3-1. **Identification**

3-1-1. *Identification of the vaccine virus*. The vaccine, diluted if necessary and mixed with a monospecific Newcastle disease virus antiserum, no longer provokes haemagglutination of chicken red blood cells or infects embryonated hens' eggs from an SPF flock (*5.2.2*) or susceptible cell cultures (*5.2.4*) into which it is inoculated.

3-1-2. *Identification of the virus strain*. The strain of vaccine virus is identified by a suitable method, for example using monoclonal antibodies.

3-2. **Bacteria and fungi**

Vaccines intended for administration by injection comply with the test for sterility prescribed in the monograph *Vaccines for veterinary use (0062)*.

Vaccines not intended for administration by injection either comply with the test for sterility prescribed in the monograph *Vaccines for veterinary use (0062)* or with the following test: carry out a quantitative test for bacterial and fungal contamination; carry out identification tests for microorganisms detected in the vaccine; the vaccine does not contain pathogenic microorganisms and contains not more than 1 non-pathogenic microorganism per dose.

Any liquid supplied with the vaccine complies with test for sterility prescribed in the monograph *Vaccines for veterinary use (0062)*.

3-3. **Mycoplasmas**. The vaccine complies with the test for mycoplasmas (*2.6.7*).

3-4. **Extraneous agents**. The vaccine complies with the tests for extraneous agents in batches of finished product (*2.6.25*).

3-5. **Safety**. For vaccines recommended for use in chickens, use not fewer than 10 chickens from an SPF flock (*5.2.2*) and of the youngest age recommended for vaccination. For vaccines recommended for use only in avian species other than the chicken, use not fewer than 10 birds of the species likely to be most sensitive to Newcastle disease, that do not have antibodies against Newcastle disease virus and of the minimum age recommended for vaccination. Administer to each bird by eye-drop, or parenterally if only parenteral administration is recommended, 10 doses of the vaccine in a volume suitable for the test. Observe the birds at least daily for 21 days. The test is not valid if more than 20 per cent of the birds show abnormal clinical signs or die from causes not attributable to the vaccine. The vaccine complies with the test if no bird shows notable clinical signs of disease or dies from causes attributable to the vaccine.

3-6. **Virus titre**. Titrate the vaccine virus by inoculation into embryonated hens' eggs from an SPF flock (*5.2.2*) or into suitable cell cultures (*5.2.4*). The vaccine complies with the test if 1 dose contains not less than the minimum virus titre stated on the label.

3-7. **Potency**. Depending on the indications, the vaccine complies with 1 or both of the tests prescribed under Immunogenicity (section 2-4-5) when administered according to the recommended schedule by a recommended route and method. If the test in section 2-4-5-2. *Vaccine for use in avian species other than the chicken* is conducted and the vaccine is recommended for use in more than 1 avian species, the test is carried out with birds of that species for which the vaccine is recommended which is likely to be the most susceptible to avian paramyxovirus 1. It is not necessary

Vaccines

to carry out the potency test for each batch of the vaccine if it has been carried out on a representative batch using a vaccinating dose containing not more than the minimum virus titre stated on the label.

01/2005:2072

PASTEURELLA VACCINE (INACTIVATED) FOR SHEEP

Vaccinum pasteurellae inactivatum ad ovem

DEFINITION

Pasteurella vaccine (inactivated) for sheep is a preparation of one or more suitable strains of *Pasteurella trehalosi*. This monograph applies to vaccines intended for administration to sheep to protect against disease caused by *P. trehalosi*.

PRODUCTION

Production of the vaccine is based on a seed-lot system. The seed material is cultured in a suitable medium; each strain is cultivated separately and identity is verified using a suitable method. During production, various parameters such as growth rate are monitored by suitable methods; the values are within the limits approved for the particular product. Purity and identity of the harvest are verified using suitable methods. After cultivation, the bacterial suspensions are collected separately and inactivated by a suitable method. The vaccine may contain an adjuvant and may be freeze-dried.

CHOICE OF VACCINE COMPOSITION

The choice of composition and the strains to be included in the vaccine is based on epidemiological data on the prevalence of the different serovars of *P. trehalosi*. The vaccine is shown to be satisfactory with respect to safety (*5.2.6*) and efficacy (*5.2.7*) in sheep. As part of the studies to demonstrate the suitability of the vaccine with respect to these characteristics the following tests may be carried out.

Safety

A. The test is carried out for each of the routes of administration to be stated on the label and in animals of each category (for example, young sheep, pregnant ewes) for which the vaccine is intended.

   For each test, use not fewer than 10 animals that preferably do not have antibodies against the serovars of *P. trehalosi* or against leucotoxin present in the vaccine. Where justified, animals with a known history of no previous pasteurella vaccination and with low antibody titres (measured in a sensitive test system such as an ELISA) may be used.

   Administer to each animal a double dose of vaccine containing not less than the maximum potency that may be expected in a batch of vaccine. Administer a single dose of vaccine to each animal after the recommended interval. Observe the animals for at least 14 days after the last administration. Record body temperature the day before vaccination, at vaccination, 2 h, 4 h and 6 h later and then daily for 4 days; note the maximum temperature increase for each animal. No abnormal local or systemic reaction occurs; the average body temperature increase for all animals does not exceed 1.5 °C and no animal shows a rise greater than 2 °C. If the vaccine is intended for use or may be used in pregnant ewes, vaccinate the ewes at the relevant stages of pregnancy and prolong the observation period until 1 day after lambing.

   The vaccine complies with the test if no animal shows abnormal local reactions or clinical signs of disease or dies from causes attributable to the vaccine. In addition, if the vaccine is intended for use in pregnant ewes, no significant effects on the pregnancy and offspring are demonstrated.

B. The animals used for the field trials are also used to evaluate safety. Carry out a test in each category of animals for which the vaccine is intended. Use not fewer than 3 groups of 20 animals with corresponding groups of not fewer than 10 controls in 3 different locations. Examine the injection sites for local reactions after vaccination. Record body temperatures the day before vaccination, at vaccination and on the 2 days following vaccination. The vaccine complies with the test if no animal shows abnormal local or systemic reactions or clinical signs of disease or dies from causes attributable to the vaccine. The average body temperature increase for all animals does not exceed 1.5 °C and no animal shows a rise greater than 2 °C. In addition, if the vaccine is intended for use in pregnant ewes, no significant effects on the pregnancy and offspring are demonstrated.

Immunogenicity. As part of the studies to demonstrate the suitability of the vaccine with respect to immunogenicity, the test described under Potency may be carried out for each proposed route of administration and using vaccine of minimum potency.

BATCH TESTING

Batch potency test. The test described under Potency is not carried out for routine testing of batches of vaccine. It is carried out, for a given vaccine, on one or more occasions, as decided by or with the agreement of the competent authority. Where the test is not carried out, a suitable validated batch potency test is carried out, the criteria for acceptance being set with reference to the results obtained with a batch of vaccine that has given satisfactory results in the test described under Potency.

Bacterial endotoxins. A test for bacterial endotoxins (*2.6.14*) is carried out on the final lot or, where the nature of the adjuvant prevents performance of a satisfactory test, on the bulk antigen or the mixture of bulk antigens immediately before addition of the adjuvant. The maximum acceptable amount of bacterial endotoxins is that found for a batch of vaccine that has been shown satisfactory in safety test A given under Choice of vaccine composition or in the safety test described under Tests, carried out using 10 animals. Where the latter test is used, note the maximum temperature increase for each animal; the average body temperature increase for all animals does not exceed 1.5 °C. The method chosen for determining the amount of bacterial endotoxin present in the vaccine batch used in the safety test for determining the maximum acceptable level of endotoxin is used subsequently for testing of each batch.

IDENTIFICATION

When injected into healthy seronegative animals, the vaccine stimulates the production of specific antibodies against the serovars of *P. trehalosi* and/or against the leucotoxin present in the vaccine.

TESTS

Safety. Use 2 sheep of the minimum age recommended for vaccination or, if not available, of an age as close as possible to the minimum recommended age, and that have not been vaccinated against Pasteurella. Administer a double dose of vaccine to each animal by a recommended route. Observe the animals for 14 days. Record body temperature the day before vaccination, at vaccination, 2 h, 4 h and 6 h later and then daily for 2 days. The animals remain in good health and no abnormal local or systemic reaction occurs; a transient temperature increase not exceeding 2 °C may occur.

Sterility. It complies with the test for sterility prescribed in the monograph on *Vaccines for veterinary use (0062)*.

POTENCY

Carry out a test for each serovar of *P. trehalosi* for which protection is claimed on the label.

Use not fewer than 20 lambs of the minimum age recommended for vaccination, free from antibodies against *P. trehalosi* and against the leucotoxin of *P. trehalosi*. Vaccinate not fewer than 10 of the animals by a recommended route and according to the recommended schedule. Keep 10 animals as controls. 21 days after the last vaccination, infect all the lambs by injection, using the subcutaneous or other suitable route, with a suitable quantity of a low-passage, virulent strain of a serovar of *P. trehalosi*. Observe the animals for a further 7 days; to avoid unnecessary suffering, severely ill animals are killed and are then considered to have died from the disease. During the observation period, the animals are examined for any signs of disease (for example, severe dullness, excess salivation) and the mortality is recorded. Kill surviving animals at the end of the observation period. Post-mortem examination is carried out on any animal that dies and those killed at the end of the observation period. The lungs, pleura, liver and spleen are examined for haemorrhages and the extent of lung consolidation due to pasteurellosis is evaluated. Samples of lung, liver and spleen tissue are collected for re-isolation of the challenge organisms. The mortality, clinical observations and the post-mortem lesions are scored and the results obtained for these parameters and the bacterial re-isolation results compared for the 2 groups.

The test is invalid if clinical signs or lesions of *P. trehalosi* infection occur in less than 70 per cent of the control lambs.

The vaccine complies with the requirements of the test if there is a significant difference between the scores obtained for the clinical and post-mortem observations in the vaccinates compared to the controls. For vaccines with a claim for a beneficial effect on the extent of infection against the serovar, the results for the infection rates are also significantly better for the vaccinates compared to the controls.

LABELLING

The label states:

– the serovar(s) of *P. trehalosi* against which protection is claimed,
– the serovar(s) of *P. trehalosi* and/or the leucotoxin present in the vaccine.

01/2005:1360

PORCINE ACTINOBACILLOSIS VACCINE (INACTIVATED)

Vaccinum actinobacillosis inactivatum ad suem

DEFINITION

Porcine actinobacillosis vaccine (inactivated) is a liquid preparation which has one or more of the following components: inactivated *Actinobacillus pleuropneumoniae* of a suitable strain or strains; toxins, proteins or polysaccharides derived from suitable strains of *A. pleuropneumoniae*, and treated to render them harmless; fractions of toxins derived from suitable strains of *A. pleuropneumoniae* and treated if necessary to render them harmless. This monograph applies to vaccines intended for protection of pigs against actinobacillosis.

PRODUCTION

The seed material is cultured in a suitable medium; each strain is cultivated separately. During production, various parameters such as growth rate, protein content and quantity of relevant antigens are monitored by suitable methods; the values are within the limits approved for the particular product. Purity and identity are verified on the harvest using suitable methods. After cultivation, the bacterial suspensions are collected separately and inactivated by a suitable method. They may be detoxified, purified and concentrated. The vaccine may contain an adjuvant.

CHOICE OF VACCINE COMPOSITION

The choice of strains is based on epidemiological data. The vaccine is shown to be satisfactory with respect to safety (*5.2.6*) and efficacy (*5.2.7*) in pigs. The following tests may be used during demonstration of safety and immunogenicity.

Safety

A. Carry out a test in each category of animals for which the vaccine is intended and by each of the recommended routes of administration. Use animals that do not have antibodies against the serotypes of *A. pleuropneumoniae* or its toxins present in the vaccine. Administer a double dose of vaccine by a recommended route to each of not fewer than 10 animals. Administer a single dose of vaccine to each of the animals after the interval recommended in the instructions for use. Observe the animals for 14 days after vaccination. Record body temperature the day before vaccination, at vaccination, 2 h, 4 h and 6 h later and then daily for 4 days; note the maximum temperature increase for each animal. No abnormal local or systemic reaction occurs; the average temperature increase for all animals does not exceed 1.5 °C and no animal shows a rise greater than 2 °C. If the vaccine is intended for use in pregnant sows, for the test in this category of animals, prolong the observation period up to farrowing and note any effects on gestation or the offspring.

B. The animals used for field trials are also used to evaluate safety. Carry out a test in each category of animals for which the vaccine is intended. Use not fewer than 3 groups each of not fewer than 20 animals with corresponding groups of not fewer than 10 controls. Examine the injection site for local reactions after vaccination. Record body temperature the day before vaccination, at vaccination, at the time interval after which a rise in temperature, if any, was seen in test A, and daily during the 2 days following vaccination; note the maximum temperature increase for each animal. No abnormal local or systemic reaction occurs; the average temperature increase for all animals does not exceed 1.5 °C and no animal shows a rise greater than 2 °C.

Immunogenicity. The test described under Potency may be used to demonstrate the immunogenicity of the vaccine.

BATCH TESTING

Batch potency test. The test described under Potency is not carried out for routine testing of batches of vaccine. It is carried out, for a given vaccine, on one or more occasions, as decided by or with the agreement of the competent authority; where the test is not carried out, a suitable validated test is carried out, the criteria for acceptance being set with reference to a batch of vaccine that has given satisfactory results in the test described under Potency. The following test may be used after a satisfactory correlation with the test described under Potency has been established.

Inject a suitable dose subcutaneously into each of 5 seronegative mice, weighing 18-20 g. Where the schedule stated on the label requires a booster injection to be given, a booster vaccination may also be given in this test provided it has been demonstrated that this will still provide a suitably sensitive test system. Before the vaccination and at a given interval within the range of 14-21 days after the last injection, collect blood from each animal and prepare serum samples. Determine individually for each serum the titre of specific antibodies against each antigenic component stated on the label, using a suitable validated test such as enzyme-linked immunosorbent assay (*2.7.1*). The vaccine complies with the test if the antibody levels are not significantly lower than those obtained for a batch that has given satisfactory results in the test described under Potency.

Bacterial endotoxins. A test for bacterial endotoxins (*2.6.14*) is carried out on the final bulk or, where the nature of the adjuvant prevents performance of a satisfactory test, on the bulk antigen or mixture of bulk antigens immediately before addition of the adjuvant. The maximum acceptable amount of bacterial endotoxins is that found for a batch of vaccine that has been shown satisfactory in safety test A described under Choice of vaccine composition or the safety test described under Tests, carried out using 10 pigs. Where the latter test is used, note the maximum temperature increase for each animal; the average temperature increase for all animals does not exceed 1.5 °C. The method chosen for determining the amount of bacterial endotoxin present in the vaccine batch used in the safety test for determining the maximum acceptable level of endotoxin is used subsequently for batch testing.

IDENTIFICATION

When injected into healthy seronegative animals, the vaccine stimulates the production of specific antibodies against the antigenic components of *A. pleuropneumoniae* stated on the label.

TESTS

Safety. Use 2 pigs of the minimum age stated for vaccination and which do not have antibodies against the serotypes of *A. pleuropneumoniae* or its toxins present in the vaccine. Administer to each pig a double dose of vaccine by a recommended route. Observe the animals for 14 days. Record body temperature the day before vaccination, at vaccination, 2 h, 4 h and 6 h later and then daily for 2 days. No abnormal local or systemic reaction occurs; a transient temperature increase not exceeding 2 °C may occur.

Sterility. The vaccine complies with the test for sterility prescribed in the monograph on *Vaccines for veterinary use (0062)*.

POTENCY

The challenge strain for the potency test is chosen to ensure challenge with each Ap toxin (1) produced by the serotypes stated on the label; it may be necessary to carry out more than one test using a different challenge strain for each test.

Vaccinate according to the recommended schedule not fewer than 7 pigs, of the minimum age recommended for vaccination, which do not have antibodies against *A. pleuropneumoniae* and Ap toxins. Keep not fewer than 7 unvaccinated pigs of the same age as controls. 3 weeks after the last vaccination, challenge all the pigs intranasally or intratracheally or by aerosol with a suitable quantity of a serotype of *A. pleuropneumoniae*. Observe the animals for 7 days; to avoid unnecessary suffering, severely ill control animals are killed and are then considered to have died from the disease. Kill all surviving animals at the end of the observation period. Carry out a post-mortem examination on all animals. Examine the lungs, the tracheobronchial lymph nodes and the tonsils for the presence of *A. pleuropneumoniae*. Evaluate the extent of lung lesions at post-mortem examination. Each of the 7 lobes of the lungs is allotted a maximum possible lesion score (2) of 5. The area showing pneumonia and/or pleuritis of each lobe is assessed and expressed on a scale of 0 to 5 to give the pneumonic score per lobe (the maximum total score possible for each complete lung is 35). Calculate separately for the vaccinated and the control animals the total score (the maximum score per group is 245, if 7 pigs are used per group).

The vaccine complies with the test if the vaccinated animals, when compared with controls, show lower incidence of: mortality; typical clinical signs (dyspnoea, coughing and vomiting); typical lung lesions; re-isolation of *A. pleuropneumoniae* from the lungs, the tracheobronchial lymph nodes and the tonsils. Where possible, the incidence is analysed statistically and shown to be significantly lower for vaccinates.

LABELLING

The label states:

- the antigens present in the vaccine,
- the serotypes of *A. pleuropneumoniae* for which the vaccine affords protection.

01/2005:0963

PORCINE INFLUENZA VACCINE (INACTIVATED)

Vaccinum influenzae inactivatum ad suem

DEFINITION

Porcine influenza vaccine (inactivated) is an aqueous suspension, an oily emulsion or a freeze-dried preparation of one or more inactivated strains of swine or human influenza virus. Suitable strains contain both haemagglutinin and neuraminidase.

PRODUCTION

The virus is propagated in the allantoic cavity of fertilised hen eggs from a healthy flock or in suitable cell cultures (*5.2.4*). Each virus strain is cultivated separately. After cultivation, the viral suspensions are collected separately and inactivated by a method that avoids destruction of the immunogenicity. If necessary, they may be purified.

An amplification test for residual infectious influenza virus is carried out on each batch of antigen immediately after inactivation by passage in the same type of substrate as that used for production (eggs or cell cultures) or a substrate shown to be at least as sensitive. The quantity of inactivated virus used in the test is equivalent to not less than 10 doses of the vaccine. No live virus is detected.

The vaccine may contain one or more suitable adjuvants; it may be freeze-dried.

(1) The nomenclature of the toxins of *A. pleuropneumoniae* is described by J. Frey *et al., Journal of General Microbiology*, 1993, 139, 1723-1728.
(2) The system of lung scores is described in detail by P.C.T. Hannan, B.S. Bhogal, J.P. Fish, *Research in Veterinary Science*, 1982, 33, 76-88.

CHOICE OF VACCINE COMPOSITION

The choice of strains is based on the antigenic types and sub-types observed in Europe. The vaccine is shown to be satisfactory with respect to safety and immunogenicity for pigs. The following tests may be used during demonstration of safety (*5.2.6*) and efficacy (*5.2.7*).

Safety

A. A test is carried out in each category of animal for which the vaccine is intended (sows, fattening pigs). The animals used do not have antibodies against swine influenza virus. 2 doses of vaccine are injected by the intended route into each of not fewer than 10 animals. After 14 days, 1 dose of vaccine is injected into each of the animals. The animals are observed for a further 14 days. During the 28 days of the test, no abnormal local or systemic reaction is produced.

B. The animals used in the test for immunogenicity are also used to evaluate safety. The rectal temperature of each vaccinated animal is measured at the time of vaccination and 24 h and 48 h later. No abnormal effect on rectal temperature is noted nor other systemic reactions (for example, anorexia). The injection site is examined for local reactions at slaughter. No abnormal local reaction occurs.

C. The animals used for field trials are also used to evaluate safety. A test is carried out in each category of animals for which the vaccine is intended (sows, fattening pigs). Not fewer than 3 groups each of not fewer than 20 animals in at least 2 locations are used with corresponding groups of not fewer than 10 controls. The rectal temperature of each animal is measured at the time of vaccination and 24 h and 48 h later. No abnormal effect on rectal temperature is noted. The injection site is examined for local reactions at slaughter. No abnormal local reaction occurs.

Immunogenicity. The test described under Potency carried out using an epidemiologically relevant challenge strain or strains is suitable to demonstrate the immunogenicity of the vaccine.

IN-PROCESS TESTS

For vaccines produced in eggs, the content of bacterial endotoxins is determined on the virus harvest to monitor production.

BATCH POTENCY TEST

The test described below under Potency is not carried out for routine testing of batches of vaccine. It is carried out, for a given vaccine, on one or more occasions, as decided by or with the agreement of the competent authority; where the test is not carried out, a suitable validated test is carried out, the criteria for acceptance being set with reference to a batch of vaccine that has given satisfactory results in the test described under Potency. The following test may be used after a satisfactory correlation with the test described under Potency has been established by a statistical evaluation.

Inject subcutaneously into each of 5 seronegative guinea-pigs, 5 to 7 weeks old, a quarter of the dose stated on the label. Collect blood samples before the vaccination and 21 days after vaccination. Determine for each sample the level of specific antibodies against each virus subtype in the vaccine by haemagglutination-inhibition or another suitable test. The vaccine complies with the test if the level of antibodies is not lower than that found for a batch of vaccine that gave satisfactory results in the potency test in pigs (see Potency).

IDENTIFICATION

When injected into healthy, susceptible animals, the vaccine stimulates the production of specific antibodies against the influenza virus subtypes included in the vaccine. The antibodies may be detected by a suitable immunochemical method (*2.7.1*).

TESTS

Safety. Use 2 pigs, free from antibodies against swine influenza virus and not older than the minimum age stated for vaccination. Inject into each pig a double dose of vaccine by the route stated on the label. Observe the animals for 14 days and then inject into each animal 1 dose of vaccine. Observe the animals for 14 days. No abnormal local or systemic reaction occurs during the 28 days of the test.

Inactivation. If the vaccine has been prepared in eggs, inoculate 0.2 ml into the allantoic cavity of each of 10 fertilised hen eggs, 9 to 11 days old. Incubate at a suitable temperature for 3 days. The death of any embryo within 24 h of inoculation is considered as non-specific mortality and the egg is discarded. The test is not valid unless at least 80 per cent of the eggs survive. Collect the allantoic fluid of each egg, pool equal quantities and carry out a second passage on fertilised eggs in the same manner. Incubate for 4 days; the allantoic fluid of these eggs shows no haemagglutinating activity.

If the vaccine has been prepared in cell cultures, carry out a suitable test for residual infectious influenza virus using 2 passages in the same type of cell culture as used in the production of vaccine. No live virus is detected. If the vaccine contains an oily adjuvant that interferes with this test, where possible separate the aqueous phase from the vaccine by means that do not diminish the capacity to detect residual infectious influenza virus.

Extraneous viruses. On the pigs used for the safety test, carry out tests for antibodies. The vaccine does not stimulate the formation of antibodies other than those against influenza virus. In particular, no antibodies against viruses pathogenic for pigs or against viruses which could interfere with the diagnosis of infectious diseases of pigs (including viruses of the pestivirus group) are detected.

Sterility. The vaccine complies with the test for sterility prescribed in the monograph on *Vaccines for veterinary use (0062)*.

POTENCY

Carry out a potency test for each subtype used in the preparation of the vaccine. Use not fewer than 20 pigs of the minimum age recommended for vaccination and that do not have antibodies against swine influenza virus. Vaccinate not fewer than 10 pigs as recommended on the label and keep not fewer than 10 pigs as unvaccinated controls. Take a blood sample from all control pigs immediately before challenge. 3 weeks after the last administration of vaccine, challenge all the pigs with a suitable quantity of a virulent influenza field virus by the intratracheal route. Kill half of the vaccinated and control pigs 24 h after challenge and the other half 72 h after challenge. For each pig, measure the quantity of influenza virus in 2 lung tissue homogenates, one from the left apical, cardiac and diaphragmatic lobes, and the other from the corresponding right lung lobes. Take equivalent samples from each animal. The test is invalid if antibodies against influenza virus are found in any control pig immediately before challenge. The vaccine complies with the test if, at both times of measurement, the mean virus titre in the pooled lung tissue samples of vaccinated pigs is significantly lower than that for control pigs, when analysed by a suitable statistical method such as the Wilcoxon Mann-Whitney test.

01/2005:0965

PORCINE PARVOVIROSIS VACCINE (INACTIVATED)

Vaccinum parvovirosis inactivatum ad suem

DEFINITION

Inactivated porcine parvovirosis vaccine consists of a suspension of inactivated porcine parvovirus or of a noninfectious fraction of the virus.

PRODUCTION

The virus is grown in suitable cell cultures (*5.2.4*). The viral suspension is harvested; the virus is inactivated by a method that avoids destruction of the immunogenicity and may be fragmented (inactivation may be by fragmentation); the virus or viral fragments may be purified and concentrated at a suitable stage of the process.

A test for residual infectious porcine parvovirus is carried out on each batch of antigen immediately after inactivation and on the final bulk or, if the vaccine contains an adjuvant, on the bulk antigen or the mixture of bulk antigens immediately before the addition of adjuvant. The quantity used in the test is equivalent to not less than 100 doses of the vaccine. The bulk harvest is inoculated into suitable non-confluent cells; after incubation for 7 days, a subculture is made using trypsinised cells. After incubation for a further 7 days, the cultures are examined for residual live parvovirus by an immunfluorescence test. No live virus is detected.

The vaccine may contain one or more suitable adjuvants.

CHOICE OF VACCINE COMPOSITION

The vaccine is shown to be satisfactory with respect to safety (including absence of adverse effects on fertility, gestation, farrowing or offspring) and immunogenicity in pigs. The following tests may be used during demonstration of safety (*5.2.6*) and efficacy (*5.2.7*).

Safety

A. A test is carried out in each category of animals for which the vaccine is intended and by each of the recommended routes. The animals used do not have antibodies against porcine parvovirus or against a fraction of the virus. Two doses of vaccine are injected by the intended route into each of not fewer than ten animals. After 14 days, one dose of vaccine is injected into each of the animals. The animals are observed for a further 14 days. During the 28 days of the test, no abnormal local or systemic reaction occurs. If the vaccine is intended for use in pregnant sows, for the test in this category of animal, the observation period is prolonged up to farrowing and any effects on gestation or the offspring are noted.

B. The animals used in the test for immunogenicity are also used to evaluate safety. The rectal temperature of each vaccinated animal is measured at the time of vaccination and 24 h and 48 h later. No abnormal effect on body temperature is noted nor other systemic reactions (for example, anorexia). The injection site is examined for local reactions after vaccination and at slaughter. No abnormal local reaction occurs.

C. The animals used for field trials are also used to evaluate safety. A test is carried out in each category of animals for which the vaccine is intended (sows, gilts). Not fewer than three groups each of not fewer than twenty animals are used with corresponding groups of not fewer than ten controls. The rectal temperature of each animal is measured at the time of vaccination and 24 h and 48 h later. No abnormal effect on body temperature is noted. The injection site is examined for local reactions after vaccination and at slaughter. No abnormal local reaction occurs.

Immunogenicity. The test described under Potency may be used to demonstrate the immunogenicity of the vaccine.

BATCH POTENCY TEST

The test described below is not carried out for routine testing of batches of vaccine. It is carried out, for a given vaccine, on one or more occasions, as decided by or with the agreement of the competent authority; where the test is not carried out,a suitable validated test is carried out, the criteria for acceptance being set with reference to a batch of vaccine that has given satisfactory results in the test described underPotency. The following test may be used after a satisfactory correlation with the test described under Potency has been established by a statistical evaluation.

Vaccinate subcutaneously not fewer than five guinea-pigs, 5 to 7 weeks old, according to the vaccination scheme stated on the label using one-fourth of the prescribed dose volume. Take blood samples after the period corresponding to maximum antibody production and carry out tests on the serum for specific antibodies by a haemagglutination-inhibition test or other suitable test. The antibody titres are not less than those obtained with a batch of vaccine shown to be satisfactory in the test in pigs (see Potency).

IDENTIFICATION

The vaccine stimulates the formation of specific antibodies against porcine parvovirus or the fraction of the virus used in the production of the vaccine when injected into susceptible animals on one or, if necessary, more than one occasion.

TESTS

Safety. Use two pigs 6 weeks to 6 months old and having no antibodies against porcine parvovirus virus or against a fraction of the virus. Inject into each animal by one of the routes stated on the label a double dose of vaccine. Observe the animals for 14 days and then inject a single dose of vaccine into each pig. Observe the animals for a further 14 days. No abnormal local or systemic reaction occurs during the 28 days of the test.

Inactivation. *This test may be omitted by the manufacturer if a test for inactivation has been carried out on the bulk vaccine, immediately before the addition of the adjuvant, where applicable.* Use a quantity of vaccine equivalent to ten doses. If the vaccine contains an oily adjuvant, break the emulsion and separate the phases. If the vaccine contains a mineral adjuvant, carry out an elution to liberate the virus. Concentrate the viral suspension 100 times by ultrafiltration or ultracentrifugation. None of the above procedures must be such as to inactivate or otherwise interfere with detection of live virus. Carry out a test for residual live virus in suitable non-confluent cells; after incubation for 7 days, make a subculture using trypsinised cells. After incubation for a further 7 days, examine the cultures for residual live parvovirus by an immunfluorescence test. No live virus is detected.

Extraneous viruses. On the pigs used for the safety test carry out tests for antibodies. The vaccine does not stimulate the formation of antibodies - other than those against porcine parvovirus - against viruses pathogenic for pigs or against viruses which could interfere with the diagnosis of infectious diseases in pigs (including the viruses of the pestivirus group).

Sterility. The vaccine complies with the test for sterility prescribed in the monograph on *Vaccines for veterinary use (0062)*.

POTENCY

Vaccinate according to the recommended schedule not less than seven gilts, 5 to 6 months old, which do not have antibodies against porcine parvovirus or against a fraction of the virus. The interval between vaccination and service is that stated on the label. Mate the gilts on two consecutive days immediately following signs of oestrus. Keep not less than five unvaccinated mated gilts of the same age as controls. At about the 40th day of gestation, challenge all gilts using a suitable strain of porcine parvovirus. Slaughter the gilts at about the 90th day of gestation and examine their foetuses for infection with porcine parvovirus as demonstrated by the presence of either virus or antibodies. The vaccine complies with the test if not fewer than 80 per cent of the total number of piglets from vaccinated gilts are protected from infection. The test is not valid unless: not fewer than seven vaccinated gilts and five control gilts are challenged; not fewer than 90 per cent of piglets from the control gilts are infected; and the average number of piglets per litter for the vaccinated gilts is not less than six.

01/2005:1361

PORCINE PROGRESSIVE ATROPHIC RHINITIS VACCINE (INACTIVATED)

Vaccinum rhinitidis atrophicantis ingravescentis suillae inactivatum

DEFINITION

Porcine progressive atrophic rhinitis vaccine (inactivated) is a preparation containing either the dermonecrotic exotoxin of *Pasteurella multocida*, treated to render it harmless while maintaining adequate immunogenic activity, or a genetically modified form of the exotoxin which has adequate immunogenic activity and which is free from toxic properties; the vaccine may also contain cells and/or antigenic components of one or more suitable strains of *P. multocida* and/or *Bordetella bronchiseptica*. This monograph applies to vaccines administered to sows and gilts for protection of their progeny.

PRODUCTION

The bacterial strains used for production are cultured separately in suitable media. The toxins and/or cells are treated to render them safe.

Detoxification. A test for detoxification of the dermonecrotic exotoxin of *P. multocida* is carried out immediately after detoxification. The concentration of detoxified exotoxin used in the test is not less than that in the vaccine. The suspension complies with the test if no toxic dermonecrotic exotoxin is detected. The test for detoxification is not required where the vaccine is prepared using a toxin-like protein free from toxic properties, produced by expression of a modified form of the corresponding gene.

Antigen content. The content of the dermonecrotic exotoxin of *P. multocida* in the detoxified suspension or the toxin-like protein in the harvest is determined by a suitable immunochemical method (*2.7.1*), such as an enzyme-linked immunosorbent assay and the value found is used in the formulation of the vaccine. The content of other antigens stated on the label is also determined (*2.7.1*).

The vaccine may contain a suitable adjuvant.

CHOICE OF VACCINE COMPOSITION

The strains used for the preparation of the vaccine are shown to be satisfactory with respect to the production of the dermonecrotic exotoxin and the other antigens claimed to be protective. The vaccine is shown to be satisfactory with respect to safety (*5.2.6*) and efficacy (*5.2.7*).

Production of antigens. The production of antigens claimed to be protective is verified by a suitable bioassay or immunochemical method (*2.7.1*), carried out on the antigens obtained from each of the vaccine strains under the conditions used for the production of the vaccine.

The following tests may be used during demonstration of safety and immunogenicity.

Safety

A. Carry out the test for each route of administration stated on the label. Use pigs that do not have antibodies against the components of the vaccine, that are from a herd or herds where there are no signs of atrophic rhinitis and that have not been vaccinated against atrophic rhinitis. If the vaccine is intended for use in pregnant animals, carry out the test in pregnant sows or gilts, vaccinating them at the recommended stage of pregnancy. Administer a double dose of vaccine by a recommended route to each of not fewer than 10 sows or gilts. Administer a single dose of vaccine to each of the animals after the recommended interval. Observe the pigs until farrowing. Record body temperature the day before vaccination, at vaccination, 2 h, 4 h and 6 h later and then daily for 4 days; note the maximum temperature increase for each animal. Note any effects on gestation and the offspring. No abnormal local or systemic reaction occurs; the average temperature increase for all animals does not exceed 1.5 °C and no animal shows a rise greater than 2 °C.

B. The animals used for field trials are also used to evaluate safety. Use not fewer than 3 groups each of not fewer than 20 animals with corresponding groups of not fewer than 10 controls. Examine the injection site for local reactions after vaccination. Record body temperature the day before vaccination, at vaccination, at the time interval after which a rise in temperature, if any, was seen in test A, and daily during the 2 days following vaccination; note the maximum temperature increase for each animal. No abnormal local or systemic reaction occurs; the average temperature increase for all animals does not exceed 1.5 °C and no animal shows a rise greater than 2 °C.

Immunogenicity. The test described under Potency is suitable for demonstration of immunogenicity.

BATCH TESTING

Batch potency test. The test described under Potency is not carried out for routine testing of batches of vaccine. It is carried out, for a given vaccine, on one or more occasions, as decided by or with the agreement of the competent authority; where the test is not carried out, a suitable validated test is carried out, the criteria for acceptance being set with reference to a batch of vaccine that has given satisfactory results in the test described under Potency. The following test may be used after a satisfactory correlation with the test described under Potency has been established.

Use not fewer than 5 pigs not less than 3 weeks old and that do not have antibodies against the components of the vaccine. Vaccinate each pig by a recommended route and according to the recommended schedule. Maintain not fewer

Vaccines

than 2 pigs of the same origin as unvaccinated controls under the same conditions.

Alternatively, if the nature of the antigens allows reproducible results to be obtained, a test in susceptible laboratory animals may be carried out. To obtain a valid assay, it may be necessary to carry out a test using several groups of animals, each receiving a different quantity of vaccine. For each quantity of vaccine, carry out the test as follows: vaccinate not fewer than 5 animals with a suitable quantity of vaccine. Maintain not fewer than 2 animals of the same species and origin as unvaccinated controls. Where the schedule stated on the label requires a booster injection to be given, a booster vaccination may also be given in this test provided it has been demonstrated that this will still provide a suitably sensitive test system. At a given interval within the range of 14 to 21 days after the last administration, collect blood from each animal and prepare serum samples. Use a validated test such as an enzyme-linked immunosorbent assay to measure the antibody response to each of the antigens stated on the label. The test is not valid and must be repeated if there is a significant antibody titre in the controls. The vaccine complies with the test if the antibody responses of the vaccinated animals are not significantly less than those obtained with a batch of vaccine that has given satisfactory results in the test or tests (as applicable) described under Potency.

Where animals seronegative for the antigens stated on the label are not available, seropositive animals may be used in the above test. During the development of a test with seropositive animals, particular care will be required during the validation of the test system to establish that the test is suitably sensitive and to specify acceptable pass, fail and retest criteria. It will be necessary to take into account the range of prevaccination antibody titres and to establish the acceptable minimum antibody titre rise after vaccination in relation to these.

Bacterial endotoxins. A test for bacterial endotoxins (*2.6.14*) is carried out on the batch or, where the nature of the adjuvant prevents performance of a satisfactory test, on the bulk antigen or the mixture of bulk antigens immediately before addition of the adjuvant. The maximum acceptable amount of bacterial endotoxins is that found for a batch of vaccine shown satisfactory in safety test A given under Choice of vaccine composition or in the safety test described under Tests, carried out using 10 pigs. Where the latter test is used, note the maximum temperature increase for each animal; the average temperature increase for all animals does not exceed 1.5 °C. The method chosen for determining the amount of bacterial endotoxin present in the vaccine batch used in the safety test for determining the maximum acceptable level of endotoxin is used subsequently for testing of each batch.

IDENTIFICATION

In animals free from specific antibodies against the antigens stated on the label, the vaccine stimulates the production of antibodies against these antigens.

TESTS

Safety. Use not fewer than 2 pigs that do not have antibodies against *P. multocida* and that preferably do not have antibodies against *B. bronchiseptica*. Administer to each pig a double dose of vaccine by a recommended route. Observe the pigs for 14 days. Record body temperature the day before vaccination, at vaccination, 2 h, 4 h and 6 h later and then daily for 2 days. No abnormal local or systemic reaction occurs; a transient temperature increase not exceeding 2 °C may occur.

Sterility (*2.6.1*). The vaccine complies with the test for sterility prescribed in the monograph on *Vaccines for veterinary use (0062)*.

POTENCY

Use pigs that do not have antibodies against the components of the vaccine, that are from a herd or herds where there are no signs of atrophic rhinitis and that have not been vaccinated against atrophic rhinitis.

A. Vaccines containing dermonecrotic exotoxin of *P. multocida* (with or without cells of *P. multocida*).

Use not fewer than 12 breeder pigs. Vaccinate not fewer than 6 randomly chosen pigs at the stage of pregnancy or non-pregnancy and by the route and schedule stated on the label. Maintain not fewer than 6 of the remaining pigs as unvaccinated controls under the same conditions. From birth allow all the piglets from the vaccinated and unvaccinated breeder pigs to feed from their own dam.

Constitute from the progeny 2 challenge groups each of not fewer than 30 piglets chosen randomly, taking not fewer than 3 piglets from each litter. On the 2 consecutive days preceding challenge, the mucosa of the nasal cavity of the piglets may be treated by instillation of 0.5 ml of a solution of acetic acid (10 g/l $C_2H_4O_2$) in isotonic buffered saline pH 7.2.

Challenge each piglet at 10 days of age by the intranasal route with a sufficient quantity of a toxigenic strain of *P. multocida*.

At the age of 42 days, kill the piglets of the 2 groups and dissect the nose of each of them transversally at premolar-1. Examine the ventral and dorsal turbinates and the nasal septum for evidence of atrophy or distortion and grade the observations on the following scales:

Turbinates

0	no atrophy
1	slight atrophy
2	moderate atrophy
3	severe atrophy
4	very severe atrophy with almost complete disappearance of the turbinate

The maximum score is 4 for each turbinate and 16 for the sum of the 2 dorsal and 2 ventral turbinates.

Nasal septum

0	no deviation
1	very slight deviation
2	deviation of the septum

The maximum total score for the turbinates and the nasal septum is 18.

The test is not valid and must be repeated if fewer than 80 per cent of the progeny of each litter of the unvaccinated breeder pigs have a total score of at least 10. The vaccine complies with the test if a significant reduction in the total score has been demonstrated in the group from the vaccinated breeder pigs compared to that from the unvaccinated breeder pigs.

B. Vaccines containing *P. multocida* dermonecrotic exotoxin (with or without cells of *P. multocida*) and cells and/or antigenic components of *B. bronchiseptica*.

Use not fewer than 24 breeder pigs. Vaccinate not fewer than 12 randomly chosen pigs at the stage of pregnancy or non-pregnancy and by the route and schedule stated on the label. Maintain not fewer than 12 of the remaining

Vaccines

pigs as unvaccinated controls under the same conditions. From birth allow all the piglets from the vaccinated and unvaccinated breeder pigs to feed from their own dam.

Using groups of not fewer than 6 pigs, constitute from their progeny 2 challenge groups from vaccinated pigs and 2 groups from unvaccinated pigs each group consisting of not fewer than 30 piglets chosen randomly, taking not fewer than 3 piglets from each litter. On the 2 consecutive days preceding challenge, the mucosa of the nasal cavity of the piglets may be treated by instillation of 0.5 ml of a solution of acetic acid (10 g/l $C_2H_4O_2$) in isotonic buffered saline pH 7.2.

For a group of piglets from not fewer than 6 vaccinated pigs and a group from not fewer than 6 controls, challenge each piglet by the intranasal route at 10 days of age with a sufficient quantity of a toxigenic strain of *P. multocida*.

For the other group of piglets from not fewer than 6 vaccinated pigs and the other group from not fewer than 6 controls, challenge each piglet at 7 days of age by the intranasal route with a sufficient quantity of *B. bronchiseptica*. In addition, challenge each piglet at 10 days of age by the intranasal route with a sufficient quantity of a toxigenic strain of *P. multocida*.

At the age of 42 days, kill the piglets of the 4 groups and dissect the nose of each of them transversally at premolar-1. Examine the ventral and dorsal turbinates and the nasal septum for evidence of atrophy or distortion and grade the observations on the scale described above.

The test is not valid and must be repeated if fewer than 80 per cent of the progeny of each litter of the unvaccinated breeder pigs have a total score of at least 10. The vaccine complies with the test if a significant reduction in the total score has been demonstrated in the groups from the vaccinated breeder pigs compared to the corresponding group from the unvaccinated breeder pigs.

LABELLING

The label states the protective antigens present in the vaccine.

Vaccines

01/2005:0451

RABIES VACCINE (INACTIVATED) FOR VETERINARY USE

Vaccinum rabiei inactivatum ad usum veterinarium

DEFINITION

Rabies vaccine (inactivated) for veterinary use is a liquid or freeze-dried preparation of fixed rabies virus inactivated by a suitable method.

PRODUCTION

The vaccine is prepared from virus grown either in suitable cell lines or in primary cell cultures from healthy animals (*5.2.4*). The virus suspension is harvested on one or more occasions within 28 days of inoculation. Multiple harvests from a single production cell culture may be pooled and considered as a single harvest. The rabies virus is inactivated by a suitable method.

Inactivation. The test for residual live rabies virus is carried out by inoculation of the inactivated virus into the same type of cell culture as that used in the production of the vaccine or a cell culture shown to be at least as sensitive; the quantity of inactivated virus used in the test is equivalent to not less than 25 doses of the vaccine. After incubation for 4 days, a subculture is made using trypsinised cells; after incubation for a further 4 days, the cultures are examined for residual live rabies virus by an immunofluorescence test. No live virus is detected.

Antigen content. The content of rabies virus glycoprotein is determined by a suitable immunochemical method (*2.7.1*). The content is within the limits approved for the particular preparation.

The vaccine may contain one or more adjuvants.

CHOICE OF VACCINE COMPOSITION

The vaccine is shown to be satisfactory with respect to immunogenicity for each species for which it is recommended. The suitability of the vaccine with respect to immunogenicity for carnivores (cats and dogs) is demonstrated by direct challenge. For other species, if a challenge test has been carried out for the vaccine in cats or dogs, an indirect test is carried out by determining the antibody level following vaccination of not fewer than twenty animals according to the recommended schedule; the vaccine is satisfactory if, after the period claimed for protection, the mean rabies virus antibody level in the serum of the animals is not less than 0.5 IU/ml and if not more than 10 per cent of the animals have an antibody level less than 0.1 IU/ml. The test described below may be used to demonstrate immunogenicity in cats and dogs.

Immunogenicity. Use not fewer than 35 susceptible animals of the minimum age recommended for vaccination. Take a blood sample from each animal and test individually for antibodies against rabies virus to determine susceptibility. Administer by the recommended route to each of not fewer than 25 animals one dose of vaccine. Keep not fewer than 10 animals as controls. Observe all the animals for a period equal to the claimed duration of immunity. No animal shows signs of rabies. On the last day of the claimed period for duration of immunity or later, challenge all animals by intramuscular injection of virulent rabies virus of a strain approved by the competent authority. Observe the animals for 90 days. Animals that die from causes not attributable to rabies are eliminated. The test is not valid if the number of such deaths reduces the number of vaccinated animals in the test to fewer than 25. The test is not valid unless at least eight control animals (or a statistically equivalent number if more than 10 control animals are challenged) show signs of rabies and the presence of rabies virus in their brain is demonstrated by the fluorescent-antibody test or some other suitable method. The vaccine complies with the test if not more than 2 of the 25 vaccinated animals (or a statistically equivalent number if more than 25 vaccinated animals are challenged) show signs of rabies.

BATCH TESTING

The test described under Potency is not necessarily carried out for routine testing of batches of vaccine. It is carried out, for a given vaccine, on one or more occasions, as decided by or with the agreement of the competent authority; where the test is not carried out, a suitable validated alternative method is used, the criteria for acceptance being set with reference to a batch of vaccine that has given satisfactory results in the test described above for immunogenicity or in the test described under Potency. The following test may be used after a suitable correlation with the test described above for immunogenicity or the test described under Potency has been established.

Batch potency test. Use 5 mice each weighing 18 g to 20 g. Vaccinate each mouse subcutaneously or intramuscularly using one-fifth of the recommended dose volume. Take blood samples 14 days after the injection and test the sera individually for rabies antibody using the rapid fluorescent focus inhibition test described for *Human rabies immunoglobulin (0723)*. The amount of antibody is not less than that produced by a vaccine that has been found satisfactory with respect to immunogenicity as described above or in the test described under Potency.

Antigen content. The quantity of rabies virus glycoprotein per dose, determined by a suitable immunochemical method (*2.7.1*), is not significantly lower than that of a batch that has been found satisfactory with respect to immunogenicity as described above or in the test described under Potency.

IDENTIFICATION

When injected into animals, the vaccine stimulates the production of specific neutralising antibodies.

TESTS

Safety. If the vaccine is intended for more than one species including one belonging to the order of Carnivora, carry out the test in dogs. Otherwise use one of the species for which the vaccine is intended. Administer, by a recommended route, a double dose of vaccine to each of 2 animals having no antibodies against rabies virus. Observe the animals for 14 days. No abnormal local or systemic reaction occurs.

Inactivation. Carry out the test using a pool of the contents of 5 containers.

For vaccines which do not contain an adjuvant, carry out a suitable amplification test for residual infectious rabies virus using the same type of cell culture as that used in the production of the vaccine or a cell culture shown to be at least as sensitive. No live virus is detected.

For vaccines that contain an adjuvant, inject intracerebrally into each of not fewer than 10 mice each weighing 11 g to 15 g 0.03 ml of a pool of at least 5 times the smallest stated dose. To avoid interference from any antimicrobial preservative or the adjuvant, the vaccine may be diluted not more than 10 times before injection. In this case or if the vaccine strain is pathogenic only for unweaned mice, carry out the test on mice 1 to 4 days old. Observe the animals for 21 days. If more than 2 animals die during the first 48 h, repeat the test. From the third to the twenty-first days following the injection, the animals show no signs of rabies and immunofluorescence tests carried out on the brains of the animals show no indication of the presence of rabies virus.

Sterility. The vaccine complies with the test for sterility prescribed in the monograph on *Vaccines for veterinary use (0062)*.

POTENCY

The potency of rabies vaccine is determined by comparing the dose necessary to protect mice against the clinical effects of the dose of rabies virus defined below, administered intracerebrally, with the quantity of a reference preparation, calibrated in International Units, necessary to provide the same protection.

The International Unit is the activity of a stated quantity of the International Standard. The equivalence in International Units of the International Standard is stated by the World Health Organisation.

Rabies vaccine (inactivated) for veterinary use BRP is calibrated in International Units against the International Standard.

The test described below uses a parallel-line model with at least 3 points for the vaccine to be examined and the reference preparation. Once the analyst has experience with the method for a given vaccine, it is possible to carry out a simplified test using one dilution of the vaccine to be examined. Such a test enables the analyst to determine that the vaccine has a potency significantly higher than the required minimum but will not give full information on the validity of each individual potency determination. It allows a considerable reduction in the number of animals required for the test and should be considered by each laboratory in accordance with the provisions of the European Convention for the Protection of Vertebrate Animals used for Experimental and other Scientific Purposes.

Selection and distribution of the test animals. Use in the test healthy female mice about 4 weeks old and from the same stock. Distribute the mice into at least 10 groups of not fewer than 10 mice.

Preparation of the challenge suspension. Inoculate a group of mice intracerebrally with the CVS strain of rabies virus and when the mice show signs of rabies, but before they die, kill the mice and remove the brains and prepare a homogenate of the brain tissue in a suitable diluent. Separate gross particulate matter by centrifugation and use the supernatant liquid as challenge suspension. Distribute the suspension in small volumes in ampoules, seal and store at a temperature below − 60 °C. Thaw one ampoule of the suspension and make serial dilutions in a suitable diluent. Allocate each dilution to a group of mice and inject intracerebrally into each mouse 0.03 ml of the dilution allocated to its group. Observe the animals for 14 days and record the number in each group that, between the fifth and the fourteenth days, develop signs of rabies. Calculate the ID_{50} of the undiluted suspension.

Determination of potency of the vaccine to be examined. Prepare at least three serial dilutions of the vaccine to be examined and three similar dilutions of the reference preparation. Prepare the dilutions such that those containing the largest quantity of vaccine may be expected to protect more than 50 per cent of the animals into which they are injected and those containing the smallest quantities of vaccine may be expected to protect less than 50 per cent of the animals into which they are injected. Allocate each dilution to a different group of mice and inject intraperitoneally into each mouse 0.5 ml of the dilution allocated to its group. 14 days after the injection prepare a suspension of the challenge virus such that, on the basis of the preliminary titration, it contains about 50 ID_{50} in each 0.03 ml. Inject intracerebrally into each vaccinated mouse 0.03 ml of this suspension. Prepare 3 suitable serial dilutions of the challenge suspension. Allocate the challenge suspension and the 3 dilutions one to each of 4 groups of 10 unvaccinated mice and inject intracerebrally into each mouse 0.03 ml of the suspension or one of the dilutions allocated to its group. Observe the animals in each group for 14 days. The test is not valid if more than 2 mice of any group die within the first 4 days after challenge. Record the numbers in each group that show signs of rabies in the period 5 days to 14 days after challenge.

The test is not valid unless:

- for both the vaccine to be examined and the reference preparation the 50 per cent protective dose lies between the smallest and the largest dose given to the mice,
- the titration of the challenge suspension shows that 0.03 ml of the suspension contained at least 10 ID_{50},
- the confidence limits (P = 0.95) are not less than 25 per cent and not more than 400 per cent of the estimated potency,
- the statistical analysis shows a significant slope and no significant deviations from linearity or parallelism of the dose-response lines.

Vaccines

The vaccine complies with the test if the estimated potency is not less than 1 IU in the smallest prescribed dose.

LABELLING

The label states:

– the type of cell culture used to prepare the vaccine and the species of origin,
– the minimum number of International Units per dose,
– the minimum period for which the vaccine provides protection.

01/2005:0746

RABIES VACCINE (LIVE, ORAL) FOR FOXES

Vaccinum rabiei perorale vivum ad vulpem

DEFINITION

Rabies vaccine (live, oral) for foxes is a preparation of an immunogenic strain of an attenuated rabies virus. The vaccine is incorporated in a bait in such a manner as to enable the tests prescribed below to be performed aseptically.

PRODUCTION

The attenuated virus strain is grown in suitable cell cultures (*5.2.4*); if the cell cultures are of mammalian origin, they are shown to be free from rabies virus. The virus suspension is harvested on one or more occasions within 14 days of inoculation. Multiple harvests from a single cell lot may be pooled and considered as a single harvest. The viral suspension may be mixed with a suitable stabiliser. The vaccine may be freeze-dried or liquid. A freeze-dried vaccine has to be reconstituted before use.

CHOICE OF VACCINE STRAIN

Only a virus strain shown to be satisfactory with respect to immunogenicity (see Potency) and the following characteristics may be used in the preparation of the vaccine:

– when administered orally at the dose and by the method recommended for use to forty foxes, it causes no sign of rabies within 180 days of administration,
– when administered orally at ten times the recommended dose to each of ten foxes, it causes no sign of rabies within 180 days of administration,
– when administered orally at ten times the recommended dose to each of ten dogs, it causes no sign of rabies within 180 days of administration,
– when administered orally at ten times the recommended dose to each of ten cats, it causes no sign of rabies within 180 days of administration,
– in natural and experimental conditions, the virus strain does not spread from one animal to another in wild rodents,
– the virus strain has one or more stable genetic markers that may be used to discriminate the vaccine strain from other rabies virus strains.

BATCH TESTING

If the test for potency has been carried out with satisfactory results on a representative batch of vaccine, this test may be omitted as a routine control on other batches of vaccine prepared from the same seed lot.

IDENTIFICATION

A. When mixed with a monospecific rabies antiserum, the vaccine is no longer able to infect susceptible cell cultures into which it is inoculated.

B. A test is carried out to demonstrate the presence of the genetic marker.

TESTS

Extraneous viruses

(a) Mix the vaccine with a specific neutralising rabies virus antiserum. It no longer provokes cytopathic effects in susceptible cell cultures. It shows no evidence of haemagglutinating or haemadsorbing agents.

(b) Inoculate 1 in 10 and 1 in 1000 dilutions of the vaccine into susceptible cell cultures. Incubate at 37 °C. After 2, 4 and 6 days, stain the cells with a panel of monoclonal antibodies that do not react with the vaccine strain but that react with other strains of rabies virus (for example, street virus, Pasteur strain). The vaccine shows no evidence of contaminating rabies virus.

Bacterial and fungal contamination. The vaccine complies with the test for sterility prescribed in the monograph on *Vaccines for veterinary use (0062)*.

Mycoplasmas (*2.6.7*). The vaccine complies with the test for mycoplasmas.

Virus titre. Titrate the vaccine in suitable cell cultures. One dose of the vaccine contains not less than the quantity of virus equivalent to the minimum titre stated on the label.

POTENCY

Use not fewer than thirty-five foxes, at least three months old, free from rabies-neutralising antibodies. Administer orally and with the bait stated on the label to each of not fewer than twenty-five animals a volume of the vaccine containing a quantity of virus equivalent to the minimum titre stated on the label. Keep not fewer than ten animals as controls. Observe all the animals for 180 days. No animal shows signs of rabies. The test is not valid if fewer than twenty-five vaccinated animals survive after this observation period. On the 180th day after vaccination, challenge all foxes by the intramuscular injection of virulent rabies virus of a strain approved by the competent authority. Observe the animals for 90 days. Animals that die from causes not attributable to rabies are eliminated. The test is not valid if the number of such deaths reduces the number of vaccinated animals in the test to fewer than twenty-five. The vaccine complies with the test if not more than two of twenty-five vaccinated animals (or a statistically equivalent number if more than twenty-five vaccinated animals are challenged) show signs of rabies. The test is not valid unless at least nine control animals (or a statistically equivalent number if more than ten control animals are challenged) show signs of rabies and the presence of rabies virus in their brain is demonstrated by the fluorescent-antibody test or some other reliable method.

LABELLING

The label states the nature of the genetic marker of the virus strain.

01/2005:0064
corrected

SWINE ERYSIPELAS VACCINE (INACTIVATED)

Vaccinum erysipelatis suillae inactivatum

DEFINITION

Swine erysipelas vaccine (inactivated) is a preparation of one or more suitable strains of *Erysipelothrix rhusiopathiae (E. insidiosa)* inactivated by a suitable method. This monograph applies to vaccines intended to protect pigs against swine erysipelas.

PRODUCTION

The vaccine may contain an adjuvant.

CHOICE OF VACCINE COMPOSITION

The vaccine is shown to be satisfactory with respect to safety (*5.2.6*) and efficacy (*5.2.7*).

Immunogenicity. The test described under Potency is suitable to demonstrate immunogenicity of the vaccine with respect to *E. rhusiopathiae* serotypes 1 and 2. If claims are made concerning another serotype, then a further test to demonstrate immunogenicity against this serotype is necessary.

BATCH TESTING

Batch potency test. The test described under Potency is not carried out for routine testing of batches of vaccine. It is carried out, for a given vaccine, on one or more occasions, as decided by or with the agreement of the competent authority. Where the test is not carried out, a suitable validated alternative test is carried out, the criteria for acceptance being set with reference to a batch of vaccine that has given satisfactory results in the test described under Potency. The following test may be used after a satisfactory correlation with the test described under Potency has been established.

Use mice of a suitable strain (for example, NMRI) weighing 17-20 g, from a uniform stock and that do not have antibodies against swine erysipelas. Administer the vaccine to be examined to a group of 10 mice. Inject a suitable dose (usually 1/10 of the pig dose) subcutaneously into each mouse. At a given interval (for example, 21-28 days), depending on the vaccine to be examined, bleed the animals under anaesthesia. Pool the sera, using an equal volume from each mouse. Determine the level of antibodies by a suitable immunochemical method (*2.7.1*), for example, enzyme-linked immunosorbent assay with *erysipelas ELISA coating antigen BRP*. The antibody level is not significantly less than that obtained with a batch that has given satisfactory results in the test described under Potency.

IDENTIFICATION

Injected into animals that do not have antibodies against *E. rhusiopathiae*, it stimulates the production of such antibodies.

TESTS

Safety. Use pigs of the minimum age recommended for vaccination and preferably having no antibodies against swine erysipelas or, where justified, use pigs with a low level of such antibodies as long as they have not been vaccinated against Swine erysipelas and administration of the vaccine does not cause an anamnestic response. Administer a double dose of vaccine by a recommended route to each of 2 pigs. Observe the animals for 14 days. No abnormal local or systemic reaction occurs.

Sterility. It complies with the test for sterility prescribed in the monograph on *Vaccines for veterinary use (0062)*.

POTENCY

If the vaccine contains more than 1 serotype, a test for 2 serotypes may be carried out on a single group by injecting each challenge serotype on different flanks of the animals. Validation and acceptance criteria are applied separately to the respective injection sites. If the vaccine contains more than 1 serotype, the potency test may also be carried out using a separate group for each serotype.

Use not fewer than 15 pigs not less than 12 weeks old, weighing not less than 20 kg and that do not have antibodies against swine erysipelas. Divide the animals into 2 groups. Vaccinate a group of not fewer than 10 pigs according to the recommended schedule. Maintain a group of not fewer than 5 pigs as unvaccinated controls. 3 weeks after vaccination, challenge the vaccinated animals and the control group by separate intradermal injections of 0.1 ml of a virulent strain of each of serotype 1 and serotype 2 of *E. rhusiopathiae*. Observe the animals for 7 days. The vaccine complies with the test if not fewer than 90 per cent of the vaccinated animals remain free from diamond skin lesions at the injection site. The test is invalid if fewer than 80 per cent of control animals show typical signs of disease, i.e. diamond skin lesions at the injection sites.

Swine erysipelas bacteria serotype 1 BRP and *swine erysipelas bacteria serotype 2 BRP* are suitable for use as challenge strains.

LABELLING

The label states the serotypes of *E. rhusiopathiae* included in the vaccine.

01/2005:0065

SWINE-FEVER VACCINE (LIVE), CLASSICAL, FREEZE-DRIED

Vaccinum pestis classicae suillae vivum cryodesiccatum

DEFINITION

Freeze-dried classical swine-fever vaccine (live) is a preparation obtained from a strain of classical swine-fever virus which has lost its pathogenicity for the pig by adaptation either to cell cultures or to the rabbit.

PRODUCTION

For vaccine prepared in rabbits, the seed-lot (or the vaccine) is made from the homog-enised organs and/or blood of rabbits from healthy colonies, sacrificed at the peak of the temperature rise following intravenous inoculation of the virus. The vaccine is freeze-dried.

CHOICE OF VACCINE STRAIN

Only a virus strain shown to be satisfactory with respect to the following characteristics may be used in the preparation of the vaccine: safety; non-transmissibility; irreversibility of attenuation; and immunogenic properties. The following tests may be used during demonstration of safety (*5.2.6*) and efficacy (*5.2.7*).

The dose of vaccine used throughout the following tests is determined by the manufacturer on the basis of prior experiments.

Tests in pigs

Selection of animals. The piglets are 6 to 7 weeks old. The sows are primiparae. All animals are healthy and must have had no contact with swine-fever virus and serologically must be free from swine-fever and bovine viral diarrhoea antibodies. They must have a week in which to adapt themselves to the new quarters where the tests are to be carried out.

Safety

(a) Each of five piglets receives intramuscularly as a single injection ten doses of vaccine (group a).

(b) Five piglets are immunodepressed by the daily injection of 2 mg of prednisolone per kilogram of body mass for five consecutive days and on the third day they receive one dose of vaccine (group b).

The animals of groups (a) and (b) are observed for 21 days. They must remain in good health. The temperature curve and the weight curve must not differ significantly from those of control animals.

(c) Ten non-immune pregnant sows each receive two doses of vaccine intramuscularly as a single injection between the twenty-fifth and thirty-fifth days of gestation. Ten non-immune pregnant sows of the same age and of the same origin receive instead of the two doses of vaccine an equal volume of a 9 g/l solution of *sodium chloride R*. The vaccinal virus does not cause abnormalities in the gestation or in the piglets.

Non-transmissibility. Twelve piglets of the same origin are kept together. Six are vaccinated in the normal way and the six others are kept as contact controls. After 40 days, all the pigs are challenged by intramuscular inoculation of a sufficient quantity of the challenge virus (see Potency) to kill an unvaccinated piglet in 7 days. The vaccinated piglets resist challenge whereas the contact piglets must display the typical signs of swine fever.

Irreversibility of attenuation. Each of two piglets receives one dose of vaccine intramuscularly. Seven days later, 5 ml of blood is taken from each of the piglets and the samples are pooled. 5 ml of the pooled blood is injected intramuscularly into each of two other piglets. This operation is repeated six times. The animals must not display any sign of swine fever and must show normal growth.

Immunogenic properties. The immunogenic properties may be demonstrated by the method described for the determination of potency. The quantity of the vaccinal virus corresponding to one dose of vaccine contains at least 100 PD_{50}.

IDENTIFICATION

A. For vaccines prepared in rabbits and lapinised vaccines prepared in cell cultures, inject intravenously 0.5 ml of the vaccine reconstituted as stated on the label into one or more non-immunised rabbits and one or more rabbits immunised either with an identical dose of a vaccine of the same type injected by the same route at least 10 days and at most 2 months beforehand or with a sufficient dose of antiserum administered a few hours before the injection of the vaccine. Measure the temperature of the rabbits in the morning and the evening starting 24 h after the injection and continuing until the fifth day after the injection. The vaccine is identified by its specific pyrogenic character leading to a rise in temperature of at least 1.5 °C in the non-immunised rabbits only.

B. For non-lapinised vaccines prepared in cell cultures, the serum of pigs immunised with the vaccine neutralises the virus used in the preparation of the vaccine.

TESTS

Safety. Use three piglets complying with the requirements prescribed for the selection of animals under Choice of Vaccine Strain. Inject intramuscularly into each piglet ten doses of the reconstituted vaccine as a single injection. Observe the animals for 21 days. The temperature curve remains normal and the animals remain in apparent good health and display normal growth.

Extraneous viruses. Mix the vaccine with a monospecific antiserum and inoculate into susceptible cell cultures. No cytopathic effect is produced.

Carry out a haemagglutination test using chicken red blood cells and the supernatant liquid of the cell cultures. The test is negative. Carry out a haemadsorption test on the cell cultures. The test is negative.

Use ten mice each weighing 11 g to 15 g. Inject intracerebrally into each mouse 0.03 ml of the vaccine reconstituted so that 1 ml contains 1 dose. Observe the animals for 21 days. If more than two mice die within the first 48 h, repeat the test. From the third to the twenty-first day after the injection, the mice show no abnormalities attributable to the vaccine.

Bacterial and fungal contamination. The vaccine to be examined complies with the test for sterility prescribed in the monograph on *Vaccines for veterinary use (0062)*.

Mycoplasmas (*2.6.7*). The vaccine complies with the test for mycoplasmas.

POTENCY

The potency is expressed as the number of 50 per cent protective doses (PD_{50}) for pigs contained in the dose indicated on the label. The vaccine contains at least 100 PD_{50} per dose.

Use piglets complying with the requirements for selection of animals described under Choice of Vaccine Strain. To two groups of five piglets inject intramuscularly:

- 1/40 of a dose of the vaccine to be examined into each piglet of the first group,
- 1/160 of a dose of the vaccine to be examined into each piglet of the second group.

Use two piglets as controls.

Prepare the dilutions using *buffered salt solution pH 7.2 R*. On the fourteenth day after the injection, inoculate intramuscularly into each vaccinated and control animal a sufficient quantity of challenge virus to kill an unvaccinated piglet in 7 days. The challenge virus preparation consists of blood of pigs infected experimentally by virus that has not been submitted to passage in cell cultures. The control animals die within the seven days of inoculation. Observe the vaccinated animals for 14 days. From the number of animals which survive without showing any sign of swine fever, calculate the number of PD_{50} contained in the vaccine using the usual statistical methods.

LABELLING

The label states that the vaccine has been prepared in cell cultures or in rabbits as appropriate.

01/2005:0697
corrected

TETANUS VACCINE FOR VETERINARY USE

Vaccinum tetani ad usum veterinarium

DEFINITION

Tetanus vaccine for veterinary use is a preparation of the neurotoxin of *Clostridium tetani* treated in a manner that eliminates toxicity while maintaining adequate immunogenic properties.

PRODUCTION

The *C. tetani* strain used for production is cultured in a suitable medium. The toxin is purified and then detoxified or it may be detoxified before purification. The antigenic purity is determined in Lf units of tetanus toxoid per milligram of protein and shown to be not less than the value approved for the particular product.

CHOICE OF VACCINE COMPOSITION

The *C. tetani* strain used in the preparation of the vaccine is shown to be satisfactory with respect to the production of the neurotoxin. The vaccine is shown to be satisfactory with respect to safety and immunogenicity for each species of animal for which it is intended. As part of the studies to demonstrate these characteristics, the tests described below may be used.

Production of antigens. The production of the neurotoxin of *C. tetani* is verified by a suitable immunochemical method (*2.7.1*) carried out on the neurotoxin obtained from the vaccine strain under the conditions used for the production of the vaccine.

Safety. Carry out the test for each recommended route of administration and species of animal for which the vaccine is intended; use animals of the minimum age recommended for vaccination and of the most sensitive category for the species.

Use not fewer than 15 animals, free from antitoxic antibodies for each test. Administer a double dose of vaccine to each animal. Administer a single dose of vaccine to each animal after the interval stated on the label. Observe the animals until 14 days after the last administration. If the vaccine is intended for use in pregnant animals, vaccinate the animals at the stage of pregnancy and according to the scheme stated on the label and prolong the observation period until 1 day after parturition. The vaccine complies with the test if no animal shows abnormal local or systemic signs of disease or dies from causes attributable to the vaccine. If the vaccine is intended for use in pregnant animals, in addition no significant effects on the gestation and the offspring are demonstrated.

Immunogenicity. The test described under Potency may be used to demonstrate immunogenicity. It shall also be demonstrated for each target species that the vaccine, administered by the recommended route, stimulates an immune response consistent with the claims for the product (for example, induction of antitoxic antibodies or induction of protective levels of antitoxic antibodies).

DETOXIFIED HARVEST

Absence of toxin and irreversibility of toxoid: carry out a test for reversion to toxicity on the detoxified harvest using 2 groups of 5 guinea-pigs, each weighing 350 g to 450 g; if the vaccine is adsorbed, carry out the test with the shortest practical time interval before adsorption. Prepare a dilution of the detoxified harvest so that the guinea-pigs each receive 10 times the amount of toxoid (measured in Lf units) that will be present in a dose of vaccine. Divide the dilution into 2 equal parts. Keep one part at 5 ± 3 °C and the other at 37 °C for 6 weeks. Attribute each dilution to a separate group of guinea-pigs and inject into each guinea-pig the dilution attributed to its group. Observe the animals for 21 days. The toxoid complies with the test if no guinea-pig shows clinical signs of disease or dies from causes attributable to the neurotoxin of *C. tetani*.

BATCH POTENCY TEST

Where the test described under Potency is used as the batch potency test, the vaccine complies with the test if the antibody titre in International Units is not less than that found for a batch of vaccine shown to be satisfactory with respect to immunogenicity in the target species.

IDENTIFICATION

If the nature of the adjuvant allows it, carry out test A. Otherwise carry out test B.

A. Dissolve in the vaccine sufficient *sodium citrate R* to give a 100 g/l solution. Maintain the solution at 37 °C for about 16 h and centrifuge until a clear supernatant liquid is obtained. The supernatant reacts with a suitable tetanus antitoxin, giving a precipitate.

B. When injected into susceptible animals, the vaccine provokes the formation of antibodies against the neurotoxin of *C. tetani*.

TESTS

Safety. Inject 5 ml of the vaccine subcutaneously as 2 equal divided doses, at separate sites into each of 5 healthy guinea-pigs, each weighing 350 g to 450 g, that have not previously been treated with any material that will interfere with the test. No abnormal local or systemic reaction occurs. If within 21 days of the injection any of the animals shows signs of or dies from tetanus, the vaccine does not comply with the test. If more than 1 animal dies from non-specific causes, repeat the test. If any animal dies in the second test, the vaccine does not comply with the test.

Sterility. The vaccine complies with the test for sterility prescribed in the monograph on *Vaccines for veterinary use (0062)*.

POTENCY

Administer 1 dose of vaccine subcutaneously to each of at least 5 susceptible guinea-pigs. After 28 days, administer again 1 dose subcutaneously to each guinea-pig. 14 days after the second dose, collect blood from each guinea-pig and prepare serum samples. Determine for each serum the titre of antibodies against the neurotoxin of *C. tetani* using a suitable immunochemical method (*2.7.1*) such as a toxin-binding-inhibition test (ToBI test) and a homologous reference serum. Determine the average antibody titre of the serum samples.

Clostridia (multicomponent) rabbit antiserum BRP, *Clostridium tetani guinea-pig antiserum for vaccines for veterinary use BRP* and *Clostridium tetani rabbit antiserum BRP* are suitable as reference sera.

Tetanus vaccine intended for use in animals other than horses complies with the test if the average antibody titre is not less than 7.5 IU/ml.

Tetanus vaccine intended for use in horses complies with the test if the average antibody titre is not less than 30 IU/ml.

For tetanus vaccine presented as a combined vaccine for use in animals other than horses, the above test may be carried out in susceptible rabbits instead of guinea-pigs. The vaccine complies with the test if the average antibody titre of the sera of the vaccinated rabbits is not less than 2.5 IU/ml.

01/2005:1580

VIBRIOSIS (COLD-WATER) VACCINE (INACTIVATED) FOR SALMONIDS

Vaccinum vibriosidis aquae frigidae inactivatum ad salmonidas

DEFINITION

Cold-water vibriosis vaccine (inactivated) for salmonids is prepared from cultures of one or more suitable strains of *Vibrio salmonicida*.

PRODUCTION

The strains of *V. salmonicida* are cultured and harvested separately. The harvests are inactivated by a suitable method. They may be purified and concentrated. Whole or disrupted cells may be used and the vaccine may contain extracellular products of the bacterium released into the growth medium.

CHOICE OF VACCINE COMPOSITION

The strain or strains of *V. salmonicida* used are shown to be suitable with respect to production of antigens of assumed immunological importance. The vaccine is shown to be satisfactory with respect to safety (*5.2.6*) and immunogenicity (*5.2.7*) in the species of fish for which it is intended. The following tests may be used during demonstration of safety and immunogenicity.

Safety. Safety is tested in three different batches using test A, test B or both, depending on the recommendations for use.

A. *Vaccines intended for administration by injection.* A test is carried out in each species of fish for which the vaccine is intended. The fish used are from a population that does not have specific antibodies against *V. salmonicida* and which has not been vaccinated against nor exposed to cold-water vibriosis. The test is carried out in the conditions recommended for the use of the vaccine with a water temperature not less than 10 °C. An amount of vaccine corresponding to twice the recommended dose per mass unit for fish of the minimum body mass recommended for vaccination is administered intraperitoneally to each of not fewer than fifty fish of the minimum recommended body mass. The fish are observed for 21 days. No abnormal local or systemic reaction occurs. The test is invalid if more than 6 per cent of the fish die from causes not attributable to the vaccine.

B. *Vaccines intended for administration by immersion.* A test is carried out in each species of fish for which the vaccine is intended. The fish used are from a population that does not have specific antibodies against *V. salmonicida* and which has not been vaccinated against nor exposed to cold-water vibriosis. The test is carried out in the conditions recommended for the use of the vaccine with a water temperature not less than 10 °C. Prepare an immersion bath at twice the recommended concentration. Not fewer than fifty fish, having not less than the minimum body mass recommended for vaccination are used. The fish are bathed for twice the recommended time. The fish are observed for 21 days. No abnormal local or systemic reaction occurs. The test is invalid if more than 6 per cent of the fish die from causes not attributable to the vaccine.

C. Safety is demonstrated in addition in field trials by administering the intended dose to a sufficient number of fish distributed in not fewer than two sets of premises. No abnormal reaction occurs.

*Immunogenicity.*The test described under Potency, carried out for each recommended route of administration, is suitable to demonstrate immunogenicity of the vaccine.

BATCH TESTING

Batch potency test. For routine testing of batches of vaccine, the test described under Potency may be carried out using groups of not fewer than thirty fish of one of the species for which the vaccine is intended; alternatively, a suitable validated test based on antibody response may be carried out, the criteria being set with reference to a batch of vaccine that has given satisfactory results in the test described under Potency. The following test may be used after a satisfactory correlation with the test described under Potency has been established.

Use fish from a population that does not have specific antibodies against *V. salmonicida* and that are within specified limits for body mass. Carry out the test at a defined temperature. Inject into each of not fewer than twenty-five fish one dose of vaccine, according to the instructions for use. Perform mock vaccination on a control group of not fewer than ten fish. Collect blood samples at a defined time after vaccination. Determine for each sample the level of specific antibodies against *V. salmonicida* by a suitable immunochemical method (*2.7.1*). The vaccine complies with the test if the mean level of antibodies is not significantly lower than that found for a batch that gave satisfactory results in the test described under Potency. The test is not valid if the control group shows antibodies against *V. salmonicida.*

IDENTIFICATION

When injected into fish that do not have specific antibodies against *V. salmonicida,* the vaccine stimulates the production of such antibodies.

TESTS

Safety. Use not fewer than ten fish of one of the species for which the vaccine is intended, having, where possible, the minimum body mass recommended for vaccination; if fish of the minimum body mass are not available, use fish not greater than twice this mass. Use fish from a population that does not have specific antibodies against *V. salmonicida* and that has not been vaccinated against nor exposed to cold-water vibriosis. Carry out the test in the conditions recommended for use of the vaccine with a water temperature not less than 10 °C. For vaccines administered by injection or immersion, inject intraperitoneally into each fish an amount of vaccine corresponding to twice the recommended dose per mass unit. For vaccines administered by immersion only, use a bath with double the recommended concentration and bathe the fish for twice the recommended immersion time. Observe the animals for 21 days. No abnormal local or systemic reaction attributable to the vaccine occurs. The test is invalid if more than 10 per cent of the fish die from causes not attributable to the vaccine.

Sterility. The vaccine complies with the test for sterility prescribed in the monograph on *Vaccines for veterinary use (0062).*

POTENCY

Carry out the test according to a protocol defining limits of body mass for the fish, water source, water flow and temperature limits, and preparation of a standardised challenge. Vaccinate not fewer than one hundred fish by a recommended route, according to the instructions for use. Perform mock vaccination on a control group of not fewer than one hundred fish; mark vaccinated and control fish for identification. Keep all the fish in the same tank or mix equal numbers of controls and vaccinates in each tank if more than one tank is used. Carry out challenge by injection at a fixed time interval after vaccination, defined according to the statement regarding development of immunity. Use for challenge a culture of *V. salmonicida* whose virulence has been verified. Observe the fish daily until at least 60 per cent specific mortality is reached in the control group. Plot for both vaccinates and controls a curve of specific mortality against time from challenge and determine by interpolation the time corresponding to 60 per cent specific mortality in controls. The test is invalid if the specific mortality is less than 60 per cent in the control group 21 days after the first death in the fish. Read from the curve for vaccinates the mortality (*M*) at the time corresponding to 60 per cent mortality in controls. Calculate the relative percentage survival (RPS) from the expression:

$$\left(1 - \frac{M}{60}\right) \times 100$$

The vaccine complies with the test if the RPS is not less than 60 per cent for vaccines administered by immersion and 90 per cent for vaccines administered by injection.

LABELLING

The label states information on the time needed for development of immunity after vaccination under the range of conditions corresponding to the recommended use.

01/2005:1581

VIBRIOSIS VACCINE (INACTIVATED) FOR SALMONIDS

Vaccinum vibriosidis ad salmonidas inactivatum

DEFINITION

Vibriosis vaccine (inactivated) for salmonids is prepared from cultures of one or more suitable strains or serovars of *Vibrio anguillarum*; the vaccine may also include *Vibrio ordalii*.

PRODUCTION

The strains of *V. anguillarum* and *V. ordalii* are cultured and harvested separately. The harvests are inactivated by a suitable method. They may be purified and concentrated. Whole or disrupted cells may be used and the vaccine may contain extracellular products of the bacterium released into the growth medium.

CHOICE OF VACCINE COMPOSITION

The strains of *V. anguillarum* and *V. ordalii* used are shown to be suitable with respect to production of antigens of assumed immunological importance. The vaccine is shown to be satisfactory with respect to safety (*5.2.6*) and immunogenicity (*5.2.7*) in the species of fish for which it is intended. The following tests may be used during demonstration of safety and immunogenicity.

Safety. Safety is tested in three different batches using test A, test B or both, depending on the recommendations for use.

A. *Vaccines intended for administration by injection.* A test is carried out in each species of fish for which the vaccine is intended. The fish used are from a population that does not have specific antibodies against the relevant serovars of *V. anguillarum* or where applicable *V. ordalii* and which has not been vaccinated against nor exposed to vibriosis. The test is carried out in the conditions recommended for the use of the vaccine with a water temperature not less than 10 °C. An amount of vaccine corresponding to twice the recommended dose per mass unit for fish of the minimum body mass recommended for vaccination is administered intraperitoneally to each of not fewer than fifty fish of the minimum recommended body mass. The fish are observed for 21 days. No abnormal local or systemic reaction occurs. The test is invalid if more than 6 per cent of the fish die from causes not attributable to the vaccine.

B. *Vaccines intended for administration by immersion.* A test is carried out in each species of fish for which the vaccine is intended. The fish used are from a population that does not have specific antibodies against the relevant serovars of *V. anguillarum* or where applicable *V. ordalii* and which has not been vaccinated against nor exposed to vibriosis. The test is carried out in the conditions recommended for the use of the vaccine with a water temperature not less than 10 °C. Prepare an immersion bath at twice the recommended concentration. Not fewer than fifty fish having the minimum body mass recommended for vaccination are used. The fish are bathed for twice the recommended time. The fish are observed for 21 days. No abnormal local or systemic reaction occurs. The test is invalid if more than 6 per cent of the fish die from causes not attributable to the vaccine.

C. Safety is also demonstrated in field trials by administering the intended dose to a sufficient number of fish distributed in not fewer than two sets of premises. No abnormal reaction occurs.

*Immunogenicity.*The test described under Potency, carried out for each recommended route of administration is suitable to demonstrate immunogenicity of the vaccine.

BATCH TESTING

Batch potency test. For routine testing of batches of vaccine, the test described under Potency may be carried out using groups of not fewer than thirty fish of one of the species for which the vaccine is intended; alternatively, a suitable validated test based on antibody response may be carried out, the criteria being set with reference to a batch of vaccine that has given satisfactory results in the test described under Potency. The following test may be used after a satisfactory correlation with the test described under Potency has been established.

Use fish from a population that does not have specific antibodies against the relevant serovars of *V. anguillarum* and where applicable *V. ordalii* and that are within specified limits for body mass. Carry out the test at a defined temperature. Inject into each of not fewer than twenty-five fish one dose of vaccine, according to the instructions for use. Perform mock vaccination on a control group of not fewer than ten fish. Collect blood samples at a defined time after vaccination. Determine for each sample the level of specific antibodies against the different serovars of *V. anguillarum* and against *V. ordalii* included in the vaccine by a suitable immunochemical method (*2.7.1*). The vaccine complies with the test if the mean levels of antibodies are not significantly lower than those found for a batch that gave satisfactory results in the test described under Potency. The test is not valid if the control group shows antibodies against the relevant serovars of *V. anguillarum* or, where applicable, against *V. ordalii*.

IDENTIFICATION

When injected into fish that do not have specific antibodies against *V. anguillarum* and, where applicable, *V. ordalii*, the vaccine stimulates the production of such antibodies.

TESTS

Safety. Use not fewer than ten fish of one of the species for which the vaccine is intended, having, where possible, the minimum body mass recommended for vaccination; if fish of the minimum body mass are not available, use fish not greater than twice this mass. Use fish from a population that does not have specific antibodies against the relevant serovars of *V. anguillarum* and, where applicable, *V. ordalii* and which has not been vaccinated against nor exposed to vibriosis. Carry out the test in the conditions recommended for the use of the vaccine with a water temperature not less than 10 °C. For vaccines administered by injection or immersion, inject intraperitoneally into each fish an amount of vaccine corresponding to twice the recommended dose per mass unit. For vaccines administered by immersion only, use a bath with double the recommended concentration and bathe the fish for twice the recommended immersion time. Observe the animals for 21 days. No abnormal local or systemic reaction attributable to the vaccine occurs. The test is invalid if more than 10 per cent of the fish die from causes not attributable to the vaccine.

Sterility. The vaccine complies with the test for sterility prescribed in the monograph on *Vaccines for veterinary use (0062)*.

POTENCY

Carry out a separate test for each species and each serovar included in the vaccine. Carry out the test according to a protocol defining limits of body mass for the fish, water source, water flow and temperature limits, and preparation of a standardised challenge. Vaccinate not fewer than one hundred fish by a recommended route, according to the instructions for use. Perform mock vaccination on a control group of not fewer than one hundred fish; mark vaccinated and control fish for identification. Keep all the fish in the same tank or mix equal numbers of controls and vaccinates in each tank if more than one tank is used. Carry out challenge by injection at a fixed time interval after vaccination, defined according to the statement regarding development of immunity. Use for challenge cultures of *V. anguillarum* or *V. ordalii* whose virulence has been verified. Observe the fish daily until at least 60 per cent specific mortality is reached in the control group. Plot for both vaccinates and controls a curve of specific mortality against time from challenge and determine by interpolation the time corresponding to 60 per cent specific mortality in controls. The test is invalid if the specific mortality is less than 60 per cent in the control group 21 days after the first death in the fish. Read from the curve for vaccinates the mortality (M) at the time corresponding to 60 per cent mortality in controls. Calculate the relative percentage survival (RPS) from the expression:

$$\left(1 - \frac{M}{60}\right) \times 100$$

The vaccine complies with the test if the RPS is not less than 60 per cent for vaccines administered by immersion and 75 per cent for vaccines administered by injection.

LABELLING

The label states:

- the serovar or serovars of *V. anguillarum* included in the vaccine,
- where applicable, that the vaccine includes *V. ordalii*,
- information on the time needed for development of immunity after vaccination under the range of conditions corresponding to the recommended use.

IMMUNOSERA FOR HUMAN USE

01/2005:0085

BOTULINUM ANTITOXIN

Immunoserum botulinicum

DEFINITION

Botulinum antitoxin is a preparation containing antitoxic globulins that have the power of specifically neutralising the toxins formed by *Clostridium botulinum* type A, type B or type E, or any mixture of these types.

PRODUCTION

It is obtained by fractionation from the serum of horses, or other mammals, that have been immunised against *Cl. botulinum* type A, type B and type E toxins.

IDENTIFICATION

It specifically neutralises the types of *Cl. botulinum* toxins stated on the label, rendering them harmless to susceptible animals.

POTENCY

Not less than 500 IU of antitoxin per millilitre for each of types A and B and not less than 50 IU of antitoxin per millilitre for type E.

The potency of botulinum antitoxin is determined by comparing the dose necessary to protect mice against the lethal effects of a fixed dose of botulinum toxin with the quantity of the standard preparation of botulinum antitoxin necessary to give the same protection. For this comparison a reference preparation of each type of botulinum antitoxin, calibrated in International Units, and suitable preparations of botulinum toxins, for use as test toxins, are required. The potency of each test toxin is determined in relation to the specific reference preparation; the potency of the botulinum antitoxin to be examined is determined in relation to the potency of the test toxins by the same method.

International Units of the antitoxin are the specific neutralising activity for botulinum toxin type A, type B and type E contained in stated amounts of the International Standards which consist of dried immune horse sera of types A, B and E. The equivalence in International Units of the International Standard is stated from time to time by the World Health Organisation.

Selection of animals. Use mice having body masses such that the difference between the lightest and the heaviest does not exceed 5 g.

Preparation of test toxins. CAUTION: Botulinum toxin is extremely toxic: exceptional care must be taken in any procedure in which it is employed. Prepare type A, B and E toxins from sterile filtrates of approximately 7-day cultures in liquid medium of *Cl. botulinum* types A, B and E. To the filtrates, add 2 volumes of glycerol, concentrate, if necessary, by dialysis against glycerol and store at or slightly below 0 °C.

Selection of test toxins. Select toxins of each type for use as test toxins by determining for mice the L+/10 dose and the LD_{50}, the observation period being 96 h. The test toxins contain at least 1000 LD_{50} in an L+/10 dose.

Determination of test doses of the toxins (L+/10 dose). Prepare solutions of the reference preparations in a suitable liquid such that each contains 0.25 IU of antitoxin per millilitre. Using each solution in turn, determine the test dose of the corresponding test toxin.

Prepare mixtures of the solution of the reference preparation and the test toxin such that each contains 2.0 ml of the solution of the reference preparation, one of a graded series of volumes of the test toxin and sufficient of a suitable liquid to bring the total volume to 5.0 ml. Allow the mixtures to stand at room temperature, protected from light, for 60 min. Using four mice for each mixture, inject a dose of 1.0 ml intraperitoneally into each mouse. Observe the mice for 96 h.

The test dose of toxin is the quantity in 1.0 ml of the mixture made with the smallest amount of toxin capable of causing, despite partial neutralisation by the reference preparation, the death of all four mice injected with the mixture within the observation period.

Determination of potency of the antitoxin. Prepare solutions of each reference preparation in a suitable liquid such that each contains 0.25 IU of antitoxin per millilitre.

Prepare solutions of each test toxin in a suitable liquid such that each contains 2.5 test doses per millilitre.

Using each toxin solution and the corresponding reference preparation in turn, determine the potency of the antitoxin. Prepare mixtures of the solution of the test toxin and the antitoxin to be examined such that each contains 2.0 ml of the solution of the test toxin, one of a graded series of volumes of the antitoxin to be examined, and sufficient of a suitable liquid to bring the total volume to 5.0 ml. Also prepare mixtures of the solution of the test toxin and the solution of the reference preparation such that each contains 2.0 ml of the solution of the test toxin, one of a graded series of volumes of the solution of the reference preparation centred on that volume (2.0 ml) that contains 0.5 IU, and sufficient of a suitable liquid to bring the total volume to 5.0 ml. Allow the mixtures to stand at room temperature, protected from light, for 60 min. Using four mice for each mixture, inject a dose of 1.0 ml intraperitoneally into each mouse. Observe the mice for 96 h.

The mixture that contains the largest volume of antitoxin that fails to protect the mice from death contains 0.5 IU. This quantity is used to calculate the potency of the antitoxin in International Units per millilitre.

The test is not valid unless all the mice injected with mixtures containing 2.0 ml or less of the solution of the reference preparation die and all those injected with mixtures containing more survive.

LABELLING

The label states the types of *Cl. botulinum* toxin neutralised by the preparation.

01/2005:0086

DIPHTHERIA ANTITOXIN

Immunoserum diphthericum

DEFINITION

Diphtheria antitoxin is a preparation containing antitoxic globulins that have the power of specifically neutralising the toxin formed by *Corynebacterium diphtheriae*.

PRODUCTION

It is obtained by fractionation from the serum of horses, or other mammals, that have been immunised against diphtheria toxin.

IDENTIFICATION

It specifically neutralises the toxin formed by *C. diphtheriae*, rendering it harmless to susceptible animals.

ASSAY

Not less than 1000 IU of antitoxin per millilitre for antitoxin obtained from horse serum. Not less than 500 IU of antitoxin per millilitre for antitoxin obtained from the serum of other mammals.

The potency of diphtheria antitoxin is determined by comparing the dose necessary to protect guinea-pigs or rabbits against the erythrogenic effects of a fixed dose of diphtheria toxin with the quantity of the standard preparation of diphtheria antitoxin necessary to give the same protection. For this comparison a reference preparation of diphtheria antitoxin, calibrated in International Units, and a suitable preparation of diphtheria toxin, for use as a test toxin, are required. The potency of the test toxin is determined in relation to the reference preparation; the potency of the diphtheria antitoxin to be examined is determined in relation to the potency of the test toxin by the same method.

The International Unit of antitoxin is the specific neutralising activity for diphtheria toxin contained in a stated amount of the International Standard, which consists of a quantity of dried immune horse serum. The equivalence in International Units of the International Standard is stated by the World Health Organisation.

Preparation of test toxin. Prepare diphtheria toxin from cultures of *C. diphtheriae* in a liquid medium. Filter the culture to obtain a sterile toxic filtrate and store at 4 °C.

Selection of test toxin. Select a toxin for use as a test toxin by determining for guinea-pigs or rabbits the lr/100 dose and the minimal reacting dose, the observation period being 48 h. The test toxin has at least 200 minimal reacting doses in the lr/100 dose.

Minimal reacting dose. This is the smallest quantity of toxin which, when injected intracutaneously into guinea-pigs or rabbits, causes a small, characteristic reaction at the site of injection within 48 h.

The test toxin is allowed to stand for some months before being used for the assay of antitoxin. During this time its toxicity declines and the lr/100 dose may be increased. Determine the minimal reacting dose and the lr/100 dose at frequent intervals. When experiment shows that the lr/100 dose is constant, the test toxin is ready for use and may be used for a long period. Store the test toxin in the dark at 0 °C to 5 °C. Maintain its sterility by the addition of toluene or other antimicrobial preservative that does not cause a rapid decline in specific toxicity.

Determination of test dose of toxin (lr/100 dose). Prepare a solution of the reference preparation in a suitable liquid such that it contains 0.1 IU of antitoxin per millilitre.

Prepare mixtures of the solution of the reference preparation and of the test toxin such that each contains 1.0 ml of the solution of the reference preparation, one of a graded series of volumes of the test toxin and sufficient of a suitable liquid to bring the total volume to 2.0 ml. Allow the mixtures to stand at room temperature, protected from light, for 15 min to 60 min. Using two animals for each mixture, inject a dose of 0.2 ml intracutaneously into the shaven or depilated flanks of each animal. Observe the animals for 48 h.

The test dose of toxin is the quantity in 0.2 ml of the mixture made with the smallest amount of toxin capable of causing, despite partial neutralisation by the reference preparation, a small but characteristic erythematous lesion at the site of injection.

Determination of potency of the antitoxin. Prepare a solution of the reference preparation in a suitable liquid such that it contains 0.125 IU of antitoxin per millilitre.

Prepare a solution of the test toxin in a suitable liquid such that it contains 12.5 test doses per millilitre.

Prepare mixtures of the solution of the test toxin and of the antitoxin to be examined such that each contains 0.8 ml of the solution of the test toxin, one of a graded series of volumes of the antitoxin to be examined and sufficient of a suitable liquid to bring the total volume to 2.0 ml. Also prepare mixtures of the solution of the test toxin and the solution of the reference preparation such that each contains 0.8 ml of the solution of the test toxin, one of a graded series of volumes of the solution of the reference preparation centred on that volume (0.8 ml) that contains 0.1 IU and sufficient of a suitable liquid to bring the total volume to 2.0 ml. Allow the mixtures to stand at room temperature, protected from light, for 15 min to 60 min. Using two animals for each mixture, inject a dose of 0.2 ml intracutaneously into the shaven or depilated flanks of each animal. Observe the animals for 48 h.

The mixture that contains the largest volume of antitoxin that fails to protect the guinea-pigs from the erythematous effects of the toxin contains 0.1 IU. This quantity is used to calculate the potency of the antitoxin in International Units per millilitre.

The test is not valid unless all the sites injected with mixtures containing 0.8 ml or less of the solution of the reference preparation show erythematous lesions and at all those injected with mixtures containing more there are no lesions.

01/2005:0090

GAS-GANGRENE ANTITOXIN, MIXED

Immunoserum gangraenicum mixtum

DEFINITION

Mixed gas-gangrene antitoxin is prepared by mixing gas-gangrene antitoxin (novyi), gas-gangrene antitoxin (perfringens) and gas-gangrene antitoxin (septicum) in appropriate quantities.

IDENTIFICATION

It specifically neutralises the alpha toxins formed by *Clostridium novyi* (former nomenclature: *Clostridium oedematiens*), *Clostridium perfringens* and *Clostridium septicum*, rendering them harmless to susceptible animals.

ASSAY

Gas-gangrene antitoxin (novyi), not less than 1000 IU of antitoxin per millilitre; gas-gangrene antitoxin (perfringens), not less than 1000 IU of antitoxin per millilitre; gas-gangrene antitoxin (septicum) not less than 500 IU of antitoxin per millilitre.

Carry out the assay for each component, as prescribed in the monographs on *Gas-gangrene antitoxin (novyi) (0087)*, *Gas-gangrene antitoxin (perfringens) (0088)* and *Gas-gangrene antitoxin (septicum) (0089)*.

01/2005:0087

GAS-GANGRENE ANTITOXIN (NOVYI)

Immunoserum gangraenicum (Clostridium novyi)

DEFINITION

Gas-gangrene antitoxin (novyi) is a preparation containing antitoxic globulins that have the power of neutralising the alpha toxin formed by *Clostridium novyi* (Former nomenclature: *Clostridium oedematiens*). It is obtained by fractionation from the serum of horses, or other mammals, that have been immunised against *Cl. novyi* alpha toxin.

IDENTIFICATION

It specifically neutralises the alpha toxin formed by *Cl. novyi*, rendering it harmless to susceptible animals.

ASSAY

Not less than 3750 IU of antitoxin per millilitre.

The potency of gas-gangrene antitoxin (novyi) is determined by comparing the dose necessary to protect mice or other suitable animals against the lethal effects of a fixed dose of *Cl. novyi* toxin with the quantity of the standard preparation of gas-gangrene antitoxin (novyi) necessary to give the same protection. For this comparison a reference preparation of gas-gangrene antitoxin (novyi), calibrated in International Units, and a suitable preparation of *Cl. novyi* toxin for use as a test toxin are required. The potency of the test toxin is determined in relation to the reference preparation; the potency of the gas-gangrene antitoxin (novyi) to be examined is determined in relation to the potency of the test toxin by the same method.

The International Unit of antitoxin is the specific neutralising activity for *Cl. novyi* toxin contained in a stated amount of the International Standard, which consists of a quantity of dried immune horse serum. The equivalence in International Units of the International Standard is stated by the World Health Organisation.

Selection of animals. Use mice having body masses such that the difference between the lightest and the heaviest does not exceed 5 g.

Preparation of test toxin. Prepare the test toxin from a sterile filtrate of an approximately 5-day culture in liquid medium of *Cl. novyi.* Treat the filtrate with *ammonium sulphate R*, collect the precipitate, which contains the toxin, dry *in vacuo* over *diphosphorus pentoxide R*, powder and store dry.

Selection of test toxin. Select a toxin for use as a test toxin by determining for mice the L+ dose and the LD_{50}, the observation period being 72 h. The test toxin has an L+ dose of 0.5 mg or less and contains not less than 25 LD_{50} in each L+ dose.

Determination of test dose of toxin (L+ dose). Prepare a solution of the reference preparation in a suitable liquid such that it contains 12.5 IU of antitoxin per millilitre.

Prepare a solution of the test toxin in a suitable liquid such that 1 ml contains a precisely known amount such as 10 mg.

Prepare mixtures of the solution of the reference preparation and the solution of the test toxin such that each contains 0.8 ml of the solution of the reference preparation, one of a graded series of volumes of the solution of the test toxin and sufficient of a suitable liquid to bring the total volume to 2.0 ml. Allow the mixtures to stand at room temperature, protected from light, for 60 min. Using six mice for each mixture, inject a dose of 0.2 ml intramuscularly into each mouse. Observe the mice for 72 h.

The test dose of toxin is the quantity in 0.2 ml of the mixture made with the smallest amount of toxin capable of causing, despite partial neutralisation by the reference preparation, the death of all six mice injected with the mixture within the observation period.

Determination of potency of the antitoxin. Prepare a solution of the reference preparation in a suitable liquid such that it contains 12.5 IU of antitoxin per millilitre.

Prepare a solution of the test toxin in a suitable liquid such that it contains 12.5 test doses per millilitre.

Prepare mixtures of the solution of the test toxin and the antitoxin to be examined such that each contains 0.8 ml of the solution of the test toxin, one of a graded series of volumes of the antitoxin to be examined and sufficient of a suitable liquid to bring the total volume to 2.0 ml. Also prepare mixtures of the solution of the test toxin and the solution of the reference preparation such that each contains 0.8 ml of the solution of the test toxin, one of a graded series of volumes of the solution of the reference preparation centred on that volume (0.8 ml) that contains 10 IU and sufficient of a suitable liquid to bring the total volume to 2.0 ml. Allow the mixtures to stand at room temperature, protected from light, for 60 min. Using six mice for each mixture, inject a dose of 0.2 ml intramuscularly into each mouse. Observe the mice for 72 h.

The mixture that contains the largest volume of antitoxin that fails to protect the mice from death contains 10 IU. This quantity is used to calculate the potency of the antitoxin in International Units per millilitre.

The test is not valid unless all the mice injected with mixtures containing 0.8 ml or less of the solution of the reference preparation die and all those injected with mixtures containing a larger volume survive.

01/2005:0088

GAS-GANGRENE ANTITOXIN (PERFRINGENS)

Immunoserum gangraenicum (Clostridium perfringens)

DEFINITION

Gas-gangrene antitoxin (perfringens) is a preparation containing antitoxic globulins that have the power of specifically neutralising the alpha toxin formed by *Clostridium perfringens.* It is obtained by fractionation from the serum of horses, or other mammals, that have been immunised against *Cl. perfringens* alpha toxin.

IDENTIFICATION

It specifically neutralises the alpha toxin formed by *Cl. perfringens*, rendering it harmless to susceptible animals.

ASSAY

Not less than 1500 IU of antitoxin per millilitre.

The potency of gas-gangrene antitoxin (perfringens) is determined by comparing the dose necessary to protect mice or other suitable animals against the lethal effects of a fixed dose of *Cl. perfringens* toxin with the quantity of the standard preparation of gas-gangrene antitoxin (perfringens) necessary to give the same protection. For this comparison a reference preparation of gas-gangrene antitoxin (perfringens), calibrated in International Units, and a suitable preparation of *Cl. perfringens* toxin for use as a test toxin are required. The potency of the test toxin is determined in relation to the reference preparation; the potency of the gas-gangrene antitoxin (perfringens) to be examined is determined in relation to the potency of the test toxin by the same method.

The International Unit of antitoxin is the specific neutralising activity for *Cl. perfringens* toxin contained in a stated amount of the International Standard, which consists of a quantity of dried immune horse serum. The equivalence in International Units of the International Standard is stated by the World Health Organisation.

Selection of animals. Use mice having body masses such that the difference between the lightest and the heaviest does not exceed 5 g.

Preparation of test toxin. Prepare the test toxin from a sterile filtrate of an approximately 5-day culture in liquid medium of *Cl. perfringens.* Treat the filtrate with *ammonium sulphate R,* collect the precipitate, which contains the toxin, dry *in vacuo* over *diphosphorus pentoxide R,* powder and store dry.

Selection of test toxin. Select a toxin for use as a test toxin by determining for mice the L+ dose and the LD_{50}, the observation period being 48 h. The test toxin has an L+ dose of 4 mg or less and contains not less than 20 LD_{50} in each L+ dose.

Determination of test dose of toxin (L+ dose). Prepare a solution of the reference preparation in a suitable liquid such that it contains 5 IU of antitoxin per millilitre.

Prepare a solution of the test toxin in a suitable liquid such that 1 ml contains a precisely known amount such as 10 mg.

Prepare mixtures of the solution of the reference preparation and the solution of the test toxin such that each contains 2.0 ml of the solution of the reference preparation, one of a graded series of volumes of the solution of the test toxin and sufficient of a suitable liquid to bring the total volume to 5.0 ml. Allow the mixtures to stand at room temperature, protected from light, for 60 min. Using six mice for each mixture, inject a dose of 0.5 ml intravenously into each mouse. Observe the mice for 48 h.

The test dose of toxin is the quantity in 0.5 ml of the mixture made with the smallest amount of toxin capable of causing, despite partial neutralisation by the reference preparation, the death of all six mice injected with the mixture within the observation period.

Determination of potency of the antitoxin. Prepare a solution of the reference preparation in a suitable liquid such that it contains 5 IU of antitoxin per millilitre.

Prepare a solution of the test toxin in a suitable liquid such that it contains five test doses per millilitre.

Prepare mixtures of the solution of the test toxin and the antitoxin to be examined such that each contains 2.0 ml of the solution of the test toxin, one of a graded series of volumes of the antitoxin to be examined and sufficient of a suitable liquid to bring the total volume to 5.0 ml. Also prepare mixtures of the solution of the test toxin and the solution of the reference preparation such that each contains 2.0 ml of the solution of the test toxin, one of a graded series of volumes of the solution of the reference preparation centred on that volume (2.0 ml) that contains 10 IU and sufficient of a suitable liquid to bring the total volume to 5.0 ml. Allow the mixtures to stand at room temperature, protected from light, for 60 min. Using six mice for each mixture, inject a dose of 0.5 ml intravenously into each mouse. Observe the mice for 48 h.

The mixture that contains the largest volume of antitoxin that fails to protect the mice from death contains 10 IU. This quantity is used to calculate the potency of the antitoxin in International Units per millilitre.

The test is not valid unless all the mice injected with mixtures containing 2.0 ml or less of the solution of the reference preparation die and all those injected with mixtures containing a larger volume survive.

01/2005:0089

GAS-GANGRENE ANTITOXIN (SEPTICUM)

Immunoserum gangraenicum (Clostridium septicum)

DEFINITION

Gas-gangrene antitoxin (septicum) is a preparation containing antitoxic globulins that have the power of specifically neutralising the alpha toxin formed by *Clostridium septicum.* It is obtained by fractionation from the serum of horses, or other mammals, that have been immunised against *Cl. septicum* alpha toxin.

IDENTIFICATION

It specifically neutralises the alpha toxin formed by *Cl. septicum,* rendering it harmless to susceptible animals.

ASSAY

Not less than 1500 IU of antitoxin per millilitre.

The potency of gas-gangrene antitoxin (septicum) is determined by comparing the dose necessary to protect mice or other suitable animals against the lethal effects of a fixed dose of *Cl. septicum* toxin with the quantity of the standard preparation of gas-gangrene antitoxin (septicum) necessary to give the same protection. For this comparison a reference preparation of gas-gangrene antitoxin (septicum), calibrated in International Units, and a suitable preparation of *Cl. septicum* toxin for use as a test toxin are required. The potency of the test toxin is determined in relation to the reference preparation; the potency of the gas-gangrene antitoxin (septicum) to be examined is determined in relation to the potency of the test toxin by the same method.

The International Unit of antitoxin is the specific neutralising activity for *Cl. septicum* toxin contained in a stated amount of the International Standard, which consists of a quantity of dried immune horse serum. The equivalence in International Units of the International Standard is stated by the World Health Organisation.

Selection of animals. Use mice having body masses such that the difference between the lightest and the heaviest does not exceed 5 g.

Preparation of test toxin. Prepare the test toxin from a sterile filtrate of an approximately 5-day culture in liquid medium of *Cl. septicum.* Treat the filtrate with *ammonium sulphate R,* collect the precipitate, which contains the toxin, dry *in vacuo* over *diphosphorus pentoxide R,* powder and store dry.

Selection of test toxin. Select a toxin for use as a test toxin by determining for mice the L+ dose and the LD_{50}, the observation period being 72 h. The test toxin has an L+ dose of 0.5 mg or less and contains not less than 25 LD_{50} in each L+ dose.

Determination of test dose of toxin (L+ dose). Prepare a solution of the reference preparation in a suitable liquid such that it contains 5 IU of antitoxin per millilitre.

Prepare a solution of the test toxin in a suitable liquid such that 1 ml contains a precisely known amount such as 20 mg.

Prepare mixtures of the solution of the reference preparation and the solution of the test toxin such that each contains 2.0 ml of the solution of the reference preparation, one of a graded series of volumes of the solution of the test toxin and sufficient of a suitable liquid to bring the total volume to 5.0 ml. Allow the mixtures to stand at room temperature,

Immunosera

protected from light, for 60 min. Using six mice for each mixture, inject a dose of 0.5 ml intravenously into each mouse. Observe the mice for 72 h.

The test dose of toxin is the quantity in 0.5 ml of the mixture made with the smallest amount of toxin capable of causing, despite partial neutralisation by the reference preparation, the death of all six mice injected with the mixture within the observation period.

Determination of potency of the antitoxin. Prepare a solution of the reference preparation in a suitable liquid such that it contains 5 IU of antitoxin per millilitre.

Prepare a solution of the test toxin in a suitable liquid such that it contains five test doses per millilitre.

Prepare mixtures of the solution of the test toxin and the antitoxin to be examined such that each contains 2.0 ml of the solution of the test toxin, one of a graded series of volumes of the antitoxin to be examined and sufficient of a suitable liquid to bring the total volume to 5.0 ml. Also prepare mixtures of the solution of the test toxin and the solution of the reference preparation such that each contains 2.0 ml of the solution of the test toxin, one of a graded series of volumes of the solution of the reference preparation centred on that volume (2.0 ml) that contains 10 IU and sufficient of a suitable liquid to bring the total volume to 5.0 ml. Allow the mixtures to stand at room temperature, protected from light, for 60 min. Using six mice for each mixture, inject a dose of 0.5 ml intravenously into each mouse. Observe the mice for 72 h.

The mixture that contains the largest volume of antitoxin that fails to protect the mice from death contains 10 IU. This quantity is used to calculate the potency of the antitoxin in International Units per millilitre.

The test is not valid unless all the mice injected with mixtures containing 2.0 ml or less of the solution of the reference preparation die and all those injected with mixtures containing more survive.

01/2005:0091

TETANUS ANTITOXIN FOR HUMAN USE

Immunoserum tetanicum ad usum humanum

DEFINITION

Tetanus antitoxin for human use is a preparation containing antitoxic globulins that have the power of specifically neutralising the toxin formed by *Clostridium tetani.*

PRODUCTION

It is obtained by fractionation from the serum of horses, or other mammals, that have been immunised against tetanus toxin.

IDENTIFICATION

It specifically neutralises the toxin formed by *Cl. tetani,* rendering it harmless to susceptible animals.

POTENCY

Not less than 1000 IU of antitoxin per millilitre when intended for prophylactic use. Not less than 3000 IU of antitoxin per millilitre when intended for therapeutic use.

The potency of tetanus antitoxin is determined by comparing the dose necessary to protect guinea-pigs or mice against the paralytic effects of a fixed dose of tetanus toxin with the quantity of the standard preparation of tetanus antitoxin necessary to give the same protection. In countries where the paralysis method is not obligatory the lethal method may be used. For this method the number of animals and the procedure are identical with those described for the paralysis method but the end-point is the death of the animal rather than the onset of paralysis and the L+/10 dose is used instead of the Lp/10 dose. For this comparison a reference preparation of tetanus antitoxin, calibrated in International Units, and a suitable preparation of tetanus toxin, for use as a test toxin, are required. The potency of the test toxin is determined in relation to the reference preparation; the potency of the tetanus antitoxin to be examined is determined in relation to the potency of the test toxin by the same method.

The International Unit of antitoxin is the specific neutralising activity for tetanus toxin contained in a stated amount of the International Standard which consists of a quantity of dried immune horse serum. The equivalence in International Units of the International Standard is stated by the World Health Organisation.

Selection of animals. If mice are used, the body masses should be such that the difference between the lightest and the heaviest does not exceed 5 g.

Preparation of test toxin. Prepare the test toxin from a sterile filtrate of an approximately 9-day culture in liquid medium of *Cl. tetani.* To the filtrate add 1 to 2 volumes of glycerol and store slightly below 0 °C. Alternatively, treat the filtrate with *ammonium sulphate R,* collect the precipitate, which contains the toxin, dry *in vacuo* over *diphosphorus pentoxide R,* powder and store dry, either in sealed ampoules or *in vacuo* over *diphosphorus pentoxide R.*

Determination of test dose of toxin (Lp/10 dose). Prepare a solution of the reference preparation in a suitable liquid such that it contains 0.5 IU of antitoxin per millilitre.

If the test toxin is stored dry, reconstitute it using a suitable liquid.

Prepare mixtures of the solution of the reference preparation and the test toxin such that each contains 2.0 ml of the solution of the reference preparation, one of a graded series of volumes of the test toxin and sufficient of a suitable liquid to bring the volume to 5.0 ml. Allow the mixtures to stand at room temperature, protected from light, for 60 min. Using six mice for each mixture, inject a dose of 0.5 ml subcutaneously into each mouse. Observe the mice for 96 h. Mice that become paralysed may be killed.

The test dose of toxin is the quantity in 0.5 ml of the mixture made with the smallest amount of toxin capable of causing, despite partial neutralisation by the reference preparation, paralysis in all six mice injected with the mixture within the observation period.

Determination of potency of the antitoxin. Prepare a solution of the reference preparation in a suitable liquid such that it contains 0.5 IU of antitoxin per millilitre.

Prepare a solution of the test toxin in a suitable liquid such that it contains five test doses per millilitre.

Prepare mixtures of the solution of the test toxin and the antitoxin to be examined such that each contains 2.0 ml of the solution of the test toxin, one of a graded series of volumes of the antitoxin to be examined and sufficient of a suitable liquid to bring the total volume to 5.0 ml. Also prepare mixtures of the solution of the test toxin and the solution of the reference preparation such that each contains 2.0 ml of the solution of the test toxin, one of a graded series of volumes of the solution of the reference preparation centred on that volume (2.0 ml) that contains 1 IU and sufficient of a suitable liquid to bring the total volume to 5.0 ml. Allow the mixtures to stand at room temperature, protected from light, for 60 min. Using six mice for each mixture, inject into each mouse subcutaneously a dose of 0.5 ml. Observe the mice for 96 h. Mice that become paralysed may be killed.

The mixture that contains the largest volume of antitoxin that fails to protect the mice from paralysis contains 1 IU. This quantity is used to calculate the potency of the antitoxin in International Units per millilitre.

The test is not valid unless all the mice injected with mixtures containing 2.0 ml or less of the solution of the reference preparation show paralysis and all those injected with mixtures containing more do not.

01/2005:0145

VIPER VENOM ANTISERUM, EUROPEAN

Immunoserum contra venena viperarum europaearum

DEFINITION

European viper venom antiserum is a preparation containing antitoxic globulins that have the power of neutralising the venom of one or more species of viper. The globulins are obtained by fractionation of the serum of animals that have been immunised against the venom or venoms.

IDENTIFICATION

It neutralises the venom of *Vipera ammodytes*, or *Vipera aspis*, or *Vipera berus*, or *Vipera ursinii* or the mixture of these venoms stated on the label, rendering them harmless to susceptible animals.

ASSAY

Each millilitre of the preparation to be examined contains sufficient antitoxic globulins to neutralise not less than 100 mouse LD_{50} of *Vipera ammodytes* venom or *Vipera aspis* venom and not less than 50 mouse LD_{50} of the venoms of other species of viper.

The potency of European viper venom antiserum is determined by estimating the dose necessary to protect mice against the lethal effects of a fixed dose of venom of the relevant species of viper.

Selection of test venoms. Use venoms which have the normal physicochemical, toxicological and immunological characteristics of venoms from the particular species of vipers. They are preferably freeze-dried and stored in the dark at 5 ± 3 °C.

Select a venom for use as a test venom by determining the LD_{50} for mice, the observation period being 48 h.

Determination of the test dose of venom. Prepare graded dilutions of the reconstituted venom in a 9 g/l solution of *sodium chloride R* or other isotonic diluent in such a manner that the middle dilution contains in 0.25 ml the dose expected to be the LD_{50}. Dilute with an equal volume of the same diluent. Using at least four mice, each weighing 18 g to 20 g, for each dilution, inject 0.5 ml intravenously into each mouse. Observe the mice for 48 h and record the number of deaths. Calculate the LD_{50} using the usual statistical methods.

Determination of the potency of the antiserum to be examined. Dilute the reconstituted test venom so that 0.25 ml contains the test dose of 5 LD_{50} (test venom solution). Prepare serial dilutions of the antiserum to be examined in a 9 g/l solution of *sodium chloride R* or other isotonic diluent, the dilution factor being 1.5 to 2.5. Use a sufficient number and range of dilutions to enable a mortality curve between 20 per cent and 80 per cent mortality to be established and to permit an estimation of the statistical variation.

Prepare mixtures such that 5 ml of each mixture contains 2.5 ml of one of the dilutions of the antiserum to be examined and 2.5 ml of the test venom solution. Allow the mixtures to stand in a water-bath at 37 °C for 30 min. Using not fewer than six mice, each weighing 18 g to 20 g, for each mixture, inject 0.5 ml intravenously into each mouse. Observe the mice for 48 h and record the number of deaths. Calculate the PD_{50}, using the usual statistical methods. At the same time verify the number of LD_{50} in the test dose of venom, using the method described above. Calculate the potency of the antiserum from the expression:

$$\frac{(T_v - 1)}{PD_{50}}$$

T_v = number of LD_{50} in the test dose of venom.

In each mouse dose of the venom-antiserum mixture at the end point there is one LD_{50} of venom remaining unneutralised by the antiserum and it is this unneutralised venom that is responsible for the deaths of 50 per cent of the mice inoculated with the mixture. The amount of venom neutralised by the antiserum is thus one LD_{50} less than the total amount contained in each mouse dose. Therefore, as the potency of the antiserum is defined in terms of the number of LD_{50} of venom that are neutralised. rather than the number of LD_{50} in each mouse dose, the expression required in the calculation of potency is $T_v - 1$ rather than T_v.

Alternatively, the quantity of test venom in milligrams that is neutralised by 1 ml or some other defined volume of the antiserum to be examined may be calculated.

LABELLING

The label states the venom or venoms against which the antiserum is effective.

Warning: Because of the allergenic properties of viper venoms, inhalation of venom dust should be avoided by suitable precautions.

IMMUNOSERA FOR VETERINARY USE

01/2005:0339

CLOSTRIDIUM NOVYI ALPHA ANTITOXIN FOR VETERINARY USE

Immunoserum clostridii novyi alpha ad usum veterinarium

DEFINITION

Clostridium novyi alpha antitoxin for veterinary use is a preparation containing the globulins that have the power of specifically neutralising the alpha toxin formed by *Clostridium novyi* (Former nomenclature: *Clostridium oedematiens*). It consists of the serum or a preparation obtained from the serum of animals immunised against *Cl. novyi* alpha toxin.

IDENTIFICATION

It specifically neutralises the alpha toxin of *Cl. novyi* rendering it harmless to susceptible animals.

POTENCY

The potency of the crude serum is not less than 750 IU/ml when obtained from horses and not less than 250 IU/ml when obtained from cattle.

The potency of the concentrated serum is not less than 1500 IU/ml when obtained from horses and not less than 500 IU/ml when obtained from cattle.

The International Unit is the specific neutralising activity for *Cl. novyi* alpha toxin contained in a stated amount of the International Standard, which consists of a quantity of dried immune horse serum. The equivalence in International Units of the International Standard is stated by the World Health Organisation.

The potency of clostridium novyi alpha antitoxin is determined by comparing the dose necessary to protect mice or other suitable animals against the toxic effects of a fixed dose of *Cl. novyi* alpha toxin with the quantity of a reference preparation of clostridium novyi alpha antitoxin, calibrated in International Units, necessary to give the same protection. For this comparison, a suitable preparation of *Cl. novyi* alpha toxin for use as a test toxin is required. The dose of the test toxin is determined in relation to the reference preparation; the potency of the clostridium novyi alpha antitoxin to be examined is determined in relation to the reference preparation using the test toxin.

Preparation of test toxin. Prepare the test toxin from a sterile filtrate of an approximately 5-day culture in liquid medium of *Cl. novyi* type B and dry by a suitable method. Select the toxin by determining for mice the L+/10 dose and the LD_{50}, the observation period being 72 h. A suitable alpha toxin contains not less than one L+/10 dose in 0.05 mg and not less than 10 LD_{50} in each L+/10 dose.

Determination of test dose of toxin. Prepare a solution of the reference preparation in a suitable liquid so that it contains 1 IU/ml. Prepare a solution of the test toxin in a suitable liquid so that 1 ml contains a precisely known amount such as 1 mg. Prepare mixtures of the solution of the reference preparation and the solution of the test toxin such that each mixture contains 1.0 ml of the solution of the reference preparation (1 IU), one of a series of graded volumes of the solution of the test toxin and sufficient of a suitable liquid to bring the total volume to 2.0 ml. Allow the mixtures to stand at room temperature for 60 min. Using not fewer than two mice, each weighing 17 g to 22 g, for each mixture, inject a dose of 0.2 ml intramuscularly or subcutaneously into each mouse. Observe the mice for 72 h. If all the mice die, the amount of toxin present in 0.2 ml of the mixture is in excess of the test dose. If none of the mice dies, the amount of toxin present in 0.2 ml of the mixture is less than the test dose. Prepare similar fresh mixtures such that 2.0 ml of each mixture contains 1.0 ml of the reference preparation (1 IU) and one of a series of graded volumes of the solution of the test toxin separated from each other by steps of not more than 20 per cent and covering the expected end-point. Allow the mixtures to stand at room temperature for 60 min.

Using not fewer than two mice for each mixture, inject a dose of 0.2 ml intramuscularly or subcutaneously into each mouse. Observe the mice for 72 h. Repeat the determination at least once and combine the results of the separate tests that have been made with mixtures of the same composition so that a series of totals is obtained, each total representing the mortality due to a mixture of a given composition. The test dose of toxin is the amount present in 0.2 ml of that mixture which causes the death of one half of the total number of mice injected with it.

Determination of the potency of the antitoxin to be examined

Preliminary test. Dissolve a quantity of the test toxin in a suitable liquid so that 1 ml contains ten times the test dose. Prepare mixtures of the solution of the test toxin and of the antitoxin to be examined such that each mixture contains 1.0 ml of the solution of the test toxin, one of a series of graded volumes of the antitoxin to be examined and sufficient of a suitable liquid to bring the final volume to 2.0 ml. Allow the mixtures to stand at room temperature for 60 min. Using not fewer than two mice for each mixture, inject a dose of 0.2 ml intramuscularly or subcutaneously into each mouse. Observe the mice for 72 h. If none of the mice dies, 0.2 ml of the mixture contains more than 0.1 IU. If all the mice die, 0.2 ml of the mixture contains less than 0.1 IU.

Final test. Prepare mixtures of the solution of the test toxin and of the antitoxin to be examined such that 2.0 ml of each mixture contains 1.0 ml of the solution of the test toxin and one of a series of graded volumes of the antitoxin to be examined, separated from each other by steps of not more than 20 per cent and covering the expected end-point as determined by the preliminary test. Prepare further mixtures such that 2.0 ml of each mixture contains 1.0 ml of the solution of the test toxin and one of a series of graded volumes of the solution of the reference preparation, in order to confirm the test dose of the toxin. Allow the mixtures to stand at room temperature for 60 min. Using not fewer than two mice for each mixture, proceed as described in the preliminary test. The test mixture which contains 0.1 IU in 0.2 ml is that mixture which kills the same or almost the same number of mice as the reference mixture containing 0.1 IU in 0.2 ml. Repeat the determination at least once and calculate the average of all valid estimates. Estimates are valid only if the reference preparation gives a result within 20 per cent of the expected value.

The confidence limits (P = 0.95) have been estimated to be:

85 per cent and 114 per cent when two animals per dose are used,

91.5 per cent and 109 per cent when four animals per dose are used,

93 per cent and 108 per cent when six animals per dose are used.

LABELLING

The label states whether the product consists of crude or concentrated serum.

Immunosera

01/2005:0340

CLOSTRIDIUM PERFRINGENS BETA ANTITOXIN FOR VETERINARY USE

Immunoserum clostridii perfringentis beta ad usum veterinarium

DEFINITION

Clostridium perfringens beta antitoxin for veterinary use is a preparation containing principally the globulins that have the power of specifically neutralising the beta toxin formed by *Clostridium perfringens* (types B and C). It consists of the serum or a preparation obtained from the serum of animals immunised against *Cl. perfringens* beta toxin.

IDENTIFICATION

It specifically neutralises the beta toxin of *Cl. perfringens* rendering it harmless to susceptible animals.

POTENCY

The potency of the crude serum is not less than 1000 IU/ml when obtained from horses and not less than 250 IU/ml when obtained from cattle.

The potency of the concentrated serum is not less than 3000 IU/ml when obtained from horses and not less than 1000 IU/ml when obtained from cattle.

The International Unit is the specific neutralising activity for *Cl. perfringens* beta toxin contained in a stated amount of the International Standard, which consists of a quantity of dried immune horse serum. The equivalence in International Units of the International Standard is stated by the World Health Organisation.

The potency of clostridium perfringens beta antitoxin is determined by comparing the dose necessary to protect mice or other suitable animals against the toxic effects of a fixed dose of *Cl. perfringens* beta toxin with the quantity of a reference preparation of clostridium perfringens beta antitoxin, calibrated in International Units, necessary to give the same protection. For this comparison, a suitable preparation of *Cl. perfringens* beta toxin for use as a test toxin is required. The dose of the test toxin is determined in relation to the reference preparation; the potency of the clostridium perfringens beta antitoxin to be examined is determined in relation to the reference preparation using the test toxin.

Preparation of test toxin. Prepare the test toxin from a sterile filtrate of an early culture in liquid medium of *Cl. perfringens* type B or type C and dry by a suitable method.

Select the test toxin by determining for mice the L+ dose and the LD_{50}, the observation period being 72 h. A suitable beta toxin contains not less than one L+ dose in 0.2 mg and not less than 25 LD_{50} in each L+ dose.

Determination of test dose of toxin. Prepare a solution of the reference preparation in a suitable liquid so that it contains 5 IU/ml. Prepare a solution of the test toxin in a suitable liquid so that 1 ml contains a precisely known amount such as 10 mg. Prepare mixtures of the solution of the reference preparation and the solution of the test toxin such that each mixture contains 2.0 ml of the solution of the reference preparation (10 IU), one of a series of graded volumes of the solution of the test toxin and sufficient of a suitable liquid to bring the total volume to 5.0 ml. Allow the mixtures to stand at room temperature for 30 min. Using not fewer than two mice, each weighing 17 g to 22 g, for each mixture, inject a dose of 0.5 ml intravenously or intra-peritoneally into each mouse. Observe the mice for 72 h. If all the mice die, the amount of toxin present in 0.5 ml of the mixture is in excess of the test dose. If none of the mice dies, the amount of toxin present in 0.5 ml of the mixture is less than the test dose. Prepare fresh mixtures such that 5.0 ml of each mixture contains 2.0 ml of the solution of the reference preparation (10 IU) and one of a series of graded volumes of the solution of the test toxin separated from each other by steps of not more than 20 per cent and covering the expected end-point. Allow the mixtures to stand at room temperature for 30 min.

Using not fewer than two mice for each mixture, inject a dose of 0.5 ml intravenously or intraperitoneally into each mouse. Observe the mice for 72 h. Repeat the determination at least once and combine the results of the separate tests that have been made with mixtures of the same composition so that a series of totals is obtained, each total representing the mortality due to a mixture of a given composition. The test dose of toxin is the amount present in 0.5 ml of that mixture which causes the death of one half of the total number of mice injected with it.

Determination of the potency of the antitoxin to be examined

Preliminary test. Dissolve a quantity of the test toxin in a suitable liquid so that 2.0 ml contains 10 times the test dose. Prepare mixtures of the solution of the test toxin and the antitoxin to be examined such that each mixture contains 2.0 ml of the solution of the test toxin, one of a series of graded volumes of the antitoxin to be examined and sufficent of a suitable liquid to bring the final volume to 5.0 ml. Allow the mixtures to stand at room temperature for 30 min. Using not fewer than two mice for each mixture, inject a dose of 0.5 ml intravenously or intraperitoneally into each mouse. Observe the mice for 72 h. If none of the mice dies, 0.5 ml of the mixture contains more than 1 IU. If all the mice die, 0.5 ml of the mixture contains less than 1 IU.

Final test. Prepare mixtures of the solution of the test toxin and of the antitoxin to be examined such that 5.0 ml of each mixture contains 2.0 ml of the solution of the test toxin and one of a series of graded volumes of the antitoxin to be examined, separated from each other by steps of not more than 20 per cent and covering the expected end-point as determined by the preliminary test. Prepare further mixtures such that 5.0 ml of each mixture contains 2.0 ml of the solution of the test toxin and one of a series of graded volumes of the solution of the reference preparation, in order to confirm the test dose of the toxin. Allow the mixtures to stand at room temperature for 30 min. Using not fewer than two mice for each mixture, proceed as described in the preliminary test. The test mixture which contains, in 0.5 ml, 1 IU is that mixture which kills the same or almost the same number of mice as the reference mixture containing, in 0.5 ml, 1 IU. Repeat the determination at least once and calculate the average of all valid estimates. Estimates are valid only if the reference preparation gives a result within 20 per cent of the expected value.

The confidence limits ($P = 0.95$) have been estimated to be:

85 per cent and 114 per cent when two animals per dose are used,

91.5 per cent and 109 per cent when four animals per dose are used,

93 per cent and 108 per cent when six animals per dose are used.

LABELLING

The label states whether the product consist of crude concentrated serum.

Immunosera

01/2005:0341

CLOSTRIDIUM PERFRINGENS EPSILON ANTITOXIN FOR VETERINARY USE

Immunoserum clostridii perfringentis epsilon ad usum veterinarium

DEFINITION

Clostridium perfringens epsilon antitoxin for veterinary use is a preparation containing the globulins that have the power of specifically neutralising the epsilon toxin formed by *Clostridium perfringens* type D. It consists of the serum or a preparation obtained from the serum of animals immunised against *Cl. perfringens* epsilon toxin.

IDENTIFICATION

It specifically neutralises the epsilon toxin of *Cl. perfringens* type D, rendering it harmless to susceptible animals.

POTENCY

The potency of the crude serum is not less than 120 IU/ml when obtained from horses and not less than 100 IU/ml when obtained from cattle.

The potency of the concentrated serum is not less than 300 IU/ml when obtained from horses and not less than 150 IU/ml when obtained from cattle.

The International Unit is the specific neutralising activity for *Cl. perfringens* epsilon toxin contained in a stated amount of the International Standard, which consists of a quantity of dried immune horse serum. The equivalence in International Units of the International Standard is stated by the World Health Organisation.

The potency of clostridium perfringens epsilon antitoxin is determined by comparing the dose necessary to protect mice or other suitable animals against the toxic effects of a fixed dose of *Cl. perfringens* epsilon toxin with the quantity of a reference preparation of clostridium perfringens epsilon anti-toxin, calibrated in International Units, necessary to give the same protection. For this comparison, a suitable preparation of *Cl. perfringens* epsilon toxin for use as a test toxin is required. The dose of the test toxin is determined in relation to the reference preparation, the potency of the antitoxin to be examined is determined in relation to the reference preparation using the test toxin.

Preparation of test toxin. Prepare the test toxin from a sterile filtrate of an early culture in liquid medium of *Cl. perfringens* type D and dry by a suitable method.

Select the test toxin by determining for mice the L+/10 dose and the LD_{50}, the observation period being 72 h. A suitable epsilon toxin contains not less than one L+/10 dose in 0.005 mg and not less than 20 LD_{50} in each L+/10 dose.

Determination of test dose of toxin. Prepare a solution of the reference preparation in a suitable liquid so that it contains 0.5 IU of antitoxin per millilitre. Prepare a solution of the test toxin in a suitable liquid so that 1 ml contains a precisely known amount such as 1 mg. Prepare mixtures of the solution of the reference preparation and the solution of the test toxin such that each mixture contains 2.0 ml of the solution of the reference preparation (1 IU), one of a series of graded volumes of the solution of the test toxin and sufficient of a suitable liquid to bring the total volume to 5.0 ml. Allow the mixtures to stand at room temperature for 30 min. Using not fewer than two mice, each weighing 17 g to 22 g, for each mixture, inject a dose of 0.5 ml intravenously or intraperitoneally into each mouse. Observe the mice for 72 h. If all the mice die, the amount of toxin present in 0.5 ml of the mixture is in excess of the test dose. If none of the mice dies, the amount of toxin present in 0.5 ml of the mixture is less than the test dose.

Prepare similar fresh mixtures such that 5.0 ml of each mixture contains 2.0 ml of the solution of the reference preparation (1 IU) and one of a series of graded volumes of the solution of the test toxin, separated from each other by steps of not more than 20 per cent and covering the expected end-point. Allow the mixtures to stand at room temperature for 30 min. Using not fewer than two mice for each mixture, inject a dose of 0.5 ml intravenously or intraperitoneally into each mouse. Observe the mice for 72 h. Repeat the determination at least once and add together the results of the separ-ate tests that have been made with mixtures of the same composition so that a series of totals is obtained, each total representing the mortality due to a mixture of a given composition. The test dose of the toxin is the amount present in 0.5 ml of that mixture which causes the death of one half of the total number of mice injected with it.

Determination of the potency of the antitoxin to be examined

Preliminary test. Dissolve a quantity of the test toxin in a suitable liquid so that 2.0 ml contains 10 times the test dose (solution of the test toxin). Prepare mixtures of the solution of the test toxin and of the antitoxin to be examined such that each mixture contains 2.0 ml of the solution of the test toxin, one of a series of graded volumes of the antitoxin to be examined and sufficient of a suitable liquid to bring the final volume to 5.0 ml. Allow the mixtures to stand at room temperature for 30 min. Using not fewer than two mice for each mixture, inject a dose of 0.5 ml intravenously or intra-peritoneally into each mouse. Observe the mice for 72 h. If none of the mice dies, 0.5 ml of the mixture contains more than 0.1 IU. If all the mice die, 0.5 ml of the mixture contains less than 0.1 IU.

Final test. Prepare mixtures of the solution of the test toxin and of the antitoxin to be examined such that 5.0 ml of each mixture contains 2.0 ml of the solution of the test toxin and one of a series of graded volumes of the antitoxin to be examined, separated from each other by steps of not more than 20 per cent and covering the expected end-point as determined by the preliminary test. Prepare further mixtures such that 5.0 ml of each mixture contains 2.0 ml of the solution of the test toxin and one of a series of graded volumes of the solution of the reference preparation to confirm the test dose of the toxin. Allow the mixtures to stand at room temperature for 30 min. Using not fewer than two mice for each mixture proceed as described in the preliminary test. The test mixture which contains 0.1 IU in 0.5 ml is that mixture which kills the same or almost the same number of mice as the reference mixture containing 0.1 IU in 0.5 ml. Repeat the determination at least once and calculate the average of all valid estimates. Estimates are valid only if the reference preparation gives a result within 20 per cent of the expected value.

The confidence limits ($P = 0.95$) have been estimated to be:

85 per cent and 114 per cent when 2 animals per dose are used,

91.5 per cent and 109 per cent when 4 animals per dose are used,

93 per cent and 108 per cent when 6 animals per dose are used.

Immunosera

LABELLING

The label states whether the product consists of crude or concentrated serum.

01/2005:0343

TETANUS ANTITOXIN FOR VETERINARY USE

Immunoserum tetanicum ad usum veterinarium

DEFINITION

Tetanus antitoxin for veterinary use is a preparation containing principally the globulins that have the power of specifically neutralising the neurotoxin formed by *Clostridium tetani.* It consists of the serum or a preparation obtained from the serum of animals immunised against tetanus toxin.

IDENTIFICATION

It specifically neutralises the neurotoxin formed by *Cl. tetani,* rendering it harmless to susceptible animals.

POTENCY

The potency of the crude serum is not less than 300 IU/ml when obtained from horses and not less than 150 IU/ml when obtained from cattle.

The potency of the concentrated serum is not less than 1000 IU/ml when obtained from horses and not less than 500 IU/ml when obtained from cattle.

The International Unit is the specific neutralising activity for tetanus toxin contained in a stated amount of the International Standard which consists of a quantity of dried immune horse serum. The equivalence in International Units of the International Standard is stated by the World Health Organisation.

The potency of tetanus antitoxin is determined by comparing the dose necessary to protect mice (or guinea-pigs) against the toxic effects of a fixed dose of tetanus toxin with the quantity of a reference preparation of tetanus antitoxin, calibrated in International Units, necessary to give the same protection. In countries where the paralysis method is not obligatory, the lethal method may be used. For this method the number of animals and the procedure are identical with those described for the paralysis method but the end-point is the death of the animal rather than the onset of paralysis and the L+/10 dose and the LD_{50} are used instead of the Lp/10 dose and the paralytic dose 50 per cent. For this comparison, a suitable preparation of tetanus toxin for use as a test toxin is required. The dose of the test toxin is determined in relation to the reference preparation; the potency of the antitoxin to be examined is determined in relation to the reference preparation using the test toxin.

Preparation of test toxin. Prepare the test toxin from a sterile filtrate of an 8 to 10 day culture in liquid medium of *Cl. tetani.* A test toxin may be prepared by adding this filtrate to *glycerol R* in the proportion of 1 volume of filtrate to 1 to 2 volumes of *glycerol R.* The solution of test toxin may be stored at or slightly below 0 °C. The toxin may also be dried by a suitable method.

Select the test toxin by determining for mice the Lp/10 dose and the paralytic dose 50 per cent. A suitable toxin contains not less than 1000 times the paralytic dose 50 per cent in one Lp/10 dose.

Lp/10 dose (Limes paralyticum). This is the smallest quantity of toxin which when mixed with 0.1 IU of antitoxin and injected subcutaneously into mice (or guinea-pigs) causes tetanic paralysis in the animals on or before the fourth day after injection.

Paralytic dose 50 per cent. This is the quantity of toxin which when injected subcutaneously into mice (or guinea-pigs) causes tetanic paralysis in one half of the animals on or before the fourth day after injection.

Determination of test dose of toxin. Reconstitute or dilute the reference preparation with a suitable liquid so that it contains 0.5 IU per millilitre. Measure or weigh a quantity of the test toxin and dilute with or dissolve in a suitable liquid. Prepare mixtures of the solution of the reference preparation and the solution of the test toxin so that each mixture will contain 0.1 IU of antitoxin in the volume chosen for injection and one of a series of graded volumes of the solution of the test toxin, separated from each other by steps of not more than 20 per cent and covering the expected end-point. Adjust each mixture with a suitable liquid to the same final volume (0.4 ml to 0.6 ml if mice are used for the test or 4.0 ml if guinea-pigs are used). Allow the mixtures to stand at room temperature for 60 min. Using not fewer than two animals for each mixture, inject the chosen volume subcutaneously into each animal. Observe the animals for 96 h and make daily records of the degree of tetanus developing in each group of animals. Repeat the test at least once and calculate the test dose as the mean of the different tests. The test dose of the toxin is the amount present in that mixture which causes tetanic paralysis in one half of the total number of animals injected with it.

When the test dose of the toxin has been determined a concentrated solution of the test toxin may be prepared in a mixture consisting of 1 volume of a 9 g/l solution of *sodium chloride R* and 1 or 2 volumes of *glycerol R.* This concentrated solution may be stored frozen and diluted as required. The specific activity of such a solution should be redetermined at frequent intervals.

Determination of the potency of the antitoxin to be examined

Preliminary test. Measure or weigh a quantity of the test toxin and dilute with or dissolve in a suitable liquid so that the solution contains five test doses per millilitre (solution of the test toxin). Prepare mixtures of the solution of the test toxin and the antitoxin to be examined so that for each mixture the volume chosen for injection contains the test dose of toxin and one of a series of graded volumes of the antitoxin to be examined. Adjust each mixture to the same final volume with a suitable liquid. Allow the mixtures to stand at room temperature for 60 min. Using not fewer than two animals for each mixture, inject the chosen volume subcutaneously into each animal. Observe the animals for 96 h and make daily records of the degree of tetanus developing in each group of animals. Using the results, select suitable mixtures for the final test.

Final test. Prepare mixtures of the solution of the test toxin and the antitoxin to be examined so that for each mixture the volume chosen for the injection contains the test dose of toxin and one of a series of graded volumes of the antitoxin to be examined, separated from each other by steps of not more than 20 per cent and covering the expected end-point as determined in the preliminary test. Prepare further mixtures with the same amount of test toxin and graded volumes of the reference preparation, centred on 0.1 IU in the volume chosen for injection, to confirm the test dose of the toxin. Adjust each mixture to the same final volume with a suitable liquid. Allow the mixtures to stand at room temperature for

60 min. Using not fewer than two animals for each mixture, inject the chosen volume subcutaneously into each animal. Observe the animals for 96 h and make daily records of the degree of tetanus developing in each group of animals. The test mixture which contains 0.1 IU in the volume injected is that mixture which causes tetanic paralysis in the same, or almost the same, number of animals as the reference mixture containing 0.1 IU in the volume injected.

Repeat the determination at least once and calculate the mean of all valid estimates. Estimates are valid only if the reference preparation gives a result within 20 per cent of the expected value.

The confidence limits ($P = 0.95$) have been estimated to be:

85 per cent and 114 per cent when 2 animals per dose are used,

91.5 per cent and 109 per cent when 3 animals per dose are used,

93 per cent and 108 per cent when 6 animals per dose are used.

LABELLING

The label states whether the product consists of crude or concentrated serum.

Immunosera

RADIOPHARMACEUTICAL PREPARATIONS

01/2005:1492

AMMONIA (^{13}N) INJECTION

Ammoniae (^{13}N) solutio iniectabilis

DEFINITION

Ammonia (^{13}N) injection is a sterile solution of [^{13}N]ammonia for diagnostic use. The injection contains not less than 90.0 per cent and not more than 110.0 per cent of the declared nitrogen-13 radioactivity at the date and time stated on the label. Not less than 99 per cent of the total radioactivity corresponds to nitrogen-13 in the form of [^{13}N]ammonia. Not less than 99.0 per cent of the total radioactivity corresponds to nitrogen-13.

PRODUCTION

RADIONUCLIDE PRODUCTION

Nitrogen-13 is a radioactive isotope of nitrogen which may be produced by various nuclear reactions, such as proton irradiation of carbon-13 or oxygen-16, or deuteron irradiation of carbon-12.

RADIOCHEMICAL SYNTHESIS

[^{13}N]Ammonia may be prepared by proton irradiation of water followed by the reduction of the resulting [^{13}N]nitrates/nitrites mixture with a reducing agent. The [^{13}N]ammonia formed is distilled from the reaction mixture and trapped in a slightly acidic solution.

Other methods may produce [^{13}N]ammonia "in-target" by proton irradiation of water containing a small amount of ethanol or acetic acid, or by proton irradiation of a slurry of [^{13}C]carbon powder in water. The resulting solution can be purified, to remove radionuclidic and radiochemical impurities, using anion and cation exchange columns.

CHARACTERS

A clear, colourless solution.

Nitrogen-13 has a half-life of 9.96 min and emits positrons with a maximum energy of 1.198 MeV, followed by annihilation gamma radiation of 0.511 MeV.

IDENTIFICATION

A. Record the gamma-ray spectrum using a suitable instrument. The only gamma photons have an energy of 0.511 MeV and, depending on the measurement geometry, a sum peak of 1.022 MeV may be observed.

B. It complies with test (a) for radionuclidic purity (see Tests).

C. Examine the chromatograms obtained in the test for radiochemical purity. The principal peak in the radiochromatogram obtained with the test solution has approximately the same retention time as the principal peak in the radiochromatogram obtained with the reference solution.

TESTS

pH (*2.2.3*). The pH of the injection is 5.5 to 8.5.

Sterility. It complies with the test for sterility prescribed in the monograph on *Radiopharmaceutical preparations (0125)*. The injection may be released for use before completion of the test.

Bacterial endotoxins (*2.6.14*): less than 175/*V* IU/ml, *V* being the maximum recommended dose in millilitres. The injection may be released for use before completion of the test.

CHEMICAL PURITY

Aluminium. In a test-tube about 12 mm in internal diameter, mix 1 ml of *acetate buffer solution pH 4.6 R* and 2 ml of a 1 in 20 dilution of the preparation to be examined in *water R*. Add 0.05 ml of a 10 g/l solution of *chromazurol S R*. After 3 min, the colour of the solution is not more intense than that of a standard prepared at the same time and in the same manner using 2 ml of a 1 in 20 dilution of *aluminium standard solution (2 ppm Al) R* (2 ppm).

The injection may be released for use before completion of the test.

RADIONUCLIDIC PURITY

(a) *Half-life*. The half-life is between 9 min and 11 min.

(b) *Gamma emitting impurities*. Retain a sample of the preparation to be examined for 2 h. Examine the gamma-ray spectrum of the decayed material for the presence of radionuclidic impurities, which should, where possible, be identified and quantified. The total gamma radioactivity due to these impurities does not exceed 1.0 per cent of the total radioactivity.

The injection may be released for use before completion of tests (a) and (b).

RADIOCHEMICAL PURITY

Examine by liquid chromatography (*2.2.29*).

Test solution. The preparation to be examined.

Reference solution. Dilute 1.0 ml of *dilute ammonia R2* to 10.0 ml with *water R*.

The chromatographic procedure may be carried out using:

- a column 0.04 m long and 4.0 mm in internal diameter packed with *cation exchange resin R* (10 μm),
- as mobile phase at a flow rate of 2 ml/min *0.002 M nitric acid*,
- a suitable radioactivity detector,
- a conductivity detector,
- a loop injector,

maintaining the column at a constant temperature between 20 °C and 30 °C.

Inject separately the test solution and the reference solution. The chromatogram obtained with the radioactivity detector and the test solution shows a principal peak with approximately the same retention time as the peak in the chromatogram obtained with the reference solution and the conductivity detector. Not less than 99 per cent of the total radioactivity corresponds to nitrogen-13 in the form of ammonia.

The injection may be released for use before completion of the test.

RADIOACTIVITY

Measure the radioactivity using suitable equipment by comparison with a standardised fluorine-18 solution or by using an instrument calibrated with the aid of such a solution. Standardised fluorine-18 solutions are available from laboratories recognised by the competent authority.

IMPURITIES

A. [^{13}N]O_2^-,

B. [^{13}N]O_3^-,

C. [18F$^-$],

D. H_2[^{15}O].

01/2005:1607

CARBON MONOXIDE (^{15}O)

Carbonei monoxidum (^{15}O)

DEFINITION

Mixture of carbon [^{15}O]monoxide in the gaseous phase and a suitable vehicle such as *Medicinal air (1238)*, for diagnostic use.

Purity:

- minimum 99 per cent of the total radioactivity corresponds to oxygen-15,
- minimum 97 per cent of the total radioactivity corresponds to oxygen-15 in the form of carbon monoxide (CO).

PRODUCTION

RADIONUCLIDE PRODUCTION

Oxygen-15 is a radioactive isotope of oxygen which may be produced by various nuclear reactions such as proton irradiation of nitrogen-15 or deuteron irradiation of nitrogen-14.

RADIOCHEMICAL SYNTHESIS

In order to recover oxygen-15 as molecular oxygen from the nitrogen target gas, carrier oxygen is added at concentrations generally ranging from 0.2 per cent *V/V* to 1.0 per cent *V/V*. After irradiation, the target gas is usually reacted with activated charcoal at a temperature of about 950 °C. The activated charcoal is preconditioned before use by flushing an inert gas at the production flow rate at a temperature of about 950 °C for not less than 1 h. The carbon [^{15}O]monoxide obtained is purified by passage through a carbon dioxide scavenger, such as soda lime, before mixing with the vehicle.

CHARACTERS

Appearance: colourless gas.

Half-life and nature of radiation of oxygen-15: see Table of physical characteristics of radionuclides (*5.7*).

IDENTIFICATION

A. Gamma spectrometry.
   Results: the only gamma photons have an energy of 0.511 MeV and, depending on the measurement geometry, a sum peak of 1.022 MeV may be observed.

B. It complies with the test for radionuclidic purity (see Tests).

C. Examine the chromatograms obtained in the test for radiochemical purity.
   Results: the principal peaks in the chromatogram obtained with the test gas using the radioactivity detector are similar in retention times to the principal peaks corresponding to carbon monoxide in the chromatogram obtained with reference gas (a) using the thermal conductivity detector.

TESTS

The following tests are performed on carbon [^{15}O]monoxide as described under radiochemical synthesis before mixing with the vehicle.

Carbon monoxide. Gas chromatography (*2.2.28*) as described in the test for radiochemical purity.

The concentration of carbon monoxide in the test sample is determined before administration and is used to calculate the amount of carbon monoxide to be administered to the patient.

Injection: test sample, reference gas (b).

Examine the chromatogram obtained with the thermal conductivity detector and calculate the content of carbon monoxide.

RADIONUCLIDIC PURITY

Oxygen-15: minimum 99 per cent of the total radioactivity.

A. Gamma spectrometry.
   Comparison: standardised fluorine-18 solution, or by using an instrument calibrated with the aid of such a solution. Standardised fluorine-18 solutions and/or standardisation services are available from the competent authority.
   Results: the spectrum obtained with the solution to be examined does not differ significantly from that obtained with a standardised fluorine-18 solution.

B. Half-life: 1.9 min to 2.2 min.

The preparation may be released for use before completion of the test.

RADIOCHEMICAL PURITY

Carbon [^{15}O]monoxide. Gas chromatography (*2.2.28*): use the normalisation procedure.

Test sample. Carbon [^{15}O]monoxide as described under radiochemical synthesis.

Reference gas (a). Nitrogen gas mixture R.

Reference gas (b). Nitrogen R, containing 2.0 per cent *V/V* of *carbon monoxide R1*.

Column:

- *size*: l = 1.8 m, Ø1 = 6.3 mm and Ø2 = 3.2 mm,
- *stationary phase*: *GC concentrical column R*,

Carrier gas: *helium for chromatography R*.

Flow rate: 65 ml/min.

Temperature:

- *column*: 40 °C,
- *injection port*: 40 °C,
- *thermal conductivity detector*: 70 °C.

Detection: thermal conductivity detector and radioactivity detector connected in series.

Injection: loop injector.

Run time: 10 min.

Retention times: oxygen, nitrogen and carbon monoxide eluting from the inner column = about 0.4 min; carbon dioxide eluting from the inner column = about 0.8 min; oxygen eluting from the outer column = about 2.1 min; nitrogen eluting from the outer column = about 3.1 min; carbon monoxide eluting from the outer column = about 6.2 min.

System suitability: reference gas (a):

- 5 clearly separated principal peaks are observed in the chromatogram obtained using the thermal conductivity detector,
- *resolution*: minimum of 1.5 between the peaks due to carbon dioxide eluting from the inner column and oxygen eluting from the outer column, in the chromatogram obtained using the thermal conductivity detector.

Limits: examine the chromatogram obtained with the radioactivity detector and calculate the percentage content of oxygen-15 substances from the peak areas.

- *carbon [^{15}O]monoxide*: minimum 97 per cent of the total radioactivity.
- *disregard* the first peak corresponding to components co-eluting from the inner column.

Radiopharmaceutical preparations

RADIOACTIVITY

The radioactive concentration is determined before administration.

Measure the radioactivity using suitable equipment by comparison with a standardised fluorine-18 solution or by measurement in an instrument calibrated with the aid of such a solution.

01/2005:0266

CHROMIUM (^{51}Cr) EDETATE INJECTION

Chromii (^{51}Cr) edetatis solutio iniectabilis

DEFINITION

Chromium (^{51}Cr) edetate injection is a sterile solution containing chromium-51 in the form of a complex of chromium(III) with ethylenediaminetetraacetic acid, the latter being present in excess. It may be made isotonic by the addition of sodium chloride and may contain a suitable antimicrobial preservative such as benzyl alcohol. Chromium-51 is a radioactive isotope of chromium and may be prepared by the neutron irradiation of chromium, either of natural isotopic composition or enriched in chromium-50. The injection contains not less than 90.0 per cent and not more than 110.0 per cent of the declared chromium-51 radioactivity at the date and hour stated on the label. Not less than 95 per cent of the radioactivity corresponds to chromium-51 in the form of chromium edetate. The injection contains a variable quantity of chromium (Cr) not exceeding 1 mg per millilitre.

CHARACTERS

A clear, violet solution.

Chromium-51 has a half-life of 27.7 days and emits gamma radiation.

IDENTIFICATION

A. Record the gamma-ray spectrum using a suitable instrument. The spectrum does not differ significantly from that of a standardised chromium-51 solution. Standardised chromium-51 solutions are available from laboratories recognised by the competent authority. The gamma photon has an energy of 0.320 MeV.

B. Examine the electropherogram obtained in the test for radiochemical purity. The distribution of radioactivity contributes to the identification of the preparation.

TESTS

pH (*2.2.3*). The pH of the solution is 3.5 to 6.5.

Chromium. Prepare a reference solution (1 mg per millilitre of Cr) as follows: dissolve 0.96 g of *chromic potassium sulphate R* and 2.87 g of *sodium edetate R* in 50 ml of *water R*, boil for 10 min, cool, adjust to pH 3.5 to 6.5 using *dilute sodium hydroxide solution R* and dilute to 100.0 ml with *water R*. Measure the absorbance (*2.2.25*) of the injection to be examined and the reference solution at the absorption maximum at 560 nm. The absorbance of the injection to be examined is not greater than that of the reference solution.

Sterility. It complies with the test for sterility prescribed in the monograph on *Radiopharmaceutical preparations (0125)*. The injection may be released for use before completion of the test.

RADIONUCLIDIC PURITY

Record the gamma-ray spectrum using a suitable instrument. The spectrum does not differ significantly from that of a standardised chromium-51 solution.

RADIOCHEMICAL PURITY

Examine by zone electrophoresis (*2.2.31*), using a paper strip as the support and a solution containing 0.2 g/l of *barbital sodium R* and 10 g/l of *sodium nitrate R* as the electrolyte solution. A paper with the following characteristics is suitable: mass per unit area 120 g/m^2; thickness 0.22 mm; capillary rise 105 mm to 115 mm per 30 min.

Apply to the paper 10 µl of the injection as a 3 mm band at a position 10 cm from the cathode. Apply an electric field of about 30 V per centimetre for 30 min using a stabilised current. [^{51}Cr]chromium edetate moves about 5 cm towards the anode. [^{51}Cr]Chromate moves about 10 cm towards the anode and [^{51}Cr]chromic ion moves about 7 cm towards the cathode. Determine the distribution of the radioactivity using a suitable detector. Not less than 95 per cent of the total radioactivity is found in the band corresponding to [^{51}Cr]chromium edetate.

RADIOACTIVITY

Measure the radioactivity using suitable equipment by comparison with a standardised chromium-51 solution or by measurement in an instrument calibrated with the aid of such a solution.

01/2005:0710

CYANOCOBALAMIN (^{57}Co) CAPSULES

Cyanocobalamini (^{57}Co) capsulae

DEFINITION

Cyanocobalamin (^{57}Co) capsules contain [^{57}Co]-α-(5,6-dimethylbenzimidazol-1-yl)cobamide cyanide and may contain suitable auxiliary substances. Cobalt-57 is a radioactive isotope of cobalt and may be produced by proton irradiation of nickel. Cyanocobalamin (^{57}Co) may be prepared by the growth of suitable micro-organisms on a medium containing (^{57}Co) cobaltous ion. Not less than 90 per cent of the cobalt-57 is in the form of cyanocobalamin. The capsules comply with the requirements for hard capsules in the monograph on *Capsules (0016)*, unless otherwise justified and authorised.

CHARACTERS

Hard gelatin capsules.

Cobalt-57 has a half-life of 271 days and emits gamma radiation.

IDENTIFICATION

A. Record the gamma-ray spectrum using a suitable instrument. The spectrum does not differ significantly from that of a standardised cobalt-57 solution. Standardised cobalt-57 and cobalt-58 solutions are available from laboratories recognised by the competent authority. The most prominent gamma photon of cobalt-57 has an energy of 0.122 MeV.

B. Examine the chromatograms obtained in the test for radiochemical purity. The principal peak in the radio-chromatogram obtained with the test solution has a retention time similar to that of the peak in the chromatogram obtained with the reference solution.

TESTS

Disintegration. The capsules comply with the test for disintegration of tablets and capsules (*2.9.1*) except that one capsule is used in the test instead of six.

Uniformity of content. Determine by measurement in a suitable counting assembly and under identical geometrical conditions the radioactivity of each of not less than ten capsules. Calculate the average radioactivity per capsule. The radioactivity of no capsule differs by more than 10 per cent from the average. The relative standard deviation is less than 3.5 per cent.

RADIONUCLIDIC PURITY

Record the gamma-ray spectrum using a suitable instrument calibrated with the aid of standardised cobalt-57 and cobalt-58 solutions. The spectrum does not differ significantly from that of the stan-dardised cobalt-57 solution. Determine the relative amounts of cobalt-57, cobalt-56 and cobalt-58 present. Cobalt-56 has a half-life of 78 days and its presence is shown by gamma photons of energy 0.847 MeV. Cobalt-58 has a half-life of 70.8 days and its presence is shown by gamma photons of energy 0.811 MeV. Not more than 0.1 per cent of the total radioactivity is due to cobalt-56, cobalt-58 and other radionuclidic impurities.

RADIOCHEMICAL PURITY

Examine by liquid chromatography (*2.2.29*).

Test solution. Dissolve the contents of a capsule in 1.0 ml of *water R* and allow to stand for 10 min. Centrifuge at 2000 r/min for 10 min. Use the supernatant.

Reference solution. Dissolve 10 mg of *cyanocobalamin CRS* in the mobile phase and dilute to 100 ml with the mobile phase. Dilute 2 ml of the solution to 100 ml with the mobile phase. Use within 1 h.

The chromatographic procedure may be carried out using:

- a stainless steel column 0.25 m long and 4 mm in internal diameter packed with *octylsilyl silica gel for chromatography R* (5 μm),
- as mobile phase at a flow rate of 1.0 ml/min a mixture prepared as follows: mix 26.5 volumes of *methanol R* and 73.5 volumes of a 10 g/l solution of *disodium hydrogen phosphate R* adjusted to pH 3.5 using *phosphoric acid R* and use within 2 days,
- a radioactivity detector adjusted for cobalt-57,
- as detector a spectrophotometer set at 361 nm,
- a loop injector.

Inject 100 μl of the test solution and record the chromatogram for three times the retention time of cyanocobalamin. Determine the peak areas and calculate the percentage of cobalt-57 present as cyanocobalamin. Inject 100 μl of the reference solution and record the chromatogram for 30 min.

RADIOACTIVITY

The average radioactivity determined in the test for uniformity of content is not less than 90.0 per cent and not more than 110.0 per cent of the declared cobalt-57 radioactivity, at the date stated on the label.

STORAGE

Store in an airtight container, protected from light, at a temperature of 2 °C to 8 °C.

01/2005:0269

CYANOCOBALAMIN (^{57}Co) SOLUTION

Cyanocobalamini (^{57}Co) solutio

DEFINITION

Cyanocobalamin (^{57}Co) solution is a solution of [^{57}Co]-α-(5,6-dimethylbenzimidazol-1-yl)cobamide cyanide and may contain a stabiliser and an antimicrobial preservative. Cobalt-57 is a radioactive isotope of cobalt and may be produced by the irradiation of nickel with protons of suitable energy. Cyanocobalamin (^{57}Co) may be prepared by the growth of suitable micro-organisms on a medium containing (^{57}Co) cobaltous ion. The solution contains not less than 90.0 per cent and not more than 110.0 per cent of the declared cobalt-57 radioactivity at the date stated on the label. Not less than 90 per cent of the cobalt-57 is in the form of cyanocobalamin.

CHARACTERS

A clear, colourless or slightly pink solution. Cobalt-57 has a half-life of 271 days and emits gamma radiation.

IDENTIFICATION

A. Record the gamma-ray spectrum using a suitable instrument. The spectrum does not differ significantly from that of a standardised cobalt-57 solution. Standardised cobalt-57 and cobalt-58 solutions are available from laboratories recognised by the competent authority. The most prominent gamma photon of cobalt-57 has an energy of 0.122 MeV.

B. Examine the chromatograms obtained in the test for radiochemical purity. The principal peak in the radiochromatogram obtained with the solution to be examined has a retention time similar to that of the peak in the chromatogram obtained with the reference solution.

TESTS

pH (*2.2.3*). The pH of the solution is 4.0 to 6.0.

RADIONUCLIDIC PURITY

Record the gamma-ray spectrum using a suitable instrument calibrated with the aid of standardised cobalt-57 and cobalt-58 solutions. The spectrum does not differ significantly from that of the standardised cobalt-57 solution. Determine the relative amounts of cobalt-57, cobalt-56 and cobalt-58 present. Cobalt-56 has a half-life of 78 days and its presence is shown by gamma photons of energy 0.847 MeV. Cobalt-58 has a half-life of 70.8 days and its presence is shown by gamma photons of energy 0.811 MeV. Not more than 0.1 per cent of the total radioactivity is due to cobalt-56, cobalt-58 and other radionuclidic impurities.

RADIOCHEMICAL PURITY

Examine by liquid chromatography (*2.2.29*).

Reference solution. Dissolve 10 mg of *cyanocobalamin CRS* in the mobile phase and dilute to 100 ml with the mobile phase. Dilute 2 ml of the solution to 100 ml with the mobile phase. Use within 1 h.

The chromatographic procedure may be carried out using:

- a stainless steel column 0.25 m long and 4 mm in internal diameter packed with *octylsilyl silica gel for chromatography R* (5 μm),

- as mobile phase at a flow rate of 1.0 ml/min a mixture prepared as follows: mix 26.5 volumes of *methanol R* and 73.5 volumes of a 10 g/l solution of *disodium hydrogen phosphate R* adjusted to pH 3.5 using *phosphoric acid R* and use within 2 days,
- a radioactivity detector adjusted for cobalt-57,
- as detector a spectrophotometer set at 361 nm,
- a loop injector.

Inject 100 µl of the solution to be examined and record the chromatogram for three times the retention time of cyanocobalamin. Determine the peak areas and calculate the percentage of cobalt-57 present as cyanocobalamin. Inject 100 µl of the reference solution and record the chromatogram for 30 min.

RADIOACTIVITY

Measure the radioactivity using suitable counting equipment by comparison with a standardised cobalt-57 solution.

STORAGE

Store protected from light at a temperature of 2 °C to 8 °C.

01/2005:1505

CYANOCOBALAMIN (^{58}Co) CAPSULES

Cyanocobalamini (^{58}Co) capsulae

DEFINITION

Cyanocobalamin (^{58}Co) capsules contain [^{58}Co]-α-(5,6-dimethylbenzimidazol-1-yl)cobamide cyanide and may contain suitable auxiliary substances. Cobalt-58 is a radioactive isotope of cobalt and may be produced by neutron irradiation of nickel. Cyanocobalamin (^{58}Co) may be prepared by the growth of suitable micro-organisms on a medium containing (^{58}Co) cobaltous ion. Not less than 84 per cent of the cobalt-58 is in the form of cyanocobalamin. The capsules comply with the requirements for hard capsules in the monograph on *Capsules (0016)*, unless otherwise justified and authorised. The average radioactivity is not less than 90.0 per cent and not more than 110.0 per cent of the declared cobalt-58 radioactivity at the date stated on the label.

CHARACTERS

Hard gelatin capsules.

Cobalt-58 has a half-life of 70.9 days and emits beta (β^+) radiation and gamma radiation.

IDENTIFICATION

A. Record the gamma-ray spectrum using a suitable instrument. The spectrum does not differ significantly from that of a standardised cobalt-58 solution. Standardised cobalt-58 solutions are available from laboratories recognised by the competent authority. The most prominent gamma photons of cobalt-58 have energies of 0.511 MeV (annihilation radiation) and 0.811 MeV.

B. Examine the chromatograms obtained in the test for radiochemical purity. The principal peak in the radiochromatogram obtained with the test solution has a retention time similar to that of the peak in the chromatogram obtained with the reference solution.

TESTS

Disintegration. The capsules comply with the test for disintegration of tablets and capsules (*2.9.1*) except that one capsule is used in the test instead of six.

Uniformity of content. Determine by measurement in a suitable counting assembly and under identical geometrical conditions the radioactivity of each of not less than ten capsules. Calculate the average radioactivity per capsule. The radioactivity of no capsule differs by more than 10 per cent from the average. The relative standard deviation is less than 3.5 per cent.

RADIONUCLIDIC PURITY

Record the gamma-ray spectrum using a suitable instrument calibrated with the aid of standardised cobalt-58, cobalt-57 and cobalt-60 solutions. The spectrum does not differ significantly from that of the standardised cobalt-58 solution. Standardised cobalt-58, cobalt-57 and cobalt-60 solutions are available from laboratories recognised by the competent authority. Determine the relative amounts of cobalt-58, cobalt-57 and cobalt-60 present. Cobalt-57 has a half-life of 272 days and its presence is shown by gamma photons of energy 0.122 MeV. Cobalt-60 has a half-life of 5.27 years and its presence is shown by gamma photons of energies 1.173 MeV and 1.333 MeV. Not more than 1 per cent of the total radioactivity is due to cobalt-60 and not more than 2 per cent of the total radioactivity is due to cobalt-57, cobalt-60 and other radionuclidic impurities.

RADIOCHEMICAL PURITY

Examine by liquid chromatography (*2.2.29*).

Test solution. Dissolve the contents of a capsule in 1.0 ml of *water R* and allow to stand for 10 min. Centrifuge at 2000 r/min for 10 min. Use the supernatant.

Reference solution. Dissolve 10 mg of *cyanocobalamin CRS* in the mobile phase and dilute to 100 ml with the mobile phase. Dilute 2 ml of the solution to 100 ml with the mobile phase. Use within 1 h of preparation.

The chromatographic procedure may be carried out using:

- a stainless steel column 0.25 m long and 4 mm in internal diameter packed with *octylsilyl silica gel for chromatography R* (5 µm),
- as mobile phase at a flow rate of 1.0 ml/min a mixture prepared as follows: mix 26.5 volumes of *methanol R* and 73.5 volumes of a 10 g/l solution of *disodium hydrogen phosphate R*, adjusted to pH 3.5 with *phosphoric acid R* and use within 2 days,
- a radioactivity detector adjusted for cobalt-58,
- as detector a spectrophotometer set at 361 nm,
- a loop injector.

Inject 100 µl of the test solution and record the chromatogram for three times the retention time of cyanocobalamin. Determine the peak areas and calculate the percentage of cobalt-58 present as cyanocobalamin. Inject 100 µl of the reference solution and record the chromatogram for 30 min.

RADIOACTIVITY

The average radioactivity determined in the test for uniformity of content is not less than 90.0 per cent and not more than 110.0 per cent of the declared cobalt-58 radioactivity, at the date stated on the label.

STORAGE

Store in an airtight container, protected from light, at a temperature of 2 °C to 8 °C.

01/2005:0270

CYANOCOBALAMIN (^{58}Co) SOLUTION

Cyanocobalamini (^{58}Co) solutio

DEFINITION

Cyanocobalamin (^{58}Co) solution is a solution of [^{58}Co]-α-(5,6-dimethylbenzimidazol-1-yl)cobamide cyanide and may contain a stabiliser and an antimicrobial preservative. Cobalt-58 is a radioactive isotope of cobalt and may be produced by neutron irradiation of nickel. Cyanocobalamin (^{58}Co) may be prepared by the growth of suitable micro-organisms on a medium containing (^{58}Co) cobaltous ion. The solution contains not less than 90.0 per cent and not more than 110.0 per cent of the declared cobalt-58 radioactivity at the date stated on the label. Not less than 90 per cent of the cobalt-58 is in the form of cyanocobalamin.

CHARACTERS

A clear, colourless or slightly pink solution.

Cobalt-58 has a half-life of 70.8 days and emits beta (β+) radiation and gamma radiation.

IDENTIFICATION

A. Record the gamma-ray spectrum using a suitable instrument. The spectrum does not differ significantly from that of a standardised cobalt-58 solution. Standardised cobalt-58, cobalt-57 and cobalt-60 solutions are available from laboratories recognised by the competent authority. The most prominent gamma photons of cobalt-58 have energies of 0.511 MeV (annihilation radiation) and 0.811 MeV.

B. Examine the chromatograms obtained in the test for radiochemical purity. The principal peak in the radiochromatogram obtained with the solution to be examined has a retention time similar to that of the peak in the chromatogram obtained with the reference solution.

TESTS

pH (*2.2.3*). The pH of the solution is 4.0 to 6.0.

RADIONUCLIDIC PURITY

Record the gamma-ray spectrum using a suitable instrument having adequate resolution and calibrated with the aid of standardised cobalt-58, cobalt-57 and cobalt-60 solutions. The spectrum does not differ significantly from that of the standardised cobalt-58 solution. Determine the relative amounts of cobalt-58, cobalt-57 and cobalt-60 present. Cobalt-57 has a half-life of 271 days and its presence is shown by gamma photons of energy 0.122 MeV. Cobalt-60 has a half-life of 5.27 years and its presence is shown by gamma photons of energies 1.173 MeV and 1.332 MeV. Not more than 1 per cent of the total radioactivity is due to cobalt-60 and not more than 2 per cent of the total radioactivity is due to cobalt-57, cobalt-60 and other radionuclidic impurities.

RADIOCHEMICAL PURITY

Examine by liquid chromatography (*2.2.29*).

Reference solution. Dissolve 10 mg of *cyanocobalamin CRS* in the mobile phase and dilute to 100 ml with the mobile phase. Dilute 2 ml of the solution to 100 ml with the mobile phase. Use within 1 h.

The chromatographic procedure may be carried out using:

– a stainless steel column 0.25 m long and 4 mm in internal diameter packed with *octylsilyl silica gel for chromatography R* (5 µm),
– as mobile phase at a flow rate of 1.0 ml/min a mixture prepared as follows: mix 26.5 volumes of *methanol R* and 73.5 volumes of a 10 g/l solution of *disodium hydrogen phosphate R* adjusted to pH 3.5 using *phosphoric acid R* and use within 2 days,
– a radioactivity detector adjusted for cobalt-58,
– as detector a spectrophotometer set at 361 nm,
– a loop injector.

Inject 100 µl of the solution to be examined and record the chromatogram for three times the retention time of cyanocobalamin. Determine the peak areas and calculate the percentage of cobalt-58 present as cyanocobalamin. Inject 100 µl of the reference solution and record the chromatogram for 30 min.

RADIOACTIVITY

Measure the radioactivity using suitable counting equipment by comparison with a standardised cobalt-58 solution or by measurement in an instrument calibrated with the aid of such a solution.

STORAGE

Store protected from light at a temperature of 2 °C to 8 °C.

01/2005:1325

FLUDEOXYGLUCOSE (^{18}F) INJECTION

Fludeoxyglucosi (^{18}F) solutio iniectabilis

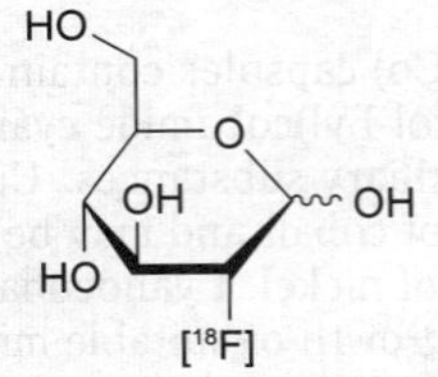

DEFINITION

Fludeoxyglucose (^{18}F) injection is a sterile solution of 2-[^{18}F]fluoro-2-deoxy-D-glucopyranose (2-[^{18}F]fluoro-2-deoxy-D-glucose) for diagnostic use. The injection contains not less than 90.0 per cent and not more than 110.0 per cent of the declared fluorine-18 radioactivity at the date and time stated on the label. Not less than 95 per cent of the radioactivity corresponds to fluorine-18 in the form of 2-[^{18}F]fluoro-2-deoxy-D-glucose and 2-[^{18}F]fluoro-2-deoxy-D-mannose, with the 2-[^{18}F]fluoro-2-deoxy-D-mannose fraction not exceeding 10 per cent of the total radioactivity. Not less than 99.0 per cent of the radioactivity corresponds to fluorine-18. The content of 2-fluoro-2-deoxy-D-glucose is not more than 10 mg per maximum recommended dose of injection.

PRODUCTION

RADIONUCLIDE PRODUCTION

Fluorine-18 is a radioactive isotope of fluorine which may be produced by various nuclear reactions induced by proton irradiation of oxygen-18, deuteron irradiation of neon-20, helium-3 or helium-4 irradiation of oxygen-16.

RADIOCHEMICAL SYNTHESIS

2-[^{18}F]Fluoro-2-deoxy-D-glucose may be prepared by various chemical synthetic pathways, which lead to different products in terms of specific radioactivity, by-products and possible impurities.

Radiopharmaceutical preparations

Most widely used is the method of phase transfer catalysed nucleophilic substitution of 1,3,4,6-tetra-*O*-acetyl-2-*O*-trifluoromethanesulphonyl-β-D-mannopyranose with [^{18}F]fluoride. Generally, [^{18}F]fluoride is adsorbed on an anion-exchange resin and eluted with a solution of potassium carbonate which is then evaporated to dryness. Addition of a phase transfer catalyst such as an aminopolyether in dry acetonitrile may be used to enhance the nucleophilicity of the [^{18}F]fluoride so that it reacts easily with the tetra-acetylated mannosyltriflate at elevated temperature. Hydrolysis under either alkaline or acidic conditions yields 2-[^{18}F]fluoro-2-deoxy-D-glucose. Hydrolysis using hydrochloric acid may lead to the formation of 2-chloro-2-deoxy-D-glucose. Hydrolysis under alkaline conditions may lead to the formation of 2-[^{18}F]fluoro-2-deoxy-D-mannose as a by-product.

Variations of the method substitute the aminopolyether by a tetra-alkyl ammonium salt, or use solid phase catalysed nucleophilic substitution on derivatised anion-exchange resin, e.g. derivatised with 4-(4-methylpiperidino)pyridine.

Electrophilic pathways for production of 2-[^{18}F]fluoro-2-deoxy-D-glucose proceed by the reaction of molecular [^{18}F]fluorine or [^{18}F]acetylhypofluorite with 3,4,6-tri-*O*-acetyl-D-glucal. [^{18}F]Acetylhypofluorite is obtained by conversion of molecular [^{18}F]fluorine on a solid complex of acetic acid and potassium acetate. The production of molecular [^{18}F]fluorine requires the addition of small amounts of fluorine to the neon target gas, usually from 0.1 per cent to 1 per cent, resulting in the reduction of the specific radioactivity of the end-product. Hydrolysis of the *O*-acetyl protected [^{18}F]fluorinated sugar yields 2-[^{18}F]fluoro-2-deoxy-D-glucose and usually small amounts of 2-[^{18}F]fluoro-2-deoxy-D-mannose.

The preparation can be purified by serial chromatography on combinations of ion-retardation resin, ion-exchange resin, alumina and octadecyl derivatised silica gel. Removal of the phase transfer catalyst can be achieved by different methods, all using combinations of separation cartridges.

Production systems and their performance comply with the requirements set by the competent authority.

STARTING MATERIALS

1. Target materials

Each batch of target material must be tested in special production runs before its use in routine fluorine-18 production and manufacture of the preparation, to ensure that under specified conditions, the target yields fluorine-18 in the desired quantity and quality.

2. Precursors for organic synthesis

It is recommended to test the precursors in production runs before their use for the manufacture of the preparation, to ensure that under specified production conditions, the precursors yield the preparation in the desired quantity and quality.

1,3,4,6-Tetra-O-acetyl-2-O-trifluoromethanesulphonyl-β-D-mannopyranose. Examine by infrared absorption spectrophotometry (*2.2.24*), comparing with the *Ph. Eur. reference spectrum of 1,3,4,6-tetra-O-acetyl-2-O-trifluoromethanesulphonyl-β-D-mannopyranose.*

Melting point (*2.2.14*): 119 °C to 122 °C.

3,4,6-Tri-O-acetyl-D-glucal. Examine by infrared absorption spectrophotometry (*2.2.24*), comparing with the *Ph. Eur. reference spectrum of 3,4,6-tri-O-acetyl-D-glucal.*

Melting point (*2.2.14*): 53 °C to 55 °C.

CHARACTERS

A clear, colourless or slightly yellow solution.

Fluorine-18 has a half-life of 109.8 min and emits positrons with a maximum energy of 0.633 MeV, followed by annihilation gamma radiation of 0.511 MeV.

IDENTIFICATION

A. Record the gamma-ray spectrum using a suitable instrument. The only gamma photons have an energy of 0.511 MeV; and depending on the measurement geometry, a sum peak of 1.022 MeV may be observed.

B. It complies with the test for radionuclidic purity (see Tests).

C. Examine the chromatograms obtained in test (a) for radiochemical purity. The principal peak in the radiochromatogram obtained with the test solution has approximately the same retention time as the principal peak in the chromatogram obtained with reference solution (b).

TESTS

pH (*2.2.3*). The pH of the injection is 4.5 to 8.5.

Sterility. It complies with the test for sterility prescribed in the monograph on *Radiopharmaceutical preparations (0125)*. The injection may be released for use before completion of the test.

Bacterial endotoxins (*2.6.14*): less than 175/*V* IU/ml, *V* being the maximum recommended dose in millilitres. The injection may be released for use before completion of the test.

CHEMICAL PURITY

Particular tests for chemical purity may be omitted if the substances mentioned are not used or cannot be formed in the production process

(a) 2-Fluoro-2-deoxy-D-glucose and 2-chloro-2-deoxy-D-glucose. Examine by liquid chromatography (*2.2.29*).

Test solution. The preparation to be examined.

Reference solution (a). Dissolve 10 mg of *glucose R* in *water R* and dilute to 100 ml with the same solvent.

Reference solution (b). Dissolve 10 mg of *2-fluoro-2-deoxy-D-glucose R* in *water R* and dilute to *V* with the same solvent, *V* being the maximum recommended dose in millilitres.

Reference solution (c). Dissolve 1.0 mg of *2-chloro-2-deoxy-D-glucose R* in *water R* and dilute to 2.0 ml with the same solvent. Dilute 1 ml of this solution to *V* with the same solvent, *V* being the maximum recommended dose in millilitres.

The chromatographic procedure may be carried out using:

- a column 0.25 m long and 4.0 mm in internal diameter packed with *strongly basic anion-exchange resin for chromatography R* (10 μm),
- as mobile phase at a flow rate of 1 ml/min *0.1 M sodium hydroxide* protected against contamination by carbon dioxide,
- a suitable radioactivity detector for radiochemical purity testing,
- a detector suitable for carbohydrates in the required concentration range,
- a loop injector,

maintaining the column at a constant temperature between 20 °C and 30 °C.

Equilibrate the column with the mobile phase until a stable baseline is achieved.

Inject separately reference solutions (a), (b) and (c). If the validation studies exclude the formation of 2-chloro-2-deoxy-D-glucose inject separately reference solutions (a) and (b). Continue the chromatography for twice the retention time of D-glucose, 2-fluoro-2-deoxy-D-glucose and when required, 2-chloro-2-deoxy-D-glucose respectively.

Inject the test solution. The chromatogram obtained with the detector for carbohydrates shows a principal peak corresponding to D-glucose (test solutions from nucleophilic pathways) or 2-fluoro-2-deoxy-D-glucose (test solutions from electrophilic pathways). When the chromatograms are recorded in the prescribed conditions, 2-chloro-2-deoxy-D-glucose elutes after 2-fluoro-2-deoxy-D-glucose, but their corresponding peaks may not be completely resolved. In the chromatogram obtained with the test solution, the areas of the peaks corresponding to 2-fluoro-2-deoxy-D-glucose and 2-chloro-2-deoxy-D-glucose are not greater than the areas of the peaks in the chromatograms obtained with reference solution (b) and/or reference solution (c) (10 mg of 2-fluoro-2-deoxy-D-glucose per *V* and 0.5 mg of 2-chloro-2-deoxy-D-glucose per *V* respectively).

(b) Aminopolyether. This test is performed only on the bulk solution before addition of sodium chloride by the producer and it is not intended for the final preparation to be injected. Examine by thin-layer chromatography (*2.2.27*), using a *TLC silica gel plate R*.

Test solution. The preparation to be examined.

Reference solution. Dissolve 0.110 g of *aminopolyether R* in *water R* and dilute to 10.0 ml with the same solvent. Dilute 0.2 ml of this solution to *V* with the same solvent, *V* being the maximum recommended dose in millilitres.

Apply separately to the plate 2 µl of the test solution and 2 µl of the reference solution. Develop over a path of about 8 cm using a mixture of 1 volume of *ammonia R* and 9 volumes of *methanol R*. Allow the plate to dry in air for 15 min. Expose the plate to iodine vapour for at least 10 min. In the chromatogram obtained with the test solution the spot corresponding to aminopolyether is not more intense than the spot in the chromatogram obtained with the reference solution (2.2 mg per *V*).

(c) Tetra-alkyl ammonium salts. Examine by liquid chromatography (*2.2.29*).

Test solution. The preparation to be examined.

Reference solution. Dilute 2.1 ml of *0.1 M tetrabutylammonium hydroxide* to 20 ml with *water R*. Dilute 1 ml of this solution to *V* with the same solvent, *V* being the maximum recommended dose in millilitres.

The chromatographic procedure may be carried out using:

- a column 0.125 m long and 4.0 mm in internal diameter packed with *octadecylsilyl silica gel for chromatography R* (5 µm),
- as mobile phase at a flow rate of 0.6 ml/min a mixture of 25 volumes of a 0.95 g/l solution of *toluenesulphonic acid R* and 75 volumes of *acetonitrile R*,
- as detector a spectrophotometer set at 254 nm,
- a loop injector,

maintaining the column at a constant temperature between 20 °C and 30 °C.

Equilibrate the column with the mobile phase until a stable baseline is obtained.

Inject the reference solution. Continue the chromatography for twice the retention time of tetrabutylammonium ions.

Inject the test solution. In the chromatogram obtained with the test solution, the area of the peak corresponding to tetrabutylammonium ions is not greater than the area of the peak in the chromatogram obtained with the reference solution (2.75 mg per *V*).

(d) Solid phase derivatisation agent 4-(4-methylpiperidino)pyridine. Examine by ultraviolet spectrophotometry (*2.2.25*).

Test solution. The preparation to be examined.

Reference solution. Dissolve 20 mg of *4-(4-methylpiperidino)pyridine R* in *water R* and dilute to 100.0 ml with the same solvent. Dilute 0.1 ml of this solution to *V* with the same solvent, *V* being the maximum recommended dose in millilitres.

Measure the absorbance of the test solution and the reference solution at the maximum of 263 nm. The absorbance of the test solution is not greater than that of the reference solution (0.02 mg per *V*).

(e) Residual solvents (*2.4.24*). The concentration of acetonitrile does not exceed 4.1 mg per *V*, *V* being the maximum recommended dose in millilitres. The injection may be released for use before completion of the test.

RADIONUCLIDIC PURITY

Record the gamma-ray spectrum using a suitable instrument. The half-life is between 105 min and 115 min. The injection may be released for use before completion of the test.

RADIOCHEMICAL PURITY

A. Examine by liquid chromatography (*2.2.29*) as described in test (a) for chemical purity.

   When the chromatograms obtained with the radioactivity detector are recorded in the prescribed conditions, the principal peak in the chromatogram obtained with the test solution has the same retention time as the peak obtained with reference solution (b) using the carbohydrate detector. The retention times of 2-[^{18}F]fluoro-2-deoxy-D-mannose and [^{18}F]fluoride are approximately 90 per cent and approximately 50 per cent of that of 2-[^{18}F]fluoro-2-deoxy-D-glucose respectively. Other peaks in the chromatogram may be due to partially acetylated 2-[^{18}F]fluoro-2-deoxy-D-glucose derivatives.

   Calculate the percentage content of [^{18}F]fluorinated substances from the areas of the peaks in the chromatogram obtained with the test solution. The sum of the percentages of radioactivity corresponding to 2-[^{18}F]fluoro-2-deoxy-D-glucose and 2-[^{18}F]fluoro-2-deoxy-D-mannose is not less than 95 per cent of the total radioactivity with the 2-[^{18}F]fluoro-2-deoxy-D-mannose fraction not exceeding 10 per cent of the total radioactivity.

   The method may underestimate or miss unhydrolysed or partially hydrolysed 2-[^{18}F]fluoro-2-deoxytetra-acetyl-D-glucose, since these intermediate reaction products may further hydrolyse to the desired end-product under the chromatographic conditions.

B. Examine by thin-layer chromatography (*2.2.27*) using a *TLC silica gel plate R*.

   Test solution. The preparation to be examined.

   Apply 2 µl to 10 µl to the plate. Develop over a path of 8 cm using a mixture of 5 volumes of *water R* and 95 volumes of *acetonitrile R*. Allow the plate to dry in air for 15 min. Determine the distribution of radioactivity using a suitable detector. Not less than 95 per cent of the total radioactivity is found in the spot corresponding to 2-fluoro-2-deoxy-D-glucose (R_f about 0.45).

   Possible contaminants are [^{18}F]fluoride (R_f 0.0); partially acetylated 2-[^{18}F]fluoro-2-deoxy-D-glucose derivatives (R_f about 0.8-0.95).

Radiopharmaceutical preparations

RADIOACTIVITY

Measure the radioactivity using suitable counting equipment by comparison with a standardised fluorine-18 solution or using an instrument calibrated with the aid of such a solution. Standardised fluorine-18 solutions are available from laboratories recognised by the competent authority.

LABELLING

The accompanying information specifies the particular synthetic pathway of production. The label on the actual container states the maximum recommended dose in millilitres.

01/2005:1917

FLUMAZENIL (*N*-[^{11}C]METHYL) INJECTION

Flumazenil (*N*-[^{11}C]methyl) solutio iniectabilis

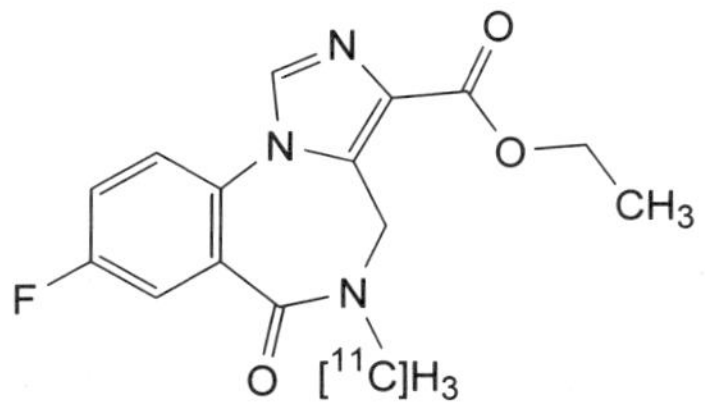

DEFINITION

Sterile solution of ethyl 8-fluoro-5-[^{11}C]methyl-6-oxo-5,6-dihydro-4*H*-imidazo[1,5-*a*][1,4]benzodiazepine-3-carboxylate which may contain a stabiliser such as ascorbic acid.

Content: 90 per cent to 110 per cent of the declared carbon-11 radioactivity at the date and time stated on the label.

Content of flumazenil: maximum 50 μg in the maximum recommended dose in millilitres.

PRODUCTION

RADIONUCLIDE PRODUCTION

Carbon-11 is a radioactive isotope of carbon which is most commonly produced by proton irradiation of nitrogen. Depending on the addition of either trace amounts of oxygen or small amounts of hydrogen, the radioactivity is obtained as [^{11}C]carbon dioxide or [^{11}C]methane, respectively.

RADIOCHEMICAL SYNTHESIS

[5-Methyl-^{11}C]flumazenil may be prepared by *N*-alkylation of ethyl 8-fluoro-6-oxo-5,6-dihydro-4*H*-imidazo[1,5-*a*][1,4]benzodiazepine-3-carboxylate (demethylflumazenil) with iodo[^{11}C]methane or [^{11}C]methyl trifluoromethanesulphonate.

Synthesis of iodo[^{11}C]methane

Iodo[^{11}C]methane may be produced from [^{11}C]carbon dioxide or from [^{11}C]methane. The most frequently used method is reduction of [^{11}C]carbon dioxide with lithium aluminium hydride. The [^{11}C]methanolate formed is reacted with hydriodic acid. Alternatively [^{11}C]methane, either obtained directly in the target or by on-line processes from [^{11}C]carbon dioxide, is reacted with iodine.

Synthesis of [^{11}C]methyl trifluoromethanesulphonate

[^{11}C]methyl trifluoromethanesulphonate may be prepared from iodo[^{11}C]methane using a solid support such as graphitised carbon, impregnated with silver trifluoromethanesulphonate.

Synthesis of [5-methyl-^{11}C]flumazenil

The most widely used method to obtain [5-methyl-^{11}C]flumazenil is the *N*-alkylation of demethylflumazenil with iodo[^{11}C]methane in alkaline conditions in a solvent such as dimethylformamide or acetone. The resulting [5-methyl-^{11}C]flumazenil can be purified by semi-preparative liquid chromatography. For example, a column packed with octadecylsilyl silica gel for chromatography eluted with a mixture of ethanol and water is suitable.

PRECURSOR FOR SYNTHESIS

Demethylflumazenil

Melting point (*2.2.14*): 286 °C to 289 °C.

Infrared absorption spectrophotometry (*2.2.24*).

Comparison: *Ph. Eur. reference spectrum of demethylflumazenil.*

CHARACTERS

Appearance: clear, colourless solution.

Half-life and nature of radiation of carbon-11: see *Table of physical characteristics of radionuclides* (*5.7*).

IDENTIFICATION

A. Gamma-ray spectrometry.

Results: the only gamma photons have an energy of 0.511 MeV and, depending on the measurement geometry, a sum peak of 1.022 MeV may be observed.

B. It complies with test B for radionuclidic purity (see Tests).

C. Examine the chromatograms obtained in the test for radiochemical purity.

Results: the principal peak in the radiochromatogram obtained with the test solution is similar in retention time to the principal peak in the chromatogram obtained with reference solution (a).

TESTS

pH (*2.2.3*): 6.0 to 8.0.

Sterility. It complies with the test for sterility prescribed in the monograph on *Radiopharmaceutical preparations (0125)*. The injection may be released for use before completion of the test.

Bacterial endotoxins (*2.6.14*): less than 175/*V* IU/ml, *V* being the maximum recommended dose in millilitres. The injection may be released for use before completion of the test.

Flumazenil and impurity A. Liquid chromatography (*2.2.29*).

Test solution. The preparation to be examined.

Reference solution (a). Dissolve 2.5 mg of *flumazenil R* in 5 ml of *methanol R*.

Reference solution (b). Dissolve 2.5 mg of *demethylflumazenil R* in 50 ml of *methanol R*.

Reference solution (c). To 0.1 ml of reference solution (a) add 0.1 ml of reference solution (b) and dilute to *V* with a 0.9 g/l solution of *sodium chloride R*, *V* being the maximum recommended dose in millilitres.

Reference solution (d). Dilute 0.1 ml of reference solution (a) to 50 ml with *methanol R*. Dilute 1.0 ml of this solution to *V* with a 0.9 g/l solution of *sodium chloride R*, *V* being the maximum recommended dose in millilitres.

Column:

- *size*: l = 0.15 m, Ø = 3.9 mm,
- *stationary phase*: spherical *octadecylsilyl silica gel for chromatography R* (5 μm) with a specific surface area of 440 m^2/g, a pore size of 100 nm and a carbon loading of 19 per cent,

Radiopharmaceutical preparations

– *temperature*: maintain at a constant temperature between 20-30 °C.

Mobile phase: *methanol R, water R* (45:55 *V/V*).

Flow rate: 1 ml/min.

Detection: spectrophotometer at 260 nm and radioactivity detector connected in series.

Injection: 100 µl.

Run time: 10 min.

Relative retention with reference to flumazenil: impurity A = about 0.74.

System suitability: reference solution (c):

– *resolution*: minimum 2.5 between the peaks due to flumazenil and impurity A.

Limits: examine the chromatogram obtained with the spectrophotometer:

– *flumazenil*: not more than the area of the corresponding peak in the chromatogram obtained with reference solution (c) (50 µg/*V*),

– *impurity A*: not more than the area of the corresponding peak in the chromatogram obtained with reference solution (c) (5 µg/*V*),

– *any other impurity*: not more than the area of the principal peak in the chromatogram obtained with reference solution (d) (1 µg/*V*).

Residual solvents are limited according to the principles defined in the general chapter (*5.4*), using the general method (*2.4.24*). The preparation may be released for use before completion of the test.

RADIONUCLIDIC PURITY

Carbon-11: minimum 99 per cent of the total radioactivity.

The preparation may be released for use before completion of the test.

A. Gamma-ray spectrometry.

Results: the spectrum obtained with the solution to be examined does not differ significantly from that obtained with a standardised fluorine-18 solution.

B. Half-life: 19.9 min to 20.9 min.

RADIOCHEMICAL PURITY

Liquid chromatography (*2.2.29*) as described in the test for flumazenil and impurity A, with the following modifications.

Injection: test solution and reference solution (a); if necessary, dilute the test solution to a radioactivity concentration suitable for the detector.

Limit: examine the chromatogram obtained with the radioactivity detector:

– *[5-methyl-^{11}C]flumazenil*: minimum 95 per cent of the total radioactivity.

RADIOACTIVITY

Determine the radioactivity using a calibrated instrument.

LABELLING

The label states the maximum recommended dose in millilitres.

IMPURITIES

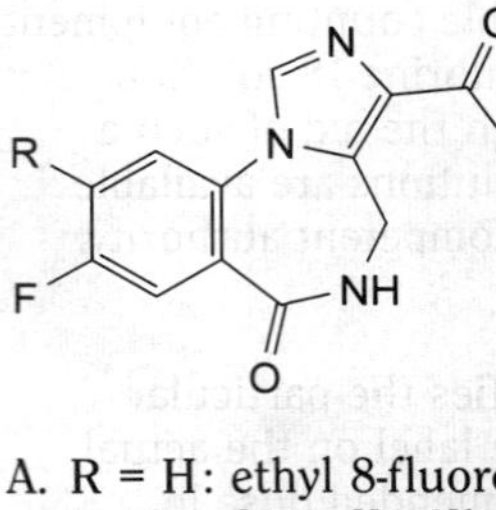

A. R = H: ethyl 8-fluoro-6-oxo-5,6-dihydro-4*H*-imidazo[1,5-*a*][1,4]benzodiazepine-3-carboxylate (demethylflumazenil),

B. R = CH_2-CO-CH_3: ethyl 8-fluoro-6-oxo-9-(2-oxopropyl)-5,6-dihydro-4*H*-imidazo[1,5-*a*][1,4]benzodiazepine-3-carboxylate (acetone addition compound of demethylflumazenil).

01/2005:0555

GALLIUM (^{67}Ga) CITRATE INJECTION

Gallii (^{67}Ga) citratis solutio iniectabilis

DEFINITION

Gallium (^{67}Ga) citrate injection is a sterile solution of gallium-67 in the form of gallium citrate. It may be made isotonic by the addition of sodium chloride and sodium citrate and may contain a suitable antimicrobial preservative such as benzyl alcohol. Gallium-67 is a radioactive isotope of gallium and may be obtained by the irradiation, with protons of suitable energy, of zinc which may be enriched in zinc-68. Gallium-67 may be separated from zinc by solvent extraction or column chromatography. The injection contains not less than 90.0 per cent and not more than 110.0 per cent of the declared gallium-67 radioactivity at the date and hour stated on the label. Not more than 0.2 per cent of the total radioactivity is due to gallium-66.

CHARACTERS

A clear, colourless solution.

Gallium-67 has a half-life of 3.26 days and emits gamma radiation.

IDENTIFICATION

A. Record the gamma-ray spectrum using a suitable instrument. The spectrum does not differ significantly from that of a standardised gallium-67 solution when measured either by direct comparison or by use of an instrument calibrated with the aid of such a solution. Standardised gallium-67 solutions are available from laboratories recognised by the competent authority. The most prominent gamma photons have energies of 0.093 MeV, 0.185 MeV and 0.300 MeV.

B. To 0.2 ml of the injection to be examined add 0.2 ml of a solution containing 1 g/l of *ferric chloride R* and 0.1 per cent *V/V* of *hydrochloric acid R* and mix. Compare the colour with that of a solution containing 9 g/l of *benzyl alcohol R* and 7 g/l of *sodium chloride R* treated in the same manner. A yellow colour develops in the test solution only.

TESTS

pH (*2.2.3*). The pH of the injection is 5.0 to 8.0.

Zinc. To 0.1 ml of the injection to be examined add 0.9 ml of *water R*, 5 ml of *acetate buffer solution pH 4.7 R*, 1 ml of a 250 g/l solution of *sodium thiosulphate R* and 5.0 ml of a dithizone solution prepared as follows: dissolve 10 mg of *dithizone R* in 100 ml of *methyl ethyl ketone R* allow to stand for 5 min, filter and immediately before use dilute the solution to ten times its volume with *methyl ethyl ketone R*. Shake vigorously for 2 min and separate the organic layer. Measure the absorbance (*2.2.25*) of the organic layer at 530 nm, using the organic layer of a blank solution as the compensation liquid. The absorbance is not greater than that of the organic layer obtained with 0.1 ml of *zinc standard solution (5 ppm Zn) R* treated in the same manner.

Sterility. It complies with the test for sterility prescribed in the monograph on *Radiopharmaceutical preparations (0125)*. The injection may be released for use before completion of the test.

RADIONUCLIDIC PURITY

Record the gamma-ray spectrum using a suitable instrument. The spectrum does not differ significantly from that of a standardised gallium-67 solution, apart from any differences attributable to the presence of gallium-66. Gallium-66 has a half-life of 9.4 h and its most prominent gamma photon has an energy of 1.039 MeV. Not more than 0.2 per cent of the total radioactivity is due to gallium-66.

RADIOACTIVITY

Measure the radioactivity using suitable counting equipment by comparison with a standardised gallium-67 solution or by measurement in an instrument calibrated with the aid of such a solution.

01/2005:1922

HUMAN ALBUMIN INJECTION, IODINATED (^{125}I)

Iodinati (^{125}I) humani albumini solutio iniectabilis

DEFINITION

Sterile, endotoxin-free solution of human albumin labelled with iodine-125. It may contain a suitable buffer and an antimicrobial preservative. The human albumin used complies with the requirements of the monograph on *Human albumin solution (0255)*.

Content: 90 per cent to 110 per cent of the declared iodine-125 radioactivity at the date stated on the label.

Purity:

- minimum of 99.0 per cent of the total radioactivity corresponds to iodine-125,
- minimum of 80 per cent of the total radioactivity is associated with the albumin fractions II to V,
- maximum of 5 per cent of the total radioactivity corresponds to unbound iodide.

Content of albumin: 95 per cent to 105 per cent of the declared albumin content stated on the label.

CHARACTERS

Appearance: clear, colourless to yellowish solution.

Half-life and nature of radiation of iodine-125: see Table of physical characteristics of radionuclides (*5.7*).

IDENTIFICATION

A. Gamma-ray and X-ray spectrometry.

Comparison: standardised iodine-125 solution, or by using a calibrated instrument. Standardised iodine-125 solutions and/or standardisation services are available from the competent authority.

Results: the spectrum obtained with the preparation to be examined does not differ significantly from that obtained with a standardised iodine-125 solution, apart from any differences attributable to the presence of iodine-126. The most prominent photon has an energy of 0.027 MeV, corresponding to the characteristic X-ray of tellurium, gamma photons of an energy of 0.035 MeV are also present. Iodine-126 has a half-life of 13.11 days and its most prominent gamma photons have energies of 0.388 MeV and 0.666 MeV.

B. Examine by a suitable immunoelectrophoresis technique (*2.7.1*). Using antiserum to normal human serum, compare normal human serum and the preparation to be examined, both diluted if necessary. The main component of the preparation to be examined corresponds to the main component of the normal human serum. The diluted solution may show the presence of small quantities of other plasma proteins.

TESTS

pH (*2.2.3*): 5.0 to 9.0.

Albumin

Reference solution. Dilute *human albumin solution R* with a 9 g/l solution of *sodium chloride R* to a concentration of 5 mg of albumin per millilitre.

To 1.0 ml of the preparation to be examined and to 1.0 ml of the reference solution add 4.0 ml of *biuret reagent R* and mix. After exactly 30 min, measure the absorbance (*2.2.25*) of each solution at 540 nm, using as the compensation liquid a 9 g/l solution of *sodium chloride R* treated in the same manner. From the absorbances measured, calculate the content of albumin in the injection to be examined in milligrams per millilitre.

Sterility. It complies with the test for sterility prescribed in the monograph on *Radiopharmaceutical preparations (0125)*.

Bacterial endotoxins (*2.6.14*): less than 175/*V* IU/ml, *V* being the maximum recommended dose in millilitres.

RADIONUCLIDIC PURITY

Iodine-125: minimum 99.0 per cent of the total radioactivity.

Gamma-ray and X-ray spectroscopy.

Comparison: standardised solution of iodine-125.

Determine the relative amounts of iodine-125 and iodine-126 present.

RADIOCHEMICAL PURITY

Iodine-125 in albumin fractions II to V, iodine-125 corresponding to unbound iodide. Size-exclusion chromatography (*2.2.30*).

Test solution. Mix 0.25 ml of the preparation to be examined with 0.25 ml of the mobile phase. Use immediately after mixing.

Reference solution. Human albumin solution R or another appropriate human albumin standard diluted with the mobile phase to a suitable albumin concentration.

Column:

- *size*: l = 0.6 m, Ø = 7.5 mm,
- *stationary phase*: *silica gel for size-exclusion chromatography R*,
- *temperature*: 25 °C.

Mobile phase: dissolve 11.24 g of *potassium dihydrogen phosphate R*, 42.0 g of *disodium hydrogen phosphate R*, 11.70 g of *sodium chloride R* in 2000 ml of *water R*.

Flow rate: 0.6 ml/min.

Detection: spectrophotometer at 280 nm and radioactivity detector set for iodine-125 connected in series.

Injection: loop injector.

Run time: 85 min.

Retention times:

Peak No.	Fraction	Description of the compound	Retention time (min)
1	I	High molecular mass compound	18 - 20
2	II	Poly III albumin	23 - 24
3	III	Poly II albumin	25 - 26
4	IV	Poly I albumin	28
5	V	Human serum albumin	29 - 31
6	VI	Iodide	43 - 45

The main peak in the chromatogram obtained with the reference solution corresponds to fraction V.

Limits:

- *radioactivity in fractions II to V*: minimum 80 per cent of the total radioactivity applied to the column,
- *iodine-125 in fraction VI*: maximum 5 per cent of the total radioactivity.

RADIOACTIVITY

Measure the radioactivity using suitable equipment by comparison with a standardised iodine-125 solution or by measurement with a calibrated instrument.

LABELLING

The label states:

- the amount of albumin,
- the maximum volume to be injected.

01/2005:1227

INDIUM (^{111}In) CHLORIDE SOLUTION

Indii (^{111}In) chloridi solutio

DEFINITION

Indium (^{111}In) chloride solution is a sterile solution of indium-111 as the chloride in aqueous hydrochloric acid containing no additives. Indium-111 is a radioactive isotope of indium and may be produced by the irradiation of cadmium with protons of suitable energy. The solution contains not less than 90.0 per cent and not more than 110.0 per cent of the declared indium-111 radioactivity at the date and hour stated on the label. Not more than 0.25 per cent of the total radioactivity is due to radionuclides other than indium-111. Not less than 95 per cent of the radioactivity corresponds to indium-111 in the form of ionic indium(III). The method of preparation is such that no carrier is added and the specific radioactivity is not less than 1.85 GBq of indium-111 per microgram of indium.

CHARACTERS

A clear, colourless solution.

Indium-111 has a half-life of 2.8 days and emits gamma radiation and X-rays.

IDENTIFICATION

A. *Carry out the test after allowing sufficient time for short-lived impurities such as indium-110m to decay.* Record the gamma-ray and X-ray spectrum using a suitable instrument. The spectrum does not differ significantly from that of a standardised indium-111 solution apart from any differences due to the presence of indium-114m, when measured either by direct comparison or by using an instrument calibrated with the aid of such a solution. Standardised indium-111 and indium-114m solutions are available from laboratories recognised by the competent authority. The most prominent gamma photons of indium-111 have energies of 0.171 MeV and 0.245 MeV.

B. To 100 µl of *silver nitrate solution R2* add 50 µl of the solution. A white precipitate is formed.

C. It complies with the test for pH (see Tests).

D. Examine the chromatogram obtained in the test for radiochemical purity. The principal peak has an R_f value of 0.5 to 0.8.

TESTS

pH (*2.2.3*). The pH of the solution is 1.0 to 2.0.

Cadmium. Not more than 0.40 µg/ml, determined by electrothermal atomic absorption spectrometry (*2.2.23, Method I*).

Test solution. Dilute 0.05 ml of the solution to be examined to a suitable volume with a suitable concentration of *hydrochloric acid R*.

Reference solutions. Prepare the reference solutions using *cadmium standard solution (0.1 per cent Cd) R*, diluted as necessary with the same concentration of *hydrochloric acid R* as in the solution to be examined.

Measure the absorbance at 228.8 nm using a cadmium hollow-cathode lamp as source of radiation.

Copper. Not more than 0.15 µg/ml, determined by electrothermal atomic absorption spectrometry (*2.2.23, Method I*).

Test solution. Dilute 0.1 ml the solution to be examined to a suitable volume with a suitable concentration of *hydrochloric acid R*.

Reference solutions. Prepare the reference solutions using *copper standard solution (0.1 per cent) R* diluted as necessary with the same concentration of *hydrochloric acid R* as the solution to be examined.

Measure the absorbance at 324.8 nm using a copper hollow-cathode lamp as source of radiation.

Iron. Not more than 0.60 µg/ml, determined by electrothermal atomic absorption spectrometry (*2.2.23, Method I*).

Test solution. Dilute 0.1 ml of the solution to be examined to a suitable volume with a suitable concentration of *hydrochloric acid R*.

Reference solutions. Prepare the reference solutions using *iron standard solution (0.1 per cent Fe) R* diluted as necessary with the same concentration of *hydrochloric acid R* as the solution to be examined.

Measure the absorbance at 248.3 nm using an iron hollow-cathode lamp as source of radiation.

Sterility. It complies with the test for sterility prescribed in the monograph on *Radiopharmaceutical preparations (0125)*. The solution may be released for use before completion of the test.

RADIONUCLIDIC PURITY

Record the gamma-ray and X-ray spectrum using a suitable instrument. The spectrum does not differ significantly from that of a standardised solution of indium-111 apart from any differences due to the presence of indium-114m.

Indium-114m. *Carry out the test after allowing sufficient time for short-lived impurities such as indium-110m to decay.* Take a volume equivalent to 30 MBq and record the gamma-ray spectrum using a suitable detector with a shield of lead, 6 mm thick, placed between the sample and the detector. The response in the region corresponding to the 0.558 MeV photon and the 0.725 MeV photon of indium-114m does not exceed that obtained using 75 kBq of a standardised solution of indium-114m (0.25 per cent) measured under the same conditions, when all measurements are calculated with reference to the date and hour of administration. Standardised indium-111 and indium-114m solutions are available from laboratories recognised by the competent authority.

RADIOCHEMICAL PURITY

Examine by thin-layer chromatography (*2.2.27*) using silica gel as the coating substance on a glass-fibre sheet.

Apply to the plate 5 μl of the solution to be examined. Develop immediately over a path of 15 cm using a 9.0 g/l solution of *sodium chloride R* adjusted to pH 2.3 ± 0.05 with *dilute hydrochloric acid R*. Allow the plate to dry in a current of cold air. Determine the distribution of radioactivity using a suitable detector. Indium-111 chloride migrates with an R_f value of 0.5 to 0.8. Not less than 95 per cent of the total radioactivity of the chromatogram corresponds to indium-111 chloride.

RADIOACTIVITY

Measure the radioactivity using suitable counting equipment by comparison with a standardised indium-111 solution or by measurement in an instrument calibrated with the aid of such a solution.

01/2005:1109

INDIUM (^{111}In) OXINE SOLUTION

Indii (^{111}In) oxini solutio

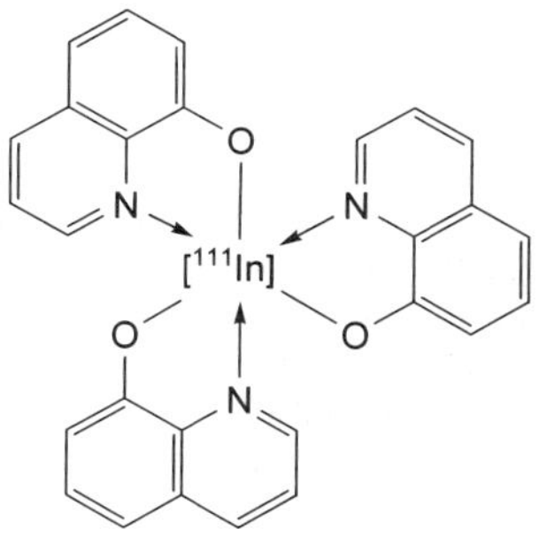

$C_{27}H_{18}[^{111}In]N_3O_3$ M_r 547.2

DEFINITION

Indium (^{111}In) oxine solution is a sterile solution of indium-111 in the form of a complex with 8-hydroxyquinoline. It may contain suitable surface active agents and may be made iso-tonic by the addition of sodium chloride and a suitable buffer. Indium-111 is a radioactive isotope of indium and may be produced by the irradiation of cadmium with protons of suitable energy. The solution contains not less than 90.0 per cent and not more than 110.0 per cent of the declared indium-111 radioactivity at the date and hour stated on the label. Not more than 0.25 per cent of the total radioactivity is due to radionuclides other than indium-111. Not less than 90 per cent of the radioactivity corresponds to indium-111 complexed with oxine. The method of preparation is such that no carrier is added and the specific radioactivity is not less than 1.85 GBq of indium-111 per microgram of indium.

CHARACTERS

A clear, colourless solution.

Indium-111 has a half-life of 2.8 days and emits gamma radiation and X-rays.

IDENTIFICATION

A. *Carry out the test after allowing sufficient time for short-lived impurities such as indium-110m to decay.* Record the gamma-ray and X-ray spectrum using a suitable instrument. The spectrum does not differ significantly from that of a standardised indium-111 solution apart from any differences due to the presence of indium-114m, when measured either by direct comparison or by using an instrument calibrated with the aid of such a solution. Standardised indium-111 and indium-114m solutions are available from laboratories recognised by the competent authority. The most prominent gamma photons of indium-111 have energies of 0.171 MeV and 0.245 MeV.

B. Place 5 mg to 10 mg of *magnesium oxide R* in a glass container of approximately 20 mm in internal diameter. Add 20 μl of the solution to be examined. Examine in ultraviolet light at 365 nm. Bright yellow fluorescence is produced.

C. The distribution of radioactivity between the organic and aqueous phases in the test for radiochemical purity contributes to the identification of the preparation.

TESTS

pH (*2.2.3*). The pH of the solution is 6.0 to 7.5.

Sterility. It complies with the test for sterility prescribed in the monograph on *Radiopharmaceutical preparations (0125)*. The solution may be released for use before completion of the test.

RADIONUCLIDIC PURITY

Record the gamma-ray and X-ray spectrum using a suitable instrument. The spectrum does not differ significantly from that of a standardised solution of indium-111, apart from any differences due to the presence of indium-114m.

Indium-114m. *Carry out the test after allowing sufficient time for short-lived impurities such as indium-110m to decay.* Take a volume equivalent to 30 MBq and record the gamma-ray spectrum using a suitable detector with a shield of lead, 6 mm thick, placed between the sample and the detector. The response in the region corresponding to the 0.558 MeV photon and the 0.725 MeV photon of indium-114m does not exceed that obtained using 75 kBq of a standardised solution of indium-114m (0.25 per cent) measured under the same conditions, when all measurements are calculated with reference to the date and hour of administration. (It should be noted that indium (^{111}In) oxine solution is a precursor used in the *in vitro* labelling of white blood cells or platelets prior to their re-injection into the patient. It is not intended for direct administration). Standardised indium-111 and indium-114m solutions are available from laboratories recognised by the competent authority.

RADIOCHEMICAL PURITY

To a silanised separating funnel containing 3 ml of a 9 g/l solution of *sodium chloride R* add 100 μl of the solution to be examined and mix. Add 6 ml of *octanol R* and shake vigorously. Allow the phases to separate and then run the lower layer into a suitable vial for counting. Allow the upper layer to drain completely into a similar vial. Add 1 ml of *octanol R* to the funnel, shake vigorously and drain into the vial containing the organic fraction. Add 5 ml of *dilute hydrochloric acid R* to the funnel, shake vigorously and drain these rinsings into a third vial. Seal each vial and, using a suitable instrument, measure the radioactivity in each. Calculate the radiochemical purity by expressing the radioactivity of the indium-111 oxine complex, found in the organic phase, as a percentage of the radioactivity measured in the three solutions. Not less than 90 per cent of the radioactivity corresponds to indium-111 complexed with oxine.

RADIOACTIVITY

Measure the radioactivity using suitable counting equipment by comparison with a standardised indium-111 solution or by measurement in an instrument calibrated with the aid of such a solution.

01/2005:0670

INDIUM (^{111}In) PENTETATE INJECTION

Indii (^{111}In) pentetatis solutio iniectabilis

DEFINITION

Indium (^{111}In) pentetate injection is a sterile and apyrogenic solution containing indium-111 in the form of indium diethylenetriaminepenta-acetate. It may contain calcium and may be made isotonic by the addition of sodium chloride and a suitable buffer. Indium-111 is a radioactive isotope of indium which may be obtained by proton irradiation, of appropriate energy, of cadmium which may be enriched with cadmium-111 or cadmium-112. The injection contains not less than 90 per cent and not more than 110 per cent of the declared indium-111 radioactivity at the date and hour stated on the label. The radioactivity due to indium-114m is not greater than 0.2 per cent of the total radioactivity at the date and hour of administration. Not less than 95 per cent of the radioactivity corresponds to indium-111 complexed with pentetate.

CHARACTERS

A clear, colourless solution.

Indium-111 has a half-life of 2.8 days and emits gamma radiation and X-rays.

IDENTIFICATION

A. Record the gamma-ray and X-ray spectrum using a suitable instrument. The spectrum does not differ significantly from that of a standardised indium-111 solution apart from any differences due to the presence of indium-114m, when measured either by direct comparison or by using an instrument calibrated with the aid of such a solution. Standardised indium-111 and indium-114m solutions are available from laboratories recognised by the competent authority. The most prominent gamma photons of indium-111 have energies of 0.171 MeV and 0.245 MeV.

B. Examine the chromatogram obtained in the test for radiochemical purity. The distribution of radioactivity contributes to the identification of the preparation.

TESTS

pH (*2.2.3*). The pH of the injection is 7.0 to 8.0.

Cadmium. Not more than 5 µg of Cd per millilitre, determined by atomic absorption spectrometry (*2.2.23, Method II*).

Test solution. Mix 0.1 ml of the injection to be examined with 0.9 ml of a mixture of 1 volume of *hydrochloric acid R* and 99 volumes of *water R*.

Reference solutions. Prepare the reference solutions using *cadmium standard solution (0.1 per cent Cd) R* and diluting with a mixture of 1 volume of *hydrochloric acid R* and 99 volumes of *water R*.

Measure the absorbance at 228.8 nm using a cadmium hollow-cathode lamp as source of radiation and an air-acetylene flame.

Uncomplexed diethylenetriaminepenta-acetic acid. In a micro test-tube, mix 100 µl of the injection to be examined with 100 µl of a freshly prepared 1 g/l solution of *hydroxynaphthol blue, sodium salt R* in *1 M sodium hydroxide*. Add 50 µl of a 0.15 g/l solution of *calcium chloride R*. The solution remains pinkish-violet or changes from blue to pinkish-violet (0.4 mg/ml).

Sterility. It complies with the test for sterility prescribed in the monograph on *Radiopharmaceutical preparations (0125)*. The injection may be released for use before completion of the test.

Bacterial endotoxins (*2.6.14*): less than 14/*V* IU/ml, *V* being the maximum recommended dose in millilitres.

RADIONUCLIDIC PURITY

Record the gamma-ray and X-ray spectrum using a suitable instrument. The spectrum does not differ significantly from that of a standardised solution of indium-111 apart from any differences due to the presence of indium-114m.

Indium-114m. Retain a sample of the injection to be examined for a sufficient time to allow the indium-111 radioactivity to decay to a sufficiently low level to permit the detection of radionuclidic impurities. Record the gamma-ray spectrum of the decayed material in a suitable instrument calibrated with the aid of a standardised indium-114m solution. Indium-114m has a half-life of 49.5 days and its most prominent gamma photon has an energy of 0.190 MeV. The radioactivity due to indium-114m is not greater than 0.2 per cent of the total radioactivity at the date and hour of administration.

RADIOCHEMICAL PURITY

Examine by thin-layer chromatography (*2.2.27*) using silica gel as the coating substance on a glass-fibre sheet. Heat the plate at 110 °C for 10 min. Use a plate such that during development the mobile phase migrates over a distance of 10 cm to 15 cm in about 10 min.

Apply to the plate 5 µl to 10 µl of the injection to be examined and allow to dry. Develop over a path of 10 cm to 15 cm using a 9 g/l solution of *sodium chloride R*. Allow the plate to dry in air. Determine the distribution of radioactivity using a suitable detector. Indium pentetate complex migrates near to the solvent front. The radioactivity of the spot corresponding to indium pentetate complex represents not less than 95 per cent of the total radioactivity of the chromatogram.

RADIOACTIVITY

Measure the radioactivity using suitable counting equipment by comparison with a standardised indium-111 solution or by measurement in an instrument calibrated with the aid of such a solution.

01/2005:1113
corrected

IOBENGUANE (^{123}I) INJECTION

Iobenguani (^{123}I) solutio iniectabilis

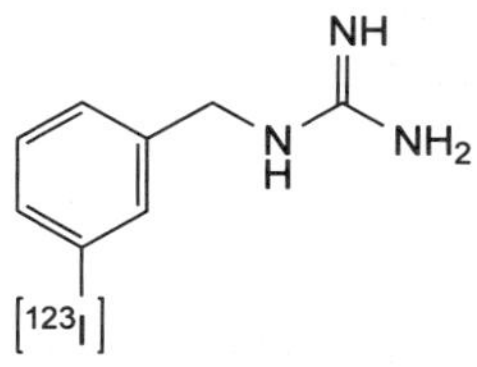

$C_8H_{10}[^{123}I]N_3$

DEFINITION

Iobenguane (^{123}I) injection is a sterile, bacterial-endotoxin free solution of 1-(3-[^{123}I]iodobenzyl)guanidine or its salts. It may contain a suitable buffer, a suitable labelling catalyst such as ionic copper, a suitable labelling stabiliser such as ascorbic acid and antimicrobial preservatives. Iodine-123 is a radioactive isotope of iodine and may be obtained by proton irradiation of xenon enriched in xenon-124 (not less than 98 per cent) followed by the decay of caesium-123 formed via xenon-123. The injection contains not less than 90.0 per cent and not more than 110.0 per cent of the declared iodine-123 radioactivity at the date and hour stated on the label. Not less than 95 per cent of the radioactivity corresponds to iodine-123 in the form of iobenguane. The specific radioactivity is not less than 10 GBq of iodine-123 per gram of iobenguane base. Not more than 0.35 per cent of the total radioactivity is due to radionuclides other than iodine-123.

CHARACTERS

A clear, colourless or slightly yellow solution.

Iodine-123 has a half-life of 13.2 h and emits gamma radiation and X-rays.

IDENTIFICATION

A. Record the gamma-ray and X-ray spectrum using a suitable instrument. The spectrum does not differ significantly from that of a standardised iodine-123 solution apart from any differences attributable to the presence of iodine-125, tellurium-121 and other radionuclidic impurities. The most prominent gamma photon of iodine-123 has an energy of 0.159 MeV. Iodine-125 has a half-life of 59.4 days and emits an X-ray of 0.027 MeV and a photon of 0.035 MeV. Tellurium-121 has a half-life of 19.2 days and the most prominent photons have energies of 0.507 MeV and 0.573 MeV. Standardised iodine-123, iodine-125 and tellurium-121 solutions are available from laboratories recognised by the competent authority.

B. Examine the chromatogram obtained in the test for radiochemical purity. The distribution of the radioactivity contributes to the identification of the preparation.

TESTS

pH (*2.2.3*). The pH of the solution is 3.5 to 8.0.

Specific radioactivity. The specific radioactivity is calculated from the results obtained in the test for radiochemical purity. Determine the content of iobenguane sulphate from the areas of the peaks corresponding to iobenguane in the chromatograms obtained with the test solution and reference solution (b). Calculate the concentration as iobenguane base by multiplying the result obtained in the assay by 0.85.

Sterility. It complies with the test for sterility prescribed in the monograph on *Radiopharmaceutical preparations (0125)*. The injection may be released for use before completion of the test.

Bacterial endotoxins (*2.6.14*): less than 175/*V* IU/ml, *V* being the maximum recommended dose in millilitres.

RADIONUCLIDIC PURITY

Record the gamma-ray spectrum using a suitable instrument. Determine the relative amounts of iodine-125, tellurium-121 and other radionuclidic impurities present. No radionuclides with longer half-lives than iodine-125 are detected. For the determination of iodine-125, tellurium-121 and other radionuclidic impurities, retain the solution to be examined for a sufficient time to allow the radioactivity of iodine-123 to decrease to a level which permits the detection of radionuclidic impurities. Record the gamma-ray spectrum and the X-ray spectrum of the decayed material using a suitable instrument. Not more than 0.35 per cent of the total radioactivity is due to radionuclides other than iodine-123. The injection may be released for use before completion of the test.

RADIOCHEMICAL PURITY

Examine by liquid chromatography (*2.2.29*).

Test solution. The injection to be examined.

Reference solution (a). Dissolve 0.100 g of *sodium iodide R* in the mobile phase and dilute to 100 ml with the mobile phase.

Reference solution (b). Dissolve 20.0 mg of *iobenguane sulphate CRS* in 50 ml of the mobile phase and dilute to 100.0 ml with the mobile phase.

The chromatographic procedure may be carried out using:

- a stainless steel column 0.25 m long and 4.0 mm in internal diameter packed with *silica gel for chromatography R* (5 µm),
- as mobile phase at a flow rate of 1.0 ml/min a mixture of 1 volume of an 80 g/l solution of *ammonium nitrate R*, 2 volumes of *dilute ammonia R2* and 27 volumes of *methanol R*,
- a suitable radioactivity detector,
- a spectrophotometer set at 254 nm and provided with a flow-cell,
- a 10 µl loop injector.

Inject the test solution and the reference solutions. Not less than 95 per cent of the radioactivity of the chromatogram is found in the peak corresponding to iobenguane. Not more than 4 per cent of the radioactivity is found in the peak corresponding to iodide and not more than 1 per cent of the radioactivity is found in other peaks.

RADIOACTIVITY

Measure the radioactivity using a suitable counting apparatus by comparison with a standardised iodine-123 solution or by measurement in an instrument calibrated with the aid of such a solution.

STORAGE

Store protected from light.

LABELLING

The label states the specific radioactivity expressed in GBq of iodine-123 per gram of iobenguane base.

01/2005:1111

IOBENGUANE (^{131}I) INJECTION FOR DIAGNOSTIC USE

Iobenguani (^{131}I) solutio iniectabilis ad usum diagnosticum

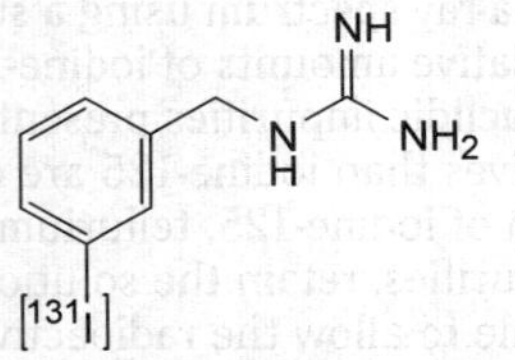

$C_8H_{10}[^{131}I]N_3$

DEFINITION

Iobenguane (^{131}I) injection for diagnostic use is a sterile, bacterial endotoxin-free solution of 1-(3-[^{131}I]iodobenzyl)guanidine or its salts. It may contain a suitable buffer. It may also contain a suitable labelling catalyst such as ionic copper and a suitable labelling stabiliser such as ascorbic acid. It may contain antimicrobial preservatives. Iodine-131 is a radioactive isotope of iodine and may be obtained by neutron irradiation of tellurium or by extraction of uranium fission products. The injection contains not less than 90.0 per cent and not more than 110.0 per cent of the declared iodine-131 radioactivity at the date and hour stated on the label. Not less than 94 per cent of the radioactivity corresponds to iodine-131 in the form of iobenguane. The specific radioactivity is not less than 20 GBq of iodine-131 per gram of iobenguane base.

CHARACTERS

A clear, colourless or slightly yellow solution.

Iodine-131 has a half-life of 8.04 days and emits beta and gamma radiation.

IDENTIFICATION

A. Record the gamma-ray spectrum using a suitable instrument. The spectrum does not differ significantly from that of a standardised iodine-131 solution by direct comparison with such a solution. Standardised iodine-131 solutions are available from laboratories recognised by the competent authority. The most prominent gamma photon of iodine-131 has an energy of 0.365 MeV.

B. Examine the chromatogram obtained in the test for radiochemical purity. The distribution of the radioactivity contributes to the identification of the preparation.

TESTS

pH (*2.2.3*). The pH of the solution is 3.5 to 8.0.

Specific radioactivity. The specific radioactivity is calculated from the results obtained in the test for radiochemical purity. Determine the content of iobenguane sulphate from the areas of the peaks corresponding to iobenguane in the chromatograms obtained with the test solution and reference solution (b). Calculate the concentration as iobenguane base by multiplying the result obtained in the assay by 0.85.

Sterility. It complies with the test for sterility prescribed in the monograph on *Radiopharmaceutical preparations (0125)*. The injection may be released for use before completion of the test.

Bacterial endotoxins (*2.6.14*): less than 175/*V* IU/ml, *V* being the maximum recommended dose in millilitres.

RADIONUCLIDIC PURITY

Record the gamma-ray spectrum using a suitable instrument. The spectrum does not differ significantly from that of a standardised iodine-131 solution. Determine the relative amounts of iodine-131, iod-ine-133, iodine-135 and other radionuclidic impurities present. Iodine-133 has a half-life of 20.8 h and its most prominent gamma photons have energies of 0.530 MeV and 0.875 MeV. Iodine-135 has a half-life of 6.55 h and its most prominent gamma photons have energies of 0.527 MeV, 1.132 MeV and 1.260 MeV. Not less than 99.9 per cent of the total radioactivity is due to iodine-131.

RADIOCHEMICAL PURITY

Examine by liquid chromatography (*2.2.29*).

Test solution. The injection to be examined.

Reference solution (a). Dissolve 0.100 g of *sodium iodide R* in the mobile phase and dilute to 100 ml with the mobile phase.

Reference solution (b). Dissolve 20.0 mg of *iobenguane sulphate CRS* in 50 ml of the mobile phase and dilute to 100.0 ml with the mobile phase.

The chromatographic procedure may be carried out using:

- a stainless steel column 0.25 m long and 4.0 mm in internal diameter packed with *silica gel for chromatography R* (5 µm),
- as mobile phase at a flow rate of 1.0 ml/min a mixture of 1 volume of an 80 g/l solution of *ammonium nitrate R,* 2 volumes of *dilute ammonia R2* and 27 volumes of *methanol R,*
- a suitable radioactivity detector,
- a spectrophotometer set at 254 nm and provided with a flow-cell,
- a 10 µl loop injector.

Inject the test solution and the reference solutions. Not less than 94 per cent of the radioactivity of the chromatogram is found in the peak corresponding to iobenguane. Not more than 5 per cent of the radioactivity is found in the peak corresponding to iodide and not more than 1 per cent of the radioactivity is found in other peaks.

RADIOACTIVITY

Measure the radioactivity using a suitable counting apparatus by comparison with a standardised iodine-131 solution or by measurement in an instrument calibrated with the aid of such a solution.

STORAGE

Store protected from light.

LABELLING

The label states the specific radioactivity expressed in gigabecquerels of iodine-131 per gram of iobenguane base.

Radiopharmaceutical preparations

01/2005:1112

IOBENGUANE (^{131}I) INJECTION FOR THERAPEUTIC USE

Iobenguani (^{131}I) solutio iniectabilis ad usum therapeuticum

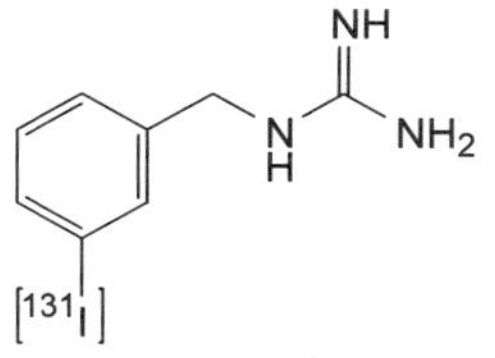

$C_8H_{10}[^{131}I]N_3$

DEFINITION

Iobenguane (^{131}I) injection for therapeutic use is a sterile, bacterial endotoxin-free solution of 1-(3-[^{131}I]iodobenzyl)guanidine or its salts. It may contain a suitable buffer, a suitable labelling catalyst such as ionic copper, a suitable labelling stabiliser such as ascorbic acid and antimicrobial preservatives. Iodine-131 is a radioactive isotope of iodine and may be obtained by neutron irradiation of tellurium or by extraction of uranium fission products. The injection contains not less than 90.0 per cent and not more than 110.0 per cent of the declared iodine-131 radioactivity at the date and hour stated on the label. Not less than 92 per cent of the radioactivity corresponds to iodine-131 in the form of iobenguane. The specific radioactivity is not less than 400 GBq of iodine-131 per gram of iobenguane base.

CHARACTERS

A clear, colourless or slightly yellow solution.

Iodine-131 has a half-life of 8.04 days and emits beta and gamma radiation.

IDENTIFICATION

A. Record the gamma-ray spectrum using a suitable instrument. The spectrum does not differ significantly from that of a standardised iodine-131 solution by direct comparison with such a solution. Standardised iodine-131 solutions are available from laboratories recognised by the competent authority. The most prominent gamma photon of iodine-131 has an energy of 0.365 MeV.

B. Examine the chromatogram obtained in the test for radio-chemical purity. The distribution of the radioactivity contributes to the identification of the preparation.

TESTS

pH (*2.2.3*). The pH of the solution is 3.5 to 8.0.

Specific radioactivity. The specific radioactivity is calculated from the results obtained in the test for radiochemical purity. Determine the content of iobenguane sulphate from the areas of the peaks corresponding to iobenguane in the chromatograms obtained with the test solution and reference solution (b). Calculate the concentration as iobenguane base by multiplying the result obtained in the assay by 0.85.

Sterility. It complies with the test for sterility prescribed in the monograph on *Radiopharmaceutical preparations (0125)*. The injection may be released for use before completion of the test.

Bacterial endotoxins (*2.6.14*): less than 175/V IU/ml, V being the maximum recommended dose in millilitres.

RADIONUCLIDIC PURITY

Record the gamma-ray spectrum using a suitable instrument. The spectrum does not differ significantly from that of a standardised iodine-131 solution. Determine the relative amounts of iodine-131, iodine-133, iodine-135 and other radionuclidic impurities present. Iodine-133 has a half-life of 20.8 h and its most prominent gamma photons have energies of 0.530 MeV and 0.875 MeV. Iodine-135 has a half-life of 6.55 h and its most prominent gamma photons have energies of 0.527 MeV, 1.132 MeV and 1.260 MeV. Not less than 99.9 per cent of the total radioactivity is due to iodine-131.

RADIOCHEMICAL PURITY

Examine by liquid chromatography (*2.2.29*).

Test solution. The injection to be examined.

Reference solution (a). Dissolve 0.100 g of *sodium iodide R* in the mobile phase and dilute to 100 ml with the mobile phase.

Reference solution (b). Dissolve 20.0 mg of *iobenguane sulphate CRS* in 50 ml of the mobile phase and dilute to 100.0 ml with the mobile phase.

The chromatographic procedure may be carried out using:

- a stainless steel column 0.25 m long and 4.0 mm in internal diameter packed with *silica gel for chromatography R* (5 μm),
- as mobile phase at a flow rate of 1.0 ml/min a mixture of 1 volume of an 80 g/lsolution of *ammonium nitrate R*, 2 volumes of *dilute ammonia R2* and 27 volumes of *methanol R*,
- a suitable radioactivity detector,
- a spectrophotometer set at 254 nm and provided with a flow-cell,
- a 10 μl loop injector.

Inject the test solution and the reference solutions. Not less than 92 per cent of the radioactivity of the chromatogram is found in the peak corresponding to iobenguane. Not more than 7 per cent of the radioactivity is found in the peak corresponding to iodide and not more than 1 per cent of the radioactivity is found in other peaks.

RADIOACTIVITY

Measure the radioactivity using a suitable counting apparatus by comparison with a standardised iodine-131 solution or by measurement in an instrument calibrated with the aid of such a solution.

STORAGE

Store protected from light.

LABELLING

The label states the specific radioactivity expressed in gigabecquerels of iodine-131 per gram of iobenguane base.

01/2005:1533

KRYPTON (^{81m}Kr) INHALATION GAS

Kryptonum (^{81m}Kr) ad inhalationem

DEFINITION

Krypton (^{81m}Kr) inhalation gas is a mixture of krypton-81m and a suitable vehicle such as air.

Krypton-81m is formed by decay of its parent radionuclide rubidium-81. Rubidium-81 has a half-life of 4.58 h.

The krypton-81m formed is separated from the rubidium-81 with a flow of a suitable gas in a rubidium/krypton generator. Rubidium-81 is produced by proton irradiation of krypton isotopes or by helium-3 or helium-4 irradiation of bromine. After separation of rubidium-81 from the target, it is retained by a suitable support.

Krypton-81m is eluted at a suitable flow rate with a vehicle such as air. The level of moisture required in the eluent depends on the type of generator used. The transport tube for administration has a defined length and inner diameter. The radioactivity concentration is determined before administration.

The radioactivity due to radionuclides other than krypton-81m is not greater than 0.1 per cent, expressed as a percentage of the total radioactivity in the preparation and calculated with reference to the date and time of administration.

CHARACTERS

A clear, colourless gas.

Krypton-81m has a half-life of 13.1 s and emits gamma radiation.

IDENTIFICATION

A. Record the gamma-ray and X-ray spectrum using a suitable instrument. The gamma photon of krypton-81m has an energy of 0.190 MeV.

B. The half-life is 11.8 s to 14.4 s.

TESTS

RADIONUCLIDIC PURITY

Elute the generator as prescribed. Pass a sufficient amount (2 litres to 10 litres) of eluate at a suitable flow rate through a suitable absorber such as water. Determine the amount of radioactivity eluted. Allow the krypton-81m to decay for 5 min and record the gamma and X-ray spectrum of the residual radioactivity on the absorber using a suitable instrument. Examine the gamma-ray and X-ray spectrum of the absorber for the presence of radioactive impurities, which must be identified and quantified. The absorbed radioactivity is not more than 0.1 per cent of the radioactivity passed through the absorber, calculated with reference to the date and time of administration.

RADIOACTIVITY

Determine the radioactive concentration of the preparation using suitable equipment such as an ionisation chamber or a gamma ray spectrometer. The measurement equipment may be calibrated by reference to a primary calibrated instrument at a laboratory recognised by the competent authority. The radioactivity is measured under defined operating conditions, such as gas flow rate and measurement geometry, that are identical to those used for the calibration of the instrument.

STORAGE

The storage conditions apply to the generator.

LABELLING

The labelling conditions apply to the generator.

01/2005:1617
corrected

L-METHIONINE ([^{11}C]METHYL) INJECTION

L-Methionini ([^{11}C]methyl) solutio iniectabilis

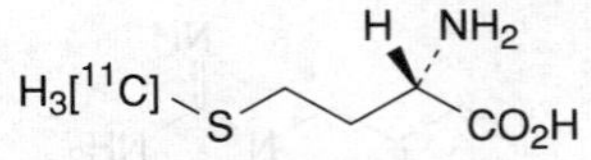

DEFINITION

Sterile solution of (2*S*)-2-amino-4-([^{11}C]methylsulphanyl)butanoic acid for diagnostic use.

Content: 90 per cent to 110 per cent of the declared carbon-11 radioactivity at the date and time stated on the label.

Purity:

- minimum of 99 per cent of the total radioactivity corresponds to carbon-11,
- minimum of 95 per cent of the total radioactivity corresponds to carbon-11 in the form of L-[*methyl*-^{11}C]methionine and D-[*methyl*-^{11}C]methionine,
- maximum of 10 per cent of the total radioactivity corresponds to carbon-11 in the form of D-[*methyl*-^{11}C]methionine.

Content of methionine: maximum of 2 mg per maximum recommended dose in millilitres.

PRODUCTION

RADIONUCLIDE PRODUCTION

Carbon-11 is a radioactive isotope of carbon which is most commonly produced by proton irradiation of nitrogen. Depending on the addition of either trace amounts of oxygen or small amounts of hydrogen, the radioactivity is obtained as [^{11}C]carbon dioxide or [^{11}C]methane.

RADIOCHEMICAL SYNTHESIS

L-[*Methyl*-^{11}C]methionine can be prepared by various chemical synthetic pathways. All methods rely on the alkylation of the sulphide anion of L-homocysteine with [^{11}C]methyl iodide or [^{11}C]methyl triflate. Variations in the procedures used to generate the sulphide anion of L-homocysteine and methods to obtain [^{11}C]methyl iodide lead to negligible differences with respect to quality in terms of specific radioactivity, enantiomeric purity and possible chemical and radiochemical impurities.

Synthesis of [^{11}C]methyl iodide

[^{11}C]Methyl iodide can be obtained either starting from [^{11}C]carbon dioxide or from [^{11}C]methane. The most frequently used method is the reduction of [^{11}C]carbon dioxide with lithium aluminium hydride. The formed [^{11}C]methanol is reacted with hydroiodic acid. Alternatively [^{11}C]methane, either obtained directly in the target or by on-line processes from [^{11}C]carbon dioxide, is reacted with iodine.

Synthesis of [^{11}C]methyl triflate

[^{11}C]methyl triflate can be prepared from [^{11}C]methyl iodide using a silver triflate-impregnated solid support such as graphitised carbon.

Synthesis of L-[*methyl*-^{11}C]methionine

The most widely used method to obtain L-[*methyl*-^{11}C]methionine is the alkylation of the sulphide anion, generated from L-homocysteine thiolactone, with

[^{11}C]methyl iodide or [^{11}C]methyl triflate in alkaline conditions in a solvent such as acetone. The L-[*methyl*-^{11}C]methionine obtained can be purified by semi-preparative liquid chromatography. For example, a column packed with octadecylsilyl silica gel for chromatography eluted with a 9 g/l solution of sodium chloride is suitable.

L-Homocysteine thiolactone hydrochloride

Specific optical rotation (*2.2.7*): + 20.5 to + 21.5, determined on a 10 g/l solution at 25 °C.

Infrared absorption spectrophotometry (*2.2.24*).

Comparison: *Ph. Eur. reference spectrum of L-homocysteine thiolactone hydrochloride.*

CHARACTERS

Appearance: clear, colourless solution.

Half-life and nature of radiation of carbon-11: see *Table of physical characteristics of radionuclides* (*5.7*).

IDENTIFICATION

A. Gamma-ray spectrometry.

Results: the only gamma photons have an energy of 0.511 MeV and, depending on the measurement geometry, a sum peak of 1.022 MeV may be observed.

B. It complies with the test for radionuclidic purity (see Tests).

C. Examine the chromatograms obtained in the test for radiochemical purity.

Results: the principal peak in the radiochromatogram obtained with the test solution is similar in retention time to the principal peak in the chromatogram obtained with reference solution (b).

TESTS

pH (*2.2.3*): 4.5 to 8.5.

Sterility. It complies with the test for sterility prescribed in the monograph on *Radiopharmaceutical preparations (0125)*. The injection may be released for use before completion of the test.

Bacterial endotoxins (*2.6.14*): less than 175/*V* IU/ml, *V* being the maximum recommended dose in millilitres. The injection may be released for use before completion of the test.

CHEMICAL PURITY

Impurity A, impurity B and methionine. Liquid chromatography (*2.2.29*).

Test solution. The preparation to be examined.

Reference solution (a). Dissolve 0.6 mg of *L-homocysteine thiolactone hydrochloride R*, 2 mg of *DL-homocysteine R* and 2 mg of *DL-methionine R* in *water R* and dilute to *V*, *V* being the maximum recommended dose in millilitres.

Reference solution (b). Dissolve 2 mg of *L-methionine R* in the same solvent as used in the test solution and dilute to 10 ml with the same solvent.

Column:

- *size*: *l* = 0.25 m, Ø = 4.6 mm,
- *stationary phase*: spherical *octadecylsilyl silica gel for chromatography R* (5 µm) with a specific surface of 220 m²/g, a pore size of 8 nm and a carbon loading of 6.2 per cent,
- *temperature*: 25 °C.

Mobile phase: 1.4 g/l solution of *potassium dihydrogen phosphate R*.

Flow rate: 1 ml/min.

Detection: spectrophotometer at 225 nm and radioactivity detector connected in series.

Injection: loop injector.

Run time: 10 min.

Relative retention with reference to methionine (retention time = about 2.6 min): impurity B = about 0.8, impurity A = about 2.7.

System suitability: reference solution (a):

- *resolution*: minimum of 2.5 between the peaks due to methionine and impurity B.

Limits: examine the chromatogram obtained with the spectrophotometer:

- *impurity A*: not more than the area of the corresponding peak in the chromatogram obtained with reference solution (a) (0.6 mg/*V*),
- *impurity B*: not more than the area of the corresponding peak in the chromatogram obtained with reference solution (a) (2 mg/*V*),
- *methionine*: not more than the area of the corresponding peak in the chromatogram obtained with reference solution (a) (2 mg/*V*).

Residual solvents (*2.4.24*): maximum 50 mg/*V* for the concentration of acetone, *V* being the maximum recommended dose in millilitres. The preparation may be released for use before completion of the test.

RADIONUCLIDIC PURITY

Carbon-11: minimum 99 per cent of the total radioactivity.

A. Gamma-ray spectroscopy.

Comparison: standardised fluorine-18 solution, or by using an instrument calibrated with the aid of such a solution. Standardised fluorine-18 solutions and/or standardisation services are available from the competent authority.

Results: the spectrum obtained with the solution to be examined does not differ significantly from that obtained with a standardised fluorine-18 solution.

B. Half-life: 19.9 min to 20.9 min.

The preparation may be released for use before completion of the test.

RADIOCHEMICAL PURITY

L-[Methyl-^{11}C]methionine and impurity E. Liquid chromatography (*2.2.29*) as described in the test for impurity A, impurity B and methionine.

Injection: test solution and reference solution (b).

Limits: examine the chromatogram obtained with the radioactivity detector:

- *total of L-[methyl-^{11}C]methionine and impurity E*: minimum of 95 per cent of the total radioactivity,
- other peaks in the chromatogram may be due to impurity C, impurity D and impurity F.

ENANTIOMERIC PURITY

Impurity E. Thin-layer chromatography (*2.2.27*).

Test solution. The preparation to be examined.

Reference solution (a). Dissolve 2 mg of *L-methionine R* in *water R* and dilute to 10 ml with the same solvent.

Reference solution (b). Dissolve 4 mg of *DL-methionine R* in *water R* and dilute to 10 ml with the same solvent.

Plate: *TLC octadecysilyl silica gel plate for chiral separations R.*

Mobile phase: *methanol R, water R* (50:50 *V/V*).

Application: 2-10 µl.

Development: over a path of 8 cm.

Radiopharmaceutical preparations

Drying: in air for 5 min.

Detection: spray with a 2 g/l solution of *ninhydrin R* in *ethanol R* and heat at 60 °C for 10 min. Determine the distribution of radioactivity using a suitable detector.

Retention factors: L-[*methyl*-^{11}C]methionine = about 0.58; impurity E = about 0.51.

System suitability: the chromatogram obtained with reference solution (b) shows 2 clearly separated spots.

Limits:

– *total of L-[methyl-^{11}C]methionine and impurity E*: minimum 95 per cent of the total radioactivity,

– *impurity E*: maximum 10 per cent of the total radioactivity.

The preparation may be released for use before completion of the test.

RADIOACTIVITY

Measure the radioactivity using suitable equipment by comparison with a standardised fluorine-18 solution or by measurement in an instrument calibrated with the aid of such a solution.

LABELLING

The accompanying information specifies the maximum recommended dose in millilitres.

IMPURITIES

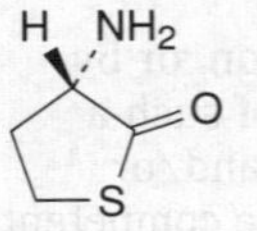

A. (3*S*)-3-aminodihydrothiophen-2(3*H*)-one (L-homocysteine thiolactone),

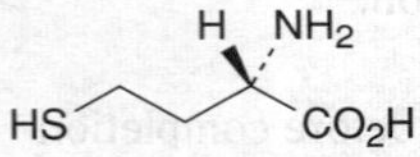

B. (2*S*)-2-amino-4-sulphanylbutanoic acid (L-homocysteine),

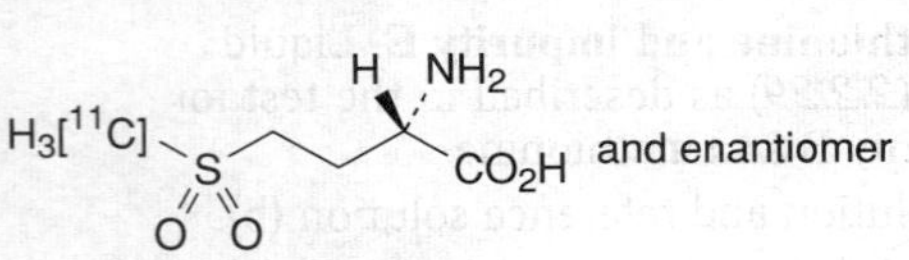

C. (2*RS*)-2-amino-4-([^{11}C]methylsulphonyl)butanoic acid (DL-[*methyl*-^{11}C]methionine *S,S*-dioxide),

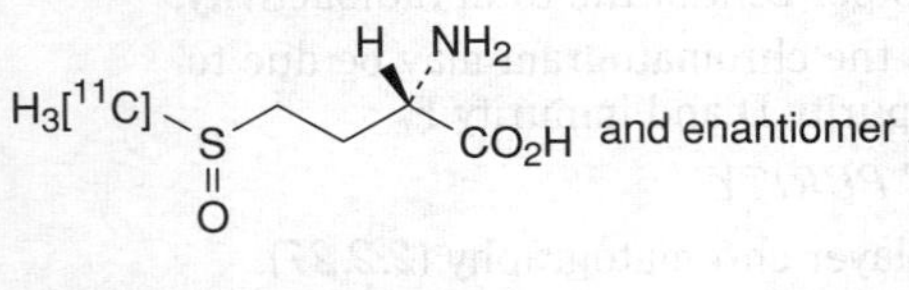

D. (2*RS*)-2-amino-4-([^{11}C]methylsulphinyl)butanoic acid (DL-[*methyl*-^{11}C]methionine *S*-oxide),

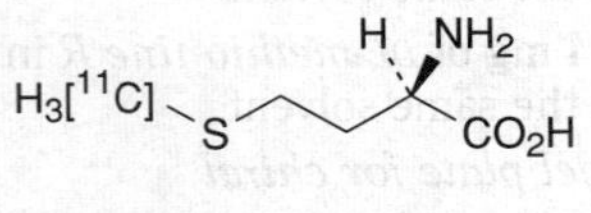

E. (2*R*)-2-amino-4-([^{11}C]methylsulphanyl)butanoic acid (D-[*methyl*-^{11}C]methionine),

F. [^{11}C]methanol

01/2005:0939

NORCHOLESTEROL INJECTION, IODINATED (^{131}I)

Norcholesteroli iodinati (^{131}I) solutio iniectabilis

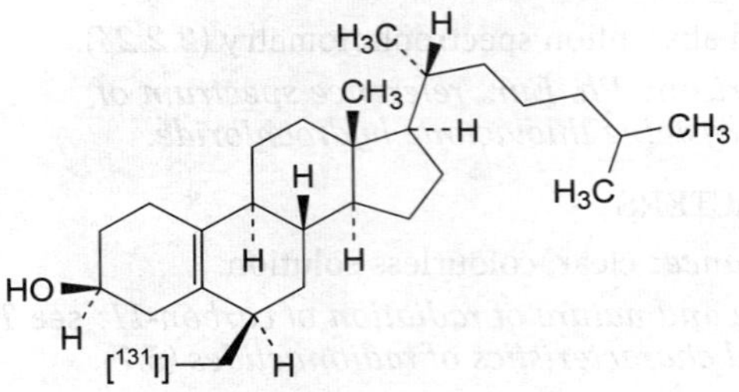

DEFINITION

Iodinated (^{131}I) norcholesterol injection is a sterile, bacterial endotoxin-free solution of 6β-[^{131}I]iodomethyl-19-norcholest-5(10)-en-3β-ol. It may contain a suitable emulsifier such as polysorbate 80 and a suitable antimicrobial preservative such as benzyl alcohol. Iodine-131 is a radioactive isotope of iodine and may be obtained by neutron irradiation of tellurium or by extraction from uranium fission products. The injection contains not less than 90.0 per cent and not more than 110.0 per cent of the declared iodine-131 radioactivity at the date and hour stated on the label. Not less than 85 per cent of the radioactivity corresponds to iodine-131 in the form of 6β-[^{131}I]iodomethyl-19-norcholest-5(10)-en-3β-ol. Not more than 5 per cent of the radioactivity corresponds to iodine-131 in the form of iodide. The specific radioactivity is 3.7 GBq to 37 GBq per gram of 6β-iodomethylnorcholesterol.

CHARACTERS

A clear or slightly turbid, colourless or pale yellow solution.

Iodine-131 has a half-life of 8.04 days and emits beta and gamma radiation.

IDENTIFICATION

A. Record the gamma-ray spectrum using a suitable instrument. The spectrum does not differ significantly from that of a standardised iodine-131 solution by direct comparison with such a solution. The most prominent photon of iodine-131 has an energy of 0.365 MeV. Standardised iodine-131 solutions are available from laboratories recognised by the competent authority.

B. Examine the chromatogram obtained in test (a) for radiochemical purity. The distribution of radioactivity contributes to the identification of the preparation.

TESTS

pH (*2.2.3*). The pH of the solution is between 3.5 and 8.5.

Sterility. It complies with the test for sterility prescribed in the monograph on *Radiopharmaceutical preparations (0125)*. The injection may be released for use before completion of the test.

Bacterial endotoxins (*2.6.14*): less than 175/*V* IU/ml, *V* being the maximum recommended dose in millilitres.

RADIONUCLIDIC PURITY

Record the gamma-ray spectrum using a suitable instrument. The spectrum does not differ significantly from that of a standardised iodine-131 solution. Determine the relative amounts of iodine-131, iodine-133, iodine-135 and other radionuclidic impurities present. Iodine-133 has a half-life of 20.8 h and its most prominent gamma photons have energies of 0.530 MeV and 0.875 MeV. Iodine-135 has a half-life of 6.55 h and its most prominent gamma photons have energies of 0.527 MeV, 1.132 MeV and 1.260 MeV. Not less than 99.9 per cent of the total radioactivity is due to iodine-131.

RADIOCHEMICAL PURITY

a) Examine by thin-layer chromatography (*2.2.27*) using *silica gel GF_{254} R* as the coating substance.

Test solution. The injection to be examined.

Carrier solution. Dissolve 10 mg of *potassium iodide R*, 20 mg of *potassium iodate R* and 0.1 g of *sodium hydrogen carbonate R* in *distilled water R* and dilute to 10 ml with the same solvent.

Apply to the plate up to 5 µl of the test solution and 10 µl of the carrier solution on the same spot. Develop over a path of 15 cm (about 60 min) using *chloroform R*. Allow the plate to dry in air and examine in ultraviolet light at 254 nm. Determine the distribution of radioactivity using a suitable detector. In the chromatogram obtained, not less than 85 per cent of the total radioactivity is found in the spot corresponding to 6β-iodomethyl-19-norcholest-5(10)-en-3β-ol at an R_f value of about 0.5. Iodide ion remains near the starting-line.

b) Examine by thin-layer chromatography (*2.2.27*) using *silica gel GF_{254} R* as the coating substance.

Test solution. The injection to be examined.

Carrier solution. Dissolve 10 mg *potassium iodide R*, 20 mg of *potassium iodate R* and 0.1 g of *sodium hydrogen carbonate R* in *distilled water R* and dilute to 10 ml with the same solvent.

Apply to the plate 10 µl of the carrier solution and then up to 5 µl of the test solution on the same spot. Develop over a path of 15 cm (about 90 min) using a mixture of equal volumes of *chloroform R* and *ethanol R*. Allow the plate to dry in air. Expose the plate to ultraviolet light at 254 nm for 5 min. A yellow spot corresponding to iodide develops at an R_f value of about 0.5. Determine the distribution of radio- activity using a suitable detector. The main peak of radio-activity is near to the solvent front. Other iodocholesterols migrate near the solvent front. In the chromatogram obtained, not more than 5 per cent of the total radioactivity is found in the spot corresponding to iodide.

RADIOACTIVITY

Measure the radioactivity using suitable counting equipment by comparison with a standardised iodine-131 solution or by measurement in an instrument calibrated with the aid of such a solution.

STORAGE

Store protected from light at a temperature not exceeding − 18 °C.

01/2005:1620

OXYGEN (^{15}O)

Oxygenium (^{15}O)

DEFINITION

Mixture of [^{15}O]oxygen in the gaseous phase and a suitable vehicle such as *Medicinal air (1238)*, for diagnostic use.

Purity:

– minimum 99 per cent of the total radioactivity corresponds to oxygen-15,
– minimum 97 per cent of the total radioactivity corresponds to oxygen-15 in the form of oxygen (O_2).

PRODUCTION

RADIONUCLIDIC PRODUCTION

Oxygen-15 is a radioactive isotope of oxygen which may be produced by various nuclear reactions such as proton irradiation of nitrogen-15 or deuteron irradiation of nitrogen-14.

RADIOCHEMICAL SYNTHESIS

In order to recover oxygen-15 as molecular oxygen from the nitrogen target gas, carrier oxygen is added at concentrations generally ranging from 0.2 per cent *V/V* to 1.0 per cent *V/V*. After irradiation, the target gas is usually passed through activated charcoal and a carbon dioxide scavenger, such as soda lime, before mixing with the vehicle.

CHARACTERS

Appearance: colourless gas.

Half-life and nature of radiation of oxygen-15: see *Table of physical characteristics of radionuclides* (*5.7*).

IDENTIFICATION

A. Gamma spectrometry.

Results: the only gamma photons have an energy of 0.511 MeV and, depending on the measurement geometry, a sum peak of 1.022 MeV may be observed.

B. It complies with the test for radionuclidic purity (see Tests).

C. Examine the chromatograms obtained in the test for radiochemical purity.

Results: the retention times of the principal peaks in the chromatogram obtained with the test gas using the radioactivity detector are similar to those of the principal peaks corresponding to oxygen in the chromatogram obtained with the reference gas using the thermal conductivity detector.

TESTS

The following tests are performed on [^{15}O]oxygen as described under radiochemical synthesis before mixing with the vehicle.

RADIONUCLIDIC PURITY

Oxygen-15: minimum 99 per cent of the total radioactivity.

A. Gamma spectrometry.

Comparison: standardised fluorine-18 solution, or by using an instrument calibrated with the aid of such a solution. Standardised fluorine-18 solutions and/or standardisation services are available from the competent authority.

Results: the spectrum obtained with the solution to be examined does not differ significantly from that obtained with a standardised fluorine-18 solution.

B. Half-life: 1.9 min to 2.2 min.

The preparation may be released for use before completion of the test.

RADIOCHEMICAL PURITY

Oxygen-15 in the form of O_2. Gas chromatography (*2.2.28*): use the normalisation procedure.

Test sample. [^{15}O]oxygen as described under radiochemical synthesis.

Reference gas. Nitrogen gas mixture R.

Column:

– *size*: l = 1.8 m, Ø1 = 6.3 mm and Ø2 = 3.2 mm,

Radiopharmaceutical preparations

– *stationary phase*: *GC concentrical column R*.

Carrier gas: *helium for chromatography R*.

Flow rate: 65 ml/min.

Temperature:

– *column*: 40 °C,
– *injection port*: 40 °C,
– *thermal conductivity detector*: 70 °C.

Detection: thermal conductivity detector and radioactivity detector connected in series.

Injection: loop injector.

Run time: 10 min.

Retention times: oxygen, nitrogen and carbon monoxide eluting from the inner column = about 0.4 min; carbon dioxide eluting from the inner column = about 0.8 min; oxygen eluting from the outer column = about 2.1 min; nitrogen eluting from the outer column = about 3.1 min; carbon monoxide eluting from the outer column = about 6.2 min.

System suitability: reference gas:

– 5 clearly separated principal peaks are observed in the chromatogram obtained using the thermal conductivity detector,
– *resolution*: minimum of 1.5 between the peaks due to carbon dioxide eluting from the inner column and oxygen eluting from the outer column, in the chromatogram obtained using the thermal conductivity detector.

Limits: examine the chromatogram obtained with the radioactivity detector and calculate the percentage content of oxygen-15 substances from the peak areas.

– *oxygen-15 gas in the form of* O_2: minimum 97 per cent of the total radioactivity,
– disregard the first peak corresponding to components co-eluting from the inner column.

RADIOACTIVITY

The radioactive concentration is determined before administration.

Measure the radioactivity using suitable equipment by comparison with a standardised fluorine-18 solution or by measurement in an instrument calibrated with the aid of such a solution.

01/2005:1924

RACLOPRIDE ([^{11}C]METHOXY) INJECTION

Raclopridi ([^{11}C]methoxy) solutio iniectabilis

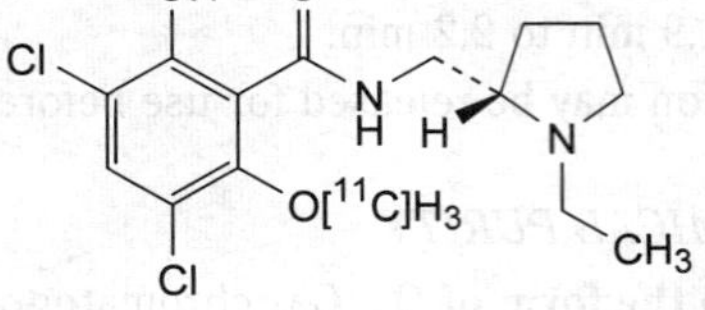

DEFINITION

Sterile solution of 3,5-dichloro-*N*-[[(2*S*)-1-ethylpyrrolidin-2-yl]methyl]-2-hydroxy-6-([^{11}C]methoxy)benzamide.

Content: 90 per cent to 110 per cent of the declared carbon-11 radioactivity at the date and time stated on the label.

Purity:

– minimum of 99 per cent of the total radioactivity corresponds to carbon-11,
– minimum of 95 per cent of the total radioactivity corresponds to carbon-11 in the form of [*methoxy*-^{11}C]raclopride.

Content of raclopride: maximum of 10 µg per maximum recommended dose in millilitres.

PRODUCTION

RADIONUCLIDE PRODUCTION

Carbon-11 is a radioactive isotope of carbon most commonly produced by proton irradiation of nitrogen. Depending on the addition of either trace amounts of oxygen or small amounts of hydrogen, the radioactivity is obtained as [^{11}C]carbon dioxide or [^{11}C]methane, respectively.

RADIOCHEMICAL SYNTHESIS

[*Methoxy*-^{11}C]raclopride may be prepared by *O*-alkylation of the corresponding phenolate anion (*S*)-3,5-dichloro-2,6-dihydroxy-*N*-[(1-ethylpyrrolidin-2-yl)methyl]benzamide with iodo[^{11}C]methane or [^{11}C]methyl trifluoromethanesulphonate.

Synthesis of iodo[^{11}C]methane

Iodo[^{11}C]methane may be produced from [^{11}C]carbon dioxide or from [^{11}C]methane. The most frequently used method is reduction of [^{11}C]carbon dioxide with lithium aluminium hydride. The lithium aluminium [^{11}C]methanolate formed is reacted with hydroiodic acid to iodo[^{11}C]methane via [^{11}C]methanol. Alternatively [^{11}C]methane, either obtained directly in the target or by on-line processes from [^{11}C]carbon dioxide, is reacted with iodine.

Synthesis of [^{11}C]methyl trifluoromethanesulphonate

[^{11}C]Methyl trifluoromethanesulphonate may be prepared from iodo[^{11}C]methane using a solid support such as graphitised carbon impregnated with silver trifluoromethanesulphonate.

Synthesis of [*methoxy*-^{11}C]raclopride

Methylation with iodo[^{11}C]methane is performed under alkaline conditions in a solvent such as dimethyl sulphoxide. The methylation with [^{11}C]methyl trifluoromethanesulphonate is performed in a solvent such as dimethylformamide or acetone. The resulting [*methoxy*-^{11}C]raclopride may be purified by semi-preparative liquid chromatography using, for example, a column packed with octadecylsilyl silica gel for chromatography eluted with a mixture of 25 volumes of acetonitrile and 75 volumes of 0.01 M phosphoric acid.

PRECURSOR FOR SYNTHESIS

(*S*)-3,5-Dichloro-2,6-dihydroxy-*N*-[(1-ethylpyrrolidin-2-yl)methyl]benzamide hydrobromide

Melting point (*2.2.14*): 211 °C to 213 °C.

Specific optical rotation (*2.2.7*): + 11.3 to + 11.5, determined on a 15.0 g/l solution in *ethanol R* at 22 °C.

CHARACTERS

Appearance: clear, colourless solution.

Half-life and nature of radiation of carbon-11: see *Table of physical characteristics of radionuclides* (*5.7*).

IDENTIFICATION

A. Gamma-ray spectrometry.
Results: the only gamma photons have an energy of 0.511 MeV and, depending on the measurement geometry, a sum peak of 1.022 MeV may be observed.

B. It complies with test B for radionuclidic purity (see Tests).

C. Examine the chromatograms obtained in the test for radiochemical purity.

Results: the principal peak in the radiochromatogram obtained with the test solution is similar in retention time to the principal peak in the chromatogram obtained with reference solution (d).

TESTS

pH (*2.2.3*): 4.5 to 8.5.

Sterility. It complies with the test for sterility prescribed in the monograph on *Radiopharmaceutical preparations (0125)*. The injection may be released for use before completion of the test.

Bacterial endotoxins (*2.6.14*): less than 175/*V* IU/ml, *V* being the maximum recommended dose in millilitres. The injection may be released for use before completion of the test.

CHEMICAL PURITY

Raclopride and impurity A. Liquid chromatography (*2.2.29*).

Test solution. The preparation to be examined.

Reference solution (a). Dissolve 7.2 mg of *raclopride tartrate R* in *water R* and dilute to 50 ml with the same solvent.

Reference solution (b). Dissolve 1.2 mg of *(S)-3,5-dichloro-2,6-dihydroxy-N-[(1-ethylpyrrolidin-2-yl)methyl]benzamide hydrobromide R* in *methanol R* and dilute to 100 ml with the same solvent.

Reference solution (c). To 0.1 ml of reference solution (a) add 0.1 ml of reference solution (b) and dilute to *V* with *water R*, *V* being the maximum recommended dose in millilitres.

Reference solution (d). Dilute 1.0 ml of reference solution (a) to 10.0 ml with *water R*.

Column:

- *size*: l = 0.05 m, Ø = 4.6 mm,
- *stationary phase*: spherical *end-capped octadecylsilyl silica gel for chromatography R* (3.5 μm) with a specific surface area of 175 m^2/g, a pore size of 12.5 nm, a pore volume of 0.7 cm^3/g and a carbon loading of 15 per cent,
- *temperature*: 30 °C.

Mobile phase: dissolve 2 g of *sodium heptanesulphonate R* in 700 ml of *water R*, adjust to pH 3.9 with *phosphoric acid R* and dilute to 1000 ml with *acetonitrile R*.

Flow rate: 1 ml/min.

Detection: spectrophotometer at 220 nm and radioactivity detector connected in series.

Injection: loop injector; inject the test solution and reference solutions (b) and (c).

Run time: 10 min.

Relative retention with reference to raclopride: impurity A = about 0.46.

System suitability: reference solution (c):

- *resolution*: minimum of 5 between the peaks due to raclopride and to impurity A.

Limits: examine the chromatogram obtained with the spectrophotometer:

- *raclopride*: not more than the area of the corresponding peak in the chromatogram obtained with reference solution (c) (10 μg/*V*),
- *impurity A*: not more than the area of the corresponding peak in the chromatogram obtained with reference solution (c) (1 μg/*V*).

Residual solvents are limited according to the principles defined in the general chapter (*5.4*), using the general method (*2.4.24*). The preparation may be released for use before completion of the test.

RADIONUCLIDIC PURITY

Carbon-11: minimum 99 per cent of the total radioactivity.

The preparation may be released for use before completion of the test.

A. Gamma-ray spectrometry.

Comparison: standardised fluorine-18 solution, or by using a calibrated instrument. Standardised fluorine-18 solutions and/or standardisation services are available from the competent authority.

Results: the spectrum obtained with the solution to be examined does not differ significantly from that obtained with a standardised fluorine-18 solution.

B. Half-life. 19.9 min to 20.9 min.

RADIOCHEMICAL PURITY

Liquid chromatography (*2.2.29*) as described in the test for raclopride and impurity A with the following modifications.

Injection: test solution and reference solution (d).

Limits: examine the chromatogram obtained with the radioactivity detector:

- *[Methoxy-^{11}C] raclopride*: minimum of 95 per cent of the total radioactivity.

RADIOACTIVITY

Mesure the radioactivity using suitable equipment by comparison with a standardised fluorine-18 solution or by using a calibrated instrument.

LABELLING

The accompanying information specifies the maximum recommended dose in millilitres.

IMPURITIES

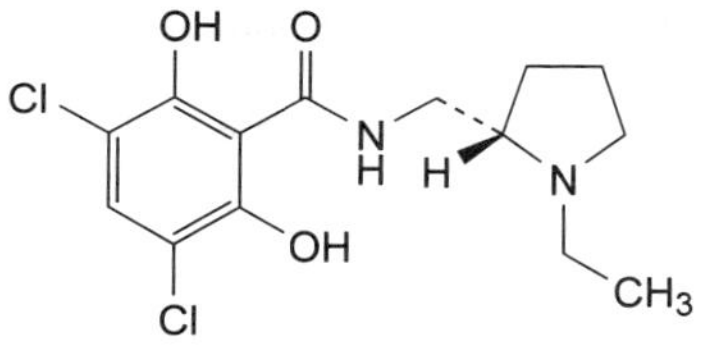

A. 3,5-dichloro-*N*-[[(2*S*)-1-ethylpyrrolidin-2-yl]methyl]-2,6-dihydroxybenzamide.

Radiopharmaceutical preparations

01/2005:1920

SODIUM ACETATE ([1-^{11}C]) INJECTION

Natrii acetatis ([1-^{11}C]) solutio iniectabilis

$CH_3{}^{11}COONa$

DEFINITION

Sterile solution of sodium [1-^{11}C]acetate, in equilibrium with [1-^{11}C]acetic acid.

Content: 90 per cent to 110 per cent of the declared carbon-11 radioactivity at the date and time stated on the label.

PRODUCTION

RADIONUCLIDE PRODUCTION

Carbon-11 is a radioactive isotope of carbon which is most commonly produced by proton irradiation of nitrogen. By the addition of trace amounts of oxygen, the radioactivity is obtained as [^{11}C]carbon dioxide.

RADIOCHEMICAL SYNTHESIS

[^{11}C]Carbon dioxide may be separated from the target gas mixture by cryogenic trapping or by trapping on a molecular sieve at room temperature. [^{11}C]Carbon dioxide is then released from the trap using an inert gas such as nitrogen at a temperature higher than the trapping temperature.

[1-^{11}C]Acetate is usually prepared by reaction of [^{11}C]carbon dioxide with methylmagnesium bromide in organic solvents such as ether or tetrahydrofuran.

Hydrolysis of the product yields [1-^{11}C]acetic acid. It is purified by chromatographic procedures. The eluate is diluted with sodium chloride solution.

PRECURSOR FOR SYNTHESIS

Methylmagnesium bromide. The reactivity of methylmagnesium bromide is tested by decomposition of a defined amount with water. The amount of hydrogen released during this reaction is not less than 90 per cent of the theoretical value.

CHARACTERS

Appearance: clear, colourless solution.

Half-life and nature of radiation of carbon-11: see *Table of physical characteristics of radionuclides* (*5.7*).

IDENTIFICATION

A. Gamma-ray spectrometry.

Results: the only gamma photons have an energy of 0.511 MeV and, depending on the measurement geometry, a sum peak of 1.022 MeV may be observed.

B. It complies with test B for radionuclidic purity (see Tests).

C. Examine the chromatograms obtained in the test for radiochemical purity.

Results: the principal peak in the radiochromatogram obtained with the test solution is similar in retention time to the principal peak in the chromatogram obtained with the reference solution.

TESTS

pH (*2.2.3*): 4.5 to 8.5.

Sterility. It complies with the test for sterility prescribed in the monograph on *Radiopharmaceutical preparations (0125)*. The injection may be released for use before completion of the test.

Bacterial endotoxins (*2.6.14*): less than 175/*V* IU/ml, *V* being the maximum recommended dose in millilitres. The injection may be released for use before completion of the test.

CHEMICAL PURITY

Acetate. Liquid chromatography (*2.2.29*).

Test solution. The preparation to be examined.

Reference solution. Dissolve 28 mg of *sodium acetate R* in *water R* and dilute to *V*, *V* being the maximum recommended dose in millilitres.

Column:
- *size*: l = 0.25 m, Ø = 4.0 mm,
- *stationary phase*: *strongly basic anion exchange resin for chromatography R* (10 µm),
- *temperature*: 25 °C.

Mobile phase: *0.1 M sodium hydroxide* protected from atmospheric carbon dioxide.

Flow rate: 1 ml/min.

Detection: spectrophotometer at 220 nm and radioactivity detector connected in series.

Injection: loop injector.

Run time: 10 min.

System suitability: reference solution:
- *resolution*: minimum 4.0 between the peaks due to hold-up volume and acetate.

Limit: examine the chromatograms obtained with the spectrophotometer:
- *acetate*: not more than the area of the corresponding peak in the chromatogram obtained with the reference solution (20 mg per *V*).

Residual solvents are limited according to the principles defined in the general chapter (*5.4*), using the general method (*2.4.24*). The preparation may be released for use before completion of the test.

RADIONUCLIDIC PURITY

Carbon-11: minimum 99 per cent of the total radioactivity. The preparation may be released for use before completion of the tests.

A. Gamma-ray spectrometry.

Comparison: standardised fluorine-18 solution, or by using a calibrated instrument. Standardised fluorine-18 solutions and/or standardisation services are available from laboratories recognised by the competent authority.

Results: the spectrum obtained with the solution to be examined does not differ significantly from that obtained with a standardised fluorine-18 solution.

B. Half-life: 19.9 min to 20.9 min.

RADIOCHEMICAL PURITY

[1-^{11}C]Acetate. Liquid chromatography (*2.2.29*) as described in the test for acetate.

Limit: examine the chromatograms obtained with the spectrophotometer and the radioactivity detector:
- *total of [1-^{11}C]acetate*: minimum 95 per cent of the total radioactivity.

RADIOACTIVITY

Measure the radioactivity using suitable equipment by comparison with a standardised fluorine-18 solution or by measurement with a calibrated instrument.

LABELLING

The accompanying information specifies the maximum recommended dose in millilitres.

01/2005:0279

SODIUM CHROMATE (^{51}Cr) STERILE SOLUTION

Natrii chromatis (^{51}Cr) solutio sterilis

DEFINITION

Sodium chromate (^{51}Cr) sterile solution is a sterile solution of sodium [^{51}Cr]chromate made isotonic by the addition of sodium chloride. Chromium-51 is a radioactive isotope of chromium and may be prepared by neutron irradiation of chromium, either of natural isotopic composition or enriched in chromium-50. The solution contains not less than 90.0 per cent and not more than 110.0 per cent of

Radiopharmaceutical preparations

the declared chromium-51 radioactivity at the date and hour stated on the label. Not less than 90 per cent of the radioactivity corresponds to chromium-51 in the form of chromate. The specific radioactivity is not less than 370 MBq of chromium-51 per milligram of chromate ion.

CHARACTERS

A clear, colourless or slightly yellow solution.

Chromium-51 has a half-life of 27.7 days and emits gamma radiation.

IDENTIFICATION

A. Record the gamma-ray spectrum using a suitable instrument. The spectrum does not differ significantly from that of a standardised chromium-51 solution. Standardised chromium-51 solution are available from laboratories recognised by the competent authority. The gamma photon has an energy of 0.320 MeV.

B. Examine the chromatogram obtained in the test for radiochemical purity. The distribution of radioactivity contributes to the identification of the preparation.

TESTS

pH (*2.2.3*). The pH of the solution is 6.0 to 8.5.

Total chromate. Not more than 2.7 µg of chromate ion (CrO_4^{2-}) per megabecquerel. Measure the absorbance of the solution (*2.2.25*) at the absorption maximum at 370 nm. Calculate the content of chromate using the absorbance of a standard consisting of a 1.7 mg/l solution of *potassium chromate R*. If necessary, adjust the solution to be examined and the standard to pH 8.0 by adding *sodium hydrogen carbonate solution R*.

Sterility. It complies with the test for sterility prescribed in the monograph on *Radiopharmaceutical preparations (0125)*. The solution may be released for use before completion of the test.

RADIONUCLIDIC PURITY

Record the gamma-ray spectrum using a suitable instrument. The spectrum does not differ significantly from that of a standardised chromium-51 solution.

RADIOCHEMICAL PURITY

Examine by ascending paper chromatography (*2.2.26*). Apply to the paper a quantity of the solution sufficient for the detection method. Begin the development immediately and develop for 2.5 h using a mixture of 25 volumes of *ammonia R*, 50 volumes of *alcohol R* and 125 volumes of *water R*. Chromic ions remain on the starting line. Determine the distribution of the radioactivity using a suitable detector. Not less than 90 per cent of the total radioactivity of the chromatogram is found in the spot with an R_f value of about 0.9, corresponding to sodium chromate.

RADIOACTIVITY

Measure the radioactivity using suitable counting equipment by comparison with a standardised chromium-51 solution or by measurement in an instrument calibrated with the aid of such a solution.

01/2005:2100

SODIUM FLUORIDE (^{18}F) INJECTION

Natrii fluoridi (^{18}F) solutio iniectabilis

DEFINITION

Sterile solution containing fluorine-18 in the form of sodium fluoride. It may contain carrier fluoride and a suitable buffer.

Content:

- *fluorine-18*: 90 per cent to 110 per cent of the declared fluorine-18 radioactivity at the date and hour stated on the label,
- *fluoride*: maximum 4.52 mg per maximum recommended dose in millilitres.

PRODUCTION

The radionuclide fluorine-18 is most commonly produced by proton irradiation of water enriched in oxygen-18. Fluorine-18 in the form of fluoride is recovered from the target water, generally by adsorption and desorption from anion-exchange resins or electrochemical deposition and redissolution.

CHARACTERS

Appearance: clear, colourless solution.

Half-life and nature of radiation of fluorine-18: see *Table of physical characteristics of radionuclides* (*5.7*).

IDENTIFICATION

A. Gamma-ray spectrometry.

Results: the only gamma photons have an energy of 0.511 MeV and, depending on the measurement geometry, a sum peak of 1.022 MeV may be observed.

B. It complies with test B for radionuclidic purity (see Tests).

C. Examine the chromatograms obtained in the test for radiochemical purity (see Tests).

Results: the principal peak in the radiochromatogram obtained with the test solution is similar in retention time to the principal peak in the chromatogram obtained with the reference solution. In the chromatogram obtained with the reference solution, the peak due to fluoride is negative.

TESTS

pH (*2.2.3*): 5.0 to 8.5.

Fluoride. Liquid chromatography (*2.2.29*).

Test solution. The preparation to be examined.

Reference solution. Dissolve 10 mg of *sodium fluoride R* in *water R* and dilute to *V* with the same solvent, *V* being the maximum recommended dose in millilitres.

Column:

- *size*: l = 0.25 m, Ø = 4 mm,
- *stationary phase*: *strongly basic anion-exchange resin for chromatography R* (10 µm),
- *temperature*: constant, between 20 °C and 30 °C.

Mobile phase: 4 g/l solution of *sodium hydroxide R*, protected from atmospheric carbon dioxide.

Flow rate: 1 ml/min.

Detection: spectrophotometer at 220 nm and a radioactivity detector connected in series.

Injection: 20 µl.

Run time: 15 min.

System suitability: examine the chromatogram obtained with the reference solution using the spectrophotometer:

- *signal-to-noise ratio*: minimum 10 for the principal peak,
- *retention time of fluoride*: minimum 3 times the hold-up time.

Limit: examine the chromatogram obtained with the spectrophotometer:

- *fluoride*: not more than the area of the corresponding peak in the chromatogram obtained with the reference solution (4.52 mg/*V*).

Sterility. It complies with the test for sterility prescribed in the monograph on *Radiopharmaceutical preparations (0125)*. The injection may be released for use before completion of the test.

Bacterial endotoxins (*2.6.14*): less than 175/*V* IU/ml, *V* being the maximum recommended dose in millilitres. The injection may be released for use before completion of the test.

RADIONUCLIDIC PURITY

Fluorine-18: minimum 99.9 per cent of the total radioactivity.

The preparation may be released for use before completion of the tests.

A. Gamma-ray spectrometry.

Determine the amount of fluorine-18 and radionuclidic impurities with a half-life longer than 2 h. For the detection and quantification of impurities, retain the preparation to be examined for a sufficient time to allow the fluorine-18 to decay to a level which permits the detection of impurities.

Results: the spectrum obtained with the preparation to be examined does not differ significantly from that of a background spectrum.

B. Half-life: 105 min to 115 min.

RADIOCHEMICAL PURITY

[^{18}F]fluoride. Liquid chromatography (*2.2.29*) as described in the test for fluoride. If necessary, dilute the test solution with *water R* to obtain a radioactivity concentration suitable for the radioactivity detector.

Limit: examine the chromatogram obtained with the radioactivity detector:

– *[^{18}F]fluoride*: minimum 98.5 per cent of the total radioactivity.

RADIOACTIVITY

Determine the radioactivity using a calibrated instrument.

LABELLING

The label states the maximum recommended dose in millilitres.

01/2005:0563

SODIUM IODIDE (^{123}I) INJECTION

Natrii iodidi (^{123}I) solutio iniectabilis

DEFINITION

Sterile solution containing iodine-123 in the form of sodium iodide; it may contain sodium thiosulphate or some other suitable reducing agent and a suitable buffer.

Content: 90 per cent to 110 per cent of the declared iodine-123 radioactivity at the date and hour stated on the label.

PRODUCTION

Iodine-123 is obtained by proton irradiation of xenon enriched in xenon-124 (minimum 98 per cent) followed by the decay of xenon-123 which is formed directly and by the decay of caesium-123. No carrier iodide is added.

CHARACTERS

Appearance: clear, colourless solution.

Half-life and nature of radiation of iodine-123: see *Table of physical characteristics of radionuclides (5.7)*.

IDENTIFICATION

A. Gamma-ray spectrometry.

Results: the spectrum obtained with the preparation to be examined does not differ significantly from that of a standardised iodine-123 solution. The most prominent gamma photon has an energy of 0.159 MeV and is accompanied by the principal X-ray of 0.027 MeV.

B. Examine the chromatograms obtained in the test for radiochemical purity.

Results: the principal peak in the radiochromatogram obtained with the test solution is similar in retention time to the principal peak in the chromatogram obtained with reference solution (a).

TESTS

pH (*2.2.3*): 7.0 to 10.0.

Sterility. It complies with the test for sterility prescribed in the monograph on *Radiopharmaceutical preparations (0125)*. The preparation may be released for use before completion of the test.

RADIONUCLIDIC PURITY

Iodine-123: minimum 99.65 per cent of the total radioactivity.

Gamma-ray spectrometry.

Determine the relative amounts of iodine-123, iodine-125, tellurium-121 and other radionuclidic impurities present. For the detection of tellurium-121 and iodine-125, retain the preparation to be examined for a sufficient time to allow iodine-123 to decay to a level which permits the detection of radionuclidic impurities. No radionuclides with a half-life longer than that of iodine-125 are detected.

The preparation may be released for use before completion of the test.

RADIOCHEMICAL PURITY

[^{123}I]iodide. Liquid chromatography (*2.2.29*).

Test solution. Dilute the preparation to be examined with a 2 g/l solution of *sodium hydroxide R* to a radioactive concentration suitable for the detector. Add an equal volume of a solution containing 1 g/l of *potassium iodide R*, 2 g/l of *potassium iodate R* and 10 g/l of *sodium hydrogen carbonate R* and mix.

Reference solution (a). Dilute 1 ml of a 26.2 mg/l solution of *potassium iodide R* to 10 ml with *water R*.

Reference solution (b). Dilute 1 ml of a 24.5 mg/l solution of *potassium iodate R* to 10 ml with *water R*. Mix equal volumes of this solution and reference solution (a).

Column:

– *size*: l = 0.25 m, Ø = 4.0 mm,

– *stationary phase*: *octadecylsilyl silica gel for chromatography R* (5 µm),

– *temperature*: constant between 20 °C and 30 °C.

Mobile phase: dissolve 5.85 g of *sodium chloride R* in 1000 ml of *water R*, add 0.65 ml of *octylamine R* and adjust to pH 7.0 with *dilute phosphoric acid R*; add 50 ml of *acetonitrile R* and mix.

Flow rate: 1.5 ml/min.

Detection: spectrophotometer at 220 nm and a radioactivity detector connected in series.

Injection: 20 µl.

Run time: 12 min.

Relative retention with reference to iodide (retention time = about 5 min): iodate = 0.2 to 0.3.

Radiopharmaceutical preparations

System suitability: reference solution (b):

- *resolution*: minimum 2 between the peaks due to iodide and iodate in the chromatogram recorded with the spectrophotometer.

Limit: examine the chromatogram obtained with the test solution using the radioactivity detector and locate the peak due to iodide by comparison with the chromatogram obtained with reference solution (a) using the spectrophotometer:

- *[^{123}I]iodide*: minimum 95 per cent of the total radioactivity.

RADIOACTIVITY

Determine the radioactivity using a calibrated instrument.

LABELLING

The label states any substance added.

IMPURITIES

A. [^{123}I]iodate ion.

01/2005:0938

SODIUM IODIDE (^{131}I) CAPSULES FOR DIAGNOSTIC USE

Natrii iodidi (^{131}I) capsulae ad usum diagnosticum

DEFINITION

Capsules for diagnostic use containing iodine-131 in the form of sodium iodide on a solid support; they may contain sodium thiosulphate or some other suitable reducing agents and a suitable buffering substance. A package contains 1 or more capsules.

Content:

- iodine-131: maximum 37 MBq per capsule; the average radioactivity determined in the test for uniformity of content is 90 per cent to 110 per cent of the declared iodine-131 radioactivity at the date and hour stated on the label;
- iodide: maximum 20 µg per capsule.

PRODUCTION

Iodine-131 is obtained by neutron irradiation of tellurium or by extraction from uranium fission products. No carrier iodide is added.

CHARACTERS

Half-life and nature of radiation of iodine-131: see *Table of physical characteristics of radionuclides (5.7)*.

IDENTIFICATION

A. Gamma-ray spectrometry.

Results: the spectrum obtained with the preparation to be examined does not differ significantly from that of a standardised iodine-131 solution. The most prominent gamma photon has an energy of 0.365 MeV.

B. Examine the chromatograms obtained in the test for radiochemical purity.

Results: the principal peak in the radiochromatogram obtained with test solution (b) is similar in retention time to the principal peak in the chromatogram obtained with reference solution (a).

TESTS

Disintegration: the contents of the capsule dissolve completely within 15 min.

In a water-bath at 37 °C, warm in a small beaker about 20 ml of a 2.0 g/l solution of *potassium iodide R*. Add a capsule to be examined. Stir magnetically at 20 r/min.

Uniformity of content. Determine the radioactivity of each of not fewer than 10 capsules. Calculate the average radioactivity per capsule. The radioactivity of no capsule differs by more than 10 per cent from the average, the relative standard deviation is not greater than 3.5 per cent.

Iodide. Liquid chromatography (*2.2.29*).

Test solution (a). Dissolve a capsule to be examined in 10 ml of *water R*. Filter through a 0.2 µm filter.

Test solution (b). Dissolve a capsule to be examined in *water R*. Filter through a 0.2 µm filter and dilute the filtrate with a 2 g/l solution of *sodium hydroxide R* to a radioactive concentration suitable for the detector. Add an equal volume of a solution containing 1 g/l of *potassium iodide R*, 2 g/l of *potassium iodate R* and 10 g/l of *sodium hydrogen carbonate R* and mix.

Reference solution (a). Dilute 1 ml of a 26.2 mg/l solution of *potassium iodide R* to 10 ml with *water R*.

Reference solution (b). Dilute 1 ml of a 24.5 mg/l solution of *potassium iodate R* to 10 ml with *water R*. Mix equal volumes of this solution and reference solution (a).

Blank solution. Prepare a solution containing 2 mg/ml of each constituent stated on the label, apart from iodide.

Column:

- *size*: l = 0.25 m, Ø = 4.0 mm,
- *stationary phase*: *octadecylsilyl silica gel for chromatography R* (5 µm),
- *temperature*: constant between 20 °C and 30 °C.

Mobile phase: dissolve 5.85 g of *sodium chloride R* in 1000 ml of *water R*, add 0.65 ml of *octylamine R* and adjust to pH 7.0 with *dilute phosphoric acid R*; add 50 ml of *acetonitrile R* and mix.

Flow rate: 1.5 ml/min.

Detection: spectrophotometer at 220 nm and radioactivity detector connected in series.

Injection: 20 µl of test solution (a), reference solutions (a) and (b) and the blank solution.

Run time: 12 min.

Relative retention with reference to iodide (retention time = about 5 min): iodate = 0.2 to 0.3.

System suitability:

- in the chromatogram obtained with the blank solution, none of the peaks has a retention time similar to that of the peak due to iodide,
- *resolution*: minimum 2 between the peaks due to iodide and iodate in the chromatogram obtained with reference solution (b) recorded with the spectrophotometer.

Limit: examine the chromatograms obtained with the spectrophotometer:

- *iodide*: not more than the area of the corresponding peak in the chromatogram obtained with reference solution (a) (20 µg/capsule).

RADIONUCLIDIC PURITY

Iodine-131: minimum 99.9 per cent of the total radioactivity.

Gamma-ray spectrometry.

Determine the relative amounts of iodine-131, iodine-133, iodine-135 and other radionuclidic impurities present.

RADIOCHEMICAL PURITY

[^{131}I]iodide. Liquid chromatography (*2.2.29*) as described in the test for iodide with the following modifications.

Injection: 20 µl of test solution (b) and reference solution (a).

Limit: examine the chromatogram obtained with the test solution using the radioactivity detector and locate the peak due to iodide by comparison with the chromatogram obtained with reference solution (a) using the spectrophotometer:

– *[^{131}I]iodide*: minimum 95 per cent of the total radioactivity.

RADIOACTIVITY

Determine the radioactivity of the package using a calibrated instrument.

LABELLING

The label states any substance added and the number of capsules in the package.

IMPURITIES

A. [^{131}I]iodate ion.

01/2005:0281

SODIUM IODIDE (^{131}I) SOLUTION

Natrii iodidi (^{131}I) solutio

DEFINITION

Solution containing iodine-131 in the form of sodium iodide and also sodium thiosulphate or some other suitable reducing agent. It may contain a suitable buffer.

Content:

– *iodine-131*: 90 per cent to 110 per cent of the declared radioactivity at the date and hour stated on the label,
– *iodide*: maximum 20 µg in the maximum recommended dose in millilitres.

PRODUCTION

Iodine-131 is a radioactive isotope of iodine and may be obtained by neutron irradiation of tellurium or by extraction from uranium fission products. No carrier iodide is added.

CHARACTERS

Appearance: clear, colourless solution.

Half-life and nature of radiation of iodine-131: see *Table of physical characteristics of radionuclides* (*5.7*).

IDENTIFICATION

A. Gamma-ray spectrometry.

Results: the spectrum obtained with the preparation to be examined does not differ significantly from that of a standardised iodine-131 solution. The most prominent gamma photon has an energy of 0.365 MeV.

B. Examine the chromatograms obtained in the test for iodide.

Results: the principal peak in the radiochromatogram obtained with test solution (a) is similar in retention time to the principal peak in the chromatogram obtained with reference solution (a).

TESTS

pH (*2.2.3*): 7.0 to 10.0.

Sterility. If intended for parenteral use, it complies with the test for sterility prescribed in the monograph on *Radiopharmaceutical preparations (0125)*. The solution may be released for use before completion of the test.

Iodide. Liquid chromatography (*2.2.29*).

Test solution (a). The preparation to be examined.

Test solution (b). Dilute the preparation to be examined with *0.05 M sodium hydroxide* until the radioactivity is equivalent to about 74 MBq/ml. Add an equal volume of a solution containing 1 g/l of *potassium iodide R*, 2 g/l of *potassium iodate R* and 10 g/l of *sodium hydrogen carbonate R* and mix.

Reference solution (a). Dilute 1 ml of a 26.2 mg/l solution of *potassium iodide R* to *V* with *water R*, *V* being the maximum recommended dose in millilitres.

Reference solution (b). Dilute 1 ml of a 24.5 mg/l solution of *potassium iodate R* to *V* with *water R*, *V* being the maximum recommended dose in millilitres. Mix equal volumes of this solution and of reference solution (a).

Blank solution. Prepare a solution containing 2 mg/ml of each of the components stated on the label, apart from iodide.

Column:

– *size*: l = 0.25 m, Ø = 4.0 mm,
– *stationary phase*: *octadecylsilyl silica gel for chromatography R* (5 µm),
– *temperature*: maintain at a constant temperature between 20 °C and 30 °C.

Use stainless steel tubing.

Mobile phase: dissolve 5.844 g of *sodium chloride R* in 1000 ml of *water R*, add 650 µl of *octylamine R* and adjust to pH 7.0 with *phosphoric acid R*; add 50 ml of *acetonitrile R* and mix.

Flow rate: 1.5 ml/min.

Detection: spectrophotometer at 220 nm and radioactivity detector connected in series.

Injection: 25 µl; inject test solution (a), the blank solution and reference solutions (a) and (b).

Run time: 12 min.

Relative retention with reference to iodide (retention time = about 5 min): iodate = 0.2 to 0.3.

System suitability:

– in the chromatogram obtained with the blank solution, none of the peaks shows a retention time similar to that of the peak due to iodide,
– *resolution*: minimum 2 between the peaks due to iodide and iodate in the chromatogram obtained with reference solution (b) recorded with the spectrophotometer.

Limit: examine the chromatogram obtained with the spectrophotometer; locate the peak due to iodide by comparison with the chromatogram obtained with reference solution (a):

– *iodide*: not more than the area of the corresponding peak in the chromatogram obtained with reference solution (a).

RADIONUCLIDIC PURITY

Iodine-131: minimum 99.9 per cent of the total radioactivity.

Gamma-ray spectrometry.

Determine the relative amounts of iodine-131, iodine-133, iodine-135 and other radionuclidic impurities present.

RADIOCHEMICAL PURITY

[^{131}I]Iodide. Liquid chromatography (*2.2.29*) as described in the test for iodide with the following modification.

Injection: test solution (b).

Radiopharmaceutical preparations

Limit: examine the chromatogram obtained with the radioactivity detector:

- *[^{131}I]iodide*: minimum 95 per cent of the total radioactivity.

RADIOACTIVITY

Measure the radioactivity using suitable equipment by comparison with a standardised iodine-131 solution or by using a calibrated instrument.

LABELLING

The label states:

- any substance added,
- the maximum recommended dose, in millilitres,
- where applicable, that the preparation is suitable for use in the manufacture of parenteral dosage forms.

IMPURITIES

A. [^{131}I]iodate ion.

01/2005:2121

SODIUM IODIDE (^{131}I) SOLUTION FOR RADIOLABELLING

Natrii iodidi (^{131}I) solutio ad radio-signandum

DEFINITION

Strongly alkaline solution containing iodine-131 in the form of sodium iodide. It does not contain a reducing agent.

Content: 90 per cent to 110 per cent of the declared iodine-131 radioactivity at the date and hour stated on the label.

PRODUCTION

Iodine-131 may be obtained by neutron irradiation of tellurium or by extraction from uranium fission products. No carrier iodide is added.

CHARACTERS

Appearance: clear, colourless solution.

Half-life and nature of radiation of iodine-131: see *Table of physical characteristics of radionuclides (5.7)*.

IDENTIFICATION

A. Gamma-ray spectrometry.

Results: the spectrum obtained with the preparation to be examined does not differ significantly from that of a standardised iodine-131 solution. The most prominent gamma photon of iodine-131 has an energy of 0.365 MeV.

B. Examine the chromatograms obtained in the test for radiochemical purity (see Tests).

Results: the principal peak in the radiochromatogram obtained with the test solution is similar in retention time to the principal peak in the chromatogram obtained with reference solution (a).

TESTS

Alkalinity (*2.2.4*). The preparation is strongly alkaline.

RADIONUCLIDIC PURITY

Iodine-131: minimum 99.9 per cent of the total radioactivity. Gamma-ray spectrometry.

Determine the relative amounts of iodine-130, iodine-131, iodine-133, iodine-135 and other radionuclidic impurities present.

RADIOCHEMICAL PURITY

[^{131}I]iodide. Liquid chromatography (*2.2.29*).

Test solution. Dilute the preparation to be examined with an equal volume of a solution containing 1 g/l of *potassium iodide R*, 2 g/l of *potassium iodate R* and 10 g/l of *sodium hydrogen carbonate R* and mix. If necessary, first dilute the preparation to be examined with a 2 g/l solution of *sodium hydroxide R* to ensure that the final mixture has a radioactivity concentration suitable for the radioactivity detector.

Reference solution (a). Dissolve 10 mg of *potassium iodide R* in *water R* and dilute to 10 ml with the same solvent.

Reference solution (b). Dissolve 20 mg of *potassium iodate R* in *water R* and dilute to 10 ml with the same solvent. Mix equal volumes of this solution and reference solution (a).

Column:

- *size*: l = 0.25 m, Ø = 4.0 mm,
- *stationary phase*: *octadecylsilyl silica gel for chromatography R* (5 µm),
- *temperature*: constant, between 20 °C and 30 °C.

Use stainless steel tubing.

Mobile phase: dissolve 5.85 g of *sodium chloride R* in 1000 ml of *water R*, add 0.65 ml of *octylamine R* and adjust to pH 7.0 with *dilute phosphoric acid R*; add 50 ml of *acetonitrile R* and mix.

Flow rate: 1.5 ml/min.

Detection: spectrophotometer at 220 nm and a radioactivity detector connected in series.

Injection: 20 µl.

Run time: 12 min.

Relative retention with reference to iodide (retention time = about 5 min): iodate = 0.2 to 0.3.

System suitability: reference solution (b):

- *resolution*: minimum 2 between the peaks due to iodide and iodate in the chromatogram recorded with the spectrophotometer.

Limit: examine the chromatogram obtained with the radioactivity detector:

- *[^{131}I]iodide*: minimum 95 per cent of the total radioactivity.

RADIOACTIVITY

Determine the radioactivity using a calibrated instrument.

LABELLING

The label states:

- the method of production of iodine-131,
- the vehicle and any substance added,
- that the preparation is not for direct human use.

IMPURITIES

A. [^{131}I]iodate ion.

01/2005:0564

SODIUM IODOHIPPURATE (^{123}I) INJECTION

Natrii iodohippurati (^{123}I) solutio iniectabilis

DEFINITION

Sodium iodohippurate (^{123}I) injection is a sterile solution of sodium (2-[^{123}I]iodobenzamido)acetate. It may contain a suitable buffer and a suitable antimicrobial preservative such as benzyl alcohol. Iodine-123 is a radioactive isotope of iodine and may be obtained by proton irradiation of xenon enriched in xenon-124 (not less than 98 per cent) followed by the decay of caesium-123 formed via xenon-123. The injection contains not less than 90.0 per cent and not more than 110.0 per cent of the declared iodine-123 radioactivity at the date and hour stated on the label. Not less than 96 per cent of the radioactivity corresponds to iodine-123 in the form of sodium 2-iodohippurate. The specific radioactivity is 0.74 GBq to 10.0 GBq of iodine-123 per gram of sodium 2-iodohippurate. Not more than 0.35 per cent of the total radioactivity is due to radionuclides other than iodine-123.

CHARACTERS

A clear, colourless liquid.

Iodine-123 has a half-life of 13.2 h and emits gamma radiation and X-rays.

IDENTIFICATION

A. Record the gamma-ray and X-ray spectrum using a suitable instrument. The spectrum does not differ significantly from that of a standardised iodine-123 solution apart from any differences attributable to the presence of iodine-125, tellurium-121 and other radionuclidic impurities. Standardised iodine-123, iodine-125 and tellurium-121 solutions are available from laboratories recognised by the national authorities. The most prominent gamma photon of iodine-123 has an energy of 0.159 MeV and is accompanied by an X-ray of 0.027 MeV. Iodine-125 has a half-life of 59.4 days and emits an X-ray of 0.027 MeV and a photon of 0.035 MeV. Tellurium-121 has a half-life of 19.2 days and the most prominent photons have energies of 0.507 MeV and 0.573 MeV.

B. Examine the chromatograms obtained in the test for radiochemical purity. The spot corresponding to the main peak of radioactivity in the chromatogram obtained with the test solution is similar in position to the spot corresponding to 2-iodohippuric acid in the chromatogram obtained with the reference solution.

TESTS

pH (*2.2.3*). The pH of the solution is 3.5 to 8.5.

Sterility. It complies with the test for sterility prescribed in the monograph on *Radiopharmaceutical preparations (0125)*. The injection may be released for use before completion of the test.

RADIONUCLIDIC PURITY

Record the gamma-ray spectrum using a suitable instrument. Determine the relative amounts of iodine-125, tellurium-121 and other radionuclidic impurities present. No radionuclides with longer half lives than iodine-125 are detected. For the determination of iodine-125, tellurium-121 and other radionuclidic impurities, retain the solution to be examined for a sufficient time to allow the radioactivity of iodine-123 to decrease to a level which permits the detection of radionuclidic impurities. Record the gamma-ray spectrum and X-ray spectrum of the decayed material using a suitable instrument. Not more than 0.35 per cent of the total radioactivity is due to radionuclides other than iodine-123. The injection may be released for use before completion of the test.

RADIOCHEMICAL PURITY

Examine by thin-layer chromatography (*2.2.27*) using *silica gel GF_{254} R* as the coating substance.

Test solution. Dissolve 1 g of *potassium iodide R* in 10 ml of *water R*, add 1 volume of this solution to 10 volumes of the injection to be examined and use within 10 min of mixing. If necessary, dilute with the reference solution (carrier) to give a radioactive concentration sufficient for the detection method, for example 3.7 MBq per millilitre.

Reference solution (*carrier*). Dissolve 40 mg of *2-iodohippuric acid R* and 40 mg of *2-iodobenzoic acid R* in 4 ml of *0.1 M sodium hydroxide*, add 10 mg of *potassium iodide R* and dilute to 10 ml with *water R*.

Apply separately to the plate 10 µl of each solution. Develop over a path of 12 cm (about 75 min) using a mixture of 1 volume of *water R*, 4 volumes of *glacial acetic acid R*, 20 volumes of *butanol R* and 80 volumes of *toluene R*. Allow the plate to dry in air and examine in ultraviolet light at 254 nm. The chromatogram obtained with the reference solution shows a spot corresponding to 2-iodohippuric acid and nearer to the solvent front a spot corresponding to 2-iodobenzoic acid. Iodide ion remains near the starting-line. Determine the distribution of radioactivity using a suitable detector. In the chromatogram obtained with the test solution, not less than 96 per cent of the total radioactivity is found in the spot corresponding to 2-iodohippuric acid and not more than 2 per cent of the total radioactivity is found in either of the spots corresponding to 2-iodobenzoic acid and to iodide ion.

RADIOACTIVITY

Measure the radioactivity using suitable counting equipment by comparison with a standardised iodine-123 solution or by measurement in an instrument calibrated with the aid of such a solution.

STORAGE

Store protected from light.

LABELLING

The label states whether or not the preparation is suitable for renal plasma-flow studies.

01/2005:0282

SODIUM IODOHIPPURATE (^{131}I) INJECTION

Natrii iodohippurati (^{131}I) solutio iniectabilis

DEFINITION

Sodium iodohippurate (^{131}I) injection is a sterile solution of sodium 2-(2-[^{131}I]iodobenzamido)acetate. It may contain a suitable buffer and a suitable antimicrobial preservative such as benzyl alcohol. Iodine-131 is a radioactive isotope of iodine and may be obtained by neutron irradiation of tellurium or by extraction from uranium fission products. The injection contains not less than 90.0 per cent and not more than 110.0 per cent of the declared iodine-131 radioactivity at the date and hour stated on the label. Not less than 96 per cent of the iodine-131 is in the form of sodium 2-iodohippurate. The specific radioactivity is 0.74 GBq to 7.4 GBq of iodine-131 per gram of sodium 2-iodohippurate.

CHARACTERS

A clear, colourless liquid.

Iodine-131 has a half-life of 8.04 days and emits beta and gamma radiation.

IDENTIFICATION

A. Record the gamma-ray spectrum using a suitable instrument. The spectrum does not differ significantly from that of a standardised iodine-131 solution. Standardised iodine-131 solutions are available from

Radiopharmaceutical preparations

laboratories recognised by the competent authority. The most prominent gamma photon of iodine-131 has an energy of 0.365 MeV.

B. Examine the chromatograms obtained in the test for radiochemical purity. The main peak of radioactivity in the chromatogram obtained with the test solution is similar in position to the spot corresponding to 2-iodohippuric acid in the chromatogram obtained with the reference solution.

TESTS

pH (*2.2.3*). The pH of the injection is 6.0 to 8.5.

Sterility. It complies with the test for sterility prescribed in the monograph on *Radiopharmaceutical preparations (0125)*. The injection may be released for use before completion of the test.

RADIONUCLIDIC PURITY

Record the gamma-ray spectrum using a suitable instrument. The spectrum does not differ significantly from that of a standardised iodine-131 solution. Determine the relative amounts of iodine-131, iodine-133, iodine-135 and other radionuclidic impurities present. Iodine-133 has a half-life of 20.8 h and its most prominent gamma photons have energies of 0.530 MeV and 0.875 MeV. Iodine-135 has a half-life of 6.55 h and its most prominent gamma photons have energies of 0.527 MeV, 1.132 MeV and 1.260 MeV. Not less than 99.9 per cent of the total radioactivity is due to iodine-131.

RADIOCHEMICAL PURITY

Examine by thin-layer chromatography (*2.2.27*) using *silica gel GF_{254} R* as the coating substance.

Test solution. Dissolve 1 g of *potassium iodide R* in 10 ml of *water R*, add 1 volume of this solution to 10 volumes of the injection to be examined and use within 10 min of mixing. If necessary dilute with the reference solution (carrier) to give a radioactive concentration sufficient for the detection method, for example 3.7 MBq per millilitre.

Reference solution (carrier). Dissolve 40 mg of *2-iodohippuric acid R* and 40 mg of *2-iodobenzoic acid R* in 4 ml of *0.1 M sodium hydroxide*, add 10 mg of *potassium iodide R* and dilute to 10 ml with *water R*.

Apply separately to the plate 10 µl of each solution. Develop over a path of 12 cm (about 75 min) using a mixture of 1 volume of *water R*, 4 volumes of *glacial acetic acid R*, 20 volumes of *butanol R* and 80 volumes of *toluene R*. Allow the plate to dry in air and examine in ultraviolet light at 254 nm. The chromatogram obtained with the reference solution shows a spot corresponding to 2-iodohippuric acid and nearer to the solvent front a spot corresponding to 2-iodobenzoic acid. Iodide ion remains near the starting-line. Determine the distribution of radioactivity using a suitable detector. In the chromatogram obtained with the test solution, not less than 96 per cent of the total radioactivity is found in the spot corresponding to 2-iodohippuric acid and not more than 2 per cent of the total radioactivity is found in either of the spots corresponding to 2-iodobenzoic acid and to iodide ion.

RADIOACTIVITY

Measure the radioactivity using suitable counting equipment by comparison with a standardised iodine-131 solution or by measurement in an instrument calibrated with the aid of such a solution.

STORAGE

Store protected from light.

LABELLING

The label states that the preparation is not necessarily suitable for renal plasma-flow studies.

01/2005:0124

SODIUM PERTECHNETATE (^{99m}Tc) INJECTION (FISSION)

Natrii pertechnetatis (^{99m}Tc) fissione formati solutio iniectabilis

This monograph applies to sodium pertechnetate (^{99m}Tc) injection obtained from molybdenum-99 extracted from fission products of uranium. Sodium pertechnetate (^{99m}Tc) injection obtained from molybdenum-99 produced by the neutron irradiation of molybdenum is described in the monograph on Sodium pertechnetate (^{99m}Tc) injection (non-fission) (0283).

DEFINITION

Sodium pertechnetate (^{99m}Tc) injection (fission) is a sterile solution containing technetium-99m in the form of pertechnetate ion and made isotonic by the addition of sodium chloride. Technetium-99m is a radionuclide formed by the decay of molybdenum-99. Molybdenum-99 is a radioactive isotope of molybdenum extracted from uranium fission products. The injection contains not less than 90.0 per cent and not more than 110.0 per cent of the declared technetium-99m radioactivity at the date and hour stated on the label. Not less than 95 per cent of the radioactivity corresponds to technetium-99m in the form of pertechnetate ion.

The radioactivity due to radionuclides other than technetium-99m, apart from that due to technetium-99 resulting from the decay of technetium-99m, is not greater than that shown below, expressed as a percentage of the total radioactivity and calculated with reference to the date and hour of administration.

molybdenum-99	0.1 per cent
iodine-131	5×10^{-3} per cent
ruthenium-103	5×10^{-3} per cent
strontium-89	6×10^{-5} per cent
strontium-90	6×10^{-6} per cent
alpha-emitting impurities	1×10^{-7} per cent
other gamma-emitting impurities	0.01 per cent

The injection may be prepared from a sterile preparation of molybdenum-99 under aseptic conditions.

CHARACTERS

A clear, colourless solution.

Technetium-99m has a half-life of 6.02 h and emits gamma radiation.

IDENTIFICATION

Record the gamma-ray spectrum using a suitable instrument. The spectrum does not differ significantly from that of a standardised technetium-99m solution either by direct comparison or by measurement in an instrument calibrated with the aid of such a solution. Standardised technetium-99m, molybdenum-99, iodine-131, ruthenium-103, strontium-89 and strontium/yttrium-90 solutions are available from laboratories recognised by the competent authority. The most prominent gamma photon of technetium-99m has an energy of 0.140 MeV.

TESTS

pH (*2.2.3*). The pH of the injection is 4.0 to 8.0.

Aluminium. In a test tube about 12 mm in internal diameter, mix 1 ml of *acetate buffer solution pH 4.6 R* and 2 ml of a 1 in 2.5 dilution of the injection in *water R*. Add 0.05 ml of a 10 g/l solution of *chromazurol S R*. After 3 min, the colour of the solution is not more intense than that of a standard prepared at the same time and in the same manner using 2 ml of *aluminium standard solution (2 ppm Al) R* (5 ppm).

Sterility. It complies with the test for sterility prescribed in the monograph on *Radiopharmaceutical preparations (0125)*. The injection may be released for use before completion of the test.

RADIONUCLIDIC PURITY

Preliminary test. To obtain an approximate estimate before use of the injection, take a volume equivalent to 37 MBq and determine the gamma-ray spectrum using a sodium iodide detector with a shield of lead, of thickness 6 mm, interposed between the sample and the detector. The response in the region corresponding to the 0.740 MeV photon of molybdenum-99 does not exceed that obtained using 37 kBq of a standardised molybdenum-99 solution measured under the same conditions, when all measurements are expressed with reference to the date and hour of administration.

Definitive test. Retain a sample of the injection for a sufficient time to allow the technetium-99m radioactivity to decay to a sufficiently low level to permit the detection of radionuclidic impurities. All measurements of radioactivity are expressed with reference to the date and hour of administration.

- *Molybdenum-99*. Record the gamma-ray spectrum of the decayed material in a suitable instrument calibrated with the aid of a standardised molybdenum-99 solution. The most prominent photons have energies of 0.181 MeV, 0.740 MeV and 0.778 MeV. Molybdenum-99 has a half-life of 66.0 h. Not more than 0.1 per cent of the total radioactivity is due to molybdenum-99.
- *Iodine-131*. Record the gamma-ray spectrum of the decayed material in a suitable instrument calibrated with the aid of a standardised iodine-131 solution. The most prominent photon has an energy of 0.365 MeV. Iodine-131 has a half-life of 8.04 days. Not more than 5×10^{-3} per cent of the total radioactivity is due to iodine-131.
- *Ruthenium-103*. Record the gamma-ray spectrum of the decayed material in a suitable instrument calibrated using a standardised ruthenium-103 solution. The most prominent photon has an energy of 0.497 MeV. Ruthenium-103 has a half-life of 39.3 days. Not more than 5×10^{-3} per cent of the total radioactivity is due to ruthenium-103.
- *Strontium-89*. Determine the presence of strontium-89 in the decayed material with an instrument suitable for the detection of beta rays, by comparison with a standardised strontium-89 solution. It is usually necessary first to carry out chemical separation of the strontium so that the standard and the sample may be compared in the same physical and chemical form. Strontium-89 decays with a beta emission of 1.492 MeV maximum energy and has a half-life of 50.5 days. Not more than 6×10^{-5} per cent of the total radioactivity is due to strontium-89.
- *Strontium-90*. Determine the presence of strontium-90 in the decayed material with an instrument suitable for the detection of beta rays. To distinguish strontium-90 from strontium-89, compare the radioactivity of yttrium-90, the daughter nuclide of strontium-90, with an yttrium-90 standard after the chemical separation of the yttrium. If prior chemical separation of the strontium is necessary, the conditions of radioactive equilibrium must be ensured. The yttrium-90 standard and the sample must be compared in the same physical and chemical form. Strontium-90 and yttrium-90 decay with respective beta emissions of 0.546 MeV and 2.284 MeV maximum energy and half-lives of 29.1 years and 64.0 h. Not more than 6×10^{-6} per cent of the total radioactivity is due to strontium-90.
- *Other gamma-emitting impurities*. Examine the gamma-ray spectrum of the decayed material for the presence of other radionuclidic impurities, which should, where possible, be identified and quantified. The total gamma radioactivity due to these impurities does not exceed 0.01 per cent of the total radioactivity.
- *Alpha-emitting impurities*. Measure the alpha radioactivity of the decayed material to detect any alpha-emitting radionuclidic impurities, which should, where possible, be identified and quantified. The total alpha radioactivity due to these impurities does not exceed 1×10^{-7} per cent of the total radioactivity.

RADIOCHEMICAL PURITY

Examine by descending paper chromatography (*2.2.26*).

Test solution. Dilute the preparation to be examined with *water R* to a suitable radioactive concentration.

Apply 5 µl of the test solution. Develop for 2 h using a mixture of 20 volumes of *water R* and 80 volumes of *methanol R*. Allow the paper to dry. Determine the distribution of radioactivity using a suitable detector. Not less than 95 per cent of the total radioactivity is in the spot corresponding to pertechnetate ion, which has an R_f value of about 0.6.

RADIOACTIVITY

Measure the radioactivity using suitable counting equipment by comparison with a standardised technetium-99m solution or by measurement in an instrument calibrated with the aid of such a solution.

01/2005:0283

SODIUM PERTECHNETATE (^{99m}Tc) INJECTION (NON-FISSION)

Natrii pertechnetatis (^{99m}Tc) sine fissione formati solutio iniectabilis

This monograph applies to sodium pertechnetate (^{99m}Tc) injection obtained from molybdenum-99 produced by neutron irradiation of molybdenum. Sodium pertechnetate (^{99m}Tc) injection obtained from molybdenum-99 extracted from fission products of uranium is described in the monograph on Sodium pertechnetate(^{99m}Tc) injection (fission) (0124).

DEFINITION

Sodium pertechnetate (^{99m}Tc) injection (non-fission) is a sterile solution containing technetium-99m in the form of pertechnetate ion and made isotonic by the addition of sodium chloride. Technetium-99m is a radionuclide formed by the decay of molybdenum-99. Molybdenum-99 is a radioactive isotope of molybdenum produced by neutron irradiation of molybdenum. The injection contains not less than 90.0 per cent and not more than 110.0 per cent of the declared technetium-99m radioactivity at the date and

Radiopharmaceutical preparations

hour stated on the label. Not less than 95 per cent of the radioactivity corresponds to technetium-99m in the form of pertechnetate ion.

The radioactivity due to radionuclides other than technetium-99m, apart from that due to technetium-99 resulting from the decay of technetium-99m is not greater than that shown below, expressed as a percentage of the total radioactivity and calculated with reference to the date and hour of administration.

Molybdenum-99	0.1 per cent
Other radionuclidic impurities	0.01 per cent

The injection may be prepared from a sterile preparation of molybdenum-99 under aseptic conditions.

CHARACTERS

A clear, colourless solution.

Technetium-99m has a half-life of 6.02 h and emits gamma radiation.

IDENTIFICATION

A. Record the gamma-ray spectrum using a suitable instrument. The spectrum does not differ significantly from that of a standardised technetium-99m solution either by direct comparison or by using an instrument calibrated with the aid of such a solution. Standardised technetium-99m and molybdenum-99 solutions are available from laboratories recognised by the competent authority. The most prominent gamma photon of technetium-99m has an energy of 0.140 MeV.

B. Examine the chromatogram obtained in the test for radiochemical purity. The distribution of radioactivity contributes to the identification of the preparation.

TESTS

pH (*2.2.3*). The pH of the injection is 4.0 to 8.0.

Aluminium. In a test tube about 12 mm in internal diameter, mix 1 ml of *acetate buffer solution pH 4.6 R* and 2 ml of a 1 in 2.5 dilution of the injection in *water R*. Add 0.05 ml of a 10 g/l solution of *chromazurol S R*. After 3 min, the colour of the solution is not more intense than that of a standard prepared at the same time in the same manner using 2 ml of *aluminium standard solution (2 ppm Al) R* (5 ppm).

Sterility. It complies with the test for sterility prescribed in the monograph on *Radiopharmaceutical preparations (0125)*. The injection may be released for use before completion of the test.

RADIONUCLIDIC PURITY

Preliminary test. To obtain an approximate estimate before use of the injection, take a volume equivalent to 37 MBq and record the gamma-ray spectrum using a sodium iodide detector with a shield of lead, of thickness 6 mm, interposed between the sample and the detector. The response in the region corresponding to the 0.740 MeV photon of molybdenum-99 does not exceed that obtained using 37 kBq of a standardised solution of molybdenum-99 measured under the same conditions, when all measurements are expressed with reference to the date and hour of administration.

Definitive test. Retain a sample of the injection for a sufficient time to allow the technetium-99m radioactivity to decay to a sufficiently low level to permit the detection of radionuclidic impurities. All measurements of radioactivity are expressed with reference to the date and hour of administration.

- *Molybdenum-99.* Record the gamma-ray spectrum of the decayed material in a suitable instrument calibrated using a standardised molybdenum-99 solution. The most prominent gamma photons have energies of 0.181 MeV, 0.740 MeV and 0.778 MeV. Molybdenum-99 has a half-life of 66.0 h. Not more than 0.1 per cent of the total radioactivity is due to molybdenum-99.
- *Other gamma-emitting impurities.* Examine the gamma-ray spectrum of the decayed material for the presence of other radionuclidic impurities, which should, where possible, be identified and quantified. The total radioactivity due to other radionuclidic impurities does not exceed 0.01 per cent of the total radioactivity.

RADIOCHEMICAL PURITY

Examine by descending paper chromatography (*2.2.26*).

Test solution. Dilute the injection with *water R* to a suitable radioactive concentration.

Apply 5 µl of the test solution. Develop for 2 h using a mixture of 20 volumes of *water R* and 80 volumes of *methanol R*. Allow the paper to dry in air. Determine the distribution of radioactivity using a suitable detector. Not less than 95 per cent of the total radioactivity is found in the spot corresponding to pertechnetate ion, which has an R_f value of about 0.6.

RADIOACTIVITY

Measure the radioactivity using suitable counting equipment by comparison with a standardised technetium-99m solution or by measurement in an instrument calibrated with the aid of such a solution.

01/2005:0284

SODIUM PHOSPHATE (^{32}P) INJECTION

Natrii phosphatis (^{32}P) solutio iniectabilis

DEFINITION

Sodium phosphate (^{32}P) injection is a sterile solution of disodium and monosodium (^{32}P) orthophosphates made isotonic by the addition of sodium chloride. Phosphorus-32 is a radioactive isotope of phosphorus and may be produced by neutron irradiation of sulphur. The injection contains not less than 90.0 per cent and not more than 110.0 per cent of the declared phosphorus-32 radioactivity at the date and hour stated on the label. Not less than 95 per cent of the radioactivity corresponds to phosphorus-32 in the form of orthophosphate ion. The specific radioactivity is not less than 11.1 MBq of phosphorus-32 per milligram of orthophosphate ion.

CHARACTERS

A clear, colourless solution.

Phosphorus-32 has a half-life of 14.3 days and emits beta radiation.

IDENTIFICATION

A. Record the beta-ray spectrum or the beta-ray absorption curve using a suitable method. The spectrum or curve does not differ significantly from that of a standardised phosphorus-32 solution obtained under the same conditions. Standardised phosphorus-32 solutions are available from laboratories recognised by the competent authority. The maximum energy of the beta radiation is 1.71 MeV.

B. Examine the chromatogram obtained in the test for radiochemical purity. The distribution of radioactivity contributes to the identification of the preparation.

TESTS

pH (*2.2.3*). The pH of the injection is 6.0 to 8.0.

Phosphates. Dilute the injection with *water R* to give a radioactive concentration of 370 kBq of phosphorus-32 per millilitre. Mix in a volumetric flask, with shaking, 1.0 ml of the solution with a mixture of 0.5 ml of a 2.5 g/l solution of *ammonium vanadate R*, 0.5 ml of *ammonium molybdate solution R* and 1 ml of *perchloric acid R* and dilute to 5.0 ml with *water R*. After 30 min, the solution is not more intensely coloured than a standard prepared at the same time in the same manner using 1.0 ml of a solution containing 33 mg of orthophosphate ion per litre.

Sterility. It complies with the test for sterility prescribed in the monograph on *Radiopharmaceutical preparations (0125)*. The injection may be released for use before completion of the test.

RADIONUCLIDIC PURITY

Record the beta-ray spectrum or the beta-ray absorption curve using a suitable method. The spectrum or curve does not differ significantly from that of a standardised phosphorus-32 solution obtained under the same conditions.

RADIOCHEMICAL PURITY

Examine by ascending paper chromatography (*2.2.26*).

Test solution. Dilute the injection with *water R* until the radioactivity is equivalent to 10 000 to 20 000 counts per minute per 10 µl

Reference solution. Prepare a solution of *phosphoric acid R* containing 2 mg of phosphorus per millilitre.

Using a strip of paper 25 mm wide and about 300 mm long, apply 10 µl of the reference solution. Apply to the same starting-point 10 µl of the test solution. Develop for 16 h using a mixture of 0.3 ml of *ammonia R*, 5 g of *trichloroacetic acid R*, 25 ml of *water R* and 75 ml of *2-propanol R*. Allow the paper to dry in air. Determine the position of the inactive phosphoric acid by spraying with a 50 g/l solution of *perchloric acid R* and then with a 10 g/l solution of *ammonium molybdate R*. Expose the paper to *hydrogen sulphide R*. A blue colour develops. Determine the position of the radioactive spot by autoradiography or by measuring the radioactivity over the whole length of the chromatogram. Not less than 95 per cent of the total radioactivity of the chromatogram is found in the spot corresponding to phosphoric acid.

RADIOACTIVITY

Measure the radioactivity using suitable counting equipment by comparison with a standardised phosphorus-32 solution or by measurement in an instrument calibrated with the aid of such a solution.

01/2005:1475

STRONTIUM (^{89}Sr) CHLORIDE INJECTION

Strontii (^{89}Sr) chloridi solutio iniectabilis

DEFINITION

Strontium (^{89}Sr) chloride injection is a sterile solution of [^{89}Sr]strontium chloride. Strontium-89 is a radioactive isotope of strontium and is produced by neutron irradiation of strontium enriched in strontium-88. The injection contains not less than 90.0 per cent and not more than 110.0 per cent of the declared strontium-89 radioactivity at the date stated on the label. Not more than 0.6 per cent of the total radioactivity is due to radionuclides other than strontium-89. The specific radioactivity is not less than 1.8 MBq of strontium-89 per milligram of strontium. The injection contains 6.0 mg/ml to 12.5 mg/ml of strontium.

CHARACTERS

A clear, colourless solution.

Strontium-89 has a half-life of 50.5 days and emits beta radiation with a maximum energy of 1.492 MeV.

IDENTIFICATION

A. Record the gamma-ray and X-ray spectrum using a suitable instrument. The spectrum does not differ significantly from that of a standardised strontium-89 solution, when measured either by direct comparison or by using an instrument calibrated with the aid of such a solution. Standardised strontium-89 solutions are available from laboratories recognised by the competent authority. The gamma photon detected has an energy of 0.909 MeV and is due to the short-lived daughter product, yttrium-89m (formed in 0.01 per cent of the disintegrations), in equilibrium with the strontium-89.

B. To 0.1 ml of the injection to be examined, add 1 ml of a freshly prepared 1 g/l solution of *sodium rhodizonate R*. Mix and allow to stand for 1 min. A reddish-brown precipitate is formed.

C. To 0.1 ml of *silver nitrate solution R2* add 50 µl of the injection to be examined. A white precipitate is formed.

TESTS

pH (*2.2.3*). The pH of the solution is 4.0 to 7.5.

Note: the following tests for aluminium, iron and lead may be carried out simultaneously with the test for strontium. If this is not the case, the reference solutions are prepared such that they contain strontium at approximately the same concentration as in the test solution.

Aluminium. Not more than 2 µg/ml, determined by atomic emission spectrometry (plasma or arc method) (*2.2.22, Method I*).

Test solution. Dilute 0.2 ml of the injection to be examined to a suitable volume with *dilute nitric acid R*.

Reference solutions. Prepare the reference solutions using *aluminium standard solution (10 ppm Al) R* diluted as necessary with *dilute nitric acid R*.

Iron. Not more than 5 µg/ml, determined by atomic emission spectrometry (plasma or arc method) (*2.2.22, Method I*).

Test solution. Dilute 0.2 ml of the injection to be examined to a suitable volume with *dilute nitric acid R*.

Reference solutions. Prepare the reference solutions using *iron standard solution (20 ppm Fe) R* diluted as necessary with *dilute nitric acid R*.

Lead. Not more than 5 µg/ml, determined by atomic emission spectrometry (plasma or arc method) (*2.2.22, Method I*).

Test solution. Dilute 0.2 ml of the injection to be examined to a suitable volume with *dilute nitric acid R*.

Reference solutions. Prepare the reference solutions using *lead standard solution (10 ppm Pb) R* diluted as necessary with *dilute nitric acid R*.

Strontium. 6.0 mg/ml to 12.5 mg/ml. Examine by atomic emission spectrometry (*2.2.22, Method I*).

Test solution. Dilute 0.2 ml of the injection to be examined to a suitable volume with *dilute nitric acid R*.

Reference solutions. Prepare the reference solutions using *strontium standard solution (1.0 per cent Sr) R* diluted as necessary with *dilute nitric acid R*.

Sterility. It complies with the test for sterility prescribed in the monograph on *Radiopharmaceutical preparations (0125)*.

RADIONUCLIDIC PURITY

Gamma emitters. Record the gamma-ray and X-ray spectrum of the injection to be examined using a suitable instrument. Not more than 0.4 per cent of the total radioactivity in the preparation to be examined is due to gamma emitting radionuclides other than yttrium-89m.

Beta emitters. Evaporate to dryness 100 µl of the injection to be examined under a radiant heat source. Dissolve the residue in 2 ml of *47 per cent hydrobromic acid R*, evaporate to dryness under the radiant heat source and dissolve the residue in 2 ml of *dilute hydrobromic acid R1*. Transfer the solution to the top of a column, 5 mm to 6 mm in diameter, packed with approximately 2 ml of *cationic exchange resin R1* (100 µm to 250 µm), previously conditioned with *dilute hydrobromic acid R1* and elute the column with the same solvent until 10 ml of eluate has been collected into a container containing 50 µl of a 15 g/l solution of *anhydrous sodium sulphate R* in *1 M hydrochloric acid*.

To a liquid scintillation vial add an appropriate volume of scintillation liquid followed by 1 ml of *water R*, 0.1 ml of a 15 g/l solution of *anhydrous sodium sulphate R* in *1 M hydrochloric acid* and 100 µl of eluate. Shake to obtain a clear solution. Using suitable counting equipment determine the radioactivity due to sulphur-35 and phosphorus-32 in the sample.

Taking into account the recovery efficiency of the separation, counting efficiency and radioactive decay, determine the radioactive concentration of sulphur-35 and phosphorus-32 in the sample and hence the percentage of total beta emitting impurities in the injection to be examined. Not more than 0.2 per cent of the total radioactivity in the injection to be examined is due to the sum of sulphur-35 and phosphorus-32 radioactivities.

RADIOACTIVITY

Measure the radioactivity using suitable equipment by comparison with a standardised strontium-89 solution or by measurement in an instrument calibrated with the aid of such a solution.

01/2005:0126

TECHNETIUM (^{99m}Tc) COLLOIDAL RHENIUM SULPHIDE INJECTION

Rhenii sulfidi colloidalis et technetii (^{99m}Tc) solutio iniectabilis

DEFINITION

Technetium (^{99m}Tc) colloidal rhenium sulphide injection is a sterile, apyrogenic colloidal dispersion of rhenium sulphide the micelles of which are labelled with technetium-99m. It is stabilised with gelatin. The injection contains not less than 90.0 per cent and not more than 110.0 per cent of the declared technetium-99m radioactivity at the date and hour stated on the label. Not less than 92 per cent of the radioactivity corresponds to technetium-99m in colloidal form. The pH of the injection may be adjusted by the addition of a suitable buffer such as a citrate buffer solution. The injection contains a variable amount of colloidal rhenium sulphide, not exceeding 0.22 mg of rhenium (Re) per millilitre, according to the method of preparation.

It is prepared from sodium pertechnetate (^{99m}Tc) injection (fission or non-fission) using suitable sterile, apyrogenic ingredients and calculating the ratio of radionuclidic impurities with reference to the date and hour of administration.

CHARACTERS

A light-brown liquid.

Technetium-99m has a half-life of 6.02 h and emits gamma radiation.

IDENTIFICATION

A. Record the gamma-ray spectrum using a suitable instrument. The spectrum does not differ significantly from that of a standardised technetium-99m solution either by direct comparison or by using an instrument calibrated with the aid of such a solution. Standardised technetium-99m and molybdenum-99 solutions are available from laboratories recognised by the competent authority. The most prominent gamma photon of technetium-99m has an energy of 0.140 MeV.

B. Examine the chromatogram obtained in the test for radiochemical purity. The distribution of radioactivity contributes to the identification of the injection.

C. To 1 ml add 5 ml of *hydrochloric acid R*, 5 ml of a 50 g/l solution of *thiourea R* and 1 ml of a 200 g/l solution of *stannous chloride R* in *hydrochloric acid R*. A yellow colour is produced.

TESTS

pH (*2.2.3*). The pH of the injection is 4.0 to 7.0.

Rhenium

Test solution. Use 1 ml of the injection to be examined.

Reference solutions. Using a solution containing 100 µg of *potassium perrhenate R* (equivalent to 60 ppm of Re) and 240 µg of *sodium thiosulphate R* per millilitre, prepare a suitable range of solutions and dilute to the same final volume with *water R*.

To the test solution and to 1 ml of each of the reference solutions add 5 ml of *hydrochloric acid R*, 5 ml of a 50 g/l solution of *thiourea R* and 1 ml of a 200 g/l solution of *stannous chloride R* in *hydrochloric acid R* and dilute to 25.0 ml with *water R*. Allow to stand for 40 min and measure the absorbance (*2.2.25*) of each solution at 400 nm, using a reagent blank as the compensation liquid. Using the absorbances obtained with the reference solutions, draw a calibration curve and calculate the concentration of rhenium in the injection to be examined.

Physiological distribution. Inject a volume not greater than 0.2 ml into the caudal vein of each of three mice each weighing 20 g to 25 g. Sacrifice the mice 20 min after the injection, remove the liver, spleen and lungs and measure the radioactivity in the organs using a suitable instrument. Measure the radioactivity in the rest of the body after having removed the tail. Determine the percentage of radioactivity in the liver, the spleen and the lungs from the expression:

$$\frac{A}{B} \times 100$$

A = radioactivity of the organ concerned,

B = total radioactivity in the liver, the spleen, the lungs and the rest of the body.

In each of the three mice at least 80 per cent of the radioactivity is found in the liver and spleen and not more than 5 per cent in the lungs. If the distribution of radioactivity in one of the three mice does not correspond to the prescribed proportions, repeat the test on a further three mice. The preparation complies with the test if the prescribed distribution of radioactivity is found in five of the six mice used. The injection may be released for use before completion of the test.

Sterility. It complies with the test for sterility prescribed in the monograph on *Radiopharmaceutical preparations (0125)*. The injection may be released for use before completion of the test.

Pyrogens. It complies with the test for pyrogens prescribed in the monograph on *Radiopharmaceutical preparations (0125)*. Inject not less than 0.1 ml per kilogram of the rabbit's mass. The injection may be released for use before completion of the test.

RADIOCHEMICAL PURITY

Examine by ascending paper chromatography (*2.2.26*). Apply to the paper 10 µl of the injection. Develop immediately over a path of 10 cm to 15 cm using a 9 g/l solution of *sodium chloride R*. Allow the paper to dry. Determine the distribution of radioactivity using a suitable detector. Technetium-99m in colloidal form remains at the starting-point and pertechnetate ion migrates with an R_f of about 0.6. There may be other impurities with an R_f of 0.8 to 0.9. The radioactivity corresponding to technetium-99m in colloidal form represents not less than 92 per cent of the total radioactivity of the chromatogram.

RADIOACTIVITY

Measure the radioactivity using suitable counting equipment by comparison with a standardised technetium-99m solution or by measurement in an instrument calibrated with the aid of such a solution.

LABELLING

The label states, in particular, the quantity of rhenium per millilitre.

01/2005:0131

TECHNETIUM (^{99m}Tc) COLLOIDAL SULPHUR INJECTION

Sulfuris colloidalis et technetii (^{99m}Tc) solutio iniectabilis

DEFINITION

Technetium (^{99m}Tc) colloidal sulphur injection is a sterile, apyrogenic colloidal dispersion of sulphur, the micelles of which are labelled with technetium-99m. It may be stabilised with a colloid-protecting substance based on gelatin. The injection contains not less than 90.0 per cent and not more than 110.0 per cent of the declared technetium-99m radioactivity at the date and hour stated on the label. Not less than 92 per cent of the radioactivity corresponds to technetium-99m in colloidal form. The pH of the injection may be adjusted by the addition of a suitable buffer, such as an acetate, citrate or phosphate buffer solution. The injection contains a variable amount of colloidal sulphur, according to the method of preparation.

It is prepared from sodium pertechnetate (^{99m}Tc) injection (fission or non-fission) using suitable sterile, apyrogenic ingredients and calculating the ratio of radionuclidic impurities with reference to the date and hour of administration.

CHARACTERS

A clear to opalescent, colourless to yellowish liquid.

Technetium-99m has a half-life of 6.02 h and emits gamma radiation.

IDENTIFICATION

A. Record the gamma-ray spectrum using a suitable instrument. The spectrum does not differ significantly from that of a standardised technetium-99m solution either by direct comparison or by using an instrument calibrated with the aid of such a solution. Standardised technetium-99m and molybdenum-99 solutions are available from laboratories recognised by the competent authority. The most prominent gamma photon of technetium-99m has an energy of 0.140 MeV.

B. Examine the chromatogram obtained in the test for radiochemical purity. The distribution of radioactivity contributes to the identification of the injection.

C. In a test-tube 100 mm long and 16 mm in internal diameter, evaporate 0.2 ml of the injection to dryness. Dissolve the sulphur by shaking the residue with 0.2 ml of *pyridine R* and add about 20 mg of *benzoin R*. Cover the open end of the tube with a filter paper moistened with *lead acetate solution R*. Heat the test-tube in a bath containing glycerol at 150 °C. The paper slowly becomes brown.

TESTS

pH (*2.2.3*). The pH of the injection is 4.0 to 7.0.

Physiological distribution. Inject a volume not greater than 0.2 ml into the caudal vein of each of 3 mice, each weighing 20 g to 25 g. Sacrifice the mice 20 min after the injection, remove the liver, spleen and lungs and measure the radioactivity in the organs using a suitable instrument. Measure the radioactivity in the rest of the body after having removed the tail. Determine the percentage of radioactivity in the liver, the spleen and the lungs from the expression:

$$\frac{A}{B} \times 100$$

A = radioactivity of the organ concerned,

B = total radioactivity in the liver, the spleen, the lungs and the rest of the body.

In each of the 3 mice at least 80 per cent of the radioactivity is found in the liver and spleen and not more than 5 per cent in the lungs. If the distribution of radioactivity in 1 of the 3 mice does not correspond to the prescribed proportions, repeat the test on a further 3 mice. The preparation complies with the test if the prescribed distribution of radioactivity is found in 5 of the 6 mice used. The injection may be released for use before completion of the test.

Sterility. It complies with the test for sterility prescribed in the monograph on *Radiopharmaceutical preparations (0125)*. The injection may be released for use before completion of the test.

Pyrogens. It complies with the test for pyrogens prescribed in the monograph on *Radiopharmaceutical preparations (0125)*. Inject not less than 0.1 ml per kilogram of the rabbit's mass. The injection may be released for use before completion of the test.

RADIOCHEMICAL PURITY

Examine by ascending paper chromatography (*2.2.26*). Apply to the paper 10 µl of the injection. Develop immediately over a path of 10 cm to 15 cm with a 9 g/l solution of *sodium chloride R*. Allow the paper to dry. Determine the distribution of radioactivity using a suitable detector. Technetium-99m in colloidal form remains at the starting-point and pertechnetate ion migrates with an R_f

of 0.6. There may be other impurities of R_f 0.8 to 0.9. The radioactivity corresponding to technetium-99m in colloidal form represents not less than 92 per cent of the total radioactivity of the chromatogram.

RADIOACTIVITY

Measure the radioactivity using suitable counting equipment by comparison with a standardised technetium-99m solution or by measurement in an instrument calibrated with the aid of such a solution.

01/2005:0689

TECHNETIUM (^{99m}Tc) COLLOIDAL TIN INJECTION

Stanni colloidalis et technetii (^{99m}Tc) solutio iniectabilis

DEFINITION

Technetium (^{99m}Tc) colloidal tin injection is a sterile, colloidal dispersion of tin labelled with technetium-99m. The injection contains a variable quantity of tin not exceeding 1 mg of Sn per millilitre; it contains fluoride ions, it may be stabilised with a suitable, apyrogenic colloid-protecting substance and it may contain a suitable buffer. The injection contains not less than 90.0 per cent and not more than 110.0 per cent of the declared technetium-99m radioactivity at the date and hour stated on the label. Not less than 95 per cent of the radioactivity corresponds to technetium-99m in colloidal form.

It is prepared from sodium pertechnetate (^{99m}Tc) injection (fission or non-fission) using suitable sterile ingredients and calculating the ratio of radionuclidic impurities with reference to the date and hour of administration. Syringes for handling the eluate intended for labelling of the final product, or the final product, should not contain rubber parts.

CHARACTERS

A clear or opalescent, colourless liquid.

Technetium-99m has a half life of 6.02 h and emits gamma radiation.

IDENTIFICATION

A. Record the gamma-ray spectrum using a suitable instrument. The spectrum does not differ significantly from that of a standardised technetium-99m solution either by direct comparison or by using an instrument calibrated with the aid of such a solution. Standardised technetium-99m and molybdenum-99 solutions are available from laboratories recognised by the competent authority. The most prominent gamma photon of technetium-99m has an energy of 0.140 MeV.

B. Mix 0.05 ml of *zirconyl nitrate solution R* with 0.05 ml of *alizarin S solution R*. Add 0.05 ml of the injection to be examined. A yellow colour is produced.

TESTS

pH (*2.2.3*). The pH of the injection to be examined is 4.0 to 7.0.

Tin

Test solution. Dilute 3.0 ml of the injection to be examined to 50.0 ml with *1 M hydrochloric acid*.

Reference solution. Dissolve 0.115 g of *stannous chloride R* in *1 M hydrochloric acid* and dilute to 1000.0 ml with the same acid.

To 1.0 ml of each solution add 0.4 ml of a 20 g/l solution of *sodium laurilsulfate R*, 0.05 ml of *thioglycollic acid R*, 0.1 ml of *dithiol reagent R* and 3.0 ml of *0.2 M hydrochloric acid*. Mix. Measure the absorbance (*2.2.25*) of each solution at 540 nm, using *0.2 M hydrochloric acid* as the compensation liquid. The absorbance of the test solution is not greater than that of the reference solution (1 mg of Sn per millilitre).

Physiological distribution. Inject not more than 0.2 ml into a caudal vein of each of three mice, each weighing 20 g to 25 g. Kill the mice 20 min after the injection and remove the liver, spleen and lungs. Measure the radioactivity in the organs using a suitable instrument. Measure the radioactivity in the rest of the body, after having removed the tail. Determine the percentage of radioactivity in the liver, the spleen and the lungs with respect to the total radioactivity of all organs and the rest of the body excluding the tail.

In each of the three mice at least 80 per cent of the radioactivity is found in the liver and spleen and not more than 5 per cent in the lungs. If the distribution of radioactivity in one of the three mice does not correspond to the prescribed proportions, repeat the test on a further three mice. The preparation complies with the test if the prescribed distribution of radioactivity is found in five of the six mice used.

Sterility. It complies with the test for sterility prescribed in the monograph on *Radiopharmaceutical preparations (0125)*. The injection may be released for use before completion of the test.

RADIOCHEMICAL PURITY

Examine by thin-layer chromatography (*2.2.27*) using silica gel as the coating substance on a glass-fibre sheet. Heat the plate at 110 °C for 10 min. Use a plate such that during development the mobile phase migrates over a distance of 10 cm to 15 cm in about 10 min.

Apply to the plate 5 µl to 10 µl of the injection to be examined. Develop immediately over a path of 10 cm to 15 cm using a 9 g/l solution of *sodium chloride R* purged with *nitrogen R*. Allow the plate to dry. Determine the distribution of radioactivity using a suitable detector. Technetium-99m in colloidal form remains at the starting point and pertechnetate ion migrates near to the solvent front. Not less than 95 per cent of the technetium-99m radioactivity corresponds to technetium in colloidal form.

RADIOACTIVITY

Measure the radioactivity using suitable counting equipment by comparison with a standardised technetium-99m solution or by measurement in an instrument calibrated with the aid of such a solution.

01/2005:0585

TECHNETIUM (^{99m}Tc) ETIFENIN INJECTION

Technetii (^{99m}Tc) et etifenini solutio iniectabilis

DEFINITION

Technetium (^{99m}Tc) etifenin injection is a sterile solution which may be prepared by mixing sodium pertechnetate (^{99m}Tc) injection (fission or non-fission) with solutions of etifenin [[(2,6-diethylphenyl)carbamoylmethylimino]di-acetic acid; $C_{16}H_{22}N_2O_5$] and stannous chloride. The injection contains a variable quantity of tin (Sn) not exceeding 0.2 mg/ml. The injection contains not less than 90.0 per cent and not more than 110.0 per cent of the declared technetium-99m radioactivity at the date and hour stated on the label. Not less than 95.0 per cent of the radioactivity corresponds to technetium-99m complexed with etifenin.

It is prepared from sodium pertechnetate (^{99m}Tc) injection (fission or non-fission) using suitable, sterile ingredients and calculating the ratio of radionuclidic impurities with reference to the date and hour of administration.

CHARACTERS

A clear, colourless solution.

Technetium-99m has a half-life of 6.02 h and emits gamma radiation.

IDENTIFICATION

A. Record the gamma-ray spectrum using a suitable instrument. The spectrum does not differ significantly from that of a standardised technetium-99m solution either by direct comparison or by using an instrument calibrated with the aid of such a solution. Standardised technetium-99m and molybdenum-99 solutions are available from laboratories recognised by the competent authority. The most prominent gamma photon of technetium-99m has an energy of 0.140 MeV.

B. Examine by liquid chromatography (*2.2.29*).

Test solution. Dilute the injection to be examined with *methanol R* to obtain a solution containing about l mg of etifenin per millilitre.

Reference solution. Dissolve 5.0 mg of *etifenin CRS* in *methanol R* and dilute to 5.0 ml with the same solvent.

The chromatographic procedure may be carried out using:

– a column 0.25 m long and 4.6 mm in internal diameter packed with *octadecylsilyl silica gel for chromatography R* (5 µm to 10 µm),

– as mobile phase at a flow rate of 1 ml/min a mixture of 20 volumes of *methanol R* and 80 volumes of a 14 g/l solution of *potassium dihydrogen phosphate R* adjusted to pH 2.5 by the addition of *phosphoric acid R*,

– a spectrophotometer set at 230 nm.

Inject 20 µl of each solution. The principal peak in the chromatogram obtained with the test solution has a similar retention time to the principal peak in the chromatogram obtained with the reference solution.

TESTS

pH (*2.2.3*). The pH of the injection is 4.0 to 6.0.

Physiological distribution. Inject 0.1 ml (equivalent to about 3.7 MBq) into a caudal vein of each of three mice, each weighing 20 g to 25 g. Kill the mice l h after the injection. Remove the liver, gall-bladder, small intestine, large intestine and kidneys, collecting excreted urine. Measure the radioactivity in the organs using a suitable instrument. Measure the radioactivity of the rest of the body, after having removed the tail. Determine the percentage of radioactivity in each organ from the expression:

$$\frac{A}{B} \times 100$$

A = radioactivity of the organ concerned,

B = radioactivity of all organs and the rest of the body, excluding the tail.

In not fewer than two mice the sum of the percentages of radioactivity in the gall-bladder and small and large intestine is not less than 80 per cent. Not more than 3 per cent of the radioactivity is present in the liver, and not more than 2 per cent in the kidneys

Tin

Test solution. Dilute 1.0 ml of the injection to be examined to 5.0 ml with *1 M hydrochloric acid.*

Reference solution. Prepare a reference solution containing 0.075 mg of *stannous chloride R* per millilitre in *1 M hydrochloric acid.*

To 1.0 ml of each solution add 0.4 ml of a 20 g/l solution of *sodium laurilsulfate R*, 0.05 ml of *thioglycollic acid R*, 0.1 ml of *dithiol reagent R* and 3.0 ml of *0.2 M hydrochloric acid.* Mix. Measure the absorbance (*2.2.25*) of each solution at 540 nm, using *0.2 M hydrochloric acid* as the compensation liquid. The absorbance of the test solution is not greater than that of the reference solution (0.2 mg of Sn per millilitre).

Sterility. It complies with the test for sterility prescribed in the monograph on *Radiopharmaceutical preparations (0125)*. The injection may be released for use before completion of the test.

RADIOCHEMICAL PURITY

Examine by thin-layer chromatography (*2.2.27*) using silicic acid as the coating substance on a glass-fibre sheet. Heat the plate at 110 °C for l0 min. The plate used should be such that during development the mobile phase moves over a distance of 10 cm to 15 cm in about 15 min.

Apply to the plate 5 µl to 10 µl of the injection to be examined. Develop immediately over a path of 10 cm to 15 cm using a 9 g/l solution of *sodium chloride R*. Allow the plate to dry. Determine the distribution of radioactivity using a suitable detector. Technetium-99m complexed with etifenin migrates almost to the middle of the chromatogram and pertechnetate ion migrates with the solvent front. Impurities in colloidal form remain at the starting point. The radioactivity corresponding to technetium-99m complexed with etifenin represents not less than 95.0 per cent of the total radioactivity of the chromatogram.

RADIOACTIVITY

Measure the radioactivity using suitable counting equipment by comparison with a standardised technetium-99m solution or by measurement in an instrument calibrated with the aid of such a solution.

01/2005:1925

TECHNETIUM (^{99m}TC) EXAMETAZIME INJECTION

Technetii (^{99m}Tc) exametazimi solutio iniectabilis

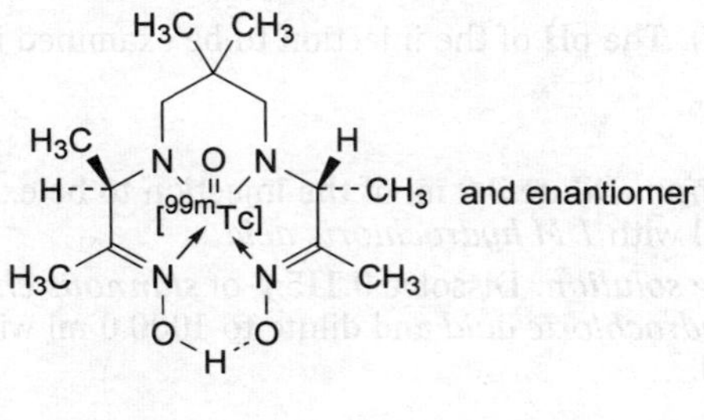

DEFINITION

Sterile solution of lipophilic technetium-99m exametazime which may be prepared by dissolving a racemic mixture of (3*RS*,9*RS*)-4,8-diaza-3,6,6,9-tetramethylundecane-2,10-dione bisoxime in the presence of a stannous salt in *Sodium pertechnetate (^{99m}Tc) injection (fission) (0124)* or *Sodium pertechnetate (^{99m}Tc) injection (non-fission) (0283)*. It may contain stabilisers and inert additives.

Content: 90 per cent to 110 per cent of the declared technetium-99m radioactivity at the date and time stated on the label.

Purity: minimum of 80 per cent of the total radioactivity corresponds to lipophilic technetium-99m exametazime and its *meso* isomer.

CHARACTERS

Appearance: clear solution.

Half-life and nature of radiation of technetium-99m: see *Table of physical characteristics of radionuclides (5.7)*.

IDENTIFICATION

A. Gamma-ray spectrometry.

Comparison: standardised technetium-99m solution, or by using a calibrated instrument. Standardised technetium-99m solutions and/or standardisation services are available from the competent authority.

Results: the spectrum obtained with the solution to be examined does not differ significantly from that obtained with a standardised technetium-99m solution. The most prominent gamma photon has an energy of 0.141 MeV.

B. Examine the chromatograms obtained in the test Impurity A under Radiochemical purity.

Results: the principal peak in the chromatogram obtained with the test solution is similar in retention time to the peak due to lipophilic technetium-99m exametazime in the chromatogram obtained with the reference solution.

TESTS

pH (*2.2.3*): 5.0 to 10.0.

Sterility. It complies with the test for sterility prescribed in the monograph on *Radiopharmaceutical preparations (0125)*. The injection may be released for use before completion of the test.

RADIOCHEMICAL PURITY

Impurity C. Thin-layer chromatography (*2.2.27*).

Test solution. The preparation to be examined.

Plate: *TLC silica gel plate R*; use a glass-fibre plate.

Mobile phase: 9 g/l solution of *sodium chloride R*.

Application: about 5 µl.

Development: immediate, over 2/3 of the plate.

Drying: in air.

Detection: determine the distribution of radioactivity using a suitable detector.

Retention factors: impurity C = 0.8 to 1.0; lipophilic technetium-99m exametazime and impurities A, B, D and E do not migrate.

Limits:

– *impurity C*: maximum 10 per cent of the total radioactivity.

Total of lipophilic technetium-99m exametazime and impurity A. Thin-layer chromatography (*2.2.27*).

Test solution. The preparation to be examined.

Plate: *TLC silica gel plate R*; use a glass-fibre plate.

Mobile phase: *methyl ethyl ketone R*.

Application: about 5 µl.

Development: immediate, over 2/3 of the plate.

Drying: in air.

Detection: determine the distribution of radioactivity using a suitable detector.

Retention factors: lipophilic technetium-99m exametazime = 0.8 to 1.0, impurity A = 0.8 to 1.0, impurity C = 0.8 to 1.0; impurities B, D and E do not migrate.

Limits: calculate the percentage of radioactivity due to impurities B, D and E from test B (*B*) and the percentage of the radioactivity due to impurity C from test A (*A*). Calculate the total percentage of lipophilic technetium-99m exametazime and impurity A from the expression:

$$100 - A - B$$

– *total of lipophilic technetium-99m exametazime and impurity A*: minimum 80 per cent of the total radioactivity.

Impurity A. Liquid chromatography (*2.2.29*).

Test solution. The preparation to be examined.

Reference solution. Dissolve the contents of a vial of *meso-rich exametazime CRS* in 0.5 ml of a 9 g/l solution of *sodium chloride R* and transfer to a lead-shielded, nitrogen-filled vial. Add 6 µl of a freshly prepared 1 g/l solution of *stannous chloride R* in *0.05 M hydrochloric acid* and 2.5 ml of sodium pertechnetate (^{99m}Tc) injection (fission or non-fission) containing 370-740 MBq. Mix carefully and use within 30 min of preparation.

Column:

– *size*: l = 0.25 m, Ø = 4.6 mm,

– *stationary phase*: *spherical base-deactivated end-capped octadecylsilyl silica gel for chromatography R* (5 µm) with a pore size of 13 nm and a carbon loading of 11 per cent.

Mobile phase: mix 33 volumes of *acetonitrile R* and 67 volumes of *0.1 M phosphate buffer solution pH 3.0 R*.

Flow rate: 1.5 ml/min.

Detection: radioactivity detector.

Injection: loop injector.

Run time: 20 min.

Relative retention with reference to lipophilic technetium-99m exametazime: impurity A = about 1.2.

System suitability: reference solution:

– chromatogram similar to the chromatogram provided with *meso-rich exametazime CRS*,

– *resolution*: minimum of 2 between the peaks due to lipophilic technetium-99m exametazime and to impurity A.

Limits:

– *impurity A*: maximum 5 per cent of the radioactivity due to lipophilic technetium-99m exametazime and impurity A.

RADIOACTIVITY

Measure the radioactivity using suitable equipment by comparison with a standardised technetium-99m solution or by using a calibrated instrument.

IMPURITIES

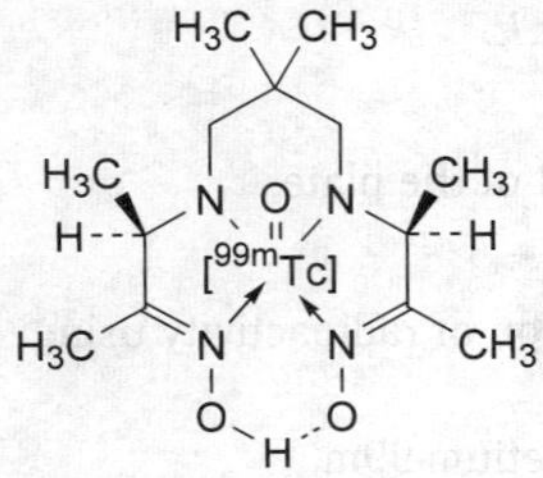

A. *meso* isomer of lipophilic technetium-99m exametazime,

B. technetium-99m in colloidal form,

C. [^{99m}Tc]pertechnetate ion,

D. non lipophilic technetium-99m exametazime complex,

E. *meso* isomer of non lipophilic technetium-99m exametazime complex.

01/2005:1047

TECHNETIUM (^{99m}Tc) GLUCONATE INJECTION

Technetii (^{99m}Tc) gluconatis solutio iniectabilis

DEFINITION

Technetium (99^mTc) gluconate injection is a sterile solution, which may be prepared by mixing solutions of calcium gluconate and a stannous salt or other suitable reducing agent with sodium pertechnetate (99^mTc) injection (fission or non-fission). The injection contains not less than 90.0 per cent and not more than 110.0 per cent of the declared technetium-99m radioactivity at the date and hour stated on the label. Not less than 90 per cent of the radioactivity corresponds to technetium-99m gluconate complex.

It is prepared from sodium pertechnetate (99^mTc) injection (fission or non-fission) using suitable sterile ingredients and calculating the ratio of radionuclidic impurities with reference to the date and hour of administration.

CHARACTERS

A slightly opalescent solution.

Technetium-99m has a half-life of 6.02 h and emits gamma radiation.

IDENTIFICATION

A. Record the gamma-ray spectrum using a suitable instrument. The spectrum does not differ significantly from that of a standardised technetium-99m solution either by direct comparison or by using an instrument calibrated with the aid of such a solution. Standardised technetium-99m and molybdenum-99 solutions are available from laboratories recognised by the competent authority. The most prominent gamma photon of technetium-99m has an energy of 0.140 MeV.

B. 5 µl of the solution complies with identification A prescribed in the monograph on *Calcium gluconate (0172)*.

C. Examine the chromatograms obtained in the test for radiochemical purity. The distribution of the radioactivity contributes to the identification of the preparation.

TESTS

pH (*2.2.3*). The pH of the solution is 6.0 to 8.5.

Physiological distribution. Inject a volume not greater than 0.2 ml into the caudal vein of each of three rats weighing 150 g to 250 g. Measure the radioactivity of the syringe before and after injection. Sacrifice the rats 30 min after the injection. Remove at least 1 g of blood by a suitable method and remove the kidneys, the liver, the bladder plus voided urine and the tail. Weigh the sample of blood.

Determine the radioactivity in the organs, the blood sample and the tail using a suitable instrument. Calculate the percentage of radioactivity in each organ and in 1 g of blood with respect to the total radioactivity calculated as the difference between the two measurements made on the syringe minus the activity in the tail. Correct the blood concentration by multiplying by a factor of $m/200$ where m is the body mass of the rat in grams.

In not fewer than two of the three rats used, the radioactivity in the kidneys is not less than 15 per cent, that in the bladder plus voided urine is not less than 20 per cent and that in the liver is not more than 5 per cent. The radioactivity in the blood, after correction, is not more than 0.50 per cent.

Sterility. It complies with the test for sterility prescribed in the monograph on *Radiopharmaceutical preparations (0125)*. The injection may be released for use before completion of the test.

RADIOCHEMICAL PURITY

Examine by thin-layer chromatography (*2.2.27*) using silica gel as the coating substance on a glass-fibre sheet. Heat the plate at 110 °C for 10 min. Use a plate such that during development the mobile phase migrates over a distance of 10 cm to 15 cm in about 10 min.

a) Apply to the plate 5 µl to 10 µl of the solution to be examined. Develop immediately over a path of 10 cm to 15 cm using a 9 g/l solution of *sodium chloride R*. Allow the plate to dry. Determine the distribution of radioactivity using a suitable detector. Impurities in colloidal form remain at the starting point. Technetium gluconate complex and pertechnetate ion migrate near to the solvent front.

b) Apply to the plate 5 µl to 10 µl of the solution to be examined and allow to dry. Develop over a path of 10 cm to 15 cm using *methyl ethyl ketone R*. Dry in a current of warm air. Determine the distribution of radioactivity using a suitable detector. Pertechnetate ion impurity migrates near to the solvent front. Technetium gluconate complex and technetium in colloidal form remain at the starting point.

The sum of the percentages of radioactivity corresponding to impurities in the chromatograms obtained in test (a) and (b) does not exceed 10 per cent.

RADIOACTIVITY

Measure the radioactivity using suitable counting equipment by comparison with a standardised technetium-99m solution or by measurement in an instrument calibrated with the aid of such a solution.

01/2005:0640

TECHNETIUM (^{99m}Tc) HUMAN ALBUMIN INJECTION

Technetii (^{99m}Tc) humani albumini solutio iniectabilis

DEFINITION

Technetium (^{99m}Tc) human albumin injection is a sterile, apyrogenic solution of human albumin labelled with technetium-99m. It contains a reducing substance, such as a tin salt in an amount not exceeding 1 mg of Sn per millilitre;

it may contain a suitable buffer and an antimicrobial preservative. Although, at present, no definite value for a maximum limit of tin can be fixed, available evidence tends to suggest the importance of keeping the ratio of tin to albumin as low as possible. The human albumin used complies with the requirements of the monograph on *Human albumin solution (0255)*. The injection contains not less than 90.0 per cent and not more than 110.0 per cent of the declared technetium-99m radioactivity at the date and hour stated on the label. The injection contains not less than 90.0 per cent and not more than 110.0 per cent of the quantity of albumin stated on the label. Not less than 80 per cent of the radioactivity is associated with the albumin fractions II to V. Not more than 5.0 per cent of the radioactivity due to technetium-99m corresponds to free pertechnetate, as determined by the method described in the test for radiochemical purity.

It is prepared from sodium pertechnetate (^{99m}Tc) injection (fission or non-fission) using suitable sterile and apyrogenic ingredients and calculating the ratio of radionuclidic impurities with reference to the date and hour of administration.

CHARACTERS

A clear, colourless or pale-yellow solution.

Technetium-99m has a half-life of 6.02 h and emits gamma radiation.

IDENTIFICATION

A. Record the gamma-ray spectrum using a suitable instrument. The spectrum does not differ significantly from that of a standardised technetium-99m solution either by direct comparison or by using an instrument calibrated with the aid of such a solution. Standardised technetium-99m and molybdenum-99 solutions are available from laboratories recognised by the competent authority. The most prominent gamma photon of technetium-99m has an energy of 0.140 MeV.

B. Using a suitable range of species-specific antisera, carry out precipitation tests on the preparation to be examined. The test is to be carried out using antisera specific to the plasma proteins of each species of domestic animal currently used in the preparation of materials of biological origin in the country concerned. The injection is shown to contain proteins of human origin and gives negative results with antisera specific to plasma proteins of other species.

C. Examine by a suitable immunoelectrophoresis technique. Using antiserum to normal human serum, compare normal human serum and the injection to be examined, both diluted if necessary. The main component of the injection to be examined corresponds to the main component of the normal human serum. The diluted solution may show the presence of small quantities of other plasma proteins.

TESTS

pH (*2.2.3*). The pH of the injection is 2.0 to 6.5.

Albumin

Reference solution. Dilute *human albumin solution R* with a 9 g/l solution of *sodium chloride R* to a concentration of 5 mg of albumin per millilitre.

To 1.0 ml of the injection to be examined and to 1.0 ml of the reference solution add 4.0 ml of *biuret reagent R* and mix. After exactly 30 min, measure the absorbance (*2.2.25*) of each solution at 540 nm, using as the compensation liquid a 9 g/l solution of *sodium chloride R* treated in the same manner. From the absorbances measured, calculate the content of albumin in the injection to be examined in milligrams per millilitre.

Tin

Test solution. To 1.0 ml of the injection to be examined add 1.0 ml of *2 M hydrochloric acid*. Heat in a water-bath at 100 °C for 30 min. Cool and centrifuge at 300 *g* for 10 min. Dilute 1.0 ml of the supernatant liquid to 10 ml with *1 M hydrochloric acid*.

Reference solution. Dissolve 95 mg of *stannous chloride R* in *1 M hydrochloric acid* and dilute to 1000.0 ml with the same acid.

To 1.0 ml of each solution add 0.4 ml of a 20 g/l solution of *sodium laurilsulfate R*, 0.05 ml of *thioglycollic acid R*, 0.1 ml of *dithiol reagent R* and 3.0 ml of *0.2 M hydrochloric acid*. Mix. Measure the absorbance (*2.2.25*) of each solution at 540 nm, using *0.2 M hydrochloric acid* as the compensation liquid. The absorbance of the test solution is not greater than that of the reference solution (1 mg of Sn per millilitre).

Physiological distribution. Inject a volume not greater than 0.5 ml and containing not more than 1.0 mg of albumin into a suitable vein such as a caudal vein or a saphenous vein of each of three male rats, each weighing 150 g to 250 g. Measure the radioactivity in the syringe before and after the injection. Kill the rats 30 min after the injection. Take one millilitre of blood by a suitable method and remove the liver and, if a caudal vein has been used for the injection, the tail. Using a suitable instrument determine the radioactivity in 1 ml of blood, in the liver and, if a caudal vein has been used for the injection, in the tail. Determine the percentage of radioactivity in the liver and in 1 ml of blood with respect to the total radioactivity calculated as the difference between the measurements made on the syringe minus the activity in the tail (if a caudal vein has been used for the injection). Correct the blood concentration by multiplying by a factor of $m/200$ where m is the body mass of the rat in grams. In not fewer than two of the three rats used, the radioactivity in the liver is not more than 15 per cent and that in blood, after correction, is not less than 3.5 per cent.

Sterility. It complies with the test for sterility prescribed in the monograph on *Radiopharmaceutical preparations (0125)*. The injection may be released for use before completion of the test.

Bacterial endotoxins (*2.6.14*): less than $175/V$ IU/ml, V being the maximum recommended dose in millilitres.

RADIOCHEMICAL PURITY

A. Examine by thin-layer chromatography (*2.2.27*) using silica gel as the coating substance on a glass-fibre sheet. Heat the plate at 110 °C for 10 min. Use a plate such that during development the mobile phase migrates over a distance of 10 cm to 15 cm in about 10 min.

   Apply to the plate 5 µl to 10 µl of the injection to be examined and allow to dry. Develop over a path of 10 cm to 15 cm using *methyl ethyl ketone R*. Allow the plate to dry. Determine the distribution of radioactivity using a suitable detector. The technetium-99m human albumin complex remains at the starting-point and pertechnetate ion migrates near to the solvent front. Not more than 5.0 per cent of the technetium-99m radioactivity corresponds to technetium in the form of pertechnetate ion.

B. Examine by size-exclusion chromatography (*2.2.30*).

   Mobile phase (concentrated). Dissolve 1.124 g of *potassium dihydrogen phosphate R*, 4.210 g of *disodium hydrogen phosphate R*, 1.17 g of *sodium chloride R* and 0.10 g of *sodium azide R* in 100 ml of *water R*.

Test solution. Mix 0.25 ml of the injection to be examined with 0.25 ml of the mobile phase (concentrated). Use immediately after dilution.

The chromatographic procedure may be carried out using:
- a stainless steel column 0.6 m long and 7.5 mm in internal diameter, packed with *silica gel for size-exclusion chromatography R*,
- as the mobile phase at a flow rate of 0.6 ml/min a mixture of equal volumes of mobile phase (concentrated) and *water R*,
- a radioactivity detector set for technetium-99m,
- a loop injector.

Inject 200 µl of the test solution. Continue the chromatography for at least 10 min after background level is reached.

Peaks are eluted with the following retention times:

I	High molecular mass compound	19-20 min
II	Poly III-albumin	23-24 min
III	Poly II-albumin	25-27 min
IV	Poly I-albumin	28-29 min
V	Human serum albumin	32-33 min
VI	Tin colloid	40-47 min
VII	Pertechnetate	48 min

At least 80 per cent of the radioactivity applied to the column is associated with the albumin fractions II to V.

RADIOACTIVITY

Measure the radioactivity using suitable counting equipment by comparison with a standardised technetium-99m solution or by measurement in an instrument calibrated with the aid of such a solution.

LABELLING

The label states:
- the amount of albumin,
- the amount of tin, if any.

01/2005:0296

TECHNETIUM (^{99m}Tc) MACROSALB INJECTION

Technetii (^{99m}Tc) macrosalbi suspensio iniectabilis

DEFINITION

Technetium (^{99m}Tc) macrosalb injection is a sterile, apyrogenic suspension of human albumin in the form of irregular insoluble aggregates obtained by denaturing human albumin in aqueous solution; the particles are labelled with technetium-99m. The injection contains reducing substances, such as tin salts in an amount not exceeding 3 mg of Sn per millilitre; it may contain a suitable buffer such as acetate, citrate or phosphate buffer and also non-denatured human albumin and an antimicrobial preservative such as benzyl alcohol. The human albumin employed complies with the requirements prescribed in the monograph on *Human albumin solution (0255)*. The injection contains not less than 90.0 per cent and not more than 110.0 per cent of the declared technetium-99m radioactivity at the date and hour stated on the label. Not less than 90 per cent of the technetium-99m is bound to the particles of the suspension as determined by the test for non-filterable radioactivity. The particles have a typical diameter between 10 µm and 100 µm. The specific radioactivity is not less than 37 MBq of technetium-99m per milligram of aggregated albumin at the date and hour of administration.

It is prepared from sodium pertechnetate (^{99m}Tc) injection (fission or non-fission) using suitable sterile and apyrogenic ingredients and calculating the ratio of radionuclidic impurities with reference to the date and hour of administration.

CHARACTERS

A white suspension which may separate on standing.

Technetium-99m has a half-life of 6.02 h and emits gamma radiation.

IDENTIFICATION

A. Record the gamma-ray spectrum using a suitable instrument. The spectrum does not differ significantly from that of a standardised technetium-99m solution either by direct comparison or by using an instrument calibrated with the aid of such a solution. Standardised technetium-99m and molybdenum-99 solutions are available from laboratories recognised by the competent authority. The most prominent gamma photon of technetium-99m has an energy of 0.140 MeV.

B. The tests for non-filterable radioactivity and particle size contribute to the identification of the preparation.

C. Transfer 1 ml of the injection to a centrifuge tube and centrifuge at 2500 *g* for 5 min to 10 min. Decant the supernatant liquid. To the residue add 5 ml of *cupri-tartaric solution R2*, mix and allow to stand for 10 min. If necessary, heat to dissolve the particles and allow to cool. Add rapidly 0.5 ml of *dilute phosphomolybdotungstic reagent R*, mixing immediately. A blue colour develops.

TESTS

pH (*2.2.3*). The pH of the injection is 3.8 to 7.5.

Non-filterable radioactivity. Use a polycarbonate membrane filter 13 mm to 25 mm in diameter, 10 µm thick and with circular pores 3 µm in diameter. Fit the membrane into a suitable holder. Place 0.2 ml of the injection on the membrane and filter, adding 20 ml of a 9 g/l solution of *sodium chloride R* during the filtration. The radioactivity remaining on the membrane represents not less than 90 per cent of the total radioactivity of the injection.

Particle size. Examine using a microscope. Dilute the injection if necessary so that the number of particles is just low enough for individual particles to be distinguished. Using a syringe fitted with a needle having a calibre not less than 0.35 mm, place a suitable volume in a suitable counting chamber such as a haemocytometer cell, taking care not to overfill the chamber. Allow the suspension to settle for 1 min and carefully add a cover slide without squeezing the sample. Scan an area corresponding to at least 5000 particles. Not more than 10 particles have a maximum dimension greater than 100 µm. No particle having a maximum dimension greater than 150 µm is present.

Aggregated albumin

Test solution. Transfer a volume of the injection expected to contain about 1 mg of aggregated albumin to a centrifuge tube and centrifuge at about 2500 *g* for 5 min to 10 min. Decant the supernatant liquid. Resuspend the sediment in 2.0 ml of a 9 g/l solution of *sodium chloride R*. Centrifuge at 2500 *g* for 5 min to 10 min. Decant the supernatant liquid.

Radiopharmaceutical preparations

Resuspend the sediment in 5.0 ml of *sodium carbonate solution R1*. Heat in a water-bath at 80 °C to 90 °C to dissolve the aggregated albumin. Allow to cool, transfer to a volumetric flask and dilute to 10.0 ml with *sodium carbonate solution R1*.

Reference solutions. Prepare a range of reference solutions containing 0.05 mg to 0.2 mg of human albumin per millilitre in *sodium carbonate solution R1*.

Introduce 3.0 ml of each solution separately into 25 ml flasks. To each flask add 15.0 ml of *cupri-tartaric solution R2*, mix and allow to stand for 10 min. Add rapidly 1.5 ml of *dilute phosphomolybdotungstic reagent R* and mix immediately. Allow to stand for 30 min and measure the absorbance (*2.2.25*) at 750 nm using *sodium carbonate solution R1* as the compensation liquid. Using the absorbances obtained with the reference solutions, draw a calibration curve and calculate the content of aggregated albumin in the injection.

Tin

Test solution. To 1.0 ml of the injection add 1.0 ml of *2 M hydrochloric acid*. Heat in a water-bath for 30 min. Cool and centrifuge for 10 min at 300 *g*. Dilute 1.0 ml of the supernatant liquid to 25.0 ml with *1 M hydrochloric acid*.

Reference solution. Dissolve 0.115 g of *stannous chloride R* in *1 M hydrochloric acid* and dilute to 1000.0 ml with the same acid.

To 1.0 ml of each solution add 0.4 ml of a 20 g/l solution of *sodium laurilsulfate R*, 0.05 ml of *thioglycollic acid R*, 0.1 ml of *dithiol reagent R* and 3.0 ml of *0.2 M hydrochloric acid*. Mix. Measure the absorbance (*2.2.25*) of each solution at 540 nm, using *0.2 M hydrochloric acid* as the compensation liquid. The absorbance of the test solution is not greater than that of the reference solution (3 mg of Sn per millilitre).

Physiological distribution. Inject a volume not greater than 0.2 ml into the caudal vein of each of three rats weighing 150 g to 250 g. Kill the rats 15 min after the injection, remove the liver, the spleen and the lungs and measure the radioactivity in the organs using a suitable instrument. Measure the radioactivity in the rest of the body, including the blood, after having removed the tail. Determine the percentage of radioactivity in the lungs, the liver and the spleen from the expression:

$$\frac{A}{B} \times 100$$

A = radioactivity of the organ concerned,

B = total radioactivity in the liver, the spleen, the lungs and the rest of the body.

In not fewer than two of the three rats used, at least 80 per cent of the radioactivity is found in the lungs and not more than a total of 5 per cent in the liver and spleen. The injection may be released for use before completion of the test.

Sterility. It complies with the test for sterility prescribed in the monograph on *Radiopharmaceutical preparations (0125)*. The injection may be released for use before completion of the test.

Pyrogens. It complies with the test for pyrogens prescribed in the monograph on *Radiopharmaceutical preparations (0125)*. Inject into the animals not less than 0.1 ml per kilogram of the rabbit's mass. The injection may be released for use before completion of the test.

RADIOACTIVITY

Measure the radioactivity using suitable counting equipment by comparison with a standardised technetium-99m solution or by measurement in an instrument calibrated with the aid of such a solution.

LABELLING

The label states:

- that the preparation should be shaken before use,
- the quantity of tin per millilitre, if any,
- that the preparation is not to be used if after shaking, the suspension does not appear homogeneous.

01/2005:0641

TECHNETIUM (^{99m}Tc) MEDRONATE INJECTION

Technetii (^{99m}Tc) medronati solutio iniectabilis

DEFINITION

Technetium (^{99m}Tc) medronate injection is a sterile solution which may be prepared by mixing solutions of sodium methylenediphosphonate and a stannous salt with sodium pertechnetate (^{99m}Tc) injection (fission or non-fission). The injection contains a variable quantity of tin (Sn) not exceeding 3 mg/ml; it may contain antimicrobial preservatives, antioxidants, stabilisers and buffers. The injection contains not less than 90.0 per cent and not more than 110.0 per cent of the declared technetium-99m radioactivity at the date and hour stated on the label. Radioactivity present as chemical forms other than technetium-99m medronate complex is not greater than 5.0 per cent of the total radioactivity.

It is prepared from sodium pertechnetate (^{99m}Tc) injection (fission or non-fission) using suitable sterile ingredients and calculating the ratio of radionuclidic impurities with reference to the date and hour of administration.

CHARACTERS

A clear, colourless solution.

Technetium-99m has a half-life of 6.02 h and emits gamma radiation.

IDENTIFICATION

A. Record the gamma-ray spectrum using a suitable instrument. The spectrum does not differ significantly from that of a standardised technetium-99m solution either by direct comparison or by using an instrument calibrated with the aid of such a solution. Standardised technetium-99m and molybdenum-99 solutions are available from laboratories recognised by the competent authority. The most prominent gamma photon of technetium-99m has an energy of 0.140 MeV.

B. Examine the chromatograms obtained in the test for radiochemical purity. The distribution of the radioactivity contributes to the identification of the preparation.

C. Examine by thin-layer chromatography (*2.2.27*) using cellulose as the coating substance.

Test solution. Dilute the injection to be examined with *water R* to obtain a solution containing about 0.1 mg to 0.5 mg of sodium medronate per millilitre.

Reference solution. Dissolve a suitable quantity (1 mg to 5 mg) of *medronic acid CRS* in a mixture of a 9.0 g/l solution of *sodium chloride R* and *water R* and dilute to

Radiopharmaceutical preparations

10 ml with the same solvent so as to obtain a solution similar to the test solution with regard to medronate and sodium chloride concentrations.

Apply separately to the plate 10 µl of each solution. Develop over a path of 12 cm to 14 cm (development time about 4 h) using a mixture of 20 volumes of *2-propanol R*, 30 volumes of *1 M hydrochloric acid* and 60 volumes of *methyl ethyl ketone R*. Allow the plate to dry in air and spray with *ammonium molybdate solution R4*. Expose the plate to ultraviolet light at 254 nm for about 10 min. The principal spot in the chromatogram obtained with the test solution is similar in position and colour to the spot in the chromatogram obtained with the reference solution.

TESTS

pH (*2.2.3*). The pH of the solution is 3.5 to 7.5.

Tin

Test solution. Dilute 1.0 ml of the solution to 50.0 ml with *1 M hydrochloric acid.*

Reference solution. Dissolve 0.115 g of *stannous chloride R* in *1 M hydrochloric acid* and dilute to 1000.0 ml with the same acid.

To 1.0 ml of each solution add 0.4 ml of a 20 g/l solution of *sodium laurilsulfate R*, 0.05 ml of *thioglycollic acid R*, 0.1 ml of *dithiol reagent R* and 3.0 ml of *0.2 M hydrochloric acid*. Mix. Measure the absorbance (*2.2.25*) of each solution at 540 nm, using *0.2 M hydrochloric acid* as compensation liquid. The absorbance of the test solution is not greater than that of the reference solution (3 mg of Sn per millilitre).

Physiological distribution. Inject a volume not greater than 0.2 ml, equivalent to not more than 0.05 mg of sodium medronate into a suitable vein such as a caudal vein or the saphenous vein of each of three rats, each weighing 150 g to 250 g. Measure the radioactivity in the syringe before and after injection. Kill the rats 2 h after the injection. Remove one femur, the liver, and some blood. Weigh the blood. Remove the tail if a caudal vein has been used for the injection. Using a suitable instrument measure the radioactivity in the femur, liver, and blood, and in the tail if a caudal vein has been used for the injection. Determine the percentage of radioactivity in each sample from the expression:

$$\frac{A}{B} \times 100$$

A = radioactivity of the sample concerned,

B = total radioactivity, which is equal to the difference between the two measurements made on the syringe minus the radioactivity in the tail if a caudal vein has been used for the injection.

Calculate the radioactivity per unit mass in the blood. Correct the blood concentration by multiplying by a factor $m/200$ where m is the body mass of the rat in grams.

In not fewer than two of the three rats: not less than 1.5 per cent of the radioactivity is found in the femur; not more than 1.0 per cent is found in the liver and not more than 0.05 per cent per gram is found in the blood.

Sterility. It complies with the test for sterility prescribed in the monograph on *Radiopharmaceutical preparations (0125)*. The injection may be released for use before completion of the test.

RADIOCHEMICAL PURITY

Examine by thin-layer chromatography (*2.2.27*) using silica gel as the coating substance on a glass-fibre sheet. Use plates such that during development, the mobile phase migrates 10 cm to 15 cm in about 10 min. Determine hydrolysed technetium and technetium in colloidal form by test (a) and pertechnetate ion by test (b).

(a) Apply to the plate 5 µl to 10 µl of the injection. Develop immediately over a path of 10 cm to 15 cm using a 136 g/l solution of *sodium acetate R*. Allow the plate to dry in air. Determine the distribution of radioactivity using a suitable detector. Hydrolysed technetium and technetium in colloidal form remain at the starting point. Technetium medronate complex and pertechnetate ion migrate near to the solvent front.

(b) Apply to the plate 5 µl to 10 µl of the injection and dry quickly. Develop over a path of 10 cm to 15 cm using *methyl ethyl ketone R*. Allow the plate to dry. Determine the distribution of radioactivity using a suitable detector. Pertechnetate ion migrates near to the solvent front. Technetium medronate complex and technetium in colloidal form remain at the starting-point.

The percentage of radioactivity corresponding to pertechnetate ion in the chromatogram obtained in test (b) is not greater than 2.0 per cent and the sum of the percentages of radioactivity corresponding to impurities in the chromatograms obtained in test (a) and test (b) (including pertechnetate ion) is not greater than 5.0 per cent.

RADIOACTIVITY

Measure the radioactivity using suitable counting equipment by comparison with a standardised technetium-99m solution or by measurement in an instrument calibrated with the aid of such a solution.

01/2005:1372

TECHNETIUM (^{99m}Tc) MERTIATIDE INJECTION

Technetii (^{99m}Tc) mertiatidi solutio iniectabilis

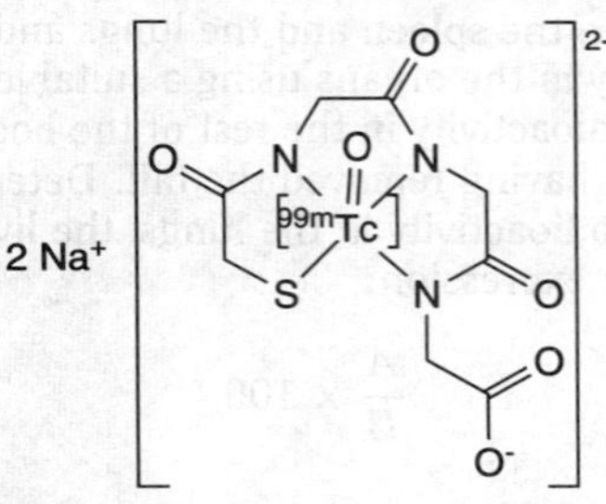

DEFINITION

Technetium (^{99m}Tc) mertiatide injection is a sterile solution which may be prepared by either heating a mixture containing *S*-benzoylmercaptoacetyltriglycine (betiatide), a weak chelating agent such as tartrate, a stannous salt and sodium pertechnetate (^{99m}Tc) injection (fission or non-fission), or by mixing solutions of mercaptoacetyltriglycine (mertiatide), a stannous salt and sodium pertechnetate (^{99m}Tc) injection (fission or non-fission) at alkaline pH. It may contain stabilisers and a buffer. The injection contains not less than 90.0 per cent and not more than 110.0 per cent of the declared technetium-99m radioactivity at the date and time stated on the label. Not less than 94 per cent of the radioactivity corresponds to technetium-99m in the form of [^{99m}Tc]technetium mertiatide.

CHARACTERS

A clear, colourless solution.

Radiopharmaceutical preparations

01/2005:0643

TECHNETIUM (^{99m}Tc) SUCCIMER INJECTION

Technetii (^{99m}Tc) succimeri solutio iniectabilis

DEFINITION

Technetium (^{99m}Tc) succimer injection is a sterile solution of *meso*-2,3-dimercaptosuccinic acid labelled with technetium-99m. It contains a reducing substance, such as a tin salt in an amount not exceeding 1 mg of Sn per millilitre, and may contain stabilisers, antioxidants such as ascorbic acid, and inert additives. The injection contains not less than 90.0 per cent and not more than 110.0 per cent of the declared technetium-99m radioactivity at the date and hour stated on the label. Not less than 95.0 per cent of the radioactivity corresponds to technetium-99m succimer complex.

It is prepared from sodium pertechnetate (^{99m}Tc) injection (fission or non-fission) using suitable sterile ingredients and calculating the ratio of radionuclidic impurities with reference to the date and hour of administration. Syringes for handling the eluate intended for labelling of the final product, or for handling the final product should not contain rubber parts.

CHARACTERS

A clear, colourless solution.

Technetium-99m has a half life of 6.02 h and emits gamma radiation.

IDENTIFICATION

A. Record the gamma-ray spectrum using a suitable instrument. The spectrum does not differ significantly from that of a standardised technetium-99m solution either by direct comparison or by using an instrument calibrated with the aid of such a solution. Standardised technetium-99m and molybdenum-99 solutions are available from laboratories recognised by the competent authority. The most prominent gamma photon of technetium-99m has an energy of 0.140 MeV.

B. Examine the chromatogram obtained in the test for radiochemical purity. The distribution of the radioactivity contributes to the identification of the preparation.

C. Place 1 ml of the injection to be examined in a test-tube and add 1 ml of a 20 g/l solution of *sodium nitroprusside R* and 0.1 ml of *glacial acetic acid R*. Mix. Place carefully at the top of the solution a layer of *concentrated ammonia R*. A violet ring develops between the layers.

TESTS

pH (*2.2.3*). The pH of the injection is 2.3 to 3.5.

Tin

Test solution. Dilute 1.5 ml of the injection to be examined to 25.0 ml with *1 M hydrochloric acid*.

Reference solution. Dissolve 0.115 g of *stannous chloride R* in *1 M hydrochloric acid* and dilute to 1000.0 ml with the same acid.

To 1.0 ml of each solution add 0.4 ml of a 20 g/l solution of *sodium laurilsulfate R*, 0.05 ml of *thioglycollic acid R*, 0.1 ml of *dithiol reagent R* and 3.0 ml of *0.2 M hydrochloric acid*. Mix. Allow to stand for 60 min. Measure the absorbance (*2.2.25*) of each solution at 540 nm, using *0.2 M hydrochloric acid* as the compensation liquid. The absorbance of the test solution is not greater than that of the reference solution (1 mg of Sn per millilitre).

Physiological distribution. Inject a volume not greater than 0.2 ml and containing not more than 0.1 mg of dimercaptosuccinic acid into a suitable vein, such as a caudal vein or a saphenous vein, of each of three rats each weighing 150 g to 250 g. Measure the radioactivity in the syringe before and after the injection. Kill the rats 1 h after the injection. Remove the kidneys, the liver, the stomach, the lungs and, if a caudal vein has been used for the injection, the tail. Using a suitable instrument determine the radioactivity in the organs and, if a caudal vein has been used for injection, in the tail. Determine the percentage of radioactivity in each organ with respect to the total radioactivity calculated as the difference between the two measurements made on the syringe minus the activity in the tail (if a caudal vein has been used for the injection).

In not fewer than two of the three rats used, the radioactivity in the kidneys is not less than 40 per cent, that in the liver is not more than 10.0 per cent, that in the stomach is not more than 2.0 per cent and that in the lungs is not more than 5.0 per cent.

Sterility. It complies with the test for sterility prescribed in the monograph on *Radiopharmaceutical preparations (0125)*. The injection may be released for use before completion of the test.

RADIOCHEMICAL PURITY

Examine by thin-layer chromatography (*2.2.27*) using silica gel as the coating substance on a glass-fibre sheet. Heat the plate at 110 °C for 10 min. Use a plate such that during development the mobile phase migrates over a distance of 10 cm to 15 cm in about 10 min.

Apply to the plate 5 µl to 10 µl of the injection to be examined. Develop immediately over a path of 10 cm to 15 cm using *methyl ethyl ketone R*. Allow the plate to dry. Determine the distribution of radioactivity using a suitable detector. Technetium succimer complex remains at the starting point. Pertechnetate ion migrates near to the solvent front. Not less than 95.0 per cent of the total radioactivity is found in the spot corresponding to technetium succimer complex. The radioactivity corresponding to pertechnetate ion represents not more than 2.0 per cent of the total radioactivity.

RADIOACTIVITY

Measure the radioactivity using suitable counting equipment by comparison with a standardised technetium-99m solution or by measurement in an instrument calibrated with the aid of such a solution.

STORAGE

Store protected from light.

01/2005:0129

TECHNETIUM (^{99m}Tc) TIN PYROPHOSPHATE INJECTION

Stanni pyrophosphatis et technetii (^{99m}Tc) solutio iniectabilis

DEFINITION

Technetium (^{99m}Tc) tin pyrophosphate injection is a sterile, apyrogenic solution which may be prepared by mixing solutions of sodium pyrophosphate and stannous chloride with sodium pertechnetate (^{99m}Tc) injection (fission or non-fission). The injection contains not less than 90.0 per cent and not more than 110.0 per cent of the declared technetium-99m radioactivity at the date and hour stated on the label. Not less than 90 per cent of the radioactivity corresponds to technetium-99m complexed with tin pyrophosphate. The injection contains a quantity of sodium pyrophosphate ($Na_4P_2O_7,10H_2O$) that may vary from 1 mg to 50 mg per millilitre and a variable quantity of tin (Sn) not exceeding 3.0 mg per millilitre.

It is prepared from sodium pertechnetate (^{99m}Tc) injection (fission or non-fission) using suitable sterile, apyrogenic ingredients and calculating the ratio of radionuclidic impurities with reference to the date and hour of administration.

CHARACTERS

A clear, colourless solution.

Technetium-99m has a half-life of 6.02 h and emits gamma radiation.

IDENTIFICATION

A. Record the gamma-ray spectrum using a suitable instrument. The spectrum does not differ significantly from that of a standardised technetium-99m solution either by direct comparison or by using an instrument calibrated with the aid of such a solution. Standardised technetium-99m and molybdenum-99 solutions are available from laboratories recognised by the competent authority. The most prominent gamma photon of technetium-99m has an energy of 0.140 MeV.

B. Examine the chromatograms obtained in the test for radiochemical purity. The distribution of radioactivity contributes to the identification of the injection.

C. To 1 ml add 1 ml of *acetic acid R*. Heat on a water-bath for 1 h. After cooling, add 10 ml of *nitro-vanadomolybdic reagent R* and allow to stand for 30 min. A yellow colour develops.

D. To 1 ml add 2 ml of a 30 per cent *V/V* solution of *sulphuric acid R*, 1 ml of *hydrochloric acid R*, 0.05 ml of *thioglycollic acid R*, 0.4 ml of a 20 g/l solution of *sodium laurilsulfate R* and 0.1 ml of *dithiol reagent R* and allow to stand for 30 min. A pink colour develops.

TESTS

pH (*2.2.3*). The pH of the injection is 6.0 to 7.0.

Sodium pyrophosphate

Test solution. Use 1 ml of the injection to be examined or a suitable dilution of it.

Reference solutions. Using a solution containing *sodium pyrophosphate R* and *stannous chloride R* in the same proportions as in the injection to be examined, prepare a range of solutions and dilute to the same final volume with *water R*.

To the test solution and to 1 ml of each of the reference solutions add successively 10 ml of a 1 g/l solution of *disodium hydrogen phosphate R*, 10 ml of *iron standard solution (8 ppm Fe) R*, 5 ml of *glacial acetic acid R* and 5 ml of a 1 g/l solution of *hydroxylamine hydrochloride R*. Dilute each solution to 40 ml with *water R* and heat in a water-bath at 40 °C for 1 h. To each solution add 4 ml of a 1 g/l solution of *phenanthroline hydrochloride R* and dilute to 50.0 ml with *water R*. Measure the absorbance (*2.2.25*) of each solution at 515 nm using as the compensation liquid a reagent blank containing hydrochloric acid (1.1 g/l HCl) instead of the *iron standard solution (8 ppm Fe) R*. Using the absorbances obtained with the reference solutions, draw a calibration curve and calculate the concentration of sodium pyrophosphate in the injection to be examined.

Tin

Test solution. Use 1 ml of the injection to be examined or a suitable dilution of it.

Reference solutions. Using a solution in hydrochloric acid (6.2 g/l HCl) containing *sodium pyrophosphate R* and *stannous chloride R* in the same proportions as in the injection to be examined, prepare a range of solutions and dilute to the same volume with hydrochloric acid (6.2 g/l HCl).

To the test solution and to 1 ml of each of the reference solutions add 2 ml of a 300 g/l solution of *sulphuric acid R*, 1 ml of *hydrochloric acid R*, 0.05 ml of *thioglycollic acid R*, 0.4 ml of a 20 g/l solution of *sodium laurilsulfate R* and 0.1 ml of *dithiol reagent R* and dilute to 15 ml with hydrochloric acid (6.2 g/l HCl). Allow the solutions to stand for 30 min and measure the absorbance (*2.2.25*) of each solution at 530 nm, using as the compensation liquid a reagent blank containing the same quantity of *sodium pyrophosphate R* as the injection to be examined. Using the absorbances obtained with the reference solutions, draw a calibration curve and calculate the concentration of tin in the injection to be examined.

Sterility. It complies with the test for sterility prescribed in the monograph on *Radiopharmaceutical preparations (0125)*. The injection may be released for use before completion of the test.

Pyrogens. It complies with the test for pyrogens prescribed in the monograph on *Radiopharmaceutical preparations (0125)*. Inject not less than 0.1 ml per kilogram of the rabbit's mass. The injection may be released for use before completion of the test.

RADIOCHEMICAL PURITY

(a) Examine by thin-layer chromatography (*2.2.27*) using silica gel as the coating substance on a glass-fibre sheet. Heat the plate at 110 °C for 10 min. The plate used should be such that during development the mobile phase migrates over a distance of 10 cm to 15 cm in about 10 min.

Apply to the plate 5 µl to 10 µl of the injection and dry in a stream of nitrogen. Develop over a path of 10 cm to 15 cm using *methyl ethyl ketone R* through which nitrogen has been bubbled in the chromatography tank for 10 min immediately before the chromatography. Allow the plate to dry. Determine the distribution of radioactivity using a suitable detector. The technetium-99m tin pyrophosphate complex remains at the starting-point and pertechnetate ion migrates with an R_f of 0.95 to 1.0.

(b) Examine by thin-layer chromatography (*2.2.27*) using silica gel as the coating substance on a glass-fibre sheet. Heat the plate at 110 °C for 10 min. The plate used should be such that during development the mobile phase migrates over a distance of 10 cm to 15 cm in about 10 min.

Apply to the plate 5 µl to 10 µl of the injection. Develop immediately over a path of 10 cm to 15 cm using a 136 g/l solution of *sodium acetate R*. Allow the plate to dry and measure the distribution of radioactivity using a suitable detector. Impurities in colloidal form remain at the starting-point and technetium-99m tin pyrophosphate complex and pertechnetate ion migrate with an R_f of 0.9 to 1.0.

Add together the percentages of radioactivity corresponding to impurities in the chromatograms obtained in test (a) and test (b). The sum does not exceed 10 per cent.

RADIOACTIVITY

Measure the radioactivity using suitable counting equipment by comparison with a standardised technetium-99m solution or by measurement in an instrument calibrated with the aid of such a solution.

LABELLING

The label states, in particular, the quantity of sodium pyrophosphate per millilitre and the quantity of tin per millilitre.

01/2005:0571

THALLOUS (^{201}Tl) CHLORIDE INJECTION

Thallosi (^{201}Tl) chloridi solutio iniectabilis

DEFINITION

Thallous (^{201}Tl) chloride injection is a sterile solution of thallium-201 in the form of thallous chloride. It may be made isotonic by the addition of *Sodium chloride (0193)* and may contain a suitable antimicrobial preservative such as *Benzyl alcohol (0256)*. Thallium-201 is a radioactive isotope of thallium formed by the decay of lead-201. Lead-201 is a radioactive isotope of lead and may be obtained by irradiation, with protons of suitable energy, of thallium which may be enriched in thallium-203. Thallium-201 may be separated from lead-201 by passing through a column of an ion-exchange resin. The injection contains not less than 90.0 per cent and not more than 110.0 per cent of the declared thallium-201 radioactivity at the date and hour stated on the label. Not more than 2.0 per cent of the total radioactivity is due to thallium-202 and not less than 97.0 per cent is due to thallium-201. Not less than 95.0 per cent of the radioactivity is due to thallium in the form of thallous ions. The specific radioactivity is not less than 3.7 GBq per milligram of thallium.

CHARACTERS

A clear, colourless solution.

Thallium-201 has a half-life of 3.05 days and emits gamma radiation and X-rays.

IDENTIFICATION

A. Record the gamma-ray and X-ray spectrum using a suitable instrument. The spectrum does not differ significantly from that of a standardised thallium-201 solution when measured either by direct comparison or by use of an instrument calibrated with the aid of such a solution. Standardised thallium-201 and thallium-202 solutions are available from laboratories recognised by the competent authority. The most prominent gamma photons have energies of 0.135 MeV, 0.166 MeV and 0.167 MeV. The X-rays have energies of 0.069 MeV to 0.083 MeV.

B. Examine the electropherogram obtained in the test for radiochemical purity. The distribution of radioactivity contributes to the identification of the preparation.

TESTS

pH (*2.2.3*). The pH of the injection is 4.0 to 7.0.

Thallium. To 0.5 ml of the injection add 0.5 ml of hydrochloric acid (220 g/l HCl) and 0.05 ml of *bromine water R* and mix. Add 0.1 ml of a 30 g/l solution of *sulphosalicylic acid R*. After decolorisation add 1.0 ml of a 1 g/l solution of *rhodamine B R*. Add 4 ml of *toluene R* and shake for 60 s. Separate the toluene layer. The toluene layer is not more intensely coloured than the toluene layer of a standard prepared at the same time in the same manner using 0.5 ml of *thallium standard solution (10 ppm Tl) R*.

Sterility. It complies with the test for sterility prescribed in the monograph on *Radiopharmaceutical preparations (0125)*. The injection may be released for use before completion of the test.

RADIONUCLIDIC PURITY

Record the gamma-ray and X-ray spectrum using a suitable instrument calibrated with the aid of standardised thallium-201 and thallium-202 solutions. The spectrum does not differ significantly from that of the standardised thallium-201 solution. Determine the relative amounts of thallium-201 and thallium-202 and other radionuclidic impurities present. Thallium-202 has a half-life of 12.2 days and its most prominent gamma photon has an energy of 0.440 MeV. Thallium-200 has a half-life of 1.09 days and its most prominent gamma photons have energies of 0.368 MeV, 0.579 MeV, 0.828 MeV and 1.206 MeV. Lead-201 has a half-life of 9.4 h and its most prominent gamma photon has an energy of 0.331 MeV. Lead-203 has a half-life of 2.17 days and its most prominent gamma photon has an energy of 0.279 MeV. Not more than 2.0 per cent of the total radioactivity is due to thallium-202 and not less than 97.0 per cent is due to thallium-201.

RADIOCHEMICAL PURITY

Examine by zone electrophoresis (*2.2.31*), using a suitable strip of cellulose acetate, as the support and a 18.6 g/l solution of *sodium edetate R* as the electrolyte solution. Soak the strip in the electrolyte solution for 45-60 min. Remove the strip with forceps taking care to handle the outer edges only. Place the strip between 2 absorbent pads and blot to remove excess solution.

Test solution. Mix equal volumes of the injection to be examined and the electrolyte solution.

Apply not less than 5 µl of the test solution to the centre of the strip and mark the point of application. Apply an electric field of 17 V/cm for at least 10 min. Allow the strip to dry in air. Determine the distribution of radioactivity using suitable equipment. Not less than 95.0 per cent of the radioactivity migrates towards the cathode.

RADIOACTIVITY

Measure the radioactivity using suitable counting equipment by comparison with a standardised thallium-201 solution or by measurement in an instrument calibrated with the aid of such a solution.

01/2005:0112

TRITIATED (^{3}H) WATER INJECTION

Aquae tritiatae (^{3}H) solutio iniectabilis

DEFINITION

Tritiated (^{3}H) water injection is water for injections in which some of the water molecules contain tritium atoms in place of protium atoms. It may be made isotonic by the addition of sodium chloride. Tritium (^{3}H) may be obtained by the neutron irradiation of lithium. The injection contains not less than 90.0 per cent and not more than 110.0 per cent of the declared tritium activity at the date stated on the label.

CHARACTERS

A clear, colourless liquid.

Tritium has a half-life of 12.3 years and emits beta radiation.

IDENTIFICATION

Record the beta-ray spectrum by the method prescribed in the test for radionuclidic purity. The spectrum does not differ significantly from that of a standardised tritiated (^3H) water. Standardised tritiated (^3H) water is available from laboratories recognised by the competent authority. The maximum energy of the beta radiation is 0.019 MeV.

TESTS

pH (*2.2.3*). The pH of the injection is 4.5 to 7.0.

Sterility. It complies with the test for sterility prescribed in the monograph on *Radiopharmaceutical preparations (0125)*.

RADIONUCLIDIC PURITY

(a) Mix 100 µl of a suitable dilution of the injection with 10 ml of a scintillation liquid consisting of 1000 ml of *dioxan R*, 100 g of *naphthalene R*, 7 g of *diphenyloxazole R* and 0.3 g of *methylphenyloxazolylbenzene R*, the reagents being of an analytical grade suitable for liquid scintillation. Measure the radioactivity of the mixture in a liquid scintillation counter fitted with a discriminator. The count should be about 5000 impulses per second at the lowest setting of the discriminator. Record the count at different discriminator settings. For each measurement count at least 10 000 impulses over a period of at least 1 min. Immediately determine in the same conditions the count for a standardised tritiated (^3H) water having approximately the same activity.

Plot the counts at each discriminator setting, correcting for background activity, on semi-logarithmic paper, the discriminator settings being in arbitrary units as the abscissae.The vertical distance between the two curves obtained is constant. They obey the mathematical relationship:

$$\frac{\frac{A_1}{B_1} - \frac{A_2}{B_2}}{\frac{A_1}{B_1}} \times 100 < 20$$

A_1 = radioactivity recorded for the standardised preparation at the lowest discriminator setting,

B_1 = radioactivity recorded for the preparation to be examined at the lowest discriminator setting,

A_2 = radioactivity recorded for the standard at the discriminator setting such that $A_2 \approx A_1 \times 10^{-3}$,

B_2 = radioactivity recorded for the preparation to be examined at the latter discriminator setting.

(b) Record the gamma-ray spectrum. The instrument registers only background activity.

RADIOCHEMICAL PURITY

Place a quantity of the injection equivalent to about 2 µCi (74 kBq), diluted to 50 ml with *water R*, in an all-glass distillation apparatus of the type used for the determination of distillation range (*2.2.11*). Determine the radioactive concentration. Distil until about 25 ml of distillate has been collected. Precautions must be taken to avoid contamination of the air. If the test is carried out in a fume cupboard, the equipment must be protected from draughts. Determine the radioactive concentration of the distillate and of the liquid remaining in the distillation flask. Neither of the radioactive concentrations determined after distillation differs by more than 5 per cent from the value determined before distillation.

RADIOACTIVITY

Determine the radioactivity using a liquid scintillation counter.

01/2005:1582

WATER (^{15}O) INJECTION

Aquae (^{15}O) solutio iniectabilis

DEFINITION

Water (^{15}O) injection is a sterile solution of [^{15}O]water for diagnostic use. The injection contains not less than 90.0 per cent and not more than 110.0 per cent of the declared oxygen-15 radioactivity at the date and time stated on the label. Not less than 99 per cent of the total radioactivity corresponds to oxygen-15 in the form of water.

PRODUCTION

RADIONUCLIDE PRODUCTION

Oxygen-15 is a radioactive isotope of oxygen which may be produced by various nuclear reactions such as proton irradiation of nitrogen-15 or deuteron irradiation of nitrogen-14.

RADIOCHEMICAL SYNTHESIS

In order to recover oxygen-15 as molecular oxygen from the nitrogen target gas, carrier oxygen is added at concentrations generally ranging from 0.2 per cent *V/V* to 1.0 per cent *V/V*. [^{15}O]Water can be prepared from [^{15}O]oxygen by reaction with hydrogen using a suitable catalyst.

An alternative method is to produce [^{15}O]water "in-target" by adding hydrogen to the irradiated target gas at a concentration generally ranging from 2 per cent *V/V* to 5 per cent *V/V*.

The [^{15}O]water vapour contained in the gas-stream is either bubbled through a reservoir of a sterile 9 g/l solution of sodium chloride, or is exchanged by diffusion into such a solution through a membrane filter for dialysis.

Ammonia is a possible chemical impurity in [^{15}O]water. This may arise either from catalytic conversion of hydrogen and nitrogen on the catalyst or by radiolysis if "in-target" production is used. In addition, there is the possibility of contamination by oxygen-15-labelled oxides of nitrogen. Although these contaminants can be effectively removed from the gas phase by soda lime and charcoal adsorbers, they may break through and be present in the final preparation.

CHARACTERS

A clear, colourless solution.

Oxygen-15 has a half-life of 2.04 min and emits positrons with a maximum energy of 1.732 MeV, followed by annihilation gamma radiation of 0.511 MeV.

IDENTIFICATION

A. Record the gamma-ray spectrum using a suitable instrument. The only gamma photons have an energy of 0.511 MeV and, depending on the measurement geometry, a sum peak of 1.022 MeV may be observed.

B. It complies with the test for radionuclidic purity (see Tests).

C. Examine the chromatogram obtained in the test for radiochemical purity. The retention time of the second peak is due to the radioactivity eluting in the void volume.

TESTS

pH (*2.2.3*). The pH of the injection is 5.5 to 8.5.

Sterility. It complies with the test for sterility prescribed in the monograph on *Radiopharmaceutical preparations (0125)*. The injection may be released for use before completion of the test.

Bacterial endotoxins (*2.6.14*): less than 175/*V* IU/ml, *V* being the maximum administered volume in millilitres. The injection may be released for use before completion of the test.

CHEMICAL PURITY

(a) Ammonium (*2.4.1*). 1 ml complies with the limit test for ammonium (10 ppm).

(b) Nitrates. To 1 ml add 49 ml of *nitrate-free water R*. Place 5 ml of this solution in a test-tube immersed in iced water, add 0.4 ml of a 100 g/l solution of *potassium chloride R*, 0.1 ml of *diphenylamine solution R* and, dropwise with shaking, 5 ml of *sulphuric acid R*. Transfer the tube to a water-bath at 50 °C. After 15 min, any blue colour in the solution is not more intense than that in a standard prepared at the same time in the same manner using a mixture of 4.5 ml of *nitrate-free water R* and 0.5 ml of *nitrate standard solution (2 ppm NO_3) R* (10 ppm).

The injection may be released for use before completion of tests (a) and (b).

RADIONUCLIDIC PURITY

Record the gamma-ray spectrum using a suitable instrument. The spectrum does not differ significantly from that of a standardised fluorine-18 solution. Standardised fluorine-18 solutions are available from the laboratories recognised by the competent authority.

The half-life is between 1.9 min and 2.2 min. Not less than 99 per cent of total radioactivity corresponds to oxygen-15.

The injection may be released for use before completion of the test.

RADIOCHEMICAL PURITY

Examine by liquid chromatography (*2.2.29*).

Test solution. The preparation to be examined.

The chromatographic procedure may be carried out using:

- a column 0.25 m long and 4.0 mm in internal diameter packed with *aminopropylsilyl silica gel for chromatography R* (10 µm),
- as mobile phase at a flow rate of 1 ml/min a 10 g/l solution of *potassium dihydrogen phosphate R* adjusted to pH 3 with *phosphoric acid R*,
- a suitable radioactivity detector,
- a loop injector,
- an internal recovery detection system, consisting of a loop of the chromatographic tubing between the injector and the column through the radioactivity detector, which has been calibrated for count recovery,

maintaining the column at a constant temperature between 20 °C and 30 °C.

Inject the test solution. Continue the chromatography for 10 min. In the chromatogram obtained, the first peak corresponds to the injected radioactivity of the test solution, the second peak corresponds to the amount of radioactivity as [^{15}O]water. Calculate the percentage content of [^{15}O]water from the areas of the peaks in the chromatogram obtained with the test solution. Not less than 99 per cent of the total radioactivity injected corresponds to oxygen-15 in the form of water.

The injection may be released for use before completion of the test.

RADIOACTIVITY

Measure the radioactivity using suitable equipment by comparison with a standardised fluorine-18 solution or by using an instrument calibrated with the aid of such a solution.

01/2005:0133

XENON (^{133}Xe) INJECTION

Xenoni (^{133}Xe) solutio iniectabilis

DEFINITION

Xenon (^{133}Xe) injection is a sterile solution of xenon-133 that may be made isotonic by the addition of sodium chloride. Xenon-133 is a radioactive isotope of xenon and is obtained by separation from the other products of uranium fission. The injection contains not less than 80 per cent and not more than 130 per cent of the declared xenon-133 radioactivity at the date and hour stated on the label.

The injection is presented in a container that allows the contents to be removed without introducing air bubbles. The container is filled as completely as possible and any gas bubble present does not occupy more than 1 per cent of the volume of the injection as judged by visual comparison with a suitable standard.

CHARACTERS

A clear, colourless solution.

Xenon-133 has a half-life of 5.29 days and emits beta and gamma radiation and X-rays.

IDENTIFICATION

Record the gamma-ray and X-ray spectrum using a suitable instrument. The spectrum does not differ significantly from that of a standardised xenon-133 solution in a 9 g/l solution of *sodium chloride R*, apart from any differences attributable to the presence of xenon-131m and xenon-133m. If standardised xenon-133 solutions are not readily available, suitable standardised ionisation chambers are obtainable from laboratories recognised by the relevant competent authority. The most prominent gamma photon of xenon-133 has an energy of 0.081 MeV and there is an X-ray (resulting from internal conversion) of 0.030 MeV to 0.035 MeV. Xenon-131m has a half-life of 11.9 days and emits a gamma photon of 0.164 MeV. Xenon-133m has a half-life of 2.19 days and emits a gamma photon of 0.233 MeV.

TESTS

pH (*2.2.3*). The pH of the injection is 5.0 to 8.0.

Sterility. It complies with the test for sterility prescribed in the monograph on *Radiopharmaceutical preparations (0125)*. The injection may be released for use before completion of the test.

RADIONUCLIDIC PURITY

(a) Record the gamma-ray and X-ray spectrum using a suitable instrument. The spectrum does not differ significantly from that of a standardised xenon-133 solution in a 9 g/l solution of *sodium chloride R*, apart from any differences attributable to the presence of xenon-131m and xenon-133m.

(b) Transfer 2 ml of the injection to an open flask and pass a current of air through the solution for 30 min, taking suitable precautions concerning the dispersion of radioactivity. Measure the residual beta and gamma activity of the solution. The activity does not differ significantly from the background activity detected by the instrument.

RADIOACTIVITY

Weigh the container with its contents. Determine its total radioactivity using suitable counting equipment by comparison with a standardised xenon-133 solution or by measurement in an instrument calibrated with the aid of such a solution, operating in strictly identical conditions. If an ionisation chamber is used its inner wall should be such that the radiation is not seriously attenuated. Remove at least half the contents and re-weigh the container. Measure the radioactivity of the container and the remaining contents as described above. From the measurements, calculate the radioactive concentration of xenon-133 in the injection.

CAUTION

Significant amounts of xenon-133 may be present in the closures and on the walls of the container. This must be taken into account in applying the rules concerning the transport and storage of radioactive substances and in disposing of used containers

Radiopharmaceutical preparations

SUTURES FOR HUMAN USE

01/2005:90004

INTRODUCTION

The following monographs apply to sutures for human use: Catgut, sterile (0317), Sutures, sterile non-absorbable (0324), Sutures, sterile synthetic absorbable braided (0667) and Sutures, sterile synthetic absorbable monofilament (0666). They cover performance characteristics of sutures and may include methods of identification. Sutures are medical devices as defined in Directive 93/42/EEC.

These monographs can be applied to show compliance with essential requirements as defined in Article 3 of Directive 93/42/EEC covering the following:

Physical performance characteristics: diameter, breaking load, needle attachment, packaging, sterility, information supplied by the manufacturer (see Section 13 of Annex 1 of Directive 93/42/EEC), labelling.

To show compliance with other essential requirements, the application of appropriate harmonised standards as defined in Article 5 of Directive 93/42/EEC may be considered.

01/2005:0317

CATGUT, STERILE

Chorda resorbilis sterilis

DEFINITION

Sterile catgut consists of sutures prepared from collagen taken from the intestinal membranes of mammals. After cleaning, the membranes are split longitudinally into strips of varying width, which, when assembled in small numbers, according to the diameter required, are twisted under tension, dried, polished, selected and sterilised. The sutures may be treated with chemical substances such as chromium salts to prolong absorption and glycerol to make them supple, provided such substances do not reduce tissue acceptability.

Appropriate harmonised standards may be considered when assessing compliance with respect to origin and processing of raw materials and with respect to biocompatibility.

Sterile catgut is a surgical wound-closure device. Being an absorbable suture it serves to approximate tissue during the healing period and is subsequently metabolised by proteolytic activity.

PRODUCTION

Production complies with relevant regulations on the use of animal tissues in medical devices notably concerning the risk of transmission of animal spongiform encephalopathy agents.

Appropriate harmonised standards may apply with respect to appropriate validated methods of sterilisation, environmental control during manufacturing, labelling and packaging.

It is essential for the effectiveness and the performance characteristics during use and during the functional lifetime of catgut that the following physical properties are specified: consistent diameter, sufficient initial strength and firm needle attachment.

The requirements outlined below have been established, taking into account stresses which occur during normal conditions of use. These requirements can be used to demonstrate that individual production batches of sterile catgut are suitable for wound closure according to usual surgical techniques.

TESTS

If stored in a preserving liquid, remove the sutures from the sachet and measure promptly and in succession the length, diameter and breaking load. If stored in the dry state, immerse the sutures in alcohol R or a 90 per cent V/V solution of 2-propanol R for 24 h and proceed with the measurements as indicated below.

Length. Measure the length without applying to the suture more tension than is necessary to keep it straight. The length of each suture is not less than 90 per cent of the length stated on the label and does not exceed 350 cm.

Diameter. Carry out the test on 5 sutures. Use a suitable instrument capable of measuring with an accuracy of at least 0.002 mm and having a circular pressor foot 10 mm to 15 mm in diameter. The pressor foot and the moving parts attached to it are weighted so as to apply a total load of 100 ± 10 g to the suture being tested. When making the measurement, lower the pressor foot slowly to avoid crushing the suture. Measure the diameter at intervals of 30 cm over the whole length of the suture. For a suture less than 90 cm in length, measure at 3 points approximately evenly spaced along the suture. The suture is not subjected to more tension than is necessary to keep it straight during measurement. The average of the measurements carried out on the sutures being tested and not less than two-thirds of the measurements taken on each suture are within the limits given in the columns under A in Table 0317.-1 for the gauge number concerned. None of the measurements is outside the limits given in the columns under B in Table 0317.-1 for the gauge number concerned.

Table 0317.-1.– *Diameters and Breaking Loads*

Gauge number	Diameter (millimetres)				Breaking load (newtons)	
	A		B		C	D
	min.	max.	min.	max.		
0.1	0.010	0.019	0.005	0.025	-	-
0.2	0.020	0.029	0.015	0.035	-	-
0.3	0.030	0.039	0.025	0.045	0.20	0.05
0.4	0.040	0.049	0.035	0.060	0.30	0.10
0.5	0.050	0.069	0.045	0.085	0.40	0.20
0.7	0.070	0.099	0.060	0.125	0.70	0.30
1	0.100	0.149	0.085	0.175	1.8	0.40
1.5	0.150	0.199	0.125	0.225	3.8	0.70
2	0.200	0.249	0.175	0.275	7.5	1.8
2.5	0.250	0.299	0.225	0.325	10	3.8
3	0.300	0.349	0.275	0.375	12.5	7.5
3.5	0.350	0.399	0.325	0.450	20	10
4	0.400	0.499	0.375	0.550	27.5	12.5
5	0.500	0.599	0.450	0.650	38.0	20.0
6	0.600	0.699	0.550	0.750	45.0	27.5
7	0.700	0.799	0.650	0.850	60.0	38.0
8	0.800	0.899	0.750	0.950	70.0	45.0

Minimum breaking load. The minimum breaking load is determined over a simple knot formed by placing one end of a suture held in the right hand over the other end held in the left hand, passing one end over the suture and through the loop so formed (see Figure 0317.-1) and pulling the knot tight. Carry out the test on 5 sutures. Submit sutures of length greater than 75 cm to 2 measurements and shorter sutures to one measurement. Determine the breaking load using a suitable tensilometer. The apparatus has 2 clamps for holding the suture, one of which is mobile and is driven at a constant rate of 30 cm/min. The clamps are designed so that the suture being tested can be attached without any possibility of slipping. At the beginning of the test the length of suture between the clamps is 12.5 cm to 20 cm and the knot is midway between the clamps. Set the mobile clamp in motion and note the force required to break the suture. If the suture breaks in a clamp or within 1 cm of it, the result is discarded and the test repeated on another suture. The average of all the results, excluding those legitimately discarded, is equal to or greater than the value given in column C in Table 0317.-1 and no individual result is less than that given in column D for the gauge number concerned.

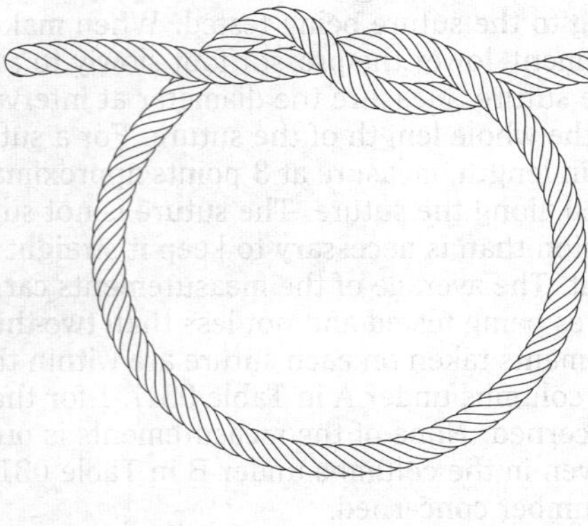

Figure 0317.-1. – *Simple knot*

Soluble chromium compounds. Place 0.25 g in a conical flask containing 1 ml of *water R* per 10 mg of catgut. Stopper the flask, allow to stand at 37 ± 0.5 °C for 24 h, cool and decant the liquid. Transfer 5 ml to a small test tube and add 2 ml of a 10 g/l solution of *diphenylcarbazide R* in *alcohol R* and 2 ml of *dilute sulphuric acid R*. The solution is not more intensely coloured than a standard prepared at the same time using 5 ml of a solution containing 2.83 µg of *potassium dichromate R* per millilitre, 2 ml of *dilute sulphuric acid R* and 2 ml of a 10 g/l solution of *diphenylcarbazide R* in *alcohol R* (1 ppm of Cr).

Needle attachment. If the catgut is supplied with an eyeless needle attached that is not stated to be detachable, it complies with the test for needle attachment. Carry out the test on 5 sutures. Use a suitable tensilometer, such as that described for the determination of the minimum breaking load. Fix the needle and suture (without knot) in the clamps of the apparatus in such a way that the swaged part of the needle is completely free of the clamp and in line with the direction of pull on the suture. Set the mobile clamp in motion and note the force required to break the suture or to detach it from the needle. The average of the 5 determinations and all individual values are not less than the respective values given in Table 0317.-2 for the gauge number concerned. If not more than one individual value fails to meet the individual requirement, repeat the test on an additional 10 sutures. The catgut complies with the test if none of these 10 values is less than the individual value in Table 0317.-2 for the gauge number concerned.

STORAGE (PACKAGING)

Sterile catgut sutures are presented in individual sachets that maintain sterility and allow the withdrawal and use of the sutures in aseptic conditions. Sterile catgut may be stored dry or in a preserving liquid to which an antimicrobial agent but not an antibiotic may be added.

Sutures in their individual sachets (primary packaging) are kept in a protective cover (box) which maintains the physical and mechanical properties until the time of use.

The application of appropriate harmonised standards for packaging of medical devices shall be considered.

Table 0317.-2. – *Minimum Strengths of Needle Attachment*

Gauge number	Mean value (newtons)	Individual values (newtons)
0.5	0.50	0.25
0.7	0.80	0.40
1	1.7	0.80
1.5	2.3	1.1
2	4.5	2.3
2.5	5.6	2.8
3	6.8	3.4
3.5	11.0	4.5
4	15.0	4.5
5	18.0	6.0

LABELLING

Reference may be made to the appropriate harmonised standards for labelling of medical devices.

The details strictly necessary for the user to identify the product properly are indicated on or in each sachet (primary packaging) and on the protective cover (box) and include at least:

- gauge number,
- length in centimetres or metres,
- if appropriate, that the needle is detachable,
- name of the product,
- intended use (surgical suture, absorbable).

01/2005:0324

SUTURES, STERILE NON-ABSORBABLE

Fila non resorbilia sterilia

DEFINITION

Sterile non-absorbable sutures are sutures which, when introduced into a living organism, are not metabolised by that organism. Sterile non-absorbable sutures vary in origin, which may be animal, vegetable, metallic or synthetic. They occur as cylindrical monofilaments or as multifilament sutures consisting of elementary fibres which are assembled by twisting, cabling or braiding; they may be sheathed; they may be treated to render them non-capillary, and they may be coloured.

Appropriate harmonised standards may be considered when assessing compliance with respect to origin and processing of raw materials and with respect to biocompatibility.

Sterile non-absorbable surgical sutures serve to approximate tissue during the healing period and provide continuing wound support.

Commonly used materials include the following:

Silk (Filum bombycis)

Sterile braided silk suture is obtained by braiding a number of threads, according to the diameter required, of degummed silk obtained from the cocoons of the silkworm *Bombyx mori* L.

Sutures

Linen (Filum lini)

Sterile linen thread consists of the pericyclic fibres of the stem of *Linum usitatissimum* L. The elementary fibres, 2.5 cm to 5 cm long, are assembled in bundles 30 cm to 80 cm long and spun into continuous lengths of suitable diameter.

Poly(ethylene terephthalate) (Filum ethyleni polyterephthalici)

Sterile poly(ethylene terephthalate) suture is obtained by drawing poly(ethylene terephthalate) through a suitable die. The suture is prepared by braiding very fine filaments in suitable numbers, depending on the gauge required.

Polyamide-6 (Filum polyamidicum-6)

Sterile polyamide-6 suture is obtained by drawing through a suitable die a synthetic plastic material formed by the polymerisation of ε-caprolactam. It consists of smooth, cylindrical monofilaments or braided filaments, or lightly twisted sutures sheathed with the same material.

Polyamide-6/6 (Filum polyamidicum-6/6)

Sterile polyamide-6/6 suture is obtained by drawing through a suitable die a synthetic plastic material formed by the polycondensation of hexamethylenediamine and adipic acid. It consists of smooth, cylindrical monofilaments or braided filaments, or lightly twisted sutures sheathed with the same material.

Polypropylene (Filum polypropylenicum)

Polypropylene suture is obtained by drawing polypropylene through a suitable die. It consists of smooth cylindrical mono-filaments.

Monofilament and multifilament stainless steel (Filum aciei irrubiginibilis monofilamentum/multifilamentum)

Sterile stainless steel sutures have a chemical composition as specified in ISO 5832-1 - Metallic Materials for surgical implants - Part 1: Specification for wrought stainless steel and comply with ISO 10334 - Implants for surgery - Malleable wires for use as sutures and other surgical applications.

Stainless steel sutures consist of smooth, cylindrical monofilaments or twisted filaments or braided filaments.

Poly(vinylidene difluoride) (PVDF) (Filum poly(vinylideni difluoridum))

Sterile PVDF suture is obtained by drawing through a suitable die a synthetic plastic material which is formed by polymerisation of 1,1-difluorethylene. It consists of smooth cylindrical monofilaments.

IDENTIFICATION

Non-absorbable sutures may be identified by chemical tests. Materials from natural origin may also be identified by microscopic examination of the morphology of these fibres. For synthetic materials, identification by infrared spectrophotometry (*2.2.24*) or by differential scanning calorimetry may be applied.

Identification of silk

A. Dissect the end of a suture, using a needle or fine tweezers, to isolate a few individual fibres. The fibres are sometimes marked with very fine longitudinal striations parallel to the axis of the suture. Examined under a microscope, a cross-section is more or less triangular to semi-circular, with rounded edges and without a lumen.

B. Impregnate isolated fibres with *iodinated potassium iodide solution R*. The fibres are coloured pale yellow.

Identification of linen

A. Dissect the end of a suture, using a needle or fine tweezers, to isolate a few individual fibres. Examined under a microscope, the fibres are seen to be 12 µm to 31 µm wide and, along the greater part of their length, have thick walls, sometimes marked with fine longitudinal striations, and a narrow lumen. The fibres gradually narrow to a long, fine point. Sometimes there are unilateral swellings with transverse lines.

B. Impregnate isolated fibres with *iodinated zinc chloride solution R*. The fibres are coloured violet-blue.

Identification of poly(ethyleneterephthalate)

It is practically insoluble in most of the usual organic solvents, but is attacked by strong alkaline solutions. It is incompatible with phenols.

A. 50 mg dissolves with difficulty when heated in 50 ml of *dimethylformamide R*.

B. To about 50 mg add 10 ml of *hydrochloric acid R1*. The material remains intact even after immersion for 6 h.

Identification of polyamide-6

It is practically insoluble in the usual organic solvents; it is not attacked by dilute alkaline solutions (for example a 100 g/l solution of *sodium hydroxide R*) but is attacked by dilute mineral acids (for example a 20 g/l solution of *sulphuric acid R*), by hot *glacial acetic acid R* and by a 70 per cent *m/m* solution of *anhydrous formic acid R*.

A. Heat about 50 mg with 0.5 ml of *hydrochloric acid R1* in a sealed glass tube at 110 °C for 18 h and allow to stand for 6 h. No crystals appear.

B. 50 mg dissolves in 20 ml of a 70 per cent *m/m* solution of *anhydrous formic acid R*.

Identification of polyamide-6/6

It is practically insoluble in the usual organic solvents; it is not attacked by dilute alkaline solutions (for example a 100 g/l solution of *sodium hydroxide R*) but is attacked by dilute mineral acids (for example a 20 g/l solution of *sulphuric acid R*), by hot *glacial acetic acid R* and by an 80 per cent *m/m* solution of *anhydrous formic acid R*.

A. In contact with a flame it melts and burns, forming a hard globule of residue and gives off a characteristic odour resembling that of celery.

B. Place about 50 mg in an ignition tube held vertically and heat gently until thick fumes are evolved. When the fumes fill the tube, withdraw it from the flame and insert a strip of *nitrobenzaldehyde paper R*. A violet-brown colour slowly appears on the paper and fades slowly in air; it disappears almost immediately on washing with *dilute sulphuric acid R*.

C. To about 50 mg add 10 ml of *hydrochloride acid R1*. The material disintegrates in the cold and dissolves within a few minutes.

D. 50 mg does not dissolve in 20 ml of a 70 per cent *m/m* solution of *anhydrous formic acid R* but dissolves in 20 ml of an 80 per cent *m/m* solution of *anhydrous formic acid R*.

Identification of polypropylene

Polypropylene is soluble in decahydronaphthalene, 1-chloronaphthalene and trichloroethylene. It is not soluble in alcohol, in ether and in cyclohexanone.

A. It softens at temperatures between 160 °C and 170 °C. It burns with a blue flame giving off an odour of burning paraffin wax and of octyl alcohol.

B. To 0.25 g add 10 ml of *toluene R* and boil under a reflux condenser for about 15 min. Place a few drops of the solution on a disc of *sodium chloride R* slide and evaporate the solvent in an oven at 80 °C. Examine by infrared absorption spectrophotometry (*2.2.24*), comparing with the spectrum obtained with *polypropylene CRS*.

C. To 2 g add 100 ml of *water R* and boil under a reflux condenser for 2 h. Allow to cool. The relative density (*2.2.5*) of the material is 0.89 g/ml to 0.91 g/ml, determined using a hydrostatic balance.

Identification of stainless steel

Stainless steel sutures are identified by confirming that the composition is in accordance with ISO 5832 Part 1.

Identification of poly(vinylidene difluoride)

It is soluble in warm dimethylformamide. It is insoluble in ethanol, hot and cold isopropyl alcohol, ethyl acetate, tetrachlorethylene.

A. The strand melts between 170 °C and 180 °C. It melts in a flame and does not burn after removal of the flame. Place a small piece of suture on an annealed copper wire or sheet. Heat in an oxidising flame. No green colour is produced.

B. Dissolve 0.25 g of the suture in 10 ml of *dimethylformamide R* and boil under a reflux condenser for about 15 min. Place a few drops of the solution on a *sodium chloride R* slide and evaporate the solvent in an oven at 80 °C (1 h). Examine by infrared absorption spectrophotometry (*2.2.24*), comparing with the *Ph. Eur. reference spectrum of poly(vinylidene difluoride)*.

C. To 2 g of suture add 100 ml of *water R* and boil under a reflux condenser for 2 h. Allow to cool. The relative density (*2.2.5*) of the material is 1.71 to 1.78.

PRODUCTION

The appropriate harmonised standards may apply with respect to appropriate validated methods of sterilisation, environmental control during manufacturing, labelling and packaging.

It is essential for the effectiveness and the performance characteristics during use and during the functional lifetime of these sutures that the following physical properties are specified: consistent diameter, sufficient initial strength and firm needle attachment.

The requirements below have been established, taking into account stresses which occur during normal conditions of use. These requirements can be used to demonstrate that individual production batches of these sutures are suitable for wound closure in accordance with usual surgical techniques.

TESTS

Remove the sutures from the sachet and measure promptly and in succession the length, diameter and minimum load.

If linen is tested the sutures are conditioned as follows: if stored in the dry state, expose to an atmosphere with a relative humidity of 65 ± 5 per cent at 20 ± 2 °C for 4 h immediately before measuring the diameter and for the determination of minimum breaking load immerse in *water R* at room temperature for 30 min immediately before carrying out the test.

Length. Measure the length without applying more tension than is necessary to keep them straight. The length of the suture is not less than 95 per cent of the length stated on the label and does not exceed 400 cm.

Diameter. Unless otherwise prescribed, measure the diameter by the following method using 5 sutures. Use a suitable mechanical instrument capable of measuring with an accuracy of at least 0.002 mm and having a circular pressor foot 10-15 mm in diameter. The pressor foot and the moving parts attached to it are weighted so as to apply a total load of 100 ± 10 g to the suture being tested. When making the measurements, lower the pressor foot slowly to avoid crushing the suture. Measure the diameter at intervals of 30 cm over the whole length of the suture. For a suture less than 90 cm in length, measure at 3 points approximately evenly spaced along the suture. During the measurement submit monofilament sutures to a tension not greater than that required to keep them straight. Submit multifilament sutures to a tension not greater than one-fifth of the minimum breaking load shown in column C of Table 0324.-1 appropriate to the gauge number and type of material concerned or 10 N whichever is less. Stainless steel sutures do not require tension to be applied during the measurement of diameter. For multifilament sutures of gauge number above 1.5 make 2 measurements at each point, the second measurement being made after rotating the suture through 90°. The diameter of that point is the average of the 2 measurements. The average of the measurements carried out on the sutures being tested and not less than two-thirds of the measurements taken on each suture are within the limits given in the column under A in Table 0324.-1 for the gauge number concerned. None of the measurements are outside the limits given in the columns under B in Table 0324.-1 for the gauge number concerned.

Minimum breaking load. Unless otherwise prescribed, determine the minimum breaking load by the following method using sutures in the condition in which they are presented. The minimum breaking load is determined over a simple knot formed by placing one end of a suture held in the right hand over the other end held in the left hand, passing one end over the suture and through the loop so formed (see Figure 0324.-1) and pulling the knot tight. For stainless steel sutures gauges 3.5 and above, the minimum breaking load is determined on a straight pull. Carry out the test on 5 sutures. Submit sutures of length greater than 75 cm to 2 measurements and shorter sutures to 1 measurement. Determine the breaking load using a suitable tensilometer. The apparatus has 2 clamps for holding the suture, 1 of which is mobile and is driven at a constant rate of 30 cm/min. The clamps are designed so that the suture being tested can be attached without any possibility of slipping. At the beginning of the test the length of suture between the clamps is 12.5 cm to 20 cm and the knot is midway between the clamps. Set the mobile clamp in motion and note the force required to break the suture. If the suture breaks in a clamp or within 1 cm of it, the result is discarded and the test repeated on another suture. The average of all the results, excluding those legitimately discarded, is equal to or greater than the value given in column C in Table 0324.-1 and no value is less than that given in column D for the gauge number and type of material concerned.

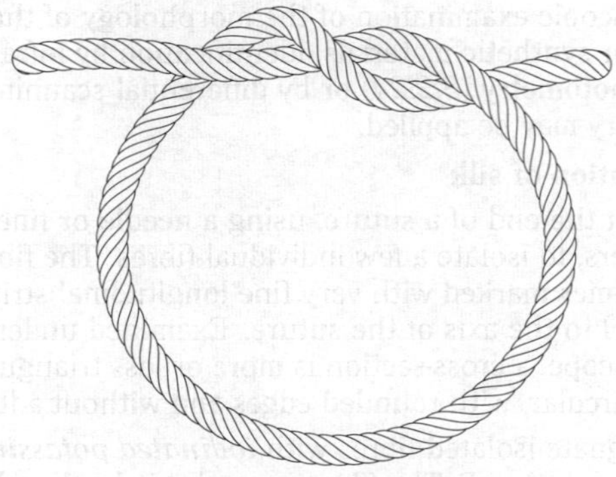

Figure 0324.-1. – *Simple knot*

Needle attachment. If the sutures are supplied with an eyeless needle attached that is not stated to be detachable, they comply with the test for needle attachment. Carry out

Table 0324.-1. – *Diameters and minimum breaking loads*

Gauge number	Diameter (millimetres)				Minimum breaking load (newtons)					
	A		B		Linen thread		All other non-absorbable strands		Stainless steel	
	min.	**max.**	**min.**	**max.**	**C**	**D**	**C**	**D**	**C**	**D**
0.05	0.005	0.009	0.003	0.012	-	-	0.01	-		
0.1	0.010	0.019	0.005	0.025	-	-	0.03	-		
0.15	0.015	0.019	0.012	0.025	-	-	0.06	0.01		
0.2	0.020	0.029	0.015	0.035	-	-	0.1	-		
0.3	0.030	0.039	0.025	0.045	-	-	0.35	0.06		
0.4	0.040	0.049	0.035	0.060	-	-	0.60	0.15	1.1	
0.5	0.050	0.069	0.045	0.085	-	-	1.0	0.35	1.6	
0.7	0.070	0.099	0.060	0.125	1.0	0.3	1.5	0.60	2.7	
1	0.100	0.149	0.085	0.175	2.5	0.6	3.0	1.0	5.3	4.0
1.5	0.150	0.199	0.125	0.225	5.0	1.0	5.0	1.5	8.0	6.0
2	0.200	0.249	0.175	0.275	8.0	2.5	9.0	3.0	13.3	10.0
2.5	0.250	0.299	0.225	0.325	9.0	5.0	13.0	5.0	15.5	11.6
3	0.300	0.349	0.275	0.375	11.0	8.0	15.0	9.0	17.7	13.3
3.5	0.350	0.399	0.325	0.450	15.0	9.0	22.0	13.0	33.4	25.0
4	0.400	0.499	0.375	0.550	18,0	11.0	27.0	15.0	46.7	35.0
5	0.500	0.599	0.450	0.650	26.0	15.0	35.0	22.0	57.9	43.4
6	0.600	0.699	0,.550	0.750	37.0	18.0	50.0	27.0	89.4	67.0
7	0.700	0.799	0.650	0.850	50.0	26.0	62.0	35.0	111.8	83.9
8	0.800	0.899	0.750	0.950	65.0	37.0	73.0	50.0	133.4	100.1
9	0.900	0.999	0.850	1.050					156.0	117.0
10	1.000	1.099	0.950	1.150					178.5	133.9

the test on 5 sutures. Use a suitable tensilometer, such as that described for the determination of the minimum breaking load. Fix the needle and suture (without knot) in the clamps of the apparatus in such a way that the swaged part of the needle is completely free of the clamp and in line with the direction of pull on the suture. Set the mobile clamp in motion and note the force required to break the suture or to detach it from the needle. The average of the 5 determinations and all individual values are not less than the respective values given in Table 0324.-2 for the gauge number concerned. If not more than 1 individual value fails to meet the individual requirement, repeat the test on an additional 10 sutures. The attachment complies with the test if none of these 10 values is less than the individual value in Table 0324.-2 for the gauge number concerned.

Extractable colour. Sutures that are dyed and intended to remain so during use comply with the test for extractable colour. Place 0.25 g of the suture to be examined in a conical flask, add 25.0 ml of *water R* and cover the mouth of the flask with a short-stemmed funnel. Boil for 15 min, cool and adjust to the original volume with *water R*. Depending on the colour of the suture, prepare the appropriate reference solution as described in Table 0324.-3 using the primary colour solutions (*2.2.2*).

The test solution is not more intensely coloured than the appropriate reference solution.

Table 0324.-2. – *Minimum strengths of needle attachment*

Gauge number	Mean value (newtons)	Individual value (newtons)
0.4	0.50	0.25
0.5	0.80	0.40
0.7	1.7	0.80
1	2.3	1.1
1.5	4.5	2.3
2	6.8	3.4
2.5	9.0	4.5
3	11.0	4.5
3.5	15.0	4.5
4	18.0	6.0
5	18.0	7.0
6	25.0	12.5
7	25.0	12.5
8	50.0	25
9	50.0	25
10	75.0	37.5

Table 0324.-3. – *Colour reference solutions*

Colour of strand	Composition of reference solution (parts by volume)			
	Red primary solution	**Yellow primary solution**	**Blue primary solution**	***Water R***
Yellow-brown	0.2	1.2	-	8.6
Pink-red	1.0	-	-	9.0
Green-blue	-	-	2.0	8.0
Violet	1.6	-	8.4	-

Monomer and oligomers. Polyamide-6 suture additionally complies with the following test for monomer and oligomers. In a continuous-extraction apparatus, treat 1.00 g with 30 ml of *methanol R* at a rate of at least 3 extractions per hour for 7 h. Evaporate the extract to dryness, dry the residue at 110 °C for 10 min, allow to cool in a desiccator and weigh. The residue weighs not more than 20 mg (2 per cent).

STORAGE (PACKAGING)

Sterile non-absorbable sutures are presented in a suitable sachet that maintains sterility and allows the withdrawal and use of a suture in aseptic conditions. They may be stored dry or in a preserving liquid to which an antimicrobial agent but no antibiotic may be added.

Sterile non-absorbable sutures are intended to be used only on the occasion when the sachet is first opened.

Sutures in their individual sachets (primary packaging) are kept in a protective cover (box) which maintains the physical and mechanical properties until the time of use.

The application of appropriate harmonised standards for packaging of medical devices shall be considered in addition.

LABELLING

Reference may be made to the appropriate harmonised standards for the labelling of medical devices.

The details strictly necessary for the user to identify the product properly are indicated on or in each sachet (primary packaging) and on the protective cover (box) and include at least:

- gauge number,
- length, in centimetres or metres,
- if appropriate, that the needle is detachable,
- name of the product,
- intended use (surgical suture, non-absorbable),
- if appropriate, that the suture is coloured,
- if appropriate, the structure (braided, monofilament, sheathed).

01/2005:0667

SUTURES, STERILE SYNTHETIC ABSORBABLE BRAIDED

Fila resorbilia synthetica torta sterilia

DEFINITION

Sterile synthetic absorbable braided sutures consist of sutures prepared from a synthetic polymer, polymers or copolymers which, when introduced into a living organism, are absorbed by that organism and cause no undue tissue irritation. They consist of completely polymerised material. They occur as multifilament sutures consisting of elementary fibres which are assembled by braiding. The sutures may be treated to facilitate handling and they may be coloured.

Appropriate harmonised standards may be considered when assessing compliance with respect to origin and processing of raw materials and with respect to biocompatibility.

Sterile synthetic absorbable braided sutures are wound-closure devices. Being absorbable they serve to approximate tissue during the healing period and subsequently lose tensile strength by hydrolysis.

PRODUCTION

Appropriate harmonised standards may apply with respect to appropriate validated methods of sterilisation, environmental control during manufacturing, labelling and packaging.

It is essential for the effectiveness and the performance characteristics during use and during the functional lifetime of these sutures that the following physical properties are specified: consistent diameter, sufficient initial strength and firm needle attachment.

The requirements below have been established, taking into account stresses which occur during normal conditions of use. These requirements can be used to demonstrate that individual production batches of these sutures are suitable for wound closure according to usual surgical techniques.

TESTS

Carry out the following tests on the sutures in the state in which they are removed from the sachet.

Length. Measure the length of the suture without applying more tension than is necessary to keep it straight. The length of each suture is not less than 95 per cent of the length stated on the label and does not exceed 400 cm.

Diameter. Unless otherwise prescribed, measure the diameter by the following method, using five sutures in the condition in which they are presented. Use a suitable instrument capable of measuring with an accuracy of at least 0.002 mm and having a circular pressor foot 10 mm to 15 mm in diameter. The pressor foot and the moving parts attached to it are weighted so as to apply a total load of 100 ± 10 g to the suture being tested. When making the measurements, lower the pressor foot slowly to avoid crushing the suture. Measure the diameter at intervals of 30 cm over the whole length of the suture. For a suture less than 90 cm in length, measure at three points approximately evenly spaced along the suture. During the measurement, submit the sutures to a tension not greater than one-fifth of the minimum breaking load shown in column C of Table 0667.-1 appropriate to the gauge number and type of material or 10 N whichever is less. For sutures of gauge number above 1.5 make two measurements at each point, the second measurement being made after rotating the suture through 90°. The diameter of that point is the average of the two measurements. The average of the measurements carried out on the sutures being tested and not less than two-thirds of the measurements taken on each suture are within the limits given in the columns under A in Table 0667.-1 for the gauge number concerned. None of the measurements is outside the limits given in the columns under B in Table 0667.-1 for the gauge number concerned.

Table 0667.-1. – *Diameters and breaking loads*

Gauge number	Diameter (millimetres)				Breaking load (newtons)	
	A		B		C	D
	min.	max.	min.	max.		
0.01	0.001	0.004	0.0008	0.005	-	-
0.05	0.005	0.009	0.003	0.012	-	-
0.1	0.010	0.019	0.005	0.025	-	-
0.2	0.020	0.029	0.015	0.035	-	-
0.3	0.030	0.039	0.025	0.045	0.45	0.23
0.4	0.040	0.049	0.035	0.060	0.70	0.35
0.5	0.050	0.069	0.045	0.085	1.4	0.7
0.7	0.070	0.099	0.060	0.125	2.5	1.3
1	0.100	0.149	0.085	0.175	6.8	3.4
1.5	0.150	0.199	0.125	0.225	9.5	4.8
2	0.200	0.249	0.175	0.275	17.7	8.9
2.5	0.250	0.299	0.225	0.325	21.0	10.5
3	0.300	0.349	0.275	0.375	26.8	13.4
3.5	0.350	0.399	0.325	0.450	39.0	18.5
4	0.400	0.499	0.375	0.550	50.8	25.4
5	0.500	0.599	0.450	0.650	63.5	31.8
6	0.600	0.699	0.550	0.750	-	-
7	0.700	0.799	0.650	0.850	-	-

Minimum breaking load. The minimum breaking load is determined over a simple knot formed by placing one end of a suture held in the right hand over the other end held in the left hand, passing one end over the suture and through the loop so formed (see Figure 0667.-1) and pulling the knot tight.

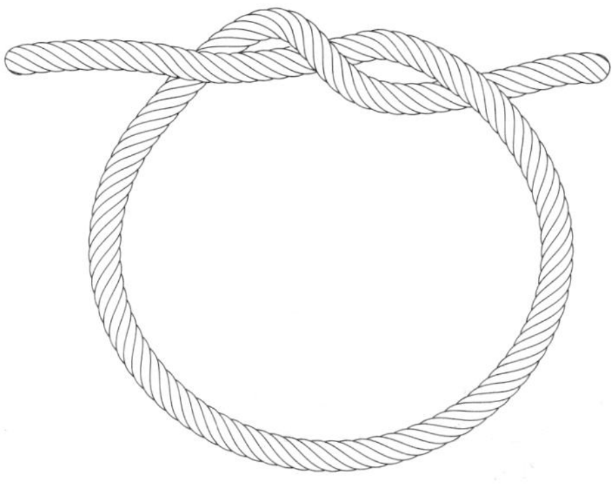

Figure 0667.-1. – *Simple knot*

Carry out the test on five sutures. Submit sutures of length greater than 75 cm to two measurements and shorter sutures to one measurement. Determine the breaking load using a suitable tensilometer. The apparatus has two clamps for holding the suture, one of which is mobile and is driven at a constant rate of 25 cm to 30 cm per minute. The clamps are designed so that the suture being tested can be attached without any possibility of slipping. At the beginning of the test the length of suture between the clamps is 12.5 cm to 20 cm and the knot is midway between the clamps. Set the mobile clamp in motion and note the force required to break the suture. If the suture breaks in a clamp or within 1 cm of it, the result is discarded and the test repeated on another suture. The average of all the results excluding those legitimately discarded is equal to or greater than the value given in column C in Table 0667.-1 and no individual result is less than that given in column D for the gauge number concerned.

Needle attachment. If the suture is supplied with an eyeless needle attached that is not stated to be detachable the attachment, it complies with the test for needle attachment. Carry out the test on five sutures. Use a suitable tensilometer, such as that described for the determination of the minimum breaking load. Fix the needle and suture (without knot) in the clamps of the apparatus in such a way that the swaged part of the needle is completely free of the clamp and in line with the direction of pull on the suture. Set the mobile clamp in motion and note the force required to break the suture or to detach it from the needle. The average of the five deter-minations and all individual values are not less than the respective values given in Table 0667.-2 for the gauge number concerned. If not more than one individual value fails to meet the individual requirement, repeat the test on an additional ten sutures. The attachment complies with the test if none of the ten values is less than the individual value in Table 0667.-2 for the gauge number concerned.

Table 0667.-2. – *Minimum strengths of needle attachment*

Gauge number	Mean value (newtons)	Individual value (newtons)
0.4	0.50	0.25
0.5	0.80	0.40
0.7	1.7	0.80
1	2.3	1.1
1.5	4.5	2.3
2	6.8	3.4
2.5	9.0	4.5
3	11.0	4.5
3.5	15.0	4.5
4	18.0	6.0
5	18.0	7.0

STORAGE (PACKAGING)

Sterile synthetic absorbable braided sutures are presented in a suitable sachet that maintains sterility and allows the withdrawal and use of the sutures in aseptic conditions. The sutures must be stored dry.

They are intended to be used only on the occasion when the sachet is first opened.

Sutures in their individual sachets (primary packaging) are kept in a protective cover (box) which maintains the physical and mechanical properties until the time of use.

The application of appropriate harmonised standards for packaging of medical devices may be considered in addition.

LABELLING

Reference may be made to the appropriate harmonised standards for the labelling of medical devices.

The details strictly necessary for the user to identify the product properly are indicated on or in each sachet (primary packaging) and on the protective cover (box) and include at least:

– gauge number,
– length in centimetres or metres,
– if appropriate, that the needle is detachable,

- name of the product,
- intended use (surgical absorbable suture),
- if appropriate, that the suture is coloured,
- the structure (braided).

01/2005:0666

SUTURES, STERILE SYNTHETIC ABSORBABLE MONOFILAMENT

Fila resorbilia synthetica monofilamenta sterilia

DEFINITION

Sterile synthetic absorbable monofilament sutures consist of sutures prepared from a synthetic polymer, polymers or copolymers which, when introduced into a living organism, are absorbed by that organism and cause no undue tissue irritation. They consist of completely polymerised material. They occur as monofilament sutures. The sutures may be treated to facilitate handling and they may be coloured.

Appropriate harmonised standards may be considered when assessing compliance with respect to origin and processing of raw materials and with respect to biocompatibility.

Sterile synthetic absorbable monofilament sutures are wound- closure devices. Being absorbable they serve to approximate tissue during the healing period and subsequently lose tensile strength by hydrolysis.

PRODUCTION

The appropriate harmonised standards may apply with respect to appropriate validated methods of sterilisation, environmental control during manufacturing, labelling and packaging.

It is essential for the effectiveness and the performance characteristics during use and during the functional lifetime of these sutures that the following physical properties are specified: consistent diameter, sufficient initial strength and firm needle attachment.

The requirements below have been established, taking into account stresses which occur during normal conditions of use. These requirements can be used to demonstrate that individual production batches of these sutures are suitable for wound closure according to usual surgical techniques.

TESTS

Carry out the following tests on the sutures in the state in which they are removed from the sachet.

Length. Measure the length of the suture without applying more tension than is necessary to keep it straight. The length of each suture is not less than 95 per cent of the length stated on the label and does not exceed 400 cm.

Diameter. Unless otherwise prescribed, measure the diameter by the following method, using five sutures in the condition in which they are presented. Use a suitable instrument cap-able of measuring with an accuracy of at least 0.002 mm and having a circular pressor foot 10 mm to 15 mm in diameter. The pressor foot and the moving parts attached to it are weighted so as to apply a total load of 100 ± 10 g to the suture being tested. When making the measurements, lower the pressor foot slowly to avoid crushing the suture. Measure the diameter at intervals of 30 cm over the whole length of the suture. For a suture less than 90 cm in length, measure at three points approximately evenly spaced along the suture. During the measurement, submit the sutures to a tension not greater than that required to keep them straight. The average of the measurements carried out on the sutures being tested and not less than two-thirds of the measurements taken on each suture are within the limits given in the columns under A in Table 0666.-1 for the gauge number concerned. None of the measurements is outside the limits given in the columns under B in Table 0666.-1 for the gauge number concerned.

Table 0666.-1. – *Diameters and breaking loads*

Gauge number	Diameter (millimetres)				Breaking load (newtons)	
	A		B		C	D
	min.	max.	min.	max.		
0.5	0.050	0.094	0.045	0.125	1.4	0.7
0.7	0.095	0.149	0.075	0.175	2.5	1.3
1	0.150	0.199	0.125	0.225	6.8	3.4
1.5	0.200	0.249	0.175	0.275	9.5	4.7
2	0.250	0.339	0.225	0.375	17.5	8.9
3	0.340	0.399	0.325	0.450	26.8	13.4
3.5	0.400	0.499	0.375	0.550	39.0	18.5
4	0.500	0.570	0.450	0.600	50.8	25.4
5	0.571	0.610	0.500	0.700	63.5	31.8

Minimum breaking load. The minimum breaking load is determined over a simple knot formed by placing one end of a suture held in the right hand over the other end held in the left hand, passing one end over the suture and through the loop so formed (see Figure 0666.-1) and pulling the knot tight.

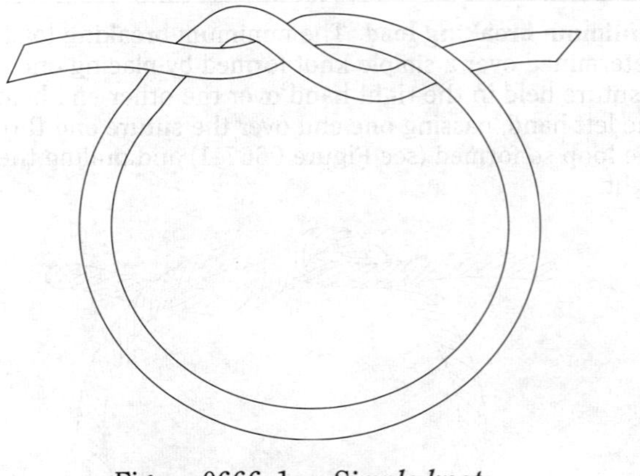

Figure 0666.-1. – *Simple knot*

Carry out the test on five sutures. Submit sutures of length greater than 75 cm to two measurements and shorter sutures to one measurement. Determine the breaking load using a suitable tensilometer. The apparatus has two clamps for holding the suture, one of which is mobile and is driven at a constant rate of 25 cm to 30 cm per minute. The clamps are designed so that the suture being tested can be attached without any possibility of slipping. At the beginning of the test the length of suture between the clamps is 12.5 cm to 20 cm and the knot is midway between the clamps. Set the mobile clamp in motion and note the force required to break the suture. If the suture breaks in a clamp or within 1 cm of it, the result is discarded and the test repeated on another suture. The average of all the results excluding those legitimately discarded is equal to or greater than the value given in column C in Table 0666.-1 and no individual result is less than that given in column D for the gauge number concerned.

Needle attachment. If the suture is supplied with an eyeless needle attached that is not stated to be detachable, the attachment complies with the test for needle attachment. Carry out the test on five sutures. Use a suitable tensilometer, such as that described for the determination of the minimum breaking load. Fix the needle and suture (without knot) in the clamps of the apparatus in such a way that the swaged part of the needle is completely free of the clamp and in line with the direction of pull on the suture. Set the mobile clamp in motion and note the force required to break the suture or to detach it from the needle. The average of the five determinations and all individual values are not less than the respective values given in Table 0666.-2 for the gauge number concerned. If not more than one individual value fails to meet the individual requirement, repeat the test on an additional ten sutures. The attachment complies with the test if none of the ten values is less than the individual value in Table 0666.-2 for the gauge number concerned.

Table 0666.-2. – *Minimum strengths of needle attachment*

Gauge number	Mean value (newtons)	Individual value (newtons)
0.5	0.80	0.40
0.7	1.7	0.80
1	2.3	1.1
1.5	4.5	2.3
2	6.8	3.4
2.5	9.0	4.5
3	11.0	4.5
3.5	15.0	4.5
4	18.0	6.0
5	18.0	7.0

STORAGE (PACKAGING)

Sterile synthetic absorbable monofilament sutures are presented in a suitable sachet that maintains sterility and allows the withdrawal and use of the sutures in aseptic conditions. The sutures must be stored dry.

They are intended to be used only on the occasion when the sachet is first opened.

Sutures in their individual sachets (primary packaging) are kept in a protective cover (box) which maintains the physical and mechanical properties until the time of use.

The application of appropriate harmonised standards for packaging of medical devices may be considered in addition.

LABELLING

Reference may be made to appropriate harmonised standards for the labelling of medical devices.

The details strictly necessary for the user to identify the product properly are indicated on or in each sachet (primary packaging) and on the protective cover (box) and include at least:

- gauge number,
- length in centimetres or metres,
- if appropriate, that the needle is detachable,
- name of the product,
- intended use (surgical absorbable suture),
- if appropriate, that the suture is coloured,
- the structure (monofilament).

SUTURES FOR VETERINARY USE

01/2005:0660

CATGUT, STERILE, IN DISTRIBUTOR FOR VETERINARY USE

Chorda resorbilis sterilis in fuso ad usum veterinarium

DEFINITION

Sterile catgut in distributor for veterinary use consists of strands prepared from collagen taken from the intestinal membranes of mammals. After cleaning, the membranes are split longitudinally into strips of varying width, which, when assembled in small numbers, according to the diameter required, are twisted under tension, dried, polished, selected and sterilised. The strands may be treated with chemical substances such as chromium salts to prolong absorption and glycerol to make them supple, provided such substances do not reduce tissue acceptability.

The strand is presented in a distributor that allows the withdrawal and use of all or part of it in aseptic conditions. The design of the distributor is such that with suitable handling the sterility of the content is maintained even when part of the strand has been withdrawn. It may be stored dry or in a preserving liquid to which an antimicrobial preservative but not an antibiotic may be added.

TESTS

If stored in a preserving liquid, remove the strand from the distributor and measure promptly and in succession the length, diameter and breaking load. If stored in the dry state, immerse the strand in alcohol R or a 90 per cent *V/V* solution of *2-propanol R* for 24 h and proceed with the measurements as indicated above.

Length. Measure the length without applying to the strand more tension than is necessary to keep it straight. The length is not less than 95 per cent of the length stated on the label. If the strand consists of several sections joined by knots, the length of each section is not less than 2.5 m.

Diameter. Carry out the test using a suitable instrument capable of measuring with an accuracy of at least 0.002 mm and having a circular pressor foot 10 mm to 15 mm in diameter. The pressor foot and the moving parts attached to it are weighted so as to apply a total load of 100 ± 10 g to the strand being tested. When making the measurements, lower the pressor foot slowly to avoid crushing the strand. Make not fewer than one measurement per 2 m of length. If the strand consists of several sections joined by knots, make not fewer than three measurements per section. In any case make not fewer than twelve measurements. Make the measurements at points evenly spaced along the strand or along each section. The strand is not subjected to more tension than is necessary to keep it straight during measurement. The average of the measurements carried out on the strand being tested and not less than two-thirds of the individual measurements are within the limits given in the column under A in Table 0660.-1 for the gauge number concerned. None of the measurements is outside the limits given in the columns under B in Table 0660.-1 for the gauge number concerned.

Table 0660.-1. – *Diameters and breaking loads*

Gauge number	Diameter (millimetres)				Breaking load (newtons)	
	A		B		C	D
	min.	max.	min.	max.		
1	0.100	0.149	0.085	0.175	1.8	0.4
1.5	0.150	0.199	0.125	0.225	3.8	0.7
2	0.200	0.249	0.175	0.275	7.5	1.8
2.5	0.250	0.299	0.225	0.325	10	3.8
3	0.300	0.349	0.275	0.375	12.5	7.5
3.5	0.350	0.399	0.325	0.450	20	10
4	0.400	0.499	0.375	0.550	27.5	12.5
5	0.500	0.599	0.450	0.650	38.4	20.0
6	0.600	0.699	0.550	0.750	45.0	27.5
7	0.700	0.799	0.650	0.850	60.0	38.0
8	0.800	0.899	0.750	0.950	70.0	45.0

Minimum breaking load. The minimum breaking load is determined over a simple knot formed by placing one end of a strand held in the right hand over the other end held in the left hand, passing one end over the strand and through the loop so formed (see Figure 0660.-1) and pulling the knot tight.

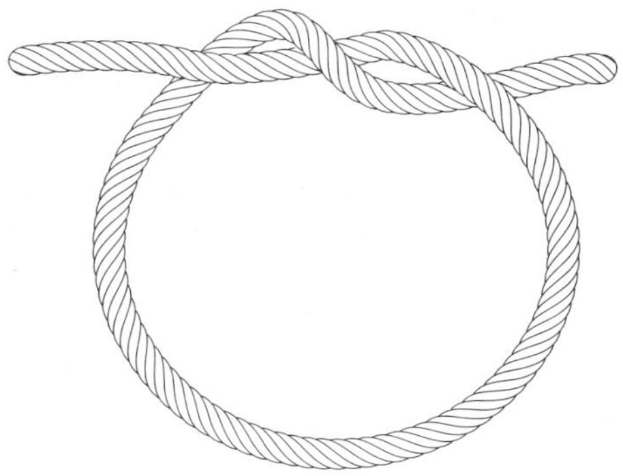

Figure 0660.-1. – *Simple knot*

Make not fewer than one measurement per 2 m of length. If the strand consists of several sections joined by knots, make not fewer than three measurements per section and, in any case, not fewer than one measurement per 2 m of length at points evenly spaced along the strand or along each section. Determine the breaking load using a suitable tensilometer. The apparatus has two clamps for holding the strand, one of which is mobile and is driven at a constant rate of 30 cm per minute. The clamps are designed so that the strand being tested can be attached without any possibility of slipping. At the beginning of the test the length of strand between the clamps is 12.5 cm to 20 cm and the knot is midway between the clamps. Set the mobile clamp in motion and note the force required to break the strand. If the strand breaks in a clamp or within 1 cm of it, the result is discarded and the test repeated on another part of the strand. The average of all the results, excluding those legitimately discarded, is equal to or greater than the value in column C and no value is less than that given in column D in Table 0660.-1 for the gauge number concerned.

Soluble chromium compounds. Place 0.25 g in a conical flask containing 1 ml of *water R* per 10 mg of catgut. Stopper the flask, allow to stand at 37 ± 0.5 °C for 24 h, cool and decant the liquid. Transfer 5 ml to a small test tube and add 2 ml of a 10 g/l solution of *diphenylcarbazide R* in *alcohol R* and 2 ml of *dilute sulphuric acid R*. The solution is not more intensely coloured than a standard prepared at the same time using 5 ml of a solution containing 2.83 µg of *potassium dichromate R* per millilitre, 2 ml of *dilute sulphuric acid R* and 2 ml of a 10 g/l solution of *diphenylcarbazide R* in *alcohol R* (1 ppm of Cr).

Sterility (*2.6.1*). It complies with the test for sterility as applied to catgut and other surgical sutures. Carry out the test on three sections, each 30 cm long, cut off respectively from the beginning, the centre and the end of the strand.

STORAGE

Store protected from light and heat.

LABELLING

The label states:

– the gauge number,

– the length in centimetres or in metres.

01/2005:0608

LINEN THREAD, STERILE, IN DISTRIBUTOR FOR VETERINARY USE

Filum lini sterile in fuso ad usum veterinarium

DEFINITION

Sterile linen thread in distributor for veterinary use consists of the pericyclic fibres of the stem of *Linum usitatissimum* L. The elementary fibres, 2.5 cm to 5 cm long, are assembled in bundles 30 cm to 80 cm long and spun into continuous lengths of suitable diameter. The thread may be creamy-white or may be coloured with colouring matter authorised by the competent authority. The thread is sterilised.

IDENTIFICATION

A. Dissect the end of a thread, using a needle or fine tweezers, to isolate a few individual fibres. Examined under a microscope, the fibres are seen to be 12 µm to 31 µm wide and, along the greater part of their length, have thick walls, sometimes marked with fine longitudinal striations, and a narrow lumen. The fibres gradually narrow to a long, fine point. Sometimes there are unilateral swellings with transverse lines.

B. Impregnate isolated fibres with *iodinated zinc chloride solution R*. The fibres are coloured violet-blue.

TESTS

It complies with the tests prescribed in the monograph on *Strands, sterile non-absorbable, in distributor for veterinary use (0605)*.

If stored in a dry state, expose to an atmosphere with a relative humidity of 65 ± 5 per cent at 20 ± 2 °C for 4 h immediately before measuring the diameter and for the determination of minimum breaking load immerse in water R at room temperature for 30 min immediately before carrying out the test.

STORAGE

See the monograph on *Strands, sterile non-absorbable, in distributor for veterinary use (0605)*.

LABELLING

See the monograph on *Strands, sterile non-absorbable, in distributor for veterinary use (0605)*.

01/2005:0609

POLYAMIDE 6 SUTURE, STERILE, IN DISTRIBUTOR FOR VETERINARY USE

Filum polyamidicum-6 sterile in fuso ad usum veterinarium

DEFINITION

Sterile polyamide 6 suture in distributor for veterinary use is obtained by drawing through a suitable die a synthetic plastic material formed by the polymerisation of ε-caprolactam. It consists of smooth, cylindrical monofilaments or braided filaments, or lightly twisted strands sheathed with the same material. It may be coloured with colouring matter authorised by the competent authority. The suture is sterilised.

CHARACTERS

It is practically insoluble in the usual organic solvents; it is not attacked by dilute alkaline solutions (for example a 100 g/l solution of sodium hydroxide) but is attacked by dilute mineral acids (for example 20 g/l sulphuric acid), by hot glacial acetic acid and by 70 per cent *m/m* formic acid.

IDENTIFICATION

A. Heat about 50 mg with 0.5 ml of *hydrochloric acid R1* in a sealed glass tube at 110 °C for 18 h and allow to stand for 6 h. No crystals appear.

B. To about 50 mg add 10 ml of *hydrochloric acid R1*. The material disintegrates in the cold and dissolves completely within a few minutes.

C. It dissolves in a 70 per cent *m/m* solution of *anhydrous formic acid R*.

TESTS

It complies with the tests prescribed in the monograph on *Strands, sterile non-absorbable, in distributor for veterinary use (0605)* and with the following test:

Monomer and oligomers. In a continuous-extraction apparatus, treat 1.00 g with 30 ml of *methanol R* at a rate of at least three extractions per hour for 7 h. Evaporate the extract to dryness, dry the residue at 110 °C for 10 min, allow to cool in a desiccator and weigh. The residue weighs not more than 20 mg (2 per cent).

STORAGE

See the monograph on *Strands, sterile non-absorbable, in distributor for veterinary use (0605)*.

LABELLING

See the monograph on *Strands, sterile non-absorbable, in distributor for veterinary use (0605)*.

The label states whether the suture is braided, monofilament or sheathed.

01/2005:0610

POLYAMIDE 6/6 SUTURE, STERILE, IN DISTRIBUTOR FOR VETERINARY USE

Filum polyamidicum-6/6 sterile in fuso ad usum veterinarium

DEFINITION

Sterile polyamide 6/6 suture in distributor for veterinary use is obtained by drawing through a suitable die a synthetic plastic material formed by the polycondensation of hexamethylene-diamine and adipic acid. It consists of smooth, cylindrical monofilaments or braided filaments, or lightly twisted strands sheathed with the same material. It may be coloured with authorised colouring matter or pigments authorised by the competent authority. The suture is sterilised.

CHARACTERS

It is practically insoluble in the usual organic solvents; it is not attacked by dilute alkaline solutions (for example a 100 g/l solution of sodium hydroxide) but is attacked by dilute mineral acids (for example 20 g/l sulphuric acid), by hot glacial acetic acid and by 80 per cent *m/m* formic acid.

IDENTIFICATION

A. In contact with a flame it melts and burns, forming a hard globule of residue and gives off a characteristic odour resembling that of celery.

B. Place about 50 mg in an ignition tube held vertically and heat gently until thick fumes are evolved. When the fumes fill the tube, withdraw it from the flame and insert a strip of *nitrobenzaldehyde paper R*. A violet-brown colour slowly appears on the paper and fades slowly in air; it disappears immediately on washing with *dilute sulphuric acid R*.

C. To about 50 mg add 10 ml of *hydrochloric acid R1*. The material disintegrates in the cold and dissolves within a few minutes.

D. It does not dissolve in a 70 per cent *m/m* solution of *anhydrous formic acid R* but dissolves in an 80 per cent *m/m* solution of *anhydrous formic acid R*.

TESTS

It complies with the tests prescribed in the monograph on *Strands, sterile non-absorbable, in distributor for veterinary use (0605).*

STORAGE

See the monograph on *Strands, sterile non-absorbable, in distributor for veterinary use (0605).*

LABELLING

See the monograph on *Strands, sterile non-absorbable, in distributor for veterinary use (0605).*

The label states whether the suture is braided, monofilament or sheathed.

01/2005:0607

POLY(ETHYLENE TEREPHTHALATE) SUTURE, STERILE, IN DISTRIBUTOR FOR VETERINARY USE

Filum ethyleni polyterephthalici sterile in fuso ad usum veterinarium

DEFINITION

Sterile poly(ethylene terephthalate) suture in distributor for veterinary use is obtained by drawing poly(ethylene terephthalate) through a suitable die. The suture is prepared by braiding very fine filaments in suitable numbers, depending on the gauge required. It may be whitish in colour, or may be coloured with authorised colouring matter or pigments authorised by the competent authority. The suture is sterilised.

CHARACTERS

It is practically insoluble in most of the usual organic solvents, but is attacked by strong alkaline solutions. It is incompatible with phenols.

IDENTIFICATION

A. It dissolves with difficulty when heated in *dimethylformamide R* and in *dichlorobenzene R*.

B. To about 50 mg add 10 ml of *hydrochloric acid R1*. The material remains intact even after immersion for 6 h.

TESTS

It complies with the tests prescribed in the monograph on *Strands, sterile non-absorbable, in distributor for veterinary use (0605).*

STORAGE

See the monograph on *Strands, sterile non-absorbable, in distributor for veterinary use (0605).*

LABELLING

See the monograph on *Strands, sterile non-absorbable, in distributor for veterinary use (0605).*

01/2005:0606

SILK SUTURE, STERILE, BRAIDED, IN DISTRIBUTOR FOR VETERINARY USE

Filum bombycis tortum sterile in fuso ad usum veterinarium

DEFINITION

Sterile braided silk suture in distributor for veterinary use is obtained by braiding a variable number of threads, according to the diameter required, of degummed silk obtained from the cocoons of the silkworm *Bombyx mori* L. It may be coloured with colouring matter authorised by the competent authority. The suture is sterilised.

IDENTIFICATION

A. Dissect the end of a strand, using a needle or fine tweezers, to isolate a few individual fibres. The fibres are sometimes marked with very fine longitudinal striations parallel to the axis of the strand. Examined under a microscope, a cross-section is more or less triangular or semi-circular, with rounded edges and without a lumen.

B. Impregnate isolated fibres with *iodinated potassium iodide solution R*. The fibres are coloured pale yellow.

TESTS

It complies with the tests prescribed in the monograph on *Strands, sterile non-absorbable, in distributor for veterinary use (0605)*.

STORAGE

See the monograph on *Strands, sterile non-absorbable, in distributor for veterinary use (0605)*.

LABELLING

See the monograph on *Strands, sterile non-absorbable, in distributor for veterinary use (0605)*.

01/2005:0605

STRANDS, STERILE NON-ABSORBABLE, IN DISTRIBUTOR FOR VETERINARY USE

Fila non resorbilia sterilia in fuso ad usum veterinarium

DEFINITION

The statements in this monograph are intended to be read in conjunction with the individual monographs on sterile non-absorbable strands in distributor for veterinary use in the Pharmacopoeia. The requirements do not necessarily apply to sterile non-absorbable strands which are not the subject of such monographs.

Sterile non-absorbable strands in distributor for veterinary use are strands which, when introduced into a living organism, are not metabolised by that organism. Sterile non- absorbable strands vary in origin, which may be animal, vegetable or synthetic. They occur as cylindrical monofilaments or as multifilament strands. Multifilament strands consist of elementary fibres which are assembled by twisting, cabling or braiding. Such strands may be sheathed. Sterile non- absorbable strands may be treated to render them non-capillary, and they may be coloured with colouring matter or pigments authorised by the competent authority. The strands are sterilised.

They are presented in a suitable distributor that allows the withdrawal and use of all or part of the strand in aseptic conditions. The design of the distributor is such that with suitable handling the sterility of the content is maintained even when part of the strand has been removed. They may be stored dry or in a preserving liquid to which an antimicrobial preservative but not an antibiotic may be added.

TESTS

Remove the strand from the distributor and measure promptly and in succession the length, diameter and minimum breaking load.

Length. Measure the length in the condition in which the strand is presented and without applying more tension than is necessary to keep it straight. The length of the strand is not less than 95 per cent of the length stated on the label.

Diameter. Unless otherwise prescribed, measure the diameter by the following method using the strand in the condition in which it is presented. Use a suitable instrument capable of measuring with an accuracy of at least 0.002 mm and having a circular pressor foot 10 mm to 15 mm in diameter. The pressor foot and the moving parts attached to it are weighted so as to apply a total load of 100 ± 10 g to the strand being tested. When making the measurements, lower the pressor foot slowly to avoid crushing the strand. Make not fewer than one measurement per 2 m of length and in any case not fewer than 12 measurements at points evenly spaced along the strand. During the measurement submit monofilament strands to a tension not greater than that required to keep them straight. Submit multifilament strands to a tension not greater than one-fifth of the minimum breaking load shown in column C of Table 0605.-1 appropriate to the gauge number and type of material concerned or 10 N whichever is less. For multifilament strands of gauge number above 1.5 make two measurements at each point, the second measurement being made after rotating the strand through 90°. The diameter of that point is the average of the two measurements. The average of the measurements carried out on the strand being tested and not less than two-thirds of the individual measurements are within the limits given in the columns under A in Table 0605.-1 for the gauge number concerned. None of the measurements is outside the limits given in the columns under B in Table 0605.-1 for the gauge number concerned.

Table 0605.-1. – *Diameters and minimum breaking loads*

Gauge number	Diameter (millimetres)				Minimum breaking load (newtons)			
	A		B		Linen thread		All other non-absorbable strands	
	min.	max.	min.	max.	C	D	C	D
0.5	0.050	0.069	0.045	0.085	-	-	1.0	0.35
0.7	0.070	0.099	0.060	0.125	1.0	0.3	1.5	0.60
1	0.100	0.149	0.085	0.175	2.5	0.6	3.0	1.0
1.5	0.150	0.199	0.125	0.225	5.0	1.0	5.0	1.5
2	0.200	0.249	0.175	0.275	8.0	2.5	9.0	3.0
2.5	0.250	0.299	0.225	0.325	9.0	5.0	13.0	5.0
3	0.300	0.349	0.275	0.375	11.0	8.0	15.0	9.0
3.5	0.350	0.399	0.325	0.450	15.0	9.0	22.0	13.0
4	0.400	0.499	0.375	0.550	18.0	11.0	27.0	15.0
5	0.500	0.599	0.450	0.650	26.0	15.0	35.0	22.0
6	0.600	0.699	0.550	0.750	37.0	18.0	50.0	27.0
7	0.700	0.799	0.650	0.850	50.0	26.0	62.0	35.0
8	0.800	0.899	0.750	0.950	65.0	37.0	73.0	50.0

Minimum breaking load. Unless otherwise prescribed, determine the minimum breaking load by the following method using the strand in the condition in which it is presented. The minimum breaking load is determined over a simple knot formed by placing one end of a strand held in the right hand over the other end held in the left hand, passing one end over the strand and through the loop so formed (see Figure 0605.-1) and pulling the knot tight.

Make not fewer than one measurement per 2 m of length at points evenly spaced along the strand. Determine the breaking load using a suitable tensilometer. The apparatus has two clamps for holding the strand, one of which is mobile and is driven at a constant rate of 30 cm per minute. The clamps are designed so that the strand being tested can be attached with-out any possibility of slipping. At the beginning of the test the length of strand between the clamps is 12.5 cm to 20 cm and the knot is midway between the clamps. Set the mobile clamp in motion and note the force required to break the strand. If the strand breaks in a clamp or within 1 cm of it, the result is discarded and the test repeated on another part of the strand. The average of all the results, excluding those legitimately dis-carded, is equal to or greater than the value in column C and no value is less than that given in column D in Table 0605.-1 for the gauge number and type of material concerned.

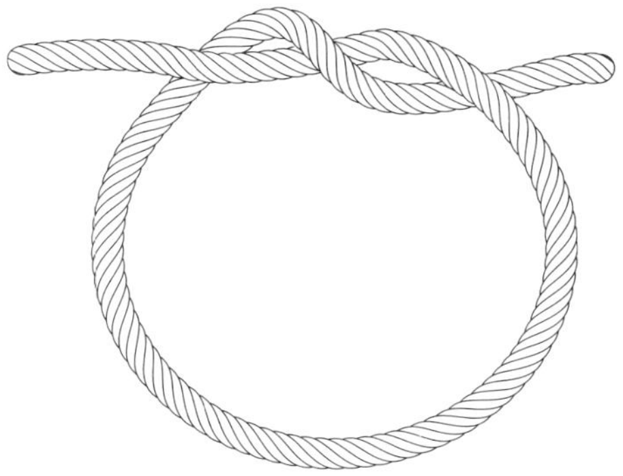

Figure 0605.-1. – *Simple knot*

Sterility (*2.6.1*). They comply with the test for sterility as applied to catgut and other surgical sutures. Carry out the test on three sections each 30 cm long, cut off respectively from the beginning, the centre and the end of the strand.

Extractable colour. Strands that are dyed and intended to remain so during use comply with the test for extractable colour. Place 0.25 g of the strand to be examined in a conical flask, add 25.0 ml of *water R* and cover the mouth of the flask with a short-stemmed funnel. Boil for 15 min, cool and adjust to the original volume with *water R*. Depending on the colour of the strand, prepare the appropriate reference solution as described in Table 0605.-2 using the primary colour solutions (*2.2.2*).

Table 0605.-2. – *Colour reference solutions*

Colour of strand	**Composition of reference solution (parts by volume)**			
	Red primary solution	**Yellow primary solution**	**Blue primary solution**	**Water**
Yellow - brown	0.2	1.2	–	8.6
Pink - red	1.0	–	–	9.0
Green - blue	–	–	2.0	8.0
Violet	1.6	–	8.4	–

The test solution is not more intensely coloured than the appropriate reference solution.

STORAGE

Store protected from light and heat.

LABELLING

The label states:

– the gauge number,

– the length in centimetres or in metres,

– where appropriate, that the strand is coloured and intended to remain so during use.

Sutures

Figure 0605.-1. – *Surgical knot*

HOMOEOPATHIC PREPARATIONS

01/2005:90006

INTRODUCTION

All general texts and other monographs of the European Pharmacopoeia that are relevant to homoeopathy are applicable.

The "Homoeopathy" chapter of the European Pharmacopoeia contains general monographs and individual monographs describing starting materials and preparations used virtually exclusively for homoeopathic medicines. Reference to these monographs for other purposes may be authorised by licensing authorities.

01/2005:2045

HERBAL DRUGS FOR HOMOEOPATHIC PREPARATIONS

Plantae medicinales ad praeparationes homoeopathicas

DEFINITION

Herbal drugs for homoeopathic preparations are mainly whole, fragmented or cut, plants, parts of plants including algae, fungi or lichens in an unprocessed state, usually in fresh form but sometimes dried. Certain exudates that have not been subjected to a specific treatment are also considered to be herbal drugs for homoeopathic preparations. Herbal drugs for homoeopathic preparations are precisely defined by the botanical scientific name of the source species according to the binomial system (genus, species, variety and author).

PRODUCTION

Herbal drugs for homoeopathic preparations are obtained from cultivated or wild plants. Suitable cultivation, harvesting, collection, sorting, drying, fragmentation and storage conditions are essential to guarantee the quality of herbal drugs for homoeopathic preparations.

Herbal drugs for homoeopathic preparations are, as far as possible, free from impurities such as soil, dust, dirt and other contaminants such as fungal, insect and other animal contaminants. They do not present signs of decay.

If a decontaminating treatment has been used, it is necessary to demonstrate that the constituents of the plant are not affected and that no harmful residues remain. The use of ethylene oxide is prohibited for the decontamination of herbal drugs for homoeopathic preparations.

Adequate measures have to be taken in order to ensure that the microbiological quality of homoeopathic preparations containing one or more herbal drugs comply with the recommendations given in the text on *Microbiological quality of pharmaceutical preparations* (*5.1.4*).

IDENTIFICATION

Herbal drugs for homoeopathic preparations are identified using their macroscopic and, where necessary, microscopic descriptions and any further tests that may be required (for example, thin-layer chromatography).

TESTS

When a fresh plant is used as a starting material for the manufacture of homoeopathic preparations, the content of foreign matter is as low as possible; if necessary, the maximum content of foreign matter is indicated in the individual monographs. When a dried plant is used as a starting material for the manufacture of homoeopathic preparations, a test for foreign matter (*2.8.2*) is carried out, unless otherwise prescribed in the individual monographs.

A specific appropriate test may apply to herbal drugs for homoeopathic preparations liable to be falsified.

If appropriate, the herbal drugs for homoeopathic preparations comply with other tests, for example, total ash (*2.4.16*) and bitterness value (*2.8.15*).

The test for loss on drying (*2.2.32*) is carried out on dried herbal drugs for homoeopathic preparations. A determination of water (*2.2.13*) is carried out on herbal drugs for homoeopathic preparations with a high essential oil content. The water content of fresh herbal drugs for homoeopathic preparations is determined by an appropriate method.

Herbal drugs for homoeopathic preparations comply with the requirements for pesticide residues (*2.8.13*). The requirements take into account the nature of the plant, where necessary the preparation in which the plant might be used, and where available the knowledge of the complete record of treatment of the batch of the plant. The content of pesticide residues may be determined by the method described in the annex to the general method.

The risk of contamination of herbal drugs for homoeopathic preparations by heavy metals must be considered. If an individual monograph does not prescribe limits for heavy metals or specific elements, such limits may be required if justified.

Limits for aflatoxins may be required.

In some specific circumstances, the risk of radioactive contamination is to be considered.

ASSAY

Where applicable, herbal drugs for homoeopathic preparations are assayed by an appropriate method.

STORAGE

Fresh herbal drugs are processed as rapidly as possible after harvesting; they may also be stored deep-frozen or in ethanol (96 per cent *V/V*) or in alcohol of a given concentration. Store dried herbal drugs protected from light.

01/2005:1038

HOMOEOPATHIC PREPARATIONS

Praeparationes homoeopathicas

DEFINITION

Homoeopathic preparations are prepared from substances, products or preparations called stocks, in accordance with a homoeopathic manufacturing procedure. A homoeopathic preparation is usually designated by the Latin name of the stock, followed by an indication of the degree of dilution.

Raw materials

Raw materials for the production of homoeopathic preparations may be of natural or synthetic origin.

For raw materials of zoological or human origin, adequate measures are taken to minimise the risk of agents of infection in the homoeopathic preparations. For this purpose, it is demonstrated that:

– the method of production includes a step or steps that have been shown to remove or inactivate agents of infection,

- where applicable, raw materials of zoological origin comply with the monograph on *Products with risk of transmitting agents of animal spongiform encephalopathies (1483)*,
- where applicable, the animals and the tissues used to obtain the raw materials comply with the health requirements of the competent authorities for animals for human consumption,
- for materials of human origin, the donor follows the recommendations applicable to human blood donors and to donated blood (see *Human plasma for fractionation (0853)*), unless otherwise justified and authorised.

A raw material of botanical, zoological or human origin may be used either in the fresh state or in the dried state. Where appropriate, fresh material may be kept deep-frozen. Raw materials of botanical origin comply with the requirements of the monograph on *Herbal drugs for homoeopathic preparations (2045)*.

Where justified and authorised for transportation or storage purposes, fresh plant material may be kept in ethanol (96 per cent *V/V*) or in alcohol of a suitable concentration, provided the whole material including the storage medium is used for processing.

Raw materials comply with any requirements of the relevant monographs of the European Pharmacopoeia.

Vehicles

Vehicles are excipients used for the preparation of certain stocks or for the potentisation process. They may include for example: purified water, alcohol of a suitable concentration, glycerol and lactose.

Vehicles comply with any requirements of the relevant monographs of the European Pharmacopoeia.

Stocks

Stocks are substances, products or preparations used as starting materials for the production of homoeopathic preparations. A stock is usually one of the following: a mother tincture or a glycerol macerate, for raw materials of botanical, zoological or human origin, or the substance itself, for raw materials of chemical or mineral origin.

Mother tinctures comply with the requirements of the monograph on *Mother tinctures for homoeopathic preparations (2029)*.

Glycerol macerates are liquid preparations obtained from raw materials of botanical, zoological or human origin by using glycerol or a mixture of glycerol and either alcohol of a suitable concentration or a solution of sodium chloride of a suitable concentration.

Potentisation

Dilutions and triturations are obtained from stocks by a process of potentisation in accordance with a homoeopathic manufacturing procedure: this means successive dilutions and succussions, or successive appropriate triturations, or a combination of the 2 processes.

The potentisation steps are usually one of the following:

- 1 part of the stock plus 9 parts of the vehicle; they may be designated as "D", "DH" or "X" (decimal),
- 1 part of the stock plus 99 parts of the vehicle; they may be designated as "C" or "CH" (centesimal).

The number of potentisation steps defines the degree of dilution; for example, "D3", "3 DH" or "3X" means 3 decimal potentisation steps, and "C3", "3 CH" or "3C" means 3 centesimal potentisation steps.

"LM-" (or "Q-") potencies are manufactured according to a specific procedure.

Dosage forms

A dosage form of a homoeopathic preparation complies with any relevant dosage form monograph in the European Pharmacopoeia and with the following:

- for the purpose of dosage forms for homoeopathic use "active substances" are considered to be "dilutions or triturations of homoeopathic stocks",
- these dosage forms are prepared using appropriate excipients,
- the test for uniformity of content is normally not appropriate. However, in certain circumstances, it is required.

Homoeopathic dosage form "pillule"

Pillules for homoeopathic use are solid preparations obtained from sucrose, lactose or other suitable excipients. They may be prepared by impregnation of preformed pillules with a dilution or dilutions of homoeopathic stocks or by progressive addition of these excipients and the addition of a dilution or dilutions of homoeopathic stocks. They are intended for oral or sublingual use.

Homoeopathic dosage form "tablet"

Tablets for homoeopathic use are solid preparations obtained from sucrose, lactose or other suitable excipients according to the monograph on *Tablets (0478)*. They may either be prepared by compressing one or more solid active substances with the excipients or by impregnating preformed tablets with a dilution or dilutions of homoeopathic stocks. The preformed tablets for impregnation are obtained from sucrose, lactose or other suitable excipients according to the monograph on *Tablets (0478)*. They are intended for oral or sublingual use.

01/2005:2029

MOTHER TINCTURES FOR HOMOEOPATHIC PREPARATIONS

Tincturae maternae ad praeparationes homoeopathicas

DEFINITION

Mother tinctures for homoeopathic preparations are liquid preparations obtained by the solvent action of a suitable vehicle upon raw materials. The raw materials are usually in the fresh form but may be dried. Mother tinctures for homoeopathic preparations may also be obtained from plant juices, with, or without the addition of a vehicle. For some preparations, the matter to be extracted may undergo a preliminary treatment.

PRODUCTION

Mother tinctures for homoeopathic preparations are prepared by maceration, digestion, infusion, decoction, fermentation or as described in the individual monographs, usually using alcohol of suitable concentration.

Mother tinctures for homoeopathic preparations are obtained using a fixed proportion of raw material to solvent, taking the moisture content of the raw material into account, unless otherwise justified and authorised.

If fresh plants are used, suitable procedures are used to ensure freshness. The competent authorities may require that the freshness is demonstrated by means of a suitable test.

Mother tinctures for homoeopathic preparations are usually clear. A slight sediment may form on standing and that is acceptable as long as the composition of the tincture is not changed significantly.

The manufacturing process is defined so that it is reproducible.

Production by maceration. Unless otherwise prescribed, reduce the matter to be extracted to pieces of suitable size, mix thoroughly and extract according to the prescribed extraction method with the prescribed extraction solvent. Allow to stand in a closed vessel for the prescribed time. The residue is separated from the extraction solvent and, if necessary, pressed out. In the latter case, the 2 liquids obtained are combined.

Adjustment of the contents. Adjustment of the content of constituents may be carried out if necessary, either by adding the extraction solvent of suitable concentration, or by adding another mother tincture for homoeopathic preparations of the vegetable or animal matter used for the preparation.

IDENTIFICATION

Where applicable, at least 1 chromatographic identification test is carried out.

TESTS

The limits in an individual monograph are set to include official methods of production. Specific limits will apply to each defined method of production.

If the test for relative density is carried out, the test for ethanol need not be carried out, and vice versa.

Relative density (*2.2.5*). The mother tincture for homoeopathic preparations complies with the limits prescribed in the monograph.

Ethanol (*2.9.10*). The ethanol content complies with that prescribed in the monograph.

Methanol and 2-propanol (*2.9.11*): maximum 0.05 per cent *V/V* of methanol and maximum 0.05 per cent *V/V* of 2-propanol, unless otherwise prescribed.

Dry residue (*2.8.16*). Where applicable, the mother tincture for homoeopathic preparations complies with the limits prescribed in the monograph.

Pesticides (*2.8.13*). Where applicable, the mother tincture for homoeopathic preparations complies with the test. This requirement is met if the herbal drug has been shown to comply with the test.

ASSAY

Where applicable, an assay with quantitative limits is performed.

STORAGE

Protected from light. A maximum storage temperature may be specified.

LABELLING

The label states:

- that the product is a mother tincture for homoeopathic preparations (designated as "TM" or "Ø"),
- the name of the raw material using the Latin title of the European Pharmacopoeia monograph where one exists,
- the method of preparation,
- the ethanol content or other solvent content, in per cent *V/V*, in the mother tincture,
- the ratio of raw material to mother tincture,
- where applicable, the storage conditions.

01/2005:1599

ARSENIOUS TRIOXIDE FOR HOMOEOPATHIC PREPARATIONS

Arsenii trioxidum ad praeparationes homoeopathicas

As_2O_3 M_r 197.8

DEFINITION

Content: 99.5 per cent to 100.5 per cent of As_2O_3.

CHARACTERS

Appearance: white or almost white powder.

Solubility: practically insoluble to sparingly soluble in water. It dissolves in solutions of alkali hydroxides and carbonates.

IDENTIFICATION

A. Dissolve 20 mg in 1 ml of *dilute hydrochloric acid R*, add 4 ml of *water R* and 0.1 ml of *sodium sulphide solution R*. The resulting yellow precipitate is soluble in *dilute ammonia R1*.

B. Dissolve 20 mg in 1 ml of *hydrochloric acid R1*, add 5 ml of *hypophosphorous reagent R* and heat for 15 min on a water-bath. A black precipitate develops.

TESTS

Appearance of solution. A 100 g/l solution in *dilute ammonia R1* is clear (*2.2.1*) and colourless (*2.2.2, Method II*).

Sulphides. Dissolve 1.0 g in 10.0 ml of *dilute sodium hydroxide solution R*. Add 0.05 ml of *lead acetate solution R*. Any colour in the test solution is not more intense than that in a standard prepared at the same time and in the same manner using a mixture of 10.0 ml of a 0.015 g/l solution of *sodium sulphide R* in *dilute sodium hydroxide solution R* and 0.05 ml of *lead acetate solution R* (20 ppm).

ASSAY

Dissolve 40.0 mg in a mixture of 10 ml of *water R* and 10 ml of *dilute sodium hydroxide solution R*. Add 10 ml of *dilute hydrochloric acid R* and 3 g of *sodium hydrogen carbonate R* and mix. Add 1 ml of *starch solution R* and titrate with *0.05 M iodine*.

1 ml of *0.05 M iodine* is equivalent to 4.946 mg of As_2O_3.

01/2005:2030

COMMON STINGING NETTLE FOR HOMOEOPATHIC PREPARATIONS

Urtica dioica ad praeparationes homoeopathicas

DEFINITION

Whole, fresh, flowering plant of *Urtica dioica* L.

CHARACTERS

Macroscopic characters described under Identification A.

The plant causes an itching, burning sensation on the skin.

IDENTIFICATION

A. Common stinging nettle is perennial. The taproot sends out creeping subterranean rhizomes, more or less 4-angled in transverse section, from which extend adventious secondary roots and very numerous brownish hairy rootlets. The stipes are erect, generally unbranched, 3 mm to 5 mm in diameter and 0.3 m to 1.5 m high, rarely up to 2.5 m high, 4-angled, greyish-green and covered in short hairs and stinging hairs.

The decussate leaves are 30 mm to 150 mm long and 20 mm to 80 mm wide. The petiole is hispid and usually slightly less than one-third the length of the lamina. The leaf blade is ovate, acuminate, cordate or rounded at the base, and coarsely dentate; the apical tooth is distinctly larger than the lateral teeth. The upper side of the leaves is dark green and usually matt, both sides bear short serried hairs intermingled with long stinging hairs. The 2 stipules are linear-subulate and free. The inflorescences growing from the leaf axils are complex, the flowers unisexual, and, particularly in male plants, generally distinctly longer than the petiole. After shedding their pollen, male inflorescences are erect at an oblique angle or horizontal; female inflorescences are pendent when the fruit is ripe. All flowers have long stalks. The perianth of the male flowers is divided half-way down into equal green lobes, widest at their base, with short bristles and stinging hairs at the margins. The stamens are equal and opposite to the perianth segments, each with a long, whitish filament that curves inwards before pollen is shed and spreads out afterwards. The ovary is rudimentary, button or cup-shaped. The perianth of the female flowers is downy or bristly on the outside and consists of outer, and 2 inner segments; the inner segments are about twice the length of the outer ones. The hypogynous, ovate, unilocular ovary bears a large capitate stigma with a brush-like shock of hair. As the one-seeded fruit grows ripe, the 2 inner segments of the perianth fold around it like wings.

B. It complies with the test for *Urtica urens* (see Tests).

TESTS

Urtica urens. The margin of the lamina is not serrate with teeth twice as long as wide. The clusters of flowers in the axils are longer than the petiole of the leaf. Unisexual, apetalous flowers are not together on the same plant and in the same cluster.

Foreign matter (*2.8.2*): maximum 5 per cent.

Loss on drying (*2.2.32*): minimum 65.0 per cent, determined on 5.0 g of finely cut drug by drying in an oven at 100-105 °C for 2 h, if performed to demonstrate the freshness of the drug.

Mother tincture

The mother tincture complies with the requirements of the general monograph on *Mother tinctures for homoeopathic preparations (2029).*

PRODUCTION

The mother tincture of *Urtica dioica* L. is prepared by maceration using alcohol of a suitable concentration.

CHARACTERS

Appearance: greenish-brown or orange-brown liquid.

IDENTIFICATION

Thin-layer chromatography (*2.2.27*).

Test solution. The mother tincture to be examined.

Reference solution. Dissolve 10 mg of *phenylalanine R* and 10 mg of *serine R* in a mixture of equal volumes of *methanol R* and *water R* and dilute to 10 ml with the same mixture of solvents.

Plate: *TLC silica gel plate R.*

Mobile phase: *glacial acetic acid R, water R, acetone R, butanol R* (10:20:35:35 *V/V/V/V*).

Application: 20 µl, as bands.

Development: over a path of 10 cm.

Drying: in air.

Detection: spray with a 1 g/l solution of *ninhydrin R* in *alcohol R.* Heat the plate at 105-110 °C for 5-10 min then examine in daylight within 10 min.

Results: see below the sequence of the zones present in the chromatograms obtained with the reference solution and the test solution.

Top of the plate	
Phenylalanine: a violet to reddish-brown zone	
	4 red to violet zones
_______	
Serine: a reddish-violet zone	A violet zone
	A violet zone
Reference solution	**Test solution**

TESTS

Relative density (*2.2.5*): 0.930 to 0.950.

Ethanol (*2.9.10*): 40 per cent *V/V* to 56 per cent *V/V.*

Dry residue (*2.8.16*): minimum 1.1 per cent.

01/2005:1610

COPPER FOR HOMOEOPATHIC PREPARATIONS

Cuprum ad praeparationes homoeopathicas

Cu A_r 63.5

DEFINITION

Content: 99.0 per cent to 101.0 per cent of Cu.

CHARACTERS

Appearance: reddish-brown powder.

Solubility: practically insoluble in water, soluble in hydrochloric acid and in nitric acid, practically insoluble in alcohol.

IDENTIFICATION

A. To 2 ml of solution S (see Tests) add 0.5 ml of *potassium ferrocyanide solution R.* A reddish-brown precipitate is formed.

B. To 5 ml of solution S add 0.6 ml of *ammonia R.* A blue precipitate is formed. Add 2 ml of *ammonia R.* The precipitate disappears; the solution has an intense blue colour.

TESTS

Solution S. Dissolve 2.0 g in 10 ml of *nitric acid R.* After nitrous fumes are no longer evolved, dilute to 60 ml with *distilled water R.*

Acidity or alkalinity. To 5.0 g add 20 ml of *carbon dioxide-free water R.* Boil for 1 min. Cool. Filter and dilute to 25.0 ml with *carbon dioxide free water R.* To 10 ml of the solution add 0.1 ml of *bromothymol blue solution R1.*

Homoeopathic preparations

Not more than 0.5 ml of *0.01 M hydrochloric acid* or *0.01 M sodium hydroxide* is required to change the colour of the indicator.

Chlorides (*2.4.4*): maximum 100 ppm.

15 ml of solution S complies with the limit test for chlorides.

Sulphates (*2.4.13*): maximum 300 ppm.

15 ml of solution S complies with the limit test for sulphates.

Iron: maximum 50 ppm.

Atomic absorption spectrometry (*2.2.23, Method I*).

Test solution. Dissolve 1.00 g in 5 ml of *nitric acid R* and dilute to 50.0 ml with *water R.*

Reference solutions. Prepare the reference solutions using *iron standard solution (20 ppm Fe) R,* diluted as necessary with a 1 per cent *V/V* solution of *nitric acid R.*

Source: iron hollow-cathode lamp.

Wavelength: 248.3 nm.

Flame: air-acetylene.

Lead: maximum 100 ppm.

Atomic absorption spectrometry (*2.2.23, Method I*).

Test solution. Use the test solution prepared for the test for iron.

Reference solutions. Prepare the reference solutions using *lead standard solution (0.1 per cent Pb) R,* diluted as necessary with a 1 per cent *V/V* solution of *nitric acid R.*

Source: lead hollow-cathode lamp.

Wavelength: 283.3 nm.

Flame: air-acetylene.

Zinc: maximum 50 ppm.

Atomic absorption spectrometry (*2.2.23, Method I*).

Test solution. Use the test solution prepared for the test for iron.

Reference solutions. Prepare the reference solutions using *zinc standard solution (100 ppm Zn) R,* diluted as necessary with a 1 per cent *V/V* solution of *nitric acid R.*

Source: zinc hollow-cathode lamp.

Wavelength: 213.9 nm.

Flame: air-acetylene.

ASSAY

Dissolve 0.100 g in 5 ml of *nitric acid R.* Heat to expel the nitrous fumes. Add 200 ml of *water R* and neutralise (*2.2.3*) with *dilute ammonia R1.* Add 1 g of *ammonium chloride R* and 3 mg of *murexide R.* Titrate with *0.1 M sodium edetate* until the colour changes from green to violet.

1 ml of *0.1 M sodium edetate* is equivalent to 6.354 mg of Cu.

01/2005:2023

GARLIC FOR HOMOEOPATHIC PREPARATIONS

Allium sativum ad praeparationes homoeopathicas

DEFINITION

Fresh bulb of *Allium sativum* L.

CHARACTERS

Macroscopic characters described under identification.

It has a characteristic odour after cutting.

IDENTIFICATION

The bulb is generally 3 cm to 5 cm broad and almost spherical; the flat base bears the remnants of numerous short greyish-brown adventitious roots. The bulb consists of about 10 daughter bulbs (cloves) arranged roughly in a circle around a central axis. Individual daughter bulbs are 1 cm to 3 cm long, laterally compressed and convex on the dorsal side. Each daughter bulb has a tough, white or reddish skin around a fleshy tubular leaf, investing a more or less rounded elongated cone of leaf primordia and vegetative apex.

TESTS

Foreign matter (*2.8.2*). It complies with the test for foreign matter.

Water (*2.2.13*): minimum 55.0 per cent, determined on 10.0 g of the finely cut drug, if performed to demonstrate the freshness of the drug.

Mother tincture

The mother tincture complies with the requirements of the general monograph on *Mother tinctures for homoeopathic preparations (2029).*

PRODUCTION

The mother tincture of *Allium sativum* L. is prepared by maceration of the cut drug using alcohol of a suitable concentration.

CHARACTERS

Appearance: brownish-yellow liquid.

It has a peculiar and unpleasant aromatic odour.

IDENTIFICATION

A. To 2 ml of the mother tincture to be examined, add 0.2 ml of *dilute sodium hydroxide solution R.* A yellowish-white precipitate develops.

B. Thin-layer chromatography (*2.2.27*).

Test solution. Extract 5 ml of the mother tincture to be examined with 2 quantities, each of 10 ml, of *ether R.* Combine the ether layers and dry over *anhydrous sodium sulphate R.* Filter and evaporate the filtrate in a water-bath at low temperature. Dissolve the residue in 0.4 ml of *methanol R.*

Reference solution. Dissolve 10 mg of *resorcinol R,* 10 mg of *thymol R* and 30 mg of *gallic acid R* in 10 ml of *methanol R.*

Plate: *TLC silica gel F_{254} plate R.*

Mobile phase: *anhydrous formic acid R, toluene R, di-isopropyl ether R* (10:40:50 *V/V/V*).

Application: 40 µl of the test solution and 10 µl of the reference solution.

Development: over a path of 10 cm.

Drying: in air.

Detection: examine in ultraviolet light at 254 nm and identify gallic acid; spray with *anisaldehyde solution R,* heat to 105-110 °C for 5-10 min. Examine in daylight within 10 min.

Results: see below the sequence of the zones present in the chromatograms obtained with the reference solution and the test solution. Other zones may also be visible in the chromatogram obtained with the test solution.

Top of the plate	
	An intense reddish-violet zone
Thymol: an orange-red zone	
	An intense reddish-violet zone
	A violet zone
	A yellowish or greenish zone
———	
Resorcinol: an intense orange-red zone	
Gallic acid: a yellow zone	A violet zone
(UV at 254 nm: a fluorescent quenching zone)	A greenish-yellow zone
	A violet zone may be present
Reference solution	**Test solution**

TESTS

Relative density (*2.2.5*): 0.885 to 0.960.

Ethanol (*2.9.10*): 50 per cent *V/V* to 70 per cent *V/V*.

Dry residue (*2.8.16*): minimum 4.0 per cent.

STORAGE

In an airtight container, protected from light.

01/2005:2024

HONEY BEE FOR HOMOEOPATHIC PREPARATIONS

Apis mellifera ad praeparationes homoeopathicas

DEFINITION

Live worker honey bee (*Apis mellifera* L.).

CHARACTERS

Characters described under Identification.

PRODUCTION

If the bee has been exposed to treatment to prevent or cure diseases, appropriate steps are taken to ensure that the levels of residues are as low as possible.

IDENTIFICATION

The body of a honey bee is about 15 mm long, black, with a silky sheen, and covered with red hairs with a touch of grey. The broad tibiae are without spines. The posterior margins of the segments and legs are brown, with gradual transition to orange-red. The claws are two-membered, the maxillary palps single-membered. On the hind legs are baskets or scoops invested with bristles. The wings have 3 complete cubital cells, with the radial cell twice as long as it is wide; the 3 cells on the lower margin and the 3 middle cells are closed. A duct connects the barbed sting with the poison sac.

Mother tincture

The mother tincture complies with the requirements of the general monograph on *Mother tinctures for homoeopathic preparations (2029)*.

PRODUCTION

The mother tincture of *Apis mellifera* L. is prepared by maceration using alcohol of a suitable concentration.

CHARACTERS

Pale yellow liquid that may darken on storage.

IDENTIFICATION

Thin-layer chromatography (*2.2.27*).

Test solution. The mother tincture to be examined.

Reference solution. Dissolve 12 mg of *4-aminobutanoic acid R*, 12 mg of *leucine R* and 12 mg of *proline R* in 5 ml of *water R* and dilute to 50 ml with *alcohol R*.

Plate: *TLC silica gel plate R*.

Mobile phase: *water R, ethanol R* (17:63 *V/V*).

Application: 20 µl, as bands.

Development: over a path of 10 cm.

Drying: in air.

Detection: spray with *ninhydrin solution R* and heat at 100-105 °C for 10 min; examine in daylight.

Results: see below the sequence of the zones present in the chromatograms obtained with the reference and test solutions. Other zones may also be visible.

Top of the plate	
———	
	A pink zone
Leucine: a pink zone	A pink zone
	A pink zone
	A pink zone
———	———
Proline: an orange-yellow zone	An orange-yellow zone
4-Aminobutanoic acid: a pink zone	A pink zone
Reference solution	**Test solution**

TESTS

Relative density (*2.2.5*): 0.890 to 0.910.

Ethanol (*2.9.10*): 60 per cent *V/V* to 70 per cent *V/V*.

Dry residue (*2.8.16*): minimum 0.30 per cent.

01/2005:2028

HYPERICUM FOR HOMOEOPATHIC PREPARATIONS

Hypericum perforatum ad praeparationes homoeopathicas

DEFINITION

Whole, fresh plant of *Hypericum perforatum* L., at the beginning of the flowering period.

CHARACTERS

Macroscopic characters described under Identification.

IDENTIFICATION

The perennial plant consists of a spindle-shaped root and a branched rhizome, giving rise to long, decumbent runners. The cylindrical, erect stem is woody at the base, 0.2 m to 1 m long, branched in the upper part, with 2 raised longitudinal lines.

The leaves are opposite, sessile, exstipulate, oblong-oval and 15 mm to 30 mm long. The leaf margins show black glandular dots, and many small translucent oil glands are present on the entire surface and are visible by transmitted light.

The flowers are regular and form corymbose clusters at the apex of the stem. They have 5 green, lanceolate sepals with acuminate apices, and black oil glands near the entire margins; 5 orange-yellow petals, much longer than the sepals, with black oil glands near the terminal margins only; 3 staminal blades, each divided into many orange-yellow stamens and 3 carpels surmounted by red styles. Each petal is asymmetrically linear-ovate in shape, with one of the margin entire and the other dentate.

TESTS

Foreign matter (*2.8.2*): maximum 4 per cent of fruits and maximum 1 per cent of other foreign matter.

Loss on drying (*2.2.32*): if performed to demonstrate the freshness of the drug, minimum 55 per cent, determined on 5.0 g of finely cut drug by drying in an oven at 100-105 °C.

Mother tincture

The mother tincture complies with the requirements of the general monograph on *Mother tinctures for homoeopathic preparations (2029)*.

PRODUCTION

The mother tincture of *Hypericum perforatum* L. is prepared by maceration using alcohol of a suitable concentration.

CHARACTERS

Dark red to brownish red liquid.

IDENTIFICATION

Thin-layer chromatography (*2.2.27*).

Test solution. The mother tincture to be examined.

Reference solution. Dissolve 5 mg of *rutin R*, 1 mg of *hypericin R* and 5 mg of *hyperoside R* in *methanol R* and dilute to 5 ml with the same solvent.

Plate: *TLC silica gel plate R.*

Mobile phase: *anhydrous formic acid R, water R, ethyl acetate R* (6:9:90 *V/V/V*).

Application: 10 µl of the test solution and 5 µl of the reference solution, as 10 mm bands.

Development: over a path of 10 cm.

Drying: at 100-105 °C for 10 min.

Detection: spray with a 10 g/l solution of *diphenylboric acid aminoethyl ester R* in *methanol R* and then a 50 g/l solution of *macrogol 400 R* in *methanol R*. Examine the plates after 30 min in ultraviolet light at 365 nm.

Results: see below the sequence of the zones present in the chromatograms obtained with the reference solution and the test solution. In the chromatogram obtained with the test solution, the zone due to rutin may be weak or even absent. The chromatogram obtained with the test solution shows a group of zones that may be blue or yellow, with a Rf similar to that of the zone due to hyperoside in the chromatogram obtained with the reference solution. Other weak zones may also be visible.

Top of the plate	
	A yellow to blue zone
Hypericin: a red zone	2 red zones
_______	_______
	Several zones
_______	_______
Hyperoside: a yellow to orange zone	Blue or yellow zones
Rutin: a yellow to orange zone	A yellow to orange zone
Reference solution	**Test solution**

TESTS

Relative density (*2.2.5*): 0.900 to 0.920.

Ethanol (*2.9.10*): 60 per cent *V/V* to 75 per cent *V/V*.

Dry residue (*2.8.16*): minimum 1.3 per cent.

01/2005:2026
corrected

IRON FOR HOMOEOPATHIC PREPARATIONS

Ferrum ad praeparationes homoeopathicas

Fe A_r 55.85

DEFINITION

Obtained by reduction or sublimation as a fine blackish-grey powder.

Content: 97.5 per cent to 101.0 per cent.

CHARACTERS

Appearance: fine, blackish-grey powder, without metallic lustre.

Solubility: practically insoluble in water and in alcohol. It dissolves with heating in dilute mineral acids.

IDENTIFICATION

Dissolve 50 mg in 2 ml of *dilute sulphuric acid R* and dilute to 10 ml with *water R*. The solution gives reaction (a) of iron (*2.3.1*).

TESTS

Solution S. To 10.0 g add 40 ml of *water R*. Boil for 1 min. Cool, filter and dilute to 50.0 ml with *water R*.

Alkalinity. To 10 ml of solution S add 0.1 ml of *bromothymol blue solution R1*. Not more than 0.1 ml of *0.01 M hydrochloric acid* is required to change the colour of the indicator to yellow.

Substances insoluble in hydrochloric acid. Dissolve 2.00 g in 40 ml of *hydrochloric acid R*. Heat on a water-bath. As soon as fumes are no longer evolved, filter through a sintered-glass filter No. 16 (*2.1.2*). Rinse with *water R*. Dry the residue in an oven at 100-105 °C for 1 h. The residue weighs a maximum of 20 mg (1.0 per cent).

Substances soluble in water. Evaporate 10.0 ml of solution S on a water-bath and dry at 100-105 °C for 1 h. The residue weighs a maximum of 2 mg (0.1 per cent).

Chlorides (*2.4.4*): maximum 50 ppm.

Dilute 5 ml of solution S to 15 ml with *water R*. The solution complies with the limit test for chlorides.

Sulphides and phosphides. In a 100 ml conical flask carefully mix 1.0 g with 10 ml of *dilute hydrochloric acid R*. Within 30 s *lead acetate paper R* moistened with *water R* and placed over the mouth of the flask is not coloured more intensely than light brown by the resulting fumes.

Arsenic (*2.4.2*): maximum 5 ppm.

Boil 0.2 g in 25 ml of *dilute hydrochloric acid R* until completely dissolved. The solution complies with limit test A.

Copper: maximum 50 ppm.

Atomic absorption spectrometry (*2.2.23, Method I*).

Test solution. Dissolve 1.00 g in a mixture of 60 ml of *dilute hydrochloric acid R* and 10 ml of *dilute hydrogen peroxide solution R*. Reduce to a volume of 5 ml and dilute to 50.0 ml with *water R*.

Reference solutions. Prepare the reference solutions using *copper standard solution (0.1 per cent Cu) R*, diluted as necessary with a 1 per cent *V/V* solution of *hydrochloric acid R*.

Source: copper hollow-cathode lamp.

Wavelength: 324.8 nm.

Flame: air-acetylene.

Lead: maximum 50 ppm.

Atomic absorption spectrometry (*2.2.23, Method I*).

Test solution. In a separating funnel, place 20 ml of the test solution prepared for the test for copper. Add 25 ml of *lead-free hydrochloric acid R*. Stir with 3 quantities, each of 25 ml, of *di-isopropyl ether R*. Collect the aqueous layer. Add 0.10 g of *sodium sulphate decahydrate R*. Evaporate to dryness. Take up the residue with 1 ml of *lead-free nitric acid R* and dilute to 20 ml with *water R*.

Reference solutions. Prepare the reference solutions using *lead standard solution (0.1 per cent Pb) R*, diluted as necessary with a 10 per cent *V/V* solution of *nitric acid R* containing 5 g/l of *sodium sulphate decahydrate R*.

Source: lead hollow-cathode lamp.

Wavelength: 217 nm.

Flame: air-acetylene.

ASSAY

Stir for 10 min 0.100 g in a hot solution of 1.25 g of *copper sulphate R* in 20 ml of *water R* in a 100 ml conical flask with a ground-glass stopper. Filter rapidly and wash the filter. Combine the filtrate and the washings, acidify with *dilute sulphuric acid R* and titrate with *0.02 M potassium permanganate* until a pink colour is obtained.

1 ml of *0.02 M potassium permanganate* is equivalent to 5.585 mg of Fe.

LABELLING

The label indicates whether the iron for homoeopathic preparations is obtained by reduction or sublimation.

01/2005:1624

SAFFRON FOR HOMOEOPATHIC PREPARATIONS

Croci stigma ad praeparationes homoeopathicas

DEFINITION

Dried stigmas of *Crocus sativus* L. usually joined by the base to a short style.

CHARACTERS

Saffron has a characteristic, aromatic odour.

It has the macroscopic and microscopic characters described under identification tests A and B.

IDENTIFICATION

A. The dark brick-red stigmas, when dry, are 20 mm to 40 mm long and after soaking with water, about 35 mm to 50 mm long. The tubes, gradually widening at the top, are incised on one side, the upper margin is open and finely crenated. The style connecting the 3 stigmas is pale yellow and not more than 5 mm long.

B. Examine under a microscope using *chloral hydrate solution R*. It shows the following diagnostic characters: elongated epidermal cells, frequently with a short, central papilla; in water they release a yellow colouring matter; the upper border of the stigma has finger-shaped papillae, up to 150 µm long; between them are single, globular pollen grains, about 100 µm wide, with a finely pitted exine, vascular bundles with small spirally thickened vessels and no fibres.

C. Carefully crush pieces of the drug to coarse particles and moisten with 0.2 ml of *phosphomolybdic acid solution R*. The particles turn blue within 1-2 min or they have a blue areole around them.

D. Examine by thin-layer chromatography (*2.2.27*).

Test solution. Carefully crush 0.1 g of the drug with a glass rod and moisten with 0.2 ml of *water R*. After 3 min add 5 ml of *methanol R*, allow to stand for 20 min, protected from light, and filter through a plug of glass wool.

Reference solution. Dissolve 5 mg of *naphthol yellow R* in 5 ml of *methanol R* and add a solution of 5 mg of *Sudan red G R* in 5 ml of *methylene chloride R*.

Plate: *TLC silica gel F_{254} plate R*.

Mobile phase: *water R, 2-propanol R, ethyl acetate R* (10:25:65 *V/V/V*).

Application: 10 µl of the test solution and 5 µl of the reference solution as bands.

Development: over a path of 10 cm.

Drying: in air.

Detection: examine in daylight.

Results: see below the sequence of the zones present in the chromatograms obtained with the reference and test solutions.

Top of the plate	
A red zone	
A yellow zone	
	2 yellow zones
	An intense yellow zone (crocine)
Reference solution	**Test solution**

Detection: in ultraviolet light at 254 nm.

Results: see below the sequence of the zones present in the chromatograms obtained with the reference and test solutions.

Top of the plate	
A red zone	1 or 2 quenching zones
A yellow zone	A quenching zone
Reference solution	**Test solution**

Homoeopathic preparations

Detection: spray with *anisaldehyde solution R* and examine in daylight while heating at 100-105 °C for 5-10 min.

Results: see below the sequence of the zones present in the chromatograms obtained with the reference and test solutions.

Top of the plate	
A red zone	1 or 2 red to reddish-violet zones
A blue to bluish-green zone	A red to reddish-violet zone
	2 blue to bluish-green zones
	An intense blue to bluish-green zone (crocine)
Reference solution	**Test solution**

E. Dilute 0.1 ml of the test solution (see Identification test D) with 1 ml of *methanol R*. Deposit 0.1 ml of this solution on a filter paper, allow to dry and spray with a 10 g/l solution of *diphenylboric acid aminoethyl ester R* in *methanol R*. Examine in ultraviolet light at 365 nm. The spot shows an intense orange-yellow fluorescence.

TESTS

Colouring power. Introduce 0.10 g into a 5 ml volumetric flask and add to 5.0 ml with *distilled water R*. Close the flask and shake every 30 min for 8 h. Then allow to stand for 16 h. Dilute 1.0 ml to 500.0 ml with *distilled water R*. The absorbance (*2.2.25*) measured at 440 nm using *distilled water R* as the compensation liquid, is not less than 0.44.

Foreign matter. Examine the drug microscopically. No parts with rough walls, no crystals and no pollen grains containing 3 germinal pores are present.

Loss on drying (*2.2.32*): maximum 10.0 per cent, determined on 0.200 g by drying in an oven at 100-105 °C.

Total ash (*2.4.16*): maximum 7.0 per cent, determined on the residue obtained in the test for loss on drying.

Members of the European Pharmacopoeia Commission: Austria, Belgium, Bosnia and Herzegovina, Croatia, Cyprus, Czech Republic, Denmark, Estonia, Finland, France, Germany, Greece, Hungary, Iceland, Ireland, Italy, Latvia, Luxembourg, Netherlands, Norway, Portugal, Romania, Serbia and Montenegro, Slovak Republic, Slovenia, Spain, Sweden, Switzerland, "The former Yugoslav Republic of Macedonia", Turkey, United Kingdom and the European Union.

Observers to the European Pharmacopoeia Commission: Albania, Algeria, Australia, Bulgaria, Canada, China, Georgia, Lithuania, Malaysia, Malta, Morocco, Poland, Senegal, Syria, Tunisia, Ukraine and WHO (World Health Organisation).

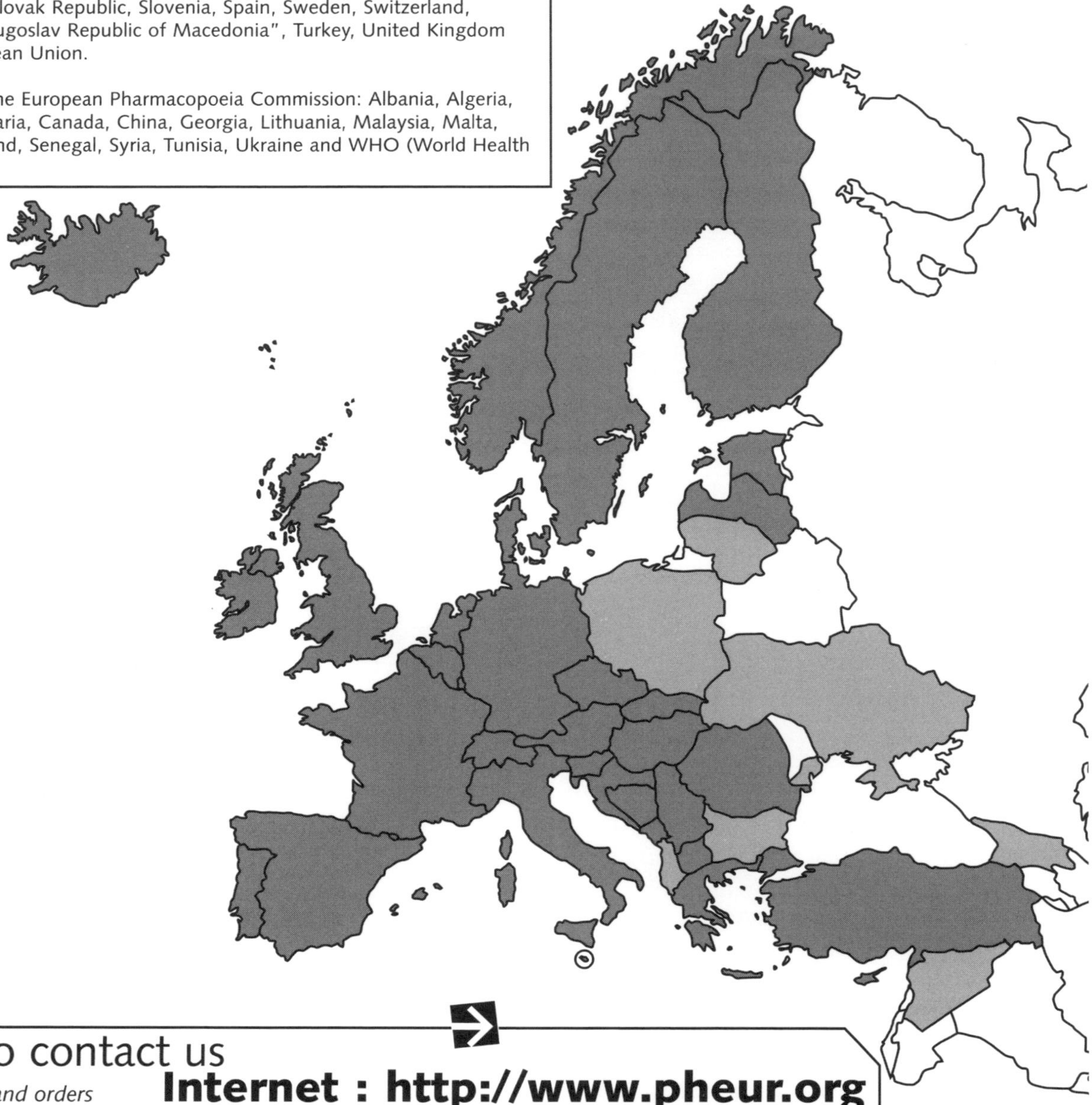

How to contact us

Information and orders **Internet : http://www.pheur.org**

European Directorate for the Quality of Medicines
Council of Europe - 226 avenue de Colmar BP 907
F-67029 STRASBOURG Cedex 1, FRANCE
Tel: +33 (0)3 88 41 30 30*
Fax: +33 (0)3 88 41 27 71*

	E-mail
CD-ROM	cdromtech@pheur.org
Certification	certification@pheur.org
Monographs	monographs@pheur.org
Publications	publications@pheur.org
Reference substances	crs@pheur.org
Conferences	publicrelations@pheur.org
All other correspondence	info@pheur.org

*: Do not dial 0 if calling from outside France.

All reference substances required for application of the monographs are available from the EDQM. A catalogue of reference substances is available on request; the catalogue is included in the Pharmeuropa subscription; it can also be consulted on the EDQM internet site.

EUROPEAN PHARMACOPOEIA

5th Edition

published 15 June 2004

replaces the 4th Edition on 1 January 2005

Volumes 1 and 2 of this publication 5.0 constitute the 5th Edition of the European Pharmacopoeia. They will be complemented by **non-cumulative supplements** that are to be kept for the duration of the 5th Edition. 2 supplements will be published in 2004 and 3 supplements in each of the years 2005 and 2006. A cumulative list of reagents will be published in supplements 5.4 and 5.7.

If you are using the 5th Edition at any time later than 1 April 2005, make sure that you have all the published supplements and consult the index of the most recent supplement to ensure that you use the latest versions of the monographs and general chapters.

EUROPEAN PHARMACOPOEIA ELECTRONIC VERSION

The 5th Edition is also available in an electronic format (CD-ROM and internet version) with all the monographs and general chapters contained in the book. With the publication of each supplement the electronic version is replaced by a new fully updated cumulative version.

PHARMEUROPA

Quarterly Forum Publication

Pharmeuropa contains preliminary drafts of all new and revised monographs proposed for inclusion in the European Pharmacopoeia and gives an opportunity for all interested parties to comment on the specifications before they are finalised. Pharmeuropa also contains information on the work programme and on certificates of suitability to monographs of the European Pharmacopoeia issued by the EDQM, scientific articles on pharmacopoeial matters and other articles of general interest. Pharmeuropa is available on subscription from the EDQM.

INTERNATIONAL HARMONISATION

Refer to information given in chapter *5.8. Pharmacopoeial Harmonisation.*

WEBSITE

http://www.pheur.org
http://book.pheur.org (for prices and orders)

KEY TO MONOGRAPHS

Carbimazole EUROPEAN PHARMACOPOEIA 5.0

Version date of the text

01/2005:0884

corrected

Text reference number

CARBIMAZOLE

Carbimazolum

Modification to be taken into account from the publication date of volume 5.0

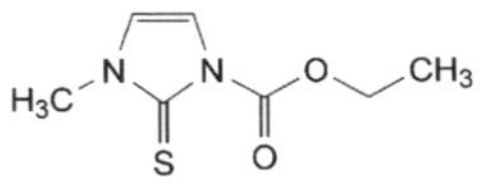

$C_7H_{10}N_2O_2S$ M_r 186.2

Chemical name in accordance with IUPAC nomenclature rules

DEFINITION

Ethyl 3-methyl-2-thioxo-2,3-dihydro-1*H*-imidazole-1-carboxylate.

Content: 98.0 per cent to 102.0 per cent (dried substance).

CHARACTERS

Appearance: white or yellowish-white, crystalline powder.

Solubility: slightly soluble in water, soluble in acetone and in alcohol.

Application of the first and second identification is defined in the General Notices (chapter 1)

IDENTIFICATION

First identification: B.

Second identification: A, C, D.

A. Melting point (*2.2.14*): 122 °C to 125 °C.

B. Infrared absorption spectrophotometry (*2.2.24*).

Preparation: discs.

Comparison: *carbimazole CRS*.

Chemical reference substance available from the Secretariat (see www.pheur.org)

C. Thin-layer chromatography (*2.2.27*).

Test solution. Dissolve 10 mg of the substance to be examined in *methylene chloride R* and dilute to 10 ml with the same solvent.

Reference solution. Dissolve 10 mg of *carbimazole CRS* in *methylene chloride R* and dilute to 10 ml with the same solvent.

Plate: *TLC silica gel GF_{254} plate R*.

Mobile phase: *acetone R*, *methylene chloride R* (20:80 *V/V*).

Reagents described in chapter 4

Application: 10 µl.

Development: over a path of 15 cm.

Drying: in air for 30 min.

Detection: examine in ultraviolet light at 254 nm.

Results: the principal spot in the chromatogram obtained with the test solution is similar in position and size to the principal spot in the chromatogram obtained with the reference solution.

D. Dissolve about 10 mg in a mixture of 50 ml of *water R* and 0.05 ml of *dilute hydrochloric acid R*. Add 1 ml of *potassium iodobismuthate solution R*. A red precipitate is formed.

TESTS

Impurity A and other related substances. Liquid chromatography (*2.2.29*).

Reference to a general chapter

Test solution. Dissolve 5.0 mg of the substance to be examined in 10.0 ml of a mixture of 20 volumes of *acetonitrile R* and 80 volumes of *water R*. Use this solution within 5 min of preparation.

Reference solution (a). Dissolve 5 mg of *thiamazole R* and 0.10 g of *carbimazole CRS* in a mixture of 20 volumes of *acetonitrile R* and 80 volumes of *water R* and dilute to 100.0 ml with the same mixture of solvents. Dilute 1.0 ml of this solution to 10.0 ml with a mixture of 20 volumes of *acetonitrile R* and 80 volumes of *water R*.

Reference solution (b). Dissolve 5.0 mg of *thiamazole R* in a mixture of 20 volumes of *acetonitrile R* and 80 volumes of *water R* and dilute to 10.0 ml with the same mixture of solvents. Dilute 1.0 ml of this solution to 100.0 ml with a mixture of 20 volumes of *acetonitrile R* and 80 volumes of *water R*.

Column:

- *size*: *l* = 0.15 m, Ø = 3.9 mm,
- *stationary phase*: *octadecylsilyl silica gel for chromatography R* (5 µm).

Mobile phase: *acetonitrile R*, *water R* (10:90 *V/V*).

Flow rate: 1 ml/min.

Detection: spectrophotometer at 254 nm.

Injection: 10 µl.

Run time: 1.5 times the retention time of carbimazole.

Retention time: carbimazole = about 6 min.

System suitability: reference solution (a):

- *resolution*: minimum 5.0 between the peaks due to impurity A and carbimazole.

Limits:

- *impurity A*: not more than half the area of the principal peak in the chromatogram obtained with reference solution (b) (0.5 per cent),
- *any other impurity*: not more than 0.1 times the area of the principal peak in the chromatogram obtained with reference solution (b) (0.1 per cent).

Loss on drying (*2.2.32*): maximum 0.5 per cent, determined on 1.000 g by drying in a desiccator over *diphosphorus pentoxide R* at a pressure not exceeding 0.7 kPa for 24 h.

Sulphated ash (*2.4.14*): maximum 0.1 per cent, determined on 1.0 g.

ASSAY

Dissolve 50.0 mg in *water R* and dilute to 500.0 ml with the same solvent. To 10.0 ml add 10 ml of *dilute hydrochloric acid R* and dilute to 100.0 ml with *water R*. Measure the absorbance (*2.2.25*) at the maximum at 291 nm. Calculate the content of $C_7H_{10}N_2O_2S$ taking the specific absorbance to be 557.

IMPURITIES

Specified impurities: A.

Other detectable impurities: B.

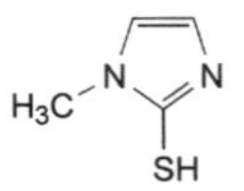

A. 1-methyl-1*H*-imidazole-2-thiol (thiamazole).

List of impurities detected by the tests (see the general monograph Substances for pharmaceutical use (2034) and chapter 5.10. Control of impurities in substances for pharmaceutical use)

See the information section on general monographs (cover pages)

General Notices (1) apply to all monographs and other texts